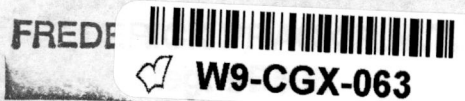

FREDE

PHYSICIAN'S
DRUG
HANDBOOK
5TH EDITION

PHYSICIAN'S DRUG HANDBOOK

5TH EDITION

Springhouse Corporation
Springhouse, Pennsylvania

Staff

Executive Director, Editorial
Stanley Loeb

Publisher
Barbara F. McVan

Editorial Director
Helen Klusek Hamilton

Art Director
John Hubbard

Drug Information Editor
George J. Blake, RPh, MS

Copy Editors
Jane V. Cray (supervisor), Mary T. Durkin, Traci A.
Ginnona, Christina P. Ponczek

Editorial Assistants
Maree DeRosa, Beverly Lane, Mary Madden

Designers
Stephanie Peters (associate art director),
Jacalyn Bove Facciolo (book designer), Maryanne
Buschini, Laurie Mirijanian, Leslie Weisman-Cook

Typography
David Kosten (director), Diane Paluba (manager),
Liz Bergman, Joyce Rossi Biletz, Phyllis Marron, Robin
Mayer, Valerie Rosenberger

Manufacturing
Deborah Meiris (manager), T.A. Landis

Production Coordination
Margaret A. Rastiello

Contents

Generic drugs and pharmacologic classes

Appendices, selected references, and index

Contributors

Steven L. Barriere, PharmD, FCCP, Specialist in Infectious Diseases, Department of Pharmaceutical Services; Adjunct Professor, Departments of Medicine and Pharmacology, School of Medicine, UCLA Center for the Health Services, Los Angeles: antibiotics.

Edward M. Bednarczyk, RPh, PharmD, Research Fellow, University Hospitals of Cleveland (Ohio), Division of Cardiology: GI drugs

Keith A. Burechson, RPh, Assistant Director of Pharmacy, Roxborough Memorial Hospital, Philadelphia: topical agents.

James B. Caldwell, RPh, PharmD, Clinical Pharmacist, Anne Arundel General Hospital, Annapolis, Md.: cephalosporins, sulfonamides, and tetracyclines.

Mark A. Campbell, RPh, MS, Pharmacist Specialist, Kaiser Foundation Hospital, San Diego Medical Center: cancer chemotherapy.

Deborah B. Cooper, RPh, PharmD, Clinical Pharmacist, The Sinai Hospital of Baltimore: ACE inhibitors, beta-adrenergic blocking agents, and rauwolfia alkaloids.

Sandra Harley Counts, RPh, PharmD, Clinical Coordinator, Pharmacy Department, Anderson Memorial Hospital, Anderson, S.C.: anticonvulsants and amphetamines.

H. Edward Davidson, RPh, PharmD, Director of Clinical Services, HPI Health Care Services, Atlanta: nitrates, cardiac glycosides, and calcium channel blocking agents.

Linda J. Dawson, RPh, PharmD, Fellow in Drug Information, University of Kentucky Medical Center, Lexington: antidepressants and phenothiazines.

Jerri O. Edwards, RPh, PharmD, Clinical Pharmacist, Baker Hospital, Charleston, S.C.: nonsteroidal anti-inflammatory agents.

Marcy Portnoff Gever, RPh, MEd, Pharmacist Consultant, West Chester, Pa.: antihistamines.

Joe N. Gibson, RPh, Assistant Director Pharmacy and I.V. Therapy, Nash General Hospital, Rocky Mount, N.C.: systemic and miotic cholinergics.

Margaret R. Glessner, RPh, PharmD, Pharmacy Consultant, Bryn Mawr, Pa.: mydriatic agents.

Edwin L. Gutshall, RPh, PharmD, Director of Pharmacy Services, John Randolph Hospital, Hopewell, Va.: gold salts.

Sarah Johnston-Miller, RPh, MS, PharmD, Advanced Resident in Pharmacy Nutrition Support, Hospital of the University of Pennsylvania, Philadelphia: aminoquinolines.

Patricia C. Kienle, RPh, MPA, Assistant Director of Pharmacy, Mercy Hospital, Wilkes-Barre, Pa.: iron supplements, thrombolytics, and anticoagulants.

Thomas H. Kramer, RPh, PharmD, Research Associate, Department of Pharmacology, College of Medicine, University of Arizona, Tucson, Ariz.: hormones.

Michael Lease, RPh, MS, Director of Pharmacy, Montgomery Hospital, Norristown, Pa.: xanthines and pancreatic enzymes.

Robert J. Lipsy, RPh, PharmD, Drug Information Resident, Arizona Poison and Drug Information Center, Tucson: anesthetic agents, barbiturates, and benzodiazepines.

Jan-Elian Markind, RPh, Staff Pharmacist, Graduate Hospital, Philadelphia: vitamins and calorics.

Barbara L. McHenry, RPh. PharmD, Clinical Pharmacist, Anne Arundel General Hospital, Annapolis, Md.: sulfonamides, tetracyclines, and cephalosporins.

Mary L. Miller, RPh, PharmD, Clinical Pharmacy Fellow in Ambulatory Care, Audie Murphy Memorial V.A. Medical Center, San Antonio, Tex.: steroids.

John Ostrosky, RPh, PharmD, Medical College of Virginia Hospital, Richmond: vaccines and toxins.

Doris M. Sherpinsky, RPh, Staff Pharmacist, Holy Redeemer Hospital and Medical Center, Meadowbrook, Pa.: cardiovascular drugs.

Joanne M. Sica, RPh, MS, Director of Pharmacy, Roxborough Memorial Hospital, Philadelphia: adrenergics and several recently approved drugs.

Thomas Simpson, RPh, PharmD, Director of Pharmacy, CPC Santa Ana (Calif.) Psychiatric Hospital: opioids.

Lilliam Sklaver, PharmD, Coordinator of Clinical Research Service, University of Miami (Fla.) School of Medicine, Papanicolaou Comprehensive Cancer Center: diuretics.

Lisa Marie Stevenson, RPh, PharmD, Clinical Pharmacy Resident, University of Kentucky Medical Center, Lexington: antidiabetic agents and thyroid hormones.

Paul J. Vitale, RPh, PharmD, Assistant Director Pharmacy/Clinical Services, Anne Arundel General Hospital, Annapolis, Md.: aminoglycosides, penicillins, and other anti-infectives.

Clinical reviewers and consultants

Douglas R. Allington, PharmD, Assistant Professor, School of Pharmacy and Allied Health, University of Montana, Missoula.

Mark J. Ellison, PharmD, FCP, BCPS, Associate Professor of Family Medicine, Department of Family Medicine, East Carolina University School of Medicine, Greenville, N.C.

Jimmi Hatton, PharmD, Assistant Professor of Pharmacy, University of Kentucky, College of Pharmacy, Lexington.

James R. Hildebrand III, PharmD, Director, Drug Information Center, Philadelphia College of Pharmacy and Science.

Cary E. Johnson, PharmD, Assistant Professor of Pharmacy, University of Michigan College of Pharmacy; Clinical Pharmacist – Pediatrics, University of Michigan Medical Center, Ann Arbor.

Gordon E. Johnson, PhD, Professor, Department of Pharmacology, University of Saskatchewan, Saskatoon, Canada.

Mary Y. Ma, PharmD, Antimicrobial Clinical Specialist, VA West Los Angeles Medical Center; Assistant Professor of Clinical Pharmacy, VA West Los Angeles Medical Center School of Pharmacy.

William A. Mahon, MD, FRCPC, Professor of Pharmacology and Medicine, Toronto General Hospital, Ontario.

Lea Anne O'Brien, PharmD, Clinical Coordinator of Critical Care, Department of Pharmacy Services, New York Hospital-Cornell Medical Center.

Andrew T. Pennell, PharmD, Assistant Professor, Clinical Pharmacy Practice, School of Pharmacy, Auburn (Ala.) University.

David R. Pipher, RPh, PharmD, Assistant Director for Clinical Services, Forbes Regional Health Center, Monroeville, Pa.

Marc S. Roth, RPh, MS, Clinical Coordinator for Critical Nutrition Support, New York Hospital-Cornell Medical Center.

Joel Shuster, PharmD, Clinical Assistant Professor, Temple University School of Pharmacy, Philadelphia; Clinical Pharmacist, Medical College Hospitals – Main Clinical Campus, Philadelphia.

J. Michael Spivey, PharmD, Assistant Professor of Family Medicine, Department of Family Medicine, East Carolina University School of Medicine, Greenville, N.C.

Joseph F. Steiner, RPh, PharmD, Professor of Clinical Pharmacy, Schools of Human Medicine and Pharmacy, College of Health Sciences, University of Wyoming, Casper.

Lisa J. Woodard, RPh, MPH, Pharmacist, Providence Community Pharmacy, Providence Medical Center, Seattle, Wash.

Special thanks to the following, who have made contributions to recent past editions: Robert D. Baker, MD, PhD, University of Massachusetts Medical Center, Worcester; Susan S. Baker, MD, PhD, University of Massachusetts Medical Center, Worcester; Marla Bartolozzi, MD, Temple University Hospital, Philadelphia; David Burton, MD, Temple University School of Medicine, Philadelphia; A. Bruce Cambell, PhD, MD, Scripps Memorial Hospitals, La Jolla, Calif.; Robert L. Danner, MD, National Institutes of Health, Bethesda, Md.; Nancy S. Day, MD, Frankford Hospital, Philadelphia; Brian B. Doyle, MD, Georgetown University Medical School, Washington, D.C.; Stephen C. Duck, MD, Marc Fund Research Center, Milwaukee; Bruce M. Frey, RPh, PharmD, Thomas Jefferson University Hospital, Philadelphia; Sarah Mendell Gilmour, MD, St. Margaret Memorial Hospital, Pittsburgh; Kevin Gleeson, MD, The Pennsylvania State University School of Medicine, Hershey; David W. Hawkins, PharmD, The University of Georgia College of Pharmacy, Athens; Kelly J. Henrickson, MD, Medical College of Wisconsin, Milwaukee; Nina E. Jakobowski, PharmD, Thomas Jefferson University Hospital, Philadelphia; Ronald N. Jones, MD, University of Iowa College of Medicine, Iowa City; Rosaline R. Joseph, MD, Medical College of Pennsylvania, Philadelphia; Joseph Patrick Kleaveland, MD, Temple University School of Medicine, Philadelphia; Peter G. Lavine, MD, FACC, Crozier-Chester Medical Center, Upland, Pa.; Herbert A. Luscombe, MD, Thomas Jefferson University Hospital, Philadelphia; Roger M. Morrell, MD, PhD, FACP, FAIC, Greater Ann Arbor (Mich.) Neurology Associates; Walter Orenstein, MD, Centers for Disease Control and Prevention, Atlanta; John J. O'Shea, MD, National Institutes of Health, Bethesda, Md.; Daniel W. Rahn, MD, Yale University School of Medicine, New Haven, Conn.; Raymond Rodriguez, MD, Thomas Jefferson University, Philadelphia; Grannum R. Sant, MD, FACS, New England Medical Center, Boston; Joanne M. Sica, RPh, MHA, Greater Atlantic Health Service, Philadelphia; J. Andrew Solis, MD, Internal Medicine, Richboro, Pa.; Kerri J. Vandel, RPh, PharmD, University of Wyoming School of Pharmacy, Wyoming Medical Center, Caspar; Paul J. Vitale, PharmD, FASCP, The Anne Arundel Medical Center, Annapolis, Md.; Charles I. Wagner, MD, University of Pennsylvania School of Medicine, Abington (Pa.) Memorial Hospital, and Holy Redeemer Hospital, Meadowbrook, Pa.

How to use this book

Physician's Drug Handbook, 5th Edition, provides exhaustively reviewed, completely updated drug information on virtually every drug in current clinical use. It covers all aspects of drug information from fundamental pharmacology to specific management of toxicity and overdose. It also includes several unique features—individual entries that describe major pharmacologic classes, a comprehensive listing of indications that includes clinically approved but unlabeled uses, and specific recommendations for use in renal failure.

Generic drug entries

The individual drug entries provide detailed information on virtually all drugs in current clinical use, all arranged alphabetically by generic name for easy access. Drug entries that describe investigational drugs are clustered in a separate section for easier access. A guide word at the top of each page identifies the generic drug or pharmacologic class presented on that page. Each generic and class entry is complete where it falls alphabetically and does not require cross-referencing to other sections of the book.

In each drug entry, the generic name (with alternate generic names following in parentheses) precedes an alphabetically arranged list of current trade names. (An asterisk signals products available only in Canada.) Several drugs available solely as combinations (such as heparin with dihydroergotamine) are listed according to the first generic in the combination.

Next, the pharmacologic and therapeutic classifications identify the drug's pharmacologic or chemical category and its major clinical uses. Listing both classifications helps the reader grasp the multiple, varying, and sometimes overlapping uses of drugs within a single pharmacologic class and among different classes. If appropriate, the next line identifies any drug that the Drug Enforcement Agency (DEA) lists as a controlled substance and specifies the schedule of control as II, III, IV, or V.

The pregnancy risk category identifies the potential risk to the fetus. Categories listed were determined by application of the Food and Drug Administration (FDA) definitions to available clinical data in order to define a drug's potential to cause birth defects or fetal death. These categories, labeled A, B, C, D, and X, are listed below with an explanation of each. Drugs in category A usually are considered safe to use in pregnancy; drugs in category X usually are contraindicated.

A: Adequate studies in pregnant women have failed to show a risk to the fetus in the first trimester of pregnancy—and there is no evidence of risk in later trimesters.

B: Animal studies have not shown an adverse effect on the fetus, but there are no adequate clinical studies in pregnant women.

C: Animal studies have shown an adverse effect on the fetus, but there are no adequate studies in humans. The drug may be useful in pregnant women despite its potential risks.

D: There is evidence of risk to the human fetus, but the potential benefits of use in pregnant women may be acceptable despite potential risks.

X: Studies in animals or humans show fetal abnormalities, or adverse reaction reports indicate evidence of fetal risk. The risks involved clearly outweigh potential benefits.

Pregnancy risk classifications were assigned for all appropriate generic drugs according to the above criteria.

How supplied lists the preparations available for each drug (for example, tablets, capsules, solution, or injection), specifying available dosage forms and strengths.

Indications, route, and dosage presents all clinically accepted indications for use with general dosage recommendations for adults and children; specific recommendations for infants, elderly patients, or other special patient groups are included when appropriate. A preceding dagger signals clinically accepted but unlabeled uses. Dosage instructions reflect current clinical trends in therapeutics and should not be considered as absolute and universal recommendations. For individual application, dosage must be considered according to the patient's condition.

Pharmacodynamics explains the mechanism and effects of the drug's physiologic action.

Pharmacokinetics describes absorption, distribution, metabolism, and excretion of the drug; it specifies onset and duration of action and half-life as appropriate.

Contraindications and precautions lists conditions that are associated with special risks in patients who receive the drug, and includes the rationale for each warning.

Interactions specifies the clinically significant additive, synergistic, or antagonistic effects that result from combined use of the drug with other drugs.

Effects on diagnostic tests lists significant interference with a diagnostic test or its result by direct effects on the test itself or by systemic drug effects that lead to misleading test results.

Adverse reactions lists the undesirable effects that may follow use of the drug; these effects are arranged by body systems (CNS, CV, DERM, EENT, GI, GU, HEMA, Hepatic, Metabolic, Respiratory, Local, and Other). Local effects occur at the site of drug administration (by application, infusion, or injection); adverse reactions not specific to a single body system (for example, the effects of hypersensitivity) are listed under *Other*. Throughout, life-threatening reactions are italicized. At the end of this section, *Note* signals a list of severe and hazardous reactions that mandate discontinuation of the drug.

Overdose and treatment summarizes the clinical manifestations of drug overdose and recommends specific treatment as appropriate. Usually, this segment recommends emesis or gastric lavage, followed by activated charcoal to reduce the amount of drug absorbed and possibly a cathartic to eliminate the toxin. This section specifies antidotes, drug therapy, and other special care, if known. It also specifies the effects of hemodialysis or peritoneal dialysis for dialyzable drugs.

Special considerations offers detailed recommendations specific to the drug for preparation and administration; for care and teaching of the patient during therapy; and for use in elderly patients, children, and breast-feeding women. This section includes recommendations for monitoring the effects of drug therapy, for preventing and treating adverse reactions, for promoting patient comfort, and for storing the drug. Recommendations that are common to all members of the drug's pharmacologic class are listed only in the relevant *class* entry. Thus, if specific considerations are unknown for geriatric, pediatric, or breast-feeding use of the generic drug, or if known information is listed in the class entry or elsewhere in the generic entry, these headings are omitted. For example, if the *Indications, route, and dosage* section lists detailed instructions for use in children and no additional considerations apply, the generic entry omits the heading *Pediatric use*. However, relevant information that applies to all drugs in the drug's pharmacologic class may exist in the class entry.

Pharmacologic class entries

Interwoven alphabetically among the generic drug entries, 61 entries describe the pharmacology, clinical indications and actions, adverse effects, and special implications of drugs that fall into a major pharmacologic group (for example, benzodiazepines, phenothiazines, or thiazide diuretics). This allows the reader to compare the effects and uses of drugs within each class. Pharmacologic class entries list special considerations that are common to all generic members of the class, and include geriatric, pediatric, and breast-feeding use. If specific considerations are unknown, these headings are omitted.

Representative combinations at the end of each class entry lists major combinations of generic drugs in the class with other generics of the same or of another class, followed by trade names of products that contain each combination of generics.

Graphic enhancement

Selected charts and tables compare uses, effects, or dosages of drugs within a class.

Investigational drugs

Subsections vary within these entries according to the amount of information available. For example, they commonly omit sections on Pharmacokinetics, Interactions, and Effects on diagnostic tests, because such data have not yet been reported.

Appendix

The appendix provides a charted summary of recommended protocols for cancer chemotherapy, and of the effectiveness of antibiotics against susceptible pathogens, specifying primary and alternate therapy for each organism. It lists designated orphan drugs and biologicals with their trade names and indications, lists antidotes to poisoning or overdose, provides a table of equivalents, and organizes information about topical drugs in a comprehensive chart. Selected references lists sources of additional information.

Index

The index lists trade names of generic drugs and combination products, alternate and former generic names, and both pharmacologic and therapeutic drug classes.

ABBREVIATIONS

Abbreviation	Meaning
ALT	serum alanine aminotransferase, formerly SGPT
AST	serum aspartate aminotransferase, formerly SGOT
ATP	adenosine triphosphate
AV	atrioventricular
b.i.d.	twice a day
BUN	blood urea nitrogen
cAMP	cyclic 3′, 5′ adenosine monophosphate
CHF	congestive heart failure
CNS	central nervous system
CPK	creatinine phosphokinase
CPR	cardiopulmonary resuscitation
CSF	cerebrospinal fluid
CV	cardiovascular
CVP	central venous pressure
DNA	deoxyribonucleic acid
ECG	electrocardiogram
EEG	electroencephalogram
FDA	Food and Drug Administration
g	gram
G	gauge
GI	gastrointestinal
GU	genitourinary
h.s.	at bedtime
I.M.	intramuscular
IU	International Unit
I.V.	intravenous
kg	kilogram
L	liter
m^2	square meter
mm^3	cubic millimeter
MAO	monoamine oxidase
mcg or μg	microgram
mEq	milliequivalent
mg	milligram
MI	myocardial infarction
ml	milliliter
ng	nanogram (millimicrogram)
OTC	over-the-counter
P.O.	by mouth
p.r.n.	as needed
q	every
q.i.d.	four times a day
RBC	red blood cell
RNA	ribonucleic acid
SA	sinoatrial
S.C.	subcutaneous
SGOT	serum glutamic oxaloacetic transaminase
SGPT	serum glutamic pyruvic transaminase
t.i.d.	three times a day
WBC	white blood cell

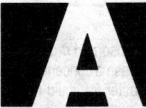

acebutolol
Sectral

- Pharmacologic classification: beta-adrenergic blocking agent
- Therapeutic classification: antihypertensive, antiarrhythmic
- Pregnancy risk category B

How supplied
Available by prescription only
Capsules: 200 mg, 400 mg

Indications, route, and dosage
Hypertension
Adults: 400 mg P.O. either as a single daily dose or divided b.i.d. Patients may receive as much as 1,200 mg daily.
Ventricular arrhythmias
Adults: 400 mg P.O. daily divided b.i.d. Dosage is then increased to provide an adequate clinical response. Usual daily dosage is 600 to 1,200 mg.
Angina
Adults: 200 mg b.i.d. Usual daily dosage is 400 to 800 mg divided b.i.d.

Pharmacodynamics
- *Antihypertensive action:* The exact mechanism of acebutolol's antihypertensive effect is unknown. Acebutolol has cardioselective beta₁-adrenergic blocking properties and mild intrinsic sympathomimetic activity.
- *Antiarrhythmic action:* Acebutolol decreases heart rate and prevents exercise-induced increases in heart rate; it also decreases myocardial contractility, cardiac output, and sinoatrial (SA) and atrioventricular (AV) nodal conduction velocity.

Pharmacokinetics
- *Absorption:* Acebutolol is absorbed well after oral administration. Peak plasma levels occur at about 2½ hours.
- *Distribution:* Acebutolol is about 26% protein-bound; minimal quantities are detected in CSF.
- *Metabolism:* Acebutolol undergoes extensive first-pass metabolism in the liver; peak levels of its major active metabolite, diacetolol, occur at about 3½ hours.
- *Excretion:* From 30% to 40% of a given dose of acebutolol is excreted in urine; remainder is excreted in feces and bile. Half-life of acebutolol is about 3 to 4 hours; half-life of diacetolol is 8 to 13 hours.

Contraindications and precautions
Acebutolol is contraindicated in patients with known hypersensitivity to the drug; in patients with persistent severe bradycardia or overt cardiac failure because drug may worsen these conditions; and in patients with second- or third-degree AV block or cardiogenic shock.

Acebutolol should be used cautiously in patients with impaired hepatic or renal function (decrease dosage if creatinine clearance falls below 50 ml/minute); in patients with coronary insufficiency because beta-adrenergic blockade may precipitate congestive heart failure (CHF); in patients with diabetes mellitus or hyperthyroidism because acebutolol may mask tachycardia (but not dizziness or sweating) caused by hypoglycemia or hyperthyroidism; and in patients with bronchospastic diseases, such as asthma or emphysema, because higher doses of the drug may inhibit bronchodilating effects of endogenous catecholamines.

Interactions
Concomitant use with cardiac glycosides may cause excessive bradycardia and increased myocardial depression.

Acebutolol may potentiate hypotensive effects of other antihypertensive agents; it also may alter insulin or oral hypoglycemic dosage requirements in stable diabetic patients. Hypotensive effects of acebutolol may be antagonized by indomethacin, nonsteroidal anti-inflammatory agents, and alpha-adrenergic stimulants, such as those contained in nonprescription cold remedies.

Effects on diagnostic tests
Acebutolol may cause positive antinuclear antibody titers.

Adverse reactions
- CNS: fatigue, headache, dizziness, insomnia.
- CV: chest pain, edema, bradycardia, CHF, *hypotension.*
- DERM: rash.
- EENT: dry eye, eye pain, abnormal vision, conjunctivitis.
- GI: nausea, constipation, diarrhea, dyspepsia.
- GU: impotence.
- Metabolic: hypoglycemia without tachycardia.
- Other: fever, wheezing, *dyspnea,* cough.
   Note: Drug should be discontinued if patient develops signs of CHF.

Overdose and treatment
Clinical signs of overdose include severe hypotension, bradycardia, heart failure, and bronchospasm.

After acute ingestion, empty stomach by emesis or gastric lavage; follow with activated charcoal to reduce absorption. Thereafter, treat symptomatically and supportively.

▶ Special considerations
Besides those relevant to all *beta-adrenergic blocking agents,* consider the following recommendation.
- Do not discontinue acebutolol abruptly.

Information for the patient
Advise patient to report wheezing promptly.

Geriatric use
Elderly patients may require lower maintenance dosages of acebutolol because of increased bioavailability. Do not exceed 800 mg/day.

Pediatric use
Safety and efficacy of acebutolol in pediatric patients have not been established; use only if potential benefit outweighs risk.

Breast-feeding
Both acebutolol and its metabolite, diacetolol, are distributed into breast milk; breast-feeding is not recommended for women receiving this drug.

---

acetaminophen
Acephen, Anacin-3, Bromo-Seltzer, Datril, Datril-500, Tempra, Tylenol, Valadol, Valorin

- Pharmacologic classification: para-aminophenol derivative
- Therapeutic classification: nonnarcotic analgesic, antipyretic
- Pregnancy risk category B

How supplied
Available without prescription
Tablets: 160 mg, 325 mg, 500 mg, 650 mg
Tablets (chewable): 80 mg
Capsules: 325 mg, 500 mg
Suppositories: 120 mg, 125 mg, 135 mg, 650 mg
Solution: 100 mg/ml
Elixir: 120 mg/5 ml, 160 mg/5 ml, 320 mg/5 ml
Liquid: 160 mg/5 ml; 500 mg/15 ml
Wafers: 120 mg
Effervescent granules: 325 mg/capful

Indications, route, and dosage
Mild pain or fever
Adults and children over age 12: 325 to 650 mg P.O. or rectally q 4 hours, p.r.n. Maximum dose should not exceed 4 g daily. Dosage for long-term therapy should not exceed 2.6 g daily.
Children under age 12: 1.5g/m^2 P.O. daily in divided doses or as shown below.
Children age 11 to 12: 480 mg/dose q 4 to 6 hours.
Children age 9 to 11: 400 mg/dose q 4 to 6 hours.
Children age 6 to 9: 320 mg/dose q 4 to 6 hours.
Children age 4 to 6: 240 mg/dose q 4 to 6 hours.
Children age 2 to 4: 160 mg/dose q 4 to 6 hours.
Children age 12 to 23 months: 120 mg/dose q 4 to 6 hours.
Children age 4 to 11 months: 80 mg/dose q 4 to 6 hours.
Children age 3 months or younger: 40 mg/dose q 4 to 6 hours.

Pharmacodynamics
The mechanism and site of action is unclear and may be related to inhibition of prostaglandin synthesis in the CNS.
- *Antipyretic action:* Acetaminophen is believed to exert its antipyretic effect by direct action on the hypothalamic heat-regulating center to block the effects of endogenous pyrogen. This results in increased heat dissipation through sweating and vasodilation.
- *Analgesic action:* Its analgesic effect may be related to an elevation of the pain threshold.

Pharmacokinetics
- *Absorption:* Acetaminophen is absorbed rapidly and completely via the GI tract. Peak plasma concentrations occur in ½ to 2 hours, slightly faster for liquid preparations.
- *Distribution:* The drug is 25% protein-bound. Plasma concentrations do not correlate well with analgesic effect, but do correlate with toxicity.
- *Metabolism:* Approximately 90% to 95% is metabolized in the liver.
- *Excretion:* Acetaminophen is excreted in urine. The average elimination half-life ranges from 1 to 4 hours. In acute overdose, prolongation of elimination half-life is correlated with toxic effects. Half-life greater than 4 hours is associated with hepatic necrosis; greater than 12 hours is associated with coma.

Contraindications and precautions
Acetaminophen is contraindicated in patients with known hypersensitivity to this compound. Administer drug cautiously to patients with anemia or hepatic or renal disease because it has been known to induce these disorders; and to patients with a history of GI disease, increased risk of GI bleeding, or decreased renal function. Acetaminophen may mask the signs and symptoms of acute infection (fever, myalgia, erythema); patients with high infection risk (such as those with diabetes) should be carefully evaluated.

Interactions
Concomitant use of acetaminophen may potentiate the effects of anticoagulants and thrombolytic drugs, but this effect appears to be clinically insignificant. Antacids and food delay and decrease the absorption of acetaminophen. Combined caffeine and acetaminophen may enhance the therapeutic effect of acetaminophen. Concomitant use of phenothiazines and acetaminophen in large doses may result in hypothermia.

Effects on diagnostic tests
Acetaminophen may cause a false-positive test result for urinary 5-hydroxyindoleacetic acid (5-HIAA).

Adverse reactions
- CNS: mental changes, stupor, confusion, agitation (with toxic doses), weakness.
- DERM: rash, urticaria, itching, unusual bruising, erythema.
- EENT: unexplained sore throat.
- GI: nausea, vomiting, diarrhea, abdominal cramps, abdominal pain, loss of appetite.
- GU: bloody or cloudy urine, difficult or painful urination, sudden decrease in amount of urine.
- HEMA: unusual bleeding, tiredness or weakness, *hemolytic anemia,* neutropenia, leukopenia, pancytopenia, thrombocytopenia, methemoglobinemia.
- Hepatic: *severe liver damage* (toxic doses).
- Other: hypoglycemia, jaundice, unexplained fever.
  Note: Drug should be discontinued if hypersensitivity or signs and symptoms of hepatic toxicity occur.

Overdose and treatment
In acute overdose, plasma levels of 300 mcg/ml 4 hours postinjection or 50 mcg/ml 12 hours postinjection are associated with hepatotoxicity. Clinical manifestations of overdose include cyanosis, anemia, jaundice, skin eruptions, fever, emesis, CNS stimulation, delirium, methemoglobinemia progressing to depression, coma,

---

vascular collapse, convulsions, and death. Acetaminophen poisoning develops in stages:

Stage 1 (12 to 24 hours after ingestion): nausea, vomiting, diaphoresis, anorexia.

Stage 2 (24 to 48 hours after ingestion): clinically improved but elevated liver function tests.

Stage 3 (72 to 96 hours after ingestion): peak hepatotoxicity.

Stage 4 (7 to 8 days after ingestion): recovery.

To treat toxic overdose of acetaminophen, empty stomach immediately by inducing emesis with ipecac syrup if patient is conscious, or by gastric lavage. Administer activated charcoal via nasogastric tube. Oral acetylcysteine (Mucomyst) is a specific antidote for acetaminophen poisoning and is most effective if started within 10 to 12 hours after ingestion, but can help if started within 24 hours after ingestion. Administer a Mucomyst loading dose of 140 mg/kg P.O., followed by maintenance doses of 70 mg/kg P.O. every 4 hours for an additional 17 doses. Doses vomited within 1 hour of administration must be repeated. Remove charcoal before administering acetylcysteine because it may interfere with this antidote's absorption.

Acetylcysteine minimizes hepatic injury by supplying sulphydryl groups that bind with acetaminophen metabolites. Hemodialysis may be helpful to remove acetaminophen from the body. Monitor laboratory parameters and vital signs closely. Cimetidine has been used investigationally to block acetaminophen's metabolism to toxic intermediates. Provide symptomatic and supportive measures (respiratory support, correction of fluid and electrolyte imbalances). Determine plasma acetaminophen levels at least 4 hours after overdose. If plasma acetaminophen levels indicate hepatotoxicity, perform liver function tests every 24 hours for at least 96 hours.

▶ **Special considerations**
● Acetaminophen has no significant anti-inflammatory effect. In spite of this, studies have shown substantial benefit in patients with osteoarthritis of the knee. Therapeutic benefits may stem from the drug's analgesic effects.
● Many nonprescription products contain acetaminophen. Be aware of this when calculating total daily dose.
● Patients unable to tolerate aspirin may be able to tolerate acetaminophen.
● Use this medication cautiously in the presence of alcoholism, hepatic disease, viral infection, renal function impairment, or cardiovascular disease.
● Monitor vital signs, especially temperature, to evaluate drug's effectiveness.
● Assess patient's level of pain and response before and after administration of acetaminophen.
● Store suppository form in refrigerator.

Information for the patient
● Instruct patient in proper administration of prescribed form.
● Advise the patient on chronic high-dose acetaminophen therapy to arrange for monitoring of laboratory parameters, especially BUN, serum creatinine, liver function tests, and CBC.
● Warn the patient with current or history of rectal bleeding to avoid using rectal acetaminophen suppositories. If they are used, they must be retained in the rectum for at least 1 hour.
● Warn patient that high doses or unsupervised chronic use of acetaminophen can cause liver damage. Use of alcoholic beverages increases the risk of liver toxicity.
● Tell the patient to avoid use for self-medication of a fever above 103.1° F. (39.5° C.), a fever persisting longer than 3 days, or a recurrent fever.
● When prescribing buffered acetaminophen effervescent granules, consider sodium content for sodium-restricted patients.
● Tell the patient not to take nonsteroidal anti-inflammatory drugs together with acetaminophen on a regular basis.
● Warn the patient to avoid taking tetracycline antibiotics within 1 hour after taking buffered acetaminophen effervescent granules.
● Tell the patient not to use this medication for arthritic or rheumatic conditions without medical approval. This medication may relieve pain but not other symptoms.
● Tell the adult patient not to take this medication more than 10 days without medical approval.
● Tell the patient to call if symptoms do not improve or if fever lasts more than 3 days.
● Tell the patient on high-dose or long-term therapy that regular follow-up visits are essential.

Geriatric use
Elderly patients are more sensitive to this drug. Use with caution.

Pediatric use
Children should not take more than five doses per day or take the drug for more than 5 days unless specifically prescribed.

Breast-feeding
Excreted into breast milk in low concentrations. No adverse effects have been reported.

acetazolamide
acetazolamide sodium
Ak-Zol, Diamox, Diamox Sequels

● Pharmacologic classification: carbonic anhydrase inhibitor
● Therapeutic classification: adjunctive treatment for open-angle glaucoma and perioperative treatment for acute angle-closure glaucoma, anticonvulsant, management of edema, prevention and treatment of acute high-altitude sickness
● Pregnancy risk category C

How supplied
Available by prescription only
Tablets: 125 mg, 250 mg
Capsules (extended-release): 500 mg
Injection: 500 mg

Indications, route, and dosage
Perioperative management of acute angle-closure glaucoma
Adults: 250 mg P.O. q 4 hours; or 250 mg b.i.d. P.O., I.M., or I.V. for short-term therapy. I.M. injection is very painful and may cause sterile abscesses from alkalinity of drug; I.V. administration (100 to 500 mg/minute) is preferred.

Edema, in congestive heart failure
Adults: 250 to 375 mg P.O., I.M., or I.V. daily in a.m.
Children: 5 mg/kg P.O., I.M., or I.V. daily in a.m.

Open-angle glaucoma
Adults: 250 mg to 1 g P.O., I.M., or I.V. daily, divided q.i.d.

Prevention or amelioration of acute mountain sickness
Adults: 250 mg P.O. q 8 to 12 hours or 500 mg extended-release capsules q 12 to 24 hours.

Myoclonic seizures, refractory generalized tonic-clonic (grand mal) or absence (petit mal) seizures, mixed seizures
Adults: 375 mg P.O., I.M., or I.V. daily up to 250 mg q.i.d. Or, Diamox Sequels 250 to 500 mg daily or b.i.d. Initial dosage when used with other anticonvulsants usually is 250 mg daily.
Children: 8 to 30 mg/kg P.O., I.M., or I.V. daily, divided t.i.d. or q.i.d. Maximum dosage is 1.5 g daily, or 300 to 900 mg/m² daily.

†Diuresis and alkalization of urine in the treatment of toxicity associated with weakly acidic drugs
Adults: 5 mg/kg I.V. p.r.n.
Children: 5 mg/kg I.V. or 150 mg/m² I.V. for 1 to 2 days (in the a.m.).

†Prevention of cystine or uric acid nephrolithiasis
Adults: 250 mg P.O. h.s.

Pharmacodynamics
● *Diuretic action:* Acetazolamide and acetazolamide sodium act by noncompetitive reversible inhibition of the enzyme carbonic anhydrase, which is responsible for formation of hydrogen and bicarbonate ions from carbon dioxide and water. This inhibition results in decreased hydrogen concentration in the renal tubules, promoting excretion of bicarbonate, sodium, potassium, and water; because carbon dioxide is not eliminated as rapidly, systemic acidosis may occur.
● *Antiglaucoma action:* In open-angle glaucoma and perioperatively for acute angle-closure glaucoma, acetazolamide and acetazolamide sodium decrease the formation of aqueous humor, lowering intraocular pressure.
● *Anticonvulsant action:* The mechanism is unknown. Other actions: Acetazolamide is used with other anticonvulsants in various types of epilepsy, particularly petit mal.
● Acetazolamide shortens the period of high-altitude acclimatization; by inhibiting conversion of carbon dioxide to bicarbonate, it may increase carbon dioxide tension in tissues and decrease it in the lungs. The resultant metabolic acidosis may also increase oxygenation during hypoxia.

Pharmacokinetics
● *Absorption:* Acetazolamide is well absorbed from the GI tract after oral administration.
● *Distribution:* Acetazolamide is distributed throughout body tissues.
● *Metabolism:* None.
● *Excretion:* Acetazolamide is excreted primarily in urine via tubular secretion and passive reabsorption.

Contraindications and precautions
Acetazolamide is contraindicated in patients with hepatic insufficiency because the drug may precipitate hepatic coma; in patients with low potassium or sodium concentration level or hyperchloremic acidosis because it may worsen electrolyte imbalance; and in patients with severe renal impairment because nephrotoxicity has been reported.

Acetazolamide should be used cautiously in patients with respiratory acidosis or other severe respiratory problems because the drug may produce acidosis; in patients with diabetes because it may cause hyperglycemia and glycosuria; in patients taking cardiac glycosides because they are more susceptible to digitalis toxicity from acetazolamide-induced hypokalemia; and in patients taking diuretics.

Interactions
Acetazolamide alkalizes urine and thus may decrease excretion of amphetamines, procainamide, quinidine, and flecainide. Acetazolamide may increase excretion of salicylates, phenobarbital, and lithium, lowering plasma levels of these drugs and possibly necessitating dosage adjustments.

Effects on diagnostic tests
Because it alkalinizes urine, acetazolamide may cause false-positive proteinuria in Albustix or Albutest. Acetazolamide may also decrease thyroid iodine uptake.

Adverse reactions
● CNS: drowsiness, paresthesias, confusion.
● DERM: rash.
● EENT: transient myopia.
● GI: nausea, vomiting, anorexia.
● GU: crystalluria, renal calculi, hematuria.
● HEMA: *aplastic anemia,* hemolytic anemia, leukopenia.
● Metabolic: *hyperchloremic acidosis,* hypokalemia, asymptomatic hyperuricemia.
● Local: pain at injection site, sterile abscesses.
   Note: Drug should be discontinued if blood pH is below 7.2.

Overdose and treatment
Specific recommendations are unavailable. Treatment is supportive and symptomatic. Acetazolamide increases bicarbonate excretion and may cause hypokalemia and hyperchloremic acidosis. Induce emesis or perform gastric lavage. Do not induce catharsis because this may exacerbate electrolyte disturbances. Monitor fluid and electrolyte levels.

▶ Special considerations
Besides those relevant to all *carbonic anhydrase inhibitors,* consider the following recommendations.
● For patients who have difficulty swallowing tablets, a single dose may be prepared by softening 1 tablet in 2 teaspoons of warm water and adding 2 teaspoonfuls of honey or syrup (chocolate, cherry) and then taken immediately.
● Suspensions containing 250 mg/5 ml of syrup are the most palatable and can be made by a pharmacist. These will remain stable for about 1 week. Tablets will not dissolve in fruit juice.
● Reconstitute powder by adding at least 5 ml sterile water for injection.
● I.M. injection is painful because of alkalinity of solution. Direct I.V. administration is preferred if drug must be given parenterally.
● Acetazolamide has been used for periodic paralysis in dosages up to 1.5 g daily in divided doses b.i.d. or t.i.d.

Geriatric use
Elderly and debilitated patients require close observation, as they are more susceptible to drug-induced diuresis. Excessive diuresis promotes rapid dehydration, leading to hypovolemia, hypokalemia, and hyponatremia, and may cause circulatory collapse. Reduced dosages may be indicated.

Breast-feeding
Safety of acetazolamide in breast-feeding women has not been established.

acetic acid
Domeboro Otic, VōSol Otic Solution

- Pharmacologic classification: acid
- Therapeutic classification: antibacterial, antifungal
- Pregnancy risk category C

How supplied
Available by prescription only
Otic solution: 2% in aluminum acetate, 2% in propylene glycol, 3%

Indications, route, and dosage
External ear canal infection
Adults and children: 4 to 6 drops into ear canal t.i.d. or q.i.d.; or insert saturated wick for first 24 hours, then continue with instillations.
Prophylaxis of swimmer's ear
Adults and children: 2 drops in each ear b.i.d.

Pharmacodynamics
Antibacterial and antifungal action: Inhibits or destroys bacteria and fungi in the ear canal by increasing acidity of normal skin, creating an undesirable environment for the growth of these organisms, particularly *Pseudomonas*. Can be used as both an otic and topical anti-infective.

Pharmacokinetics
Unknown.

Contraindications and precautions
Acetic acid is contraindicated in patients with hypersensitivity to any component of the preparation. Otic preparations should be used with caution in the presence of perforated eardrum.

Interactions
None reported.

Effects on diagnostic tests
None significant.

Adverse reactions
- DERM: urticaria.
- Ear: irritation or itching.
- Other: overgrowth of nonsusceptible organisms.
  Note: Drug should be discontinued if severe irritation or sensitivity develops.

Overdose and treatment
To treat accidental ingestion, dilute drug but do not induce vomiting, and evaluate for burns. Treat accidental ocular exposure by flushing the eye with warm water for at least 15 minutes. Treat accidental dermal exposure by washing affected area twice with soap and water.

▶ **Special considerations**
- Reculture persistent otic drainage.
- Avoid contact with eyes and mucous membranes.
- Apply to freshly cleansed area free of other medications.
- Topical application is especially useful for treating superficial gram-negative infections.
- Use aseptic technique to prevent infection.
- To administer eardrops to adults, pull the earlobe up and back.

Information for the patient
Teach patient correct and safe procedures for using acetic acid and administering eardrops.

Pediatric use
To administer eardrops to children, pull the earlobe down and back.

acetohexamide
Dymelor

- Pharmacologic classification: sulfonylurea
- Therapeutic classification: antidiabetic agent
- Pregnancy risk category D

How supplied
Available by prescription only
Tablets: 250 mg, 500 mg

Indications, route, and dosage
Adjunct to diet to lower blood glucose levels in patients with non-insulin-dependent diabetes mellitus (type II)
Adults: Initially, 250 mg P.O. daily before breakfast; may increase dose q 5 to 7 days (by 250 to 500 mg) as needed to a maximum of 1.5 g daily, divided b.i.d. or t.i.d. before meals.
To replace insulin therapy
Adults: If insulin dosage is less than 20 units daily, insulin may be stopped and oral therapy started with 250 mg P.O. daily before breakfast, increased as above, if needed. If insulin dosage is 20 or more units daily, start oral therapy with 250 mg P.O. daily before breakfast, while reducing the insulin dosage 25% to 30% daily or every other day, depending on response to oral therapy.

Pharmacodynamics
Antidiabetic action: Acetohexamide lowers blood glucose levels by stimulating insulin release from functioning beta cells in the pancreas. After prolonged administration, the drug's hypoglycemic effects appear to reflect extrapancreatic effects, possibly including reduction of basal hepatic glucose production and enhanced peripheral sensitivity to insulin. The latter may result either from an increase in the number of insulin receptors or from changes in events subsequent to insulin binding. Acetohexamide has a moderate uricosuric effect.

Pharmacokinetics
• *Absorption:* Acetohexamide is absorbed rapidly from the GI tract. Onset of action occurs within 1 hour, with a maximum decrease in serum glucose levels within 2 hours.
• *Distribution:* Acetohexamide's distribution is not fully understood, but probably is similar to that of the other sulfonylureas; it is highly protein-bound.
• *Metabolism:* Acetohexamide is metabolized in the liver, primarily to a potent active metabolite.
• *Excretion:* Acetohexamide and its metabolites are excreted primarily (80%) in urine. The duration of action is 12 to 24 hours. Half-life of acetohexamide and its metabolite is approximately 6 hours.

Contraindications and precautions
Acetohexamide is contraindicated in patients with known hypersensitivity to sulfonylureas or thiazides; in patients with burns, acidosis, diabetic coma, severe infection, ketosis, severe trauma, or major surgery because such conditions of severe physiologic stress require insulin for adequate control of serum glucose levels; and in patients with nonfunctioning beta cells.

This drug should be used with caution in patients with hepatic or renal insufficiency because it is metabolized in the liver and excreted in urine; and in those with adrenal, pituitary, or thyroid dysfunction.

Interactions
Concomitant use of acetohexamide with alcohol may produce a disulfiram-like reaction consisting of nausea, vomiting, abdominal cramps, and headaches. Concomitant use with anticoagulants may produce an increase in plasma levels of both drugs and, after continued therapy, reduced plasma levels and anticoagulant effects. Concomitant use with chloramphenicol, guanethidine, insulin, monoamine oxidase inhibitors, oxyphenbutazone, phenylbutazone, probenecid, salicylates, or sulfonamides may enhance the hypoglycemic effect by displacing acetohexamide from its protein-binding sites.

Concomitant use of acetohexamide with beta-adrenergic blocking agents (including ophthalmics) may increase the risk of hypoglycemia by masking symptoms of developing hypoglycemia, such as rising pulse rate and blood pressure, and by blocking gluconeogenesis, thereby prolonging hypoglycemia. Use with drugs that may increase blood glucose levels (adrenocorticoids, glucocorticoids, amphetamines, baclofen, corticotropin, epinephrine, ethacrynic acid, furosemide, oral contraceptives, phenothiazines, phenytoin, thiazide diuretics, triamterene, or thyroid hormones) may require dosage adjustments for either or both drugs.

Concomitant use of acetohexamide may increase the hypoglycemic effects of anabolic steroids, cimetidine, clofibrate, NSAIDs, and miconazole; and may decrease the hypoglycemic effects of isoniazid, nicotinic acid, calcium channel blockers, and rifampin.

Because smoking increases corticosteroid release, patients who smoke may require a higher dosage of acetohexamide.

Effects on diagnostic tests
Acetohexamide therapy alters serum uric acid concentration, cholesterol, alkaline phosphatase, bilirubin, and blood urea nitrogen levels.

Adverse reactions
• CNS: weakness, paresthesia.
• DERM: eczema, pruritus, facial flushing, erythema, urticaria, morbilliform or maculopapular eruptions, photosensitivity.
• GI: cholestatic jaundice, nausea, vomiting, epigastric fullness, heartburn.
• HEMA: leukopenia, thrombocytopenia, mild anemia, *agranulocytosis.*
• Metabolic: sodium loss, hypoglycemia.
• Other: *hypersensitivity reactions.*
Note: Drug should be discontinued if signs or symptoms of hypersensitivity, including jaundice, skin eruptions, blood dyscrasias, and severe diarrhea, occur, or if serial and progressive increases in serum alkaline phosphatase levels occur.

Overdose and treatment
Clinical manifestations of overdose include low blood glucose levels, tingling of lips and tongue, hunger, nausea, decreased cerebral function (lethargy, yawning, confusion, agitation, and nervousness), increased sympathetic activity (tachycardia, sweating, and tremor), and ultimately convulsions, stupor, and coma.

Mild hypoglycemia (without loss of consciousness or neurologic findings) can be treated with oral glucose and dosage adjustments. In severe hypoglycemia, the patient should be hospitalized immediately. If patient loses consciousness or experiences neurologic symptoms, patient should receive rapid injection of dextrose 50%, followed by a continuous infusion of dextrose 10% at a rate to maintain blood glucose levels greater than 100 mg/dl. Monitor for 24 to 48 hours.

▶ **Special considerations**
Besides those relevant to all *sulfonylureas,* consider the following recommendations.
• To avoid GI intolerance in patients taking dosages of 1 g/day or more and to improve control of hyperglycemia, divided doses are recommended. These are given before the morning and evening meals.
• Patients switching from chlorpropamide to acetohexamide should be monitored closely for 1 week because of chlorpropamide's prolonged retention in the body.
• Elderly, debilitated, or malnourished patients and those with impaired renal or hepatic function usually require a lower initial dosage.
• The manufacturer recommends against using acetohexamide in pregnancy complicated by diabetes.
• Oral hypoglycemic agents have been associated with an increased risk of cardiovascular mortality as compared to diet or diet and insulin treatments.

Information for the patient
• Emphasize the importance of following prescribed diet, exercise, and medical regimen.
• Tell patient to take medication at the same time each day. If a dose is missed, it should be taken immediately, unless it's almost time for the next dose. Patient should never take double doses.
• Advise patient to avoid alcohol; disulfiram-like reaction is possible with moderate to large intake.
• Advise patient to wear a Medic Alert bracelet or necklace.
• Tell patient to take acetohexamide with food if the drug causes GI upset.
• Teach patient to recognize signs and symptoms of hypoglycemia and hyperglycemia and what to do if they occur.

● Teach patient to monitor blood glucose, urine glucose, or ketone levels, as prescribed.

Geriatric use
Elderly patients may be more sensitive to the effects of this medication because of reduced metabolism and elimination and are more likely to develop neurologic symptoms of hypoglycemia.

Pediatric use
Acetohexamide is ineffective in insulin-dependent (type I, juvenile-onset) diabetes.

acetohydroxamic acid
Lithostat

● Pharmacologic classification: urease inhibitor
● Therapeutic classification: antiurolithic, adjunctive agent in treatment of urinary tract infection
● Pregnancy risk category X

How supplied
Available by prescription only
Tablets (scored): 250 mg

Indications, route, and dosage
Prophylaxis of struvite renal calculi; adjunctive agent in treating chronic urinary tract infections caused by urease-producing bacteria
Adults: 250 mg P.O. t.i.d. or q.i.d. Administer at 6- to 8-hour intervals at a time when the stomach is empty. Maximum daily dose is 1.5 g.
Children: Initially, 10 mg/kg P.O. daily in two or three divided doses; titrate to clinical condition and hematologic effects.

Pharmacodynamics
● *Antiurolithic action:* Acetohydroxamic acid causes irreversible, noncompetitive inhibition of the enzyme urease, thus inhibiting the hydrolysis of urea and the subsequent production of ammonia in urine infected with urease-producing bacterial flora. Acetohydroxamic acid decreases urine pH and indirectly reduces the formation and growth of urine calculi or crystals. Acetohydroxamic acid is most effective at a urine pH of 7, but will inhibit urease production within a pH range of 5 to 9.
● *Antibacterial action:* Acetohydroxamic acid does not have a direct antibacterial effect at normal concentrations, but the reduction of pH and urinary ammonia concentrations may act synergistically with some antibacterials.

Pharmacokinetics
● *Absorption:* An oral dose is absorbed rapidly, primarily in the upper GI tract.
● *Distribution:* Acetohydroxamic acid is distributed widely in body water. The drug crosses the placenta; its distribution in human breast milk is unknown.
● *Metabolism:* Acetohydroxamic acid is metabolized to a non-urease-inhibiting compound, acetamide, through a saturable or rate-limited process. Unchanged ace-

tohydroxamic acid in the urine is the active form of the drug.
● *Excretion:* Acetohydroxamic acid is excreted principally in urine. In patients with normal renal function, approximately 35% to 65% of an oral dose is excreted unchanged in the urine within 24 to 48 hours. Less than 10% is excreted as acetamide. In patients with impaired or reduced renal function, a smaller fraction of the dose is excreted unchanged. The plasma half-life of acetohydroxamic acid increases with increasing dose and ranges from 3.5 to 10 hours. It is not known if the drug is dialyzable. The urinary acetohydroxamic acid concentration for optimal response has not been established. Therapeutic effect has been observed with urine concentration between 8 and 70 mcg/ml, but best results occur with levels above 30 mcg/ml.

Contraindications and precautions
Acetohydroxamic acid is contraindicated in patients with non-urease producing organisms, and in those with serum creatinine greater than 2.5 mg or creatinine clearance below 20 ml/minute, because the drug may accumulate in patients with renal failure. It should be used only in carefully selected patients, usually concomitantly with effective antimicrobial therapy or surgical removal of renal calculi. It is contraindicated in women who are or may become pregnant. Women of childbearing age should not receive this drug unless they have an effective method of birth control.

Patients treated with acetohydroxamic acid should have a complete blood count (CBC) with reticulocyte count after 2 weeks of therapy and every 3 months thereafter. If the CBC reveals a reticulocyte count greater than 6%, dosage should be reduced.

Interactions
Concomitant use of acetohydroxamic acid with alcohol may cause a macular rash on the upper extremities and face, typically within 30 to 45 minutes after alcohol ingestion. When used concurrently with iron, acetohydroxamic acid may chelate and interfere with both iron and acetohydroxamic acid absorption; with methenamine, acetohydroxamic acid produces a synergistic reaction, potentiating the antibacterial effects of methenamine in chronic urinary tract infections.

Effects on diagnostic tests
None reported.

Adverse reactions
● CNS: headache, depression, anxiety, nervousness.
● CV: phlebitis, deep vein thrombosis, pulmonary embolism, palpitation.
● DERM: macular rash, scalp tenderness, alopecia, excessive perspiration.
● GI: nausea, vomiting, anorexia, diarrhea, constipation.
● HEMA: reticulocytosis, hypochromic anemia, Coombs'-negative hemolytic anemia, decreased platelet count, decreased white blood cell count.
● Other: malaise, lethargy, fatigue.

Overdose and treatment
Overdose with acetohydroxamic acid may cause anorexia, tremulousness, hematologic toxicity, nausea, and vomiting. Treatment is mainly supportive and symptomatic; it may include blood transfusions as necessary.

▶ **Special considerations**
● Administer on an empty stomach 1 hour before or 2 hours after a meal to ensure maximum drug absorption.
● Review cardiopulmonary, cardiovascular, and hematologic status, including CBC and platelet count. Obtain a baseline and check every 2 weeks initially, then every 3 months, for possible adverse reactions.
● Monitor renal and hepatic function studies to check for possible impairment. Check intake and output and watch for signs and symptoms of decreased renal function.
● Watch for signs and symptoms of phlebitis as a possible side effect.
● If patient needs iron, administer it parenterally; oral iron intake may interfere with absorption of drug because of chelate formation.
● Do not administer to fertile female until pregnancy has been ruled out and appropriate contraception is in effect.

Information for the patient
● Advise patient to avoid alcohol, which can cause a skin rash in patients who are taking acetohydroxamic acid.
● Warn patient to avoid pregnancy during treatment because drug is teratogenic.
● Warn patient to avoid oral iron supplements and all other oral preparations containing iron because drug can chelate iron and decrease absorption.

Geriatric use
Lower doses may be required for elderly patients with decreased renal function.

Pediatric use
Safe use has not been established in children under age 8.

Breast-feeding
It is not known whether acetohydroxamic acid enters breast milk, but use should be avoided in breast-feeding women.

---

acetophenazine maleate
Tindal

● Pharmacologic classification: phenothiazine (piperazine derivative)
● Therapeutic classification: antipsychotic
● Pregnancy risk category C

How supplied
Available by prescription only
Tablets: 20 mg

Indications, route, and dosage
Psychotic disorders
Adults: Initially, 20 mg P.O. t.i.d. or q.i.d. Daily dosage ranges from 40 to 80 mg in outpatients or 80 to 120 mg in hospitalized patients; however, in severe psychotic states, up to 600 mg daily has been administered safely. Smallest effective dose should be used at all times.

Pharmacodynamics
Antipsychotic action: Acetophenazine is thought to exert its antipsychotic effects by postsynaptic blockade of CNS dopamine receptors, thereby inhibiting dopamine-mediated effects.
Acetophenazine has many other central and peripheral effects; it produces alpha and ganglionic blockade and counteracts histamine- and serotonin-mediated activity. Its most prominent adverse reactions are extrapyramidal.

Pharmacokinetics
● *Absorption:* Oral tablet absorption is erratic and variable, with onset of action ranging from ½ to 1 hour.
● *Distribution:* Acetophenazine is distributed widely into the body, including breast milk. CNS concentrations are higher than plasma concentrations. Drug is 91% to 99% protein-bound. Peak effect occurs at 2 to 4 hours; steady-state serum levels are achieved within 4 to 7 days.
● *Metabolism:* Acetophenazine is metabolized extensively by the liver, but no active metabolites are formed; duration of action is about 4 to 6 hours.
● *Excretion:* Most of the drug is excreted in urine as inactive metabolites; some is excreted in feces via the biliary tract.

Contraindications and precautions
Acetophenazine is contraindicated in patients with known hypersensitivity to phenothiazines and related compounds, including allergic reactions involving hepatic function; in patients with blood dyscrasias and bone marrow depression because it may cause agranulocytosis; in patients in coma or with brain damage, CNS depression, circulatory collapse, or cerebrovascular disease because of its hypotensive effects; and in patients with adrenergic blocking agents or spinal or epidural anesthetics because of the potential for additive adrenergic blocking effects.
Acetophenazine should be used cautiously in patients with cardiac disease (arrhythmias, congestive heart failure, angina pectoris, valvular disease, or heart block), encephalitis, Reye's syndrome, head injury, respiratory disease, epilepsy and other seizure disorders, glaucoma, prostatic hypertrophy, urinary retention, hepatic or renal dysfunction, Parkinson's disease, pheochromocytoma, or hypocalcemia.

Interactions
Concomitant use of acetophenazine with sympathomimetics, including epinephrine, phenylephrine, phenylpropanolamine, and ephedrine (often found in nasal sprays), and appetite suppressants may decrease their stimulatory and pressor effects. Concomitant use of epinephrine as a pressor agent may cause epinephrine reversal because of its alpha-adrenergic blocking effects.
Acetophenazine may inhibit blood pressure response to centrally acting antihypertensive drugs such as guanethidine, guanabenz, guanadrel, clonidine, methyldopa, and reserpine. Additive effects are likely after concomitant use of acetophenazine with CNS depressants (including alcohol, analgesics, barbiturates, narcotics, tranquilizers, and general, spinal, or epidural anesthetics) and parenteral magnesium sulfate (oversedation, respiratory depression, and hypotension); antiarrhythmic agents, quinidine, disopyramide, or procainamide (increased incidence of cardiac dysrhythmias and conduction defects); atropine and other an-

ticholinergic drugs (including antidepressants, monoamine oxidase inhibitors, phenothiazines, antihistamines, meperidine, and antiparkinsonian agents [oversedation, paralytic ileus, visual changes, and severe constipation]); nitrates (hypotension); or metrizamide (increased risk of convulsions).

Beta-blocking agents may inhibit acetophenazine metabolism, increasing plasma levels and toxicity.

Concomitant use with propylthiouracil increases risk of agranulocytosis; concomitant use with lithium may result in severe neurologic toxicity with an encephalitis-like syndrome, and a decreased therapeutic response to acetophenazine.

Pharmacokinetic alterations and subsequent decreased therapeutic response to acetophenazine may follow concomitant use with phenobarbital (enhanced renal excretion), aluminum- and magnesium-containing antacids and antidiarrheals (decreased absorption), or caffeine, and with heavy smoking (increased metabolism).

Acetophenazine may antagonize the therapeutic effects of bromocriptine on prolactin secretion; it may also decrease the vasoconstricting effects of high-dose dopamine and may decrease the effectiveness and increase toxicity of levodopa (by dopamine blockade). Acetophenazine may inhibit metabolism and increase toxicity of phenytoin.

Effects on diagnostic tests
Acetophenazine may cause false-positive test results for urinary porphyrins, urobilinogen, amylase, and 5-hydroxyindoleacetic acid (5-HIAA), because of darkening of urine by metabolites; it also causes false-positive results in urine pregnancy tests using human chorionic gonadotropin (HCG).

Acetophenazine elevates results of tests for liver function and protein-bound iodine and causes quinidine-like effects on the ECG.

Adverse reactions
● CNS: extrapyramidal symptoms, such as dystonia, akathisia, torticollis, and tardive dyskinesia (usually dose-related with long-term therapy but it can develop quickly); sedation (low incidence), pseudoparkinsonism, drowsiness (frequent); *neuroleptic malignant syndrome* (dose-related; fatal *respiratory failure* in over 10% of patients if untreated); dizziness, headache, insomnia, exacerbation of psychotic symptoms.
● CV: orthostatic hypotension, *asystole,* tachycardia, dizziness, fainting, arrhythmias, ECG changes, increased anginal pain (after I.M. injection).
● EENT: blurred vision, tinnitus, mydriasis, increased intraocular pressure, ocular changes (retinal pigmentary change with long-term use).
● GI: dry mouth, constipation, nausea, vomiting, anorexia, diarrhea.
● GU: urinary retention, gynecomastia, hypermenorrhea, inhibited ejaculation.
● HEMA: transient leukopenia, *agranulocytosis,* thrombocytopenia, anemia (within 30 to 90 days).
● Local: contact dermatitis from concentrate or injectable form, muscle necrosis from I.M. injection.
● Other: hyperprolactinemia, photosensitivity, increased appetite and weight gain, hypersensitivity (rash, urticaria, drug fever, edema, cholestatic jaundice [in 2% to 4% of patients within first 30 days]).

After abrupt withdrawal of long-term therapy, gastritis, nausea, vomiting, dizziness, tremors, feeling of heat or cold, sweating, tachycardia, headache, or insomnia may occur.

Note: Drug should be discontinued if the following reactions occur: hypersensitivity, jaundice, agranulocytosis, neuroleptic malignant syndrome (marked hyperthermia, extrapyramidal effects, autonomic dysfunction), and severe extrapyramidal symptoms that persist after dosage is lowered. Drug should be discontinued 48 hours before and 24 hours after myelography using metrizamide because of the risk of convulsions. When feasible, drug should be withdrawn slowly and gradually; many drug effects persist after withdrawal.

Overdose and treatment
Acetophenazine overdose causes CNS depression characterized by deep, unarousable sleep and possible coma, hypotension or hypertension, extrapyramidal symptoms, dystonia, abnormal involuntary muscle movements, agitation, seizures, arrhythmias, ECG changes, hypothermia or hyperthermia, and autonomic nervous system dysfunction.

Treatment is symptomatic and supportive, including maintaining vital signs, airway, stable body temperature, and fluid and electrolyte balance.

Do not induce vomiting: drug inhibits cough reflex, and aspiration may occur. Use gastric lavage, then activated charcoal and saline cathartics; drug is not dialyzable. Regulate body temperature as needed. Treat hypotension with I.V. fluids: *do not give epinephrine.* Treat seizures with parenteral diazepam or barbiturates; arrhythmias with parenteral phenytoin (1 mg/kg with rate titrated to blood pressure); extrapyramidal reactions with benztropine or parenteral diphenhydramine at 2 mg/kg/minute.

▶ Special considerations
Besides those relevant to all *phenothiazines,* consider the following recommendations.
● Drug may cause a pink-brown discoloration of the patient's urine.
● Acetophenazine causes a high incidence of extrapyramidal effects and photosensitivity reactions. Patient should avoid exposure to sunlight or heat lamps.
● Oral tablet may cause stomach upset; administer with food or fluid.
● Sugarless chewing gum or hard candy, ice chips, or artificial saliva may help to alleviate dry mouth.
● Monitor blood pressure before and after oral administration.

Information for the patient
● Explain risks of dystonic reactions and tardive dyskinesia, and tell patient to report abnormal body movements.
● Tell patient to avoid sun exposure and to wear sunscreen when going outdoors, to prevent photosensitivity reactions. (Note that heat lamps and tanning beds also may cause burning of the skin or skin discoloration.)
● Warn patient to avoid extremely hot or cold baths and exposure to temperature extremes, sunlamps, or tanning beds. Drug may cause thermoregulatory changes.
● Tell patient to take the drug exactly as prescribed, not to double dose for missed ones, and not to discontinue the drug suddenly.
● Explain that most adverse reactions can be relieved

by a dosage reduction. Patient should promptly report difficulty urinating, sore throat, dizziness, or fainting.
● Tell patient that many drug interactions are possible. Patient should seek medical approval before taking *any* self-prescribed medications.
● Inform patient that he should become tolerant to the drug's sedative effects in several weeks.
● Tell patient to avoid hazardous activities that require alertness until the drug's effect is established.
● Tell patient to avoid alcohol and other medications that may cause excessive sedation.
● Suggest sugarless hard candy or chewing gum, or ice to relieve dry mouth.

Geriatric use
Elderly patients may require only 30% to 50% of regular adult dose. They are more likely to develop adverse reactions, especially tardive dyskinesia and other extrapyramidal effects.

Pediatric use
Drug is not recommended for pediatric use.

Breast-feeding
Acetophenazine enters into the breast milk. Drug should be used with caution. The potential benefits to the mother should outweigh the potential harm to the breast-feeding infant.

acetylcholine chloride
Miochol

● Pharmacologic classification: cholinergic agonist
● Therapeutic classification: miotic
● Pregnancy risk category C

How supplied
Available by prescription only
Ophthalmic solution: 1%

Indications, route, and dosage
Anterior segment surgery
Adults and children: 0.5 to 2 ml of 1% solution instilled gently in anterior chamber of eye. Drug is used during ophthalmic surgery to cause rapid, complete miosis.

Pharmacodynamics
Miotic action: The cholinergic activity of acetylcholine causes contraction of the sphincter muscles of the iris, resulting in miosis and contraction of the ciliary muscle, leading to accommodation. It also acts to deepen the anterior chamber and vasodilates conjunctival vessels of the outflow tract.

Pharmacokinetics
● *Absorption:* Action begins within seconds.
● *Distribution:* Unknown.
● *Metabolism:* Probably local, by cholinesterases.
● *Excretion:* Duration of activity is 10 to 20 minutes.

Contraindications and precautions
Acetylcholine is contraindicated in patients with hypersensitivity to the drug and in patients in whom miosis is undesirable (acute iritis). Although systemic effects are uncommon at usual doses, caution is advised in patients with acute cardiac failure, bronchial asthma, peptic ulcer, hyperthyroidism, GI spasm, urinary tract obstruction, or Parkinson's disease, because drug may worsen these conditions.

Interactions
None reported.

Effects on diagnostic tests
None significant.

Adverse reactions
● Eye: transient lenticular opacities, iris atrophy (drug concentrations greater than 1%).
Note: Drug should be discontinued if signs of systemic absorption occur; these include bradycardia, hypotension, flushing, breathing difficulties, and sweating.

Overdose and treatment
Overdose is extremely rare after ophthalmic use but may cause miosis, flushing, vomiting, bradycardia, bronchospasm, increased bronchial secretion, sweating, tearing, involuntary urination, hypotension, and seizures. Flush eyes with normal saline solution or sterile water. If drug was accidentally swallowed, vomiting is usually spontaneous; if not, induce emesis with activated charcoal or a cathartic. Treat accidental dermal exposure by washing the area twice with water. Epinephrine may be used to treat adverse cardiovascular reactions.

▶ Special considerations
Besides those relevant to all *cholinergic agonists,* consider the following recommendations.
● Solutions of acetylcholine chloride are unstable; prepare solution immediately before use, and discard any solution that is not clear and colorless or any unused solution.
● If the center rubber plug seal does not go down or is already down when reconstituting, do not use the vial.
● Do not gas-sterilize vial. Ethylene oxide may produce formic acid.

acetylcysteine
Airbron*, Mucomyst, Mucosol, Parvolex*

● Pharmacologic classification: amino acid (L-cysteine) derivative
● Therapeutic classification: mucolytic agent, antidote for acetaminophen overdose
● Pregnancy risk category B

How supplied
Available by prescription only
Solution: 10%, 20%
Injection*: 200 mg/ml

Indications, route, and dosage
Acute and chronic bronchopulmonary disease, tracheostomy care, pulmonary complications of surgery, diagnostic bronchial studies

---

Administer by nebulization, direct application, or intratracheal instillation.

Adults and children: 1 to 2 ml of 10% or 20% solution by direct instillation into trachea as often as every hour; or 3 to 5 ml of 20% solution or 6 to 10 ml of 10% solution administered by nebulizer every 2 to 3 hours. For instillation via percutaneous intratracheal catheter, administer 1 to 2 ml of 20% solution or 2 to 4 ml of 10% solution; via tracheal catheter to treat a specific bronchopulmonary tree segment, administer 2 to 5 ml of 20% solution. For diagnostic bronchial studies (administered before procedure), administer 1 to 2 ml of 20% solution or 2 to 4 ml of 10% solution for 2 or 3 doses.

Acetaminophen toxicity
Adults and children: Initially, 140 mg/kg P.O., followed by 70 mg/kg q 4 hours for 17 doses (a total of 1,330 mg/kg) or until acetaminophen assay reveals nontoxic level. Alternatively may be administered intravenously: Loading dose 150 mg/kg I.V. in 200 ml D_5W over 15 minutes, followed by 50 mg/kg I.V. in 500 ml D_5W over 4 hours, followed by 100 mg/kg I.V. in 100 ml D_5W over 16 hours.

Pharmacodynamics
● *Mucolytic action:* Acetylcysteine produces its mucolytic effect by splitting the disulfide bonds of mucoprotein, the substance responsible for increased viscosity of mucus secretions in the lungs; thus, pulmonary secretions become less viscous and more liquid.
● *Acetaminophen antidote:* The mechanism by which acetylcysteine reduces acetaminophen toxicity is not fully understood; it is thought that acetylcysteine restores hepatic stores of glutathione or inactivates the toxic metabolite of acetaminophen via a chemical interaction, thereby preventing liver damage.

Pharmacokinetics
● *Absorption:* Most inhaled acetylcysteine acts directly on the mucus in the lungs; the remainder is absorbed by pulmonary epithelium. Action begins within 1 minute after inhalation, and immediately upon direct intratracheal instillation; peak effect occurs in 5 to 10 minutes. After oral administration, acetylcysteine is absorbed from the GI tract.
● *Distribution:* Unknown.
● *Metabolism:* Acetylcysteine is metabolized in the liver.
● *Excretion:* Unknown.

Contraindications and precautions
Acetylcysteine is contraindicated in patients with known hypersensitivity to the drug; however, it may be given to hypersensitive patients to treat acetaminophen overdose if the allergic symptoms are controlled. It should be used with caution in patients with asthma because bronchospasm may occur; if it does, discontinue acetylcysteine immediately. It also should be used with caution in geriatric or debilitated patients with respiratory insufficiency, because it may increase airway obstruction; and in all patients who exhibit inadequate cough during therapy, because secretions may occlude airways.

Interactions
Activated charcoal adsorbs orally administered acetylcysteine, preventing its absorption.

Acetylcysteine is incompatible with oxytetracycline, tetracycline, chlortetracycline, erythromycin lactobionate, amphotericin B, ampicillin, iodized oil, chymotryp-

sin, trypsin, and hydrogen peroxide; drug should be administered separately.

Effects on diagnostic tests
None reported.

Adverse reactions
● CNS: drowsiness.
● EENT: rhinorrhea, hemoptysis.
● GI: stomatitis, vomiting, nausea.
● Other: clammy skin, *bronchospasm,* sensitization (rare), fever and chills (rare).
● Long-term use: transient maculopapular rash.

Overdose and treatment
No information available.

▶ Special considerations
● Acetylcysteine solutions release hydrogen sulfide and discolor on contact with rubber and some metals (especially iron, nickel, and copper); drug tarnishes silver (this does not affect drug potency).
● Solution may turn light purple; this does not affect drug's safety or efficacy. Use plastic, stainless steel, or other inert metal when administering drug by nebulization. Do not use hand-held bulb nebulizers; output is too small and particle size too large.
● After opening, store in refrigerator or use within 96 hours.
● Monitor cough type and frequency; for maximum effect, instruct patient to clear airway by coughing before aerosol administration. Many clinicians pretreat with bronchodilators before administration of acetylcysteine. Keep suction equipment available; if patient has insufficient cough to clear increased secretions, suction will be needed to maintain open airway.
● When used orally for acetaminophen overdose, dilute with cola, fruit juice, or water to a 5% concentration and administer within 1 hour.
● Do not place directly in the chamber of a heated (hot pot) nebulizer.

Information for the patient
Warn patient of unpleasant odor (rotten egg odor of hydrogen sulfide), and explain that increased amounts of liquefied bronchial secretion plus unpleasant odor may cause nausea and vomiting; have patient rinse mouth with water after nebulizer treatment because it may leave a sticky coating on the oral cavity.

Geriatric use
Elderly patients may have inadequate cough and be unable to clear airway completely of mucus. Keep suction equipment available, and monitor patient closely.

Pediatric use
Acetylcysteine may be given by tent or croupette. A sufficient volume (up to 300 ml) of a 10% or 20% solution should be used to maintain a heavy mist in the tent for the time prescribed. Administration may be continuous or intermittent.

Breast-feeding
It is unknown if acetylcysteine is excreted in breast milk.

activated charcoal
Actidose-Aqua, Arm-a-char,
Charcoaide, Charcocaps, Insta-Char,
Liquid-Antidose

- Pharmacologic classification: adsorbent
- Therapeutic classification: antidote, antidiarrheal, antiflatulent
- Pregnancy risk category C

How supplied
Available without prescription
Tablets: 325 mg, 650 mg
Capsules: 260 mg
Powder: 30 g, 50 g
Suspension: 0.625 g/5 ml, 0.83 g/5 ml, 1 g/5 ml,
1.25 g/5 ml

Indications, route, and dosage
Flatulence or dyspepsia
Adults: 600 mg to 5 g P.O. t.i.d. or q.i.d.
Poisoning
Adults and children: 5 to 10 times estimated weight of
drug or chemical ingested. Minimum dose is 30 g in
250 ml water to make a slurry.

Give orally, preferably within 30 minutes of ingestion.
Larger doses are necessary if food is in the stomach.
Drug is used adjunctively in treating poisoning or overdose with acetaminophen, amphetamines, aspirin, antimony, atropine, arsenic, barbiturates, camphor, cocaine, cardiac glycosides, glutethimide, ipecac, malathion, morphine, poisonous mushrooms, opium, oxalic
acid, parathion, phenol, phenothiazines, potassium
permanganate, propoxyphene, quinine, strychnine, sulfonamides, or tricyclic antidepressants.

Activated charcoal may be given 30 g q 6 hours for
1 to 2 days (gastric dialysis) to enhance removal of
some drugs from the bloodstream.

Pharmacodynamics
- *Antidote action:* Activated charcoal adsorbs ingested
toxins, thereby inhibiting GI absorption.
- *Antidiarrheal action:* Activated charcoal adsorbs toxic
and nontoxic irritants that cause diarrhea or GI discomfort.
- *Antiflatulent action:* Activated charcoal adsorbs intestinal gas to relieve discomfort.

Pharmacokinetics
- *Absorption:* Activated charcoal is not absorbed from
the GI tract.
- *Distribution:* None.
- *Metabolism:* None.
- *Excretion:* Activated charcoal is excreted in feces.

Contraindications and precautions
Activated charcoal is contraindicated in patients with
poisoning resulting from ingestion of cyanide, mineral
acids, strong bases, methanol, and ethanol because it
is relatively ineffective. It may produce vomiting, or may
obstruct endoscopic evaluation of GI lesions.

Interactions
Milk products decrease the effectiveness of activated
charcoal. Activated charcoal inactivates syrup of ipecac
and also adsorbs and inactivates many oral medica-
tions when used concomitantly, including orally administered acetylcysteine; charcoal should be removed by
gastric lavage before acetylcysteine is administered.

Effects on diagnostic tests
None reported.

Adverse reactions
- GI: vomiting (especially with high doses), constipation or diarrhea, black stools.

Overdose and treatment
No information available.

▶ Special considerations
- Do not give activated charcoal to a semiconscious
or unconscious patient.
- Because activated charcoal absorbs and inactivates
syrup of ipecac, give only after emesis is complete.
- Activated charcoal is most effective when used within
30 minutes of toxin ingestion; a cathartic is commonly
administered with or after activated charcoal to speed
removal of the toxin/charcoal complex.
- Do not give in ice cream, milk, or sherbert; dairy
products reduce drug's absorptive capacity.
- Powder form is most effective. Mix with tap water to
form consistency of thick syrup. A small amount of fruit
juice or flavoring may be added to make mixture more
palatable.
- May need to repeat dose if patient vomits shortly
after administration.
- Prolonged use (over 72 hours) may impair patient's
nutritional status.
- If administering this drug for any indication other than
poisoning, be sure to give other medications 1 hour
before or 2 hours after activated charcoal.
- Activated charcoal may be used orally to decrease
colostomy odor.

Information for the patient
- Tell patient to call poison information center or hospital emergency department before taking activated
charcoal as an antidote.
- If patient is using activated charcoal as an antidiarrheal or antiflatulent, instruct him to take medications
1 hour before or 2 hours after activated charcoal. For
antidiarrheal use, advise him to report diarrhea that
persists after 2 days of therapy, fever or flatulence that
persists after 7 days.
- Warn patient that activated charcoal turns stools
black.
- Advise patient not to mix drug with milk products,
which may lessen its effectiveness.

---

*Canada only   †Unlabeled clinical use   Italicized adverse reactions are life-threatening.

acyclovir (acycloguanosine)
acyclovir sodium
Zovirax

- Pharmacologic classification: synthetic purine nucleoside
- Therapeutic classification: antiviral agent
- Pregnancy risk category C

How supplied
Available by prescription only
Tablets: 800 mg
Capsules: 200 mg
Oral suspension: 200 mg/5 ml
Injection: 500 mg/vial, 1g/vial
Ointment: 5%

Indications, route, and dosage
Initial and recurrent mucocutaneous herpes simplex virus (HSV-I and HSV-II) or severe initial genital herpes in immunocompromised patient
Adults and children over age 11: 5 mg/kg, given at a constant rate over a period of 1 hour by I.V. infusion q 8 hours for 7 days (5 days for genital herpes).
Children under age 12: 250 mg/m², given at a constant rate over a period of 1 hour by I.V. infusion q 8 hours for 7 days (5 days for genital herpes).
†*Treatment of disseminated herpes zoster*
Adults: 5 to 10 mg/kg I.V. q 8 hours for 7 to 10 days. Infuse over at least 1 hour.
Treatment of initial genital herpes
Adults: 200 mg P.O. q 4 hours while awake (a total of five capsules daily). Treatment should continue for 10 days.
Treatment of acute herpes zoster infections
Adults: 800 mg P.O. five times daily for 7 to 10 days. Initiate therapy within 48 hours of rash onset.
Intermittent therapy for recurrent genital herpes
Adults: 200 mg P.O. q 4 hours while awake (a total of five capsules daily). Treatment should continue for 5 days. Initiate therapy at the first sign of recurrence.
Chronic suppressive therapy for recurrent genital herpes
Adults: 200 mg P.O. t.i.d. for up to 6 months.
Herpes genitalis; non-life-threatening herpes simplex infection in immunocompromised patient
Adults and children: Apply sufficient quantity of ointment to adequately cover all lesions q 3 hours, six times a day for 7 days.
Treatment of acute varicella (chicken pox) infections
Adults and children: 20 mg/kg (not to exceed 800 mg) P.O. q.i.d. for 5 days. Initiate therapy at first sign or symptom.
Dosage in renal failure
Oral dose
200 mg q 12 hours if creatinine clearance drops below 10 ml/minute.
I.V. dose
5 mg/kg q 8 hours if creatinine clearance exceeds 50 ml/minute; 5 mg/kg q 12 hours if it ranges from 25 to 50 ml/minute; 5 mg/kg q 24 hours if it ranges from 10 to 25 ml/minute; 2.5 mg/kg q 24 hours if it falls below 10 ml/minute.
Note: In patients undergoing hemodialysis, 5 mg/kg may be given after each dialysis treatment.

Pharmacodynamics
Antiviral action: Acyclovir is converted by the viral cell into its active form (triphosphate) and inhibits viral DNA polymerase.

In vitro, acyclovir is active against herpes simplex virus Type I, herpes simplex virus Type II, varicella-zoster virus, Epstein-Barr virus, and cytomegalovirus. In vivo, acyclovir may reduce the duration of acute infection and speed lesion healing in initial genital herpes episodes. Patients with frequent herpes recurrences (more than six episodes a year) may receive oral acyclovir prophylactically for 4 to 6 months to prevent recurrences or reduce their frequency.

Pharmacokinetics
- *Absorption:* With oral administration, acyclovir is absorbed slowly and incompletely (15% to 30%). Peak concentrations occur in 1½ to 2 hours. Absorption is not affected by food. With topical administration, absorption is minimal.
- *Distribution:* Acyclovir is distributed widely to organ tissues and body fluids. CSF concentrations equal approximately 50% of serum concentrations. About 9% to 33% of a dose binds to plasma proteins.
- *Metabolism:* Acyclovir is metabolized inside the viral cell to its active form. Approximately 10% of a dose is metabolized extracellularly.
- *Excretion:* Up to 92% of systemically absorbed acyclovir is excreted as unchanged drug by the kidneys by glomerular filtration and tubular secretion. In patients with normal renal function, half-life is 2 to 3½ hours. Renal failure may extend half-life to 19 hours.

Contraindications and precautions
Acyclovir is contraindicated in patients with known hypersensitivity to the drug.

Acyclovir should be administered cautiously to patients with dehydration, renal dysfunction, or preexisting neurologic dysfunction, because it may aggravate these disorders.

The risk of neurologic abnormalities may increase in patients who experience neurologic reactions to interferon or intrathecal methotrexate.

Interactions
Concomitant use with probenecid may result in reduced renal tubular secretion of acyclovir, leading to increased drug half-life, reduced elimination rate, and decreased urinary excretion. This reduced clearance causes more sustained serum drug levels. Concomitant use with zidovudine may result in increased levels of acyclovir, causing toxicity.

Effects on diagnostic tests
Serum creatinine and blood urea nitrogen (BUN) levels may increase during acyclovir therapy.

Adverse reactions
- CNS: headache, encephalopathic signs (lethargy, obtundation, tremor, confusion, hallucinations, agitation, *seizures, coma*).
- CV: hypotension.
- DERM: rash, transient burning and stinging, pruritus.
- GI: nausea, vomiting, diarrhea.

- GU: hematuria, crystalluria, reversible renal dysfunction
- Local: inflammation, vesicular eruptions and phlebitis at injection site.
- Other: arthralgia, resistant viruses (with prolonged or repeated use).
  Note: Drug should be discontinued if hypersensitivity or encephalopathic reactions occur.

Overdose and treatment
Overdose has followed I.V. bolus administration in patients with unmonitored fluid status or in patients receiving inappropriately high parenteral dosages. Acute toxicity has not been reported after high oral dosage. Hemodialysis removes acyclovir.

Clinical effects of overdose include signs of nephrotoxicity, including elevated serum creatinine and BUN levels, progressing to renal failure.

▶ **Special considerations**
- Drug should not be administered subcutaneously, I.M., by I.V. bolus, or ophthalmically.
- Intravenous dose should be infused over at least 1 hour to prevent renal tubular damage.
- Acyclovir's solubility in urine is low. Ensure that patient taking the systemic form of the drug is well hydrated to prevent nephrotoxicity.
- Monitor serum creatinine level. If level does not return to normal within a few days after therapy begins, may increase hydration, adjust dose, or discontinue drug.
- Encephalopathic signs are more likely in patients who have experienced neurologic reactions to cytotoxic drugs.

Information for the patient
- Warn patient that although drug helps manage the disease, it does not cure it or prevent it from spreading to others.
- For best results, tell patient to begin taking drug when early infection symptoms (such as tingling, itching, or pain) occur.
- Instruct patient who is taking ointment to use a finger cot or rubber glove and to apply about a ½" (1 cm) ribbon of ointment for every 4 in² (26 cm²) of surface area to be covered. Ointment should thoroughly cover each lesion. Warn patient to avoid getting ointment in the eye.
- Warn patient to avoid sexual intercourse during active genital infection.

Geriatric use
Administer drug cautiously to elderly patients because they may suffer from renal dysfunction or dehydration.

Pediatric use
Safety and effectiveness of oral and topical acyclovir in children have not been established. I.V. acyclovir has been used with only a limited number of children. To reconstitute acyclovir for children, do not use bacteriostatic water for injection containing benzyl alcohol.

adenosine
Adenocard

- Pharmacologic classification: nucleoside
- Therapeutic classification: antiarrhythmic
- Pregnancy risk category C

How supplied
Available by prescription only
Injection: 3 mg/ml in 2-ml vials

Indications, route, and dosage
Conversion of paroxysmal supraventricular tachycardia (PSVT) to sinus rhythm
Adults: 6 mg I.V. by rapid bolus injection (over 1 to 2 seconds). If PSVT is not eliminated in 1 to 2 minutes, give 12 mg by rapid I.V. push. Repeat 12-mg dose if necessary. Single doses over 12 mg are not recommended.

Pharmacodynamics
Antiarrhythmic action: Adenosine is a naturally occurring nucleoside. In the heart, it acts on the AV node to slow conduction and inhibit reentry pathways. Adenosine is also useful for the treatment of PSVT associated with accessory bypass tracts (Wolff-Parkinson-White syndrome).

Pharmacokinetics
- *Absorption:* Adenosine is administered by rapid I.V. injection.
- *Distribution:* Adenosine is rapidly taken up by erythrocytes and vascular endothelial cells.
- *Metabolism:* Adenosine is metabolized within tissues to inosine and adenosine monophosphate.
- *Excretion:* Unknown; circulating plasma half-life is less than 10 seconds.

Contraindications and precautions
Adenosine is contraindicated in patients with atrial flutter, atrial fibrillation, and ventricular tachycardia because the drug is ineffective in treating these arrhythmias. It is also contraindicated in patients allergic to the drug.

Because it decreases conduction through the AV node, adenosine may produce a transient first-, second-, or third-degree heart block. For this reason, it is contraindicated in patients with second- or third-degree heart block or sick sinus syndrome, unless the patient has an artificial pacemaker. Because the drug has a very short half-life, these effects are usually transient; however, patients who develop significant block after a dose of adenosine should not receive additional doses.

More than half of the patients in clinical trials developed new arrhythmias when adenosine was used to convert to normal sinus rhythm. Such arrhythmias are usually transient, but may include sinus bradycardia or tachycardia, atrial premature contractions, various degrees of AV block, premature ventricular contractions, and skipped beats.

Inhaled adenosine will cause bronchoconstriction in asthmatic patients. Asthma attacks have not been reported, but the potential for bronchoconstriction exists. According to some experimental evidence, high concentrations of adenosine may induce chromosomal damage. The clinical significance of this effect is not known.

Interactions
Higher degrees of heart block occur in patients receiving concomitant carbamazepine. Dipyridamole may potentiate the drug's effects, and smaller doses may be necessary. Methylxanthines antagonize effects of adenosine. Therefore, patients receiving theophylline or caffeine may require higher doses or may not respond to adenosine therapy.

Effects on diagnostic tests
None reported.

Adverse reactions
● CNS: apprehension, back pain, blurred vision, burning sensation, dizziness, heaviness in arms, light-headedness, neck pain, numbness, tingling in arms.
● CV: chest pain, facial flushing, headache, hypotension, palpitations, sweating.
● GI: metallic taste, nausea.
● Respiratory: chest pressure, dyspnea, shortness of breath, hyperventilation.
● Other: tightness in throat, groin pressure.

Overdose and treatment
Because the half-life of adenosine is less than 10 seconds, the adverse effects of overdosage usually dissipate rapidly and are self-limiting. Treat any lingering adverse effects symptomatically.

▶ Special considerations
● Rapid I.V. injection is necessary for drug action. Administer directly into a vein if possible; if an I.V. line is used, use the most proximal port and follow with a rapid saline flush to ensure that the drug reaches the systemic circulation rapidly.
● Check solution for crystals, which may occur if solution is cold. If crystals are visible, gently warm solution to room temperature. Do not use solutions that aren't clear.
● Discard unused drug because it contains no preservatives.

Information for the patient
Warn the patient that facial flushing may occur.

PHARMACOLOGIC CLASS

adrenergics, direct and indirect acting

albuterol sulfate
bitolterol mesylate
dobutamine hydrochloride
dopamine hydrochloride
ephedrine
ephedrine hydrochloride
ephedrine sulfate
epinephrine
epinephrine bitartrate
epinephrine hydrochloride
epinephryl borate
isoetharine hydrochloride
isoetharine mesylate
isoproterenol
isoproterenol hydrochloride
isoproterenol sulfate
metaproterenol sulfate
metaraminol bitartrate
metaxalone
naphazoline hydrochloride
norepinephrine bitartrate
phenylephrine hydrochloride
pirbuterol
pseudoephedrine hydrochloride
pseudoephedrine sulfate
terbutaline sulfate
tetrahydrozoline
xylometazoline

Beta-receptor activation is associated with the activation of adenylate cyclase and the accumulation of cyclic 3',5'-monophosphate (cyclic AMP); the cellular consequences of alpha-receptor activation are less well understood.

Over the years, more specific alpha- and beta-receptor agonists and antagonists have been synthesized and studied, and these agents have permitted the subclassification of these receptors. Alpha$_1$ receptors are located on smooth muscle and glands and are excitatory; alpha$_2$ receptors are prejunctional regulatory receptors in the CNS and postjunctional receptors in many peripheral tissues. Beta$_1$ receptors are located in cardiac tissues and are excitatory; beta$_2$ receptors are located primarily on smooth muscle and glands and are inhibitory.

Adrenergic drugs may mimic the naturally occurring catecholamines norepinephrine, epinephrine, and dopamine, or they may function indirectly by stimulating the release of norepinephrine.

Pharmacology
Most of the actions of the clinically useful adrenergic agents involve peripheral excitatory actions on glands and vascular smooth muscle; cardiac excitatory actions; CNS excitatory actions; peripheral inhibitory actions on smooth muscle of the bronchial tree, blood vessels supplying skeletal muscle, and gut; and metabolic and endocrine effects. Because different tissues respond in varying degrees to adrenergic agonists, differences in the actions of catecholamines are attributed to the presence of different receptor types within the tissues (alpha and beta).

Clinical indications and actions
Most agents act on two or more receptor sites; the net effect is the sum of alpha and beta activity. Dopaminergic and serotonergic activity may occur as well, possibly stimulating receptors in the CNS to release histamine.

Temporary appetite suppression is another of their effects, often resulting in a reboundlike weight gain after patient develops tolerance to the anorexic effect, or after withdrawal of the drug. Other uses include support of blood pressure, suppression of urinary incontinence and enuresis, and relief from pain of dysmenorrhea.

Hypotension
Alpha agonists (norepinephrine, metaraminol, phenylephrine, and pseudoephedrine) cause arteriolar and venous constriction, resulting in increased blood pressure. This action is useful in supporting blood pressure in hypotensive states and in management of various serious allergic conditions. Topical formulations are used to induce local vasoconstriction (decongestion), to ar-

---

rest superficial hemorrhage (styptic), to stimulate radial smooth muscle of the iris (mydriasis), and in combination with local anesthetics to localize anesthesia and prolong duration of action.

Cardiac stimulation

The $beta_1$ agonists (dobutamine) act primarily in the heart, producing a positive inotropic effect. Because they increase heart rate, enhance atrioventricular (AV) conduction, and increase the strength of the heartbeat, $beta_1$ agonists may be used to restore heartbeat in cardiac arrest and for heart block in syncopal seizures (not treatment of choice), or to treat acute heart failure and cardiogenic or other types of shock. Their use in shock is somewhat controversial, because $beta_1$ agonists induce lipolysis (increase of free fatty acids in plasma), which promotes a metabolic acidosis, and because they favor arrhythmias, which pose a special threat in cardiogenic shock.

Bronchodilation

$Beta_2$ agonists (albuterol, bitolterol, isoetharine, metaproterenol, and terbutaline) act primarily on smooth muscle of the bronchial tree, vasculature, intestine, and uterus. They also induce hepatic and muscle glycogenolysis, which results in hyperglycemia (sometimes useful in insulin overdose) and hyperlactic acidemia.

Some are used as bronchodilators; some as vasodilators. They are also used to relax the uterus and delay delivery in premature labor and for dysmenorrhea. Some degree of cardiostimulation may occur, because all $beta_2$ agonists have some degree of $beta_1$ activity.

Shock

Dopamine is currently the only commercially available sympathomimetic with significant dopaminergic activity, although some other sympathomimetics appear to act on dopamine receptors in the CNS. Dopamine receptors are prominent in the periphery (splanchnic and renal vasculature), where they mediate vasodilation, which is useful in treating shock and acute heart failure. Renal vasodilation may induce diuresis.

Overview of adverse reactions

As expected, the multiple activities of sympathomimetics can produce numerous adverse reactions. However, certain precautions apply to all. Patients known to be more sensitive to the effects of these drugs include elderly persons, infants, and patients with thyrotoxicosis or cardiovascular disease.

The alpha agonists commonly produce cardiovascular reactions. An excessive increase in blood pressure is a major adverse reaction of systemically administered alpha agonists. Exaggerated pressor response may occur in hypertensive or elderly patients, which may evoke vagal reflex responses resulting in bradycardia and various degrees of AV block. Alpha agonists also interfere with lactation and may cause nausea, vomiting, sweating, piloerection, rebound congestion, rebound miosis, difficult urination, and headache. Ophthalmic use may cause mydriasis and photophobia.

The beta agonists most frequently cause tachycardia, palpitations, and other arrhythmias. Their other effects include premature atrial and ventricular contraction; tachyarrhythmias, and myocardial necrosis. Reflex tachycardia and palpitations occur with $beta_2$ agonists because of decreased blood pressure.

Metabolic reactions to beta agonists include hyperglycemia, increased metabolic rate, hyperlactic acidosis, local and systemic acidosis (decreases bronchodilator response).

Respiratory reactions include increased perfusion of nonfunctioning portions of lungs (in chronic obstructive pulmonary disease); mucus plugs may develop as a result of increased mucus secretion.

Other reactions include tremors, vertigo, insomnia, sweating, headache, nausea, vomiting, and anxiety.

The centrally acting adrenergics have similar effects, which may also be associated with dry mouth, flushing, diarrhea, impotence, hyperthermia (excessive doses), agitation, anorexia, dizziness, dyskinesia, and changes in libido. Chronic use of adrenergics in children may cause endocrine disturbances that arrest growth; however, growth usually rebounds after withdrawal of drug.

▶ Special considerations
Parenteral preparations

● If used as a pressor agent, correct fluid volume depletion before administration. Adrenergics are not a substitute for blood, plasma, fluid, or electrolytes.
● Monitor blood pressure, pulse, and respiratory and urinary output carefully during therapy.
● Tachyphylaxis or tolerance may develop after prolonged or excessive use.

For inhalation therapy

● The preservative sodium bisulfite is present in many adrenergic formulations. Patients with a history of allergy to sulfites should avoid preparations that contain this preservative.
● Therapy should be administered when patient arises in morning and before meals to reduce fatigue by improving lung ventilation.
● For unknown reasons, paradoxical airway resistance (manifested by sudden increase in dyspnea) may result from repeated excessive use of isoetharine. If this occurs, patient should discontinue drug and use alternative therapy (such as epinephrine).
● Adrenergic inhalation may be alternated with other drug administration (steroids, other adrenergics) if necessary, but should not be administered simultaneously because of danger of excessive tachycardia.
● Do not use discolored or precipitated solutions.
● Protect solutions from light, freezing, and heat. Store at controlled room temperature.
● Systemic absorption can follow applications to nasal and conjunctival membranes, though infrequently. If symptoms of systemic absorption occur, patient should stop the drug.
● Prolonged or too-frequent use may cause tolerance to bronchodilating and cardiac stimulant effect. Rebound bronchospasm may follow end of drug effect.

Information for the patient
Inhalation

● Dosage and recommended method of inhaling may vary with type of nebulizer and formulation used. Carefully instruct patient in correct use of nebulizer and warn him to use lowest effective dose.
● Instruct patient to wait 1 full minute after initial 1 to 2 inhalations of adrenergic to be sure of necessity for another dose. Drug action should begin immediately and peak within 5 to 15 minutes.
● Teach patient or family that a single aerosol treatment is usually enough to control an asthma attack and to call promptly if the patient requires a significant increase in dosage to prevent an attack. Explain that overuse of adrenergic bronchodilators may cause

tachycardia, palpitations, headache, nausea and dizziness, loss of effectiveness, possible paradoxical reaction, and cardiac arrest.

• Tell patient to call if bronchodilator causes dizziness, chest pain, or lack of therapeutic response to usual dose.

• Tell patient to avoid other adrenergic medications unless they are prescribed.

• Inform patient that saliva and sputum may appear pink after inhalation treatment.

• Information and instructions are furnished with the aerosol forms of these drugs. Urge patient to read them carefully and ask questions if necessary.

• Treatment should start with first symptoms of bronchospasm.

• Caution patient to keep spray away from eyes.

• Tell patient that increased fluid intake facilitates clearing of secretions.

• Teach patient how to accomplish postural drainage, to cough productively, and to clap and vibrate to promote good respiratory hygiene.

• Tell patient not to discard drug applicator. Refill units are available.

• Inform patient taking repeated doses (and responsible family members) about adverse reactions, and advise them to report such reactions promptly.

Nasal

• Instruct patient to blow nose gently (with both nostrils open) to clear nasal passages well, before administration of medication.

• Instruct patient on proper method of instillation.

— Drops: Tell patient to tilt head back while sitting or standing up, or to lie on bed with head over side. Stay in position a few minutes to permit medication to spread through nose.

— Spray: With head upright, squeeze bottle quickly and firmly to produce 1 or 2 sprays into each nostril; wait 3 to 5 minutes, blow nose, and repeat dose.

— Jelly: Place in each nostril and sniff it well back into nose.

Ophthalmic

• To avoid excessive systemic absorption of ophthalmic preparations, tell patient to apply pressure to lacrimal sac during and for 1 to 2 minutes after instillation of drops.

• Inform patient that after instillation of ophthalmic preparation, pupils of eyes will be very large and eyes may be more sensitive to light than usual. Advise patient to use dark glasses until pupils return to normal.

• Warn patient to use drug only as directed.

• Tell patient to call if no relief occurs or condition worsens.

• Tell patient to store drug away from heat and light and out of reach of children.

Geriatric use

Elderly patients may be more sensitive to therapeutic and adverse effects of some adrenergics and may require lower dose.

Pediatric use

Lower doses of adrenergics are recommended for use in children.

Breast-feeding

The use of adrenergics during breast-feeding usually is not recommended.

Representative combinations

Ephedrine sulfate with guaifenesin and theophylline: Bronkaid, Bronkolixir; with guaifenesin, theophylline, and phenobarbital: Bronkotabs; with belladonna extract, boric acid, zinc oxide, bismuth oxyiodide, bismuth subcarbonate, balsam peru, beeswax, and cocoa butter: Wyanoids.

Epinephrine with lidocaine: Ardecaine; with benzalkonium chloride: Mytrate, Glaucon; with pilocarpine: E-Pilo, Epicar, E-Carpine.

Isoproterenol hydrochloride with phenylephrine bitartrate: Duo-Medihaler.

Naphazoline with antazoline phosphate, boric acid, phenylmercuric acetate, carbonate anhydrous: Vasocon-A Ophthalmic; with antazoline and polyvinyl alcohol: Albalon-A Liquifilm; with methapyrilene hydrochloride, cetylpyridinium chloride, and thimerosal: Vapocyn II Nasal Spray; with pheniramine maleate: Naphcon A; with phenylephrine hydrochloride, pyrilamine maleate, and phenylpropanolamine hydrochloride: 4-Way Nasal Spray; with polyvinyl alcohol: Albalon Ophthalmic Solution.

Phenylephrine and pilocarpine: Pilofrin.

Pseudoephedrine with chlorpheniramine: Chlortrimeton; with codeine phosphate and guaifenesin: Alamine Expectorant, Bazhistine Expectorant, C-Tussin, Deproist Expectorant with Codeine, Isoclar Expectorant, Novohistine Expectorant, Robitussin-DAC; with dextromethorphan: Contac Cough, Mediquell Decongestant, Sudafed DM; with dextromethorphan and acetaminophen: Viro-Med Liquid; with dextromethorphan, acetaminophen, and guaifenesin: Day-Care, Vicks Formula 44M; with dextromethorphanamine: Disophrol, Drixoral; with dexchlorpheniramine: Polaramine; with guaifenesin: Robitussin-P.E., Sudafed Expectorant*, Zephrex, Pseudo-Bid, Head and Chest; with hydrocordone bitartrate: Bay Cotussend Liquid, De-Tuss, De-tussin Liquid, Entuss-D, Tussend; with triprolidine: Actacin, Actagen, Actamine, Actifed, Actihist, Allerfrin OTC, Aprodine, Cerafed Plus, Norafed, Trifed, Triphed, Tripodrine, Triposed.

See also antihistamines, barbiturates, xanthines.

adrenocorticoids (nasal and oral inhalation)

Nasal
beclomethasone dipropionate
dexamethasone sodium phosphate
flunisolide

Oral
triamcinolone acetonide

Topical administration via oral aerosol and nasal spray delivers adrenocorticoids to sites of inflammation in the nasal passages or the tracheobronchial tree. Because smaller doses are administered, less drug is absorbed systemically, with fewer systemic adverse effects.

Pharmacology

Inhaled glucocorticoid is absorbed through the nasal mucosa or through the trachea, bronchi, and alveoli. The anti-inflammatory effects of the glucocorticoids depend upon the direct local action of the steroid. Glucocorticoids stimulate transcription of messenger RNA in individual cell nuclei to synthesize enzymes that decrease inflammation. These enzymes stimulate biochemical pathways that decrease the inflammatory response by stabilizing leukocyte lysosomal membranes, which prevent the release of destructive acid hydrolases from leukocytes; inhibiting macrophage accumulation in inflamed areas; reducing leukocyte adhesion to the capillary endothelium; reducing capillary wall permeability and edema formation; decreasing complement components; antagonizing histamine activity and release of kinin from substrates; reducing fibroblast proliferation, collagen deposition, and subsequent scar tissue formation; and by other unknown mechanisms.

Clinical indications and actions
Nasal inflammation
Nasal solutions are used to relieve symptoms of seasonal or perennial rhinitis when antihistamines and decongestants are ineffective; to treat inflammatory conditions of the nasal passages; and to prevent recurrence after surgical removal of nasal polyps.
Chronic bronchial asthma
Aerosols are used to treat chronic bronchial asthma not controlled by bronchodilators and other nonsteroidal medications.

Overview of adverse reactions
● Nasal: local sensations of nasal burning and irritation in about 10% of patients; sneezing attacks immediately after the nasal application in about 10% of patients; and transient mild nosebleeds in 10% to 15% of patients, but it is unknown whether this is an effect of the nasal solution or of the dryness it induces in the nasal passages. Localized candidal infections of the nose or pharynx have occurred rarely.
● Oral: localized infections with *Candida albicans* or *Aspergillus niger*, which have occurred commonly in the mouth and pharynx and occasionally in the larynx. These infections may require treatment with appropriate antifungal therapy or discontinuation of treatment with the inhaled corticosteroid.
● Systemic absorption may occur, potentially leading to hypothalamic-pituitary-adrenal (HPA) axis suppression. This is more likely with large doses or with combined nasal and oral corticosteroid therapy.
● Other: Hypersensitivity reactions are possible. Also, some patients may be intolerant of the fluorocarbon propellants in the preparations.

▶ Special considerations
● The therapeutic effects of intranasal inhalants, unlike those of sympathomimetic decongestants, are not immediate. Full therapeutic benefit requires regular use and is usually evident within a few days, although a few patients may require up to 3 weeks of therapy for maximum benefit.
● Use of nasal or oral inhalation therapy may occasionally allow a patient to discontinue systemic corticosteroid therapy. Systemic corticosteroid therapy should be discontinued by gradually tapering the dosage while carefully observing the patient for signs of adrenal insufficiency (joint pain, lassitude, depression).
● After the desired clinical effect is obtained, maintenance dose should be reduced to the smallest amount necessary to control symptoms.
● The drug should be discontinued if the patient develops signs of systemic absorption (including Cushing's syndrome, hyperglycemia, or glucosuria), mu-

cosal irritation or ulceration, hypersensitivity, or infection. (If antifungals or antibiotics are being used with corticosteroids and the infection does not respond immediately, discontinue corticosteroids until the infection is controlled.)

Information for the patient
For patients using a *nasal* inhaler
● Instruct patient to use only as directed. Inform him that full therapeutic effect is not immediate but requires regular use of inhaler.
● Encourage patient with blocked nasal passsages to use an oral decongestant ½ hour before intranasal corticosteroid administration to ensure adequate penetration. Advise patient to clear nasal passages of secretions before using the inhaler.
● Ask patient to read manufacturer's instructions and demonstrate use of inhaler. Assist patient until proper use of inhaler is demonstrated.
● Instruct patient to clean inhaler according to manufacturer's instructions.

For patients using an *oral* inhaler
● Instruct patient to use only as directed.
● Advise patient receiving bronchodilators by inhalation to use the bronchodilator *before* the corticosteroid inhalant to enhance penetration of the corticosteroid into the bronchial tree. Patient should wait several minutes to allow time for the bronchodilator to relax the smooth muscle.
● Ask patient to read manufacturer's instructions and demonstrate use of inhaler. Assist patient until proper use of inhaler is demonstrated.
● Instruct patient to hold breath for a few seconds to enhance placement and action of the drug and to wait 1 minute before taking subsequent puffs of medication.
● Tell patient to rinse mouth with water after using the inhaler to decrease the chance of oral fungal infections. Tell him to check nasal and oral mucous membranes frequently for signs of fungal infection.
● Instruct patient to clean inhaler according to manufacturer's instructions.
● Warn asthma patients not to increase use of corticosteroid inhaler during a severe asthma attack, but to call for adjustment of therapy possibly by adding a systemic steroid.

For patients using *either* type of inhaler
● Tell patient to report decreased response; an adjustment in dosage or discontinuation of the drug may be necessary.
● Instruct patient to observe for adverse effects, and if fever or local irritation develops, to discontinue use and report the effect promptly.

Geriatric use
Many elderly patients suffer from hyperglycemia, impaired wound healing from circulatory disorders, edema, cataracts, insomnia, or osteoporosis; these conditions could be aggravated by the excessive use of corticosteroid inhalant therapy. Because elderly patients also have a reduced ability to metabolize and eliminate drugs, they may have higher plasma drug levels and a higher incidence of adverse reactions. Monitor these patients closely for adverse effects.

Pediatric use
In children, systemic corticosteroid therapy may be successfully substituted for nasal or oral inhalant corti-

costeroid therapy, thus reducing the risk of adverse systemic effects. However, the risk of HPA axis suppression and Cushing's syndrome still exists, particularly if excessive dosages are used. Manifestations of adrenal suppression in children include retardation of linear growth, delayed weight gain, low plasma cortisol concentrations, and lack of response to corticotropin stimulation.

Breast-feeding
Whether systemic absorption of inhaled corticosteroid is sufficient to produce quantities detectable in breast milk is not known. Systemic corticosteroids are secreted into breast milk, but the small quantities are not likely to harm the infant. However, inhalant corticosteroids should be used with caution in breast-feeding women.

Representative combinations
None.

PHARMACOLOGIC CLASS

adrenocorticoids (ophthalmic)

dexamethasone
dexamethasone sodium phosphate
fluorometholone
medrysone
prednisolone acetate
prednisolone sodium phosphate

Ophthalmic preparations provide a simple method of applying medication directly to the site of an ocular disorder. Topical ophthalmic steroids can be used in much smaller doses than those required in oral therapy, thus minimizing the risk of adverse effects. They are effective for treating most external inflammatory conditions of the conjunctiva, sclera, cornea, and anterouveal tract. Ophthalmic corticosteroid preparations are available as sterile ointments, solutions, and suspensions. Solutions or suspensions, which cause minimal interference with vision and have minimal effect on corneal reepithelialization, usually are used during the day. Ointments provide longer contact with the eye and usually are used at night or to treat inflammatory conditions of the eyelid.

Pharmacology
The anti-inflammatory effects of the adrenocorticoids depend on the direct local action of the steroid. Adrenocorticoids stimulate transcription of messenger RNA in individual cell nuclei to synthesize enzymes that decrease inflammation. These enzymes stimulate biochemical pathways that decrease the inflammatory response by stabilizing leukocyte lysosomal membranes, which prevent the release of destructive acid hydrolases from leukocytes; inhibiting macrophage accumulation in inflamed areas; reducing leukocyte adhesion to the capillary endothelium; reducing capillary wall permeability and edema formation; decreasing complement components; antagonizing histamine activity and release of kinin from substrates; reducing fibroblast proliferation, collagen deposition, and subsequent scar tissue formation; and by other unknown mechanisms.

Clinical indications and actions
Inflammation
Ophthalmic adrenocorticoids provide symptomatic relief of allergic disorders involving the eyelid, conjunctiva, cornea, iris, or ciliary body. These disorders include nonpurulent blepharitis, nonpurulent phlyctenular keratoconjunctivitis, vernal conjunctivitis, acne rosacea, iritis, superficial punctate keratitis, cyclitis, contact dermatitis of the conjunctiva and eyelid, episcleritis, and uveitis.

Ophthalmic adrenocorticoids are used to treat corneal injuries from chemical, radiation, or thermal burns, or penetration by foreign bodies.

In combination with anti-infective agents, they are effective in treating eye infections.

Overview of adverse reactions
Topical ophthalmic corticosteroids may cause increased intraocular pressure. The magnitude of increase in intraocular pressure depends on the corticosteroid used, its concentration, and the frequency and duration of administration. A significant increase in intraocular pressure may develop after 1 to 6 weeks of therapy and is usually reversible within a few weeks after discontinuation. Prolonged use (usually longer than a year) may result in open-angle glaucoma, optic nerve damage, or defects in visual acuity and field of vision.

Patients with diabetes mellitus, preexisting glaucoma, or significant myopia are at much greater risk for increased intraocular pressure. In those patients susceptible to intraocular hypertension, a clinically significant increase in intraocular pressure occurs rarely with 1% medrysone; 0.1% fluorometholone is less likely to cause hypertension than 0.5% hydrocortisone or 0.1% prednisolone; and 0.5% hydrocortisone or 0.1% prednisolone is less likely to cause ocular hypertension than 0.1% dexamethasone.

Transient burning and stinging may occur after application. Rarely, mydriasis, ptosis, epithelial punctate keratitis, and possible corneal or scleral malacia may develop. Hypersensitivity has occurred rarely with topical corticosteroid therapy.

Prolonged use (more than 2 years) may result in posterior subcapsular cataracts that do not regress when the drugs are discontinued.

▶ Special considerations
● Ophthalmic products may initially cause sensitivity to bright light. This may be minimized by wearing sunglasses.
● Monitor the patient's response by observing the area of inflammation and eliciting patient comments concerning pruritus and vision. Inspect the eye and surrounding tissues for infection and additional irritation.
● Discontinue the drug if the patient develops signs of systemic absorption (including Cushing's syndrome, hyperglycemia, or glucosuria), skin irritation or ulceration, hypersensitivity, or infection. (If antivirals or antibiotics are being used with corticosteroids and the infection does not respond immediately, corticosteroids should be stopped until the infection is controlled.)

Information for the patient
Method for administering eye drops
● Wash hands well.
● Shake solution or suspension well.
● Tilt head back or lie down.
● Lightly pull lower eyelid down by applying gentle pressure at the lid base at the bony rim of orbit.

- Approach the eye from below with the dropper; do not touch dropper to any tissue.
- Holding dropper no more than 1″ above the eye, drop medication inside lower lid while looking up.
- Try to keep eye open for 30 seconds.
- Apply light finger pressure inward and down to the side of the bridge of the nose (the lacrimal canaliculi) for 1 to 2 minutes after instillation to prevent drainage of solution into nasal passages, where more of the drug is absorbed systemically.
- If using more than one kind of drug at the same time, wait at least 5 minutes before applying the other drops.

Method for administering ophthalmic ointments
- Wash hands well. Hold the tube in your hand several minutes before use to warm it and improve flow of ointment.
- When opening the ointment tube for the first time, squeeze out the first ¼″ of ointment and discard (using sterile gauze) because it may be too dry.
- Apply a small "ribbon" or strip of ointment (¼″ to ½″) to the inside of the lower eyelid. Do not touch any part of the eye with the tip of the tube. Close the eye gently and roll the eyeball in all directions to spread the ointment.
- If using a second eye ointment, wait at least 10 minutes before applying it.

For patients taking any form of eye medication
- Instruct patient to observe for adverse effects. The patient should call if no improvement occurs after 7 to 8 days, if the condition worsens, or if pain, itching, or swelling of the eye occurs.
- Warn patient not to use nonprescription ophthalmic preparations other than those specifically recommended. Nonprescription ophthalmic solutions should not be used for more than 7 days or in children under age 2.
- Warn the patient not to use leftover medication for a new eye inflammation and never to share eye medication with others. Tell him to store all eye medications in original container.
- Patient should call for specific instructions before discontinuing therapy.

Geriatric use
Visual changes become more pronounced as persons age, but 80% to 85% of elderly adults have good to adequate visual acuity up to age 90. However, with advancing age, persons become more vulnerable to pathologic conditions such as cataracts, glaucoma, and macular degeneration. Unfortunately, chronic use of systemic drugs for other medical problems also affects the eyes. Drugs that are especially problematic include antidepressants, cardiovascular drugs, anticholinergic agents, and phenothiazines. Be aware of the visual adverse effects of various drugs in order to advise the patient and other health care practitioners.

In elderly patients, loss of collagen leads to more friable and transparent skin with increased epidermal permeability to water and certain chemicals. Thus, topically applied drugs, such as steroid ointments, may have a greater effect in the elderly. Elderly patients' ability to metabolize and eliminate drugs is also reduced; therefore, they may have higher drug plasma levels and an increased risk of adverse reactions. Monitor these patients closely for adverse effects.

Pediatric use
Because of their greater ratio of skin surface area to body weight, children may be more susceptible than adults to topical corticosteroid-induced hypothalamic-pituitary-adrenal axis suppression and Cushing's syndrome. Although such reactions occur extremely rarely with ophthalmic therapy, it is still advisable to limit corticosteroid therapy in children to the minimum amount necessary for therapeutic efficacy.

Breast-feeding
Whether systemic absorption of ophthalmic corticosteroids is sufficient to produce quantities detectable in breast milk is unknown. Systemic corticosteroids are secreted into breast milk, but the quantities are not likely to harm the infant. However, ophthalmic corticosteroids should be used with caution in breast-feeding women.

Representative combinations
Dexamethasone with neomycin sulfate: NeoDecadron Ocumeter Ophthalmic Solution, NeoDecadron Ophthalmic Ointment; with neomycin sulfate and polymixin B sulfate: Maxitrol Ophthalmic Suspension; with neomycin and polymixin B sulfate: Dexaridin Ophthalmic Suspension.

Hydrocortisone with neomycin sulfate: NeoCortef Ophthalmic Suspension; with neomycin sulfate and polymyxin B sulfate: Cortisporin

Prednisolone acetate with neomycin sulfate: Neo-Delta-Cortef; with chloramphenicol: Chloroptic-P Ophthalmic Ointment; with sulfacetamide sodium: Cetapred Ophthalmic Ointment, Blephamide Liquifilm, Blephamide S.O.P., Metimyd Ophthalmic Ointment or Suspension, Pred-Forte, Predamide, Vasocidin; with phenylephrine: Predulose; with sulfacetamide and phenylephrine hydrochloride: Sulfapred; with atropine sulfate: Mydrapred.

Prednisolone sodium phosphate with neomycin sulfate: Neo-Hydeltrasol; with sodium sulfacetamide: Optimyd.

PHARMACOLOGIC CLASS

adrenocorticoids (systemic)

Glucocorticoids
betamethasone
betamethasone sodium phosphate
**betamethasone sodium phosphate
  and betamethasone acetate**
cortisone acetate
dexamethasone
dexamethasone acetate
dexamethasone sodium phosphate
hydrocortisone
hydrocortisone acetate
hydrocortisone cypionate
hydrocortisone sodium phosphate
hydrocortisone sodium succinate
methylprednisolone
methylprednisolone acetate
**methylprednisolone sodium
  succinate**
paramethasone acetate
prednisolone
prednisolone acetate
prednisolone sodium phosphate
prednisolone tebutate
prednisone

triamcinolone
triamcinolone acetonide
triamcinolone diacetate
triamcinolone hexacetonide

Mineralocorticoids
fludrocortisone acetate

Active adrenocortical extracts were first prepared in 1930; by 1942, chemists had isolated 28 steroids from the adrenal cortex. The adrenocortical hormones are classified according to their activity into two groups: the mineralocorticoids and the glucocorticoids. The mineralocorticoids regulate electrolyte homeostasis. The glucocorticoids regulate carbohydrate, lipid, and protein metabolism; inflammation; and the body's immune responses to diverse stimuli. Many corticosteroids exert both kinds of activity.

Pharmacology

The corticosteroids dramatically affect almost all body systems. They are thought to act by controlling the rate of protein synthesis; they react with receptor proteins in the cytoplasm of sensitive cells to form a steroid-receptor complex. Steroid receptors have been identified in many tissues. The steroid-receptor complex migrates into the nucleus of the cell, where it binds to chromatin. Information carried by the steroid of the receptor protein directs the genetic apparatus to transcribe RNA, resulting in the synthesis of specific proteins that serve as enzymes in various biochemical pathways. Because the maximum pharmacologic activity lags behind peak blood concentrations, corticosteroids' effects may result from modification of enzyme activity rather than from direct action by the drugs.

Mineralocorticoids act renally at the distal tubules to enhance the reabsorption of sodium ions (and thus water) from the tubular fluid into the plasma, and the urinary excretion of both potassium and hydrogen ions. The primary features of excess mineralocorticoid activity are positive sodium balance and expansion of the extracellular fluid volume; normal or slight increase in the concentration of sodium in the plasma; hypokalemia; and alkalosis. In contrast, deficiency of mineralocorticoids produces sodium loss, hyponatremia, hyperkalemia, contraction of the extracellular fluid volume, and cellular dehydration.

Clinical indications and actions
Inflammation

A major pharmacologic use of the glucocorticoids is treatment of inflammation. The anti-inflammatory effects depend on the direct local action of the steroids. Glucocorticoids decrease the inflammatory response by stabilizing leukocyte lysosomal membranes, which prevent the release of destructive acid hydrolases from leukocytes; inhibiting macrophage accumulation in inflamed areas; reducing leukocyte adhesion to the capillary endothelium; reducing capillary wall permeability and edema formation; decreasing complement components; antagonizing histamine activity and release of kinin from substrates; reducing fibroblast proliferation, collagen deposition, and subsequent scar tissue formation; and by other unknown mechanisms.
Immunosuppression

Another major pharmacologic use of the glucocorticoids is immunosuppression. The complete mechanisms of action are unknown, but glucocorticoids reduce activity and volume of the lymphatic system, producing lymphocytopenia, decreasing immunoglobulin and complement concentrations, decreasing passage of immune complexes through basement membranes, and possibly depressing reactivity of tissue to antigen-antibody interaction.
Adrenal insufficiency

Combined mineralocorticoid and glucocorticoid therapy is used in treating adrenal insufficiency and in salt-losing forms of congenital adrenogenital syndrome.
Rheumatic and collagen diseases; other severe diseases

Glucocorticoids are used to treat rheumatic and collagen diseases (arthritis, polyarteritis nodosa, systemic lupus erythematosus); thyroiditis; severe dermatologic diseases, such as pemphigus, exfoliative dermatitis, lichen planus, and psoriasis; allergic reactions; ocular disorders (such as inflammations); respiratory diseases (asthma, sarcoidosis, lipid pneumonitis); hematologic diseases (autoimmune hemolytic anemia, idiopathic thrombocytopenia); neoplastic diseases (leukemias, lymphomas); and GI diseases (ulcerative colitis, regional enteritis, celiac disease). Other indications include myasthenia gravis, organ transplants, nephrotic syndrome, and septic shock.

Overview of adverse reactions

Suppression of the hypothalamic-pituitary-adrenal (HPA) axis is the major effect of systemic therapy with corticosteroids. When administered in high doses or for prolonged therapy, the glucocorticoids suppress release of adrenocorticotropic hormone (ACTH) from the pituitary gland; subsequently, the adrenal cortex stops secreting endogenous corticosteroids. The degree and duration of HPA axis suppression produced by the drugs is highly variable among patients and depends on the dose, frequency and time of administration, and duration of therapy. Patients with a suppressed HPA axis resulting from exogenous glucocorticoid administration who abruptly discontinue therapy may experience severe withdrawal symptoms such as fever, myalgia, arthralgia, malaise, anorexia, nausea, desquamation of skin, orthostatic hypotension, dizziness, fainting, dyspnea, and hypoglycemia. Therefore, corticosteroid therapy should always be withdrawn gradually. Adrenal suppression may persist for as long as 12 months in patients who have received large doses for prolonged periods. Until complete recovery occurs, such patients subjected to stress may show signs and symptoms of adrenal insufficiency; they may require replacement therapy with both a glucocorticoid and a mineralocorticoid.

Cushingoid symptoms, the effects of excessive glucocorticoid therapy, may develop in patients receiving large doses of glucocorticoids over a period of several weeks or longer. These include moon face, central obesity, striae, hirsutism, acne, ecchymoses, hypertension, osteoporosis, muscle atrophy, sexual dysfunction, diabetes, cataracts, hyperlipidemia, peptic ulcer, increased susceptibility to infection, and fluid and electrolyte imbalance.

Other adverse reactions to normal or high dosages of corticosteroids may include CNS effects (euphoria, insomnia, psychotic behavior, pseudotumor cerebri, mental changes, nervousness, restlessness); cardiovascular effects (congestive heart failure, hypertension, edema); GI effects (peptic ulcer, irritation, increased appetite); metabolic effects (hypokalemia, sodium retention, fluid retention, weight gain, hyperglycemia, osteoporosis); dermatologic effects (delayed wound healing, acne, skin eruptions, muscle atrophy, striae); and immunosuppression (increased susceptibility to infection).

▶ Special considerations
● Establish baseline blood pressure, fluid intake and output, weight, and electrolyte status. Watch for any sudden patient weight gain, edema, change in blood pressure, or change in electrolyte status.
● During times of physiologic stress (trauma, surgery, infection), the patient may require additional steroids and may experience signs of steroid withdrawal; patients who were previously steroid-dependent may need systemic corticosteroids to prevent adrenal insufficiency.
● After long-term therapy, the drug should be reduced gradually. Rapid reduction may cause withdrawal symptoms.
● Be aware of the patient's psychological history and watch for any behavioral changes.
● Observe for signs of infection or delayed wound healing.

Information for the patient
● Be sure that the patient understands the need to take the adrenocorticosteroid as prescribed. Give the patient instructions on what to do if a dose is inadvertently missed.
● Warn the patient not to discontinue the drug abruptly.
● Inform the patient of the possible therapeutic and adverse effects of the drug, so that he may report any complications as soon as possible.
● The patient should carry a medical identification card indicating the need for supplemental adrenocorticoids during stress.

Geriatric use
Many elderly patients suffer from hyperglycemia, impaired wound healing from circulatory disorders, edema, cataracts, insomnia, or osteoporosis. These medical conditions could easily be aggravated by corticosteroid therapy. Elderly patients also have a reduced ability to metabolize and eliminate drugs; therefore, they may have higher plasma drug levels and an increased risk of adverse reactions. Monitor these patients closely.

Pediatric use
If possible, avoid long-term administration of pharmacologic dosages of glucocorticoids in children because these drugs may retard bone growth. Manifestations of adrenal suppression in children include retardation of linear growth, delayed weight gain, low plasma cortisol concentrations, and lack of response to corticotropin stimulation. In children who require prolonged therapy, closely monitor growth and development. Alternate-day therapy is recommended to minimize growth suppression.

Breast-feeding
Systemic corticosteroids are secreted into breast milk and could harm the infant. Manufacturers recommend that women who are taking pharmacologic dosages of corticosteroids should not breast-feed.

Representative combinations
Betamethasone sodium phosphate with betamethasone acetate: Celestone Soluspan.

Dexamethasone sodium phosphate with lidocaine hydrochloride: Decadron with Xylocaine.
Prednisolone sodium phosphate with prednisolone acetate: Dual-Pred, Soluject.

PHARMACOLOGIC CLASS

adrenocorticoids (topical)

alclometasone dipropionate
amcinonide
betamethasone benzoate
betamethasone dipropionate
betamethasone valerate
clobetasol propionate
clocortolone pivalate
desonide
desoximetasone
dexamethasone
dexamethasone sodium phosphate
diflorasone diacetate
fluocinolone acetonide
fluocinonide
flurandrenolide
fluticasone propionate
halcinonide
halobetasol propionate
hydrocortisone
hydrocortisone acetate
hydrocortisone butyrate
hydrocortisone valerate
methylprednisolone acetate
mometasone furoate
triamcinolone acetonide

Since topical hydrocortisone was introduced in the 1950s, numerous analogues have been developed to provide a wide range of potencies in creams, ointments, lotions, and gels.

Pharmacology
The anti-inflammatory effects of topical glucocorticoids depend on the direct local action of the steroid. Although the exact mechanism of action is unclear, many researchers believe that glucocorticoids stimulate transcription of messenger RNA in individual cell nuclei to synthesize enzymes that decrease inflammation. These enzymes stimulate biochemical pathways that decrease the inflammatory response by stabilizing leukocyte lysosomal membranes, which prevent the release of destructive acid hydrolases from leukocytes; inhibiting macrophage accumulation in inflamed areas; reducing leukocyte adhesion to the capillary endothelium; reducing capillary wall permeability and edema formation; decreasing complement components; antagonizing histamine activity and release of kinin from substrates; reducing fibroblast proliferation, collagen deposition, and subsequent scar tissue formation; and by other unknown mechanisms.

Topical corticosteroids are minimally absorbed systemically and cause fewer adverse effects than systemically administered corticosteroids. Fluorinated derivatives are absorbed to a greater extent than other topical steroids. The degree of absorption depends on the site of application, the amount applied, the relative potency, the presence of an occlusive dressing (may increase penetration by 10%), the condition of the skin, and the vehicle carrying the drug. Topical corticoste-

COMPARATIVE POTENCY OF TOPICAL CORTICOSTEROIDS

Topical corticosteroid preparations can be grouped according to relative anti-inflammatory activity. The following list arranges groups of topical corticosteroids in decreasing order of potency (based mainly on vasoconstrictor assay or clinical effectiveness in psoriasis). Preparations within each group are approximately equivalent.

GROUP	DRUG	CONCENTRATION (%)
I	betamethasone dipropionate (Diprolene)	0.05
	betamethasone dipropionate (Diprolene AF)	0.05
	clobetasol propionate (Temovate)	0.05
	diflorasone diacetate (Psorcon)	0.05
II	amcinonide (Cyclocort)	0.1
	betamethasone dipropionate ointment (Diprosone)	0.05
	desoximetasone (Topicort)	0.05, 0.25
	diflorasone diacetate (Florone, Maxiflor)	0.05
	fluocinonide (Lidex)	0.05
	fluocinonide gel	0.05
	halcinonide (Halog)	0.1
III	betamethasone benzoate gel	0.025
	betamethasone dipropionate cream (Diprosone)	0.05
	betamethasone valerate ointment (Valisone)	0.1
	diflorasone diacetate cream (Florone, Maxiflor)	0.05
	mometasone furoate (Elocon)	0.1
	triamcinolone acetonide cream (Artistocort)	0.5
IV	desoximetasone (Topicort LP)	0.05
	fluocinolone acetonide (Synalar-HP)	0.2
	fluocinolone acetonide ointment (Synalar)	0.025
	flurandrenolide (Cordran)	0.05
	fluticasone propionate (Cutivate)	0.005, 0.05
	triamcinolone acetonide ointment (Aristocort, Kenalog)	0.1
V	betamethasone benzoate cream	0.025
	betamethasone dipropionate lotion (Diprosone)	0.05
	betamethasone valerate cream or lotion (Valisone)	0.1
	fluocinolone acetonide cream (Synalar)	0.025
	flurandrenolide (Cordran)	0.05
	hydrocortisone butyrate (Locoid)	0.1
	hydrocortisone valerate (Westcort)	0.2
	triamcinolone acetonide cream or lotion (Kenalog)	0.1
VI	alclometasone dipropionate (Aclovate)	0.05
	desonide (Tridesilon)	0.05
	fluocinolone acetonide solution (Synalar)	0.01

roids are used to relieve pruritus, inflammation, and other signs of corticosteroid-responsive dermatoses.

Among the several dosage forms available, ointments are preferred for dry, scaly areas; solutions, gels, aerosols, and lotions for hairy areas. Creams can be used for most areas except those in which additional dampness may cause maceration. Gels and lotions can be used for moist lesions; however, gels may contain alcohol, which can be drying and irritating to the skin. The topical preparations are classified by potency into six groups: group I is the most potent, group VI the least potent.

Clinical indications and actions
Inflammatory disorders of skin and mucous membranes

The topical adrenocorticoids relieve inflammatory and pruritic skin disorders, including localized neurodermatitis, psoriasis, atopic or seborrheic dermatitis, the inflammatory phase of xerosis, anogenital pruritus, discoid lupus erythematosus, lichen planus, granuloma annulare, and lupus erythematosus.

These drugs may also relieve irritant or allergic contact dermatitis; however, relief of acute dermatosis may require systemic adrenocorticoids.

Rectal disorders responsive to this class of drugs include ulcerative colitis, cryptitis, inflamed hemorrhoids, post-irradiation or factitial proctitis, and pruritus ani.

Oral lesions, such as nonherpetic oral inflammatory and ulcerative lesions and routine gingivitis, may respond to treatment with topical adrenocorticoids.

Nonprescription formulations of the topical corticosteroids are indicated for minor skin irritation such as itching; rashes due to eczema, dermatitis, insect bites, poison ivy, poison oak, or poison sumac; or dermatitis resulting from exposure to soaps, detergents, cosmetics, and jewelry.

Overview of adverse reactions

Local effects include burning, itching, irritation, dryness, folliculitis, striae, miliaria, acne, perioral dermatitis, hypopigmentation, hypertrichosis, allergic contact dermatitis, secondary infection, and atrophy.

Systemic absorption may occur, leading to hypothalamic-pituitary-adrenal (HPA) axis suppression.

The risk of adverse reactions increases with the use of occlusive dressings or more potent steroids, in patients with liver disease, and in children (because of their greater ratio of skin surface to body weight).

Prolonged application around the eyes may lead to cataracts or glaucoma.

▶ Special considerations
Method for applying topical preparations
● Wash your hands before and after applying the drug.
● Gently cleanse the area of application. Washing or soaking the area before application may increase drug penetration.
● Apply sparingly in a light film; rub in lightly. Avoid contact with patient's eyes, unless using an ophthalmic product.
● Avoid prolonged application in areas near the eyes, genitals, rectum, on the face, and in skin folds. High-potency topical corticosteroids are more likely to cause striae and atrophy in these areas because of their higher rates of absorption.
● Monitor patient response. Observe area of inflammation and elicit patient comments concerning pruritus. Inspect skin for infection, striae, and atrophy. Skin atrophy is common and may be clinically significant within 3 to 4 weeks of treatment with high-potency preparations; it also occurs more readily at sites where percutaneous absorption is high.
● Do not apply occlusive dressings over topical steroids because this may lead to secondary infection, maceration, atrophy, striae, or miliaria caused by increasing steroid penetration and potency.
● To use with an occlusive dressing if necessary: Apply cream, then cover with a thin, pliable, noninflammable plastic film; seal to adjacent unaffected skin with hypoallergenic tape. Minimize adverse reactions by using occlusive dressing intermittently. Do not leave it in place longer than 16 hours each day.
● For patients with eczematous dermatitis who may develop irritation from adhesive material, hold dressings in place with gauze, elastic bandages, stockings, or stockinette.
● Stop drug if the patient develops signs of systemic absorption (including Cushing's syndrome, hyperglycemia, or glucosuria), skin irritation or ulceration, hypersensitivity, or infection. (If antifungals or antibiotics are being used with corticosteroids and the infection does not respond immediately, corticosteroids should be stopped until infection is controlled.)

Information for the patient
● Instruct patient in use of drug.
● Demonstrate proper application of cream. Observe return demonstration to determine patient's ability to carry out procedure properly at home.
● Instruct patient to discontinue drug and report local or systemic adverse reactions, worsening condition, or persistent symptoms.
● Warn patient not to use nonprescription topical preparations other than those specifically recommended.

Geriatric use
In elderly patients, loss of collagen may lead to more friable and transparent skin with increased epidermal permeability to water and certain chemicals. In these patients, topically applied drugs, such as steroid creams, may have a greater effect locally. Elderly patients also have a reduced ability to metabolize and eliminate drugs and may have higher plasma drug levels and a higher incidence of adverse reactions. Monitor these patients closely.

Pediatric use
Because they have a higher ratio of skin surface area to body weight than adults, children are more susceptible to the systemic effects of topical corticosteroids. This may result in HPA axis suppression, manifested by retardation of linear growth, delayed weight gain, low plasma concentrations, and lack of response to corticotropin stimulation. To minimize the risk, limit topical corticosteroid therapy in children to the minimum amount necessary for therapeutic efficacy. Advise parents not to use tight-fitting diapers or plastic pants on a child being treated in the diaper area, since such garments may serve as occlusive dressings.

Breast-feeding
Whether systemic absorption of topical corticosteroids is sufficient to produce quantities detectable in breast milk is unknown. Systemic corticosteroids are secreted into breast milk, but the quantities are not likely to harm the infant. However, topical corticosteroids should be used with caution in breast-feeding women.

Representative combinations
Betamethasone with clotrimazole: Lotrisone.

Betamethasone dipropionate with clotrimazole: Lotrisone.

Dexamethasone with neomycin sulfate: Neo-Decadron Cream; with neomycin sulfate and polymixin B sulfate: Dexacidin Ointment.

Fluocinolone acetonide with neomycin: Neo-Synalar.
Flurandrenolide with neomycin: Cordran-N.

Hydrocortisone with iodoquinol: Vytone; with iodochlorhydroxyquin: Racet, Vioform-hydrocortisone, AP, Caquin, Corque, Cortin, Lanvisone, Pedi-Cort-V, Viodo HC, Hysone; with pramoxine: Pramosone, FEP, Zone-A; with iodochlorhydroxyquin and pramoxine: Vipramosone, Dermarex, Stera-Foam, Vio-Hydrosone; with neomycin: Neo-Cortef, Neo-Cort-Dome; with neomycin and polymixin B: Cortisporin Cream; with neomycin, bacitracin, and polymyxin B sulfate: Cortisporin Ointment; with neomycin sulfate and polymyxin B sulfate: Cortisporin; with dibucaine: Corticaine; with pyrilamine maleate, pheniramine maleate, and chlorpheniramine: HC Derma-PAX Liquid; with benzocaine, oxyquinoline, ephedrine, menthol, ichthammol, and zinc oxide: Derma Medicone-HC Ointment; with chlorcyclizine: Mantadil Cream; with benzoyl peroxide and mineral oil: Vanoxide HC; with lidocaine and glycerin: Lida-Mantle-HC Cream; with sulfur and salicylic acid: Theracort Lotion; with sodium thiosulfate, salicylic acid, isopropyl alcohol, menthol, and camphor: Komed HC Lotion; with diperodone and zinc oxide: Allersone Ointment.

Methylprednisolone with neomycin: Neo-Medrol.

Prednisolone acetate with neomycin: Neo-Delta-Cortef.

Triamcinolone acetonide with nystatin: Mykacet, Mycogen II, Mycolog II, Myco-Triacet II, Mytrex F, N.G.T.; with neomycin, gramicidin, and nystatin: MycoTricet, Tri-Statin.

---

albumin, human (normal serum albumin, human)
Albuminar-5, Albuminar-25, Albutein 5%, Albutein 25%, Buminate 5%, Buminate 25%, Plasbumin-5, Plasbumin-25

- Pharmacologic classification: blood derivative
- Therapeutic classification: plasma volume expander
- Pregnancy risk category C

How supplied
Injection: 5% (50 mg/ml) in vials of 50 ml, 250 ml, 500 ml, 1,000 ml; 25% (250 mg/ml) in vials of 20 ml, 50 ml, 100 ml

Indications, route, and dosage
Shock
Adults: Initially, 500 ml (5% solution) by I.V. infusion, repeated p.r.n. Dose varies with patient's condition and response. Do not give more than 250 g/48 hours.
Children: 25% to 50% of adult dose in nonemergency.
Hypoproteinemia
Adults: 1,000 to 1,500 ml 5% solution by I.V. infusion daily, maximum rate 5 to 10 ml/minute; or 25 to 100 g 25% solution by I.V. infusion daily, maximum rate 3 ml/minute. Dose varies with patient's condition and response.
Burns
Dosage varies according to extent of burn and patient's condition. Usually maintain plasma albumin level at 2 to 3 g/dl.
Hyperbilirubinemia
Infants: 1 g albumin (4 ml of 25% solution)/kg before transfusion.

Pharmacodynamics
Plasma volume-expanding action: Albumin, 5%, supplies colloid to the blood and expands plasma volume. Albumin, 25%, provides intravascular oncotic pressure at 5:1, causing fluid to shift from interstitial space to the circulation and slightly increasing plasma protein concentration.

Pharmacokinetics
- *Absorption:* Albumin is not adequately absorbed from the GI tract.
- *Distribution:* Albumin accounts for approximately 50% of plasma proteins; it is distributed into the intravascular space and extravascular sites, including skin, muscle, and lungs. In patients with reduced circulating blood volume, hemodilution secondary to albumin administration persists for many hours; in patients with normal blood volume, excess fluid and protein are lost.
- *Metabolism:* Although albumin is synthesized in the liver, liver is not involved in clearance of albumin from plasma in healthy individuals.
- *Excretion:* Little is known about excretion in healthy individuals. Administration of albumin decreases hepatic albumin synthesis and increases albumin clearance if plasma oncotic pressure is high. In certain pathologic states, the liver, kidneys, or intestines may provide elimination mechanisms for albumin.

Contraindications and precautions
Albumin is contraindicated in patients with severe anemia and heart failure because of potential for fluid overload.

Administer albumin cautiously to patients without albumin deficiency or to those with low cardiac reserve, severely restricted salt intake, hepatic or renal failure, dehydration, or pulmonary disease, because of potential for hypervolemia.

Interactions
None significant.

Effects on diagnostic tests
Preparations of albumin derived from placental tissue may increase serum alkaline phosphatase level; all products may slightly increase plasma albumin level.

Adverse reactions
- CV: *vascular overload after rapid infusion,* hypotension, tachycardia, flushing, dilutional anemia (with large doses).
- DERM: urticaria.
- GI: increased salivation, nausea, vomiting.
- Other: chills, fever, altered respiration, *pulmonary edema with rapid infusions,* headache.

Overdose and treatment
Clinical manifestations of overdose include signs of circulatory overload, such as increased venous pressure and distended neck veins, or pulmonary edema; slow flow to a keep-vein-open rate and re-evaluate therapy.

▶ Special considerations
- Solution should be a clear amber color; do not use if cloudy or contains sediment. Store at room temperature; freezing may break bottle.
- Use opened solution promptly, discarding unused portion after 4 hours; solution contains no preservatives and becomes unstable.
- One volume of 25% albumin produces the same hemodilution and relative anemia as five volumes of 5% albumin; reference to "1 unit" albumin usually indicates 50 ml of the 25% concentration, containing 12.5 grams of albumin.
- Dilute if necessary with normal saline solution or 5% dextrose injection. Use 5-micron or larger filter; do not give through 0.22-micron I.V. filter.
- Be certain patient is properly hydrated before starting infusion; product may be administered without regard to blood typing and crossmatching.
- Avoid rapid I.V. infusion; rate is individualized according to patient's age, condition, and diagnosis. In patients with hypovolemic shock, infuse 5% solution at a rate not exceeding 2 to 4 ml/minute, and 25% solution (diluted or undiluted) at a rate not exceeding 1 ml/minute; in patients with normal blood volume, infuse 5% solution at a rate not exceeding 5 to 10 ml/minute, and 25% solution (diluted or undiluted), at a rate not exceeding 2 to 3 ml/minute. Do not give more than 250 g in 48 hours.
- Monitor vital signs carefully; observe patient for adverse reactions.
- Monitor intake and output, hemoglobin, hematocrit, and serum protein and electrolyte levels to help determine continuing dosage.
- Each liter contains 130 to 160 mEq of sodium before dilution with any additional I.V. fluids; a 50-ml bottle of

solution contains 7 to 8 mEq sodium. This preparation was once known as "salt-poor albumin."

Pediatric use
Premature infants with low serum protein concentrations may receive 1.4 to 1.8 ml of a 25% albumin solution (350 to 450 mg albumin).

albuterol sulfate
Proventil, Proventil Repetabs, Proventil Syrup, Ventolin, Ventolin Syrup

- Pharmacologic classification: adrenergic
- Therapeutic classification: bronchodilator
- Pregnancy risk category C

How supplied
Available by prescription only
Tablets: 2 mg, 4 mg
Tablets (sustained-release): 4 mg
Solution: 2 mg/5 ml
Aerosol inhaler: 90 mcg/metered spray
Solution for nebulization: 0.083%, 0.5%

Indications, route, and dosage
To prevent and treat bronchospasm in patients with reversible obstructive airway disease
Adults and children age 12 and over: One to two inhalations q 4 to 6 hours. More frequent administration or a greater number of inhalations is not usually recommended. However, because deposition of inhaled medications is variable, higher doses are occasionally used, especially in patients with acute bronchospasm.

For tablets, give 2 to 4 mg (immediate-release) P.O. t.i.d. or q.i.d.; maximum dosage, 8 mg q.i.d. Alternatively, use sustained-release tablets. Usual starting dosage is 4 mg q 12 hours. Increase to 8 mg q 12 hours if patient fails to respond. Cautiously increase stepwise as needed and tolerated to 16 mg q 12 hours.
Children age 6 to 11: Administer 2 mg P.O. t.i.d. or q.i.d.
Children age 2 to 5: Administer 0.1 mg/kg P.O. t.i.d., not to exceed 2 mg t.i.d.
Adults over age 65: Administer 2 mg P.O. t.i.d. or q.i.d.
To prevent exercise-induced bronchospasm
Adults and children age 12 and over: Two inhalations 15 minutes before exercise.

Pharmacodynamics
Bronchodilator action: Albuterol selectively stimulates beta$_2$-adrenergic receptors of the lungs, uterus, and vascular smooth muscle. Bronchodilation results from relaxation of bronchial smooth muscles, which relieves bronchospasm and reduces airway resistance.

Pharmacokinetics
- *Absorption:* After oral inhalation, albuterol appears to be absorbed gradually (over several hours) from the respiratory tract; however, most of the dose is swallowed and absorbed through the GI tract. Onset of action occurs within 5 to 15 minutes, peaks in ½ to 2 hours, and lasts 3 to 6 hours. After oral administration, albuterol is well-absorbed through the GI tract. Onset of action occurs within 30 minutes and peaks in 2 to 3 hours. Drug effect lasts 4 to 6 hours with regular release tablets and 12 hours with extended release tablets.

- *Distribution:* Albuterol does not cross the blood-brain barrier.
- *Metabolism:* Albuterol is extensively metabolized in the liver to inactive compounds.
- *Excretion:* Albuterol is rapidly excreted in urine and feces. After oral inhalation, 70% of a dose is excreted in urine unchanged and as metabolites within 24 hours; 10% in feces. Elimination half-life is about 4 hours. After oral administration, 75% of a dose is excreted in urine within 72 hours as metabolites; 4% in feces.

Contraindications and precautions
Albuterol is contraindicated in patients with known hypersensitivity to the drug. Administer with caution to patients with hyperthyroidism, diabetes mellitus, cardiovascular disorders (coronary insufficiency or hypertension), or sensitivity to sympathomimetic amines, as drug may worsen these conditions.

Interactions
Concomitant use of orally inhaled albuterol with epinephrine and other orally inhaled sympathomimetic amines may increase sympathomimetic effects and risk of toxicity. Serious cardiovascular effects may follow concomitant use with monoamine oxidase inhibitors and tricyclic antidepressants.

Propranolol and other beta-adrenergic blockers may antagonize the effects of albuterol.

Effects on diagnostic tests
Albuterol may decrease the sensitivity of spirometry used for the diagnosis of asthma.

Adverse reactions
- CNS: tremor, nervousness, sweating, vertigo, central stimulation, hyperactivity, excitement, irritable behavior, insomnia, weakness, dizziness, drowsiness, headache.
- CV: tachycardia, palpitations, peripheral vasodilation, increased or decreased blood pressure, angina.
- EENT: drying and irritation of nose (inhaled form), dilated pupils, epistaxis.
- GI: nausea, vomiting, unusual taste, irritation of oropharynx, increased appetite, heartburn.
- Other: difficult urination, cough, muscle cramps, urticaria, rash, allergic reactions.
Note: Drug should be discontinued if hypersensitivity or paradoxical bronchospasm occurs.

Overdose and treatment
Clinical manifestations of overdose include exaggeration of common adverse reactions, particularly angina, hypertension, hypokalemia, and seizures.

To treat, use selective beta$_2$-adrenergic blockers (such as metoprolol) with extreme caution; these may induce asthmatic attack. *Dialysis is not appropriate.* Monitor vital signs and electrolyte levels closely.

▶ Special considerations
Besides those relevant to all *adrenergics*, consider the following recommendations.
- Small, transient increases in blood glucose level may occur after oral inhalation.
- Serum potassium levels may decrease after I.V. administration, but potassium supplementation is usually unnecessary.
- Effectiveness of treatment is measured by periodic monitoring of the patient's pulmonary function.

Canada only   †Unlabeled clinical use   Italicized adverse reactions are life-threatening.

Information for the patient
• Instruct the patient in proper use of inhaler. Tell patient to read directions before use, that dryness of mouth and throat may occur, and that rinsing with water after each dose may help.
—Administration by metered-dose nebulizers: Shake canister thoroughly to activate; place mouthpiece well into mouth, aimed at back of throat. Close lips and teeth around mouthpiece. Exhale through nose as completely as possible, then inhale through mouth slowly and deeply while actuating the nebulizer to release dose. Hold breath 10 seconds (count "1-100, 2-100, 3-100," until "10-100" is reached); remove mouthpiece, and then exhale slowly.
—Administration by metered powder inhaler: Caution patient not to take forced deep breath, but to breathe with normal force and depth. Observe patient closely for exaggerated systemic drug action.
—Administration by oxygen aerosolization: Administer over 15- to 20-minute period, with oxygen flow rate adjusted to 4 liters/minute. Turn on oxygen supply before patient places nebulizer in mouth. Lips need not be closed tightly around nebulizer opening. Placement of Y tube in rubber tubing permits patient to control administration. Advise patient to rinse mouth immediately after inhalation therapy to help prevent dryness and throat irritation. Rinse mouthpiece thoroughly with warm running water at least once daily to prevent clogging. (It is not dishwasher-safe.) After cleaning, wait until mouthpiece is completely dry before storing. Do not place near artificial heat (dishwasher or oven). Replace reservoir bag every 2 to 3 weeks or as needed; replace mouthpiece every 6 to 9 months or as needed.
Note: Replacement of bags or mouthpieces may require a prescription.
• Tell patient that repeated use may result in paradoxical bronchospasm. The patient should discontinue drug immediately and report this effect immediately.
• Tell patient to call if troubled breathing persists 1 hour after using medication, if symptoms return within 4 hours, if condition worsens, or if new (refill) canister is needed within 2 weeks.
• Tell patient to wait 15 minutes after using inhalational albuterol before using adrenocorticoids (beclomethasone, dexamethasone, flunisolide, or triamcinolone).
• Warn patient to use only as directed, and not to use more than prescribed amount or more often than prescribed.

Geriatric use
Lower dose may be required, because elderly patients are more sensitive to sympathomimetic amines.

Pediatric use
Safety and efficacy of extended release tablets in children under age 12 or regular release tablets in children under age 6 has not been established.

Breast-feeding
It is unknown if albuterol is excreted in breast milk. Alternative feeding methods are recommended.

alclometasone dipropionate
Aclovate

• Pharmacologic classification: topical adrenocorticoid
• Therapeutic classification: anti-inflammatory
• Pregnancy risk category C

How supplied
Available by prescription only
Cream, ointment: 0.05%

Indications, route, and dosage
Inflammation of corticosteroid-responsive dermatoses
Adults: Apply a thin film to affected areas b.i.d. or t.i.d. Gently massage until the medication disappears.

Pharmacodynamics
Anti-inflammatory action: Alclometasone stimulates the synthesis of enzymes needed to decrease the inflammatory response. Alclometasone is a group V nonfluorinated topical glucocorticoid with greater anti-inflammatory activity than hydrocortisone 0.25% to 2.5%. It is similar in potency to desonide 0.05% and fluocinolone acetonide, 0.01%. Applied topically, alclometasone may be used for refractory lesions of psoriasis and other deep-seated dermatoses, such as localized neurodermatitis.

Pharmacokinetics
• *Absorption:* The amount of drug absorbed depends on the amount applied and on the nature of the skin at the application site. It ranges from about 1% in areas with thick stratum corneum (such as the palms, soles, elbows, and knees) to as high as 36% in areas of the thinnest stratum corneum (face, eyelids, and genitals). Absorption increases in areas of skin damage, inflammation, or occlusion. Some systemic absorption of topical steroids may occur, especially through the oral mucosa.
• *Distribution:* After topical application, alclometasone is distributed throughout the local skin. If the drug is absorbed into the circulation, it is rapidly removed from the blood and distributed into muscle, liver, skin, intestines, and kidneys.
• *Metabolism:* After topical administration, alclometasone is metabolized primarily in the skin. The small amount that is absorbed into systemic circulation is metabolized primarily in the liver to inactive compounds.
• *Excretion:* Inactive metabolites are excreted by the kidneys, primarily as glucuronides and sulfates, but also as unconjugated products. Small amounts of the metabolites are also excreted in feces.

Contraindications and precautions
Alclometasone is contraindicated in patients who are hypersensitive to any component of the preparation and in patients with viral, fungal, or tubercular skin lesions.
Alclometasone should be used with extreme caution in patients with impaired circulation because it may increase the risk of skin ulceration.

Interactions
None reported.

Effects on diagnostic tests
None significant.

Adverse reactions
● Local: burning, itching, irritation, dryness, folliculitis, hypertrichosis, acneiform eruptions, hypopigmentation, perioral dermatitis, allergic contact dermatitis, maceration, secondary infection, atrophy, striae, miliaria.

Significant systemic absorption may produce the following reactions.
● CNS: euphoria, insomnia, headache, psychotic behavior, pseudotumor cerebri, mental changes, nervousness, restlessness.
● CV: congestive heart failure, hypertension, edema.
● EENT: cataracts, glaucoma, thrush.
● GI: peptic ulcer, GI irritation, increased appetite.
● Immune: immunosuppression, increased susceptibility to infection.
● Metabolic: hypokalemia, sodium retention, fluid retention, weight gain, hyperglycemia, osteoporosis, growth suppression in children.
● Musculoskeletal: muscle atrophy.
● Other: withdrawal syndrome (nausea, fatigue, anorexia, dyspnea, hypotension, hypoglycemia, myalgia, arthralgia, fever, dizziness, and fainting).

Note: Drug should be discontinued if local irritation, infection, systemic absorption, or hypersensitivity reaction occurs.

Overdose and treatment
No information available.

▶ Special considerations
Recommendations for use of alclometasone, for care and teaching of patients during therapy, and for use in elderly patients, children, and during breast-feeding are the same as those for all *topical adrenocorticoids.*

aldesleukin (interleukin-2, IL-2)
Proleukin

● Pharmacologic classification: lymphokine
● Therapeutic classification: immunoregulatory agent
● Pregnancy risk category C

How supplied
Available by prescription only
Injection: 22 million IU/vial

Indications, route, and dosage
Metastatic renal cell carcinoma
Adults: 600,000 IU/kg (0.037 mg/kg) I.V. q 8 hours for 5 days (a total of 14 doses). After a 9-day rest, repeat the sequence for another 14 doses. Repeat courses may be administered after a rest period of at least 7 weeks from hospital discharge.

Pharmacodynamics
Immunoregulatory action: Aldesleukin is a lymphokine, a highly purified immunoregulatory protein synthesized using genetically engineered *Escherichia coli.* The drug produced is similar to human interleukin-2 (IL-2): it enhances lymphocyte mitogenesis, stimulates long-term growth of IL-2-dependent cell lines, enhances lymphocyte cytotoxicity, induces both lymphokine-activated and natural killer cell activity, and induces the production of interferon gamma.

Pharmacokinetics
● *Absorption:* Onset of aldesleukin is rapid after I.V. administration.
● *Distribution:* Peak serum levels are proportional to dose. About 30% of drug rapidly distributes to the plasma; the balance is rapidly distributed to the liver, kidneys, and lungs. Initial studies indicate that the distribution half-life is 13 minutes after a 5-minute I.V. infusion.
● *Metabolism:* Drug is metabolized by the kidneys to amino acids within the cells lining the proximal convoluted tubules.
● *Excretion:* Drug is excreted through the kidneys by peritubular extraction and glomerular filtration. Peritubular extraction ensures drug clearance as renal function diminishes and serum creatinine rises. Elimination half-life is 85 minutes.

Contraindications and precautions
Aldesleukin is contraindicated in patients with hypersensitivity to the drug or any of its components; drug contains sodium dodecyl sulfate as a solubilizing agent. Aldesleukin is also contraindicated in patients who have received organ allografts because it may increase the risk of allograft rejection in transplant recipients and in patients with abnormal cardiac (thallium) stress test or pulmonary function tests. Retreatment is contraindicated in patients who experienced any of these toxicities from the drug: pericardial tamponade; abnormal cardiac rhythms that were uncontrolled or unresponsive to intervention; sustained ventricular tachycardia (5 beats or more); chest pain accompanied by ECG changes, indicated MI or angina pectoris; renal dysfunction requiring dialysis for 72 hours or more; coma or toxic psychosis lasting 48 hours or more; seizures that were repetitive or difficult to control; ischemia or perforation of the bowel; and GI bleeding requiring surgery.

Do not use this drug unless the patient has had definitive tests documenting normal cardiac and pulmonary function. Use with extreme caution in patients with normal test results if they have a history of cardiac or pulmonary disease. Also use with extreme caution in patients with a history of seizure disorders because the drug may cause seizures.

Use cautiously and with close clinical monitoring because severe adverse effects generally accompany therapy at the recommended dosage. This drug should be used only in a hospital setting under the direction of a physician experienced in the use of anticancer agents. An intensive care facility and specialists skilled in intensive care or cardiopulmonary medicine must be readily available.

Aldesleukin is associated with impaired neutrophil function, which can lead to disseminated infection. Many studies employed prophylactic antibiotic therapy with oxacillin, nafcillin, ciprofloxacin, or vancomycin. Monitor for infection. Patients with bacterial infections should be treated before therapy with aldesleukin.

Aldesleukin has also been associated with capillary leak syndrome (CLS), a condition that results from loss of vascular tone, which allows plasma proteins and fluids to escape into the extravascular space. Mean arterial blood pressure begins to drop within 2 to 12 hours of treatment, edema and effusions may be severe, and death can result from hypoperfusion of major organs. Other conditions that accompany CLS include cardiac arrhythmias, MI, angina, mental status changes, renal insufficiency, respiratory distress or failure, and GI bleeding or infarction.

Interactions

Patients receiving antihypertensives may be at increased risk for hypotension. Concomitant use with corticosteroids may decrease antitumor effectiveness of aldesleukin. Aldesleukin may enhance the toxicity of hepatotoxic, nephrotoxic, cardiotoxic, or myelotoxic drugs. Because aldesleukin can alter CNS function, use cautiously with psychotropic agents.

Effects on diagnostic tests

No direct laboratory test interference has been reported. Toxic effects of the drug may be seen in decreasing hepatic, renal, and thyroid function tests; abnormal serum electrolytes; or abnormal cardiac or pulmonary function tests.

Adverse reactions

● CNS: mental status changes, dizziness, sensory dysfunction, special senses disorders, syncope, motor dysfunction, headache, *coma.*
● CV: hypotension, sinus tachycardia, *arrhythmias,* bradycardia, *PVCs,* premature atrial contractions, *myocardial ischemia, MI, CHF, cardiac arrest, myocarditis, endocarditis, CVA,* pericardial effusion, thrombosis.
● DERM: pruritus, erythema, rash, dryness, *exfoliative dermatitis,* purpura, alopecia, petechiae.
● GI: nausea, vomiting, diarrhea, stomatitis, anorexia, *GI bleeding,* dyspepsia, constipation, abdominal pain.
● GU: oliguria, *anuria,* proteinuria, hematuria, dysuria, urine retention, urinary frequency, urinary tract infection.
● HEMA: anemia, thrombocytopenia, *leukopenia,* coagulation disorders, leukocytosis, eosinophilia.
● Respiratory: *pulmonary congestion,* dyspnea, *pulmonary edema, respiratory failure, pleural effusion, apnea, pneumothorax,* tachypnea.
● Other: jaundice; ascites; hepatomegaly; elevated bilirubin, BUN, serum creatinine, transaminase, and alkaline phosphatase levels; *hypomagnesemia; acidosis; hypocalcemia; hypophosphatemia; hypokalemia;* hyperuricemia; *hypoalbuminemia; hypoproteinemia; hyponatremia; hyperkalemia;* arthralgia; myalgia; fever; chills; chest or back pain; fatigue; weakness; malaise; edema; infections of the catheter tip or injection site; phlebitis; sepsis; weight gain; weight loss, conjunctivitis.

Overdose and treatment

Administration of high doses will produce rapid onset of expected adverse reactions, including cardiac, renal, and hepatic toxicity.

Drug toxicity is dose-related. Treatment is supportive. Because aldesleukin's serum half-life is short, discontinuing the drug may ameliorate many of the adverse effects. Dexamethasone may decrease drug's toxicity but may also impair effectiveness.

▶ Special considerations

● Perform standard hematologic tests, including CBC, differential, and platelet counts; serum electrolytes; and

renal and hepatic function tests before therapy. Also obtain chest X-ray. Repeat daily during drug administration.
● Discontinue drug if patient develops moderate to severe lethargy or somnolence because continued administration can result in coma.
● Patients should be neurologically stable with a negative computed tomography scan for CNS metastases. Drug may exacerbate symptoms in patients with unrecognized or undiagnosed CNS metastases.
● Renal and hepatic impairment occur during treatment. Avoid administering other hepatotoxic or nephrotoxic drugs because toxicity may be additive. Also be prepared to adjust dosage of other drugs to compensate for this impairment. Dosage modification because of toxicity is usually accomplished by holding a dose or interrupting therapy rather than by reducing the dose to be administered.
● Severe anemia or thrombocytopenia may occur. Packed RBCs or platelets may be necessary.
● Treat CLS with careful monitoring of fluid status, pulse, mental status, urine output, and organ perfusion. Central venous pressure monitoring is necessary.
● Because fluid management or administration of pressor agents may be essential to treat CLS, use cautiously in patients who require large volumes of fluid (such as patients with hypercalcemia).
● To avoid altering the drug's pharmacologic properties, reconstitute and dilute carefully, and follow manufacturer's recommendations. Do not mix with other drugs or albumin.
● Reconstitute the vial containing 22 million IU (1.3 mg) with 1.2 ml sterile water for injection. Do not use bacteriostatic water or 0.9% sodium chloride injection because these diluents cause increased aggregation of drug. Direct the stream at the sides of the vial and gently swirl to reconstitute. Do not shake.
● The reconstituted solution will have a concentration of 18 million IU (1.1 mg)/ml. The reconstituted drug should be particle-free and colorless to slightly yellow.
● Add the correct dose of reconstituted drug to 50 ml dextrose 5% in water and infuse over 15 minutes. Do not use an in-line filter. Plastic infusion bags are preferred because they provided consistent drug delivery in early clinical trials.
● Vials are for single-use only and contain no preservative. Discard unused drug.
● Powder for injection or reconstituted solutions must be stored in the refrigerator. After reconstitution and dilution, drug must be administered within 48 hours. Be sure that solutions are returned to room temperature before administering drug to patient.
● Preliminary studies indicate that a high percentage of patients (> 75%) develop nonneutralizing antibodies to aldesleukin when treated with the every-8-hour dosing regimen. A small number (< 1%) develop neutralizing antibodies. The clinical significance of this finding is not yet known.
● Aldesleukin has been investigated for various cancers, including Kaposi's sarcoma, metastatic melanoma, colorectal cancer, and non-Hodgkin's lymphoma.

Information for the patient

Make sure patient understands the serious toxicity that accompanies this drug. Adverse effects are expected with normal doses, and serious toxicity may occur despite close clinical monitoring.

Pediatric use
Safety and effectiveness have not been established in children under age 18.

Breast-feeding
It is unknown if drug is excreted in breast milk. Consider risk/benefit and decide whether to discontinue the drug or discontinue breast-feeding because of the risk of serious adverse effects on the infant.

alfentanil hydrochloride
Alfenta

- Pharmacologic classification: opioid
- Therapeutic classification: analgesic, adjunct to anesthesia, anesthetic
- Controlled substance schedule II
- Pregnancy risk category C

How supplied
Available by prescription only
Injection: 500 mcg/ml in 2, 5, 10, and 20 ml ampules.

Indications, route, and dosage
Adjunct to general anesthetic in the maintenance of general anesthesia with barbiturate, nitrous oxide, and oxygen
Adults: Initially, 8 to 50 mcg/kg I.V., then increments of 3 to 15 mcg/kg I.V. Alternatively, may be administered as a continuous infusion of 0.5 to 3 mcg/kg/minute.
Primary anesthetic for induction of anesthesia when endotracheal intubation and mechanical ventilation are required
Adults: Initially, 130 to 245 mcg/kg I.V., then 0.5 to 1.5 mcg/kg/minute I.V.

Pharmacodynamics
Analgesic and anesthetic action: Alfentanil is a potent opiate receptor agonist with a quick onset and short duration of action.

Pharmacokinetics
- *Absorption:* Administered I.V., alfentanil has an immediate onset of action.
- *Distribution:* Redistributed quickly after absorption, alfentanil is highly (> 90%) protein-bound.
- *Metabolism:* Alfentanil is metabolized in the liver. It has a short half-life (about 1.5 hours).
- *Excretion:* Alfentanil is excreted in urine.

Contraindications and precautions
Alfentanil is contraindicated in patients with known hypersensitivity to any phenylpiperidine (diphenoxylate, fentanyl, meperidine, or sufentanil).

Administer alfentanil with extreme caution to patients with supraventricular arrhythmias; avoid, or administer drug with extreme caution to patient with head injury or increased intracranial pressure, because drug obscures neurologic parameters; or during pregnancy and labor, because drug readily crosses placenta (premature infants are especially sensitive to respiratory and CNS depressant effects of narcotic agonists).

Administer alfentanil cautiously to patients with renal or hepatic dysfunction, because drug accumulation or prolonged duration of action may occur; to patients with pulmonary disease (asthma, chronic obstructive pulmonary disease), because drug depresses respiration and suppresses cough reflex; to patients undergoing biliary tract surgery, because drug may cause biliary spasm; to patients with convulsive disorders, because drug may precipitate seizures; to elderly or debilitated patients, who are more sensitive to both therapeutic and adverse drug effects; and to patients prone to physical or psychic addiction, because of the high risk of addiction to this drug.

In patients weighing more than 20% above their ideal body weight, determine dosage based on ideal body weight.

Alfentanil may produce bradycardia (which may be treated with atropine); administer with particular caution to patients with preexisting bradyarrhythmias.

Interactions
Concomitant use with other CNS depressants (narcotic analgesics, general anesthetics, antihistamines, phenothiazines, barbiturates, benzodiazepines, sedative-hypnotics, tricyclic antidepressants, alcohol, and muscle relaxants) potentiates alfentanil's respiratory and CNS depression, sedation, and hypotensive effects. Concomitant use with cimetidine may also increase respiratory and CNS depression, causing confusion, disorientation, apnea, or seizures.

Drug accumulation and enhanced effects may result if drug is given concomitantly with other drugs that are extensively metabolized in the liver (rifampin, phenytoin, digitoxin); combined use with anticholinergics may cause paralytic ileus.

Patients who become physically dependent on this drug may experience acute withdrawal syndrome if given high doses of a narcotic agonist-antagonist or a single dose of a narcotic antagonist.

Severe cardiovascular depression may result from concomitant use with general anesthetics. Diazepam may produce cardiovascular depression when given concomitantly with high doses of alfentanil – administration before or after high doses of alfentanil decreases blood pressure secondary to vasodilation; therefore, recovery may be prolonged.

Alfentanil may produce muscle rigidity involving all the skeletal muscles (incidence and severity are dose-related).

Effects on diagnostic tests
None reported.

Adverse reactions
- CNS: euphoria, insomnia, agitation, confusion, headache, tremor, miosis, *seizures,* psychic dependence, blurred vision.
- CV: tachycardia, *asystole,* bradycardia (may be treated with atropine), palpitations, chest wall rigidity, hypertension, hypotension, syncope, edema.
- GI: dry mouth, anorexia, biliary spasms (colic).
- GU: urinary retention or hesitancy, decreased libido.
- DERM: flushing, rash, pruritus, pain at injection site.
- Respiratory: *respiratory depression,* delayed apnea, hypercapnea.
- Other: intraoperative muscle movement, skeletal muscle rigidity (dose-related), shivering.
Note: Drug should be discontinued if hypersensitivity, seizures, or cardiac arrhythmias occur.

Overdose and treatment
The most common signs and symptoms of alfentanil overdose are CNS depression, respiratory depression,

and miosis (pinpoint pupils). Other acute toxic effects include hypotension, bradycardia, hypothermia, shock, apnea, cardiopulmonary arrest, circulatory collapse, pulmonary edema, and convulsions.

To treat acute overdose, first establish adequate respiratory exchange through a patent airway and ventilation as needed; administer a narcotic antagonist (naloxone) to reverse respiratory depression. (Because the duration of action of alfentanil may be longer than that of naloxone, repeated naloxone dosing may be necessary.) Do not give unless the patient has clinically significant respiratory or cardiovascular depression. Monitor vital signs closely.

Provide symptomatic and supportive treatment (continued respiratory support, correction of fluid or electrolyte imbalance). Closely monitor laboratory parameters, vital signs, and neurologic status.

▶ **Special considerations**
Besides those relevant to all *opioids*, consider the following recommendations.
● Assisted or controlled ventilation is required.
● Use a tuberculin syringe (or equivalent) to administer small volume of alfentanil accurately; alternatively, use infusion pump for controlled delivery.

Geriatric use
Lower doses are usually indicated for elderly patients, because they may be more sensitive to the therapeutic and adverse effects (especially apnea) of the drug.

Pediatric use
Safe use in children under age 12 has not been established.

Breast-feeding
Alfentanil is excreted in breast milk. Administer cautiously to breast-feeding women.

**alglucerase
(glucocerebrosidase,
glucosylceramidase,
glucocerebrosidase-beta-
glucosidase)**
Ceredase

● Pharmacologic classification: glycosidase
● Therapeutic classification: replacement enzyme
● Pregnancy risk category C

How supplied
Available by prescription only
Injection: 80 IU/ml

Indications, route, and dosage
Long-term endogenous enzyme (glucosylceramidase) replacement therapy in confirmed Type I Gaucher's disease
Adults: Dosage should be individualized; initial dose of up to 60 units/kg/infusion may be used. Frequency of infusion may be adjusted based on severity of disease or patient convenience; initial frequency is once q 2 weeks. After response is established, reduce dosage downward for maintenance at intervals of 3 to 6 months.

Pharmacodynamics
Enzymatic action: Alglucerase appears to reduce glycolipid accumulation by acting as a catalyst for the hydrolysis of glucocerebroside to glucose and ceramide – part of the normal degradation pathway for lipids.

Pharmacokinetics
● *Absorption:* After I.V. administration, steady-state enzymatic activity is achieved within 60 minutes.
● *Distribution:* Gaucher's cells in liver, spleen, bone marrow, lung, kidney, and intestine.
● *Metabolism:* Unknown.
● *Excretion:* Unknown.

Contraindications and precautions
Alglucerase is contraindicated in patients with known hypersensitivity reactions to it.

Alglucerase is purified from a large pool of human placental tissue collected from selected donors. The risk of viral contamination has been reduced but cannot be totally eliminated. Although the risk of viral contamination from slow-acting or latent viruses is considered remote, risk-benefit must be assessed before administration.

Interactions
No known interactions.

Effects on diagnostic tests
None reported.

Adverse reactions
● GI: abdominal discomfort, nausea, vomiting.
● Other: chills, slight fever, discomfort, burning, swelling at injection site.

Overdose and treatment
No toxicity detected.

▶ **Special considerations**
● Infusion should run over 1 to 2 hours and be given once every 2 weeks.
● Monitor response parameters to utilize lowest effective dose.
● There is no age restriction for receiving alglucerase.
● Hemoglobin levels may normalize after 6 months of therapy.
● Improved mineralization of bone may also follow prolonged treatment.
● *Do not shake bottle.* Shaking may denature the glycoprotein and render it biologically inactive.
● Store drug at 39.2° F. (4° C.). Do not use if the solution is discolored or contains particles.
● Alglucerase is preservative-free. Do not store for subsequent use after opening.
● Prepare fresh solution by diluting the appropriate amount of alglucerase with normal saline to a final volume not to exceed 100 ml. Use an in-line particulate filter during administration.

Pediatric use
There are no age restrictions for the use of alglucerase.

Breast-feeding
Excretion in breast milk is unknown. Use with caution in breast-feeding women.

---

alkylating agents

altretamine
busulfan
carboplatin
carmustine
chlorambucil
cisplatin
cyclophosphamide
dacarbazine
ifosfamide
lomustine
mechlorethamine
melphalan
pipobroman
streptozocin
thiotepa
uracil mustard

Alkylating antineoplastic agents are cycle-phase nonspecific. They appear to act independently of the specific phase of the cell cycle. Varying degrees of specificity exist among the different agents. They are polyfunctional compounds which can be divided chemically into five groups: nitrogen mustards, ethylenimines, alkylsulfonates, triazenes, and nitrosureas. They are often effective against tumors with large volumes and slow cell turnover rate.

Pharmacology
Alkylating agents are highly reactive, primarily targeting nucleic acids and forming covalent linkages with the nucleophilic centers in many different kinds of molecules. Their polyfunctional character allows them to cross-link double-stranded DNA, preventing the strands from separating for replication, which appears to contribute more to the cytotoxic effects of these agents than other results of alkylation.

Clinical indications and actions
Alkylating agents are useful alone or in combination with other types of antineoplastic agents for the treatment of a variety of tumors. See individual agents for specific uses.

Overview of adverse reactions
The most frequent adverse reactions include bone marrow depression, leukopenia, thrombocytopenia, fever, chills, sore throat, nausea, vomiting, diarrhea, flank or joint pain, anxiety, swelling of feet or lower legs, loss of hair, and redness or pain at injection site.

▶ **Special considerations**
● Follow all established procedures for the safe and proper handling, administration, and disposal of chemotherapeutic agents.
● Vital signs and patency of catheter or I.V. line throughout administration should be monitored.
● Treat extravasation promptly.
● Attempt to alleviate or reduce anxiety in patient and family before treatment.
● Monitor BUN, hematocrit, platelet count, ALT (SGPT), AST (SGOT), LDH, serum bilirubin, serum creatinine, uric acid total and differential leukocyte, and other levels as required per specific agent.
● Immunizations should be avoided if possible.

Information for the patient
● Tell patient to avoid exposure to persons with bacterial or viral infections because chemotherapy can increase susceptibility to infection. Patient should report any signs of infection promptly.
● Instruct patient in proper oral hygiene, including caution when using toothbrush, dental floss, and toothpicks.
● Tell patient to complete dental work before initiation of therapy whenever possible, or to delay it until blood counts are normal.
● Warn patient that he may bruise easily because of drug's effect on blood count.

Representative combinations
None.

allopurinol
Lopurin, Zurinol, Zyloprim

● Pharmacologic classification: xanthine oxidase inhibitor
● Therapeutic classification: antigout
● Pregnancy risk category C

How supplied
Available by prescription only
Tablets (scored): 100 mg, 300 mg

Indications, route, and dosage
Gout, primary or secondary hyperuricemia
Gout may be secondary to diseases such as acute or chronic leukemia, polycythemia vera, multiple myeloma, or psoriasis or after administration of chemotherapeutic agents. Dosage varies with severity of disease; can be given as single dose or divided, but doses larger than 300 mg should be divided.
Adults: Mild gout, 200 to 300 mg P.O. daily; severe gout with large tophi, 400 to 600 mg P.O. daily. Same dose for maintenance in secondary hyperuricemia.
Hyperuricemia secondary to malignancies
Children age 6 to 10: 300 mg P.O. daily (100 mg t.i.d.).
Children under age 6: 150 mg P.O. daily (50 mg t.i.d.).
To prevent acute gouty attacks
Adults: 100 mg P.O. daily; increase at weekly intervals by 100 mg without exceeding maximum dose (800 mg), until serum uric acid level falls to 6 mg/100 ml or less.
To prevent uric acid nephropathy during cancer chemotherapy
Adults: 600 to 800 mg P.O. daily for 2 to 3 days, with high fluid intake.
Recurrent calcium oxalate calculi
Adults: 200 to 300 mg P.O. daily in single dose or divided doses.
Dosage in renal failure
Adults: 100 mg q 3 days if creatinine clearance is 0 to 9 ml/minute; 100 mg q 2 days, 10 to 19 ml/minute; 100 mg daily, 20 to 39 ml/minute; 150 mg daily, 40 to 59 ml/minute; 200 mg daily, 60 to 79 ml/minute; 250 mg daily, 80 ml/minute.

Pharmacodynamics
Antigout action: Allopurinol inhibits xanthine oxidase, the enzyme catalyzing the conversion of hypoxanthine to xanthine, and the conversion of xanthine to uric acid. By blocking this enzyme, allopurinol and its metabolite,

oxypurinol, prevent the conversion of oxypurines (xanthine and hypoxanthine) to uric acid, thus decreasing serum and urine concentrations of uric acid. The drug has no analgesic, anti-inflammatory, or uricosuric action.

Pharmacokinetics
● *Absorption:* After oral administration, approximately 80% to 90% of a dose of allopurinol is absorbed. Peak concentrations of allopurinol are achieved 2 to 6 hours after a usual dose.
● *Distribution:* Allopurinol is distributed widely throughout the body except in the brain, where concentrations of the drug are 50% of those found in the rest of the body. Allopurinol and oxypurinol are not bound to plasma proteins.
● *Metabolism:* Allopurinol is metabolized to oxypurinol by xanthine oxidase. The half-life of allopurinol is 1 to 2 hours; of oxypurinol, approximately 15 hours.
● *Excretion:* 5% to 7% of an allopurinol dose is excreted in urine unchanged within 6 hours of ingestion. After this, it is excreted by the kidneys as oxypurinol, allopurinol, and oxypurinol ribonucleosides. About 70% of the administered daily dose is excreted in urine as oxypurinol and an additional 2% appears in feces as unchanged drug within 48 to 72 hours.

Contraindications and precautions
Allopurinol is contraindicated in patients with hypersensitivity to the drug and in those with idiopathic hemochromatosis. It should be used cautiously in pregnant and breast-feeding women. Patients with impaired renal function must be carefully monitored while receiving allopurinol. Dosage adjustments may be necessary in patients with bone marrow depression, lower GI tract disease, and impaired renal function.

Interactions
In patients with decreased renal function, the concomitant use of allopurinol and a thiazide diuretic may increase the risk of allopurinol-induced hypersensitivity reactions.

Concomitant use with azathioprine and mercaptopurine may increase these drugs' toxic effects, particularly bone marrow depression. Combined use of these drugs requires reduction of initial doses of azathioprine or mercaptopurine to 25% to 33% of the usual dose, with subsequent doses adjusted according to patient response and toxic effects.

Concomitant use of allopurinol with cyclophosphamide may increase the incidence of bone marrow depression through an unknown mechanism. Allopurinol inhibits hepatic microsomal metabolism of dicumarol, thus increasing the half-life of dicumarol; patients receiving the two drugs concomitantly should be observed for increased anticoagulant effects.

Concomitant use of allopurinol with ampicillin or amoxicillin may increase the incidence of skin rash.

Because allopurinol or its metabolites may compete with chlorpropamide for renal tubular secretion, patients who receive these drugs concomitantly should be observed for signs of excessive hypoglycemia.

Concomitant use of co-trimoxazole with allopurinol has been associated with thrombocytopenia.

Effects on diagnostic tests
Increased alkaline phosphatase, AST (SGOT), and ALT (SGPT) levels have been reported in patients on allopurinol therapy.

Adverse reactions
● CNS: headache, peripheral neuropathy, neuritis, paresthesia, somnolence.
● DERM: rash, *Stevens-Johnson syndrome, toxic epidermal necrolysis,* alopecia, erythema multiforme, ichthyosis, purpuric lesions, vesicular bullous dermatitis, eczematoid dermatitis, pruritus, urticaria, onycholysis, lichen planus.
● EENT: cataracts, retinopathy, severe furunculosis of nose.
● GI: nausea, vomiting, diarrhea, intermittent abdominal pain, gastritis, dyspepsia, metallic taste, loss of taste.
● GU: renal failure, uremia.
● HEMA: *agranulocytosis,* anemia, *aplastic anemia,* bone marrow depression, leukopenia, pancytopenia, thrombocytopenia, ecchymosis.
● Hepatic: increased alkaline phosphatase, AST (SGOT), ALT (SGPT) levels; hepatomegaly; hyperbilirubinemia; cholestatic jaundice; granulomatous hepatitis; hepatic necrosis.
● Other: acute attacks of gout, fever, myopathy, epistaxis, loss or perversion of taste, hypersensitivity (fever, chills, leukopenia, leukocytosis, eosinophilia, arthralgia, nausea, vomiting), renal failure, uremia.
Note: Drug should be discontinued at first sign of rash, which may precede severe hypersensitivity reaction or any other adverse reaction.

Overdose and treatment
No information available.

▶ Special considerations
● Skin rash occurs most often in patients taking diuretics and in those with renal disorders.
● Monitor patient's intake and output. Daily urine output of at least 2 liters and maintenance of neutral or slightly alkaline urine is desirable.
● If renal insufficiency exists at any time during treatment, allopurinol dose should be reduced.
● Monitor CBC, serum uric acid levels, and hepatic and renal function at start of therapy and periodically thereafter.
● Acute gout attacks may occur in first 6 weeks of therapy; concurrent use of colchicine or another anti-inflammatory agent may be prescribed prophylactically.
● Minimize GI adverse reactions by administering with meals or immediately after. Tablets may be crushed and administered with fluid or food.
● Allopurinol may predispose patient to ampicillin-induced rash.
● Allopurinol-induced rash may occur weeks after discontinuation of drug.

Information for the patient
● Encourage patient to drink plenty of fluids (10 to 12 8-oz [240 ml] glasses a day) while taking this drug unless otherwise contraindicated.
● When using to treat recurrent calcium oxalate stones, advise patient to reduce dietary intake of animal protein, sodium, refined sugars, vitamin C, oxalate-rich foods, and calcium.
● Advise patient to avoid hazardous activities requiring alertness until CNS response to drug is known, because drug may cause drowsiness.
● Advise patient to avoid alcohol, because it decreases effectiveness of allopurinol.
● Tell patient to report all adverse reactions immediately.

• Advise patient to take a missed dose when remembered unless it is time for next scheduled dose and not to double the doses.

Geriatric use
Follow dosage recommendations for adults. Watch for renal disorders or impaired renal function and treat according to dosage recommendations for patients with impaired renal function.

Pediatric use
Allopurinol should not be used in children except to treat hyperuricemia secondary to malignancies.

Breast-feeding
Because oxypurinol and allopurinol are distributed into breast milk, allopurinol should be used with extreme caution in breast-feeding women.

alpha-adrenergic blocking agents

dihydroergotamine mesylate
doxazosin mesylate
ergotamine tartrate
phenoxybenzamine hydrochloride
phentolamine mesylate
prazosin hydrochloride
terazosin hydrochloride
tolazoline hydrochloride

Drugs that block the effects of neurohormonal transmitters (norepinephrine, epinephrine, and related sympathomimetic amines) on adrenergic receptors in various effector systems are designated as adrenergic blocking agents. As adrenoreceptors are classified into two subtypes – alpha and beta – so too are the blocking agents. Essentially, those agents that antagonize mydriasis, cause vasoconstriction, nonvascular smooth muscle excitation, and other adrenergic responses due to alpha receptor stimulation are termed alpha-adrenergic blocking agents.

Pharmacology
Nonselective alpha antagonists
Ergotamine, phentolamine, and phenoxybenzamine antagonize both alpha$_1$ and alpha$_2$ receptors. Generally, alpha blockade results in tachycardia, palpitations, and increased secretion of renin due to the abnormally large amounts of norepinephrine (transmitter "overflow") released from adrenergic nerve endings as a result of the concurrent blockade of alpha$_1$ and alpha$_2$ receptors. The effects of norepinephrine are clinically counterproductive to the major uses of nonselective alpha blockers, which include treating peripheral vascular disorders such as Raynaud's disease, acrocyanosis, frost bite, acute atrial occlusion, phlebitis, phlebothrombosis, diabetic gangrene, shock, and pheochromocytoma.

Selective alpha antagonists
Alpha$_1$ blockers have readily observable effects and are currently the only alpha-adrenergic agents with known clinical uses. They decrease vascular resistance and increase venous capacitance, thereby lowering blood pressure and causing pink warm skin, nasal and scleroconjunctival congestion, ptosis, postural and exercise hypotension, mild to moderate miosis, and interference with ejaculation. Because alpha$_1$ blockers

do not block alpha$_2$ receptors, they do not cause transmitter overflow. In theory, alpha$_1$ blockers should be useful in the same conditions as nonselective alpha blockers; however, doxazosin, prazosin, and terazosin are approved only for treating hypertension. Prazosin also has proven useful in refractory heart failure because of its ability to decrease cardiac afterload.

Alpha$_2$ blockers produce more subtle physiologic effects and currently have no therapeutic applications. Yohimbine is one such agent.

Clinical indications and actions
Peripheral vascular disorders
Alpha-adrenergic blocking agents are indicated for treating peripheral vascular disorders including Raynaud's disease, acrocyanosis, frost bite, acute atrial occlusion, phlebitis, and diabetic gangrene. Dihydroergotamine and ergotamine have been used to treat vascular headaches. Prazosin has been used to treat Raynaud's disease. Phentolamine is indicated to treat dermal necrosis caused by extravasation of norepinephrine.

Hypertension
Phenoxybenzamine is used to treat pheochromocytoma. Tolazoline is indicated to treat persistent pulmonary hypertension in neonates. Prazosin and terazosin are used in managing essential hypertension. Phentolamine is used to control hypertension and is a useful adjunct in surgical treatment of pheochromocytoma.

Overview of adverse reactions
Nonselective alpha antagonists typically cause postural hypotension, tachycardia, palpitations, fluid retention (from excess renin secretion), nasal and ocular congestion, and aggravation of the signs and symptoms of respiratory infection. Use of these agents is contraindicated in patients with severe cerebral and coronary atherosclerosis and in those with renal insufficiency.

Selective alpha antagonists typically cause severe postural hypotension and syncope, especially during early treatment, which are the most common side effects of alpha$_1$ blockade. Excessive tachycardia, stroke volume, and plasma renin levels may result from alpha$_2$ blockade.

▶ Special considerations
• Monitor vital signs, especially blood pressure.
• Administer dose at bedtime to reduce potential of dizziness or light-headedness.

Information for the patient
• Warn patient about postural hypotension. Tell patient to avoid sudden changes to upright position.
• Tell patient to promptly report dizziness or irregular heartbeat.
• Advise patient to take dose at bedtime to reduce potential for dizziness or light-headedness.
• Warn patient to avoid driving and other hazardous tasks that require mental alertness until effects of medication are established.
• Reassure patient that adverse effects should lessen after several doses.
• Tell patient that the use of alcohol, excessive exercise, prolonged standing, and exposure to heat will intensify adverse effects.
• Advise patient against taking any other medication, including any that can be purchased without a prescription.

Geriatric use
Hypotensive effects may be more pronounced in the elderly.

Representative combinations
None.

---

alpha₁-proteinase inhibitor (human) (alpha₁-PI)
Prolastin

- Pharmacologic classification: enzyme inhibitor
- Therapeutic classification: orphan drug
- Pregnancy risk category: C

How supplied
Available by prescription only
Injection: 500 mg and 1,000 mg activity per vial.

Indications, route, and dosage
For chronic replacement of alpha₁-antitrypsin in patients with clinically demonstrable panacinar emphysema and PiZZ, PiZ (null) or Pi (null) (null) phenotype
Adults: 60 mg/kg I.V. once weekly to increase and maintain functional alpha₁-PI level in the epithelial lining of the lower respiratory tract providing adequate anti-elastase activity in the lungs of patients with alpha₁-antitrypsin deficiency.

Pharmacodynamics
Enzyme inhibiting action: Alpha₁-PI inhibits the elastase released by inflammatory cells in the lung parenchyma. Persons with congenital alpha₁-antitrypsin deficiency develop emphysema in the third or fourth decade of life as a result of chronic degradation of elastin tissues.

Pharmacokinetics
- *Absorption:* Alpha₁-PI must be administered intravenously.
- *Distribution:* I.V. alpha₁-PI appears to distribute to lung tissues; however, distribution is not well documented.
- *Metabolism:* unknown.
- *Excretion:* unknown.

Contraindications and precautions
There are no known contraindications to the use of alpha₁-PI. Because alpha₁-PI is derived from large pools of fresh human plasma obtained from many paid donors, the presence of hepatitis viruses in such pools must be assumed. No cases of hepatitis, either hepatitis B or non-A, non-B have been reported; however, all patients who received alpha₁-PI also received prophylaxis against hepatitis B.

Interactions
None reported.

Effects on diagnostic tests
None reported.

Adverse reactions
- HEMA: possible transmission of viruses.
- Other: delayed fever.

Overdose and treatment
No information available.

▶ Special considerations
- Only patients with early evidence of clinically demonstrable panacinar emphysema should be considered for chronic replacement therapy with alpha₁-PI. Subjects with the PiMZ or PiMS phenotypes of alpha₁-antitrypsin deficiency appear to be at small risk for panacinar emphysema and should not receive treatment with alpha₁-PI.
- Alpha₁-proteinase inhibitor is not indicated for use in patients other than those with PiZZ, PiZ(null) or Pi (null) (null) phenotypes.
- For I.V. use only. May be given at a rate of 0.08 ml/kg/minute or greater.
- Refrigerate at 2° to 8° C. (35° to 46° F.). Avoid freezing.
- Factors that could diminish alpha₁-PI effectiveness or cause adverse effects include improper storage and handling or method of administration, incorrect diagnosis, and individual biological differences.
- Manufacturers' directions for use must be followed carefully.
- Consider the risk of transmitting viruses before prescribing this agent. Prophylaxis against hepatitis B is recommended.
- Commercial assays of antigenic activity may be used to monitor alpha₁-PI serum levels in patients receiving this agent; however, results of such tests do not reflect the functional activity (potency; the capacity to neutralize pancreatic elastase) of alpha₁-PI and cannot be used to determine therapeutic dosage.

Pediatric use
Alpha₁-PI has been used only in adults.

Breast-feeding
No information available.

---

alprazolam
Xanax

- Pharmacologic classification: benzodiazepine
- Therapeutic classification: antianxiety agent
- Controlled substance schedule IV
- Pregnancy risk category D

How supplied
Available by prescription only
Tablets: 0.25 mg, 0.5 mg, 1 mg, 2 mg

Indications, route, and dosage
Anxiety and tension
Adults: Usual starting dose is 0.25 to 0.5 mg t.i.d. Maximum total daily dosage is 4 mg in divided doses. In elderly or debilitated patients, usual starting dose is 0.25 mg b.i.d. or t.i.d.

Panic disorder

Adults: Initially, 0.5 mg P.O. t.i.d. Increase as needed and tolerated at intervals of 3 or 4 days in increments of 1 mg daily. Most patients require more than 4 mg daily; however, dosages from 1 to 10 mg daily have been reported.

Pharmacodynamics

Anxiolytic action: Alprazolam depresses the CNS at the limbic and subcortical levels of the brain. It produces an antianxiety effect by enhancing the effect of the neurotransmitter gamma-aminobutyric acid (GABA) on its receptor in the ascending reticular activating system, which increases inhibition and blocks both cortical and limbic arousal.

Pharmacokinetics

● *Absorption:* When administered orally, alprazolam is well absorbed. Onset of action occurs within 15 to 30 minutes, with peak action in 1 to 2 hours.
● *Distribution:* Alprazolam is distributed widely throughout the body. Approximately 80% to 90% of an administered dose is bound to plasma protein.
● *Metabolism:* Alprazolam is metabolized in the liver equally to alpha-hydroxyalprazolam and inactive metabolites.
● *Excretion:* Alpha-hydroxyalprazolam and other metabolites are excreted in urine. Alprazolam's half-life is 12 to 15 hours.

Contraindications and precautions

Alprazolam is contraindicated in patients with known hypersensitivity to the drug; in patients with acute narrow-angle glaucoma or untreated open-angle glaucoma, because of its possible anticholinergic effect; in patients in coma; and in patients with acute alcohol intoxication who have depressed vital signs, because the drug will worsen CNS depression.

Use alprazolam cautiously in patients with psychoses, because the drug is rarely beneficial in such patients and may induce paradoxical reactions; in patients with myasthenia gravis or Parkinson's disease, because it may exacerbate the disorder; in patients with impaired renal or hepatic function, which prolongs elimination of the drug; and in elderly or debilitated patients, who are usually more sensitive to the drug's CNS effects. Abrupt withdrawal may precipitate seizures in some patients. Alprazolam may produce additive CNS depression in patients with acute alcohol intoxication.

Use cautiously in individuals prone to addiction or drug abuse.

Interactions

Alprazolam potentiates the CNS depressant effects of phenothiazines, narcotics, barbiturates, alcohol, general anesthetics, antihistamines, monoamine oxidase inhibitors, and antidepressants.

Concomitant use with cimetidine and possibly disulfiram diminishes hepatic metabolism of alprazolam, increasing its plasma concentration.

Heavy smoking accelerates alprazolam metabolism, thus lowering clinical effectiveness.

Benzodiazepines may decrease serum levels of haloperidol.

Effects on diagnostic tests

Alprazolam therapy may elevate liver function test results. Minor changes in EEG patterns, usually low-voltage, fast activity, may occur during and after alprazolam therapy.

Adverse reactions

● CNS: confusion, depression, drowsiness, lethargy, light-headedness, headache, confusion, hostility, hangover effect, ataxia, dizziness, syncope, nightmares, fatigue, slurred speech, tremors, vertigo.
● CV: hypotension, bradycardia, palpitations, shortness of breath.
● DERM: rash, urticaria, jaundice, flushing.
● EENT: diplopia, blurred vision, photosensitivity, nystagmus.
● GI: constipation, dry mouth, metallic taste, hiccups, nausea, vomiting, abdominal discomfort.
● GU: urinary incontinence or retention.
● Other: *respiratory depression,* dysarthria, hepatic dysfunction, changes in libido.
  Note: Drug should be discontinued if hypersensitivity or the following paradoxical reactions occur: acute hyperexcited state, anxiety, hallucinations, increased muscle spasticity, insomnia, or rage.

Overdose and treatment

Clinical manifestations of overdose include somnolence, confusion, coma, hypoactive reflexes, dyspnea, labored breathing, hypotension, bradycardia, slurred speech, unsteady gait, and impaired coordination.

Support blood pressure and respiration until drug effects subside; monitor vital signs. Flumazenil, a specific benzodiazepine antagonist, may be useful. Mechanical ventilatory assistance via endotracheal tube may be required to maintain a patent airway and support adequate oxygenation. As needed, use I.V. fluids and vasopressors such as dopamine and phenylephrine to treat hypotension. If the patient is conscious, induce emesis. Use gastric lavage if ingestion was recent, but only if an endotracheal tube is in place to prevent aspiration. After emesis or lavage, administer activated charcoal with a cathartic as a single dose. Dialysis is of limited value. Do not use barbiturates if excitation occurs because of possible exacerbation of excitation or CNS depression.

▶ Special considerations

Besides those relevant to all *benzodiazepines,* consider the following recommendations.
● Patients receiving prolonged therapy with high doses should be weaned from the drug gradually to prevent withdrawal symptoms.
● Lower doses are effective in elderly patients and patients with renal or hepatic dysfunction.
● Anxiety associated with depression is also responsive to alprazolam but may require more frequent dosing.
● Store in a cool, dry place away from direct light.

Information for the patient

● Be sure patient understands that the potential exists for physical and psychological dependence with chronic use of alprazolam.
● Instruct patient not to alter drug regimen in any way.
● Warn patient that sudden changes in position can cause dizziness. Advise patient to dangle legs for a few minutes before getting out of bed to prevent falls and injury.

Geriatric use
● Lower doses are usually effective in elderly patients because of decreased elimination.
● During initiation of therapy or after an increase in dose, elderly patients who receive this drug require supervision with ambulation and activities of daily living.

Pediatric use
● Closely observe a neonate for withdrawal symptoms if mother took alprazolam during pregnancy. Use of alprazolam during labor may cause neonatal flaccidity.
● Safety has not been established in children under age 18.

Breast-feeding
The breast-fed infant of a woman who uses alprazolam may become sedated, have feeding difficulties, or lose weight. Avoid use in breast-feeding women.

alprostadil
Prostin VR Pediatric

● Pharmacologic classification: prostaglandin
● Therapeutic classification: ductus arteriosus patency adjunct

How supplied
Available by prescription only
Injection: 500 mcg/ml

Indications, route, and dosage
Temporary maintenance of patency of ductus arteriosus until surgery can be performed
Infants: Initial I.V. infusion of 0.05 to 0.1 mcg/kg/minute via infusion pump. After satisfactory response is achieved, reduce infusion rate to the lowest dosage that will maintain response. Maintenance dosage is usually one-hundredth to one-tenth the initial dose. I.V. route is preferred but intraarterial or intraaortic route may be used.

Pharmacodynamics
Ductus arteriosus patency adjunct action: Alprostadil, also known as prostaglandin E_1 or PGE_1, is a prostaglandin that relaxes or dilates the rings of smooth muscle of the ductus arteriosus and maintains patency in neonates when infused before natural closure.

Pharmacokinetics
● *Absorption:* Alprostadil is administered I.V.
● *Distribution:* Alprostadil is distributed rapidly throughout the body.
● *Metabolism:* 68% of a dose is metabolized in one pass through the lung, primarily by oxidation; 100% is metabolized within 24 hours.
● *Excretion:* All metabolites are excreted in urine within 24 hours.

Contraindications and precautions
Alprostadil is contraindicated in infants with respiratory distress syndrome because of the potential for adverse cardiovascular effects. It should be used cautiously in infants with bleeding tendencies because it inhibits platelet aggregation.

Interactions
None reported.

Effects on diagnostic tests
None reported.

Adverse reactions
● CNS: *seizures,* hyperpyrexia, *cerebral bleeding,* fever, apnea.
● CV: flushing, bradycardia, hypotension, tachycardia, edema in lower extremities, *damage to the ductus pulmonary artery and aorta* (with prolonged infusion).
● GI: diarrhea, gastric regurgitation.
● HEMA: *disseminated intravascular coagulation (DIC),* anemia, thrombocytopenia, bleeding, hyperbilirubinemia.
● Respiratory: bradypnea, wheezing, hypercapnia, tachypnea, *respiratory distress.*
● Other: sepsis, hypokalemia, hyperkalemia, hypoglycemia, cortical hyperostosis (with long-term use).

Overdose and treatment
Clinical manifestations are similar to the adverse reactions and include apnea, bradycardia, pyrexia, hypotension, and flushing. Apnea most frequently occurs in neonates weighing less than 2 kg at birth and usually develops during the first hour of drug therapy.

Treatment of apnea or bradycardia requires discontinuance of the infusion and appropriate supportive therapy, including mechanical ventilation as needed. Pyrexia or hypotension may be treated by reducing the infusion rate. Flushing may be corrected by repositioning the intraarterial catheter.

▶ Special considerations
● Adding a 500-mcg solution to 50 ml of dextrose 5% in water or normal saline solution provides a concentration of 10 mcg/ml. At this concentration, a 0.01 ml/kg/minute infusion rate will deliver 0.1 mcg alprostadil/kg/minute.
● Drug must be diluted before administration. Discard prepared solution after 24 hours.
● Assess all vital functions closely and frequently to prevent adverse effects.
● Monitor arterial pressure by umbilical artery catheter, auscultation, or Doppler transducer. Slow the rate of infusion if arterial pressure falls significantly.
● In infants with restricted pulmonary blood flow, measure drug's effectiveness by monitoring blood oxygenation. In infants with restricted systemic blood flow, measure drug's effectiveness by monitoring systemic blood pressure and blood pH.
● Apnea and bradycardia may reflect drug overdose. Stop the infusion immediately if they occur.
● Monitor respiratory status throughout treatment; have ventilatory assistance immediately available.
● Peripheral arterial vasodilation (flushing) may respond to repositioning of the catheter.
● This drug should be administered only by personnel trained in pediatric intensive care.
● Store alprostadil ampules in refrigerator.

---

alteplase (recombinant alteplase, tissue plasminogen activator)
Activase

- Pharmacologic classification: enzyme
- Therapeutic classification: thrombolytic enzyme
- Pregnancy risk category C

How supplied
Available by prescription only
Injection: 20-mg (11.6 million IU), 50-mg (29 million IU) vials

Indications, route, and dosage
Lysis of thrombi obstructing coronary arteries in management of acute MI
Adults (over 65 kg): 60 mg in the first hour, with 6 to 10 mg I.V. bolus over the first 1 to 2 minutes; then 20 mg/hour for an additional 2 hours. Total dose is 100 mg.
Adults (65 kg or less): 1.25 mg/kg with 60% of the drug administered in the first hour (10% of the first hour's dose to be given over the first 1 to 2 minutes).
Pulmonary embolism
Adults: 100 mg by I.V. infusion over 2 hours. Heparin therapy should be initiated at the end of the infusion.

Pharmacodynamics
Thrombolytic action: Alteplase is an enzyme that catalyzes the conversion of tissue plasminogen to plasmin in the presence of fibrin. This fibrin specificity produces local fibrinolysis in the area of recent clot formation, with limited systemic proteolysis. In patients with acute MI, this allows for reperfusion of ischemic cardiac muscle and improved left ventricular function with a decreased incidence of congestive heart failure after an MI.

Pharmacokinetics
- *Absorption:* Alteplase must be given intravenously.
- *Distribution:* Alteplase is rapidly cleared from the plasma by the liver. 80% of a dose is cleared within 10 minutes after infusion is discontinued.
- *Metabolism:* Primarily hepatic.
- *Excretion:* Over 85% of drug is excreted in the urine, 5% in the feces. Plasma half-life is less than 10 minutes.

Contraindications and precautions
Alteplase is contraindicated in patients with active internal bleeding, bleeding diathesis, aneurysm, arteriovenous malformation, history of cerebrovascular accident, recent intraspinal or intracranial surgery or trauma, brain tumor, or severe uncontrolled hypertension, because of the potential for uncontrolled bleeding.

Use with extreme caution in patients with acute pericarditis, cerebrovascular disease, diabetic hemorrhagic retinopathy, significant hepatic disease, marked hypertension, subacute bacterial endocarditis, septic thrombophlebitis, or in patients who are at risk for left heart thrombi (mitral stenosis with atrial fibrillation), because bleeding problems (the most common adverse effects of alteplase therapy) may pose a substantial risk to these patients.

Interactions
Concomitant use of alteplase with drugs that antagonize platelet function (such as aspirin and dipyridamole) is associated with an increased risk of bleeding; however, many clinicians employ aspirin or dipyridamole during or after heparin therapy (which usually follows alteplase).

Effects on diagnostic tests
Altered results may be expected in coagulation and fibrinolytic tests. The use of aprotinin (150 to 200 units/ml) in the blood sample may attenuate this interference.

Adverse reactions
- CV: arrhythmias (associated with reperfusion of ischemic myocardium).
- DERM: urticaria.
- GI: *bleeding*, nausea, vomiting.
- GU: hematuria.
- HEMA: excessive fibrinolysis leading to bleeding from disturbed sites (punctures, recent wounds), *intracranial* or *retroperitoneal bleeding*.
- Other: *hypersensitivity reactions*, fever.
  Note: Drug should be discontinued if anaphylactoid reaction occurs.

Overdose and treatment
No information is available regarding accidental ingestion.

Excessive I.V. dosage can lead to bleeding problems. Doses of 150 mg have been associated with an increased incidence of intracranial bleeding. Discontinue infusion immediately if signs or symptoms of bleeding are observed.

▶ Special considerations
- Expect to begin alteplase infusions within 6 hours after onset of MI symptoms (angina pain or equivalent, greater than 30 minutes duration, angina that is unresponsive to nitroglycerin, or ECG evidence of MI).
- Heparin is usually administered during or after alteplase as part of the treatment regimen.
- Monitor ECG for transient arrhythmias (sinus bradycardia, ventricular tachycardia, accelerated idioventricular rhythm, ventricular premature depolarizations) associated with reperfusion after coronary thrombolysis. Have antiarrhythmic agents available.
- Avoid I.M. injections, venipuncture, and arterial puncture during therapy. Use pressure dressings or ice packs on recent puncture sites to prevent bleeding. If arterial puncture is necessary, select a site on the arm and apply pressure for 30 minutes afterward.
- Prepare solution using supplied sterile water for injection. Do not use bacteriostatic water for injection.
- Do not mix other drugs with alteplase. Use 18G needle for preparing solution – aim water stream at lyphilized cake. Expect a slight foaming to occur. Do not use if vacuum is not present.
- Drug may be further diluted with normal saline solution injection or D_5W. Reconstituted or diluted solutions are stable for up to 8 hours at room temperature.

Information for the patient
- Teach patient signs and symptoms of internal bleeding. Tell patient to report these immediately.
- Advise patient about proper dental care to avoid excessive gum trauma.

altretamine
(hexamethylmelamine)
Hexalen, Hexastat*

- Pharmacologic classification: alkylating agent
- Therapeutic classification: antineoplastic
- Pregnancy risk category D

How supplied
Available by prescription only
Capsules: 50 mg

Indications, route, and dosage
Palliative treatment of persistent or recurrent ovarian cancer after first-line therapy with cisplatin or alkylating agent combination
Single agent therapy
Adults: 260 mg/m²/day P.O. in four divided doses (after meals and h.s.) for 14 to 21 consecutive days in a 28-day cycle.
Combination therapy
Adults: 150 mg/m²/day P.O. in four divided doses (after meals and h.s.) administered on days 1 to 14 of a 28-day cycle. Used with cyclophosphamide and doxorubicin, with or without cisplatin.

Pharmacodynamics
Antineoplastic action: The precise mechanism of action is unknown. Metabolism in the liver is required for cytotoxicity.

Pharmacokinetics
- *Absorption:* Altretamine is well-absorbed from the GI tract after oral administration; however, rapid and extensive demethylation causes variations in plasma levels.
- *Distribution:* Altretamine does not cross the blood-brain barrier to a significant extent. The drug and its metabolites show binding to plasma proteins.
- *Metabolism:* Rapid and extensive demethylation in the liver.
- *Excretion:* Metabolites are excreted primarily in the urine. A small amount is eliminated through the lungs in expired air; trace amounts are excreted in feces.

Contraindications and precautions
Altretamine is contraindicated in patients with known hypersensitivity to the drug and in patients with pre-existing severe bone marrow depression or severe neurologic toxicity.

Unresponsive GI intolerance, WBC count below 2,000/mm³ or granulocytes below 1,000/mm³, platelets below 7,500/mm³, and progressive neurotoxicity require temporary discontinuation for 14 days or more and a dosage reduction to 200 mg/m²/day when restarted.

Interactions
Concurrent administration of MAO inhibitors may cause severe orthostatic hypotension. Concurrent use with cimetidine increases altretamine's half-life and potential for toxicity because cimetidine inhibits microsomal drug metabolism.

Effects on diagnostic tests
Blood and urine uric acid concentrations may be increased; serum creatinine and BUN levels may be altered.

Adverse reactions
- CNS: mild to moderate neurotoxicity, peripheral neuropathy, mood disorders, ataxia, dizziness, vertigo, consciousness disorders, fatigue, *seizures.*
- GI: mild to severe dose-related nausea and vomiting, increased alkaline phosphatase, anorexia.
- HEMA: mild to *severe anemia,* leukopenia, *thrombocytopenia.*
- Other: *hepatic toxicity,* skin rash, pruritus, alopecia.

Overdose and treatment
Clinical manifestations of overdose include myelosuppression and severe nausea and vomiting unresponsive to usual treatment.

Symptoms are more likely to occur in patients receiving continuous high-dose daily altretamine. Neurologic toxicity appears reversible and may be diminished by concurrent administration of pyridoxine.

Treatment is usually supportive and may include antiemetics and transfusion of blood components.

▶ Special considerations
- Monitor peripheral blood counts at least monthly and before each course of therapy.
- Premedication with antiemetics may decrease incidence or severity of nausea and vomiting.
- Tolerance to GI effects may develop after several weeks of therapy. If severity is uncontrolled with antiemetics, dosage reduction may be required.
- Perform neurologic examinations regularly during administration to check for neurotoxicities. Concomitant administration of 100 mg pyridoxine may diminish neurotoxicity.

Information for the patient
- Tell patient to call physician if vomiting occurs shortly after the dose is taken.
- Emphasize importance of continuing to take medication despite occasional nausea and vomiting.
- Encourage fluid intake to increase urine output and facilitate excretion of uric acid.
- Instruct patient to report any signs of neurotoxicity.
- Instruct patient to avoid exposure to people with infections.

Pediatric use
Safety and efficacy in children have not been established.

Breast-feeding
It is unknown if altretamine is excreted in breast milk; however, it is recommended that breast-feeding be discontinued during treatment because of the risk of toxicity to the infant.

aluminum carbonate
Basaljel

- Pharmacologic classification: inorganic aluminum salt
- Therapeutic classification: antacid, hypophosphatemic agent
- Pregnancy risk category C

How supplied
Available without prescription
Tablets or capsules: aluminum hydroxide equivalent 500 mg
Suspension: aluminum hydroxide equivalent 400 mg/5 ml, 1 g/5 ml

Indications, route, and dosage
Antacid
Adults: 5 to 10 ml suspension p.r.n.; 2.5 to 5 ml extra-strength suspension p.r.n.; or 1 to 2 tablets or capsules p.r.n.
To prevent formation of urinary phosphate stones (with low-phosphate diet)
Adults: 15 to 30 ml suspension in water or juice 1 hour after meals and h.s.; 5 to 15 ml extra-strength suspension in water or juice 1 hour after meals and h.s.; or 2 to 6 tablets or capsules 1 hour after meals and h.s.

Pharmacodynamics
- *Antacid action:* Aluminum carbonate exerts its antacid effect by neutralizing gastric acid; this increases pH, thereby decreasing pepsin activity.
- *Hypophosphatemic action:* Aluminum carbonate reduces serum phosphate levels by complexing with phosphate in the gut. This results in formation of insoluble, nonabsorbable aluminum phosphate, which is then excreted in feces. Calcium absorption increases secondary to reduced phosphate absorption.

Pharmacokinetics
- *Absorption:* Aluminum carbonate is largely unabsorbed; small amounts may be absorbed systemically.
- *Distribution:* None.
- *Metabolism:* None.
- *Excretion:* Aluminum carbonate is excreted in feces; some may be excreted in breast milk.

Contraindications and precautions
Aluminum carbonate is contraindicated in patients with hypophosphatemia, appendicitis, impaired renal function, undiagnosed rectal or GI bleeding, constipation, fecal impaction, chronic diarrhea, gastric outlet obstruction, and intestinal obstruction, because the drug may exacerbate these conditions.

Aluminum carbonate should be used cautiously in patients with hemorrhoids because constipation associated with drug use may be irritating; and in patients with decreased GI motility, such as elderly patients and those receiving anticholinergics or antidiarrheals.

Interactions
Aluminum carbonate may decrease absorption of many drugs, including tetracycline, quinolones, coumarin anticoagulants, phenothiazines (especially chlorpromazine), chenodiol, antimuscarinics, diazepam, chlordi-

azepoxide, isoniazid, vitamin A, digoxin, iron salts, and sodium or potassium phosphate, thereby lessening their effectiveness. Separate administration by at least 2 hours. Use with enterically coated drugs causes premature drug release.

Effects on diagnostic tests
Aluminum carbonate may interfere with imaging techniques using sodium pertechnetate Tc 99m and thus impair evaluation of Meckel's diverticulum. It may also interfere with reticuloendothelial imaging of liver, spleen, or bone marrow using technetium Tc 99m sulfur colloid. It may antagonize pentagastrin's effect during gastric acid secretion tests.

Aluminum carbonate may increase serum gastrin levels and decrease serum phosphate levels.

Adverse reactions
- GI: constipation, intestinal obstruction, appetite loss, decreased bowel motility.
- Metabolic: hypophosphatemia, mildly elevated alkaline phosphatase, transient hypercalciuria early in therapy, osteomalacia.
  Note: Drug should be discontinued if anorexia, malaise, muscle weakness, or other signs of hypophosphatemia develop.

Overdose and treatment
No specific information available. Patients with impaired renal function are at a higher risk of aluminum toxicity to brain, bone, and parathyroid glands.

▶ **Special considerations**
- When administering suspension (especially extra-strength suspension), shake well and give with small amounts of water or fruit juice.
- After administration through a nasogastric tube, tube should be flushed with water to prevent obstruction.
- When administering drug as an antiurolithic, encourage increased fluid intake to enhance drug effectiveness.
- Constipation may be managed with stool softeners or bulk laxatives, or administer alternately with magnesium-containing antacids (unless patient has renal disease). Aluminum hydroxide may also help.
- Monitor serum calcium and phosphate levels periodically; reduced serum phosphate levels may lead to increased serum calcium levels.
- Long-term aluminum carbonate use can lead to calcium resorption and subsequent bone demineralization.

Information for the patient
- Advise patient to take drug only as directed and not to take more than 24 capsules or tablets, 120 ml (24 tsp) of regular suspension, or 60 ml (12 tsp) of extra-strength suspension in a 24-hour period. Instruct patient to shake suspension well.
- As needed, advise patient to restrict sodium intake, to drink plenty of fluids, and to follow a low-phosphate diet.
- Advise patient not to switch antacids without medical approval.

Geriatric use
Because elderly patients commonly have decreased GI motility, they may become constipated from this drug.

Pediatric use
Aluminum carbonate should be used cautiously in children under age 6.

aluminum hydroxide
Alagel, ALternaGEL, Alu-Cap, Aluminett, Alu-Tab, Amphojel, Dialume, Hydroxal, Nephrox, Nutrajel

- Pharmacologic classification: aluminum salt
- Therapeutic classification: antacid, hypophosphatemic agent, adsorbent
- Pregnancy risk category C

How supplied
Available without prescription
Tablets: 300 mg, 600 mg
Capsules: 475 mg, 500 mg
Suspension: 320 mg/5 ml, 600 mg/5 ml, 675 mg/5 ml

Indications, route, and dosage
Antacid
Adults: 500 to 1,800 mg P.O. (5 to 15 ml of most products) 1 hour after meals and h.s.; or 300- or 600-mg tablet, chewed before swallowing, taken with milk or water five to six times daily after meals and h.s.; or one to three capsules 1 hour after meals and h.s. (maximum nine capsules/day).
Hyperphosphatemia in renal failure
Adults: 500 mg to 2 g b.i.d. to q.i.d.

Pharmacodynamics
- *Antacid action:* Aluminum hydroxide neutralizes gastric acid, reducing the direct acid irritant effect. This increases pH, thereby decreasing pepsin activity.
- *Hypophosphatemic action:* Aluminum hydroxide reduces serum phosphate levels by complexing with phosphate in the gut, resulting in insoluble, nonabsorbable aluminum phosphate, which is then excreted in feces. Calcium absorption increases secondary to decreased phosphate absorption.

Pharmacokinetics
- *Absorption:* Aluminum hydroxide is absorbed minimally; small amounts may be absorbed systemically.
- *Distribution:* None.
- *Metabolism:* None.
- *Excretion:* Aluminum hydroxide is excreted in feces; some drug may be excreted in breast milk.

Contraindications and precautions
Aluminum hydroxide is contraindicated in patients with hypophosphatemia, appendicitis, impaired renal function, undiagnosed rectal or GI bleeding, constipation, fecal impaction, chronic diarrhea, gastric outlet obstruction, or intestinal obstruction, because the drug may exacerbate these symptoms.

Aluminum hydroxide should be used cautiously in patients with hemorrhoids and in patients with decreased GI motility, such as elderly patients and those receiving anticholinergics or antidiarrheals, because constipation associated with drug use may be irritating.

Interactions
Aluminum hydroxide may decrease absorption of many drugs, including quinolones, tetracycline, phenothiazines (especially chlorpromazine), coumarin anticoagulants, chenodiol, antimuscarinics, diazepam, chlordiazepoxide, isoniazid, vitamin A, digoxin, iron salts, and sodium or potassium phosphate, thereby decreasing their effectiveness; separate doses by at least 2 hours. Drug causes premature release of enterically coated drugs; separate doses by 1 hour.

Effects on diagnostic tests
Aluminum hydroxide therapy may interfere with imaging techniques using sodium pertechnetate Tc 99m and thus impair evaluation of Meckel's diverticulum. It may also interfere with reticuloendothelial imaging of liver, spleen, and bone marrow using technetium Tc 99m sulfur colloid. It may antagonize pentagastrin's effect during gastric acid secretion tests.

Aluminum hydroxide may elevate serum gastrin levels and reduce serum phosphate levels.

Adverse reactions
- GI: constipation, appetite loss, decreased bowel motility.
- Metabolic: hypophosphatemia, osteomalacia.
- Other: aluminum toxicity.
Note: Drug should be discontinued if anorexia, malaise, muscle weakness, or other signs and symptoms of hypophosphatemia develop.

Overdose and treatment
No specific information available. Patients with impaired renal function are at a higher risk of aluminum toxicity to brain, bone, and parathyroid glands.

▶ Special considerations
- Shake suspension well (especially extra-strength suspension) and give with small amounts of water or fruit juice.
- After administration through nasogastric tube, tube should be flushed with water to prevent obstruction.
- When administering drug as an antiurolithic, encourage increased fluid intake to enhance drug effectiveness.
- Constipation may be managed with stool softeners or bulk laxatives. Also, alternate aluminum hydroxide with magnesium-containing antacids (unless patient has renal disease).
- Periodically monitor serum calcium and phosphate levels; decreased serum phosphate levels may lead to increased serum calcium levels. Observe patient for hypophosphatemia signs and symptoms (anorexia, muscle weakness, and malaise).

Information for the patient
- Caution patient to take aluminum hydroxide only as directed; to shake suspension well or chew tablets thoroughly; and to follow with sips of water or juice.
- As indicated, instruct patient to restrict sodium intake, drink plenty of fluids, or follow a low-phosphate diet.
- Advise patient not to switch to another antacid without medical approval.

Geriatric use
Because elderly patients commonly have decreased GI motility, they may become constipated from this drug.

Pediatric use
Use with caution in children under age 6.

Breast-feeding
Although aluminum hydroxide may be excreted in breast milk, no problems have been associated with its use in breast-feeding women.

aluminum phosphate
Phosphaljel

- Pharmacologic classification: aluminum salt
- Therapeutic classification: phosphate replacement
- Pregnancy risk category C

How supplied
Available without prescription
Suspension: 233 mg/5 ml

Indications, route, and dosage
Phosphate replacement
Adults: 15 to 30 ml undiluted q 2 hours between meals and h.s.

Pharmacodynamics
Phosphate replacement: Aluminum phosphate reduces fecal excretion of phosphate.

Pharmacokinetics
- *Absorption:* Small amounts of aluminum phosphate may be absorbed systemically.
- *Distribution:* None.
- *Metabolism:* None.
- *Excretion:* Aluminum phosphate is excreted in feces; some may be excreted in breast milk.

Contraindications and precautions
Aluminum phosphate is contraindicated in patients with impaired renal function, appendicitis, constipation, fecal impaction, undiagnosed rectal or GI bleeding, chronic diarrhea, gastric outlet obstruction, or intestinal obstruction, because drug may exacerbate these conditions.

Aluminum phosphate should be used cautiously in patients who must restrict sodium intake because of the sodium content of the suspension; and in patients who have hemorrhoids and in patients with decreased GI motility, such as elderly patients and those receiving anticholinergics or antidiarrheals, because it may cause constipation and increase irritation.

Interactions
Aluminum phosphate may decrease absorption of many drugs, including phenothiazines (especially chlorpromazine), quinolones, tetracycline, coumarin anticoagulants, chenodiol, antimuscarinics, diazepam, chlordiazepoxide, isoniazid, vitamin A, digoxin, and iron salts, thereby lessening their effectiveness; separate drug use by at least 2 hours. Drug may cause premature release of enterically coated drugs; separate dose by 1 hour.

Effects on diagnostic tests
Aluminum phosphate may interfere with imaging techniques using sodium pertechnetate Tc 99m and thus impair evaluation of Meckel's diverticulum, reticuloendothelial imaging of liver, spleen, and bone marrow using technetium Tc 99m sulfur colloid. It may antagonize pentagastrin's effect during gastric acid secretion tests.

Adverse reactions
GI: constipation, decreased GI motility, anorexia.

Overdose and treatment
No specific information available.

▶ Special considerations
- Shake suspension well and give alone or with small amounts of water or milk.
- After administration through nasogastric tube, tube should be flushed with water to prevent obstruction.
- Constipation may be managed with stool softeners or bulk laxatives. Aluminum phosphate may be alternated with magnesium-containing antacids (unless patient has renal disease).
- Closely observe patient who is dehydrated, has restricted fluid intake, or has suspected intestinal obstruction; during long-term use, observe sodium-restricted patients.
- Drug may be used to reverse hypophosphatemia induced by other aluminum-containing antacids.
- Aluminum phosphate is a weak antacid that contains no sugar.

Information for the patient
- Caution patient to take drug only as directed.
- Instruct patient to shake suspension well.
- Tell patient to take other medications 1 or 2 hours before or after aluminum phosphate.
- Advise patient not to switch antacids without medical approval.

Geriatric use
Because elderly patients commonly have decreased GI motility, they may become constipated from this drug.

Pediatric use
Use with caution in children under age 6.

Breast-feeding
Although aluminum phosphate may be excreted in breast milk, no problems have been associated with its use in breast-feeding women.

amantadine hydrochloride
Symmetrel

- Pharmacologic classification: synthetic cyclic primary amine
- Therapeutic classification: antiviral, antiparkinsonism agent
- Pregnancy risk category D

How supplied
Available by prescription only
Capsules: 100 mg
Syrup: 50 mg/5 ml

Indications, route, and dosage

Prophylaxis or symptomatic treatment of influenza type A virus, respiratory tract illnesses in elderly or debilitated patients

Adults to age 64 and children age 10 and over: 200 mg P.O. daily in a single dose or divided b.i.d.

Children age 1 to 9: 4.4 to 8.8 mg/kg P.O. daily, divided b.i.d. or t.i.d. Do not exceed 150 mg/day.

Adults over age 64: 100 mg P.O. once daily.

Treatment should continue for 24 to 48 hours after symptoms disappear. Prophylaxis should start as soon as possible after initial exposure and continue for at least 10 days after exposure. Prophylactic treatment may be continued up to 90 days for repeated or suspected exposures if influenza virus vaccine is unavailable. If used with influenza virus vaccine, continue dose for 2 to 3 weeks until protection from vaccine develops.

Treatment of drug-induced extrapyramidal reactions

Adults: 100 mg P.O. b.i.d., up to 300 mg/day in divided doses. Patient may benefit from as much as 400 mg/day, but doses over 200 mg must be closely supervised.

Treatment of idiopathic parkinsonism, parkinsonian syndrome

Adults: 100 mg P.O. b.i.d.; in patients who are seriously ill or receiving other antiparkinsonian drugs, 100 mg/day for at least 1 week, then 100 mg b.i.d., p.r.n.

Patients with renal dysfunction require dosage reduction.

Dosage in renal failure

Base dosage on creatinine clearance value, as follows:

Creatinine clearance value (ml/minute/1.73 m²) determines maintenance dosage. Thus, if creatinine clearance is > 80 ml/minute, maintenance dosage is 100 mg twice daily; if 60 to 80 ml/minute, 200 mg or 100 mg on alternate days; 40 to 60 ml/minute, 100 mg once daily; 30 to 40 ml/minute, 200 mg twice weekly; 20 to 30 ml/minute, 100 mg three times weekly; 10 to 20 ml/minute, 200 mg or 100 mg alternating every 7 days.

Note: Patients on chronic hemodialysis should receive 200 mg or 100 mg alternating every 7 days.

Pharmacodynamics

● *Antiviral action:* Amantadine interferes with penetration of influenza A virus into susceptible cells and blocks viral uncoating by ribonucleic acid (RNA). In vitro, amantadine is active only against influenza type A virus. (However, spontaneous resistance frequently occurs.) In vivo, amantadine may protect against influenza type A virus in 70% to 90% of patients; when administered within 24 to 48 hours of onset of illness, it reduces duration of fever and other systemic symptoms.

● *Antiparkinsonism action:* Amantadine is thought to cause the release of dopamine in the substantia nigra.

Pharmacokinetics

● *Absorption:* With oral administration, amantadine is well absorbed from the GI tract. Peak serum levels occur in 1 to 8 hours; usual serum level is 0.2 to 0.9 mcg/ml. (Neurotoxicity may occur at levels exceeding 1.5 mcg/ml.)

● *Distribution:* Amantadine is distributed widely throughout the body and crosses the blood-brain barrier.

● *Metabolism:* About 10% of dose is metabolized.

● *Excretion:* About 90% of dose is excreted unchanged in urine, primarily by tubular secretion. Portion of drug may be excreted in breast milk. Excretion rate depends on urine pH (acidic pH enhances excretion). In patients with normal renal function, elimination half-life is approximately 24 hours. In patients with renal dysfunction, elimination half-life may be prolonged to 10 days.

Contraindications and precautions

Amantadine is contraindicated in patients with known hypersensitivity to the drug.

Amantadine should be administered cautiously to patients with a history of hepatic disease, seizures, psychosis, renal disease, recurrent eczematoid dermatitis, epilepsy, cardiovascular disease (especially congestive heart failure), peripheral edema, or orthostatic hypotension, because the drug may exacerbate these disorders. Do not administer to pregnant women or women of childbearing age without adequate contraceptive measures because animal studies have demonstrated embryotoxic and teratogenic potential.

Interactions

When used concomitantly, amantadine may potentiate anticholinergic adverse effects of trihexyphenidyl and benztropine (when these drugs are given in high doses), possibly causing confusion and hallucinations. Concomitant use with a combination of hydrochlorothiazide and triamterene may decrease urinary amantadine excretion, resulting in increased serum amantadine levels and possible toxicity.

Concomitant use with CNS stimulants may cause additive stimulation. Concomitant use with alcohol may result in light-headedness, confusion, fainting, and hypotension.

Effects on diagnostic tests

None reported.

Adverse reactions

● CNS: depression, fatigue, confusion, dizziness, psychosis, hallucinations, anxiety, irritability, ataxia, insomnia, weakness, headache, light-headedness, difficulty concentrating.

● CV: peripheral edema, orthostatic hypotension, *congestive heart failure.*

● DERM: livedo reticularis (with prolonged use).

● GI: anorexia, nausea, constipation, vomiting, dry mouth.

● GU: urinary retention.

Note: Drug should be discontinued if patient develops hypersensitivity reaction.

Overdose and treatment

Clinical effects of overdose include nausea, vomiting, anorexia, hyperexcitability, tremors, slurred speech, blurred vision, lethargy, anticholinergic symptoms, convulsions, and possible *ventricular arrhythmias,* including *torsade de pointes* and *ventricular fibrillation.*

Note: CNS effects result from increased levels of dopamine in the brain.

Treatment includes immediate gastric lavage or emesis induction along with supportive measures, forced fluids, and, if necessary, I.V. administration of fluids. Urine acidification may be used to increase drug excretion. Physostigmine may be given (1 to 2 mg by slow I.V. infusion at 1- to 2-hour intervals) to counteract CNS toxicity. Seizures or arrhythmias may be treated with conventional therapy. Patient should be monitored closely.

▶ Special considerations

• To prevent orthostatic hypotension, instruct patient to move slowly when changing position (especially when rising to standing position).

• If patient experiences insomnia, administer dose several hours before bedtime.

• Prophylactic drug use is recommended for selected high-risk patients who cannot receive influenza virus vaccine. Manufacturer recommends prophylactic therapy lasting up to 90 days with possible repeated or unknown exposure.

Information for the patient

• Warn patient that drug may impair mental alertness.

• Advise patient to take drug after meals to ensure best absorption.

• Caution patient to avoid abrupt position changes because these may cause light-headedness or dizziness.

• If patient is taking drug to treat parkinsonism, warn him not to discontinue it abruptly, because that might precipitate a parkinsonian crisis.

• Warn patient to avoid alcohol while taking drug.

• Instruct patient to report adverse effects promptly, especially dizziness, depression, anxiety, nausea, and urinary retention.

Geriatric use

Elderly patients are more susceptible to adverse neurologic effects; dividing daily dosage into two doses may reduce this risk.

Pediatric use

Amantadine's safety and effectiveness in children under age 1 have not been established.

Breast-feeding

Amantadine is excreted in breast milk. Breast-feeding should be avoided during therapy with amantadine.

---

ambenonium chloride
Mytelase

• Pharmacologic classification: cholinesterase inhibitor
• Therapeutic classification: antimyasthenic agent
• Pregnancy risk category C

How supplied

Available by prescription only
Tablets: 10 mg

Indications, route, and dosage
Symptomatic treatment of myasthenia gravis
Adults: Dose must be individualized for each patient, but usually ranges from 5 to 25 mg P.O. t.i.d. to q.i.d. Starting dose usually 5 mg P.O. t.i.d. to q.i.d., increased gradually and adjusted at 2-day intervals to avoid drug accumulation and overdose. Maintenance dosage may range from 5 mg to as much as 75 mg per dose.
Children: Initially, 0.3 mg/kg/day or 10 mg/m²/day up to 1.5 mg/kg/day or 50 mg/m²/day in three or four doses.

Pharmacodynamics
Muscle stimulant action: Ambenonium blocks hydrolysis of acetylcholine by cholinesterase, resulting in

acetylcholine accumulation at cholinergic synapses. That leads to increased stimulation of cholinergic receptors at the myoneural junction.

Because of its toxic potential, ambenonium chloride is usually used only in patients who cannot tolerate neostigmine or pyridostigmine (such as those who are hypersensitive to bromides).

Pharmacokinetics

• *Absorption:* Ambenonium is poorly absorbed from the GI tract. Onset of action usually occurs in 20 to 30 minutes.
• *Distribution:* Largely unknown.
• *Metabolism:* The exact metabolic fate is unknown; however, drug is not hydrolyzed by cholinesterases. Duration of effect is usually 3 to 8 hours, depending on patient's physical and emotional status and severity of disease.
• *Excretion:* Unknown.

Contraindications and precautions

Ambenonium is contraindicated in patients with mechanical obstruction of the intestinal or urinary tract because of its stimulatory effect on smooth muscle and in patients with bradycardia and hypotension because it may exacerbate these conditions.

Administer ambenonium cautiously to patients with epilepsy because of the drug's possible CNS stimulatory effects; to patients with recent coronary occlusion or cardiac arrhythmias, because the drug stimulates the cardiovascular system; to patients with peptic ulcer, because the drug may stimulate gastric acid secretion; and to patients with bronchial asthma, because the drug may precipitate asthma attacks. Avoid giving large doses to patients with megacolon or decreased GI motility because intoxication may occur after gastric motility has been restored. Other cholinergic drugs should be discontinued before ambenonium administration begins to avoid additive cholinergic effects.

Interactions

Procainamide and quinidine may reverse ambenonium's cholinergic effects on muscle. Use with corticosteroids also may decrease ambenonium's cholinergic effects; however, after corticosteroids are stopped, cholinergic effects may increase, possibly altering muscle strength. Combined use with succinylcholine may cause prolonged respiratory depression from plasma esterase inhibition and resulting delay in succinylcholine hydrolysis. Use with ganglionic blockers, such as mecamylamine, may critically decrease blood pressure; effect is usually preceded by abdominal symptoms. Concomitant use of magnesium may antagonize beneficial effects of anticholinesterase therapy through a direct depressant effect on skeletal muscle.

Effects on diagnostic tests
None reported.

Adverse reactions
• CNS: headache, dizziness, convulsions, confusion, nervousness.
• CV: *arrhythmias (especially bradycardia)*, decreased cardiac output, hypotension.
• Eye: miosis, lacrimation, diplopia, blurred vision, conjunctival hyperemia.
• GI: nausea, vomiting, diarrhea, increased peristalsis, increased abdominal cramps, increased salivation, increased GI secretions, dysphagia.

- GU: urinary frequency and urgency, incontinence.
- Musculoskeletal: muscle weakness, muscle cramps, fasciculations.
- Respiratory: increased tracheobronchial secretions, laryngospasm, bronchiolar constriction, bronchospasm, *respiratory muscle paralysis.*
- Other: fever.

Note: Drug should be discontinued if hypersensitivity, difficulty breathing, incoordination, paralysis, or restlessness or agitation develops.

Overdose and treatment
Clinical signs of overdose include nausea, vomiting, diarrhea, excessive salivation, increased bronchial secretions, excessive sweating, muscle weakness, fasciculations, paralysis, hypotension, and bradycardia.

Treatment consists mainly of respiratory support and bronchial suctioning. Discontinue drug immediately. Atropine (0.5 to 4 mg I.V.) will block ambenonium's muscarinic effects but will not counter paralytic effects on skeletal muscle. Avoid atropine overdose, because it may cause bronchial plug formation.

▶ Special considerations
Besides those relevant to all *cholinesterase inhibitors,* consider the following recommendations.
- Give ambenonium with food or milk to reduce the chance of GI adverse effects.
- Observe and record variations in patient's muscle strength.
- If muscle weakness is severe, determine if this problem results from drug toxicity or exacerbation of myasthenia gravis. A test dose of edrophonium I.V. will aggravate drug-induced weakness but will temporarily relieve weakness that results from the disease.
- Consider providing hospitalized patients with bedside supply of tablets to take themselves.
- Patients may develop resistance to this drug.

Information for the patient
Teach patient how to evaluate muscle strength and to report changes; also advise him to report any skin rash or extreme fatigue.

---

amcinonide
Cyclocort

- Pharmacologic classification: topical adrenocorticoid
- Therapeutic classification: anti-inflammatory
- Pregnancy risk category C

How supplied
Available by prescription only
Cream, ointment: 0.1%
Lotion: 0.1%

Indications, route, and dosage
Inflammation of corticosteroid-responsive dermatoses

Adults and children: Apply a light film to affected areas b.i.d. or t.i.d. Rub cream in gently and thoroughly until it disappears.

Pharmacodynamics
Anti-inflammatory action: Amcinonide stimulates the synthesis of enzymes needed to decrease the inflammatory response. Amcinonide is a group II fluorinated corticosteroid with much greater anti-inflammatory activity than hydrocortisone 0.25% to 2.5%. It has vasoconstrictor, antipruritic, and anti-inflammatory actions equal to those of betamethasone dipropionate 0.05% and triamcinolone acetonide 0.5%.

Pharmacokinetics
- *Absorption:* The amount of drug absorbed depends on the amount applied and on the nature of the skin at the application site. It ranges from about 1% in areas with a thick stratum corneum (such as the palms, soles, elbows, and knees) to as high as 36% in areas of the thinnest stratum corneum (face, eyelids, and genitals). Absorption increases in areas of skin damage, inflammation, or occlusion. Some systemic absorption of topical steroids may occur, especially through the oral mucosa.
- *Distribution:* After topical application, amcinonide is distributed throughout the local skin. Any drug that is absorbed into circulation is removed rapidly from the blood and distributed into muscle, liver, skin, intestines, and kidneys.
- *Metabolism:* After topical administration, amcinonide is metabolized primarily in the skin. The small amount that is absorbed into systemic circulation is metabolized primarily in the liver to inactive compounds.
- *Excretion:* Inactive metabolites are excreted by the kidneys, primarily as glucuronides and sulfates, but also as unconjugated products. Small amounts of the metabolites are also excreted in feces.

Contraindications and precautions
Amcinonide is contraindicated in patients who are hypersensitive to any component of the preparation and in patients with viral diseases of the skin, such as varicella or herpes simplex, because it suppresses the patient's immune response.

Amcinonide should be used with extreme caution in patients with impaired circulation because it may increase the risk of skin ulceration.

Avoid applying to the face or genital area because increased absorption may result in striae.

Interactions
None significant.

Effects on diagnostic tests
None reported.

Adverse reactions
- Local: burning, itching, irritation, dryness, folliculitis, hypertrichosis, acneiform eruptions, hypopigmentation, perioral dermatitis, allergic contact dermatitis, maceration, secondary infection, atrophy, striae, miliaria.

Significant systemic absorption may produce the following reactions.
- CNS: euphoria, insomnia, headache, psychotic behavior, pseudotumor cerebri, mental changes, nervousness, restlessness.
- CV: congestive heart failure, hypertension, edema.
- EENT: cataracts, glaucoma, thrush.
- GI: peptic ulcer, irritation, increased appetite.
- Immune: immunosuppression, increased susceptibility to infection.
- Metabolic: hypokalemia, sodium retention, fluid re-

---

tention, weight gain, hyperglycemia, osteoporosis, growth suppression in children.
● Musculoskeletal: muscle atrophy.
● Other: withdrawal syndrome (nausea, fatigue, anorexia, dyspnea, hypotension, hypoglycemia, myalgia, arthralgia, fever, dizziness, and fainting).

Note: Drug should be discontinued if local irritation, infection, systemic absorption, or hypersensitivity reaction occurs.

Overdose and treatment
No information available.

▶ Special considerations
Recommendations for use of amcinonide, for care and teaching of patients during therapy, and for use in elderly patients, in children, and during breast-feeding are the same as those for all *topical adrenocorticoids.*

---

amikacin sulfate
Amikin

● Pharmacologic classification: aminoglycoside
● Therapeutic classification: antibiotic
● Pregnancy risk category D

How supplied
Available by prescription only
Injection: 50 mg/ml, 250 mg/ml

Indications, route, and dosage
Serious infections caused by susceptible organisms
Adults and children with normal renal function: 15 mg/kg/day divided q 8 to 12 hours I.M. or I.V. (in 100 to 200 ml dextrose 5% in water administered over 30 to 60 minutes). May be given by direct I.V. push if necessary.
Neonates with normal renal function: Initially, 10 mg/kg I.M. or I.V. (in dextrose 5% in water administered over 1 to 2 hours), q 12 hours for 2 days, then 10 mg/kg q 8 hours.
Meningitis
Adults: Systemic therapy as above; may also use up to 20 mg intrathecally or intraventricularly daily.
Children: Systemic therapy as above; may also use 1 to 2 mg intrathecally daily.
Uncomplicated urinary tract infections
Adults: 250 mg I.M. or I.V. b.i.d.
Dosage in renal failure
Initially, 7.5 mg/kg. Subsequent doses and frequency determined by blood amikacin concentrations and renal function studies. One method is to administer additional 7.5 mg/kg doses and alter dosing interval based upon steady state serum creatinine:

$$\frac{\text{creatinine}}{\text{(mg/100 ml)}} \times 9 = \frac{\text{dosing interval}}{\text{(in hours)}}$$

Keep peak serum concentrations between 15 and 30 mcg/ml, and trough serum concentrations should not exceed 5 to 10 mcg/ml.

Pharmacodynamics
Antibiotic action: Amikacin is bactericidal; it binds directly to the 30S ribosomal subunit, thus inhibiting bacterial protein synthesis. Its spectrum of activity includes many aerobic gram-negative organisms (including most strains of *Pseudomonas aeruginosa*) and some aerobic gram-positive organisms. Amikacin may act against some organisms resistant to other aminoglycosides, such as *Proteus, Pseudomonas,* and *Serratia;* some strains of these may be resistant to amikacin. It is ineffective against anerobes.

Pharmacokinetics
● *Absorption:* Amikacin is absorbed poorly after oral administration and is given parenterally; after I.M. administration, peak serum concentrations occur in 45 minutes to 2 hours.
● *Distribution:* Amikacin is distributed widely after parenteral administration; intraocular penetration is poor. Factors that increase volume of distribution (burns, peritonitis) may increase dosage requirements. CSF penetration is low, even in patients with inflamed meninges. Intraventricular administration produces high concentrations throughout the CNS. Protein binding is minimal. Amikacin crosses the placenta.
● *Metabolism:* Not metabolized.
● *Excretion:* Amikacin is excreted primarily in urine by glomerular filtration; small amounts may be excreted in bile and breast milk. Elimination half-life in adults is 2 to 3 hours. In patients with severe renal damage, half-life may extend to 30 to 86 hours. Over time, amikacin accumulates in inner ear and kidneys; urine concentrations approach 800 mcg/ml 6 hours after a 500-mg I.M. dose.

Contraindications and precautions
Amikacin is contraindicated in patients with known hypersensitivity to amikacin or any other aminoglycoside.

Amikacin should be used cautiously in patients with decreased renal function; in patients with tinnitus, vertigo, or high-frequency hearing loss, who are susceptible to ototoxicity; in patients with dehydration, because of potential for increased nephrotoxicity with decreased urinary output; in patients with myasthenia gravis, parkinsonism, and hypocalcemia, because the drug may exacerbate symptoms associated with these disorders; in neonates and other infants; and in elderly patients.

Interactions
Concomitant use with the following drugs may increase the hazard of nephrotoxicity, ototoxicity, and neurotoxicity: amphotericin B, loop diuretics, methoxyflurane, polymyxin B, capreomycin, cisplatin, cephalosporins, and other aminoglycosides; hazard of ototoxicity is also increased during use with ethacrynic acid, furosemide, bumetanide, urea, or mannitol. Dimenhydrinate and other antiemetics and antivertigo drugs may mask amikacin-induced ototoxicity.

Amikacin may potentiate neuromuscular blockade from general anesthetics or neuromuscular blocking agents such as succinylcholine and tubocurarine.

Concomitant use with penicillins results in a synergistic bactericidal effect against *Pseudomonas aeruginosa, Escherichia coli, Klebsiella, Citrobacter, Enterobacter, Serratia,* and *Proteus mirabilis.* However, the drugs are physically and chemically incompatible and are inactivated when mixed or given together. In vivo inactivation has also been reported when aminoglycosides and penicillins are used concomitantly.

Effects on diagnostic tests
Amikacin-induced nephrotoxicity may elevate BUN, nonprotein nitrogen, or serum creatinine levels, and increase urinary excretion of casts.

Adverse reactions
• CNS: headache, lethargy, *neuromuscular blockade with respiratory depression.*
• EENT: *ototoxicity (tinnitus, vertigo, hearing loss).*
• GI: diarrhea.
• GU: *nephrotoxicity (cells or casts in urine, oliguria, proteinuria, decreased creatinine clearance, increased BUN, serum creatinine, and nonprotein nitrogen levels).*
• Other: hypersensitivity reactions (eosinophilia, fever, rash, urticaria, pruritus), bacterial or fungal superinfections.
   Note: Drug should be discontinued if signs of ototoxicity, nephrotoxicity, or hypersensitivity occur.

Overdose and treatment
Clinical signs of overdose include ototoxicity, nephrotoxicity, and neuromuscular toxicity. Drug can be removed by hemodialysis or peritoneal dialysis. Treatment with calcium salts or anticholinesterases reverses neuromuscular blockade.

▶ Special considerations
Besides those relevant to all *aminoglycosides,* consider the following recommendations.
• Because amikacin is dialyzable, patients undergoing hemodialysis may need dosage adjustments.
• Recommendations for care and teaching of patients during therapy and use in elderly patients and breast-feeding women are the same as for all *aminoglycosides.*

Pediatric use
Because the potential for ototoxicity is unknown, amikacin should only be used in infants when other drugs are ineffective or contraindicated. Patient should be closely monitored during therapy.

amiloride hydrochloride
Midamor

• Pharmacologic classification: potassium-sparing diuretic
• Therapeutic classification: diuretic, antihypertensive
• Pregnancy risk category B

How supplied
Available by prescription only
Tablets: 5 mg

Indications, route, and dosage
Hypertension; edema associated with congestive heart failure, usually in patients who are also taking thiazide or other potassium-wasting diuretics
Adults: Usually 5 mg P.O. daily. Dosage may be increased to 10 mg daily, if necessary. Do not exceed 20 mg daily.

Pharmacodynamics
• *Diuretic action:* Amiloride acts directly on the distal renal tubule to inhibit sodium reabsorption and potassium excretion, thereby reducing potassium loss.
• *Antihypertensive action:* Amiloride is frequently used in combination with more effective diuretics to manage edema associated with congestive heart failure, hepatic cirrhosis, and hyperaldosteronism. The mechanism of amiloride's hypotensive effect is unknown.

Pharmacokinetics
• *Absorption:* About 50% of an amiloride dose is absorbed from the GI tract. Food decreases absorption to 30%. Diuresis usually begins in 2 hours and peaks in 6 to 10 hours.
• *Distribution:* Amiloride has wide extravascular distribution.
• *Metabolism:* Insignificant.
• *Excretion:* Most of the amiloride dose is excreted in urine; half-life is 6 to 9 hours in patients with normal renal function.

Contraindications and precautions
Amiloride is contraindicated in patients whose serum potassium levels are over 5.5 mEq/liter or who are receiving other potassium-sparing diuretics or potassium supplements; in patients with anuria, acute or chronic renal insufficiency, or diabetic nephropathy because of the potential for hyperkalemia; and in patients with known hypersensitivity to the drug.
   Amiloride should be used cautiously in patients with severe hepatic insufficiency, because electrolyte imbalance may precipitate hepatic encephalopathy, and in patients with diabetes, who are at increased risk of hyperkalemia.

Interactions
Amiloride may potentiate hypotensive effects of other antihypertensive agents; this may be used to therapeutic advantage.
   Amiloride increases the risk of hyperkalemia when administered with other potassium-sparing diuretics, angiotensin-converting enzyme inhibitors (captopril or enalapril), potassium supplements, potassium-containing medications (parenteral penicillin G), or salt substitutes. Amiloride may reduce renal clearance of lithium and increase lithium blood levels.
   Nonsteroidal anti-inflammatory agents, such as indomethacin or ibuprofen, may alter renal function and thus affect potassium excretion.

Effects on diagnostic tests
Transient abnormal renal and hepatic function tests have been noted. Amiloride therapy causes severe hyperkalemia in diabetic patients following I.V. glucose tolerance testing; discontinue amiloride at least 3 days before testing.

Adverse reactions
• CNS: headache, weakness, dizziness.
• CV: orthostatic hypotension.
• GI: nausea, anorexia, diarrhea, vomiting, abdominal pain, constipation.
• GU: impotence.
• Metabolic: *hyperkalemia.*
   Note: Drug should be discontinued if hyperkalemia occurs.

Overdose and treatment

Clinical manifestations of overdose are consistent with dehydration and electrolyte disturbance.

Treatment is supportive and symptomatic. In acute ingestion, empty stomach by emesis or lavage. In severe hyperkalemia (≥ 6.5 mEq/liter), reduce serum potassium levels with I.V. sodium bicarbonate or glucose with insulin. A cation exchange resin, sodium polystyrene sulfonate (Kayexalate), given orally or as a retention enema, may also reduce serum potassium levels.

▶ **Special considerations**
Recommendations for the use of amiloride and for care and teaching of the patient during therapy are the same as those for all *potassium-sparing diuretics.*

Geriatric use
Elderly and debilitated patients require close observation because they are more susceptible to drug-induced diuresis and hyperkalemia. Reduced dosages may be indicated.

Pediatric use
Safety and efficacy in children have not been established.

Breast-feeding
Amiloride is excreted in breast milk in animals; human data are unavailable.

amino acid solution
Aminosyn, Aminosyn with dextrose, Aminosyn with electrolytes, Aminosyn-PF, Aminosyn (pH6), Aminosyn II, Aminosyn II in dextrose, Aminosyn II with electrolytes, Aminosyn II with electrolytes in dextrose, FreAmine III, FreAmine III with electrolytes, Novamine, Novamine without electrolytes, ProcalAmine, Travasol with electrolytes, Travasol without electrolytes, TrophAmine 6%

amino acid solutions for renal failure
Aminess 5.2%, Aminosyn-RF 5.2%, NephrAmine 5.4%, RenAmine

amino acid solutions for high metabolic stress
Aminosyn-HBC 7%, BranchAmin 4%, FreAmine HBC 6.9%

amino acid solutions for hepatic failure or hepatic encephalopathy
HepatAmine

- Pharmacologic classification: protein substrates
- Therapeutic classification: parenteral nutritional therapy and caloric agent
- Pregnancy risk category C

How supplied
Available by prescription only
Injection: without electrolytes – 1,000 ml (3.5%, 5%, 8.5%, 10%; 10% with 60 mg potassium metabisulfite, 11.4%); 500 ml (5%, 5.5% with sodium bisulfite, 7%, 8.5%, 8.5% with sodium bisulfite, 10%, 10% with sodium bisulfite, 11.4%); 250 ml (5%, 10% with sodium bisulfite, 11.4%)
Injection: with electrolytes – 1,000 ml (3% with 50 mg potassium metabisulfite and 3 mEq calcium/liter, 3% with potassium metabisulfite, 3.5%, 3.5% with 60 mg sodium hydrosulfite), 500 ml (3.5%, 5.5% with 3 mEq sodium bisulfite/liter, 7% with potassium bisulfite, 8% in 1,000-ml container with potassium metabisulfite, 8.5% with potassium metabisulfite, 8.5% with 3 mEq sodium bisulfite/liter)

Indications, route, and dosage
Hepatic encephalopathy in patients with cirrhosis or hepatitis; nutritional support
Adults: 80 to 120 g of amino acids (12 to 18 g of nitrogen)/day. Use formulation specifically for hepatic failure or encephalopathy (HepatAmine). Typically, 500 ml amino acid injection is mixed with 500 ml dextrose 50% in water and administered over a 24-hour period. Add electrolytes, vitamins, and trace elements needed.
Total supportive, or supplemental and protein-sparing parenteral nutrition to maintain normal nutrition and metabolism (amino acid solution)
Adults: 1 to 1.5 g/kg I.V. daily.
Children: 2 to 3 g/kg I.V. daily.
Note: Individualize dosage to metabolic and clinical response as determined by nitrogen balance and body weight corrected for fluid balance. Add electrolytes, vitamins, trace elements, and nonprotein caloric solutions as needed.

Pharmacodynamics
Nutritional action: Amino acid injection and solution provide a substrate for protein synthesis in the protein-depleted patient or enhance conservation of body protein.

Pharmacokinetics
Amino acid solution is administered directly into the vascular system. No information is available regarding systemic distribution, metabolism, or excretion.

Contraindications and precautions
Amino acids are contraindicated in patients with decreased circulating blood volume, inborn errors of amino acid metabolism, or hypersensitivity to any component. General amino acid formulations are contraindicated in patients with severe renal failure, severe liver disease, hepatic coma, hepatic encephalopathy, or hyperammonemia. Renal failure formulations are contraindicated in patients with severe electrolyte and acid-base imbalance and hyperammonemia. Hepatic failure and hepatic encephalopathy formulations are contraindicated in patients with anuria. High metabolic stress formulations are contraindicated in patients with anuria, hepatic coma, or severe electrolyte or acid-base imbalances.

Electrolytes should be administered cautiously in patients with cardiac insufficiency, renal impairment, or pulmonary disease. Administering sodium to patients with chronic heart failure, renal failure, or edema with sodium retention requires special precautions. Admin-

---

istering potassium requires caution in patients with hyperkalemia, severe renal failure, or potassium retention. Acetate must be used cautiously in patients with alkalosis or hepatic insufficiency.

Amino acid infusions should be used with special caution in patients with elevated BUN levels, which usually result from increased protein intake; discontinue infusion if BUN levels continue to rise. Renal failure or GI bleeding may also increase BUN levels. Azotemia patients should avoid amino acid administration unless total nitrogen concentration is considered.

When used as protein-sparing therapy, if daily BUN levels increase for more than 3 days, protein-sparing therapy should be discontinued and a nonprotein regimen substituted. Circulatory overload should be avoided in patients with cardiac dysfunction. Amino acids should always be administered with dextrose in patients with myocardial infarction.

Hypertonic solutions containing more than 12.5% dextrose should not be administered peripherally. Hyperosmolar solutions should not be used in dehydrated patients with intracranial or intraspinal hemorrhage or delirium tremens.

Patients should be monitored carefully for glucose imbalance; glucose intolerance is quite common, especially in septic or hypermetabolic patients and in patients with renal failure. Metabolic adaptation to a large glucose load takes up to 72 hours. Reducing the administration rate may help prevent glucose intolerance. Excessive carbohydrates may cause fatty infiltration of the liver. Excessive glucose may precipitate respiratory failure. Abrupt discontinuation of concentrated dextrose solutions may result in rebound hypoglycemia; a dextrose 5% solution should be administered during gradual withdrawal.

Intravenous nutritional therapy requires continuous monitoring. Amino acid metabolism may result in hyperchloremic metabolic acidosis; therefore, chloride content must be minimized. Conservative doses of amino acid injection must be administered to patients with impaired liver function. Hyperammonemia requires discontinuation and reevaluation of amino acid therapy. This occurs most often in children or adults with renal or hepatic disease with a diminished ability to handle the protein load. Hyperammonemia is particularly significant in infants, who may develop mental retardation as a result.

Interactions

Concurrent tetracycline administration may reduce the protein-sparing effects of infused amino acids.

Because of the potential for incompatibility, other drugs should not be mixed with amino acid-carbohydrate solutions. Mixture with folic acid precipitates calcium salts as calcium folate. Mixture with sodium bicarbonate may precipitate calcium and magnesium and decreases the activity of insulin and vitamin B complex with vitamin C. Acidic I.V. solutions for total parenteral nutrition (TPN) may release bicarbonate as gas. When vitamin K is indicated, administer it separately. Supplementary vitamins, electrolytes, trace minerals, heparin, or insulin may be added cautiously when necessary; other medications should not be administered via the central venous catheter. Simultaneous administration with blood may cause pseudoagglutination.

Effects on diagnostic tests

None reported.

Adverse reactions

● CNS: mental confusion, unconsciousness, headache, dizziness.
● CV: hypervolemia related to congestive heart failure (in susceptible patients), *pulmonary edema*, exacerbation of hypertension (in predisposed patients).
● DERM: chills, flushing, feeling of warmth, papular and erythematous rashes.
● GI: nausea, vomiting.
● GU: glycosuria, osmotic diuresis.
● Hepatic: fatty liver, elevated liver enzyme levels.
● Metabolic: *rebound hypoglycemia* (when long-term infusions are stopped abruptly), *hyperglycemia*, hypocalcemia, metabolic acidosis, metabolic alkalosis, hypophosphatemia, *hyperosmolar hyperglycemic nonketotic coma (HHNC)*, hyperammonemia, hypovitaminosis, dehydration (if hyperosmolar solutions are used), osteoporosis.
● Local: tissue sloughing at infusion site from extravasation, catheter sepsis, thrombophlebitis, *thrombosis*.
● Systemic: fever.
● Other: allergic reactions, vertigo, diaphoresis.

Overdose and treatment

No information available.

▶ Special considerations

● Consult pharmacist about compatibility before combining amino acid solutions with other substances.
● Begin I.V. infusion slowly and increase over 1 to 2 days to prevent hyperglycemia. Taper off over 1 to 2 days to prevent rebound hypoglycemia.
● All I.V. equipment (I.V. lines, filter, and bottle) should be replaced every 24 hours.
● Observe infusion site for signs of infection, drainage, edema, and extravasation. Check for fever or other possible signs of infection or hypersensitivity.
● TPN line should be used solely for providing nutrition, not for collecting blood samples, transfusing blood, or administering drugs.
● Vital signs should be checked at least every 4 hours.
● Monitor intake, output, and pattern, as well as caloric intake for significant changes.
● Patient should be weighed daily at the same time (preferably in the morning after urinating), in the same clothing, and on the same scale. After the patient's weight has stabilized, weighing him twice or three times weekly is sufficient.
● Patient's urine should be tested for glucose, acetone, and specific gravity every 6 hours until infusion rate is stabilized, then twice daily.
● Test for urine glucose with Clinistix, Keto-Diastix, or Tes-Tape. These tests do not react with the reducing substances in IVH solutions.
● High blood glucose levels may require supplementary insulin to prevent dehydration and coma.
● Essential fatty acid deficiency may result from long-term fat-free I.V. feedings. Providing 500 ml of fat emulsion per week may be necessary.
● If IVH must be interrupted, administer dextrose 5% or 10% in water by peripheral vein to prevent rebound hypoglycemia.
● Watch for signs of circulatory overload.
● Regularly monitor the following laboratory values throughout IVH therapy: CBC with differential and platelet count, serum electrolytes, blood glucose, urine glucose and ketones, prothrombin time, renal and hepatic function tests, trace elements, and plasma lipids.
● In patients receiving protein-sparing therapy, check

BUN determinations daily. If BUN levels increase 10 to 15 mg/dl for more than 3 days, therapy adjustment is usually required.
• Carefully monitor BUN and creatinine ratios. A BUN-to-creatinine ratio exceeding 1:10 may indicate that patient is receiving too much protein per unit of glucose. Reportedly, 100 to 150 g carbohydrate calories per gram of nitrogen are required to use amino acids effectively.
• Frequent, meticulous mouth care is important to prevent parotitis.
• Administer 10 mg of phytonadione weekly to prevent vitamin K deficiency.

Information for the patient
• Patients receiving TPN often imagine they taste or smell food. Explain that these sensations are common, and suggest some distracting activity during mealtimes.
• Encourage patient to take special care with mouth hygiene. Recommend that he use a soft toothbrush with a fluoride toothpaste and floss teeth daily.
• Inform patient that he will have fewer bowel movements while receiving TPN.

Pediatric use
• The effect of amino acid infusions without dextrose on the carbohydrate metabolism of children is unknown.
• Take special precautions in children with acute renal failure and especially in low-birth-weight infants. In these patients, laboratory and clinical monitoring must be extensive and frequent.
• Monitor serum calcium levels frequently to check for signs of bone demineralization.

---

aminocaproic acid
Amicar

• Pharmacologic classification: carboxylic acid derivative
• Therapeutic classification: fibrinolysis inhibitor
• Pregnancy risk category C

How supplied
Available by prescription only
Tablets: 500 mg
Syrup: 250 mg/ml
Injection: 5 g/20 ml for dilution; 24 g/96 ml for infusion

Indications, route, and dosage
Excessive acute bleeding from hyperfibrinolysis
Adults: 4 to 5 g I.V. or P.O. over first hour, followed with constant infusion of 1 g/hour for about 8 hours or until bleeding is controlled; plasma level should be 130 mcg/ml. Maximum dosage is 30 g/24 hours.
Chronic bleeding tendency
Adults: 5 to 30 g/day P.O. in divided doses at 3- to 6-hour intervals.
Children: 100 mg/kg I.V., or 3 g/m² I.V. first hour, followed by constant infusion of 33.3 mg/kg/hour or 1 g/m²/hour. Maximum dosage is 18 g/m² for 24 hours.

†*Antidote for excessive thrombolysis due to administration of streptokinase or urokinase*
Adults: 4 to 5 g I.V. in the first hour, followed by continuous infusion of 1 g/hr. Treatment is continued for 8 hours or until hemorrhage is controlled.

Pharmacodynamics
Hemostatic action: Aminocaproic acid inhibits plasminogen activators; to a lesser degree, it blocks antiplasmin activity by inhibiting fibrinolysis.

Pharmacokinetics
• *Absorption:* Aminocaproic acid is rapidly and completely absorbed from the GI tract. Peak plasma level occurs in 2 hours; sustained plasma levels are achieved by repeated oral doses or continuous I.V. infusion.
• *Distribution:* Aminocaproic acid readily permeates human blood cells and other body cells. It is not protein-bound.
• *Metabolism:* Insignificant.
• *Excretion:* Duration of action of a single parenteral dose is less than 3 hours; 40% to 60% of a single oral dose is excreted unchanged in urine in 12 hours.

Contraindications and precautions
Aminocaproic acid is contraindicated in patients with active intravascular clotting; do not use in patients with disseminated intravascular coagulation (DIC) without concomitant heparin therapy, because aminocaproic acid may induce thrombus formation.
Contraindicated in neonates because it contains benzyl alcohol, which has been associated with toxicity.
Administer drug cautiously to patients with thrombophlebitis or cardiac disease because of potential for clotting abnormalities, and to patients with hepatic or renal disease because of potential for drug accumulation.

Interactions
Concomitant use with estrogens and oral contraceptives containing estrogen increases risk of hypercoagulability; use with caution.

Effects on diagnostic tests
Drug may elevate serum potassium level in some patients with decreased renal function; it may increase creatinine phosphokinase (CPK), serum glutamic-oxaloacetic transaminase (SGOT), and serum glutamic-pyruvic transaminase (SGPT) levels.

Adverse reactions
• CNS: dizziness, malaise, headache, delirium, hallucinations, seizures.
• CV: hypotension, bradycardia, arrhythmias (especially with rapid I.V. infusion).
• DERM: rash.
• EENT: tinnitus, nasal stuffiness, conjunctival suffusion.
• GI: nausea, cramps, diarrhea.
• GU: diuresis, dysuria, inhibition of ejaculation, prolonged menses, red-brown urine.
• HEMA: generalized thrombosis, thrombophlebitis.
• Other: malaise; hepatic failure; skeletal myopathy; elevated CPK, ALT (SGPT), AST (SGOT) levels.
Note: Drug should be discontinued if signs of allergy or thrombosis appear.

Overdose and treatment

Clinical manifestations of overdose may include nausea, diarrhea, delirium, thrombotic episodes, and cardiac and hepatic necrosis. Discontinue drug immediately. Animal studies have demonstrated subendocardial hemorrhagic lesions after long-term high-dose administration.

▶ Special considerations

• To prepare an I.V. infusion, use normal saline injection, 5% dextrose injection, or lactated Ringer's injection for dilution. Dilute doses up to 5 g with 250 ml of solution, doses of 5 g or greater with at least 500 ml.
• Avoid rapid I.V. infusion to minimize risk of CV adverse reactions; use infusion pump to ensure constancy of infusion.
• Monitor coagulation studies, heart rhythm, and blood pressure. Chronic use of this agent requires routine CPK determinations. Be alert for signs of phlebitis.

Information for the patient

• Tell patient to change positions slowly to minimize dizziness.
• With long-term use, tell patient that routine CPK determinations will be necessary.
• Teach patient signs and symptoms of thrombophlebitis, and advise him to report them promptly.

aminoglutethimide
Cytadren

• Pharmacologic classification: antiadrenal hormone
• Therapeutic classification: antineoplastic
• Pregnancy risk category D

How supplied

Available by prescription only
Tablets: 250 mg

Indications, route, and dosage

Dosage and indications may vary. Check current literature for recommended protocol.
Adrenal hyperplasia from ectopic ACTH-producing tumors; †medical adrenalectomy in postmenopausal metastatic breast cancer; †prostate cancer; suppression of adrenal function in Cushing's syndrome
Adults: Initiate therapy at 250 mg P.O. b.i.d. or t.i.d. for 2 weeks. Maintenance dose is 250 mg P.O. q.i.d. at 6-hour intervals. Dosage may be increased in increments of 250 mg daily q 1 to 2 weeks to a maximum total daily dose of 2 g.

Pharmacodynamics

Antineoplastic action: Aminoglutethimide interferes with the enzymatic conversion of cholesterol to delta-5-pregnenolone, effectively inhibiting the synthesis of corticosteroids, androgens, and estrogens. Therefore, by suppressing the adrenals, aminoglutethimide inhibits the growth of tumors that need estrogen to thrive.

Pharmacokinetics

• *Absorption:* Aminoglutethimide is well absorbed across the GI tract after oral administration.

• *Distribution:* Aminoglutethimide is distributed widely into body tissues.
• *Metabolism:* Aminoglutethimide is metabolized extensively in the liver.
• *Excretion:* Aminoglutethimide and its metabolites are primarily eliminated through the kidneys, mostly as unchanged drug.

Contraindications and precautions

Aminoglutethimide is contraindicated in patients with a history of hypersensitivity to the drug or to glutethimide, as cross-sensitivity may exist. Drug should be used cautiously in elderly patients because these patients may be more sensitive to the CNS adverse effects of this drug, and in those with serious infections or hypothyroidism because the drug may worsen the symptoms of these disorders.

Interactions

Concomitant use of aminoglutethimide with dexamethasone decreases the half-life and therapeutic effect of dexamethasone by increasing the metabolism of dexamethasone.

By a similar mechanism, aminoglutethimide may diminish the effects of warfarin, theophylline, digitoxin, and medroxyprogesterone.

Effects on diagnostic tests

Aminoglutethimide therapy may decrease plasma cortisol, serum thyroxine, and urinary aldosterone levels, and may increase serum alkaline phosphatase, SGOT, and thyroid-stimulating hormone concentrations.

Adverse reactions

• CNS: drowsiness, headache, dizziness, nystagmus.
• CV: hypotension, tachycardia.
• DERM: morbilliform skin rash, pruritus, urticaria.
• Endocrine: adrenal insufficiency, masculinization, hirsutism, hypothyroidism.
• GI: nausea, vomiting, anorexia, cholestatic jaundice.
• HEMA: transient leukopenia, *severe pancytopenia.*
• Other: fever, myalgia, hypothyroidism.

Overdose and treatment

Clinical manifestations of overdose include exaggerated skin rash, hypotension, nausea, and vomiting.

Treatment usually is supportive and includes induction of emesis, gastric lavage, antiemetics, and symptomatic treatment of abnormal vital signs. Aminoglutethimide is removable by dialysis.

▶ Special considerations

• Give in divided doses, two to three times per day, to reduce the incidence of nausea and vomiting.
• Most adverse effects will decrease in incidence and severity after the first 2 to 6 weeks of therapy because of accelerated metabolism of the drug with continued use.
• Some clinicians advocate routine hydrocortisone supplementation as glucocorticoid replacement (in patients with metastatic breast cancer).
• Adrenal hypofunction may develop under stressful conditions such as surgery, trauma, or acute illness. Additional steroids may be required to assure a normal response to stress.
• Aminoglutethimide therapy does not require gradually tapered withdrawal because the adrenal cortex rapidly returns to normal responsiveness following cessation of therapy.

• Up to 50% of patients will require mineralocorticoid replacement with fludrocortisone at a dosage of 0.1 mg daily or three times per week.
• Monitor blood pressure frequently.
• Perform baseline hematologic studies and monitor CBC periodically. Also monitor thyroid function studies because drug may decrease thyroid hormone production.

Information for the patient
• Emphasize importance of continuing medication despite nausea and vomiting, which usually subsides as therapy continues.
• Warn patient that drowsiness may occur. Patient should avoid hazardous activities that require alertness until sedative effect subsides. Patient usually develops tolerance within a month.
• If a skin rash develops when starting therapy, patient should call if it persists for 5 to 8 days. Therapy may be discontinued temporarily until rash clears.
• Advise patient to stand up slowly to avoid dizziness.

Geriatric use
Elderly patients are more sensitive to CNS adverse effects and are more likely to be lethargic. Safety precautions are recommended.

Pediatric use
Aminoglutethimide may induce precocious sexual development in males and masculinization in females.

Breast-feeding
It is not known whether aminoglutethimide distributes into breast milk. However, because of potential for serious adverse reactions in the infant, breast-feeding during aminoglutethimide therapy is not recommended.

PHARMACOLOGIC CLASS

aminoglycosides

amikacin sulfate
gentamicin sulfate
kanamycin sulfate
neomycin sulfate
netilmicin sulfate
streptomycin sulfate
tobramycin sulfate

Aminoglycoside antibiotics were discovered during the search for drugs to treat serious penicillin-resistant gram-negative infections. Streptomycin, derived from soil actinomycetes, was the first therapeutically useful aminoglycoside. Bacterial resistance to this prototype and adverse reactions soon led to the development of kanamycin, gentamicin, neomycin, netilmicin, tobramycin, and amikacin.

The basic structure of aminoglycosides is a hexose nucleus joined to at least two amino sugars by glycosidic linkage—hence the name aminoglycosides.

The aminoglycosides share certain pharmacokinetic properties, such as poor oral absorption, poor CNS penetration, and renal excretion, as well as serious adverse reactions and toxicity; their clinical use requires close monitoring of serum levels.

Pharmacology
Aminoglycosides are bactericidal. They bind directly and irreversibly to 30S ribosomal subunits, inhibiting bacterial protein synthesis. Bacterial resistance to aminoglycosides may be from decreased bacterial cell wall permeability, low affinity of the drug for ribosomal binding sites, or enzymatic degradation by microbial enzymes.

Aminoglycosides are active against many aerobic gram-negative organisms and some aerobic gram-positive organisms; they do not kill fungi, viruses, or anaerobic bacteria.

Gram-negative organisms susceptible to aminoglycosides include *Acinetobacter, Citrobacter, Enterobacter, Escherichia coli, Klebsiella,* indole-positive and indole-negative *Proteus, Providencia, Pseudomonas aeruginosa, Salmonella, Serratia,* and *Shigella.* Streptomycin is active against *Brucella, Calymmatobacterium granulomatis, Pasteurella multocida,* and *Yersinia pestis.*

Susceptible aerobic gram-positive organisms include *Staphylococcus aureus* and *S. epidermidis.* Streptomycin is active against *Nocardia, Erysipelothrix,* and some mycobacteria, including *Mycobacterium tuberculosis, M. marinum,* and certain strains of *M. kansasii* and *M. leprae.*

Aminoglycosides are not systemically absorbed after oral administration to patients with intact GI mucosa and, with few exceptions, are used parenterally for systemic infections; intraventricular or intrathecal administration is necessary for CNS infections. Kanamycin and neomycin are given orally for bowel sterilization.

Aminoglycosides are distributed widely throughout the body after parenteral administration; CSF concentrations are minimal even in patients with inflamed meninges. Over time, aminoglycosides accumulate in body tissue, especially the kidney and inner ear, causing drug saturation. The drug is released slowly from these tissues. Most aminoglycosides are minimally proteinbound, and are not metabolized. They don't penetrate abscesses well.

Aminoglycosides are excreted primarily in urine, chiefly by glomerular filtration; neomycin is chiefly excreted unchanged in feces when taken orally. Elimination half-life ranges between 2 and 4 hours and is prolonged in patients with decreased renal function.

Clinical indications and actions
Infection caused by susceptible organisms
Aminoglycosides are used as sole therapy for:
• infections caused by susceptible aerobic gram-negative bacilli, including septicemia; postoperative, pulmonary, intra-abdominal, and urinary tract infections; and infections of skin, soft tissue, bones, and joints
• infections from aerobic gram-negative bacillary meningitis (not susceptible to other antibiotics); because of poor CNS penetration, drugs are given intrathecally or intraventricularly (in ventriculitis).

Aminoglycosides are combined with other antibacterials in many other types of infection, including:
• serious staphylococcal infections (with an antistaphylococcal penicillin)
• serious *P. aeruginosa* infections (with such drugs as an antipseudomonal penicillin or cephalosporin)
• enterococcal infections, including endocarditis (with such drugs as penicillin G, ampicillin, or vancomycin)
• as initial empiric therapy in febrile, leukopenic compromised host (with an antipseudomonal penicillin and/ or cephalosporin)

AMINOGLYCOSIDES: RENAL FUNCTION AND HALF-LIFE

As the chart shows, the aminoglycosides, which are excreted by the kidneys, have significantly prolonged half-lives in patients with end-stage renal disease. Knowing this can help you assess the patient's potential for drug accumulation and toxicity. Nephrotoxicity, a major hazard of therapy with aminoglycosides, is clearly linked to serum concentrations that exceed the therapeutic concentrations listed in the chart below. Therefore, monitoring peak and trough levels is essential for safe use of these drugs.

DRUG AND ADMINISTRATION	HALF-LIFE		THERAPEUTIC CONCENTRATIONS (mcg/ml)	
	NORMAL RENAL FUNCTION	END-STAGE RENAL DISEASE	PEAK	TROUGH
amikacin I.M., I.V.	2 to 3 hr	30 to 86 hr	15 to 30	<5
gentamicin I.M., I.V., topical	2 to 3 hr	24 to 60 hr	4 to 10	<2
kanamycin I.M., I.V., topical	2 to 4 hr	27 to 80 hr	8 to 16	<5
neomycin oral, topical	2 to 3 hr	12 to 24 hr	Not applicable	Not applicable
netilmicin I.M., I.V.	2 to 2½ hr	18 to 30 hr	0.5 to 10	<4
streptomycin I.M., I.V.	2 to 3 hr	4 to 110 hr	5 to 25	1 to 5
tobramycin I.M., I.V., topical	2 to 3 hr	24 to 60 hr	4 to 8	<2

- serious *Klebsiella* infections (with a cephalosporin)
- nosocomial pneumonia (with a cephalosporin)
- anaerobic infections involving *Bacteroides fragilis* (with such drugs as clindamycin, metronidazole, cefoxitin, doxycycline, chloramphenicol, or ticarcillin)
- tuberculosis (concomitant use of parenteral kanamycin or streptomycin with other antitubercular agents).

Overview of adverse reactions

Systemic reactions: Ototoxicity and nephrotoxicity are the most serious complications of aminoglycoside therapy. Ototoxicity involves both vestibular and auditory functions and usually is related to persistently high serum drug levels. The number of affected sensory hair cells determines the degree of permanent dysfunction; cumulative hair cell destruction can cause permanent deafness. Elderly patients, patients taking other ototoxic drugs, and those with preexisting auditory loss are most susceptible as are patients taking other potentially ototoxic drugs. In addition, tobramycin, gentamicin, and streptomycin primarily affect vestibular function; amikacin, kanamycin, and neomycin are primarily audiotoxic. Damage is reversible only if detected early and if drug is discontinued promptly.

Any aminoglycoside may cause usually reversible nephrotoxicity; the incidence of reported reactions ranges from 2% to 10%. The damage results in tubular necrosis. Mild proteinuria and granular cylindruria are early signs of declining renal function; elevated serum creatinine levels follow several days after the decline has begun. Nephrotoxicity usually begins on the 4th to 7th day of therapy and appears to be dose-related. The best management is preventive monitoring of urinary cast excretion and serum drug levels, especially in pa-

tients at maximum risk: elderly patients, patients with hypovolemia or preexisting renal dysfunction, and patients requiring extended therapy.

Neuromuscular blockade results in skeletal weakness and respiratory distress similar to that seen with the use of neuromuscular blocking agents like tubocurarine and succinylcholine. It is most likely to occur in patients receiving those blocking agents; in patients with preexisting neuromuscular disease such as myasthenia gravis; in patients receiving general anesthetics; and in patients with hypocalcemia.

Oral aminoglycoside therapy most often causes nausea, vomiting, and diarrhea. Less common adverse reactions include hypersensitivity reactions (ranging from mild rashes, fever, and eosinophilia to *fatal anaphylaxis*); hematologic reactions include hemolytic anemia, transient neutropenia, leukopenia, and thrombocytopenia. Transient elevations of liver function values also occur.

Local reactions: Parenterally administered forms of aminoglycosides may cause vein irritation, phlebitis, and sterile abscess.

▶ Special considerations

- Assess patient's allergic history; do not give an aminoglycoside to a patient with a history of hypersensitivity reactions to any aminoglycoside; monitor patient continuously for this and other adverse reactions.
- Obtain results of culture and sensitivity tests before first dose; however, therapy may begin before tests are completed. Repeat tests periodically to assess drug efficacy.
- Monitor vital signs, electrolyte levels, and renal function studies before and during therapy; be sure patient

is well hydrated to minimize chemical irritation of renal tubules; watch for signs of declining renal function.

● Keep peak serum levels and trough serum levels at recommended concentrations, especially in patients with decreased renal function. Draw blood for peak level 1 hour after I.M. injection (30 minutes to 1 hour after I.V. infusion); for trough level, draw sample just before the next dose. Time and date all blood samples. Do not use heparinized tube to collect blood samples; it interferes with results.

● Evaluate patient's hearing before and during therapy; monitor for complaints of tinnitus, vertigo, or hearing loss.

● Avoid concomitant use of aminoglycosides with other ototoxic or nephrotoxic drugs.

● Usual duration of therapy is 7 to 10 days; if no response occurs in 3 to 5 days, drug should be discontinued and cultures repeated for reevaluation of therapy.

● Closely monitor patients on long-term therapy—especially elderly and debilitated patients and others receiving immunosuppressant or radiation therapy—for possible bacterial or fungal superinfection; monitor especially for fever.

● Do not add or mix other drugs with I.V. infusions—particularly penicillins, which will inactivate aminoglycosides; the two groups are chemically and physically incompatible. If other drugs must be given I.V., temporarily stop infusion of primary drug.

● Oral aminoglycoside may be absorbed systemically in patients with ulcerative GI lesions; significant absorption may endanger patients with decreased renal function.

Oral and parenteral administration
● Consult manufacturer's directions for reconstitution, dilution, and storage of drugs; check expiration dates.
● Shake oral suspensions well before administering, to assure correct dosage.
● Administer I.M. dose deep into large muscle mass (gluteal or midlateral thigh); rotate injection sites to minimize tissue injury; do not inject more than 2 g of drug per injection site. Apply ice to injection site for pain.
● Too-rapid I.V. administration may cause neuromuscular blockade. Infuse I.V. drug continuously or intermittently over 30 to 60 minutes for adults, 1 to 2 hours for infants; dilution volume for children is determined individually.
● Solutions should always be clear, colorless to pale yellow (in most cases, darkening indicates deterioration), and free of particles; do not give solutions containing precipitates or other foreign matter.
● Amikacin, gentamicin (without preservatives), kanamycin, and tobramycin have been administered intrathecally or intraventricularly. Many clinicians prefer intraventricular administration to ensure adequate CSF levels in the treatment of ventriculitis.

Information for the patient
● Teach signs and symptoms of hypersensitivity and other adverse reactions to aminoglycosides; urge patient to report *any* unusual effects promptly.
● Teach signs and symptoms of bacterial or fungal superinfection to elderly and debilitated patients and others with low resistance from immunosuppressants or irradiation; emphasize need to report them promptly.
● Be sure patient understands how and when to take drug; urge patient to complete entire prescribed regimen, to comply with instructions for around-the-clock dosage, and to keep follow-up appointments.

Geriatric use
Elderly patients often have decreased renal function and, thus, are at greater risk for nephrotoxicity; they often require lower drug dosage and longer dosing intervals. They are also susceptible to ototoxicity and superinfection.

Pediatric use
The half-life of aminoglycosides is prolonged in neonates and premature infants because of immaturity of their renal systems; dosage alterations may be necessary in infants and children.

Breast-feeding
Small amounts of aminoglycosides are excreted in breast milk; safety has not been established in breast-feeding women. An alternative feeding method is recommended during therapy.

Representative combinations
Neomycin with polymyxin B sulfates and bacitracin: Neosporin, Mycitracin, Foille, Neo-Polycin; with polymyxin B sulfates and gramicidin: Neosporin; with polymyxin B sulfates and hydrocortisone: Corticosporin, Drotic, Octicair, Ortega Otic-M, Otocart, Otoreid-HC; with dexamethasone sodium phosphate: Neo-decadron; with flurandrenolide: Cordron-N.

See also adrenocorticoids, topical.

---

aminophylline
Amoline, Phyllocontin, Somophylline, Truphylline

● Pharmacologic classification: xanthine derivative
● Therapeutic classification: bronchodilator
● Pregnancy risk category C

How supplied
Available by prescription only
Tablets: 100 mg, 200 mg
Tablets (controlled-release): 225 mg
Liquid: 105 mg/5 ml
Injection: 250-mg, 500-mg vials and ampules
Rectal suppositories: 250 mg, 500 mg
Rectal solution: 300 mg/5 ml

Indications, route and dosage
Symptomatic relief of bronchospasm
Patients not currently receiving theophylline who require rapid relief of symptoms: Loading dose is 6 mg/kg (equivalent to 4.7 mg/kg anhydrous theophylline) I.V. slowly (less than or equal to 25 mg/minute), then maintenance infusion.
Adults (nonsmokers): 0.7 mg/kg/hour for 12 hours; then 0.5 mg/kg/hour.
Otherwise healthy adult smokers: 1 mg/kg/hour for 12 hours; then 0.8 mg/kg/hour.
Older patients; adults with cor pulmonale: 0.6 mg/kg/hour for 12 hours; then 0.3 mg/kg/hour.
Adults with congestive heart failure (CHF) or liver disease: 0.5 mg/kg/hour for 12 hours; then 0.1 to 0.2 mg/kg/hour.
Children age 9 to 16: 1 mg/kg/hour for 12 hours; then 0.8 mg/kg/hour.

Children age 6 months to 9 years: 1.2 mg/kg/hour for 12 hours; then 1 mg/kg/hour.

Patients currently receiving theophylline: Aminophylline infusions of 0.63 mg/kg (0.5 mg/kg anhydrous theophylline) will increase plasma levels of theophylline by 1 mcg/ml. Some clinicians recommend a loading dose of 3.1 mg/kg (2.5 mg/kg anhydrous theophylline) if no obvious signs of theophylline toxicity are present.

Chronic bronchial asthma

Adults: 600 to 1600 mg P.O. daily divided t.i.d. or q.i.d.
Children: 12 mg/kg P.O. daily divided t.i.d. or q.i.d.

Monitor serum levels to ensure that theophylline concentrations range from 10 to 20 mcg/ml. However, some patients may respond with adequate bronchodilation at 5 to 10 mcg/ml.

†Adjunctive treatment of neonatal apnea

Loading dose 3 to 6 mg/kg I.V. over at least 20 minutes, followed by maintenance dose of 1 to 2 mg/kg q 8 or 12 hours P.O. or I.V. Alternatively, maintenance dose of 7 to 12 mg/kg/day divided q 6 hours or q 12 hours. Peak serum concentrations should be 6 to 15 mcg/ml.

Pharmacodynamics

Bronchodilating action: Aminophylline acts at the cellular level after it is converted to theophylline. (Aminophylline [theophylline ethylenediamine] is 79% theophylline). Theophylline acts by either inhibiting phosphodiesterase or blocking adenosine receptors in the bronchi, resulting in relaxation of the smooth muscle. The drug also stimulates the respiratory center in the medulla and prevents diaphragmatic fatigue.

Pharmacokinetics

● *Absorption:* Most dosage forms are absorbed well; absorption of the suppository, however, is unreliable and slow. The rate and onset of action also depend upon the dosage form selected. Food may alter the rate, but not the extent of absorption, of oral doses.
● *Distribution:* Aminophylline is distributed in all tissues and extracellular fluids except fatty tissue.
● *Metabolism:* Aminophylline is converted to theophylline, then metabolized to inactive compounds.
● *Excretion:* Aminophylline is excreted in the urine as theophylline (10%).

Contraindications and precautions

Aminophylline is contraindicated in patients with hypersensitivity to xanthines or ethylenediamine. It should be used cautiously in patients with compromised cardiac or circulatory function, diabetes, glaucoma, hypertension, hyperthyroidism, peptic ulcer, or gastroesophageal reflux, because drug may worsen these conditions.

Interactions

Aminophylline increases the excretion of lithium. Concomitant cimetidine, allopurinol (high dose), propranolol, erythromycin, or troleandomycin may increase serum concentration of aminophylline by decreasing hepatic clearance. Phenobarbital, tobacco, marijuana, and aminoglutethimide decrease effects of aminophylline. Alkali-sensitive drugs reduce activity of aminophylline. Do not add these drugs to I.V. fluids containing aminophylline.

Effects on diagnostic tests

Aminophylline may alter the assay for uric acid, depending on method used, and increases plasma-free fatty acids and urinary catecholamines. Theophylline

levels are falsely elevated in the presence of furosemide, phenylbutazone, probenecid, theobromine, caffeine, tea, chocolate, cola beverages, and acetaminophen, depending on type of assay used.

Adverse reactions

● CNS: irritability, restlessness, headache, insomnia, dizziness, convulsions, depression, light-headedness, muscle twitching.
● CV: palpitations, marked flushing, hypotension, sinus tachycardia, *ventricular tachycardia* and other life-threatening arrhythmias, extrasystoles, *circulatory failure.*
● DERM: urticaria.
● GI: nausea, vomiting, epigastric pain, discomfort, dyspepsia, bitter aftertaste, loss of appetite, diarrhea.
● Respiratory: tachypnea, *respiratory arrest.*
● Local: rectal irritation from suppositories.
● Other: fever, urinary retention, hyperglycemia.
  Note: Drug should be discontinued if an adverse reaction intensifies; this signals impending overdose.

Overdose and treatment

Clinical manifestations of overdose include nausea, vomiting, insomnia, irritability, tachycardia, extrasystoles, tachypnea, and tonic/clonic seizures. Onset of toxicity may be sudden and severe; arrhythmias and seizures are the first signs. Induce emesis, except in convulsing patients, then use activated charcoal and cathartics. Charcoal hemoperfusion may be beneficial. Treat arrhythmias with lidocaine and seizures with I.V. benzodiazepine; support respiratory and cardiovascular systems.

▶ Special considerations

● Before giving loading dose, check that patient has not had recent theophylline therapy.
● Do not combine in fluids for I.V. infusion with the following: ascorbic acid, chlorpromazine, codeine phosphate, dimenhydrinate, epinephrine, erythromycine gluceptate, hydralazine, insulin, levorphanol tartrate, meperidine, methadone, methicillin, morphine sulfate, norepinephrine bitartrate, oxytetracycline, penicillin G potassium, phenobarbital, phenytoin, prochlorperazine, promazine, promethazine, tetracycline, vancomycin, vitamin B complex with C.
● Do not crush controlled-release tablets.
● I.V. drug administration includes I.V. push at a very slow rate or an infusion with 100 to 200 ml of dextrose 5% or 0.9% sodium chloride.
● GI symptoms may be relieved by taking oral drug with full glass of water at meals, although food in stomach delays absorption. Enteric-coated tablets may also delay absorption. There is no evidence that antacids reduce GI adverse reactions.
● Suppositories are slowly and erractically absorbed; retention enemas may be absorbed more rapidly. Rectally administered preparations can be given when patient cannot take drug orally. Schedule after evacuation, if possible; may be retained better if given before meal. Advise patient to remain recumbent 15 to 20 minutes after insertion.
● Individuals metabolize xanthines at different rates. Adjust dose by monitoring response, tolerance, pulmonary function, and theophylline blood levels. Therapeutic level is 10 to 20 mcg/ml, but some patients may respond at lower levels; toxicity occurs at levels over 20 mcg/ml.
● Plasma clearance may be decreased in patients with

CHF, hepatic dysfunction, or pulmonary edema. Smokers show accelerated clearance. Dose adjustments necessary.

Information for the patient
• Teach patient rationale for therapy and importance of compliance with prescribed regimen; if a dose is missed, patient should take it as soon as possible, but not double up on doses. Advise patient to avoid taking extra "breathing pills".
• Advise the patient of the adverse effects and possible signs of toxicity.
• Tell patient not to eat or drink large quantities of xanthine-containing foods and beverages.
• Warn that nonprescription remedies may contain ephedrine in combination with theophylline salts; excessive CNS stimulation may result. Tell patient to seek medical approval before taking *any* other medications.

Geriatric use
Use reduced doses, and monitor the patient closely. Warn elderly patients of dizziness, a common adverse reaction at start of therapy.

Pediatric use
Drug is not recommended for use in infants younger than age 6 months.

Breast-feeding
Drug is excreted in breast milk and may cause irritability, insomnia, or fretfulness in the breast-fed infant.

PHARMACOLOGIC CLASS

aminoquinolines

chloroquine hydrochloride
chloroquine phosphate
hydroxychloroquine sulfate
primaquine phosphate

The 4-aminoquinolines and 8-aminoquinolines were developed during World War II after an intensive search for more potent, less toxic antimalarial agents than those compounds previously used. After testing of hundreds of compounds, the 4-aminoquinolines, chloroquine and hydroxychloroquine, and the 8-aminoquinoline, primaquine, have emerged as the most effective and the least likely to cause adverse effects.

Pharmacology
The aminoquinolines are synthetic antimalarial agents. Although their precise mechanism of action is unknown, the 4-aminoquinolines appear to exert their effects by intercalation into DNA and therefore ultimately by interfering with RNA and protein synthesis in susceptible organisms; they inhibit DNA and RNA polymerases. The 4-aminoquinolines also appear to concentrate in parasites' digestive vacuoles, disrupting their function and resulting in increased pH levels. The 8-aminoquinoline, primaquine, acts primarily through disruption of parasitic mitochondria. These differing mechanisms explain the different antimalarial properties of these two subclasses of aminoquinolines.

Also, the 4-aminoquinolines have an anti-inflammatory effect, which may result from antagonism of histamine, serotonin, or prostaglandin or from inhibition of chemotaxis by various white blood cell types.

Chloroquine acts as an amebicide through an unknown mechanism.

Clinical indications and actions
Malaria
Chloroquine phosphate and hydroxychloroquine sulfate do not prevent infection; they are used to suppress and treat acute attacks of malaria caused by *Plasmodium vivax, P. malariae, P. ovale,* and susceptible strains of *P. falciparum.* Chloroquine hydrochloride is used when parenteral therapy is required.

Primaquine is used with either chloroquine or hydroxychloroquine for the radical cure of *P. vivax* or *P. ovale.* Primaquine is indicated for returning travelers who were exposed to malaria in areas where *P. vivax* and *P. ovale* are endemic.

Inflammation
Hydroxychloroquine is indicated in rheumatoid arthritis resistant to salicylates and other nonsteroidal anti-inflammatory drugs (NSAIDs). The NSAIDs may be continued during treatment with hydroxychloroquine. Hydroxychloroquine also is indicated in discoid or systemic lupus erythematosus that is treated concomitantly with topical or systemic corticosteroids and/or salicylates.

Amebiasis
Chloroquine is used to treat extraintestinal amebiasis caused by *Entamoeba histolytica;* it is often used with other amebicides to treat hepatic abscess caused by this organism.

Overview of adverse reactions
Therapeutic dosage of the aminoquinolines may cause GI distress and headache. Long-term therapy with these agents may cause reversible and irreversible ophthalmologic changes, or muscle weakness. Serious hematologic changes may occur, particularly in patients with G6PD deficiency or NADH methemoglobin reductase deficiency. Chloroquine may cause an irreversible cardiomyopathy that is histologically distinct. CNS changes and cardiovascular or respiratory depression may indicate overdose.

▶ Special considerations
• Give drug immediately before or after meals to minimize GI side effects.
• Obtain a baseline ECG, blood counts, and an ophthalmologic examination, and check periodically for changes.
• Monitor patient for signs of cumulative effects, such as blurred vision, increased sensitivity to light, muscle weakness, impaired hearing, tinnitus, fever, sore throat, unusual bleeding or bruising, unusual pigmentation of the oral mucous membranes, and jaundice. Maximal effects may not occur for 6 months.
• Muscle weakness and alterations of deep tendon reflexes may require discontinuing the drug.

Information for the patient
• Tell patient to report any visual or hearing changes, muscle weakness, or darkening of urine immediately.
• Tell patient to take these drugs after meals to help prevent GI distress and to report any pronounced GI distress. Recommend that the patient separate use of magnesium or kaolin compounds from drug by at least 4 hours.
• Advise patient to wear sunglasses in bright light or sunlight to reduce risk of ocular damage, and to avoid prolonged exposure to sunlight to avoid exacerbation of drug-induced dermatoses.

- Counsel patient to complete the entire prescribed course of therapy.
- Instruct patient about the need for follow-up blood tests and examinations.
- Warn patient to keep drugs out of the reach of children.

Pediatric use
Children are especially susceptible to overdose with aminoquinolines and should not receive long-term therapy.

Breast-feeding
Aminoquinolines are excreted in breast milk and should be used with caution in breast-feeding women.

Representative combinations
None.

---

amiodarone hydrochloride
Cordarone

- Pharmacologic classification: benzofuran derivative
- Therapeutic classification: ventricular and supraventricular antiarrhythmic
- Pregnancy risk category C

How supplied
Available by prescription only
Tablets: 100 mg*, 200 mg

Indications, route, and dosage
Ventricular and †supraventricular arrhythmias (†recurrent supraventricular tachycardia, atrial fibrillation and flutter, †ventricular tachycardia)
Adults: Loading dose of 800 to 1,600 mg P.O. daily for 1 to 3 weeks until initial therapeutic response occurs. Maintenance dosage is 200 to 600 mg P.O. daily. Alternatively, loading dose is 5 to 10 mg/kg by I.V. infusion via central line, followed by I.V. infusion of 10 mg/kg/day for 3 to 5 days.
Note: Intravenous use of amiodarone is investigational.
Children: 10 mg/kg P.O. per day or 800 mg/1.73 m² P.O. per day for 10 days or until response is seen. Then 5 mg/kg or 400 mg/1.73 m²; usual maintenance dose is 2.5 mg/kg or 200 mg/1.73 m² per day.

Pharmacodynamics
Ventricular antiarrhythmic action: Although it has mixed Class Ic and Class III antiarrhythmic effects, amiodarone generally is considered a Class III agent. It widens the action potential duration (repolarization inhibition). With prolonged therapy, the effective refractory period (ERP) increases in the atria, ventricles, AV node, His-Purkinje system, and bypass tracts and conduction slows in the atria, AV node, His-Purkinje system, and ventricles; sinus node automaticity decreases. Amiodarone also noncompetitively blocks beta-adrenergic receptors. Clinically, it has little, if any, negative inotropic effect. Coronary and peripheral vasodilator effects may occur with long-term therapy. Amiodarone is among the most effective antiarrhythmic agents, but its therapeutic applications are somewhat limited by its severe adverse reactions.

Pharmacokinetics
- *Absorption:* Amiodarone has slow, variable absorption. Bioavailability is approximately 22% to 86%. Peak plasma levels occur 3 to 7 hours after oral administration; however, onset of action may be delayed from 2 to 3 days to 2 to 3 months—even with loading doses.
- *Distribution:* Amiodarone is distributed widely because it accumulates in adipose tissue and in organs with marked perfusion, such as the lungs, liver, and spleen. It is also highly protein-bound (96%). The therapeutic serum level is not well-defined but probably ranges from 1 to 2.5 mcg/ml.
- *Metabolism:* Amiodarone is metabolized extensively in the liver to a pharmacologically active metabolite, desethyl amiodarone.
- *Excretion:* Amiodarone's main excretory route is hepatic, through the biliary tree (with enterohepatic recirculation). Because no renal excretion occurs, patients with impaired renal function do not require dosage reduction. Terminal elimination half-life—25 to 110 days—is the longest of any antiarrhythmic; in most patients, half-life ranges from 40 to 50 days.

Contraindications and precautions
Amiodarone is contraindicated in patients with preexisting sinus-node dysfunction and bradycardia causing syncope or second- or third-degree heart block (except if patient has artificial pacemaker), because of its potent effects on the AV conduction system. It should be used with caution in patients with CHF because of the potential for adverse hemodynamic effects; in patients with liver disease because metabolism may be reduced; and in patients with hypokalemia, because drug may be ineffective.

Interactions
Concomitant use of amiodarone with quinidine, disopyramide, tricyclic antidepressants, or phenothiazines may cause additive effects that lead to a prolonged QT interval, possibly resulting in torsades de pointes ventricular tachycardia.

Concomitant use with warfarin may cause prolonged prothrombin time, as a result of enhanced drug displacement from protein-binding sites. Concomitant use with digoxin, quinidine, phenytoin, or procainamide may lead to increased serum levels of these drugs, resulting in enhanced effects.

Effects on diagnostic tests
Amiodarone alters thyroid function test results, causing increased serum thyroxine (T_4) and decreased triiodothyronine (T_3) levels. (However, most patients maintain normal thyroid function during therapy.)

Adverse reactions
- CNS: peripheral neuropathy and extrapyramidal symptoms, headache, malaise, fatigue.
- CV: bradycardia, hypotension, *arrhythmia*.
- DERM: photosensitivity, blue-gray pigmentation.
- EENT: corneal microdeposits, visual disturbances.
- Endocrine: hypothyroidism and hyperthyroidism.
- GI: nausea, vomiting, constipation.
- Hepatic: altered liver enzyme levels, hepatic dysfunction.
- Metabolic: electrolyte disturbances.

- Respiratory: *severe pulmonary toxicity* (pneumonitis, alveolitis) with high doses, *pulmonary fibrosis*.
- Other: muscle weakness.
  Note: Drug should be discontinued if signs or symptoms of pulmonary toxicity or epididymitis occur.

Overdose and treatment
Clinical effects of overdose include bradyarrhythmias. Treatment may involve beta-adrenergic agonists (such as isoproterenol) or artificial pacing to help restore an acceptable heart rate. To treat hypotension, positive inotropic agents (such as dopamine or dobutamine) or vasopressors (such as epinephrine or norepinephrine) may be administered. General supportive measures should be used, as necessary. Amiodarone cannot be removed by dialysis.

▶ Special considerations
- Amiodarone has proved effective in treating arrhythmias resistant to other drug therapy. However, high incidence of adverse effects limits drug's use.
- Divide loading dose into three equal doses, and give with meals to minimize GI intolerance. Maintenance dose may be given once daily but may be divided into two doses taken with meals if GI intolerance occurs.
- Monitor blood pressure and heart rate and rhythm frequently for significant change.
- Periodically monitor hepatic and thyroid function tests. Perform periodic ophthalmologic evaluations to assess corneal microdeposits.
- Monitor for signs and symptoms of pneumonitis, such as exertional dyspnea, nonproductive cough, and pleuritic chest pain. Also check pulmonary function tests and chest X-ray. (Pulmonary toxicity is more common with daily doses exceeding 600 mg.) Pulmonary complications require discontinuation of amiodarone and possibly, treatment with corticosteroids.
- Digoxin, quinidine, phenytoin, and procainamide doses should be decreased during amiodarone therapy to avoid toxicity.
- Adverse effects are more prevalent with high doses but usually resolve within about 4 months after drug therapy stops.

Information for the patient
- Advise patient to use sunscreen lotion to prevent photosensitivity, which may result in sunburn and blistering.
- Although corneal microdeposits typically appear 1 to 4 months after therapy begins, only 2% to 3% of patients have actual visual disturbances. To minimize this complication, recommend frequent instillation of methylcellulose ophthalmic solution.

Geriatric use
Drug should be used with caution in elderly patients because they may experience ataxia.

Pediatric use
Children receiving amiodarone concomitantly with digoxin may experience more acute effects of interaction. Children may experience faster onset of action and shorter duration of effect than adults.

Breast-feeding
Amiodarone is excreted in breast milk and should not be used in breast-feeding women.

amitriptyline hydrochloride
Amitril*, Amitriptylene, Elavil, Emitrip, Endep, Enovil, Levate*, Mevaril*, Novotriptyn*, SK-Amitriptyline

- Pharmacologic classification: tricyclic antidepressant
- Therapeutic classification: antidepressant
- Pregnancy risk category D

How supplied
Available by prescription only
Tablets: 10 mg, 25 mg, 50 mg, 75 mg, 100 mg, 150 mg
Injection: 10 mg/ml

Indications, route, and dosage
Depression; †anorexia or bulimia associated with depression
Adults: 50 to 100 mg P.O. daily, divided t.i.d. or may be given h.s. Increase to 200 mg daily (average adult dose); maximum dosage is 300 mg daily if needed; or 20 to 30 mg I.M. t.i.d. Alternatively, the entire dosage can be given at bedtime.
Elderly patients and adolescents: 30 mg P.O. daily in divided doses; may be increased to 150 mg.
Parenteral therapy should be changed to oral route as soon as possible.

†Adjunctive treatment of neurogenic pain
Adults: Initially, 25 mg b.i.d. or q.i.d. Increase dosage as needed and tolerated up to 300 mg/day.

Pharmacodynamics
Antidepressant action: Amitriptyline is thought to exert its antidepressant effects by inhibiting reuptake of norepinephrine and serotonin in CNS nerve terminals (presynaptic neurons), resulting in increased concentrations and enhanced activity of these neurotransmitters in the synaptic cleft. Amitriptyline more actively inhibits reuptake of serotonin than norepinephrine; it carries a high incidence of undesirable sedation, but tolerance to this effect usually develops within a few weeks.

Pharmacokinetics
- *Absorption:* Amitriptyline is absorbed rapidly from the GI tract after oral administration and from muscle tissue after I.M. administration.
- *Distribution:* Amitriptyline is distributed widely into the body, including the CNS and breast milk. Drug is 96% protein-bound. Peak effect occurs 2 to 12 hours after a given dose, and steady state is achieved within 4 to 10 days; full therapeutic effect usually occurs in 2 to 4 weeks.
- *Metabolism:* Amitriptyline is metabolized by the liver to the active metabolite nortriptyline; a significant first-pass effect may account for variability of serum concentrations in different patients taking the same dosage.
- *Excretion:* Most of drug is excreted in urine.

Contraindications and precautions
Amitriptyline is contraindicated in patients with known hypersensitivity to tricyclic antidepressants, trazodone, and related compounds; in the acute recovery phase of myocardial infarction because of its arrhythmogenic potential; in patients in coma or with severe respiratory depression because of additive depressant effects on

---

CNS; and during or within 14 days of therapy with mono-amine oxidase inhibitors.

Amitriptyline should be used with caution in patients with other cardiac disease (arrhythmias, congestive heart failure [CHF], angina pectoris, valvular disease, or heart block); respiratory disorders; alcoholism, epilepsy and other seizure disorders; scheduled electro-convulsive therapy (ECT); bipolar disease; glaucoma; hyperthyroidism, or in those taking thyroid replacement; Type I and Type II diabetes; prostatic hypertrophy, paralytic ileus, or urinary retention; hepatic or renal dysfunction; Parkinson's disease; and in those under-going surgery with general anesthesia.

Interactions
Concomitant use of amitriptyline with sympathomimetics, including epinephrine, phenylephrine, phenylpropanolamine, and ephedrine (often found in nasal sprays) may increase blood pressure; use with warfarin may increase prothrombin time and cause bleeding.

Concomitant use with thyroid hormones, pimozide, or antiarrhythmic agents (quinidine, disopyramide, procainamide) may increase incidence of cardiac dys-rhythmias and conduction defects.

Amitriptyline may decrease hypotensive effects of centrally acting antihypertensive drugs, such as guanethidine, guanabenz, guanadrel, clonidine, methyldopa, and reserpine. Concomitant use with disulfiram or ethchlorvynol may cause delirium and tachycardia.

Additive effects are likely after concomitant use of amitriptyline with CNS depressants, including alcohol, analgesics, barbiturates, narcotics, tranquilizers, and anesthetics (oversedation); atropine or other anticho-linergic drugs, including phenothiazines, antihistamines, meperidine, and antiparkinsonian agents (oversedation, paralytic ileus, visual changes, and severe constipation); or metrizamide (increased risk of convulsions).

Barbiturates and heavy smoking induce amitriptyline metabolism and decrease therapeutic efficacy; phenothiazines and haloperidol decrease its metabolism, decreasing therapeutic efficacy; methylphenidate, cimetidine, oral contraceptives, propoxyphene, and beta blockers may inhibit amitriptyline metabolism, increasing plasma levels and toxicity.

Effects on diagnostic tests
Amitriptyline may prolong conduction time (elongation of Q-T and PR intervals, flattened T waves on ECG); it also may elevate liver function test results, decrease white blood cell counts, and decrease or increase serum glucose levels.

Adverse reactions
● CNS: drowsiness, dizziness, sedation, excitation, tremors, weakness, headache, nervousness, *seizures*, peripheral neuropathy, extrapyramidal symptoms, anxiety, vivid dreams, decreased libido, confusion (more marked in elderly patients).
● CV: orthostatic hypotension, tachycardia, *arrhythmias, MI, stroke, heart block, CHF*, palpitations, hypertension, ECG changes.
● EENT: blurred vision, tinnitus, mydriasis, increased intraocular pressure.
● GI: dry mouth, constipation, abdominal cramping, nausea, vomiting, anorexia, diarrhea, paralytic ileus, jaundice.
● GU: urine retention.

● Other: sweating, photosensitivity, hypersensitivity (rash, urticaria, drug fever, edema).

After abrupt withdrawal of long-term therapy, nausea, headache, malaise (does not indicate addiction) may occur.

Note: Drug should be discontinued (not abruptly) if signs of hypersensitivity occur. Reevaluate therapy if the following signs and symptoms occur: urine retention, extreme dry mouth, rash, excessive sedation, seizures, tachycardia, sore throat, fever, or jaundice.

Overdose and treatment
The first 12 hours after acute ingestion are a stimulatory phase characterized by excessive anticholinergic activity (agitation, irritation, confusion, hallucinations, hyperthermia, parkinsonian symptoms, seizure, urine retention, dry mucous membranes, pupillary dilatation, constipation, and ileus). This is followed by CNS depressant effects, including hypothermia, decreased or absent reflexes, sedation, hypotension, cyanosis, and cardiac irregularities, including tachycardia, conduction disturbances, and quinidine-like effects on the ECG.

Severity of overdose is best indicated by widening of the QRS complex and usually represents a serum level in excess of 1,000 mg/ml; metabolic acidosis may follow hypotension, hypoventilation, and convulsions. Delayed cardiac anomalies and death may occur.

Treatment is symptomatic and supportive, including maintaining airway, stable body temperature, and fluid and electrolyte balance. Induce emesis with ipecac if gag reflex is intact; follow with gastric lavage and activated charcoal to prevent further absorption. Dialysis is of little use. Treatment of seizures may include parenteral diazepam or phenytoin; treatment of arrhythmias, parenteral phenytoin or lidocaine; and treatment of acidosis, sodium bicarbonate. *Do not give barbiturates;* these may enhance CNS and respiratory depressant effects.

▶ Special considerations
Besides those relevant to all *tricyclic antidepressants,* consider the following recommendations.
● Amitriptyline also may be used to prevent migraine and cluster headaches, intractable hiccups and post-herpetic neuralgia.
● Amitriptyline causes a high incidence of sedative effect. Tolerance to sedative effects usually develops over several weeks but may never occur.
● The full dose may be given at bedtime to help offset daytime sedation.
● The oral administration route should be substituted for the parenteral route as soon as possible.
● Intramuscular administration may result in a more rapid onset of action than oral administration.
● The drug should not be withdrawn abruptly.
● The drug should be discontinued at least 48 hours before surgical procedures.
● Chewing gum, sugarless hard candy, or ice may alleviate dry mouth. Stress the importance of regular dental hygiene, as dry mouth can increase the incidence of dental caries.

Information for the patient
● Tell patient to take amitriptyline exactly as prescribed and not to double dose for missed ones.
● The full dose may be taken at bedtime to alleviate daytime sedation. Alternatively, it may be taken in the early evening to avoid morning "hangover."

---

*Canada only   †Unlabeled clinical use   Italicized adverse reactions are life-threatening.

- Explain that full effects of the drug may not become apparent for up to 4 weeks after initiation of therapy.
- Warn that drug may cause drowsiness or dizziness. Patient should avoid hazardous activities that require alertness until the full effects of the drug are known.
- Warn patient not to drink alcoholic beverages while taking this drug.
- Suggest taking drug with food or milk if it causes stomach upset and chewing gum or sucking hard candy to relieve dry mouth.
- After initial doses, patient should lie down for about 30 minutes and rise to upright position slowly to prevent dizziness or fainting.
- Warn patient not to stop taking drug suddenly.
- Encourage patient to report troublesome or unusual effects, especially confusion, movement disorders, rapid heartbeat, dizziness, fainting, or difficulty urinating.
- Tell patient to store drug safely away from children.

Geriatric use
Elderly patients may be at greater risk for adverse cardiac effects.

Pediatric use
Drug is not recommended for children under age 12.

Breast-feeding
Amitriptyline is excreted in breast milk in concentrations equal to or greater than those in maternal serum. Approximately 1% of the ingested dose appears in the breast-feeding infant's serum. The potential benefit to the mother should outweigh the possible adverse reactions in the infant.

ammonium chloride

- Pharmacologic classification: acid-forming salt
- Therapeutic classification: acidifying agent, expectorant
- Pregnancy risk category C

How supplied
Available with or without prescription
Tablets: 500 mg
Tablets (enteric coated): 500 mg, 1,000 mg
Injection: 2.14% (0.4 mEq/ml), 26.75% (5 mEq/ml)

Indications, route, and dosage
Metabolic alkalosis
Adults and children: Dosage is calculated by amount of chloride deficit. Infusion rate is 0.9 to 1.3 ml/minute of 2.14% solution; do not exceed 2 ml/minute. Hypodermoclysis has been used in infants and young children. One-half the calculated volume should be given, then patient should be reassessed.
As acidifying agent and diuretic
Adults: 4 to 12 g P.O. daily in divided doses every 4 to 6 hours.
Children: 75 mg/kg daily P.O. in four divided doses.
As expectorant
Adults: 250 to 500 mg P.O. q 2 to 4 hours.

Pharmacodynamics
- *Acidifying action:* Ammonium chloride increases acidity by increasing free hydrogen ion (H^+) concentration.
- *Expectorant action:* Ammonium chloride acts as an expectorant by irritating the mucosa, causing reflex stimulation of bronchial mucosal glands.

Pharmacokinetics
- *Absorption:* Ammonium chloride is absorbed rapidly from the GI tract; absorption is complete in 3 to 6 hours.
- *Distribution:* Unknown.
- *Metabolism:* Ammonium chloride is metabolized in the liver to urea and hydrochloric acid.
- *Excretion:* Ammonium chloride is excreted in urine.

Contraindications and precautions
Ammonium chloride is contraindicated in patients with severe hepatic dysfunction (cirrhosis or hepatitis), because of the hazard of drug retention and subsequent ammonia intoxication and hepatic coma; and in patients with primary acidosis and high carbon dioxide and buffer base, because of the potential for severe acidosis.

Ammonium chloride should not be used as the sole therapy for metabolic alkalosis in patients with severe renal dysfunction in whom metabolic alkalosis has followed marked sodium loss from vomiting, because sodium depletion will not be corrected. It should be used with caution in patients with pulmonary insufficiency or cardiac edema because of potential for severe acid-base disturbances.

Interactions
Concomitant use with spironolactone or carbonic anhydrase inhibitors increases risk of systemic acidosis. Ammonium chloride is incompatible with milk or other alkaline solutions.

Effects on diagnostic tests
None reported.

Adverse reactions
- CNS: headache, confusion, progressive drowsiness, excitement alternating with *coma*, hyperventilation, muscle twitching, asterixis, hyperreflexia, EEG abnormalities.
- CV: bradycardia, *arrhythmias.*
- DERM: rash, pallor.
- GI: (with oral dose) gastric irritation, nausea, vomiting, thirst, anorexia, diarrhea.
- GU: glycosuria, diuresis.
- Metabolic: hyperchloremia, hypokalemia, hyperglycemia, hypercalciuria, hypocalcemia, tetany, hyponatremia, hypomagnesemia.
- Respiratory: *irregular respirations* with periods of apnea.
- Local: pain at injection site.
  Note: Adverse reactions usually result from ammonia toxicity or too-rapid I.V. administration. Such reactions may include hyperammonemia, vomiting, pallor, sweating, irregular breathing, bradycardia, asterixis, hyperreflexia, tonic convulsions, and coma.

Overdose and treatment
Symptoms of overdose include muscle twitching, tonic convulsions, progressive drowsiness, mental confusion, pallor, sweating, irregular breathing, bradycardia, cardiac arrhythmias, and coma. Treat acidosis with I.V. sodium bicarbonate (or sodium lactate or acetate).

▶ **Special considerations**

● Do not give injectable ammonium chloride intraperitoneally, subcutaneously, or rectally.

● Concentrated solutions of ammonium chloride crystallize when exposed to low temperatures; dissolve crystals by warming solution in a water bath before use. Dilute concentrated solutions by adding 20 to 40 ml of 26.75% solution or 500 to 1,000 ml of normal saline solution.

● Decrease infusion rate to allow ammonium ion metabolism by the liver and reduce the pain of I.V. injection.

● Determine CO_2-combining power and serum electrolyte levels before and during therapy to prevent acidosis.

● Monitor urine pH levels and output; diuresis for the first 2 days is normal.

● May cause metabolic acidosis if used continuously for more than 3 to 4 days, especially in patients with renal failure.

● Monitor rate and depth of respirations. Shortness of breath and increased ventilation indicate acidosis.

● If used, hypodermoclysis should involve lateral aspect of thigh, which is less sensitive than the frontal aspect; discontinue infusion immediately if pain occurs.

● Give oral drug after meals to decrease GI side effects; enteric-coated tablets minimize GI symptoms, but absorption is erratic.

● When using drug as an expectorant, give with a full glass of water.

● Drug produces most effective diuretic action when given for 3 to 4 days, discontinued for several days, then resumed.

● If appropriate, advise patient on diuretic therapy to follow a diet high in potassium – oranges, bananas, cantaloupe, honeydew melon, milk (all types), yogurt, spinach, tomatoes, mushrooms, and potatoes – to replace potassium lost from acidosis.

Geriatric use
Aggressive diuresis may precipitate urinary retention in elderly males with prostatic hypertrophy, and acute sodium and potassium depletions or incontinence in both sexes.

Monitor urine specific gravity; elevation with mild diuresis in elderly patients suggests renal failure.

Pediatric use
Safety of ammonium chloride for injection in children has not been established.

Breast-feeding
Safe use in breast-feeding women has not been established.

amobarbital, amobarbital sodium
Amytal

● Pharmacologic classification: barbiturate
● Therapeutic classification: sedative-hypnotic, anticonvulsant
● Controlled substance schedule II
● Pregnancy risk category D

How supplied
Available by prescription only
Tablets: 30 mg, 50 mg, 100 mg
Capsules: 65 mg, 200 mg
Powder for injection: 250 mg, 500 mg/vial
Powder (bulk): 15 g, 30 g

Indications, route, and dosage
Sedation
Adults: Usually 30 to 50 mg P.O. b.i.d. or t.i.d. but may range from 15 to 120 mg b.i.d. to q.i.d.
Children: 3 to 6 mg/kg P.O. daily divided into four equal doses.
Insomnia
Adults: 65 to 200 mg P.O. or deep I.M. h.s.; I.M. injection not to exceed 5 ml in any one site. Maximum dosage is 500 mg.
Children over age 6: 3 to 5 mg/kg deep I.M. h.s.; I.M. injection not to exceed 5 ml in any one site.
Preanesthetic sedation
Adults and children over age 6: 200 mg P.O. or I.M. 1 to 2 hours before surgery.
Adjunct in psychotherapy ("amobarbital interview")
Adults: 50 mg/minute by slow, continuous I.V. infusion. Continue until patient shows drowsiness or sustained rapid lateral nystagmus (commonly after 150 to 350 mg). Proceed with interview using supplemental doses of 25 to 50 mg every 5 minutes.
Anticonvulsant
Adults: 65 to 500 mg by slow I.V. injection (rate not exceeding 100 mg/minute). Maximum dose is 1 g.
Children under age 6: 3 to 5 mg/kg slow I.V.

Pharmacodynamics
● Anticonvulsant action: The exact cellular site and mechanism(s) of action are unknown. Parenteral amobarbital suppresses the spread of seizure activity produced by epileptogenic foci in the cortex, thalamus, and limbic systems by enhancing the effect of gamma-aminobutyric acid (GABA). Both presynaptic and postsynaptic excitability are decreased.

● Sedative-hypnotic action: Amobarbital acts throughout the CNS as a nonselective depressant with an intermediate onset and duration of action. Particularly sensitive to this drug is the mesencephalic reticular activating system, which controls CNS arousal. Amobarbital decreases both presynaptic and postsynaptic membrane excitability by facilitating the action of GABA.

Pharmacokinetics
● Absorption: Amobarbital is absorbed well after oral administration. Absorption after I.M. administration is 100%. Onset of action is 45 to 60 minutes.
● Distribution: Amobarbital is distributed well throughout body tissues and fluids.

---

*Canada only   †Unlabeled clinical use   Italicized adverse reactions are life-threatening.

• *Metabolism:* Amobarbital is metabolized in the liver by oxidation to a tertiary alcohol.
• *Excretion:* Less than 1% of a dose is excreted unchanged in the urine. The rest is excreted as metabolites. The half-life is biphasic, with a first phase half-life of about 40 minutes and a second phase of about 20 hours. Duration of action is 6 to 8 hours.

Contraindications and precautions
Amobarbital is contraindicated in patients with known hypersensitivity to barbiturates and in patients with bronchopneumonia, status asthmaticus, or other severe respiratory distress because of the potential for respiratory depression.

Amobarbital should not be used in patients who are depressed or have suicidal ideation, because the drug can worsen depression; in patients with uncontrolled acute or chronic pain, because paradoxical excitement can occur; or in patients with porphyria, because this drug can trigger symptoms of this disease.

Amobarbital should be used cautiously in patients who must perform hazardous tasks requiring mental alertness, because the drug causes drowsiness. Administer parenteral amobarbital slowly and with extreme caution to patients with hypotension or severe pulmonary or cardiovascular disease because of potential adverse hemodynamic effects. Because tolerance and physical or psychological dependence may occur, prolonged use of high doses should be avoided.

Use cautiously in patients with renal or hepatic disease, as drug accumulation may occur. CNS depression may be exacerbated in patients with shock or uremia. Use parenteral amobarbital cautiously in patients with cardiovascular disease. Prenatal exposure to barbiturates is associated with an increased incidence of fetal abnormalities, and possibly brain tumors. Use of barbiturates in the third trimester may be associated with physical dependence in neonates. Risk to benefit ratio must be considered.

Interactions
Amobarbital may add to or potentiate CNS and respiratory depressant effects of other sedative-hypnotics, antihistamines, narcotics, antidepressants, monoamine oxidase inhibitors, tranquilizers, and alcohol.

Amobarbital enhances the enzymatic degradation of warfarin and other oral anticoagulants; patients may require increased doses of the anticoagulants. Amobarbital also enhances hepatic metabolism of digitoxin (not digoxin), corticosteroids, theophylline and other xanthines, oral contraceptives and other estrogens, and doxycycline. Amobarbital impairs the effectiveness of griseofulvin by decreasing absorption from the GI tract. Amobarbital may cause unpredictable fluctuations in serum phenytoin levels.

Valproic acid, phenytoin, monoamine oxidase inhibitors, and disulfiram decrease the metabolism of amobarbital and can increase its toxicity.

Rifampin may decrease amobarbital levels by increasing metabolism.

Effects on diagnostic tests
Amobarbital may cause a false-positive phentolamine test. The physiologic effects of amobarbital may impair the absorption of cyanocobalamin ^{57}Co; it may decrease serum bilirubin concentrations in neonates, epileptic patients, and in patients with congenital nonhemolytic unconjugated hyperbilirubinemia. EEG patterns are altered, with a change in low-voltage, fast activity; changes persist for a time after discontinuation of therapy.

Adverse reactions
• CNS: drowsiness, lethargy, vertigo, headache, CNS depression, mental depression, paradoxical excitement; confusion and agitation (especially in elderly patients).
• CV: hypotension (after rapid I.V. administration), bradycardia, syncope, *circulatory collapse.*
• DERM: urticaria, rash, *exfoliative dermatitis, Stevens-Johnson syndrome.*
• EENT: laryngospasm, *bronchospasm,* miosis, mydriasis (with severe toxicity).
• GI: nausea, vomiting, diarrhea, constipation, epigastric pain.
• Local: thrombophlebitis, pain and possible tissue damage at extravascular injection site.
• Other: *respiratory depression,* blood dyscrasias, rebound insomnia, increased dreams or nightmares, possibly *seizures* (after acute withdrawal or reduction in dosage). Vitamin K deficiency and bleeding have occurred in newborns of mothers treated during pregnancy. Hyperalgesia occurs with low doses or in patients with chronic pain.
Note: Drug should be discontinued if hypersensitivity reaction, profound CNS or respiratory depression, or skin eruption occurs.

Overdose and treatment
Clinical manifestations of overdose include unsteady gait, slurred speech, sustained nystagmus, somnolence, confusion, respiratory depression, pulmonary edema, areflexia, and coma. Oliguria, jaundice, hypothermia, fever, and shock with tachycardia and hypotension may occur.

Maintain and support ventilation as necessary; support circulation with vasopressors and I.V. fluids as needed.

Treatment is aimed to maintain and support ventilation and pulmonary function as necessary; support cardiac function and circulation with vasopressors and I.V. fluids as needed. If patient is conscious with a functioning gag reflex and ingestion has been recent, then induce emesis by administering ipecac syrup. Gastric lavage may be performed if a cuffed endotracheal tube is in place to prevent aspiration when emesis is inappropriate. Follow with administration of activated charcoal or saline cathartic. Measure fluid intake and output, vital signs, and laboratory parameters. Maintain body temperature.

Alkalinization of urine may be helpful in removing amobarbital from the body; hemodialysis may be useful in severe overdose.

▶ Special considerations
Besides those relevant to all *barbiturates,* consider the following recommendations.
• Not commonly used as a sedative or aid to sleeping; barbiturates have been replaced by safer benzodiapines for such use.
• Administer oral amobarbital before meals or on an empty stomach to enhance the rate of absorption.
• Reconstitute powder for injection with sterile water for injection. Roll vial in hands; do not shake. Use 2.5 or 5 ml (for 250 or 500 mg of amobarbital) to make 10% solution. For I.M. use, prepare 20% solution by using 1.25 ml or 2.5 ml of sterile water for injection.

• Administer reconstituted parenteral solution within 30 minutes after opening the vial.

• Do not administer any amobarbital solution that is cloudy or forms a precipitate after 5 minutes of reconstitution.

• Administer I.V. dose at a rate no greater than 100 mg/minute in adults or 60 mg/m²/minute in children to prevent possible hypotension and respiratory depression. Have emergency resuscitative equipment available.

• Administer I.M. dose deep into large muscle mass, giving no more than 5 ml in any one injection site. Sterile abscess or tissue damage may result from inadvertent superficial I.M. or S.C. injection.

• Administering full loading doses over short periods of time to treat status epilepticus may require ventilatory support in adults.

• Assess cardiopulmonary status frequently for possible alterations. Monitor blood counts for potential adverse reactions.

• Assess renal and hepatic laboratory studies to ensure adequate drug removal.

• Monitor prothrombin times carefully when patient on amobarbital starts or ends anticoagulant therapy. Anticoagulant dosage may need to be adjusted.

Information for the patient
Warn patient of possible physical or psychological dependence with prolonged use.

Geriatric use
Elderly patients usually require lower doses. Confusion, disorientation, and excitability may occur in elderly patients. Use with caution.

Pediatric use
Safe use in children under age 6 has not been established. Use of amobarbital may cause paradoxical excitement in some children.

Breast-feeding
Amobarbital passes into breast milk and may cause drowsiness in the infant. If so, dosage adjustment or discontinuation of drug or of breast-feeding may be necessary. Use with caution.

---

amoxapine
Asendin

• Pharmacologic classification: dibenzox-azepine, tricyclic antidepressant
• Therapeutic classification: antidepressant
• Pregnancy risk category C

How supplied
Available by prescription only
Tablets: 25 mg, 50 mg, 100 mg, 150 mg

Indications, route, and dosage
Depression
Adults: Initial dosage is 50 mg P.O. t.i.d; may increase to 100 mg t.i.d. on 3rd day of treatment. Increases above 300 mg daily should be made only if this dosage has been ineffective during a trial period of at least 2 weeks. When effective dosage is established, entire dosage

(not exceeding 300 mg) may be given at bedtime. Maximum dosage is 600 mg in hospitalized patients.

Do not give more than 300 mg in a single dose.

Pharmacodynamics
Antidepressant action: Amoxapine is thought to exert its antidepressant effects by inhibiting reuptake of norepinephrine and serotonin in CNS nerve terminals (presynaptic neurons), which results in increased concentrations and enhanced activity of these neurotransmitters in the synaptic cleft. Amoxapine has a greater inhibitory effect on norepinephrine reuptake than on serotonin. Amoxapine also blocks CNS dopamine receptors, which may account for the higher incidence of movement disorders during amoxapine therapy.

Pharmacokinetics
• *Absorption:* Amoxapine is absorbed rapidly and completely from the GI tract after oral administration.
• *Distribution:* Amoxapine is distributed widely into the body, including the CNS and breast milk. Drug is 92% protein-bound. Peak effect occurs in 8 to 10 hours; steady state, within 2 to 7 days. Proposed therapeutic plasma levels (parent drug and metabolite) range from 200 ng/ml to 400 ng/ml.
• *Metabolism:* Amoxapine is metabolized by the liver to the active metabolite 8-hydroxyamoxapine; a significant first-pass effect may explain variability of serum concentrations in different patients taking the same dosage.
• *Excretion:* Amoxapine is excreted in urine and feces (7% to 18%); about 60% of a given dose is excreted as the conjugated form within 6 days.

Contraindications and precautions
Amoxapine is contraindicated in patients with known hypersensitivity to tricyclic antidepressants, trazodone, or related compounds; in the acute recovery phase of myocardial infarction (MI) because of its potential arrhythmogenic effects; in patients in coma or severe respiratory depression because of additive CNS depression; and during or within 14 days of monoamine oxidase therapy.

Amoxapine should be used cautiously in patients with other cardiac disease (arrhythmias, congestive heart failure [CHF], angina pectoris, valvular disease, or heart block); respiratory disorders; epilepsy and other seizure disorders; scheduled electroconvulsive therapy (ECT); bipolar disease; glaucoma; hyperthyroidism or in those taking thyroid replacement; Type I and Type II diabetes; prostatic hypertrophy, paralytic ileus, or urinary retention; hepatic or renal dysfunction; Parkinson's disease; and in those undergoing surgery with general anesthesia. Caution also is recommended in patients with tardive dyskinesia, because amoxapine may induce or exacerbate this disorder.

Interactions
Concomitant use of amoxapine with sympathomimetics, including epinephrine, phenylephrine, phenylpropanolamine, and ephedrine (often found in nasal sprays) may increase blood pressure; use with warfarin may increase prothrombin time and cause bleeding.

Concomitant use with thyroid medication, pimozide, and antiarrhythmic agents (quinidine, disopyramide, procainamide) may increase the incidence of cardiac arrhythmias and conduction defects.

Amoxapine may decrease hypotensive effects of centrally acting antihypertensive drugs such as gua-

---

*Canada only   †Unlabeled clinical use   Italicized adverse reactions are life-threatening.

nethidine, guanabenz, guanadrel, clonidine, methyldopa, and reserpine.

Concomitant use with disulfiram or ethchlorvynol may cause delirium and tachycardia.

Additive effects are likely after concomitant use of amoxapine with CNS depressants, including alcohol, analgesics, barbiturates, narcotics, tranquilizers, and anesthetics (oversedation); atropine or other anticholinergic drugs, including phenothiazines, antihistamines, meperidine, and antiparkinsonian agents (oversedation, paralytic ileus, visual changes, and severe constipation); or metrizamide (increased risk of convulsions).

Barbiturates and heavy smoking induce amoxapine metabolism and decrease therapeutic efficacy; phenothiazines and haloperidol decrease its metabolism, decreasing therapeutic efficacy. Methylphenidate, cimetidine, oral contraceptives, propoxyphene, and beta blockers may inhibit amoxapine metabolism, increasing plasma levels and toxicity.

Effects on diagnostic tests

Amoxapine may prolong conduction time (elongation of Q-T and PR intervals, flattened T waves on ECG); it also may elevate liver function test results, decrease white blood cell counts, and decrease or increase serum glucose levels.

Adverse reactions

● CNS: drowsiness, dizziness, sedation, excitation, tremors, weakness, headache, nervousness, *seizures* (especially pronounced with this drug), peripheral neuropathy, extrapyramidal symptoms (numbness, tingling, ataxia, tardive dyskinesia, in 1% of patients), anxiety, vivid dreams, confusion (more marked in elderly patients), decreased libido.
● CV: orthostatic hypotension, tachycardia, *dysrhythmias, MI, stroke, heart block, CHF,* palpitations, hypertension, ECG changes.
● EENT: blurred vision, tinnitus, mydriasis, increased intraocular pressure.
● Endocrine: breast enlargement or gynecomastia, testicular edema, sexual dysfunction.
● GI: dry mouth, constipation, nausea, vomiting, anorexia, diarrhea, paralytic ileus, jaundice.
● GU: urinary retention.
● Other: sweating, photosensitivity, hypersensitivity (rash, urticaria, drug fever, edema).

After abrupt withdrawal of long-term therapy, nausea, headache, malaise (does not indicate addiction).

Note: Drug should be discontinued (not abruptly) if signs of hypersensitivity occur. Reevaluate therapy if the following reactions occur: urinary retention, extreme dry mouth, rash, excessive sedation, seizures, tachycardia, sore throat, fever, tardive dyskinesia, or jaundice.

Overdose and treatment

The first 12 hours after acute ingestion are a stimulatory phase characterized by excessive anticholinergic activity (agitation, irritation, confusion, hallucinations, hyperthermia, parkinsonian symptoms, seizures, urinary retention, dry mucous membranes, pupillary dilatation, constipation, and ileus). This is followed by CNS depressant effects, including hypothermia, decreased or absent reflexes, sedation, hypotension, cyanosis, and cardiac irregularities, including tachycardia, conduction disturbances, and quinidine-like effects on the ECG.

Overdose with amoxapine produces a much higher incidence of CNS toxicity than do other antidepressants. Acute deterioration of renal function (evidenced by myoglobin in urine) occurs in 5% of overdosed patients; this is most likely to occur in patients with repeated seizures after the overdose. Seizures may progress to status epilepticus within 12 hours.

Severity of overdose is best indicated by widening of the QRS complex, which generally represents a serum level in excess of 1,000 ng/ml; serum concentrations are not usually helpful. Metabolic acidosis may follow hypotension, hypoventilation, and convulsions.

Treatment is symptomatic and supportive, including maintaining airway, stable body temperature, and fluid and electrolyte balance; monitor renal status because of the risk of renal failure. Induce emesis with ipecac if patient is conscious; follow with gastric lavage and activated charcoal to prevent further absorption. Dialysis is of little use. Treat seizures with parenteral diazepam or phenytoin; arrhythmias, with parenteral phenytoin or lidocaine; and acidosis, with sodium bicarbonate. *Do not give barbiturates;* these may enhance CNS and respiratory depressant effects.

▶ Special considerations

Besides those relevant to all *tricyclic antidepressants,* consider the following recommendations.
● Amoxapine is associated with a high incidence of seizures.
● The full dose may be given at bedtime to help reduce daytime sedation.
● The full dose should not be withdrawn abruptly.
● Tolerance to sedative effects usually develops over the first few weeks of therapy.
● The drug should be discontinued at least 48 hours before surgical procedures.
● Chewing gum, hard candy, or ice may alleviate dry mouth.
● Tardive dyskinesia and other extrapyramidal effects may occur because of amoxapine's dopamine-blocking activity. Elderly patients appear to be more susceptible to these effects.
● Watch for gynecomastia in males and females since amoxapine may increase cellular division in breast tissue.

Information for the patient

● Explain that the full effects of the drug may not become apparent for at least 2 weeks or more after initiation of therapy, perhaps not for 4 to 6 weeks.
● Tell patient to take the medication exactly as prescribed; however, the full dose may be taken at bedtime to alleviate daytime sedation. Patient should not double dose for missed ones.
● Warn patient that drug may cause drowsiness or dizziness. Patient should avoid hazardous activities that require alertness until the full effects of the drug are known.
● Tell patient not to drink alcoholic beverages while taking this drug.
● Suggest taking drug with food or milk if it causes stomach upset and relieving dry mouth with gum or hard candy.
● After initial doses, patient should lie down for about 30 minutes and rise slowly to prevent dizziness.
● Warn patient not to discontinue drug suddenly.
● Encourage patient to report any unusual or troublesome reactions immediately, especially confusion, movement disorders, rapid heartbeat, dizziness, fainting, or difficulty urinating.

● Warn patient of the risks of tardive dyskinesia. Tell patient what symptoms to look for.
● Tell patient that exposure to sunlight, sunlamps, or tanning beds may cause burning of the skin or abnormal pigmentary changes.
● Tell patient to store drug safely away from children.

Geriatric use
● Lower doses are indicated because older patients are more sensitive to the therapeutic and adverse effects of the drug. Recommended starting dose is 25 mg t.i.d.
● Elderly patients are much more susceptible to tardive dyskinesia and extrapyramidal symptoms.

Pediatric use
Not recommended for patients younger than age 16.

Breast-feeding
Amoxapine is excreted in breast milk in concentrations of 20% of maternal serum as parent drug and 30% as metabolites. The potential benefits to the mother should outweigh the possible adverse reactions in the infant.

---

amoxicillin trihydrate
Amoxil, Polymox, Trimox, Utimox, Wymox

● Pharmacologic classification: aminopenicillin
● Therapeutic classification: antibiotic
● Pregnancy risk category B

How supplied
Available by prescription only
Capsules: 250 mg, 500 mg
Suspension: 125 mg/5 ml, 250 mg/5 ml, 50 mg/5 ml (after reconstitution, pediatric drops)
Tablets (chewable): 125 mg, 250 mg

Indications, route, and dosage
Systemic infections, acute and chronic urinary or respiratory tract infections caused by susceptible organisms
Adults: 750 mg to 1.5 g P.O. daily, divided into doses given q 8 hours.
Children: 20 to 40 mg/kg P.O. daily, divided into doses given q 8 hours.
Uncomplicated gonorrhea
Adults: 3 g P.O. with 1 g probenecid given as a single dose.
Uncomplicated urinary tract infections caused by susceptible organisms
Adults: 3 g P.O. given as a single dose.
Dosage in renal failure
Patients who require repeated doses may need adjustment of dosing interval. If creatinine clearance is 10 to 50 ml/min, increase interval to q 12 hours; if creatinine clearance is < 10 ml/min, administer q 12 to 16 hours. Supplemental doses may be necessary after hemodialysis.

Pharmacodynamics
Antibacterial action: Amoxicillin is bactericidal; it adheres to bacterial penicillin-binding proteins, thus inhibiting bacterial cell wall synthesis.

Amoxicillin's spectrum of action includes nonpenicillinase-producing gram-positive bacteria, Streptococcus group B, *Neisseria gonorrheae, Proteus mirabilis, Salmonella,* and *H. influenzae.* It is also effective against non-penicillinase producing *S. aureus, S. pyogenes, S. bovis, S. pneumoniae, S. viridans, N. meningitidis, E. coli, S. typhi, B. pertussis, G. vaginalis, Peptococcus,* and *Peptostreptococcus.*

Pharmacokinetics
● *Absorption:* Amoxicillin is approximately 80% absorbed after oral administration; peak serum concentrations occur at 1.0 to 2.5 hours after an oral dose.
● *Distribution:* Amoxicillin distributes into pleural peritoneal and synovial fluids, and into the lungs, prostate, muscle, liver, and gallbladder; it also penetrates middle ear, maxillary sinus and bronchial secretions, tonsils, and sputum. Amoxicillin readily crosses the placenta. Amoxicillin is 17% to 20% protein-bound.
● *Metabolism:* Amoxicillin is metabolized only partially.
● *Excretion:* Amoxicillin is excreted principally in urine by renal tubular secretion and glomerular filtration; it is also excreted in breast milk. Elimination half-life in adults is 1 to 1½ hours; severe renal impairment increases half-life to 7½ hours.

Contraindications and precautions
Amoxicillin is contraindicated in patients with known hypersensitivity to any other penicillin or to cephalosporins.
Amoxicillin should not be used in patients with infectious mononucleosis, because many patients develop a rash during therapy.
Amoxicillin should be used cautiously in patients with renal impairment because it is excreted by the kidney; decreased dosage is required in moderate to severe renal failure.

Interactions
Concomitant use with allopurinol appears to increase the incidence of skin rash from both drugs.
Concomitant use with clavulanate potassium enhances effect of amoxicillin against certain beta-lactamase-producing bacteria.
Probenecid blocks renal tubular secretion of amoxicillin, raising its serum concentrations.
Large doses of penicillins may interfere with renal tubular secretion of methotrexate, thus delaying elimination and prolonging elevated serum concentrations of methotrexate.
Concomitant use with an aminoglycoside antibiotic causes a synergistic bactericidal effect against some strains of enterococci and group B streptococci; however, the drugs are physically and chemically incompatible and are inactivated if mixed or given together.

Effects on diagnostic tests
Amoxicillin may alter results of urine glucose tests that use cupric sulfate (Benedict's reagent or Clinitest). Make urine glucose determinations with glucose oxidase methods (Clinistix or Tes-Tape).
Amoxicillin may falsely decrease serum aminoglycoside concentrations.

Adverse reactions
● GI: nausea, vomiting, diarrhea, *pseudomembranous colitis.*
● GU: *acute interstitial nephritis.*

---

*Canada only   †Unlabeled clinical use   Italicized adverse reactions are life-threatening.

● HEMA: anemia, thrombocytopenia, thrombocytopenic purpura, eosinophilia, leukopenia.
● Other: *hypersensitivity* (erythematous maculopapular rash, urticaria, *anaphylaxis*), bacterial or fungal superinfection.

Note: Drug should be discontinued if immediate hypersensitivity reactions occur or if bone marrow toxicity or acute interstitial nephritis develops.

Overdose and treatment
Clinical signs of overdose include neuromuscular sensitivity or seizures. After recent ingestion (4 hours or less), empty the stomach by induced emesis or gastric lavage; follow with activated charcoal to reduce absorption. Amoxicillin can be removed by hemodialysis.

▶ Special considerations
Besides those relevant to all *penicillins*, consider the following recommendations.
● Oral dosage is maximally absorbed from an empty stomach, but food does not cause significant loss of potency.
● Pediatric drops may be placed on child's tongue or added to formula, milk, fruit juice, or soft drink. Be sure child ingests all of prepared dose.
● Suspension and drops are stable for 7 days at room temperature and 14 days in refrigerator after reconstitution.
● Amoxicillin may cause less diarrhea than ampicillin.

Information for the patient
● Tell patient to chew tablets thoroughly or crush before swallowing and wash down with liquid to ensure adequate absorption of drug; capsule may be emptied and contents swallowed with water.
● Encourage patient to report diarrhea promptly.

Geriatric use
Because of diminished renal tubular secretion, half-life may be prolonged in elderly patients.

Breast-feeding
Amoxicillin is distributed readily into breast milk; safe use in breast-feeding women has not been established. Alternative feeding method is recommended during therapy.

amoxicillin/clavulanate potassium
Augmentin, Clavulin*

● Pharmacologic classification: aminopenicillin and beta-lactamase inhibitor
● Therapeutic classification: antibiotic
● Pregnancy risk category B

How supplied
Available by prescription only
Oral suspension: 125 mg amoxicillin trihydrate and 31.25 mg clavulanic acid/5 ml (after reconstitution)
Suspension: 250 mg amoxicillin trihydrate and 62.5 mg clavulanic acid/5 ml (after reconstitution)
Chewable tablets: 125 mg amoxicillin trihydrate, 31.25 mg clavulanic acid; 250 mg amoxicillin trihydrate, 62.5 mg clavulanic acid
Film-coated tablets: 250 mg amoxicillin trihydrate, 125 mg clavulanic acid; 500 mg amoxicillin trihydrate, 125 mg clavulanic acid

Indications, route, and dosage
Lower respiratory infections, otitis media, sinusitis, skin and skin structure infections, and urinary tract infections caused by susceptible organisms
Adults: 250 mg (based on the amoxicillin component) P.O. q 8 hours. For more severe infections, 500 mg q 8 hours.
Children: 20 to 40 mg/kg/day (based on the amoxicillin component) given in divided doses q 8 hours.

Pharmacodynamics
Antibiotic action: Amoxicillin is bactericidal; it adheres to bacterial penicillin-binding proteins, thus inhibiting bacterial cell wall synthesis.

Clavulanate has only weak antibacterial activity and does not affect mechanism of action of amoxicillin. However, clavulanic acid has a beta-lactam ring and is structurally similar to penicillin and cephalosporins; it binds irreversibly with certain beta-lactamases and prevents them from inactivating amoxicillin, enhancing its bactericidal activity.

This combination acts against penicillinase- and nonpenicillinase-producing gram-positive bacteria, *Neisseria gonorrhoeae, N. meningitidis, Haemophilus influenzae, Escherichia coli, Proteus mirabilis, Citrobacter diversus, Klebsiella pneumoniae, P. vulgaris, Salmonella,* and *Shigella.*

Pharmacokinetics
● *Absorption:* Amoxicillin and clavulanate potassium are well absorbed after oral administration; peak serum levels occur at 1 to 2½ hours.
● *Distribution:* Both amoxicillin and clavulanate potassium distribute into pleural fluid, lungs, and peritoneal fluid; high urine concentrations are attained. Amoxicillin also distributes into synovial fluid, liver, prostate, muscle, and gallbladder; and penetrates into middle ear effusions, maxillary sinus secretions, tonsils, sputum, and bronchial secretions. Amoxicillin and clavulanate cross the placenta and low concentrations occur in breast milk. Amoxicillin and clavulanate potassium have minimal protein-binding of 17% to 20% and 22% to 30%, respectively.
● *Metabolism:* Amoxicillin is metabolized only partially. The metabolic fate of clavulanate potassium is not completely identified, but it appears to undergo extensive metabolism.
● *Excretion:* Amoxicillin is excreted principally in urine by renal tubular secretion and glomerular filtration; the drug is also excreted in breast milk.

Clavulanate potassium is excreted by glomerular filtration. Elimination half-life of amoxicillin in adults is 1 to 1½ hours; it is prolonged to 7½ hours in patients with severe renal impairment. Half-life of clavulanate in adults is about 1 to 1½ hours, prolonged to 4½ hours in patients with severe renal impairment.

Both drugs are removed readily by hemodialysis and minimally removed by peritoneal dialysis.

Contraindications and precautions
Amoxicillin/potassium clavulanate is contraindicated in patients with known hypersensitivity to any other penicillin or to cephalosporins.

Amoxicillin clavulanate potassium should not be used

in patients with mononucleosis because many patients develop a rash during therapy.

The combination should be used cautiously in patients with renal impairment because it is excreted in urine; decreased dosage is required in moderate to severe renal failure.

Interactions
Concomitant use with an aminoglycoside antibiotic causes a synergistic bactericidal effect against some strains of enterococci and group B streptococci. However, the drugs are physically and chemically incompatible and are inactivated if mixed or given together. In vivo inactivation of aminoglycosides has also been reported when aminoglycosides and penicillins are used concomitantly; however, they are clinically synergistic against some bacteria.

Concomitant use with allopurinol appears to increase incidence of skin rash from both drugs.

Probenecid blocks tubular secretion of amoxicillin, raising its serum concentrations; it has no effect on clavulanate.

Large doses of penicillins may interfere with renal tubular secretion of methotrexate, thus delaying elimination and prolonging elevated serum concentrations of methotrexate.

Effects on diagnostic tests
Amoxicillin/potassium clavulanate alters results of urine glucose tests that use cupric sulfate (Benedict's reagent or Clinitest). Make urine glucose determinations with glucose oxidase methods (Clinistix or Tes-Tape). Positive Coombs' tests have been reported with other clavulanate combinations.

Amoxicillin may falsely decrease serum aminoglycoside concentrations.

Adverse reactions
Adverse reactions to this combination are similar to those occurring with amoxicillin; however, GI reactions may occur more frequently, due to greater absorption of clavulanate.
- GI: nausea, vomiting, diarrhea, *pseudomembranous colitis* (may be indicated by severe diarrhea).
- GU: *acute interstitial nephritis.*
- Other: *hypersensitivity* (erythematous maculopapular rash, urticaria, *anaphylaxis*), bacterial and fungal superinfection.

Note: Drug should be discontinued if immediate hypersensitivity reactions occur, or if bone marrow toxicity or acute interstitial nephritis develops.

Overdose and treatment
Clinical signs of overdose include neuromuscular sensitivity or seizures. After recent ingestion (4 hours or less), empty the stomach by induced emesis or gastric lavage; follow with activated charcoal to reduce absorption. Amoxicillin/potassium clavulanate can be removed by hemodialysis.

▶ Special considerations
Besides those relevant to all *penicillins*, consider the following recommendations.
- Oral dosage is maximally absorbed from an empty stomach, but food does not cause significant impairment of absorption.
- Pediatric drops may be placed on child's tongue or added to formula, milk, fruit juice, or soft drink. Be sure child ingests all of prepared dose.
- Suspension and drops are stable for 7 days at room temperature and 14 days in refrigerator after reconstitution.
- When using film-coated tablets, be aware that both dosages contain different amounts of amoxicillin, but the *same amount* of clavulanate; therefore two "250-mg" tablets are not the equivalent of one "500-mg" tablet.
- Because ampicillin/potassium clavulanate is dialyzable, patients undergoing hemodialysis may need dosage adjustments.

Information for the patient
- Tell patient to chew tablets thoroughly or crush before swallowing and wash down with liquid to ensure adequate absorption of drug; capsule may be emptied and contents swallowed with water.
- Encourage patient to report diarrhea promptly.

Geriatric use
In elderly patients, diminished renal tubular secretion may prolong half-life of amoxicillin.

Breast-feeding
Both amoxicillin and potassium clavulanate are excreted in breast milk; drug should be used with caution in breast-feeding women.

PHARMACOLOGIC CLASS

amphetamines

amphetamine sulfate
benzphetamine hydrochloride
dextroamphetamine sulfate
diethylpropion hydrochloride
fenfluramine hydrochloride
methamphetamine hydrochloride
phendimetrazine hydrochloride
phenmetrazine hydrochloride
phentermine hydrochloride

Amphetamines were the first drugs widely prescribed as anorexigenics. They no longer are used for this purpose because dependence can develop. The Food and Drug Administration has found no advantage to their use as compared with other, safer anorexigenics. Amphetamines now are used chiefly to control narcolepsy in adults and attention deficit disorder in hyperactive children.

Pharmacology
Amphetamines are sympathomimetic amines with CNS stimulant activity; in children with hyperkinesia, they have a paradoxical calming effect. Their mechanisms of action for narcolepsy, attention deficit disorder, and appetite control are unknown; anorexigenic effects are thought to occur in the hypothalamus, where decreased smell and taste acuity decreases appetite.

The cerebral cortex and reticular activating system appear to be the primary sites of activity; amphetamines release nerve terminal stores of norepinephrine, promoting nerve impulse transmission. At high doses, effects are mediated by dopamine.

Peripheral effects include elevated blood pressure, respiratory stimulation, and weak bronchodilation. At therapeutic dosage levels, cardiac output and cerebral

---

blood flow remain unchanged; high doses may cause arrhythmias.

Clinical indications and actions
Narcolepsy; attention deficit disorders
Amphetamines may be used to treat narcolepsy and as adjuncts to psychosocial measures in attention deficit disorder in children.
Adjuncts in managing obesity
Amphetamines may be tried for short-term control of refractory obesity, with caloric restriction and behavior modification; anorexigenic effects persist only a few weeks, and patient must be encouraged to learn modification of eating habits rapidly.

Overview of adverse reactions
Adverse reactions to the amphetamines reflect excessive sympathomimetic and CNS stimulation and commonly include insomnia, tremor, and restlessness; toxic dosage levels can induce psychosis, mydriasis, hypertension, arrhythmias, coma, circulatory collapse, and death.

Tolerance to amphetamines can occur within a few weeks, necessitating increased dosages to produce desired effects; abusers take an average of 1 to 2 g/ day. Both physical tolerance and psychological dependence may occur. Symptoms of chronic abuse include mental impairment, loss of appetite, somnolence, social withdrawal, and occupational and emotional problems; prolonged abuse may cause schizoid syndromes and hallucinations.

▶ Special considerations
● Amphetamines are contraindicated in patients with symptomatic cardiovascular disease, hyperthyroidism, nephritis, angina pectoris, any degree of hypertension, arteriosclerosis-induced parkinsonism, certain types of glaucoma, advanced arteriosclerosis, agitated states, or a history of substance abuse.
● Amphetamines should be used cautiously in patients with diabetes mellitus; in elderly, debilitated, or hyperexcitable patients; and in children with Gilles de la Tourette's syndrome. Avoid long-term therapy when possible because of the risk of psychic dependence or habituation.
● Patient should receive lowest effective dose with dosage adjusted individually according to response; after long-term use, dosage should be lowered gradually to prevent acute rebound depression.
● Amphetamines may impair ability to perform tasks requiring mental alertness, such as driving a car.
● Vital signs should be checked regularly for increased blood pressure or other signs of excessive stimulation; avoid late-day or evening dosing, especially of long-acting dosage forms, to minimize insomnia.
● Amphetamines are not recommended as first-line therapy for obesity; be sure patients taking amphetamines for weight reduction are on reduced-calorie diet; also monitor calorie intake.
● Amphetamine therapy should be discontinued when tolerance to anorexigenic effects develops; dosage should not be increased.
● Encourage patient to get adequate rest; unusual, compensatory fatigue may result as drug wears off.
● Amphetamine use for analeptic effect is discouraged; CNS stimulation superimposed on CNS depression may cause neuronal instability and seizures.
● Carefully follow manufacturer's directions for reconstitution, storage, and administration of all preparations.

● Prolonged administration of CNS stimulants to children with attention deficit disorders may be associated with temporary decreased growth.
● Amphetamines have a high potential for abuse; they are not recommended to combat the fatigue of exhaustion or the need for sleep, but are often abused for this purpose by students, athletes, and truck drivers.
● In the event of overdose, protect patient from excessive noise or stimulation.

Information for the patient
● Explain rationale for therapy and the potential risks and benefits.
● Tell patient to avoid drinks containing caffeine, to prevent added CNS stimulation; and not to increase dosage.
● Advise narcoleptic patients to take first dose on awakening.
● Advise patients on weight reduction programs to take last dose several hours before bedtime to avoid insomnia.
● Tell patient not to chew or crush sustained-release dosage forms.
● Warn patient not to use drug to mask fatigue, to be sure to obtain adequate rest, and to report excessive CNS stimulation.
● Advise diabetic patients to monitor blood glucose levels carefully, as drug may alter insulin needs.
● Advise patient to avoid tasks that require mental alertness until degree of cognitive impairment is determined.

Geriatric use
Use amphetamines with caution. Elderly patients are usually more sensitive to drugs' effects and may obtain therapeutic effect from lower dosages.

Pediatric use
Amphetamines are not recommended for weight reduction in children under age 12; amphetamine use for hyperactivity is contraindicated in children under age 3.

Breast-feeding
Safety has not been established. An alternative feeding method is recommended during therapy.

Representative combinations
Amphetamine sulfate with dextroamphetamine sulfate: Biphetamine, Obetrol.

    Methamphetamine hydrochloride with amobarbital and homatropine: Obe-Slim; with dl-methamphetamine and butabarbital: Span-RD; with Pamabrom, pyrilamine, homatropine, hyoscyamine sulfate, and scopolamine hydrobromide: Aridol; with pentobarbital: Fetamin; with phenobarbital and ascorbic acid: Obetrim-T.

See also barbiturates.

amphetamine sulfate

- Pharmacologic classification: amphetamine
- Therapeutic classification: CNS stimulant, short-term adjunctive anorexigenic agent, sympathomimetic amine
- Controlled substance schedule II
- Pregnancy risk category D

How supplied
Available by prescription only
Tablets: 5 mg, 10 mg
Capsules: 6.25 mg, 10 mg

Indications, route, and dosage
Attention deficit disorder with hyperactivity
Children age 6 and older: 5 mg P.O. daily. Increase at 5-mg increments weekly until desired response. Dosage rarely exceeds 40 mg/day.
Children age 3 to 5: 2.5 mg P.O. daily, increase at 2.5-mg increments weekly until desired response.
Narcolepsy
Adults: 5 to 60 mg P.O. daily in divided doses.
Children over age 12: 10 mg P.O. daily, with 10-mg increments weekly, p.r.n.
Children age 6 to 12: 5 mg P.O. daily, with 5-mg increments weekly, p.r.n.
Children under age 6: Dosage seldom exceeds 40 mg daily.
Short-term adjunct in exogenous obesity
Adults: Single 10-mg or 15-mg long-acting capsule daily, or two if needed, up to 30 mg daily; or 5 to 30 mg daily in divided doses 30 to 60 minutes before meals. Not recommended for children under age 12.
†Short-term treatment of depression in patients intolerant of tricyclic antidepressants
Adults: 5 to 10 mg P.O. b.i.d. 30 minutes before meals.

Pharmacodynamics
- *CNS stimulant action:* Amphetamines are sympathomimetic amines with CNS stimulant activity; in hyperactive children, they have a paradoxical calming effect.
  Amphetamines are used to treat narcolepsy and as adjuncts to psychosocial measures in attention deficit disorder in children. The cerebral cortex and reticular activating system appear to be their primary sites of activity; amphetamines release nerve terminal stores of norepinephrine, promoting nerve impulse transmission. At high dosages, effects are mediated by dopamine.
- *Anorexigenic action:* Anorexigenic effects are thought to occur in the hypothalamus, where decreased smell and taste acuity decreases the appetite. They may be tried for short-term control of refractory obesity, with caloric restriction and behavior modification.

Pharmacokinetics
- *Absorption:* Amphetamine sulfate is absorbed completely within 3 hours after oral administration; therapeutic effects persist for 4 to 24 hours.
- *Distribution:* Amphetamine sulfate is distributed widely throughout the body, with high concentrations in the brain. Therapeutic plasma levels are 5 to 10 mcg/dl.

- *Metabolism:* Amphetamine sulfate is metabolized by hydroxylation and deamination in the liver.
- *Excretion:* Amphetamine sulfate is excreted in urine.

Contraindications and precautions
Amphetamines are contraindicated in patients with hypersensitivity or idiosyncratic reaction to sympathomimetic amines; in those with symptomatic cardiovascular disease, hyperthyroidism, nephritis, angina pectoris, hypertension, glaucoma, advanced arteriosclerosis, or agitated states; and in patients with a history of drug or alcohol abuse. They also are contraindicated for concomitant use with monoamine oxidase (MAO) inhibitors or within 14 days of discontinuing MAO inhibitors.
  Amphetamines should be used with caution in patients with diabetes mellitus; in elderly, debilitated, or hyperexcitable patients; and in children with Gilles de la Tourette's syndrome. Avoid long-term therapy, when possible, because of the risk of psychic or physical dependence.

Interactions
Concomitant use with MAO inhibitors (or drugs with MAO-inhibiting effects such as furazolidone) or within 14 days of such therapy may cause hypertensive crisis; concomitant use with antihypertensives may antagonize their hypertensive effects.
  Concomitant use with antacids, sodium bicarbonate, or acetazolamide may enhance reabsorption of amphetamine and prolong its duration of action, whereas concomitant use with ammonium chloride or ascorbic acid enhances amphetamine excretion or shortens duration of action. Use with phenothiazines or haloperidol decreases amphetamine effects; barbiturates counteract amphetamine by CNS depression, whereas caffeine or other CNS stimulants produce additive effects.
  Amphetamines may alter insulin requirements.

Effects on diagnostic tests
Amphetamines may elevate plasma corticosteroid levels and also may interfere with urinary steroid determinations.

Adverse reactions
- CNS: restlessness, tremor, hyperactivity, talkativeness, insomnia, irritability, dizziness, headache, chills, over-stimulation, dysphoria, psychosis, paranoid ideation.
- CV: tachycardia, palpitations, hypertension, hypotension.
- GI: nausea, vomiting, cramps, dry mouth, diarrhea, constipation, metallic taste, anorexia, weight loss.
- GU: changes in libido, impotence.
- Other: urticaria, tolerance, psychological and physical dependence.
  Note: Drug should be discontinued if signs of hypersensitivity or idiosyncrasy occur.

Overdose and treatment
Symptoms of acute overdose include increasing restlessness, irritability, insomnia, tremor, hyperreflexia, diaphoresis, mydriasis, flushing, confusion, hypertension, tachypnea, fever, delirium, self-injury, dysrhythmias, convulsions, coma, circulatory collapse, and death.
  Treat overdose symptomatically and supportively: if ingestion is recent (within 4 hours) use gastric lavage or emesis; activated charcoal, saline catharsis, and

---

urinary acidification may enhance excretion. Forced fluid diuresis may help. In massive ingestion, hemodialysis or peritoneal dialysis may be needed. Keep patient in a cool room, monitor his temperature, and minimize external stimulation. Haloperidol may be used for psychotic symptoms; diazepam, for hyperactivity.

▶ **Special considerations**
Recommendations for administration of amphetamine sulfate, for care and teaching of the patient during therapy, and for use in elderly or breast-feeding patients are the same as those for all *amphetamines*.
● Avoid administration late in the day (after 4 p.m.) to prevent insomnia.
● First dose is usually given upon awakening, additional doses at 4 to 6 hour intervals.
● Amphetamine capsules should not be used for initial or subsequent titration of dosage; however, once dosage has been established the capsules can be substituted if once-daily dosing is required.

Pediatric use
Amphetamines are not recommended for weight reduction in children under age 12; use of amphetamines for hyperactivity is contraindicated in children under age 3. A pediatric elixir is available; temporary suppression of normal growth has followed its long-term use; such use must be monitored carefully.

---

amphetericin B
Fungizone

● Pharmacologic classification: polyene macrolide
● Therapeutic classification: antifungal
● Pregnancy risk category B

How supplied
Available by prescription only
Injection: 50-mg lyophilized cake
Cream: 3%
Lotion: 3%
Ointment: 3%

Indications, route, and dosage
Systemic (potentially fatal) fungal infections, caused by susceptible organisms; †fungal endocarditis; fungal septicemia
Adults and children: Some clinicians recommend an initial dose of 1 mg I.V. in 250 ml dextrose 5% in water infused over 2 to 4 hours. If this test dose is tolerated, 5 mg in 500 ml dextrose 5% in water is given I.V. on the next day, followed by 10 mg in 1 liter dextrose 5% in water on day 3. Additional increases of 5 to 10 mg per day are administered as tolerated. Total daily dosage may be as high as 1 mg/kg. Once dosage is stabilized, alternate-day therapy at 1.5 mg/kg may be possible. Do not exceed a total daily dosage of 1.5 mg/kg. Duration of therapy is dependent upon the severity and nature of the infection:
Histoplasmosis, cryptococcosis, and *blastomycosis:* Total I.V. dose is 2 to 4 g.
Sporotrichosis: 20 mg amphotericin B daily I.V. for up to 9 months.
Aspergillosis: Total I.V. dosage of 3.6 g over 11 months
Chronic pulmonary histoplasmosis: Total I.V. dosage of

35 mg/kg; disseminated histoplasmosis may require up to 40 mg/kg.
†*Topical fungal infections (3% cream, lotion, ointment)*
Adults and children: Apply liberally and rub well into affected area b.i.d. to q.i.d.
†*Fungal meningitis*
Adults: Intrathecal injection of 25 mcg/0.1 ml diluted with 10 to 20 ml of cerebrospinal fluid (CSF) and administered by barbotage two or three times weekly. Initial dose should not exceed 100 mcg.
†*Coccidioidal arthritis*
Adults: 5 to 15 mg into joint spaces.
Cutaneous or mucocutaneous candidal infections
Adults and children: Apply topical product b.i.d., t.i.d., or q.i.d. for 1 to 3 weeks; apply up to several months for interdigital or paronychial lesions.
Note: Intrathecal and intra-articular uses are unapproved.

Pharmacodynamics
Antifungal action: Amphotericin B is *fungistatic* or *fungicidal,* depending on the concentrations available in body fluids and on the susceptibility of the fungus. It binds to sterols in the fungal cell membrane, increasing membrane permeability of fungal cells causing subsequent leakage of intracellular components; it also may interfere with some human cell membranes that contain sterols.
    The spectrum of activity includes *Histoplasma capsulatum, Coccidioides immitis, Blastomyces dermatitidis, Cryptococcus neoformans, Candida* species, *Aspergillus fumigatus, Mucor* species, *Rhizopus* species, *Absidia* species, *Entomophthora* species, *Basidiobolus* species, *Paracoccidioides brasiliensis, Sporothrix schenckii,* and *Rhodotorula* species.

Pharmacokinetics
● *Absorption:* Amphotericin B is absorbed poorly from the GI tract.
● *Distribution:* Amphotericin distributes well into inflamed pleural cavities and joints; in low concentrations into aqueous humor, bronchial secretions, pancreas, bone, muscle, and parotids. CSF concentrations reach about 3% of serum concentrations. The drug is 90% to 95% bound to plasma proteins. It reportedly crosses the placenta.
● *Metabolism:* The metabolic fate of amphotericin B is not well defined.
● *Excretion:* Amphotericin B's elimination is biphasic; second phase half-life is about 15 days. About 2% to 5% of the drug is excreted unchanged in urine. Amphotericin B is not readily removed by hemodialysis.

Contraindications and precautions
Amphotericin B is contraindicated in patients with known hypersensitivity to the drug, unless no other therapy is effective. It should be used with caution in patients taking other nephrotoxic drugs.

Interactions
Concomitant use with aminoglycosides, cisplatin, and other nephrotoxic drugs should be avoided, when possible, because of added nephrotoxic effects.
    Because amphotericin B induces hypokalemia, concomitant use with digoxin increases the risk of digitalis toxicity. Because of added potassium depletion, concomitant use with corticosteroids requires careful mon-

---

itoring of serum electrolyte levels and cardiac function.

Amphotericin B-induced hypokalemia may enhance effects of skeletal muscle relaxants. It potentiates the effects of flucytosine and other antibiotics, presumably by increasing cell membrane permeability.

Effects on diagnostic tests

Amphotericin B therapy may increase BUN, serum creatinine, alkaline phosphatase, and bilirubin levels.

Amphotericin B may cause hypokalemia and hypomagnesemia and may decrease white blood cell, red blood cell, and platelet counts.

Adverse reactions

● CNS: headache, peripheral neuropathy; with intrathecal administration – peripheral nerve pain, paresthesias.
● CV: hypotension.
● DERM: with topical application – possible dryness, erythema, burning pruritus, contact dermatitis.
● GI: anorexia, weight loss, nausea, vomiting, dyspepsia, diarrhea, epigastric cramps.
● GU: abnormal renal function with *hypokalemia, azotemia, hyposthenuria,* renal tubular acidosis, nephrocalcinosis; with large doses – permanent renal impairment, anuria, oliguria.
● HEMA: normochromic, normocytic anemia.
● Local: burning, stinging, irritation, tissue damage with extravasation, *thrombophlebitis,* pain at injection site.
● Other: arthralgia, myalgia, muscle weakness secondary to hypokalemia, *fever, chills,* anaphylactoid reactions, hypomagnesemia, malaise, generalized pain.

Overdose and treatment

Overdose may affect cardiovascular and respiratory function. Treatment is largely supportive.

▶ Special considerations

● Cultures and histologic and sensitivity testing must be completed and diagnosis confirmed before starting therapy in nonimmunocompromised patient.
● Prepare infusion as manufacturer directs, with strict aseptic technique, using *only* 10 ml of sterile water to reconstitute. To avoid precipitation, do not mix with solutions containing sodium chloride, other electrolytes, or bacteriostatic agents, such as benzyl alcohol.
● Lyophilized cake contains no preservatives. Do not use if solution contains a precipitate or other foreign particles. Store cake at 35.6° to 46.4° F. (2° to 8° C.). Protect drug from light, and check expiration date.
● For I.V. infusion, use an in-line membrane with a mean pore diameter larger than 1 micron.
● Infuse slowly; rapid infusion may cause cardiovascular collapse.
● Do not mix or piggyback antibiotics with amphotericin B infusion; the I.V. solution appears compatible with small amounts of heparin sodium, hydrocortisone sodium succinate, and methylprednisolone sodium succinate.
● Give in distal veins, and monitor site for discomfort or thrombosis; if thrombosis occurs, alternate-day therapy may be considered.
● Vital signs should be checked every 30 minutes for at least 4 hours after start of I.V. infusion; fever may appear in 1 to 2 hours but should subside within 4 hours of discontinuing drug.
● Monitor intake/output and check for changes in urine appearance or volume; renal damage may be reversible if drug is stopped at earliest sign of dysfunction.

● Monitor potassium and magnesium levels closely; monitor calcium and magnesium levels twice weekly; perform liver and renal function studies and CBCs weekly.
● Severity of some adverse reactions can be reduced by premedication with aspirin, acetaminophen, antihistamines, antiemetics, meperidine, or small doses of corticosteroids; by addition of phosphate buffer to the solution; and by alternate-day dosing. If reactions are severe, drug may have to be discontinued for varying periods.
● Use topical products for folds of groin, neck, or armpit; avoid occlusive dressing with ointment, and discontinue if signs of hypersensitivity develop.
● Topical products may stain skin or clothes.
● Store at room temperature. Solution is stable at room temperature and in indoor light for 24 hours or in refrigerator for 1 week.

Information for the patient

● Teach patient signs and symptoms of hypersensitivity and other adverse reactions, especially those associated with I.V. therapy. Warn them that they are likely to have fever and chills, which can be quite severe when therapy is initiated. These symptoms usually subside with repeated doses. Encourage patient feedback during infusion.
● Warn patient that therapy may take several months; teach personal hygiene and other measures to prevent spread and recurrence of lesions.
● Urge patient to adhere to regimen and to return as instructed for follow-up.
● Tell patient that topical products may stain skin and clothing; cream or lotion may be removed from clothing with soap and water.

Breast-feeding

Safety has not been established.

---

ampicillin

Amcill, Apo-Ampi*, Novoampicillin*, Omnipen, Penbritin*, Polycillin, Principen, Roampicillin, Super Totacillin

ampicillin sodium

Ampicin*, Ampilean*, NaMPICIL, Omnipen-N, Pen A/N, Penbritin* Polycillin-N, Totacillin-N

ampicillin trihydrate

D-Amp, Polycillin, Principen (capsules and suspension), Totacillin (capsules and suspension)

● Pharmacologic classification: aminopenicillin
● Therapeutic classification: antibiotic
● Pregnancy risk category B

How supplied

Available by prescription only
Capsules: 250 mg, 500 mg
Suspension: 100 mg/ml (pediatric drops), 125 mg/5 ml, 250 mg/5 ml, 500 mg/5 ml (after reconstitution)
Parenteral: 125 mg, 250 mg, 500 mg, 1 g, 2 g

Pharmacy bulk package: 10 g vial
Infusion: 500 mg, 1 g, 2 g

Indications, route, and dosage
Systemic infections, acute and chronic urinary tract infections caused by susceptible organisms
Adults: 1 to 4 g P.O. daily, divided into doses given q 6 hours; or 2 to 12 g I.M. or I.V. daily, divided into doses given q 4 to 6 hours.
Children: 50 to 100 mg/kg P.O. daily, divided into doses given q 6 hours; or 100 to 200 mg/kg I.M. or I.V. daily, divided into doses given q 6 hours.
Meningitis
Adults: 8 to 14 g I.V. daily for 3 days; then 8 to 14 g I.M. divided q 3 to 4 hours.
Children: Up to 400 mg/kg I.V. daily for 3 days; then up to 300 mg/kg I.M. divided q 4 hours. May be given concurrently with chloramphenicol, pending culture results.
Uncomplicated gonorrhea
Adults: 3.5 g P.O. with 1 g probenecid given as a single dose.
Dosage in renal failure
Dosing interval should be increased to q 12 hours in patients with severe renal impairment (creatinine clearance ≤10 ml/min).

Pharmacodynamics
Antibiotic action: Ampicillin is bactericidal; it adheres to bacterial penicillin-binding proteins, thus inhibiting bacterial cell wall synthesis.

Ampicillin's spectrum of action includes nonpenicillinase-producing gram-positive bacteria. It is also effective against many gram-negative organisms, including: *Neisseria gonorrhoeae, N. meningitidis, Haemophilus influenzae, Escherichia coli, Proteus mirabilis, Salmonella,* and *Shigella.* Ampicillin should be used in gram-negative systemic infections only when organism sensitivity is known.

Pharmacokinetics
● *Absorption:* Approximately 42% of ampicillin is absorbed after an oral dose; peak serum concentrations occur at 1 to 2 hours. After I.M. administration, peak serum concentrations occur at 1 hour.
● *Distribution:* Ampicillin distributes into pleural, peritoneal and synovial fluids, lungs, prostate, liver, and gallbladder; it also penetrates middle ear effusions, maxillary sinus and bronchial secretions, tonsils, and sputum. Ampicillin readily crosses the placenta; it is minimally protein-bound at 15% to 25%.
● *Metabolism:* Ampicillin is metabolized only partially.
● *Excretion:* Ampicillin is excreted in urine by renal tubular secretion and glomerular filtration. It is also excreted in breast milk. Elimination half-life is about 1 hour to 1½ hours; in patients with extensive renal impairment, half-life is extended to 10 to 24 hours.

Contraindications and precautions
Ampicillin is contraindicated in patients with known hypersensitivity to any other penicillin or to cephalosporins.

Ampicillin should not be used in patients with infectious mononucleosis because many patients develop a rash during therapy.

Ampicillin should be used cautiously in patients with renal impairment because it is excreted in urine; decreased dosage is required in moderate to severe renal failure.

Interactions
Concomitant use with an aminoglycoside antibiotic causes a synergistic bactericidal effect against some strains of enterococci and group B streptococci. However, the drugs are physically and chemically incompatible and are inactivated if mixed or given together.

Concomitant use with allopurinol appears to increase incidence of skin rash from both drugs.

Concomitant use with clavulanate results in increased bactericidal effects, because clavulanic acid is a beta-lactamase inhibitor.

Probenecid inhibits renal tubular secretion of ampicillin, raising its serum concentrations.

Large doses of penicillins may interfere with renal tubular secretion of methotrexate, thus delaying elimination and elevating serum concentrations of methotrexate.

Effects on diagnostic tests
Ampicillin alters results of urine glucose tests that use cupric sulfate (Benedict's reagent or Clinitest). Make urine glucose determinations with glucose oxidase methods (Clinistix or TesTape).

Ampicillin may falsely decrease serum aminoglycoside concentrations.

Adverse reactions
● GI: nausea, vomiting, *diarrhea,* glossitis, stomatitis, *pseudomembranous colitis.*
● GU: acute interstitial nephritis.
● HEMA: anemia, thrombocytopenia, thrombocytopenic purpura, eosinophilia, leukopenia.
● Local: pain at injection site, vein irritation, thrombophlebitis.
● Other: *hypersensitivity (erythematous maculopapular rash, urticaria, anaphylaxis),* bacterial and fungal superinfection.
Note: Drug should be discontinued if immediate hypersensitivity reaction occurs or if bone marrow toxicity, pseudomembranous colitis, or acute interstitial nephritis develops.

Overdose and treatment
Clinical signs of overdose include neuromuscular sensitivity or seizures. After recent ingestion (within 4 hours), empty the stomach by induced emesis or gastric lavage; follow with activated charcoal to reduce absorption. Ampicillin can be removed by hemodialysis.

▶ Special considerations
Besides those relevant to all *penicillins,* consider the following recommendation.
● Administer I.M. or I.V. only when patient is too ill to take oral drug.

Information for the patient
Encourage patient to report diarrhea promptly.

Geriatric use
Because of diminished renal tubular secretion in elderly patients, half-life of drug may be prolonged.

Breast-feeding
Use cautiously. Ampicillin is distributed readily into breast milk; safety in breast-feeding women has not been established.

---

*Canada only   †Unlabeled clinical use   Italicized adverse reactions are life-threatening.

ampicillin sodium/sulbactam sodium
Unasyn

- Pharmacologic classification: aminopenicillin/beta-lactamase inhibitor combination
- Therapeutic classification: antibiotic
- Pregnancy risk category B

How supplied
Available by prescription only
Injection: Vials and piggyback vials containing 1.5 g (1 g ampicillin sodium with 500 mg sulbactam sodium) and 3 g (2 g ampicillin sodium with 1 g sulbactam sodium)

Indications, route, and dosage
Skin and skin-structure infections, intra-abdominal and gynecologic infections caused by susceptible beta-lactamase-producing strains of Staphylococcus aureus, Escherichia coli, Klebsiella *(including* K. pneumoniae*),* Proteus mirabilis, Bacteroides *(including* B. fragilis*),* Enterobacter, *and* Acinetobacter calcoaceticus
Adults: 1.5 to 3 g I.M. or I.V. q 6 hours. Do not exceed 4 g/day sulbactam sodium.
Dosage in renal failure

Creatinine clearance (ml/min/ 1.73 m²)	Half-life (hours)	Recommended dosage
≥30	1	1.5 to 3 g q 6 to 8 hr
15 to 29	5	1.5 to 3 g q 12 hr
5 to 14	9	1.5 to 3 g q 24 hr

Pharmacodynamics
Antibiotic action: Ampicillin is bactericidal; it adheres to bacterial penicillin-binding proteins, thus inhibiting bacterial cell wall synthesis. Sulbactam inhibits beta-lactamase, an enzyme produced by ampicillin-resistant bacteria that degrades ampicillin.

Pharmacokinetics
- *Absorption:* Peak plasma levels occur immediately after I.V. infusion and within 1 hour after I.M. injection.
- *Distribution:* Both drugs distribute into pleural, peritoneal and synovial fluids, lungs, prostate, liver, and gallbladder; they also penetrate middle ear effusions, maxillary sinus and bronchial secretions, tonsils, and sputum. Ampicillin readily crosses the placenta; it is minimally protein-bound at 15% to 25%; sulbactam is about 38% bound.
- *Metabolism:* Both drugs are metabolized only partially; only 15% to 25% of both drugs are metabolized.
- *Excretion:* Both ampicillin and sulbactam are excreted in the urine by renal tubular secretion and glomerular filtration. It is also excreted in breast milk. Elimination half-life is 1 to 1½ hours; in patients with extensive renal impairment, half-life can be as long as 10 to 24 hours.

Contraindications and precautions
Ampicillin/sulbactam is contraindicated in patients with a history of hypersensitivity to any penicillin because this combination may cause a serious anaphylactoid reaction. Patients with mononucleosis may develop a skin rash after treatment with ampicillin; avoid ampicillin/sulbactam therapy in these patients.

Interactions
Concomitant use with probenecid decreases excretion of both ampicillin and sulbactam; with allopurinol may lead to an increased incidence of skin rash. The ampicillin component may cause *in vitro* inactivation of aminoglycosides if these antibiotics are mixed in the same infusion container.

Effects on diagnostic tests
Ampicillin alters results of urine glucose tests that use cupric sulfate (Benedict's reagent or Clinitest). Make urine glucose determinations with glucose oxidase methods (Clinistix or Tes-Tape).
In pregnant women, transient decreases in serum estradiol, conjugated estrone, conjugated estriol, and estriol glucuronide may occur.

Adverse reactions
- DERM: *exfoliative dermatitis.*
- GI: nausea, vomiting, *diarrhea,* glossitis, stomatitis, *pseudomembranous colitis.*
- HEMA: anemia, thrombocytopenia, thrombocytopenic purpura, eosinophilia, leukopenia.
- Local: pain at injection site, vein irritation, thrombophlebitis.
- Other: *hypersensitivity (erythematous maculopapular rash, urticaria, anaphylaxis),* bacterial and fungal superinfection.
  Note: Drug should be discontinued if immediate hypersensitivity reaction, bone marrow toxicity, pseudomembranous colitis, or acute interstitial nephritis develops.

Overdose and treatment
Neurologic adverse reactions, including seizures, are likely. Treatment is supportive. Although confirming data is lacking, ampicillin and sulbactam are likely to be removed by hemodialysis.

Special considerations
- I.V. administration should be given by slow injection over at least 10 to 15 minutes or infused in greater dilutions with 50 to 100 ml of a compatible diluent over 15 to 30 minutes.
- For I.V. use, reconstitute powder in piggyback units to desired concentrations with sterile water for injection, 0.9% sodium chloride injection, 5% dextrose injection, lactated Ringer's injection, M/6 sodium lactate injection, 5% dextrose in 0.45% saline, or 10% invert sugar.
- If piggyback bottles are unavailable, reconstitute standard vials of sterile powder with sterile water for injection to yield solutions of 375 mg/ml (250 mg ampicillin/125 mg sulbactam). Then immediately dilute an appropriate volume with a suitable diluent to yield solutions of 3 to 45 mg/ml (2 to 30 mg ampicillin/1 to 15 mg sulbactam per ml).
- For I.M. injection, reconstitute with sterile water for injection, or 0.5% or 2% lidocaine HCl injection. To obtain 375 mg/ml solutions (250 mg ampicillin/125 mg sulbactam/ml), add contents of the 1.5-g vial to 3.2 ml of diluent to produce 4 ml withdrawal volume; add 3-g

---

*Canada only   †Unlabeled clinical use   Italicized adverse reactions are life-threatening.

vial to 6.4 ml of diluent to produce 8 ml withdrawal volume.
• Reconstituted solutions are stable for varying periods (from 2 hours to 72 hours) depending on diluent used. Check with pharmacist. For patients on sodium restriction, note that a 1.5-g dose of ampicillin sodium/sulbactam sodium yields 5 mEq of sodium.

Geriatric use
Because of diminished renal tubular secretion in elderly patients, half-life of drug may be prolonged.

Pediatric use
Safe use in children under age 12 is not established.

Breast-feeding
Ampicillin is distributed readily into breast milk; safety in breast-feeding women has not been established. Alternative feeding method is recommended during therapy.

amrinone lactate
Inocor Lactate Injection

• Pharmacologic classification: bipyridine derivative
• Therapeutic classification: inotropic, vasodilator
• Pregnancy risk category C

How supplied
Available by prescription only
Injection: 5 mg/ml

Indications, route, and dosage
Short-term management of congestive heart failure
Adults: Initially, 0.75 mg/kg I.V. bolus over 2 to 3 minutes; then, begin maintenance infusion of 5 to 10 mcg/kg/minute. Additional bolus of 0.75 mg/kg may be given 30 minutes after therapy starts. Maximum daily dose is 10 mg/kg.

Pharmacodynamics
• *Vasodilating action:* The primary vasodilating effect of amrinone seems to stem from a direct effect on peripheral vessels.
• *Inotropic action:* The mechanism of action responsible for the apparent inotropic effect is not fully understood; however, it may be associated with inhibition of phosphodiesterase activity, resulting in increased cellular levels of adenosine 3',5'-cyclic phosphate; this, in turn, may alter intracellular and extracellular calcium levels. The role of calcium homeostasis has not been determined. Clinical effects include increased cardiac output mediated by reduced afterload and, possibly, inotropism.

Pharmacokinetics
• *Absorption:* With I.V. administration, onset of action occurs in 2 to 5 minutes, with peak effects in about 10 minutes. Cardiovascular effects may persist for 1 to 2 hours.
• *Distribution:* Distribution volume is 1.2 liters/kg. Distribution sites are unknown. Protein binding ranges from 10% to 49%. Therapeutic steady-state serum levels

range from 0.5 to 7 mcg/ml (ideal concentration: 3 mcg/ml).
• *Metabolism:* Amrinone is metabolized in the liver to several metabolites of unknown activity.
• *Excretion:* In normal patients, amrinone is excreted in the urine, with a terminal elimination half-life of about 4 hours. Half-life may be prolonged slightly in patients with congestive heart failure.

Contraindications and precautions
Amrinone is contraindicated in patients with known hypersensitivity to amrinone or sulfites (because sodium metabisulfite is used as a preservative). In patients with severe aortic or pulmonary valvular disease, amrinone should not be used in place of surgery. It should be used with caution in patients with hypertrophic subaortic stenosis, because it may exacerbate outflow tract obstruction; in patients recovering from acute myocardial infarction (in acute phase), because it may be arrhythmogenic; in patients with hepatic disease, because it may be hepatotoxic; and in patients with renal impairment, because of the potential for drug accumulation.

Interactions
Concomitant use with disopyramide may cause severe hypotension.

Effects on diagnostic tests
The physiologic effects of amrinone may decrease serum potassium or increase serum hepatic enzymes.

Adverse reactions
• CV: *arrhythmias,* hypotension.
• GI: nausea, vomiting, cramps, dyspepsia, diarrhea.
• HEMA: reversible thrombocytopenia.
• Hepatic: enzyme elevation, possible hepatotoxicity.
• Local: burning at injection site.
• Other: hypersensitivity.
 Note: Drug should be discontinued if thrombocytopenia becomes clinically significant.

Overdose and treatment
Clinical effects of overdose include severe hypotension. Treatment may include administration of a potent vasopressor, such as norepinephrine, as well as other general supportive measures, including cautious fluid volume replacement.

▶ Special considerations
• Administer drug as supplied or dilute in normal or half-normal saline solution to concentration of 1 to 3 mg/ml. Do not dilute drug with solutions containing dextrose because slow chemical reaction occurs over 24 hours. However, amrinone can be injected into running dextrose infusions through Y-connector or directly into tubing. Use diluted solution within 24 hours.
• Do not administer furosemide in I.V. lines containing amrinone, as a chemical reaction occurs immediately.
• Monitor blood pressure and heart rate throughout infusion. Infusion should be slowed or stopped if patient's blood pressure falls or if cardiac arrhythmias (ventricular or supraventricular) occur. Dosage may need to be reduced.
• Monitor platelet counts. A count below 150,000 mm³ usually necessitates dosage reduction.
• Monitor electrolyte levels (especially potassium) because drug increases cardiac output, which may cause diuresis.

● Monitor liver function tests to detect hepatic damage (rare).
● Observe for adverse gastrointestinal effects (such as nausea, vomiting, and diarrhea); reduce dosage or discontinue drug.
● Amrinone is prescribed primarily for patients who have not responded to therapy with digitalis, diuretics, and vasodilators.

Pediatric use
Safety and effectiveness in children under age 18 has not been established.

Breast-feeding
Drug may be excreted in breast milk. Safety in breast-feeding women has not been established.

amsacrine (m-AMSA)
Amsa P-D*

● Pharmacologic classification: acridine dye derivative
● Therapeutic classification: antineoplastic
● Pregnancy risk category C

How supplied
Available only through investigational protocols
Injection: 50 mg/ml

Indications, route, and dosage
Dosage and indications may vary. Check current literature for recommended protocol.
†*Acute lymphocytic leukemia*
Adults: Induction, 75, 100, or 125 mg/m² I.V. daily infusion (over 60 to 90 minutes) for 5 days. Repeat q 3 to 4 weeks. Maintenance dose, one-half the induction dose, repeated q 7 to 8 weeks.

Pharmacodynamics
Antineoplastic action: Amsacrine exerts its cytotoxic activity by intercalating between DNA base pairs, thus inhibiting DNA synthesis.

Pharmacokinetics
● *Absorption:* Drug is administered I.V. only and is immediately absorbed.
● *Distribution:* Amsacrine is distributed mainly in the liver. The drug probably does not cross the blood-brain barrier to a significant extent.
● *Metabolism:* Amsacrine is metabolized extensively in the liver.
● *Excretion:* The elimination of amsacrine from the plasma appears to be biphasic, with a half-life of 12 minutes in the initial phase and 2½ hours in the terminal phase. The metabolites of amsacrine are excreted in urine and bile.

Contraindications and precautions
There are no reported contraindications for amsacrine. Drug should be used cautiously in patients with impaired liver function.

Interactions
Amsacrine and heparin are physically incompatible. Admixture of these two agents results in the formation of a precipitate.

Effects on diagnostic tests
Amsacrine therapy may increase serum concentrations of bilirubin and alkaline phosphatase, indicating drug-induced cholestasis or hepatotoxicity.

Adverse reactions
● CNS: *seizures* at doses as low as 40 mg/m²/day.
● CV: *ventricular arrhythmias* and *cardiac arrest* (rare), possibly caused by the diluent.
● GI: mild nausea and vomiting, stomatitis at higher doses.
● HEMA: *leukopenia* (usually dose-limiting), mild thrombocytopenia; *bone marrow depression* (dose-limiting).
● Local: vein irritation, phlebitis.

Overdose and treatment
Clinical manifestations of overdose include myelosuppression, nausea, and vomiting.
Treatment is usually supportive and includes transfusion of blood components and antiemetics.

▶ Special considerations
● To prepare solution for administration, two sterile liquids are combined. Add 1.5 ml from the amsacrine ampule (50 mg/ml) to the vial containing 13.5 ml of lactic acid. The combined solution will contain 5 mg/ml of amsacrine.
● Use a glass syringe for preparation of amsacrine, because the alcohol diluent quickly melts plastic unless buffer is added.
● Solutions for infusion are stable at least 48 hours at room temperature. Use undiluted mixture within 8 hours; it does not contain a preservative.
● The solution may be further diluted for infusion with dextrose 5% in water (D₅W) to minimize vein irritation. Administer doses of less than 100 mg in at least 100 ml of D₅W, doses from 100 to 199 mg in 250 ml D₅W, and doses 200 mg or greater in a minimum of 500 ml D₅W.
● Solutions should be infused slowly over several hours to minimize vein irritation.
● Do not add amsacrine to normal saline or other chloride-containing solution. Precipitation may occur.
● Do not administer amsacrine through membrane-type in-line filters. The diluent may dissolve the filter.
● Monitor CBC and liver function tests.
● Patient's urine will appear orange.
● Monitor patient closely for CNS and cardiac toxicity during administration.
● Avoid direct contact of amsacrine with skin because of possible sensitization.

Information for the patient
● Encourage adequate fluid intake to increase urine output, and to facilitate excretion of uric acid.
● Tell patient to avoid exposure to people with infections.
● Warn patient that the drug will turn urine orange.

Pediatric use
Safety not established.

Breast-feeding
It is not known whether amsacrine distributes into breast milk. However, because of the potential for serious adverse reactions, mutagenicity, and carcinogenicity in the infant, breast-feeding is not recommended.

---

*Canada only   †Unlabeled clinical use   Italicized adverse reactions are life-threatening.

amyl nitrite

- Pharmacologic classification: nitrate
- Therapeutic classification: vasodilator, cyanide poisoning adjunct
- Pregnancy risk category C

How supplied
Available by prescription only
Nasal inhalant: 0.18 ml, 0.3 ml

Indications, route, and dosage
Angina pectoris
Adults: 0.18 to 0.3 ml by inhalation (one glass ampule inhaler), p.r.n.
†*Adjunct treatment of cyanide poisoning*
Adults and children: 0.3 ml by inhalation for 15 to 30 seconds; repeat every 60 seconds until I.V. sodium nitrite infusion and I.V. sodium thiosulfate infusion are available.

Pharmacodynamics
Vasodilating action: Amyl nitrite reduces myocardial oxygen demand by decreasing left ventricular end-diastolic pressure (preload) and systemic vascular resistance and arterial pressure (afterload). It also increases collateral coronary blood flow. By relaxing vascular smooth muscle, it produces generalized vasodilation. Amyl nitrite also relaxes all other smooth muscle, including bronchial and biliary smooth muscle. In cyanide poisoning, it converts hemoglobin to methemoglobin which reacts with cyanide to form cyanmet-hemoglobin.

Pharmacokinetics
- *Absorption:* Inhaled amyl nitrite is absorbed readily through the respiratory tract; action begins in 30 seconds and lasts 3 to 5 minutes.
- *Distribution:* Not available.
- *Metabolism:* Amyl nitrite, an organic nitrite, is metabolized by the liver to form inorganic nitrites, which are much less potent vasodilators than the parent drug.
- *Excretion:* One third of the inhaled dose is excreted in urine.

Contraindications and precautions
Amyl nitrite is contraindicated in patients with severe anemia or hypersensitivity, head trauma, or cerebral hemorrhage because it dilates the meningeal vessels. Use cautiously in patients with hypotension or glaucoma. Because it reduces maternal blood pressure and blood flow to the placenta, amyl nitrite could harm the fetus if administered to a pregnant woman.

Interactions
Concomitant use of alcohol, phenothiazines, beta blockers, or antihypertensives may cause excessive hypotension.

Effects on diagnostic tests
Amyl nitrite therapy alters the Zlatkis-Zak color reaction, causing a false decrease in serum cholesterol levels.

Adverse reactions
- CNS: severe, persistent (sometimes throbbing) headache; dizziness; weakness; muscle twitching.
- CV: orthostatic hypotension, tachycardia, palpitations, fainting.
- DERM: cutaneous vasodilation, visible flushing on face and neck; perspiration; cold sweats.
- GI: nausea, vomiting.
- HEMA: methemoglobinemia.
  Note: Drug should be discontinued if a severe drop in blood pressure occurs or if patient faints.

Overdose and treatment
Clinical signs of overdose include methemoglobinemia, characterized by blue skin and mucous membranes, hypotension, tachycardia, palpatations, skin changes, diaphoresis, dizziness, syncope, vertigo, headache, nausea, vomiting, anorexia, increased intracranial pressure, confusion, moderate fever, and paralysis. Hypoxia may lead to metabolic acidosis, cyanosis, convulsions, coma, and cardiac collapse. Treat with high flow oxygen and methylene blue. Usual dose of methylene blue for adults and children is 1 to 2 mg/kg I.V. given slowly over several minutes. In severe cases, this dose may be repeated only once; doses exceeding 4 mg/kg may produce methemoglobinemia.

▶ Special considerations
- Rarely used as an antianginal.
- Keep patient sitting or lying down during and immediately after inhalation. Crush ampule (has a woven gauze covering) between fingers, and hold to nose for inhalation.
- Monitor for orthostatic hypotension; do not allow patient to make rapid postural changes while inhaling drug.
- Amyl nitrite is highly flammable; keep away from open flame and extinguish all cigarettes before use.
- Amyl nitrite is used illegally to enhance sexual pleasure, chiefly by homosexuals. Street names include "Amy" and "poppers."

Information for the patient
- Explain that ampule must be crushed to release drug.
- Warn patient to use drug only when seated or lying down.

Geriatric use
Orthostatic hypotensive effects may be more likely to occur in elderly patients.

Pediatric use
Safety and efficacy have not been established.

Breast-feeding
It is unknown whether amyl nitrite is excreted in breast milk; risk and benefit must be considered.

PHARMACOLOGIC CLASS

anabolic steroids

nandrolone decanoate
nandrolone phenpropionate
oxandrolone
oxymetholone
stanozolol
testolactone

The anabolic steroids are closely related to the naturally occurring androgen testosterone. They result from efforts to produce drugs with the anabolic (tissue-building) properties of testosterone, but without testosterone's androgenic properties. While the anabolic steroids have a higher ratio of anabolic to androgenic activity than testosterone, they all retain some androgenic activity.

Pharmacology
The anabolic steroids enhance anabolic (tissue-building) processes and reverse catabolic (tissue breakdown) processes. They improve nitrogen balance in the presence of an adequate diet and have antianemic effects related to stimulation of erythropoietin production. The exact mechanism of action of the anabolic steroids is not known. These compounds also have androgenic effects similar to those of the androgens.

Clinical indications and actions
Catabolic states
In patients suffering significant weight loss from chronic infection, severe trauma, or corticosteroid-induced catabolism, the anabolic steroids may promote weight gain, provided an adequate diet is maintained. These agents can only be considered adjunctive therapy for this purpose and do not replace specific therapy.
Anemias
Anabolic steroids may be used to treat certain anemias refractory to conventional therapy. Nandrolone decanoate is indicated to treat anemia associated with renal insufficiency. Oxymetholone is indicated to treat aplastic and hypoplastic anemias and myelofibrosis.
Osteoporosis
Anabolic steroids are indicated to treat bone pain, weakness, and weight loss associated with osteoporosis.
Breast cancer
Nandrolone phenpropionate is indicated to treat metastatic breast cancer, especially hormone-responsive tumors. Testolactone is indicated for adjunctive use in the palliative treatment of advanced or disseminated breast carcinoma in postmenopausal women.
†Hereditary angioedema
Stanozolol is indicated as a prophylactic agent to decrease the frequency and severity of attacks in this disorder.
†Precocious puberty
Testolactone is used in the management of precocious puberty in girls with McCune-Albright syndrome.

Overview of adverse reactions
Virilization is the most common adverse effect associated with use of the anabolic steroid agents. In prepubertal males, enlargement of the penis and an increased frequency of erection are to be expected. Hirsutism and increased skin pigmentation also may occur. In postpubertal males, priapism, bladder irritability (frequency and urgency), testicular atrophy, receding hairline, or gynecomastia may occur. Oligospermia and decreased libido occur with prolonged use.

In females, deepening of the voice, hair growth, clitoral enlargement, and irregular or absent menstrual cycles may occur. Vocal and clitoral changes commonly do not revert to normal, even after discontinuation of the drug. Oily skin and acne may occur in all age-groups of both sexes.

Metabolic reactions are also common and may include retention of fluid and electrolytes (resulting in weight gain and sometimes edema) and increases in serum calcium (hypercalcemia may occur in women with metastatic breast cancer), creatinine, phosphorous, and cholesterol levels. Serum glucose levels are commonly decreased. Paresthesia, aches and edema of extremeties, glossitis, anorexia, hot flashes, nausea, vomiting, and diarrhea have occurred in patients receiving testolactone.

Hepatic dysfunction, sometimes severe, has occasionally been linked to use of anabolic steroids.

▶ Special considerations
● Anabolic steroids are contraindicated in patients with hypersensitivity to the drug; in patients with prostatic hypertrophy with obstruction; prostatic and male breast cancer; cardiac, hepatic, or renal decompensation; and nephrosis; and in premature infants. Use cautiously in prepubertal males; in patients with diabetes or coronary diseases; and in patients taking adrenocorticotropic hormone, corticosteroids, or anticoagulants.
● *Anabolic steroids should not be used to improve athletic performance.* Risks associated with their use for this purpose far outweigh any possible benefits. Proof of anabolic steroid use is grounds for disqualification in many athletic events. Some states impose criminal penalties on physicians who prescribe anabolic steroids for this purpose. Anabolic steroids are now classified as schedule III controlled substances and their distribution is regulated by the Drug Enforcement Agency.
● Hypercalcemia symptoms may be difficult to distinguish from symptoms of condition being treated unless anticipated and thought of as a cluster. Hypercalcemia is most likely to occur in metastatic breast cancer and may indicate bone metastases.
● Watch female patients for signs of virilization. If possible, discontinue therapy when virilization first becomes apparent because some adverse effects (deepening of voice, clitoral enlargement) are irreversible.
● Edema usually is controllable with salt restriction, diuretics, or both. Monitor weight routinely.
● Watch for symptoms of jaundice. Dosage adjustment may reverse condition. Periodic liver function tests are recommended.
● Observe patient on concomitant anticoagulant therapy for ecchymotic areas, petechiae, or abnormal bleeding. Monitor prothrombin time.
● Watch for symptoms of hypoglycemia in patients with diabetes. Change of antihypoglycemic drug dosage may be required.
● Patients with metastatic breast cancer should have regular determinations of serum calcium levels to identify potential for serious hypercalcemia.
● Anabolic steroids may alter many laboratory studies during therapy and for 2 to 3 weeks after therapy is stopped.
● Use with diet high in calories and protein unless contraindicated. Give small, frequent meals.

Information for the patient
● Tell patient to take drug with food or meals if GI upset occurs.
● Tell female patient to report menstrual irregularities; therapy should be discontinued pending etiologic determination.

Geriatric use
Elderly male patients should be observed carefully for signs of prostatic hypertrophy or cancer.

Pediatric use
Anabolic steroids should be used with caution in prepubertal children. Boys should be closely observed for precocious development of male sexual characteristics.

Girls should be closely observed for signs and symptoms of virilization. In children, X-rays of wrist bones should establish level of bone maturation before therapy is initiated. During treatment, bone maturation may proceed more rapidly than linear growth. Intermittent dosage and periodic X-rays are recommended to monitor skeletal effects.

Breast-feeding

The degree of excretion of anabolic steroids into breast milk is unknown; because of the risk of adverse effects to the infant, women receiving anabolic steroids should not breast-feed.

Representative combinations
None.

androgens

danazol
fluoxymesterone
methyltestosterone
testosterone
testosterone cypionate
testosterone enanthate
testosterone propionate

Testosterone is the endogenous androgen (male sex hormone). The testosterone esters (cypionate, enanthate, propionate), methyltestosterone, and fluoxymesterone are synthetic derivatives with greater potency or longer duration of action than testosterone.

Pharmacology

Testosterone promotes maturation of the male sexual organs and the development of secondary sexual characteristics (facial and body hair, vocal cord thickening). Testosterone also causes the growth spurt of adolescence and terminates growth of the long bones by closing the epiphyses (growth plates at the ends of bones). Testosterone promotes retention of calcium, nitrogen, phosphorus, sodium, and potassium and enhances anabolism (tissue building). Through negative feedback on the pituitary, exogenously administered testosterone (and other androgenic drugs) decreases endogenous testosterone production and to some degree inhibits spermatogenesis in males. Androgens repeatedly stimulate production of erythrocytes, apparently by enhancing the production of erythropoietic stimulating factor.

Clinical indications and actions
Androgen deficiency

Androgens (testosterone, all testosterone esters, methyltestosterone, fluoxymestrerone) are indicated to treat androgen deficiency resulting from testicular failure or castration, or gonadotropin or luteinizing hormone releasing hormone deficiency of pituitary origin. Methyltestosterone and testosterone cypionate are also indicated to treat male climacteric symptoms and impotence when these are caused by androgen deficiency.

Delayed male puberty

All androgens may be used to stimulate the onset of puberty when it is significantly delayed and psychological support proves insufficient.

Breast cancer

Testosterone, all testosterone esters, and fluoxymesterone are indicated for palliative treatment of metastatic breast cancer in women during the first 5 postmenopausal years. Androgens also may be used in premenopausal women with metastatic disease if the tumor is hormone-responsive.

Postpartum breast engorgement

Fluoxymesterone, testosterone, methyltestosterone, and testosterone propionate are indicated to treat painful postpartum breast engorgement in non-breast-feeding women.

†Hereditary angioedema

Danazol is indicated in the prophylaxis of angioedema attacks.

Endometriosis

Danazol is indicated for palliative treatment of endometriosis. Danazol relieves pain and helps resolve endometrial lesions in 30% to 80% of patients who receive it. Endometriosis usually recurs 8 to 12 months after danazol is discontinued.

Fibrocystic breast disease

Danazol is indicated for palliative treatment of fibrocystic breast disease unresponsive to simple therapy. It usually relieves pain before it reduces nodularity. Fibrocystic breast disease recurs in about half of patients treated successfully with danazol, usually 1 year after discontinuing the drug.

Overview of adverse reactions

The most common side effects associated with androgen therapy are extensions of the hormonal action. In males, frequent and prolonged erections, bladder irritability (causing frequent urination), and gynecomastia (swelling or tenderness of breast tissue) may occur. In females, clitoral enlargement, deepening of the voice, growth of facial or body hair, unusual hair loss, and irregular or absent menses may occur. Note that deepening of the voice may be irreversible even with prompt discontinuation of the drug. Oily skin or acne occurs commonly in both sexes.

Metabolic side effects include retention of fluid and electrolytes (occasionally resulting in edema), increased serum calcium levels (hypercalcemia may occur, especially in women receiving the drug for breast cancer metastatic to bone), decreased blood glucose levels, and increased serum cholesterol levels.

Long-term administration of androgens may cause loss of libido and suppression of spermatogenesis in males. Serious, although rare, hepatic dysfunction, including hepatic necrosis and hepatocellular carcinoma, has been reported in prolonged androgen administration.

▶ Special considerations

● Do not administer androgens to males with breast or prostatic cancer, or symptomatic prostatic hypertrophy; to patients with severe cardiac, renal, or hepatic disease; or to patients with undiagnosed abnormal genital bleeding.

● Administration of androgens during pregnancy may cause masculinization of the female fetus and is therefore contraindicated.

● Hypercalcemia symptoms may be difficult to distinguish from symptoms of the condition being treated unless anticipated and thought of as a cluster. Hypercalcemia is most likely to occur in women with breast cancer, particularly when metastatic to bone.

● Priapism in males indicates that dosage is excessive.

Serious acute toxicities from large overdoses have not been reported.

• Yellowing of the sclera of the eyes, or of the skin, may indicate hepatic dysfunction resulting from administration of androgens.

Information for the patient
• *Androgens should not be used to improve athletic performance.* Risks associated with their use for this purpose far outweigh any possible benefits. Proof of androgen use is grounds for disqualification in many athletic events. Some states impose criminal penalties on physicians who prescribe androgens for this purpose. Androgens are now classified as schedule III controlled substances and their distribution is regulated by the Drug Enforcement Agency.
• Tell patient to report GI upset, which may be caused by the drug.
• Virilization, including *hirsutism*, deepening of voice, or clitoral enlargement, may not be reversible upon discontinuation of drug.
• Explain to female patients that medication may cause menstrual cycle irregularities in premenopausal women and withdrawal bleeding in postmenopausal women.

Geriatric use
Elderly male patients receiving androgens may be at increased risk for prostatic hypertrophy and prostatic carcinoma. Androgens are contraindicated in the presence of prostatic hypertrophy with obstruction because they can aggravate this condition.

Pediatric use
Children receiving androgens must be observed carefully for excessive virilization and precocious puberty. Androgen therapy may cause premature epiphyseal closure and short stature. Regular X-ray examinations of hand bones may be used to monitor skeletal maturation during therapy.

Breast-feeding
The degree of androgen excretion in breast milk is unknown. Because androgens may induce premature sexual development (in males) or virilization (in females), women who are receiving androgens should not breast-feed their infants.

Representative combinations
Testosterone cypionate with estradiol cypionate: Andro/Fem, De-Comberol, depAndrogyn, Depo-Testadiol, Depotestogen, Duo Cyp, Duratestrin, Menoject-L.A., Testadiate-Depo, Test-Estro Cypionate.

Testosterone enanthate with estradiol valerate: Andrest, Andro-Estro, Androgyn L.A., Deladumone, Deladumone OB, Ditate DS, Duo-Gen L.A., Duogex L.A.*, Duoval PA, Estrand*, Estra-Testrin, Neo-Pause*, Teev, Testradiol L.A., Valertest.

Fluoxymesterone with ethinyl estradiol: Halodrin.

angiotensin-converting enzyme inhibitors

captopril
enalapril maleate
fosinopril sodium
lisinopril
quinapril
ramipril

Angiotensin-converting enzyme (ACE) inhibitors are relatively new therapeutic agents used to manage hypertension and congestive heart failure.

Pharmacology
ACE inhibitors prevent the conversion of angiotensin I to angiotensin II, a potent vasoconstrictor. Besides decreasing vasoconstriction, and thus reducing peripheral arterial resistance, inhibition of angiotensin II decreases adrenocortical secretion of aldosterone. This results in decreased sodium and water retention and extracellular fluid volume.

Clinical indications and actions
Hypertension, CHF
ACE inhibitors are used to treat hypertension; their antihypertensive effects are secondary to decreased sodium and water retention.

Captopril and enalapril are used to manage congestive heart failure; they decrease systemic vascular resistance (afterload) and pulmonary capillary wedge pressure (preload). ACE inhibitors may also increase cardiac output.

Overview of adverse reactions
The most common adverse effects of therapeutic doses of ACE inhibitors are headache, fatigue, tachycardia, dysgeusia, proteinuria, hyperkalemia, rash, cough, and angioedema of the face and extremities. Severe hypotension usually occurs at toxic drug levels. ACE inhibitors should be used cautiously in patients with impaired renal function or serious autoimmune disease, and in patients taking other drugs known to depress white blood cell (WBC) count or immune response. Proteinuria and nephrotic syndrome may occur; reevaluate therapy if proteinuria is persistent or exceeds 1 g/day.

▶ Special considerations
• Discontinue diuretic therapy 2 to 3 days before beginning ACE inhibitor therapy to reduce risk of hypotension; if drug does not adequately control blood pressure, reinstate diuretics.
• Perform WBC and differential counts before treatment, every 2 weeks for 3 months, and periodically thereafter.
• Lower dosage is necessary in patients with impaired renal function.
• Use potassium supplements with caution because ACE inhibitors may cause potassium retention.

Information for the patient
• Tell patient to report feelings of light-headedness, especially in first few days, so dose can be adjusted; signs of infection such as sore throat and fever, because drugs may decrease WBC count; facial swelling or dif-

ficulty breathing, because drugs may cause angio-edema; and loss of taste, which may necessitate discontinuation of the drug.
• Advise patient to avoid sudden position changes to minimize orthostatic hypotension.
• Warn patient to seek medical approval before taking self-prescribed cold preparations.
• Tell patient to contact physician if troublesome cough develops.

Geriatric use
Elderly patients may need lower doses because of impaired drug clearance.

Pediatric use
Safety and efficacy of ACE inhibitors in children have not been established; use only if potential benefit outweighs risk.

Breast-feeding
Captopril and enalapril are distributed into breast milk, but their effect on infants is unknown. An alternative feeding method is recommended during therapy.

Representative combinations
Captopril with hydrochlorothiazide: Capozide.
Enalapril with hydrochlorothiazide: Vaseretic.

---

anisotropine methylbromide
Valpin 50

• Pharmacologic classification: anticholinergic, synthetic belladonna alkaloid derivative
• Therapeutic classification: antimuscarinic, gastrointestinal antispasmodic
• Pregnancy risk category C

How supplied
Available by prescription only
Tablets: 50 mg

Indications, route, and dosage
Adjunctive treatment of peptic ulcer
Adults: 50 mg P.O. t.i.d. To be effective, should be titrated to individual patient needs.

Pharmacodynamics
Anticholinergic action: Anisotropine competitively blocks acetylcholine at cholinergic neuroeffector sites, inhibiting gastric acid secretion.

Pharmacokinetics
• *Absorption:* Anisotropine is poorly absorbed from the GI tract; less than 10% of the drug is absorbed when taken orally.
• *Distribution:* Unknown.
• *Metabolism:* Unknown.
• *Excretion:* Absorbed drug is excreted in the urine as unchanged drug and metabolites.

Contraindications and precautions
Anisotropine is contraindicated in patients with narrow-angle glaucoma, because drug-induced cycloplegia and mydriasis may increase intraocular pressure; in patients with obstructive uropathy, obstructive GI tract

disease, severe ulcerative colitis, myasthenia gravis, paralytic ileus, intestinal atony, or toxic megacolon, because the drug may exacerbate these conditions; and in patients with known hypersensitivity to anticholinergics.

Administer anisotropine cautiously to patients with autonomic neuropathy, hyperthyroidism, coronary artery disease, cardiac arrhythmias, congestive heart failure, or ulcerative colitis, because drug can exacerbate symptoms of these disorders; to patients with hepatic or renal disease, because toxic accumulation can occur; to patients over age 40, because the drug may increase the risk of glaucoma; to patients with hiatal hernia associated with reflux esophagitis, because the drug may decrease lower esophageal sphincter tone; and in hot or humid environments, because the drug may contribute to heatstroke.

Interactions
Concurrent administration of antacids decreases oral absorption of anticholinergics. Administer anisotropine at least 1 hour before antacids.

Concomitant administration of drugs with anticholinergic effects may cause additive toxicity.

Decreased GI absorption of many drugs has been reported after the use of anticholinergics (for example, levodopa and ketoconazole). Conversely, slowly dissolving digoxin tablets may yield higher serum digoxin levels when administered with anticholinergics.

Use cautiously with oral potassium supplements (especially wax-matrix formulations) because the incidence of potassium-induced GI ulcerations may be increased.

Effects on diagnostic tests
None reported.

Adverse reactions
• CNS: headache, insomnia, drowsiness, dizziness, confusion or excitement (in elderly patients), nervousness, weakness.
• CV: palpitations, tachycardia, orthostatic hypertension.
• DERM: urticaria, decreased sweating or anhidrosis, other dermal manifestations.
• EENT: blurred vision, mydriasis, increased ocular pressure, cycloplegia, photophobia.
• GI: dry mouth, dysphagia, heartburn, loss of taste, nausea, vomiting, paralytic ileus, constipation.
• GU: urinary hesitancy and retention, impotence.
• Other: fever, allergic reactions.
Note: Drug should be discontinued if hypersensitivity, urinary retention, confusion or excitement, curare-like symptoms, or skin rash develops.

Overdose and treatment
Clinical signs of overdose may include dilated, nonreactive pupils; blurred vision; flushed, hot, dry skin; dryness of mucous membranes; dysphagia; decreased or absent bowel sounds; urinary retention; hyperthermia; tachycardia; hypertension; and increased respiration.

Treatment is primarily symptomatic and supportive. If the patient is alert, induce emesis (or use gastric lavage) and follow with activated charcoal and a saline cathartic to prevent further absorption. In severe overdose, physostigmine may be administered to block antimuscarinic effects. Give fluids, as needed, to treat shock.

---

*Canada only   †Unlabeled clinical use   Italicized adverse reactions are life-threatening.

If urinary retention occurs, catheterization may be necessary.

▶ **Special considerations**
Recommendations for use of anisotropine, care and teaching of the patient during therapy, and for use in children are the same as those for any *anticholinergic*.

Geriatric use
Anisotropine should be administered cautiously to elderly patients. Lower doses are indicated.

Breast-feeding
Anisotropine may be excreted in breast milk, possibly resulting in infant toxicity. Breast-feeding women should avoid this drug. The drug may also decrease milk production.

anistreplase (anisoylated plasminogen-streptokinase activator complex; APSAC)
Eminase

- Pharmacologic classification: thrombolytic enzyme
- Therapeutic classification: thrombolytic enzyme
- Pregnancy risk category C

How supplied
Available by prescription only
Injection: 30 units/single-dose vial

Indications, route, and dosage
Treatment of acute coronary arterial thrombosis
Adults: 30 units by direct I.V. injection over 2 to 5 minutes.

Pharmacodynamics
Enzymatic action: Anistreplase is derived from Lys-plasminogen and streptokinase. It activates the endogenous fibrinolytic system to produce plasmin, which degrades fibrin clots, fibrinogen, and other plasma proteins, including procoagulant factors V and VIII.

Pharmacokinetics
- *Absorption:* Anistreplase is administered I.V.
- *Distribution:* Information not available.
- *Metabolism:* Immediately after injection, anistreplase is deacylated by a nonenzymatic process to form the active streptokinase-plasminogen complex. The half-life of acylated and deacylated anistreplase is 88 to 112 minutes.
- *Excretion:* Unknown. The duration of fibrinolytic activity is 4 to 6 hours and is limited by the deacylation of the anistreplase.

Contraindications and precautions
Anistreplase is contraindicated in patients with history of hypersensitivity to streptokinase; with confirmed or suspected dissecting or intracranial aneurysm; active bleeding; arteriovenous malformation; active bleeding; brain tumor or neoplasm metastatic to CNS; history of cerebrovascular accident; recent thoracic, intracranial, or intraspinal surgery; recent trauma to CNS; or severe uncontrolled hypertension.

Caution should be used and risk-benefit assessed in patients with history of mild allergic reaction to anistreplase or streptokinase or in use of either drug within past 5 days to 6 months; recent streptococcal infection; childbirth within past 10 days; uncontrolled coagulation defects; subacute bacterial endocarditis; severe GI bleeding within past 10 days; history of GI ulcer or other lesion; hemorrhagic ophthalmic conditions; neurosurgical procedure within past 2 months; organ biopsy within past 10 days; mitral stenosis with atrial fibrillation; and acute pericarditis and in patients age 75 and over.

Observe patient closely for bleeding. Fibrin deposits are lysed wherever they exist because the drug promotes conversion of plasminogen to plasmin within or upon the thrombus or embolus as well as in circulating blood. Lysis of fibrin deposits responsible for homeostasis is also promoted.

Interactions
Concurrent use with heparin, oral anticoagulants, and drugs that alter platelet function (including aspirin and dipyridamole) may increase the risk of bleeding. Use with adrenocorticoids, glucocorticoids, or chronic therapeutic corticotropin or ethacrynic acid may increase risk of severe hemorrhage. Antihypertensive agents may increase risk of severe hypotension. Cefamandole, cefoperazone, cefotetan, moxalactam, plicamycin, and valproic acid may increase risk of severe hemorrhage because of their ability to cause hypoprothrombinemia, inhibit platelet aggregation, or cause irreversible platelet damage. Nonsteroidal anti-inflammatory drugs or sulfinpyrazone may increase the risk of bleeding.

Effect on diagnostic tests
Anistreplase prolongs activated partial thromboplastin time (APTT), prothrombin time (PT), and thrombin time; the drug remains active in vitro and can cause degradation of fibrinogen in blood samples drawn for analysis. Decreases in alpha$_2$-antiplasmin activity, Factor V activity, Factor VIII activity, fibrinogen activity, and plasminogen activity have been reported, as well as moderate reductions in hematocrit and hemoglobin. Concentrations of fibrinogen- and fibrin-degradation products are increased.

Adverse reactions
- CNS: *intracranial hemorrhage.*
- CV: *arrhythmias,* conduction disorders, hypotension.
- DERM: hematomas, urticaria, itching, flushing, delayed (2 weeks after treatment) purpuric rash.
- EENT: hemoptysis, gum or mouth hemorrhage.
- GI: bleeding.
- GU: hematuria.
- Local: bleeding at injection site.
- Other: *anaphylactoid reactions* (rare).

▶ **Special considerations**
- Before and after administration, the following tests may be warranted: APTT, PT, thrombin time, hemoglobin, hematocrit, fibrinogen determination, platelet count, fibrin-fibrinogen degradation products.
- Coronary angiography may be useful to monitor effectiveness.
- ECG monitoring is recommended to detect arrhythmias associated with acute MI or reperfusion and may help determine effectiveness of treatment.

- Initiate therapy as soon as possible after onset of clinical symptoms of acute MI.
- Monitor vital signs, mental status, and neurologic status.
- Anistreplase is derived from human plasma. No cases of hepatitis or human immunodeficiency virus infection have been reported to date.
- Reconstitute by slowly adding 5 ml sterile water for injection. Direct the stream against the side of the vial, not at the drug itself. Gently roll the vial to mix the dry powder and water. To avoid excessive foaming, *Do not shake vial.* Solution should be colorless to pale yellow.
- Do not mix with other medications or further dilute after reconstitution.
- Discard any drug that is not administered within 30 minutes of reconstituting.
- To decrease risk of rethrombosis, heparin therapy may be initiated after administration.
- Addition of fibrinolysis inhibitor (for example, aprotinin) or aminocaproic acid to blood samples drawn to obtain specific measurement of fibrinogen will attenuate the degradation of fibrinogen associated with thrombolytic-treated patients.
- Keep patient on strict bed rest and apply pressure dressings to recently invaded sites. To minimize risk of bleeding, avoid nonessential handling or moving of patient, invasive procedures such as biopsies, and I.M. injections.

Information for the patient
- Instruct patient and caregiver to recognize and report signs and symptoms of internal bleeding.
- Instruct patient about importance of strict bed rest.

Geriatric use
No age-specific problems have been reported to date. Risk-benefit must be assessed in patients age 75 and over because preexisting conditions increase the risk of hemorrhagic complications.

Pediatric use
Safety and efficacy have not been established.

Breast-feeding
It is unknown if anistreplase is excreted in breast milk. Use with caution in breast-feeding women.

---

anthralin
Anthra-Derm, Drithocreme, Drithocreme HP 1%, Lasan

- Pharmacologic classification: germicide
- Therapeutic classification: topical antipsoriatic
- Pregnancy risk category C

How supplied
Available by prescription only
Ointment: 0.1%, 0.25%, 0.5%, 1%
Cream: 0.1%, 0.25%, 0.5%, 1%

Indications, route, and dosage
Quiescent or chronic psoriasis
Adults and children: Apply thinly daily or as directed. Start with lowest concentration and increase, p.r.n.

Pharmacodynamics
Antipsoriatic action: Although the mechanism of action is not fully known, it is thought that anthralin decreases the mitotic rate and reduces the proliferation of epidermal cells in psoriasis by inhibiting the synthesis of nucleic protein in psoriatic cell tissue.

Pharmacokinetics
- *Absorption:* Limited absorption with topical use.
- *Distribution:* None.
- *Metabolism:* None.
- *Excretion:* None.

Contraindications and precautions
Anthralin is contraindicated in patients with hypersensitivity to the drug. Drug should not be used on acute or inflammatory eruptions or applied to the face or genitalia. Avoid contact with the eyes or mucous membranes. Use cautiously in patients with renal disease because renal abnormalities may occur.

Interactions
None reported.

Effects on diagnostic tests
None reported.

Adverse reactions
- DERM: contact dermatitis, irritation, erythema.
  Note: Drug should be discontinued if sensitization develops.

Overdose and treatment
If accidental oral ingestion occurs, force fluids and contact local or regional poison information center.

▶ Special considerations
- Avoid use on eyes and mucous membranes.
- Drug may stain skin, hair, and fabrics.
- Gloves may be worn when applying drug, as drug may stain skin.
- Patients with renal disease and those having extensive or prolonged applications should have periodic urine tests for albuminuria.

Information for the patient
- Advise patient how to apply drug. At the end of the treatment period, patient should bathe or shower to remove any excess cream.
- Tell patient anthralin may stain skin, clothing, or bed linens a red-brown to purple-brown color. To prevent staining of clothing and linen, advise patient to use protective dressings.
- If patient shampoos with anthralin, advise him to avoid applying cream to uninvolved scalp areas.
- Tell patient to always wash hands thoroughly after use.
- Avoid applying to normal skin by coating area surrounding lesion with petrolatum.
- Advise patient to decrease the frequency of application if redness develops on adjacent normal skin.

Breast-feeding
Because the drug may be excreted in breast milk, a decision should be made to discontinue breast-feeding or to discontinue the drug, depending on the importance of the drug to the mother.

---

antibiotic antineoplastics

bleomycin sulfate
dactinomycin
daunorubicin hydrochloride
doxorubicin hydrochloride
idarubicin
mitomycin
mitoxantrone
plicamycin
procarbazine hydrochloride
streptozocin

Although classified as antibiotics, these agents exert cytotoxic effects, ruling out their use as antimicrobial agents. These agents interfere with proliferation of malignant cells through several mechanisms. Their action may be cycle-phase nonspecific, cycle-phase specific, or both. Some even demonstrate activity resembling alkylating agents or antimetabolites; for example, streptozocin is considered an alkylating agent because of its therapeutic activity.

Pharmacology
By binding to or complexing with DNA, antineoplastic antibiotics inhibit DNA and RNA synthesis. They inhibit protein synthesis by one of the following mechanisms: inhibiting DNA-dependent RNA synthesis, directly inhibiting RNA synthesis, altering DNA and thus inhibiting RNA synthesis, or reacting with DNA to cause strand breakage.

Clinical indications and actions
Antibiotic antineoplastics are useful alone or in combination with other types of antineoplastics for treating various tumors. See individual agents for specific uses.

Overview of adverse reactions
The most frequent adverse reactions include nausea, vomiting, diarrhea, fever, chills, sore throat, anxiety, confusion, flank or joint pain, swelling of feet or lower legs, loss of hair, redness or pain at injection site, bone marrow depression, and leukopenia.

▶ Special considerations
● Vital signs and patency of catheter or I.V. line should be monitored throughout administration.
● Carefully follow all established procedures for the safe and proper handling, administration, and disposal of chemotherapeutic agents.
● Treat extravasation promptly.
● Attempt to ease anxiety in patient and family before treatment.
● Monitor BUN, hematocrit, platelet count, ALT (SGPT), AST (SGOT), LDH, serum bilirubin, serum creatinine, uric acid, and total and differential leukocytes.
● Avoid immunizations if possible. Warn patient to avoid close contact with persons who have taken oral poliovirus vaccine.

Information for the patient
● Tell patient to avoid exposure to persons with bacterial or viral infections as chemotherapy can make the patient more susceptible to infection. Urge patient to report infection immediately.
● Advise patient to use proper hygiene and caution when using toothbrush, dental floss, and toothpicks. Chemotherapy can increase incidence of microbial infection, delayed healing, and bleeding gums.
● Tell patient that dental work should be completed before initiation of therapy whenever possible, or delayed until blood counts are normal.
● Warn patient that he may bruise easily because of drug's effects on blood count.
● Tell patient to immediately report redness, pain, or swelling at injection site. Local tissue injury and scarring may result if I.V. infiltrates.

Representative combinations
None.

anticholinergics

Belladonna alkaloids
atropine sulfate
hyoscyamine sulfate
scopolamine
scopolamine hydrobromide

Semisynthetic belladonna derivative
methscopolamine bromide

Synthetic quaternary anticholinergics
anisotropine methylbromide
clidinium bromide
glycopyrrolate
hexocyclium methylsulfate
isopropamide iodide
mepenzolate bromide
methantheline bromide
oxyphenonium bromide
propantheline bromide

Tertiary synthetic (antispasmodic) derivatives
dicyclomine hydrochloride
oxyphencyclimine hydrochloride

Antiparkinsonism agents
benztropine mesylate
biperiden hydrochloride
biperiden lactate
procyclidine hydrochloride
trihexyphenidyl hydrochloride

Anticholinergics are used to treat various spastic conditions, including acute dystonic reactions, muscle rigidity, parkinsonism, and extrapyramidal disorders. They also are used to reverse neuromuscular blockade, to prevent nausea and vomiting resulting from motion sickness, as adjunctive treatment for peptic ulcer disease and other GI disorders, and preoperatively to decrease secretions and block cardiac reflexes. Belladonna alkaloids are naturally occurring anticholinergics that have been used for centuries. Many semisynthetic alkaloids and synthetic anticholinergic compounds are available; however, most offer few advantages over naturally occurring alkaloids.

Pharmacology
Anticholinergics competitively antagonize the actions of acetylcholine and other cholinergic agonists within

the parasympathetic nervous system. Lack of specificity for site of action increases the hazard of adverse effects in association with therapeutic effects.

Antispasmodics are structurally similar to anticholinergics; however, their anticholinergic activity usually occurs only at high doses. They are believed to directly relax smooth muscle.

Clinical indications and actions
Hypersecretory conditions
Many anticholinergics (anisotropine, atropine, belladonna leaf, clidinium, glycopyrrolate, hexocyclium, hyoscyamine, isopropamide, levorotatory alkaloids of belladonna, mepenzolate, and methantheline) are used therapeutically for their antisecretory properties; these properties derive from competitive blockade of cholinergic receptor sites, causing decreased gastric acid secretion, salivation, bronchial secretions, and sweating.
GI tract disorders
Some anticholinergics (atropine, belladonna leaf, glycopyrrolate, hexocyclium, hyoscyamine, isopropamide, levorotatory alkaloids of belladonna, mepenzolate, methantheline, and propantheline), as well as the antispasmodics dicyclomine and oxyphencyclimine, treat spasms and other GI tract disorders. These drugs competitively block acetylcholine's actions at cholinergic receptor sites. Antispasmodics presumably act by a nonspecific, direct spasmolytic action on smooth muscle. These agents are useful in treating pylorospasm, ileitis, and irritable bowel syndrome.
Sinus bradycardia
Atropine is used to treat sinus bradycardia caused by drugs, poisons, or sinus node dysfunction. It blocks normal vagal inhibition of the SA node and causes an increase in heart rate.
Dystonia and parkinsonism
Benztropine, biperiden, and procyclidine are used to treat acute dystonic reactions and drug-induced extrapyramidal adverse effects. They act centrally by blocking cholinergic receptor sites, balancing cholinergic activity.
Perioperative use
Atropine, glycopyrrolate, and hyoscyamine are used postoperatively with anticholinesterase agents to reverse nondepolarizing neuromuscular blockade. These agents block muscarinic effects of anticholinesterase agents by competitively blocking muscarinic receptor sites.

Atropine, glycopyrrolate, and scopolamine are used preoperatively to decrease secretions and block cardiac vagal reflexes. They diminish secretions by competitively inhibiting muscarinic receptor sites; they block cardiac vagal reflexes by preventing normal vagal inhibition of the sinoatrial node.
Motion sickness
Scopolamine is effective in preventing nausea and vomiting associated with motion sickness. Its exact mechanism of action is unknown, but it is thought to affect neural pathways originating in the labyrinth of the ear.

Overview of adverse reactions
Dry mouth, decreased sweating or anhidrosis, headache, mydriasis, blurred vision, cycloplegia, urinary hesitancy and retention, constipation, palpitations, and tachycardia most commonly occur with therapeutic doses and usually disappear once the drug is discontinued. Signs of drug toxicity include CNS signs resembling psychosis (disorientation, confusion, halluci-

nations, delusions, anxiety, agitation, and restlessness) and such peripheral effects as dilated, nonreactive pupils; blurred vision; hot, dry, flushed skin; dry mucous membranes; dysphagia; decreased or absent bowel sounds; urinary retention; hyperthermia; tachycardia; hypertension; and increased respiration.

▶ Special considerations
● Give medication 30 minutes to 1 hour before meals and at bedtime to maximize therapeutic effects. In some instances, drugs should be administered with meals; always follow dosage recommendations.
● Monitor patient's vital signs, urine output, visual changes, and for signs of impending toxicity.
● Give ice chips, cool drinks, or hard candy to relieve dry mouth.
● Constipation may be relieved by stool softeners or bulk laxatives.
● The safety of anticholinergic therapy during pregnancy has not been determined. Use by pregnant women is indicated only when the drug's benefits outweigh potential risks to the fetus.

Information for the patient
● Teach patient how and when to take drug for his particular condition; caution patient to take drug only as prescribed and not to take other medications with drug except as prescribed.
● Warn patient to avoid driving and other hazardous tasks if he experiences dizziness, drowsiness, or blurred vision.
● Advise patient to avoid alcoholic beverages, because they may cause additive CNS effects.
● Advise patient to consume plenty of fluids and dietary fiber to help avoid constipation.
● Tell patient to promptly report dry mouth, blurred vision, skin rash, eye pain, or any significant change in urine volume, or pain or difficulty on urination.
● Warn patient that drug may cause increased sensitivity or intolerance to high temperatures, resulting in dizziness.
● Instruct patient to report confusion and rapid or pounding heartbeat.
● Advise women patients to report pregnancy or the intent to conceive.

Geriatric use
Administer anticholinergics cautiously to elderly patients. Lower doses are usually indicated. Patients over age 40 may be more sensitive to the effects of these drugs.

Pediatric use
Safety and effectiveness not established.

Breast-feeding
Some anticholinergics may be excreted in breast milk, possibly resulting in infant toxicity. Breast-feeding women should avoid these drugs. Anticholinergics may decrease milk production.

Representative combinations
Atropine with meperidine: Atropine/Demerol injection; with scopolamine hydrobromide (hyoscine hydrobromide), hyoscyamine sulfate, and phenobarbital: Atrosed, Barbella, Barbeloid, Brobella-P.B., Belbutal, Bellaphen, Donnacin, Donnatal, Haponal, Hyatal, Hybephen, Kinesed, Nilspasm, Sedamine, Sedapar, Sedralex, Seds, Spasdel, Spasidon, Spasloids, Spasmolin,

---

Spastolate, Stannitol; with scopolamine hydrobromide (hyoscine hydrobromide), hyoscyamine sulfate, kaolin, pectin, sodium benzoate, alcohol, and powdered opium: Donnagel PB; with scopolamine hydrobromide (hyoscine hydrobromide), hyoscyamine sulfate, and pentobarbital sodium: Eldonal; with hyoscyamine hydrobromide, scopolamine hydrobromide; acetaminophen, chlorpheniramine maleate, phenylephrine hydrochloride, and phenylpropanolamine: Koryza; with phenazopyridine, hyoscyamine, and scopolamine: Urogesic; with hyoscyamine sulfate, scopolamine hydrobromide (hyoscine hydrobromide) and butabarbital: Zemarine; with hyoscyamine, methenamine, phenyl salicylate, methylene blue, and benzoic acid: Urised.

Anisotropine methylbromide with phenobarbital: Valpin 50 PB.

Belladonna alkaloids with phenylpropanolamine, chlorpheniramine maleate, and pheniramine maleate: Decobel Lanacaps, Fitacol Stankaps; with ergotamine tartrate, caffeine, and phenacetin: Wigraine.

Belladonna Extract with ephedrine, boric acid, zinc oxide, bismuth subcarbonate, peruvian balsam, and cocoa butter in a suppository: Wyanoids; with amobarbital: Amobell; with phenobarbital: Belap; with phenobarbital and activated charcoal: Bellachar; with phenylephrine hydrochloride, pyrilamine maleate, and chlorpheniramine maleate: Bellafedrol; with butabarbital: Butibel.

Dicyclomine with phenobarbital: Bentyl with phenobarbital, Dicyclon No.2, Dicyclon No.3; with pyrilamine maleate and pyridoxine hydrochloride: Dicyclon-M.

---

antihemophilic factor (AHF)
Factorate, Hemofil M, Humafac, Humate-P, Koāte-HP, Koāte-HS, Monoclate, Profilate

- Pharmacologic classification: blood derivative
- Therapeutic classification: antihemophilic
- Pregnancy risk category C

How supplied
Available by prescription only
Injection: Vials, with diluent. Number of units on label. A new porcine product is now available for patients with congenital hemophilia A who have antibodies to human Factor VIII:C.

Indications, route, and dosage
Hemophilia A (Factor VIII deficiency)
Adults and children: 10 to 20 units/kg I.V. push or infusion q 8 to 24 hours. Maintenance doses may be less. Administer solutions containing less than 34 AHF units/ml at a rate of 10 to 20 ml over 3 minutes; administer solutions containing 34 or more AHF units/ml at a maximum of 2 ml/minute. Dosage varies with individual needs.

One AHF unit is equal to the activity present in 1 ml normal pooled human plasma less than 1 hour old.

Do not confuse commercial product with blood bank-produced cryoprecipitated Factor VIII from individual human donors.

AHF is designed for I.V. use only; use plastic syringe, because solution adheres to glass surfaces.

Pharmacodynamics
Antihemophilic action: AHF replaces deficient clotting factor that converts prothrombin to thrombin.

Pharmacokinetics
- Absorption: AHF must be given parenterally for systemic effect.
- Distribution: AHF equilibrates intravascular and extravascular compartments; it does not readily cross placenta.
- Metabolism: AHF is cleared rapidly from plasma.
- Excretion: AHF is consumed during blood clotting. Half-life ranges from 4 to 24 hours (average 12 hours).

Contraindications and precautions
Administer AHF cautiously to patients with hepatic disease and to neonates and infants because of susceptibility to hepatitis, which it may transmit.

The risk potential for viral transmission has been considerably reduced by heat treatment of all available AHF products, using a newer method similar to pasteurization.

Monoclonal antibody-derived AHF is contraindicated in patients with hypersensitivity to mouse protein.

Interactions
None significant.

Effects on diagnostic tests
None reported.

Adverse reactions
- CNS: headache, paresthesia, clouding or loss of consciousness.
- CV: tachycardia; hypotension; possible intravascular hemolysis in patients with blood type A, B, or AB.
- DERM: erythema, urticaria.
- EENT: disturbed vision.
- GI: nausea, vomiting, viral hepatitis.
- Other: chills, fever, backache, flushing, cough, chest pain, hypersensitivity reactions (erythema, urticaria, bronchospasm), stinging at infusion site.

Note: Drug should be discontinued if signs of allergic reaction occur.

Overdose and treatment
Large or frequently repeated doses of AHF in patients with blood group A, B, or AB may cause intravascular hemolysis; monitor complete blood count and direct Coombs' test, and if intravascular hemolysis occurs, give serologically compatible type O red blood cells.

▶ Special considerations
- Refrigerate concentrate until needed; before reconstituting, warm concentrate and diluent bottles to room temperature. To mix, gently roll vial between your hands; do not shake or mix with other I.V. solutions. Keep product away from heat (but do not refrigerate because that may cause precipitation of active ingredient), and use within 3 hours.
- Take baseline pulse rate before I.V. administration. If pulse rate increases significantly during administration, flow rate should be reduced or drug discontinued. Adverse reactions are usually related to too-rapid infusion.
- Monitor coagulation studies before and during therapy; monitor vital signs regularly, and be alert for allergic reactions.
- Prophylactic oral diphenhydramine may be pre-

scribed if patient has history of transient allergic reactions to AHF.

● All products are now heat-treated by special method similar to pasteurization to decrease risk of transmitting hepatitis. Patient should be immunized with hepatitis B vaccine to decrease the risk of transmission of hepatitis.

Information for the patient
● Teach patient how to use, inject, and store prescribed product.
● Advise patient not to take salicylates or other drugs that inhibit platelet formation.

Pediatric use
Administer cautiously to neonates and older infants because of susceptibility to hepatitis.

PHARMACOLOGIC CLASS

antihistamines

astemizole
azatadine maleate
brompheniramine maleate
buclizine hydrochloride
carbinoxamine maleate
chlorpheniramine maleate
clemastine fumarate
cyclizine hydrochloride
cyclizine lactate
cyproheptadine hydrochloride
dexchlorpheniramine maleate
dimenhydrinate
diphenhydramine hydrochloride
meclizine hydrochloride
methdilazine
methdilazine hydrochloride
promethazine hydrochloride
pyrilamine maleate
terfenadine
trimeprazine tartrate
tripelennamine citrate
tripelennamine hydrochloride
triprolidine hydrochloride

Antihistamines, synthetically produced histamine H_1-receptor antagonists, were discovered in the late 1930s and proliferated rapidly during the next decade. They have many applications related specifically to chemical structure, their widespread use testifying to their versatility and relative safety. Some antihistamines are used primarily to treat rhinitis or pruritus, whereas others are used more often for their antiemetic and antivertigo effects; still others are used as sedative-hypnotics, local anesthetics, and antitussives.

Pharmacology
Antihistamines are structurally related chemicals that compete with histamine for histamine H_1-receptor sites on the smooth muscle of the bronchi, GI tract, uterus, and large blood vessels, binding to the cellular receptors and preventing access and subsequent activity of histamine. They do not directly alter histamine or prevent its release.

Clinical indications and actions
Allergy
Most antihistamines (azatadine, brompheniramine, carbinoxamine, chlorpheniramine, clemastine, cyproheptadine, dexchlorpheniramine, diphenhydramine, promethazine, terfenadine, tripelennamine, and triprolidine) are used to treat allergic symptoms, such as rhinitis and urticaria. By preventing access of histamine to H_1-receptor sites, they suppress histamine-induced allergic symptoms.
Pruritus
Cyproheptadine, hydroxyzine, methdilazine, tripelennamine, and trimeprazine are used systemically. It is believed that these drugs counteract histamine-induced pruritus by a combination of peripheral effects on nerve endings and local anesthetic and sedative activity.

Tripelennamine and diphenhydramine are used topically to relieve itching associated with minor skin irritation. Structurally related to local anesthetics, these compounds prevent initiation and transmission of nerve impulses.
Vertigo; nausea and vomiting
Buclizine, cyclizine, dimenhydrinate, and meclizine are used only as antiemetic and antivertigo agents; their antihistaminic activity has not been evaluated. Diphenhydramine and promethazine are used as antiallergic and antivertigo agents and as antiemetics and antinauseants. Although the mechanisms are not fully understood, antiemetic and antivertigo effects probably result from central antimuscarinic activity.
Sedation
Diphenhydramine and promethazine are used for their sedative action; the mechanism of antihistamine-induced CNS depression is unknown.
Suppression of cough
Diphenhydramine syrup is used as an antitussive. The cough reflex is suppressed by a direct effect on the medullary cough center.
Dyskinesia
The central antimuscarinic action of diphenhydramine reduces drug-induced dyskinesias and parkinsonism via inhibition of acetylcholine (anticholinergic effect).

Overview of adverse reactions
At therapeutic dosage levels, all antihistamines except astemizole and terfenadine are likely to cause drowsiness and impaired motor function during initial therapy. Also, their anticholinergic action usually causes dry mouth and throat, blurred vision, and constipation. Antihistamines that are also phenothiazines, such as promethazine, may cause other adverse effects, including cholestatic jaundice (thought to be a hypersensitivity reaction) and may predispose patients to photosensitivity; patients taking such drugs should avoid prolonged exposure to sunlight.

Toxic doses elicit a combination of CNS depression and excitation as well as atropine-like symptoms, including sedation, reduced mental alertness, apnea, cardiovascular collapse, hallucinations, tremors, convulsions, dry mouth, flushed skin, and fixed, dilated pupils. Toxic effects reverse when medication is discontinued. Used appropriately, in correct dosages, antihistamines are safe for prolonged use.

▶ Special considerations
● Antihistamines are contraindicated during an acute asthma attack, because they may not alleviate the symptoms and antimuscarinic effects can cause thickening of secretions.

• Use antihistamines with caution in elderly patients and in those with increased intraocular pressure, hyperthyroidism, cardiovascular or renal disease, diabetes, hypertension, bronchial asthma, urinary retention, prostatic hypertrophy, bladder neck obstruction, or stenosing peptic ulcers.

• Monitor blood counts during long-term therapy; watch for signs of blood dyscrasias.

• Reduce GI distress by giving antihistamines with food; give sugarless gum, sour hard candy, or ice chips to relieve dry mouth; increase fluid intake (if allowed) or humidify air to decrease adverse effect of thickened secretions.

• If tolerance develops to one antihistamine, another may be substituted.

• Some antihistamines may mask ototoxicity from high doses of aspirin and other salicylates.

Information for the patient

• Advise patient to take drug with meals or snack to prevent gastric upset and to use any of the following measures to relieve dry mouth: warm water rinses, artificial saliva, ice chips, or sugarless gum or candy. Patient should avoid overusing mouthwash, which may add to dryness (alcohol content) and destroy normal flora.

• Warn patient to avoid hazardous activities, such as driving a car or operating machinery, until extent of CNS effects are known and to seek medical approval before using alcoholic beverages, tranquilizers, sedatives, pain relievers, or sleeping medications.

• Warn patient to stop taking antihistamines 4 days before diagnostic skin tests, to preserve accuracy of tests. In the case of terfenadine, discontinue drug at least 2 days before the test.

Geriatric use

Elderly patients are usually more sensitive to adverse effects of antihistamines and are especially likely to experience a greater degree of dizziness, sedation, hypotension, and urinary retention than younger patients.

Pediatric use

Children, especially those under age 6, may experience paradoxical hyperexcitability with restlessness, insomnia, nervousness, euphoria, tremors, and seizures.

Breast-feeding

Antihistamines should not be used during breast-feeding; many of these drugs are secreted in breast milk, exposing the infant to hazards of unusual excitability; neonates, especially premature infants, may experience convulsions.

Representative combinations

Carbinoxamine maleate with acetaminophen: Clistin-D; with ammonium chloride: Clistin Expectorant; with pseudoephedrine and dextromethorphan: Baydec DM Drops, Carbodec DM, Pseudocar DM, Rondec-DM, Tussafed; with pseudoephedrine hydrochloride: Rondec, Rondec-TR; with pseudoephedrine and guaifenesin: Brexin.

Chlorpheniramine with atropine: Histunex; with phenylephrine and phenylpropanolamine: Naldecon; with phenylephrine, analgesics, and vitamin C: Corico; with dextromethorphan: "Vicks Formula 44" Cough Mixture; with dextromethorphan and acetaminophen: Remcol-C; with codeine and guaifenesin: Tussar-2 Cough, Tussar SF; with acetaminophen: Remcol-C; with pseudoephedrine and dextromethorphan: Cremacoat, Histolet DM, Novahistine, Pediacare, Rhinosyn DM; with pseudoephedrine, dextromethorphan, and acetaminophen: Co-Apap, Contac Severe Cold Formula, CoTylenol, Dristan Ultra Colds Formula; with phenylpropanolamine: Contac 12-hour Caplets, Oragest, Ornade, Resaid S.R., Triaminic-12, Duravent, Rta-Tuss II.

Cyclizine with ergotamine tartrate and caffeine: Migral.

Dexchlorpheniramine maleate with pseudoephedrine sulfate: Anafed, Anamine, Brexin L.A., Chlorafed, Chlor-Trimeton, Codimal-L.A., Co-Pyronil, Deconamine, Fedahist, Histalet, Isoclor, Novafed A Novahistex*, Pseudo-Hist, Sudafed Plus.

Diphenhydramine with codeine and ammonium chloride: Benylin with Codeine*, Calmylin with Codeine*; with dextromethorphan and ammonium chloride: Benlin-DM*; with pseudoephedrine: Benadryl Decongestant, Benylin D.

Promethazine with codeine: Phenergan with codeine; with dextromethorphan: Phenergan with Dextromethorphan; with phenylephrine: My-K, Phenergan VC; with phenylephrine and codeine: Phenergan VC with codeine; with pseudoephedrine: Phenergan-D.

Pyrilamine maleate with codeine and terpin hydrate: Tricodene; with phenylephrine and codeine: Codimal; with phenylephrine and dextromethorphan: Codimal DM; with phenylephrine, dextromethorphan, and acetaminophen: Robitussin Night Relief Colds Formula; with phenylephrine and hydrocodone: Codimal; with phenylephrine, hydrocodone, and ammonium chloride: Hycomine*, Hycomine-S Pediatric*; with phenylpropanolamine, dextromethorphan, and sodium salicylate: Kolephrin NN Liquid.

Triprolidine with pseudoephedrine and codeine: Actifed with Codeine Cough, CoActifed*, Pseudodine C Cough; with pseudoephedrine: Actacin, Actagen, Actamine, Actifed, Actahist, Allerfrin, Norafed, Pseudodine, Rofed, Tagafed, Triacin, Triafed, Trifed, Tri-fed, Trilitron, Triphed, Triprodrine, Triposed.

PHARMACOLOGIC CLASS

antimetabolites

cytarabine
floxuridine
fludarabine phosphate
fluorouracil
hydroxyurea
mercaptopurine
methotrexate
thioguanine
trimetrexate

Antimetabolites are structural analogs of normally occurring metabolites and can be divided into three subcategories: purine analogs, pyrimidine analogs, and folinic acid analogs. Most of these agents interrupt cell reproduction at a specific phase of the cell cycle and are most effective against tumors with a high growth fraction (that is, high numbers/proportion of cells dividing at any one time).

Pharmacology

The mechanism of action of each subcategory differs according to function with which the drug interferes. The purine analogs are incorporated into DNA and RNA,

---

interfering with nucleic acid synthesis (via miscoding) and replication. They may also inhibit the synthesis of purine bases through pseudofeedback mechanisms. Pyrimidine analogs inhibit enzymes in metabolic pathways which interfere with the biosynthesis of uridine and thymine. Folic acid antagonists prevent conversion of dehydrofolate to tetrahydrofolate by inhibiting the enzyme dihydrofolic acid reductase.

Antimetabolites may slow the entry of some cells into the "S" phase, thus sparing these cells from the drug's cytotoxic effects. As most antimetabolites act in the "S" phase of the cell cycle, this slowing effect may limit their cytoxicity.

Clinical indications and actions
Antimetabolites are useful alone or in combination with other types of antineoplastic agents for treating various tumors. See individual agents for specific uses.

Overview of adverse reactions
The most frequent adverse effects include nausea, vomiting, diarrhea, fever, chills, possible loss of hair, flank or joint pain, redness or pain at injection site, anxiety, bone marrow depression, leukopenia, and swelling of feet or lower legs.

▶ Special considerations
● Follow all established procedures for the safe and proper handling, administration, and disposal of chemotherapy.
● Monitor vital signs and patency of catheter or I.V. line throughout administration.
● Extravasations should be treated promptly.
● Attempt to alleviate or reduce anxiety in patient and family before treatment.
● Monitor BUN, hematocrit, platelet count, ALT (SGPT), AST (SGOT), LDH, serum bilirubin, serum creatinine, uric acid, total and differential leukocyte, and others as required.
● Avoid immunizations if possible.

Information for the patient
● Instruct patient in proper oral hygiene including caution when using toothbrush, dental floss, and toothpicks. Chemotherapy can increase incidence of microbial infection, delayed healing, and bleeding gums.
● Tell patient that dental work should be completed before initiation of therapy whenever possible, or delayed until blood counts are normal.
● Warn patient that he may bruise easily because of drug's effect on platelets.
● Warn patient to avoid close contact with persons who have taken oral poliovirus vaccine and to avoid exposure to persons with bacterial or viral infection, because chemotherapy may increase susceptibility to infection. Instruct him to report signs of infection immediately.
● Tell patient to report immediately any redness, pain, or swelling occur at injection site. Local tissue injury and scarring may result from tissue infiltration at the infusion site.

Representative combinations
None.

antirabies serum

● Pharmacologic classification: immune serum
● Therapeutic classification: rabies prophylaxis product
● Pregnancy risk category C

How supplied
Available by prescription only
Injection: 125 IU/ml in 1,000-unit vials

Indications, route, and dosage
Rabies exposure
Adults and children: 40 units/kg at time of first dose of rabies vaccine. Use half dose to infiltrate wound area. Give remainder I.M. Don't give rabies vaccine and antirabies serum in same syringe or at same site.

For wounds on mucous membranes, the entire dose should be administered I.M. This immune serum should be administered to a patient only once.

Pharmacodynamics
Rabies prophylaxis: Antirabies serum provides passive immunity to rabies by supplying antibodies to the rabies virus.

Pharmacokinetics
No information available.

Contraindications and precautions
Antirabies serum is contraindicated in patients with a history of allergic symptoms or hypersensitivity to horse serum.

Interactions
Concomitant use of antirabies serum with corticosteroids or immunosuppressants may interfere with the immune response to antirabies serum. Whenever possible, avoid concomitant use of these agents, or institute serologic testing to determine if sufficient antibody response to antirabies serum has occurred. Also, because antirabies serum may partially suppress the normal antibody response to rabies vaccine, use only the recommended dosage of antirabies serum.

Effects on diagnostic tests
None reported.

Adverse reactions
● Local: pain, erythema, and urticaria at injection site.
● Systemic: immediate – itching, sneezing, coughing, wheezing, generalized urticaria, marked hypotension; delayed – serum sickness within 6 to 12 days in at least 40% of adult patients (reaction rates for children are lower). Symptoms include skin eruptions, arthralgia, pruritus, lymphadenopathy, fever, headache, malaise, abdominal pain, and *anaphylaxis.*

Overdose and treatment
No information available.

▶ Special considerations
● Obtain a thorough history of animal bite, asthma, angioedema, allergies (especially to horse serum), connective tissue disease, and reactions to immunizations.

• Epinephrine solution 1:1,000 should be available to treat allergic reactions.
• Perform a sensitivity test before giving I.M. dose. Dilute antirabies serum to 1:100 or 1:1,000 with normal saline solution for injection. Inject intradermally 0.1 ml of 1:100 dilution (or 0.05 ml of 1:1,000 dilution in patient with a history of allergy) on inner forearm. Inject other arm with 0.1 ml of normal saline solution intradermally as a control. Read within 30 minutes.
Positive reaction: wheal of 10 mm or more and erythematous flare of 20 x 20 mm. For patients hypersensitive to horse serum, use human rabies immune globulin instead.
• This immune serum provides immediate short-term passive immunity.
• Do not confuse this drug with rabies vaccine, which is a suspension of attenuated or killed microorganisms used to confer long-term active immunity. These two drugs frequently are administered together prophylactically after exposure to known or suspected rabid animals.
• Ask the date of the patient's last tetanus immunization to determine need for a booster.
• Because untreated rabies can be fatal, use of antirabies serum during pregnancy appears justified. No fetal risk from antirabies serum use has been reported to date.
• Store between 2° and 8° C. (36° to 46° F.). Do not freeze.
• Equine antirabies serum is used primarily only when human rabies immune globulin is unavailable.

Information for the patient
• Explain to patient that the body takes approximately 1 week to develop immunity to rabies after the vaccine is given. He is receiving antirabies serum to provide antibodies in his blood for immediate protection against rabies.
• Tell patient that reactions to antirabies serum may develop up to 12 days after administration and are related to the product's source, namely horses. Have patient immediately report skin changes, difficulty breathing, headache, swollen lymph nodes, or joint pain.
• Tell patient that acetaminophen may relieve headache, joint pain, or other minor discomfort after injection of antirabies serum.

antithrombin III (heparin cofactor I)
ATnativ

• Pharmacologic classification: glycoprotein
• Therapeutic classification: anticoagulant, antithrombotic
• Pregnancy risk category C

How supplied
Available by prescription only
Injection: 500 IU

Indications, route, and dosage
Prophylaxis and adjunct treatment of thromboembolism associated with hereditary antithrombin III deficiency
Adults, adolescents, and children: Initial dose is individualized to the quantity required to increase antithrombin III activity to 120% of normal activity as determined 30 minutes after administration. Usual dose is 50 to 100 IU/minute I.V., not to exceed 100 IU/minute. Dose is calculated based on anticipated 1% increase in plasma antithrombin III activity produced by 1 IU/kg of body weight using the formula:

$$\text{Dose} = \frac{\text{desired}}{\text{level}} - \frac{\text{baseline}}{\text{level}} \times \frac{\text{body weight (kg)}}{1\%/\text{IU/kg}}$$

Maintenance: Dose is individualized to quantity required to increase antithrombin III activity to 80% of normal activity and is administered at 24-hour intervals. Dose is calculated as follows:

$$\text{Dose} = \frac{\text{desired}}{\text{level}} - \frac{\text{baseline}}{\text{level}} \times \frac{\text{body weight (kg)}}{\text{actual increase}}$$

produced by 1 IU/kg as determined 30 minutes after administration of initial dose.
Treatment is usually continued for 2 to 8 days except in pregnancy or when used with surgery or prolonged immobilization, when more prolonged administration may be needed.

Pharmacodynamics
Antithrombotic action: Administration of exogenous antithrombin III corrects hereditary antithrombin III deficiency, normalizing coagulation-inhibiting capability and inhibiting formation of thromboemboli. It also inactivates plasmin, but to a lesser extent than the clotting factor.

Pharmacokinetics
• *Absorption:* Drug is administered intravenously.
• *Distribution:* Binding to epithelium and redistribution into the extravascular compartment removes antithrombin III from the blood. Special receptors on hepatocytes bind antithrombin III clotting factor complexes, rapidly removing them from circulation.
• *Metabolism:* Unknown.
• *Excretion:* Unknown.

Contraindications and precautions
Because the drug is prepared from pooled plasma from human donors, it carries with it a minimal risk of transmission of viruses, including hepatitis and human immunodeficiency virus. Plasma used in the manufacturing process is screened for these viruses, and the product is heat-treated for 10 hours at 140° F. (60° C.) to further reduce the risk of viral transmission.
Because of the risk of neonatal thromboembolism in children of parents with hereditary antithrombin III deficiency, measure antithrombin III levels immediately after birth. Fatal neonatal thromboembolism has been reported.

Interactions
Concurrent administration with heparin increases the anticoagulant effect of both; heparin dosage reduction may be necessary.

Effects on diagnostic tests
Plasma levels of antithrombin III may be measured with clotting assays or amidolytic assays using synthetic chromogenic substrates. Immunoassays may not detect all congenital antithrombin III deficiencies.

Adverse reactions
None reported.

Overdose and treatment
None reported. Patients with antithrombin III levels of 150% to 210% remained asymptomatic.

▶ Special considerations
● Transmission of viral disease by drug has not been reported to date.
● Determinations of antithrombin III activity should be performed twice daily until the dosage requirement has stabilized, then performed daily, immediately before dose. Functional assays are preferable because quantitative immunologic test results may be normal despite decreased drug activity.
● 1 IU is equivalent to the quantity of endogenous antithrombin III present in 1 ml of normal human plasma.
● Dyspnea and increased blood pressure may result from too-rapid administration (1,500 IU in 5 minutes).
● Heparin binds to antithrombin III lysine-binding sites in a 1:1 molar ratio, which results in increased efficacy of heparin.
● Not recommended for long-term prophylaxis of thrombotic episodes.
● Store at 36° to 46° F. (2° to 8° C.).
● Reconstitute using 10 ml sterile water (provided), normal saline, or 5% dextrose. *Do not shake vial.* Further dilution in same diluent solution is acceptable.
● Solutions should be at room temperature for administration and should be used within 3 hours of reconstitution.

Geriatric use
No specific problems have been reported to date.

Pediatric use
No specific problems have been reported to date.

Breast-feeding
Distribution into breast milk is unlikely because of the drug's large molecular size. No problems in breast-fed infants have been reported.

---

apomorphine hydrochloride

● Pharmacologic classification: semisynthetic alkaloidal salt
● Therapeutic classification: emetic
● Pregnancy risk category C

How supplied
Available by prescription only
Tablets: 6 mg (soluble) for injection

Indications, route, and dosage
To induce vomiting in acute oral overdoses or poisoning
Adults: 2 to 10 mg S.C. or I.M. followed by oral administration of 200 to 300 ml water. Alternatively, 0.01 mg/kg I.V.
Children: 0.07 to 0.1 mg/kg or 3 mg/m² S.C. or I.M. followed by oral administration of water.

Pharmacodynamics
Emetic action: Apomorphine induces vomiting by directly stimulating the chemoreceptor trigger zone (vomiting center). Onset of emesis occurs in 5 to 10 minutes in adults, 1 to 2 minutes in children.

Pharmacokinetics
● *Absorption:* Unknown.
● *Distribution:* Unknown.
● *Metabolism:* Apomorphine is metabolized in the liver.
● *Excretion:* Unknown.

Contraindications and precautions
Apomorphine is contraindicated in unconscious patients and those with poisoning caused by alkalis, corrosives, or petroleum distillates; in patients with narcosis resulting from opiates, barbiturates, or other CNS depressants, and in severely inebriated patients or in patients with narcotic sensitivity or a depressed gag reflex because of the potential for aspiration pneumonia; in patients who are in shock because drug may cause circulatory failure; and in patients with strychnine poisoning or seizures because of the potential for aspiration and loss of airway.

Apomorphine should be used cautiously in elderly or debilitated patients and in children because these patients have a greater risk of hazardous reactions to this drug.

Interactions
Apomorphine may fail to induce emesis in patients with a narcotic overdose because the drug depresses the chemoreceptor trigger zone.

Concomitant use with antiemetics may decrease emetic response to apomorphine and, if antiemetic is a CNS depressant, may prolong sleep or exacerbate respiratory depression or circulatory effects.

Effects on diagnostic tests
Apomorphine may decrease serum prolactin levels.

Adverse reactions
● CNS: confusion, euphoria, restlessness, tremors, drowsiness.
● CV: hypotension, bradycardia, tachycardia, *acute CV failure* in elderly or debilitated patients.
● GI: nausea, vomiting.
● Other: shortness of breath, difficulty breathing (caused by depressed respiration with large or repeated dosage), unusual sweating and salivation.

Overdose and treatment
Clinical effects of overdose may include continual vomiting and retching, hypotension, circulatory failure, and death.

Treat with naloxone to antagonize apomorphine's emetic CNS and respiratory depressant effects.

▶ **Special considerations**
• Apomorphine is generally not recommended as the drug of choice to induce vomiting.
• Do not administer drug to unconscious or semiconscious patient.
• To prepare drug, dissolve tablet in 1 to 2 ml of normal saline solution or sterile water for injection. Filter before administering. Protect solution from light and air; do not use drug if solution is discolored green or brown.
• Administer water after giving dose. Emetic action is increased if dose is followed immediately by water.
• Monitor frequency and quantity of emesis. Vomiting occurs in 5 to 10 minutes in adults. If vomiting does not occur within 15 minutes, gastric lavage should begin. *Never repeat dose.* Stomach contents are usually expelled completely; vomitus may also contain material from upper portion of intestinal tract.
• Keep narcotic antagonist, such as naloxone, readily available to reverse apomorphine's effects, if necessary.

Geriatric use
Use drug with caution if patient is debilitated or has a cardiac disorder.

Pediatric use
Use with caution.

---

apraclonidine hydrochloride
Iopidine

• Pharmacologic classification: alpha-adrenergic agonist
• Therapeutic classification: ocular hypotensive agent
• Pregnancy risk category C

How supplied
Available by prescription only
Ophthalmic solution: 1%

Indications, route, and dosage
Prevention or control of intraocular pressure elevations after argon laser trabeculoplasty or iridotomy
Adults: Instill 1 drop in the eye 1 hour before initiation of laser surgery on the anterior segment, followed by 1 drop immediately upon completion of surgery.

Pharmacodynamics
Ocular hypotensive action: Apraclonidine is an alpha-adrenergic agonist that reduces intraocular pressure, possibly by decreasing aqueous humor production.

Pharmacokinetics
No information is available. Onset of action is within 1 hour after instillation, and maximum effect on intraocular pressure reduction occurs in 3 to 5 hours.

Contraindications and precautions
Apraclonidine is contraindicated in patients allergic to either apraclonidine or clonidine. Patients who tend to develop exaggerated decreases in intraocular pressure after drug therapy should be monitored closely.
Systemic effects of the drug (altered heart rate and blood pressure) are uncommon after usual dosage, but

patients with severe systemic disease, including hypertension, should be monitored closely.
Observe patient closely for vasovagal attack during laser surgery.

Interactions
Topical beta-adrenergic blocking agents or pilocarpine may produce additive lowering of intraocular pressure.

Effects on diagnostic tests
None reported.

Adverse reactions
Eye: upper eyelid elevation, conjunctival blanching, mydriasis.

Overdose and treatment
No information available.

▶ **Special considerations**
Protect stored drug from light.

Pediatric use
Safety and efficacy have not been established.

Breast-feeding
There is no information regarding the excretion of apraclonidine in breast milk. Consider discontinuing breast-feeding on the day of surgery.

---

aprobarbital
Alurate

• Pharmacologic classification: barbiturate
• Therapeutic classification: sedative-hypnotic
• Controlled substance schedule III
• Pregnancy risk category D

How supplied
Available by prescription only
Elixir: 40 mg/5 ml

Indications, route, and dosage
Sedation
Adults: 40 mg P.O. t.i.d.
Mild insomnia
Adults: 40 to 80 mg P.O. h.s.
Severe insomnia
Adults: 80 to 160 mg P.O. h.s.

Pharmacodynamics
Sedative action: The exact cellular site and mechanism(s) of action are unknown. Aprobarbital acts throughout the CNS as a nonselective depressant with intermediate onset and duration of action. Particularly sensitive to this drug is the recticular activating system, which controls CNS arousal. Aprobarbital decreases both presynaptic and postsynaptic membrane excitability by facilitating the action of gamma-aminobutyric acid (GABA).

Pharmacokinetics
• *Absorption:* Aprobarbital is absorbed well after oral administration. Peak serum levels are reached within

---

3 hours, and onset of action occurs 45 to 60 minutes after dosing.

● *Distribution:* Aprobarbital is distributed widely throughout body tissues and fluids. Drug is 35% protein-bound.

● *Metabolism:* Aprobarbital is metabolized in the liver by oxidation to inactive metabolites.

● *Excretion:* Aprobarbital and metabolites are eliminated in urine; about 15% to 25% of a dose is excreted as unchanged drug. Half-life ranges from 14 to 34 hours. Its duration of action is 6 to 8 hours.

Contraindications and precautions

Aprobarbital is contraindicated in patients with known hypersensitivity to barbiturates and in patients with bronchopneumonia, status asthmaticus, or other severe respiratory distress because of the potential for respiratory depression. Aprobarbital should not be used in patients who are depressed or have suicidal ideation, because the drug can worsen depression; in patients with uncontrolled acute or chronic pain, because paradoxical excitement can occur; or in patients with porphyria, because this drug can trigger symptoms of this disease.

Aprobarbital should be used cautiously in patients who must perform hazardous tasks requiring mental alertness because the drug causes drowsiness and in patients with impaired renal function because up to 25% of aprobarbital is excreted unchanged in urine. Prolonged use of high doses should be avoided because tolerance and physical or psychological dependence may occur.

Prenatal exposure to barbiturates is associated with an increased incidence of fetal abnormalities and, possibly, brain tumors. Use of barbiturates in the third trimester may be associated with physical dependence in neonates. Risk-benefit must be considered.

Interactions

Concomitant use with other sedative-hypnotics, antihistamines, narcotics, antidepressants, tranquilizers, and alcohol may potentiate or add to their CNS and respiratory depressant actions.

Aprobarbital enhances the enzymatic degradation of warfarin and other oral anticoagulants; patients may require increased doses of the anticoagulants. Drug also enhances hepatic metabolism of digitoxin (not digoxin), corticosteroids, theophylline and other xanthines, oral contraceptives and other estrogens, and doxycycline. Aprobarbital may inhibit absorption of griseofulvin.

Valproic acid, phenytoin, disulfiram, and monoamine oxidase inhibitors decrease the metabolism of aprobarbital and can increase its toxicity; rifampin may decrease aprobarbital levels by increasing metabolism.

Effects on diagnostic tests

Aprobarbital may cause a false-positive phentolamine test. The physiologic effects of the drug may impair the absorption of cyanocobalamin [57]Co; it may decrease serum bilirubin concentrations in neonates, epileptic patients, and patients with congenital nonhemolytic unconjugated hyperbilirubinemia. EEG patterns are altered, with a change in low-voltage, fast activity; changes persist for a time after discontinuation of therapy.

Adverse reactions

● CNS: drowsiness, lethargy, vertigo, headache, CNS depression, mental depression, paradoxical excitement, confusion and agitation (especially in elderly patients).

● CV: bradycardia, hypotension, syncope.

● DERM: urticaria, rash, *exfoliative dermatitis, Stevens-Johnson syndrome.*

● EENT: laryngospasm or *bronchospasm,* miosis.

● GI: nausea, vomiting, diarrhea, constipation.

● Other: *respiratory depression,* blood dyscrasias, rebound insomnia, increased dreams or nightmares, possibly *seizures* (after acute withdrawal or reduction in dosage). Vitamin K deficiency and bleeding have occurred in newborns of mothers treated during pregnancy. Hyperalgesia may occur with the use of low doses or in patients with chronic pain.

Note: Drug should be discontinued if hypersensitivity reaction, profound CNS or respiratory depression, or skin eruption occurs.

Overdose and treatment

Clinical manifestations of overdose include somnolence, confusion, respiratory depression, pulmonary edema, areflexia, and coma. Typical shock syndrome with tachycardia and hypotension may occur. Jaundice, oliguria and hypothermia may occur, followed by fever, unsteady gait, slurred speech, and sustained nystagmus.

Maintain and support ventilation and pulmonary function, as necessary; support cardiac function and circulation with vasopressors and I.V. fluids, as needed. If patient is conscious with a functioning gag reflex and ingestion is recent, induce emesis by administering ipecac syrup. Gastric lavage may be performed as long as a cuffed endotracheal tube is in place to prevent aspiration when emesis is inappropriate. Follow by administering activated charcoal or saline cathartic. Measure intake and output, vital signs, and laboratory parameters. Maintain body temperature. Alkalinization of urine may be helpful in removing drug from the body; hemodialysis may be useful in severe overdose.

▶ Special considerations

Besides those relevant to all *barbiturates,* consider the following recommendations.

● Available as elixir only, with alcohol 20%.

● Assess cardiopulmonary status frequently. Monitor vital signs and report any changes.

● Assess renal and hepatic function studies, and blood counts to detect abnormalities.

● Monitor prothrombin times carefully when patient on aprobarbital starts or ends anticoagulant therapy. Anticoagulant dosage may need to be adjusted.

● Watch for signs of barbiturate toxicity (coma, pupillary constriction, cyanosis, clammy skin, hypotension). Overdose can be fatal.

Information for the patient

● Warn patient not to change dose or frequency of use, or to discontinue drug abruptly without medical approval. Rebound insomnia, increased dreams or nightmares, or seizures may occur.

● Warn patient that psychological and physical dependence may result from prolonged use.

● Tell the patient to avoid alcohol ingestion while taking this drug. Excessive depressant effects can occur even if drug is taken the evening before ingestion of alcohol.

Geriatric use
● Elderly patients usually require lower doses.
● Elderly patients are more susceptible to CNS depressant effects of aprobarbital: Confusion, disorientation, and excitability may occur.

Pediatric use
Barbiturates may cause paradoxical excitement in children. Use with caution.

Breast-feeding
Aprobarbital passes into breast milk and may cause drowsiness in the infant. If so, dosage adjustment, or discontinuation of the drug or of breast-feeding may be necessary. Use with caution.

artificial tears
Adapettes, Adsorbotear, Artificial Tears, Hypotears, Isopto Alkaline, Isopto Plain, Isopto Tears, Lacril Artificial Tears, Lacrisert, Liquifilm Forte, Liquifilm Tears, Lyteers, Moisture Drops, Murocel Solution, Muro Tears Solution, Neotears, Tearisol, Tears Naturale, Tears Plus

● Pharmacologic classification: derivatives of polyvinyl alcohol or cellulose
● Therapeutic classification: demulcent
● Pregnancy risk category C

How supplied
Available without prescription except Lacrisert, which is available by prescription only

Indications, route, and dosage
Insufficient tear production
Adults and children: Instill 1 to 2 drops in eye t.i.d., q.i.d., or p.r.n.
Moderate to severe dry eye syndromes, including keratoconjunctivitis sicca
Adults: Insert 1 Lacrisert rod daily into inferior cul-de-sac. Some patients may require twice-daily dosage.

Pharmacodynamics
Demulcent action: Provides ocular lubrication when patient has insufficient tear production; also used as a lubricant for artificial eyes.

Pharmacokinetics
Unknown.

Contraindications and precautions
Artificial tear solutions are contraindicated in patients with hypersensitivity to their active components or preservative and in patients with hard or soft contact lenses in place. Use only solutions indicated for such use.

Interactions
Artificial tear products containing polyvinyl alcohol used with borate external irrigation solutions may leave gummy deposits on the lids.

Effects on diagnostic tests
None reported.

Adverse reactions
● Eye: discomfort, burning, pain on instillation, blurred vision (especially with Lacrisert), crust formation on eyelids and eyelashes (with high-viscosity products).
Note: Drug should be discontinued if eye pain, change in vision, or continued redness or irritation of the eye occurs, or if the condition worsens or is not relieved within 72 hours.

Overdose and treatment
Local manifestations of overdose include severe irritation or sensitivity. If these effects occur, flush eye with normal saline solution or sterile water.
  If accidentally swallowed, may cause hypotension, shock, restlessness, weakness, seizures, nausea, vomiting, diarrhea, oliguria, hypothermia, hyperthermia, and erythematous rash. Substantial ingestion should be treated with induced emesis followed by a cathartic unless the patient is comatose or obtunded. Treat hypotension with fluids. Treat seizures with I.V. diazepam.

▶ Special considerations
● Artificial tear products can be used as often as desired. There are no known toxic effects unless patient is allergic to the preservative or is sensitive to boric acid found in some preparation.
● Do not instill when contact lens is in place unless the product is specifically designed for use with contact lens.
● Patient's eyelids should be kept clean. Some products cause gummy deposit to form on the lids.
● Lacrisert rod should be inserted with special applicator included in the package.

Information for the patient
● Reassure patient that artificial tear products may be used as often as desired.
● Tell patient that product should not be shared with others.
● Show patient how to instill eye drops.
● Warn patient not to touch tip of container to eye or surrounding tissue.

ascorbic acid (vitamin C)
Arco-Cee, Ascorbicap, Cebid Timecelles, Cecon Solution, Cemill-500, Cemill-1000, Cetane, Cevalin, Cevi-Bid, Ce-Vi-Sol, Cevita, C-Long, C-Span, Dull-C, Flavorcee, Vitacee

● Pharmacologic classification: water-soluble vitamin
● Therapeutic classification: vitamin
● Pregnancy risk category A (C if > recommended daily allowance [RDA])

How supplied
Available by prescription only
Injection: 100 mg/ml in 2-ml and 10-ml ampules; 250 mg/ml in 10-ml ampules and 10-ml, 30-ml, and 50-ml vials; 500 mg/ml in 2-ml and 5-ml ampules and 50-ml vials; 500 mg/ml (with monothioglycerol) in 1-ml ampules

Available without prescription, as appropriate
Tablets: 25 mg, 50 mg, 100 mg, 250 mg, 500 mg, 1,000 mg, 1,500 mg; effervescent – 1,000 mg sugar-free;

chewable – 100 mg, 250 mg, 500 mg; timed-release – 500 mg, 750 mg, 1,000 mg, 1,500 mg
Capsules (timed-release): 500 mg
Crystals: 100 g (4 g/tsp), 1,000 g (4 g/tsp, sugar-free)
Powder: 100 g (4 g/tsp), 500 g (4 g/tsp), 1,000 g (4 g/tsp, sugar-free)
Liquid: 50 ml (35 mg/0.6 ml)
Solution: 50 ml (100 mg/ml)
Syrup: 20 mg/ml in 120 ml and 480 ml; 500 mg/5ml in 5 ml, 10 ml, 120 ml, and 473 ml

Indications, route, and dosage
Frank and subclinical scurvy
Adults: 100 to 250 mg, depending on severity, P.O., S.C., I.M., or I.V. daily or b.i.d., then at least 50 mg/day for maintenance.
Children: 100 to 300 mg, depending on severity, P.O., S.C., I.M., or I.V. daily, then at least 35 mg/day for maintenance.
Infants: 50 to 100 mg P.O., I.M., I.V., or S.C. daily.
Extensive burns, delayed fracture or wound healing, postoperative wound healing, severe febrile or chronic disease states
Adults: 200 to 500 mg P.O., S.C., I.M., or I.V. daily.
Children: 100 to 200 mg P.O., S.C., I.M., or I.V. daily.
Prevention of ascorbic acid deficiency in those with poor nutritional habits or increased requirements
Adults: 45 to 60 mg P.O., S.C., I.M., or I.V. daily.
Pregnant or lactating women: At least 60 mg P.O., S.C., I.M., or I.V. daily.
Children: At least 40 mg P.O., S.C., I.M., or I.V. daily.
Infants: At least 35 mg P.O., S.C., I.M., or I.V. daily.
†*Potentiation of methenamine in urine acidification*
Adults: 4 to 12 g daily in divided doses.
Before gastrectomy
Adults: 1 g daily for 4 to 7 days.
†*Adjunctive therapy in the treatment of idiopathic methemoglobinemia*
Adults: 300 to 600 mg P.O. daily in divided doses.

Pharmacodynamics
Nutritional action: Ascorbic acid, an essential vitamin, is involved with the biological oxidations and reductions used in cellular respiration. It is essential for the formation and maintenance of intracellular ground substance and collagen. In the body, ascorbic acid is reversibly oxidized to dehydroascorbic acid and influences tyrosine metabolism, conversion of folic acid to folinic acid, carbohydrate metabolism, resistance to infections, and cellular respiration. Ascorbic acid deficiency causes scurvy, a condition marked by degenerative changes in the capillaries, bone, and connective tissues. Restoring adequate ascorbic acid intake completely reverses symptoms of ascorbic acid deficiency. Data regarding the use of ascorbic acid as a urinary acidifier are conflicting.

Pharmacokinetics
● *Absorption:* After oral administration, ascorbic acid is absorbed readily. After very large doses, absorption may be limited because absorption is an active process. Absorption also may be reduced in patients with diarrhea or GI diseases. Normal plasma concentrations of ascorbic acid are about 10 to 20 mcg/ml. Plasma concentrations below 1.5 mcg/ml are associated with scurvy. However, leukocyte concentrations (although not usually measured) may better reflect ascorbic acid

tissue saturation. Approximately 1.5 g of ascorbic acid is stored in the body. Within 3 to 5 months of ascorbic acid deficiency, clinical signs of scurvy become evident.
● *Distribution:* Ascorbic acid is distributed widely in the body, with large concentrations found in the liver, leukocytes, platelets, glandular tissues, and lens of the eye. Ascorbic acid crosses the placenta; cord blood concentrations are usually two to four times the maternal blood concentrations. Ascorbic acid is distributed into breast milk.
● *Metabolism:* Ascorbic acid is metabolized in the liver.
● *Excretion:* Ascorbic acid is reversibly oxidized to dehydroascorbic acid. Some is metabolized to inactive compounds that are excreted in urine. The renal threshold is approximately 14 mcg/ml. When the body is saturated and blood concentrations exceed the threshold, unchanged ascorbic acid is excreted in urine. Renal excretion is directly proportional to blood concentrations. Ascorbic acid is also removed by hemodialysis.

Contraindications and precautions
Ascorbic acid products containing tartrazine can cause allergic reactions, including bronchial asthma, in susceptible individuals (many are also allergic to aspirin). Prolonged use of large doses of ascorbic acid may increase its metabolism. If intake is then reduced to normal levels, rebound scurvy may occur. Ingestion of large doses of this vitamin during pregnancy has caused scurvy in neonates.

Patients on salt-restricted diets must consider that each gram of sodium ascorbate contains approximately 5 mEq of sodium.

Interactions
Concomitant use of ascorbic acid with acidic drugs in large doses (more than 2 g/day) may lower urine pH, causing renal tubular reabsorption of acidic drugs. Conversely, concomitant use with basic drugs (for example, amphetamines or tricyclic antidepressants) may cause decreased reabsorption and therapeutic effect.

Concurrent use of ascorbic acid with sulfonamides may cause crystallization. Concomitant use with iron maintains it in the ferrous state and increases iron absorption in the GI tract, but this increase may not be significant. A combination of 30 mg of iron with 200 mg of ascorbic acid is sometimes recommended.

Concomitant use of ascorbic acid with dicumarol influences the intensity and duration of the anticoagulant effect; use with warfarin may inhibit the anticoagulant effect; use with ethinyl estradiol may increase plasma levels of ethinyl estradiol.

Smoking may decrease serum ascorbic acid levels, thus increasing dosage requirements of this vitamin.

Salicylates inhibit ascorbic acid uptake by leukocytes and platelets. Although no evidence exists that salicylates precipitate ascorbic acid deficiency, patients receiving high doses of salicylates with ascorbic acid supplements must be observed for symptoms of ascorbic acid deficiency.

Effects on diagnostic tests
Ascorbic acid is a strong reducing agent; it alters results of tests that are based on oxidation-reduction reactions.

Large doses of ascorbic acid (more than 500 mg) may cause false-negative glucose determinations using the glucose oxidase method, or false-positive results using the copper reduction method or Benedict's reagent.

Ascorbic acid should not be used for 48 to 72 hours

---

before an amine-dependent test for occult blood in the stool is conducted. A false-negative result may occur.

Depending on the reagents used, ascorbic acid may also cause interactions with other diagnostic tests.

Adverse reactions
● CNS: faintness or dizziness with rapid I.V. administration, fatigue, headache, insomnia.
● DERM: discomfort at injection site.
● GI: diarrhea, epigastric burning, nausea, vomiting, cramps.
● GU: oxalate or urate renal calculi.
● Other: dental erosion after prolonged use of chewable tablets.

Overdose and treatment
Excessively high doses of parenteral ascorbic acid are excreted renally after tissue saturation and rarely accumulate. Serious adverse effects or toxicity is very uncommon. Severe effects require discontinuation of therapy.

▶ Special considerations
● Administer large doses of ascorbic acid (1,000 mg/day) in divided amounts because the body uses only a limited amount and excretes the rest in urine. Large doses may increase small-intestine pH and impair vitamin B_{12} absorption. The recommended RDA of ascorbic acid is as follows:
Adults: 60 mg/day
Smokers: 100 mg/day
Infants and children: 30 mg/day.
● Administer oral solutions of ascorbic acid directly into the mouth or mix with food. Effervescent tablets should be dissolved in a glass of water immediately before ingestion.
● Administer the I.V. solution slowly.
● Conditions that raise the metabolic rate (hyperthyroidism, fever, infection, burns and other severe trauma, postoperative states, neoplastic disease, and chronic alcoholism) significantly raise ascorbic acid requirements.
● Reportedly, patients taking oral contraceptives require ascorbic acid supplements.
● Smokers appear to have increased requirements for ascorbic acid because the vitamin is oxidized and excreted more rapidly than in nonsmokers.
● Use ascorbic acid cautiously in patients with renal insufficiency because the vitamin is normally excreted in urine.
● Persons whose diets are chemically deficient in fruits and vegetables can develop subclinical ascorbic acid deficiency. Observe for such deficiency in elderly and indigent patients, patients on restricted diets, those receiving long-term treatment with I.V. fluids or hemodialysis, and drug addicts or alcoholics.
● Overt symptoms of ascorbic acid deficiency include irritability; emotional disturbances; general debility; pallor; anorexia; sensitivity to touch; limb and joint pain; follicular hyperkeratosis (particularly on thighs and buttocks); easy bruising; petechiae; bloody diarrhea; delayed healing; loosening of teeth; sensitive, swollen, and bleeding gums; and anemia.
● Protect ascorbic acid solutions from light.

Information for the patient
● Teach patient about good dietary sources of ascorbic acid, such as citrus fruits, leafy vegetables, tomatoes, green peppers, and potatoes.
● Teach patient to cover foods and fruit juices tightly and to use them promptly.
● Advise patients with ascorbic acid deficiency to decrease or stop smoking. Replacement ascorbic acid dosages will be greater for the smoker.
● Tell patients who are prone to renal calculi, who have diabetes, who are undergoing tests for occult blood in stools, or who are on sodium-restricted diets or anticoagulant therapy to avoid high doses of ascorbic acid.

Pediatric use
Infants fed on cow's milk alone require supplemental ascorbic acid.

Breast-feeding
Administer with caution to breast-feeding women because ascorbic acid is distributed into breast milk.

asparaginase
Elspar, Kidrolase

● Pharmacologic classification: enzyme (L-asparagine amidohydrolase) (cell cycle-phase specific, G_1 phase)
● Therapeutic classification: antineoplastic
● Pregnancy risk category C

How supplied
Available by prescription only
Injection: 10,000-IU vials

Indications, route, and dosage
Dosage and indications may vary. Check current literature for recommended protocol.
Acute lymphocytic leukemia
Adults and children: When used alone, 200 IU/kg daily I.V. for 28 days. When used in combination with other chemotherapeutic agents, dosage is highly individualized.

Pharmacodynamics
Antineoplastic action: Asparaginase exerts its cytotoxic activity by inactivating the amino acid, asparagine, which is required by tumor cells to synthesize proteins. Because the tumor cells cannot synthesize their own asparagine, protein synthesis and eventually synthesis of DNA and RNA are inhibited.

Pharmacokinetics
● *Absorption:* Asparaginase is not absorbed across the GI tract after oral administration; therefore the drug must be given I.V. or I.M.
● *Distribution:* Asparaginase distributes primarily within the intravascular space, with detectable concentrations in the thoracic and cervical lymph. The drug crosses the blood-brain barrier to a minimal extent.
● *Metabolism:* The metabolic fate of asparaginase is unclear; hepatic sequestration by the reticuloendothelial system may occur.
● *Excretion:* The plasma elimination half-life, which is not related to dose, sex, age, or hepatic or renal function, ranges from 8 to 30 hours.

Contraindications and precautions

Asparaginase is contraindicated in patients with a history of anaphylactoid reactions to the drug or in patients with pancreatitis or a history of pancreatitis.

Drug should be used cautiously in patients with impaired liver function, infections, or recent therapy with antineoplastics or radiation because of risk of increased adverse effects.

Interactions

Concomitant use of asparaginase with methotrexate decreases the effectiveness of methotrexate, because asparaginase destroys the actively replicating cells that methotrexate requires for its cytotoxic action. Concomitant use of asparaginase and vincristine can cause additive neuropathy and disturbances of erythropoiesis. When asparaginase is used with prednisone, hyperglycemia may result from an additive effect on the pancreas.

Effects on diagnostic tests

Asparaginase therapy alters the results of thyroid function tests by decreasing concentrations of serum thyroxine-binding globulin.

Adverse reactions

● CNS: lethargy, somnolence, headache, confusion, agitation, tremor.
● DERM: rash, urticaria.
● GI: vomiting (may last up to 24 hours), anorexia, nausea, cramps, weight loss, stomatitis.
● GU: azotemia, *renal failure,* uric acid nephropathy, glycosuria, polyuria.
● HEMA: hypofibrinogenemia and depression of other clotting factors, *thrombocytopenia, leukopenia,* depression of serum albumin.
● Hepatic: elevated SGOT and SGPT levels; hepatotoxicity.
● Metabolic: elevated alkaline phosphatase and bilirubin (direct and indirect) levels; increase or decrease in total lipids; hyperglycemia; increased blood ammonia.
● Other: *hemorrhagic pancreatitis, anaphylaxis* (relatively common).
   Note: Drug should be discontinued at the first sign of renal failure or pancreatitis.

Overdose and treatment

Clinical manifestations of overdose include nausea and diarrhea.

Treatment is generally supportive and includes antiemetics and antidiarrheals.

▶ **Special considerations**
● Reconstitute drug for I.M. administration with 2 ml unpreserved normal saline or sterile water for injection. Do not use if precipate forms.
● I.M. injections should not contain more than 2 ml per injection. Multiple injections may be used for each dose.
● For I.V. administration: Reconstitute with 5 ml of sterile water for injection or sodium chloride injection. Solution will be clear or slightly cloudy. May further dilute with sodium chloride injection or dextrose 5% in water and administer I.V. over 30 minutes. Filtration through a 5-micron in-line filter during administration will remove particulate matter that may develop on standing; filtration through a 0.22-micron filter will result in a loss of potency. Do not use if precipate forms.

● Shake vial gently when reconstituting. Vigorous shaking will result in a decrease of potency.
● Refrigerate unopened dry powder. Reconstituted solution is stable 6 hours at room temperature, 24 hours refrigerated.
● Don't use as sole agent to induce remission unless combination therapy is inappropriate. Not recommended for maintenance therapy.
● Should be administered in hospital setting with close supervision.
● I.V. administration of asparaginase with or immediately before vincristine or prednisone may increase toxicity reactions.
● Conduct skin test before initial dose. Observe site for 1 hour. Erythema and wheal formation indicate a positive reaction.
● Risk of hypersensitivity increases with repeated doses. Patient may be desensitized, but this doesn't rule out risk of allergic reactions. Routine administration of 2-unit I.V. test dose may identify high-risk patients.
● Because of vomiting, patient may need parenteral fluids for 24 hours or until oral fluids are tolerated.
● Monitor CBC and bone marrow function. Bone marrow regeneration may take 5 to 6 weeks.
● Obtain frequent serum amylase determinations to check pancreatic status. If elevated, asparaginase should be discontinued.
● Tumor lysis can result in uric acid nephropathy. Prevent occurrence by increasing fluid intake. Allopurinol should be started before therapy begins.
● Watch for signs of bleeding, such as petechiae and melena.
● Monitor blood glucose and test urine before and during therapy. Watch for signs of hyperglycemia, such as glycosuria and polyuria.
● Keep epinephrine, diphenhydramine, and I.V. corticosteroids available for treatment of anaphylaxis.

Information for the patient

● Encourage adequate intake of fluids to increase urine output and facilitate excretion of uric acid.
● Tell patient drowsiness may occur during therapy or for several weeks after treatment has ended. Patient should avoid hazardous activities requiring mental alertness.

Pediatric use

Asparaginase toxicity appears to be less severe in children than in adults.

Breast-feeding

It is not known whether asparaginase distributes into breast milk. However, because of the potential for serious adverse reactions and carcinogenicity in the infant, breast-feeding is not recommended.

---

aspirin
A.S.A., A.S.A. Enseals, Aspergum, Bayer Timed-Release, Buffinol, Easprin, Ecotrin, Empirin, Encaprin, Entrophen, Measurin, Novasen*, Sal-Adult*, Sal-Infant*, Supasa*, Zorprin

- Pharmacologic classification: salicylate
- Therapeutic classification: nonnarcotic analgesic, antipyretic, anti-inflammatory, antiplatelet
- Pregnancy risk category D

How supplied
Available without prescription
Tablets: 65 mg, 81 mg, 325 mg (5 grains), 500 mg, 600 mg, 650 mg
Tablets (enteric-coated): 325 mg, 500 mg, 650 mg
Tablets (extended-release): 650 mg
Capsules: 325 mg, 500 mg
Chewing gum: 227.5 mg
Suppositories: 60 to 120 mg

Available by prescription only
Tablets (enteric-coated): 975 mg
Tablets (extended-release): 800 mg

Indication, route, and dosage
Arthritis
Adults: 2.6 to 5.2 g P.O. daily in divided doses.
Children: 90 to 130 mg/kg P.O. daily divided q 4 to 6 hours.
Mild pain or fever
Adults: 325 to 650 mg P.O. or rectally q 4 hours, p.r.n.
Mild pain
Children: 65 to 100 mg/kg P.O. or rectally daily divided q 4 to 6 hours, p.r.n.
Fever
Children: 40 to 80 mg/kg P.O. or rectally daily divided q 6 hours, p.r.n.
Thromboembolic disorders
Adults: 325 to 650 mg P.O. daily or b.i.d.
Transient ischemic attacks
Adults: 650 mg P.O. b.i.d. or 325 mg q.i.d.
To reduce the risk of heart attack in patients with previous myocardial infarction or unstable angina
Adults: 325 mg P.O. once daily.
Treatment of Kawasaki (mucocutaneous lymph node) syndrome
Adults: 80 to 100 mg/kg P.O. daily in four divided doses. Some patients may require up to 120 mg/kg daily to maintain acceptable serum salicylate concentrations of over 200 mcg/ml during the febrile phase. After the fever subsides, reduce dosage to 3 to 8 mg/kg once daily. Therapy is usually continued for 6 to 10 weeks.

Pharmacodynamics
- *Analgesic action:* Aspirin produces analgesia by an ill-defined effect on the hypothalamus (central action) and by blocking generation of pain impulses (peripheral action). The peripheral action may involve blocking of prostaglandin synthesis via inhibition of cyclo-oxygenase enzyme.
- *Anti-inflammatory effects:* Although the exact mechanism is unknown, aspirin is believed to inhibit prostaglandin synthesis; it may also inhibit the synthesis or action of other mediators of inflammation.
- *Antipyretic effect:* Aspirin relieves fever by acting on the hypothalamic heat-regulating center to produce peripheral vasodilation. This increases peripheral blood supply and promotes sweating, which leads to loss of heat and to cooling by evaporation.
- *Anticoagulant effects:* Aspirin appears to impede clotting by blocking prostaglandin synthetase action, which prevents formation of the platelet-aggregating substance thromboxane A_2. This interference with platelet activity is irreversible and can prolong bleeding time.

Pharmacokinetics
- *Absorption:* Aspirin is absorbed rapidly and completely from the GI tract. Therapeutic blood salicylate concentrations for analgesia and anti-inflammatory effect are 15 to 50 mg/100 ml; responses vary with the patient.
- *Distribution:* Aspirin is distributed widely into most body tissues and fluids. Protein-binding to albumin is concentration dependent, ranges from 75% to 90%, and decreases as serum concentration increases. Severe toxic side effects may occur at serum concentrations greater than 400 mcg/ml.
- *Metabolism:* Aspirin is hydrolyzed partially in the GI tract to salicylic acid with almost complete metabolism in the liver.
- *Excretion:* Aspirin is excreted in urine as salicylate and its metabolites. Elimination half-life ranges from 15 to 20 minutes.

Contraindications and precautions
Children or teenagers who have chicken pox or flu symptoms should avoid aspirin and salicytes because they have been associated with Reye's syndrome, a rare but life-threatening condition. Aspirin is contraindicated in patients with known hypersensitivity to aspirin or other nonsteroidal anti-inflammatory drugs (NSIADs). Aspirin-induced bronchospasm is commonly associated with asthma, nasal polyps, and chronic urticaria. Patients sensitive to yellow tartrazine dye should avoid aspirin.

Aspirin is also contraindicated in patients with GI ulcer or GI bleeding because the drug's irritant effects may worsen these conditions.

Administer cautiously to patients with hypoprothrombinemia, vitamin K deficiency, bleeding disorders, renal impairment, or liver disease, because the drug may cause bleeding. Patients should avoid aspirin during pregnancy, especially during the third trimester, because of potential adverse maternal and fetal effects.

Interactions
When used concomitantly, anticoagulants and thrombolytic drugs may to some degree potentiate the platelet-inhibiting effects of aspirin. Concomitant use of aspirin with drugs that are highly protein-bound (phenytoin, sulfonylureas, warfarin) may cause displacement of either drug and adverse effects. Monitor therapy closely for both drugs. Concomitant use with other GI-irritant drugs such as alcohol, steroids, antibiotics, and other NSAIDs may potentiate the aspirin's adverse GI effects. Use together with caution. Concomitant use with other ototoxic drugs, such as aminoglycosides, bumetanide, capreomycin, ethacrynic acid, furosemide, cisplatin, vancomycin, or erythromycin, may potentiate ototoxic effects. Aspirin decreases renal clearance of lithium carbonate, thus increasing serum lithium

levels and the risk of adverse effects. Aspirin is antagonistic to the uricosuric effect of phenylbutazone, probenecid, and sulfinpyrazone.

Ammonium chloride and other urine acidifiers increase aspirin blood levels; monitor for aspirin toxicity. Furosemide may impair aspirin excretion. Antacids in high doses, and other urine alkalizers, decrease aspirin blood levels; monitor for decreased salicylate effect. Corticosteroids enhance aspirin elimination. Food and antacids delay and decrease absorption of aspirin.

Effects on diagnostic tests
Aspirin will cause an increased bleeding time. Aspirin interferes with urinary glucose analysis performed with Clinistix, Tes-Tape, Clinitest, and Benedict's solution, and with urinary 5-hydroxyindoleacetic acid (5-HIAA) and vanillylmandelic acid (VMA) tests. Serum uric acid levels may be falsely increased. Aspirin may interfere with the Gerhardt test for urine acetoacetic acid.

Adverse reactions
● DERM: rash, bruising.
● EENT: tinnitus, hearing loss.
● GI: nausea, vomiting, GI distress, anorexia, dyspepsia, heartburn, occult bleeding.
● GU: reduced creatinine clearance, albuminuria, proteinuria.
● Other: hypersensitivity manifested by anaphylaxis or asthma, elevated liver enzymes, hepatitis, prolonged bleeding time.
Note: Drug should be discontinued if the following occur: hypersensitivity, salicylism, tinnitus, headache, dizziness, confusion, impaired vision.

Overdose and treatment
Clinical manifestations of overdose include metabolic acidosis with respiratory alkalosis, hyperpnea, and tachypnea, because of increased CO_2 production and direct stimulation of the respiratory center.

To treat aspirin overdose, empty the patient's stomach immediately by inducing emesis with ipecac syrup if patient is conscious, or by gastric lavage. Administer activated charcoal via nasogastric tube. Provide symptomatic and supportive measures (respiratory support and correction of fluid and electrolyte imbalances). Closely monitor laboratory parameters and vital signs. Enhance renal excretion by administering sodium bicarbonate to alkalinize urine. Use cooling blanket or sponging if patient's rectal temperature is above 104° F. (40° C.). Hemodialysis is effective in removing aspirin, but is only used in severely poisoned individuals or those at risk for pulmonary edema.

▶ Special considerations
Besides those relevant to all *salicylates,* consider the following recommendations.
● Enteric-coated products are absorbed slowly and are not suitable for acute therapy. They are better suited for long-term therapy such as for arthritis.
● There is no evidence that aspirin reduces the incidence of transient ischemic attacks in women.
● Avoid giving effervescent aspirin preparations to sodium-restricted patients.
● Stop aspirin therapy 1 week before elective surgery, if possible.
● Moisture may cause aspirin to lose potency. Store in a cool, dry place, and avoid using if tablets smell like vinegar.

Information for the patient
● Tell parents to keep aspirin out of childrens' reach; encourage use of child-resistant closures because aspirin is a leading cause of poisoning.
● Advise patients receiving high-dose, long-term aspirin therapy to watch for petechiae, bleeding gums, and signs of GI bleeding.
● Instruct patient to avoid use of aspirin if allergic to tartrazine dye.

Geriatric use
● Patients over age 60 may be more susceptible to the toxic effects of aspirin. Use with caution.
● The effects of aspirin on renal prostaglandins may cause fluid retention and edema, a significant drawback for elderly patients and those with congestive heart failure.

Pediatric use
● Because of epidemiologic association with Reye's syndrome, the Centers for Disease Control recommend that children with chicken pox or flulike symptoms not be given aspirin or other salicylates.
● Do not use long-term salicylate therapy in children under age 14; safety of this use has not been established.

Breast-feeding
Salicylates are distributed into breast milk; use of aspirin should be avoided during breast-feeding.

---

astemizole
Hismanal

● Pharmacologic classification: histamine₁-receptor antagonist
● Therapeutic classification: antiallergy agent
● Pregnancy risk category C

How supplied
Available by prescription only
Tablets: 10 mg

Indications, route, and dosage
Relief of symptoms associated with chronic idiopathic urticaria and seasonal allergic rhinitis
Adults and children age 12 and older: 10 mg P.O. daily. A loading dose may be given to achieve steady state plasma levels quickly. Initiate therapy at 30 mg on the first day, 20 mg on the second, followed thereafter by 10 mg daily.
Children age 6 to 12: 5 mg P.O. daily.

Pharmacodynamics
Antihistamine action: Astemizole blocks the effects of histamine at histamine₁ (H_1) receptors. Astemizole is a nonsedating antihistamine because its chemical structure prevents entry into the CNS.

Pharmacokinetics
● *Absorption:* Astemizole is rapidly absorbed from the GI tract. Peak plasma levels occur within 1 hour.
● *Distribution:* About 96% of the drug is bound to plasma proteins.

● *Metabolism:* Hepatic.
● *Excretion:* Primarily in the feces. Elimination half-life is 1 to 2½ days.

Contraindications and precautions
Contraindicated in patients hypersensitive to astemizole. Use cautiously in patients with hepatic or renal disease.

Because antihistamines may possess anticholinergic effects, use cautiously in patients with lower airway diseases, including asthma, to avoid excessive drying and bronchial mucus plug formation.

Interactions
None reported.

Effects on diagnostic tests
None reported.

Adverse reactions
● CNS: headache, weight increase, nervousness, dizziness.
● EENT: dry mouth, pharyngitis, conjunctivitis.
● GI: nausea, diarrhea, abdominal pain, appetite increase.
● Other: arthralgia, weight increase.

Overdose and treatment
Cases of serious ventricular arrhythmias have been reported with overdoses of 200 mg or more. Careful observation and constant ECG monitoring is recommended. Treatment is supportive. Some patients may require an antiarrhythmic agent.

▶ Special considerations
Besides those relevant to all *antihistamines,* consider the following recommendations.
● Because of its potential for anticholinergic effects, use this drug cautiously in patients with lower airway diseases (including asthma) because drying effects can increase the risk of bronchial mucus plug formation.
● Use with caution in patients with hepatic or renal disease. Astemizole is not believed to be dialyzable.

Information for the patient
Instruct patient to take this drug on an empty stomach at least 2 hours after a meal and to avoid eating for at least 1 hour after each dose.

Breast-feeding
Animal studies indicate that astemizole may be excreted in breast milk.

atenolol
Tenormin

● Pharmacologic classification: beta-adrenergic blocking agent
● Therapeutic classification: antihypertensive, antianginal
● Pregnancy risk category C

How supplied
Available by prescription only
Tablets: 50 mg, 100 mg

Indications, route, and dosage
Hypertension
Adults: Initially, 50 mg P.O. as a single daily dose. Dosage may be increased to 100 mg/day after 7 to 14 days. Higher dosages are unlikely to produce further benefit. Adjust dosage in patients with creatinine clearance below 35 ml/minute.
Chronic stable angina pectoris
Adults: 50 mg P.O. once daily; may be increased to 100 mg/day after 7 days for optimal effect. Maximum daily dosage is 200 mg/day.
To reduce risk of cardiovascular mortality in patients with acute myocardial infarction
Adults: 5 mg I.V., followed by another 5 mg I.V. 10 minutes later. Initiate oral therapy 10 minutes after the final dose in patients who tolerate the full I.V. dose.
Dosage in renal failure
In patients with creatinine clearance of 15 to 35 ml/min/1.73m^2, 50 mg per day; in patients with creatinine clearance < 15 ml/min/1.73m^2, 50 mg on alternate days; in patients undergoing hemodialysis, 50 mg after each treatment with close supervision.

Pharmacodynamics
● *Antihypertensive action:* Atenolol may reduce blood pressure by adrenergic receptor blockade, thus decreasing cardiac output by decreasing sympathetic outflow from the CNS and by suppressing renin release. At low doses, atenolol, like metoprolol, selectively inhibits cardiac beta$_1$-receptors; it has little effect on beta$_2$-receptors in bronchial and vascular smooth muscle.
● *Antianginal action:* Atenolol aids in treating chronic stable angina by decreasing myocardial contractility and heart rate (negative inotropic and chronotropic effect), thus reducing myocardial oxygen consumption.
● *Cardioprotective action:* The mechanism whereby atenolol improves survival in patients with MI is unknown. However, it reduces the frequency of ventricular premature beats, chest pain, and enzyme elevation.

Pharmacokinetics
● *Absorption:* About 50% to 60% of a dose of atenolol is absorbed. An effect on heart rate usually occurs within 60 minutes, with peak effect at 2 to 4 hours. Antihypertensive effect persists for about 24 hours.
● *Distribution:* Atenolol distributes into most tissues and fluids except the brain and CSF. Drug is approximately 5% to 15% protein-bound.
● *Metabolism:* Minimal.
● *Excretion:* Approximately 40% to 50% of a given dose is excreted unchanged in urine; remainder is excreted as unchanged drug and metabolites in feces. In patients with normal renal function, plasma half-life is 6 to 7 hours; half-life increases as renal function decreases.

Contraindications and precautions
Atenolol is contraindicated in patients with known hypersensitivity to the drug; and in patients with overt cardiac failure, second- or third-degree AV block, or cardiogenic shock, because the drug may worsen these conditions.

Atenolol should be used cautiously in patients with impaired renal function because drug elimination may be impaired; in patients with coronary insufficiency because beta-adrenergic blockade may precipitate congestive heart failure (CHF); in patients with diabetes mellitus or hyperthyroidism, because atenolol may mask tachycardia (but not dizziness or sweating) caused by hypoglycemia or hyperthyroidism; and in patients with bronchospastic diseases, such as asthma or emphysema, because dosages exceeding 100 mg/day may inhibit bronchodilating effects of endogenous catecholamines.

Interactions
Concomitant use with cardiac glycosides may cause excessive bradycardia and increased myocardial depression.

Atenolol may potentiate the antihypertensive effects of other antihypertensive agents; it also may alter insulin or oral hypoglycemic dosage requirements in stable diabetic patients.

Antihypertensive effects of atenolol may be antagonized by indomethacin, nonsteroidal anti-inflammatory agents, and alpha-adrenergic agents, such as those found in nonprescription cold remedies.

Effects on diagnostic tests
Atenolol may increase or decrease serum glucose levels in diabetic patients; it does not potentiate insulin-induced hypoglycemia or delay recovery of serum glucose to normal levels.

Atenolol also may cause changes in exercise tolerance and ECG; it has reportedly elevated platelet count as well as serum levels of potassium, uric acid, transaminase, alkaline phosphatase, lactate dehydrogenase, creatinine, and BUN.

Adverse reactions
● CNS: fatigue, lethargy.
● CV: bradycardia, hypotension, CHF, peripheral vascular disease.
● DERM: rash.
● GI: nausea, vomiting, diarrhea.
● GU: impotence.
● Other: fever, wheezing, dyspnea.
  Note: Drug should be discontinued if signs of cardiac failure develop.

Overdose and treatment
Clinical signs of overdose include severe hypotension, bradycardia, heart failure, and bronchospasm.

After acute ingestion, empty stomach by emesis or gastric lavage; follow with activated charcoal to reduce absorption. Thereafter, treat symptomatically and supportively.

▶ Special considerations
Besides those relevant to all beta-adrenergic blocking agents, consider the following recommendations.
● Give oral single daily dose at same time each day.
● Dosage may need to be reduced in patients with renal insufficiency.
● I.V. atenolol affords a rapid onset of the protective effects of beta-adrenergic blockade against reinfarction.
● The patient who cannot tolerate I.V. atenolol after an MI may be a candidate for oral atenolol therapy. Some evidence suggests that gastric absorption of atenolol may be delayed in the early phase of MI. This may result from the physiologic changes that accompany MI or from the effects of morphine, which is commonly administered to treat chest pain. However, oral therapy alone may still provide benefits. Clinical trials suggest giving 100 mg of atenolol daily P.O. (either as 50 mg b.i.d. or 100 mg once a day) for at least 7 days. In the

absence of contraindications, some clinicians may continue therapy for 1 to 3 years.
● Although such use is controversial, atenolol has been used adjunctively to treat alcohol withdrawal.
● Stress importance of not missing doses, but tell patient not to double the dose if one is missed, especially if taking once a day.
● Advise patient to seek medical approval before taking nonprescription cold preparations.

Geriatric use
Elderly patients may require lower maintenance dosages of atenolol because of increased bioavailability or delayed metabolism; they also may experience enhanced adverse effects.

Pediatric use
Safety and efficacy of atenolol in children have not been established; use only if potential benefit outweighs risk.

Breast-feeding
Safety has not been established. An alternative feeding method is recommended during therapy.

---

atracurium besylate
Tracrium

● Pharmacologic classification: nondepolarizing neuromuscular blocking agent
● Therapeutic classification: skeletal muscle relaxant
● Pregnancy risk category C

How supplied
Available by prescription only
Injection: 10 mg/ml

Indications, route, and dosage
Adjunct to general anesthesia, to facilitate endotracheal intubation, and to provide skeletal muscle relaxation during surgery or mechanical ventilation
Dose depends on anesthetic used, individual needs, and response. Doses are representative and must be adjusted.
Adults and children over age 2: Initially, 0.4 to 0.5 mg/kg by I.V. bolus. Maintenance dose of 0.08 to 0.10 mg/kg within 20 to 45 minutes of initial dose should be administered during prolonged surgical procedures. Maintenance doses may be administered q 12 to 25 minutes in patients receiving balanced anesthesia.
Children age 1 month to 2 years: Initially, 0.3 to 0.4 mg/kg by I.V. bolus when under halothane anesthesia. Frequent maintenance doses may be needed.

Pharmacodynamics
Skeletal muscle relaxant action: Atracurium produces skeletal muscle paralysis by causing a decreased response to acetylcholine (ACh) at the neuromuscular junction. Because of its high affinity to ACh receptor sites, atracurium competitively blocks access of ACh to the motor end-plate, thus blocking depolarization. At usual doses (0.45 mg/kg), atracurium produces minimal cardiovascular effects and does not affect intraocular pressure, lower esophageal sphincter pressure, barrier pressure, heart rate or rhythm, mean arterial pressure,

---

systemic vascular resistance, cardiac output, or central venous pressure. Cardiovascular effects such as decreased peripheral vascular resistance, usually seen at doses greater than 0.5 mg/kg, are caused by histamine release.

Pharmacokinetics

● *Absorption:* Onset of action is within 2 minutes, with maximum neuromuscular blockade within 3 to 5 minutes. The maximum neuromuscular blockade increases with increasing dose. Repeated administration does not appear to be cumulative, nor is recovery time prolonged. Recovery from neuromuscular blockade under balanced anesthesia usually begins 20 to 35 minutes after dose is injected.
● *Distribution:* Atracurium is distributed into the extracellular space after I.V. administration. It is approximately 82% protein-bound.
● *Metabolism:* In plasma, atracurium is rapidly metabolized by Hofmann elimination and by nonspecific enzymatic ester hydrolysis. The liver does not appear to play a major role.
● *Excretion:* Atracurium and its metabolites are excreted in urine and feces by biliary elimination.

Contraindications and precautions

Atracurium is contraindicated in patients with myasthenia gravis, because the drug may induce prolonged paralysis; in patients with conditions in which histamine release would be hazardous; known hypersensitivity to the drug; severe electrolyte disturbances; or asthma. Administer cautiously to elderly or debilitated patients; those with hepatic or renal disease because of potential for drug accumulation; to patients with pulmonary impairment or those with respiratory depression because of potential for further respiratory impairment; those with bronchogenic carcinoma because these patients may exhibit a myasthenic syndrome and prolonged neuromuscular blockade; and those with dehydration or hypotension because of risk of further cardiovascular impairment.

Also administer cautiously to pregnant women receiving magnesium sulfate because dosage may need to be decreased. In severely obese patients, airway maintenance and ventilation support may be necessary.

Interactions

The neuromuscular blockade associated with atracurium may be enhanced by concomitant use with many general anesthetics, particularly enflurane and isoflurane, or with aminoglycoside antibiotics, clindamycin, lincomycin, polymyxin antibiotics, furosemide, lithium, beta-adrenergic blockers, depolarizing neuromuscular blocking agents, other nondepolarizing neuromuscular blocking agents, parenteral magnesium salts, quinidine, quinine, thiazide diuretics, and potassium-depleting drugs. Concomitant use of opioid analgesics may cause additive respiratory depression and should be used with extreme caution during surgery and immediately postoperatively.

Effects on diagnostic tests

None significant.

Adverse reactions

● CV: hypotension, tachycardia.
● DERM: flushing, erythema, pruritus, urticaria, rash.
● Other: hypothermia, increased pulmonary function

impairment, *respiratory depression*, wheezing, increased bronchial secretions, *bronchospasm*.
Note: Drug should be discontinued if hypersensitivity or cardiovascular collapse occurs.

Overdose and treatment

Clinical manifestations of overdose include prolonged respiratory depression or apnea and cardiovascular collapse. A sudden release of histamine may also occur.

A peripheral nerve stimulator is recommended to monitor response and to determine the nature and degree of neuromuscular block. Maintain an adequate airway and manual or mechanical ventilation until patient can maintain respiration unassisted.

For treatment of overdose, administer cholinesterase inhibitors, such as edrophonium, neostigmine, or pyridostigmine, to reverse neuromuscular blockade; and atropine or glycopyrrolate to counteract muscarinic adverse effects of cholinesterase inhibitors. Monitor vital signs at least every 15 minutes until patient is stable, then every ½ hour for the next 2 hours. Observe airway until patient has fully recovered from drug effects. Note rate, depth, and pattern of respirations.

▶ Special considerations

● Atracurium must be administered by I.V. injection (I.M. injection causes tissue irritation).
● Reduce dose and administration rate in patients in whom histamine release may be hazardous.
● Prior administration of succinylcholine does not prolong duration of action of atracurium, but it quickens onset and may deepen neuromuscular blockade.
● Atracurium has a longer duration of action than succinylcholine and a shorter duration than tubocurarine or pancuronium.
● Atracurium has little or no effect on heart rate and will not counteract or reverse the bradycardia caused by anesthetics or vagal stimulation. Thus, bradycardia is seen more frequently with atracurium than with other neuromuscular blocking agents. Pretreatment with anticholinergics (atropine or glycopyrrolate) is advised.
● If bradycardia occurs during atracurium administration, treat by administration of I.V. atropine.
● Alkaline solutions such as barbiturates should not be admixed in the same syringe or given through the same needle with atracurium.
● Peripheral nerve stimulator may be used to detect residual paralysis during recovery and to avoid atracurium overdose.
● Atracurium should be used only if endotracheal intubation, administration of oxygen under positive pressure, artificial respiration, and assisted or controlled ventilation are immediately available.
● To evaluate patient for recovery from neuromuscular blocking effect, observe for ability to breathe, to cough, to protrude tongue, to keep eyes open, to lift head keeping mouth closed, and to show adequate strength of hand-grip. Assess for adequate negative inspiratory force (− 25 cm H$_2$O).
● Until head and neck muscles recover from blockade effects, patient may find speech difficult.
● If indicated, assess for need for pain medication or sedation. Drug does not affect consciousness or relieve pain.

Geriatric use

Elderly patients may be more sensitive to the drug's effects.

Pediatric use
Safety and efficacy have not been established for children under age 1 month.

Breast-feeding
It is unknown if atracurium is excreted in breast milk; therefore, use with caution in breast-feeding women.

atropine sulfate

- Pharmacologic classification: anticholinergic, belladonna alkaloid
- Therapeutic classification: antiarrhythmic, vagolytic
- Pregnancy risk category C

How supplied
Available by prescription only
Injection: 0.05 mg/ml, 0.1 mg/ml, 0.3 mg/ml, 0.4 mg/ml, 0.5 mg/ml, 0.6 mg/ml, 0.8 mg/ml, 1 mg/ml, and 1.2 mg/ml
Tablets: 0.4 mg, 0.6 mg

Indications, route, and dosage
Symptomatic bradycardia, bradyarrhythmia (junctional or escape rhythm)
Adults: Usually 0.5 to 1 mg by I.V. push; repeat q 5 minutes, to a maximum of 2 mg. Lower doses (less than 0.5 mg) may cause bradycardia.
Children: 0.01 mg/kg up to maximum 0.4 mg; or 0.3 mg/m²; may repeat q 4 to 6 hours.
Preoperatively for diminishing secretions and blocking cardiac vagal reflexes
Adults: 0.4 to 0.6 mg I.M. 45 to 60 minutes before anesthesia.
Children: 0.01 mg/kg I.M. up to a maximum dose of 0.4 mg 45 to 60 minutes before anesthesia.
Antidote for anticholinesterase insecticide poisoning
Adults and children: 2 mg I.M. or I.V. repeated every 20 to 30 minutes until muscarinic symptoms disappear. Severe cases may require up to 6 mg I.M. or I.V q 1 hour.

Pharmacodynamics
Antiarrhythmic action: An anticholinergic (parasympatholytic) agent with many uses, atropine remains the mainstay of pharmacologic treatment for bradyarrhythmias. It blocks acetylcholine's effects on the SA and AV nodes, thereby increasing SA and AV node conduction velocity. It also increases sinus node discharge rate and decreases the AV node's effective refractory period. These changes result in an increased heart rate (both atrial and ventricular).

Atropine has variable – and clinically negligible – effects on the His-Purkinje system. Small doses (< 0.5 mg) and occasionally larger doses may lead to a paradoxical slowing of the heart rate, which may be followed by a more rapid rate.

As a cholinergic blocking agent, atropine decreases the action of the parasympathetic nervous system on certain glands (bronchial, salivary, and sweat), resulting in decreased secretions. It also decreases cholinergic effects on the iris, ciliary body, and intestinal and bronchial smooth muscle.

As an antidote for cholinesterase poisoning, atropine blocks the cholinomimetic effects of these pesticides.

Pharmacokinetics
- *Absorption:* I.V. administration is the most common route for bradyarrhythmia treatment. With endotracheal administration, atropine is well absorbed from the bronchial tree (drug has been used in 1-mg doses in acute bradyarrhythmia when an I.V. line has not been established). Effects on heart rate peak within 2 to 4 minutes after I.V. administration. Atropine is well absorbed after oral and I.M. administration, and peak inhibitory effects on salivation occur in 30 minutes to 1 hour after either route.
- *Distribution:* Atropine is well distributed throughout the body, including the CNS. Only 18% of the drug binds with plasma protein (clinically insignificant).
- *Metabolism:* Atropine is metabolized in the liver to several metabolites. About 30% to 50% of a dose is excreted by the kidneys as unchanged drug.
- *Excretion:* Drug is excreted primarily through the kidneys; however, small amounts may be excreted in the feces and expired air. Elimination half-life is biphasic, with an initial 2-hour phase followed by a terminal half-life of about 12½ hours.

Contraindications and precautions
Atropine should be used with caution in patients with acute myocardial infarction because it may promote arrhythmias, including ventricular fibrillation and tachycardia as well as atrial fibrillation; the resulting increase in heart rate may increase myocardial oxygen consumption and worsen myocardial ischemia.

Atropine should be used cautiously in patients with narrow-angle glaucoma, obstructive uropathy, obstructive gastrointestinal tract disease, myasthenia gravis, paralytic ileus, intestinal atony, unstable cardiovascular status from acute hemorrhage, and toxic megacolon, because the drug may worsen these symptoms or disorders.

Interactions
Concomitant use of atropine and other anticholinergics or drugs with anticholinergic effects produce additive effects.

Effects on diagnostic tests
None reported.

Adverse reactions
- CNS: headache; restlessness; ataxia; disorientation; hallucinations; delirium; coma; insomnia; dizziness; excitement, agitation, confusion (especially in elderly patients).
- CV: tachycardia (possibly extreme), palpitations, angina.
- DERM: hot, flushed skin.
- EENT: mydriasis, photophobia (with 1-mg dose); blurred vision, mydriasis (with 2-mg dose).
- GI: dry mouth, thirst, constipation, nausea, vomiting.
- GU: urinary retention.
- HEMA: leukocytosis.
- Other: hyperpyrexia.

Overdose and treatment
Clinical signs of overdose reflect excessive anticholinergic activity, especially cardiovascular and CNS stimulation.

Treatment includes physostigmine administration, to

---

reverse excessive anticholinergic activity, and general supportive measures, as necessary.

▶ **Special considerations**
● Observe for tachycardia if patient has cardiac disorder.
● With I.V. administration, drug may cause paradoxical initial bradycardia, which usually disappears within 2 minutes.
● Monitor patient's fluid intake and output; drug causes urinary retention and hesitancy. If possible, patient should void before taking drug.
● High doses may cause hyperpyrexia, urinary retention, and CNS effects, including hallucinations and confusion (anticholinergic delirium). Other anticholinergic drugs may increase vagal blockage.
● Adverse reactions vary considerably with dose.

Geriatric use
Monitor closely for urinary retention in elderly males with benign prostatic hypertrophy.

---

auranofin
Ridaura

● Pharmacologic classification: gold salt
● Therapeutic classification: antiarthritic
● Pregnancy risk category C

How supplied
Available by prescription only
Capsules: 3 mg

Indications, route, and dosage
Rheumatoid arthritis
Adults: 6 mg P.O. daily, administered either as 3 mg b.i.d. or 6 mg once daily. After 4 to 6 months, may be increased to 9 mg daily. If response remains inadequate after 3 months at 9 mg daily, discontinue the drug.

Pharmacodynamics
Antiarthritic action: Auranofin suppresses or prevents, but does not cure, adult or juvenile arthritis and synovitis. It is anti-inflammatory in active arthritis. This drug is thought to reduce inflammation by altering the immune system. Auranofin has been shown to decrease high serum concentrations of immunoglobulins and rheumatoid factors in patients with arthritis. However the exact mechanism of action remains unknown.

Pharmacokinetics
● *Absorption:* When administered P.O., 25% of auranofin is absorbed through the GI tract. Time to peak plasma concentration is 1 to 2 hours.
● *Distribution:* The drug is 60% protein-bound and is distributed widely in body tissues. Oral gold from auranofin is bound to a higher degree than gold from the injectable form. Synovial fluid levels are approximately 50% of blood concentrations. No correlation between blood-gold concentrations and safety or efficacy has been determined.
● *Metabolism:* The metabolic fate of auranofin is not known, but it is believed that the drug is not broken down into elemental gold.
● *Excretion:* 60% of the absorbed auranofin (15% of the administered dose) is excreted in the urine and the

remainder in the feces. The average plasma half-life is 26 days, compared with about 6 days for gold sodium thiomalate.

Contraindications and precautions
Auranofin is contraindicated in patients with a known hypersensitivity to gold or other heavy metals or with a history of blood dyscrasias, because the drug may induce blood dyscrasias; in patients with severe diabetes, congestive heart failure, hemorrhagic conditions, systemic lupus erythematosus, tuberculosis, or exfoliative dermatitis because it may exacerbate these conditions; in patients with colitis, because the drug can precipitate GI distress; and in patients with impaired renal or hepatic function.

Auranofin should be used cautiously in patients with decreased cerebral or cardiovascular circulation, a history of drug rash, a history of hepatic or renal disease, or severe hypertension.

Interactions
Concomitant use of auranofin with other drugs that may cause blood dyscrasias can produce additive hematologic toxicity.

Effects on diagnostic tests
Serum protein-bound iodine test, especially when done by the chloric acid digestion method, gives false readings during and for several weeks after gold therapy.

Adverse reactions
● GI: abdominal pain, diarrhea, nausea, vomiting, stomatitis, enterocolitis, anorexia, metallic taste, dyspepsia, flatulence.
● GU: transient proteinuria, hematuria, nephrotic syndrome.
● HEMA: *thrombocytopenia* (with or without purpura), aplastic anemia, agranulocytosis, leukopenia, eosinophilia.
● Hepatic: jaundice, elevated liver enzymes.
● Other: hypersensitivity (syncope [rarely], bradycardia, *anaphylactic shock*), interstitial pneumonitis, sore throat, sensory change in the hands and feet (with long-term use).

Overdose and treatment
When severe reactions to gold occur, corticosteroids, dimercaprol (a chelating agent), or penicillamine may be given to aid recovery. Prednisone 40 to 100 mg daily in divided doses is recommended to manage severe renal, hematologic, pulmonary, or enterocolitic reactions to gold. Dimercaprol may be used concurrently with steroids to facilitate the removal of the gold when steroid treatment alone is ineffective. Use of chelating agents is controversial, and caution is recommended.

▶ **Special considerations**
Besides those relevant to all *gold salts*, consider the following recommendations.
● Auranofin should be discontinued if the platelet count falls below 100,000/mm³.
● When switching from injectable gold, start auranofin at 6 mg P.O. daily.

Information for the patient
● Emphasize the importance of monthly follow-up to monitor patient's platelet count.
● Reassure patient that beneficial drug effect may be delayed for 3 months. However, if response is inade-

---

quate after 6 to 9 months, auranofin will probably be discontinued.

● Encourage the patient to take the drug as prescribed and not to alter the dosage schedule.

● Diarrhea is the most common adverse reaction. Tell patient to continue taking the drug if he experiences mild diarrhea; however, if he notes blood in his stool, he should call immediately.

● Tell patient to continue taking concomitant drug therapy, such as nonsteroidal anti-inflammatory drugs, if prescribed.

● Dermatitis is a common adverse reaction. Advise patient to report any rashes or other skin problems immediately.

● Stomatitis is another common adverse reaction. Tell patient that stomatitis is often preceded by a metallic taste. Advise him to report this symptom immediately.

Geriatric use
Administer usual adult dose. Use cautiously in patients with decreased renal function.

Pediatric use
Safe dosage has not been established; use in children under age 6 is not recommended.

Breast-feeding
Auranofin is not recommended for use during breast-feeding.

---

aurothioglucose
Solganal

● Pharmacologic classification: gold salt
● Therapeutic classification: antiarthritic
● Pregnancy risk category C

How supplied
Available by prescription only
Injection: 50 mg/ml suspension in sesame oil with aluminum monostearate 2% and propylparaben 0.1% in a 10-ml container

Indications, route, and dosage
Rheumatoid arthritis
Adults: Initially, 10 mg I.M., followed by 25 mg for second and third doses at weekly intervals. Then, 50 mg weekly until 1 g has been given. If improvement occurs without toxicity, continue 25 to 50 mg at 3- to 4-week intervals indefinitely as maintenance therapy.
Children age 6 to 12: One-quarter usual adult dose. Alternatively, 1 mg/kg I.M. (not to exceed 25 mg per dose) once weekly for 20 weeks.

Pharmacodynamics
Antiarthritic action: Aurothioglucose is thought to be effective against rheumatoid arthritis by altering the immune system to reduce inflammation. Although the exact mechanism of action remains unknown, these compounds have reduced serum concentrations of immunoglobulins and rheumatoid factors in patients with arthritis.

Pharmacokinetics
● *Absorption:* Absorption of aurothioglucose is slow and erratic because it is in oil suspension.

● *Distribution:* Higher tissue concentrations occur with parenteral gold salts, with a mean steady-state plasma level of 1 to 5 mcg/ml. Drug is distributed widely throughout the body in lymph nodes, bone marrow, kidneys, liver, spleen, and tissues. About 85% to 90% is protein-bound.

● *Metabolism:* Aurothioglucose is not broken down into its elemental form. The half-life with cumulative dosing is 14 to 40 days.

● *Excretion:* About 70% of the drug is excreted in the urine, 30% in the feces.

Contraindications and precautions
Gold compounds are contraindicated in patients with uncontrolled diabetes mellitus, systemic lupus erythematosus, Sjögren's syndrome, agranulocytosis, or blood dyscrasias; in patients who recently received radiation therapy; in breast-feeding patients, because the drug distributes into breast milk; and in patients with a history of sensitivity to gold compounds. They should be administered cautiously to patients with marked hypertension, compromised cerebral or cardiovascular function, or renal or hepatic dysfunction, because gold may exacerbate these conditions. They should be used with caution in women of childbearing age, because gold compounds are teratogenic in high doses in animals.

Interactions
Concomitant use with other drugs known to cause blood dyscrasias causes an additive risk of hematologic toxicity.

Effects on diagnostic tests
Serum protein-bound iodine test, especially when done by the chloric acid digestion method, gives false readings during and for several weeks after gold therapy.

Adverse reactions
● CNS: dizziness, syncope, sweating.
● CV: bradycardia.
● DERM: rash, pruritus, dermatitis, *exfoliative dermatitis.*
● EENT: corneal gold deposition, corneal ulcers.
● GI: diarrhea, abdominal pain, nausea, vomiting, stomatitis, enterocolitis, anorexia, metallic taste, dyspepsia, flatulence.
● GU: albuminuria, proteinuria, nephrotic syndrome, nephritis, acute tubular necrosis.
● HEMA: thrombocytopenia (with or without purpura), *aplastic anemia, agranulocytosis,* leukopenia, eosinophilia.
● Hepatic: jaundice, elevated liver enzymes.
● Other: gold bronchitis and interstitial pneumonitis, partial or complete loss of hair, fever, *anaphylaxis,* angioneurotic edema.

Overdose and treatment
When severe reactions to gold occur, corticosteroids, dimercaprol (a chelating agent), or penicillamine may be given to aid in the recovery. Prednisone 40 to 100 mg/day in divided doses is recommended to manage severe renal, hematologic, pulmonary, or enterocolitic reactions to gold. Dimercaprol may be used concurrently with steroids to facilitate the removal of the gold when the steroid treatment alone is ineffective. Use of chelating agents is controversial, and caution is recommended.

▶ **Special considerations**

Besides those relevant to all *gold salts,* consider the following recommendations.

● Gold salts should be administered only under constant supervision and careful consideration of the drug's toxicities and benefits.

● Most adverse reactions are readily reversible if drug is discontinued immediately.

● Administer all gold salts I.M., preferably intragluteally. Normal color of drug is pale yellow; do not use if it darkens.

● Observe patient for 30 minutes after administration because of possible anaphylactic reaction.

● Aurothioglucose is a suspension. Immerse vial in warm water and shake vigorously before injecting.

● Urine should be analyzed for protein and sediment changes before each injection.

● Platelet counts should be performed if patient develops purpura or ecchymoses.

● If adverse reactions are mild, some rheumatologists order resumption of gold therapy after 2 to 3 weeks' rest.

Information for the patient

● Emphasize the importance of monthly follow-up to monitor platelet count. Drug should be stopped if the platelet count falls below 100,000/mm³.

● Reassure patient that beneficial drug effect may be delayed for 3 months. However, if response is inadequate after 6 months, aurothioglucose will probably be discontinued.

● Explain that vasomotor adverse reactions – faintness, weakness, dizziness, flushing, nausea, vomiting, diaphoresis – may occur immediately after injection. Advise patient to lie down until symptoms subside and to report persistent symptoms.

● Tell patient to continue taking the drug if he experiences mild diarrhea; however, if diarrhea persists, or if he notes blood in his stool, he should call immediately.

● Tell patient that stomatitis is often preceded by a metallic taste. Advise him to report this symptom immediately.

● Advise patient to report any rashes or other skin problems immediately.

● Encourage patient to take the drug as prescribed and not to alter the dosage schedule.

● Tell patient to continue taking concomitant drug therapy, such as nonsteroidal anti-inflammatory drugs, as prescribed.

Geriatric use

Administer usual adult dose. Use cautiously in patients with decreased renal function.

Pediatric use

Use in children younger than age 6 is not recommended. Children age 6 to 12 may receive one-fourth the usual adult dose.

Breast-feeding

Aurothioglucose is not recommended for use in breast-feeding women.

azacytidine (5-azacytidine)

● Pharmacologic classification: antimetabolite (cell cycle-phase specific, S phase)
● Therapeutic classification: antineoplastic
● Pregnancy risk category C

How supplied

Available only through investigational protocols
Injection: 100-mg vials

Indications, route, and dosage

Dosage and indications may vary. Check current literature for appropriate protocol.

†*Refractory acute lymphocytic and acute myelogenous leukemia*

Adults and children: 200 to 300 mg/m² I.V. daily for 5 to 10 days, repeated at 2- to 3-week intervals.

Pharmacodynamics

Antimetabolic action: The primary mechanism of action for azacytidine has not been defined. However, azacytidine may act as an antimetabolite, interfering with pyrimidine synthesis. Azacytidine is incorporated into DNA and RNA, thereby inhibiting protein synthesis.

Pharmacokinetics

● *Absorption:* Azacytidine is rapidly and completely absorbed following subcutaneous administration.
● *Distribution:* Azacytidine does not cross the blood-brain barrier to a significant extent.
● *Metabolism:* Azacytidine is metabolized in the liver.
● *Excretion:* Azacytidine and its metabolites are excreted primarily in urine. The plasma elimination half-life is reported to be about 4 hours.

Contraindications and precautions

Azacytidine is contraindicated in patients with liver disease, particularly hepatic metastases, because the drug may be hepatotoxic; and in patients with a serum albumin level below 3 g/100 ml or with bone marrow depression, because the drug may exacerbate these conditions.

Interactions

None reported.

Effects on diagnostic tests

Azacytidine therapy increases blood uric acid concentrations.

Adverse reactions

● CNS: infrequent neurologic toxicities, including generalized muscle pain and weakness, confusion, somnolence.
● CV: hypotension from rapid infusion.
● GI: severe nausea and vomiting, diarrhea, stomatitis.
● GU: azotemia, nephrotoxicity, polyuria.
● HEMA: *bone marrow depression* (dose-limiting), *leukopenia, thrombocytopenia.*
● Local: pain on injection.
● Other: hepatotoxicity (rare), drug fever, hypophosphatemia.

Overdose and treatment
Clinical manifestations of overdose include myelosuppression, nausea, and vomiting.

Treatment is usually supportive and includes antiemetics and transfusion of blood components.

▶ Special considerations
● Follow all established procedures for the safe and proper handling, administration, and disposal of chemotherapeutic agents.
● Reconstitute powder with 19.9 ml of sterile water for injection to yield a concentration of 5 mg/ml. Within 30 minutes, dilute further with lactated Ringer's solution for I.V. infusion. Drug is stable for up to 3 hours once diluted.
● For stability reasons, azacytidine should be infused only in lactated Ringer's solutions.
● The drug should be given by slow I.V. infusion to prevent severe hypotension.
● I.V. push administration is not recommended.
● If necessary, the drug may be given subcutaneously. The drug should be mixed in a smaller quantity of diluent (3 to 5 ml for a 100-mg vial) for subcutaneous administration.
● Blood pressure should be monitored before infusion and at 30-minute intervals during infusion. If systolic blood pressure falls below 90 mm Hg, infusion should be stopped and therapy reevaluated.
● Nausea and vomiting may be reduced with continuous infusions. Tolerance to nausea and vomiting develops during extended course of treatment.
● Instruct patient to report any signs of neurotoxicity such as muscle pain or weakness.
● Monitor temperature, CBC, and liver function tests.

Information for the patient
● Encourage adequate fluid intake to increase urine output and facilitate excretion of uric acid.
● Tell patient to avoid exposure to people with infections.
● Tell patient to report any unusual bruising or bleeding.

Breast-feeding
It is not known whether azacytidine distributes into breast milk. However, because of the risk of serious adverse reactions, mutagenicity, and carcinogenicity in the infant, breast-feeding is not recommended.

azatadine maleate
Optimine

● Pharmacologic classification: piperidine antihistamine
● Therapeutic classification: antihistamine
● Pregnancy risk category B

How supplied
Available by prescription only
Tablets: 1 mg

Indications, route, and dosage
Rhinitis, allergy symptoms, chronic urticaria
Adults: 1 to 2 mg P.O. b.i.d. Maximum dosage is 4 mg daily.

Drug is not intended for children under age 12.

Pharmacodynamics
Antihistamine action: Azatadine competes with histamine for histamine H_1-receptor sites on the smooth muscle of the bronchi, GI tract, uterus, and large blood vessels; by binding to cellular receptors, they prevent access of histamine and suppress histamine-induced allergic symptoms, even though they do not prevent its release.

Pharmacokinetics
● *Absorption:* Azatadine is well absorbed from the GI tract; its effects begin in 15 to 30 minutes, and peak effect occurs at about 4 hours.
● *Distribution:* The distribution of azatadine is not fully known; it apparently crosses the blood-brain barrier, resulting in CNS effects. Azatadine is minimally protein-bound.
● *Metabolism:* 80% of azatadine is metabolized by the liver.
● *Excretion:* Drug and metabolites are excreted in urine; about 20% of drug is excreted unchanged. Half-life of drug is about 9 to 12 hours.

Contraindications and precautions
Azatadine is contraindicated in patients with known hypersensitivity to this drug or antihistamines with similar chemical structures (cyproheptadine); in patients experiencing asthmatic attacks, because azatadine thickens bronchial secretions; and in patients who have taken monoamine oxidase (MAO) inhibitors within the previous 2 weeks, because these drugs prolong and intensify sedative and anticholinergic effects of antihistamines.

Azatadine should be used with caution in patients with narrow-angle glaucoma; in those with pyloroduodenal obstruction or urinary bladder obstruction from prostatic hyperthrophy or narrowing of the bladder neck, because of their marked anticholinergic effects; in patients with cardiovascular disease, hypertension, or hyperthyroidism, because of the risk of palpitations and tachycardia; and in patients with renal disease, diabetes, bronchial asthma, urinary retention, or stenosing peptic ulcers.

Pregnant women should avoid antihistamines, especially in the third trimester, as should breast-feeding women; although most antihistamines have not been studied in such patients, convulsions have occurred in premature infants and other neonates.

Interactions
MAO inhibitors interfere with detoxification of antihistamines and thus prolong and intensify their sedative and anticholinergic effects; additive CNS depression may occur when azatadine is administered with other CNS depressants, such as alcohol, barbiturates, tranquilizers, sleeping aids, or antianxiety agents.

Effects on diagnostic tests
Discontinue azatadine 4 days before performing diagnostic skin tests; antihistamines can prevent or reduce positive skin reactions, thereby masking a response to the test.

Adverse reactions
● CNS: (especially in elderly patients) drowsiness, dizziness, vertigo, disturbed coordination.
● CV: hypotension, palpitations.
● DERM: urticaria, rash.
● GI: anorexia, nausea, vomiting, dry mouth and throat.

- GU: urinary retention.
- HEMA: thrombocytopenia.
- Respiratory: thick bronchial secretions.

Overdose and treatment

Clinical manifestations of overdose may include either CNS depression (sedation, reduced mental alertness, apnea, and cardiovascular collapse) or CNS stimulation (insomnia, hallucinations, tremors, or convulsions). Anticholinergic symptoms, such as dry mouth, flushed skin, fixed and dilated pupils, tonic-clonic seizures, and postictal depression, are common, especially in children.

Treat overdose by inducing emesis with ipecac syrup (in conscious patient), followed by activated charcoal to reduce further drug absorption. Use gastric lavage if patient is unconscious, is experiencing seizures, or has lost the gag reflex or if ipecac fails. Treat hypotension with vasopressors, and control seizures with diazepam or phenytoin I.V. *Do not give stimulants.*

▶ Special considerations

Besides those relevant to all *antihistamines,* consider the following recommendation.
- Azatadine causes less drowsiness than some antihistamines.

Information for the patient

Recommendations for patient teaching are the same as those for all antihistamines.

Geriatric use

Elderly patients are usually more sensitive to adverse effects of azatadine and are especially likely to experience a greater degree of dizziness, sedation, hyperexcitability, dry mouth, and urinary retention than younger patients.

Pediatric use

The safety of azatadine in children under age 12 has not been established; pediatric patients, especially those under age 6, may experience paradoxical hyperexcitability.

Breast-feeding

Although it is unknown if azatadine is excreted in breast milk, patients should use an alternative feeding method during therapy. Many antihistamines are excreted in breast milk and expose the infant to risk of unusual excitability; newborns and premature infants may experience convulsions.

azathioprine
Imuran

azathioprine sodium
Imuran

- Pharmacologic classification: purine antagonist
- Therapeutic classification: immunosuppressive
- Pregnancy risk category D

How supplied
Available by prescription only
Tablets: 50 mg
Injection: 100 mg

Indications, route, and dosage
Prevention of the rejection of kidney transplants
Adults and children: Initially, 3 to 5 mg/kg P.O. daily beginning on the day of (or 1 to 3 days before) transplantation. After transplantation, dosage may be administered I.V., until patient is able to tolerate oral dosage. Usual maintenance dosage is 1 to 3 mg/kg daily. Dosage varies with patient response.
Severe, refractory rheumatoid arthritis
Adults: Initially, 1 mg/kg (about 50 to 100 mg) P.O. taken as a single dose or in divided doses. If patient response is unsatisfactory after 6 to 8 weeks, dosage may be increased by 0.5 mg/kg daily (up to a maximum of 2.5 mg/kg daily) at 4-week intervals.

Pharmacodynamics
Immunosuppressant action: The mechanism of azathioprine's immunosuppressive activity is unknown; however, the drug may inhibit RNA and DNA synthesis, mitosis, or (in patients undergoing renal transplantation) coenzyme formation and functioning. Azathioprine suppresses cell-mediated hypersensitivity and alters antibody production.

Pharmacokinetics
- *Absorption:* Azathioprine is well absorbed orally.
- *Distribution:* Azathioprine and its major metabolite, mercaptopurine, are distributed throughout the body; both are 30% protein-bound. Azathioprine and its metabolites cross the placenta.
- *Metabolism:* Azathioprine is metabolized primarily to mercaptopurine.
- *Excretion:* Small amounts of azathioprine and mercaptopurine are excreted in urine intact; most of a given dose is excreted in urine as secondary metabolites.

Contraindications and precautions
Azathioprine is contraindicated in patients with known hypersensitivity to the drug and in pregnant patients. It should be used cautiously in patients with hepatic or renal dysfunction; in patients receiving cadaveric kidneys, who may have decreased elimination; and in rheumatoid arthritis patients previously treated with alkylating agents – cyclophosphamide, chlorambucil, or melphalan – who are at increased risk of neoplasia.

Interactions

Azathioprine's major metabolic pathway is inhibited by allopurinol, which competes for the oxidative enzyme xanthine oxidase; concomitant use with allopurinol is potentially hazardous and should be avoided.

Azathioprine may reverse neuromuscular blockade resulting from use of the nondepolarizing muscle relaxants tubocurarine and pancuronium.

Effects on diagnostic tests

Azathioprine alters CBC and differential blood counts, decreases serum uric acid levels, and elevates liver enzymes test results.

Adverse reactions

● GI: nausea, vomiting, anorexia, diarrhea, oral mucous membrane ulceration, esophagitis with possible ulceration.
● HEMA: *leukopenia, macrocytic anemia,* pancytopenia, thrombocytopenia, bone marrow depression.
● Hepatic: jaundice, biliary stasis, hepatic veno-occlusive disease.
● Other: skin rash, hair loss, drug fever, arthralgias, increased risk of infection and malignancy.

Note: Drug should be discontinued or dosage reduced if patient develops signs of hypersensitivity, leukopenia, pancytopenia, or thrombocytopenia, jaundice, or hepatic veno-occlusive disease; or if WBC falls below 3,000/mm³, to prevent progression to irreversible bone marrow depression.

Overdose and treatment

Clinical signs of overdose include nausea, vomiting, diarrhea, and extension of hematologic effects. Supportive treatment may include treatment with blood products if necessary.

▶ Special considerations

● Monitor patient for signs of hepatic damage: clay-colored stools, dark urine, jaundice, pruritus, and elevated liver enzyme levels.
● If infection occurs, drug dosage should be reduced and infection treated.
● If nausea and vomiting occur, divide dose and/or give with or after meals.
● Monitor for unusual bleeding or bruising, fever, or sore throat.
● If used to treat rheumatoid arthritis, nonsteroidal anti-inflammatory agents should be continued when azathiprine therapy is initiated.
● Hematologic status should be monitored while patient is receiving azathioprine. CBCs, including platelet counts, should be taken at least weekly during the 1st month, twice monthly for the 2nd and 3rd months, then monthly.
● Chronic immunosuppression with azathioprine is associated with an increased risk of neoplasia.

Information for the patient

● Teach patient about disease and rationale for therapy; explain possible side effects and importance of reporting them, especially any unusual bleeding or bruising, fever, sore throat, mouth sores, abdominal pain, pale stools, or dark urine.
● Encourage compliance with therapy and follow-up visits.
● Advise patient to avoid pregnancy during therapy and for 4 months after stopping therapy.

● Tell patients with rheumatoid arthritis that clinical response may not be apparent for up to 12 weeks.
● Suggest taking drug with or after meals or in divided doses to prevent nausea.

azithromycin
Zithromax

● Pharmacologic classification: azalide macrolide
● Therapeutic classification: antibiotic
● Pregnancy risk category B

How supplied

Available by prescription only
Capsules: 250 mg

Indications, route and dosage

Acute bacterial exacerbations of chronic obstructive pulmonary disease caused by Haemophilus influenzae, Moraxella (Branhamella) catarrhalis, *or* Streptococcus pneumoniae; *mild community-acquired pneumonia caused by* H. influenzae *or* S. pneumoniae; *uncomplicated skin and skin structure infections caused by* Staphylococcus aureus, Streptococcus pyogenes, *or* S. agalactiae; *and second-line therapy of pharyngitis or tonsillitis caused by* S. pyogenes
Adults and adolescents age 16 and older: Initially, 500 mg P.O. as a single dose on day 1, followed by 250 mg daily on days 2 through 5. Total cumulative dose is 1.5 g.
Nongonococcal urethritis or cervicitis caused by Chlamydia trachomatis
Adults and adolescents age 16 and older: 1 g P.O. as a single dose.

Pharmacodynamics

Antibiotic action: Azithromycin, a derivative of erythromycin, binds to the 50S subunit of bacterial ribosomes, blocking protein synthesis. It is bacteriostatic or bactericidal, depending on concentration.

Pharmacokinetics

● *Absorption:* Azithromycin is rapidly absorbed from the GI tract; food decreases both maximum plasma concentrations and amount of drug absorbed.
● *Distribution:* Azithromycin is rapidly distributed throughout the body and readily penetrates cells; it does not readily enter the CNS. Drug concentrates in fibroblasts and phagocytes. Significantly higher levels of drug are reached in the tissues as compared with the plasma. Uptake and release of the drug from tissues contributes to the long half-life. With a loading dose, peak and trough blood levels are stable within 48 hours. Without a loading dose, 5 to 7 days are required before steady state is reached.
● *Metabolism:* Drug is not metabolized.
● *Excretion:* Drug is excreted mostly in the feces after excretion into the bile. Less than 10% is excreted in the urine. Terminal elimination half-life is 68 hours.

Contraindications and precautions

Azithromycin is contraindicated in patients with hypersensitivity to the drug, erythromycin, or other macrolides.

Drug has been shown safe and effective only in treatment of mild, community-acquired pneumonia caused by *Streptococcus pneumoniae* or *Haemophilus influenzae*. Do not use azithromycin to treat moderate to severe pneumonia in patients for whom outpatient oral therapy is inappropriate or who have risk factors, such as a nosocomial infection or known or suspected bacteremia including a condition requiring hospitalization; elderly or debilitated patients; or patients with illness (such as AIDS or functional asplenia) that may compromise their ability to respond to treatment.

Use cautiously in patients with impaired hepatic function.

Interactions
Concomitant administration with aluminum- and magnesium-containing antacids may result in lower peak plasma levels of azithromycin. Separate administration times by at least 2 hours.

Other macrolides interact with several drugs. Until the effect of azithromycin is known, use cautiously. Macrolides may increase plasma theophylline levels by decreasing theophylline clearance. Concomitant administration with drugs metabolized by the hepatic cytochrome P450 system (such as phenytoin, barbiturates, carbamazepine, and cyclosporine) may result in impaired metabolism of these agents and increased risk of toxicity. Clearance of triazolam may be decreased, increasing the risk of triazolam toxicity. Acute ergot toxicity has been reported when macrolides have been administered with ergotamine or dihydroergotamine.

Also use cautiously with warfarin because other macrolides may increase prothrombin time; effect of azithromycin is unknown. Monitor prothrombin time carefully.

Effects on diagnostic tests
None reported.

Adverse reactions
● CNS: dizziness, vertigo, headache, fatigue, somnolence.
● CV: palpitations, chest pain.
● DERM: rash, photosensitivity.
● GI: nausea, vomiting, diarrhea, abdominal pain, dyspepsia, flatulence, melena, cholestatic jaundice, pseudomembranous colitis.
● GU: monilia, vaginitis, nephritis.
● Other: angioedema.

Overdose and treatment
Specific information is not available. Treat symptomatically.

▶ Special considerations
● Obtain culture and sensitivity tests before first dose. Therapy can begin before results are obtained.
● Drug may cause overgrowth of nonsusceptible bacteria or fungi. Watch for signs and symptoms of superinfection.

Information for the patient
● Tell patient to take all of the medication prescribed, even if he feels better.
● Remind patient that drug should always be taken on an empty stomach because food or antacids will decrease absorption. He should take drug 1 hour before or 2 hours after a meal and should not take antacids.

● Instruct patient to promptly report adverse reactions.
● Serologic tests for syphilis and cultures for gonorrhea should be taken from patients diagnosed with sexually transmitted urethritis or cervicitis. Drug should not be used to treat gonorrhea or syphilis.

Geriatric use
In clinical trials of patients with normal hepatic and renal function, in using the 5-day dosage regimen, no significant pharmacokinetic differences were seen in those between ages 65 and 85.

Pediatric use
Safety and efficacy have not been established in children age 16 and under.

Breast-feeding
It is unknown if drug is excreted in breast milk. Use cautiously in breast-feeding women.

---

azlocillin sodium
Azlin

● Pharmacologic classification: extended-spectrum penicillin, acylaminopenicillin
● Therapeutic classification: antibiotic
● Pregnancy risk category B

How supplied
Available by prescription only
Injection: 2 g, 3 g, 4 g per vial

Indications, route, and dosage
Serious infections caused by susceptible organisms
Adults: 200 to 350 mg/kg I.V. daily in four to six divided doses. Usual dose is 3 g q 4 hours (18 g/day). Maximum daily dosage is 24 g. May be administered by I.V. intermittent infusion or by direct slow I.V. injection.
Children with acute exacerbation of cystic fibrosis: 75 mg/kg q 4 hours (450 mg/kg daily). Maximum daily dosage is 24 g.

Not recommended for use in neonates.
Dosage in renal failure
Reduced dosage is required in patients with creatinine clearance below 30 ml/minute. Measurement of serum level may be necessary.

Pharmacodynamics
Antibiotic action: Azlocillin is bactericidal; it adheres to bacterial penicillin-binding proteins, thus inhibiting bacterial cell wall synthesis. Extended-spectrum penicillins are more resistant to inactivation by certain beta-lactamases, especially those produced by gram-negative organisms, but are still liable to inactivation by certain others.

Azlocillin's spectrum of activity includes many gram-negative aerobic and anaerobic bacilli; many gram-positive and gram-negative aerobic cocci; and some gram-positive aerobic and anaerobic bacilli. Azlocillin may be effective against some strains of carbenicillin-resistant and ticarcillin-resistant gram-negative bacilli. Azlocillin is less active against *Enterobacteriaceae* than other members of this class, such as mezlocillin and piperacillin, but it is more effective against *Pseudomonas aeruginosa*.

Pharmacokinetics

● *Absorption:* No appreciable absorption occurs after oral administration. After an I.M. dose, peak plasma concentrations occur at ½ to 2 hours.

● *Distribution:* Azlocillin is distributed widely after parenteral administration, with good penetration into various organs, tissues, and secretions. It penetrates minimally into uninflamed meninges and slightly into bone and sputum. Volume of distribution is between 0.14 and 0.3 L/kg. Azlocillin is 20% to 46% protein-bound; it crosses the placenta.

● *Metabolism:* Azlocillin is metabolized partially; 15% of a dose is metabolized to inactive metabolites.

● *Excretion:* Azlocillin is excreted primarily (50% to 70%) in urine by glomerular filtration and tubular secretion. It is also excreted in bile and in breast milk. Elimination half-life in adults is about 1 to 1½ hours; in patients with extensive renal impairment, half-life is extended to 4 to 8½ hours. Azlocillin is removed by hemodialysis but not by peritoneal dialysis.

Contraindications and precautions

Azlocillin is contraindicated in patients with known hypersensitivity to any other penicillin or to cephalosporins.

Azlocillin should be used with caution in patients with renal impairment because it is excreted in urine; decreased dosage is required in moderate to severe renal failure.

Interactions

Concomitant use with aminoglycoside antibiotics results in synergistic bactericidal effect against *P. aeruginosa, Escherichia coli, Klebsiella, Citrobacter, Enterobacter, Serratia,* and *Proteus mirabilis.* However, the drugs are physically and chemically incompatible and are inactivated if mixed or given together. In vivo inactivation of aminoglycosides has also been reported when aminoglycosides and extended spectrum penicillins are used concomitantly.

Concomitant use of azlocillin (and other extended-spectrum penicillins) with clavulanic acid also produces a synergistic bactericidal effect against certain beta-lactamase-producing bacteria.

Probenecid blocks tubular secretion of azlocillin, raising its serum concentration levels.

Large doses of penicillins may interfere with renal tubular secretion of methotrexate, delaying elimination and elevating serum concentrations of methotrexate.

Effects on diagnostic tests

Azlocillin alters results of tests for urinary or serum proteins; it interferes with turbidimetric methods that use sulfosalicylic acid, trichloracetic acid, acetic acid, or nitric acid. Azlocillin does not interfere with tests using bromphenal blue (Albustix, Albutest, MultiStix).

Azlocillin may falsely decrease serum aminoglycoside concentrations. Systemic effects of azlocillin may cause hypokalemia and hypernatremia and may prolong prothrombin times; azlocillin may also cause transient elevations in liver function study results and transient reductions in red blood cell, white blood cell, and platelet counts.

Adverse reactions

● CNS: neuromuscular irritability, headache, dizziness.
● GI: nausea, diarrhea, vomiting.
● HEMA: *bleeding with high doses,* neutropenia, eosinophilia, leukopenia, *thrombocytopenia.*

● Metabolic: *hypokalemia.*
● Local: pain at injection site, vein irritation, phlebitis.
● Other: *hypersensitivity* (edema, fever, chills, rash, pruritus, urticaria, *anaphylaxis*), overgrowth of nonsusceptible organisms.

Note: Drug should be discontinued if immediate hypersensitivity reactions or bleeding complications occur and if severe diarrhea occurs, because that may indicate pseudomembranous colitis.

Overdose and treatment

Clinical signs of overdose include neuromuscular hypersensitivity or seizures resulting from CNS irritations by high drug concentrations: a 4- to 6-hour hemodialysis will remove 6% to 50% of azlocillin.

▶ **Special considerations**

Besides those relevant to all *penicillins,* consider the following recommendations.

● Azlocillin is almost always used with another antibiotic, such as an aminoglycoside, in life-threatening situations.

● Azlocillin may be more suitable than carbenicillin or ticarcillin for patients on salt-free diets; azlocillin contains only 2.17 mEq of sodium per gram.

● Azlocillin may be administered by direct I.V. injection, given slowly over at least 5 minutes; chest discomfort occurs if injection is given too rapidly.

● Monitor serum electrolyte levels to avoid adverse effects.

● Because azlocillin is partially dialyzable, patients undergoing hemodialysis may need dosage adjustments.

● Some clinicians administer 3 g I.V. after each dialysis treatment, then every 12 hours.

Geriatric use

Half-life may be prolonged in elderly patients because of decreased renal function.

Pediatric use

Elimination half-life is prolonged in neonates; safety of azlocillin in neonates has not been established.

Breast-feeding

Azlocillin is readily distributed into breast milk; safety in breast-feeding women has not been established.

---

aztreonam
Azactam

● Pharmacologic classification: monobactam
● Therapeutic classification: antibiotic
● Pregnancy risk category B

How supplied

Available by prescription only
Injection: 500-mg, 1-g, 2-g vials

Indications, route, and dosage

Urinary tract, respiratory tract, intra-abdominal, gynecologic, or skin infections; or septicemia caused by gram-negative bacteria
Adults: 500 mg to 2 g I.V. or I.M. q 8 to 12 hours. For severe systemic or life-threatening infections, 2 g q 6 to 8 hours may be given. Maximum dose is 8 g daily.

Children: 90 to 120 mg/kg/day I.M. or I.V. in divided doses q 6 to 8 hours.

Dosage in renal failure
In patients with a creatinine clearance of 10 to 30 ml/min/1.73 m², reduce dose by one half after an initial dose of 1 to 2 g. In patients with a creatinine clearance < 10 ml/min/1.73 m², an initial dose of 500 mg to 2 g should be followed by one quarter of the usual dose at the usual intervals; give one eighth the initial dose after each session of hemodialysis.

Pharmacodynamics
Antibacterial action: Aztreonam is a monobactam that inhibits mucopeptide synthesis of the bacterial cell wall. It preferentially binds to penicillin-binding protein 3 (PBP 3) of susceptible organisms and often causes cell lysis and cell death.

Aztreonam has a narrow spectrum of activity and is usually bactericidal in action. Aztreonam is effective against *Escherichia coli, Enterobacter, Klebsiella pneumoniae, Proteus mirabilis,* and *Pseudomonas aeruginosa.* It has limited activity against *Citrobacter, Haemophilus influenzae, K. oxytoca, Hafnia, Serratia marcescens, E. aerogenes, Morganella morganii, P. vulgaris, Providencia, Branhamella catarrhalis,* and *Neisseria gonorrhoeae.* It does not induce beta-lactamase activity and is highly stable in the presence of beta-lactamases. It does not bind to any essential PBPs in gram-positive or anaerobic organisms.

Pharmacokinetics
● *Absorption:* The drug is absorbed poorly from the GI tract after oral administration but is absorbed rapidly and completely after I.M. or I.V. administration; peak concentrations occur in 60 minutes.
● *Distribution:* The drug is distributed rapidly and widely to all body fluids and tissues, including bile, breast milk, and CSF. It crosses the placental barrier and is found in fetal circulation.
● *Metabolism:* From 6% to 16% is metabolized to inactive metabolites by nonspecific hydrolysis of the beta-lactam ring; 56% to 60% is protein-bound, less if renal impairment is present.
● *Excretion:* Aztreonam is excreted principally in urine as unchanged drug by glomerular filtration and tubular secretion; 1.5% to 3.5% is excreted in feces as unchanged drug. Half-life averages 1.7 hours. The drug is excreted in breast milk; it may be removed by hemodialysis and peritoneal dialysis.

Contraindications and precautions
Aztreonam is contraindicated in patients with known hypersensitivity to the drug.

It should be used cautiously in patients with a history of hypersensitivity or allergic reactions to other beta-lactam antibiotics and in patients with impaired hepatic or renal function (dosage reductions may be required).

Interactions
When used concomitantly, probenecid may prolong the rate of tubular secretion of aztreonam. Synergistic or additive effects occur when the drug is used concomitantly with aminoglycosides, or other beta-lactam antibiotics, including azlocillin, piperacillin, moxalactam, cefoperazone, cefotaxime, clindamycin, or metronidazole. Potent inducers of beta-lactamase production (cefoxitin, imipenem) may inactivate aztreonam. Chloramphenicol is antagonistic; give the two preparations several hours apart.

Use with clavulanic acid may be synergistic or antagonistic, depending on organism involved. Furosemide increases serum aztreonam levels, but this is clinically unimportant.

Effects on diagnostic tests
Aztreonam therapy alters urinary glucose determinations using cupric sulfate (Clinitest or Benedict's reagent) but not Diastix, Tes-Tape, and other glucose oxidase tests.

Coombs' test may become positive during therapy. The drug may prolong prothrombin time and partial thromboplastin time and may transiently increase ALT (SGPT), AST (SGOT), LDH, and serum creatinine concentrations.

Adverse reactions
● CNS: weakness, headache, malaise, *seizure,* confusion, vertigo, paresthesia, insomnia, dizziness.
● CV: hypotension, transient ECG changes, ventricular bigeminy and PVCs.
● DERM: purpura, erythema multiforme, urticaria, *exfoliative dermatitis,* petechiae, pruritus, diaphoresis.
● EENT: nasal congestion, tinnitus, diplopia.
● GI: abdominal cramps, *Clostridium difficile*-associated diarrhea, nausea, vomiting, altered taste sensation, halitosis, tongue numbness, mouth ulcers.
● HEMA: neutropenia, leukocytosis, anemia.
● Hepatic: hepatitis, jaundice.
● Local: thrombophlebitis at I.V. site, discomfort and swelling at I.M. injection site.
● Other: dyspnea, vaginal candidiasis, vaginitis, breast tenderness, *anaphylaxis,* muscular aches.

Overdose and treatment
No information is available on the symptoms of overdose. Hemodialysis or peritoneal dialysis will increase elimination of aztreonam.

▶ Special considerations
Aztreonam also has been used to treat bone and joint infection caused by susceptible aerobic, gram-negative bacteria.
● To reconstitute for I.M. use, dilute with at least 3 ml of sterile water for injection, bacteriostatic water for injection, normal saline solution, or bacteriostatic normal saline solution for each gram of aztreonam (15-ml vial).
● To reconstitute for I.V. use, add 6 to 10 ml of sterile water for injection to each 15-ml vial; for I.V. infusion, prepare as for I.M. solution. May be further diluted by adding to normal saline, Ringer's solution, lactated Ringer's solution, 5% or 10% dextrose, or other electrolyte-containing solutions. For I.V. piggyback (100-ml bottles), add at least 50 ml of diluent for each gram of aztreonam. Final concentration should not exceed 20 mg/ml.
● I.V. route is preferred for doses larger than 1 g or in patients with bacterial septicemia, localized parenchymal abscesses, peritonitis, or other life-threatening infections; administer by direct I.V. push over 3 to 5 minutes or by intermittent infusion over 20 to 60 minutes.
● After addition of diluent, shake vigorously and immediately; not intended for multiple-dose use.
● Solutions may be colorless or light straw yellow. On standing, they may develop a slight pink tint; potency is not affected.
● Admixtures of aztreonam and nafcillin, cephradine, or metronidazole are incompatible; in general, do not

mix aztreonam with other medications. Check with pharmacy for compatibility.
● Reduced dose may be required in patients with impaired renal function, cirrhosis, or other hepatic impairment.
● May be stored at room temperature for 48 hours or in refrigerator for 7 days.

Information for the patient
Tell patient to call immediately if skin rash, redness, or itching develops.

Geriatric use
Studies in elderly males (age 65 to 75) have shown that the half-life of aztreonam may be prolonged in elderly patients because of their diminished renal function.

Breast-feeding
Aztreonam is excreted in breast milk, but is not absorbed from the infant's GI tract and is unlikely to cause serious problems in breast-feeding infants.

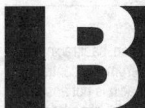

bacampicillin hydrochloride
Spectrobid

- Pharmacologic classification: aminopenicillin
- Therapeutic classification: antibiotic
- Pregnancy risk category B

How supplied
Available by prescription only
Suspension: 125 mg/5 ml (after reconstitution)
Tablets: 400 mg

Indications, route, and dosage
Upper and lower respiratory tract, urinary tract, and skin infections caused by susceptible organisms
Adults and children weighing more than 25 kg: 400 to 800 mg P.O. q 12 hours.
Children weighing less than 25 kg: 25 to 50 mg/kg P.O. q 12 hours.
Gonorrhea
Adults and children weighing more than 25 kg: Usual dosage is 1.6 g plus 1 g probenecid given as a single dose.

Pharmacodynamics
Antibiotic action: Bacampicillin is precursor of ampicillin with no innate bactericidal activity; ampicillin is the active metabolite. Ampicillin is bactericidal; it adheres to bacterial penicillin-binding proteins, thus inhibiting bacterial cell wall synthesis. Each milligram of bacampicillin yields 623 to 727 mcg of ampicillin.

Ampicillin's spectrum of activity includes nonpenicillinase-producing gram-positive bacteria, *Neisseria gonorrhoeae, N. meningitidis, Haemophilus influenzae, Escherichia coli, Proteus mirabilis, Salmonella,* and *Shigella.*

Pharmacokinetics
- *Absorption:* Bacampicillin is hydrolyzed rapidly to ampicillin after oral administration, both in GI tract and plasma; peak plasma concentrations occur 30 to 90 minutes after an oral dose.
- *Distribution:* No unchanged bacampicillin is found in serum after oral administration; ampicillin distributes into pleural, peritoneal, and synovial fluids; lungs, prostate, muscle, liver, and gallbladder; it also penetrates middle ear effusions, maxillary sinus and bronchial secretions, tonsils, and sputum. Ampicillin crosses the placenta; it is 15% to 25% protein-bound.
- *Metabolism:* Bacampicillin is hydrolyzed to ampicillin; ampicillin is metabolized partially.
- *Excretion:* Ampicillin and metabolites are excreted in urine by renal tubular secretion and glomerular filtration; they are also excreted in breast milk. Elimination half-life in adults is 1 to 1½ hours, extended to 7½ hours in patients with severe renal impairment.

Contraindications and precautions
Bacampicillin is contraindicated in patients with known hypersensitivity to any other penicillin or to cephalosporins.

Bacampicillin should not be used in patients with infectious mononucleosis because many patients develop a rash during therapy.

Bacampicillin should be used cautiously in patients with renal impairment, because it is excreted in urine; decreased dosage is required in moderate to severe renal failure.

Interactions
Concomitant use with an aminoglycoside antibiotic causes a synergistic bactericidal effect against some strains of enterococci and group B streptococci. However, the drugs are physically and chemically incompatible and are inactivated if mixed or given together.

Concomitant use with allopurinol may increase incidence of rash from either drug.

Probenecid inhibits renal tubular secretion of ampicillin, increasing its serum concentrations. Large doses of penicillins may interfere with renal tubular secretion of methotrexate, delaying elimination and elevating serum concentrations of methotrexate.

Effects on diagnostic tests
Bacampicillin alters results of urine glucose tests that use cupric sulfate (Benedict's reagent or Clinitest). Make urine glucose determinations with glucose oxidase methods (Clinistix or Tes-Tape).

Bacampicillin may falsely decrease serum aminoglycoside concentrations.

Adverse reactions
- GI: nausea, vomiting, diarrhea, glossitis, stomatitis, *pseudomembranous colitis.*
- GU: *acute interstitial nephritis.*
- HEMA: anemia, thrombocytopenia, thrombocytopenic purpura, eosinophilia, leukopenia.
- Other: *hypersensitivity* (erythematous maculopapular rash, urticaria, *anaphylaxis*), bacterial or fungal superinfection.

Note: Drug should be discontinued if immediate hypersensitivity reaction, bone marrow toxicity, acute interstitial nephritis, or pseudomembranous colitis occurs.

Overdose and treatment
Clinical signs of overdose include neuromuscular sensitivity or seizures. After recent ingestion (4 hours or less), empty the stomach by induced emesis or gastric lavage; follow with activated charcoal to reduce absorption. Bacampicillin and ampicillin can be removed by hemodialysis.

▶ Special considerations
Besides those relevant to all *penicillins,* consider the following recommendations.
- Oral dosage is maximally absorbed from an empty stomach, but food does not cause significant loss of

---

potency of bacampicillin tablets; food impairs absorption of bacampicillin suspension.
● Because the active metabolite of bacampicillin (ampicillin) is dialyzable, patients undergoing hemodialysis may need dosage adjustments.

Information for the patient
● Tell patient to call if rash, fever, or chills develop. A rash is the most common allergic reaction.
● Patient should report diarrhea promptly.

Geriatric use
In elderly patients, diminished renal tubular secretion may prolong half-life of bacampicillin.

Breast-feeding
Ampicillin is distributed readily into breast milk; drug should be used with caution in breast-feeding women.

bacitracin
Ak-tracin, Baciguent

● Pharmacologic classification: polypeptide antibiotic
● Therapeutic classification: antibiotic
● Pregnancy risk category C

How supplied
Available without prescription in topical ointment combination products containing neomycin, polymyxin B, and bacitracin

Available by prescription only
Injection: 10,000-unit and 50,000-unit vials
Ophthalmic ointment: 500 units/g
Topical ointment: 500 units/g

Indications, route, and dosage
Pneumonia or empyema caused by susceptible staphylococci
Infants over 2.5 kg: 1,000 units/kg I.M. daily, divided q 8 to 12 hours. Do not give for more than 12 days.
Infants under 2.5 kg: 900 units/kg I.M. daily, divided q 8 to 12 hours. Do not give for more than 12 days.
  Although current labelling indicates bacitracin is only used in infants, adults with susceptible staphylococcal infections may receive 10,000 to 25,000 units I.M. q 6 hours (maximum 25,000 units/dose, 100,000 units daily).
Topical infections, impetigo, abrasions, cuts, and minor wounds
Adults and children: Apply thin film b.i.d., t.i.d., or more often, depending on severity of condition.
† Treatment of antibiotic-associated pseudomembranous colitis caused by Clostridium difficile
Adults: 20,000 to 25,000 units P.O. q 6 hours for 7 to 10 days.

Pharmacodynamics
Antibacterial action: Bacitracin impairs bacterial cell-wall synthesis, damaging the bacterial plasma membrane and making the cell more vulnerable to osmotic pressure. Drug is effective against many gram-positive organisms, including *Clostridium difficile*. Drug is only minimally active against gram-negative organisms.

Pharmacokinetics
● *Absorption:* With I.M. administration, bacitracin is absorbed rapidly and completely; serum concentrations range from 0.2 to 2 mcg/ml. Bacitracin is not absorbed from the GI tract and not significantly absorbed from intact or denuded skin wounds or mucous membranes.
● *Distribution:* Bacitracin is distributed widely throughout all body organs and fluids except CSF (unless meninges are inflamed). Bacitracin binds to plasma protein only minimally.
● *Metabolism:* Bacitracin is not significantly metabolized.
● *Excretion:* When administered I.M., 10% to 40% of dose is excreted by the kidneys.

Contraindications and precautions
Bacitracin is contraindicated in patients with known hypersensitivity or previous toxic reactions to the agent. Bacitracin should be administered cautiously (if at all) to patients with preexisting renal dysfunction because it is nephrotoxic. Topical ointment is contraindicated for application in external ear canal if eardrum is perforated.

Interactions
Systemically administered bacitracin may induce additive damage when given concomitantly with other nephrotoxic drugs. It also may prolong or increase neuromuscular blockade induced by anesthetics or neuromuscular blocking agents.

Effects on diagnostic tests
Urinary sediment tests may show increased protein and cast excretion. Serum creatinine and blood urea nitrogen (BUN) levels may increase during bacitracin therapy.

Adverse reactions
● DERM: urticaria; rash; stinging and other allergic reactions, such as itching, burning, and swelling of lips or face (with topical application).
● EENT: ototoxicity.
● GI: nausea, vomiting, anorexia, diarrhea, rectal itching or burning.
● GU: *nephrotoxicity* (albuminuria, cylindruria, oliguria, anuria, increased BUN level, tubular and glomerular necrosis).
● HEMA: blood dyscrasias, eosinophilia.
● Local: pain at injection site.
● Other: superinfection, fever, *anaphylaxis*, neuromuscular blockade, allergic reactions, chest tightness, hypotension, overgrowth of nonsusceptible organisms.
Note: Drug should be discontinued if renal toxicity occurs or if patient develops hypersensitivity reaction.

Overdose and treatment
With parenteral administration over several days, bacitracin may cause nephrotoxicity. Acute oral overdose may cause nausea, vomiting, and minor GI upset.
  Treatment is supportive.

▶ Special considerations
● Culture and sensitivity tests should be done before treatment starts.
● Obtain baseline renal function studies before starting therapy, and monitor results daily for signs of deterioration.
● Patients allergic to neomycin may also be allergic to bacitracin.

• Injectable forms of the drug may be used for I.M. administration only. I.V. administration may cause severe thrombophlebitis. Dilute injectable drug in solution containing sodium chloride and 2% procaine hydrochloride (if hospital policy permits). After reconstitution, bacitracin concentration should range from 5,000 to 10,000 units/ml. Inject deeply into upper outer quadrant of buttocks (may be painful). Do not give if patient is sensitive to procaine or para-aminobenzoic acid (PABA) derivatives.

• Ensure adequate fluid intake and monitor output closely.

• Monitor patient's urine pH. It should be kept above 6 with good hydration, and alkalinizing agents. (such as sodium bicarbonate), if necessary, to limit nephrotoxicity.

• Drug may be used orally with neomycin as bowel preparation or in solution as wound irrigating agent.

Information for the patient

• Advise patient to discontinue topical use of the drug and to call promptly if his condition worsens or does not respond to the drug.

• Warn patient with a skin infection to avoid sharing washcloths and towels with family members.

• Instruct patient to wash hands before and after applying ointment.

• Advise patient using ophthalmic ointment to cleanse eye area of excess exudate before applying ointment. Warn him not to touch tip of tube to any part of eye or surrounding tissue.

• Warn patient that ophthalmic ointment may cause blurred vision. Tell him to stop drug immediately and report signs of sensitivity, such as itchy eyelids or constant burning.

• Instruct patient to store ophthalmic ointment in tightly closed, light-resistant container.

• Caution patient not to share eye medications with other persons.

---

baclofen
Lioresal

• Pharmacologic classification: chlorophenyl derivative
• Therapeutic classification: skeletal muscle relaxant
• Pregnancy risk category C

How supplied
Available by prescription only
Tablets: 10 mg, 20 mg

Indications, route, and dosage
Spasticity in multiple sclerosis and other spinal cord lesions
Adults: Initially, 5 mg P.O. t.i.d. for 3 days. Dosage may be increased (based on response) at 3-day intervals by 15 mg daily up to maximum of 80 mg daily.

Pharmacodynamics
Skeletal muscle relaxant action: Precise mechanism of action is unknown, but drug appears to act at the spinal cord level to inhibit transmission of monosynaptic and polysynaptic reflexes, possibly through hyperpolarization of afferent fiber terminals. It may also act at su-

praspinal sites, because baclofen at high doses produces generalized CNS depression. Baclofen decreases the number and severity of spasms and relieves associated pain, clonus, and muscle rigidity, and therefore improves mobility.

Pharmacokinetics
• *Absorption:* Baclofen is rapidly and extensively absorbed from the GI tract, but is subject to individual variation. Peak plasma levels occur at 2 to 3 hours. Also, as dose increases, rate and extent of absorption decreases. Onset of therapeutic effect may not be immediately evident; varies from hours to weeks. Peak effect is seen at 2 to 3 hours.

• *Distribution:* Studies indicate that baclofen is widely distributed throughout the body, with small amounts crossing the blood-brain barrier. It is about 30% plasma protein-bound.

• *Metabolism:* About 15% is metabolized in the liver via deamination.

• *Excretion:* 70% to 80% is excreted in urine unchanged or as its metabolites; remainder, in feces.

Contraindications and precautions
Baclofen is contraindicated in patients with known hypersensitivity to the drug. Administer cautiously to patients with impaired renal function, peptic ulcer disease, cerebral lesions, cerebrovascular accident (increased risk of CNS, respiratory, or cardiac depression), diabetes (may increase blood glucose levels), epilepsy (may cause deterioration of seizure control and EEG), or in patients who need spasticity to maintain upright posture and balance.

Interactions
Concomitant use with CNS depressant drugs, including alcohol, narcotics, antipsychotics, anxiolytics, and general anesthetics, may add to drug's CNS effects. Use with tricyclic antidepressants or monoamine oxidase inhibitors may cause CNS depression, respiratory depression, and hypotension. Baclofen may increase blood glucose levels and require dosage adjustments of hypoglycemic drug or insulin.

Effects on diagnostic tests
Baclofen therapy increases blood glucose, SGOT, and alkaline phosphatase levels.

Adverse reactions
• CNS: transient drowsiness, dizziness, weakness, headache, confusion, fatigue, insomnia.
• CV: hypotension, dyspnea, palpitations, chest pain, syncope.
• DERM: rash, pruritus.
• EENT: blurred vision, miosis, nystagmus, strabismus, mydriasis, diplopia, nasal congestion.
• GI: nausea, constipation, vomiting, dry mouth, taste disorders, diarrhea, anorexia, abdominal pain, positive tests for occult blood in stools.
• GU: urinary frequency or retention, enuresis, dysuria, nocturia, hematuria, inability to ejaculate, impotence.
• Musculoskeletal: muscle pain, paresthesia, coordination disorders (tremor, rigidity, dystonia, ataxia).
• Other: ankle edema, excessive perspiration, weight gain without edema.

Overdose and treatment
Clinical manifestations of overdose include absence of reflexes, vomiting, muscular hypotonia, marked sali-

---

vation, drowsiness, visual disorders, seizures, respiratory depression, and coma.

Treatment requires supportive measures, including endotracheal intubation and positive-pressure ventilation. If patient is conscious, remove drug by inducing emesis followed by gastric lavage.

If patient is comatose, *do not induce emesis*. Gastric lavage may be performed after endotracheal tube is in place with cuff inflated. Do not use respiratory stimulants. Monitor vital signs closely.

▶ **Special considerations**
● The incidence of adverse reactions may be reduced by slowly decreasing the dosage. Abrupt withdrawal can result in hallucinations or seizures and acute exacerbation of spasticity.
● Watch for increased incidence of seizures in patients with epilepsy.
● Watch for increased blood glucose levels in diabetic patients.
● Baclofen is used investigationally to reduce choreiform movements in Huntington's chorea; to reduce rigidity in Parkinson's disease; to reduce spasticity in cerebrovascular accident, cerebral lesions, cerebral palsy, and rheumatic disorders; for analgesia in trigeminal neuralgia; and for treatment of unstable bladder.
● In some patients, smoother response may be obtained by giving daily dose in four divided doses.
● Patient may need supervision during walking. The initial loss of spasticity induced by baclofen may affect patient's ability to stand or walk. (In some patients, spasticity helps patient to maintain upright posture and balance.)
● Observe patient's response to drug. Signs of effective therapy may appear in a few hours to 1 week and may include diminished frequency of spasms and severity of foot and ankle clonus, increased ease and range of joint motion, and enhanced performance of daily activities.
● Drug should be discontinued if signs of improvement do not occur within 1 to 2 months.
● Closely monitor patients with epilepsy by EEG, clinical observation, and interview for possible loss of seizure control.

Information for the patient
● Advise patient to report adverse reactions promptly. Most can be reduced by decreasing dosage. Reportedly, drowsiness, dizziness, and ataxia are more common in patients over age 40.
● Warn patient of additive effects with use of other CNS depressants, including alcohol.
● Caution patient to avoid hazardous activities that require mental alertness.
● Tell diabetic patient that baclofen may raise blood glucose levels and may require adjustment of insulin dosage during treatment with baclofen. Urge patient to promptly report changes in urine or blood glucose tests.
● Caution patient against taking any nonprescription drug without medical approval. Explain that hazardous drug interactions are possible.
● Inform patient that drug should be withdrawn gradually over 1 to 2 weeks. Abrupt withdrawal after prolonged use of this drug may cause anxiety, agitated behavior, auditory and visual hallucinations, severe tachycardia, and acute spasticity.

Geriatric use
Elderly patients are especially sensitive to this drug. Observe carefully for adverse reactions, such as mental confusion, depression, and hallucinations. Lower doses are usually indicated.

Pediatric use
Not recommended for children under age 12.

PHARMACOLOGIC CLASS

barbiturates

amobarbital
amobarbital sodium
aprobarbital
butabarbital
mephobarbital
metharbital
pentobarbital sodium
phenobarbital
phenobarbital sodium
primidone
secobarbital sodium

Barbituric acid was compounded over 100 years ago in 1864. The first hypnotic barbiturate, barbital, was introduced into medicine in 1903. Although barbiturates have been used extensively as sedative-hypnotics and antianxiety agents, benzodiazepines are the current drugs of choice for sedative-hypnotic effects. Phenobarbital remains a cornerstone of anticonvulsant therapy. A few short-acting barbiturates are used as general anesthetics.

Pharmacology
Barbiturates are structurally related compounds that act throughout the central CNS, particularly in the mesencephalic reticular activating system, which controls the CNS arousal mechanism. Barbiturates decrease both presynaptic and postsynaptic membrane excitability.

The exact mechanism(s) of action of barbiturates at these sites is not known, nor is it clear which cellular and synaptic actions result in sedative-hypnotic effects. Barbiturates can produce all levels of CNS depression, from mild sedation to coma to death. Barbiturates exert their effects by facilitating the actions of gamma-aminobutyric acid (GABA). Barbiturates also exert a central effect, which depresses respiration and GI motility. The principal anticonvulsant mechanism of action is reduction of nerve transmission and decreased excitability of the nerve cell. Barbiturates also raise the seizure threshold. After oral or rectal administration all barbiturates act within 20 to 60 minutes.

Clinical indications and actions
Seizure disorders
Phenobarbital is used in the prophylactic treatment of seizure disorders. It is used mainly in tonic-clonic (grand mal) and partial seizures. At anesthetic doses, all barbiturates have anticonvulsant activity.

Barbiturates suppress the spread of seizure activity produced by epileptogenic foci in the cortex, thalamus, and limbic systems by enhancing the effects of GABA.

Sedation, hypnosis

All currently available barbiturates are used as sedative-hypnotics for short-term (up to 2 weeks) treatment of insomnia because of their nonspecific CNS effects.

Barbiturates are not used as routinely as sedatives because of excess sedation, short-term efficacy, and the potential for severe adverse reactions upon withdrawal or overdose; they have been replaced for such use by benzodiazepines and nonspecific sedatives. Barbiturate-induced sleep differs from physiologic sleep by decreasing the rapid-eye-movement (REM) sleep cycles.

Overview of adverse reactions

Drowsiness, lethargy, vertigo, headache, and CNS depression are common with barbiturates. After hypnotic doses, a hangover effect, subtle distortion of mood, and impairment of judgment or motor skills may continue for many hours. After a decrease in dosage or discontinuation of barbiturates used for hypnosis, rebound insomnia or increased dreaming or nightmares may occur. Barbiturates cause hyperalgesia in subhypnotic doses. Hypersensitivity reactions (rash, fever, serum sickness) are not common, and are more likely to occur in patients with a history of asthma or allergies to other drugs; reactions include urticaria, rash, angioedema, and Stevens-Johnson syndrome. Barbiturates can cause paradoxical excitement at low doses, confusion in elderly patients, and hyperactivity in children. High fever, severe headache, stomatitis, conjunctivitis, or rhinitis may precede skin eruptions. Because of the potential for fatal consequences, discontinue barbiturates if dermatologic reactions occur.

Withdrawal symptoms may occur after as little as 2 weeks of uninterrupted therapy. Symptoms of abstinence usually occur within 8 to 12 hours after the last dose, but may be delayed up to 5 days. They include weakness, anxiety, nausea, vomiting, insomnia, hallucinations, and possibly seizures.

▶ **Special considerations**
● Dosage of barbiturates must be individualized for each patient, because different rates of metabolism and enzyme induction occur.
● Parenteral solutions are highly alkaline; avoid extravasation, which may cause local tissue damage and tissue necrosis; inject I.V. or deep I.M. only. Do not exceed 5 ml per I.M. injection site to avoid tissue damage.
● Too-rapid I.V. administration of barbiturates may cause respiratory depression, apnea, laryngospasm, or hypotension. Have resuscitative measures available. Assess I.V. site for signs of infiltration or phlebitis.
● May be given rectally if oral or parenteral route is inappropriate.
● Assess level of consciousness before and frequently during therapy to evaluate effectiveness of drug. Monitor neurologic status for possible alterations or deteriorations. Monitor seizure character, frequency, and duration for changes. Institute seizure precautions, as necessary.
● Vital signs should be checked frequently, especially during I.V. administration.
● Assess patient's sleeping patterns before and during therapy to ensure effectiveness of drug.
● Institute safety measures – side rails, assistance when out of bed, call light within reach – to prevent falls and injury.

● Anticipate possible rebound confusion and excitatory reactions in patient.
● Assess bowel elimination patterns; monitor for complaints of constipation. Advise diet high in fiber, if indicated.
● Monitor prothrombin time carefully in patients taking anticoagulants; dosage of anticoagulant may require adjustment to counteract possible interaction.
● Observe patient to prevent hoarding or self-dosing, especially in depressed or suicidal patients, or those who are or have a history of being drug-dependent.
● Abrupt discontinuation may cause withdrawal symptoms; discontinue slowly.
● Death is common with an overdose of 2 to 10 g; it may occur at much smaller doses if alcohol is also ingested.
● Avoid administering barbiturates to patients with status asthmaticus.

Information for the patient
● Warn patient to avoid concurrent use of other drugs with CNS depressant effects, such as antihistamines, analgesics, and alcohol, because they will have additive effects and result in increased drowsiness. Instruct patient to seek medical approval before taking any nonprescription cold or allergy preparations.
● Caution patient not to increase or decrease dose or frequency without medical approval; abrupt discontinuation of medication may trigger rebound insomnia, with increased dreaming, nightmares, or seizures.
● Advise patient against driving and other hazardous tasks that require alertness while taking barbiturates. Instruct patient in safety measures to prevent injury.
● Be sure patient understands that barbiturates are capable of causing physical or psychological dependence (addiction), and that these effects may be transmitted to the fetus; withdrawal symptoms can occur in neonates whose mothers took barbiturates in the third trimester.
● Instruct patient to report any skin eruption or other marked adverse effect.
● Explain that a morning hangover is common after therapeutic use of barbiturates.

Geriatric use
Elderly patients and patients receiving subhypnotic doses may experience hyperactivity, excitement, or hyperalgesia. Use with caution.

Pediatric use
Premature infants are more susceptible to the depressant effects of barbiturates because of immature hepatic metabolism. Children receiving barbiturates may experience hyperactivity, excitement, or hyperalgia.

Breast-feeding
Barbiturates are excreted in breast milk and may result in infant CNS depression. Use with caution.

Representative combinations
Amobarbital with ephedrine hydrochloride, theophylline, and chlorpheniramine maleate: Theo-Span; with secobarbital: Amsc, Compobarb, Dusotal, Lanabarb, Tuinal; with dextroamphetamine: Amodex

Butabarbital with acetaminophen: Constalgesic, G-3, Sedapap, Sedapap 10, Amino-Bar, Minotal; with acetaminophen and mephenesin: T-caps; with acetaminophen, phenacetin, and caffeine: Windolor; with aminophylline, phenylpropanolamine hydrochloride, chlorpheniramine maleate, aluminum hydroxide, and magnesium hydrobromide: Pedo-Sol; with acetaminophen, salicylamide, d-amphetamine Sedragesic; with amphetamine sulfate: Bontril; with belladonna: Butibel, Quiebel; with secobarbital and phenobarbital: Tri-Barbs.

Pentobarbital sodium with acetaminophen, salicylamide, and codeine: Tega-Code; with adiphenine hydrochloride: Spasmasorb; with atropine sulfate, hyoscine hydrobromide, and hyoscyamine: Eldonal; with carbromal: Carboprent; with ephedrine: Ephedrine and Nembutal; with ergotamine tartrate, caffeine, and bellafoline: Cafergot-P.B.; with homatropine methylbromide, dehydrocholic acid, and ox bile extract: Homachol; with pyrilamine maleate: A-N-R, Rectorette; with secobarbital, butabarbital, and phenobarbital: Quadrabarb; with vitamin compounds and d-methamphetamine hydrochloride: Fetamin.

Phenobarbital with CNS stimulants: Amodrine, Aristrate, Asminyl, Belkatal, Bellophen, Bowdrin, Bronkolixir, Bronkatab, Duovent, Ephenyllin, Luasmin, Phelantin, Phyldrox, Quadrinal, Sedamine, Spabelin, Synophedal, T.E.P.; with mannitol hexanitrate: Hyrunal, Manotensin, Ruhexatal, Vascused, Vermantin; with veratrum viride: Hyperlon, Hyrunal, Verabar; with theobromine: Harbolin, Theocardone, T.P.K.I.; with hyoscyamus: Anaspaz PB, Elixiral, Floramine, Gylanphenb, Neoquess, Nevrotose, Restophen, Sedajen.

See also Anticholinergics (belladonna alkaloids), Salicylates, Xanthine derivatives.

bacillus Calmette-Guérin, live intravesical (BCG)
TheraCys, TICE BCG

- Pharmacologic classification: bacterial agent
- Therapeutic classification: antineoplastic agent
- Pregnancy risk category C

How supplied
Available by prescription only

TheraCys
Suspension (freeze-dried) for bladder instillation: 27 mg/vial

TICE BCG
Suspension (freeze-dried) for bladder instillation: approximately 50 mg/ampule

Indications, route, and dosage
Treatment of in situ carcinoma of the urinary bladder (primary and relapsed)
Adults: Administer 3 reconstituted and diluted vials intravesically once weekly for 6 weeks (induction) followed by additional treatments at 3, 6, 12, 18, and 24 months (TheraCys); 1 bladder instillation (1 ampule suspended in 50 ml sterile, preservative-free saline solution) once weekly for 6 weeks, then once monthly for 6 to 12 months (TICE BCG).

Pharmacodynamics
Antitumor action: Exact mechanism unknown. Instillation of the live bacterial suspension causes a local inflammatory response. Local infiltration of histiocytes and leukocytes is followed by a decrease in the superficial tumors within the bladder.

Pharmacokinetics
No information available.

Contraindications and precautions
Because of the risk of bacterial infection, the drug is contraindicated in patients with compromised immune systems and in patients receiving immunosuppressive therapy. Persons with immune deficiency should not handle the product.

BCG is contraindicated in patients with fever of unknown origin. If the fever is caused by an infection, the drug should be withheld until the patient has recovered. It is also contraindicated in patients with urinary tract infection because of the risk of increased bladder irritation or disseminated BCG infection.

Drug should not be used as an immunizing agent for the prevention of cancer or tuberculosis. Do not confuse the drug with BCG vaccine.

Carefully monitor patient's urinary status because the drug causes an inflammatory response in the bladder. It has been associated with bacterial urinary tract infection, hematuria, dysuria, and urinary frequency.

Closely monitor patients for evidence of systemic BCG infection. Withhold therapy if systemic infection is suspected (short-term high fever above 103 F. [39.4 C.]; persistent fever above 101 F. [38.3 C.] over 2 days or with severe malaise). Contact infectious disease specialist for initiation of antituberculosis therapy. BCG infections are rarely evidenced by positive cultures.

Patients with a small bladder capacity may experience increased local irritation with the usual dose of BCG live.

BCG intravesical should not be administered within 1 week of transurethral resection. Fatal disseminated BCG infection has occurred after traumatic catheterization.

The drug has the potential to cause hypersensitivity reactions. Manage such reactions symptomatically.

Interactions
Concomitant antimicrobial therapy for other infections may attenuate the response to BCG live.

Drugs that depress the bone marrow, radiation therapy, and immunosuppressants may impair the response to BCG intravesical because these treatments can decrease the patient's immune response. These treatments may also increase the risk of osteomyelitis or disseminated BCG infection.

Effects on diagnostic tests
Tuberculin sensitivity may be rendered positive by BCG intravesical treatment. Determine patients reactivity to tuberculin before initiating therapy.

Adverse reactions
- GI: nausea, vomiting, anorexia, diarrhea, mild abdominal pain.
- GU: dysuria, urinary frequency, hematuria, cystitis, urinary urgency, urinary incontinence, urinary tract infection, cramps, pain, decreased bladder capacity, local infection, renal toxicity, genital pain.
- HEMA: anemia, leukopenia, thrombocytopenia.

- Other: malaise, fever (above 101 F.), chills, myalgia, arthralgia, elevated liver enzymes.

Overdose and treatment
No information available.

▶ Special considerations
- Reconstitute the drug just before use, only with the diluent provided. All persons handling the product should wear masks and gloves.
- Handle the drug and all material used for instillation of the drug as infectious material because it contains live attenuated mycobacteria. Dispose of all associated materials (syringes, catheters, and containers) as biohazardous waste.
- Each vial of TheraCys should be reconstituted with 1 ml of the supplied diluent. Do not remove the rubber stopper to prepare the solution. The contents of the three reconstituted vials are to be added to 50 ml of sterile, preservative-free saline (final volume, 53 ml). A urethral catheter is instilled into the bladder under aseptic conditions, the bladder is drained, and then 53 ml of the prepared solution is added by gravity feed. The catheter is then removed.
- To administer TICE BCG, use thermosetting plastic or sterile glass containers and syringes. Draw 1 ml of sterile, preservative-free saline solution into a 3-ml syringe. Add to one ampule of the drug; gently expel back into the ampule three times to ensure thorough mixing. Dispense the cloudy suspension into the top end of a catheter-tipped syringe that contains 49 ml saline. Gently rotate the syringe.
- Use strict aseptic technique to administer the drug, thus minimizing the trauma to the GU tract and preventing introduction of other contaminants to the area.
- If there is evidence of traumatic catheterization, do not administer the drug and delay treatment for at least 1 week. Subsequent treatment may resume as if no interruption of the schedule has occurred.
- Bladder irritation can be treated symptomatically with phenazopyridine, acetaminophen, and propantheline bromide. Systemic adverse reactions that are caused by hypersensitivity can be treated with diphenhydramine hydrochloride.

Information for the patient
- Tell the patient that after installation he is to retain the fluid in his bladder for 2 hours (if possible). For the first hour he should lie 15 minutes prone, 15 minutes supine, and 15 minutes on each side. He may be up for the second hour.
- For safety, the patient should be seated when voiding. Instruct patient to disinfect urine for 6 hours after instillation of the drug. Tell patient to add undiluted household bleach (5% sodium hypochlorite solution) in equal volume to voided urine to the toilet; allow to stand for 15 minutes before flushing.
- Tell the patient to call physician if the symptoms worsen or if any of the following symptoms occur: blood in the urine, fever and chills, frequent urge to urinate or painful urination, nausea, vomiting, joint pain, rash, or cough.

Pediatric use
Safe use in children has not been established.

Breast-feeding
It is not known if the drug is excreted in breast milk. Use with caution in breast-feeding women.

---

bacillus Calmette-Guérin (BCG) vaccine

- Pharmacologic classification: vaccine
- Therapeutic classification: bacterial vaccine
- Pregnancy risk category C

How supplied
Available by prescription only
Percutaneous injection: 1 to 8 × 10⁸ colony-forming units (CFU) per ml of Tice-Chicago or Tice-University of Illinois strain BCG per ml, equivalent to approximately 50 mg
Intradermal injection: 8 to 26 million CFU/ml of live attenuated Danish substrain of BCG per ml

Indications, route, and dosage
Tuberculosis exposure
Intradermal injection
Adults and children: 0.1 ml intradermally.
Neonates: 0.05 ml intradermally.
Percutaneous injection
Adults and children over 1 month: Apply 0.2 to 0.3 ml of prepared vaccine on the cleansed surface of the skin; apply multiple-puncture disk through vaccine. The vaccine should flow into the wound and dry. Keep site dry for 24 hours.
Repeat dosage in all patients who have a negative tuberculin test at 2- to 3-month follow-up. ACIP/ACET suggests revaccination with a full dose at 1 year of age if skin test is negative.
Neonates under 1 month: Reduce dosage to one-half by using 2 ml of sterile water when reconstituting.

Pharmacodynamics
Immunostimulant action: BCG vaccine promotes active immunity to tuberculosis. Immunity is not permanent or entirely predictable.

Pharmacokinetics
No information available.

Contraindications and precautions
BCG vaccine is contraindicated in patients with recent smallpox vaccinations, extensive burns, or positive tuberculin (PPD) skin tests as well as in immunosuppressed patients (those with congenital immunodeficiencies, cancer, or acquired immune deficiency syndrome and those being treated with corticosteroids, antineoplastic agents, or radiation).

Interactions
Concomitant use of BCG vaccine with antitubercular drugs (isoniazid, rifampin, or streptomycin) inhibits the multiplication of BCG and impairs the vaccine's efficacy. Concomitant use with corticosteroids or immunosuppressants may alter the immune response to BCG vaccine and should be avoided.

Effects on diagnostic tests
BCG vaccination may affect the interpretation of subsequent tuberculin skin test reactions.

Adverse reactions
● Local: lymphangitis, lymph node and skin abscesses, ulceration at injection site (2 to 3 weeks after injection), lupus reaction.
● Other: urticaria of trunk and limbs, lymphadenitis, granulomas, osteomyelitis, *anaphylaxis*, disseminated BCG disease.

Overdose and treatment
No information available.

▶ **Special considerations**
● Obtain thorough history of allergies and reactions to immunizations.
● Epinephrine solution 1:1,000 should be available to treat allergic reactions.
● Severe or prolonged reactions may be treated with antitubercular drugs.
● To prepare intradermal injection, add 1 ml sterile water (without preservatives) to each vial of vaccine. Do not shake vial after reconstitution, to avoid foaming. Allow to stand for 1 minute; withdrawing solution into syringe will create a uniform suspension.
● To prepare percutaneous injection, add 1 ml sterile water (without preservatives) to each vial of vaccine. Draw mixture into syringe and expel into ampule three times to ensure adequate mixing.
● If alcohol is used to swab the skin, allow it to evaporate before vaccination. Otherwise, it could inactivate the virus.
● Vaccinate patients with chronic skin diseases in area of healthy skin.
● BCG vaccine is of no value as an immunoprophylactic in patients with a positive PPD test.
● Expected lesion forms 7 to 10 days after vaccination with intradermal form and reaches a maximum diameter of 8 mm in 5 weeks.
● Articles contaminated with this live vaccine must be autoclaved or treated with formaldehyde before disposal.
● Store vaccine at 2° to 8° C. (36° to 46° F.). Avoid exposure to light.
● BCG vaccine has shown some value in treating various cancers, including malignant melanoma, multiple myeloma, leukemia, bladder cancer, some lung cancers, and some breast tumors. Consult other references and published protocols for appropriate dosage regimens.

Information for the patient
● Tell patient to expect swollen lymph nodes or a body rash after vaccination. A lesion at the injection site will develop within 7 to 10 days of vaccination and may persist for up to 6 months.
● Tell patient to report any distressing adverse reactions.
● Tell patient that a tuberculin skin test will be performed 2 to 3 months after vaccination, to confirm development of delayed hypersensitivity.

beclomethasone dipropionate
beclomethasone dipropionate
monohydrate

Nasal inhalants
Beconase, Vancenase

Nasal sprays
Beconase AQ, Vancenase AQ

Oral inhalants
Beclovent, Becotide∗, Vanceril

● Pharmacologic classification: glucocorticoid
● Therapeutic classification: anti-inflammatory, antiasthmatic
● Pregnancy risk category C

How supplied
Available by prescription only
Nasal aerosol: 42 mcg/metered spray
Nasal spray: 42 mcg/metered spray
Oral inhalation aerosol: 42 mcg/metered spray

Indications, route, and dosage
Steroid-dependent asthma
Oral inhalation
Adults: Two to four inhalations t.i.d. or q.i.d. Maximum of 20 inhalations daily.
Children age 6 to 12: One to two inhalations t.i.d. or q.i.d. Maximum of 10 inhalations daily.
Perennial or seasonal rhinitis; prevention of recurrence of nasal polyps after surgical removal
Nasal inhalation
Adults and children over age 12: One spray (42 mcg) in each nostril b.i.d. to q.i.d. Usual total dosage is 168 to 400 mcg daily.
Children age 6 to 12: One spray in each nostril t.i.d. (252 mcg daily).

Pharmacodynamics
● *Anti-inflammatory action:* Beclomethasone stimulates the synthesis of enzymes needed to decrease the inflammatory response. The anti-inflammatory and vasoconstrictor potency of topically applied beclomethasone is, on a weight basis, about 5,000 times greater than that of hydrocortisone, 500 times greater than that of betamethasone or dexamethasone, and about five times greater than fluocinolone or triamcinolone.
● *Antiasthmatic action:* Beclomethasone is used as a nasal inhalant to treat symptoms of seasonal or perennial rhinitis and to prevent the recurrence of nasal polyps after surgical removal, and as an oral inhalant to treat bronchial asthma in patients who require chronic administration of corticosteroids to control symptoms.

Pharmacokinetics
● *Absorption:* After nasal inhalation, the drug is absorbed primarily through the nasal mucosa, with minimal systemic absorption. After oral inhalation, the drug is absorbed rapidly from the lungs and GI tract. Greater systemic absorption is associated with oral inhalation, but systemic effects do not occur at usual doses because of rapid metabolism in the liver and local me-

tabolism of drug that reaches the lungs. Onset of action usually occurs in a few days but may take as long as 3 weeks in some patients.

• *Distribution:* Distribution after intranasal administration has not been described. There is no evidence of tissue storage of beclomethasone or its metabolites. About 10% to 25% of a nasal spray or orally inhaled dose is deposited in the respiratory tract. The remainder, deposited in the mouth and oropharynx, is swallowed. When absorbed, it is 87% bound to plasma proteins.

• *Metabolism:* Beclomethasone that is swallowed undergoes rapid metabolism in the liver or GI tract to a variety of metabolites, some of which have minor glucocorticoid activity. The portion that is inhaled into the respiratory tract is partially metabolized before absorption into systemic circulation. Most of the drug is metabolized in the liver.

• *Excretion:* Excretion of beclomethasone administered by inhalation has not been described; however, when the drug is administered systemically, its metabolites are excreted mainly in feces via biliary elimination and to a lesser extent in urine. The biological half-life of beclomethasone averages 15 hours.

Contraindications and precautions
Beclomethasone is contraindicated in patients with acute status asthmaticus and in patients who are hypersensitive to any component of the preparation.

Drug should be used with caution in patients receiving systemic corticosteroids, because of increased risk of hypothalamic-pituitary-adrenal axis suppression; when substituting inhalation for oral systemic administration, because withdrawal symptoms may occur; and in patients with tuberculosis, healing nasal septal ulcers, oral or nasal surgery or trauma, or bacterial, fungal, or viral respiratory infection.

Interactions
None reported.

Effects on diagnostic tests
None reported.

Adverse reactions
• EENT: (after oral inhalation) flushing, rash, dry mouth, hoarseness, irritation of the tongue or throat, and impaired sense of taste; (after nasal inhalation) itchy nose, dryness, burning, irritation and sneezing, infrequent epistaxis, bloody mucus.
• Immune: immunosuppression (may allow fungal overgrowth and infections of the nose, mouth, or throat).

Note: Drug should be discontinued if no improvement is evident after 3 weeks, or if nasal or oral infections develop.

Overdose and treatment
No information available.

▶ Special considerations
Recommendations for use of beclomethasone and for care and teaching of patients during therapy are the same as those for all *inhalant adrenocorticoids.*

Pediatric use
Beclomethasone is not recommended for children under age 6.

bendroflumethiazide
Naturetin

• Pharmacologic classification: thiazide diuretic
• Therapeutic classification: diuretic, antihypertensive
• Pregnancy risk category B

How supplied
Available by prescription only
Tablets: 2.5 mg, 5 mg, 10 mg

Indications, route, and dosage
Edema, hypertension
Adults: 2.5 to 20 mg P.O. daily as a single morning dose or in two divided doses.
Children: Initially, 0.1 to 0.4 mg/kg daily in one or two doses. Maintenance dosage is 0.05 to 0.1 mg/kg daily in one or two doses.

Pharmacodynamics
• *Diuretic action:* Bendroflumethiazide increases urinary excretion of sodium and water by inhibiting sodium reabsorption in the cortical diluting tubule of the nephron, thus relieving edema.
• *Antihypertensive action:* The exact mechanism of bendroflumethiazide's antihypertensive effect is unknown; its effect may partially result from direct arteriolar vasodilation and a decrease in total peripheral resistance.

Pharmacokinetics
• *Absorption:* Bendroflumethiazide is well absorbed from the GI tract.
• *Distribution:* Extent of distribution is unknown.
• *Metabolism:* Insignificant.
• *Excretion:* Bendroflumethiazide is excreted unchanged in urine.

Contraindications and precautions
Bendroflumethiazide is contraindicated in patients with anuria and in those with known sensitivity to the drug or to other sulfonamide derivatives. Bendroflumethiazide should be used cautiously in patients with severe renal disease because it may decrease glomerular filtration rate and precipitate azotemia; in patients with impaired hepatic function or liver disease because electrolyte changes may precipitate coma; and in patients taking digoxin because hypokalemia may predispose patients to digitalis toxicity.

Naturetin contains tartrazine, which may cause allergic reactions such as bronchospasm in asthmatic and aspirin-sensitive patients.

Interactions
Bendroflumethiazide potentiates the hypotensive effects of most other antihypertensive drugs; this may be used to therapeutic advantage.

Bendroflumethiazide may potentiate hyperglycemic, hypotensive, and hyperuricemic effects of diazoxide, and its hyperglycemic effect may increase insulin or sulfonylurea requirements in diabetic patients.

Bendroflumethiazide may reduce renal clearance of lithium, elevating serum lithium levels, and may necessitate a 50% reduction in lithium dosage.

Bendroflumethiazide turns urine slightly more alkaline and may decrease urinary excretion of some amines such as amphetamine and quinidine; alkaline urine may also decrease therapeutic efficacy of methenamine compounds such as methenamine mandelate.

Cholestyramine and colestipol may bind bendroflumethiazide, preventing its absorption; administer drugs 1 hour apart.

Effects on diagnostic tests

Bendroflumethiazide therapy may alter serum electrolyte levels and may increase serum urate, glucose, cholesterol, and triglyceride levels.

Bendroflumethiazide may interfere with tests for parathyroid function and should be discontinued before such tests.

Adverse reactions
● CV: volume depletion and dehydration, orthostatic hypotension, hypercholesterolemia, hypertriglyceridemia.
● DERM: dermatitis, photosensitivity, rash.
● GI: anorexia, nausea, pancreatitis.
● HEMA: *aplastic anemia, agranulocytosis,* leukopenia, thrombocytopenia.
● Hepatic: hepatic encephalopathy.
● Metabolic: *asymptomatic hyperuricemia; gout; hyperglycemia and impairment of glucose tolerance;* fluid and electrolyte imbalances, including hypokalemia, dilutional hyponatremia and hypochloremia, and hypercalcemia; metabolic acidosis.
● Other: hypersensitivity reactions, such as pneumonitis and vasculitis.
Note: Drug should be discontinued if rising BUN and serum creatinine levels indicate renal impairment or if patient shows signs of impending coma.

Overdose and treatment

Clinical signs of overdose include GI irritation and hypermotility, diuresis, and lethargy, which may progress to coma.

Treatment is mainly supportive; monitor and assist respiratory, cardiovascular, and renal function as indicated. Monitor fluid and electrolyte balance. Induce vomiting with ipecac syrup in conscious patient; otherwise, use gastric lavage to avoid aspiration. Do not give cathartics; these promote additional loss of fluids and electrolytes.

▶ Special considerations
Besides those relevant to all *thiazide diuretics,* consider the following recommendation.
● Diuretic effect lasts more than 18 hours, permitting longer dosage intervals.

Geriatric use
Elderly and debilitated patients require close observation and may require reduced dosages. They are more sensitive to excess diuresis because of age-related changes in cardiovascular and renal function. Excess diuresis promotes orthostatic hypotension, dehydration leading to hypovolemia, hyponatremia, hypomagnesemia, and hypokalemia.

Pediatric use
Safety and effectiveness have not been established.

Breast-feeding
Bendroflumethiazide is distributed in breast milk; its safety and effectiveness in breast-feeding women have not been established.

---

bentiromide
Chymex

● Pharmacologic classification: para-aminobenzoic acid (PABA) derivative
● Therapeutic classification: pancreatic function test
● Pregnancy risk category B

How supplied
Available by prescription only
Solution: 500 mg/17.5 ml

Indications, route, and dosage
Screening test for pancreatic exocrine insufficiency
Adults and children over age 12: Following overnight fast and morning void, administer a single 500-mg dose P.O. and follow with an 8-oz glass of water.
Children under age 12: Dose is 14 mg/kg followed with an 8-oz glass of water.

Give patient another glass of water 2 hours after dose. An additional two glasses of water are recommended during postdosing hours 2 to 6.

Pharmacodynamics
Pancreatic function testing action: Following oral administration, bentiromide is cleaved by the pancreatic enzyme chymotrypsin, causing the release of PABA (para-aminobenzoic acid). This test is not conclusive, because a negative result does not rule out pancreatic disease and a positive result is only a strong indicator of a problem. Confirmatory tests are required.

Pharmacokinetics
● *Absorption:* The absorption process depends on the presence of chymotrypsin in the small intestine. PABA is absorbed after hydrolysis of bentiromide by chymotrypsin; the extent of absorption may be altered by other conditions, including gastric stasis, maldigestion, and malabsorption. The mean peak plasma level in healthy adults is about 6 mcg/ml and occurs in 2 to 3 hours. In patients with chronic pancreatitis, mean peak plasma levels are reduced to 3 mcg/ml and occur in 2 to 6 hours.
● *Distribution:* The distribution into body tissues and fluids has not been determined for bentiromide or PABA.
● *Metabolism:* Bentiromide is hydrolyzed in the small intestine and the metabolites are further broken down in the liver.
● *Excretion:* PABA and its metabolites are excreted in urine.

Contraindications and precautions
Bentiromide is contraindicated in patients with hypersensitivity to bentiromide or PABA; such patients may have an anaphylactic reaction. Drug should be used with caution in pregnancy and breast-feeding, because safety of such use has not been established.

Interactions
When used concomitantly, bentiromide may displace methotrexate from PABA binding sites. Pancreatic enzyme preparations may yield a false-negative result; they should be discontinued 5 days before testing with bentiromide.

Effects on diagnostic tests
Bentiromide therapy alters no other tests, but several factors may invalidate bentiromide test results. Various drugs, including acetaminophen, benzocaine, chloramphenicol, thiazides, lidocaine, PABA preparations, procainamide, procaine, and sulfonamides, are metabolized into arylamines, which increase the PABA content in urine. Foods such as apples, plums, prunes, and cranberries have a similar effect. All of these drugs and foods should be discontinued at least 3 days before testing with bentiromide.

Adverse reactions
- CNS: headache.
- GI: diarrhea, gas, nausea, vomiting.
- Respiratory: shortness of breath (rare).
- Other: weakness.

Overdose and treatment
No information available.

▶ Special considerations
- A pre-test urine sample may help determine dietary PABA levels.
- Hydrate the patient after administration of bentiromide by giving 250 ml of water immediately and 250 to 750 ml during the next 6 hours.
- Patient's urine should be collected for exactly 6 hours after administration for analysis.
- Monitor blood glucose for possible adjustment of insulin in diabetic patients during fast.

Information for the patient
- Tell patient to avoid the medications and foods listed in "Interactions" and "Effects on diagnostic tests" sections for the specified times.
- Instruct patient to fast after midnight the night before test.
- Have patient void just prior to testing to ensure accurate results.

Pediatric use
The dose for children ages 6 to 12 is 14 mg/kg, to a maximum dose of 500 mg.

---

benzocaine
Americaine, Hurricaine, Orabase with Benzocaine, Orajel, Rid-A-Pain

- Pharmacologic classification: local anesthetic (ester)
- Therapeutic classification: anesthetic
- Pregnancy risk category C

How supplied
Available without prescription
Gel: 20%
Ointment, cream, and dental paste: 1% to 20%
Topical solution: 20%
Topical solution (aerosol): 20%
Lotion: 0.5% to 8%

Indications, route, and dosage
Local anesthetic for dental pain or dental procedures
Adults and children: Apply topical gel (20%) or dental paste to area as needed.
Local anesthetic for pruritic dermatoses, pruritus, or other irritations
Adults: Apply topical preparation (1% to 20%) to affected area as needed.

Pharmacodynamics
Analgesic action: Acts at sensory neurons to produce a local anesthetic effect.

Pharmacokinetics
Unknown.

Contraindications and precautions
Benzocaine is contraindicated in patients with hypersensitivity to any component of the preparation or related substances and in patients with secondary infection in the area or serious burns.

Interactions
None significant.

Effects on diagnostic tests
None reported.

Adverse reactions
- DERM: urticaria.
- Ear: irritation or itching.
- Other: edema.
  Note: Drug should be discontinued if symptoms of hypersensitivity occur.

Overdose and treatment
Maximum recommended dose is 5 g/day. Overdose is unlikely; however, methemoglobinemia has been reported after topical application for teething pain. Treat symptomatically; if necessary, administer methylene blue 1% 0.1 ml/kg I.V. over at least 10 minutes.

▶ Special considerations
- Use with antibiotic to treat underlying cause of pain, because using alone may mask more serious condition.
- Use cautiously in patients with severely traumatized mucosa or local sepsis.
- Keep container tightly closed and away from moisture.

Information for the patient
- Tell patient to call if pain lasts longer than 48 hours, if burning or itching occurs, or if the condition persists.
- Tell patient to keep container tightly closed and away from moisture.
- Advise patient not to eat or chew gum until effect of local anesthetic has worn off to avoid the risk of bite trauma.

Pediatric use
Excessive use may cause methemoglobinemia in infants. Do not use in children younger than age 1.

---

benzodiazepines

alprazolam
chlordiazepoxide hydrochloride
clonazepam
clorazepate dipotassium
diazepam
estazolam
flurazepam hydrochloride
halazepam
lorazepam
midazolam
oxazepam
prazepam
quazepam
temazepam
triazolam

Benzodiazepines, synthetically produced sedative-hypnotics, gained popularity in the early 1960s, replacing barbiturates as the treatment of choice for anxiety, convulsive disorders, and sedation. These drugs are preferred over barbiturates because therapeutic doses produce less drowsiness and impairment of motor function and toxic doses are less likely to be fatal.

Pharmacology
Benzodiazepines are a group of structurally related chemicals that selectively act on polysynaptic neuronal pathways throughout the CNS. Their precise sites and mechanisms of action are not completely known. However, the benzodiazepines enhance or facilitate the action of gamma-aminobutyric acid (GABA), an inhibitory neurotransmitter in the CNS. All of the benzodiazepines have CNS-depressant activities; however, individual derivatives act more selectively at specific sites, allowing them to be subclassified into five categories based on their predominant clinical use.

Clinical indications and actions
Convulsive disorders
Four of the benzodiazepines (diazepam, clonazepam, clorazepate, and parenteral lorazepam) are used as anticonvulsants. Their anticonvulsant properties are derived from an ability to suppress the spread of seizure activity produced by epileptogenic foci in the cortex, thalamus, and limbic systems by enhancing presynaptic inhibition. Clonazepam is particularly useful in the adjunctive treatment of petit mal variant (Lennox-Gastaut syndrome), myoclonic, or akinetic seizures. Parenteral diazepam is indicated to treat status epilepticus.
Anxiety, tension, and insomnia
Most benzodiazepines (alprazolam, chlordiazepoxide, clorazepate, diazepam, estazolam, flurazepam, halazepam, lorazepam, oxazepam, prazepam, quazepam, temazepam, and triazolam) are useful as antianxiety agents and sedative-hypnotic agents. They have a similar mechanism of action: they are believed to facilitate the effects of GABA in the ascending reticular activating system, increasing inhibition and blocking both cortical and limbic arousal.

They are used to treat anxiety and tension that occur alone or as a side effect of a primary disorder. They are not recommended for tension associated with everyday stress. The choice of a specific benzodiazepine depends on individual metabolic characteristics of the

drug. For instance, in patients with depressed renal or hepatic function, alprazolam, lorazepam, or oxazepam may be selected because they have a relatively short duration of action and have no active metabolites. The sedative-hypnotic properties of chlordiazepoxide, clorazepate, diazepam, lorazepam, and oxazepam make these the drugs of choice as preoperative medication and as an adjunct in the rehabilitation of alcoholics.
Surgical adjuncts for conscious sedation or amnesia
Diazepam, midazolam, and lorazepam have amnesic effects. The mechanism of such action is not known. Parenteral administration before such procedures as endoscopy or elective cardioversion causes impairment of recent memory and interferes with the establishment of memory trace, producing anterograde amnesia.
Skeletal muscle spasm, tremor
Because oral forms of diazepam and chlordiazepoxide have skeletal muscle relaxant properties, they are often used to treat neurologic conditions involving muscle spasms and tetanus. The mechanism of such action is unknown, but they are believed to inhibit spinal polysynaptic and monosynaptic afferent pathways.

Overview of adverse reactions
Therapeutic dosage of the benzodiazepines usually causes drowsiness and impaired motor function, which should be monitored early in treatment. It may or may not be persistent. GI discomfort, such as constipation, diarrhea, vomiting, and changes in appetite, with urinary alterations also have been reported. Visual disturbances and cardiovascular irregularities also are common. Continuing problems with short-term memory, confusion, severe depression, shakiness, vertigo, slurred speech, staggering, bradycardia, shortness of breath or difficulty breathing, and severe weakness usually indicate a toxic dose level. Prolonged or frequent use of benzodiazepines can cause physical dependency and withdrawal syndrome when use is discontinued.

▶ Special considerations
● Crush tablet or empty capsule and mix with food if patient has difficulty swallowing.
● Assess level of consciousness and neurologic status before and frequently during therapy for changes. Monitor for paradoxical reactions, especially early in therapy.
● Assess sleep patterns and quality. Institute seizure precautions. Assess for changes in seizure character, frequency, or duration.
● Assess vital signs frequently during therapy. Significant changes in blood pressure and heart rate may indicate impending toxicity.
● Administer with milk or immediately after meals to prevent GI upset. Give antacid, if needed, at least 1 hour before or after dose to prevent interaction and ensure maximum drug absorption and effectiveness.
● Monitor renal and hepatic function periodically to ensure adequate drug removal and prevent cumulative effects.
● Comfort measures – such as back rubs and relaxation techniques – may enhance drug effectiveness.
● As needed, institute safety measures – raised side rails and ambulatory assistance – to prevent injury. Anticipate possible rebound excitement reactions.
● Patient should be observed to prevent drug hoarding or self-dosing, especially in depressed or suicidal patients or those who are, or who have a history of being,

drug-dependent. Patient's mouth should be checked to be sure tablet or capsule was swallowed.
• After prolonged use, abrupt discontinuation may cause withdrawal symptoms; discontinue gradually.

Information for the patient
• Warn patient to avoid use of alcohol or other CNS depressants, such an antihistamines, analgesics, monoamine oxidase inhibitors, antidepressants, and barbiturates, while taking benzodiazepines to prevent additive depressant effects.
• Caution patient not to take the drug except as prescribed and not to give medication to others. Tell patient not to increase the dose or frequency and to call before taking any nonprescription cold or allergy preparations that may potentiate CNS depressant effects.
• Warn patient to avoid activities requiring alertness and good psychomotor coordination until the CNS response to the drug is determined. Instruct patient in safety measures to prevent injury.
• Tell patient to avoid using antacids, which may delay drug absorption, unless prescribed.
• Be sure patient understands that benzodiazepines are capable of causing physical and psychological dependence with prolonged use.
• Warn patient not to stop taking the drug abruptly to prevent withdrawal symptoms after prolonged therapy.
• Tell patient that smoking decreases the drug's effectiveness. Encourage patient to stop smoking during therapy.
• Tell patient to report any adverse effects. These are often dose-related and can be relieved by dosage adjustments.
• Inform women who are taking the drug to report if they suspect they are pregnant or intend to become pregnant.

Geriatric use
• Because they are sensitive to their CNS effects, elderly patients receiving benzodiazepines require lower doses. Use with caution.
• Parenteral administration of these drugs is more likely to cause apnea, hypotension, bradycardia, and cardiac arrest in elderly patients.
• Geriatric patients may show prolonged elimination of benzodiazepines, except possibly for oxazepam, lorazepam, temazepam, and triazolam.

Pediatric use
• Because children, particularly very young ones, are sensitive to the CNS depressant effects of benzodiazepines, caution must be exercised. A neonate whose mother took a benzodiazepine during pregnancy may exhibit withdrawal symptoms.
• Use of benzodiazepines during labor may cause neonatal flaccidity.

Breast-feeding
The breast-fed infant of a mother who uses a benzodiazepine drug may show sedation, feeding difficulties, and weight loss. Safe use has not been established.

Representative combinations
Chlordiazepoxide with amitriptyline hydrochloride: Limbitrol, Mylan; with clidinium bromide: Librax; with esterified estrogens: Menrium.

benzonatate
Tessalon

• Pharmacologic classification: local anesthetic (ester)
• Therapeutic classification: nonnarcotic antitussive agent

How supplied
Available by prescription only
Capsules: 100 mg

Indications, route, and dosage
Cough suppression
Adults and children over age 10: 100 mg P.O. t.i.d.; up to 600 mg daily.
Children under age 10: 8 mg/kg P.O. in three to six divided doses.

Pharmacodynamics
Antitussive action: Benzonatate suppresses the cough reflex at its source by anesthetizing peripheral stretch receptors located in the respiratory passages, lungs, and pleura.

Pharmacokinetics
• *Absorption:* Action begins within 15 to 20 minutes and lasts for 3 to 8 hours.
• *Distribution, metabolism, and excretion* have not been established.

Contraindications and precautions
Benzonatate is contraindicated in patients with a known hypersensitivity to the drug or to related compounds, such as tetracaine.

Interactions
None significant.

Effects on diagnostic tests
None reported.

Adverse reactions
• CNS: dizziness, headache, sedation.
• DERM: rash, eruptions, pruritus.
• EENT: nasal congestion, sensation of burning in eyes.
• GI: nausea, constipation, GI upset.
• Other: chills, chest numbness, hypersensitivity.

Overdose and treatment
CNS stimulation from overdose of drug may cause restlessness and tremors, which may lead to chronic convulsions followed by profound CNS depression.
Empty stomach by gastric lavage and follow with activated charcoal. Treat convulsions with a short-acting barbiturate given I.V; do not use CNS stimulants. Mechanical respiratory support may be necessary in severe cases.

▶ **Special considerations**
Monitor cough type and frequency and volume and quality of sputum. Encourage fluid intake to help liquefy sputum.

Information for the patient
● Instruct patient never to chew or dissolve capsules in the mouth, as local anesthesia will result.
● Teach patient comfort measures for a nonproductive cough: limit talking and smoking; use a cold mist or steam vaporizer; use sugarless hard candy to increase saliva flow.

Breast-feeding
Safe use during breast-feeding has not been established.

---

benzphetamine hydrochloride
Didrex

● Pharmacologic classification: amphetamine
● Therapeutic classification: short-term adjunctive anorexigenic agent for refractory exogenous obesity, sympathomimetic amine
● Controlled substance schedule III
● Pregnancy risk category X

How supplied
Available by prescription only
Tablets: 25 mg, 50 mg

Indications, route, and dosage
Short-term adjunct in exogenous obesity
Adults: 25 to 50 mg P.O. daily given midmorning and midafternoon. My be increased to a maximum of 50 mg t.i.d.

Pharmacodynamics
Anorexigenic action: The precise mechanism of action for appetite control is unknown; anorexigenic effects are thought to occur in the hypothalamus, where decreased smell and taste acuity decreases appetite. The cerebral cortex and reticular activating system appear to be the primary sites of activity; amphetamines release nerve terminal stores of norepinephrine, promoting nerve impulse transmission. At high doses, effects are mediated by dopamine.

Benzphetamine is used as an adjunct in the short-term control of refractory obesity, with caloric restriction and behavior modification.

Pharmacokinetics
● *Absorption:* Benzphetamine hydrochloride is readily absorbed from the GI tract; effects persist for about 4 hours after oral administration.
● *Distribution:* Widely distributed throughout the body.
● *Metabolism:* Metabolized by the liver.
● *Excretion:* Excreted in urine.

Contraindications and precautions
Benzphetamine is contraindicated in patients with hypersensitivity or idiosyncratic reaction to sympathomimetic amines; in those with hyperthyroidism, nephritis, glaucoma, any degree of hypertension, angina pectoris, other symptomatic cardiovascular disease, arteriosclerosis-induced parkinsonism, advanced arteriosclerosis, or agitated states; and in patients with a history of substance abuse. It also is contraindicated for concomitant use with monoamine oxidase (MAO) in-

hibitors or within 14 days of discontinuing MAO inhibitors.

The 25-mg tablet contains tartrazine and is contraindicated in patients with asthma or aspirin allergy. Benzphetamine should be used with caution in patients with diabetes mellitus and in elderly, debilitated, or hyperexcitable patients.

Interactions
Concomitant use of benzphetamine with MAO inhibitors (or drugs with MAO-inhibiting activity, such as furazolidone) or within 14 days of such therapy may cause hypertensive crisis; use with antihypertensives may antagonize the antihypertensive effects.

Concomitant use with antacids, sodium bicarbonate, or acetazolamide enhances renal reabsorption of benzphetamine and prolongs its duration of action. Use with phenothiazines or haloperidol may decrease benzphetamine effects. Concomitant use with barbiturates antagonize benzphetamine, resulting in CNS depression; use with caffeine or other CNS stimulants produces additive effects.

Amphetamines may alter insulin requirements.

Effects on diagnostic tests
Benzphetamine may elevate plasma corticosteroid levels and may interfere with urinary steroid determinations.

Adverse reactions
● CNS: restlessness, tremor, hyperactivity, talkativeness, insomnia, irritability, dizziness, headache, chills, over-stimulation, dysphoria, *psychotic episodes.*
● CV: *tachycardia,* palpitations, hypertension, hypotension.
● DERM: urticaria.
● GI: nausea, vomiting, cramps, dry mouth, diarrhea, constipation, metallic taste, anorexia, weight loss.
● GU: changes in libido, impotence.
● Other: tolerance, psychological or physical dependence.
Note: Drug should be discontinued if signs of hypersensitivity or idiosyncrasy occur.

Overdose and treatment
Clinical manifestations of overdose include flushing, pallor, palpitations, changing pulse rate and blood pressure levels, heart block, chest pain, hyperpyrexia, confusion, delirium, psychoses, and hallucinations.

Treat overdose symptomatically and supportively: if ingestion is recent (within 4 hours), use gastric lavage or emesis and sedate with barbiturate; monitor vital signs and fluid and electrolyte balance. Urinary acidification may enhance excretion. Specific treatment to lower body temperature or intracranial pressure may be necessary.

▶ Special considerations
Recommendations for administration of benzphetamine, for care and teaching of patient during therapy, and for use in elderly or breast-feeding patients are the same as those for all *amphetamines.*
● The use of benzamphetamine for weight control is highly controversial because the drug's appetite suppression effects are transient.
● In managing benzphetamine withdrawal, place patient in a quiet room with low stimulation and allow him to sleep.
● Monitor vital signs; institute suicide precautions.

---

*Canada only   †Unlabeled clinical use   Italicized adverse reactions are life-threatening.

Pediatric use
Benzphetamine is not recommended for weight reduction in children.

---

benzquinamide hydrochloride
Emete-Con

- Pharmacologic classification: benzoquinolizine derivative
- Therapeutic classification: antiemetic
- Pregnancy risk category C

How supplied
Available by prescription only
Injection: 50 mg/vial

Indications, route, and dosage
Nausea and vomiting associated with anesthesia and surgery
Adults: 50 mg I.M. (0.5 to 1 mg/kg); may repeat in 1 hour and thereafter q 3 to 4 hours, p.r.n. Or 25 mg (0.2 to 0.4 mg/kg) I.V. as single dose, administered slowly.

Pharmacodynamics
Antiemetic action: Benzquinamide probably acts directly at the chemoreceptor trigger zone (vomiting center). The exact mechanism is unknown, but the drug has anticholinergic, antihistamine, and antiseritonergic activity.

Pharmacokinetics
- *Absorption:* Unknown. Onset of action occurs in about 15 minutes.
- *Distribution:* Benzquinamide is distributed rapidly in body tissues, with highest concentration in the liver and kidneys. About 58% of the drug is plasma protein-bound.
- *Metabolism:* Most drug (90% to 95%) is metabolized in the liver.
- *Excretion:* About 5% to 10% of drug is excreted unchanged in urine. Metabolites are excreted in urine, bile, and feces.

Contraindications and precautions
Benzquinamide is contraindicated in patients who are hypersensitive to this drug, and in patients receiving drugs that cause arrhythmias or that increase heart rate or blood pressure, because the drug may exacerbate these symptoms. I.V. administration is contraindicated in patients with cardiovascular disease and within 15 minutes of preanesthetics or cardiovascular drugs because it may cause premature atrial or ventricular contractions or a sudden rise in blood pressure.

Drug may mask signs of overdose of toxic agents or of intestinal obstruction or brain tumor.

Interactions
When used concomitantly, benzquinamide may enhance response to drugs that increase blood pressure, such as epinephrine.

Effects on diagnostic tests
Benzquinamide increases free fatty acid serum levels.

Adverse reactions
- CNS: drowsiness (most common), fatigue, restlessness, dizziness, headache, insomnia.
- CV: *hypertension,* hypotension, *arrhythmias,* flushing.
- DERM: rash, allergic reaction.
- EENT: dry mouth, salivation, blurred vision.
- GI: anorexia, nausea, hiccups.
- Musculoskeletal: tremors, weakness.
- Other: sweating, fever, chills.
  Note: Drug should be discontinued if patient experiences cardiac arrhythmias or sudden blood pressure increase.

Overdose and treatment
No information available.

▶ **Special considerations**
- I.M administration is the preferred route. Cardiovascular adverse reactions are more likely to occur with I.V. administration.
- Reconstitute with 2.2 ml sterile water for injection or bacteriostatic water for injection. Solution remains stable for 14 days at room temperature. Protect stored drug from light.
- Give I.M. injection into large muscle mass; use deltoid muscle only if well developed. Be especially careful to avoid inadvertent I.V. injection.
- Monitor patient's blood pressure. (Patient who is receiving drugs that increase blood pressure may require a lower dose.)

Information for the patient
Warn patient that drug may cause dry mouth.

Geriatric use
Because elderly patients commonly have cardiovascular problems, including hypertension, they may require a decreased dose.

Pediatric use
Not approved for use in children.

---

benzthiazide
Aquatag, Exna, Hydrex, Marazide, Proaqua

- Pharmacologic classification: thiazide diuretic
- Therapeutic classification: diuretic, antihypertensive
- Pregnancy risk category C

How supplied
Available by prescription only
Tablets: 50 mg

Indications, route, and dosage
Edema
Adults: 50 to 200 mg P.O. daily or in divided doses.
Children: 1 to 4 mg/kg P.O. daily in three divided doses.
Hypertension
Adults: 50 mg P.O. daily b.i.d., t.i.d., or q.i.d., adjusted to patient's response.

Pharmacodynamics
- *Diuretic action:* Benzthiazide increases urinary excretion of sodium and water by inhibiting sodium reab-

---

sorption in the cortical diluting tubule of the nephron, thereby relieving edema.

• *Antihypertensive action:* The exact mechanism of benzthiazide's antihypertensive effect is unknown; it may be partially because of direct arteriolar vasodilation and a decrease in total peripheral resistance.

Pharmacokinetics
• *Absorption:* Benzthiazide is well absorbed from the GI tract. Diuresis begins within 2 hours.
• *Distribution:* Benzthiazide, like other thiazide diuretics, is thought to enter extracellular space. Peak effect occurs in 3 to 6 hours.
• *Metabolism:* Insignificant.
• *Excretion:* Benzthiazide is excreted unchanged in urine.

Contraindications and precautions
Benzthiazide is contraindicated in anuria and in patients with known sensitivity to the drug or other sulfonamide derivatives. Benzthiazide should be used cautiously in patients with severe renal disease because it may decrease glomerular filtration rate and precipitate azotemia; in patients with impaired hepatic function or liver disease because electrolyte changes may precipitate coma; and in patients taking digoxin, because hypokalemia may predispose patients to digitalis toxicity.

Aquatag and Exna contain tartrazine, which may cause allergic reactions such as bronchospasm in asthmatic and aspirin-sensitive patients.

Interactions
Benzthiazide potentiates the hypotensive effects of most other antihypertensive drugs; this may be used to therapeutic advantage.

Benzthiazide may potentiate hyperglycemic, hypotensive, and hyperuricemic effects of diazoxide, and its hyperglycemic effect may increase insulin or sulfonylurea requirements in diabetic patients.

Benzthiazide may reduce renal clearance of lithium, elevating serum lithium levels, and may necessitate reduction in lithium dosage by 50%.

Benzthiazide turns urine slightly more alkaline and may decrease urinary excretion of some amines such as amphetamine and quinidine; alkaline urine may also decrease therapeutic efficacy of methenamine compounds such as methenamine mandelate.

Cholestyramine and colestipol may bind benzthiazide, preventing its absorption; give drugs 1 hour apart.

Effects on diagnostic tests
Benzthiazide therapy may alter serum electrolyte levels and may increase serum urate, glucose, cholesterol, and triglyceride levels.

Benzthiazide may interfere with tests for parathyroid function and should be discontinued before such tests.

Adverse reactions
• CV: *volume depletion and dehydration,* orthostatic hypotension, hypercholesterolemia, hypertriglyceridemia.
• DERM: dermatitis, photosensitivity, rash.
• HEMA: *aplastic anemia, agranulocytosis,* leukopenia, thrombocytopenia.
• GI: anorexia, nausea, pancreatitis.
• Hepatic: hepatic encephalopathy.
• Metabolic: *asymptomatic hyperuricemia;* gout; *hyperglycemia* and *impairment of glucose tolerance;* fluid and electrolyte imbalances, including hypokalemia, hy-

ponatremia, hypochloremia, and hypercalcemia; metabolic alkalosis.
• Other: hypersensitivity reactions, such as pneumonitis and vasculitis.

Note: Drug should be discontinued if rising BUN and serum creatinine levels indicate renal impairment or if patient shows signs of hypersensitivity reaction or impending coma.

Overdose and treatment
Clinical signs of overdose include GI irritation and hypermotility, diuresis, and lethargy, which may progress to coma.

Treatment is mainly supportive; monitor and assist respiratory, cardiovascular, and renal function as indicated. Monitor fluid and electrolyte balance. Induce vomiting with ipecac in conscious patient; otherwise, use gastric lavage to avoid aspiration. Do not give cathartics; these promote additional loss of fluids and electrolytes.

▶ **Special considerations**
Recommendations for use of benzthiazide and care and teaching of the patient during therapy are the same as those for all *thiazide diuretics.*

Geriatric use
Elderly and debilitated patients require close observation and may require reduced dosages. They are more sensitive to excess diuresis because of age-related changes in cardiovascular and renal function. Excess diuresis promotes orthostatic hypotension, dehydration leading to hypovolemia, hyponatremia, hypomagnesemia, and hypokalemia.

Breast-feeding
Benzthiazide is distributed in breast milk; its safety and effectiveness in breast-feeding women have not been established.

---

benztropine mesylate
Cogentin

• Pharmacologic classification: anticholinergic
• Therapeutic classification: antiparkinsonian agent
• Pregnancy risk category C

How supplied
Available by prescription only
Tablets: 0.5 mg, 1 mg, 2 mg
Injection: 1 mg/ml in 2-ml ampule

Indications, route, and dosage
Acute dystonic reaction
Adults: 2 mg I.V. followed by 1 to 2 mg P.O. b.i.d. to prevent recurrence.
Parkinsonism
Adults: 0.5 to 6 mg P.O. daily. Initially, 0.5 mg to 1 mg, increased 0.5 mg every 5 to 6 days. Adjust dosage to meet individual requirements.
Drug-induced extrapyramidal reactions
Adults: 1 to 4 mg P.O. or I.V. daily or b.i.d. Alternatively, 1 to 2 mg b.i.d. to t.i.d. usually provides relief within 1 to 2 days. Reevaluate use after 1 to 2 weeks of therapy.

---

*Canada only   †Unlabeled clinical use   Italicized adverse reactions are life-threatening.

Pharmacodynamics

Antiparkinsonian action: Benztropine blocks central cholinergic receptors, helping to balance cholinergic activity in the basal ganglia. It may also prolong dopamine's effects by blocking dopamine reuptake and storage at central receptor sites.

Pharmacokinetics

● *Absorption:* Benztropine is absorbed from the GI tract.
● *Distribution:* Largely unknown; however, the drug crosses the blood-brain barrier and may cross the placenta.
● *Metabolism:* Unknown.
● *Excretion:* Like other muscarinics, benztropine is excreted in the urine as unchanged drug and metabolites. After oral therapy, small amounts are probably excreted in feces as unabsorbed drug.

Contraindications and precautions

Benztropine is contraindicated in patients with narrow-angle glaucoma, because drug-induced cycloplegia and mydriasis may increase intraocular pressure.

Administer benztropine cautiously to patients with prostatic hypertrophy, because the drug may exacerbate urinary retention; to patients with tachycardia, because the drug may block vagal inhibition of the sinoatrial node pacemaker and exacerbate tachycardia; and to elderly patients and young children, because they may be more susceptible to the drug's effects.

Interactions

Concomitant use with amantadine may amplify such adverse anticholinergic effects as confusion and hallucinations. Benztropine dosage should be decreased before giving amantadine. Concomitant use with haloperidol and phenothiazines may decrease their effect, possibly reflecting direct CNS antagonism. Concomitant use with phenothiazines increases the risk of adverse anticholinergic effects.

Alcohol and other CNS depressants increase benztropine's sedative effects. Antacids and antidiarrheals may decrease benztropine absorption. Administer benztropine at least 1 hour prior to these agents.

Effects on diagnostic tests

None reported.

Adverse reactions

● CNS: disorientation, restlessness, agitation, confusion, excitement, memory loss, giddiness, psychoses, paranoia, delirium, delusions, euphoria, paresthesia, heaviness of extremities, hallucinations, headache, depression, weakness.
● CV: palpitations, tachycardia, paradoxical bradycardia.
● DERM: urticaria, hypersensitivity rash, decreased sweating.
● EENT: dilated pupils, blurred vision, photophobia.
● GI: constipation, dry mouth, nausea, vomiting, epigastric distress, dysphagia.
● GU: dysuria, urinary hesitancy or retention.
Note: Drug should be discontinued if hypersensitivity; urinary retention; confusion; hallucinations; dilated and nonreactive pupils; or hot, dry, flushed skin occurs.

Overdose and treatment

Clinical manifestations of overdose include central stimulation followed by depression and psychotic symptoms such as disorientation, confusion, hallucinations, delusions, anxiety, agitation, and restlessness. Peripheral effects may include dilated, nonreactive pupils; blurred vision; hot, flushed, dry skin; dryness of mucous membranes; dysphagia; decreased or absent bowel sounds; urinary retention; hyperthermia; tachycardia; hypertension; and increased respiration.

Treatment is primarily symptomatic and supportive, as necessary. Maintain a patent airway. If patient is alert, induce emesis (or use gastric lavage) and follow with a saline cathartic and activated charcoal to prevent further absorption. In severe cases, physostigmine may be administered to block benztropine's antimuscarinic effects. Give fluids as needed to treat shock, diazepam to control psychotic symptoms, and pilocarpine (instilled into the eyes) to relieve mydriasis. If urinary retention occurs, catheterization may be necessary.

▶ **Special considerations**

Besides those relevant to all *anticholinergics,* consider the following recommendations.
● To help prevent gastric irritation, administer drug after meals.
● Never discontinue drug abruptly.
● Monitor patient for intermittent constipation and abdominal distention and pain, which may indicate paralytic ileus.

Information for the patient

● Explain that drug's full effect may not occur for 2 to 3 days after therapy begins.
● Caution patient not to discontinue drug suddenly; dosage should be reduced gradually.
● Tell patient that drug may increase sensitivity of his eyes to light.

Pediatric use

Benztropine is not recommended for children younger than age 3.

Breast-feeding

Benztropine may be excreted in breast milk, possibly causing infant toxicity. Breast-feeding women should avoid this drug. Benztropine may decrease milk production.

bepridil hydrochloride
Vascor

● Pharmacologic classification: calcium channel blocker
● Therapeutic classification: antianginal
● Pregnancy risk category C

How supplied

Available by prescription only
Tablets: 200 mg, 300 mg, 400 mg

Indications, route, and dosage

Treatment of chronic stable angina (classic effort-associated angina) in patients who are unresponsive or inadequately responsive to other antianginals

Adults: Initially, 200 mg P.O. daily; adjust dosage according to patient tolerance and response. Maximum daily dose is 400 mg. Most common maintenance dose is 300 mg daily.

Pharmacodynamics

Antianginal action: Precise mechanism of action is unknown. It is believed to reduce heart rate and arterial pressure by dilating peripheral arterioles and reducing total peripheral resistance (afterload). The effects are dose-dependent. Bepridil has dose-related Class I antiarrhythmic properties affecting electrophysiologic changes, such as prolongation of QT and QTc intervals. It inhibits calcium ion influx into cardiac and vascular smooth muscle and also inhibits the sodium inward influx, resulting in reductions in the maximal upstroke velocity and amplitude of the action potential.

Pharmacokinetics

● *Absorption:* Bepridil is rapidly and completely absorbed after oral administration; peak concentrations occur in 2 to 3 hours.
● *Distribution:* Over 99% of the drug is plasma protein-bound.
● *Metabolism:* Bepridil is metabolized in the liver.
● *Excretion:* Elimination is biphasic. Bepridil has a distribution half-life of 2 hours. Over 10 days, 70% is excreted in urine, 22% in feces as metabolites. Terminal half-life after multiple dosing averaged 42 hours (range 26 to 64 hours).

Contraindications and precautions

Bepridil is contraindicated in patients with known hypersensitivity to the drug and in patients with a history of serious ventricular arrhythmias, sick sinus syndrome, second- or third-degree atrioventricular (AV) block (except those with a functioning ventricular pacemaker), hypotension (below 90 mm Hg systolic), uncompensated cardiac insufficiency, congenital QT interval prolongation, and in patients who are taking other drugs that prolong the QT interval.

Use with caution in patients with left bundle branch block or sinus bradycardia and serious renal or hepatic disorders.

Interactions

Concurrent administration with quinidine, procainamide, or tricyclic antidepressants is contraindicated because of additive prolongation of the QT interval. Also avoid potassium-wasting diuretics because of their potential for causing hypokalemia, which increases the risk of serious ventricular arrhythmias. Use with caution with cardiac glycosides, which could exaggerate depression of AV nodal conduction. Modest increases in steady-state serum digoxin concentrations have also been observed with concurrent use of bepridil, although data are insufficient to determine clinical significance in patients with cardiac conduction abnormalities.

Effects on diagnostic tests

Increased ALT (SGPT) levels and abnormal liver function test results have been observed.

Adverse reactions

● CNS: dizziness, headache, drowsiness, tremor, parasthesia, insomnia, nervousness, syncope, depression, vertigo, akathisia.
● CV: arrhythmias, sinus tachycardia, sinus bradycardia, hypertension, prolonged QT interval, vasodilation, palpitations.
● GI: dyspepsia, nausea, diarrhea, dry mouth, anorexia, abdominal pain, constipation, flatulence, gastritis, increased appetite.
● GU: impotence, decreased libido.

● Respiratory: rhinitis, cough, pharyngitis, dyspnea.
● Other: agranulocytosis, flulike syndrome, superinfection, fever, pain, myalgic asthenia, rash, sweating, skin irritation, blurred vision, tinnitus, taste change, edema.

Overdose and treatment

Exaggerated adverse reactions, especially clinically significant hypotension, high-degree AV block, and ventricular tachycardia, have been observed. Treat with appropriate supportive measures, including gastric lavage, beta-adrenergic stimulation, parenteral calcium solutions, vasopressor agents, and cardioversion, as necessary. Close observation in a cardiac care facility for a minimum of 48 hours is recommended.

▶ Special considerations

● Careful patient selection and monitoring are essential. Use the following selection criteria: Diagnosis of chronic stable angina with failure to respond or inadequate response to other therapies, QTc interval below 0.44 seconds, absence of hypokalemia, hypotension, severe left ventricular dysfunction, serious ventricular arrhythmias, unpacked sick sinus syndrome, second- or third-degree AV block, and no concomitant use of other drugs that prolong the QT interval.
● Monitor serum potassium levels and correct hypokalemia before initiating therapy. Use potassium-sparing diuretics for patients who require diuretic therapy.
● Monitor QTc interval before and during therapy. Reduced dosage is required if QTc prolongation is greater than 0.52 seconds or increases more than 25%. If prolongation of QTc interval persists, discontinue bepridil.
● Beta blockers, nitrates, digoxin, insulin, and oral hypoglycemics may be used with bepridil.
● Food does not interfere with absorption of bepridil.
● Elderly patients may require more frequent monitoring.
● Use cautiously in patients with renal or hepatic disorders. No clinical data are available.
● Tell patient to report any signs of infection (for example, sore throat, fever). If infection is suspected, obtain WBC count.

Information for the patient

● Instruct patient to recognize signs and symptoms of hypokalemia.
● Tell patient to report any signs of infection.
● Instruct patient to take drug with food or at bedtime if nausea occurs.

Geriatric use

Recommended starting dose is same as in adult patients; however, more frequent monitoring may be required.

Pediatric use

Safety and efficacy have not been established.

Breast-feeding

Bepridil is excreted in breast milk; risk-benefit must be assessed because of the potential for serious adverse reactions in the infant.

---

beractant (natural lung surfactant)
Survanta

- Pharmacolgic classification: bovine lung extract
- Therapeutic classification: lung surfactant

How supplied
Available by presciption only
Suspension: 25 mg of phospholipids/ml suspended in 0.9% sodium chloride in 8-ml single-dose vials

Indications, route, and dosage
Prevention and treatment (rescue) of respiratory distress syndrome (hyaline membrane disease) in premature infants
Infants: 100 mg of phospholipids/kg of birth weight (4 ml/kg) administered by intratracheal instillation through a #5 French end-hole catheter inserted into the infant's endotracheal tube with the tip of the catheter protruding just beyond the end of the tube above the carina. Shorten the length of the catheter before inserting it through the tube. Beractant should not be instilled into a mainstem bronchus. Use the dosing chart below as a guide.

BERACTANT DOSING CHART

WEIGHT IN GRAMS	TOTAL DOSE (ML)
600 to 650	2.6
651 to 700	2.8
701 to 750	3
751 to 800	3.2
801 to 850	3.4
851 to 900	3.6
901 to 950	3.8
951 to 1000	4
1001 to 1050	4.2
1051 to 1100	4.4
1101 to 1150	4.6
1151 to 1200	4.8
1201 to 1250	5
1251 to 1300	5.2
1301 to 1350	5.4
1351 to 1400	5.6
1401 to 1450	5.8
1451 to 1500	6
1501 to 1550	6.2
1551 to 1600	6.4
1601 to 1650	6.6
1651 to 1700	6.8
1701 to 1750	7
1751 to 1800	7.2
1801 to 1850	7.4
1851 to 1900	7.6
1901 to 1950	7.8
1951 to 2000	8

Pharmacodynamics
Beractant is a natural bovine lung extract containing phospholipids, neutral lipids, fatty acids, and surfactant-associated proteins to which dipalmitoylphosphatidylcholine, palmitic acid, and tripalmitin are added to standardize and to mimic surface tension-lowering properties of natural lung surfactant. Endogenous lung surfactant lowers surface tension on alveolar surfaces during respiration and stabilizes the alveoli against collapse at resting transpulmonary pressures. Beractant lowers minimum surface tension, restores pulmonary surfactant, and restores surface activity to the lungs of premature infants with respiratory distress syndrome (RDS).

Pharmacokinetics
- *Absorption:* Most of the administered dose becomes lung-associated within hours.
- *Distribution:* Across the alveolar surface.
- *Metabolism:* Lipids enter endogenous surfactant pathway of recycling and reutilization.
- *Excretion:* Alveolar clearance of lipid components is rapid.

Adverse reactions
- CV: transient bradycardia, vasoconstriction, hypotension, hypertension.
- Respiratory: apnea.
- Other: endotracheal tube reflux, pallor, endotracheal tube blockage, hypocarbia, hypercarbia.

Overdose and treatment
Overdose may result in acute airway obstruction. Treatment should be supportive and symptomatic.

▶ Special considerations
- Rales and moist breath sounds can occur transiently after beractant administration. Endotracheal suctioning or other remedial action is not required unless clear-cut signs of airway obstruction are present.
- There is an increased probability of post-treatment nosocomial sepsis.
- Frequently monitor infant. Transient bradycardia and decreased oxygen saturation have occurred during dosing. Initiate appropriate corrective measures.
- Marked improvements in oxygenation may occur within minutes of administration and significant improvements may be sustained for 48 to 72 hours.
- Ensure proper placement and patency of endotracheal tube before administration. Suction endotracheal tube if needed, and allow infant to stabilize before administration of beractant.
- Determine total dose and slowly withdraw entire contents of vial into syringe through at least a 20G needle. Attach premeasured French catheter to syringe and fill with beractant. Discard any excess through the catheter so that syringe contains only the total dose to be given.
- To ensure homogeneous distribution of beractant, each dose is divided into quarter doses and administered with the infant in a different position: head and body inclined slightly down, head turned to the right; head and body inclined slightly down, head turned to the left; head and body inclined slightly up, head turned to the right; head and body inclined slightly up, head turned to the left. Four doses may be administered within the first 48 hours of life at intervals no greater than q 6 hours.
- Refrigerate stored beractant; warm to room temper-

ature before administration (standing, at least 20 minutes; in hand, at least 8 minutes). Do not use artificial warming methods.
● Begin preparation before infant's birth if preventive dose is to be given.
Prevention strategy: Weigh, intubate, and stabilize infant. Dose should be administered as soon as possible after birth, within 15 minutes. Position infant and gently instill first quarter dose through catheter over 2 to 3 seconds; remove catheter and manually ventilate with sufficient oxygen to prevent cyanosis, at a rate of 60 breaths/minute and with sufficient positive pressure to provide adequate air exchange and chest wall excursion.
Rescue strategy: First dose should be given as soon as possible after the infant is placed on a ventilator for management of RDS. Position infant and gently instill first quarter dose through catheter over 2 to 3 seconds; remove catheter and return infant to mechanical ventilator.
Both strategies: Ventilate infant for at least 30 seconds or until stable. Reposition infant and instill next quarter dose. Remaining doses should be instilled using same procedure. After final quarter dose is administered, remove catheter without flushing. Do not suction for 1 hour unless signs of significant airway obstruction occur. Resume usual ventilator management and clinical care once dosing procedure is completed.
Repeat doses: Need for repeat doses is determined by evidence of continuing respiratory distress. Dosage is 100 mg phospholipids/kg based on infant's birth weight. Infant should not be reweighed.

PHARMACOLOGIC CLASS

beta-adrenergic blockers

beta₁ blockers
acebutolol
atenolol
metoprolol tartrate

beta₁ and beta₂ blockers
betaxolol hydrochloride
carteolol hydrochloride
esmolol
labetalol
levobunolol
metipranolol hydrochloride
nadolol
penbutolol
pindolol
propranolol
timolol maleate

Beta-adrenergic blocking agents were first used clinically in the early 1960s; they are now widely used in the management of hypertension, angina pectoris, and arrhythmias. These agents are well tolerated by most patients.

Pharmacology
Beta blockers are chemicals that compete with beta agonists for available beta-receptor sites; individual agents differ in their ability to affect beta receptors. Most available agents are considered nonselective; that is, they block both beta₁ receptors in cardiac muscle and beta₂ receptors in bronchial and vascular smooth mus-

cle. Several agents are cardioselective and in lower doses primarily inhibit beta₁ receptors. Some beta blockers have intrinsic sympathomimetic activity and simultaneously stimulate and block beta receptors, decreasing cardiac output; still others also have membrane-stabilizing activity, which affects cardiac action potential.

Clinical indications and actions
Hypertension
All currently available beta blockers are used to treat hypertension. Although the exact mechanism of their antihypertensive effect is unknown, the action is thought to result from decreased cardiac output, decreased sympathetic outflow from the CNS, and suppression of renin release.
Angina
Propranolol and nadolol are used to treat angina pectoris; they decrease myocardial oxygen requirements via blockade of catecholamine-induced increases in heart rate, blood pressure, and the extent of myocardial contraction.
Arrhythmia
Propranolol, acebutolol, and esmolol are used to treat arrhythmias; they prolong the refractory period of the atrioventricular (AV) node and slow AV conduction.
Glaucoma
The mechanism by which betaxolol, levobunolol, metipranolol, and timolol reduce intraocular pressure is unknown, but the drug effect is at least partially caused by decreased production of aqueous humor.
Myocardial infarction
Timolol, propranolol, and metoprolol are used to prevent myocardial infarction (MI) in susceptible patients; the mechanism of this protective effect is unknown.
Migraine prophylaxis
Propranolol is used to prevent recurrent attacks of migraine and other vascular headaches. The exact mechanism by which propranolol decreases the incidence of migraine headache attacks is unknown, but it is thought to result from inhibition of vasodilation of cerebral vessels.
Other uses
Beta blockers have been used as antianxiety agents, as adjunctive therapy of bleeding esophageal varices, and to treat portal hypertension.

Overview of adverse reactions
Therapeutic doses of beta-adrenergic blockers usually cause bradycardia, fatigue, and dizziness; some may cause other CNS disturbances such as nightmares, depression, memory loss, and hallucinations. Impotence, cold extremities, and elevated serum cholesterol levels have been reported. Severe hypotension, bradycardia, heart failure, or bronchospasm usually indicates toxic dosage levels.

▶ **Special considerations**
● Check apical pulse rate daily; discontinue and reevaluate therapy if extremes occur (for example, a pulse rate below 60 beats/minute).
● Monitor blood pressure, ECG, and heart rate and rhythm frequently; be alert for progression of AV block or severe bradycardia.
● Weigh patients with congestive heart failure regularly; watch for gains of more than 5 lb (2.25 kg) per week.
● Signs of hypoglycemic shock are masked; watch diabetic patients for sweating, fatigue, and hunger.

COMPARING BETA-ADRENERGIC BLOCKING AGENTS

DRUG	HALF-LIFE (HR)	LIPID SOLUBILITY	MEMBRANE-STABILIZING ACTIVITY	INTRINSIC SYMPATHOMIMETIC ACTIVITY
Nonselective				
carteolol	6	low	0	+ +
labetalol	6 to 8	moderate	0	0
metipranolol	4	low to moderate	0	0
nadolol	20	low	0	0
penbutolol	5	high	0	+
pindolol	3 to 4	moderate	+	+ + +
propranolol	4	high	+ +	0
timolol	4	low to moderate	0	0
Beta₁-selective				
acebutolol	3 to 4	low	+	+
atenolol	6 to 7	low	0	0
betaxolol	14 to 22	low	+	0
esmolol	0.15	low	0	0
metoprolol	3 to 7	moderate	*	0

* = only in higher-than-usual doses

● *Do not discontinue these drugs before surgery for pheochromocytoma;* before any surgical procedure, notify anesthesiologist that patient is taking a beta-adrenergic blocking agent.
● Glucagon may be prescribed to reverse signs and symptoms of beta blocker overdose.
● Don't prescribe for patients with asthma.

Information for the patient
● Explain rationale for therapy, and emphasize importance of taking drugs as prescribed, even when patient is feeling well.
● Warn patient not to discontinue these drugs suddenly; abrupt discontinuation can exacerbate angina or precipitate MI.
● Explain potential adverse effects and importance of reporting any unusual effects.
● Teach patient to minimize dizziness from orthostatic hypotension by taking dose at bedtime, and by rising slowly and avoiding sudden position changes.
● Advise patient to seek medical approval before taking nonprescription cold preparations.

Geriatric use
Elderly patients may require lower maintenance doses of beta-adrenergic blocking agents because of increased bioavailability or delayed metabolism; they also may experience enhanced adverse effects.

Pediatric use
Safety and efficacy of beta-adrenergic blocking agents in children have not been established; they should be used only if potential benefit outweighs risk.

Breast-feeding
Beta-adrenergic blocking agents are distributed into breast milk. Recommendations for breast-feeding vary with individual drugs.

Representative combinations
Atenolol with chlorthalidone: Tenoretic.
Metoprolol with hydrochlorothiazide: Lopressor HCT.
Nadolol with bendroflumethiazide: Corzide.
Pindolol with hydrochlorothiazide: Viskazide.
Propranolol with hydrochlorothiazide: Inderide, Inderide LA.
Timolol with hydrochlorothiazide: Timolide.

betamethasone (systemic)
Betnelan★, Celestone

betamethasone sodium phosphate
Betnesol★, BSP, Celestone Phosphate, Prelestone, Selestoject

betamethasone sodium phosphate and betamethasone acetate
Celestone Soluspan

● Pharmacologic classification: glucocorticoid
● Therapeutic classification: anti-inflammatory
● Pregnancy risk category C

How supplied
Available by prescription only
Betamethasone
Syrup: 600 mcg/5 ml
Tablets: 600 mcg
Tablets (extended-release): 1 mg
Betamethasone sodium phosphate
Effervescent tablets★: 500 mcg
Injection: 4 mg (3 mg base)/ml in 5-ml vials

Enema*: 5 mg (base)

Betamethasone sodium phosphate and betamethasone acetate suspension

Injection: betamethasone acetate 3 mg and betamethasone sodium phosphate (equivalent to 3 mg base) per ml

Indications, route, and dosage

Severe inflammation or immunosuppression

Adults: 0.6 to 7.2 mg or 2 to 6 mg (extended-release) P.O. daily.

Betamethasone sodium phosphate

Adults: 0.5 to 9 mg I.M., I.V., or into joint or soft tissue daily.

Betamethasone sodium phosphate and betamethasone acetate suspension

Adults: 1.5 to 12 mg into joint or soft tissue q 1 to 2 weeks, p.r.n.

Children: 0.0625 to 0.25 mg/kg P.O. divided t.i.d. or q.i.d.; or 21 to 125 mcg/kg I.M. or 625 mcg to 3.75 mg/m² q 12 to 24 hours.

Adrenocortical insufficiency

Adults: 0.6 to 7.2 mg P.O. daily, or up to 9 mg I.M. or I.V. daily.

Children: 17.5 mcg/kg P.O. daily or 500 mcg/m² P.O. daily in three or four divided doses; or 17.5 mcg/kg or 500 mg/m² I.M. q 3 days.

Pharmacodynamics

Anti-inflammatory action: Betamethasone stimulates the synthesis of enzymes needed to decrease the inflammatory response. Betamethasone is a long-acting steroid with an anti-inflammatory potency 25 times that of an equal weight of hydrocortisone. It has essentially no mineralocorticoid activity. Betamethasone tablets and syrup are used as oral anti-inflammatory agents. Betamethasone sodium phosphate is highly soluble, has a prompt onset of action, and may be given I.V. Betamethasone sodium phosphate and betamethasone acetate (Celestone Soluspan) combines the rapid-acting phosphate salt and the slightly soluble, slowly released acetate salt to provide rapid anti-inflammatory effects with a sustained duration of action. It is a suspension and should not be given I.V. It is particularly useful as an anti-inflammatory agent in intra-articular, intradermal, and intralesional injections.

Pharmacokinetics

● *Absorption:* Betamethasone is absorbed readily after oral administration. After oral and I.V. administration, peak effects occur in 1 to 2 hours. Onset and duration of action of the suspensions for injection vary, depending on whether they are injected into an intra-articular space or a muscle, and on the local blood supply. Systemic absorption occurs slowly following intra-articular injections.

● *Distribution:* Betamethasone is removed rapidly from the blood and distributed to muscle, liver, skin, intestines, and kidneys. Betamethasone is bound weakly to plasma proteins (transcortin and albumin). Only the unbound portion is active. Adrenocorticoids are distributed into breast milk and through the placenta.

● *Metabolism:* Betamethasone is metabolized in the liver to inactive glucuronide and sulfate metabolites.

● *Excretion:* The inactive metabolites and small amounts of unmetabolized drug are excreted by the kidneys. Insignificant quantities of drug are also excreted in feces. The biological half-life of betamethasone is 36 to 54 hours.

Contraindications and precautions

Betamethasone is contraindicated in patients with hypersensitivity to ingredients of adrenocorticoid preparations or with systemic fungal infections. Patients who are receiving betamethasone should not be given live virus vaccines because betamethasone suppresses the immune response.

Betamethasone should be used with extreme caution in patients with GI ulceration, renal disease, hypertension, osteoporosis, diabetes mellitus, thromboembolic disorders, idiopathic thrombocytopenic purpura, seizures, myasthenia gravis, congestive heart failure (CHF), tuberculosis, hypoalbuminemia, hypothyroidism, cirrhosis of the liver, emotional instability, psychotic tendencies, hyperlipidemias, glaucoma, or cataracts, because the drug may exacerbate these conditions.

Because adrenocorticoids increase susceptibility to and mask symptoms of infection, betamethasone should not be used (except in life-threatening situations) in patients with viral or bacterial infections not controlled by anti-infective agents.

Interactions

When used concomitantly, betamethasone may decrease the effects of oral anticoagulants (rarely); increase the metabolism of isoniazid and salicylates; and cause hyperglycemia, requiring dosage adjustment of insulin or oral hypoglycemic agents in diabetic patients. Use with barbiturates, phenytoin, and rifampin may cause decreased corticosteroid effects because of increased hepatic metabolism. Use with cholestyramine, colestipol, and antacids decreases betamethasone's effect by adsorbing the corticosteroid, decreasing the amount absorbed.

Betamethasone may enhance hypokalemia associated with diuretic or amphotericin B therapy. The hypokalemia may increase the risk of toxicity in patients concurrently receiving digitalis glycosides.

Concomitant use with estrogens may reduce the metabolism of corticosteroids by increasing the concentrations of transcortin. The half-life of the corticosteroid is then prolonged because of increased protein binding. Concomitant administration of ulcerogenic drugs such as nonsteroidal anti-inflammatory agents may increase the risk of GI ulceration.

Effects on diagnostic tests

Adrenocorticoid therapy suppresses reactions to skin tests; causes false-negative results in the nitroblue tetrazolium tests for systemic bacterial infections; and decreases ¹³¹I uptake and protein-bound iodine concentrations in thyroid function tests.

It may increase glucose and cholesterol levels; decrease serum potassium, calcium, thyroxine, and triiodothyronine levels; and increase urine glucose and calcium levels.

Adverse reactions

When administered in high doses or for prolonged therapy, betamethasone suppresses release of adrenocorticotropic hormone (ACTH) from the pituitary gland; the adrenal cortex then stops secreting endogenous corticosteroids. The degree and duration of hypothalamic-pituitary-adrenal (HPA) axis suppression produced is highly variable among patients and depends on the dose, time and frequency of administration, and duration of glucocorticoid therapy.

● *CNS:* euphoria, insomnia, headache, psychotic be-

---

havior, pseudotumor cerebri, mental changes, nervousness, restlessness.
● CV: CHF, hypertension, edema.
● DERM: delayed healing, acne, skin eruptions, striae.
● EENT: cataracts, glaucoma, thrush.
● GI: peptic ulcer, irritation, increased appetite.
● Immune: immunosuppression, increased susceptibility to infection.
● Metabolic: hypokalemia, sodium retention, fluid retention, weight gain, hyperglycemia, osteoporosis, growth suppression in children.
● Musculoskeletal: muscle atrophy, weakness.
● Other: pancreatitis, hirsutism, cushingoid symptoms, withdrawal syndrome (nausea, fatigue, anorexia, dyspnea, hypotension, hypoglycemia, myalgia, arthralgia, fever, dizziness, and fainting). Sudden withdrawal may be fatal or may exacerbate the underlying disease. Acute adrenal insufficiency may follow increased stress (infection, surgery, trauma) or abrupt withdrawal after long-term therapy.

Overdose and treatment
Acute ingestion, even in massive doses, is rarely a clinical problem. Toxic signs and symptoms rarely occur if drug is used for less than 3 weeks, even at large doses. However, chronic use causes adverse physiologic effects, including suppression of the HPA axis, cushingoid appearance, muscle weakness, and osteoporosis.

▶ **Special considerations**
Investigational use includes prevention of respiratory distress syndrome in premature infants (hyaline membrane disease). Give 6 mg (2 ml) of Celestone Soluspan I.M. once daily 24 to 36 hours before induced delivery.
    Recommendations for use of betamethasone and for care and teaching of patients during therapy are the same as those for all systemic adrenocorticoids.

Pediatric use
Chronic use of betamethasone in children and adolescents may delay growth and maturation.

---

betamethasone benzoate
Beben*, Benisone, Uticort

betamethasone dipropionate
Alphatrex, Diprolene AF, Diprolene Ointment, Diprosone, Maxivate, Psorion

betamethasone valerate
Betacort*, Betaderm*, Betatrex, Beta-Val, Betnovate*, Celestoderm-V*, Ectosone*, Metaderm*, Novobetamet*, Valisone in U.S.

● Pharmacologic classification: topical glucocorticoid
● Therapeutic classification: anti-inflammatory
● Pregnancy risk category C

How supplied
Available by prescription only
Betamethasone benzoate
Lotion, ointment, gel, cream: 0.025%

Betamethasone dipropionate
Lotion, ointment, cream: 0.05%
Aerosol: 0.1%
Betamethasone valerate
Lotion, ointment: 0.1%;
Cream: 0.01%, 0.1%
Aerosol solution: 0.1%

Indications, route, and dosage
Inflammation of corticosteroid-responsive dermatoses
Betamethasone benzoate
Betamethasone valerate
Adults and children: Apply cream, lotion, ointment, or gel sparingly once daily to q.i.d.
Betamethasone dipropionate
Adults and children: Apply cream, lotion, or ointment sparingly daily or b.i.d. The dosage of Diprolene Ointment 0.05% should not exceed 45 g per week. To apply aerosol, direct spray onto affected area from a distance of 6″ (15 cm) for only 3 seconds t.i.d. to q.i.d.

Pharmacodynamics
Anti-inflammatory action: Betamethasone stimulates the synthesis of enzymes needed to decrease the inflammatory response. Betamethasone, a fluorinated derivative, has the advantage of availability in various bases to vary the potency for individual conditions.

Pharmacokinetics
● Absorption: The amount absorbed depends on the potency of the preparation, the amount applied, and the nature of the skin at the application site. It ranges from about 1% in areas with a thick stratum corneum (such as the palms, soles, elbows, and knees) to as high as 36% in areas with a thin stratum corneum (face, eyelids, and genitals). Absorption increases in areas of skin damage, inflammation, or occlusion. Some systemic absorption of topical steroids occurs, especially through the oral mucosa.
● Distribution: After topical application, betamethasone is distributed throughout the local skin. Any drug absorbed into circulation is removed rapidly from the blood and distributed into muscle, liver, skin, intestines, and kidneys.
● Metabolism: After topical administration, betamethasone is metabolized primarily in the skin. The small amount that is absorbed into systemic circulation is metabolized primarily in the liver to inactive compounds.
● Excretion: Inactive metabolites are excreted by the kidneys, primarily as glucuronides and sulfates, but also as unconjugated products. Small amounts of the metabolites are also excreted in feces.

Contraindications and precautions
Betamethasone is contraindicated in patients who are hypersensitive to any component of the preparation and in patients with viral, fungal, or tubercular skin lesions.
    Betamethasone should be used with extreme caution in patients with impaired circulation, because it may increase the risk of skin ulceration.

Interactions
None significant.

Effects on diagnostic tests
None reported.

Adverse reactions
● Local: burning, itching, irritation, dryness, folliculitis, hypertrichosis, acneiform eruptions, hypopigmentation, perioral dermatitis, allergic contact dermatitis, maceration, secondary infection, skin atrophy, striae, miliaria.
  Systemic absorption may produce the following reactions.
● CNS: euphoria, insomnia, headache, psychotic behavior, pseudotumor cerebri, mental changes, nervousness, restlessness.
● CV: congestive heart failure, hypertension, edema.
● EENT: cataracts, glaucoma, thrush.
● GI: peptic ulcer, irritation, increased appetite.
● Immune: immunosuppression, increased susceptibility to infection.
● Metabolic: hypokalemia, sodium retention, fluid retention, weight gain, hyperglycemia, osteoporosis, growth suppression in children.
● Musculoskeletal: muscle atrophy.
● Other: withdrawal syndrome (nausea, fatigue, anorexia, dyspnea, hypotension, hypoglycemia, myalgia, arthralgia, fever, dizziness, and fainting). *Sudden withdrawal may be fatal or may exacerbate the underlying disease.*
  Note: Drug should be discontinued if local irritation, infection, systemic absorption, or hypersensitivity reaction occurs.

Overdose and treatment
No information available.

▶ **Special considerations**
Besides those relevant to all *topical adrenocorticoids,* consider the following recommendation.
● Diprolene Ointment may suppress the hypothalamic-pituitary-adrenal axis at doses as low as 7 g per day. Patient should not use more than 45 g per week and should not use occlusive dressings.

Pediatric use
Treatment with Diprolene Ointment is not recommended in children under age 12.

betaxolol hydrochloride
Betoptic, Kerlone

● Pharmacologic classification: beta-adrenergic blocking agent
● Therapeutic classification: antiglaucoma agent, antihypertensive
● Pregnancy risk category C

How supplied
Available by prescription only
Tablets: 10 mg, 20 mg
Ophthalmic solution: 5 mg/ml (0.5%) in 5-ml and 10-ml dropper bottles

Indications, route, and dosage
Chronic open-angle glaucoma and ocular hypertension
Adults: Instill 1 drop in eyes b.i.d.

Management of hypertension (used alone or with other antihypertensives)
Adults: Initially, 10 mg P.O. once daily. After 7 to 14 days full antihypertensive effect should be seen. If necessary, double dosage to 20 mg P.O. once daily.

Pharmacodynamics
● *Ocular hypotensive action:* Betaxolol hydrochloride is a cardioselective beta$_1$ blocker that reduces intraocular pressure (IOP), possibly by reducing production of aqueous humor.
● *Antihypertensive action:* The cardioselective adrenergic blocking effects of betaxolol slow heart rate and decrease cardiac output.

Pharmacokinetics
● *Absorption:* Essentially complete after oral administration; minimal after ophthalmic use. A small first-pass effect reduces bioavailability by about 10%. Absorption is not affected by food or alcohol.
● *Distribution:* Peak concentrations in plasma occur about 3 hours (range 1.5 to 6) after a single oral dose. The drug is about 50% bound to plasma proteins.
● *Metabolism:* Hepatic; about 85% of the drug is recovered in the urine as metabolites. Elimination half-life is prolonged in patients with hepatic disease, but clearance is not affected, so dosage adjustment in unnecessary.
● *Excretion:* Primarily renal (about 80%). Plasma half-life is 14 to 22 hours.

Contraindications and precautions
Betaxolol is contraindicated in patients with bronchial asthma, a history of bronchial asthma, or severe chronic obstructive pulmonary disease, sinus bradycardia, second- or third-degree AV block, CHF, cardiac failure, or cardiogenic shock because the drug may worsen these symptoms or conditions and in hypersensitivity to any components of the preparation.
  Drug should be used cautiously in patients with angle-closure glaucoma (use with miotic), muscle weakness (myasthenic-like symptoms), or a history of heart failure or restricted pulmonary function because the drug may worsen these symptoms or conditions; or in patients with diabetes mellitus because the drug may mask some signs of hypoglycemia, such as tachycardia.
  Betaxolol may be used cautiously in patients with CHF controlled by digitalis and diuretics because beta-adrenergic blocking agents do not block the inotropic effects of digitalis.
  Note that patients with a history of CHF but no overt symptoms may exhibit signs of cardiac decompensation with oral beta blocker therapy.
  Patients with bronchospastic disease (asthma, chronic bronchitis, emphysema) should avoid beta-blocker-receptor antagonism from cardioselective agents such as betaxolol. However, some clinicians will use cardioselective beta blockers for such patients who cannot tolerate other antihypertensives.
  Patients with unrecognized coronary artery disease may exhibit signs of angina pectoris upon rapid withdrawal of the drug.
  Beta blockade may block the signs and symptoms of hypoglycemia (such as tachycardia and blood pressure changes) and may inhibit glycogenolysis.
  Beta blocking agents may mask tachycardia associated with hyperthyroidism. In patients suspected of

having thyrotoxicosis, beta blocker therapy should be withdrawn gradually to avoid thyroid storm.

The anesthesiologist should be advised that the patient is receiving a beta blocking agent so that isoproterenol or dobutamine is made readily available for the reversal of the drug's cardiac effects.

Interactions
When used concomitantly, ophthalmic betaxolol may increase the systemic effect of oral beta blockers, enhance the hypotensive and bradycardiac effect of reserpine and catecholamine-depleting agents, and enhance the lowering of IOP with pilocarpine, epinephrine, and carbonic anhydrase inhibitors.

Concomitant use of oral betaxolol with reserpine and catecholamine-depleting drugs may have an additive effect when administered with a beta blocker. Use with general anesthetics may cause increased hypotensive effects. Observe carefully for excessive hypotension, bradycardia, or orthostatic hypotension. Use with calcium channel blocking agents increases risk of hypotension, left ventricular failure, and AV conduction disturbances. I.V. calcium antagonists should be used with caution. Concomitant use with beta blockers may increase the effects of lidocaine.

Effects on diagnostic tests
Although oral beta blockers have been reported to decrease serum glucose levels from blockage of normal glycogen release after hypoglycemia, no such effect has been reported with the use of ophthalmic beta blockers.

Oral beta blockers may alter the results of glucose tolerance tests.

Adverse reactions
Ophthalmic betaxolol
● Eye: brief discomfort, tearing, erythema, itching, photophobia, corneal sensitivity, corneal staining, keratitis, and anisocoria.
● Systemic: insomnia, depressive neurosis.
Note: Drug should be discontinued if symptoms of systemic toxicity occur.

Systemic betaxolol
● CV: bradycardia, chest pain, hypotension, worsening of angina, peripheral vascular insufficiency, *CHF*, edema, syncope, postural hypotension, conduction disturbances.
● CNS: dizziness, fatigue, headache, lethargy, anxiety.
● DERM: rash.
● GI: flatulence, constipation, nausea, diarrhea, dry mouth, vomiting, anorexia.
● Respiratory: dyspnea, wheezing, *bronchospasm*.

Overdose and treatment
Clinical manifestations of overdose, which are extremely rare with ophthalmic use, may include diplopia, bradycardia, heart block, hypotension, shock, increased airway resistance, cyanosis, fatigue, sleepiness, headache, sedation, coma, respiratory depression, seizures, nausea, vomiting, diarrhea, hypoglycemia, hallucinations, and nightmares. Discontinue drug and flush eye with normal saline solution or water. For treatment of accidental substantial ingestion, emesis is most effective if initiated within 30 minutes, providing the patient is not obtunded, comatose, or having seizures. Activated charcoal may be used. Treat bradycardia, conduction defects, and hypotension with I.V.

fluids, glucagon, atropine, or isoproterenol; refractory bradycardia may require a transvenous pacemaker. Treat bronchoconstriction with I.V. aminophylline; seizures, with I.V. diazepam.

▶ Special considerations
Ophthalmic use
● Betaxolol is a cardioselective beta-adrenergic blocker. Its pulmonary and systemic effects are considerably milder than those of timolol or levobunolol.
● Ophthalmic betaxolol is intended for twice-daily dosage. Encourage patient to comply with this regimen.
● In some patients, a few weeks' treatment may be required to stabilize pressure-lowering response. Determine IOP during the first 4 weeks of drug therapy.

Systemic use
● Withdrawal of beta blocker therapy before surgery is controversial. Some clinicians advocate withdrawal to prevent any impairment of cardiac responsiveness to reflex stimuli and to prevent any decreased responsiveness to exogenous catecholamines.
● In patients with renal failure, dosage adjustments are usually not necessary, but therapy should begin with 5 mg daily. Dosage may be increased at 2-week intervals by 5 mg/day increments to a total of 20 mg/day.
● To withdraw the drug, dosage should be gradually reduced over at least 2 weeks.

Information for the patient
Ophthalmic use
● Instruct patient to tilt his head back and, while looking up, drop the drug into the lower lid.
● Warn patient not to touch dropper to eye or surrounding tissue.
● Instruct the patient not to close his eyes tightly or blink more than usual after instillation.
● Remind the patient to wait at least 5 minutes before using other eye drops.
● Advise patient to wear sunglasses or avoid exposure to bright lights.

Systemic use
Advise the patient to take the drug exactly as prescribed, and warn against discontinuing the drug suddenly. Advise patient to report shortness of breath or difficulty breathing, unusually fast heartbeat, cough, or fatigue with exertion.

Geriatric use
Use with caution in elderly patients with cardiac or pulmonary disease.

Breast-feeding
Use with caution. After oral administration, betaxolol is excreted in breast milk in sufficient amounts to exert an effect on the breast-feeding infant.

bethanechol chloride
Duvoid, Myotonachol, Urabeth, Urecholine

- Pharmacologic classification: cholinergic agonist
- Therapeutic classification: urinary tract and GI tract stimulant
- Pregnancy risk category C

How supplied
Available by prescription only
Tablets: 5 mg, 10 mg, 25 mg, 50 mg
Injection: 5 mg/ml

Indications, route, and dosage
Acute postoperative and postpartum nonobstructive (functional) urinary retention, neurogenic atony of urinary bladder with retention, abdominal distention, megacolon
Adults: 10 to 50 mg P.O. b.i.d., t.i.d., or q.i.d. Or 2.5 to 10 mg S.C. *Never give I.M. or I.V.* When used for urinary retention, some patients may require 50 to 100 mg P.O. per dose. Use such doses with extreme caution. Test dose: 2.5 mg S.C. repeated at 15- to 30-minute intervals to total of four doses to determine the minimal effective dose; then use minimal effective dose q 6 to 8 hours. Adjust dosage to meet individual requirements.
Children: 0.6 mg/kg/day P.O. or 0.15 to 0.20 mg/kg S.C. t.i.d. or q.i.d.

Pharmacodynamics
- *Urinary tract stimulant action:* Bethanechol directly binds to and stimulates muscarinic receptors of the parasympathetic nervous system. That increases tone of the bladder's detrusor muscle, usually resulting in contraction, decreased bladder capacity, and subsequent urination.
- *GI tract stimulant action:* Bethanechol directly stimulates cholinergic receptors, leading to increased gastric tone and motility and peristalsis restoration in patients with abdominal distention or megacolon. Bethanechol improves lower esophageal sphincter tone by directly stimulating cholinergic receptors, thereby alleviating gastric reflux.

Pharmacokinetics
- *Absorption:* Bethanechol is poorly absorbed from the GI tract (absorption varies considerably among patients). After oral administration, action usually begins in 30 to 90 minutes; after S.C. administration, in 5 to 15 minutes.
- *Distribution:* Largely unknown; however, therapeutic doses do not penetrate the blood-brain barrier.
- *Metabolism:* Unknown. Usual duration of effect after oral administration is 1 hour; after S.C. administration, up to 2 hours.
- *Excretion:* Unknown.

Contraindications and precautions
Bethanechol is contraindicated in patients with uncertain bladder wall strength or integrity; in patients for whom increased muscular activity of the GI or urinary tract poses a risk; in patients with mechanical obstruction of the GI or urinary tract because of drug's stimulatory effect on smooth muscle; in patients with bra-

dycardia, vagotonia, hyperthyroidism, hypotension, or Parkinson's disease, because the drug may exacerbate these conditions; in patients with epilepsy because of the drug's possible CNS stimulatory effects; in patients with cardiac or coronary artery disease because of stimulatory effects on the cardiovascular system; in patients with peptic ulcer, because drug may stimulate gastric acid secretion; and in patients with asthma, because the drug may precipitate asthma attacks.

Administer bethanechol cautiously to patients with hypertension and vasomotor instability, because of its stimulatory effects, and to patients with peritonitis or other acute GI inflammatory conditions, because the drug may aggravate these conditions.

Interactions
Concomitant use with procainamide and quinidine may reverse bethanechol's cholinergic effect on muscle. Concomitant use with ganglionic blockers, such as mecamylamine, may cause a critical blood pressure decrease; this effect is usually preceded by abdominal symptoms.

Effects on diagnostic tests
Bethanechol increases serum levels of amylase, lipase, bilirubin, and AST (SGOT), and increases sulfobromophthalein retention time.

Adverse reactions
- CNS: headache, malaise.
- CV: bradycardia, orthostatic hypotension, *cardiac arrest,* reflex tachycardia, transient syncope, complete heart block, and decreased diastolic blood pressure.
- DERM: flushing, sweating.
- EENT: lacrimation, miosis.
- GI: abdominal cramps, diarrhea, salivation, nausea, vomiting, belching, borborygmus, involuntary defecation, colicky pain.
- GU: urinary retention, urinary urgency.
- Other: increased bronchial secretions, asthma attack, substernal pressure or pain from bronchoconstriction or esophageal spasm.
Note: Drug should be discontinued if difficulty breathing, restlessness or agitation, incoordination, blood pressure changes, hypersensitivity, or skin rash occurs.

Overdose and treatment
Clinical signs of overdose include nausea, vomiting, abdominal cramps, diarrhea, involuntary defecation, urinary urgency, excessive salivation, miosis, excessive tearing, bronchospasm, increased bronchial secretions, hypotension, excessive sweating, bradycardia or reflex tachycardia, and substernal pain.

Treatment requires discontinuation of the drug and administration of atropine by S.C., I.M., or I.V. route. (Atropine must be administered cautiously; an overdose could cause bronchial plug formation.) Contact local or regional poison control center for more information.

▶ Special considerations
Besides those relevant to all *cholinergics,* consider the following recommendations.
- Never give bethanechol I.M. or I.V., because that could cause circulatory collapse, hypotension, severe abdominal cramps, bloody diarrhea, shock, or cardiac arrest. Give only by subcutaneous route when giving parenterally.

- For administration to treat urinary retention, bedpan should be readily available.
- For administration to prevent abdominal distention and GI distress, insertion of a rectal tube will facilitate passage of gas.
- Give bethanechol on an empty stomach; eating soon after drug administration may cause nausea and vomiting.
- Patients with hypertension receiving bethanechol may experience a precipitous drop in blood pressure.

biperiden hydrochloride
biperiden lactate
Akineton

- Pharmacologic classification: anticholinergic
- Therapeutic classification: antiparkinsonian agent
- Pregnancy risk category C

How supplied
Available by prescription only
Tablets: 2 mg
Injection: 5 mg/ml in 1-ml ampule

Indications, route, and dosage
Extrapyramidal disorders
Adults: 2 mg P.O. daily, b.i.d., or t.i.d., depending on severity. Usual dose is 2 mg daily, or 2 mg I.M. or I.V. q ½ hour, not to exceed four doses or 8 mg daily.
Parkinsonism
Adults: 2 mg P.O. t.i.d. to q.i.d. For prolonged therapy, titrate dose to maximum of 16 mg daily.

Pharmacodynamics
Antiparkinsonian action: Biperiden blocks central cholinergic receptors, helping to balance cholinergic activity in the basal ganglia. It may also prolong dopamine's effects by blocking dopamine reuptake and storage at central receptor sites.

Pharmacokinetics
- *Absorption:* Biperiden is well absorbed from the GI tract.
- *Distribution:* Biperiden is well distributed throughout the body.
- *Metabolism:* Exact metabolic fate is unknown.
- *Excretion:* Biperiden is excreted in the urine as unchanged drug and metabolites. After oral therapy, small amounts are probably excreted as unabsorbed drug.

Contraindications and precautions
Administer biperiden cautiously to patients with prostatic hypertrophy, because the drug may exacerbate urinary retention; to patients with cardiac arrhythmias, because it may block vagal inhibition of the sinoatrial node pacemaker; and to patients with narrow-angle glaucoma, because drug-induced cycloplegia and mydriasis may increase intraocular pressure.

Interactions
Amantadine may amplify biperiden's anticholinergic adverse effects, such as confusion and hallucinations. Decrease biperiden dosage before amantadine administration.

Concomitant use with haloperidol or phenothiazines may decrease the antipsychotic effectiveness of these drugs, possibly by direct CNS antagonism. Concomitant use with phenothiazines increases risk of anticholinergic adverse effects.

Alcohol and other CNS depressants increase biperiden's sedative effects. Antacids and antidiarrheals may decrease biperiden absorption. Administer biperiden at least 1 hour before these drugs.

Effects on diagnostic tests
None reported.

Adverse reactions
- CNS: headache, disorientation, temporary euphoria, restlessness, drowsiness, confusion and excitement (in elderly), dizziness, transient psychosis, agitation, disturbed behavior.
- CV: transient postural hypotension.
- EENT: blurred vision.
- GI: constipation, dry mouth, nausea, vomiting, epigastric distress, abdominal distention.
- GU: urinary hesitancy or retention.
Note: Drug should be discontinued if hypersensitivity; urinary retention; confusion; hallucinations; dilated, nonreactive pupils; or hot, dry, flushed skin occurs.

Overdose and treatment
Clinical effects of overdose include central stimulation followed by depression and psychotic symptoms such as disorientation, confusion, hallucinations, delusions, anxiety, agitation, and restlessness. Peripheral effects may include dilated, nonreactive pupils; blurred vision; hot, dry, flushed skin; dry mucous membranes; dysphagia; decreased or absent bowel sounds; urinary retention; hyperthermia; headache; tachycardia; hypertension; and increased respiration.

Treatment is primarily symptomatic and supportive, as necessary. Maintain patent airway. If the patient is alert, induce emesis (or use gastric lavage)and follow with a saline cathartic and activated charcoal to prevent further absorption of orally administered drug. In severe cases, physostigmine may be administered to block biperiden's antimuscarinic effects. Give fluids, as needed, to treat shock; diazepam to control psychotic symptoms; and pilocarpine (instilled into the eyes) to relieve mydriasis. If urinary retention occurs, catheterization may be necessary.

▶ Special considerations
Besides those relevant to all *anticholinergics,* consider the following recommendations.
- When giving drug parenterally, keep patient supine; parenteral administration may cause transient postural hypotension and disturbed coordination.
- When giving biperiden I.V., inject the drug slowly.
- Because biperiden may cause dizziness, patient may need assistance when walking.
- In patients with severe parkinsonism, tremors may increase when drug is administered to relieve spasticity.

Information for the patient
- With chronic biperiden administration, tolerance to therapeutic and adverse effects can occur.
- Tell patient that drug may increase sensitivity of his eyes to light.

Geriatric use
Biperiden should be administered cautiously to elderly patients. Lower doses are indicated.

Pediatric use
Biperiden is not recommended for children.

Breast-feeding
Biperiden may be excreted in breast milk, possibly resulting in infant toxicity. It may also decrease milk production. Breast-feeding women should avoid this drug.

bisacodyl
Biscolax, Carter's Little Pills, Dacodyl Tabs, Deficol, Dulcolax, Theralax Suppositories

bisacodyl tannex
Clysodrast

- Pharmacologic classification: diphenylmethane derivative
- Therapeutic classification: stimulant laxative
- Pregnancy risk category C

How supplied
Available without prescription
Tablets: 5 mg
Suppositories: 5 mg, 10 mg
Suspension (enema): 0.33 mg/dl
Powder for rectal solution (bisacodyl tannex): 1.5 mg bisacodyl and 2.5 g tannic acid

Indications, route, and dosage
Constipation; preparation for delivery, surgery, or rectal or bowel examination
Adults: 10 to 15 mg P.O. in evening or before breakfast. Up to 30 mg may be used for thorough evacuation needed for examinations or surgery. Alternatively, give one suppository (10 mg), as needed, or contents of one retention enema.
Children over age 3: 5 mg P.O., or one suppository (10 mg); alternatively, may give half the contents of microenema.
Children age 3 and under: 5 mg suppository.

Pharmacodynamics
Laxative action: Bisacodyl has a direct stimulant effect on the colon, increasing peristalsis and enhancing bowel evacuation.

Pharmacokinetics
- *Absorption:* Absorption is minimal; action begins 6 to 8 hours after oral administration and 15 to 60 minutes after rectal administration.
- *Distribution:* Bisacodyl is distributed locally.
- *Metabolism:* Up to 15% of an oral dose may enter the enterohepatic circulation.
- *Excretion:* Bisacodyl is excreted primarily in feces; some is excreted in urine.

Contraindications and precautions
Bisacodyl is contraindicated in patients with fluid and electrolyte disturbances, appendicitis, any abdominal condition necessitating immediate surgery, ulcerative colitis, rectal fissures, ulcerated hemorrhoids, fecal impaction, and intestinal obstruction because the drug may exacerbate these conditions. Chronic use may decrease serum potassium levels.

Bisacodyl tannex should not be used if multiple enemas are to be administered because significant absorption of tannic acid may result in hepatotoxicity.

Interactions
Antacids, milk, and other drugs that increase gastric pH levels may cause premature dissolution of the enteric coating, resulting in intestinal or gastric irritation or cramping.

Effects on diagnostic tests
None reported.

Adverse reactions
- GI: nausea, vomiting, abdominal cramps, diarrhea (with high doses); burning sensation in rectum (with suppositories).
- Other: laxative dependence with long-term or excessive use.
Note: Drug should be discontinued if severe abdominal pain or laxative dependence occurs.

Overdose and treatment
No cases of overdose have been reported.

▶ Special considerations
Patients should swallow tablets whole rather than crushing or chewing them, to avoid GI irritation. Administer with full glass (8 oz) of fluid.

Information for the patient
- Instruct patient about medication and dosage schedule.
- Tell patient to take only as directed to avoid laxative dependence.

Pediatric use
Do not give bisacodyl tannex (Clysodrast) to children under age 10.

Breast-feeding
Bisacodyl may be used as directed by breast-feeding women.

bismuth subgallate
Devron

bismuth subsalicylate
Pepto-Bismol

- Pharmacologic classification: adsorbent
- Therapeutic classification: antidiarrheal
- Pregnancy risk category C (D in third trimester)

How supplied
Available without prescription
Chewable tablets: 262 mg
Suspension: 262 mg/15 ml

Indications, route, and dosage
Mild, nonspecific diarrhea
Adults: 1 to 2 tablets chewed or swallowed whole t.i.d. (subgallate); or 30 ml or 2 tablets q ½ to 1 hour up to a maximum of 8 doses and for no longer than 2 days (subsalicylate).
Children age 9 to 12: 20 ml.
Children age 6 to 9: 10 ml.
Children age 3 to 6: 5 ml.
Prevention and treatment of traveler's diarrhea
Adults: Prophylactically, 60 ml (Pepto-Bismol) q.i.d. during the first 2 weeks of travel. During acute illness, 30 to 60 ml q 30 minutes for a total of 8 doses. Alternatively, 2 tablets P.O. q.i.d. for up to 3 weeks.

Drug is useful for indigestion without causing constipation; nausea; and relief of flatulence and abdominal cramps.

Pharmacodynamics
Antidiarrheal action: Bismuth adsorbs extra water in the bowel during diarrhea. It also adsorbs toxins and forms a protective coating for the intestinal mucosa.

Pharmacokinetics
● *Absorption:* Bismuth is absorbed poorly; significant salicylate absorption may occur after using bismuth subsalicylate.
● *Distribution:* Bismuth is distributed locally in the gut.
● *Metabolism:* Drug is metabolized minimally.
● *Excretion:* Bismuth subsalicylate is excreted in urine.

Contraindications and precautions
Bismuth subsalicylate is contraindicated in patients with known hypersensitivity to salicylates.

Interactions
Bismuth subsalicylate and bismuth subgallate may impair tetracycline absorption. Bismuth subsalicylate may impair sulfinpyrazone's uricosuric effect and may increase the risk of aspirin toxicity.

Effects on diagnostic tests
Because bismuth is radiopaque, it may interfere with radiologic examination of the GI tract.

Adverse reactions
● GI: temporary tongue and stool darkening, fecal impaction in infants and debilitated patients.
● Other: salicylism (with high doses of bismuth subsalicylate).
Note: Drug should be discontinued if abdominal pain occurs.

Overdose and treatment
Overdose has not been reported. However, overdose is more likely with bismuth subsalicylate; probable clinical effects include CNS effects, such as tinnitus, and fever.

▶ Special considerations
● Monitor hydration status and serum electrolyte levels; record number and consistency of stools.
● If administered by tube, tube should be flushed via nasogastric tube, to clear it and ensure drug's passage to stomach.
● If patient is also receiving tetracycline, administer bismuth at least 1 hour apart; to avoid decreased drug absorption, dosages or schedules of other medications may require adjustment.

● Bismuth subsalicylate has been used investigationally to treat peptic ulcer. Doses of 600 mg t.i.d. may be as effective as cimetidine 800 mg once a day.
● Drug has shown some effectiveness in the treatment of pyloric *Helicobacter* infections, either alone or with an antibiotic.

Information for the patient
● Advise patients who are taking anticoagulants or medication for diabetes or gout to seek medical approval before taking this drug.
● Instruct patient to chew tablets well or to shake suspension well before using.
● Tell patient to report persistent diarrhea.
● Warn patient that bismuth may temporarily darken stools and tongue.

Breast-feeding
Small amounts of bismuth subsalicylate are excreted in breast milk. Patient should seek medical approval before using.

bitolterol mesylate
Tornalate

● Pharmacologic classification: adrenergic, beta₂ agonist
● Therapeutic classification: bronchodilator
● Pregnancy risk category C

How supplied
Available by prescription only
Aerosol inhaler: 370 mcg/metered spray

Indications, route, and dosage
To prevent and treat bronchial asthma and bronchospasm
Adults and children over age 12: For symptomatic relief of bronchospasm, two inhalations at an interval of at least 1 to 3 minutes followed by a third inhalation, if needed; to prevent bronchospasm, two inhalations q 8 hours. Usually, dose should not exceed three inhalations q 6 hours or two inhalations q 4 hours. However, because deposition of inhaled medications is variable, higher doses are occasionally used, especially in patients with acute bronchospasm.

Pharmacodynamics
Bronchodilator action: Bitolterol selectively stimulates beta₂-adrenergic receptors of the lungs. Bronchodilation results from relaxation of bronchial smooth muscles, which relieves bronchospasm and reduces airway resistance. Some cardiovascular stimulation may occur as a result of beta₁-adrenergic stimulation, including mild tachycardia, palpitations, and changes in blood pressure or heart rate.

Pharmacokinetics
● *Absorption:* After oral inhalation, bronchodilation results from local action on the bronchial tree, with most of the inhaled dose being swallowed. Onset of action occurs within 3 to 5 minutes, peaks in ½ to 2 hours, and lasts 4 to 8 hours.
● *Distribution:* Bitolterol is widely distributed throughout the body.

- *Metabolism:* Bitolterol is hydrolyzed by esterases to active metabolites.
- *Excretion:* After oral administration, bitolterol and its metabolites are excreted primarily in urine.

Contraindications and precautions
Bitolterol is contraindicated in patients with known hypersensitivity to drug. Administer cautiously to patients with cardiovascular disorders (ischemic heart disease, hypertension, or cardiac arrhythmias), hyperthyroidism, diabetes, seizure disorders, or sensitivity to other sympathomimetic amines.

Interactions
Concomitant use with other orally inhaled beta-adrenergic agonists may produce additive sympathomimetic effects. Evidence suggests that cardiotoxic effects may be increased when bitolterol is used with a theophylline salt such as aminophylline.

Propranolol and other beta blockers may antagonize the effects of bitolterol.

Effects on diagnostic tests
Bitolterol therapy may increase AST (SGOT) levels and decrease platelet or leukocyte count. Proteinuria may also occur. Drug may also render spirometry insensitive for the diagnosis of asthma.

Adverse reactions
- CNS: tremor, nervousness, dizziness, headache, insomnia, light-headedness, hyperkinesia.
- CV: palpitations, tachycardia, chest discomfort, premature ventricular contractions, flushing, changes in blood pressure.
- EENT: throat irritation.
- GI: nausea, vomiting, unusual taste, irritation of oropharynx, increased appetite, heartburn.
- Other: dyspnea, cough, dyspepsia, *bronchospasm.*
  Note: Drug should be discontinued if hypersensitivity or bronchoconstriction occurs.

Overdose and treatment
Clinical manifestations of overdose include exaggeration of common adverse reactions, especially arrhythmias, extreme tremor, nausea, and vomiting.

Treatment requires supportive measures. To reverse effects, use selective beta$_1$-adrenergic blockers (acebutolol, atenolol, metoprolol) with extreme caution (may induce asthmatic attack). Monitor vital signs and ECG closely.

▶ Special considerations
Besides those relevant to all *adrenergics,* consider the following recommendation.
- Repeated use may result in paradoxical bronchospasm. Discontinue immediately if this occurs.

Information for the patient
- Tell patient to use only as directed and not to use more than prescribed amount or more often than prescribed.
- Teach patient to use drug correctly. Tell patient to ensure proper delivery of dose by cleaning plastic mouthpiece with warm tap water and drying thoroughly at least once daily. Tell patient that dryness of mouth and throat may occur, but that rinsing with water after each dose may help.
- Tell patient to call promptly if troubled breathing persists 1 hour after using drug, if symptoms return within

4 hours, if condition worsens, or if new (refill) canister is needed within 2 weeks.
- Tell patient to wait 15 minutes after use of bitolterol before using adrenocorticoid inhaler.
- Give patient instructions on proper use of inhaler:
Administration by metered-dose nebulizers: Shake canister to activate; place mouthpiece well into mouth, aimed at back of throat. Close lips and teeth around mouthpiece. Exhale through nose, then inhale through mouth slowly and deeply, while actuating the nebulizer, to release dose. Hold breath 10 seconds (count "1-100, 2-100, 3-100" to "10-100"); remove mouthpiece, then exhale slowly.
Administration by metered powder inhaler: Caution patient not to take forced deep breaths, but to breathe normally. Observe patient closely for exaggerated systemic drug action. Patients requiring more than three aerosol treatments within 24 hours should be under close medical supervision.
Administration by oxygen aerosolization: Administer over 15 to 20 minutes, with oxygen flow rate adjusted to 4 liters/minute. Turn on oxygen supply before patient places nebulizer in mouth. (Patient need not close lips tightly around nebulizer opening.) Placement of Y tube in rubber tubing permits patient to control administration. Advise patient to rinse mouth immediately after inhalation therapy to help prevent dryness and throat irritation. Rinse mouthpiece with warm running water at least once daily to prevent clogging. (It is not dishwasher-safe.) Wait until mouthpiece is dry before storing. Do not place near artificial heat (dishwasher or oven). Replace reservoir bag every 2 to 3 weeks or as needed; replace mouthpiece every 6 to 9 months or as needed. Replacement of bags or mouthpieces may require a prescription.

Geriatric use
Lower doses are indicated in elderly patients, who may be more sensitive to the drug's effects.

Pediatric use
Not recommended for use in children under age 12.

Breast-feeding
Administer cautiously to breast-feeding women. It is unknown if bitolterol is distributed into breast milk.

black widow spider *(Latrodectus mactans)* antivenin

- Pharmacologic classification: antivenin
- Therapeutic classification: black widow spider antivenin
- Pregnancy risk category C

How supplied
Available by prescription only
Injection: combination package–1 vial of antivenin (6,000 units/vial), one 2.5-ml vial of diluent (sterile water for injection), and one 1-ml vial of normal equine (horse) serum (1:10 dilution) for sensitivity testing

Indications, route, and dosage
Black widow spider bite
Adults and children: 2.5 ml (1 vial) I.M. in anterolateral thigh or deltoid muscle. If symptoms do not subside in

1 to 3 hours, an equal dose may be repeated. Antivenin also may be given I.V. in 10 to 50 ml of normal saline solution over 15 minutes (the preferred route for severe cases, such as patients in shock or those under age 12).

Pharmacodynamics
Antivenin action: Black widow spider antivenin provides immune globulins that specifically bind black widow spider venom.

Pharmacokinetics
No information available.

Contraindications and precautions
This product is derived from horses immunized with black widow spider venom. Observe patient for signs and symptoms of allergic reactions to this product.

Interactions
None significant.

Effects on diagnostic tests
None reported.

Adverse reactions
● Local: pain, erythema, urticaria.
● Systemic: hypersensitivity, *anaphylaxis,* serum sickness.
  Note: Drug should be discontinued if severe systemic reactions occur.

Overdose and treatment
No information available.

▶ Special considerations
● Immobilize patient immediately. Splint the bitten limb to prevent spread of venom.
● If possible, hospitalize patient.
● Obtain a thorough patient history of allergies, especially to horses and horse immune serum, and previous reactions to immunizations.
● Test patient for sensitivity (against a control of normal saline solution in opposing extremity) before giving antivenin. Give 0.2 ml of the 1:10 dilution of horse serum intradermally. Read results after 5 to 30 minutes.
Positive reaction: Wheal with or without pseudopodia and surrounding erythema. If skin sensitivity test is positive, consider a conjunctival test and desensitization schedule.
● Early use of antivenin is recommended for best results.
● Apply tourniquet above site of I.M. injection if systemic reaction to antivenin occurs.
● Epinephrine solution 1:1,000 should be available to treat allergic reactions.
● Black widow spider venom is neurotoxic and may cause ascending motor convulsions. Watch patient carefully for 2 to 3 days for signs of neurotoxicity.
● A black widow spider bite induces painful muscle spasms. Patient may need analgesia and prolonged warm baths.
● Administer a 10-ml injection of 10% calcium gluconate to control muscle spasm p.r.n.
● Vital signs should be checked every 30 minutes for 1 to 3 hours.
● Find out when the patient received last tetanus immunization; many clinicians order a booster at this time.

Information for the patient
● Inform patient that allergic reactions to the antivenin may cause a rash, joint swelling or pain, fever, or difficulty breathing.
● Encourage patient to report any unusual effects he experiences while hospitalized
● Explain that residual effects of the spider bite (general weakness, tingling of the extremities, nervousness, and muscle spasm) may persist for weeks or months after recovery from the acute phase.

Breast-feeding
Patient should discontinue breast-feeding temporarily until effects of the venom subside or if symptoms of serum sickness develop.

---

bleomycin sulfate
Blenoxane

● Pharmacologic classification: antibiotic, antineoplastic (cell cycle-phase specific, G_2 and M phase)
● Therapeutic classification: antineoplastic
● Pregnancy risk category D

How supplied
Available by prescription only
Injection: 15-unit ampules (1 unit = 1 mg)

Indications, route, and dosage
Dosage and indications may vary. Check literature for current protocol.
Hodgkin's disease, squamous cell carcinoma, non-Hodgkin's lymphoma, or testicular carcinoma
Adults: 10 to 20 units/m² (0.25 to 0.5 units/kg) I.V., I.M., or S.C., one or two times weekly. After 50% response, maintenance dose of 1 unit daily or 5 units weekly.
†*Malignant pleural effusion*
Adults: 50 to 60 units by intracavitary administration.

Pharmacodynamics
Antineoplastic action: The exact mechanism of bleomycin's cytotoxicity is unknown. Its action may be through scission of single- and double-stranded DNA and inhibition of DNA, RNA, and protein synthesis. Bleomycin also appears to inhibit cell progression out of the G_2 phase.

Pharmacokinetics
● *Absorption:* Bleomycin is poorly absorbed across the GI tract following oral administration. I.M. administration results in lower serum levels than those occurring after equivalent I.V. doses.
● *Distribution:* Bleomycin distributes widely into total body water, mainly in the skin, lungs, kidneys, peritoneum, and lymphatic tissue.
● *Metabolism:* The metabolic fate of bleomycin is undetermined; however, extensive tissue inactivation occurs in the liver and kidney and much less in the skin and lungs.
● *Excretion:* Bleomycin and its metabolites are excreted primarily in urine. The terminal plasma elimination phase half-life is reported at 2 hours.

Contraindications and precautions

Bleomycin is contraindicated in patients with a history of hypersensitivity or idiosyncratic reaction to the drug. Use with caution in patients with renal impairment because drug accumulation may occur; also use cautiously in patients with pulmonary impairment and monitor the patient carefully for signs of pulmonary toxicity, because pulmonary fibrosis may occur. Patient should have chest X-rays every 1 to 2 weeks during therapy, and evaluation of pulmonary diffusion capacity for carbon dioxide every month.

Interactions

Concomitant use may decrease serum levels of phenytoin and digoxin.

Effects on diagnostic tests

Bleomycin therapy may increase blood and urine concentrations of uric acid.

Adverse reactions

- CNS: hyperesthesia of scalp and fingers, headache.
- DERM: erythema, vesiculation, and hardening and discoloration of palmar and plantar skin in 8% of patients; desquamation of hands, feet, and pressure areas; hyperpigmentation; acne.
- GI: stomatitis, prolonged anorexia in 13% of patients, nausea, vomiting, diarrhea.
- Respiratory: fine crackles, fever, dyspnea, nonproductive cough; dose-limiting pulmonary fibrosis in 10% of patients.
- Other: reversible alopecia, swelling of interphalangeal joints, leukocytosis, *allergic reaction* (fever up to 106 F. [41.1 C.] with chills up to 5 hours after injection; *anaphylaxis* in 1% to 6% of patients).

  Note: Drug should be discontinued if patient develops signs of pulmonary fibrosis or mucocutaneous toxicity.

Overdose and treatment

Clinical manifestations of overdose include pulmonary fibrosis, fever, chills, vesiculation, and hyperpigmentation.

Treatment is usually supportive and includes antipyretics for fever.

▶ Special considerations

- To prepare solution for I.M. administration, reconstitute the drug with 1 to 5 ml of normal saline solution, sterile water for injection, or dextrose 5% in water.
- For I.V. administration, dilute with a minimum of 5 ml of diluent and administer over 10 minutes as I.V. push injection.
- Prepare infusions of bleomycin in glass bottles, as absorption of drug to plastic occurs with time. Plastic syringes do not interfere with bleomycin activity.
- Use precautions in preparing and handling drug; wear gloves and wash hands after preparing and administering.
- Drug can be administered by intracavitary, intraarterial, or intratumoral injection. It can also be instilled into bladder for bladder tumors.
- Cumulative lifetime dosage should not exceed 400 units.
- Pulmonary function tests may be useful in predicting fibrosis.
- Response to therapy may take 2 to 3 weeks.
- Administer a 1-unit test dose before therapy to assess hypersensitivity to bleomycin. If no reaction occurs, then

follow the dosing schedule. The test dose can be incorporated as part of the total dose for the regimen.
- Have epinephrine, diphenhydramine, I.V. corticosteroids, and oxygen available in case of anaphylactic reaction.
- Premedication with aspirin, steroids, and diphenhydramine may reduce drug fever and risk of anaphylaxis.
- Dosage should be reduced in patients with renal or pulmonary impairment.
- Drug concentrates in keratin of squamous epithelium. To prevent linear streaking, don't use adhesive dressings on skin.
- Allergic reactions may be delayed especially in patients with lymphoma.
- Pulmonary function tests should be performed to establish a baseline and then monitored periodically.
- Monitor chest X-rays and auscultate the lungs.
- Bleomycin is stable for 24 hours at room temperature and 48 hours under refrigeration. Refrigerate unopened vials containing dry powder.

Information for the patient

Explain that hair should grow back after treatment is discontinued.

Geriatric use

Use with caution in patients over age 70. They are at increased risk for pulmonary toxicity.

Breast-feeding

It is not known whether bleomycin distributes into breast milk. However, because of the risk of serious adverse reactions, mutagenicity, and carcinogenicity in infants, breast-feeding is not recommended.

---

boric acid
Borofax, Collyrium, Ear-Dry, Neo-Flo, Ocu-Bath, Swim Ear, Ting

- Pharmacologic classification: acid
- Therapeutic classification: topical anti-infective

How supplied

Available without prescription
Ophthalmic ointment: 5%, 10%
Otic solution: 2.75% boric acid in isopropyl alcohol
Topical ointment: 5%, 10%

Indications, route, and dosage
External ear canal infection

Adults and children: Fill ear canal with solution and plug with cotton. Repeat t.i.d. or q.i.d.
Relief of abrasions, dry skin, minor burns, insect bites, and other skin irritations

Adults and children: Apply 5% or 10% ointment to affected area t.i.d. or q.i.d.
Eyelid inflammation and irritation

Adults and children: Apply 5% or 10% ophthalmic ointment to inner surface of lower eyelid b.i.d. or t.i.d.

Pharmacodynamics

Local anti-infection action: Boric acid destroys or inhibits the growth of microorganisms. It is indicated to treat irritated and inflamed eyelids and to inhibit or destroy bacteria present in the ear canal.

Pharmacokinetics
Unknown.

Contraindications and precautions
Boric acid is contraindicated in patients with hypersensitivity to any components of the preparations. Otic preparation is contraindicated in patients with perforated eardrum or excoriated membranes in the ear. Ophthalmic preparation is contraindicated in patients with eye lacerations or abraded cornea. Topical form is contraindicated for use in patients with abraded skin or granulating wounds, because significant absorption may occur and cause systemic symptoms.

Interactions
Do not use with eye drops or contact lens wetting solutions containing polyvinyl alcohol; concomitant use with boric acid for ophthalmic use may form insoluble complexes with polyvinyl alcohol. Avoid concomitant use with idoxuridine to prevent local irritation.

Effects on diagnostic tests
None reported.

Adverse reactions
- CNS: restlessness, delirium, convulsions, headache.
- CV: *circulatory collapse*, tachycardia.
- DERM: urticaria.
- Ear: irritation or itching.
- GI: nausea, vomiting, diarrhea, irritation.
- GU: *renal damage*, hypothermia.
- Other: overgrowth of nonsusceptible organisms

Note: Drug should be discontinued if ophthalmic use causes eye pain, changes in vision, continued redness or irritation of the eye; if the condition worsens or persists; or if signs of hypersensitivity or systemic toxicity occur.

Overdose and treatment
Clinical manifestations of overdose include hypotension, shock, restlessness, weakness, seizures, nausea, vomiting, diarrhea, oliguria, hypothermia, hyperthermia, and erythematous rash.

To treat accidental substantial ingestion, induce emesis, then administer activated charcoal and a saline cathartic unless the patient is comatose or obtunded. Treat hypotension with fluids. Treat seizures with I.V. diazepam.

▶ Special considerations
- When used topically, drug is a mild antiseptic and astringent.
- Avoid long-term use.
- Ophthalmic use is not recommended when soft contact lenses are in place.
- Drug is weak bacteriostatic, fungistatic agent.
- Boric acid ointments for topical use are contraindicated for ophthalmic use.
- When used as an otic, watch for signs of superinfection (continual pain, inflammation, fever).

Information for the patient
- Advise patient using boric acid as an otic to moisten cotton plug with medication when using cotton plug in ear and not to touch dropper to ear.
- Tell patient not to use ophthalmic preparation when contact lenses are in place.
- Advise patient to avoid long-term topical use or use on abraded skin.

Pediatric use
Use with caution in children, who are at increased risk for systemic absorption. Topical application is contraindicated in children under age 2 unless directed by a physician.

---

botulinum toxin type A
Oculinum

- Pharmacologic classification: neurotoxin
- Therapeutic classification: muscle relaxant
- Pregnancy risk category C

How supplied
Available by prescription only
Powder for injection: 100 units/vial

Indications, route, and dosage
Treatment of strabismus
Adults and children age 12 and over: Injections should be made only by physicians familiar with the technique, which involves surgical exposure of the region as well as electromyographic guidance of the injection needle.

Dosage varies with the degree of deviation (lower doses are used for small deviations). For vertical muscles and for horizontal strabismus of < 20 prism diopters, the usual dose is 1.25 to 2.5 units in any one muscle. For horizontal strabismus of 20 to 50 prism diopters, dosage is 2.5 to 5 units injected into any one muscle. For persistent VI nerve palsy greater than 1 month's duration, dosage is 1.25 to 2.5 units injected into the medial rectus muscle.

Subsequent doses for recurrent or residual strabismus should not be administered unless 7 to 14 days have elapsed after the initial dose and substantial function has returned to the injected and adjacent muscles. Dosage may be increased to twice the initial dose for patients experiencing incomplete paralysis; patients with adequate response should receive a similar dose. The maximum single dose for any one muscle is 25 units.

Treatment of blepharospasm
Adults: Initially, 1.25 to 2.5 units injected into the medial and lateral pretarsal orbicularis oculi of the upper and lower lids. Effects should be apparent within 3 days and peak in 1 to 2 weeks after treatment. At subsequent treatments, dosage may be doubled if inadequate paralysis is achieved, but exceeding 5 units per site produces no apparent benefit. The effect of each treatment lasts about 3 months. Treatment can be repeated indefinitely.

The cumulative dosage of botulinum toxin type A should not exceed 200 units per month.

Pharmacodynamics
Neuromuscular blocking action: Botulinum toxin type A produces a neuromuscular paralysis by binding to acetylcholine receptors on the motor end plate. It may also inhibit the release of acetylcholine from the presynaptic nerve ending.

Pharmacokinetics
- *Absorption:* Unknown.
- *Distribution:* Unknown.
- *Metabolism:* Unknown.

• *Excretion:* Unknown. However, patients treated for blepharospasm did not require retreatment for an average of 12.5 weeks after injection. Over half of the patients treated for strabismus maintained improvements over 6 months.

Contraindications and precautions
Contraindicated in patients hypersensitive to any ingredient in the formulation (which includes human albumin). Because the drug is a protein, epinephrine should be readily available in the event of an anaphylactic reaction.

Safe and effective use of the drug requires knowledge of certain specialized administration techniques, including electromyography. Particular attention should be paid to proper storage, reconstitution, and dilution of the drug.

Needle penetrations into the orbit have occurred during administration. An ophthalmoscope should be available to diagnose globe penetrations. Retrobulbar hemorrhages should be treated appropriately.

Injection into the orbicular muscle may lead to reduced blinking and subsequent corneal exposure and ulceration. Test corneal sensation in previously operated eyes, and avoid injection into the lower lid to prevent ectropion. Treat any epithelial defect (using drops, ointment, or an eye patch as needed).

Effectiveness of therapy can be reduced if the patient develops antibodies to the toxin. To avoid this, keep doses as low as possible (preferably less than 200 units in any 1-month period).

Interactions
Muscle paralysis may be potentiated by concomitant use of aminoglycoside antibiotics.

Effects on diagnostic tests
None reported.

Adverse reactions
• EENT: double vision, blurred vision, spatial disorientation, ptosis, vertical deviation (after treatment of strabismus), irritation (after treatment of blepharospasm).
• Local: diffuse skin rash, swelling of eyelid, ecchymosis.

Overdose and treatment
Information may be obtained from the manufacturer, Allergan Pharmaceuticals, at 1-800-347-5063 (8 a.m. to 4 p.m. Pacific time), or at other times at 1-714-724-5954 for a recorded message.

▶ **Special considerations**
• The drug should be stored in the freezer at or below 23° F. (− 5° C.).
• Reconstitute the drug with normal saline (0.9% sodium chloride) solution without a preservative. The vacuum in the vial should be noticeable when reconstituting. Inject the diluent into the vial gently, because severe agitation can denature the protein.
• Reconstituting with 1 ml produces a concentration of 10 units/0.1 ml; adding 2 ml yields 5 units/0.1 ml. Adding more diluent (such as 4 ml to produce 2.5 units/0.1 ml or 8 ml to yield 1.25 units/0.1 ml) or using different injection volumes are methods commonly used to adjust dosage.
• Reconstituted drug should be clear, colorless, and free of particles. It must be administered within 4 hours

of removal from the freezer. Reconstituted drug should be refrigerated until use. Be sure to record the date and time of reconstitution.
• When treating strabismus, injection volume should be 0.05 to 0.15 ml per muscle. When treating blepharospasm, injection volumes are maintained at 0.05 to 0.1 ml per site. Dosage adjustments are made by altering the volume of diluent used to reconstitute the drug.
• When treating strabismus, several drops of an ocular decongestant and a topical anesthetic should be applied before the procedure.
• Prepare injection by drawing slightly more volume than needed into a sterile 1-ml syringe. Expel air bubbles in the barrel of the syringe, and attach an electromyographic injection needle (if treating strabismus), such as a 1½″, 27G needle. Expel unnecessary drug (into an appropriate waste container) while checking for leakage around the needle. Be sure to use a new needle and syringe for each injection.

Information for the patient
• Many patients with blepharospasm may have been sedentary for extended periods of time. Recommend caution as they resume normal activity.
• Explain to the patient that muscle paralysis becomes evident 1 or 2 days after injection and increases in intensity over the first week. The paralysis lasts for 2 to 6 weeks and eventually resolves.

Pediatric use
Safety and efficacy in children under age 12 have not been established.

Breast-feeding
It is not known if the drug is excreted in breast milk. Use with caution in breast-feeding women.

botulism antitoxin, trivalent (ABE) equine

• Pharmacologic classification: antitoxin
• Therapeutic classification: botulism antitoxin
• Pregnancy risk category C

How supplied
Available through your state health department or the office of the state epidemiologist

Indications, route, and dosage
Botulism
Adults and children: 2 vials I.V. Dilute antitoxin 1:10 in dextrose 5% or 10% in water or normal saline solution before giving. Give first 10 ml of dilution over 5 minutes; after 15 minutes, rate may be increased.

Pharmacodynamics
Antitoxin action: Botulism antitoxin neutralizes and binds toxin.

Pharmacokinetics
No information available.

Contraindications and precautions
Use with caution in patients with a history of sensitivity to horses or horse serums and of severe reactions to immunizations.

Interactions
None reported.

Effects on diagnostic tests
None reported.

Adverse reactions
● Systemic: hypersensitivity, *anaphylaxis*, serum sickness (marked by urticaria, pruritus, fever, malaise, and arthralgia occurring 5 to 13 days after administration).
Note: Drug should be discontinued if severe systemic reactions occur.

Overdose and treatment
No information available.

▶ Special considerations
● Obtain a thorough patient history of allergies, especially to horses and horse immune serum, and previous reactions to immunizations.
● Epinephrine solution 1:1,000 should be available to treat allergic reactions.
● This product is derived from horses immunized with *Clostridium botulinum* toxin. Therefore, test patient for sensitivity (against a control of normal saline solution) before giving it. Read results after 5 to 30 minutes. Instructions for an eye test or skin test are provided in the package insert. *Positive reaction:* wheal with or without pseudopodia and surrounding erythema. If skin sensitivity test is positive, desensitization is required.
● Earliest possible use of antitoxin is recommended for best results.
● Monitor vital signs every 30 minutes until patient's condition improves.
● Assess for evidence of neurotoxicity, respiratory depression, and change in comfort level.

Information for the patient
● Tell patient that this product is derived from horse serum and that he may experience allergic reactions, such as rash, joint swelling or pain, fever, or difficulty breathing. Explain that he will be monitored closely and will be given medications, as needed, to ease such effects.
● Encourage patient to report any unusual symptoms while hospitalized.
● Warn patient that delayed adverse effects may occur 5 to 13 days after the acute phase of botulism. Urge him to report any allergic reactions or other unusual symptoms.

Breast-feeding
Patient should discontinue breast-feeding temporarily until signs of botulism subside or if symptoms of serum sickness develop.

bretylium tosylate
Bretylate*, Bretylol

● Pharmacologic classification: adrenergic blocking agent
● Therapeutic classification: ventricular antiarrhythmic
● Pregnancy risk category C

How supplied
Available by prescription only
Injection: 50 mg/ml

Indications, route, and dosage
Ventricular fibrillation
Adults: 5 mg/kg undiluted by rapid I.V. injection. If necessary, increase dose to 10 mg/kg and repeat q 15 to 30 minutes until 30 mg/kg has been given.
Unstable ventricular tachycardia and other ventricular arrhythmias
Adults: Initially, 500 mg diluted to 50 ml with dextrose 5% in water or normal saline solution and infused I.V. over more than 8 minutes at 5 to 10 mg/kg. Dosage may be repeated in 1 to 2 hours. Thereafter, give q 6 to 8 hours. Infused in diluted solution of 500 ml dextrose 5% in water or normal saline solution at 1 to 2 mg/minute. For I.M. injection, administer 5 to 10 mg/kg undiluted. Repeat in 1 to 2 hours if needed. Thereafter, repeat q 6 to 8 hours.
†*Children:* 2 to 5 mg/kg I.M. as a single dose. Alternatively, give 5 mg/kg I.V. Follow with 10 mg/kg I.V. if fibrillation persists.

Pharmacodynamics
Ventricular antiarrhythmic action: Bretylium is a Class III antiarrhythmic used to treat ventricular fibrillation and tachycardia. Like other Class III antiarrhythmics, it widens the action potential duration (repolarization inhibition) and increases the effective refractory period (ERP); it does not affect conduction velocity. These actions follow a transient increase in conduction velocity and shortening of the action potential duration and ERP.
Initial effects stem from norepinephrine release from sympathetic ganglia and postganglionic adrenergic neurons immediately after drug administration. Norepinephrine release also accounts for an increased threshold for successful defibrillation, increased blood pressure, and increased heart rate. This initial phase of drug's action is brief (up to 1 hour).
Bretylium also alters the disparity in action potential duration between ischemic and nonischemic myocardial tissue; its antiarrhythmic action may result from this activity.
Hemodynamic drug effects include increased blood pressure, heart rate, and possible cardiac irritability (all resulting from initial norepinephrine release). The drug-induced adrenergic blockade ultimately predominates, leading to vasodilation and a subsequent blood pressure drop (primarily orthostatic). This effect has been referred to as chemical sympathectomy.

Pharmacokinetics
● *Absorption:* Bretylium is incompletely and erratically absorbed from the gastrointestinal tract; it is well absorbed after I.M. administration. With I.M. administra-

---

tion, the drug's antiarrhythmic (ventricular tachycardia and ectopy) action begins within about 20 to 60 minutes but may not reach maximal level for 6 to 9 hours when given by this route (for this reason, I.M. administration is not recommended for treating life-threatening ventricular fibrillation).

With I.V. administration, antifibrillatory action begins within a few minutes. However, suppression of ventricular tachycardia and other ventricular arrhythmias occurs more slowly – usually within 20 minutes to 2 hours; peak antiarrhythmic effects may not occur for 6 to 9 hours.

• *Distribution:* Bretylium is distributed widely throughout the body. It does not cross the blood-brain barrier. Only about 1% to 10% is plasma protein-bound.
• *Metabolism:* No metabolites have been identified.
• *Excretion:* Bretylium is excreted in the urine mostly as unchanged drug; half-life ranges from 5 to 10 hours (longer in patients with renal impairment). Duration of effect ranges from 6 to 24 hours and may increase with continued dosage increases. (Patients with ventricular fibrillation may require continuous infusion to maintain desired effect.)

Contraindications and precautions
Bretylium is contraindicated in patients with digitalis-induced arrhythmias, because the resulting release of norepinephrine may aggravate digitalis toxicity.

Bretylium should be used with extreme caution in patients with aortic stenosis and/or pulmonary hypertension, because these patients may be unable to compensate for the fall in blood pressure; and in patients with fixed cardiac output, aortic stenosis, and pulmonary hypertension, because the drug may cause sudden severe hypotension.

Interactions
Concomitant use of bretylium with other antiarrhythmic agents may cause additive toxic effects and additive or antagonistic cardiac effects. Concomitant use with digitalis may exacerbate ventricular tachycardia associated with digitalis toxicity. When used concomitantly with pressor amines (sympathomimetics), bretylium may potentiate the action of these drugs.

Effects on diagnostic tests
None reported.

Adverse reactions
• CNS: vertigo, dizziness, light-headedness, syncope (usually secondary to hypotension).
• CV: severe hypotension (especially orthostatic), bradycardia, anginal pain.
• GI: severe nausea, vomiting (with rapid infusion).

Overdose and treatment
Clinical effects of overdose primarily involve severe hypotension.

Treatment includes administration of vasopressors (such as dopamine or norepinephrine), to support blood pressure, and general supportive measures, as necessary. Volume expanders and positional changes also may be effective.

▶ **Special considerations**
• Administer I.V. infusion at appropriate rate to avoid or minimize adverse reactions.
• For I.M. injection, do not exceed 5-ml volume in any one site and rotate sites.

• Patient should remain supine and avoid sudden postural changes until tolerance to hypotension develops.
• Simultaneous initiation of therapy with digitalis and bretylium should be avoided.
• Monitor ECG and blood pressure throughout therapy for any significant change. If supine systolic pressure falls below 75 mm Hg, norepinephrine, dopamine, or volume expanders may be prescribed to raise blood pressure.
• Monitor patient closely if he is receiving pressor amines (sympathomimetics) to correct hypotension; bretylium potentiates these drugs' effects.
• Observe for increased anginal pain in susceptible patients.
• Because bretylium is excreted exclusively by the kidneys, patients with renal impairment require dosage modification. Dosage interval should be increased because the elimination half-life increases three to sixfold.
• Subtherapeutic doses (less than 5 mg/kg) may cause hypotension.
• Drug is not a first-line agent, according to American Heart Association advanced cardiac life-support guidelines. With ventricular fibrillation, drug should follow lidocaine; with ventricular tachycardia, drug should follow lidocaine and/or procainamide.
• Ventricular tachycardia and other ventricular dysrhythmias respond to drug less rapidly than ventricular fibrillation.
• Drug is ineffective against atrial arrhythmias.
• Drug has been used investigationally to treat hypertension. Usual dose is 100 to 400 mg P.O. t.i.d.

Breast-feeding
Safety has not been established.

bromocriptine
Parlodel

• Pharmacologic classification: dopamine receptor agonist
• Therapeutic classification: semisynthetic ergot alkaloid, dopaminergic agonist, antiparkinsonism agent, inhibitor of prolactin release, inhibitor of growth hormone release
• Pregnancy risk category C

How supplied
Available by prescription only
Tablets: 2.5 mg (as mesylate)
Capsules: 5 mg (as mesylate)

Indications, route, and dosage
Amenorrhea and galactorrhea associated with hyperprolactinemia; female infertility
Adults: Initially, 1.25 to 2.5 mg daily, increased by 2.5 mg daily at 3- to 7-day intervals as tolerated until optimal therapeutic effects are achieved. Maintenance dose is usually 5 to 7.5 mg daily (range 2.5 to 15 mg daily).
Prevention of postpartum lactation
Adults: 2.5 mg P.O. b.i.d., t.i.d., or q.i.d. with meals for 14 days. Treatment may be extended for up to 21 days, if necessary.

Acromegaly
Adults: Initially, 1.25 to 2.5 mg P.O. for 3 days. An additional 1.25 to 2.5 mg may be added q 3 to 7 days until patient receives therapeutic benefit. Maintenance dosage is 10 to 60 mg daily in divided doses.

Parkinson's disease
Adults: Initial dose of 1.25 mg P.O. b.i.d. with meals. Dosage may be increased every 14 to 28 days, up to 100 mg daily or until a maximal therapeutic response is achieved. Safety in dosages over 100 mg daily has not been established.

Pharmacodynamics
• *Prolactin inhibiting action:* Bromocriptine reduces prolactin concentrations by inhibiting release of prolactin from the anterior pituitary gland, a direct action on the pituitary. It may also stimulate postsynaptic dopamine receptors in the hypothalamus to release prolactin-inhibitory factor via a complicated catecholamine pathway. Bromocriptine reduces high serum prolactin concentrations and restores ovulation and ovarian function in amenorrheic women and suppresses puerperal or nonpuerperal lactation in women with adequate gonadotropin concentrations and ovarian function. The average time for reversing amenorrhea is 6 to 8 weeks, but it may take up to 24 weeks.

When therapy is started after a delivery and continued for 14 to 21 days, bromocriptine inhibits prolactin secretion to prevent physiologic lactation in women. Unlike estrogen preparations, bromocriptine has no direct action on the mammary tissues.

• *Antiparkinsonism action:* Bromocriptine activates dopaminergic receptors in the neostriatum of the CNS, which may produce its antiparkinsonism activity. Dysregulation of brain serotonin activity also may occur. The precise role of bromocriptine in treating parkinsonism syndrome requires further study of its safety and efficacy in long-term therapy.

Pharmacokinetics
• *Absorption:* Bromocriptine is 28% absorbed when given orally and reaches peak levels in about 1 to 3 hours. Plasma concentrations for therapeutic effects are unknown. After an oral dose, serum prolactin decreases within 2 hours, is decreased maximally at 8 hours, and remains decreased at 24 hours.
• *Distribution:* Bromocriptine is 90% to 96% bound to serum albumin.
• *Metabolism:* First-pass metabolism occurs with over 90% of the absorbed dose. Bromocriptine is metabolized completely in the liver, principally by hydrolysis, before excretion. The metabolites are not active or toxic.
• *Excretion:* The major route of bromocriptine excretion is through the bile. Only 2.5% to 5.5% of the dose is excreted in urine. Almost all (85%) of the dose is excreted in feces in 120 hours.

Contraindications and precautions
Bromocriptine is contraindicated in patients with a sensitivity to any ergot alkaloids and in those with severe ischemic heart disease or peripheral vascular disease because of the cardiovascular effects of the drug. Because bromocriptine prevents lactation, it should not be used by breast-feeding women.

Bromocriptine should be used cautiously in patients with Raynaud's disease, which may be exacerbated; in patients with hepatic and renal dysfunction or with a history of psychiatric disorders, because the drug may worsen these disorders; and in patients with a history

of myocardial infarction with residual arrhythmias, because drug may induce arrhythmias.

Interactions
Concomitant use of bromocriptine with drugs that increase prolactin concentrations (amitriptyline, butyrophenones, imipramine, methyldopa, phenothiazines, and reserpine) may require increased dosage of bromocriptine.

Bromocriptine may potentiate antihypertensive agents, requiring a reduction of their dosage to prevent hypotension.

Alcohol intolerance may result when high doses of bromocriptine are administered; therefore, concomitant ingestion of alcohol should be limited.

Effects on diagnostic tests
Transient elevation of BUN, ALT (SGPT), AST (SGOT), CPK, alkaline phosphatase, and uric acid levels may occur.

Adverse reactions
Incidence of adverse effects is high (68%); however, most are mild to moderate, and only 6% of patients discontinue the drug for this reason. Nausea is the most common adverse reaction, occurring in 51% of patients taking the drug. The potential for adverse effects may be decreased by reducing dosage to one half of a tablet 1 to 3 times daily initially, then gradually increasing it to the minimum effective dose.
• CNS: dizziness, headache, fatigue, mania, delusions, nervousness, insomnia, depression.
• CV: hypotension, postural hypotension, syncope.
• DERM: rash, mottling of the skin, urticaria.
• EENT: nasal congestion, tinnitus, blurred vision.
• GI: nausea, vomiting, abdominal cramps, constipation, diarrhea, metallic taste, dry mouth, dysphagia, anorexia.
• GU: urinary retention and frequency, incontinence, diuresis.
• Other: *pulmonary infiltrates* and *pleural effusions*, coolness and pallor of fingers and toes, facial pallor.

Overdose and treatment
Overdosage of bromocriptine may cause nausea, vomiting, and severe hypotension. Treatment includes emptying the stomach by aspiration and lavage, and administering I.V. fluids to treat hypotension.

▶ **Special considerations**
• Examine patients carefully for pituitary tumor (Forbes-Albright syndrome). Use of bromocriptine will not affect tumor size, although it may alleviate amenorrhea or galactorrhea.
• When administering drug to prevent physiologic lactation, start therapy only after patient's vital signs have stabilized and no sooner than 4 hours after delivery. Monitor blood pressure frequently.
• May lead to early postpartum conception. Test patient for pregnancy every 4 weeks or whenever period is missed after menses are reinitiated. If pregnancy is confirmed, discontinue bromocriptine.
• First-dose phenomenon occurs in 1% of patients. Sensitive patients may experience syncope for 15 to 60 minutes but can usually tolerate subsequent treatment without ill effects. Patient should begin therapy with lowest dosage, taken at bedtime.
• Administer with meals, milk, or snacks to diminish GI distress.

• Alcohol intolerance may occur, especially when high doses of bromocriptine are administered; therefore, alcohol intake should be limited.

• As an antiparkinsonism agent, bromocriptine is usually given with either levodopa alone or levodopa-carbidopa combination.

• Adverse reactions are more common when drug is given in high doses, as in treating parkinsonism.

Information for the patient

• Advise patient that it may take 6 to 8 weeks or longer for menses to be reinstated and for galactorrhea to be suppressed.

• Tell patient to take first dose where and when she can lie down, because drowsiness commonly occurs after initiation of therapy.

• Instruct patient to report any visual problems, severe nausea and vomiting, or acute headaches.

• Warn patient that the drug's CNS effects may impair ability to perform tasks that require alertness and coordination.

• Advise patient to use a nonhormonal contraceptive during treatment because of potential amenorrheic side effects.

• Advise patient to limit use of alcohol during treatment.

Geriatric use

• Use with caution, particularly in patients receiving long-term, high-dose therapy. Regular physical assessment is recommended, with particular attention toward changes in pulmonary function.

• Safety not established for long-term use at the doses required to treat Parkinson's disease.

Pediatric use

Drug is not recommended for children under age 15.

Breast-feeding

Because bromocriptine inhibits lactation, it should not be used in women who intend to breast-feed.

---

brompheniramine maleate
Bromamine, Brombay, Bromphen, Chlorphed, Dehist, Dimetane, Histaject Modified, Nasahist B, N-D Stat Revised, Oraminic II, Veltrane

• Pharmacologic classification: alkylamine antihistamine
• Therapeutic classification: antihistamine (H₁-receptor antagonist)
• Pregnancy risk category B

How supplied
Available with or without prescription
Tablets: 4 mg
Tablets (timed-release): 8 mg, 12 mg
Elixir: 2 mg/5 ml
Injection: 10 mg/ml, 100 mg/ml

Indications, route, and dosage
Rhinitis, allergy symptoms
Adults and children age 12 and older: 4 to 8 mg P.O. t.i.d. or q.i.d.; or (timed-release) 8 to 12 mg P.O. every 8 or 12 hours (maximum timed-release dosage is 24

mg daily); or 5 to 20 mg q 6 to 12 hours I.M., I.V., or S.C. Maximum dosage is 40 mg daily.
Children age 7 to 11: 2 to 4 mg t.i.d. or q.i.d.; or (timed-release) 8 to 12 mg q 12 hours; or 0.5 mg/kg daily I.M., I.V., or S.C. divided t.i.d. or q.i.d.
Children age 2 to 6: 0.5 mg/kg daily P.O., I.M., I.V., or S.C. divided t.i.d. or q.i.d., not to exceed 6 mg/day.

Pharmacodynamics
Antihistamine action: Antihistamines compete with histamine for histamine H₁-receptor sites on the smooth muscle of the bronchi, GI tract, uterus, and large blood vessels; by binding to cellular receptors, they prevent access of histamine and suppress histamine-induced allergic symptoms, even though they do not prevent its release.

Pharmacokinetics
• *Absorption:* Brompheniramine is absorbed readily from the GI tract; action begins within 15 to 30 minutes and peaks in 2 to 5 hours. A second lower peak effect apparently exists, possibly from drug reabsorption in the distal small intestine.
• *Distribution:* Brompheniramine is distributed widely into the body.
• *Metabolism:* Approximately 90% to 95% of brompheniramine is metabolized by the liver.
• *Excretion:* Half-life of brompheniramine ranges from about 12 to 34½ hours. Brompheniramine and its metabolites are excreted primarily in urine; a small amount is excreted in feces. About 5% to 10% of an oral dose of brompheniramine is excreted unchanged in urine.

Contraindications and precautions
Brompheniramine is contraindicated in patients with known hypersensitivity to this drug and in those taking antihistamines with similar chemical structures (chlorpheniramine, dexchlorpheniramine, and triprolidine); in patients experiencing asthmatic attacks, because brompheniramine thickens bronchial secretions; and in patients who have taken monoamine oxidase (MAO) inhibitors within the previous 2 weeks. (See Interactions.)

Brompheniramine should be used with caution in patients with narrow-angle glaucoma; in those with pyloroduodenal obstruction or urinary bladder obstruction from prostatic hypertrophy or narrowing of the bladder neck, because of their marked anticholinergic effects; in patients with cardiovascular disease, hypertension, or hyperthyroidism, because of the risk of palpitations and tachycardia; and in patients with renal disease, diabetes, bronchial asthma, urinary retention, prostatic hypertrophy, or stenosing peptic ulcers.

Brompheniramine should not be used during pregnancy (especially in the third trimester) or during breast-feeding. Antihistmines have caused convulsions and other severe reactions in premature infants and other neonates.

Interactions
MAO inhibitors interfere with the metabolism of brompheniramine and thus prolong and intensify their central depressant and anticholinergic effects; additive CNS depression may occur when brompheniramine is given concomitantly with other CNS depressants, such as alcohol, barbiturates, tranquilizers, sleeping aids, and antianxiety agents.

Brompheniramine may diminish the effects of sul-

---

fonylureas and partially may counteract the anticoagulant effects of heparin.

Effects on diagnostic tests
Brompheniramine should be discontinued 4 days before performing diagnostic skin tests; it can prevent, reduce, or mask positive skin test response.

Adverse reactions
● CNS: dizziness, tremors, irritability, insomnia, drowsiness, stimulation, impaired coordination.
● CV: hypotension, palpitations.
● DERM: urticaria, rash.
● EENT: blurred vision.
● GI: anorexia, nausea, vomiting, dry mouth and throat, constipation.
● GU: urinary retention.
● HEMA: thrombocytopenia, *agranulocytosis.*
● Respiratory: thickened bronchial secretions.
   Note: Drug should be discontinued if signs of acute hypersensitivity in the form of severe agranulocytosis occur: high fever, chills, and, possibly, gangrenous mouth and throat ulcers, pneumonia, and exhaustion.

Overdose and treatment
Clinical manifestations of overdose may include either those of CNS depression (sedation, reduced mental alertness, apnea, and cardiovascular collapse) or of CNS stimulation (insomnia, hallucinations, tremors, or convulsions). Anticholinergic symptoms, such as dry mouth, flushed skin, fixed and dilated pupils, and GI symptoms, are common, especially in children.
   Treat overdose by inducing emesis with ipecac syrup (in conscious patients), followed by activated charcoal to reduce further drug absorption. Use gastric lavage if patient is unconscious or ipecac fails. Treat hypotension with vasopressors, and control seizures with diazepam or phenytoin I.V. *Do not give stimulants.*

▶ Special considerations
Besides those relevant to all *antihistamines,* consider the following recommendations.
● Drug causes less drowsiness than some antihistamines.
● Store parenteral solutions and elixirs away from light and freezing temperatures; solution may crystallize if stored below 0° C. Crystals will dissolve when warmed to 30° C.

Information for the patient
Instruct patients who self-medicate not to exceed 24 mg/day (for adults and children age 12 and older) or 12 mg/day (for children age 6 to 11).

Geriatric use
Elderly patients are usually more sensitive to adverse effects of antihistamines and are especially likely to experience a greater degree of dizziness, sedation, hyperexcitability, dry mouth, and urinary retention than younger patients. Symptoms usually respond to a decrease in medication dosage.

Pediatric use
Brompheniramine is not indicated for use in newborns; children, especially those under age 6, may experience paradoxical hyperexcitability. Timed-release tablets are not recommended for children under age 11.

Breast-feeding
Antihistamines such as brompheniramine should not be used during breast-feeding. Many of these drugs are secreted in breast milk, exposing the infant to risks of unusual excitability, especially premature infants and other neonates, who may experience convulsions.

buclizine hydrochloride
Bucladin-S

● Pharmacologic classification: piperazine-derivative antihistamine
● Therapeutic classification: antiemetic and antivertigo agent
● Pregnancy risk category X

How supplied
Available by prescription only
Tablets: 50 mg

Indications, route, and dosage
Motion sickness (prophylaxis)
Adults: 50 mg P.O. at least ½ hour before beginning travel. If needed, may repeat another 50 mg P.O. after 4 to 6 hours.
Vertigo
Adults: 50 mg P.O.; up to 150 mg P.O. daily in severe cases. Maintenance dosage is 50 mg b.i.d.

Pharmacodynamics
● *Antiemetic action:* Buclizine probably inhibits nausea and vomiting by centrally depressing sensitivity of the labyrinth apparatus that relays stimuli to the chemoreceptor trigger zone and stimulates the vomiting center in the brain.
● *Antivertigo action:* Buclizine depresses conduction in vestibular-cerebellar pathways and reduces labyrinth excitability.

Pharmacokinetics
Duration of action is 4 to 6 hours; no other data available.

Contraindications and precautions
Buclizine is contraindicated in patients with known hypersensitivity to this drug or other antiemetic antihistamines with a similar chemical structure, such as cyclizine, meclizine, or dimenhydrinate; and in pregnancy, because it is teratogenic in animals. It should be used with caution in patients with narrow-angle glaucoma, asthma, prostatic hypertrophy, or GU or GI obstruction, because of its anticholinergic effects; drug may mask signs of intestinal obstruction or brain tumor. Bucladin-S Softabs contain tartrazine (FD&C yellow #5 dye), which may cause bronchial asthma or other allergic reactions in patients who are sensitive to tartrazine or aspirin.

Interactions
Additive sedative and CNS depressant effects may occur when buclizine is used concomitantly with other CNS depressants, such as alcohol, barbiturates, tranquilizers, sleeping agents, or antianxiety agents; drug should not be given to patients taking ototoxic medications, such as aminoglycosides, salicylates, vanco-

---

mycin, loop diuretics, and cisplatin, because buclizine may mask signs of ototoxicity.

Effects on diagnostic tests
None reported.

Adverse reactions
- CNS: drowsiness, dizziness, headache, nervousness.
- GI: dry mouth.

Overdose and treatment
Overdose and treatment for buclizine is not documented; however, symptoms may be anticipated to approximate those of other histamine H_1-receptor antagonists. Clinical manifestations of overdose may include either CNS depression (sedation, reduced mental alertness, apnea, and cardiovascular collapse) or CNS stimulation (insomnia, hallucinations, tremors, or convulsions). Anticholinergic symptoms, such as dry mouth, flushed skin, fixed and dilated pupils, and GI symptoms, are common, especially in children.

Treat overdose with gastric lavage to empty stomach contents; emesis with ipecac syrup may be ineffective. Treat hypotension with vasopressors, and control seizures with diazepam or phenytoin. *Do not give stimulants.*

▶ **Special considerations**
Besides those relevant to all *antihistamines*, consider the following recommendations.
- Tablets may be placed in mouth and allowed to dissolve without water, or they may be chewed or swallowed whole.
- Abrupt withdrawal of drug after long-term use may cause sudden reversal of improved state or paradoxical reactions.

Geriatric use
Elderly patients are usually more sensitive to adverse effects of antihistamines and are especially likely to experience a greater degree of dizziness, sedation, hyperexcitability, dry mouth, and urinary retention than younger patients.

Pediatric use
Safety and efficacy for use in children have not been established. Do not use in children under age 12; children, especially those under age 6, may experience paradoxical hyperexcitability.

Breast-feeding
Antihistamines such as buclizine should not be used during breast-feeding. Many of these drugs are secreted in breast milk, exposing the infant to risks of unusual excitability, especially premature infants, who may experience convulsions. Buclizine also may inhibit lactation.

bumetanide
Bumex

- Pharmacologic classification: loop diuretic
- Therapeutic classification: diuretic
- Pregnancy risk category C

How supplied
Available by prescription only
Tablets: 0.5 mg, 1 mg, 2 mg
Injection: 0.25 mg/ml

Indications, route, and dosage
Edema (congestive heart failure, hepatic and renal disease)
Adults: 0.5 to 2 mg P.O. once daily. If diuretic response is not adequate, give a second or third dose at 4- to 5-hour intervals. Maximum dosage is 10 mg/day. Give parenterally when oral route is not feasible. Usual initial dose is 0.5 to 1 mg I.V. or I.M. If response is not adequate, give a second or third dose at 2- to 3-hour intervals. Maximum dosage is 10 mg/day.

Pharmacodynamics
Diuretic action: Loop diuretics inhibit sodium and chloride reabsorption in the proximal part of the ascending loop of Henle, promoting the excretion of sodium, water, chloride, and potassium; bumetanide produces renal and peripheral vasodilation and may temporarily increase glomerular filtration rate and decrease peripheral vascular resistance.

Pharmacokinetics
- *Absorption:* After oral administration, 85% to 95% of a dose of bumetanide is absorbed; food delays oral absorption. I.M. bumetanide is completely absorbed. Diuresis usually begins 30 to 60 minutes after oral and 40 minutes after I.M. administration; peak diuresis occurs 1 to 2 hours after either. Diuresis begins a few minutes after I.V. administration and peaks in 15 to 30 minutes.
- *Distribution:* Bumetanide is approximately 92% to 96% protein-bound; it is unknown whether bumetanide enters CSF or breast milk or crosses the placenta.
- *Metabolism:* Bumetanide is metabolized by the liver to at least five metabolites.
- *Excretion:* Bumetanide is excreted in urine (80%) and feces (10% to 20%). Half-life ranges from 1 to 1½ hours; duration of effect is about 2 to 4 hours.

Contraindications and precautions
Bumetanide is contraindicated in patients with known hypersensitivity, anuria, hepatic coma, or electrolyte depletion, and in patients with increasing BUN and creatinine levels or oliguria, despite its use as a diuretic in patients with renal impairment.

Bumetanide should be used cautiously in patients allergic to sulfonamides, including furosemide, because cross-sensitivity may occur; in patients with hepatic cirrhosis and ascites because electrolyte alterations may precipitate hepatic encephalopathy; and in patients receiving cardiac glycosides (digoxin, digitoxin) because bumetanide-induced hypokalemia may predispose them to digitalis toxicity. Rapid I.V. administration increases hazard of ototoxicity.

Interactions

Bumetanide potentiates the hypotensive effect of most other antihypertensive agents and of other diuretics; both actions are used to therapeutic advantage.

Concomitant use of bumetanide with potassium-sparing diuretics (spironolactone, triamterene, amiloride) may decrease bumetanide-induced potassium loss; use with other potassium-depleting drugs such as steroids and amphotericin B may cause severe potassium loss.

Bumetanide may reduce renal clearance of lithium and increase lithium levels; lithium dosage may require adjustment.

Indomethacin and probenecid may reduce bumetanide's diuretic effect, and their combined use is not recommended; however, if there is no therapeutic alternative, an increased dose of bumetanide may be required.

Concomitant administration of bumetanide with ototoxic or nephrotoxic drugs may result in enhanced toxicity.

Bumetanide could prolong neuromuscular blockade by tubocurarine or gallamine, although this has not been reported.

Effects on diagnostic tests

Bumetanide therapy alters electrolyte balance and liver and renal function tests.

Adverse reactions

- CNS: dizziness, headache.
- CV: volume depletion and dehydration, orthostatic hypotension, ECG changes.
- DERM: rash.
- EENT: transient deafness.
- GI: nausea.
- HEMA: transient thrombocytopenia and leukopenia.
- Metabolic: hypochloremic alkalosis; asymptomatic hyperuricemia; fluid and electrolyte imbalances, including hyponatremia, hypokalemia, hypocalcemia, and hypomagnesemia; hyperglycemia and impairment of glucose tolerance.
- Other: muscle pain and tenderness.

Note: Drug should be discontinued if dehydration or hypotension occurs or if BUN and serum creatinine levels rise.

Overdose and treatment

Clinical manifestations of overdose include profound electrolyte and volume depletion, which may cause circulatory collapse.

Treatment of bumetanide overdose is primarily supportive; replace fluid and electrolytes as needed.

▶ Special considerations

Besides those relevant to all *loop diuretics,* consider the following recommendation.

- Give I.V. bumetanide slowly, over 1 or 2 minutes, for I.V. infusion; dilute bumetanide in dextrose 5% in water, normal saline solution, or lactated Ringer's solution; and use within 24 hours.

Geriatric use

Elderly and debilitated patients require close observation, as they are more susceptible to drug-induced diuresis. Excessive diuresis promotes rapid dehydration, hypovolemia, hypokalemia, and hyponatremia in these patients, and may cause circulatory collapse. Reduced dosages may be indicated.

Pediatric use

Safety and efficacy of bumetanide in children under age 18 have not been established. In children, the following dosage has been used: 0.015 to 0.1 mg/kg/day, given every other day. Use with extreme caution in neonates.

Breast-feeding

Bumetanide should not be used by breast-feeding women.

buprenorphine hydrochloride
Buprenex

- Pharmacologic classification: narcotic agonist-antagonist, opioid partial agonist
- Therapeutic classification: analgesic
- Controlled substance schedule V
- Pregnancy risk category C

How supplied

Available by prescription only
Injection: 0.3 mg/ml

Indications, route, and dosage
Moderate to severe pain

Adults: 0.3 mg I.M. or slow I.V. q 6 hours, p.r.n. or around the clock. May administer up to 0.6 mg per dose if necessary. S.C. administration is not recommended.

Pharmacodynamics

Analgesic action: The exact mechanisms of action of buprenorphine are unknown. It is believed to be a competitive antagonist at some, and an agonist at other opiate receptors, thus relieving moderate to severe pain.

Pharmacokinetics

- *Absorption:* Buprenorphine is absorbed rapidly after I.M. administration. Onset of action occurs in 15 minutes, with peak effect 1 hour after dosing.
- *Distribution:* Buprenorphine is about 96% protein-bound.
- *Metabolism:* Drug is metabolized in the liver.
- *Excretion:* Duration of action is 6 hours. Drug is excreted in urine and feces.

Contraindications and precautions

Buprenorphine is contraindicated in patients with known hypersensitivity to any semisynthetic opioid or thebaine derivative.

Administer buprenorphine with extreme caution to patients with supraventricular arrhythmias; avoid, or administer drug with extreme caution to patients with head injury or increased intracranial pressure, because drug obscures neurologic parameters; and during pregnancy and labor, because drug readily crosses the placenta (premature infants are especially sensitive to the drug's respiratory and CNS depressant effects).

Administer buprenorphine cautiously to patients with renal or hepatic dysfunction, because drug accumulation or prolonged duration of action may occur; to patients with pulmonary disease (asthma, chronic obstructive pulmonary disease), because drug depresses respiration and suppresses cough reflex; to patients undergoing biliary tract surgery, because drug may cause biliary spasm; to patients with convulsive dis-

---

orders, because drug may precipitate seizures; to elderly or debilitated patients, who are more sensitive to therapeutic and adverse drug effects; and to patients prone to physical or psychic addiction, because of the high risk of addiction to this drug.

Buprenorphine has lower potential for abuse than do opioid agonists.

Interactions
If administered within a few hours of barbiturate anesthetic such as thiopental, buprenorphine may produce additive CNS and respiratory depressant effects and, possibly, apnea.

Reduced doses of buprenorphine are usually necessary when drug is used concomitantly with other CNS depressants (narcotic analgesics, antihistamines; phenothiazines, barbiturates, benzodiazepines, sedative-hypnotics; alcohol), tricyclic antidepressants, and muscle relaxants, which may potentiate drug's respiratory and CNS depression, sedation, and hypotensive effects; use with general anesthesics may also cause severe cardiovascular depression.

Drug accumulation and enhanced effects may result from concomitant use with other drugs that are extensively metabolized in the liver (rifampin, phenytoin, and digitoxin).

Patients who become physically dependent on this drug may experience acute withdrawal syndrome if given an antagonist. Use with caution and monitor closely.

Use with caution if a patient is also to receive monoamine oxidase inhibitors.

There is one report of respiratory and cardiovascular collapse in a patient who received diazepam and buprenorphine in usual doses, given concomitantly ; there is one report of a suspected interaction between phenprocoumon and buprenorphine; a pruritic response was observed.

Effects on diagnostic tests
None reported.

Adverse reactions
● CNS: dizziness/vertigo, sedation (most common), euphoria, insomnia, agitation, confusion, headache, tremor, miosis, *seizures*, visual abnormalities, dysphoria.
● CV: tachycardia, bradycardia, hypertension, hypotension.
● DERM: flushing, rash, pruritus, sweating.
● GI: nausea and vomiting, anorexia, and constipation (colic).
● Other: hypoventilation, apnea, *respiratory depression*.

Note: Drug should be discontinued if hypersensitivity, seizures, or cardiac arrhythmias occur.

Overdose and treatment
To date there has been limited experience with overdosage. The safety of buprenorphine in acute overdosage is expected to be better than that of other opioid analgesics because of its antagonist properties at high doses. Overdose may cause CNS depression, respiratory depression, and miosis (pinpoint pupils). Other acute toxic effects might include hypotension, bradycardia, hypothermia, shock, apnea, cardiopulmonary arrest, circulatory collapse, pulmonary edema, and convulsion.

To treat acute overdose, first establish adequate respiratory exchange via a patent airway and ventilation as needed; administer a narcotic antagonist (naloxone) to reverse respiratory depression. (Because the duration of buprenorphine is longer than that of naloxone, repeated naloxone dosing is necessary. Naloxone should not be given unless the patient has clinically significant respiratory or cardiovascular depression. Monitor vital signs closely.

Naloxone does not completely reverse buprenorphine-induced respiratory depression; mechanical ventilation and higher than usual doses of naloxone and doxaprane may be indicated.

Provide symptomatic and supportive treatment (continued respiratory support, correction of fluid or electrolyte imbalance). Closely monitor laboratory parameters, vital signs, and neurologic status.

▶ Special considerations
Besides those relevant to all *narcotic agonist-antagonists*, consider the following recommendations.
● The adverse effects of buprenorphine may not be as readily reversed by naloxone as are those of pure agonists.
● Buprenorphine 0.3 mg is equal to 10 mg morphine or 75 mg meperidine in analgesic potency; duration of analgesia is longer than either.

Geriatric use
Administer with caution; lower doses are usually indicated for elderly patients, who may be more sensitive to the therapeutic and adverse effects of these drugs.

Breast-feeding
It is unknown whether the drug is excreted in breast milk; use with caution.

bupropion hydrochloride
Wellbutrin

● Pharmacologic classification: aminoketone
● Therapeutic classification: antidepressant
● Pregnancy risk category B

How supplied
Available by prescription only
Tablets: 75 mg, 100 mg

Indications, route, and dosage
Depression
Adults: Initially, 100 mg P.O. b.i.d. If necessary, increase after 3 days to usual dosage of 100 mg P.O. t.i.d. If there is no response after several weeks of therapy, consider increasing dosage to 150 mg t.i.d.

Pharmacodynamics
Antidepressant action: The mechanism of action is unknown. Bupropion does not inhibit monoamine oxidase (MAO); it is a weak inhibitor of norepinephrine, dopamine, and serotonin reuptake.

Pharmacokinetics
● *Absorption:* Animal studies indicate that only 5% to 20% of the drug is bioavailable. Peak plasma levels are achieved within 2 hours.

● *Distribution:* At plasma concentrations up to 200 mcg/ml, the drug appears to be about 80% bound to plasma proteins.

● *Metabolism:* Probably hepatic; several active metabolites have been identified. With prolonged use, the active metabolites are expected to accumulate in the plasma and their concentration may exceed that of the parent compound. Bupropion appears to induce its own metabolism.

● *Excretion:* Primarily renal; elimination half-life of the parent compound in single-dose studies ranged from 8 to 24 hours.

Contraindications and precautions

Bupropion is contraindicated in patients who are allergic to the drug, patients who have taken MAO inhibitors within the previous 14 days, and patients with a seizure disorder. About 0.4% of patients treated at dosages up to 450 mg/day may experience seizures. If dosage increases to 600 mg/day, the incidence of seizures increases about tenfold.

Bupropion is also contraindicated in patients with a history of bulimia or anorexia nervosa because studies have revealed a higher incidence of seizures in these patients. Studies have also shown that patients who experience seizures often have predisposing factors (including histories of head trauma, prior seizure, or CNS tumors), or they may be taking a drug that lowers the seizure threshold.

Interactions

Concomitant administration with levodopa, phenothiazines, MAO inhibitors, or tricyclic antidepressants or recent and rapid withdrawal of benzodiazepines may increase the risk of adverse effects, including seizures. Animal studies suggest that bupropion may induce drug-metabolizing enzymes.

Effects on diagnostic tests

None reported.

Adverse reactions

● CNS: headache, akathisia, agitation, anxiety, confusion, decreased libido, delusions, euphoria, hostility, impaired sleep quality, insomnia, sedation, sensory disturbance, tremor.

● CV: arrhythmias, hypertension, hypotension, palpitations, syncope, tachycardia.

● DERM: pruritus, rash, cutaneous temperature disturbance.

● GI: appetite increase, constipation, dyspepsia, nausea, vomiting, dry mouth.

● GU: impotence, menstrual complaints, urinary frequency.

● Other: arthritis, fever and chills, excessive sweating, auditory disturbance, dysgeusia, blurred vision.

Note: In a controlled study, the above adverse reactions were reported more frequently in patients taking bupropion than in control subjects and reflect events reported by at least 1% of the study population.

Overdose and treatment

Signs of overdose include labored breathing, salivation, arched back, ptosis, ataxia, and convulsions.

If the ingestion was recent, empty the stomach using gastric lavage or induce emesis with ipecac, as appropriate; follow with activated charcoal. Treatment should be supportive. Control seizures with I.V. benzodiazepines; stuporous, comatose, or convulsing patients may need intubation. There are no data to evaluate the benefits of dialysis, hemoperfusion, or diuresis.

▶ **Special considerations**

● Consider the inherent risk of suicide until significant improvement of depressive state occurs. High-risk patients should have close supervision during initial drug therapy. To reduce risk of suicidal overdose, prescribe the smallest quantity of tablets consistent with good management.

● Many patients experience a period of increased restlessness, especially at initiation of therapy. This may include agitation, insomnia, and anxiety. In clinical studies, these symptoms required sedative-hypnotic agents in some patients; about 2% had to discontinue the drug.

● Antidepressants can cause manic episodes during the depressed phase in patients with bipolar disorder.

● Clinical trials revealed that 28% of the patients experienced a weight loss of 5 lb (2.3 kg) or more. This effect should be considered if weight loss is a major factor in the patient's depressive illness.

Information for the patient

● Advise the patient to take the drug regularly as scheduled, and to take each day's dosage in three divided doses to minimize the risk of seizures.

● Warn patient to avoid the use of alcohol, which may contribute to the development of seizures.

● Advise the patient to avoid activities that require alertness and coordination until the CNS effects of the drug are known.

● Patient should not take any other medications, including OTC medications, without medical approval.

Geriatric use

No information available.

Pediatric use

Safety in children under age 18 has not been established.

Breast-feeding

Because of the potential for serious adverse reactions in the infant, breast-feeding during therapy is not recommended.

---

buspirone hydrochloride
BuSpar

● Pharmacologic classification: azaspirodecanedione derivative
● Therapeutic classification: antianxiety agent
● Pregnancy risk category B

How supplied

Available by prescription only
Tablets: 5 mg, 10 mg

Indications, route, and dosage
Management of anxiety disorders

Adults: Initially, 5 mg P.O. t.i.d. Dosage may be increased at 3-day intervals. Usual maintenance dosage is 20 to 30 mg daily in divided doses.

Pharmacodynamics

Anxiolytic action: Buspirone is an azaspirodecanedione derivative with anxiolytic activity. It suppresses conflict and aggressive behavior and inhibits conditioned avoidance responses. Its precise mechanism of action has not been determined, but it appears to depend upon simultaneous effects on several neurotransmitters and receptor sites: decreasing serotonin neuronal activity, increasing norepinephrine metabolism, and partial action as a presynaptic dopamine antagonist. Studies suggest an indirect effect on benzodiazepine GABA-chloride receptor complex or GABA receptors, or on other neurotransmitter systems.

Buspirone is not pharmacologically related to benzodiazepines, barbiturates, or other sedative and anxiolytic agents. It exhibits both a non-traditional clinical profile and is uniquely anxiolytic. It has no anticonvulsant or muscle relaxant activity and does not appear to cause physical dependence or significant sedation.

Pharmacokinetics

● *Absorption:* Buspirone is absorbed rapidly and completely after oral administration, but extensive first-pass metabolism limits absolute bioavailability to 1% to 13% of the oral dose. Food slows absorption but increases the amount of unchanged drug in systemic circulation.
● *Distribution:* The drug is 95% protein-bound; it does not displace other highly protein-bound medications such as warfarin. Onset of therapeutic effect may require 1 to 2 weeks.
● *Metabolism:* The drug is metabolized in the liver by hydroxylation and oxidation, resulting in at least one pharmacologically active metabolite – 1, pyrimidinylpiperazine (1-PP).
● *Excretion:* 29% to 63% is excreted in urine in 24 hours, primarily as metabolites; 18% to 38% is excreted in feces.

Contraindications and precautions

Buspirone is contraindicated in patients with known hypersensitivity to the drug.

The drug should be used cautiously in patients with a history of drug abuse or dependence (because of potential misuse or abuse) and in patients with impaired hepatic or renal function because impaired metabolism or excretion may result.

Interactions

When used concomitantly with monoamine oxidase inhibitors, buspirone may elevate blood pressure; avoid this combination.

Buspirone may displace digoxin from serum-binding sites when the drugs are used concomitantly.

Use cautiously with alcohol or other CNS depressants because sedation may result, especially with doses greater than 30 mg per day. Buspirone does not increase alcohol-induced impairment of mental and motor performance; however, CNS effects in individuals are not predictable.

Effects on diagnostic tests

None reported.

Adverse reactions

● CNS: dizziness, drowsiness, nervousness, headache, fatigue, weakness, insomnia, light-headedness, excitement, confusion, depression, decreased concentration, chewing movements, lip-smacking or pucker-

ing; puffing of checks or rapid, worm-like movements of tongue; *tardive dyskinesia* (with long-term use).
● CV: tachycardia, palpitations, nonspecific chest pain.
● EENT: blurred vision, tinnitus, sore throat, nasal congestion.
● GI: nausea, dry mouth, abdominal pain, gastric distress, diarrhea, constipation, vomiting.
● Other: hyperventilation, shortness of breath.

Overdose and treatment

Signs of overdose include severe dizziness, drowsiness, unusual constriction of pupils, and stomach upset, including nausea and vomiting.

Treatment of overdose is symptomatic and supportive; empty stomach with immediate gastric lavage. Monitor respiration, pulse, and blood pressure. No specific antidote is known. Effect of dialysis is unknown.

▶ Special considerations

● Although buspirone does not appear to cause tolerance or physical or psychological dependence, the possibility exists that patients prone to drug abuse may experience these effects.
● Buspirone will not block withdrawal syndrome associated with benzodiazepines or other common sedative and hypnotic agents; therefore, these agents should be withdrawn gradually before replacement with buspirone therapy.
● Monitor hepatic and renal function; hepatic and renal impairment will impede metabolism and excretion of the drug and may lead to toxic accumulation; dosage reduction may be necessary.

Information for the patient

● Advise patient to take drug exactly as prescribed; explain that therapeutic effect may not occur for 2 weeks or more. Warn patient not to double the dose if one is missed, but to take a missed dose as soon as possible, unless it is almost time for next dose.
● Caution patient to avoid hazardous tasks requiring alertness until effect of medication is known. The effects of alcohol and other CNS depressants (such as antihistamines, sedatives, tranquilizers, sleeping aids, prescription pain medication, barbiturates, seizure medicine, muscle relaxants, anesthetics, and medicines for colds, coughs, hay fever, or allergies) may be enhanced by additive sedation and drowsiness caused by buspirone.
● Tell patient to store drug away from heat and light and out of children's reach.
● Explain importance of regular follow-up visits to check progress. Urge patient to report adverse reactions immediately.

Breast-feeding

Reports of animal studies show that buspirone and its metabolites are excreted in the breast milk of rats; however, the extent of excretion in human milk is unknown. Buspirone should be avoided in breast-feeding women.

busulfan
Myleran

- Pharmacologic classification: alkylating agent (cell cycle-phase nonspecific)
- Therapeutic classification: antineoplastic
- Pregnancy risk category D

How supplied
Available by prescription only
Tablets (scored): 2 mg

Indications, route, and dosage
Dosage and indications may vary. Check current literature for recommended protocol.
Chronic myelogenous leukemia
Adults: 4 to 8 mg P.O. daily but may range from 1 to 12 mg P.O. daily (0.06 mg/kg or 1.8 mg/m²).
Children: 0.06 to 0.12 mg/kg or 1.8 to 4.6 mg/m² P.O. daily.

Pharmacodynamics
Antineoplastic action: Busulfan is an alkylating agent that exerts its cytotoxic activity by interfering with DNA replication and RNA transcription, causing a disruption of nucleic acid function.

Pharmacokinetics
- *Absorption:* Busulfan is well absorbed from the GI tract.
- *Distribution:* Distribution into the brain and CSF is unknown.
- *Metabolism:* Busulfan is metabolized in the liver.
- *Excretion:* Busulfan is cleared rapidly from the plasma. Busulfan and its metabolites are excreted in urine.

Contraindications and precautions
Busulfan is contraindicated in patients with a history of resistance to therapy with busulfan.

Busulfan should be used with caution in men and women of childbearing age because it can impair fertility, in those with a history of gout from hyperuricemic effects of the drug, and in patients whose immune system is compromised because of potential for additive toxicity. The drug can cause further myelosuppression, increasing the patient's risk of infection.

Interactions
None reported.

Effects on diagnostic tests
Drug-induced cellular dysplasia may interfere with interpretation of cytologic studies.

Busulfan therapy may increase blood and urine levels of uric acid as a result of increased purine catabolism that accompanies cell destruction.

Adverse reactions
- DERM: transient hyperpigmentation, anhidrosis.
- GI: nausea, vomiting, diarrhea, cheilosis, glossitis, stomatitis.
- GU: amenorrhea, testicular atrophy, renal calculi, uric acid nephropathy, impotence.
- HEMA: *bone marrow depression* (dose-limiting); WBC count falling after about 10 days and continuing to fall

for 2 weeks after stopping drug; *thrombocytopenia, leukopenia,* anemia.
- Hepatic: *cholestatic jaundice.*
- Metabolic: *Addison-like wasting syndrome, profound hyperuricemia from increased cell lysis.*
- Other: gynecomastia, alopecia, *irreversible pulmonary fibrosis (commonly termed "busulfan lung"),* cellular dysplasia.

Note: Consider discontinuing the drug if the leukocyte count decreases to approximately 15,000/mm³, or if patient's clinical symptoms and changes on chest X-ray support pulmonary fibrosis.

Overdose and treatment
Clinical manifestations of overdose include hematologic manifestations such as leukopenia and thrombocytopenia.

Treatment is supportive and includes transfusion of blood components and antibiotics for infections that may develop.

▶ Special considerations
- Avoid all I.M. injections when platelets are below 100,000/mm³.
- Patient response usually begins 1 to 2 weeks (increased appetite, sense of well-being, decreased total leukocyte count, reduction in size of spleen) after initiating the drug.
- Use cautiously in patients recently given other myelosuppressive drugs or radiation treatment and in those with depressed neutrophil or platelet count.
- Watch for signs of infection (fever, sore throat).
- Pulmonary fibrosis may be delayed for 4 to 6 months.
- Persistent cough and progressive dyspnea with alveolar exudate may result from drug toxicity, not pneumonia. Instruct patient to report symptoms so dose adjustments can be made.
- Monitor uric acid, CBC, and kidney function.

Information for the patient
- Advise the patient to use aspirin-containing products cautiously and to watch closely for signs of bleeding. Tell the patient to promptly report signs of bleeding.
- Tell patient to take medication at the same time each day.
- Emphasize the importance of continuing to take medication despite nausea and vomiting.
- Instruct the patient about the signs and symptoms of infection and tell him to report them promptly.

Breast-feeding
It is not known whether busulfan distributes into breast milk. However, the potential for mutagenicity, carcinogenicity, and serious adverse reactions in the infant should be taken into consideration when a decision to breast-feed is made.

butabarbital
Barbased, Butalan, Buticaps, Butisol,
Butatran, Day-Barb*, Neo-Barb*,
Sarisol No. 2

- Pharmacologic classification: barbiturate
- Therapeutic classification: sedative-hypnotic
- Controlled substance schedule III
- Pregnancy risk category D

How supplied
Available by prescription only
Tablets: 15 mg, 30 mg, 50 mg, 100 mg
Capsules: 15 mg, 30 mg
Elixir: 30 mg/5 ml, 33.3 mg/5 ml

Indications, route, and dosage
Sedation
Adults: 15 to 30 mg P.O. t.i.d. or q.i.d.
Children: 2 mg/kg P.O. divided t.i.d. or 60 mg/m² t.i.d.
Preoperative sedation
Adults: 50 to 100 mg P.O. 60 to 90 minutes before surgery.
Children: 2 to 6 mg/kg; up to a maximum of 100 mg/dose.
Insomnia
Adults: 50 to 100 mg P.O. h.s.
Children: Dosage must be individualized.

Pharmacodynamics
Sedative-hypnotic action: The exact cellular site and mechanism(s) of action are unknown. Butabarbital acts throughout the CNS as a nonselective depressant with an intermediate onset and duration of action. Particularly sensitive to the drug is the reticular activating system, which controls CNS arousal. Butabarbital decreases both presynaptic and postsynaptic membrane excitability by facilitating the action of gamma-aminobutyric acid (GABA).

Pharmacokinetics
- *Absorption:* Butabarbital is absorbed well after oral administration, with peak concentrations occurring in 3 to 4 hours. Onset of action occurs in 45 to 60 minutes. Serum concentrations needed for sedation and hypnosis are 2 to 3 mcg/ml and 25 mcg/ml, respectively.
- *Distribution:* Butabarbital is distributed well throughout body tissues and fluids.
- *Metabolism:* Butabarbital is metabolized extensively in the liver by oxidation. Its duration of action is 6 to 8 hours.
- *Excretion:* Inactive metabolites of butabarbital are excreted in urine. Only 1% to 2% of an oral dose is excreted in urine unchanged. The terminal half-life ranges from 30 to 40 hours.

Contraindications and precautions
Butabarbital is contraindicated in patients with known hypersensitivity to barbiturates and in patients with bronchopneumonia, status asthmaticus, or other severe respiratory distress because of the potential for respiratory depression. Butabarbital should not be used in patients who are depressed or have suicidal ideation, because the drug can worsen depression; in patients with uncontrolled acute or chronic pain, because ex-

acerbation of pain or paradoxical excitement can occur; or in patients with porphyria, because this drug can trigger symptoms of this disease. Some butabarbital preparations contain tartrazine, which may precipitate an allergic reaction. Do not administer butabarbital to patients with a tartrazine sensitivity.

Butabarbital should be used cautiously in patients who must perform hazardous tasks requiring mental alertness, because the drug causes drowsiness. Prolonged use of high doses should be avoided because tolerance and physical or psychological dependence may occur.

Prenatal exposure to barbiturates is associated with an increased incidence of fetal abnormalaities, including brain tumors. Use of barbiturates in the third trimester may be associated with physical dependence in neonates. Risk-benefit must be considered.

Use cautiously in patients with renal or hepatic dysfunction because of the risk of drug accumulation.

Interactions
Butabarbital may add to or potentiate the CNS and respiratory depressant effects of other sedative-hypnotics, antihistamines, narcotics, antidepressants, tranquilizers, and alcohol. Butabarbital enhances the enzymatic degradation of warfarin and other oral anticoagulants; patients may require increased doses of the anticoagulants. Drug also enhances hepatic metabolism of some drugs, including digitoxin (not digoxin), corticosteroids, oral contraceptives and other estrogens, theophylline and other xanthines, and doxycycline. Butabarbital impairs the effectiveness of griseofulvin by decreasing absorption from the GI tract.

Valproic acid, phenytoin, disulfiram, and monoamine oxidase inhibitors decrease the metabolism of butabarbital and can increase its toxicity. Rifampin may decrease butabarbital levels by increasing hepatic metabolism.

Effects on diagnostic tests
Butabarbital may cause a false-positive phentolamine test. The physiologic effects of the drug may impair the absorption of cyanocobalamin ⁵⁷Co; it may decrease serum bilirubin concentrations in neonates, epileptic patients, and patients with congenital nonhemolytic unconjugated hyperbilirubinemia. EEG patterns are altered, with a change in low-voltage, fast activity; changes persist for a time after discontinuation of therapy. Barbiturates may increase sulfobromophthalein retention.

Adverse reactions
- CNS: drowsiness, lethargy, vertigo, headache, CNS depression, paradoxical excitement, confusion and agitation (especially in elderly patients), rebound insomnia, increased dreams, nightmares, possibly *seizures* (after acute withdrawal or reduction in dosage)
- CV: hypotension, bradycardia, syncope, *circulatory collapse.*
- DERM: urticaria, rash, *exfoliative dermatitis, Stevens-Johnson syndrome.*
- EENT: miosis.
- GI: epigastric pain, nausea, vomiting, diarrhea, constipation.
- Other: laryngospasm, *bronchospasm,* blood dyscrasias. Vitamin K deficiency and bleeding have been reported in newborns of mothers treated during pregnancy. Hyperalgesia occurs with low doses or in patients with chronic pain.

---

*Canada only   †Unlabeled clinical use   Italicized adverse reactions are life-threatening.

Note: Drug should be discontinued if hypersensitivity reaction, profound CNS or respiratory depression, or skin eruption occurs.

Overdose and treatment
Clinical manifestations of overdose include unsteady gait, slurred speech, sustained nystagmus, somnolence, confusion, respiratory depression, pulmonary edema, areflexia, and coma. Jaundice, hypothermia followed by fever, oliguria, and typical shock syndrome with tachycardia and hypotension may occur.

To treat, maintain and support ventilation and pulmonary function, as necessary; support cardiac function and circulation with vasopressors and I.V. fluids, as needed. If patient is conscious with a functioning gag reflex and ingestion was recent, induce emesis by administering ipecac syrup. If emesis is contraindicated, perform gastric lavage while a cuffed endotracheal tube is in place, to prevent aspiration. Follow by administering activated charcoal or saline cathartic. Measure intake and output, vital signs, and laboratory parameters. Maintain body temperature. Alkalinization of urine may be helpful in removing drug from the body; hemodialysis may be useful in severe overdose.

▶ **Special considerations**
Besides those relevant to all *barbiturates,* consider the following recommendations.
● Tablet may be crushed and mixed with food or fluid if patient has difficulty swallowing. Capsule may be opened and contents mixed with food or fluids to aid in swallowing.
● Assess cardiopulmonary status frequently; monitor vital signs for significant changes.
● Monitor patients for possible allergic reaction resulting from tartrazine sensitivity.
● Periodically evaluate blood counts and renal and hepatic studies for abnormalities and adverse effects.
● Monitor prothrombin times carefully when patient on butabarbital starts or ends anticoagulant therapy. Anticoagulant dosage may need to be adjusted.
● Watch for signs of barbiturate toxicity (coma, pupillary constriction, cyanosis, clammy skin, hypotension). Overdose can be fatal.
● Prolonged administration is not recommended; drug has not been shown to be effective after 14 days. A drug-free interval of at least 1 week is advised between dosing periods.

Information for the patient
● Tell patient to avoid driving and other hazardous activities that require alertness because the drug may cause drowsiness.
● Warn patient that prolonged use can result in physical or psychological dependence.
● Emphasize the dangers of combining the drug with alcohol. Excessive depressant effect is possible, even if the drug is taken the evening before ingestion of alcohol.

Geriatric use
● Elderly patients are more susceptible to the CNS depressant effects of butabarbital. Confusion, disorientation, and excitability may occur.
● Elderly patients usually require lower doses.

Pediatric use
Butabarbital may cause paradoxical excitement in children. Dosage is dependent on age and weight of child and degree of sedation required. Use with caution.

Breast-feeding
Butabarbital passes into breast milk; avoid use in breast-feeding women.

butoconazole nitrate
Femstat

● Pharmacologic classification: synthetic imidazole derivative
● Therapeutic classification: topical fungistat
● Pregnancy risk category C

How supplied
Available by prescription only
Vaginal cream: 2% supplied with applicators

Indications, route, and dosage
Vulvovaginal candidiasis (moniliasis)
Adults (nonpregnant): One applicatorful intravaginally at bedtime for 3 days.
Adults (pregnant): One applicatorful intravaginally at bedtime for 6 days. Use only during 2nd or 3rd trimester.

Pharmacodynamics
Antifungal action: Although the exact mechanism is unknown, it is thought that butoconazole controls or destroys fungi by disrupting the cell membrane's permeability and reducing its osmotic pressure resistance. Butoconazole is active against many fungi, including dermatophytes and yeasts. It is also active in vitro against some gram-positive bacteria.

Pharmacokinetics
● *Absorption:* Approximately 5.5% of the medication inserted is absorbed through the vaginal walls.
● *Distribution:* Unknown.
● *Metabolism:* Systemically absorbed drug appears to be metabolized, probably in the liver.
● *Excretion:* Systemically absorbed drug appears to be excreted in the urine and feces.

Contraindications and precautions
Butoconazole is contraindicated in patients with known hypersensitivity to the drug. Butoconazole should be used with caution in the first trimester of pregnancy.

Interactions
None reported.

Effects on diagnostic tests
None reported.

Adverse reactions
● GU: vulvovaginal itching, burning, discharge, soreness, swelling.
● Other: itchy fingers, headache.

Overdose and treatment
No information available.

▶ **Special considerations**
● Ascertain that the patient understands directions for use and length of therapy.
● Butoconazole may be used concomitantly with oral contraceptives and antibiotic therapy.

Information for the patient
● Instruct patient to follow the directions enclosed in the package and to insert the applicator high into the vagina and to wash hands after use.
● Tell patient to complete the full course of therapy, including through menstrual period. However, tell patient to avoid using tampons during treatment.
● Advise patient to refrain from sexual contact or to have partner use a condom to avoid reinfection during therapy.
● Tell patient to use a sanitary napkin to prevent staining clothing and to absorb discharge.
● Tell patient to report symptoms that persist after full course of therapy.

Breast-feeding
Butoconazole should be used with caution in breast-feeding women since it is unknown whether it is distributed into breast milk.

butorphanol tartrate
Stadol, Stadol NS

● Pharmacologic classification: narcotic agonist-antagonist; opioid partial agonist
● Therapeutic classification: analgesic, adjunct to anesthesia
● Pregnancy risk category C

How supplied
Available by prescription only
Injection: 1 mg/ml, 1-ml vials; 2 mg/ml, 1-ml, 2-ml, and 10-ml vials
Nasal spray: 10 mg/ml

Indications, route, and dosage
Moderate to severe pain
Adults: 1 to 4 mg I.M. q 3 to 4 hours, p.r.n. or around the clock; or 0.5 to 2 mg I.V. q 3 to 4 hours, p.r.n. or around the clock. Alternatively, give 1 mg by nasal spray (1 spray in one nostril). Repeat if pain relief is inadequate after 60 to 90 minutes. Repeat q 3 to 4 hours.

Pharmacodynamics
Analgesic action: The exact mechanisms of action of butorphanol are unknown. Drug is believed to be a competitive antagonist at some, and an agonist at other, opiate receptors, thus relieving moderate to severe pain. Like narcotic agonists, it causes respiratory depression, sedation, and miosis.

Pharmacokinetics
● *Absorption:* Butorphanol is well absorbed after I.M. administration. Onset of analgesia after parenteral administration is less than 10 minutes, with peak analgesic effect at ½ to 1 hour. Onset of analgesia usually occurs within 15 minutes after nasal administration.
● *Distribution:* Butorphanol rapidly crosses the placenta, and neonatal serum concentrations are 0.4 to 1.4 times maternal concentrations.

● *Metabolism:* Butorphanol is metabolized extensively in the liver, primarily by hydroxylation, to inactive metabolites.
● *Excretion:* Duration of effect is 3 to 4 hours after parenteral administration; 4 to 5 hours after nasal administration. Butorphanol is excreted in inactive form, mainly by the kidneys. About 11% to 14% of a parenteral dose is excreted in feces.

Contraindications and precautions
Butorphanol is contraindicated in patients with known hypersensitivity to the drug.

Administer butorphanol with extreme caution to patients with supraventricular arrhythmias; avoid, or administer drug with extreme caution to patients with head injury or increased intracranial pressure, because neurologic parameters are obscured; and during pregnancy and labor, because drug readily crosses placenta (premature infants are especially sensitive to respiratory and CNS depressant effects). Administer butorphanol cautiously to patients with renal or hepatic dysfunction, because drug accumulation or prolonged duration of action may occur; to patients with pulmonary disease (asthma, chronic obstructive pulmonary disease), because drug depresses respiration and suppresses cough reflex; to patients undergoing biliary tract surgery, because drug may cause biliary spasm; to patients with convulsive disorders, because drug may precipitate seizures; to elderly or debilitated patients, who are more sensitive to both therapeutic and adverse drug effects; and to patients prone to physical or psychic addiction, because of the high risk of addiction to this drug.

Butorphanol has a lower potential for abuse than do narcotic agonists. Butorphanol increases the work of the heart, especially the pulmonary circuit; the use of this drug in patients with acute myocardial infarction or in cardiac patients should be limited to those hypersensitive to other agents that might be used; for example, meperidine (cross-hypersensitivity to the morphine-allergic patient must be considered with butorphanol).

Use butorphanol cautiously as a preoperative or preanesthetic drug in hypertensive patients, because it may cause increases in systolic blood pressure.

Interactions
If administered within a few hours of barbiturate anesthetics such as thiopental, butorphanol may produce additive CNS and respiratory depressant effects and, possibly, apnea. According to some reports cimetidine may potentiate butorphanol toxicity, causing disorientation, respiratory depression, apnea, and seizures. Because data are limited, this combination is not contraindicated; however, be prepared to administer a narcotic antagonist if toxicity occurs.

Reduced doses of butorphanol are usually necessary when drug is used concomitantly with other CNS depressants (narcotic analgesics, antihistamines, phenothiazines, barbiturates, benzodiazepines, sedative-hypnotics, alcohol, tricyclic antidepressants, and muscle relaxants), which may potentiate drug's respiratory and CNS depression, sedation, and hypotensive effects. Use with general anesthetics may also cause severe cardiovascular depression.

Drug accumulation and enhanced effects may result if drug is given concomitantly with other drugs that are extensively metabolized in the liver (rifampin, phenytoin, digitoxin).

Patients who become physically dependent on opioids may experience acute withdrawal syndrome if given a narcotic antagonist. Use with caution and monitor closely.

Concomitant use with pancuronium may increase conjunctival changes.

Effects on diagnostic tests
None reported.

Adverse reactions
● CNS: euphoria, sedation, somnolence, agitation, confusion, headache, lethargy, dizziness, vertigo, nervousness, blurred vision, diplopia, floating feeling, lightheadedness, unusual dreams, hallucinations.
● CV: palpitations, hypertension, hypotension.
● DERM: flushing, rash, clamminess, excessive sweating, sensitivity to cold.
● GI: dry mouth, nausea, vomiting.
● Other: *respiratory depression.*
  Note: Drug should be discontinued if hypersensitivity, seizures, or cardiac arrhythmias occur.

Overdose and treatment
No information available.

▶ **Special considerations**
Besides those relevant to all *narcotic agonist-antagonists,* consider the following recommendations.
● Patients who are using nasal formulation for severe pain may initiate therapy with 2 mg (one spray in each nostril) provided they remain recumbent. Don't repeat dosage for 3 to 4 hours.

Information for the patient
● Teach patient how to use nasal spray. Patient should use one spray in one nostril unless otherwise directed.

Geriatric use
Lower doses are usually indicated for elderly patients, because they may be more sensitive to the therapeutic and adverse effects of the drug. Plasma half-life is increased by 25% in patients over age 65.

Pediatric use
Safety and efficacy in children under age 18 has not been established.

Breast-feeding
Use of butorphanol in breast-feeding women is not recommended.

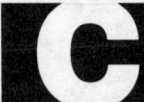

caffeine
NôDōz, Tirend, Vivarin

- Pharmacologic classification: methylxanthine
- Therapeutic classification: CNS stimulant, analeptic, respiratory stimulant
- Pregnancy risk category C

How supplied
Available without prescription
Tablets: 100 mg, 150 mg, 200 mg
Capsules (timed-release): 200 mg, 250 mg

Available by prescription only
Injection: caffeine (125 mg/ml) with sodium benzoate (125 mg/ml)

Indications, route, and dosage
CNS depression
Note: This use is strongly discouraged by many clinicians.
Adults: 100 to 200 mg P.O. q 4 hours, p.r.n.; timed-release, 200 or 250 mg q 4 to 6 hours. For emergencies – 500 mg I.M. or I.V.; maximum single dose 1 g.
Infants and children: 8 mg/kg I.M., I.V., or S.C. q 4 hours, p.r.n.
†Neonatal apnea
Neonates: 5 to 10 mg/kg (base) I.V., I.M., or P.O. as a loading dose (10 to 20 mg/kg caffeine citrate), followed by 2.5 to 5 mg/kg (base) I.V., I.M., or P.O. daily (5 to 10 mg/kg caffeine citrate). Adjust dosage according to patient tolerance and plasma caffeine levels.

Pharmacodynamics
- *CNS stimulant action:* Caffeine, like theophylline, is a xanthine derivative; it increases levels of cyclic $3':5'$-adenosine monophosphate by inhibiting phosphodiesterase. Caffeine stimulates all levels of the CNS; it hastens and clarifies thinking and improves arousal and psychomotor coordination.
- *Respiratory stimulant action:* In respiratory depression and in neonatal apnea (unlabeled use), larger doses of caffeine increase respiratory rate. Caffeine increases contractile force and decreases fatigue of skeletal muscle.

Pharmacokinetics
- *Absorption:* Caffeine is well absorbed from the GI tract; absorption after I.M. injection may be slower.
- *Distribution:* Caffeine is distributed rapidly throughout the body; it crosses the blood-brain barrier and placenta. Approximately 17% protein-bound, caffeine's plasma half-life is 3 to 4 hours in adults.
- *Metabolism:* Caffeine is metabolized by the liver; in neonates, liver metabolism is much less evident and half-life may approach 80 hours.
- *Excretion:* Excreted in urine.

Contraindications and precautions
Caffeine is contraindicated in patients with known hypersensitivity to caffeine; in patients with symptomatic cardiac arrhythmias or palpitations; and for 6 weeks after acute myocardial infarction because of its arrhythmogenic potential. It also is contraindicated in patients with a history of peptic ulcer disease; large amounts of caffeine may reactivate ulcers by stimulating gastric acid secretion. Use injectable form with caution in neonates: sodium benzoate content reportedly causes kernicterus.

Caffeine does not reverse alcohol intoxication or its depressant effects; excessive use of caffeine in patients with such conditions may deepen CNS depression. Withdrawal of caffeine may cause acute abstinence syndrome from physical tolerance.

Interactions
Concomitant use of caffeine with oral contraceptives, cimetidine, or disulfiram inhibits caffeine metabolism and increases its effects; use with other xanthine derivatives (theophylline) may increase incidence of stimulant-induced adverse reactions, such as tremor, tachycardia, insomnia, and nervousness. Concomitant use of beta agonists (terbutaline, albuterol, metaproterenol) increases incidence of cardiac effects and tremors.

Effects on diagnostic tests
Caffeine may increase blood glucose levels and cause false-positive urate levels; it also may cause false-positive test results for pheochromocytoma or neuroblastoma by increasing certain urinary catecholamines.

Adverse reactions
- CNS: stimulation, insomnia, restlessness, nervousness, mild delirium, headache, excitement, agitation, muscle tremors, twitches, tinnitus, light-headedness.
- CV: tachycardia, palpitations.
- DERM: hyperesthesia.
- GI: nausea, vomiting, diarrhea, abdominal pain.
- GU: diuresis.
  Note: Drug should be discontinued if signs of hypersensitivity, tachycardia, palpitations, or dizziness occur.

Overdose and treatment
Clinical manifestations of overdose in adults may include insomnia, dyspnea, altered states of consciousness, muscle twitching, seizure, diuresis, arrhythmias, and fever. In infants, symptoms may include alternating hypotonicity and hypertonicity, opisthotonoid posture, tremors, bradycardia, hypotension, and severe acidosis.

Treat overdose symptomatically and supportively; lavage and charcoal may help. Carefully monitor vital signs, ECG, and fluid and electrolyte balance. Seizures may be treated with diazepam or phenobarbital; diazepam can exacerbate respiratory depression.

▶ **Special considerations**
● Restrict caffeine-containing beverages in patients with arrhythmic symptoms or those who are taking aminophylline or theophylline.
● Caffeine content in beverages (mg/180 ml) is the following: cola drinks, 17 to 55; tea, 40 to 100; instant coffee, 60 to 180; brewed coffee, 100 to 150; decaffeinated coffee, 1 to 6.
● Many nonprescription pain relievers contain caffeine, but evidence concerning its analgesic effects conflicts. Caffeine (30%) may be used in a hydrophilic base or hydrocortisone cream to treat atopic dermatitis.
● Caffeine has been used to relieve headache after lumbar puncture and, in topical creams, to treat atopic dermatitis.

Information for the patient
● Advise patient to avoid excessive caffeine consumption and therefore CNS stimulation by learning caffeine content of beverages and foods.
● Warn patient not to exceed recommended dosage, not to substitute caffeine for needed sleep, and to discontinue drug if dizziness or tachycardia occurs.

Geriatric use
Elderly patients are more sensitive to caffeine and should take lower doses.

Pediatric use
● Unlabeled uses include neonatal apnea. For control of neonatal apnea, maintain plasma caffeine level at 5 to 20 mcg/ml.
● Adverse CNS effects are usually more severe in children.
● In neonates, avoid using caffeine products containing sodium benzoate because they may cause kernicterus.

Breast-feeding
Caffeine appears in breast milk. Alternative feeding method is recommended during therapy with caffeine.

---

calcifediol
Calderol

● Pharmacologic classification: vitamin D analog
● Therapeutic classification: antihypocalcemic
● Pregnancy risk category C

How supplied
Available by prescription only
Capsules: 20 mcg, 50 mcg

Indications, route, and dosage
Treatment and management of metabolic bone disease associated with chronic renal failure
Adults: Initially, 300 to 350 mcg P.O. weekly, given on a daily or alternate-day schedule. Dosage may be increased at 4-week intervals. Optimal dose must be carefully determined for each patient.

Pharmacodynamics
Antihypocalcemic action: Calcifediol is a vitamin D analog (25-hydroxycholecalciferol) that works with para-

thyroid hormone to regulate serum calcium; drug must be activated for its full effect, but it appears to have some intrinsic activity.

Pharmacokinetics
● *Absorption:* Drug is absorbed readily from the small intestine.
● *Distribution:* Drug is distributed widely and highly protein-bound.
● *Metabolism:* Drug is metabolized in the liver and kidney; half-life is 16 days. It is activated to 1,25 dihydroxycholecalciferol.
● *Excretion:* Drug is excreted in urine and bile.

Contraindications and precautions
Calcifediol is contraindicated in patients with hypercalcemia or sensitivity to vitamin D.

Interactions
Antacids may alter calcifediol absorption. Barbiturates, phenytoin, and primidone may increase metabolism and reduce activity of calcifediol. The increases in calcium produced by calcifediol may potentiate the effects of digitalis glycosides.

Effects on diagnostic tests
Calcifediol may falsely elevate cholesterol determinations made using the Zlatkis-Zak reaction. Alters concentrations of serum alkaline phosphatase concentrations and may alter electrolytes, such as magnesium, phosphate, and calcium, in the serum and urine.

Adverse reactions
● CNS: headache, irritability, somnolence.
● EENT: conjunctivitis, photophobia, rhinorrhea.
● GI: nausea, vomiting, constipation, anorexia, metallic taste.
● GU: polyuria.
● Other: bone pain, weakness, muscle pain, hyperthermia, hypertension, weight loss.
  Note: Drug should be discontinued if adverse reactions become severe.

Overdose and treatment
The only clinical manifestation of overdose is hypercalcemia. Treatment involves discontinuing therapy, instituting a low-calcium diet, and increasing fluid intake. Provide supportive measures. Severe overdose has led to death from cardiac and renal failure. Calcitonin administration may be useful in hypercalcemia.

▶ **Special considerations**
● Monitor serum calcium levels several times weekly when initiating therapy.
● There is some evidence that monitoring urine calcium and urine creatinine is very helpful in screening for hypercalciuria. The ratio of urine calcium to urine creatinine should be less than or equal to 0.18. A value > 0.2 suggests hypercalciuria, and the dose should be decreased regardless of serum calcium level.

Information for the patient
Explain the importance of a diet rich in calcium.

Pediatric use
Some infants may be hyperreactive to drug.

Breast-feeding
Very little of the drug appears in breast milk; however, the effect of vitamin D levels exceeding the RDA in infants is unknown. Drug should be used cautiously in breast-feeding women.

---

calcitonin
Calcimar (salmon), Cibacalcin (human), Miacalcin (salmon)

Pharmacologic classification: thyroid hormone
- Therapeutic classification: hypocalcemic
- Pregnancy risk category C

How supplied
Available by prescription only
Injection: Salmon – 200-IU/ml, 2-ml vials; 100-IU/ml, 1-ml ampules; Human – 0.5 mg/vial

Indications, route, and dosage
Paget's disease of bone (osteitis deformans)
Adults: Initially, 100 IU calcitonin (salmon) S.C. or I.M. daily or 0.5 mg calcitonin (human). Maintenance dose is 50 to 100 IU calcitonin (salmon) or 0.25 mg calcitonin (human) daily or every other day.
Hypercalcemia
Adults: 100 to 400 IU calcitonin (salmon) I.M. daily or b.i.d., or 4 IU/kg q 12 hours.
Postmenopausal osteoporosis
Adults: 100 IU calcitonin S.C. daily.

Pharmacodynamics
- Hypocalcemic action: Calcitonin directly inhibits the bone resorption of calcium. This effect is mediated by drug-induced increase of cyclic adenosine monophosphate concentration in bone cells, which alters transport of calcium and phosphate across the plasma membrane of the osteoclast. A secondary effect occurs in the kidneys, where calcitonin directly inhibits tubular resorption of calcium, phosphate, and sodium, thereby increasing their excretion. A clinical effect may not be seen for several months in patients with Paget's disease. Calcitonin salmon and calcitonin human are pharmacologically the same, but calcitonin salmon is more potent and has a longer duration of action.

Pharmacokinetics
- Absorption: Calcitonin must be administered parenterally. Plasma concentrations of 0.1 to 0.4 mg/ml are achieved within 15 minutes of a 200 IU S.C. dose. The maximum effect is seen in 2 to 4 hours; duration of action may be 8 to 24 hours for S.C. or I.M. doses, and ½ to 12 hours for I.V. doses.
- Distribution: Whether calcitonin enters the CNS or crosses the placenta is unknown.
- Metabolism: Rapid metabolism occurs in the kidney, with additional activity in the blood and peripheral tissues. Calcitonin salmon has a longer half-life than calcitonin human, which has a 1-hour half-life.
- Excretion: Calcitonin is excreted in urine as inactive metabolites.

Contraindications and precautions
Calcitonin is contraindicated in patients with hypersensitivity to the drug or its gelatin diluent. Interactions Calcitonin may be antagonized by calcium and vitamin D in treating hypercalcemia.

Effects on diagnostic tests
None reported.

Adverse reactions
- CNS: headaches.
- CV: flushing of face and extremities.
- GI: transient nausea with or without vomiting, diarrhea, anorexia.
- GU: transient diuresis.
- Metabolic: hyperglycemia, hypocalcemia.
- Local: pain and inflammation at injection site, rash.
- Other: hypersensitivity, urticaria, anaphylaxis, swelling, tingling and tenderness of hands, altered taste sensation.
  Note: Drug should be discontinued if allergic reaction occurs.

Overdose and treatment
Clinical manifestations of overdose include hypocalcemia and hypocalcemic tetany. This usually will occur in patients at higher risk during the first few doses. Parenteral calcium will correct the symptoms and therefore should be readily available.

▶ Special considerations
- The S.C. route is the preferred method of administration.
- If patient has allergic reactions to foreign proteins, test for hypersensitivity before therapy. Systemic allergic reactions are possible since hormone is a protein. Epinephrine should be kept readily available.
- Keep parenteral calcium available during the first doses in case of hypocalcemic tetany.
- Periodically monitor serum calcium levels during therapy.
- Observe patient for signs of hypocalcemic tetany during therapy (muscle twitching, tetanic spasms, and convulsions if hypocalcemia is severe).
- Watch for signs of hypercalcemic relapse: bone pain, renal calculi, polyuria, anorexia, nausea, vomiting, thirst, constipation, lethargy, bradycardia, muscle hypotonicity, pathologic fracture, psychosis, and coma. Patients with good initial clinical response to calcitonin who suffer relapse should be evaluated for antibody formation response to the hormone protein.
Refrigerate solution.

Information for the patient
- Instruct patient on self-administration of drug and assist patient until proper technique is achieved.
- Tell patient to handle missed doses as follows:
  –Daily dosing: take as soon as possible; do not double up on doses.
  –Every other day dosing: take as soon as possible, then restart the alternate days from this dose.
- Stress importance of regular follow-up to assess progress.
- If given for postmenopausal osteoporosis, remind patient to take adequate calcium and vitamin D supplements.

---

calcitriol
Rocaltrol

- Pharmacologic classification: vitamin D analog
- Therapeutic classification: antihypocalcemic
- Pregnancy risk category C

How supplied
Available by prescription only
Capsules: 0.25 mcg, 0.5 mcg

Indications, route, and dosage
Management of hypocalcemia in patients undergoing chronic dialysis
Adults: Initially, 0.25 mcg P.O. daily. Dosage may be increased by 0.25 mcg daily at 2- to 4-week intervals. Maintenance dose is 0.25 mcg every other day up to 0.5 to 1.25 mcg daily.
Management of hypoparathyroidism and pseudohypoparathyroidism
Adults and children over age 1: Initially, 0.25 mcg P.O. daily. Dosage may be increased at 2- to 4-week intervals. Maintenance dose is 0.25 to 2 mcg daily.

Pharmacodynamics
Antihypocalcemic action: Calcitriol is a vitamin D analog (1,25 dihydroxycholecalciferol), or activated cholecalciferol. It promotes absorption of calcium from the intestine by forming a calcium-binding protein. It reverses the signs of rickets and osteomalacia in patients who cannot activate or utilize ergocalciferol or cholecalciferol. In patients with renal failure it reduces bone pain, muscle weakness, and parathyroid serum levels.

Pharmacokinetics
- *Absorption:* Calcitriol is absorbed readily after oral administration.
- *Distribution:* Calcitriol is distributed widely and protein-bound.
- *Metabolism:* Calcitriol is metabolized in the liver and kidney, with a half-life of 3 to 8 hours. No activation step is required.
- *Excretion:* Calcitriol is excreted primarily in the feces.

Contraindications and precautions
Calcitriol is contraindicated in patients with hypercalcemia or sensitivity to vitamin D. Use cautiously in patients taking digitalis, because dyshypercalcemia may precipitate cardiac arrhythmias.

Interactions
Antacids may alter calcitriol absorption. Barbiturates, phenytoin, and primidone may increase metabolism of calcitriol and reduce activity. The increases in calcium may potentiate the effects of digitalis glycosides.

Effects on diagnostic tests
Calcitriol therapy may falsely elevate cholesterol determinations made using the Zlatkis-Zak reaction. It also alters serum alkaline phosphatase concentrations and may alter electrolytes, such as magnesium, phosphate, and calcium in serum and urine.

Adverse reactions
- CNS: headache, somnolence, irritability.
- EENT: conjunctivitis, photophobia, rhinorrhea.
- GI: nausea, vomiting, constipation, metallic aftertaste, dry mouth, anorexia.
- GU: polyuria.
- Other: weakness, bone and muscle pain, hyperthermia, hypertension, weight loss.
   Note: Drug should be discontinued if adverse reactions become severe.

Overdose and treatment
Clinical manifestation of overdose is hypercalcemia. Treatment requires discontinuation of drug, institution of a low-calcium diet, increased fluid intake, and supportive measures. Calcitonin administration may help reverse hypercalcemia. In severe cases, death has followed cardiovascular and renal failure.

▶ Special considerations
- Monitor serum calcium levels several times weekly after initiating therapy.
- Protect drug from heat and light.

Information for the patient
- Instruct patient on the importance of a diet rich in calcium.
- There is some evidence that monitoring urine calcium and urine creatinine is very helpful in screening for hypercalciuria. The ratio of urine calcium to urine creatinine should be less than or equal to 0.18. A value > 0.2 suggests hypercalciuria, and the dose should be decreased regardless of serum calcium level.
- Advise patient to report any adverse reactions immediately.
- Tell patient to avoid magnesium-containing antacids and other self-prescribed drugs.

Pediatric use
Some infants may be hyperreactive to drug.

Breast-feeding
Very little drug appears in breast milk; however, the effect of vitamin D levels exceeding the RDA in infants is not known. For this reason, large doses should not be administered to breast-feeding women.

calcium carbonate
Alka-2, Alka-Mints, Amitone, Calcilac, Calglycine, Chooz, Dicarbosil, Equilet, Mallamint, Os-Cal, P.H. Tablets, Titracid, Titralac, Tums, Tums E-X

- Pharmacologic classification: calcium salt
- Therapeutic classification: antacid
- Pregnancy risk category C

How supplied
Available without prescription
Calcium carbonate contains 40% calcium; 20 mEq calcium/g.
Tablets: 350 mg, 420 mg, 500 mg, 650 mg, 750 mg, 850 mg
Suspension: 1 g/5 ml

Indications, route, and dosage
Antacid to neutralize or reduce gastric acidity
Adults: One or two tablets, 4 to 6 times daily, chewed well and taken with water; or 1 g of suspension (5 ml of most products), 1 hour after meals and h.s.
Children: For use as an antacid, give 5 to 15 ml q 3 to 6 hours or 1 to 3 hours after meals and h.s.
To prevent GI bleeding in critical illness
Children: 5 to 15 ml q 1 to 2 hours.
Infants: 2 to 5 ml q 1 to 2 hours.
Calcium supplement
Adults: 1 to 1.5 g P.O. t.i.d., not to exceed 8 g/day.

Pharmacodynamics
Antacid action: Calcium carbonate neutralizes or reduces gastric acidity, increasing pH to 4 or above; increased pH inhibits the proteolytic activity of pepsin. Calcium carbonate may cause rebound hyperacidity and milk-alkali syndrome (hypercalcemia, metabolic alkalosis, and possibly renal impairment). Calcium carbonate is also used as a source of calcium cation to treat or prevent calcium depletion in patients with inadequate dietary intake of calcium.

Pharmacokinetics
● *Absorption:* Site of action is the GI tract. Calcium carbonate slowly dissolves in the stomach and reacts with hydrochloric acid to form calcium chloride, carbon dioxide, and water. About 90% of the calcium chloride formed is converted to insoluble calcium salts (calcium carbonate, calcium phosphate), and calcium soaps in the small intestine and is not absorbed. A limited amount of calcium and intestinal bicarbonate may be absorbed and hypercalcemia may occur.
● *Distribution:* Not well characterized.
● *Metabolism:* None significant.
● *Excretion:* Calcium is excreted by the kidneys; hypercalciuria commonly occurs in patients receiving calcium carbonate.

Contraindications and precautions
Use calcium carbonate with caution in patients with renal failure and hypercalcemia because calcium may accumulate. Patients with renal impairment or dehydration and electrolyte imbalance are predisposed to the milk-alkali syndrome. Exercise caution in patients with calcium loss secondary to decreased mobility (especially the elderly) and in patients with GI hemorrhage or obstruction.

Interactions
Calcium carbonate decreases the antibiotic effect of tetracycline. Give tetracycline 1 hour before or 2 hours after calcium carbonate.

Effects on diagnostic tests
Calcium carbonate may interfere with laboratory tests for calcium or phosphate.

Adverse reactions
● GI: constipation, gastric distention, belching, flatulence, acid-rebound, nausea, vomiting.
● Metabolic: hypercalcemia, hypophosphatemia; if taken with milk, milk-alkali syndrome, hypomagnesemia.

Overdose and treatment
Overdose produces adverse effects related to hypercalcemia. Treatment after ingestion of oral form includes removal by emesis or gastric lavage. Provide supportive therapy.

▶ Special considerations
● For use as an *antacid,* administer ½ hour to 1 hour after meals and at bedtime.
● Do not administer with milk or other foods high in vitamin D. Can cause milk-alkali syndrome (headache, confusion, distaste for food, nausea, vomiting, hypercalcemia, hypercalciuria, calcinosis, hypophosphatemia).
● May cause enteric-coated tablets to be released prematurely in stomach. Calcium carbonate and the enteric-coated tablet should be taken 1 hour apart.
● Monitor bowel function. Manage constipation with laxatives or stool softeners.
● Monitor serum and urine calcium levels, especially in mild renal impairment and with long-term use. Observe patient for symptoms of hypercalcemia (nausea, vomiting, headache, mental confusion, anorexia).

Information for the patient
● Instruct patient regarding medication and dosage schedule. Warn patient not to take calcium carbonate indiscriminately and not to switch from prescribed antacid.
● Tell patient to chew tablets completely for easier dissolution and passage to the GI tract.
● Tell patient that adverse effects become more likely if calcium carbonate is taken in large doses, over a long time, or in the presence of kidney disease.

Breast-feeding
Calcium has been shown to pass into the breast milk but not in quantities great enough to affect the breast-fed infant.

PHARMACOLOGIC CLASS

calcium channel blockers

bepridil hydrochloride
diltiazem
felodipine
isradipine
nicardipine hydrochloride
nifedipine
nimodipine
verapamil hydrochloride

Calcium channel blockers (also called slow calcium channel blockers) were introduced in the United States in the early 1980s. They have become increasingly popular as a treatment for classic and variant angina and are now the preferred drugs for Prinzmetal's variant angina (vasospastic angina). They also continue to gain acceptance as antihypertensives: nifedipine and diltiazem sustained release have both been approved for treatment of hypertension. Verapamil has proved effective in the acute treatment of supraventricular tachycardias.

Pharmacology
The main physiologic action of calcium channel blockers is to inhibit calcium influx across the slow channels of myocardial and vascular smooth muscle cells. Calcium is especially important to these cells as well as specialized cardiac conduction cells. By inhibiting cal-

COMPARING ORAL CALCIUM CHANNEL BLOCKERS

DRUG	ONSET OF ACTION	PEAK SERUM LEVEL	HALF-LIFE	THERAPEUTIC SERUM LEVEL
bepridil	1 hour	2 to 3 hours	24 hours	1 to 2 ng/ml
diltiazem	15 minutes	30 minutes	3 to 4 hours	50 to 200 ng/ml
felodipine	2 to 5 hours	2.5 to 5 hours	11 to 16 hours	unknown
nicardipine	20 minutes	1 hour	8.6 hours	28 to 50 ng/ml
nifedipine	5 to 30 minutes	30 minutes to 2 hours	2 to 5 hours	25 to 100 ng/ml
nimodipine	unknown	<1 hour	1 to 2 hours	unknown
verapamil	30 minutes	1 to 2.2 hours	6 to 12 hours	80 to 300 ng/ml

cium influx into these cells, calcium channel blockers reduce intracellular calcium concentrations. This, in turn, dilates coronary arteries, peripheral arteries, and arterioles, and slows cardiac conduction.

When used to treat Prinzmetal's variant angina, calcium channel blockers inhibit coronary spasm, increasing oxygen delivery to the heart. Peripheral artery dilation leads to a decrease in total peripheral resistance; this reduces afterload, which, in turn, decreases myocardial oxygen consumption. Inhibition of calcium influx into the specialized cardiac conduction cells (specifically, those in the sinoatrial and atrioventricular nodes) slows conduction through the heart. This effect is most pronounced with verapamil.

Structurally dissimilar, diltiazem, nifedipine, and verapamil are thought to work at different receptor sites on the calcium channel. Consequently, their pharmacologic effects vary markedly in degree.

Clinical indications and actions
Angina
Calcium channel blockers are useful in managing Prinzmetal's variant angina, chronic stable angina, and unstable angina. In Prinzmetal's variant angina, they inhibit spontaneous and ergonovine-induced coronary spasm, thereby increasing coronary blood flow and maintaining myocardial oxygen delivery. By dilating peripheral arteries, these drugs decrease total peripheral resistance, reducing afterload and, in turn, myocardial oxygen consumption. In unstable and chronic stable angina, their effectiveness presumably stems from their ability to reduce afterload.
Arrhythmias
Of the calcium channel blockers, verapamil has the greatest effect on the AV node, slowing the ventricular rate in atrial fibrillation or flutter. Parenteral diltiazem has been used investigationally to treat supraventricular tachyarrhythmias.
Hypertension
Because they dilate systemic arteries, most calcium channel blockers are useful in treating mild to moderate hypertension.
Other actions
Calcium channel blockers (especially verapamil) may also prove to be effective as a hypertrophic cardiomyopathy therapy adjunct by improving left ventricular outflow as a result of negative inotropic effects and possibly improved diastolic function. They have been used to treat peripheral vascular disorders, and as adjunctive therapy in the treatment of esophageal spasm.

Overview of adverse reactions
Adverse reactions vary in degree according to the specific drug used. Verapamil may cause adverse effects on the conduction system, including bradycardia, and various degrees of heart block, exacerbate heart failure, and cause hypotension after rapid I.V. administration. Prolonged oral verapamil therapy may cause constipation. Most adverse effects of nifedipine, such as hypotension (commonly accompanied by reflex tachycardia), peripheral edema, flushing, light-headedness, and headache, result from its potent vasodilatory properties.

Diltiazem most commonly causes anorexia and nausea. It may also induce various degrees of heart block, bradycardia, congestive heart failure, and peripheral edema.

▶ Special considerations
• Monitor cardiac rate and rhythm and blood pressure carefully when initiating therapy or increasing dose.
• Total serum calcium concentrations are not affected by calcium channel blocking agents.
• Concomitant use of calcium supplements may decrease the effectiveness of calcium channel blockers.

Information for the patient
• Tell patient not to abruptly discontinue the drug; gradual dosage reduction may be necessary.
• Instruct patient to report any of the following: irregular heartbeat, shortness of breath, swelling of hands and feet, pronounced dizziness, constipation, nausea, or hypotension.
• Advise patient that if he misses a dose, to take the dose as soon as possible, but not to take it if almost time for next dose. Warn patient not to double dose.

Pediatric use
Adverse hemodynamic effects of parenteral verapamil have been observed in neonates and infants. Safety and effectiveness of diltiazem and nifedipine have not been established.

Geriatric use
Use with caution, because the half-life of calcium channel blockers may be increased as a result of decreased clearance.

---

*Canada only   †Unlabeled clinical use   Italicized adverse reactions are life-threatening.

Breast-feeding
Calcium channel blocking agents (verapamil and diltiazem) may be excreted in breast milk. To avoid possible adverse effects in infants, breast-feeding should be discontinued during therapy with these drugs.

Representative combinations
None.

---

calcium polycarbophil
Equalactin, Fiberall, FiberCon, Mitrolan

- Pharmacologic classification: hydrophilic agent
- Therapeutic classification: bulk laxative, antidiarrheal
- Pregnancy risk category C

How supplied
Available without prescription
Tablets: 500 mg (FiberCon)
Tablets (chewable): 500 mg (Equalactin, Fiberall, Mitrolan)

Indications, route, and dosage
Constipation
Adults: 1 g P.O. q.i.d. as required. Maximum dosage is 6 g in 24-hour period.
Children age 6 to 12: 500 mg P.O. t.i.d. as required. Maximum dosage is 3 g in 24-hour period.
Children age 3 to 6: 500 mg P.O. b.i.d. as required. Maximum dosage is 1.5 g in 24-hour period.
Acute nonspecific diarrhea associated with irritable bowel syndrome
Adults: 1 g P.O. q.i.d. as required. Maximum dosage is 6 g in 24-hour period.
Children age 6 to 12: 500 mg P.O. t.i.d. as required. Maximum dosage is 3 g in 24-hour period.
Children age 3 to 6: 500 mg P.O. b.i.d. as required. Maximum dosage is 1.5 g in 24-hour period.

Pharmacodynamics
- *Laxative action:* Calcium polycarbophil absorbs water and expands, thereby increasing stool bulk and moisture and promoting normal peristalsis and bowel motility.
- *Antidiarrheal action:* Calcium polycarbophil absorbs intestinal fluid, thereby restoring normal stool consistency and bulk.

Pharmacokinetics
- *Absorption:* None.
- *Distribution:* None.
- *Metabolism:* None.
- *Excretion:* Calcium polycarbophil is excreted in feces.

Contraindications and precautions
Calcium polycarbophil is contraindicated in patients with GI obstruction because the drug may exacerbate this condition.

Interactions
When used concomitantly, calcium polycarbophil may impair tetracycline absorption.

Effects on diagnostic tests
None reported.

Adverse reactions
- GI: abdominal fullness, flatulence.
- Other: laxative dependence in long-term or excessive use.
    Note: Drug should be discontinued if abdominal pain occurs or if drug fails to relieve constipation after 1 week of therapy.

Overdose and treatment
No information available.

▶ **Special considerations**
- Patient must chew tablets (chewable) before swallowing; administer tablets with full glass (8 oz) of fluid. Administer less fluid for antidiarrheal effect.
- When using drug as an antidiarrheal, do not give if patient has high fever.

Information for the patient
- For chewable tablets: Instruct patient to chew tablets instead of swallowing them whole. If he is taking drug as a laxative, advise him to drink a full glass (8 oz) of fluid after each tablet; to take less water if he is using the drug to treat diarrhea.
- Warn patient not to take more than 12 tablets in 24-hour period (6 tablets for child age 6 to 12; 3 tablets for child age 3 to 6) and to take for length of time prescribed.
- If patient is taking drug as laxative, advise him to call promptly and discontinue drug if constipation persists after 1 week or if fever, nausea, vomiting, or abdominal pain occurs.
- For acute diarrhea, patient may repeat dose every 30 minutes but should not exceed maximum daily dosage.
- If patient notes abdominal discomfort or fullness, he may take smaller doses more frequently throughout the day, at regular intervals.

---

calcium salts

calcium carbonate
Alka-mints, Amitone, Bio-Cal, Calcilac, Calglycine, Caltrate, Cal-Sup, Chooz, Dicarbosil, Equilet, Gustalac, Os-Cal 500, PAMA No.1, Suplical, Titracid, Titralac, Tums, Tums E-X

calcium chloride

calcium citrate
Citracal

calcium glubionate
Neo-Calglucon

calcium gluceptate

calcium gluconate
Kalcinate

calcium glycerophosphate

calcium lactate

calcium phosphate, dibasic

calcium phosphate, tribasic
Posture

- Pharmacologic classification: calcium supplement
- Therapeutic classification: therapeutic agent for electrolyte balance, cardiotonic
- Pregnancy risk category C

How supplied
Available by prescription only
Calcium chloride
Injection: 10% solution (1 g/10 ml; each ml of solution provides 27.2 mg or 1.36 mEq of calcium) in 10-ml ampules, vials, and syringes
Calcium gluceptate
Injection: 1.1 g/5 ml in 5-ml ampules or 50-ml vials (each ml of solution provides 18 mg or 0.9 mEq of calcium)
Calcium gluconate
Injection: 10% solution (1 g/10 ml; each ml of solution provides 9.3 mg or 0.46 mEq of calcium) in 10-ml ampules and vials, or 20-ml vials

Available without prescription
Calcium carbonate
Tablets: 650 mg, 667 mg, 750 mg, 1.25 g, 1.5 g
Tablets (chewable): 350 mg, 420 mg, 500 mg, 625 mg, 750 mg, 850 mg, 1.25 g
Chewy squares: 1.5 g
Capsules: 1.512 g
Oral suspension: 1.25 g/5 ml (contains 400 mg of elemental calcium/g)
Calcium citrate
Tablets: 950 mg (contains 211 mg of elemental calcium/g)

Calcium glubionate
Syrup: 1.8 g/5 ml (contains 64 mg of elemental calcium/g)
Calcium gluconate
Tablets: 500 mg, 650 mg, 975 mg, 1 g (contains 90 mg of elemental calcium/g)
Calcium lactate
Tablets: 325 mg, 650 mg (contains 130 mg of elemental calcium/g)
Calcium phosphate, dibasic
Tablets: 468 mg (contains 230 mg of elemental calcium/g)
Calcium phosphate, tribasic
Tablets: 300 mg, 600 mg (contains 400 mg of elemental calcium/g)

Indications, route, and dosage
Emergency treatment of hypocalcemia
Calcium chloride
Adults: 500 mg to 1 g I.V. slowly (not to exceed 1 ml/minute).
Children: 25 mg/kg I.V. slowly.
Calcium gluceptate
Adults: 440 mg to 1.1g I.M. or I.V. slowly (not to exceed 2 ml/minute).
Children: 440 mg to 1.1 g I.M. (in lateral thigh if dose is more than 5 ml) or slow I.V. (not to exceed 2 ml/minute).
Calcium gluconate
Adults: 970 mg I.V. slowly (not to exceed 5 ml/minute).
Children: 200 to 500 mg I.V. slowly (not to exceed 5 ml/minute).
  Repeat above dosage based upon clinical laboratory value.
Cardiotonic use
Calcium chloride
Adults: 500 mg to 1 g I.V. slowly (not to exceed 1 ml/minute); or 200 to 400 mg calcium chloride intraventricularly as a single dose.
Hyperkalemia
Calcium gluconate
Adults: 1 to 2 g I.V. slowly (not to exceed 5 ml/minute). Calcium gluconate administration must be titrated based upon ECG response.
Hypermagnesemia
Calcium chloride
Adults: 500 mg I.V. initially, repeated based upon clinical response.
Calcium gluceptate
Adults: 1.2 to 2.4 g I.V. slowly, at a rate not to exceed 2 ml/minute.
Calcium gluconate
Adults: 1 to 2 g I.V. slowly, at a rate not to exceed 5 ml/minute.
During exchange transfusions
Adults and children: 0.5 ml I.V. after each 100-ml blood exchange.
Hypocalcemia
Calcium gluconate
Adults: 1 to 2 g P.O. b.i.d. or t.i.d.
Calcium lactate
Adults: 325 mg to 1.3 g P.O. t.i.d. with meals.
Children: 500 mg/kg in divided doses over 24 hours.
Osteoporosis prevention
Adults: 1 to 1.5 g P.O. daily of elemental calcium.

Pharmacodynamics
Calcium replacement: Calcium is essential for maintaining the functional integrity of the nervous, muscular,

---

and skeletal systems, and for cell-membrane and capillary permeability. Calcium salts are used as a source of calcium cation to treat or prevent calcium depletion in patients in whom dietary measures are inadequate. Conditions associated with hypocalcemia are chronic diarrhea, vitamin D deficiency, steatorrhea, sprue, pregnancy and lactation, menopause, pancreatitis, renal failure, alkalosis, hyperphosphatemia, and hypoparathyroidism.

Pharmacokinetics

● *Absorption:* The I.M. and I.V. calcium salts are absorbed directly into the bloodstream. I.V. injection gives an immediate blood level, which will decrease to previous levels in about 30 to 120 minutes. The oral dose is absorbed actively in the duodenum and proximal jejunum and, to a lesser extent, in the distal part of the small intestine. Calcium is absorbed only in the ionized form. Pregnancy and reduction of calcium intake may increase the efficiency of absorption. Vitamin D in its active form is required for calcium absorption.

● *Distribution:* Calcium enters the extracellular fluid and then is incorporated rapidly into skeletal tissue. Bone contains 99% of the total calcium; 1% is distributed equally between the intracellular and extracellular fluids. CSF concentrations are about 50% of serum calcium concentrations.

● *Metabolism:* None significant.

● *Excretion:* Calcium is excreted mainly in the feces as unabsorbed calcium that was secreted via bile and pancreatic juice into the lumen of the GI tract. Most calcium entering the kidney is reabsorbed in the loop of Henle and the proximal and distal convoluted tubules. Only small amounts of calcium are excreted in the urine.

Contraindications and precautions

Calcium chloride is contraindicated in ventricular fibrillation during cardiac resuscitation; in patients with hypercalcemia; in patients with a history of cardiac or renal insufficiency, respiratory acidosis and failure, metastatic bone disease, or hypercalcemia; and in patients with digitalis toxicity.

I.M. administration of calcium gluconate and calcium gluceptate may be tolerated, but the I.V. route is preferred in all cases except in emergencies when intravenous access cannot be established. Do not give S.C.

Interactions

Concomitant use of calcium salts with cardiac glycosides increases digitalis toxicity; administer calcium very cautiously, if at all, to digitalized patients.

Calcium may antagonize the therapeutic effects of calcium channel blocker drugs (verapamil).

Calcium should not be physically mixed with phosphates, carbonates, sulfates, or tartrates, especially at high concentrations. Calcium competes with magnesium and may compete for absorption, thus decreasing the amount of bioavailable magnesium. Concurrent administration of calcium decreases the therapeutic effect of tetracycline as a result of chelation.

Effects on diagnostic tests

I.V. calcium may produce transient elevation of plasma 11-hydroxycorticosteroid concentrations (Glen-Nelson technique) and false-negative values for serum and urine magnesium as measured by the Titan yellow method.

Adverse reactions

● CNS: hypercalcemia may cause dizziness and a change in mental status; somnolence, headache, confusion, psychosis; from I.V. use, tingling sensation, sense of oppression or "heat waves."

● CV: mild fall in blood pressure; with rapid I.V. injection, vasodilation, bradycardia, cardiac arrhythmias, *cardiac arrest.*

● GI: with oral ingestion, constipation, irritation, hemorrhage, gastric distention, nausea, vomiting; with I.V. administration, chalky taste, *GI hemorrhage,* nausea, vomiting, thirst, abdominal pain.

● GU: polyuria, renal calculi, nocturia, azotemia.

● Metabolic: hypercalcemia, hypophosphatemia.

● Local: with S.C. or I.M. injection, possible pain and irritation, burning, necrosis, sloughing of skin, cellulitis, soft-tissue calcification; with I.V. administration, venous irritation, muscle pain, cellulitis, soft-tissue necrosis and calcification, requiring skin grafting (especially after I.V. push).

Overdose and treatment

Acute hypercalcemia syndrome is characterized by a markedly elevated plasma calcium level, lethargy, weakness, nausea and vomiting, and coma, and may lead to sudden death.

In case of overdose, calcium should be discontinued immediately. After oral ingestion of calcium overdose, treatment includes removal by emesis or gastric lavage followed by supportive therapy, as needed.

▶ Special considerations

● Monitor ECG when giving calcium I.V. Such injections should not exceed 0.7 and 1.5 mEq/minute. Stop injection if patient complains of discomfort.

● Calcium chloride should be given I.V. only.

● I.V. route is recommended in children, but not by scalp vein because calcium salts can cause tissue necrosis.

● I.V. calcium should be administered slowly through a small-bore needle into a large vein to avoid extravasation and necrosis.

● After I.V. injection, patient should be recumbent for 15 minutes to prevent orthostasis.

● If perivascular infiltration occurs, discontinue I.V. immediately. Venospasm may be reduced by administering 1% procaine hydrochloride and hyaluronidase to the affected area.

● Use I.M. route only in emergencies when no I.V. route is available. Give I.M. injections in the gluteal region in adults, lateral thigh in infants.

● Monitor serum calcium levels frequently, especially in patients with renal impairment.

● Hypercalcemia may result when large doses are given to patients with chronic renal failure.

● Severe necrosis and sloughing of tissue may occur after extravasation. Calcium gluconate is less irritating to veins and tissue than calcium chloride.

● Assess Chvostek's and Trousseau's signs periodically to check for tetany.

● Crash carts usually contain both gluconate and chloride. Be sure to specify form to be administered.

● If GI upset occurs with oral calcium, give 2 to 3 hours after meals.

● Oxalic acid (found in rhubarb and spinach), phytic acid (in bran and whole-grain cereals), and phosphorus (in milk and dairy products) may interfere with absorption of calcium.

● With oral product, patient may need laxatives or stool softeners to manage constipation.

● Monitor for symptoms of hypercalcemia (nausea, vomiting, headache, mental confusion, anorexia), and report them immediately. Calcium absorption of an oral dose is decreased in patients with certain disease states such as achlorhydria, renal osteodystrophy, steatorrhea, or uremia.

Information for the patient
● Tell patient not to exceed the manufacturer's recommended dosage of calcium.
● Warn patient not to use bonemeal or dolomite as a source of calcium; they may contain lead.
● Advise patient to avoid tobacco and to limit intake of alcohol and caffeine-containing beverages.

Geriatric use
Calcium absorption (after oral administration) may be decreased in elderly patients.

Pediatric use
Calcium should be administered cautiously to children by the I.V. route (not I.M.).

Breast-feeding
Calcium has been shown to pass into the breast milk, but not in quantities large enough to affect the breast-feeding infant.

---

cantharidin
Cantharone, Verr-Canth

● Pharmacologic classification: cantharide derivative
● Therapeutic classification: keratolytic
● Pregnancy risk category C

How supplied
Available by prescription only
Liquid: 0.7%

Indications, route, and dosage
Removal of ordinary and periungual warts
Adults and children: Apply directly to lesion and cover completely. Allow to dry, then cover with nonporous adhesive tape. Remove tape in 24 hours (or less if it causes extreme pain) and replace with loose bandage. Reapply, if necessary.
Removal of moluscum contagiosum
Adults and children: Coat each lesion. Repeat in a week on new or remaining lesions, this time covering with occlusive tape. Remove tape in 4 to 6 hours.
Removal of plantar warts
Adults and children: Pare away keratin. Apply drug to wart and 1 to 3 mm around the wart. Allow to dry; then cover with nonporous tape. Debride 1 to 3 weeks after treatment. Repeat 3 times, if necessary, on large lesions.

Pharmacodynamics
Keratolytic action: Cantharidin causes exfoliation of benign epithelial growths as a consequence of acantholytic action. This action does not go beyond the epidermal cells; the basal layer remains intact.

Pharmacokinetics
● *Absorption:* Limited with use.
● *Distribution:* None.
● *Metabolism:* None.
● *Excretion:* None.

Contraindications and precautions
Cantharidin is contraindicated in patients with hypersensitivity to the drug. Avoid use near eyes or mucous membranes. Do not use on sensitive areas, such as the face or genitalia, or on moles, birthmarks, or hairgrowing warts. Drug should be used with caution in patients with diabetes or impaired peripheral circulation.

Interactions
None reported.

Effects on diagnostic tests
None reported.

Adverse reactions
● Local: irritation, burning, tingling, tenderness at site; may cause annular warts.
Note: Drug should be discontinued if sensitization develops.

Overdose and treatment
Cantharidin is a strong vesicant. If spilled on skin, wipe off at once with acetone, alcohol, or tape remover and wash with soap and water.

▶ Special considerations
● Apply directly to lesion and cover with nonporous tape. Avoid applying to normal skin tissue. Use only on affected area. Be sure to wash hands well after using drug.
● Use of mild antibacterial is recommended until tissue re-epithelializes.

Information for the patient
Advise patient that cantharidin may cause tingling, itching, or burning a few hours after application and may even cause blistering. The site of application may be extremely tender for a week after application.

Breast-feeding
Safety has not been established; therefore, use of drug in breast-feeding women is not recommended.

---

capreomycin sulfate
Capastat Sulfate

● Pharmacologic classification: polypeptide antibiotic
● Therapeutic classification: antitubercular agent
● Pregnancy risk category C

How supplied
Available by prescription only
Injection: 1 g/vial

Indications, route, and dosage
Adjunctive treatment in pulmonary tuberculosis
Adults: 15 mg/kg up to 1 g I.M. daily injected deeply into large muscle mass for 60 to 120 days; then 1 g two to three times weekly for a period of 18 to 24 months. Maximum dose should not exceed 20 mg/kg daily. Must be given concurrently with another antitubercular drug. Reduce dosage in decreased renal function.

Dosage in renal failure
Specific recommendations are unavailable.

Pharmacodynamics
Antibiotic action: Capreomycin is bacteriostatic; its mechanism of antibacterial action is unknown. Capreomycin is considered adjunctive therapy in tuberculosis and is combined with other antituberculosis agents to prevent or delay development of *Mycobacterium tuberculosis* resistance. The spectrum of activity for capreomycin include *M. tuberculosis, M. bovis, M. kansasii,* and *M. avium.*

Pharmacokinetics
• *Absorption:* Capreomycin is not absorbed after oral administration and is given by I.M. injection. Peak serum concentrations occur 1 to 2 hours and low serum concentrations occur 24 hours after I.M. injection.
• *Distribution:* Distribution is unknown.
• *Metabolism:* No metabolism reported.
• *Excretion:* Capreomycin is excreted primarily unchanged in urine by glomerular filtration. Elimination half-life in adults is 4 to 6 hours; half-life is prolonged and serum concentrations elevated in patients with renal impairment.

Contraindications and precautions
Capreomycin is contraindicated in patients with known hypersensitivity to this drug.

Use capreomycin with great caution in patients taking other ototoxic or nephrotoxic drugs; in patients with tinnitus, vertigo, and high-frequency hearing loss, who are susceptible to ototoxicity; and in patients with decreased renal function. Use drug with caution in patients with known allergies (particularly to drugs), and in patients with hepatic disease, myasthenia gravis, or parkinsonism because the drug may exacerbate the symptoms of these disorders.

Interactions
Concomitant use with the following drugs may increase the hazard of nephrotoxicity, ototoxicity, or neurotoxicity: colistin, polymyxin B, ethionamide, vancomycin, and aminoglycosides. Capreomycin may potentiate the hepatotoxicity of other antituberculars.

Capreomycin may potentiate neuromuscular blockade produced by general anesthetics or neuromuscular blocking agents such as succinylcholine and tubocurarine.

Effects on diagnostic tests
The drug's physiologic effects may decrease sulfobromophthalein (BSP) excretion. Capreomycin-induced nephrotoxicity may elevate BUN and serum creatinine levels, and increase urinary white blood cells, red blood cells, casts, and protein.

Adverse reactions
• CNS: headache, *neuromuscular blockade.*
• EENT: ototoxicity (tinnitus, vertigo, hearing loss).

• GU: *nephrotoxicity* (elevated BUN and nonprotein nitrogen, proteinuria, casts, red blood cells, leukocytes; tubular necrosis, decreased creatinine clearance).
• HEMA: eosinophilia, leukocytosis, leukopenia.
• Metabolic: hypokalemia, alkalosis.
• Local: pain, induration, excessive bleeding and sterile abscesses at injection site.
• Other: *hypersensitivity reactions,* possible hepatotoxicity.
Note: Drug should be discontinued if patient shows signs of hypersensitivity reaction; therapy should be reevaluated if signs of nephrotoxicity or ototoxicity occur.

Overdose and treatment
No information available.

▶ Special considerations
• Capreomycin should only be used in combination with other antitubercular drugs, and it should be reserved for patients refractory to or intolerant of other agents.
• Obtain results of the following laboratory tests before therapy and at intervals during therapy to assure efficacy and minimize toxicity. Therapy may begin before test results are complete. Other tests should be performed at suggested intervals: *audiometrics,* q 1 to 2 weeks; *vestibular function,* as indicated; *complete blood counts and SMA-12,* weekly; *renal function studies,* weekly; *liver function studies,* as indicated; *serum potassium,* q 30 days.
• Do not administer drug I.V.; intravenous use may cause neuromuscular blockade.
• Administer I.M. dose deep into large muscle mass (gluteal or midlateral thigh); rotate injection sites to minimize tissue injury; do not inject more than 2 g of drug per injection site.
• To minimize pain at injection site, reconstitute I.M. dose with 0.5% lidocaine hydrochloride without epinephrine or bacteriostatic water for injection with 0.9% benzyl alcohol; apply ice to injection site for pain.
• Solutions for injection should always be clear, colorless to pale yellow, and free of particles; do not give solutions containing precipitates or other foreign matter. After reconstitution, solutions may darken slightly over time without loss of potency.
• Solutions are stable for 24 hours at room temperature; concentrations up to 100 mg/ml are stable for 24 hours if refrigerated. Discard unused portions thereafter.

Information for the patient
• Explain disease process and rationale for long-term therapy.
• Teach signs and symptoms of hypersensitivity and other adverse reactions, and emphasize need to report *any* unusual effects.
• Be sure patient understands how and when to take drugs; urge patient to complete entire prescribed regimen, to comply with instructions for around-the-clock dosage, and to keep follow-up appointments.

Breast-feeding
Safe use has not been established. Alternative feeding method is recommended during therapy.

captopril
Capoten

- Pharmacologic classification: angiotensin-converting enzyme (ACE) inhibitor
- Therapeutic classification: antihypertensive, adjunctive treatment of congestive heart failure (CHF)
- Pregnancy risk category C

How supplied
Available by prescription only
Tablets: 12.5 mg, 25 mg, 37.5 mg, 50 mg, 100 mg

Indications, route, and dosage
Mild to severe hypertension
Adults: Initially, 25 mg P.O. b.i.d. or t.i.d.; if necessary, dosage may be increased to 50 mg t.i.d. after 1 to 2 weeks; if control is still inadequate after 1 to 2 weeks more, a diuretic may be added. Dosage may be raised to a maximum of 150 mg t.i.d. (450 mg/day) while continuing the diuretic. Daily dose may be given b.i.d.
CHF
Adults: Initially, 25 mg P.O. t.i.d.; may be increased to 50 mg t.i.d., with maximum of 450 mg/day. In patients taking diuretics, initial dosage is 6.25 to 12.5 mg t.i.d.

Pharmacodynamics
- *Antihypertensive action:* Captopril inhibits ACE, preventing pulmonary conversion of angiotensin I to angiotensin II, a potent vasoconstrictor. Reduced formation of angiotensin II decreases peripheral arterial resistance, which results in decreased aldosterone secretion, thus reducing sodium and water retention and lowering blood pressure.
- *Cardiac load-reducing action:* Captopril decreases systemic vascular resistance (afterload) and pulmonary capillary wedge pressure (preload), thus increasing cardiac output in patients with CHF.

Pharmacokinetics
- *Absorption:* Captopril is absorbed through the GI tract; food may reduce absorption by up to 40%. Antihypertensive effect begins in 15 minutes; peak blood levels occur at 1 hour. Maximum therapeutic effect may require several weeks.
- *Distribution:* Captopril is distributed into most body tissues except the CNS; drug is approximately 25% to 30% protein-bound.
- *Metabolism:* About 50% of captopril is metabolized in the liver.
- *Excretion:* Captopril and its metabolites are excreted primarily in urine; small amounts are excreted in feces. Duration of effect is usually 2 to 6 hours; this increases with higher doses. Elimination half-life is less than 3 hours. Duration of action may be increased in patients with renal dysfunction.

Contraindications and precautions
Captopril is contraindicated in patients with known hypersensitivity to captopril or other ACE inhibitors.

Captopril should be used cautiously in patients with impaired renal function or collagen vascular disease and in patients taking drugs known to depress leukocytes or immune response; such patients are at increased risk of developing neutropenia, especially if they have impaired renal function.

Interactions
Indomethacin, aspirin, and other nonsteroidal anti-inflammatory drugs may decrease captopril's antihypertensive effect; antacids also decrease captopril's effects and should be given at different dose intervals.

Captopril may increase antihypertensive effects of diuretics or other antihypertensive drugs.

Patients with impaired renal function or CHF and patients concomitantly receiving drugs that can increase serum potassium levels – for example, potassium-sparing diuretics, potassium supplements, or salt substitutes – may develop hyperkalemia during captopril therapy.

Captopril may increase serum digoxin concentrations by 15% to 30%. Clinical significance is unknown.

Effects on diagnostic tests
Captopril may cause false-positive results for urinary acetone; it also may cause hyperkalemia and may transiently elevate liver enzyme levels.

Adverse reactions
- CNS: dizziness, fainting.
- CV: tachycardia, hypotension, angina pectoris, *CHF, pericarditis.*
- DERM: urticarial or maculopapular rash, pruritus.
- EENT: loss of taste (dysgeusia).
- GI: anorexia.
- GU: proteinuria, nephrotic syndrome, membranous glomerulopathy, *renal failure,* urinary frequency.
- HEMA: leukopenia, *neutropenia, agranulocytosis,* pancytopenia.
- Metabolic: hyperkalemia.
- Other: fever, angioedema of face and extremities, cough.

Note: Drug should be discontinued if neutropenia or renal failure occurs.

Overdose and treatment
Overdose is manifested primarily by severe hypotension. After acute ingestion, empty stomach by induced emesis or gastric lavage. Follow with activated charcoal to reduce absorption. Subsequent treatment is usually symptomatic and supportive. In severe cases, hemodialysis may be considered.

▶ Special considerations
- Diuretic therapy is usually discontinued 2 to 3 days before beginning ACE inhibitor therapy, to reduce risk of hypotension; if drug does not adequately control blood pressure, diuretics may be reinstated.
- Perform white blood cell (WBC) and differential counts before treatment, every 2 weeks for 3 months, and periodically thereafter. Monitor serum potassium levels because potassium retention has been noted.
- Lower dosage or reduced dosing frequency is necessary in patients with impaired renal function. Titrate patient to effective levels over a 1- to 2-week interval, then reduce dosage to lowest effective level.
- Give drug 1 hour before meals; food reduces absorption.
- Several weeks of therapy may be required before the beneficial effects of captopril are seen.
- Proteinuria and nephrotic syndrome may occur in patients who are on captopril therapy.
- If patient is receiving antacids, give them at different

---

*Canada only   †Unlabeled clinical use   Italicized adverse reactions are life-threatening.

dose intervals (1 to 2 hours) because they may decrease captopril's effects.

Information for the patient
● Tell patient to report feelings of light-headedness, especially in first few days, so dosage can be adjusted; signs of infection, such as sore throat or fever, because drug may decrease WBC count; facial swelling or difficulty breathing, because drug may cause angioedema; and loss of taste, which may necessitate discontinuing drug.
● Advise patient to avoid sudden position changes, to minimize orthostatic hypotension.
● Warn patient to seek medical approval before taking nonprescription cold preparations.
● Advise patient to take drug 1 hour before meals.

Geriatric use
Elderly patients may need lower doses because of impaired drug clearance. They also may be more sensitive to captopril's hypotensive effects.

Pediatric use
Safety and efficacy of captopril in children have not been established; use only if potential benefit outweighs risk.

Breast-feeding
Captopril is distributed into breast milk, but its effect on breast-feeding infants is unknown; use drug with caution in breast-feeding women.

carbachol
Intraocular Solution, Isopto Carbachol, Miostat

● Pharmacologic classification: cholinergic agonist
● Therapeutic classification: miotic
● Pregnancy risk category C

How supplied
Available by prescription only
Intraocular injection: 0.01%
Ophthalmic solution: 0.75%, 1.5%, 2.25%, 3%

Indications, route, and dosage
Ocular surgery (to produce pupillary miosis)
Adults: Instill 0.5 ml (intraocular form) gently into the anterior chamber for production of satisfactory miosis. It may be instilled before or after securing sutures.
Open-angle or narrow-angle glaucoma
Adults: Instill 1 drop (topical form) into eye daily, b.i.d., t.i.d., or q.i.d.

Pharmacodynamics
Miotic action: Carbachol's cholinergic activity causes contraction of the sphincter muscles of the iris, producing miosis, and contraction of the ciliary muscle, resulting in accommodation. It also acts to deepen the anterior chamber and dilates conjunctival vessels of the outflow tract.

Pharmacokinetics
● *Absorption:* Action begins within 10 to 20 minutes and peaks in less than 4 hours.

● *Distribution:* Unknown.
● *Metabolism:* Unknown.
● *Excretion:* Duration of effect is usually about 8 hours.

Contraindications and precautions
Carbachol is contraindicated in patients with hypersensitivity to any components of the preparation or in patients in whom miosis is undesirable (acute iritis).

Although systemic effects are uncommon with usual doses, caution is advised in patients with acute cardiac failure, bronchial asthma, peptic ulcer, hyperthyroidism, GI spasm, urinary tract obstruction, and Parkinson's disease, because drug may worsen these conditions.

Interactions
When used concomitantly, cyclopentolate or the ophthalmic belladonna alkaloids (atropine, homatropine) may interfere with the antiglaucoma actions of carbachol.

Effects on diagnostic tests
None significant.

Adverse reactions
● CNS: headache, muscle tremors, syncope.
● CV: flushing, sweating, hypotension, bradycardia, *arrhythmias*.
● Eye: accommodative myopia, blurred vision, conjunctival irritation, ciliary congestion, fixed iris, paradoxical increased intraocular pressure, lens opacities, decreased visual acuity, ocular and periorbital pain, twitching eyelids.
● GI: abdominal cramps, diarrhea, salivation, epigastric distress.
● Respiratory: asthma, *bronchospasm*.
Note: Drug should be discontinued if signs of systemic absorption, including bradycardia, hypotension, flushing, breathing difficulties, and sweating, occur.

Overdose and treatment
Clinical manifestations of overdose include miosis, flushing, vomiting, bradycardia, bronchospasm, increased bronchial secretion, sweating, tearing, involuntary urination, hypotension, and seizures.

With accidental oral ingestion, vomiting is usually spontaneous; if not, induce emesis and follow with activated charcoal or a cathartic.

Treat dermal exposure by washing the area twice with water. Treat cardiovascular or blood pressure responses with epinephrine. Atropine has been suggested as a direct antagonist for toxicity.

▶ Special considerations
● Drug is especially useful in glaucoma patients resistant or allergic to pilocarpine hydrochloride or nitrate.
● Premixed drugs should be used for single-dose intraocular use only.
● Discard unused portions of injectable drug.

Information for the patient
● Tell patient with glaucoma that long-term use may be necessary. Stress compliance, and explain importance of medical supervision for tonometric readings before and during therapy.
● Instruct patient to apply finger pressure on the lacrimal sac 1 to 2 minutes after topical instillation of the drug.
● Reassure patient that blurred vision usually diminishes with continued use.

---

*Canada only   †Unlabeled clinical use   Italicized adverse reactions are life-threatening.

• Teach patient how to instill eye drops correctly and warn him not to touch eye or surrounding area with dropper.
• Warn patient not to drive for 1 or 2 hours after administration until effect on vision is determined.

carbamazepine
Epitol, Mazepine, Tegretol

• Pharmacologic classification: iminostilbene derivative; chemically related to tricyclic antidepressants
• Therapeutic classification: anticonvulsant, analgesic
• Pregnancy risk category C

How supplied
Available by prescription only
Tablets: 200 mg
Tablets (chewable): 100 mg
Oral suspension: 100 mg/5 ml

Indications, route, and dosage
Generalized tonic-clonic, complex-partial, mixed seizure patterns
Adults and children over age 12: 200 mg P.O. b.i.d. on day 1. May increase by 200 mg P.O. per day at weekly intervals, in divided doses at 6- to 8-hour intervals. Adjust to minimum effective level when control is achieved; do not exceed 1,000 mg/day in children age 12 to 15, or 1,200 mg/day in those over age 15. In rare instances, dosages up to 1,600 mg/day have been used in adults.
Oral loading dose for rapid seizure control is 8 mg/kg.
Children age 6 to 12: Initially, 100 mg P.O. b.i.d. increased at weekly intervals by adding 100 mg P.O. daily, using first a t.i.d. schedule, then q.i.d. if necessary. Adjust dosage based upon the response. Generally, dosage should not exceed 1,000 mg/day.
Oral loading dose for rapid seizure control is 10 mg/kg.
†*Bipolar affective disorder, intermittent explosive disorder*
Adults: Initially 200 mg P.O. b.i.d.,increased as needed every 3 to 4 days. Maintenance dosage may range from 600 to 1,600 mg/day.
†*Alcohol withdrawal*
Adults: Initially 200 mg P.O. q.i.d. Maintenance dosage is 800 to 1,000 mg/day.
†*Nonneuritic pain syndromes (such as phantom limb pain)*
Adults: Initially 100 mg P.O. b.i.d. Maintenance dosage is 600 to 1,400 mg/day usually combined with a tricyclic antidepressant.
†*Benzodiazepine withdrawal*
Adults: Initially 200 mg P.O. b.i.d. Maintenance dosage 400 to 800 mg daily.
† *Diabetes insipidus*
Adults: 200 mg P.O. b.i.d. or t.i.d.
Trigeminal neuralgia
Adults: 100 mg P.O. b.i.d. with meals on day 1. Increase by 100 mg q 12 hours until pain is relieved. Don't exceed 1.2 g daily. Maintenance dose is 200 to 400 mg P.O. b.i.d.

Pharmacodynamics
• *Anticonvulsant action:* Carbamazepine is chemically unrelated to other anticonvulsants and its mechanism of action is unknown. It appears to limit seizure propagation by reducing polysynaptic responses.
  Many clinicians consider carbamazepine the drug of choice for initial anticonvulsant therapy, especially in women and children; it is increasingly preferred to phenobarbital in children because it has less effect on alertness and behavior. In seizure disorders, carbamazepine can be used alone or with other anticonvulsants.
• *Analgesic action:* In trigeminal neuralgia, carbamazepine is a specific analgesic through its reduction of synaptic neurotransmission.

Pharmacokinetics
• *Absorption:* Carbamazepine is absorbed slowly from the GI tract; peak plasma concentrations occur at 2 to 8 hours.
• *Distribution:* Carbamazepine is distributed widely throughout the body; it crosses the placenta and accumulates in fetal tissue. The drug is approximately 75% protein-bound. Therapeutic serum levels are 3 to 14 mcg/ml; nystagmus can occur above 4 mcg/ml and ataxia, dizziness, and anorexia at or above 10 mcg/ml. Serum levels may be misleading because an unmeasured active metabolite also can cause toxicity.
• *Metabolism:* Carbamazepine is metabolized by the liver to an active metabolite. It may also induce its own metabolism; over time, higher doses are needed to maintain plasma levels.
• *Excretion:* Carbamazepine is excreted in urine (70%) and feces (30%); carbamazepine levels in breast milk approach 60% of serum levels.

Contraindications and precautions
Carbamazepine is contraindicated in patients with known hypersensitivity to carbamazepine and tricyclic antidepressants and in patients with past or present bone marrow depression; it also is contraindicated for use with monoamine oxidase (MAO) inhibitors or within 14 days of such use.
  Use carbamazepine with caution in patients with cardiovascular, renal, or hepatic damage; increased intraocular pressure; or atypical absence seizures. It also may activate latent psychosis, agitation, or confusion in elderly patients.

Interactions
Concomitant use of carbamazepine with MAO inhibitors may cause hypertensive crisis; use with calcium channel blockers (verapamil and possibly diltiazem) may increase serum levels of carbamazepine significantly (therefore, carbamazepine dosage should be decreased by 40% to 50% when given with verapamil); concomitant use with azithromycin, clarithromycin, erythromycin, cimetidine, isoniazid, or propoxyphene also may increase serum carbamazepine levels.
  Concomitant use with phenobarbital, phenytoin, or primidone lowers serum carbamazepine levels. When used with warfarin, phenytoin, haloperidol, ethosuximide, or valproic acid, carbamazepine may increase the metabolism of these drugs; it may decrease the effectiveness of theophylline and oral contraceptives.

Effects on diagnostic tests
Carbamazepine may elevate liver enzyme levels; it also may decrease values of thyroid function tests.

Adverse reactions

- CNS: dizziness, vertigo, drowsiness, fatigue, ataxia, worsening of seizures, hallucinations, speech disturbances.
- CV: congestive heart failure, hypertension, hypotension, aggravation of coronary artery disease, thrombophlebitis, *arrhythmias* (deaths have occurred).
- DERM: rash, urticaria, erythema multiforme, *Stevens-Johnson syndrome.*
- EENT: conjunctivitis, dry mouth and pharynx, blurred vision, diplopia, nystagmus.
- GI: nausea, vomiting, abdominal pain, diarrhea, anorexia, stomatitis, glossitis, dry mouth.
- GU: urinary frequency or retention, impotence, albuminuria, glycosuria, elevated blood urea nitrogen levels.
- HEMA: *aplastic anemia, agranulocytosis,* eosinophilia, leukocytosis, *thrombocytopenia.*
- Hepatic: abnormal liver function tests, hepatitis.
- Metabolic: water intoxication, hypocalcemia.
- Other: diaphoresis, fever, chills, pulmonary hypersensitivity, paralysis, abnormal movements, leg cramps, joint pain.

Note: Drug should be discontinued if signs of hypersensitivity, significant elevation of liver function tests, or hematologic abnormalities occur; or if any of the following signs of bone marrow depression appear: fever, sore throat, mouth ulcers, easy bruising, or petechial or purpuric hemorrhage.

Overdose and treatment

Symptoms of overdose may include irregular breathing, respiratory depression, tachycardia, blood pressure changes, shock, arrhythmias, impaired consciousness (ranging to deep coma), convulsions, restlessness, drowsiness, psychomotor disturbances, nausea, vomiting, anuria, or oliguria.

Treat overdose with repeated gastric lavage, especially if the patient ingested alcohol concurrently. Oral charcoal and laxatives may hasten excretion. Carefully monitor vital signs, ECG, and fluid and electrolyte balance. Diazepam may control seizures but can exacerbate respiratory depression.

▶ Special considerations

- Carbamazepine dosage should be adjusted according to individual response.
- Drug is structurally similar to tricyclic antidepressants; some risk of activating latent psychosis, confusion, or agitation in elderly patients exists.
- Hematologic toxicity is rare but serious. Routinely monitor hematologic and liver functions.
- Chewable tablets are available for children.
- Unlabeled uses of carbamazepine include neurogenic diabetes insipidus, certain psychiatric disorders, and management of alcohol withdrawal.
- For administering via a nasogastric tube, mix with an equal volume of diluent (dextrose 5% in water or 0.9% sodium chloride) and administer; then flush with 100 ml of diluent.

Information for the patient

- Reduced bioavailability has been reported with use of improperly stored carbamazepine tablets. Remind patient to store drug in a cool, dry place, not in the medicine cabinet.
- Tell patient that carbamazepine may cause GI distress. Patient should take drug with food at equally spaced intervals.

- Warn patient not to stop drug abruptly.
- Encourage patient to promptly report unusual bleeding, bruising, jaundice, dark urine, pale stools, abdominal pain, impotence, fever, chills, sore throat, mouth ulcers, edema, or disturbances in mood, alertness, or coordination.
- Emphasize importance of follow-up laboratory tests and continued medical supervision. Periodic eye examinations are recommended.
- Warn patient that drug may cause drowsiness, dizziness, and blurred vision. Patient should avoid hazardous activities that require alertness, especially during 1st week of therapy and when dosage is increased.
- Remind patients to shake suspension well before using.

Geriatric use

Carbamazepine may activate latent psychosis, confusion, or agitation in elderly patients and should be used with caution.

Pediatric use

Safety and efficacy have not been established for children under age 6.

Breast-feeding

Significant amounts of carbamazepine appear in breast milk; alternative feeding method is recommended during therapy.

carbamide peroxide

Auro Ear Drops, Cank-aid, Debrox Drops, Gly-Oxide Liquid, Murine Ear Drops, Orajel, Orajel Brace-aid Rinse, Proxigel

- Pharmacologic classification: urea hydrogen peroxide
- Therapeutic classification: ceruminolytic, topical antiseptic
- Pregnancy risk category C

How supplied

Available without prescription
Otic solution: 6.5% carbamide in glycerin or glycerin and propylene glycol
Oral solution: 10% carbamide in anhydrous glycerin
Oral gel: 11% carbamide in anhydrous glycerin

Indications, route, and dosage
Impacted cerumen

Adults and children: 5 to 10 drops otic solution into ear canal b.i.d. for 3 to 4 days.

Inflammation or irritation of lips, mouth, gums

Adults: Apply several drops oral solution on undiluted solution to affected area or place 10 drops on tongue (mix with saliva, swish for several minutes and expectorate 1 to 3 minutes) after meals and h.s.
Children: Apply undiluted gel to affected area (massage into area with finger or swab) q.i.d.

Pharmacodynamics

- *Ceruminolytic action:* Emulsifies and disperses accumulated cerumen.
- *Antiseptic action:* Releases oxygen upon contact with

---

oral mucosa, which results in a cleansing and mild anti-inflammatory action.

Pharmacokinetics
Unknown.

Contraindications and precautions
Carbamide peroxide is contraindicated in patients with ear drainage or discharge, ear pain, irritation or rash in the ear, dizziness, injured or perforated eardrum, or hypersensitivity to any component of the preparation.

Interactions
None reported.

Effects on diagnostic tests
None significant.

Adverse reactions
None reported.

Overdose and treatment
Clinical manifestations of overdose include mild irritation to mucosal tissue or, if swallowed, irritation, inflammation, and burns in the mouth, throat, esophagus, or stomach. Gastric distention may result from liberation of oxygen. Accidental ocular exposure causes immediate pain and irritation, but severe injury is rare. Irrigate eyes with large amounts of warm water for at least 15 minutes. Accidental dermal exposure bleaches the exposed area. Wash exposed skin twice with soap and water. Treat oral exposure by immediate dilution with water. Spontaneous vomiting may occur.

▶ **Special considerations**
● Do not use to treat swimmer's ear or itching of the ear canal. Also, do not use if patient has a perforated eardrum.
● Irrigation of ear may be necessary to aid removal of cerumen.
● Tip of dropper should not touch ear or ear canal when using otic preparation.
● Remove cerumen remaining after instillation by using a soft rubber-bulb otic syringe to gently irrigate the ear canal with warm water.

Information for the patient
● Teach patient correct way to use product.
● Tell patient to call if inflammation or irritation persists.
● Warn patient not to use otic preparation for more than 4 consecutive days and to avoid contact with eyes.
● Instruct patient to keep otic solution in ear for at least 15 minutes by tilting head sideways or putting cotton in ear.

Pediatric use
Use with caution in children under age 12.

carbenicillin disodium
Geopen, Pyopen

● Pharmacologic classification: extended-spectrum penicillin, alpha-carboxy-penicillin
● Therapeutic classification: antibiotic
● Pregnancy risk category B

How supplied
Available by prescription only
Injection: 1 g, 2 g, 5 g per vial
Pharmacy bulk package: 10 g, 20 g, 30 g per vial
I.V. infusion piggyback: 2 g, 5 g, 10 g

Indications, route, and dosage
Serious infections caused by susceptible organisms
Adults: 30 to 40 g daily I.V. infusion, divided into doses given q 4 to 6 hours.
Children: 400 to 600 mg/kg daily I.V. infusion, divided into doses given q 4 to 6 hours.
Urinary tract infections
Adults: 200 mg/kg daily I.M. or I.V. infusion, divided into doses given q 4 to 6 hours.
The maximum daily dosage of carbenicillin disodium in an adult is 40 g.
Dosage in renal failure (creatinine clearance < 10 ml/min)
Adults: 2 g I.V. q 8 to 12 hours. Alternatively, give the usual dose q 24 to 48 hours.
Adults undergoing hemodialysis: 2 g I.V. q 4 hours for serious infections. Alternatively, administer as above with supplemental 750 mg to 2 g I.V. after each treatment.
Adults undergoing peritoneal dialysis: 2 g I.V. q 6 to 12 hours.

Pharmacodynamics
Antibiotic action: Carbenicillin is bactericidal; it adheres to bacterial penicillin-binding proteins, thus inhibiting bacterial cell wall synthesis.
Extended-spectrum penicillins are more resistant to inactivation by certain beta-lactamases, especially those produced by gram-negative organisms, but are still liable to inactivation by certain others.
Carbenicillin's spectrum of activity includes many gram-negative aerobic and anaerobic bacilli, many gram-positive and gram-negative aerobic cocci, and some gram-positive aerobic and anaerobic bacilli.

Pharmacokinetics
● *Absorption:* No appreciable absorption occurs after oral administration. After an I.M. dose, peak plasma concentrations occur at 0.5 to 2.0 hours.
● *Distribution:* Carbenicillin disodium is distributed widely after parenteral administration; it penetrates minimally into uninflamed meninges and only slightly into bone and sputum. Carbenicillin disodium crosses the placenta and is 30% to 60% protein-bound.
● *Metabolism:* Carbenicillin disodium is metabolized partially.
● *Excretion:* Carbenicillin disodium and its metabolites are excreted primarily (79% to 99%) in urine by glomerular filtration and tubular secretion; some drug is excreted in breast milk. Elimination half-life in adults is

about 1 hour; in patients with extensive renal impairment, half-life is extended to 9½ to 23 hours. Carbenicillin disodium is removed by hemodialysis but not by peritoneal dialysis.

Contraindications and precautions

Carbenicillin disodium is contraindicated in patients with known hypersensitivity to any other penicillin or to cephalosporins.

Carbenicillin disodium should be used with caution in patients with renal impairment, because it is excreted in urine; decreased dosage is required in moderate to severe renal failure.

Interactions

Concomitant use of carbenicillin with aminoglycoside antibiotics results in synergistic bactericidal effects against *Pseudomonas aeruginosa, Escherichia coli, Klebsiella, Citrobacter, Enterobacter, Serratia,* and *Proteus mirabilis.* However, the drugs are physically and chemically incompatible and are inactivated if mixed or given together. Concomitant use of carbenicillin disodium (and other extended-spectrum penicillins) with clavulanic acid produces synergistic bactericidal effects against certain beta-lactamase-producing bacteria.

Probenecid blocks tubular secretion of carbenicillin, raising its serum concentrations.

Large doses of penicillins may interfere with renal tubular secretion of methotrexate, delaying elimination and elevating serum concentrations of methotrexate.

Effects on diagnostic tests

Carbenicillin disodium alters results of urine glucose tests that use cupric sulfate (Benedict's reagent or Clinitest). Make urine glucose determinations with glucose oxidase methods (Clinistix or Tes-Tape). Carbenicillin disodium causes increased serum uric acid values (cupric sulfate method) and false elevations of urine specific gravity in dehydrated patients with low urine output; positive Coombs' tests have been reported.

Carbenicillin may falsely decrease serum aminoglycoside concentrations.

Carbenicillin interferes with some human leukocyte antigen (HLA) tests and could cause inaccurate HLA typing. This drug's systemic effects may cause hypokalemia and hypernatremia and may prolong prothrombin times; it may also cause transient elevations in liver function study results and transient reductions in red blood cell, white blood cell, and platelet counts.

Adverse reactions

● CNS: neuromuscular irritability seizures.
● GI: nausea, vomiting.
● GU: *acute interstitial nephritis.*
● HEMA: *bleeding with high doses,* neutropenia, eosinophilia, leukopenia, thrombocytopenia, anemia.
● Local: pain at injection site, vein irritation, phlebitis.
● Metabolic: *hypokalemia.*
● Other: *hypersensitivity (edema, fever, chills, rash, pruritus, urticaria, anaphylaxis),* bacterial and fungal superinfection.

Note: Drug should be discontinued if immediate hypersensitivity reactions or bleeding complications occur; and if severe diarrhea occurs, because that may indicate pseudomembranous colitis.

Overdose and treatment

Clinical signs of overdose include neuromuscular hypersensitivity or seizures resulting from CNS irritation

by high drug concentrations. Carbenicillin disodium can be removed by hemodialysis; about 45% to 70% of a given dose is removed after 4 to 6 hours of hemodialysis.

▶ Special considerations

Besides those relevant to all *penicillins,* consider the following recommendations.
● Carbenicillin is almost always used with another antibiotic, such as an aminoglycoside, in life-threatening situations.
● Dosage reduction is not required unless the patient's creatinine clearance is below 10 ml/minute.
● Check complete blood count, differential, and platelet count frequently. Drug may cause thrombocytopenia. Observe carefully for signs of overt or occult bleeding.
● High blood concentrations of this drug may cause seizures.
● Because carbenicillin is dialyzable, patients undergoing hemodialysis may need dosage adjustments.
● Pharmacy bulk packages (10 g, 20 g, 30 g) are not intended for direct I.V. infusion.
● Use this drug cautiously in patients on sodium-restricted diets; sodium content is 4.7 to 5.3 mEq sodium per gram of carbenicillin.

Geriatric use

Half-life may be prolonged in elderly patients because of decreased renal function.

Pediatric use

Elimination half-life is prolonged in neonates.

Breast-feeding

Carbenicillin disodium is distributed into breast milk; it should be used with caution in breast-feeding women.

---

carbenicillin indanyl sodium
Geocillin

● Pharmacologic classification: extended-spectrum penicillin, alpha-carboxy-penicillin
● Therapeutic classification: antibiotic
● Pregnancy risk category B

How supplied

Available by prescription only
Tablets: 382 mg

Indications, route, and dosage
Urinary tract infection and prostatitis caused by susceptible organisms
Adults: 382 to 764 mg P.O. q.i.d.
Note: Use drug only in patients whose creatinine clearance equals or exceeds 10 ml/minute to ensure adequate bladder concentrations.

Pharmacodynamics

Antibiotic action: Carbenicillin indanyl sodium is bactericidal; it adheres to bacterial penicillin-binding proteins, thus inhibiting bacterial cell wall synthesis.

Extended-spectrum penicillins are more resistant to inactivation by certain beta-lactamases, especially those produced by gram-negative organisms, but are still liable to inactivation by certain others.

Carbenicillin indanyl sodium has an activity spectrum similar to that of carbenicillin disodium, including many gram-negative aerobic and anaerobic bacilli; some gram-positive aerobic and anaerobic bacilli; and many gram-positive and gram-negative aerobic cocci.

Pharmacokinetics

● *Absorption:* Carbenicillin indanyl sodium is stable in gastric acid, but absorbed incompletely (30% to 40%) from GI tract. Peak plasma concentrations occur at 30 minutes after oral dose; indanyl salt is completely hydrolyzed to carbenicillin in plasma within 90 minutes.

● *Distribution:* Carbenicillin indanyl sodium is distributed widely after oral administration, but concentrations are insufficient to treat systemic infections. Carbenicillin crosses the placenta and is 30% to 60% protein-bound.

● *Metabolism:* Carbenicillin indanyl sodium is hydrolyzed rapidly in plasma to carbenicillin; carbenicillin is metabolized partially.

● *Excretion:* Carbenicillin indanyl sodium and its metabolites are excreted primarily (79% to 99%) in urine by renal tubular secretion and glomerular filtration; some drug is excreted in breast milk. Elimination half-life in adults is about 1 hour. In patients with extensive renal impairment, half-life is extended to 9½ to 23 hours; urine concentrations in renal parenchyma and urine in patients with such impairment are insufficient for treating urinary tract infections.

Contraindications and precautions

Carbenicillin indanyl sodium is contraindicated in patients with known hypersensitivity to any other penicillin or to cephalosporins.

Use cautiously in patients with impaired renal function.

Interactions

Concomitant use with aminoglycoside antibiotics results in synergistic bactericidal effects against *Pseudomonas aeruginosa, Escherichia coli, Klebsiella, Citrobacter, Enterobacter, Serratia,* and *Proteus mirabilis.* However, the drugs are physically and chemically incompatible and are inactivated when mixed or given together. Concomitant use of carbenicillin indanyl sodium (and other extended-spectrum penicillins) with clavulanic acid produces synergistic bactericidal effects against certain beta-lactamase-producing bacteria.

Probenecid is used with some penicillins to achieve higher serum concentrations of drug, an undesired effect in urinary tract infection.

Large doses of penicillins may interfere with renal tubular secretion of methotrexate, delaying elimination and elevating serum concentration of methotrexate.

Effects on diagnostic tests

Carbenicillin indanyl sodium alters results of urine glucose tests that use cupric sulfate (Benedict's reagent or Clinitest). Make urine glucose determinations with glucose oxidase methods (Clinistix or Tes-Tape). It causes increased serum uric acid values (cupric sulfate method) and false elevations of urine specific gravity in dehydrated patients with low urine output.

Positive Coombs' tests have been reported after carbenicillin therapy; drug also interferes with some HLA antigen tests and could cause inaccurate HLA typing. Systemic effect of carbenicillin may alter results of electrolyte studies (hypokalemia and hypernatremia) and prolong prothrombin times; it may cause transient elevations in liver function study results and transient

reductions in red blood cell, white blood cell, and platelet counts.

Carbenicillin may also falsely decrease serum aminoglycoside concentrations.

Adverse reactions

● GI: nausea, vomiting, diarrhea, flatulence, abdominal cramps, unpleasant taste.
● GU: acute interstitial nephritis.
● HEMA: leukopenia, neutropenia, eosinophilia, anemia, thrombocytopenia, anemia.
● Other: hypersensitivity (rash, chills, fever, urticaria, pruritus, *anaphylaxis*), bacterial and fungal superinfection.

Note: Drug should be discontinued if immediate hypersensitivity reactions or bleeding complications occur; and if severe diarrhea occurs, because that may indicate pseudomembranous colitis.

Overdose and treatment

Clinical signs of overdose include neuromuscular hypersensitivity or seizures resulting from CNS irritation by high drug concentrations. No specific treatment is recommended. Treatment is supportive. After recent ingestion (within 4 hours), empty the stomach by induced emesis or gastric lavage. Follow with activated charcoal to reduce absorption. Carbenicillin indanyl sodium can be removed by hemodialysis.

▶ **Special considerations**

Besides those relevant to all *penicillins,* consider the following recommendations.
● Administer drug 1 to 2 hours before and 2 to 3 hours after meals with full glass of water to obtain maximum drug levels.
● Because carbenicillin is dialyzable, patients undergoing hemodialysis may need dosage adjustments.

Geriatric use
Half-life may be prolonged in elderly patients because of decreased renal function.

Pediatric use
Safe use in children has not been established. High incidence of nausea, vomiting, and diarrhea has been associated with its use in children.

Breast-feeding
Carbenicillin is distributed into breast milk; drug should be used with caution in breast-feeding women.

PHARMACOLOGIC CLASS

carbonic anhydrase inhibitors

acetazolamide
dichlorphenamide
methazolamide

The carbonic anhydrase inhibitors were developed in the 1940s during research aimed at synthesizing sulfonamide compounds with the carbonic anhydrase inhibitory properties of sulfanilamide. Most studies have been conducted with acetazolamide, prototype for this class of drugs. Carbonic anhydrase inhibitors have been largely replaced by thiazides and are seldom used as diuretics because their propensity for causing metabolic acidosis makes patients refractory to their diuretic effects, requiring intermittent therapy to restore effective diuresis.

Pharmacology

As their name implies, carbonic anhydrase inhibitors act by noncompetitive reversible inhibition of the enzyme carbonic anhydrase, which is responsible for formation of hydrogen and bicarbonate ions from carbon dioxide and water. This inhibition results in decreased hydrogen levels in the renal tubules, promoting excretion of bicarbonate, sodium, potassium, and water; because carbon dioxide is not eliminated as rapidly, systemic acidosis may occur.

Clinical indications and actions
Open-angle glaucoma and angle-closure glaucoma
Because carbonic anhydrase inhibitors reduce the formation of aqueous humor, lowering intraocular pressure, they are useful as adjunctive therapy in patients with glaucoma.
Epilepsy
Acetazolamide is used with other anticonvulsants in various types of epilepsy, particularly petit mal. It acts to inhibit seizures by an unknown mechanism; it may act by inducing metabolic acidosis or by increasing carbon dioxide tension within the CNS.
Diuresis
Acetazolamide, a carbonic anhydrase inhibitor, reversibly blocks the enzyme responsible for formation of hydrogen and bicarbonate ions from carbon dioxide and water. This decreases hydrogen concentration in the renal tubules, promoting excretion of bicarbonate, sodium, potassium, and water.
Mountain sickness
Acetazolamide shortens the period of high-altitude acclimatization; by inhibiting conversion of carbon dioxide to bicarbonate, it may increase carbon dioxide tension in tissues and decrease it in the lungs; the resultant etabolic acidosis may also increase oxygenation during hypoxia.

Overview of adverse reactions
Many adverse reactions associated with carbonic anhydrase inhibitors are dose-related and respond to lowered dosage; each drug has a slightly different adverse reaction profile, and patients who cannot tolerate one of the drugs may be able to tolerate another. Serious adverse effects are infrequent, because drugs are primarily given for short-term use. Some of the more common adverse effects include generalized weakness, tiredness, or discomfort; nausea; vomiting; diarrhea; loss of appetite; metallic taste in the mouth; peripheral numbness or tingling in hands, fingers, toes, or tongue.

▶ Special considerations
● Drug use in glaucoma may be limited because of the propensity for causing metabolic acidosis; signs and symptoms include weakness, malaise, headache, abdominal pain, nausea, vomiting, and poor skin turgor.
● In treating edema, intermittent dosage schedules may minimize tendency to cause metabolic acidosis and permit diuresis.
● Because they alkalize urine, these drugs may cause false-positive results on test for proteinuria.
● Establish baseline values before therapy, and monitor blood pressure and pulse rate for changes. Impose safety measures until patient's response to the diuretic is known.

● Establish baseline and periodically review laboratory tests: CBC, including white blood cell count; serum electrolyte, CO_2, BUN, and creatinine levels; and, especially, liver function tests. Patients with liver disease are especially susceptible to diuretic-induced electrolyte imbalance; in extreme cases, stupor, coma, and death can result.
● Administer diuretics in the morning so that major diuresis occurs before bedtime. To prevent nocturia, diuretics should not be administered after 6 p.m.
● Consider possible dosage adjustment: reduced dosage for patients with hepatic dysfunction and those taking other antihypertensive agents; increased dosage for patients with renal impairment, oliguria, or decreased diuresis (inadequate urine output may result in circulatory overload, causing water intoxication, pulmonary edema, and congestive heart failure); increased doses of insulin or oral hypoglycemics in diabetic patients.
● Monitor for signs of toxicity: postural hypotension; muscle weakness and cardiac dysrhythmia (signs of hypokalemia); leg cramps, nausea, muscle weakness, dry mouth, and dizziness (hyponatremia); lethargy, confusion, stupor, muscle twitching, increased reflexes, and convulsions (water intoxication); severe weakness, headache, abdominal pain, malaise, nausea, and vomiting (metabolic acidosis); sore throat, rash, or jaundice (blood dyscrasia from hypersensitivity); joint swelling, redness, and pain (hyperuricemia).
● Monitor patient for edema. Observe lower extremities of ambulatory patients and the sacral area of patients on bed rest. Check abdominal girth with tape measure to detect ascites. Dosage adjustment may be indicated. Patient's weight should be recorded each morning immediately after voiding and before breakfast; the patient should be weighed in the same type of clothing and on the same scale. Weight provides an index for dosage adjustments.
● Consult with dietitian on possible need for high-potassium diet or supplement.
● Patient should have urinal or commode readily available.

Information for the patient
● Explain rationale for therapy and diuretic effect of these drugs (increased volume and frequency of urination).
● Teach patient signs of adverse effects, especially hypokalemia (weakness, fatigue, muscle cramps, paresthesias, confusion, nausea, vomiting, diarrhea, headache, dizziness, or palpitations), and importance of reporting these symptoms promptly.
● Advise patient to eat potassium-rich foods, such as citrus fruits, potatoes, dates, raisins, and bananas; to avoid high-sodium foods, such as lunch meat, smoked meats, and processed cheeses; and not to add salt to other foods. Recommend salt substitutes.
● Counsel patient to avoid smoking because nicotine increases blood pressure.
● Tell patient to seek medical approval before taking nonprescription drugs; many contain sodium and potassium and can cause electrolyte imbalance.
● Warn patient of photosensitivity reactions. Explain that this reaction is a photoallergy in which ultraviolet radiation alters drug structure, causing allergic reactions in some persons; reactions occur 10 days to 2 weeks after initial sun exposure.
● Emphasize importance of keeping follow-up appointments to monitor effectiveness of diuretic therapy.

• Tell patient to report increased edema or weight or excess diuresis (more than 2-lb weight loss/day), and to record weight each morning after voiding and before breakfast, using the same scale and wearing the same type of clothing.
• Caution patient to change position slowly, especially when rising from lying or sitting position, to prevent dizziness from orthostatic hypotension.
• Instruct patient to immediately report chest, back, or leg pain; shortness of breath; or dyspnea.
• Tell patient to take drugs only as prescribed and at the same time each day, to prevent night diuresis and interrupted sleep.

Geriatric use
Elderly and debilitated patients require close observation, because they are more susceptible to drug-induced diuresis. In elderly patients excessive diuresis can quickly lead to rapid dehydration, hypovolemia, hypokalemia, and hyponatremia and may cause circulatory collapse. Reduced dosages may be indicated.

Pediatric use
Guidelines for safe use vary with each drug.

Breast-feeding
Safety has not been established.

Representative combinations
None.

---

carboplatin
Paraplatin

• Pharmacologic classification: alkylating agent (cell cycle-phase nonspecific)
• Therapeutic classification: antineoplastic
• Pregnancy risk category D

How supplied
Available by prescription only
Injection: 50-mg, 150-mg, and 450-mg vials

Indications, route, and dosage
Palliative treatment of ovarian carcinoma
Adults: Initial recommended dose is 360 mg/m² I.V. on day 1. Dose is repeated every 4 weeks. Dosage adjustments are based on the lowest post-treatment platelet or neutrophil value obtained in weekly blood counts.

Lowest platelet count (per mm³)	Lowest neutrophil count (per mm³)	Adjusted dose
> 100,000	> 2,000	125%
50,000 to 100,000	500 to 2,000	No adjustment
< 50,000	< 500	75%

Pharmacodynamics
Antitumor action: Carboplatin causes cross-linking of DNA strands.

Pharmacokinetics
• *Absorption:* Carboplatin is administered I.V.
• *Distribution:* Carboplatin's volume of distribution is approximately equal to total body water; no significant protein binding occurs.
• *Metabolism:* Carboplatin is hydrolyzed to form hydroxylated and aquated species.
• *Excretion:* 65% of the drug is excreted by the kidneys within 12 hours, 71% within 24 hours. Free platinum exhibits a half-life of 5 hours. Enterohepatic recirculation may occur.

Contraindications and precautions
Carboplatin is contraindicated in patients with a history of hypersensitivity to cisplatin, platinum-containing compounds, or mannitol. Avoid using drug in patients with severe bone marrow depression or bleeding. Transfusions may be necessary during treatment due to cumulative anemia. Bone marrow depression may be more severe in patients with creatinine clearance less than 60 ml/minute. Patients over age 65 are at greater risk for neurotoxicity.

Use with caution in patients with decreased renal function; use adjusted dose. Exercise extreme caution when preparing or administering carboplatin to avoid mutagenic, teratogenic, and carcinogenic risks. Use a biological containment cabinet, wear gloves and mask, and use syringes with Luer-Lok fittings to prevent leakage of drug solution. Also correctly dispose of needles, vials, and unused drug, and avoid contaminating work surfaces. Avoid inhalation of dust or vapors and contact with skin or mucous membranes.

Interactions
Concomitant use with nephrotoxic agents produces additive nephrotoxicity of carboplatin. Concomitant use with phenytoin may decrease phenytoin serum levels.

Effects on diagnostic tests
High doses of carboplatin may cause elevated bilirubin, alkaline phosphatase, AST (SGOT), serum creatinine, and blood urea levels.

Adverse reactions
• CNS: peripheral neuropathy.
• GI: constipation, diarrhea, nausea, vomiting, electrolyte loss.
• HEMA: *bone marrow depression* (thrombocytopenia, leukopenia, neutropenia, anemia).
• Hepatic: hepatotoxicity, pain.
• Local: pain at injection site.
• Other: alopecia, *hypersensitivity,* ototoxicity, pain, asthenia.

Overdose and treatment
Symptoms of overdose result from bone marrow suppression or hepatotoxicity. There is no known antidote for carboplatin overdose.

▶ Special considerations
Besides those relevant to all *alkylating agents,* consider the following recommendations.
• Reconstitute with 5% dextrose in water, normal saline solution, or sterile water for injection to make a concentration of 10 mg/ml.
• Carboplatin can be diluted with normal saline solution or 5% dextrose in water.
• Unopened vials should be stored at room temperature. Once reconstituted and diluted as directed, so-

---

*Canada only   †Unlabeled clinical use   Italicized adverse reactions are life-threatening.

lution is stable at room temperature for 8 hours. Because the drug does not contain antibacterial preservatives, unused drug should be discarded after 8 hours.
● Do not use needles or I.V. administration sets containing aluminum because carboplatin may precipitate and lose potency.
● Although drug is promoted as causing less nausea and vomiting than cisplatin, it can cause severe emesis. Administer antiemetic therapy.
● Administration of carboplatin requires the supervision of a physician who is experienced in the use of chemotherapeutic agents.

Information for the patient
● Stress importance of adequate fluid intake and increase in urine output, to facilitate uric acid excretion.
● Tell patient to report tinnitus immediately, to prevent permanent hearing loss. Patient should have audiometric test before initial and subsequent course.
● Advise patient to avoid exposure to people with infections.
● Tell patient to promptly report any unusual bleeding or bruising.

Geriatric use
Patients over age 65 are at greater risk for neurotoxicity.

Pediatric use
Safety has not been established.

Breast-feeding
It is unknown if carboplatin is distributed in breast milk.

---

carboprost tromethamine
Hemabate

● Pharmacologic classification: prostaglandin
● Therapeutic classification: oxytocic
● Pregnancy risk category C

How supplied
Available by prescription only
Injection: 250 mcg/ml

Indications, route, and dosage
Abort pregnancy between 13th and 20th weeks of gestation
Adults: Initially, 250 mcg is administered deep I.M. Subsequent doses of 250 mcg should be administered at intervals of 1½ to 3½ hours, depending on uterine response. Increments in dosage may be increased to 500 mcg if contractility is inadequate after several 250 mcg doses. Total dose should not exceed 12 mg, and therapy should not continue for more than 2 days.
Postpartum hemorrhage due to uterine atony that has not responded to conventional management
Adults: 250 mcg by deep I.M. injection. May administer repeat doses at 15- to 90-minute intervals. Maximum total dose is 2 mg.

Pharmacodynamics
Oxytocic action: Carboprost tromethamine stimulates myometrial contractions in the gravid uterus similar to the contractions of term labor. The exact mechanism

is unknown but the effect may be due to one or more of the following: direct stimulation, regulation of cellular calcium transport, or regulation of intracellular concentrations of cyclic $3',5'$-adenosine monophosphate. Uterine response increases with the length of the pregnancy. Carboprost tromethamine also facilitates cervical dilation by softening the cervix.

Pharmacokinetics
● *Absorption:* Following deep I.M. administration, peak concentrations occur in 30 minutes.
● *Distribution:* Unknown.
● *Metabolism:* Enzymatic deactivation occurs in maternal tissues.
● *Excretion:* Drug is excreted primarily in urine. The mean abortion time is 16 hours.

Contraindications and precautions
Drug is contraindicated when the fetus has reached the stage of viability and in patients with hypersensitivity to the drug, acute pelvic inflammatory disease, or active renal, cardiac, or hepatic disease, because of increased potential for adverse effects. Drug should be used cautiously in patients with asthma, epilepsy, diabetes, hypotension, or jaundice, because drug may exacerbate the symptoms or disorders; and in patients with compromised (scarred) uterus, because of contractile effects on smooth muscle.

Interactions
When used concomitantly, carboprost tromethamine will enhance the effects of oxytocin and other oxytocics; however, cervical laceration and trauma have been reported with concomitant use of oxytocin.

Effects on diagnostic tests
None reported.

Adverse reactions
● CV: hypotension, syncope, flushing, hot flashes, fainting.
● GI: nausea, vomiting, diarrhea.
● Respiratory: *bronchospasm,* wheezing, dyspnea.
● Other: chest pain, chest tightness, fever, chills, headache, abdominal pain; uterine bleeding and uterine rupture have been reported less frequently.
  Note: Drug should be discontinued if wheezing, troubled breathing, or tightness in chest occurs.

Overdose and treatment
Clinical manifestations of overdose are extensions of the adverse reactions. Because drug is metabolized rapidly, treatment involves discontinuing drug and providing supportive care.

▶ Special considerations
● Administer only in hospitals with intensive care and surgical facilities available.
● Confirmation of fetal death is imperative before administration when used for missed abortion or intrauterine fetal death.
● Premedicate with antiemetic and antidiarrheal agents to minimize GI effects.
● Meperidine may be helpful to reduce abdominal cramps.
● Store drug in refrigerator.

Information for the patient
Advise the patient of the expected adverse reactions.

---

cardiac glycosides

deslanoside
digitalis leaf
digitoxin
digoxin

The cardiac glycosides all derive from digitalis, a natural substance obtained from the foxglove plant (*Digitalis purpurea*). The effects of digitalis on the heart were described in the late 1700s by John Ferriar. However, its clinical value in treating congestive heart failure (CHF) did not become apparent until the early 1900s. Today, it remains an important agent in managing congestive heart failure and atrial tachyarrhythmias. Although the long-term benefits of cardiac glycosides in managing CHF remain controversial, these drugs are still the only useful oral inotropic agents available. Despite their inherent toxicity, these drugs can be used safely because their pharmacokinetics, adverse reactions, and interactions are well defined.

Pharmacology

Cardiac glycosides include glycoside mixtures (digitalis leaf); digitoxin, derived from *Digitalis purpurea*; and deslanoside and digoxin, derived from *Digitalis lanata*. Although they differ pharmacokinetically, these agents have similar therapeutic effects on the heart.

Note: Because the response to glycoside mixtures varies, single agents are preferred.

The effects of cardiac glycosides on the myocardium are dose-related and involve both direct and indirect mechanisms. The drugs directly increase myocardial contractile force and velocity, increase AV node refractory period, and increase total peripheral resistance. At higher doses, they enhance sympathetic outflow. They indirectly depress the SA node and prolong conduction to the AV node.

In patients with heart failure, the increased contractile force induced by cardiac glycosides enhances cardiac output, improves systolic emptying, and decreases diastolic heart size. It also reduces elevated ventricular end-diastolic pressure and, consequently, decreases pulmonary and systemic venous pressures. Increased myocardial contractility and cardiac output reflexively reduce sympathetic tone. This compensates for the drugs' direct vasoconstrictive effect, thereby reducing total peripheral resistance; it also slows increased heart rate and causes diuresis in edematous patients.

In patients without CHF, cardiac glycosides cause only minimal slowing of the heart rate, which in this case results mainly from vagal (cholinergic) and sympatholytic effects on the SA node. (However, with toxic doses, slow heart rate stems from direct depression of SA node automaticity.) Although therapeutic doses have little effect on the action potential, toxic doses increase automaticity (spontaneous diastolic depolarization) of all cardiac regions except the SA node.

Clinical indications and actions
Heart failure

Cardiac glycosides increase contractile force, in turn increasing cardiac output. This results in diuresis and symptomatic relief of both right-sided heart failure caused by systemic venous congestion and left-sided heart failure caused by pulmonary congestion. Gen-

erally, cardiac glycosides are most effective in managing low-output heart failure, somewhat less effective in managing high output heart failure, and of limited use in managing heart failure caused by mechanical disturbances.

Arrhythmias

Because of their effects on the specialized cardiac conduction system, cardiac glycosides prove valuable in acute and chronic management of atrial tachydysrhythmias. They are the preferred drugs for controlling rapid ventricular rate in patients with chronic atrial flutter. Digoxin alone or, if necessary, combined with propanolol or verapamil, is the preferred drug for controlling ventricular rate in established paroxysmal atrial fibrillation or flutter.

Paroxysmal atrial tachycardia or AV junctional rhythm

Cardiac glycosides' direct and indirect effects on the cardiac conduction system make them valuable in the acute and chronic management of paroxysmal atrial tachycardia (PAT) and AV junctional rhythm. However, if treating PAT is necessary, measures to increase vagal tone or administration of verapamil are the preferred treatments. Treatment of paroxysmal junctional rhythm may include digitalis, with measures to increase vagal tone, or cardioversion. Digitalis in conjunction with measures to increase vagal tone also may be effective in treating these tachycardias.

Myocardial infarction

The inotropic effects of cardiac glycosides may be beneficial in treating CHF after acute myocardial infarction. However, such use of these drugs is still controversial.

Other uses

Cardiac glycosides have also been used to treat cardiogenic shock in patients with pulmonary edema and/or atrial fibrillation or flutter with rapid ventricular rate; angina pectoris, in patients with cardiomegaly and heart failure; and septic shock, in patients with heart failure and systemic hypotension that persist after elevation of central venous or pulmonary artery pressure. However, support for these indications is limited; also, cardiac glycosides may adversely affect patients suffering from shock resulting from infection by gram-negative organisms.

Overview of adverse reactions

Various adverse reactions and toxic effects limit use of cardiac glycosides. These drugs have a narrow therapeutic index; also, signs and symptoms of the underlying disease may be difficult to distinguish from those indicating toxicity. Anorexia, nausea, and vomiting (probably centrally mediated) may be early indications of toxicity. Abdominal discomfort or pain and diarrhea may also occur. Drug effects on the cardiac conduction system may lead to multiple arrhythmias, ranging from various degrees of AV block to complex ventricular ectopy. Gynecomastia may occur with chronic administration. Rarely, hypersensitivity reactions, indicated by rash, eosinophilia, or thrombocytopenia, may occur. Digitalis glycosides are a major cause of poisoning in children.

▶ Special considerations

● Ask patient if he has a history of chronic or recent cardiac glycoside use before starting therapy.
● Monitor heart rate daily because of drug's effects on the cardiac conduction system. Slowing of the heart rate (60 beats/minute or less) may be an early sign of

---

*Canada only   †Unlabeled clinical use   Italicized adverse reactions are life-threatening.

toxicity (except in patients with chronically slow heart rate).

● Observe for GI adverse effects, such as nausea, anorexia, and vomiting, which may be early signs of toxicity.

● Obtain serum drug levels before administering morning dose or at least 6 to 12 hours after a dose is administered, because of drug's slow distribution.

● Discontinue drug at least 24 hours before elective cardioversion.

● Higher-than-usual doses and serum drug levels may be needed to adequately control atrial tachydysrhythmias.

● Before prescribing additional drugs for patient currently receiving cardiac glycosides, review drug interactions, which are numerous and may seriously affect therapy.

Information for the patient

● Instruct patient to take drug only as directed and at same time every day.

● Teach patient how to take pulse rate; advise him to call if rate drops below 60 beats/minute.

● Warn patient not to take missed dose with next regularly scheduled dose and to call for instructions if he misses more than two doses.

● Warn patient not to take nonprescription preparations, such as cough, cold, or allergy medications or diet drugs, except as directed.

● Instruct patient to report loss of appetite, stomach pain, nausea, vomiting, diarrhea, unusual fatigue or weakness, drowsiness, headache, blurred or yellow vision, rash or hives, or depression.

● Warn patient not to stop taking drug without medical approval.

Geriatric use

Many geriatric patients have renal or hepatic dysfunction, or electrolyte imbalances that may predispose them to toxicity. Digoxin is best for patients with liver impairment because it is cleared primarily by the kidneys. Digitoxin is best for patients with renal dysfunction because it is primarily cleared by the liver.

Pediatric use

Children over age 1 month may require proportionally larger doses than adults.

Breast-feeding

Cardiac glycosides are excreted in breast milk. Use these drugs with caution in breast-feeding women.

Representative combinations

None.

carisoprodol

Rela, Sodol, Soma, Soprodol

● Pharmacologic classification: carbamate derivative
● Therapeutic classification: skeletal muscle relaxant
● Pregnancy risk category C

How supplied

Available by prescription only
Tablets: 350 mg

Indications, route, and dosage

Adjunct for relief of discomfort in acute, painful musculoskeletal conditions

Adults and children over age 12: Administer 350 mg P.O. t.i.d. and at bedtime.

Pharmacodynamics

Skeletal muscle relaxant action: Carisoprodol does not relax skeletal muscle directly, but apparently as a result of its sedative effects. However, the exact mechanism of action is unknown. Animal studies suggest that the drug modifies central perception of pain without eliminating peripheral pain reflexes, and has slight antipyretic activity.

Pharmacokinetics

● *Absorption:* With usual therapeutic doses, onset of action occurs within 30 minutes and persists 4 to 6 hours.

● *Distribution:* Carisoprodol is widely distributed throughout the body.

● *Metabolism:* Carisoprodol is metabolized in the liver. The drug may induce microsomal enzymes in the liver.

● *Excretion:* The drug is excreted in urine mainly as its metabolites; less than 1% of a dose is excreted unchanged. The drug may be removed by hemodialysis or peritoneal dialysis.

Contraindications and precautions

Carisoprodol is contraindicated in patients with acute intermittent porphyria, because the drug may exacerbate the condition, and in those who have demonstrated allergic or idiosyncratic reactions to the drug or its related compounds (meprobamate).

Administer cautiously to patients with impaired renal or hepatic function. Patients allergic or sensitive to the dye tartrazine should avoid taking Rela tablets. Although tartrazine sensitivity is rare, it frequently occurs in patients sensitive to aspirin.

Administer cautiously to patients with CNS depression, because effects may be additive. Psychological dependence and abuse have been reported in those with a history of drug abuse or dependence. Avoid use in patients with head injury or coma.

Interactions

Concomitant use with other CNS depressants, including alcohol, produces additive CNS depression. When used with other depressant drugs (general anesthetics, opioid analgesics, antipsychotics, tricyclic antidepressants, or anxiolytics), exercise care to avoid overdose. Concurrent use with monoamine oxidase inhibitors or tricyclic antidepressants may increase CNS depression, respiratory depression, and hypotensive effects. Dosage adjustments (reduction of one or both) are required.

Effects on diagnostic tests
None significant.

Adverse reactions
● CNS: drowsiness, dizziness, vertigo, ataxia, tremor, insomnia, agitation, irritability, headache, depression, syncope.
● CV: tachycardia, postural hypotension (orthostatic), facial flushing.
● DERM: rash, erythema, urticaria, pruritus, fixed drug eruption.
● GI: nausea, vomiting, hiccups, increased bowel activity, epigastric distress.
● HEMA: eosinophilia.
● Other: asthmatic episodes, fever, angioneurotic edema, weakness, stinging or burning eyes, *anaphylaxis.*
Note: Drug should be discontinued if allergic or idiosyncratic reactions occur during therapy. May be treated with epinephrine, antihistamines, or corticosteroids as needed. Hypersensitivity possible to drug or to tartrazine in formulation.

Overdose and treatment
Clinical manifestations of overdose include exaggerated CNS depression, stupor, coma, shock, and respiratory depression.

Treatment of a conscious patient requires emptying the stomach by emesis or gastric lavage; activated charcoal may be used after gastric lavage to adsorb any remaining drug. If patient is comatose, secure endotracheal tube with cuff inflated before gastric lavage. Provide supportive therapy by maintaining adequate airway and assisted ventilation. CNS stimulants and pressor agents should be used cautiously. Monitor vital signs, fluid and electrolyte levels, and neurologic status closely.

Monitor urine output, and avoid overhydration. Forced diuresis using mannitol, peritoneal dialysis, or hemodialysis may be beneficial. Continue to monitor patient for relapse from incomplete gastric emptying and delayed absorption.

▶ **Special considerations**
● Use with caution with other CNS depressants, because effects may be cumulative.
● Initially, allergic or idiosyncratic reactions may occur (first to the fourth dose). Symptoms usually subside after several hours; treat with supportive and symptomatic measures.
● Psychological dependence may follow long-term use.
● Withdrawal symptoms (abdominal cramps, insomnia, chilliness, headache, and nausea) may occur with abrupt termination of drug after prolonged use of higher-than-recommended doses.
● Rela contains tartrazine, which may cause allergic reactions, including bronchial asthma, in susceptible individuals. Such patients also may be sensitive to aspirin.

Information for the patient
● Inform patient that carisoprodol may cause dizziness and faintness in some patients. Symptoms may be controlled by making position changes slowly and in stages. Patient should report persistent symptoms.

● Tell patient to avoid alcoholic beverages and to use cough or cold preparations containing alcohol cautiously while taking this medication. He should also avoid other CNS depressants (effects may be additive) unless prescribed.
● Warn patient drug may cause drowsiness. Avoid hazardous activities that require alertness until CNS depressant effects can be determined.
● Advise patient to discontinue drug immediately and to call if rash, diplopia, dizziness, or other unusual signs or symptoms appear.
● Tell patient to store drug away from direct heat and light (not in bathroom medicine cabinet).
● Instruct patient to take missed dose only if remembered within 1 hour. If remembered later, patient should skip that dose and go back to regular schedule. Patient should not double the dose.

Geriatric use
Elderly patients may be more sensitive to the effects of carisoprodol.

Pediatric use
Safety and efficacy have not been established in children under age 12. However, some clinicians suggest a dosage of 25 mg/kg or 750 mg/m^2 divided q.i.d. for children age 5 and older.

Breast-feeding
Carisoprodol may be distributed into breast milk at two to four times maternal plasma concentrations.

carmustine (BCNU)
BiCNU

● Pharmacologic classification: alkylating agent; nitrosourea (cell cycle-phase nonspecific)
● Therapeutic classification: antineoplastic
● Pregnancy risk category D

How supplied
Available by prescription only
Injection: 100-mg vial (lyophilized), with a 3-ml vial of absolute alcohol supplied as a diluent

Indications, route, and dosage
Dosage and indications may vary. Check current literature for recommended protocol.
Brain, colon, and stomach cancer; Hodgkin's disease; non-Hodgkin's lymphomas; melanomas; multiple myeloma; hepatoma
Adults: 75 to 100 mg/m^2 I.V. by slow infusion daily for 2 consecutive days, repeated q 6 weeks if platelet count is above 100,000/mm^3 and WBC count is above 4,000/mm^3. Reduce dosage by 50% when WBC count is below 2,000/mm^3 and platelet count is below 25,000/mm^3.
Alternate therapy: 200 mg/m^2 I.V. slow infusion as a single dose, repeated q 6 to 8 weeks; or 40 mg/m^2 I.V. slow infusion for 5 consecutive days, repeated q 6 weeks.

Pharmacodynamics
Antineoplastic action: The cytotoxic action of carmustine is mediated through its metabolites, which inhibit

---

several enzymes involved with DNA formation. This agent can also cause cross-linking of DNA. Cross-linking interferes with DNA, RNA, and protein synthesis. Cross-resistance between carmustine and lomustine has been shown to occur.

Pharmacokinetics
● *Absorption:* Carmustine is not absorbed across the GI tract.
● *Distribution:* Carmustine is cleared rapidly from the plasma. After I.V. administration, carmustine and its metabolites distribute rapidly into the CSF. Carmustine also is distributed in breast milk.
● *Metabolism:* Carmustine is metabolized extensively in the liver.
● *Excretion:* Approximately 60% to 70% of carmustine and its metabolites are excreted in urine within 96 hours, 6% to 10% is excreted as carbon dioxide by the lungs, and 1% is excreted in feces. Enterohepatic circulation and storage of the drug in adipose tissue can occur and may cause delayed hematologic toxicity.

Contraindications and precautions
Carmustine is contraindicated in patients with a history of hypersensitivity to the drug.

Drug should be withheld or dosage reduced in the presence of hepatic or renal insufficiency because drug accumulation may occur; in patients with compromised hematologic status because of the drug's adverse hematologic effects; and in patients with recent exposure to cytotoxic medications or radiation therapy.

Interactions
Concomitant use with cimetidine increases the bone marrow toxicity of carmustine. The mechanism of this interaction is unknown. Avoid concomitant use of these drugs.

Effects on diagnostic tests
Carmustine therapy may increase BUN, serum alkaline phosphatase, AST (SGOT), and bilirubin concentrations.

Adverse reactions
● DERM: hyperpigmentation upon accidental contact of drug with skin; alopecia.
● GI: nausea, possibly severe, lasting 2 to 6 hours after dose; vomiting.
● GU: nephrotoxicity.
● HEMA: *bone marrow depression* (dose-limiting, usually occurring 4 to 6 weeks after a dose), *leukopenia, thrombocytopenia,* anemia.
● Hepatic: hepatotoxicity.
● Metabolic: possible hyperuricemia in lymphoma patients when rapid cell lysis occurs.
● Local: intense pain at infusion site.
● Other: *pulmonary fibrosis.*

Overdose and treatment
Clinical manifestations of overdose include leukopenia, thrombocytopenia, nausea, and vomiting.

Treatment consists of supportive measures, including transfusion of blood components, antibiotics for infections that may develop, and antiemetics.

▶ Special considerations
● Reconstitute the 100-mg vial with the 3 ml of absolute alcohol provided by the manufacturer, then dilute further with 27 ml sterile water for injection. Resultant solution contains 3.3 mg carmustine/ml in 10% ethanol. Dilute in normal saline or dextrose 5% in water for I.V. infusion. Give at least 250 ml over 1 to 2 hours. Discard excess drug.
● Wear gloves to administer carmustine infusion and when changing I.V. tubing. Avoid contact with skin because carmustine will cause a brown stain. If drug comes into contact with skin, wash off thoroughly.
● Solution is unstable in plastic I.V. bags. Administer only in glass containers.
● Carmustine may decompose at temperatures above 80° F. (26.6° C.).
● If powder liquefies or appears oily, it is a sign of decomposition. Discard.
● Reconstituted solution may be stored in refrigerator for 24 hours.
● Don't mix with other drugs during administration.
● Avoid all I.M. injections when platelets are below 100,000/mm³.
● To reduce pain on infusion, dilute further or slow infusion rate.
● Intense flushing of the skin may occur during an I.V. infusion, but usually disappears within 2 to 4 hours.
● To reduce nausea, give antiemetic before administering.
● Monitor CBC.
● Consider that pulmonary toxicity is more likely in people who smoke.
● At first sign of extravasation, infusion should be discontinued and area infiltrated with liberal injections of 0.5 mEq/ml sodium bicarbonate solution.
● Carmustine has been applied topically in concentrations of 0.5% to 2% to treat mycosis fungoides.
● Prescribe anticoagulants and aspirin products cautiously. Monitor patient closely for signs of bleeding.
● Because carmustine crosses the blood-brain barrier, it may be used to treat primary brain tumors.

Information for the patient
● Warn patient to watch for signs of infection and bone marrow toxicity (fever, sore throat, anemia, fatigue, easy bruising, nose or gum bleeds, melena). Patient should take temperature daily.
● Remind patient to return for follow-up blood work weekly, or as needed, and to watch for signs and symptoms of infection.
● Advise patient to avoid exposure to people with infections.
● Tell patient to avoid over-the-counter products containing aspirin because they may precipitate bleeding. Advise him to report any signs of bleeding promptly.

Breast-feeding
Active metabolites of carmustine have been found in breast milk. Therefore, it is not advisable for women receiving the drug to breast-feed their infants because of the risk of serious adverse reactions, mutagenicity, and carcinogenicity in the infant.

carteolol hydrochloride
Cartrol

- Pharmacologic classification: beta-adrenergic blocking agent
- Therapeutic classification: antihypertensive
- Pregnancy risk category C

How supplied
Available by prescription only
Tablets: 2.5 mg, 5 mg

Indications, route, and dosage
Hypertension
Adults: Initially, 2.5 mg as a single daily dose. Gradually increase the dosage as required to 5 mg daily or 10 mg daily as a single dose.
Dosage in renal failure
Patients with substantial renal failure should receive the usual dose of carteolol scheduled at longer intervals as shown:

Creatinine clearance (ml/min/ 1.73 m²)	Dosage interval (hours)
>60	24
20 to 60	48
<20	72

Pharmacodynamics
Antihypertensive action: Carteolol is a nonselective beta-adrenergic blocking agent with intrinsic sympathomimetic activity (ISA). Its antihypertensive effects are probably caused by decreased sympathetic outflow from the brain and decreased cardiac output. Carteolol does not have a consistent effect on renin output.

Pharmacokinetics
- *Absorption:* Rapid, achieving peak plasma levels in 1 to 3 hours. Bioavailablity is about 85%.
- *Distribution:* Carteolol is 20% to 30% bound to plasma proteins.
- *Metabolism:* Only 30% to 50% of the drug is metabolized in the liver to 8-hydroxycarteolol, an active metabolite, and the inactive metabolite glucuronoside.
- *Excretion:* Primarily renal. Plasma half-life is about 6 hours.

Contraindications and precautions
Carteolol is contraindicated in patients with bronchial asthma, because it may block bronchodilation by endogenous catecholamines or beta-receptor agonists; in patients with severe bradycardia and those with greater than first-degree heart block, because it may further slow the heart rate; and in patients with cardiogenic shock or congestive heart failure (CHF), because it may worsen cardiac decompensation. It may be used cautiously in patients with CHF controlled by digitalis and diuretics, because beta-adrenergic blocking agents do not block the inotropic effects of digitalis. Note that currently asymptomatic patients with a history of CHF who do not currently exhibit symptoms may show signs of cardiac decompensation with beta-blocker therapy.

Patients with unrecognized coronary artery disease may exhibit signs of angina pectoris upon withdrawal of the drug.

Beta blockade may block the signs and symptoms of hypoglycemia (such as tachycardia and blood pressure changes) and inhibit glycogenolysis. It may also attenuate insulin release.

Beta-blocking agents may mask tachycardia associated with hyperthyroidism. Patients suspected of having thyrotoxicosis should undergo gradual withdrawal of beta blocker to avoid thyroid storm.

Withdrawal of beta blocker before surgery is controversial. Some clinicians advocate withdrawal to prevent any impairment of the heart's ability to respond to reflex stimuli and to prevent any decreased responsiveness to exogenous catecholamine administration. However, the beta-blocking effects of carteolol may persist for weeks, and discontinuing the drug before surgery may be impractical. The anesthesiologist should be advised that the patient is receiving a beta-blocking agent so that isoproterenol or dobutamine is made readily available for the reversal of the drug's cardiac effects.

Interactions
The dosage of insulin and oral hypoglycemic agents may have to be adjusted in patients receiving carteolol. Catecholamine-depleting drugs, such as reserpine, may have an additive effect when administered with a beta blocker. Carteolol may potentiate the hypotension produced by general anesthetics. Observe carefully for excessive hypotension or bradycardia and for orthostatic hypotension.

Avoid concurrent administration of oral calcium antagonists and beta blockers in patients with impaired cardiac function because of the risk of hypotension, left ventricular failure, and AV conduction disturbances. I.V. calcium antagonists should be used with caution.

Effects on diagnostic tests
None reported.

Adverse reactions
- CNS: weakness, lassitude, fatigue, somnolence.
- CV: *conduction disturbances.*
- Other: muscle cramps, dyspnea, wheezing.

Overdose and treatment
No specific information is available. The likely symptoms are bradycardia, bronchospasm, CHF, and hypotension.

Atropine should be used to treat symptomatic bradycardia. If no response is seen, cautiously use isoproterenol. Bronchospasm should be treated with a beta₂ agonist, such as isoproterenol, or theophylline. Digitalis or diuretics may be useful in treating CHF. Vasopressors (epinephrine, dopamine, or norepinephrine) should be given to combat hypotension.

▶ **Special considerations**
Besides those relevant to all *beta-adrenergic blocking agents,* consider the following recommendations.
- Dosage over 10 mg daily does not produce a greater response; it may actually decrease response.
- Food may slow the rate, but not the extent, of carteolol absorption.
- Steady-state levels are reached rapidly (within 1 to 2 days) in patients with normal renal function.

Information for the patient
• Advise the patient to take the drug exactly as prescribed and not to discontinue the drug suddenly.
• Advise the patient to report shortness of breath or difficulty breathing, unusually fast heartbeat, cough, or fatigue with exertion.

Geriatric use
No specific age-related recommendations are available.

Pediatric use
Safety has not been established.

Breast-feeding
Animal studies indicate that carteolol may be distributed in breast milk. Use with caution in breast-feeding women.

---

cascara sagrada

cascara sagrada aromatic fluid extract

cascara sagrada fluid extract

• Pharmacologic classification: anthraquinone glycoside mixture
• Therapeutic classification: laxative
• Pregnancy risk category C

How supplied
Available without prescription
Tablets: 325 mg
Aromatic fluid extract: 1 g/ml
Fluidextract: 1 g/ml

Indications, route, and dosage
Acute constipation; preparation for bowel or rectal examination
Adults: 1 tablet P.O. h.s.; 1 ml fluid extract daily; or 5 ml aromatic fluid extract daily.
Children age 2 to 12: One half of adult dose.
Children under age 2: One quarter of adult dose.

Pharmacodynamics
Laxative action: Cascara sagrada, obtained from the dried bark of the buckthorn tree *(Rhamnus purshiana)*, contains cascarosides A and B (barbaloin glycosides) and cascarosides C and D (chrysaloin glycosides). It exerts a direct irritant action on the colon that promotes peristalsis and bowel motility. It also enhances colonic fluid accumulation, increasing the laxative effect.

Pharmacokinetics
• *Absorption:* Minimal drug absorption occurs in the small intestine. Onset of action usually occurs in about 6 to 12 hours but may not occur for 3 or 4 days.
• *Distribution:* Cascara may be distributed in the bile, saliva, colonic mucosa, and breast milk.
• *Metabolism:* Cascara is hydrolyzed by colonic flora enzymes to active, free anthraquinones, which are metabolized in the liver.
• *Excretion:* Cascara is excreted in feces via biliary elimination, in urine, or in both.

Contraindications and precautions
Cascara is contraindicated in patients with fluid and electrolyte disturbances; appendicitis; nausea, vomiting, or abdominal pain; any abdominal condition necessitating immediate surgery; fecal impaction; rectal bleeding; or intestinal obstruction, because the drug may exacerbate these conditions.

Interactions
None reported.

Effects on diagnostic tests
Cascara turns alkaline urine pink to red, red to violet, or red to brown and turns acidic urine yellow to brown in the phenolsulfonphthalein excretion test.

Adverse reactions
• GI: nausea, vomiting, diarrhea; loss of normal bowel function with excessive use; abdominal cramps, especially in severe constipation; malabsorption of nutrients; "cathartic colon" (syndrome resembling ulcerative colitis radiologically) after chronic misuse; discoloration of rectal mucosa after long-term use.
• Metabolic: hypokalemia, protein enteropathy, electrolyte imbalance in excessive use.
• Other: laxative dependence in long-term or excessive use, weakness, dizziness, fainting, sweating.
Note: Drug should be discontinued if abdominal pain occurs.

Overdose and treatment
No information available.

▶ Special considerations
• Prescribe doses carefully; fluid extract preparation is five times as potent as aromatic fluid extract.
• Aromatic fluid extract tastes better than fluid extract.
• Drug may color urine reddish pink or brown, depending on urine pH.
• Cascara is a common ingredient in many so-called natural laxatives available without a prescription.

Information for the patient
Warn patient that drug may turn urine reddish pink or brown.

Geriatric use
Because many elderly persons use laxatives, they have a particularly high risk of developing laxative dependence. Urge them to use laxatives only for short periods.

Pediatric use
Use with caution in children.

Breast-feeding
Cascara may be excreted in breast milk. However, no adverse effects from its use have been reported.

---

castor oil
Alphamul, Emulsoil, Neoloid, Purge

- Pharmacologic classification: glyceride, *Ricinus communis* derivative
- Therapeutic classification: stimulant laxative
- Pregnancy risk category X

How supplied
Available without prescription
Capsules: (0.62 ml oil)
Liquid: 60 ml, 120 ml, 180 ml, pints, gallons

Indications, route, and dosage
Preparation for rectal or bowel examination, or surgery; acute constipation (rarely)
Adults: 15 to 60 ml P.O. as liquid or 2 to 4 capsules P.O.
Children age 2 and older: 5 to 15 ml P.O.
Children under age 2: 1.25 to 7.5 ml P.O.
Infants: Up to 4 ml P.O. Increased dose produces no greater effect.

Pharmacodynamics
Laxative action: Castor oil acts primarily in the small intestine, where it is metabolized to ricinoleic acid, which stimulates the intestine, promoting peristalsis and bowel motility.

Pharmacokinetics
- *Absorption:* Unknown; action begins in 2 to 6 hours.
- *Distribution:* Castor oil is distributed locally, primarily in the small intestine.
- *Metabolism:* Like other fatty acids, castor oil is metabolized by intestinal enzymes into its active form, ricinoleic acid.
- *Excretion:* Castor oil is excreted in feces.

Contraindications and precautions
Castor oil is contraindicated in patients with fluid or electrolyte disturbances because it may worsen the imbalance; in patients with appendicitis, acute surgical abdomen, fecal impaction, intestinal obstruction, or intestinal perforation, because excessive intestinal stimulation may exacerbate symptoms of these disorders; in pregnant women because it may induce labor; and in patients with hypersensitivity to castor beans.

Interactions
Castor oil may decrease absorption of intestinally absorbed drugs.

Effects on diagnostic tests
None reported.

Adverse reactions
- GI: nausea; vomiting; diarrhea; loss of normal bowel function in excessive use; abdominal cramps, especially in severe constipation; malabsorption of nutrients; "cathartic colon" (syndrome resembling ulcerative colitis radiologically) after chronic misuse; constipation.
- Metabolic: hypokalemia, protein enteropathy, other electrolyte imbalance in excessive use.
- Other: laxative dependence in long-term or excessive use.

Note: Drug should be discontinued if abdominal pain occurs.

Overdose and treatment
No information available.

▶ Special considerations
- Castor oil is not recommended for routine use in constipation; it is commonly used to evacuate the bowels before diagnostic or surgical procedures.
- Do not administer drug at bedtime because of rapid onset of action.
- Drug is most effective when taken on an empty stomach; shake well.
- Observe patient for signs and symptoms of dehydration.
- Flavored preparations are available.

Information for the patient
- Instruct patient not to take drug at bedtime.
- Suggest that patient chill drug or take it with juice or carbonated beverage for palatability.
- Instruct patient to shake emulsion well.
- Reassure patient that after response to drug he may not need to move bowels again for 1 or 2 days after taking drug.

Geriatric use
With chronic use, elderly patients may experience electrolyte depletion, resulting in weakness, incoordination, and orthostatic hypotension.

Breast-feeding
Breast-feeding women should seek medical approval before using castor oil.

cefaclor
Ceclor

- Pharmacologic classification: second-generation cephalosporin
- Therapeutic classification: antibiotic
- Pregnancy risk category B

How supplied
Available by prescription only
Capsules: 250 mg, 500 mg
Suspension: 125 mg/5 ml, 250 mg/5 ml

Indications, route, and dosage
Infections of respiratory or urinary tracts, skin, and soft tissue; and otitis media caused by susceptible organisms
Adults: 250 to 500 mg P.O. q 8 hours. Total daily dosage should not exceed 4 g.
Children: 40 mg/kg P.O. daily in divided doses q 8 hours, not to exceed 1 g/day.

Pharmacodynamics
Antibacterial action: Cefaclor is primarily bactericidal; however, it may be bacteriostatic. Activity depends on the organism, tissue penetration, drug dosage, and rate of organism multiplication. It acts by adhering to bacterial penicillin-binding proteins, thereby inhibiting cell wall synthesis.

Cefaclor has the same bactericidal spectrum as other

second-generation cephalosporins, except that it has increased activity against ampicillin- or amoxicillin-resistant *Haemophilus influenzae* and *Branhamella catarrhalis*.

Pharmacokinetics
● *Absorption:* Cefaclor is well absorbed from the GI tract; peak serum levels occur 30 to 60 minutes after an oral dose. Food will delay but not prevent complete GI tract absorption.
● *Distribution:* Cefaclor is distributed widely into most body tissues and fluids; CSF penetration is poor. Cefaclor crosses the placenta; it is 25% protein-bound.
● *Metabolism:* Cefaclor is not metabolized.
● *Excretion:* Cefaclor is excreted primarily in urine by renal tubular secretion and glomerular filtration; small amounts of drug are excreted in breast milk. Elimination half-life is ½ to 1 hour in patients with normal renal function; end-stage renal disease prolongs half-life to 3 to 5½ hours. Hemodialysis removes cefaclor.

Contraindications and precautions
Cefaclor is contraindicated in patients with known hypersensitivity to any cephalosporin; it should be used cautiously in patients with penicillin allergy, who usually are more susceptible to such reactions.

Interactions
Probenecid competitively inhibits renal tubular secretion of cephalosporins, resulting in higher, prolonged serum levels of these drugs.

Concomitant use with nephrotoxic agents (vancomycin, colistin, polymixin B, or aminoglycosides) or loop diuretics increases the risk of nephrotoxicity.

Concomitant use of cefaclor with bacteriostatic agents (tetracyclines, erythromycin, or chloramphenicol) may impair its bactericidal activity.

Effects on diagnostic tests
Cefaclor may cause false-positive Coombs' test results. Cefaclor also causes false-positive results in urine glucose tests utilizing cupric sulfate (Benedict's reagent or Clinitest); use glucose oxidase tests (Clinistix or Tes-Tape) instead.

Cefaclor causes false elevations in serum or urine creatinine levels in tests using Jaffé's reaction.

Adverse reactions
● CNS: dizziness, headache, somnolence, paresthesias, and seizures.
● DERM: maculopapular rash, dermatitis.
● GI: nausea, vomiting, diarrhea, anorexia, *pseudomembranous colitis*, heartburn, glossitis, dyspepsia, abdominal cramping, tenesmus, anal pruritus.
● GU: red and white cells in urine, nephrotoxicity.
● HEMA: transient leukopenia, lymphocytosis, anemia, eosinophilia.
● Other: hypersensitivity (serum sickness [erythema multiforme, rashes, urticaria, polyarthritis, fever]), bacterial and fungal superinfection.
   Note: Drug should be discontinued if signs of toxicity, immediate hypersensitivity reaction, or serum sickness occur or if severe diarrhea indicates pseudomembranous colitis; consider alternative therapy if the following symptoms occur: fever, eosinophilia, hematuria, neutropenia, or unexplained elevations in BUN or serum creatinine levels.

Overdose and treatment
Clinical signs of overdose include neuromuscular hypersensitivity; seizure may follow high CNS concentrations. Remove cefaclor by hemodialysis or peritoneal dialysis.

▶ Special considerations
Besides those relevant to all *cephalosporins*, consider the following recommendations.
● To prevent toxic accumulation, reduced dosage may be required if patient's creatinine clearance is below 40 ml/minute.
● Cefaclor may be given with food to minimize GI distress.
● Total daily dosage may be administered b.i.d. rather than t.i.d. with similar therapeutic effect.
● Stock oral suspension is stable for 14 days if refrigerated.
● Because cefaclor is dialyzable, patients who are receiving treatment with hemodialysis or peritoneal dialysis may require drug dosage adjustment.

Geriatric use
Dosage reduction may be necessary in patients with reduced renal function.

Pediatric use
Can be used safely in children.

Breast-feeding
Cefaclor distributes into breast milk and should be used with caution in breast-feeding women.

---

cefadroxil monohydrate
Duricef, Ultracef

● Pharmacologic classification: first-generation cephalosporin
● Therapeutic classification: antibiotic
● Pregnancy risk category B

How supplied
Available by prescription only
Capsules: 500 mg
Tablets: 1 g
Suspension: 125 mg/5 ml, 250 mg/5 ml, 500 mg/5 ml

Indications, route, and dosage
Urinary tract, skin, and soft-tissue infections caused by susceptible organisms
Adults: 500 mg to 2 g P.O. daily, depending on the infection treated. Usually given in once-daily or b.i.d. doses.
Children: 30 mg/kg daily in two divided doses.
Dosage in renal failure
In patients with a creatinine clearance of 10 to 50 ml/minute, extend dosing interval to every 24 hours. If creatinine clearance is less than 10 ml/minute, administer every 48 hours.

Pharmacodynamics
Antibacterial action: Cefadroxil is primarily bactericidal; however, it may be bacteriostatic. Activity depends on the organism, tissue penetration, drug dosage, and rate of organism multiplication. It acts by adhering to bac-

terial penicillin-binding proteins, thereby inhibiting cell wall synthesis.

Cefadroxil is active against many gram-positive cocci, including penicillinase-producing *Staphylococcus aureus* and *epidermidis*; *Streptococcus pneumoniae*, group B streptococci, and group A beta-hemolytic streptococci; and susceptible gram-negative organisms, including *Klebsiella pneumoniae*, *Escherichia coli*, *Proteus mirabilis*, and *Shigella*.

Pharmacokinetics
● *Absorption:* Cefadroxil is absorbed rapidly and completely from the GI tract after oral administration; peak serum levels occur at 1 to 2 hours.
● *Distribution:* Cefadroxil is distributed widely into most body tissues and fluids, including the gallbladder, liver, kidneys, bone, bile, sputum, and pleural and synovial fluids; CSF penetration is poor. Cefadroxil crosses the placenta; it is 20% protein-bound.
● *Metabolism:* Cefadroxil is not metabolized.
● *Excretion:* Cefadroxil is excreted primarily unchanged in the urine via glomerular filtration and renal tubular secretion; small amounts of drug may be excreted in breast milk. Elimination half-life is about 1 to 2 hours in patients with normal renal function; end-stage renal disease prolongs half-life to 25 hours. Cefadroxil can be removed by hemodialysis.

Contraindications and precautions
Cefadroxil is contraindicated in patients with known hypersensitivity to any cephalosporin; it should be used cautiously in patients with penicillin allergy, who usually are more susceptible to such reactions.

Interactions
Probenecid competitively inhibits renal tubular secretion of cephalosporins, resulting in higher, prolonged serum levels of these drugs.

Concomitant use with nephrotoxic agents (vancomycin, colistin, polymixin B, or aminoglycosides) or loop diuretics increases the risk of nephrotoxicity.

Concomitant use with bacteriostatic agents (tetracyclines, erythromycin, or chloramphenicol) may interfere with bactericidal activity.

Effects on diagnostic tests
Cefadroxil causes false-positive results in urine glucose tests utilizing cupric sulfate (Benedict's reagent or Clinitest); use glucose oxidase test (Clinistix or Tes-Tape) instead. Cefadroxil causes false elevations in serum or urine creatinine levels in tests using Jaffé's reaction.

Positive Coombs' test results occur in about 3% of patients taking cephalosporins.

Adverse reactions
● CNS: dizziness, headache, malaise, paresthesias, seizures.
● DERM: maculopapular and erythematous rashes, urticaria.
● GI: *pseudomembranous colitis*, nausea, anorexia, vomiting, diarrhea, glossitis, dyspepsia, abdominal cramps, anal pruritus, tenesmus.
● GU: genital pruritus, moniliasis.
● HEMA: transient neutropenia, eosinophilia, leukopenia, anemia.
● Other: dyspnea, bacterial and fungal superinfection.
Note: Drug should be discontinued if signs of toxicity or immediate hypersensitivity reaction occur or if severe diarrhea indicates pseudomembranous colitis; alter-

native therapy should be considered if the following symptoms occur: fever, eosinophilia, hematuria, neutropenia, or unexplained elevations in BUN or serum creatinine levels.

Overdose and treatment
Clinical signs of overdose include neuromuscular hypersensitivity; seizure may follow high CNS concentrations. Remove cefadroxil by hemodialysis. Other treatment is supportive.

▶ Special considerations
Besides those relevant to all *cephalosporins*, consider the following recommendations.
● Longer half-life permits once- or twice-daily dosing.
● Because cefadroxil is dialyzable, patients who are receiving treatment with hemodialysis may require dosage adjustment.

Geriatric use
Reduce dosage in elderly patients with diminished renal function.

Pediatric use
The serum half-life is prolonged in neonates and infants younger than age 1.

Breast-feeding
Cefadroxil distributes into breast milk and should be used with caution in breast-feeding women.

---

cefamandole nafate
Mandol

● Pharmacologic classification: second-generation cephalosporin
● Therapeutic classification: antibiotic
● Pregnancy risk category B

How supplied
Available by prescription only
Injectable solution: 500 mg, 1 g, 2 g, 10 g
Pharmacy bulk package: 10 g

Indications, route, and dosage
Serious respiratory, genitourinary, skin and soft-tissue, and bone and joint infections; septicemia; peritonitis from susceptible organisms
Adults: 500 mg to 1 g q 4 to 8 hours. In life-threatening infections, up to 2 g q 4 hours may be needed.
Infants and children: 50 to 100 mg/kg daily in equally divided doses q 4 to 8 hours. May be increased to total daily dosage of 150 mg/kg (not to exceed maximum adult dose) for severe infections.

Total daily dosage is same for I.M. or I.V. administration and depends on susceptibility of organism and severity of infection. Cefamandole should be injected deep I.M. into a large muscle mass, such as the gluteus or the lateral aspect of the thigh.
Dosage in renal failure
In patients with impaired renal function, doses or frequency of administration must be modified according to degree of renal impairment, severity of infection, and susceptibility of organism.

---

192 CEFAMANDOLE NAFATE

Creatinine clearance (ml/min/1.73 m²)	Severe infections	Life-threatening infections (maximum)
>80	1 to 2 g q 6 hr	2 g q 4 hr
50 to 80	750 mg to 1.5 g q 6 hr	1.5 g q 4 hr; or 2 g q 6 hr
25 to 50	750 mg to 1.5 g q 8 hr	1.5 g q 6 hr; or 2 g q 8 hr
10 to 25	500 mg to 1 g q 8 hr	1 g q 6 hr; or 1.25 g q 8 hr
2 to 10	500 to 750 mg q 12 hr	670 mg q 8 hr; or 1 g q 12 hr
<2	250 to 500 mg q 12 hr	500 mg q 8 hr; or 750 mg q 12 hr

DOSAGE IN ADULTS

Pharmacodynamics

Antibacterial action: Cefamandole is primarily bactericidal; however, it may be bacteriostatic. Activity depends on the organism, tissue penetration, drug dosage, and rate of organism multiplication. It acts by adhering to bacterial penicillin-binding proteins, thereby inhibiting cell wall synthesis.

Cefamandole is active against *Escherichia coli* and other coliform bacteria, *Staphylococcus aureus* (penicillinase- and nonpenicillinase-producing), *Staphylococcus epidermidis*, group A beta-hemolytic streptococci, *Klebsiella, Haemophilus influenzae, Proteus mirabilis*, and *Enterobacter* as the second-generation drugs. *Bacteroides fragilis* and *Acinetobacter* are resistant.

Pharmacokinetics

• *Absorption:* Cefamandole is not absorbed from the GI tract and must be given parenterally; peak serum levels occur ½ to 2 hours after an I.M. dose.
• *Distribution:* Cefamandole is distributed widely into most body tissues and fluids, including the gallbladder, liver, kidneys, bone, sputum, bile, and pleural and synovial fluids; CSF penetration is poor. Cefamandole crosses the placenta; it is 65% to 75% protein-bound.
• *Metabolism:* Cefamandole is not metabolized.
• *Excretion:* Cefamandole is excreted primarily in urine by renal tubular secretion and glomerular filtration; small amounts of drug are excreted in breast milk. Elimination half-life is about ½ to 2 hours in patients with normal renal function; severe renal disease prolongs half-life to 12 to 18 hours. Hemodialysis removes some cefamandole.

Contraindications and precautions

Cefamandole is contraindicated in patients with known hypersensitivity to any cephalosporin. It should be used with caution in patients with penicillin allergy, who usually are more susceptible to such reactions; in patients with coagulopathy; and in severely debilitated and malnourished patients, who are at greater risk of bleeding complications.

Interactions

Probenecid competitively inhibits renal tubular secretion of cephalosporins, resulting in higher, prolonged serum levels of these drugs.

Concomitant use with nephrotoxic agents (vancomycin, colistin, polymyxin B, or aminoglycosides) or loop diuretics increases the risk of nephrotoxicity.

Concomitant use of cefamandole with bacteriostatic agents (tetracyclines, erythromycin, or chloramphenicol) may impair its bactericidal activity.

Concomitant use with alcohol may cause severe disulfiram-like reactions.

Effects on diagnostic tests

Cefamandole causes false-positive results in urine glucose tests utilizing cupric sulfate (Benedict's reagent or Clinitest); use glucose oxidase tests (Clinistix or Tes-Tape) instead. Cefamandole also causes false elevations in serum or urine creatinine levels in tests using Jaffé's reaction.

Cefamandole may cause positive Coombs' test results, and may elevate liver function test results or prothrombin times.

Adverse reactions

• CNS: headache, malaise, paresthesia, dizziness, seizures.
• DERM: maculopapular and erythematous rashes, urticaria.
• GI: *pseudomembranous colitis*, nausea, anorexia, vomiting, diarrhea, glossitis, dyspepsia, abdominal cramps, tenesmus, anal pruritus.
• GU: nephrotoxicity, vaginitis.
• HEMA: transient neutropenia, eosinophilia, hemolytic anemia, *hypoprothrombinemia*, bleeding.
• Local: at injection site—pain, induration, sterile abscesses, temperature elevation, tissue sloughing; phlebitis and thrombophlebitis with I.V. injection.
• Other: hypersensitivity (serum sickness [erythema multiforme, rashes, polyarthritis, fever]), dyspnea, bacterial and fungal superinfection.

Note: Drug should be discontinued if signs of toxicity, immediate hypersensitivity reaction, serum sickness, or hypoprothrombinemia occur or if severe diarrhea indicates pseudomembranous colitis; consider alternative therapy if the following symptoms occur: fever, eosinophilia, hematuria, neutropenia, hypoprothrombinemia, or unexplained elevations in BUN or serum creatinine levels.

Overdose and treatment

Clinical signs of overdose include neuromuscular hypersensitivity. Seizure may follow high CNS concentrations. Hypoprothrombinemia and bleeding may occur; they may be treated with vitamin K or blood products. Some cefamandole may be removed by hemodialysis.

▶ Special considerations

• For most cephalosporin-sensitive organisms, cefamandole offers little advantage over others; it is less effective than cefoxitin against anaerobic infections. Some clinicians consider it inappropriate for pediatric use, especially for serious infections like *Haemophilus influenzae*.
• For I.V. use, reconstitute 1 g with 10 ml of sterile water for injection, dextrose 5%, or 0.9% sodium chloride for injection. Administer slowly, over 3 to 5 minutes,

*Canada only   †Unlabeled clinical use   Italicized adverse reactions are life-threatening.

or by intermittent infusion or continuous infusion in compatible solutions. Check package insert.

• Don't mix with I.V. infusions containing magnesium or calcium ions, which are chemically incompatible and may cause irreversible effects.

• Cefamandole injection contains 3.3 mEq of sodium per gram of drug.

• For I.M. use, dilute 1 g of cefamandole in 3 ml of sterile water for injection, bacteriostatic water for injection, 0.9% sodium chloride for injection, or 0.9% bacteriostatic sodium chloride for injection.

• Administer deeply into large muscle mass to ensure maximum absorption. Rotate injection sites.

• I.M. cefamandole is less painful than cefoxitin injection; it does not require addition of lidocaine.

• After reconstitution, solution remains stable for 24 hours at room temperature or 96 hours under refrigeration. Solution should be light yellow to amber. Do not use solution if it is discolored or contains a precipitate.

• Monitor for signs or symptoms of bleeding. Monitor patient's prothrombin times and platelet levels. Patient may require prophylactic use of vitamin K to prevent bleeding.

• Bleeding can be reversed by administering vitamin K or blood products.

• Concomitant use with alcohol will lead to disulfiram-like reaction. For patients who drink alcohol, consider alternative drugs if home I.V. antibiotic therapy is necessary.

Geriatric use
Dosage reduction may be required in patients with diminished renal function. Hypoprothrombinemia and bleeding have been reported most frequently in elderly, malnourished, and debilitated patients.

Pediatric use
Safe use in infants younger than age 1 month has not been established.

Breast-feeding
Cefamandole distributes into breast milk and should be used with caution in breast-feeding women. Safe use has not been established.

---

cefazolin sodium
Ancef, Kefzol, Zolicef

• Pharmacologic classification: first-generation cephalosporin
• Therapeutic classification: antibiotic
• Pregnancy risk category B

How supplied
Available by prescription only
Injection (parenteral): 250 mg, 500 mg, 1 g, 5 g, 10 g
Infusion: 500 mg/100 ml vial, 500-mg or 1-g Redi Vials, Faspaks, or ADD-Vantage vials

Indications, route, and dosage
Serious respiratory, genitourinary, skin and soft-tissue, and bone and joint infections; septicemia, endocarditis from susceptible organisms
Adults: 250 mg I.M. or I.V. q 8 hours to 1 g q 6 hours. Maximum dosage is 12 g/day in life-threatening situations.
Children over age 1 month: 50 to 100 mg/kg/day I.M. or I.V. in divided doses q 8 hours.

Total daily dosage is same for I.M. or I.V. administration and depends on the susceptibility of organism and severity of infection. Cefazolin should be injected deep I.M. into a large muscle mass, such as the gluteus or the lateral aspect of the thigh.

Dosage in renal failure
Dose or frequency of administration must be modified according to the degree of renal impairment, severity of infection, susceptibility of organism, and serum levels of drug.

Creatinine clearance (ml/min/1.73 m²)	Dosage in adults
≥ 55	Usual adult dose
35 to 54	Full dose q 8 hr or less frequently
11 to 34	½ usual dose q 12 hr
≤ 10	½ usual dose q 18 to 24 hr

Creatinine clearance (ml/min/1.73 m²)	Dosage in children
> 70	Usual pediatric dose
40 to 70	7.5 to 30 mg per kg of body weight q 12 hr
20 to 40	3.125 to 12.5 mg per kg of body weight q 12 hr
5 to 20	2.5 to 10 mg per kg of body weight q 24 hr

Pharmacodynamics
Antibacterial action: Cefazolin is primarily bactericidal; however, it may be bacteriostatic. Activity depends on the organism, tissue penetration, drug dosage, and rate of organism multiplication. It acts by adhering to bacterial penicillin-binding proteins, thereby inhibiting cell wall synthesis.

Cefazolin is active against *Escherichia coli, Enterobacteriaceae,* gonococci, *Haemophilus influenzae, Klebsiella, Proteus mirabilis, Staphylococcus aureus, Streptococcus pneumoniae,* and group A beta-hemolytic streptococci.

Pharmacokinetics
• *Absorption:* Cefazolin is not well absorbed from the GI tract and must be given parenterally; peak serum levels occur 1 to 2 hours after an I.M. dose.
• *Distribution:* Cefazolin is distributed widely into most body tissues and fluids, including the gallbladder, liver, kidneys, bone, sputum, bile, and pleural and synovial fluids; CSF penetration is poor. It crosses the placenta; it is 74% to 86% protein-bound.
• *Metabolism:* Cefazolin is not metabolized.

• *Excretion:* Cefazolin is excreted primarily unchanged in urine by renal tubular secretion and glomerular filtration; small amounts of drug are excreted in breast milk. Elimination half-life is about 1 to 2 hours in patients with normal renal function; end-stage renal disease prolongs half-life to 12 to 50 hours. Hemodialysis or peritoneal dialysis removes cefazolin.

Contraindications and precautions
Cefazolin is contraindicated in patients with known hypersensitivity to any cephalosporin; it should be used with caution in patients with penicillin allergy, who usually are more susceptible to such reactions.

Interactions
Probenecid competitively inhibits renal tubular secretion of cephalosporins, resulting in higher, prolonged serum levels of these drugs.

Concomitant use with nephrotoxic agents (vancomycin, colistin, polymyxin B, or aminoglycosides) or loop diuretics increases the risk of nephrotoxicity.

Concomitant use with bacteriostatic agents (tetracyclines, erythromycin, or chloramphenicol) may interfere with bactericidal activity.

Effects on diagnostic tests
Cephalosporins cause false-positive results in urine glucose tests utilizing cupric sulfate (Benedict's reagent or Clinitest); use glucose oxidase tests (Clinistix or Tes-Tape) instead. Cefazolin causes false elevations in serum or urine creatinine levels in tests using Jaffé's reaction.

Cefazolin also causes positive Coombs' test results and may elevate liver function test results.

Adverse reactions
• CNS: dizziness, headache, malaise, paresthesias, seizures.
• DERM: maculopapular and erythematous rashes, urticaria.
• GI: *pseudomembranous colitis*, nausea, anorexia, vomiting, diarrhea, glossitis, dyspepsia, abdominal cramps, anal pruritus, tenesmus.
• GU: genital pruritus, vaginitis, nephrotoxicity.
• HEMA: transient neutropenia, leukopenia, eosinophilia, anemia.
• Local: at injection site – pain, induration, sterile abscesses, tissue sloughing; phlebitis and thrombophlebitis with I.V. injection.
• Other: hypersensitivity, dyspnea, fever, bacterial and fungal superinfection.
   Note: Drug should be discontinued if signs of toxicity or immediate hypersensitivity reaction occur or if severe diarrhea indicates pseudomembranous colitis; consider alternative therapy if the following symptoms occur: fever, eosinophilia, hematuria, neutropenia, or unexplained elevations in BUN or serum creatinine levels.

Overdose and treatment
Clinical signs of overdose include neuromuscular hypersensitivity; seizure may follow high CNS concentrations. Remove cefazolin by hemodialysis.

▶ Special considerations
Besides those relevant to all *cephalosporins,* consider the following recommendations.
• For patients on sodium restrictions, note that cefazolin injection contains 2 mEq of sodium per gram of drug.

• Because of the long duration of effect, most infections can be treated with a single dose every 8 hours.
• For I.M. use, reconstitute with sterile water, bacteriostatic water, or 0.9% sodium chloride solution: 2 ml to a 250-mg vial, 2 ml to a 500-mg vial, and 2.5 ml to a 1-g vial produces concentrations of 125 mg/ml, 225 mg/ml, and 330 mg/ml respectively.
• Reconstituted solution is stable for 24 hours at room temperature; for 96 hours if refrigerated.
• I.M. cefazolin injection is less painful than that of other cephalosporins.
• Because hemodialysis removes cefazolin, patients who are undergoing hemodialysis may require dosage adjustment.

Pediatric use
Cefazolin has been used in children. However, safety in infants younger than age 1 month has not been established.

Breast-feeding
Safety has not been established. Cefazolin should be used with caution in breast-feeding women.

---

cefixime
Suprax

• Pharmacologic classification: third-generation cephalosporin
• Therapeutic classification: antibiotic
• Pregnancy risk category B

How supplied
Available by prescription only
Tablets: 200 mg, 400 mg
Powder for oral suspension: 100 mg/5 ml

Indications, route, and dosage
Otitis media; acute bronchitis; acute exacerbations of chronic bronchitis, pharyngitis, and tonsillitis
Adults: 400 mg P.O. daily in one or two doses.
Children over age 6 months: 8 mg/kg P.O. daily in one or two doses.
Dosage in renal failure

Creatinine clearance (ml/min/1.73 m^2)	Dosage in adults
>60	Usual dose
20 to 60	75% of the usual dose
<20 or patients receiving continuous ambulatory peritoneal dialysis	50% of the usual dose

Pharmacodynamics
Antibacterial action: Cefixime is primarily bactericidal; it acts by binding to penicillin-binding proteins in the bacterial cell wall, thereby inhibiting cell-wall synthesis. It is used in the treatment of otitis media caused by *Haemophilus influenzae* (penicillinase- and nonpeni-

cillinase-producing), *Moraxella (Branhamella) catarrhalis* (which is penicillinase-producing), and *Streptococcus pyogenes* (although efficacy against *S. pyogenes* was studied in fewer than 10 patients). Substantial drug resistance has been noted. Cefixime was also active in the treatment of acute bronchitis and acute exacerbations of chronic bronchitis caused by *S. pneumoniae* and *H. influenzae* (penicillinase- and non-penicillinase-producing), pharyngitis and tonsillitis caused by *S. pyogenes,* and uncomplicated urinary tract infections caused by *Escherichia coli* and *Proteus mirabilis.*

Pharmacokinetics
● *Absorption:* Cefixime is well absorbed from the GI tract. Absorption is delayed by food, but the total amount absorbed is not affected.
● *Distribution:* Cefixime is widely distributed. It enters the CSF in patients with inflamed meninges. It is about 65% bound to plasma proteins.
● *Metabolism:* About 50% of the drug is metabolized.
● *Excretion:* Cefixime is excreted primarily in the urine. The elimination half-life in patients with normal renal function is 3 to 4 hours. In patients with end-stage renal disease, half-life may be prolonged to 11½ hours.

Contraindications and precautions
Cefixime is contraindicated in patients with known allergy to cephalosporins. Use cautiously in patients with a history of hypersensitivity to penicillins or other drugs. Cross-hypersensitivity has been demonstrated in about 10% of patients with a known penicillin allergy.

As with other broad-spectrum antibiotics, pseudomembranous colitis has been reported in patients that have received cefixime. Symptoms can occur during or after therapy. Administer cautiously to patients with a history of GI disease, particularly colitis.

Interactions
None reported.

Effects on diagnostic tests
Cefixime may cause false-positive results in urine glucose tests utilizing cupric sulfate (Benedict's reagent or Clinitest); use glucose oxidase tests (Clinistix or Tes-Tape) instead. Cefixime may cause false-positive results in tests for urine ketones that utilize nitroprusside (but not nitroferricyanide).

False-positive direct Coombs' test results have been seen with other cephalosporins.

Adverse reactions
● CNS: headache, dizziness.
● DERM: rashes, urticaria, pruritus, *Stevens-Johnson syndrome, erythema multiforme, toxic epidermal necrolysis.*
● GI: diarrhea, loose stools, abdominal pain, dyspepsia, nausea, vomiting, *pseudomembranous colitis.*
● GU: vaginitis, candidiasis, transient elevations of BUN or creatinine levels, renal dysfunction.
● HEMA: transient thrombocytopenia, leukopenia, and eosinophilia; *aplastic anemia;* hemolytic anemia; hemorrhage.
● Hepatic: hepatic dysfunction; cholestasis; transient elevations of AST (SGOT), ALT (SGPT), and alkaline phosphatase levels.
● Other: hypersensitivity reactions, drug fever, *anaphylaxis,* superinfection.

Overdose and treatment
No specific antidote available. Gastric lavage and supportive treatment are recommended. Peritoneal dialysis and hemodialysis will remove substantial quantities of the drug.

Studies in volunteers revealed no unusual effects after acute ingestion of 2 g of cefixime.

▶ **Special considerations**
Besides those relevant to all *cephalosporins,* consider the following recommendations.
● Cefixime is the first orally active, third-generation cephalosporin that is effective with once-a-day dosage.
● The manufacturer suggests that tablets should not be substituted for suspension when treating otitis media.
● Patients with antibiotic-induced diarrhea should be evaluated for overgrowth of pseudomembranous colitis caused by *Clostridium difficile.* Mild cases usually respond to discontinuation of the drug; moderate to severe cases may require fluid, electrolyte, and protein supplementation. Oral vancomycin is the drug of choice for the treatment of antibiotic-associated *C. difficile* pseudomembranous colitis.
● Acute hypersensitivity reactions should be treated immediately. Emergency measures, such as airway management, pressor amines, epinephrine, oxygen, antihistamines, and corticosteroids, may be required.
● Some cephalosporins may cause seizures, especially in patients with renal failure who receive full therapeutic dosages. If seizures occur, the drug should be discontinued and anticonvulsant therapy initiated.

Information for the patient
● Advise patient to report any unpleasant effects, such as itching, rash, or severe diarrhea. Note that diarrhea is the most common adverse GI effect.
● Advise the patient that the oral suspension is stable for 14 days after reconstitution and does not require refrigeration.

Pediatric use
The incidence of adverse GI effects in children receiving oral suspension is similar to those in adults receiving tablets.

Breast-feeding
Distribution in breast milk is unknown. The manufacturer recommends that discontinuation of breast-feeding should be considered during cefixime therapy.

cefmetazole sodium
Zefazone

● Pharmacologic classification: second-generation cephalosporin
● Therapeutic classification: antibiotic
● Pregnancy risk category B

How supplied
Available by prescription only
Injection: 1 g, 2 g

Indications, route, and dosage

Serious respiratory, urinary, skin and soft-tissue, abdominal, and pelvic infections caused by susceptible organisms
Adults: 1 to 8 g I.V. total daily dose divided q 6 to 12 hours.

Surgical prophylaxis
Adults: 2 g I.V. administered 30 to 90 minutes before the procedure.

Dosage in renal failure
Adults: If creatinine clearance is 50 to 90 ml/min, dosage is 1 to 2 g I.V. q 12 hours; if 30 to 50 ml/min, 1 to 2 g I.V. q 16 hours; if 10 to 30 ml/min, 1 to 2 g I.V. q 24 hours; if < 10 ml/min, 1 to 2 g I.V. q 48 hours.

Pharmacodynamics
Antibacterial action: Cefmetazole is primarily bactericidal; however, it may be bacteriostatic. Activity depends on the organism, tissue penetration, drug dosage, and rate of organism multiplication. It acts by adhering to bacterial penicillin-binding proteins, thereby inhibiting cell wall synthesis.

Cefmetazole's spectrum of activity resembles that of other second-generation cephalosporins. It is active against many gram-positive organisms and enteric gram-negative bacilli, including *Escherichia coli* and other coliform bacteria. *Staphylococcus aureus* (penicillinase- and nonpenicillinase-producing), *Staphylococcus epidermidis,* streptococci, *Klebsiella, Haemophilus influenzae,* and *Bacteroides* species (including *B. fragilis*). *Enterobacter, Pseudomonas, Acinetobacter, Serratia marcescens, Citrobacter freundii,* and methicillin-resistant staphylococci are generally resistant to cefmetazole.

Pharmacokinetics
● *Absorption:* Cefmetazole is not absorbed from the GI tract and must be given parenterally. Peak serum levels occur 30 to 45 minutes after an I.M. dose.
● *Distribution:* Cefmetazole is distributed widely in most body tissues and fluids, including the gallbladder, liver, kidney, bone, sputum, bile, and pleural and synovial fluids. CSF penetration is poor. Cefmetazole is 65% protein-bound.
● *Metabolism:* Only about 15% of a dose is metabolized, probably in the liver.
● *Excretion:* Cefmetazole is excreted primarily in the urine by renal tubular secretion and glomerular filtration. Elimination half-life is approximately 1.5 hours in patients with normal renal function. Patients with renal dysfunction require dosage adjustment.

Contraindications and precautions
Cefmetazole is contraindicated in patients with known hypersensitivity to any cephalosporin. It should be used with caution in patients with penicillin allergy.

Interactions
Probenecid competitively inhibits renal tubular secretion of cephalosporins, resulting in higher, prolonged serum levels of these drugs.

Concomitant use of cefmetazole with nephrotoxic agents (vancomycin, colistin, polymyxin B, or aminoglycosides) or loop diuretics increases the risk of nephrotoxicity. Concomitant use with bacteriostatic agents (tetracyclines, erythromycin, or chloramphenicol) may impair cefmetazole's bactericidal activity. Concomitant use with alcohol may cause disulfiram-like reactions.

Effects on diagnostic tests
Cefmetazole causes false-positive results of urine glucose tests that use cupric sulfate (Benedict's reagent or Clinitest); use glucose oxidase tests (Clinistrix or Tes-Tape) instead.

Cefmetazole may cause positive Coombs' test results and may elevate liver function test results.

Adverse reactions
● CNS: headache, vertigo, dizziness.
● DERM: rash, pruritus, erythema.
● GI: nausea, vomiting, diarrhea, anorexia, abdominal pain, loose stools, *pseudomembranous colitis.*
● GU: nephrotoxicity.
● HEMA: thrombocytopenia, neutropenia, anemia, eosinophilia, hypoprothrombinemia.
● Other: *hypersensitivity* (erythema multiforme, rash, polyarthritis, fever, dyspnea), bacterial and fungal superinfection.

Note: Drug should be discontinued if signs of toxicity, immediate hypersensitivity reaction, serum sickness, or hypoprothrombinemia occur or if severe diarrhea indicates pseudomembranous colitis; consider alternative therapy if the following symptoms occur: fever, eosinophilia, hematuria, neutropenia, hypoprothrombinemia, or unexplained elevations in BUN or serum creatinine levels.

Overdose and treatment
Clinical signs of overdose include neuromuscular hypersensitivity. Seizure may follow high CNS concentrations. Hypoprothrombinemia and bleeding may occur; they may be treated with vitamin K or blood products. Some cefmetazole may be removed by hemodialysis.

▶ Special considerations
● For most cephalosporin-sensitive organisms, cefmetazole offers little advantage over other cephalosporins.
● Concomitant use with alcohol will lead to disulfiram-like reactions. Use cautiously with home I.V. antibiotic patients who drink alcohol, or consider alternative drug therapy.
● Cefmetazole injection contains 2 mEq of sodium per gram of drug.
● Manufacturer does not recommend I.M. dosing.
● Hypoprothrombinemia may occur. If bleeding occurs or if prothrombin time increases, this can be reversed by administering vitamin K.

Geriatric use
Dosage reduction may be required in patients with diminished renal function. Hypoprothrombinemia and bleeding have been reported most frequently in elderly, malnourished, and debilitated patients.

Pediatric use
The safety and effectiveness of cefmetazole have not been established in children.

Breast-feeding
Trace concentrations have been detected in breast milk. Consider temporarily discontinuing breast-feeding during therapy.

---

cefonicid sodium
Monocid

- Pharmacologic classification: second-generation cephalosporin
- Therapeutic classification: antibiotic
- Pregnancy risk category B

How supplied
Available by prescription only
Injection: 500 mg, 1 g
Infusion: 1 g/dl
Pharmacy bulk package: 10 g

Indications, route, and dosage
Serious lower respiratory, urinary tract, skin, and skin-structure infections; septicemia; bone and joint infections from susceptible organisms
Adults: Usual dosage is 1 g I.V. or I.M. q 24 hours. In life-threatening infections, 2 g q 24 hours.

Total daily dosage is same for I.M. or I.V. administration and depends on susceptibility of organism and severity of infection. Cefonicid should be injected deep I.M. into a large muscle mass, such as the gluteus or the lateral aspect of the thigh.
Dosage in renal failure
In patients with impaired renal function, doses or frequency of administration must be modified according to degree of renal impairment, severity of infection, and susceptibility of organism. To prevent toxic accumulation, reduced dosage may be necessary in patients with creatinine clearance below 60 ml/minute.

DOSAGE IN ADULTS		
Creatinine clearance (ml/min/ 1.73 m²)	Mild to moderate infections	Severe infections
≥ 80	Usual adult dose	Usual adult dose
60 to 79	10 mg/kg q 24 hours	25 mg/kg q 24 hours
40 to 59	8 mg/kg q 24 hours	20 mg/kg q 24 hours
20 to 39	4 mg/kg q 24 hours	15 mg/kg q 24 hours
10 to 19	4 mg/kg q 48 hours	15 mg/kg q 48 hours
5 to 9	4 mg/kg q 3 to 5 days	15 mg/kg q 3 to 5 days
< 5	3 mg/kg q 3 to 5 days	4 mg/kg q 3 to 5 days

Pharmacodynamics
Antibacterial action: Cefonicid is primarily bactericidal; however, it may be bacteriostatic. Activity depends on the organism, tissue penetration, drug dosage, and rate of organism multiplication. It acts by adhering to bacterial penicillin-binding proteins, thereby inhibiting cell wall synthesis.

Cefonicid is active against many gram-positive organisms and enteric gram-negative bacilli, including *Streptococcus pneumoniae, Klebsiella pneumoniae,* *Escherichia coli, Haemophilus influenzae, Proteus mirabilis, Staphylococcus aureus* and *epidermidis,* and *Streptococcus pyogenes;* however, *Bacteroides fragilis, Pseudomonas,* and *Acinetobacter* are resistant to cefonicid. Cefonicid is less effective than cefamandole or cefuroxime against gram-positive cocci; it is twice as effective as cefamandole against *H. influenzae* and slightly more active than cefamandole or cefoxitin against gonococci.

Pharmacokinetics
- *Absorption:* Cefonicid is not absorbed from the GI tract and must be given parenterally; peak serum levels occur 1 to 2 hours after an I.M. dose.
- *Distribution:* Cefonicid is distributed widely into most body tissues and fluids, including the gallbladder, liver, kidneys, bone, sputum, bile, and pleural and synovial fluids; CSF penetration is poor. Cefonicid is 90% to 98% protein-bound. Cefonicid crosses the placenta.
- *Metabolism:* Cefonicid is not metabolized.
- *Excretion:* Cefonicid is excreted primarily in urine by renal tubular secretion and glomerular filtration; small amounts of drug are excreted in breast milk. Elimination half-life is about 3½ to 6 hours in patients with normal renal function; 100 hours in patients with severe renal disease. Hemodialysis partially removes cefonicid.

Contraindications and precautions
Cefonicid is contraindicated in patients with known hypersensitivity to any cephalosporin. It should be used with caution in patients with penicillin allergy, who usually are more susceptible to such reactions.

Interactions
Probenecid competitively inhibits renal tubular secretion of cephalosporins, resulting in higher, prolonged serum levels of these drugs.

Concomitant use with nephrotoxic agents (vancomycin, colistin, polymyxin B, or aminoglycosides) or loop diuretics increases the risk of nephrotoxicity.

Concomitant use with bacteriostatic agents (tetracyclines, erythromycin, or chloramphenicol) may interfere with bactericidal activity.

Effects on diagnostic tests
Cefonicid causes positive Coombs' test results and may elevate liver function test results or prothrombin times. Cefonicid also causes false-positive results in urine glucose tests utilizing cupric sulfate (Benedict's reagent or Clinitest); use glucose oxidase tests (Clinistix or Tes-Tape) instead.

Cefonicid causes false elevations in serum or urine creatinine levels in tests using Jaffé's reaction.

Adverse reactions
- CNS: dizziness, headache, malaise, paresthesias, seizures.
- DERM: maculopapular and erythematous rashes, urticaria.
- GI: *pseudomembranous colitis,* nausea, anorexia, vomiting, diarrhea, glossitis, dyspepsia, abdominal cramps, anal pruritus, tenesmus.
- GU: genital pruritus, vaginitis, hematuria.
- HEMA: transient neutropenia, leukopenia, eosinophilia, anemia.
- Local: at injection site—pain, induration, sterile abscesses, tissue sloughing; phlebitis and thrombophlebitis with I.V. injection.
- Other: hypersensitivity (serum sickness [erythema

multiforme, rashes, polyarthritis, fever]), dyspnea, bacterial and fungal superinfection.

Note: Drug should be discontinued if signs of toxicity, immediate hypersensitivity reaction, or serum sickness occur or if severe diarrhea indicates pseudomembranous colitis; consider alternative therapy if the following symptoms occur: fever, eosinophilia, hematuria, neutropenia, or unexplained elevations in BUN or serum creatinine levels.

Overdose and treatment
Clinical signs of overdose include neuromuscular hypersensitivity. Seizure may follow high CNS concentrations. Some cefonicid may be removed by hemodialysis.

▶ **Special considerations**
Besides those relevant to all *cephalosporins,* consider the following recommendations.
● When cefonicid is used for surgical prophylaxis, administer 1 hour before surgery.
● For patients on sodium restrictions, note that cefonicid injection contains 3.7 mEq of sodium per gram of drug.
● Reconstitute I.M. or bolus I.V. dose with sterile water for injection. Shake well to ensure complete drug dissolution. Check for precipitate. Discard solution that contains a precipitate.
● Administer deep I.M. dose into a large muscle mass to decrease pain and local irritation. Rotate injection sites. Apply ice to site after administration to reduce pain. Do not inject more than 1 g into a single I.M. site.
● For I.V. infusion, further dilute drug in 50 to 100 ml of recommended fluid. Administer I.V. bolus slowly over 3 to 5 minutes directly or through I.V. tubing if solution is compatible.
● Reconstituted solution is stable at room temperature for 24 hours; if refrigerated, for 72 hours. Slight yellowing of solution does not indicate loss of potency.
● Because cefonicid is dialyzable, patients undergoing treatment with hemodialysis may require dosage adjustment.

Geriatric use
Reduced dosage may be required in patients with diminished renal function.

Pediatric use
Safety in children has not been established.

Breast-feeding
Cefonicid distributes into breast milk and should be used with caution in breast-feeding women.

---

cefoperazone sodium
Cefobid

● Pharmacologic classification: third-generation cephalosporin
● Therapeutic classification: antibiotic
● Pregnancy risk category B

How supplied
Available by prescription only
Parenteral: 1 g, 2 g
Infusion: 1 g, 2 g piggyback

Indications, route, and dosage
Serious respiratory tract, intra-abdominal, gynecologic, and skin infections; bacteremia; and septicemia caused by susceptible organisms
Adults: Usual dosage is 1 to 2 g q 12 hours I.M. or I.V. In severe infections or infections caused by less sensitive organisms, the total daily dosage or frequency may be increased up to 16 g/day in certain situations.
Dosage in renal failure
No dosage adjustment is usually necessary in patients with renal impairment. However, dosages of 4 g/day should be given cautiously to patients with hepatic disease. Adults with combined hepatic and renal function impairment should not receive more than 1 g (base) daily without serum determinations. In patients who are receiving hemodialysis treatments, a dose should be scheduled to follow hemodialysis.

Pharmacodynamics
Antibacterial action: Cefoperazone is primarily bactericidal; however, it may be bacteriostatic. Activity depends on the organism, tissue penetration, drug dosage, and rate of organism multiplication. It acts by adhering to bacterial penicillin-binding proteins, thereby inhibiting cell wall synthesis. Third-generation cephalosporins appear more active against some beta-lactamase-producing gram-negative organisms.

Cefoperazone is active against some gram-positive organisms and many enteric gram-negative bacilli, including *Streptococcus pneumoniae* and *Streptococcus pyogenes, Staphylococcus aureus* (penicillinase- and nonpenicillinase-producing), *Staphylococcus epidermidis,* enterococcus, *Escherichia coli, Klebsiella, Haemophilus influenzae, Enterobacter, Citrobacter, Proteus,* some *Pseudomonas* species (including *Pseudomonas aeruginosa),* and *Bacteroides fragilis. Acinetobacter* and *Listeria* usually are resistant. Cefoperazone is less effective than moxalactam, cefotaxime, or ceftizoxime against Enterobacteriaceae but is slightly more active than those drugs against *Pseudomonas aeruginosa.*

Pharmacokinetics
● *Absorption:* Cefoperazone is not absorbed from the GI tract and must be given parenterally; peak serum levels occur 1 to 2 hours after an I.M. dose.
● *Distribution:* Cefoperazone is distributed widely into most body tissues and fluids, including the gallbladder, liver, kidneys, bone, sputum, bile, and pleural and synovial fluids; CSF penetration is achieved in patients with inflamed meninges. Cefoperazone crosses the placenta. Protein binding is dose-dependent and decreases as serum levels rise; average is 82% to 93%.
● *Metabolism:* Cefoperazone is not substantially metabolized.
● *Excretion:* Cefoperazone is excreted primarily *in bile;* some drug is excreted in urine by renal tubular secretion and glomerular filtration; and small amounts, in breast milk. Elimination half-life is about 1½ to 2½ hours in patients with normal hepatorenal function; biliary obstruction or cirrhosis prolongs half-life to about 3½ to 7 hours. Hemodialysis removes cefoperazone.

Contraindications and precautions
Cefoperazone is contraindicated in patients with known hypersensitivity to any cephalosporin. It should be used with caution in patients with penicillin allergy, who usually are more susceptible to such reactions; in patients with coagulopathy; and in elderly, debilitated, or mal-

---

nourished patients who are at greater risk of bleeding complications.

Interactions
Concomitant use with aminoglycosides results in synergistic activity against *Pseudomonas aeruginosa* and *Serratia marcescens;* such combined use slightly increases the risk of nephrotoxicity.

Concomitant use with clavulanic acid results in synergistic activity against many Enterobacteriaceae, *Bacteroides fragilis, P. aeruginosa,* and *S. aureus.*

Concomitant use with alcohol may cause disulfiram-like reactions (flushing, sweating, tachycardia, headache, and abdominal cramping).

Probenicid competitively inhibits renal tubular secretions of cephalosporins, causing prolonged serum levels of these drugs.

Effects on diagnostic tests
Cephalosporins cause false-positive results in urine glucose tests utilizing cupric sulfate (Benedict's reagent or Clinitest); use glucose oxidase (Clinistix or Tes-Tape) instead.

Cefoperazone may cause positive Coombs' test results, and elevated liver function test results and prothrombin times.

Adverse reactions
● CNS: headache, malaise, paresthesias, dizziness, seizures.
● DERM: maculopapular and erythematous rashes, urticaria.
● GI: *pseudomembranous colitis,* nausea, anorexia, vomiting, *diarrhea,* glossitis, dyspepsia, abdominal cramps, tenesmus, anal pruritus.
● GU: genital pruritus, hematuria.
● HEMA: transient neutropenia, eosinophilia, hemolytic anemia, *hypoprothrombinemia, bleeding.*
● Hepatic: mildly elevated liver enzyme levels.
● Local: at injection site – pain, induration, sterile abscesses, temperature elevation, tissue sloughing; phlebitis and thrombophlebitis with I.V. injection.
● Other: hypersensitivity (serum sickness [erythema multiforme, rashes, polyarthritis, fever]), bacterial and fungal superinfection.
Note: Drug should be discontinued if signs of toxicity, immediate hypersensitivity reaction, serum sickness, or hypoprothrombinema occur or if severe diarrhea indicates pseudomembranous colitis; alternative therapy should be considered if the patient develops fever, eosinophilia, hematuria, or neutropenia.

Overdose and treatment
Clinical signs of overdose include neuromuscular hypersensitivity. Seizure may follow high CNS concentrations. Hypoprothrombinemia and bleeding may occur and may require treatment with vitamin K or blood products. Hemodialysis will remove cefoperazone.

▶ Special considerations
Besides those relevant to all *cephalosporins,* consider the following recommendations.
● Diarrhea may be more common with cefoperazone than with other cephalosporins because of the high degree of biliary excretion.
● Patients with biliary disease may need lower doses.
● For patients on sodium restriction, note that cefoperazone injection contains 1.5 mEq of sodium per gram of drug.

● To prepare I.M. injection, use the appropriate diluent, including sterile water for injection or bacteriostatic water for injection. Follow manufacturer's recommendations for mixing drug with sterile water for injection and lidocaine 2% injection. Final solution for I.M. injection will contain 0.5% lidocaine and will be less painful upon administration (recommended for concentrations of 250 mg/ml or greater). Cefoperazone should be injected deep I.M. into a large muscle mass, such as the gluteus or the lateral aspect of the thigh.
● Store drug in refrigerator and away from light before reconstituting.
● Allow solution to stand after reconstituting to allow foam to dissipate and solution to clear. Solution can be shaken vigorously to ensure complete drug dissolution.
● After reconstitution, solution is stable for 24 hours at a controlled room temperature or 5 days if refrigerated. Protecting drug from light is unnecessary.
● Because cefoperazone is dialyzable, patients undergoing treatment with hemodialysis may require dosage adjustment.
● Concomitant use with alcohol can lead to disulfiram-like reaction. Use this drug cautiously in home antibiotic therapy patients who drink alcohol, or consider alternate drug therapy.

Geriatric use
Hypoprothrombinemia and bleeding have been reported more frequently in elderly patients. Use with caution, and monitor prothrombin times and check for signs of abnormal bleeding.

Pediatric use
Safety and effectiveness in children under age 12 have not been established.

Breast-feeding
Cefoperazone distributes into breast milk and should be used with caution in breast-feeding women.

---

ceforanide
Precef

● **Pharmacologic classification:** second-generation cephalosporin
● **Therapeutic classification:** antibiotic
● **Pregnancy risk category B**

How supplied
Available by prescription only
Injection: 500 mg, 1 g
Infusion: 500 mg, 1 g piggyback

Indications, route, and dosage
Serious lower respiratory, urinary, skin, and bone and joint infections; endocarditis; and septicemia from susceptible organisms
Adults: 0.5 to 1 g I.V. or I.M. q 12 hours.
Children: 20 to 40 mg/kg/day in equally divided doses q 12 hours.
Prophylaxis of surgical infections
Adults: 0.5 to 1 g I.M. or I.V. 1 hour before surgery.

Total daily dosage is the same for I.M. or I.V. administration and depends on susceptibility of organism and severity of infection. Ceforanide should be injected deep

---

I.M. into a large muscle mass, such as the gluteus or lateral aspect of the thigh.

Dosage in renal failure

In patients with impaired renal function, doses or frequency of administration must be modified according to the degree of renal impairment, severity of infection, and susceptibility of organism. To prevent toxic accumulation, reduced dosage may be required in patients with creatinine clearance below 60 ml/minute.

Creatinine clearance (ml/min/1.73 m²)	Dosage in adults
≥60	Usual adult dose
20 to 59	500 mg to 1 g q 24 hr
5 to 19	500 mg to 1 g q 48 hr
<5	500 mg to 1 g q 48 to 72 hr

Pharmacodynamics

Antibacterial action: Ceforanide is primarily bactericidal; however, it may be bacteriostatic. Activity depends on the organism, tissue penetration, drug dosage, and rate of organism multiplication. It acts by adhering to bacterial penicillin-binding proteins, thereby inhibiting cell wall synthesis.

Ceforanide is active against many gram-positive organisms and enteric gram-negative bacilli, including *Streptococcus pneumoniae, Klebsiella pneumoniae, Escherichia coli, Haemophilus influenzae, Proteus mirabilis, Staphylococcus aureus* and *epidermidis,* and *Streptococcus pyogenes; Bacteroides fragilis, Pseudomonas,* and *Acinetobacter* are resistant. Ceforanide is less effective than cefamandole or cefuroxime against *S. aureus* or *H. influenzae.*

Pharmacokinetics

● *Absorption:* Ceforanide is not absorbed from the GI tract and must be given parenterally; peak serum levels occur 1 hour after an I.M. dose.
● *Distribution:* Ceforanide is distributed widely into most body tissues and fluids, including the gallbladder, liver, kidneys, bone, skeletal muscle, uterus, jejunum, myocardium, and bile. CSF penetration is poor. It is unknown if ceforanide crosses the placenta. Ceforanide is about 80% protein-bound.
● *Metabolism:* Ceforanide is not metabolized.
● *Excretion:* Ceforanide is excreted primarily in urine by renal tubular secretion and glomerular filtration; elimination half-life is 2½ to 3½ hours in patients with normal renal function; 5½ to 25 hours in patients with end-stage renal disease. Hemodialysis removes ceforanide.

Contraindications and precautions

Ceforanide is contraindicated in patients with known hypersensitivity to any cephalosporin. It should be used with caution in patients with penicillin allergy, who usually are more susceptible to such reactions.

Interactions

Probenecid competitively inhibits renal tubular secretion of cephalosporins, resulting in higher, prolonged serum levels of these drugs.

Concomitant use of ceforanide with nephrotoxic agents (vancomycin, colistin, polymixin B, or aminoglycosides) or loop diuretics increases the risk of nephrotoxicity. Concomitant use with bacteriostatic agents (tetracyclines, erythromycin, or chloramphenicol) may impair its bactericidal activity.

Effects on diagnostic tests

Cephalosporins cause false-positive results in urine glucose tests utilizing cupric sulfate (Benedict's reagent or Clinitest); use glucose oxidase tests (Clinistix or Tes-Tape) instead. Ceforanide causes false elevations in serum or urine creatinine levels in tests using Jaffé's reaction.

Ceforanide may elevate results of liver function tests and may cause positive Coombs' test results.

Adverse reactions

● CNS: confusion, headache, lethargy, seizures.
● DERM: maculopapular and erythematous rashes, urticaria.
● GI: *pseudomembranous colitis,* nausea, anorexia, vomiting, diarrhea, glossitis, dyspepsia, abdominal cramps.
● GU: genital pruritus, hematuria, nephrotoxicity.
● HEMA: transient neutropenia, leukopenia, eosinophilia, thrombocytopenia, anemia.
● Hepatic: transient elevation in liver enzymes.
● Local: at injection site – pain, induration, sterile abscesses, tissue sloughing; phlebitis and thrombophlebitis with I.V. injection.
● Other: hypersensitivity (dyspnea, serum sickness [erythema multiforme, rashes, polyarthritis, fever]), bacterial and fungal superinfection.

Note: Drug should be discontinued if signs of toxicity, immediate hypersensitivity reaction, or serum sickness occur or if severe diarrhea indicates pseudomembranous colitis; alternative therapy should be considered if patient develops fever, eosinophilia, hematuria, neutropenia, or unexplained elevations in BUN or serum creatinine levels.

Overdose and treatment

Clinical signs of overdose include neuromuscular hypersensitivity. Seizure may follow high CNS concentrations. Hemodialysis removes ceforanide.

▶ Special considerations

Besides those relevant to all *cephalosporins,* consider the following recommendations.
● Administer deep I.M. into a large muscle mass to prevent tissue damage.
● Administer I.V. dose slowly with compatible solution.
● Upon reconstitution, ceforanide injection may appear cloudy. Let it stand briefly to allow solution to deaerate and clarify. Check package insert for compatible diluents.
● Because ceforanide is hemodialyzable, patients undergoing treatment with hemodialysis may require dosage adjustments.

Geriatric use

Reduced dosage may be required in patients with reduced renal function.

Pediatric use

Use in infants younger under age 1 is not recommended.

Breast-feeding

Safe use has not been established. Use with caution in breast-feeding women.

---

cefotaxime sodium
Claforan

- Pharmacologic classification: third-generation cephalosporin
- Therapeutic classification: antibiotic
- Pregnancy risk category B

How supplied
Available by prescription only
Injection: 500 mg, 1 g, 2 g
Pharmacy bulk package: 10-g vial
Infusion: 1 g, 2 g

Indications, route, and dosage
Serious lower respiratory, urinary, CNS, gynecologic, and skin infections; bacteremia; septicemia caused by susceptible organisms
Adults and children weighing more than 50 kg: Usual dosage is 1 g I.V. or I.M. q 6 to 8 hours. Up to 12 g daily can be administered in life-threatening infections.

Total daily dosage is same for I.M. or I.V. administration and depends on susceptibility of organism and severity of infection. Cefotaxime should be injected deep I.M. into a large muscle mass, such as the gluteus or the lateral aspect of the thigh.
Children age 1 month to 12 years weighing less than 50 kg: 50 to 180 mg/kg/day in five or six equally divided doses. Higher doses are reserved for serious infections (such as meningitis).
Neonates age 1 to 4 weeks: 50 mg/kg I.V. q 8 hours.
Neonates age 0 to 1 week: 50 mg/kg I.V. q 12 hours.
Dosage in renal failure
In patients with impaired renal function, dose or frequency of administration must be modified according to the degree of renal impairment, severity of infection, and susceptibility of organism. To prevent toxic accumulation, reduced dosage may be required in patients with creatinine clearance below 20 ml/minute.

Pharmacodynamics
Antibacterial action: Cefotaxime is primarily bactericidal; however, it may be bacteriostatic. Activity depends on the organism, tissue penetration, drug dosage, and rate of organism multiplication. It acts by adhering to bacterial penicillin-binding proteins, thereby inhibiting cell wall synthesis.

Third-generation cephalosporins appear more active against some beta-lactamase-producing gram-negative organisms.

Cefotaxime is active against some gram-positive organisms and many enteric gram-negative bacilli, including streptococci (*Streptococcus pneumoniae* and *pyogenes*), *Staphylococcus aureus* (penicillinase- and nonpenicillinase-producing), *Staphylococcus epidermidis, Escherichia coli, Klebsiella* species, *Haemophilus influenzae, Enterobacter* species, *Proteus* species, and *Peptostreptococcus* species, and some strains of *Pseudomonas aeruginosa. Listeria* and *Acinetobacter* are often resistant. The active metabolite of cefotaxime, desacetylcefotaxime, may act synergistically with the parent drug against some bacterial strains.

Pharmacokinetics
- *Absorption:* Cefotaxime is not absorbed from the GI tract and must be given parenterally; peak serum levels occur 30 minutes after an I.M. dose.
- *Distribution:* Cefotaxime is distributed widely into most body tissues and fluids, including the gallbladder, liver, kidneys, bone, sputum, bile, and pleural and synovial fluids. Unlike most other cephalosporins, cefotaxime has adequate CSF penetration when meninges are inflamed; it crosses the placenta. Cefotaxime is 13% to 38% protein-bound.
- *Metabolism:* Cefotaxime is metabolized partially to an active metabolite, desacetylcefotaxime.
- *Excretion:* Cefotaxime and its metabolites are excreted primarily in urine by renal tubular secretion; some drug may be excreted in breast milk. About 25% of cefotaxime is excreted in urine as the active metabolite; elimination half-life in normal adults is about 1 to 1½ hours for cefotaxime and about 1½ to 2 hours for desacetylcefotaxime; severe renal impairment prolongs cefotaxime's half-life to 11½ hours and that of the metabolite to as much as 56 hours. Hemodialysis removes both the drug and its metabolites.

Contraindications and precautions
Cefotaxime is contraindicated in patients with known hypersensitivity to any cephalosporin. It should be used with caution in patients with penicillin allergy, who usually are more susceptible to such reactions.

Interactions
Concomitant use with aminoglycosides results in apparent synergistic activity against *Enterobacteriaceae* and some strains of *Pseudomonas aeruginosa* and *Serratia marcescens;* such combined use may increase the risk of nephrotoxicity slightly.

Probenecid may block renal tubular secretion of cefotaxime and prolong its half-life.

Effects on diagnostic tests
Cephalosporins cause false-positive results in urine glucose tests utilizing cupric sulfate (Benedict's reagent or Clinitest); use glucose oxidase (Clinistix or Tes-Tape) instead. Cefotaxime also causes false elevations in urine creatinine levels in tests using Jaffé's reaction.

Cefotaxime may cause positive Coombs' tests results and elevations of liver function test results.

Adverse reactions
- CNS: headache, malaise, paresthesia, dizziness, seizures.
- DERM: maculopapular and erythematous rashes, urticaria.
- GI: *pseudomembranous colitis,* nausea, anorexia, vomiting, *diarrhea,* glossitis, dyspepsia, abdominal cramps, tenesmus, anal pruritus.
- GU: genital pruritus, hematuria.
- HEMA: transient neutropenia, eosinophilia, hemolytic anemia.
- Local: at injection site – pain, induration, sterile abscesses, temperature elevation, tissue sloughing; phlebitis and thrombophlebitis with I.V. injection.
- Other: hypersensitivity (serum sickness [erythema multiforme, rashes, urticaria, polyarthritis, fever]), dyspnea, bacterial and fungal superinfection.

Note: Drug should be discontinued if signs of toxicity, immediate hypersensitivity reaction, or serum sickness occur or if severe diarrhea indicates pseudomembranous colitis; alternative therapy should be considered if

---

patient develops fever, eosinophilia, hematuria, or neutropenia.

Overdose and treatment
Clinical signs of overdose include neuromuscular hypersensitivity. Seizure may follow high CNS concentrations. Cefotaxime may be removed by hemodialysis.

▶ Special considerations
Besides those relevant to all *cephalosporins*, consider the following recommendations.
● For patients on sodium restriction, note that cefotaxime contains 2.2 mEq of sodium per gram of drug.
● For I.M. injection, add 2 ml, 3 ml, or 5 ml of sterile or bacteriostatic water for injection to each 500-mg, 1-g, or 2-g vial. Shake well to dissolve drug completely. Check solution for particles and discoloration. Color ranges from light yellow to amber.
● Do not inject more than 1 g into a single I.M. site to prevent pain and tissue reaction.
● Do not mix with any aminoglycoside or with sodium bicarbonate or any fluid with a pH above 7.5.
● For I.V. use, reconstitute all strengths of an I.V. dose with 10 ml of sterile water for injection. For infusion bottles, add 50 to 100 ml of 0.9% NaCl injection or 5% dextrose injection. May be further reconstituted to 50 to 1,000 ml with fluids recommended by manufacturer.
● Administer cefotaxime by direct intermittent I.V. infusion over 3 to 5 minutes. Cefotaxime also may be given more slowly into a flowing I.V. line of compatible solution.
● Solution is stable for 24 hours at room temperature or at least 5 days under refrigeration. Cefotaxime may be stored in disposable glass or plastic syringes.
● Because cefotaxime is hemodialyzable, patients undergoing treatment with hemodialysis may require dosage adjustment.

Geriatric use
Use with caution in elderly patients with diminished renal function.

Pediatric use
Cefotaxime may be used in neonates, infants, and children.

Breast-feeding
Cefotaxime distributes into breast milk and should be used with caution in breast-feeding women.

---

cefotetan disodium
Cefotan

● Pharmacologic classification: second-generation cephalosporin, cephamycin
● Therapeutic classification: antibiotic
● Pregnancy risk category B

How supplied
Available by prescription only
Injection: 1 g, 2 g, 10 g (pharmacy bulk package)
Infusion: 1 g, 2 g piggyback

Indications, route, and dosage
Serious urinary, lower respiratory, gynecologic, skin, intra-abdominal, and bone and joint infections caused by susceptible organisms
Adults: 1 to 2 g I.V. or I.M. q 12 hours for 5 to 10 days. Up to 6 g daily in life-threatening infections.

Total daily dosage is same for I.M. or I.V. administration and depends on the susceptibility of the organism and severity of infection. Cefotetan should be injected deep I.M. into a large muscle mass, such as the gluteus or the lateral aspect of the thigh.
Dosage in renal failure
In patients with impaired renal function, doses or frequency of administration must be modified according to the degree of renal impairment, severity of infection, and susceptibility of organism. To prevent toxic accumulation, reduced dosage may be necessary in patients with creatinine clearance below 30 ml/minute.

Creatinine clearance (ml/min/1.73 m²)	Dosage in adults
> 30	Usual adult dose
10 to 30	Usual adult dose q 24 hours; or one half the usual adult dose q 12 hours
< 10	Usual adult dose q 48 hours; or one fourth the usual adult dose q 12 hours
Hemodialysis patients	One fourth the usual adult dose q 24 hours on the days between hemodialysis sessions; and one half the usual adult dose on the day of hemodialysis

Pharmacodynamics
Antibacterial action: Cefotetan is primarily bactericidal; however, it may be bacteriostatic. Activity depends on the organism, tissue penetration, drug dosage, and rate of organism multiplication. It acts by adhering to bacterial penicillin-binding proteins, thereby inhibiting cell wall synthesis.

Cefotetan is active against many gram-positive organisms and enteric gram-negative bacilli, including streptococci, *Staphylococcus aureus* (penicillinase- and nonpenicillinase-producing), *Staphylococcus epidermidis*, *Escherichia coli*, *Klebsiella* species, *Enterobacter* species, *Proteus* species, *Haemophilus influenzae*, *Neisseria gonorrhoeae*, and *Bacteroides* species (including some strains of *B. fragilis*); however, some *B. fragilis* strains, *Pseudomonas*, and *Acinetobacter* are resistant to cefotetan. Most Enterobacteriaceae are more susceptible to cefotetan than to other second-generation cephalosporins.

Pharmacokinetics
● *Absorption:* Cefotetan is not absorbed from the GI tract and must be given parenterally; peak serum levels occur 1½ to 3 hours after an I.M. dose.
● *Distribution:* Cefotetan is distributed widely into most body tissues and fluids, including the gallbladder, liver, kidneys, bone, sputum, bile, and pleural and synovial fluids; CSF penetration is poor. Biliary concentration levels of cefotetan can be up to 20 times higher than

---

serum concentrations in patients with good gallbladder function. Cefotetan crosses the placenta; it is 75% to 90% protein-bound.
● *Metabolism:* Cefotetan is not metabolized.
● *Excretion:* Cefotetan is excreted primarily in urine by glomerular filtration and some renal tubular secretion. Small amounts of the drug are excreted in breast milk. Elimination half-life is about 3 to 4½ hours in patients with normal renal function.

Contraindications and precautions
Cefotetan is contraindicated in patients with known hypersensitivity to any cephalosporin. It should be used with caution in patients with penicillin allergy, who usually are more susceptible to such reactions, and in patients with coagulopathy, and elderly, debilitated, or malnourished patients, who are at greater risk of bleeding complications.

Interactions
Concomitant use of cefotetan with nephrotoxic agents (vancomycin, colistin, polymixin B, or aminoglycosides) or loop diuretics may increase the risk of nephrotoxicity. Concomitant use of cefotetan with bacteriostatic agents (tetracyclines, erythromycin, or chloramphenicol) may impair its bactericidal activity. Concomitant use with alcohol may cause disulfiram-like reactions (flushing, sweating, tachycardia, headache, and abdominal cramping).

Effects on diagnostic tests
Cefotetan also causes false-positive results in urine glucose tests utilizing cupric sulfate (Benedict's reagent or Clinitest); use glucose oxidase tests (Clinistix or Tes-Tape) instead. Cefotetan causes false elevations in serum or urine creatinine levels in tests using Jaffé's reaction. It may cause positive Coombs' test results and may elevate liver function test results and prothrombin times.

Adverse reactions
● CNS: headache, malaise, paresthesias, dizziness, seizures.
● DERM: maculopapular and erythematous rashes, urticaria.
● GI: *pseudomembranous colitis,* nausea, anorexia, vomiting, *diarrhea,* glossitis, dyspepsia, abdominal cramps, tenesmus, anal pruritus.
● GU: genital pruritus, vaginitis, hematuria, nephrotoxicity.
● HEMA: transient neutropenia, eosinophilia, hemolytic anemia, hypoprothrombinemia, bleeding.
● Local: at injection site – pain, induration, sterile abscesses; phlebitis and thrombophlebitis with I.V. injection.
● Other: hypersensitivity, (serum sickness [erythema multiforme, rashes, polyarthritis, fever]), bacterial or fungal superinfection.
Note: Drug should be discontinued if signs of toxicity, immediate hypersensitivity reaction, serum sickness, or hypoprothrombinemia occur or if severe diarrhea indicates pseudomembranous colitis; alternative therapy should be considered if patient develops fever, eosinophilia, hematuria, neutropenia, or unexplained elevations in BUN or serum creatinine levels.

Overdose and treatment
Clinical signs of overdose include neuromuscular hypersensitivity. Seizure may follow high CNS concentrations. Hypoprothrombinemia and bleeding may occur; they may be treated with vitamin K or blood products. Cefotetan may be removed by hemodialysis.

▶ **Special considerations**
Besides those relevant to all *cephalosporins,* consider the following recommendations.
● For I.V. use, reconstitute with sterile water for injection. Then it may be mixed with 50 to 100 ml of dextrose 5% in water or 0.9% NaCl solution. Infuse intermittently over 30 to 60 minutes.
● For I.M. injection, cefotetan may be reconstituted with sterile water or bacteriostatic water for injection or with normal saline or 0.5% or 1% lidocaine hydrochloride. Shake to dissolve and let solution stand until clear.
● Reconstituted solution remains stable for 24 hours at room temperature of for 96 hours when refrigerated.
● Assess for signs and symptoms of overt and occult bleeding. Monitor vital signs. Check complete blood count differential, platelet levels, and prothrombin time for abnormalities.
● Bleeding can be reversed promptly by administering vitamin K.
● Because cefotetan is hemodialyzable, patients undergoing treatment with hemodialysis may require dosage adjustments.
● Concomitant use with alcohol may cause severe disulfiram-like reactions.

Geriatric use
Hypoprothrombinemia and bleeding have been reported more frequently in elderly and debilitated patients.

Pediatric use
Safe use in children has not been established.

Breast-feeding
Cephalosporins distribute into breast milk and should be used with caution in breast-feeding women. Safe use has not been established.

cefoxitin sodium
Mefoxin

● Pharmacologic classification: second-generation cephalosporin, cephamycin
● Therapeutic classification: antibiotic
● Pregnancy risk category B

How supplied
Available by prescription only
Injection: 1 g, 2 g
Pharmacy bulk package: 10 g
Infusion: 1 g, 2 g in 50-ml or 100-ml container

Indications, route, and dosage
Serious respiratory, genitourinary, skin, soft-tissue, bone and joint, blood, and intra-abdominal infections caused by susceptible organisms
Adults: 1 to 2 g q 6 to 8 hours for uncomplicated forms of infection. Up to 12 g daily in life-threatening infections.
Children: 80 to 160 mg/kg daily given in four to six equally divided doses.

Total daily dosage is same for I.M. or I.V. administration and depends on susceptibility of organism and severity of infection. Cefoxitin should be injected deep I.M. into a large muscle mass, such as the gluteus or lateral aspect of the thigh.

Dosage in renal failure

In patients with impaired renal function, doses or frequency of administration must be modified according to the degree of renal impairment, severity of infection, and susceptibility of organism. To prevent toxic accumulation, reduced dosage may be required in patients with creatinine clearance below 50 ml/minute.

Creatinine clearance (ml/min/1.73 m²)	Dosage in adults
>50	Usual adult dose
30 to 50	1 to 2 g q 8 to 12 hours
10 to 29	1 to 2 g q 12 to 24 hours
5 to 9	500 mg to 1 g q 12 to 24 hours
<5	500 mg to 1 g q 24 to 48 hours

Pharmacodynamics

Antibacterial action: Cefoxitin is primarily bactericidal; however, it may be bacteriostatic. Activity depends on the organism, tissue penetration, drug dosage, and rate of organism multiplication. It acts by adhering to bacterial penicillin-binding proteins, thereby inhibiting cell wall synthesis.

Cefoxitin is active against many gram-positive organisms and enteric gram-negative bacilli, including *Escherichia coli* and other coliform bacteria, *Staphylococcus aureus* (penicillinase- and nonpenicillinase-producing), *Staphylococcus epidermidis*, streptococci, *Klebsiella*, *Haemophilus influenzae*, and *Bacteroides* species (including *B. fragilis*). *Enterobacter*, *Pseudomonas*, and *Acinetobacter* are resistant to cefoxitin.

Pharmacokinetics

• *Absorption:* Cefoxitin is not absorbed from the GI tract and must be given parenterally; peak serum levels occur 20 to 30 minutes after an I.M. dose.
• *Distribution:* Cefoxitin is distributed widely into most body tissues and fluids, including the gallbladder, liver, kidneys, bone, sputum, bile, and pleural and synovial fluids; CSF penetration is poor. Cefoxitin crosses the placenta; it is 50% to 80% protein-bound.
• *Metabolism:* About 2% of a cefoxitin dose is metabolized.
• *Excretion:* Cefoxitin is excreted primarily in urine by renal tubular secretion and glomerular filtration; small amounts of drug are excreted in breast milk. Elimination half-life is about ½ to 1 hour in patients with normal renal function; half-life is prolonged in patients with severe renal dysfunction to 6½ to 21½ hours. Cefoxitin can be removed by hemodialysis but not by peritoneal dialysis.

Contraindications and precautions

Cefoxitin is contraindicated in patients with known hypersensitivity to any cephalosporin. It should be used with caution in patients with penicillin allergy.

Interactions

Probenecid competitively inhibits renal tubular secretion of cephalosporins, resulting in higher, prolonged serum levels of these drugs.

Concomitant use of cefoxitin with nephrotoxic agents (vancomycin, colistin, polymyxin B, or aminoglycosides) or loop diuretics increases the risk of nephrotoxicity. Concomitant use with bacteriostatic agents (tetracyclines, erythromycin, or chloramphenicol) may impair cefoxitin's bactericidal activity.

Effects on diagnostic tests

Cefoxitin causes false-positive results in urine glucose tests utilizing cupric sulfate (Benedict's reagent or Clinitest); use glucose oxidase tests (Clinistix or Tes-Tape) instead. Cefoxitin also causes false elevations in serum or urine creatinine levels in tests using Jaffé's reaction.

Cefoxitin may elevate liver function test results and may cause positive Coombs' test results.

Adverse reactions

• CNS: headache, malaise, paresthesia, dizziness, *seizures*.
• DERM: maculopapular and erythematous rashes, urticaria.
• GI: *pseudomembranous colitis*, nausea, anorexia, vomiting, diarrhea, glossitis, dyspepsia, abdominal cramps, tenesmus, anal pruritus.
• GU: genital pruritus, vaginitis, hematuria, nephrotoxicity.
• HEMA: transient neutropenia, eosinophilia, *hemolytic anemia*.
• Local: at injection site – pain, induration, sterile abscesses, tissue sloughing; phlebitis and thrombophlebitis with I.V. injection.
• Other: hypersensitivity (serum sickness [erythema multiforme, rashes, polyarthritis, fever]), bacterial and fungal superinfection.

Note: Drug should be discontinued if signs of toxicity, immediate hypersensitivity reaction, or serum sickness occur or if severe diarrhea indicates pseudomembranous colitis; alternative therapy should be considered if the patient develops fever, eosinophilia, hematuria, neutropenia, or unexplained elevations in BUN or serum creatinine levels.

Overdose and treatment

Clinical signs of overdose include neuromuscular hypersensitivity. Seizure may follow high CNS concentrations. Cefoxitin may be removed by hemodialysis.

▶ Special considerations

Besides those relevant to all *cephalosporins*, consider the following recommendations.
• For I.V. use, reconstitute 1 g of cefoxitin with at least 10 ml of sterile water for injection, or 2 g of cefoxitin with 10 to 20 ml. Solutions of dextrose 5% and 0.9% NaCl for injection can also be used.
• Cefoxitin has been associated with thrombophlebitis. Assess I.V. site frequently for signs of infiltration or phlebitis. Change I.V. site every 48 to 72 hours.
• For I.M. injection, reconstitute with 0.5% to 1% lidocaine hydrochloride (without epinephrine) to minimize pain at injection site; or with sterile water for injection, as ordered.
• Administer I.M. dose deep into a large muscle mass. Aspirate before injecting to prevent inadvertent injection into a blood vessel. Rotate injection sites to prevent tissue damage.

• After reconstituting, shake vial and then let stand until clear to ensure complete drug dissolution. Solution is stable for 24 hours at room temperature or for 1 week if refrigerated or 26 weeks if frozen.
• Solution may range from colorless to light amber and may darken during storage. Slight color change does not indicate loss of potency.
• Cefoxitin injection contains 2.3 mEq of sodium per gram of drug.
• Because cefoxitin is hemodialyzable, patients undergoing treatment with hemodialysis may require dosage adjustments.

Geriatric use
Dosage reduction may be necessary in patients with diminished renal function.

Pediatric use
Reduced dosage may be indicated in infants younger than age 3 months. Safety has not been established.

Breast-feeding
Cefoxitin distributes into breast milk and should be used with caution in breast-feeding women.

---

cefprozil
Cefzil

• Pharmacologic classification: second-generation cephalosporin
• Therapeutic classification: antibiotic
• Pregnancy risk category B

How supplied
Available by prescription only
Tablets: 250 mg, 500 mg
Oral suspension: 125 mg/5 ml, 250 mg/5 ml

Indications, route, and dosage
Pharyngitis or tonsillitis caused by **Strepto-coccus pyogenes**
Adults: 500 mg P.O. daily for at least 10 days.
Otitis media caused by **S. pneumoniae, Hae-mophilus influenzae,** *and* **Moraxella (Branha-mella) catarrhalis**
Infants and children age 6 months to 12 years: 15 mg/kg P.O. q 12 hours for 10 days.
Secondary bacterial infections of acute bron-chitis and acute bacterial exacerbation of chronic bronchitis caused by **S. pneumoniae, H. influenzae,** *and* **M. (B.) catarrhalis**
Adults: 500 mg P.O. q 12 hours for 10 days.
Uncomplicated skin and skin structure infec-tions caused by **Staphylococcus aureus** *and* **Streptococcus pyogenes**
Adults: 250 mg P.O. b.i.d., or 500 mg daily to b.i.d.
Dosage adjustment for patients with renal failure
No adjustments are necessary for patients with cre-atinine clearance over 30 ml/minute. For patients with creatinine clearance of 30 ml/minute or less, dose should be reduced by 50%; however, dosing interval remains unchanged. Because drug is partially removed by hemodialysis, it should be administered after the hemodialysis session.

Pharmacodynamics
Antibiotic action: Cefprozil interferes with bacterial cell wall synthesis during cell replication, leading to osmotic instability and cell lysis. Bactericidal or bacteriostatic, depending on concentration.

Pharmacokinetics
Note: Pharmacokinetic data is derived from investi-gational studies that employed an oral capsule for-mulation which is not commercially available.
• *Absorption:* Cefprozil is approximately 95% absorbed from the GI tract. Peak levels occur within 1½ hours of a dose. Food did not interfere with the capsule for-mulation; it is unknown if food will interfere with ab-sorption of tablets or oral suspension.
• *Distribution:* Drug is about 36% protein-bound.
• *Metabolism:* Cefprozil is probably metabolized by the liver; plasma half-life increases only slightly in patients with impaired hepatic function.
• *Excretion:* About 60% of a dose is recovered un-changed in the urine. The plasma half-life is 1.3 hours in patients with normal renal function; 2 hours, impaired hepatic function; and 5.2 to 5.9 hours, end-stage renal disease. Drug is removed by hemodialysis.

Contraindications and precautions
Cefprozil is contraindicated in patients with hypersen-sitivity to the drug or any other cephalosporin. Use caution if administering to a patient with a history of hypersensitivity to penicillin because up to 10% of these patients will exhibit cross-sensitivity to a cephalosporin. Also use cautiously in patients with impaired hepatic or renal failure.

Interactions
Concomitant use with aminoglycoside antibiotics may increase the risk of nephrotoxicity of cephalosporins. Probenecid may decrease excretion of cefprozil.

Effects on diagnostic tests
Cephalosporins may produce a false-positive test for urine glucose with tests that use copper reduction method (Benedict's test, Fehling's solution, or Clinitest tablets). Instead, use enzymatic methods (such as Tes-Tape). A false-negative reaction may occur in the fer-ricyanide test for blood glucose.

Adverse reactions
• CNS: dizziness, hyperactivity, headache, nervous-ness, insomnia.
• DERM: rash, urticaria, diaper rash.
• GI: diarrhea, nausea, vomiting, abdominal pain, pseudomembranous colitis.
• GU: elevated serum creatinine level, genital pruritus, vaginitis.
• HEMA: decreased leukocyte count, eosinophilia.
• Hepatic: elevated BUN level, elevated liver enzymes, cholestatic jaundice (rare).
• Other: superinfection, hypersensitivity, *anaphylaxis*.

Overdose and treatment
Because drug is eliminated primarily by the kidneys, the manufacturer states that hemodialysis may aid in removal of drug in cases of extreme overdose, espe-cially in patients with decreased renal function.

▶ **Special considerations**
Besides those relevant to all *cephalosporins*, consider the following recommendations.

● Pseudomembranous colitis has been reported with nearly all antibacterial agents. Consider this diagnosis in patients who develop diarrhea secondary to antibiotic therapy. Although most patients respond to withdrawal of drug therapy alone, it may be necessary to institute treatment with an antibacterial agent effective against *Clostridium difficile*, an organism linked to this disorder.
● Obtain specimen for culture and sensitivity tests before first dose. Therapy may begin pending test results.
● Drug may cause overgrowth of nonsusceptible bacteria or fungi. Monitor for signs and symptoms of superinfection.

Information for the patient
Tell patient to take all of the medication prescribed, even if he feels better.

Geriatric use
Elderly volunteers (age 65 and over) exhibited higher area under the plasma-concentration-versus-time curve (AUC) and lower renal clearance as compared to younger subjects.

Pediatric use
Oral suspensions contain the drug in a bubble-gum flavored vehicle to improve palatability and compliance in children. Reconstituted suspension should be stored in the refrigerator, and unused drug should be discarded after 14 days. Shake suspension well before measuring dose.

Breast-feeding
It is unknown if drug is excreted in breast milk. Use with caution in breast-feeding women.

ceftazidime
Fortaz, Tazicef, Tazidime

● Pharmacologic classification: third-generation cephalosporin
● Therapeutic classification: antibiotic
● Pregnancy risk category B

How supplied
Available by prescription only
Injection: 500 mg, 1 g, 2 g
Pharmacy bulk package: 6 g
Infusion: 1 g, 2 g in 100-ml vials and bags

Indications, route, and dosage
Bacteremia, septicemia, and serious respiratory, urinary, gynecologic, intra-abdominal, CNS, and skin infections from susceptible organisms
Adults: 1 g I.V. or I.M. q 8 to 12 hours; up to 6 g daily in life-threatening infections.
Children age 1 month to 12 years: 30 to 50 mg/kg I.V. q 8 hours.
Neonates age 0 to 4 weeks weighing less than 1,200 g: 50 mg/kg I.V. q 12 hours.
Neonates age 0 to 4 weeks weighing 1,200 to 2,000 g: 50 mg/kg I.V. q 12 hours for 7 days; then 50 mg/kg I.V. q 8 hours.
Neonates age 0 to 4 weeks weighing more than 2,000 g: 30 mg/kg I.V. q 8 hours for 7 days; then 50 mg/kg I.V. q 8 hours.

Total daily dosage is same for I.M. or I.V. administration and depends on susceptibility of organism and severity of infection. Ceftazidime should be injected deep I.M. into a large muscle mass, such as the gluteus or lateral aspect of the thigh.
Dosage in renal failure
In patients with impaired renal function, doses or frequency of administration must be modified according to the degree of renal impairment, severity of infection, and susceptibility of organism. To prevent toxic accumulation, reduced dosage may be required in patients with creatinine clearance below 50 ml/minute.

Creatinine clearance (ml/min/1.73 m²)	Dosage in adults
>50	Usual adult dose
31 to 50	1 g q 12 hours
16 to 30	1 g q 24 hours
6 to 15	500 mg q 24 hours
<5	500 mg q 48 hours
Hemodialysis patients	1 g after each hemodialysis period
Peritoneal dialysis patients	500 mg q 24 hours

Pharmacodynamics
Antibacterial action: Ceftazidime is primarily bactericidal; however, it may be bacteriostatic. Activity depends on the organism, tissue penetration, drug dosage, and rate of organism multiplication. It acts by adhering to bacterial penicillin-binding proteins, thereby inhibiting cell wall synthesis. Third-generation cephalosporins appear more active against some beta-lactamase-producing gram-negative organisms.

Ceftazidime is active against some gram-positive organisms and many enteric gram-negative bacilli, including streptococci (*Streptococcus pneumoniae* and *S. pyogenes*); *Staphylococcus aureus* (penicillinase- and nonpenicillinase-producing); *Escherichia coli*; *Klebsiella* species; *Proteus* species; *Enterobacter species*; *Haemophilus influenzae*; *Pseudomonas* species; and some strains of *Bacteroides* species. It is more effective than any cephalosporin or penicillin derivative against *Pseudomonas*. Some other third-generation cephalosporins are more active against gram-positive organisms and anaerobes.

Pharmacokinetics
● *Absorption:* Ceftazidime is not absorbed from the GI tract and must be given parenterally; peak serum levels occur 1 hour after an I.M. dose.
● *Distribution:* Ceftazidime is distributed widely into most body tissues and fluids, including the gallbladder, liver, kidneys, bone, sputum, bile, and pleural and synovial fluids; unlike most other cephalosporins, ceftazidime has good CSF penetration; it crosses the placenta. Ceftazidime is 5% to 24% protein-bound.
● *Metabolism:* Ceftazidime is not metabolized.
● *Excretion:* Ceftazidime is excreted primarily in urine by glomerular filtration; small amounts of drug are excreted in breast milk. Elimination half-life is about 1½ to 2 hours in patients with normal renal function; up to 35 hours in patients with severe renal disease. Hemodialysis or peritoneal dialysis removes ceftazidime.

---

*Canada only   †Unlabeled clinical use   Italicized adverse reactions are life-threatening.

Contraindications and precautions

Ceftazidime is contraindicated in patients with known hypersensitivity to any cephalosporin. It should be used with caution in patients with penicillin allergy, who usually are more susceptible to such reactions.

Interactions

Concomitant use with aminoglycosides results in synergistic activity against *Pseudomonas aeruginosa* and some strains of Enterobacteriaceae; such combined use may slightly increase the risk of nephrotoxicity.

Concomitant use with clavulanic acid results in synergistic activity against some strains of *Bacteroides fragilis*.

Effects on diagnostic tests

Ceftazidime causes false-positive results in urine glucose tests utilizing cupric sulfate (Benedict's reagent or Clinitest); use glucose oxidase (Clinistix or Tes-Tape) instead. Ceftazidime also causes false elevations in urine creatinine levels in tests using Jaffé's reaction.

Ceftazidime may cause positive Coombs' test results and elevated liver function test results.

Adverse reactions

● CNS: headache, dizziness, seizures.
● DERM: maculopapular and erythematous rashes, urticaria.
● GI: *pseudomembranous enterocolitis*, nausea, vomiting, diarrhea, dysgeusia, abdominal cramps.
● GU: hematuria, genital pruritus.
● HEMA: *eosinophilia, thrombocytosis, neutropenia*, leukopenia, anemia.
● Hepatic: transient elevation in liver enzymes.
● Local: at injection site—pain, induration, sterile abscesses, tissue sloughing; phlebitis and thrombophlebitis with I.V. injection.
● Other: hypersensitivity, (dyspnea, serum sickness [erythema multiforme, rashes, polyarthritis, fever]), bacterial and fungal superinfection.

Note: Drug should be discontinued if signs of toxicity, immediate hypersensitivity reaction, or serum sickness occur or if severe diarrhea indicates pseudomembranous colitis; alternative therapy should be considered if patient develops fever, eosinophilia, hematuria, or neutropenia.

Overdose and treatment

Clinical signs of overdose include neuromuscular hypersensitivity. Seizure may follow high CNS concentrations. Ceftazidime may be removed by hemodialysis or peritoneal dialysis.

▶ Special considerations

Besides those relevant to all *cephalosporins*, consider the following recommendations.
● For patients on sodium restriction, note that ceftazidime contains 2.3 mEq of sodium per gram of drug.
● Ceftazidime powders for injection contain 118 mg sodium carbonate per gram of drug; ceftazidime sodium is more water-soluble and is formed in situ upon reconstitution.
● Ceftazidime vials are supplied under reduced pressure. When the antibiotic is dissolved, carbon dioxide is released and a positive pressure develops. Each brand of ceftazidime includes specific instructions for reconstitution. Read and follow these instructions carefully.
● Because ceftazidime is hemodialyzable, patients un-

dergoing treatments with hemodialysis or peritoneal dialysis may require dosage adjustment.

Geriatric use

Reduced dosage may be necessary in elderly patients with diminished renal function.

Pediatric use

Ceftazidime may be used in infants and children.

Breast-feeding

Ceftazidime is distributed into breast milk and should be used with caution in breast-feeding women. Safe use has not been established.

---

ceftizoxime sodium
Cefizox

● Pharmacologic classification: third-generation cephalosporin
● Therapeutic classification: antibiotic
● Pregnancy risk category B

How supplied

Available by prescription only
Injection: 1 g, 2 g
Infusion: 1 g, 2 g in 100-mg vials, or 50 ml in D_5W

Indications, route, and dosage
Bacteremia, septicemia, meningitis, and serious respiratory, urinary, gynecologic, intra-abdominal, bone and joint, and skin infections from susceptible organisms
Adults: Usual dosage is 1 to 2 g I.V. or I.M. q 8 to 12 hours. In life-threatening infections, up to 2 g q 4 hours.

Total daily dosage is same for I.M. or I.V. administration and depends on susceptibility of organism and severity of infection. Ceftizoxime should be injected deep I.M. into a large muscle mass, such as the gluteus or lateral aspect of the thigh.

Dosage in renal failure

In patients with impaired renal function, doses or frequency of administration must be modified according to the degree of renal impairment, severity of infection, and susceptibility of organism. To prevent toxic accumulation, reduced dosage may be required in patients with creatinine clearance below 80 ml/minute.

DOSAGE IN ADULTS		
Creatinine clearance (ml/min/ 1.73 m²)	Less severe infections	Life-threatening infections
>80	Usual adult dose	Usual adult dose
50 to 79	500 mg q 8 hours	750 mg to 1.5 g q 8 hours
5 to 49	250 to 500 mg q 12 hours	500 mg to 1 g q 12 hours
0 to 4	500 mg q 48 hours; or 250 mg q 24 hours	500 mg to 1 g q 48 hours; or 500 mg q 24 hours

Pharmacodynamics

Antibacterial action: Ceftizoxime is primarily bactericidal; however, it may be bacteriostatic. Activity depends on the organism, tissue penetration, drug dosage, and rate of organism multiplication. It acts by adhering to bacterial penicillin-binding proteins, thereby
inhibiting cell wall synthesis. Third-generation cephalosporins appear more active against some beta-
lactamase-producing gram-negative organisms.

Ceftizoxime is active against some gram-positive organisms and many enteric gram-negative bacilli, including streptococci (*Streptococcus pneumoniae* and
pyogenes; *Staphylococcus aureus* (penicillinase- and
non-penicillinase-producing); *Staphylococcus epidermidis*; *Escherichia coli*; *Klebsiella* species; *Haemophilus influenzae*; *Enterobacter* species; *Proteus* species;
Bacteroides species (including *Bacteroides fragilis*);
Peptostreptococcus species; some strains of *Pseudomonas* and *Acinetobacter*. Cefotaxime and moxalactam are slightly more active than ceftizoxime against
gram-positive organisms but are less active against
gram-negative organisms.

Pharmacokinetics

● *Absorption:* Ceftizoxime is not absorbed from the GI
tract and must be given parenterally; peak serum levels
occur at ½ to 1½ hours after an I.M. dose.
● *Distribution:* Ceftizoxime is distributed widely into
most body tissues and fluids, including the gallbladder,
liver, kidneys, bone, sputum, bile, and pleural and synovial fluids; unlike most other cephalosporins, ceftizoxime has good CSF penetration and achieves adequate concentration in inflamed meninges; ceftizoxime
crosses the placenta. Ceftizoxime is 28% to 31%
protein-bound.
● *Metabolism:* Ceftizoxime is not metabolized.
● *Excretion:* Ceftizoxime is excreted primarily in urine
by renal tubular secretion and glomerular filtration; small
amounts of drug are excreted in breast milk. Elimination
half-life is about 1½ to 2 hours in patients with normal
renal function; severe renal disease prolongs half-life
up to 30 hours. Hemodialysis or peritoneal dialysis removes minimal amounts of ceftizoxime.

Contraindications and precautions

Ceftizoxime is contraindicated in patients with known
hypersensitivity to any cephalosporin. It should be used
with caution in patients with penicillin allergy, who usually are more susceptible to such reactions.

Interactions

Probenecid competitively inhibits renal tubular secretion of cephalosporins, causing higher, prolonged serum
levels.

Concomitant use of ceftizoxime with bacteriostatic
agents (tetracyclines, erythromycin, or chloramphenicol) may impair its bactericidal effects. Concomitant use
with aminoglycosides may slightly increase the risk of
nephrotoxicity.

Effects on diagnostic tests

Ceftizoxime causes false-positive results in urine glucose tests utilizing cupric sulfate (Benedict's reagent
or Clinitest); use glucose oxidase (Clinistix or Tes-Tape)
instead. Ceftizoxime also causes false elevations in
urine creatinine levels using Jaffé's reaction.

Ceftizoxime may cause positive Coombs' test results
and elevated liver function test results.

Adverse reactions

● CNS: headache, malaise, paresthesias, dizziness,
seizures.
● DERM: maculopapular and erythematous rashes, urticaria.
● GI: *pseudomembranous colitis*, nausea, anorexia,
vomiting, diarrhea, glossitis, dyspepsia, abdominal
cramps, tenesmus, anal pruritus, altered taste.
● GU: genital pruritus, nephrotoxicity, vaginitis, hematuria.
● HEMA: transient neutropenia, eosinophilia, hemolytic anemia.
● Local: at injection site – pain, induration, sterile abscesses, tissue sloughing; phlebitis and thrombophlebitis with I.V. injection.
● Other: hypersensitivity, (serum sickness [erythema
multiforme, rashes, polyarthritis, fever]), bacterial and
fungal superinfection.
Note: Drug should be discontinued if signs of toxicty,
immediate hypersensitivity reaction, or serum sickness
occur or if severe diarrhea indicates pseudomembranous colitis; alternative therapy should be considered if
patient develops fever, eosinophilia, hematuria, or neutropenia.

Overdose and treatment

Clinical signs of overdose include neuromuscular hypersensitivity. Seizure may follow high CNS concentrations. Ceftizoxime may be removed by hemodialysis.

▶ Special considerations

Besides those relevant to all *cephalosporins,* consider
these recommendations.
● For patients on sodium restriction, note that ceftizoxime contains 2.6 mEq of sodium per gram of drug.
● Drug may be supplied as frozen, sterile solution in
plastic containers. Thaw at room temperature. Thawed
solution is stable for 24 hours at room temperature, or
for 10 days if refrigerated. Do not refreeze.
● For I.M. use, reconstitute with sterile water for injection. Shake vial well to ensure complete dissolution of
drug. To administer a dose that exceeds 1 g, divide the
dose and inject it into separate sites to prevent tissue
injury.
● For I.V. use, reconstitute I.V. dose with sterile water
for injection. Solution should clear after shaking well
and range in color from yellow to amber. If particles
are visible, discard solution. Reconstituted solution is
stable for 8 hours at room temperature or 48 hours if
refrigerated.
● Administer I.V. as a direct injection slowly over 3 to
5 minutes directly or through tubing of compatible infusion fluid. If given as intermittent infusion, dilute reconstituted drug in 50 to 100 ml of compatible fluid.
Check package insert.

Geriatric use

Reduced dosage may be necessary in elderly patients
with diminished renal function.

Pediatric use

Safely and efficacy have not been established in infants
younger than age 6 months.

Breast-feeding

Ceftizoxime is distributed into breast milk and should
be used with caution in breast-feeding women. Safe
use has not been established.

---

ceftriaxone sodium
Rocephin

- Pharmacologic classification: third-generation cephalosporin
- Therapeutic classification: antibiotic
- Pregnancy risk category B

How supplied
Available by prescription only
Injection: 250 mg, 500 mg, 1 g, 2 g
Pharmacy bulk package: 10 g
Infusion: 1 g, 2 g

Indications, route, and dosage
Bacteremia, septicemia, and serious respiratory, urinary, gynecologic, intra-abdominal, and skin infections from susceptible organisms
Adults: 1 to 2 g I.M. or I.V. once daily or in equally divided doses twice daily. Total daily dosage should not exceed 4 g.
Children: 50 to 75 mg/kg, given in divided doses every 12 hours.
Meningitis
Adults and children: 100 mg/kg given in divided doses every 12 hours.
May give loading dose of 75 mg/kg. Total daily dosage is same for I.M. or I.V. administration and depends on susceptibility of organism and severity of infection. Ceftriaxone should be injected deep I.M. into a large muscle mass, such as the gluteus or lateral aspect of the thigh.
†Lyme disease
Adults: 1 to 2 g I.M. or I.V. every 12 to 24 hours.

Pharmacodynamics
Antibacterial action: Ceftriaxone is primarily bactericidal; however, it may be bacteriostatic. Activity depends on the organism, tissue penetration, and drug dosage and on the rate of organism multiplication. It acts by adhering to bacterial penicillin-binding proteins, thereby inhibiting cell wall synthesis. Third-generation cephalosporins appear more active against some beta-lactamase-producing gram-negative organisms.

Ceftriaxone is active against some gram-positive organisms and many enteric gram-negative bacilli, including streptococci; *Streptococcus pneumoniae* and *pyogenes; Staphylococcus aureus* (penicillinase and non-penicillinase producing); *Staphylococcus epidermidis; Escherichia coli; Klebsiella* species; *Haemophilus influenzae, Enterobacter; Proteus;* some strains of *Pseudomonas* and *Peptostreptococcus* and spirochetes such as *Borrelia burgdorferi* (the causative organism of Lyme disease). Most strains of *Listeria, Pseudomonas,* and *Acinetobacter* are resistant. Generally, ceftriaxone's activity is most like that of cefotaxime and ceftizoxime.

Pharmacokinetics
- *Absorption:* Ceftriaxone is not absorbed from the GI tract and must be given parenterally; peak serum levels occur at 1½ to 4 hours after an I.M. dose.
- *Distribution:* Ceftriaxone is distributed widely into most body tissues and fluids, including the gallbladder, liver, kidneys, bone, sputum, bile, and pleural and synovial fluids; unlike most other cephalosporins, ceftriax-

one has good CSF penetration. Ceftriaxone crosses the placenta. Protein binding is dose-dependent and decreases as serum levels rise; average is 58% to 96%.
- *Metabolism:* Ceftriaxone is partially metabolized.
- *Excretion:* Ceftriaxone is excreted principally in urine; some drug is excreted in bile by biliary mechanisms, and small amounts are excreted in breast milk. Elimination half-life is 5½ to 11 hours in adults with normal renal function; severe renal disease prolongs half-life only moderately. Neither hemodialysis nor peritoneal dialysis will remove ceftriaxone.

Contraindications and precautions
Ceftriaxone is contraindicated in patients with known hypersensitivity to any cephalosporin. It should be used with caution in patients with penicillin allergy, who usually are more susceptible to such reactions.

Interactions
Concomitant use with aminoglycosides produces synergistic antimicrobial activity against *Pseudomonas aeruginosa* and some strains of *Enterobacteriaceae.*

Effects on diagnostic tests
Ceftriaxone causes false-positive results in urine glucose tests utilizing cupric sulfate (Benedict's reagent or Clinitest); use glucose oxidase (Clinistix or Tes-Tape) instead. Ceftriaxone also causes false elevations in urine creatinine levels in tests using Jaffe's reaction.

Ceftriaxone may cause positive Coombs' test results, and elevations in liver function test results.

Adverse reactions
- CNS: headache, dizziness, seizures.
- DERM: maculopapular and erythematous rashes, urticaria.
- GI: *pseudomembranous enterocolitis,* nausea, vomiting, diarrhea, dysgeusia, abdominal cramps.
- GU: genital pruritus, hematuria.
- HEMA: *eosinophilia, neutropenia, thrombocytosis,* leukopenia, anemia.
- Hepatic: transient elevation in liver enzymes.
- Local: at injection site – pain, induration, sterile abscesses, tissue sloughing; phlebitis and thrombophlebitis with I.V. injection.
- Other: hypersensitivity, (dyspnea, elevated temperature, serum sickness [erythema multiforme, rashes, polyarthritis, fever]).
   Note: Drug should be discontinued if signs of toxicity, immediate hypersensitivity reaction, or serum sickness occur or if severe diarrhea indicates pseudomembranous colitis; alternative therapy should be considered if patient develops fever, eosinophilia, hematuria, or neutropenia.

Overdose and treatment
Clinical signs of overdose include neuromuscular hypersensitivity. Seizure may follow high CNS concentrations. Treatment is supportive.

▶ Special considerations
Besides those relevant to all *cephalosporins,* consider the following recommendations.
- For patients on sodium restriction, note that ceftriaxone injection contains 3.6 mEq of sodium per gram of drug.
- Ceftriaxone is used commonly in home care programs for management of serious infections, such as osteomyelitis. It is frequently given I.M., and injection

---

*Canada only   †Unlabeled clinical use   Italicized adverse reactions are life-threatening.

may be painful. This may be partially alleviated by reconstituting the drug in 1% lidocaine (*without* epinephrine).

● Dosage adjustment usually is not necessary in patients with renal insufficiency because of partial biliary excretion. In patients with impaired hepatic and renal function, dosage should not exceed 2 g/day without monitoring of serum levels.

Pediatric use
Ceftriaxone may be used in neonates and children.

Breast-feeding
Ceftriaxone is distributed into breast milk. Use with caution in breast-feeding women.

---

cefuroxime axetil
Ceftin

cefuroxime sodium
Kefurox, Zinacef

● Pharmacologic classification: second-generation cephalosporin
● Therapeutic classification: antibiotic
● Pregnancy risk category B

How supplied
Available by prescription only
Cefuroxime axetil
Tablets: 125 mg, 250 mg, 500 mg
Cefuroxime sodium
Injection: 750 mg, 1.5 g
Infusion: 750 mg, 1.5-g Infusion Packets

Indications, route, and dosage
Serious lower respiratory, urinary tract, skin and skin-structure infections; septicemia; meningitis caused by susceptible organisms
Adults: Usual dosage is 750 mg to 1.5 g I.M. or I.V. q 8 hours, usually for 5 to 10 days. For life-threatening infections and infections caused by less susceptible organisms, 1.5 g I.M. or I.V. q 6 hours; for bacterial meningitis, up to 3 g I.V. q 8 hours.
Children and infants over age 3 months: 50 to 100 mg/kg I.M. or I.V. daily. Some clinicians give 100 to 150 mg/kg/day. For meningitis, the usual starting dose is 200 to 240 mg/kg/day I.V., reduced to 100 mg/kg/day when clinical improvement is seen. However, some clinicians prefer other agents for meningitis.
Total daily dosage is same for I.M. or I.V. administration and depends on susceptibility of organism and severity of infection. Cefuroxime should be injected deep I.M. into a large muscle mass, such as the gluteus or lateral aspect of the thigh.
Pharyngitis, tonsillitis, lower respiratory infection, urinary tract infection
Adults: 125 to 500 mg P.O. b.i.d.
Children under age 12: 125 mg P.O. b.i.d.
Otitis media
Infants and children under age 2: 125 mg P.O. b.i.d.
Children age 2 and over: 250 mg P.O. b.i.d.
Note: Compliance may be a problem when treating otitis media in children. The tablets are not chewable and may be difficult for a child to swallow. The drug

has an unpleasant taste so tablets should not be crushed. An alternative drug may be considered.
Dosage in renal failure
In patients with impaired renal function, dose or frequency of administration must be modified according to the degree of renal impairment, severity of infection, and susceptibility of organism. To prevent toxic accumulation, reduced dosage may be required in patients with creatinine clearance below 20 ml/minute.

Creatinine clearance (ml/min/1.73 m²)	Dosage in adults
> 20	750 mg to 1.5 g q 8 hours
10 to 20	750 mg q 12 hours
< 10	750 mg q 24 hours
Hemodialysis patients	750 mg at the end of each dialysis period

Pharmacodynamics
Antibacterial action: Cefuroxime is primarily bactericidal; however, it may be bacteriostatic. Activity depends on the organism, tissue penetration, drug dosage, and rate of organism multiplication. It acts by adhering to bacterial penicillin-binding proteins, thereby inhibiting cell wall synthesis.
Cefuroxime is active against many gram-positive organisms and enteric gram-negative bacilli, including *Streptococcus pneumoniae* and *S. pyogenes*, *Haemophilus influenzae*, *Klebsiella* species, *Staphylococcus aureus*, *Escherichia coli*, *Enterobacter*, and *Neisseria gonorrhoeae*; its spectrum is similar to that of cefamandole, but it is more stable against beta-lactamases. *Bacteroides fragilis*, *Pseudomonas*, and *Acinetobacter* are resistant to cefuroxime.

Pharmacokinetics
● *Absorption:* Cefuroxime sodium is not well absorbed from the GI tract and must be given parenterally; peak serum levels occur 15 to 60 minutes after an I.M. dose.
Cefuroxime axetil is better absorbed orally, with between 37% to 52% of an oral dose reaching the systemic circulation. Peak serum levels after oral administration occur in about 2 hours. Food appears to enhance absorption.
● *Distribution:* Cefuroxime is distributed widely into most body tissues and fluids, including the gallbladder, liver, kidneys, bone, bile, and pleural and synovial fluids; CSF penetration is greater than that of most first- and second-generation cephalosporins and achieves adequate therapeutic levels in inflamed meninges. Cefuroxime crosses the placenta; it is 33% to 50% protein-bound.
● *Metabolism:* Cefuroxime is not metabolized.
● *Excretion:* Cefuroxime is primarily excreted in urine by renal tubular secretion and glomerular filtration; elimination half-life is 1 to 2 hours in patients with normal renal function; end-stage renal disease prolongs half-life 15 to 22 hours. Some of the drug is excreted in breast milk. Hemodialysis removes cefuroxime.

Contraindications and precautions
Cefuroxime is contraindicated in patients with known hypersensitivity to any cephalosporin. It should be used with caution in patients with penicillin allergy, who usually are more susceptible to such reactions.

Interactions
Probenecid competitively inhibits renal tubular secretion of cephalosporins, resulting in higher, prolonged serum levels of these drugs.

Concomitant use of cefuroxime with nephrotoxic agents (vancomycin, colistin, polymixin B, or aminoglycosides) or loop diuretics increases the risk of nephrotoxicity. Concomitant use with bacteriostatic agents (tetracyclines, erythromycin, or chloramphenicol) may impair its bactericidal activity.

Effects on diagnostic tests
Cefuroxime causes false-positive results in urine glucose tests utilizing cupric sulfate (Benedict's reagent or Clinitest); use glucose oxidase tests (Clinistix or Tes-Tape) instead. Cefuroxime also causes false elevations in serum or urine creatinine levels in tests using Jaffé's reaction.

Cefuroxime may elevate liver function test results and may cause positive Coombs' test results.

Adverse reactions
● CNS: headache, malaise, paresthesias, dizziness, seizures.
● DERM: maculopapular and erythematous rashes, urticaria.
● GI: *pseudomembranous colitis*, nausea, anorexia, vomiting, diarrhea, glossitis, dyspepsia, abdominal cramps, tenesmus, anal pruritus.
● GU: genital pruritus, hematuria, nephrotoxicity.
● HEMA: transient neutropenia, eosinophilia, hemolytic anemia, decrease in hemoglobin and hematocrit levels.
● Local: at injection site – pain, induration, sterile abscesses, temperature elevation, tissue sloughing; phlebitis and thrombophlebitis with I.V. injection.
● Other: hypersensitivity, (dyspnea, serum sickness [erythema multiforme, rashes, polyarthritis, and fever]), bacterial and fungal superinfection.
   Note: Drug should be discontinued if signs of toxicity, immediate hypersensitivity reaction, or serum sickness occur or if severe diarrhea indicates pseudomembranous colitis; alternative therapy should be considered if the following symptoms occur: fever, eosinophilia, hematuria, neutropenia, or unexplained elevations in BUN or serum creatinine levels.

Overdose and treatment
Clinical signs of overdose include neuromuscular hypersensitivity. Seizure may follow high CNS concentrations. Hemodialysis or peritoneal dialysis will remove cefuroxime.

▶ Special considerations
Besides those relevant to all *cephalosporins,* consider the following recommendations.
● Cefuroxime is a second-generation cephalosporin similar to cefamandole. However, cefuroxime has not been associated with prothrombin deficiency and bleeding. It offers the advantage of effectiveness in treating meningitis.
● For patients on sodium restriction, note that cefuroxime contains 2.4 mEq of sodium per gram of drug.
● Check solutions for particulate matter and discoloration. Solution may range in color from light yellow to amber without affecting potency.
● Shake I.M. solution gently before administration to ensure complete drug dissolution. Administer deep I.M. in a large muscle mass, preferably the gluteus area.

Aspirate before injecting to prevent inadvertent injection into a blood vessel. Rotate injection sites to prevent tissue damage. Apply ice to injection site to relieve pain.
● For direct intermittent I.V., inject solution slowly into vein over 3 to 5 minutes or slowly through tubing of free-running, compatible I.V. solution.
● Reconstituted solution retains potency for 24 hours at room temperature or for 48 hours if refrigerated.
● Because cefuroxime is hemodialyzable, patients undergoing treatment with hemodialysis or peritoneal dialysis may require dosage adjustments.

Geriatric use
Use with caution in elderly patients.

Pediatric use
Safe use in infants younger than age 3 months has not been established.

Breast-feeding
Cefuroxime distributes into breast milk and should be used with caution in breast-feeding women.

---

cephalexin hydrochloride
Keftab

cephalexin monohydrate
Ceporex*, Keflet, Keflex, Novolexin*

● Pharmacologic classification: first-generation cephalosporin
● Therapeutic classification: antibiotic
● Pregnancy risk category B

How supplied
Available by prescription only
Cephalexin hydrochloride
Tablets: 250 mg, 500 mg
Cephalexin monohydrate
Tablets: 250 mg, 500 mg, 1 g
Capsules: 250 mg, 500 mg
Suspension: 125 mg/5 ml, 250 mg/5 ml
Drops: 100 mg/ml (pediatric)

Indications, route, and dosage
Respiratory, genitourinary, skin and soft-tissue, or bone and joint infections, and otitis media caused by susceptible organisms
Adults: 250 mg to 1 g P.O. q 6 hours.
Children: 6 to 12 mg/kg P.O. q 6 hours. Maximum 25 mg/kg q 6 hours.
Dosage in renal failure
To prevent toxic accumulation in patients with impaired renal function, those with creatinine clearance below 40 ml/minute should receive reduced dosage.

Pharmacodynamics
Antibacterial action: Cephalexin is primarily bactericidal; however, it may be bacteriostatic. Activity depends on the organism, tissue penetration, drug dosage, and rate of organism multiplication. It acts by adhering to bacterial penicillin-binding proteins, thereby inhibiting cell wall synthesis.

Cephalexin is active against many gram-positive organisms, including penicillinase-producing *Staphylococcus aureus* and *epidermidis, Streptococcus pneu-*

moniae, group B streptococci, and group A beta-hemolytic streptococci; susceptible gram-negative organisms include *Klebsiella pneumoniae, Escherichia coli, Proteus mirabilis,* and *Shigella.*

Pharmacokinetics

● *Absorption:* Cephalexin is absorbed rapidly and completely from the GI tract after oral administration; peak serum levels occur within 1 hour. The base monohydrate is probably converted to the hydrochloride in the stomach before absorption. Food delays but does not prevent complete absorption.

● *Distribution:* Cephalexin is distributed widely into most body tissues and fluids, including the gallbladder, liver, kidneys, bone, sputum, bile, and pleural and synovial fluids; CSF penetration is poor. Cephalexin crosses the placenta; it is 6% to 15% protein-bound.

● *Metabolism:* Cephalexin is not metabolized.

● *Excretion:* Cephalexin is excreted primarily unchanged in urine by glomerular filtration and renal tubular secretion; small amounts of drug may be excreted in breast milk. Elimination half-life is about ½ to 1 hour in patients with normal renal function; 7½ to 14 hours in patients with severe renal impairment. Hemodialysis or peritoneal dialysis removes cephalexin.

Contraindications and precautions

Cephalexin is contraindicated in patients with known hypersensitivity to any cephalosporin. It should be used with caution in patients with penicillin allergy, who usually are more susceptible to such reactions.

Interactions

Probenecid competitively inhibits renal tubular secretion of cephalosporins, resulting in higher, prolonged serum levels of these drugs.

Concomitant use with nephrotoxic agents (vancomycin, colistin, polymyxin B, or aminoglycosides) or loop diuretics increases the risk of nephrotoxicity.

Concomitant use with bacteriostatic agents (tetracyclines, erythromycin, or chloramphenicol) may interfere with bactericidal activity.

Effects on diagnostic tests

Cephalexin causes false-positive results in urine glucose tests utilizing cupric sulfate (Benedict's reagent or Clinitest); use glucose oxidase test (Clinistix or Tes-Tape) instead. Cephalexin also causes false elevations in serum or urine creatinine levels in tests using Jaffe's reaction.

Positive Coombs' test results occur in about 3% of patients taking cephalexin.

Adverse reactions

● CNS: dizziness, headache, malaise, paresthesias, *seizures.*

● DERM: maculopapular and erythematous rashes, urticaria.

● GI: *pseudomembranous colitis,* nausea, anorexia, vomiting, diarrhea, glossitis, dyspepsia, abdominal cramps, anal pruritus, tenesmus.

● GU: genital pruritus, vaginitis, hematuria, nephrotoxicity.

● HEMA: transient neutropenia, eosinophilia, anemia, neutropenia.

● Other: hypersensitivity, (dyspnea, serum sickness [erythema, multiforme, rashes, polyarthritis, and fever]), bacterial and fungal superinfection.

Note: Drug should be discontinued if signs of toxicity

or immediate hypersensitivity reaction occur or if severe diarrhea indicates pseudomembranous colitis; alternative therapy should be considered if the following symptoms occur: fever, eosinophilia, hematuria, neutropenia, or unexplained elevations in BUN or serum creatinine levels.

Overdose and treatment

Clinical signs of overdose include neuromuscular hypersensitivity; seizure may follow high CNS concentrations. Remove cephalexin by hemodialysis or peritoneal dialysis. Other treatment is supportive.

▶ **Special considerations**

Besides those relevant to all *cephalosporins,* consider the following recommendations.

● To prepare the oral suspension, add the required amount of water to the powder in two portions. Shake well after each addition. After mixing, store in refrigerator. Suspension is stable for 14 days without significant loss of potency. Store mixture in tightly closed container. Shake well before using.

● Because cephalexin is dialyzable, patients undergoing treatment with hemodialysis or peritoneal dialysis may require dosage adjustment.

Geriatric use

Reduce dosage in elderly patients with diminished renal function.

Pediatric use

The serum half-life is prolonged in neonates and in infants younger than age 1.

Breast-feeding

Cephalexin distributes into breast milk and should be used with caution in breast-feeding women.

PHARMACOLOGIC CLASS

cephalosporins

First-generation cephalosporins
cefadroxil monohydrate
cefazolin sodium
cephalexin monohydrate
cephalothin sodium
cephapirin sodium
cephradine

Second-generation cephalosporins
cefaclor
cefamandole nafate
cefmetazole sodium
cefonicid sodium
ceforanide
cefotetan disodium
cefoxitin sodium
cefprozil
cefuroxime axetil
cefuroxime sodium

Third-generation cephalosporins
cefixime
cefoperazone sodium
cefotaxime sodium
ceftazidime
ceftizoxime sodium
ceftriaxone sodium

Oxa-beta lactam
moxalactam

Cephalosporins are beta-lactam antibiotics first isolated in 1948 from the fungus *Cephalosporium acremonium*. Their mechanism of action is similar to that of penicillins, but their antibacterial spectra differ. Over the past 15 years, intensive research and development has resulted in the availability of many newer cephalosporins, which are now classified by generations. Generations are differentiated in terms of individual antimicrobial activity.

First-generation cephalosporins act like penicillins against gram-positive cocci, and are also effective against some gram-negative organisms. Second-generation cephalosporins have increased activity against gram-negative organisms, including beta-lactamase-producing strains, but are less effective against gram-positive cocci than are first-generation drugs. Third-generation cephalosporins have a still broader spectrum of action, especially against gram-negative organisms, including some strains resistant to first- and second-generation drugs; some effectively attack *Pseudomonas*. However, they have less gram-positive activity than do first- and second-generation drugs. Moxalactam, an oxa-beta lactam, is chemically similar to third-generation cephalosporins, and its antibacterial spectrum is similar to third-generation cephalosporins.

Pharmacology
Cephalosporins are chemically and pharmacologically similar to penicillin; their structure contains a beta-lactam ring, a dihydrothiazine ring, and side chains, and they act by inhibiting bacterial cell wall synthesis, causing rapid cell lysis.

The sites of action for cephalosporins are enzymes known as penicillin-binding proteins (PBP). The affinity of certain cephalosporins for PBP in various microorganisms helps explain the differing spectra of activity in this class of antibiotics.

Bacterial resistance to beta-lactam antibiotics is conferred most significantly by production of beta-lactamase enzymes (by both gram-negative and gram-positive bacteria) that destroy the beta-lactam ring and thus inactivate cephalosporins; decreased cell wall permeability and alteration in binding affinity to PBP also contribute to bacterial resistance.

Cephalosporins are bactericidal; they act against many gram-positive and gram-negative bacteria, and some anaerobic bacteria; they do not kill fungi or viruses.

First-generation cephalosporins act against many gram-positive cocci, including penicillinase-producing *Staphylococcus aureus* and *Staphylococcus epidermidis*; *Streptococcus pneumoniae*, group B streptococci, and group A beta-hemolytic streptococci; susceptible gram-negative organisms include *Klebsiella pneumoniae, Escherichia coli, Proteus mirabilis*, and *Shigella*.

Second-generation cephalosporins are effective against all organisms attacked by first-generation drugs and have additional activity against *Branhamella catarrhalis, Haemophilus influenzae, Enterobacter, Citrobacter, Providencia, Acinetobacter, Serratia*, and *Neisseria; Bacteroides fragilis* is susceptible to cefotetan and cefoxitin.

Third-generation cephalosporins are less active than first- and second-generation drugs against gram-positive bacteria, but more active against gram-negative organisms, including those resistant to first- and second-generation drugs; they have the greatest stability against beta-lactamases produced by gram-negative bacteria. Susceptible gram-negative organisms include *E. coli, Klebsiella, Enterobacter, Providencia, Acinetobacter, Serratia, Proteus, Morganella*, and *Neisseria;* some third-generation drugs are active against *Bacteroides fragilis* and *Pseudomonas*.

Oral absorption of cephalosporins varies widely; many must be given parenterally. Most are distributed widely into the body, the actual amount varying with individual drugs. CSF penetration by first- and second-generation drugs is minimal; third-generation drugs achieve much greater penetration. Cephalosporins cross the placenta. Degree of metabolism varies with individual drugs; some are not metabolized at all, and others are extensively metabolized.

Cephalosporins are excreted primarily in urine, chiefly by renal tubular effects; elimination half-life ranges from ½ to 10 hours in patients with normal renal function. Some drug is excreted in breast milk. Most cephalosporins can be removed by hemodialysis or peritoneal dialysis. Patients on dialysis may require dosage adjustment.

Clinical indications and actions
Infection caused by susceptible organisms
● *Parenteral cephalosporins:* Cephalosporins are used to treat serious infections of the lungs, skin, soft tissue, bones, joints, urinary tract, blood (septicemia), abdomen, and heart (endocarditis).

Third-generation cephalosporins (except moxalactam and cefoperazone) and the second-generation drug cefuroxime are used to treat CNS infections caused by susceptible strains of *N. meningitidis, H. influenzae,* and *S. pneumoniae;* meningitis caused by *E. coli* or *Klebsiella* can be treated by ceftriaxone, cefotaxime, or ceftizoxime.

First-generation, and some second-generation, cephalosporins also can be given prophylactically to reduce postoperative infection after surgical procedures classified as contaminated or potentially contaminated; third-generation drugs are not usually indicated.

Penicillinase-producing *N. gonorrhoeae* can be treated with cefoxitin, cefotaxime, ceftriaxone, ceftizoxime, or cefuroxime.

● *Oral cephalosporins:* Cephalosporins can be used to treat otitis media and infections of the respiratory tract, urinary tract, and skin and soft tissue; cefaclor is particularly effective against ampicillin-resistant middle ear infection caused by *H. influenzae.*

Overview of adverse reactions
Many cephalosporins share a similar profile of adverse effects. Hypersensitivity reactions range from mild rashes, fever, and eosinophilia to fatal anaphylaxis, and are more common in patients with penicillin allergy. Hematologic reactions include positive direct and indirect antiglobulin (Coombs' test), thrombocytopenia or thrombocythemia, transient neutropenia, and revers-

COMPARING CEPHALOSPORINS

DRUG AND ROUTE	ELIMINATION HALF-LIFE (hours)		SODIUM (mEq/g)	CEREBROSPINAL FLUID PENETRATION
	NORMAL RENAL FUNCTION	END-STAGE RENAL DISEASE		
cefaclor oral	0.5 to 1	3 to 5.5	No data available	No
cefadroxil oral	1 to 2	20 to 25	No data available	No
cefamandole I.M., I.V.	0.5 to 2	12 to 18	3.3	No
cefazolin I.M., I.V.	1.2 to 2.2	12 to 50	2.0	No
cefixime oral	3-4	11.5	No data available	Unknown
cefmetazole I.V.	1.2	Unknown	49	Unknown
cefonicid I.M., I.V.	3.5 to 5.8	100	3.7	No
cefoperazone I.M., I.V.	1.5 to 2.5	3.4 to 7	1.5	Sometimes
ceforanide I.M., I.V.	2.5 to 3.5	5.5 to 25	No data available	No
cefotaxime I.M., I.V.	1 to 1.5	11.5 to 56	2.2	Yes
cefotetan I.M., I.V.	2.8 to 4.6	13 to 35	3.5	No
cefoxitin I.M., I.V.	0.5 to 1	6.5 to 21.5	2.3	No
cefprozil oral	1 to 1.5	5.2 to 5.9	No data available	Unknown
ceftazidime I.M., I.V.	1.5 to 2	35	2.3	Yes
ceftizoxime I.M., I.V.	1.5 to 2	30	2.6	Yes
ceftriaxone I.M., I.V.	5.5 to 11	15.7	3.6	Yes
cefuroxime I.M., I.V.	1 to 2	15 to 22	2.4	Yes
cephalexin oral	0.5 to 1	7.5 to 14	No data available	No
cephalothin I.M., I.V.	0.5 to 1	19	2.8	No
cephapirin I.M., I.V.	0.5 to 1	1.0 to 1.5	2.4	No
cephradine oral, I.M., I.V.	0.5 to 2	8 to 15 hr	6	No
moxalactam I.M., I.V.	2 to 3.5	5 to 10	3.8	Yes

*Canada only   †Unlabeled clinical use   Italicized adverse reactions are life-threatening.

ible leukopenia. Adverse renal effects may occur with any cephalosporin; they are most common in older patients, those with decreased renal function, and those taking other nephrotoxic drugs. GI reactions include nausea, vomiting, diarrhea, abdominal pain, glossitis, dyspepsia, and tenesmus; minimal elevation of liver function test results occurs occasionally.

Local venous pain and irritation are common after I.M. injection; such reactions occur more often with higher doses and long-term therapy.

Disulfiram-type reactions occur when cefamandole, cefoperazone, moxalactam, cefonicid, or cefotetan are administered within 48 to 72 hours of alcohol ingestion.

Bacterial and fungal superinfection results from suppression of normal flora.

▶ **Special considerations**
● Review patient's history of allergies; do not give a cephalosporin to any patient with a history of hypersensitivity reactions to cephalosporins; administer cautiously to patients with penicillin allergy because they are more susceptible to such reactions.
● Try to determine whether previous reactions were true hypersensitivity reactions and not merely an adverse effect such as GI distress that patient has interpreted as allergy.
● Monitor continuously for possible hypersensitivity reactions or other untoward effects.
● Obtain results of cultures and sensitivity tests before first dose, but do not delay therapy; check test results periodically to assess drug efficacy.
● Monitor renal function studies; dosages of certain cephalosporins must be lowered in patients with severe renal impairment. In decreased renal function, monitor BUN levels, serum creatinine levels, and urine output for significant changes.
● Monitor prothrombin times and platelet counts and assess patient for signs of hypoprothrombinemia, which may occur, with or without bleeding, during therapy with cefamandole, cefoperazone, cefonicid, cefotetan, or moxalactam, usually in elderly, debilitated, or malnourished patients.
● Monitor patients on long-term therapy for possible bacterial and fungal superinfection, especially elderly, and debilitated patients, and others receiving immunosuppressants or radiation therapy.
● Monitor susceptible patients receiving sodium salts of cephalosporins for possible fluid retention; consult individual drug entry for sodium content.
● Cephalosporins cause false-positive results in urine glucose tests utilizing cupric sulfate solutions (Benedict's reagent or Clinitest); glucose oxidase tests (Clinistix or Tes-Tape) are not affected. Consult individual drug entries for other possible test interactions.

Administration
● Give cephalosporins at least 1 hour before giving bacteriostatic antibiotics (tetracyclines, erythromycins, and chloramphenicol); these drugs inhibit bacterial cell growth, decreasing cephalosporin uptake by bacterial cell walls.
● Give oral cephalosporin at least 1 hour before or 2 hours after meals for maximum absorption.
● Refrigerate oral suspensions (stable for 14 days); shake well before administering, to assure correct dosage.
● Always consult manufacturer's directions for reconstitution, dilution, and storage of drugs; check expiration dates.

● Administer I.M. dose deep into large muscle mass (gluteal or midlateral thigh); rotate injection sites to minimize tissue injury.
● Do not add or mix other drugs with I.V. infusions – particularly aminoglycosides, which will be inactivated if mixed with cephalosporins; if other drugs must be given I.V., temporarily stop infusion of primary drug.
● Adequate dilution of I.V. infusion and rotation of the site every 48 hours help minimize local vein irritation; use of small-gauge needle in larger available vein may be helpful.

Information for the patient
● Explain disease process and rationale for therapy.
● Teach signs and symptoms of hypersensitivity and other adverse reactions, and emphasize need to report *any* unusual effects.
● Teach signs and symptoms of bacterial and fungal superinfection to elderly and debilitated patients and others with low resistance from immunosuppressants or irradiation; emphasize need to report them promptly.
● Warn patient not to ingest alcohol in any form within 72 hours of treatment with cefamandole, cefoperazone, moxalactam, cefonicid, or cefotetan.
● Advise patient to add yogurt or buttermilk to diet to prevent intestinal superinfection resulting from suppression of normal intestinal flora.
● Advise diabetic patients to monitor urine glucose level with Clinistix or Tes-Tape and not to use Clinitest.
● Tell patient to take oral drug with food if GI irritation occurs.
● Be sure patient understands how and when to take drug; urge patient to complete entire prescribed regimen, to comply with instructions for around-the-clock dosage, and to keep follow-up appointments.
● Counsel patient to check expiration date of drug, how to store drug, and to discard unused drug.

Geriatric use
Use with caution; elderly patients are susceptible to superinfection and to coagulopathies. Elderly patients commonly have renal impairment and may require lower dosage of cephalosporins.

Pediatric use
Serum half-life is prolonged in neonates and in infants up to age 1.

Breast-feeding
Cephalosporins are excreted in breast milk; use with caution in breast-feeding women.

Representative combinations
None.

cephalothin sodium
Keflin, Seffin

- Pharmacologic classification: first-generation cephalosporin
- Therapeutic classification: antibiotic
- Pregnancy risk category B

How supplied
Available by prescription only
Injection: 1 g, 2 g, 4 g
Infusion: 1 g/50 ml, 2 g/50 ml, 1 g/dl, 2 g/dl
Pharmacy bulk package: 10 g, 20 g

Indications, route, and dosage
Serious respiratory, genitourinary, GI, skin and soft-tissue, bone and joint infections; septicemia; endocarditis; meningitis
Adults: 500 mg to 1 g I.M. or I.V. (or intraperitoneally) q 4 to 6 hours; in life-threatening infections, up to 2 g q 4 hours.
Children: 14 to 27 mg/kg I.V. q 4 hours, or 20 to 40 mg/kg q 6 hours; dosage should be proportionately less in accordance with age, weight, and severity of infection.

Cephalothin should be injected deep I.M. into a large muscle mass, such as the gluteus or lateral aspect of the thigh. I.V. route is preferable in severe or life-threatening infections.
Dosage in renal failure
Dosage schedule is determined by the degree of renal impairment, severity of infection, and susceptibility of causative organism. To prevent toxic accumulation, reduced dosage may be required in patients with creatinine clearance below 50 ml/minute.

Creatinine clearance (ml/min/1.73 m^2)	Dosage in adults
>80	Usual adult dose
50 to 80	Up to 2 g q 6 hours
25 to 50	Up to 1.5 g q 6 hours
10 to 25	Up to 1 g q 6 hours
2 to 10	Up to 500 mg q 6 hours
<2	Up to 500 mg q 8 hours

Pharmacodynamics
Antibacterial action: Cephalothin is primarily bactericidal; however, it may be bacteriostatic. Activity depends on the organism, tissue penetration, drug dosage, and rate of organism multiplication. It acts by adhering to bacterial penicillin-binding proteins, thereby inhibiting cell wall synthesis.

Like other first-generation cephalosporins, cephalothin is active mainly against gram-positive organisms and some gram-negative organisms. Susceptible organisms include *Escherichia coli* and other coliform bacteria, Enterobacteriaceae, enterococci, gonococci, group A beta-hemolytic streptococci, *Haemophilus influenzae, Klebsiella, Proteus mirabilis, Salmonella, Staphylococcus aureus, Shigella, Streptococcus pneumoniae,* staphylococci, and *Streptococcus viridans.*

Pharmacokinetics
- *Absorption:* Cephalothin is not absorbed from the GI tract and must be given parenterally; peak serum levels occur 30 minutes after an I.M. dose.
- *Distribution:* Cephalothin is distributed widely into most body tissues and fluids, including the gallbladder, liver, kidneys, bone, sputum, bile, and pleural and synovial fluids; CSF penetration is poor. Cephalothin crosses the placenta; it is 65% to 79% protein-bound.
- *Metabolism:* Cephalothin is metabolized partially by the liver and kidneys.
- *Excretion:* Cephalothin is excreted primarily in urine by renal tubular secretion and glomerular filtration. Small amounts of drug are excreted in breast milk. Elimination half-life is ½ to 1 hour in patients with normal renal function; 19 hours in patients with severe renal disease. Hemodialysis or peritoneal dialysis removes cephalothin.

Contraindications and precautions
Cephalothin is contraindicated in patients with known hypersensitivity to any cephalosporin; it should be used with caution in patients with penicillin allergy, who usually are more susceptible to such reactions.

Interactions
Probenecid competitively inhibits renal tubular secretion of cephalosporins, resulting in higher, prolonged serum levels of these drugs.

Concomitant use with nephrotoxic agents (vancomycin, colistin, polymyxin B, or aminoglycosides) or loop diuretics increases the risk of nephrotoxicity.

Concomitant use with bacteriostatic agents (tetracyclines, erythromycin, or chloramphenicol) may impair cephalothin's bactericidal activity.

Effects on diagnostic tests
Cephalothin causes false-positive results in urine glucose tests utilizing cupric sulfate (Benedict's reagent or Clinitest); use glucose oxidase tests (Clinistix or Tes-Tape) instead. Cephalothin also causes false elevations in serum or urine creatinine levels in tests using Jaffé's reaction.

Cephalothin may cause positive Coombs' test results or elevate liver function test results.

Adverse reactions
- CNS: headache, malaise, paresthesias, dizziness, seizures.
- DERM: maculopapular and erythematous rashes, urticaria.
- GI: *pseudomembranous colitis,* nausea, anorexia, vomiting, diarrhea, glossitis, dyspepsia, abdominal cramps, tenesmus, anal pruritus.
- GU: *nephrotoxicity,* genital pruritus, hematuria.
- HEMA: transient neutropenia, eosinophilia, hemolytic anemia.
- Local: at injection site – pain, induration, sterile abscesses, tissue sloughing; phlebitis and thrombophlebitis with I.V. injection.
- Other: hypersensitivity, dyspnea, fever, bacterial and fungal superinfection.
    Note: Drug should be discontinued if signs of toxicity or immediate hypersensitivity reaction occur or if severe diarrhea indicates pseudomembranous colitis; alternative therapy should be considered if the following symptoms occur: fever, eosinophilia, hematuria, neutropenia, or unexplained elevations in BUN or serum creatinine levels.

Overdose and treatment
Clinical signs of overdose include neuromuscular hypersensitivity; seizure may follow high CNS concentrations. Remove cephalothin by hemodialysis or peritoneal dialysis.

▶ **Special considerations**
Besides those relevant to all *cephalosporins*, consider the following recommendations.
● I.M. injection is painful; avoid this route if possible. Inject I.M. dose deeply into a large muscle mass to reduce pain. Apply ice to injection site. Rotate injection sites to prevent tissue irritation.
● For I.M. administration, reconstitute each gram of cephalothin with 4 ml of sterile water for injection, providing 500 mg in each 2.2 ml. If contents do not dissolve completely, add an additional 0.2 to 0.4 ml of diluent, and warm contents slightly.
● For I.V. administration, dilute contents of a 4-g vial with at least 20 ml of sterile water for injection, dextrose 5% for injection, or 0.9% sodium chloride for injection and add to one of the following I.V. solutions: lactated Ringer's injection, dextrose 5% injection, dextrose 5% in lactated Ringer's injection, Ionosol B in dextrose 5% in water, Normosol-R in dextrose 5% in water, Ringer's injection, or 0.9% sodium chloride injection. Choose solution and fluid volume according to patient's fluid and electrolyte status.
● Administer reconstituted I.M. and I.V. solutions within 12 hours. Solutions for continuous infusion should start within 12 hours and be completed within 24 hours.
● Reconstituted solutions are stable for 96 hours under refrigeration. Low temperature may cause solution to precipitate. Warm to room temperature with gentle agitation before using.
● Discoloration in solution stored at room temperature does not indicate loss of potency.
● Do not freeze drug in plastic syringes.
● Solutions reconstituted in original container and frozen immediately are stable for as long as 12 weeks at −20° C. Do not thaw solution until ready to use. Do not heat to thaw or refreeze once thawed.
● Because cephalothin is dialyzable, patients undergoing treatment with hemodialysis or peritoneal dialysis may require dosage adjustments.

Geriatric use
Dosage reduction may be required in patients with diminished renal function.

Breast-feeding
Cephalothin distributes into breast milk and should be used with caution in breast-feeding women.

cephapirin sodium
Cefadyl

● Pharmacologic classification: first-generation cephalosporin
● Therapeutic classification: antibiotic
● Pregnancy risk category B

How supplied
Available by prescription only
Injection: 500 mg, 1 g, 2 g
Infusion: 1 g, 2 g, 4 g piggyback

Pharmacy bulk package: 20 g

Indications, route, and dosage
Serious respiratory, genitourinary, GI, skin and soft-tissue, bone and joint infections (including osteomyelitis); septicemia; endocarditis
Adults: 500 mg to 1 g I.V. or I.M. q 4 to 6 hours up to 12 g daily.
Children over age 3 months: 10 to 20 mg/kg I.V. or I.M. q 6 hours; dosage depends on age, weight, and severity of infection.
Cephapirin should be injected deep I.M. into a large muscle mass, such as the gluteus or lateral aspect of the thigh.
Dosage in renal failure
Depending on the causative organism and severity of infection, patients with reduced renal function may be treated adequately with a lower dosage (7.5 to 15 mg/kg q 12 hours). Patients with severely reduced renal function and who are to be dialyzed should receive the same dosage just before dialysis and every 12 hours thereafter. To prevent toxic accumulation, reduced dosage may be required in patients with creatinine clearance below 10 ml/minute.

Pharmacodynamics
Antibacterial action: Cephapirin is primarily bactericidal; however, it may be bacteriostatic. Activity depends on the organism, tissue penetration, drug dosage, and rate of organism multiplication. It acts by adhering to bacterial penicillin-binding proteins, thereby inhibiting cell wall synthesis.
Like other first-generation cephalosporins, cephapirin is active mainly against gram-positive organisms and some gram-negative organisms. Susceptible organisms include *Streptococcus pneumoniae, Escherichia coli,* group A beta-hemolytic streptococci, *Haemophilus influenzae, Klebsiella, Proteus mirabilis, Staphylococcus aureus,* and *Streptococcus viridans.*

Pharmacokinetics
● *Absorption:* Cephapirin is not absorbed from the GI tract and must be given parenterally; peak serum levels occur 30 minutes after an I.M. dose.
● *Distribution:* Cephapirin is distributed widely into most body tissues and fluids, including the gallbladder, liver, kidneys, bone, sputum, bile, and pleural and synovial fluids; CSF penetration is poor. Cephapirin crosses the placenta; it is 44% to 50% protein-bound.
● *Metabolism:* Cephapirin is metabolized partially.
● *Excretion:* Cephapirin and metabolites are excreted primarily in urine by renal tubular secretion and glomerular filtration; small amounts of drug are excreted in breast milk. Elimination half-life is about ½ to 1 hour in patients with normal renal function; severe renal dysfunction prolongs half-life to 1 to 1½ hours. Hemodialysis removes cephapirin.

Contraindications and precautions
Cephapirin is contraindicated in patients with known hypersensitivity to any cephalosporin. It should be used with caution in patients with penicillin allergy, who usually are more susceptible to such reactions.

Interactions
Probenecid competitively inhibits renal tubular secretion of cephalosporins, resulting in higher, prolonged serum levels of these drugs.

Concomitant use with nephrotoxic agents (vancomycin, colistin, polymyxin B, or aminoglycosides) or loop diuretics increases the risk of nephrotoxicity.

Concomitant use with bacteriostatic agents (tetracyclines, erythromycin, or chloramphenicol) may impair bactericidal activity.

Effects on diagnostic tests

Cephapirin causes false-positive results in urine glucose tests utilizing cupric sulfate (Benedict's reagent or Clinitest); use glucose oxidase tests (Clinistix or Tes-Tape) instead. Cephapirin also causes false elevations in serum or urine creatinine levels in tests using Jaffé's reaction.

Cephapirin may cause positive Coombs' test results and may elevate liver function test results.

Adverse reactions

● CNS: dizziness, headache, malaise, paresthesias, seizures.
● DERM: maculopapular and erythematous rashes, urticaria.
● GI: *pseudomembranous colitis,* nausea, anorexia, vomiting, diarrhea, glossitis, dyspepsia, abdominal cramps, tenesmus, anal pruritus.
● GU: genital pruritus, vaginitis, *nephrotoxicity,* hematuria.
● HEMA: transient neutropenia, eosinophilia, anemia.
● Local: at injection site—pain, induration, sterile abscesses, tissue sloughing; phlebitis and thrombophlebitis with I.V. injection.
● Other: hypersensitivity, dyspnea, bacterial and fungal superinfection.

Note: Drug should be discontinued if signs of toxicity or immediate hypersensitivity reaction occur or if severe diarrhea indicates pseudomembranous colitis; alternative therapy should be considered if the following symptoms occur: fever, eosinophilia, hematuria, neutropenia, or unexplained elevations in BUN or serum creatinine levels.

Overdose and treatment

Clinical signs of overdose include neuromuscular hypersensitivity; seizure may follow high CNS concentrations. Remove cephapirin by hemodialysis.

▶ Special considerations

Besides those relevant to all *cephalosporins,* consider the following recommendations.
● For I.M. administration, reconstitute 1-g or 2-g vial with 1 to 2 ml respectively of sterile or bacteriostatic water for injection, so that 1.2 ml contains 500 mg of cephapirin.
● Inform patient that I.M. injection is painful. Administer deep into large muscle mass; apply ice to reduce pain. Rotate injection sites.
● For I.V. use, reconstitute 1-g or 2-g vial with 10 ml or more of 0.9% NaCl injection, bacteriostatic water for injection or dextrose injection as diluent.
● Administer direct I.V. infusion over 4 to 5 minutes. For intermittent infusion, use Y-tube administration set. Dilute 4-g vial with 40 ml of bacteriostatic water, dextrose, or NaCl for injection. Stop primary infusion during cephapirin infusion.
● Reconstituted cephapirin is stable for 10 days under refrigeration and for 12 to 48 hours at room temperature. Solution may become slightly yellow, which does not indicate loss of potency.
● Because cephapirin is dialyzable, patients undergoing treatment with hemodialysis or peritoneal dialysis may require dosage adjustments.

Pediatric use

Safe use has not been established in infants younger than age 3 months.

Breast-feeding

Cephapirin distributes into breast milk and should be used with caution in breast-feeding women. Safe use has not been established.

---

cephradine
Anspor, Velosef

● Pharmacologic classification: first-generation cephalosporin
● Therapeutic classification: antibiotic
● Pregnancy risk category B

How supplied

Available by prescription only
Capsules: 250 mg, 500 mg
Suspension: 125 mg/5 ml, 250 mg/5 ml
Injection: 250 mg, 500 mg, 1 g, 2 g, 4 g
Infusion: 2 g

Indications, route, and dosage
Serious respiratory, genitourinary, GI, skin and soft-tissue, bone and joint infections; septicemia; endocarditis; and otitis media
Adults: 500 mg to 1 g I.M. or I.V. b.i.d. to q.i.d.; do not exceed 8 g daily. Or 250 to 500 mg P.O. q 6 hours. Severe or chronic infections may require larger and/or more frequent doses (up to 1 g P.O. q 6 hours).
Children over age 1: 6 to 12 mg/kg P.O. q 6 hours. 12 to 25 mg/kg I.M. or I.V. q 6 hours.

Larger doses (up to 1 g q.i.d.) may be given for severe or chronic infections in all patients regardless of age and weight. Parenteral therapy may be followed by oral therapy. Injections should be given deep I.M. in a large muscle mass, such as the gluteus or lateral aspect of the thigh.
Dosage in renal failure
To prevent toxic accumulation, reduced dosage may be required in patients with creatinine clearance below 20 ml/minute. After an initial loading dose of 750 mg, adults with impaired renal function may require a reduction in dose as follows:

Creatinine clearance (ml/min/1.73 m^2)	Dosage in adults
> 20	500 mg q 6 hours
5 to 20	250 mg q 6 hours
< 5	250 mg q 12 hours

Pharmacodynamics
Antibacterial action: Cephradine is primarily bactericidal; however, it may be bacteriostatic. Activity depends on the organism, tissue penetration, drug dosage, and rate of organism multiplication. It acts by adhering to bacterial penicillin-binding proteins, thereby inhibiting cell wall synthesis.

Like other first-generation cephalosporins, cephradine is active against many gram-positive organisms and some gram-negative organisms. Susceptible organisms include *Escherichia coli* and other coliform bacteria, group A beta-hemolytic streptococci, *Hemophilus influenzae*, *Klebsiella*, *Proteus mirabilis*, *Staphylococcus aureus*, *Streptococcus pneumoniae*, staphylococci, and *Streptococcus viridans*.

Pharmacokinetics
● *Absorption:* Cephradine is well absorbed from the GI tract; peak serum levels occur within 1 hour after an oral dose and between 1 and 2 hours after an I.M. dose.
● *Distribution:* Cephradine is distributed widely into most body tissues and fluids, including the gallbladder, liver, kidneys, bone, sputum, bile, and pleural and synovial fluids; CSF penetration is poor. Cephradine crosses the placenta; it is 6% to 20% protein-bound.
● *Metabolism:* Cephradine is not metabolized.
● *Excretion:* Cephradine is excreted primarily in urine by renal tubular and glomerular filtration; small amounts of drug are excreted in breast milk. Elimination half-life is about ½ to 2 hours in normal renal function; end-stage renal disease prolongs half-life to 8 to 15 hours. Hemodialysis or peritoneal dialysis removes cephradine.

Contraindications and precautions
Cephradine is contraindicated in patients with known hypersensitivity to any cephalosporin. It should be used with caution in patients with penicillin allergy, who usually are more susceptible to such reactions.

Interactions
Probenecid competitively inhibits renal tubular secretion of cephalosporins, resulting in higher, prolonged serum levels of these drugs.

Concomitant use with nephrotoxic agents (vancomycin, colistin, polymyxin B, or aminoglycosides) or loop diuretics increases the risk of nephrotoxicity.

Concomitant use with bacteriostatic agents (tetracyclines, erythromycin, or chloramphenicol) may interfere with bactericidal activity.

Effects on diagnostic tests
Cephradine causes false-positive results in urine glucose tests utilizing cupric sulfate (Benedict's reagent or Clinitest); use glucose oxidase tests (Clinistix or Tes-Tape) instead. Cephradine also causes false elevations in serum or urine creatinine levels in tests using Jaffé's reaction.

Cephradine may cause positive Coombs' test results or elevate liver function test results.

Adverse reactions
● CNS: dizziness, headache, malaise, paresthesias, seizures.
● DERM: maculopapular and erythematous rashes, urticaria.
● GI: *pseudomembranous colitis,* nausea, anorexia, vomiting, heartburn, glossitis, dyspepsia, abdominal cramping, diarrhea, tenesmus, anal pruritus.
● GU: genital pruritus, vaginitis, nephrotoxicity, hematuria.
● HEMA: transient neutropenia, eosinophilia.
● Local: at injection site – pain, induration, sterile abscesses, tissue sloughing; phlebitis and thrombophlebitis with I.V. injection.

● Other: hypersensitivity, dyspnea, fever, bacterial and fungal superinfection.
Note: Drug should be discontinued if signs of toxicity or immediate hypersensitivity reaction occur or if severe diarrhea indicates pseudomembranous colitis; alternative therapy should be considered if the following symptoms occur: fever, eosinophilia, hematuria, neutropenia, or unexplained elevations in BUN or serum creatinine levels.

Overdose and treatment
Clinical signs of overdose include neuromuscular hypersensitivity; seizure may follow high CNS concentrations. Remove cephradine by hemodialysis.

▶ Special considerations
Besides those relevant to all *cephalosporins,* consider the following recommendations.
● Reconstituted oral suspension may be stored for 7 days at room temperature or for 14 days in refrigerator.
● For I.M. administration, reconstitute with sterile water for injection or with bacteriostatic water for injection as follows: 1.2 ml to 250-mg vial; 2 ml to 500-mg vial; 4 ml to 1 g-vial. I.M. solutions stored at room temperature must be used within 2 hours; if refrigerated, within 24 hours. Solutions may vary in color from light straw to yellow without affecting potency.
● A solution containing 30 mg (anhydrous base) per milliliter is approximately isotonic.
● If administration time is prolonged, infusions should be replaced every 10 hours with freshly prepared solution.
● When preparing cephradine for I.V. adminitration, use preparation specifically supplied for infusion, when available.
● I.M. injection is painful. Inject deeply into a large muscle mass; apply ice to injection site to reduce pain. Rotate injection sites to prevent tissue irritation.
● Cephradine is the only cephalosporin available in both oral and injectable forms.
● For patients on sodium restriction, note that cephradine injection contains 6 mEq of sodium per gram of drug.
● Because cephradine is dialyzable, patients undergoing treatment with hemodialysis may require dosage adjustments.

Geriatric use
Reduced dosage may be required in patients with reduced renal function. Use with caution.

Pediatric use
The serum half-life is prolonged in neonates and infants younger than age 1. Safe use has not been established.

Breast-feeding
Cephradine distributes into breast milk and should be used with caution in breast-feeding women. Safe use has not been established.

chenodiol
Chenix

- Pharmacologic classification: bile acid
- Therapeutic classification: cholelitholytic
- Pregnancy risk category X

How supplied
Available by prescription only
Tablets: 250 mg

Indications, route, and dosage
Dissolution of radiolucent cholesterol stones (gallstones) when systemic disease or age precludes surgery; to increase bile flow in patients with bile duct prostheses or stents
Adults: 250 mg b.i.d. for the first 2 weeks, followed, as tolerated, by weekly increases of 250 mg/day, up to 13 to 16 mg/kg/day for up to 18 months.

Pharmacodynamics
Cholelitholytic action: The exact mechanism of action is not fully understood; the probable methods of dissolving gallstones include altering the bile acid-to-cholesterol ratio in bile to reduce the amount of cholesterol present; suppressing the hepatic synthesis of cholesterol and cholic acid; or altering the biliary lipid content. This agent allows gradual dissolution of the radiolucent cholesterol gallstone by desaturating the bile surrounding the stone. It has no effect on radiopaque or calcified stones.

Pharmacokinetics
- *Absorption:* Absorption occurs in the small intestine and is complete in doses under 500 mg. The presence of food decreases the rate but not the extent of absorption.
- *Distribution:* Drug is 96% bound to plasma protein and is distributed primarily in enterohepatic circulation and bile.
- *Metabolism:* There is an extensive first-pass effect (60% to 80%); drug is metabolized to conjugated forms and remains in enterohepatic circulation.
- *Excretion:* Chenodiol is excreted in feces where bacteria degrade the drug to lithocholic acid.

Contraindications and precautions
Chenodiol is contraindicated in patients with hepatocyte dysfunction, bile duct abnormalities, and biliary obstruction, because the drug may be hepatotoxic; in patients with acute cholecystitis, cholangitis, gallstone pancreatitis, and biliary GI fistula, because the drug may exacerbate the symptoms of these disorders; in patients with non-visualizing gallbladder and radiopaque stones, because therapy will be ineffective; and in pregnancy, because of potential fetotoxic effects.

Interactions
Bile acid sequestering agents and aluminum-containing antacids may interfere with the absorption of chenodiol. Cholestyramine, colestipol, clofibrate, estrogens, and oral contraceptives may decrease the effectiveness of chenodiol by increasing biliary secretion of cholesterol.

Effects on diagnostic tests
Drug alters serum cholesterol and ALT (SGPT) levels.

Adverse reactions
- GI: diarrhea, constipation, gas, indigestion, loss of appetite, nausea, vomiting, stomach cramps and pain, possible liver toxicity.
Note: Drug should be discontinued if serum aminotransferase levels exceed three times the upper normal limit or if there is no response by 18 months.

Overdose and treatment
The clinical manifestation of overdose is severe diarrhea. Treatment includes gastric lavage with charcoal suspension or cholestyramine; 1 liter of lavage fluid will be necessary.

▶ Special considerations
- Administer morning and evening.
- Monitor liver function studies.

Information for the patient
- Tell patient to report diarrhea, which may require dosage adjustment.
- Inform patient that periodic liver function tests and an ultrasound or oral cholecystograms will be necessary to monitor stone dissolution.
- Tell patient that therapy may continue for up to 18 months.

Breast-feeding
It is unknown whether chenodiol appears in breast milk; it should be used with caution in breast-feeding women.

chloral hydrate
Aquachloral, Noctec, Novochlorhydrate

- Pharmacologic classification: general CNS depressant
- Therapeutic classification: sedative-hypnotic
- Controlled substance schedule IV
- Pregnancy risk category C

How supplied
Available by prescription only
Capsules: 250 mg, 500 mg
Syrup: 250 mg/5 ml, 500 mg/5 ml
Suppositories: 325 mg, 500 mg, 650 mg

Indications, route, and dosage
Sedation
Adults: 250 mg P.O. or rectally t.i.d. after meals.
Children: 8 mg/kg P.O. t.i.d. Maximum dosage is 500 mg t.i.d.
Insomnia
Adults: 500 mg to 1 g P.O. or rectally 15 to 30 minutes before bedtime.
Children: 50 mg/kg single dose. Maximum dosage is 1 g.
Premedication for EEG
Children: 25 mg/kg single dose. Maximum dosage is 1 g.
Hypnosis
Children: 50 mg/kg P.O. or 1.5 g/m² as a single dose.

Pharmacodynamics
Sedative-hypnotic action: Chloral hydrate has CNS depressant activities similar to those of the barbiturates. Nonspecific CNS depression occurs at hypnotic doses; however, respiratory drive is only slightly affected. The

drug's primary site of action is the reticular activating system, which controls arousal. The cellular site(s) of action are not known.

Pharmacokinetics
● *Absorption:* Chloral hydrate is absorbed well after oral and rectal administration. Sleep occurs 30 to 60 minutes after a 500-mg to 1-g dose.
● *Distribution:* Chloral hydrate and its active metabolite trichloroethanol are distributed throughout the body tissue and fluids. Trichloroethanol is 35% to 41% protein-bound.
● *Metabolism:* Chloral hydrate is metabolized rapidly and nearly completely in the liver and erythrocytes to the active metabolite trichloroethanol. It is further metabolized in the liver and kidneys to trichloroacetic acid and other inactive metabolites.
● *Excretion:* The inactive metabolites of chloral hydrate are excreted primarily in urine. Minor amounts are excreted in bile. The half-life of trichloroethanol is 8 to 10 hours.

Contraindications and precautions
Chloral hydrate is contraindicated in patients with known hypersensitivity to chloral derivatives; in patients with severe cardiac disease; and in patients with marked renal or hepatic failure because elimination of the drug will decrease.

Chloral hydrate should be used cautiously in patients with signs and symptoms of depression, suicidal ideation, or history of drug abuse or addiction, because the drug depresses CNS function; and in patients who need to perform hazardous tasks requiring mental alertness or physical coordination. Do not administer oral forms of chloral hydrate to patients with esophagitis, gastritis, or gastric or duodenal ulcers, because the drug is irritating to the GI tract. Rectal chloral hydrate may exacerbate proctitis or ulcerative colitis.

Interactions
Concomitant use with alcohol, sedative-hypnotics, narcotics, antihistamines, tranquilizers, tricyclic antidepressants, or other CNS depressants will add to or potentiate their effects. Concomitant use with alcohol may cause vasodilation, tachycardia, sweating, and flushing in some patients.

Administration of chloral hydrate followed by I.V. furosemide may cause a hypermetabolic state by displacing thyroid hormone from binding sites, resulting in sweating, hot flashes, tachycardia, and variable blood pressure.

Chloral hydrate may displace oral anticoagulants such as warfarin from protein-binding sites, causing increased hypoprothrombinemic effects.

Effects on diagnostic tests
Chloral hydrate therapy may produce false-positive results for urine glucose with tests using cupric sulfate, such as Benedict's reagent and possibly Clinitest. It does not interfere with Clinistix or Tes-Tape results. It will interfere with fluorometric tests for urine catecholamines; do not use drug for 48 hours before the test. Drug may also interfere with Reddy-Jenkins-Thorn test for urinary 17-hydroxycorticosteroids. It also may cause a false-positive phentolamine test.

Adverse reactions
● CNS: hangover, headache, ataxia, confusion, hallucinations, disorientation, excitement, nightmares, paranoia.
● DERM: rash, urticaria, erythema, eczematoid dermatitis, scarlatiniform exanthema.
● GI: gastric irritation, nausea, vomiting, diarrhea, flatulence, altered taste.
● GU: ketonuria.
● HEMA: leukopenia, eosinophilia.
   Note: Drug should be discontinued if hypersensitivity occurs, if patient becomes incoherent or disoriented, or if patient exhibits paranoid behavior.

Overdose and treatment
Clinical manifestations of overdose include stupor, coma, respiratory depression, pinpoint pupils, hypotension, and hypothermia. Esophageal stricture may follow gastric necrosis and perforation. GI hemorrhage has also been reported. Hepatic damage and jaundice may occur.

Treatment is supportive of respiration (including mechanical ventilation if needed), blood pressure, and body temperature. If the patient is conscious, empty stomach by emesis or gastric lavage. Hemodialysis will remove chloral hydrate and its metabolite, trichloroethanol. Peritoneal dialysis is ineffective.

▶ Special considerations
● Not a first-line drug because of potential for adverse or toxic side effects.
● Assess level of consciousness before administering drug to ensure appropriate baseline level.
● Give chloral hydrate capsules with a full glass of water to lessen GI upset; dilute syrup in a half glass of water or juice before administration to improve taste.
● Monitor vital signs frequently.
● Store in dark container away from heat and moisture to prevent breakdown of medicine. Store suppositories in refrigerator.

Information for the patient
● Advise patient to take with a full glass of water, and to dilute syrup with juice or water before taking.
● Instruct patient in proper administration of drug form prescribed.
● Warn patient not to attempt tasks that require mental alertness or physical coordination until the CNS effects of the drug are known.
● Tell patient to avoid alcohol and other CNS depressants.
● Instruct patient to call before using any nonprescription allergy or cold preparations.
● Warn patient not to increase the dose or stop the drug except as prescribed.

Geriatric use
Elderly patients may be more susceptible to the drug's CNS depressant effects because of decreased elimination. Lower doses are indicated.

Pediatric use
Chloral hydrate is safe and effective as a premedication for EEG and other procedures.

Breast-feeding
Small amounts pass into the breast milk and may cause drowsiness in breast-fed infants of mothers taking chloral hydrate; avoid use in breast-feeding women.

---

chlorambucil
Leukeran

- Pharmacologic classification: alkylating agent (cell cycle-phase nonspecific)
- Therapeutic classification: antineoplastic
- Pregnancy risk category D

How supplied
Available by prescription only
Tablets (sugar-coated): 2 mg

Indications, route, and dosage
Dosage and indications may vary. Check current literature for recommended protocol.
Chronic lymphocytic leukemia, diffuse lymphocytic lymphoma, Hodgkin's disease, autoimmune hemolytic anemias, lupus glomerulonephritis, nephrotic syndrome, polycythemia vera, macroglobulinemia, ovarian neoplasms
Adults: 100 to 200 mcg/kg P.O. daily or 3 to 6 mg/m² P.O. daily as a single dose or in divided doses; for 3 to 6 weeks. Usual dose is 4 to 10 mg daily. Reduce dose if within 4 weeks of a full course of radiation therapy.
Children: 100 to 200 mcg/kg or 4.5 mg/m² as a single daily dose.

Pharmacodynamics
Antineoplastic action: Chlorambucil exerts its cytotoxic activity by cross-linking strands of cellular DNA and RNA, disrupting normal nucleic acid function.

Pharmacokinetics
- *Absorption:* Chlorambucil is well absorbed from the GI tract.
- *Distribution:* The distribution of chlorambucil is not well understood. However, the drug and its metabolites have been shown to be highly bound to plasma and tissue proteins.
- *Metabolism:* Chlorambucil is metabolized in the liver. The primary metabolite, phenylacetic acid mustard, also possesses cytotoxic activity.
- *Excretion:* The metabolites of chlorambucil are excreted in urine. The half-life of the parent compound is 2 hours; the phenylacetic acid metabolite, 2½ hours. Chlorambucil is probably not dialyzable.

Contraindications and precautions
Chlorambucil is contraindicated in patients with a history of hypersensitivity to the drug or of resistance to previous therapy with the drug. Cross-sensitivity, which manifests as a rash, may occur between chlorambucil and other alkylating agents.
Dosage adjustments must be considered in patients with hematologic impairment because of the drug's hematologic toxicity.
Chlorambucil should be used with caution in patients with a history of seizures, head trauma, or use of epileptogenic drugs. There is a small risk of chlorambucil-induced seizure.
Patients should not receive a full dose of chlorambucil if a full course of radiation therapy or other myelosuppressive drugs were administered within the preceding 4 weeks because of the potential for additive toxicity.

Interactions
None reported.

Effects on diagnostic tests
Chlorambucil therapy may increase concentrations of serum alkaline phosphatase, AST (SGOT), and blood and urine uric acid.

Adverse reactions
- CNS: seizures (with high doses).
- DERM: rash, pruritus, peripheral neuropathy (rare).
- GI: nausea, vomiting, anorexia, abdominal pain, diarrhea.
- GU: sterile cystitis (rare).
- HEMA: *pancytopenia* (dose-limiting).
- Metabolic: hyperuricemia.
- Other: *pulmonary fibrosis,* drug fever, alopecia (rare).

Overdose and treatment
Clinical manifestations of overdose include reversible pancytopenia in adults and vomiting, ataxia, abdominal pain, muscle twitching, and major motor seizures in children. Treatment is usually supportive with transfusion of blood components if necessary and appropriate anticonvulsant therapy if seizures occur. Induction of emesis, activated charcoal, and gastric lavage may be useful in removing unabsorbed drug.

▶ Special considerations
Besides those relevant to all *alkylating agents,* consider the following recommendations.
- Oral suspension can be prepared in the pharmacy by crushing tablets and mixing powder with a suspending agent and simple syrup.
- Avoid all I.M. injections when platelets are below 100,000/mm³.
- Anticoagulants and aspirin products should be used cautiously. Watch closely for signs of bleeding.
- Chlorambucil-induced pancytopenia generally lasts 1 to 2 weeks but may persist for 3 to 4 weeks. It is reversible up to a cumulative dose of 6.5 mg/kg in a single course.
- To prevent hyperuricemia with resulting uric acid nephropathy, allopurinol may be used with adequate hydration. Monitor uric acid.
- Store tablets in a tightly closed, light-resistant container.

Information for the patient
- Emphasize importance of continuing medication despite nausea and vomiting, and of keeping appointments for periodic blood work.
- Advise patient to call if vomiting occurs shortly after taking the dose or if symptoms of infection or bleeding are present.
- Tell patient to avoid exposure to people with infections.
- Instruct patient to avoid nonprescription products containing aspirin.

Pediatric use
The safe and effective use of chlorambucil in children has not been established. The potential benefits versus risks must be evaluated.

Breast-feeding
It is unknown if chlorambucil distributes into breast milk. The risk of potential serious adverse reactions, mutagenicity, and carcinogenicity in breast-feeding infants

---

and the mother's need for the medication should be considered in deciding whether to discontinue the drug or breast-feed.

chloramphenicol
Antibiopto, Chloromycetin, Chloroptic, Econochlor, Fenicol*, Isopto-Fenicol, Novochlorocap*, Ophthochlor, Pentamycetin*

chloramphenicol palmitate
Chloromycetin Palmitate

chloramphenicol sodium succinate
Chloromycetin Sodium Succinate, Mychel S, Pentamycetin*

- Pharmacologic classification: dichloroacetic acid derivative
- Therapeutic classification: antibiotic
- Pregnancy risk category C

How supplied
Available by prescription only
Capsules: 250 mg, 500 mg
Suspension: 150 mg/5 ml
Injection: 1-g, 10-g vial
Ophthalmic solution: 0.5%
Ophthalmic ointment: 1%
Topical cream: 1%
Otic solution: 0.5%

Indications, route, and dosage
Severe meningitis, brain abscesses, bacteremia, or other serious infections
Adults and children: 50 to 100 mg/kg P.O. or I.V. daily, divided q 6 hours. Maximum dose is 100 mg/kg daily.
Premature infants and neonates: 25 mg/kg I.V. daily.
Neonates weighing more than 2,000 g and age 7 days or more: 25 mg/kg I.V. q 12 hours. I.V. route must be used to treat meningitis.
Superficial infections of the skin caused by susceptible bacteria
Adults and children: Rub into affected area b.i.d. or t.i.d.
External ear canal infection
Adults and children: 2 to 3 drops into ear canal t.i.d or q.i.d.
Surface bacterial infection involving conjunctiva or cornea
Adults and children: Instill 2 drops of solution in eye every hour until condition improves, or instill q.i.d., depending on severity of infection. Apply small amount of ointment to lower conjunctival sac at bedtime as supplement to drops. To use ointment alone, apply small amount to lower conjunctival sac q 3 to 6 hours or more frequently if necessary. Continue until condition improves.

Pharmacodynamics
Antibacterial action: Chloramphenicol palmitate and chloramphenicol sodium succinate must be hydrolyzed to chloramphenicol before antimicrobial activity can take place. The active compound then inhibits bacterial protein synthesis by binding to the ribosome's 50S subunit, thus inhibiting peptide bond formation.

Chloramphenicol usually produces bacteriostatic effects on susceptible bacteria, including *Rickettsia, Chlamydia,* and *Mycoplasma* and certain *Salmonella* strains, as well as most gram-positive and gram-negative organisms. It is used to treat *Haemophilus influenzae,* Rocky Mountain spotted fever, meningitis, lymphogranuloma, psittacosis, severe meningitis, and bacteremia.

Pharmacokinetics
- *Absorption:* After oral administration, chloramphenicol is well absorbed from the GI tract. Palmitate and sodium succinate salts are hydrolyzed quickly to chloramphenicol. Peak serum concentrations occur in 1 to 3 hours. In patients receiving chloramphenicol palmitate, mean serum concentrations resemble those achieved by the base. Recommended therapeutic range is 15 to 25 mcg/ml for peak levels and 5 to 10 mcg/ml for trough levels.
  With I.V. administration, serum concentrations vary greatly, depending on patient's metabolism.
- *Distribution:* Chloramphenicol is distributed widely to most body tissues and fluids, including CSF, liver, and kidneys; it readily crosses the placenta. Approximately 50% to 60% of the drug binds to plasma proteins.
- *Metabolism:* Parent drug is metabolized primarily by hepatic glucuronyl transferase to inactive metabolites.
- *Excretion:* About 8% to 12% of dose is excreted by the kidneys as unchanged drug; the remainder is excreted as inactive metabolites. (However, some drug may be excreted in breast milk.) Plasma half-life ranges from about 1½ to 4½ hours in adults with normal hepatic and renal function. Plasma half-life of parent drug is prolonged in patients with hepatic dysfunction. Peritoneal hemodialysis does not remove significant drug amounts. Plasma chloramphenicol levels may be elevated in patients with renal impairment after I.V. chloramphenicol administration.

Contraindications and precautions
Chloramphenicol is contraindicated in patients with minor infections (such as influenza, throat infections, and colds) or as prophylaxis against infection, because potential toxicity may outweigh therapeutic benefit; it is also contraindicated in patients with known hypersensitivity or history of toxic reaction to the drug.

Chloramphenicol should be administered cautiously to infants and to patients with renal or hepatic dysfunction, acute intermittent porphyria, or glucose-6-phosphate dehydrogenase (G6PD) deficiency because of potential for adverse hematopoietic effects (including gray syndrome).

Interactions
When used concomitantly, chloramphenicol inhibits hepatic metabolism of phenytoin, dicumarol, tolbutamide, chlorpropamide, phenobarbital, and cyclophosphamide (by inhibiting microsomal enzyme activity); that leads to prolonged plasma half-life of these drugs and possible toxicity from increased serum drug concentrations. When used concomitantly, chloramphenicol may antagonize penicillin's bactericidal activity.

Concomitant use with acetaminophen causes an elevated serum chloramphenicol level (by an unknown mechanism), possibly resulting in an enhanced pharmacologic effect. Concomitant use with iron salts, folic acid, and vitamin B_2 reduces the hematologic response to these substances.

Effects on diagnostic tests

False elevation of urinary para-aminobenzoic acid (PABA) levels will result if chloramphenicol is administered during a bentiromide test for pancreatic function. Treatment with chloramphenicol will cause false-positive results on tests for urine glucose level using cupric sulfate (Clinitest). Erythrocyte, platelet, and leukocyte counts in the blood and possibly the bone marrow may decrease during chloramphenicol therapy (from reversible or irreversible bone marrow depression). Hemoglobinuria or lactic acidosis may also occur.

Adverse reactions

● CNS: headache, mild depression, confusion, delirium, peripheral neuropathy (with prolonged therapy).
● CV: *cardiovascular collapse in newborns (gray syndrome).*
● DERM: possible contact sensitivity; itching, burning, urticaria, angioneurotic edema in patients hypersensitive to any drug components (topical application).
● EENT: itching or burning ears (with otic application); optic neuritis in patients with cystic fibrosis; glossitis; decreased visual acuity; optic atrophy in children; stinging, burning, or itching eyes (ophthalmic); urticaria; vesicular or maculopapular dermatitis (otic).
● GI: nausea, vomiting, stomatitis, diarrhea, enterocolitis, jaundice.
● HEMA: granulocytopenia, *aplastic anemia* (not dose-related, irreversible, and idiopathic), hypoplastic anemia, granulocytopenia, thrombocytopenia (dose-related, reversible).
● Other: infection by nonsusceptible organisms (with topical or systemic administration); hypersensitivity reaction (fever, rash, urticaria, *anaphylaxis*); sore throat; angioedema; *gray syndrome* in premature and newborn infants (abdominal distention, gray cyanosis, *vasomotor collapse, respiratory distress, and possible death* within a few hours of symptom onset).
  Note: Drug should be discontinued if patient develops hypersensitivity reaction, optic or peripheral neuritis, or blood dyscrasias. Systemic adverse reactions have not been reported with short-term topical use.

Overdose and treatment

Clinical effects of parenterally administered overdose include anemia and metabolic acidosis followed by hypotension, hypothermia, abdominal distention, and possible death. Clinical effects of acute oral overdose include nausea, vomiting, and diarrhea.
  Initial treatment is symptomatic and supportive. Chloramphenicol may be removed by charcoal hemoperfusion.

▶ Special considerations

● Culture and sensitivity tests may be done concurrently with first dose and then as needed.
● Use drug only when clearly indicated for severe infection. Because of chloramphenicol's potential for severe toxicity, it should be reserved for potentially life-threatening infections.
● If administering drug concomitantly with penicillin, give penicillin 1 hour or more before chloramphenicol to avoid reduction in penicillin's bactericidal activity.
● For I.V. administration, reconstitute 1-g vial of powder for injection with 10 ml of sterile water for injection; concentration will be 100 mg/ml. Solution remains stable for 30 days at room temperature; however, refrigeration is recommended. Do not use cloudy solutions.

Administer I.V. infusion slowly, over at least 1 minute. Check injection site daily for phlebitis and irritation.
● Monitor complete blood count, platelet count, reticulocyte count, and serum iron level before therapy begins and every 2 days during therapy. Discontinue immediately if test results indicate anemia, reticulocytopenia, leukopenia, or thrombocytopenia.
● Observe patient for signs and symptoms of superinfection by nonsusceptible organisms.

Information for the patient

● Instruct patient to take oral drug forms on an empty stomach 1 hour before or 2 hours after meals. (If patient develops adverse GI effects, however, advise him to take drug with food.)
● Instruct patient to report adverse reactions, especially nausea, vomiting, diarrhea, bleeding, fever, confusion, sore throat, or mouth sores.
● Tell patient to take medication for prescribed period and to take it exactly as directed, even after he feels better.
● Instruct patient to wash hands before and after applying topical ointment or solution.
● If patient is using otic solution, caution him not to touch ear with dropper.
● If patient is using topical cream, warn him to avoid sharing washcloths and towels with family members.
● If patient is using ophthalmic drug form, instruct him to cleanse eye area of excess exudate before applying drug, and show him how to instill drug in eye. Warn him not to touch applicator tip to eye or surrounding tissue. Instruct him to observe for signs and symptoms of sensitivity, such as itchy eyelids or constant burning, and to discontinue use of the drug and call immediately should any occur.

Geriatric use

Administer drug cautiously to elderly patients with impaired liver function.

Pediatric use

Use drug cautiously in children under age 2 because of risk of gray syndrome (although most cases occur in first 48 hours after birth). Drug has prolonged half-life in neonates, necessitating special dose.

Breast-feeding

Drug is excreted in breast milk in low concentrations, posing risk of bone marrow depression and slight risk of gray syndrome. Alternative feeding method is recommended during treatment with chloramphenicol.

---

*Canada only   †Unlabeled clinical use   Italicized adverse reactions are life-threatening.

chlordiazepoxide
Libritabs

chlordiazepoxide hydrochloride
Apo-Chlordiazepoxide*, Librium, Lipoxide, SK-Lygen, Medilium*, Murcil, Novopoxide*, Reposans-10, Sereen, Solium*

- Pharmacologic classification: benzodiazepine
- Therapeutic classification: antianxiety agent; anticonvulsant; sedative-hypnotic
- Controlled substance schedule IV
- Pregnancy risk category D

How supplied
Available by prescription only
Tablets: 5 mg, 10 mg, 25 mg
Capsules: 5 mg, 10 mg, 25 mg
Powder for injection: 100 mg/ampule

Indications, route, and dosage
Mild to moderate anxiety and tension
Adults: 5 to 10 mg t.i.d. or q.i.d.
Children over age 6: 5 mg P.O. b.i.d. to q.i.d. Maximum dosage is 10 mg P.O. b.i.d. to t.i.d.
Severe anxiety and tension
Adults: 20 to 25 mg t.i.d. or q.i.d.
Withdrawal symptoms of acute alcoholism
Adults: 50 to 100 mg P.O., I.M., or I.V. Maximum dosage is 300 mg/day.
Preoperative apprehension and anxiety
Adults: 5 to 10 mg P.O. t.i.d. or q.i.d. on day before surgery; or 50 to 100 mg I.M. 1 hour before surgery.
Note: Parenteral form is not recommended in children under age 12.

Pharmacodynamics
- *Anxiolytic action:* Chlordiazepoxide depresses the CNS at the limbic and subcortical levels of the brain. It produces an antianxiety effect by influencing the effect of the neurotransmitter gamma-aminobutyric acid (GABA) on its receptor in the ascending reticular activating system, which increases inhibition and blocks both cortical and limbic arousal after stimulation of the reticular formation.
- *Anticonvulsant action:* Chlordiazepoxide suppresses the spread of seizure activity produced by the epileptogenic foci in the cortex, thalamus, and limbic structures by enhancing presynaptic inhibition.

Pharmacokinetics
- *Absorption:* When given orally, chlordiazepoxide is absorbed well through the GI tract. Action begins in 30 to 45 minutes, with peak action in 1 to 3 hours. I.M. administration results in erratic absorption of the drug; onset of action usually occurs in 15 to 30 minutes. After I.V. administration, rapid onset of action occurs in 1 to 5 minutes after injection.
- *Distribution:* Chlordiazepoxide is distributed widely throughout the body. Drug is 80% to 90% protein-bound.
- *Metabolism:* Chlordiazepoxide is metabolized in the liver to several active metabolites.
- *Excretion:* Most metabolites of chlordiazepoxide are

excreted in urine as glucuronide conjugates. The half-life of chlordiazepoxide is 5 to 30 hours.

Contraindications and precautions
Chlordiazepoxide is contraindicated in patients with known hypersensitivity to the drug; in patients with acute narrow-angle glaucoma or untreated open-angle glaucoma, because of the drug's possible anticholinergic effect; in patients in shock or coma, because the drug's hypnotic or hypotensive effect may be prolonged or intensified; in patients with acute alcohol intoxication who have depressed vital signs, because the drug will worsen CNS depression; and in infants younger than age 30 days, in whom slow metabolism causes the drug to accumulate.

Chlordiazepoxide should be used cautiously in patients with psychoses, because it is rarely beneficial in such patients and may induce paradoxical reactions; in patients with myasthenia gravis or Parkinson's disease, because drug may exacerbate the disorder; in patients with impaired renal or hepatic function, which prolongs elimination of the drug; in elderly or debilitated patients, who are usually more sensitive to the drug's CNS effects; and in individuals prone to addiction or drug abuse.

Interactions
Chlordiazepoxide potentiates the CNS depressant effects of phenothiazines, narcotics, barbiturates, alcohol, antihistamines, monoamine oxidase inhibitors, general anesthetics, and antidepressants. Concomitant use with cimetidine and possibly disulfiram diminishes hepatic metabolism of chlordiazepoxide, which increases its plasma concentration. Heavy smoking accelerates chlordiazepoxide's metabolism, thus lowering clinical effectiveness. Oral contraceptives may impair the metabolism of chlordiazepoxide. Antacids may delay the absorption of chlordiazepoxide. Concomitant use with levodopa may decrease the therapeutic effects of levodopa. Benzodiazepines may decrease serum levels of haloperidol.

Effects on diagnostic tests
Chlordiazepoxide therapy may elevate results of liver function tests. Minor changes in EEG patterns, usually low-voltage, fast activity, may occur during and after chlordiazepoxide therapy. Chlordiazepoxide may cause a false-positive pregnancy test, depending on method used. It may also alter urinary 17-ketosteroids (Zimmerman reaction), urine alkaloid determination (Frings thin layer chromatography method), and urinary glucose determinations (with Clinistix and Diastix, but not Tes-Tape).

Adverse reactions
- CNS: confusion, depression, drowsiness, lethargy, hangover effect, ataxia, dizziness, syncope, nightmares, fatigue, slurred speech, tremor, vertigo, paradoxical reactions (such as hyperaggressiveness, rage), decreased libido.
- CV: *cardiovascular collapse,* transient hypotension, palpitations, bradycardia.
- DERM: rash, urticaria, hair loss.
- EENT: diplopia, blurred vision, nystagmus.
- GI: constipation, dry mouth, nausea, vomiting, difficulty swallowing, anorexia, abdominal discomfort.
- GU: urinary incontinence, urine retention.
- Local: pain, phlebitis, and desquamation at injection site.

● Other: *respiratory depression,* dysarthria, headache, hepatic dysfunction, active intermittent porphyria.

Note: Drug should be discontinued if hypersensitivity or the following paradoxical reactions occur: acute hyperexcited state, anxiety, hallucinations, increased muscle spasticity, insomnia, or rage.

Overdose and treatment
Clinical manifestations of overdose include somnolence, confusion, coma, hypoactive reflexes, dyspnea, labored breathing, hypotension, bradycardia, slurred speech, and unsteady gait or impaired coordination.

Support blood pressure and respiration until drug effects subside; monitor vital signs. Flumazenil, a specific benzodiazepine antagonist, may be useful. Mechanical ventilatory assistance via endotracheal tube may be required to maintain a patent airway and support adequate oxygenation. Use I.V. fluids and vasopressors like dopamine and phenylephrine to treat hypotension as needed. Use gastric lavage if ingestion was recent, but only if an endotracheal tube is in place to prevent aspiration. Induce emesis if the patient is conscious. After emesis or lavage, administer activated charcoal with a cathartic as a single dose. Do not administer barbiturates if excitation occurs. Dialysis is of limited value.

▶ **Special considerations**
Besides those relevant to all *benzodiazepines,* consider the following recommendations.

● I.M. administration is not recommended because of erratic and slow absorption. However, if I.M. route is used, reconstitute with special diluent only. Do not use diluent if hazy. Discard unused portion. Inject I.M. deep into large muscle mass.

● For I.V. administration, drug should be reconstituted with sterile water or normal saline solution and infused slowly, directly into a large vein, at a rate not exceeding 50 mg/minute for adults. Do not infuse chlordiazepoxide into small veins. Avoid extravasation into subcutaneous tissue. Observe the infusion site for phlebitis. Keep resuscitation equipment nearby in case of an emergency.

● Prepare solutions for I.V. or I.M. use immediately before administration. Discard any unused portions.

● Patients should remain in bed under observation for at least 3 hours after parenteral administration of chlordiazepoxide.

● Lower doses are effective in patients with renal and hepatic dysfunction. Closely monitor renal and hepatic studies for signs of dysfunction.

Information for the patient
Warn patient that sudden changes in position may cause dizziness. Advise patient to dangle legs a few minutes before getting out of bed to prevent falls and injury.

Geriatric use
● Elderly patients demonstrate a greater sensitivity to the CNS depressant effects of chlordiazepoxide. Some may require supervision with ambulation and activities of daily living during initiation of therapy or after an increase in dose.

● Lower doses are usually effective in elderly patients because of decreased elimination.

● Parenteral administration of this drug is more likely to cause apnea, hypotension, and bradycardia in elderly patients.

Pediatric use
Safety of oral use has not been established in children under age 6. Safety of parenteral use has not been established in children under age 12.

Breast-feeding
The breast-fed infant of a mother who uses chlordiazepoxide may become sedated, have feeding difficulties, or lose weight. Do not administer drug to breast-feeding women.

chloroquine hydrochloride
Aralen Hydrochloride

chloroquine phosphate
Aralen Phosphate

● Pharmacologic classification: 4-aminoquinoline
● Therapeutic classification: antimalarial, amebicide, anti-inflammatory
● Pregnancy risk category C

How supplied
Available by prescription only
Chloroquine hydrochloride
Injection: 50 mg/ml (40 mg/ml base)
Chloroquine phosphate
Tablets: 250 mg (150-mg base), 500 mg (300-mg base)

Indications, route, and dosage
Suppressive prophylaxis and treatment of acute attacks of malaria
Adults: Initially, 600 mg (base) P.O., then 300 mg P.O. at 6, 24, and 48 hours. Or 160 to 200 mg (base) I.M. initially; repeat in 6 hours if needed. Do not exceed 800 mg (base) total dose in the first 24 hours. Switch to oral therapy as soon as possible. Continue oral therapy for 3 days until approximately 1.5 g of base has been administered.
Children: Initially, 10 mg (base)/kg P.O., then 5 mg (base)/kg P.O. at 6, 24, and 48 hours (do not exceed adult dosage). Or 5 mg (base)/kg I.M. initially; repeat in 6 hours if needed. Switch to oral therapy as soon as possible.
Suppressive treatment of malaria in areas where chloroquine-resistant Plasmodium falciparum has not been reported
Adults and children: 5 mg (base)/kg P.O. (not to exceed 300 mg) weekly on same day of the week (begin 1 week before entering endemic area and continue for 4 weeks after leaving). If treatment begins after exposure, double the initial dose (600 mg for adults, 10 mg/kg for children) in two divided doses P.O. 6 hours apart.
Extraintestinal amebiasis
Adults: 160 to 200 mg of chloroquine (hydrochloride) base I.M. daily for no more than 12 days. As soon as possible, substitute 1 g (600 mg base) of chloroquine phosphate P.O. daily for 2 days; then 500 mg (300 mg base) daily for 2 to 3 weeks. Treatment is usually combined with an effective intestinal amebicide.
Children: 10 mg/kg of chloroquine (hydrochloride) base for 2 to 3 weeks. Maximum 300 mg daily.
†Rheumatoid arthritis
Adults: 250 mg of chloroquine phosphate daily with evening meal.

---

†*Lupus erythematosus*
Adults: 250 mg of chloroquine phosphate daily with evening meal; reduce dosage gradually over several months when lesions regress.

Pharmacodynamics
● *Antimalarial action:* Chloroquine binds to DNA, interfering with protein synthesis. It also inhibits both DNA and RNA polymerases.
● *Amebicidal action:* Mechanism of action is unknown.
● *Anti-inflammatory action:* Mechanism of action is unknown. Chloroquine may antagonize histamine and serotonin and inhibit prostaglandin effects by inhibiting conversion of arachidonic acid to prostaglandin F_2; it also may inhibit chemotaxis of polymorphonuclear leukocytes, macrophages, and eosinophils.

Chloroquine's spectrum of activity includes the asexual erythrocytic forms of *P. malariae, P. ovale, P. vivax,* many strains of *P. falciparum,* and *Entamoeba histolytica.*

Pharmacokinetics
● *Absorption:* Chloroquine is absorbed readily and almost completely, with peak plasma concentrations occurring at 1 to 2 hours.
● *Distribution:* Chloroquine is 55% bound to plasma proteins. It concentrates in the liver, spleen, kidneys, heart, and brain and is strongly bound in melanin-containing cells.
● *Metabolism:* About 30% of an administered dose of chloroquine is metabolized by the liver to monodesethylchloroquine and bidesethylchloroquine.
● *Excretion:* About 70% of an administered dose is excreted unchanged in urine; unabsorbed drug is excreted in feces. Small amounts of the drug may be present in urine for months after the drug is discontinued. Renal excretion is enhanced by urinary acidification. It is excreted in breast milk.

Contraindications and precautions
Chloroquine is contraindicated in patients who have experienced retinal or visual field changes or hypersensitivity reactions to 4-aminoquinoline compounds unless these compounds are the only agents to which the malarial strain is sensitive.

Chloroquine should be used cautiously in patients with psoriasis, porphyria, or G6PD deficiency because the drug may exacerbate these conditions. Because chloroquine concentrates in the liver and may cause adverse hepatic effects, it should be used cautiously in patients with hepatic disease or alcoholism and in patients receiving other hepatotoxic drugs.

Interactions
Concomitant administration of kaolin or magnesium trisilicate may decrease absorption of chloroquine. Chloroquine may interfere with antibody response to intradermal human diploid cell rabies vaccine.

Effects on diagnostic tests
Chloroquine may cause inversion or depression of the T wave or widening of the QRS complex on ECG. Rarely, it may cause decreased white blood cell, red blood cell, or platelet counts.

Adverse reactions
● CNS: mild and transient headache, neuromyopathy, psychic stimulation, fatigue, irritability, nightmares, seizures, dizziness, toxic psychosis, apathy, confusion, depression.
● CV: hypotension, ECG changes, cardiomyopathy.
● DERM: pruritus, lichen planus-like eruptions, skin and mucosal pigmentary changes, pleomorphic skin eruptions, exacerbations of psoriasis.
● EENT: *visual disturbances* (blurred vision; difficulty in focusing; reversible corneal changes; generally irreversible, sometimes progressive or delayed, retinal changes, such as narrowing of arterioles; macular lesions; pallor of optic disk; optic atrophy; patchy retinal pigmentation, often leading to blindness); ototoxicity (nerve deafness, vertigo, tinnitus).
● GI: anorexia, abdominal cramps, diarrhea, nausea, vomiting, stomatitis.
● HEMA: *agranulocytosis,* hemolytic anemia, aplastic anemia, thrombocytopenia.
● Other: bleaching of hair.
Note: Drug should be discontinued at the first sign of visual changes not explainable by difficulties of accommodation or corneal opacities or of hematologic abnormalities not attributable to the disease being treated, or if muscular weakness occurs during therapy.

Overdose and treatment
Symptoms of chloroquine overdose may appear within 30 minutes after ingestion and may include headache, drowsiness, visual changes, cardiovascular collapse, and convulsions followed by respiratory and cardiac arrest.

Treatment is symptomatic. The stomach should be emptied by emesis or lavage. After lavage, activated charcoal in an amount at least five times the estimated amount of drug ingested may be helpful if given within 30 minutes of ingestion.

Ultra-short-acting barbiturates may help control seizures. Intubation may become necessary. Peritoneal dialysis and exchange transfusions also may be useful. Forced fluids and acidification of the urine are helpful after the acute phase.

▶ Special considerations
Besides those relevant to all *aminoquinolines,* consider the following recommendations.
● Baseline and periodic ophthalmologic examinations are necessary in prolonged or high-dosage therapy.
● Patient should report blurred vision, increased sensitivity to light, hearing loss, pronounced GI disturbances, or muscle weakness promptly.
● Give immediately before or after meals on the same day each week to minimize gastric distress. Patients who cannot tolerate the drug because of GI distress may tolerate hydroxychloroquine.
● Resistance of *P. falciparum* to chloroquine has spread to most areas with malaria except the Dominican Republic, Haiti, Central America west of the Panama Canal, the Middle East, and Egypt.
● The Centers for Disease Control currently recommends weekly chloroquine prophylaxis for travellers who cannot tolerate doxycycline or mefloquine, especially children under 15 kg and pregnant women.
● It may also be advisable to provide travellers with sulfadoxine with pyrimethamine (Fansidar) to be carried during travel. Patients should be instructed to take the drug in the event of a febrile illness where professional medical care is not available. (The recommended prescriptive dose for adults is 1,500 mg sulfadoxine and 75 mg pyrimethamine, or three tablets.) Emphasize that such self-treatment is a temporary measure, and that

they must seek medical care as soon as possible. They should continue prophylaxis after the treatment dose of Fansidar.

Information for the patient
To prevent drug-induced dermatoses, warn patient to avoid excessive exposure to the sun.

Pediatric use
Children are extremely susceptible to toxicity; monitor closely for adverse effects.

Breast-feeding
Safety has not been established. Use with caution in breast-feeding women.

chlorothiazide
Diachlor, Diuril, Ro-Chlorozide, SK-Chlorothiazide

- Pharmacologic classification: thiazide diuretic
- Therapeutic classification: diuretic, antihypertensive
- Pregnancy risk category B

How supplied
Available by prescription only
Tablets: 250 mg, 500 mg
Suspension: 250 mg/5 ml
Injection: 500-mg vial

Indications, route, and dosage
Edema, hypertension
Adults: 500 mg to 2 g P.O. or I.V. daily or in two divided doses.
Diuresis
Children age 6 months or over: 20 mg/kg P.O. or I.V. daily in divided doses.
Children under age 6 months: May require 30 mg/kg P.O. or I.V. daily in two divided doses.

Pharmacodynamics
- *Diuretic action:* Chlorothiazide increases urinary excretion of sodium and water by inhibiting sodium reabsorption in the cortical diluting tubule of the nephron, thus relieving edema.
- *Antihypertensive action:* The exact mechanism of chlorothiazide's antihypertensive effect is unknown. It may partially result from direct arteriolar vasodilation and a decrease in total peripheral resistance.

Pharmacokinetics
- *Absorption:* Chlorothiazide is absorbed incompletely and variably from the GI tract.
- *Distribution:* Unknown.
- *Metabolism:* None.
- *Excretion:* Chlorothiazide is excreted unchanged in urine.

Contraindications and precautions
Chlorothiazide is contraindicated in patients with anuria and in those with known sensitivity to the drug or to other sulfonamide derivatives. Chlorothiazide should be used with caution in patients with severe renal disease because it may decrease glomerular filtration rate and precipitate azotemia; in patients with impaired hepatic function or liver disease because electrolyte changes may precipitate coma; and in patients taking digoxin, because hypokalemia may predispose them to digitalis toxicity.

Interactions
Chlorothiazide potentiates the hypotensive effects of most other antihypertensive drugs; this may be used to therapeutic advantage.

Chlorothiazide may potentiate hyperglycemic, hypotensive, and hyperuricemic effects of diazoxide, and its hyperglycemic effect may increase insulin or sulfonylurea requirements in diabetic patients.

Chlorothiazide may reduce renal clearance of lithium, elevating serum lithium levels, and may necessitate reduction in lithium dosage by 50%.

Chlorothiazide turns urine slightly more alkaline and may decrease urinary excretion of some amines, such as amphetamine and quinidine; alkaline urine may also decrease therapeutic efficacy of methenamine compounds such as methenamine mandelate.

Cholestyramine and colestipol may bind chlorothiazide, preventing its absorption; give drugs 1 hour apart.

Effects on diagnostic tests
Chlorothiazide therapy may alter serum electrolyte levels and may increase serum urate, glucose, cholesterol, and triglyceride levels. It may also interfere with tests for parathyroid function and should be discontinued before such tests.

Adverse reactions
- CV: volume depletion and dehydration, orthostatic hypotension, hypercholesterolemia, hypertriglyceridemia.
- DERM: dermatitis, photosensitivity, rash.
- GI: anorexia, nausea, pancreatitis.
- HEMA: *aplastic anemia, agranulocytosis,* leukopenia, thrombocytopenia.
- Hepatic: hepatic encephalopathy.
- Metabolic: asymptomatic hyperuricemia; gout; hyperglycemia and impairment of glucose tolerance; fluid and electrolyte imbalances, including hypokalemia, hyponatremia, hypochloremia, and hypercalcemia; metabolic alkalosis.
- Other: hypersensitivity reactions, such as pneumonitis and vasculitis.

Note: Drug should be discontinued if rising BUN and serum creatinine levels indicate renal impairment, if patient exhibits symptoms of hypersensitivity, or if patient shows signs of impending coma.

Overdose and treatment
Clinical signs of overdose include GI irritation and hypermotility, diuresis, and lethargy, which may progress to coma.

Treatment is mainly supportive; monitor and assist respiratory, cardiovascular, and renal function as indicated. Monitor fluid and electrolyte balance. Induce vomiting with ipecac in conscious patient; otherwise, use gastric lavage to avoid aspiration. Do not give cathartics; these promote additional loss of fluids and electrolytes.

▶ **Special considerations**
Besides those relevant to all *thiazide diuretics,* consider the following recommendations.

● Chlorothiazide is the only thiazide available in liquid form.

● Give chlorothiazide sodium for I.V. injection only (never I.M. or S.C.) because it is extremely irritating to tissues; do not administer with whole blood or blood products.

● Inspect skin and mucous membranes of patients on prolonged therapy for petechiae, which require reduced dosage or discontinuation of drug.

Geriatric use
Elderly and debilitated patients require close observation and may require reduced dosages. They are more sensitive to excess diuresis because of age-related changes in cardiovascular and renal function. Excess diuresis promotes orthostatic hypotension and dehydration, hypovolemia, hyponatremia, hypomagnesemia, and hypokalemia.

Breast-feeding
Chlorothiazide is distributed in breast milk; its safety and effectiveness in breast-feeding women have not been established.

chlorotrianisene
Tace

● Pharmacologic classification: estrogen
● Therapeutic classfication: estrogen replacement, antineoplastic
● Pregnancy risk category X

How supplied
Available by prescription only
Capsules: 12 mg, 25 mg

Indications, route, and dosage
Prostatic cancer
Adults: 12 to 25 mg P.O. daily.
Menopausal symptoms or management of atrophic vaginitis or kraurosis vulvae
Adults: 12 to 25 mg P.O. daily in 30-day cycles (3 weeks on, 1 week off).
Female hypogonadism
Adults: 12 to 25 mg P.O. for 21 days, followed by 1 dose of progesterone 100 mg I.M. or 5 days of oral progestogen given concurrently with last 5 days of chlorotrianisene (that is, medroxyprogesterone 5 to 10 mg). Begin on day 5 of menstrual cycle.
Atrophic vaginitis
Adults: 12 to 25 mg P.O. daily for 30 to 60 days.
Postpartum breast engorgement
Adults: 12 mg P.O. q.i.d. for 7 days or 50 mg P.O. q 6 hours for 6 doses. First dose to be administered within 8 hours after parturition.

Pharmacodynamics
Estrogenic action: Chlorotrianisene mimics the action of endogenous estrogen in treating menopausal symptoms and atrophic vaginitis. It inhibits growth of hormone-sensitive tissue in advanced, inoperable prostatic cancer.

Pharmacokinetics
Very little pharmacokinetic data is available for this compound. Chlorotrianisene appears to have a longer duration of action than the naturally occurring estrogens, possibly as a result of extensive distribution into, and subsequent release from, fatty tissue.

Contraindications and precautions
Chlorotrianisene is contraindicated in patients with thrombophlebitis or thromboembolism, estrogen-responsive carcinoma (breast or genital tract cancer), or undiagnosed abnormal genital bleeding because the drug may aggravate these disorders. The drug is also contraindicated during pregnancy and breast-feeding.

This drug should be used cautiously in patients with disorders that may be aggravated by fluid and electrolyte accumulation, such as asthma, seizure disorders, migraine, or cardiac, renal, or hepatic dysfunction. Carefully monitor female patients who have breast nodules, fibrocystic breast disease, or a family history of breast cancer. Because of the risk of thromboembolism, therapy with this drug should be discontinued at least 1 week before elective surgical procedures associated with an increased incidence of thromboembolism.

Chlorotrianisene capsules contain tartrazine, which may induce allergic reactions in aspirin-sensitive individuals.

Interactions
Concomitant administration of drugs that induce hepatic metabolism, such as rifampin, barbiturates, primidone, carbamazepine, and phenytoin, may decrease estrogenic effects from a given dose. These drugs are known to accelerate the rate of metabolism of certain other agents.

Effects on diagnostic tests
In patients with diabetes, chlorotrianisene may increase blood glucose levels, necessitating dosage adjustment of insulin or oral hypoglycemic drugs.

Chlorotrianisene has the potential to decrease the effects of warfarin-type anticoagulants.

Adverse reactions
● CNS: headache, dizziness, chorea, irritability, sudden loss of coordination, slurred speech, migraine, depression, libido changes.
● CV: thrombophlebitis; *thromboembolism;* hypertension; edema; *increased risk of stroke, pulmonary embolism, and myocardial infarction.*
● DERM: melasma, urticaria, acne, seborrhea, oily skin, hirsutism or loss of hair, photosensitivity, erythema multiforme, erythema nodosum.
● EENT: worsening of myopia or astigmatism, intolerance to contact lenses.
● GI: nausea, vomiting, abdominal cramps, bloating, diarrhea, constipation, anorexia, increased appetite, excessive thirst, weight changes.
● GU: breakthrough bleeding, altered menstrual flow, dysmenorrhea, amenorrhea, premenstrual-like syndrome, cervical erosion or abnormal secretions, enlargement of uterine fibromas, cystitis-like syndrome, vaginal candidiasis; in males: gynecomastia, testicular atrophy, impotence.
● Hepatic: cholestatic jaundice.
● Metabolic: hyperglycemia, hypercalcemia, folic acid deficiency.
● Other: leg cramps, purpura, breast changes (tenderness, enlargement, secretion), pigmentation of nipples.

Note: Drug should be discontinued if patient becomes hypertensive during therapy.

Overdose and treatment
Specific recommendations are unavailable. Chlorotrianisene overdose may cause nausea. Treatment should be supportive.

▶ Special considerations
Besides those relevant to all *estrogens,* consider the following recommendation.
● Because of its prolonged duration of action, this drug is not recommended for correcting menstrual disorders.

Information for the patient
Warn patient to report immediately abdominal pain, numbness, or stiffness in legs or buttocks; pressure or pain in chest; shortness of breath; severe headaches; visual disturbances, such as blind spots, flashing lights, or blurriness; vaginal bleeding or discharge; breast lumps; swelling of hands or feet; yellow skin and sclera; dark urine; and light-colored stools.

Geriatric use
Because of the potential for numerous adverse effects, use with caution in elderly patients. Administration of estrogens to postmenopausal women may be associated with increased incidence of endometrial or breast cancer.

Breast-feeding
Chlorotrianisene is contraindicated in breast-feeding women.

---

chlorphenesin carbamate
Maolate

● Pharmacologic classification: carbamate derivative
● Therapeutic classification: skeletal muscle relaxant
● Pregnancy risk category C

How supplied
Available by prescription only
Tablets (scored): 400 mg

Indications, route, and dosage
Adjunct for relief of discomfort in short-term, acute, painful musculoskeletal conditions
Adults: Initial dosage 800 mg P.O. t.i.d., then adjusted to lowest effective dosage. Usual dosage 400 mg P.O. q.i.d. for maximum of 8 weeks.
† *Trigeminal neuralgia*
Adults: 400 mg P.O. upon awakening and at noon and then 800 mg h.s.

Pharmacodynamics
Skeletal muscle relaxant action: Chlorphenesin does not relax skeletal muscle directly, but apparently as a result of its sedative effects. However, the exact mechanism of action is unknown. Animal studies suggest that the drug modifies central perception of pain without eliminating peripheral pain reflexes.

Pharmacokinetics
● *Absorption:* Chlorphenesin is rapidly and completely absorbed from the GI tract. Peak effect occurs in 1 to 3 hours.
● *Distribution:* Unknown.
● *Metabolism:* Chlorphenesin is partly metabolized in the liver.
● *Excretion:* Chlorphenesin is rapidly excreted in urine, mainly as the glucuronide metabolite and other metabolites.

Contraindications and precautions
Chlorphenesin is contraindicated in patients with known hypersensitivity to the drug. Administer cautiously to patients with hepatic or renal impairment, because the drug may accumulate in these patients upon chronic administration.
Patients allergic or sensitive to the dye tartrazine (FD&C Yellow No. 5) should not take chlorphenesin. Although tartrazine sensitivity is rare, it frequently occurs in patients sensitive to aspirin.

Interactions
Concomitant use with other CNS depressant drugs, including alcohol, may produce additive CNS depression. When using with other depressant drugs (general anesthetics, opioid analgesics, antipsychotics, anxiolytics, or tricyclic antidepressants), exercise care to avoid overdose.

Effects on diagnostic tests
None reported.

Adverse reactions
● CNS: drowsiness, dizziness, confusion, headache, weakness, dose-related paradoxical stimulation, agitation, insomnia, nervousness.
● GI: nausea, epigastric distress.
● HEMA: blood dyscrasia.
● Other: rash, pruritus, *anaphylaxis,* allergic reactions.
Note: Drug should be discontinued if allergic reactions to drug or tartrazine dye occur during therapy.

Overdose and treatment
Clinical manifestations of overdose include prolonged drowsiness leading to exaggerated CNS depression, mild nausea, and respiratory depression.
Treatment is supportive. Monitor vital signs and neurologic status. If ingestion is recent, induce emesis or perform gastric lavage, followed by a saline cathartic to reduce absorption.

▶ Special considerations
● Watch for allergic reactions.
● Monitor blood studies. Watch for unusual reactions (rash, unusual bleeding, or bruising).

Information for the patient
● Chlorphenesin may cause drowsiness. Tell patient to avoid hazardous activities that require alertness until CNS depressant effect is determined.
● Tell patient to avoid alcoholic beverages and to use caution with cold and cough preparations, because some contain alcohol.
● Tell patient to store drug away from direct heat and light (not in bathroom medicine cabinet) and out of children's reach.
● Tell patient to report unusual reactions immediately.
● Instruct patient to take missed dose only if remem-

---

bered within 1 hour. If remembered later, patient should skip that dose and return to regular schedule; the patient should not double dose.
• Warn patient that skeletal muscle relaxants are banned in athletic competition sponsored by the U.S. Olympics Committee and the National Collegiate Athletic Association. Use can lead to disqualification.

Geriatric use
Lower doses are recommended in elderly patients, because they may be more sensitive to the drug's effects.

Pediatric use
Not recommended for use in children under age 12.

chlorpheniramine maleate
Alermine, Aller-Chlor, Allerid O.D., Chlo-Amine, Chlor-100, Chlor-Mal, Chlor-Niramine, Chlorphen*, Chlor-Pro, Chlorspan, Chlortab, Chlor-Trimeton, Chlor-Tripolon*, Hal-Chlor, Histray, Novopheniram*, Phenetron, T.D. Alermine, Teldrin, Trymegen

• Pharmacologic classification: propylamine-derivative antihistamine
• Therapeutic classification: antihistamine (H_1-receptor antagonist)
• Pregnancy risk category B

How supplied
Available with or without prescription
Tablets (chewable): 2 mg
Tablets: 4 mg
Tablets (timed-release): 8 mg, 12 mg
Capsules (timed-release): 8 mg, 12 mg
Syrup: 2 mg/5 ml
Injection: 10 mg/ml, 100 mg/ml

Indications, route, and dosage
Rhinitis, allergy symptoms
Adults and children age 12 or older: 4 mg of tablets or syrup q 4 to 6 hours; or 8 to 12 mg of timed-release tablets b.i.d. or t.i.d. Maximum dosage is 24 mg/day.
Children age 6 to 11: 2 mg of tablets or syrup q 4 to 6 hours; or one 8-mg timed-release tablet in 24 hours. Maximum dosage is 12 mg/day.
Children age 2 to 5: 1 mg of syrup q 4 to 6 hours. Maximum dosage is 4 mg/day.

Pharmacodynamics
Antihistamine action: Antihistamines compete with histamine for histamine H_1-receptor sites on smooth muscle of the bronchi, GI tract, uterus, and large blood vessels; they bind to cellular receptors, preventing access of histamine, thereby suppressing histamine-induced allergic symptoms. They do not directly alter histamine or its release.

Pharmacokinetics
• *Absorption:* Chlorpheniramine is well absorbed from the GI tract; action begins within 30 to 60 minues, and peaks in 2 to 6 hours. Food in the stomach delays absorption but does not affect bioavailability.
• *Distribution:* Chlorpheniramine is distributed extensively into the body; drug is about 72% protein-bound.

• *Metabolism:* Drug is metabolized largely in GI mucosal cells and liver (first-pass effect).
• *Excretion:* Chlorpheniramine's half-life is 12 to 43 hours in adults and 10 to 13 hours in children; drug and metabolites are excreted in urine.

Contraindications and precautions
Chlorpheniramine is contraindicated in patients with known hypersensitivity to this medication or antihistamines with similar chemical structures, such as dexchlorpheniramine, brompheniramine, or triprolidine; during an acute asthmatic attack, because it thickens bronchial secretions; and in patients who have taken monoamine oxidase (MAO) inhibitors within the preceding 2 weeks.

Antihistamines, should be used with caution in patients with narrow-angle glaucoma; in those with pyloroduodenal obstruction or urinary bladder obstruction from prostatic hypertrophy or narrowing of the bladder neck, because of their marked anticholinergic effects; in patients with cardiovascular disease, hypertension, or hyperthyroidism, because of the risk of palpitations and tachycardia; and in patients with renal disease, diabetes, bronchial asthma, urinary retention, or stenosing peptic ulcers.

Antihistamines should not be used during pregnancy (especially in the third trimester) or during breast-feeding. Antihistamines have caused convulsions and other severe reactions, especially in premature infants.

Interactions
MAO inhibitors interfere with the detoxification of chlorpheniramine and thus prolong and intensify its central depressant and anticholinergic effects; additive sedation may occur when antihistamines are given concomitantly with other CNS depressants, such as alcohol, barbiturates, tranquilizers, sleeping aids, or antianxiety agents.

Chlorpheniramine enhances the effects of epinephrine and may diminish the effects of sulfonylureas, and partially counteract the anticoagulant action of heparin.

Effects on diagnostic tests
Discontinue chlorpheniramine 4 days before diagnostic skin tests; antihistamines can prevent, reduce, or mask positive skin test response.

Adverse reactions
• CNS: stimulation, sedation, drowsiness, dizziness, vertigo, disturbed coordination, excitability.
• CV: hypotension, palpitations.
• DERM: urticaria, rash.
• GI: anorexia, nausea, constipation, epigastric distress, vomiting, dry mouth and throat.
• GU: urinary retention.
• Respiratory: thick bronchial secretions.

Overdose and treatment
Clinical manifestations of overdose may include either CNS depression (sedation, reduced mental alertness, apnea, and cardiovascular collapse) or CNS stimulation (insomnia, hallucinations, tremors, and convulsions). Atropine-like symptoms, such as dry mouth, flushed skin, fixed and dilated pupils, and GI symptoms, are common, especially in children.

Treat overdose by inducing emesis with ipecac syrup (in conscious patient), followed by activated charcoal to reduce further drug absorption. Use gastric lavage if patient is unconscious or ipecac fails. Treat hypoten-

---

*Canada only   †Unlabeled clinical use   Italicized adverse reactions are life-threatening.

sion with vasopressors, and control seizures with diazepam or phenytoin. *Do not give stimulants.* Administering ammonium chloride or vitamin C to acidify urine will promote drug excretion.

▶ **Special considerations**
Besides those relevant to all *antihistamines,* consider the following recommendations.
● Give 100 mg/ml of injectable form S.C. or I.M. *only.* Do not give I.V.; I.V. preparation contains preservatives.
● Do not use parenteral solutions intradermally.
● Administer I.V. solution slowly, over 1 minute.

Information for the patient
● Sustained-release tablets should be swallowed whole; do not crush or permit patient to chew tablet.
● Store syrup and parenteral solution away from light.

Geriatric use
Elderly patients are usually more sensitive to adverse effects of antihistamines and are especially likely to experience a greater degree of dizziness, sedation, hyperexcitability, dry mouth, and urinary retention than younger patients. Symptoms usually respond to a decrease in medication dosage.

Pediatric use
Not indicated for use in premature or newborn infants. Children, especially those under age 6, may experience paradoxical hyperexcitability.

Breast-feeding
Antihistamines such as chlorpheniramine should not be used during breast-feeding. Many of these drugs are secreted in breast milk, exposing the infant to risks of unusual excitability; premature infants are at particular risk for convulsions.

---

chlorpromazine hydrochloride
Chlor-Promanyl*, Chlorzine, Largactil*, Novo-chlorpromazine*, Ormazine, Promapar, Promaz, Sonazine, Thorazine, Thor-Prom

● Pharmacologic classification: aliphatic phenothiazine
● Therapeutic classification: antipsychotic, antiemetic
● Pregnancy risk category C

How supplied
Available by prescription only
Tablets: 10 mg, 25 mg, 50 mg, 100 mg, 200 mg
Capsules (sustained-release): 30 mg, 75 mg, 150 mg, 200 mg, 300 mg
Syrup: 10 mg/5 ml
Oral concentrate: 30 mg/ml, 100 mg/ml
Suppositories: 25 mg, 100 mg
Injection: 25 mg/ml

Indications, route, and dosage
Psychosis
Adults: 30 to 75 mg P.O. daily in two to four divided doses. Dosage may be increased twice weekly by 20 to 50 mg until symptoms are controlled. Most patients

respond to 200 mg daily, but doses up to 800 mg may be necessary.
Children: 0.25 mg/kg P.O. q 4 to 6 hours; or 0.25 mg/kg I.M. q 6 to 8 hours; or 0.5 mg/kg rectally q 6 to 8 hours. Maximum dosage is 40 mg in children under age 5, and 75 mg in children age 5 to 12.
Acute management of psychosis in severely agitated patients
Adults: 25 mg I.M.; may be repeated with 25 to 50 mg I.M. in 1 hour. May be gradually increased over several days to a maximum of 400 mg q 4 to 6 hours.
Nausea and vomiting
Adults: 10 to 25 mg P.O. or I.M. q 4 to 6 hours, p.r.n.; or 50 to 100 mg rectally q 6 to 8 hours, p.r.n.
Children and infants: 0.25 mg/kg P.O. q 4 to 6 hours; or 0.25 mg/kg I.M. q 6 to 8 hours; or 0.5 mg/kg rectally q 6 to 8 hours.
Intractable hiccups
Adults: 25 to 50 mg P.O. or I.M. t.i.d. or q.i.d.
Mild alcohol withdrawal, acute intermittent porphyria, and tetanus
Adults: 25 mg to 50 mg I.M. t.i.d. or q.i.d.

Pharmacodynamics
Antipsychotic action: Chlorpromazine is thought to exert its antipsychotic effects by postsynaptic blockade of CNS dopamine receptors, thereby inhibiting dopamine-mediated effects; antiemetic effects are attributed to dopamine receptor blockade in the medullary chemoreceptor trigger zone (CTZ). Chlorpromazine has many other central and peripheral effects; it produces both alpha and ganglionic blockade and counteracts histamine- and serotonin-mediated activity. Its most prominent adverse reactions are antimuscarinic and sedative.

Pharmacokinetics
● *Absorption:* Rate and extent of absorption vary with route of administration. Oral tablet absorption is erratic and variable, with onset ranging from ½ to 1 hour; peak effects occur at 2 to 4 hours and duration of action is 4 to 6 hours. Sustained-release preparations have similar absorption, but action lasts for 10 to 12 hours. Suppositories act in 60 minutes and last 3 to 4 hours. Oral concentrates and syrups are much more predictable; I.M. drug is absorbed rapidly.
● *Distribution:* Chlorpromazine is distributed widely into the body, including breast milk; concentration is usually higher in CNS than plasma. Steady-state serum level is achieved within 4 to 7 days. Drug is 91% to 99% protein-bound.
● *Metabolism:* Chlorpromazine is metabolized extensively by the liver and forms 10 to 12 metabolites; some are pharmacologically active.
● *Excretion:* Most of drug is excreted as metabolites in urine; some is excreted in feces via the biliary tract. It may undergo enterohepatic circulation.

Contraindications and precautions
Antipsychotics are contraindicated in patients with known hypersensitivity to phenothiazines and related compounds, including allergic reactions involving hepatic function; in patients with blood dyscrasias and bone marrow depression because chlorpromazine may induce agranulocytosis; in patients with disorders accompanied by coma, brain damage, or CNS depression because of additive CNS depressant effects; in patients with circulatory collapse or cerebrovascular disease because of the potential for hypotensive or adverse

---

cardiac effects; and for use with adrenergic blocking agents or spinal or epidural anesthetics because of the alpha-blocking potential of chlorpromazine.

Chlorpromazine should be used cautiously in patients with cardiac disease (arrhythmias, congestive heart failure, angina pectoris, valvular disease, or heart block), encephalitis, Reye's syndrome, head injury, respiratory disease, epilepsy and other seizure disorders, glaucoma, prostatic hypertrophy, urinary retention, hepatic or renal dysfunction, Parkinson's disease, pheochromocytoma, or hypocalcemia.

Interactions
Concomitant use of chlorpromazine with sympathomimetics, including epinephrine, phenylephrine, phenylpropanolamine, and ephedrine (often found in nasal sprays), and appetite suppressants may decrease their stimulatory and pressor effects. Chlorpromazine may cause epinephrine reversal: the beta-adrenergic agonist activity of epinephrine is evident while its alpha effects are blocked, leading to decreased diastolic and increased systolic pressures and tachycardia.

Chlorpromazine may inhibit blood pressure response to centrally acting antihypertensive drugs such as guanethidine, guanabenz, guanadrel, clonidine, methyldopa, and reserpine. Additive effects are likely after concomitant use of chlorpromazine and CNS depressants (including alcohol, analgesics, barbiturates, narcotics, tranquilizers, and general, spinal, or epidural anesthetics), or parenteral magnesium sulfate (oversedation, respiratory depression, and hypotension); antiarrhythmic agents, quinidine, disopyramide, and procainamide (increased incidence of cardiac dysrhythmias and conduction defects); atropine and other anticholinergic drugs, including antidepressants, monoamine oxidase inhibitors, phenothiazines, antihistamines, meperidine, and antiparkinsonian agents (oversedation, paralytic ileus, visual changes, and severe constipation); nitrates (hypotension); and metrizamide (increased risk of convulsions).

Beta-blocking agents may inhibit chlorpromazine metabolism, increasing plasma levels and toxicity.

Concomitant use with propylthiouracil increases risk of agranulocytosis; concomitant use with lithium may cause severe neurologic toxicity with an encephalitis-like syndrome, and a decreased therapeutic response to chlorpromazine.

Pharmacokinetic alterations and subsequent decreased therapeutic response to chlorpromazine may follow concomitant use with phenobarbital (enhanced renal excretion), aluminum- and magnesium-containing antacids and antidiarrheals (decreased absorption), caffeine, and with heavy smoking (increased metabolism).

Chlorpromazine may antagonize therapeutic effect of bromocriptine on prolactin secretion; it also may decrease the vasoconstricting effects of high-dose dopamine and may decrease effectiveness and increase toxicity of levodopa (by dopamine blockade). Chlorpromazine may inhibit metabolism and increase toxicity of phenytoin.

Effects on diagnostic tests
Chlorpromazine causes false-positive test results for urinary porphyrins, urobilinogen, amylase, and 5-hydroxyindoleacetic acid (5-HIAA), because of darkening of urine by metabolites; it also causes false-positive results in urine pregnancy tests using human chorionic gonadotropin (HCG).

Chlorpromazine elevates tests for liver function and protein-bound iodine and causes quinidine-like ECG effects.

Adverse reactions
● CNS: extrapyramidal symptoms – dystonia, akathisia, torticollis, tardive dyskinesia (usually dose-related, with long-term therapy, but it can develop rapidly); sedation, pseudoparkinsonism, drowsiness (frequent); *neuroleptic malignant syndrome* (dose-related; if untreated, *fatal respiratory failure* in over 10% of patients); dizziness, headache, insomnia, exacerbation of psychotic symptoms.
● CV: *asystole*, orthostatic hypotension, tachycardia, dizziness, fainting, arrhythmias, ECG changes, increased anginal pain (after I.M. injection).
● EENT: blurred vision, tinnitus, mydriasis, increased intraocular pressure, ocular changes (retinal pigmentary change with long-term use).
● GI: dry mouth, constipation, nausea, vomiting, anorexia, diarrhea.
● GU: urinary retention, gynecomastia, hypermenorrhea, inhibited ejaculation.
● HEMA: transient leukopenia, *agranulocytosis*, thrombocytopenia, anemia (within 30 to 90 days).
● Local: contact dermatitis from concentrate or injectable, muscle necrosis from I.M. injection.
● Other: hyperprolactinemia, photosensitivity, increased appetite or weight gain, hypersensitivity (rash, urticaria, drug fever, edema, cholestatic jaundice [in 0.1% to 4% of patients within first 30 days]), decreased libido.

After abrupt withdrawal of long-term therapy, gastritis, nausea, vomiting, dizziness, tremors, feeling of heat or cold, sweating, tachycardia, headache, or insomnia may occur.

Note: Drug should be discontinued immediately if the following reactions occur: hypersensitivity, jaundice, agranulocytosis; neuroleptic malignant syndrome (marked hyperthermia, extrapyramidal effects, autonomic dysfunction); and severe extrapyramidal symptoms even after dose is lowered. Chlorpromazine should be discontinued 48 hours before and 24 hours after myelography using metrizamide, because of the risk of convulsions. When feasible, withdraw drug slowly and gradually; many drug effects persist after withdrawal.

Overdose and treatment
CNS depression is characterized by deep, unarousable sleep and possible coma, hypotension or hypertension, extrapyramidal symptoms, abnormal involuntary muscle movements, agitation, seizures, arrhythmias, ECG changes, hypothermia or hyperthermia, and autonomic nervous system dysfunction.

Treatment is symptomatic and supportive, including maintaining vital signs, airway, stable body temperature, and fluid and electrolyte balance.

Do not induce vomiting: drug inhibits cough reflex, and aspiration may occur. Use gastric lavage, then activated charcoal and saline cathartics; dialysis does not help. Regulate body temperature as needed. Treat hypotension with I.V. fluids: *do not give epinephrine*. Treat seizures with parenteral diazepam or barbiturates; dysrhythmias with parenteral phenytoin (1 mg/kg with rate titrated to blood pressure); extrapyramidal reactions with benztropine or parenteral diphenhydramine 2 mg/kg/minute.

▶ **Special considerations**

Besides those relevant to all *phenothiazines*, consider the following recommendations.

● A pink-brown discoloration of urine may be observed.

● Chlorpromazine has a high incidence of sedation, orthostatic hypotension, and photosensitivity reactions (3%). Patient should avoid exposure to sunlight or heat lamps.

● Sustained-release preparations should not be crushed or opened, but swallowed whole.

● Oral formulations may cause stomach upset and may be administered with food or fluid.

● Dilute the concentrate in 2 to 4 oz of liquid, preferably water, carbonated drinks, fruit juice, tomato juice, milk, puddings, or applesauce.

● Store the suppository form in a cool place.

● If tissue irritation occurs, chlorpromazine injection may be diluted with normal saline solution or 2% procaine.

● The I.V. form should be used only during surgery or for severe hiccups.

● Dilute the injection to 1 mg/ml with normal saline solution and administer at a rate of 1 mg/2 minutes for children and 1 mg/minute for adults.

● The I.M. injection should be given deep in the upper outer quadrant of the buttocks. Injection is usually painful; massaging the area after administration may prevent abscess formation. Do not extravasate because skin necrosis can occur.

● The liquid and injectable formulations may cause a rash if skin contact occurs.

● Solution for injection may be slightly discolored. Do not use if drug is excessively discolored or if a precipitate is evident. Monitor blood pressure before and after parenteral administration.

● Shake the syrup before administration.

Information for the patient

● Explain the risks of dystonic reactions and tardive dyskinesia, and tell the patient to report abnormal body movements.

● Tell patient to avoid sun exposure and to wear sunscreen when going outdoors, to prevent photosensitivity reactions. (Note that sunlamps and tanning beds also may cause burning of the skin or skin discoloration.)

● Warn patient to avoid extremely hot or cold baths or exposure to temperature extremes, sunlamps, or tanning beds. Drug may cause thermoregulatory changes.

● Tell patient not to spill the liquid preparation on the skin because rash and irritation may result.

● Tell patient to take the drug exactly as prescribed and not to double dose to compensate for missed ones.

● Explain that many drug interactions are possible. Patient should seek medical approval before taking *any* self-prescribed medications.

● Tell patient not to stop taking drug suddenly.

● Encourage patient to report difficulty urinating, sore throat, dizziness, or fainting.

● Tell patient to avoid hazardous activities that require alertness until the effect of the drug is established. Excessive sedative effects tend to subside after several weeks.

● Tell patient to avoid alcohol and medications that may cause excessive sedation.

● Explain what fluids are appropriate for diluting the concentrate and the dropper technique for measuring dose. Teach patient how to use the suppository form.

● Sugarless chewing gum or hard candy, ice chips, or artificial saliva may help to alleviate dry mouth.

● Tell patient to shake syrup before administration.

Geriatric use

Older patients tend to require lower doses, titrated individually. They also are more likely to develop adverse reactions, especially tardive dyskinesia and other extrapyramidal effects.

Pediatric use

Chlorpromazine is not recommended for patients under age 6 months. Sudden infant death syndrome has been reported to occur in children under age 1 receiving the drug.

Breast-feeding

Chlorpromazine enters into the breast milk. Potential benefits to the mother should outweigh the potential harm to the infant.

---

chlorpropamide

Chloronase*, Diabinese, Glucamide, Novopropamide*, Stabinol*

● Pharmacologic classification: sulfonyl-urea
● Therapeutic classification: antidiabetic agent, antidiuretic agent
● Pregnancy risk category D

How supplied

Available by prescription only
Tablets: 100 mg, 250 mg

Indications, route, and dosage

Adjunct to diet to lower blood glucose levels in patients with non-insulin-dependent diabetes mellitus (type II)

Adults: 250 mg P.O. daily with breakfast or in divided doses if GI disturbances occur. First dosage increase may be made after 5 to 7 days because of extended duration of action, then dose may be increased q 3 to 5 days by 50 to 125 mg, if needed, to a maximum of 750 mg daily. Start with dose of 100 to 125 mg in older patients.

Adults over age 65: Initial dosage should be 100 to 125 mg daily.

To change from insulin to oral therapy

Adults: If insulin dosage is less than 40 units daily, insulin may be stopped and oral therapy started as above. If insulin dosage is 40 units or more daily, start oral therapy as above, with insulin dose reduced 50% the first few days. Further insulin reductions should be made according to the patient's response.

As antidiuretic

Adults: 100 to 250 mg as a single daily dose, adjusted at 2- to 3-day intervals up to 500 mg.

Pharmacodynamics

● *Antidiabetic action:* Chlorpropamide lowers blood glucose levels by stimulating insulin release from beta cells in the pancreas. After prolonged administration, it produces hypoglycemic effects through extrapancreatic mechanisms, including reduced basal hepatic glucose production and enhanced peripheral sensitivity

---

to insulin; the latter may result either from an increased number of insulin receptors or from changes in events that follow insulin binding.

• *Antidiuretic action:* Chlorpropamide appears to potentiate the effects of minimal levels of antidiuretic hormone.

Pharmacokinetics

• *Absorption:* Chlorpropamide is absorbed readily from the GI tract. Onset of action occurs within 1 hour, with a maximum decrease in serum glucose levels at 3 to 6 hours.

• *Distribution:* Chlorpropamide's distribution is not fully understood, but probably is similar to that of the other sulfonylureas. It is highly protein-bound.

• *Metabolism:* Approximately 80% of chlorpropamide is metabolized by the liver. Whether the metabolites have hypoglycemic activity is unknown.

• *Excretion:* Chlorpropamide and its metabolites are excreted in urine. The rate of excretion depends on urinary pH; it increases in alkaline urine and decreases in acidic urine. The duration of action is up to 60 hours; half-life is 36 hours.

Contraindications and precautions

Chlorpropamide is contraindicated in patients with known hypersensitivity to sulfonylureas or thiazides; in patients with burns, acidosis, diabetic coma, severe infection, ketosis, severe trauma, and major surgery because these conditions require treatment with insulin; and in patients with nonfunctioning beta cells. During periods of stress, insulin may be required temporarily.

Chlorpropamide should be used cautiously in patients with impaired cardiac function because sodium and water retention may precipitate congestive heart failure; in patients with water retention because it may potentiate antidiuretic hormone; in patients with hepatic or renal insufficiency because it is metabolized in the liver and excreted in urine; and in patients with adrenal, pituitary, or thyroid dysfunction because of altered fluid and electrolyte balance.

Interactions

Concomitant use of chlorpropamide with alcohol may produce a disulfiram-like reaction consisting of nausea, vomiting, abdominal cramps, and headaches. Concomitant use with anticoagulants may increase plasma levels of both drugs and, after continued therapy, may reduce plasma levels and anticoagulant effects. Concomitant use with chloramphenicol, guanethidine, insulin, monoamine oxidase inhibitors, probenecid, salicylates, or sulfonamides may enhance hypoglycemic effects by displacing chlorpropamide from its protein-binding sites.

Concomitant use with nonspecific beta-adrenergic blocking agents, including ophthalmics, may increase the risk of hypoglycemia by masking its symptoms, such as rising pulse rate and blood pressure. Use with drugs that may increase blood glucose levels (acetazolamide, adrenocorticoids, glucocorticoids, amphetamines, baclofen, corticotropin, epinephrine, estrogens, ethacrynic acid, furosemide, oral contraceptives, phenytoin, thiazide diuretics, triamterene, and thyroid hormones) may require dosage adjustments. Chlorpropamide appears to potentiate the effects of minimal levels of antidiuretic hormone.

Because smoking increases corticosteroid release,

patients who smoke may require higher dosages of chlorpropamide.

Effects on diagnostic tests

Chlorpropamide therapy alters cholesterol, alkaline phosphatase, bilirubin, urine phenyl ketone, porphyrins, and protein levels, and cephalin flocculation (thymol turbidity).

Adverse reactions

• DERM: eczema, pruritus, erythema, urticaria, facial flushing, morbilliform or maculopapular eruptions, photosensitivity.

• GI: cholestatic jaundice, nausea, vomiting, epigastric fullness, heartburn.

• GU: tea-colored urine.

• HEMA: leukopenia, thrombocytopenia, mild anemia, *agranulocytosis.*

• Metabolic: hypoglycemia, dilutional hyponatremia.

• Neurologic: weakness, paresthesias.

• Other: hypersensitivity reactions.

Note: Drug should be discontinued if signs or symptoms of hypersensitivity occur (jaundice, skin eruptions, blood dyscrasias, or severe diarrhea) or if progressive increases in serum alkaline phosphatase levels occur.

Overdose and treatment

Clinical manifestations of overdose include low blood glucose levels, tingling of lips and tongue, hunger, nausea, decreased cerebral function (lethargy, yawning, confusion, agitation, and nervousness), increased sympathetic activity (tachycardia, sweating, and tremor), and ultimately convulsions, stupor, and coma.

Mild hypoglycemia (without loss of consciousness or neurologic findings) can be treated with oral glucose and dosage adjustments. If patient loses consciousness or experiences neurologic symptoms, he should receive rapid injection of dextrose 50%, followed by a continuous infusion of dextrose 10% at a rate to maintain blood glucose levels greater than 100 mg/dl. Because of chlorpropamide's long half-life, monitor patient for 3 to 5 days.

▶ **Special considerations**

Besides those relevant to all *sulfonylureas,* consider the following recommendations.

• To avoid GI intolerance in those patients who require dosages of 250 mg/day or more and to improve control of hyperglycemia, divided doses are recommended. These are given before the morning and evening meals.

• Elderly, debilitated, or malnourished patients and those with impaired renal or hepatic function usually require a lower initial dosage.

• Patients switching from chlorpropamide to another sulfonylurea should be monitored closely for 1 week because of chlorpropamide's prolonged retention in the body.

• Because of this drug's long duration of action, adverse reactions, especially hypoglycemia, may be more frequent or severe than with some other sulfonylureas.

• Patients with severe diabetes who do not respond to 500 mg usually will not respond to higher doses.

• Chlorpropamide may accumulate in patients with renal insufficiency. Watch for such signs as dysuria, anuria, and hematuria.

• Chlorpropamide may potentiate antidiuretic effect of vasopressin. Watch for drowsiness, muscle cramps, seizures, unconsciousness, water retention, and weakness.

● Oral hypoglycemic agents have been associated with an increased risk of cardiovascular mortality as compared to diet or diet and insulin treatments.

Information for the patient
● Emphasize the importance of following a prescribed diet, as well as the exercise and medical regimen.
● Tell patient to take medication at the same time each day. If a dose is missed, it should be taken immediately, unless it's almost time for the next dose. Patient should never take double doses.
● Tell patient to avoid alcohol, and remind him that many foods and nonprescription medications contain alcohol. Alcohol may cause a disulfiram-like reaction.
● Encourage patient to wear a Medic Alert bracelet or necklace.
● Instruct patient to take chlorpropamide with food if it causes GI upset.
● Teach patient how to monitor blood glucose, urine glucose, and ketone levels, as needed.
● Teach patient to recognize the signs and symptoms of hypoglycemia and hyperglycemia and what to do if they occur.
● Reassure patient that skin reactions are transient and usually subside with continuation of therapy.

Geriatric use
● Elderly patients may be more sensitive to the effects of this medication because of reduced metabolism and elimination. They are more likely to develop neurologic symptoms of hypoglycemia.
● Chlorpropamide probably should be avoided in elderly patients because of its longer duration of action.
● Elderly patients usually require a lower initial dosage.

Pediatric use
Chlorpropamide is ineffective in insulin-dependent (type I, juvenile-onset) diabetes.

Breast-feeding
Chlorpropamide is excreted in breast milk and is not recommended for use in breast-feeding women.

---

chlorprothixene, chlorprothixene hydrochloride
Taractan, Tarasan*

● Pharmacologic classification: thioxanthene
● Therapeutic classification: antipsychotic
● Pregnancy risk category C

How supplied
Available by prescription only
Tablets: 10 mg, 25 mg, 50 mg, 100 mg
Oral concentrate: 100 mg/5 ml (fruit)
Injection: 12.5 mg/ml

Indications, route, and dosage
Psychotic disorders
Adults: Initially, 10 mg P.O. t.i.d. to q.i.d.; increase gradually to maximum of 600 mg daily.
Children over age 6: 10 to 25 mg P.O. t.i.d. or q.i.d.

Agitation of severe neurosis, depression, schizophrenia
Adults: 25 to 50 mg P.O. or I.M. t.i.d. or q.i.d.; increase as needed to maximum of 600 mg daily.

Pharmacodynamics
Antipsychotic action: Chlorprothixene is thought to exert its antipsychotic effects by postsynaptic blockade of CNS dopamine receptors, thereby inhibiting dopamine-mediated effects. Chlorprothixene has many other central and peripheral effects; it also acts as an alpha-blocking agent. Its most prominent adverse reactions are extrapyramidal.

Pharmacokinetics
● *Absorption:* Oral absorption is rapid; I.M. onset of action is 10 to 30 minutes.
● *Distribution:* Chlorprothixene is distributed widely into the body. Peak effects occur at 1 to 3 hours; drug is 91% to 99% protein-bound.
● *Metabolism:* Metabolism of chlorprothixene is minimal; duration of action is 6 hours.
● *Excretion:* Most of drug is excreted as parent drug in feces via the biliary tract.

Contraindications and precautions
Chlorprothixene is contraindicated in patients with known hypersensitivity to thioxanthenes, phenothiazines, and related compounds, including that evidenced by jaundice and other allergic symptoms; in patients with blood dyscrasias and bone marrow depression because of its potential for agranulocytosis; in patients with disorders accompanied by coma, brain damage, or CNS depression because of additive CNS depressant effects; and in patients with circulatory collapse or cerebrovascular disease because of its potential for arrhythmogenic effects.

Chlorprothixene should be used cautiously in patients with cardiac disease (arrhythmias, congestive heart failure, angina pectoris, valvular disease, or heart block), encephalitis, Reye's syndrome, head injury, respiratory disease, epilepsy and other seizure disorders, glaucoma, prostatic hypertrophy, urinary retention, hepatic or renal dysfunction, Parkinson's disease, pheochromocytoma, or hypocalcemia.

Oral preparations of chlorprothixene may contain tartrazine; dye may cause allergic reaction in patients with aspirin allergy.

Interactions
Concomitant use of chlorprothixene with sympathomimetics, including epinephrine, phenylephrine, phenylpropanolamine, and ephedrine (often found in nasal sprays), or appetite suppressants may decrease their stimulatory and pressor effects.

Chlorprothixene may inhibit blood pressure response to centrally acting antihypertensive drugs, such as guanethidine, guanabenz, guanadrel, clonidine, methyldopa, and reserpine. Additive effects are likely after concomitant use of chlorprothixene with CNS depressants (including alcohol, analgesics, barbiturates, narcotics, tranquilizers, and general, spinal, or epidural anesthetics) or parenteral magnesium sulfate (oversedation, respiratory depression, and hypotension); antiarrhythmic agents, quinidine, disopyramide, or procainamide (increased incidence of cardiac dysrhythmias and conduction defects); atropine or other anticholinergic drugs including antidepressants, monoamine oxidase inhibitors, phenothiazines, antihista-

---

mines, meperidine, and antiparkinsonian agents (over-sedation, paralytic ileus, visual changes, and severe constipation); nitrates (hypotension); or metrizamide (increased risk of convulsions).

Beta-blocking agents may inhibit chlorprothixene metabolism, increasing plasma levels and toxicity.

Concomitant use with propylthiouracil increases risk of agranulocytosis; concomitant use with lithium may result in severe neurologic toxicity with an encephalitis-like syndrome, and a decreased therapeutic response to chlorprothixene.

Pharmacokinetic alterations and subsequent decreased therapeutic response to chlorprothixene may follow concomitant use with phenobarbital (enhanced renal excretion), aluminum- and magnesium-containing antacids and antidiarrheals (decreased absorption), or caffeine, and with heavy smoking (increased metabolism).

Chlorprothixene may antagonize therapeutic effect of *bromocriptine* on prolactin secretion; it also may decrease the vasoconstricting effects of high-dose dopamine, and may decrease effectiveness and increase toxicity of levodopa (by dopamine blockade). Chlorprothixene may inhibit metabolism and increase toxicity of phenytoin.

Effects on diagnostic tests
Chlorprothixene causes false-positive test results for urinary porphyrins, urobilinogen, amylase, and 5-hydroxyindoleacetic acid (5-HIAA), because of darkening of urine by metabolites; it also causes false-positive results in urine pregnancy tests using human chorionic gonadotropin.

Chlorprothixene elevates results of tests for liver enzymes and protein-bound iodine and causes quinidine-like ECG effects.

Adverse reactions
● CNS: extrapyramidal symptoms – dystonia, akathisia, torticollis, tardive dyskinesia (usually dose-related, with long-term therapy, but it can develop rapidly), sedation, pseudoparkinsonism, drowsiness (frequent), *neuroleptic malignant syndrome* (dose-related; if untreated, death follows *respiratory failure* in over 10% of patients), dizziness, headache, insomnia, exacerbation of psychotic symptoms.
● CV: *asystole*, orthostatic hypotension, tachycardia, dizziness or fainting, arrhythmias, ECG changes, increased anginal pain after I.M. injection.
● EENT: blurred vision, tinnitus, mydriasis, increased intraocular pressure, ocular changes (retinal pigmentary change with long-term use).
● GI: dry mouth, constipation, nausea, vomiting, anorexia, diarrhea.
● GU: urinary retention, gynecomastia, hypermenorrhea, inhibited ejaculation.
● HEMA: transient leukopenia, *agranulocytosis,* thrombocytopenia, anemia (within 30 to 90 days).
● Local: contact dermatitis from concentrate or injectable form, muscle necrosis from I.M. injection.
● Other: hyperprolactinemia, photosensitivity, increased appetite or weight gain, hypersensitivity (rash, urticaria, drug fever, edema, cholestatic jaundice [in 0.1% to 4% of patients within first 30 days]), decreased libido.

After abrupt withdrawal of long-term therapy, gastritis, nausea, vomiting, dizziness, tremors, feeling of heat or cold, sweating, tachycardia, headache, or insomnia may occur.

Note: Drug should be discontinued immediately if the following reactions occur: hypersensitivity, jaundice, agranulocytosis; neuroleptic malignant syndrome (marked hyperthermia, extrapyramidal effects, autonomic dysfunction); and severe extrapyramidal symptoms even after dose is lowered. Chlorprothixene should be withdrawn 48 hours before and 24 hours after myelography using metrizamide, because of the risk of seizures. When feasible, withdraw drug slowly and gradually; many drug effects persist after withdrawal.

Overdose and treatment
CNS depression is characterized by deep, unarousable sleep and possible coma, hypotension or hypertension, extrapyramidal symptoms, abnormal involuntary muscle movements, agitation, seizures, arrhythmias, ECG changes, hypothermia or hyperthermia, and autonomic nervous system dysfunction.

Treatment is symptomatic and supportive, including maintaining vital signs, airway, stable body temperature, and fluid and electrolyte balance. *Do not induce vomiting:* drug inhibits cough reflex, and aspiration may occur. Use gastric lavage, then activated charcoal and saline cathartics; dialysis does not help. Regulate body temperature as needed. Treat hypotension with I.V. fluids: *do not give epinephrine.* Treat seizures with parenteral diazepam or barbiturates; arrhythmias, with parenteral phenytoin (1 mg/kg with rate titrated to blood pressure); extrapyramidal reactions, with benztropine or parenteral diphenhydramine at 2 mg/kg/minute.

▶ Special considerations
Besides those relevant to all *phenothiazines,* consider the following recommendations.
● Chlorprothixene causes a high incidence of extrapyramidal effects and photosensitivity reactions.
● Oral formulations may cause stomach upset and may be administered with food or fluid.
● Concentrate must be diluted in 2 to 4 oz of liquid, preferably water, carbonated drinks, fruit juice, tomato juice, milk, or pudding.
● The I.M. injection should be given deep in the upper outer quadrant of the buttocks. Massaging the area after administration may prevent the formation of abscesses. Do not give I.V.
● The liquid and injectable formulations may cause a rash if skin contact occurs.
● The injection solution may be slightly discolored. Do not use if drug is excessively discolored or if a precipitate is evident. Contact pharmacist.
● Protect the liquid formulation from light.
● The concentrate should be shaken and diluted before administration.
● Monitor blood pressure before and after parenteral administration.
● Drug is stable after reconstitution for 48 hours at room temperature.

Information for the patient
● Explain the risks of dystonic reactions and tardive dyskinesia, and tell patient to report abnormal body movements promptly.
● Tell patient to avoid sun exposure and to wear sunscreen when going outdoors, to prevent photosensitivity reactions. (Note that sunlamps and tanning beds also may cause burning of the skin or skin discoloration.)
● Warn patient to avoid extremely hot or cold baths or exposure to temperature extremes, sunlamps, or tan-

ning beds because the drug may cause thermoregulatory changes.
● Tell patient not to spill the liquid preparation on the skin because rash and irritation may result.
● Tell patient to take the drug exactly as prescribed and not to double dose to compensate for missed ones.
● Tell patient that many drug interactions are possible. Patient should seek medical approval before taking *any* self-prescribed medication.
● Inform patient that he should become tolerant to the sedative effects of the drug in several weeks.
● Tell patient not to stop taking the drug suddenly.
● Encourage patient to report difficulty urinating, sore throat, dizziness, or fainting.
● Tell patient to avoid hazardous activities that require alertness until the effect of the drug is established.
● Tell patient to avoid alcohol and other medications that may cause excessive sedation.
● Sugarless chewing gum or hard candy, ice chips, or artificial saliva may alleviate dry mouth.
● Tell patient to shake and dilute the concentrate before administration.

Geriatric use
Elderly patients tend to require lower doses, titrated to individual response. They also are more likely to develop adverse effects, especially tardive dyskinesia and other extrapyramidal effects.

Pediatric use
Drug is not recommended for patients under age 12.

chlortetracycline hydrochloride
Aureomycin, Aureomycin Ophthalmic

● Pharmacologic classification: tetracycline
● Therapeutic classification: anitbiotic, anti-infective
● Pregnancy risk category D

How supplied
Available by prescription only
Ophthalmic ointment: 10 mg/g in 3.75-g tube
Suspension: 1%

Available without prescription
Topical ointment: 3% in 14.2-g and 30-g tubes

Indications, route, and dosage
Superficial infections of the skin caused by susceptible bacteria
Adults and children: Rub into affected area b.i.d.
Superficial ophthalmic bacterial infections
Adults and children: Ophthalmic ointment applied to affected area every 2 to 12 hours, or 1 to 2 drops ophthalmic suspension b.i.d., t.i.d., or q.i.d.
Ophthalmic chlamydial infections
Adults and children: Ophthalmic ointment or 2 drops ophthalmic suspension in each eye b.i.d., t.i.d., or q.i.d.
Ophthalmia neonatorum prophylaxis
Newborn: 1- to 2-cm ribbon of ophthalmic ointment or 1 to 2 drops of ophthalmic suspension applied to neonate's lower conjuctival sac shortly after birth.

Pharmacodynamics
Anitbacterial and anti-infective action: Inhibits transfer RNA binding to the messenger RNA complex at the 30S subunit, inhibiting bacterial protein synthesis. Chlortetracycline is a broad spectrum bacteriostatic agent.

Pharmacokinetics
Unknown.

Contraindications and precautions
Chlortetracycline is contraindicated in patients with hypersensitivity to any of the tetracyclines and in pregnant patients in the second and third trimesters. Use with caution to avoid overgrowth of nonsusceptible organisms during long-term use.

Interactions
None significant.

Effects on diagnostic tests
Although the oral administration of chlortetracycline has been reported to decrease serum chloresterol levels, no such effect has been reported with the topical or ophthalmic administration of chlortetracycline.

Adverse reactions
● DERM: dermatitis, drying.
● Eye: foreign body sensation, transient stinging or burning sensation, increased tearing.

Overdose and treatment
Chlortetracycline content of an entire tube of ophthalmic ointment is insufficient to cause toxicity when accidently ingested orally. Nausea, vomiting, abdominal discomfort, or headache may occur, but severe toxicity is unlikely; induced emesis is indicated only after substantial ingestion. Antacids may be used to treat gastric irritation. Treat patient symptomatically.

▶ Special considerations
Besides those relevant to all *tetracyclines,* consider the following recommendations.
● Avoid contact of topical ointment with eyes.
● Drug has lanolin base; do not use in patients allergic to wool.
● Prolonged use may result in overgrowth of nonsusceptible organisms.
● Treated skin fluoresces under ultraviolet light.
● If no improvement is seen or if condition worsens, discontinue drug.

Information for the patient
Topical ointment
● Tell patient to cleanse infected area of skin prior to application, and cover with sterile dressing if necessary.
● Tell patient to call if rash or fever develops, or if condition worsens.
● Warn patient that ointment may stain clothing.
● Explain that use may cause photosensitivity, and advise patient to avoid prolonged sun exposure during use.
● Long-term use of topical ointment may cause tooth discoloration.

Ophthalmic ointment
● Tell patient to use ointment for full period prescribed.
● Tell patient to remove excess exudate before each new application, to enhance comfort.

Breast-feeding
No data available on distribution into breast milk. Long-term use of topical ointment by breast-feeding women may cause tooth discoloration in infants.

chlorthalidone
Hygroton, Hylidone, Novothalidone*
Thalitone, Uridone*

- Pharmacologic classification: thiazide-like diuretic
- Therapeutic classification: diuretic, antihypertensive
- Pregnancy risk category B

How supplied
Available by prescription only
Tablets: 25 mg, 50 mg, 100 mg

Indications, route, and dosage
Edema
Adults: 50 to 100 mg P.O. daily, or 100 mg three times weekly or on alternate days.
Children: 2 mg/kg P.O. three times weekly.
Hypertension
Adults: 25 to 100 mg P.O. daily.
Children: 2 mg/kg P.O. three times weekly.

Pharmacodynamics
- *Diuretic action:* Chlorthalidone increases urinary excretion of sodium and water by inhibiting sodium reabsorption in the cortical diluting tubule of the nephron, thus relieving edema.
- *Antihypertensive action:* The exact mechanism of chlorthalidone's hypotensive effect is unknown. This effect may partially result from direct arteriolar vasodilation and a decrease in total peripheral resistance.

Pharmacokinetics
- *Absorption:* Chlorthalidone is absorbed from the GI tract; extent of absorption is unknown.
- *Distribution:* Chlorthalidone is 90% bound to erythrocytes.
- *Metabolism:* Data are limited.
- *Excretion:* Between 30% and 60% of a given dose of chlorthalidone is excreted unchanged in urine; half-life is 54 hours.

Contraindications and precautions
Chlorthalidone is contraindicated in patients with anuria and in those with known sensitivity to the drug or to other sulfonamide derivatives. Chlorthalidone should be used cautiously in patients with severe renal disease because it may decrease glomerular filtration rate and precipitate azotemia; in patients with impaired hepatic function or liver disease because electrolyte changes may precipitate coma; and in patients taking digoxin, because hypokalemia may predispose them to digitalis toxicity.

Interactions
Chlorthalidone potentiates the hypotensive effects of most other antihypertensive drugs; this may be used to therapeutic advantage.
Chlorthalidone may potentiate hyperglycemic, hypotensive, and hyperuricemic effects of diazoxide, and

its hyperglycemic effect may increase insulin or sulfonylurea requirements in diabetic patients. Chlorthalidone may reduce renal clearance of lithium, elevating serum lithium levels, and may necessitate reduction in lithium dosage by 50%.
Chlorthalidone turns urine slightly more alkaline and may decrease urinary excretion of some amines, such as amphetamine and quinidine; alkaline urine also may decrease therapeutic efficacy of methenamine compounds such as methenamine mandelate.
Cholestyramine and colestipol may bind chlorthalidone, preventing its absorption; give drugs 1 hour apart.

Effects on diagnostic tests
Chlorthalidone therapy may alter serum electrolyte levels and may increase serum urate, glucose, cholesterol, and triglyceride levels.
Chlorthalidone may interfere with tests for parathyroid function and should be discontinued before such tests.

Adverse reactions
- CV: volume depletion and dehydration, orthostatic hypotension, hypercholesterolemia, hypertriglyceridemia.
- DERM: dermatitis, photosensitivity, rash.
- GI: anorexia, nausea, pancreatitis.
- GU: impotence.
- HEMA: *aplastic anemia, agranulocytosis,* leukopenia, thrombocytopenia.
- Hepatic: hepatic encephalopathy.
- Metabolic: asymptomatic hyperuricemia; gout; hyperglycemia and impairment of glucose tolerance; fluid and electrolyte imbalances, including hypokalemia (may be profound), hyponatremia, hypochloremia, and hypercalcemia; metabolic alkalosis.
- Other: hypersensitivity reactions, such as pneumonitis and vasculitis.
Note: Drug should be discontinued if rising BUN and serum creatinine levels indicate renal impairment or if patient shows signs of impending coma.

Overdose and treatment
Clinical signs of overdose include GI irritation and hypermotility, diuresis, and lethargy, which may progress to coma.
Treatment is mainly supportive; monitor and assist respiratory, cardiovascular, and renal function as indicated. Monitor fluid and electrolyte balance. Induce vomiting with ipecac in conscious patient; otherwise, use gastric lavage to avoid aspiration. Do not give cathartics; these promote additional loss of fluids and electrolytes.

▶ Special considerations
Recommendations for use of chlorthalidone and for care and teaching of the patient during therapy are the same as those for all *thiazide and thiazide-like diuretics.*

Geriatric use
Elderly and debilitated patients require close observation and may require reduced dosages. They are more sensitive to excess diuresis because of age-related changes in cardiovascular and renal function. Excess diuresis promotes orthostatic hypotension, dehydration, hypovolemia, hyponatremia, hypomagnesemia, and hypokalemia.

Breast-feeding
Chlorthalidone is distributed in breast milk; its safety and effectiveness in breast-feeding women have not been established.

chlorzoxazone
Paraflex, Parafon Forte DSC
- Pharmacologic classification: benzoxazole derivative
- Therapeutic classification: skeletal muscle relaxant
- Pregnancy risk category C

How supplied
Available by prescription only
Tablets (film-coated): 250 mg, 500 mg

Indications, route, and dosage
Adjunct in acute, painful musculoskeletal conditions
Adults: 250, 500, or 750 mg P.O. t.i.d. or q.i.d. Reduce to lowest effective dose after response is obtained.
Children: 20 mg/kg or 600 mg² P.O. daily divided t.i.d. or q.i.d., or 125 to 500 mg t.i.d. or q.i.d., depending on age and weight.

Pharmacodynamics
Skeletal muscle relaxant action: Chlorzoxazone does not relax skeletal muscle directly, but apparently as a result of its sedative effects. However, the exact mechanism of action is unknown.
   Animal studies suggest that the drug modifies central perception of pain without eliminating peripheral pain reflexes.

Pharmacokinetics
- *Absorption:* Chlorzoxazone is rapidly and completely absorbed from the GI tract. Onset of action occurs within 1 hour; duration of action is 3 to 4 hours.
- *Distribution:* Chlorzoxazone is widely distributed in the body.
- *Metabolism:* Drug is metabolized in the liver to inactive metabolites.
- *Excretion:* Drug is excreted in urine as glucuronide metabolite.

Contraindications and precautions
Chlorzoxazone is contraindicated in patients with known sensitivity to the drug or impaired hepatic function, because the drug is metabolized by the liver. Use with caution in patients with allergies or a history of allergic reactions to drugs.

Interactions
Concomitant use with other CNS depressants, including alcohol, produces further CNS depression. When used with other depressant drugs (general anesthetics, opioid analgesics, antipsychotics, anxiolytics, or tricyclic antidepressants), exercise care to avoid overdose. Concurrent use with monoamine oxidase inhibitors or tricyclic antidepressants may result in increased CNS depression, respiratory depression, and hypotensive effects. Reduce dosage of one or both agents.

Effects on diagnostic tests
None reported.

Adverse reactions
- CNS: drowsiness, dizziness, tremor, insomnia, agitation, irritability, headache, depression.
- DERM: rash, pruritus, urticaria.
- GI: nausea, vomiting, constipation, diarrhea, epigastric distress.
   Note: Drug should be discontinued if signs or symptoms of hepatic dysfunction or hypersensitivity occur.

Overdose and treatment
Clinical manifestations of overdose include nausea, vomiting, diarrhea, drowsiness, dizziness, light-headedness, headache, malaise, or sluggishness, followed by loss of muscle tone, decreased or absent deep tendon reflexes, respiratory depression, and hypotension.
   To treat overdose, induce emesis or perform gastric lavage followed by activated charcoal. Closely monitor vital signs and neurologic status. Provide general supportive measures, including maintenance of adequate airway and assisted ventilation. Use caution if administering pressor agents.

▶ Special considerations
- Chlorzoxazone may cause drowsiness.
- Urine may turn orange or reddish purple.
- Be aware of other CNS depressant drugs patient is taking, because effects are cumulative.
- Monitor liver function tests in patients receiving long-term therapy.

Information for the patient
- Caution patient to avoid hazardous activities that require alertness or physical coordination until CNS depression is determined.
- Warn patient to avoid alcoholic beverages and to use caution when taking cough and cold preparations, because they may contain alcohol.
- Tell patient to store drug away from direct heat or light (not in bathroom medicine cabinet, where heat and humidity cause deterioriation of drug).
- Tell patient to take missed dose only if remembered within 1 hour of scheduled time. If beyond 1 hour, patient should skip dose and go back to regular schedule. Patient should not double-dose.
- Tell patient not to stop taking this medication without calling for specific instructions.
- Tell patient urine may turn orange or reddish purple, but this is a harmless effect.
- If patient is an athlete, warn that skeletal muscle relaxants are banned in competition sponsored by the U.S. Olympics Committee and the National Collegiate Athletic Association. Use can lead to disqualification.

Geriatric use
Elderly patients may be more sensitive to drug's effects.

Pediatric use
Tablets may be crushed and mixed with food, milk, or fruit juice to aid dosing in children.

Breast-feeding
Unknown whether excreted in breast milk. No clinical problems have been reported.

---

cholera vaccine

- Pharmacologic classification: vaccine
- Therapeutic classification: cholera prophylaxis product
- Pregnancy risk category C

How supplied
Available by prescription only
Injection: suspension of killed *Vibrio cholerae* (each milliliter contains 8 units of Inaba and Ogawa serotypes) in 1-ml, 1.5-ml, and 20-ml vials

Indications, route, and dosage
Primary immunization
Adults and children over age 10: 2 doses of 0.5 ml I.M. or 1 ml S.C., 1 week to 1 month apart, before traveling in cholera area. Booster dosage is 0.5 ml q 6 months for as long as protection is needed.
Children age 5 to 10: 0.3 ml I.M. or S.C.
Children age 6 months to 4 years: 0.2 ml I.M. or S.C. Boosters of same dose should be given q 6 months for as long as protection is needed.

Pharmacodynamics
Cholera prophylaxis: This vaccine promotes active immunity to cholera in 25% to 50% of those immunized.

Pharmacokinetics
Virus-induced immunity begins to taper off within 3 to 6 months.

Contraindications and precautions
Cholera vaccine is contraindicated in patients with acute respiratory or other active infections, immune deficiency states, or a previous serious reaction to cholera vaccine.

The simultaneous administration of cholera vaccine with yellow fever vaccine may decrease the response to both.

Interactions
Concomitant use of cholera vaccine with corticosteroids or immunosuppressants may impair the immune response to cholera vaccine and therefore should be avoided.

Effects on diagnostic tests
None reported.

Adverse reactions
- Local: erythema, swelling, pain, tenderness, induration; rarely, necrosis and ulceration at injection site.
- Systemic: malaise, low-grade fever, headache, general aches and pains, flushing, urticaria, tachycardia, *hypotension, anaphylaxis.*

Overdose and treatment
No information available.

▶ Special considerations
- Obtain a thorough history of allergies and reactions to immunizations.
- Epinephrine solution 1:1,000 should be available to treat allergic reactions.
- When possible, cholera and yellow fever vaccines

should be administered at least 3 weeks apart; however, they may be administered simultaneously if time constraints make this necessary.
- Cholera vaccine may be given intradermally, but I.M. and S.C. routes give higher levels of protection. Do not use intradermal route in children under age 5.
- Shake vial well before removing a dose.
- Administer I.M. in deltoid muscle in adults and children over age 3 and in the anterolateral thigh in children under age 3.
- Store at 2° to 8° C. (36° to 46° F.). Do not freeze.

Information for the patient
- Tell patient to report skin changes, difficulty breathing, fever, or joint pain.
- Patient may take acetaminophen to relieve minor side effects, such as pain and tenderness at injection site.

Pediatric use
Not recommended for infants under age 6 months.

Breast-feeding
Maternal vaccination with cholera vaccine may increase significantly anticholera toxin IgA titer in breast milk. The effects of maternal transfer of antibodies to breast-feeding infants are unknown.

cholestyramine
Questran, Questran-Light

- Pharmacologic classification: anion exchange resin
- Therapeutic classification: antilipemic, bile acid sequestrant
- Pregnancy risk category C

How supplied
Available by prescription only
Powder: 378-g cans, 9-g single-dose packets (Questran). 5-g single dose packets (Questran-Light). Each scoop of powder or single-dose packet contains 4 g of cholestyramine resin.

Indications, route, and dosage
Hyperlipidemia, hypercholesterolemia
Drug is indicated in primary hyperlipidemia, pruritus, and diarrhea caused by excess bile acid; as adjunctive therapy to reduce elevated serum cholesterol levels; in patients with primary hypercholesterolemia; and to reduce the risks of atherosclerotic coronary artery disease and myocardial infarction.
Adults: 4 g before meals and h.s., not to exceed 32 g daily. Can be given in two divided doses.
Children age 6 to 12: 80 mg/kg, or 2.35 g/m² t.i.d. Safe dosage has not been established for children under age 6.

Pharmacodynamics
Antilipemic action: Bile is normally excreted into the intestine to facilitate absorption of fat and other lipid materials. Cholestyramine binds with bile acid, forming an insoluble compound that is excreted in feces. With less bile available in the digestive system, less fat and lipid materials in food are absorbed, more cholesterol is used by the liver to replace its supply of bile acids, and the serum cholesterol level decreases. In partial

biliary obstruction, excess bile acids accumulate in dermal tissue, resulting in pruritus; by reducing levels of dermal bile acids, cholestyramine combats pruritus.

Cholestyramine can also act as an antidiarrheal in postoperative diarrhea caused by bile acids in the colon.

Pharmacokinetics
● *Absorption:* Cholestyramine is not absorbed. Cholesterol levels may begin to decrease 24 to 48 hours after the start of therapy and may continue to fall for up 12 months. In some patients, the initial decrease is followed by a return to or above baseline cholesterol levels on continued therapy. Relief of pruritus associated with cholestasis occurs 1 to 3 weeks after initiation of therapy. Diarrhea associated with bile acids may cease in 24 hours.
● *Distribution:* None.
● *Metabolism:* None.
● *Excretion:* Insoluble cholestyramine with bile acid complex is excreted in feces.

Contraindications and precautions
Cholestyramine is contraindicated in patients with complete biliary obstruction and in patients hypersensitive to any of its components. Cholestyramine powder contains tartrazine (FD&C Yellow No. 5), which may cause allergic reactions in susceptible individuals.

Use resin cautiously in patients with constipation because of the risk of fecal impaction; in patients with malabsorption, whose condition may deteriorate from further decreased absorption of fats and fat-soluble vitamins E, A, D, and K; and in pregnant women, because impaired maternal absorption of vitamins and other nutrients is a potential threat to the fetus. Do not prescribe Questran-Light for patients who are sensitive to aspartame.

Interactions
Cholestyramine may reduce absorption of other oral medications, such as acetaminophen, corticosteroids, thiazide diuretics, thyroid preparations, and cardiac glycosides, thus decreasing their therapeutic effects. Its binding potential may also decrease anticoagulant effects of warfarin; concurrent depletion of vitamin K may either negate this effect or increase anticoagulant activity; careful monitoring of prothrombin time is mandatory.

Dosage of any oral medication may require adjustment to compensate for possible binding with cholestyramine; give other drugs at least 1 hour before or 4 to 6 hours after cholestyramine (longer if possible); readjustment must also be made when cholestyramine is withdrawn, to prevent high-dose toxicity.

Effects on diagnostic tests
Cholestyramine therapy alters serum concentrations of alkaline phosphatase, aspartate aminotransferase, chloride, phosphorus, potassium, calcium, and sodium. Impaired calcium absorption may lead to osteoporosis. Cholecystography using iopanoic acid will yield abnormal results because iopanoic acid is also bound by cholestyramine.

Adverse reactions
● DERM: rash; irritation of skin, tongue, and perianal area.
● GI: constipation, fecal impaction, aggravation of hemorrhoids, abdominal discomfort, flatulence, nausea, vomiting, steatorrhea.

● Other: vitamin A, D, and K deficiency from decreased absorption; hyperchloremic acidosis with long-term use or very high dosage.
Note: Drug should be discontinued if constipation continues even after reduction in dosage; if a paradoxical increase in serum cholesterol level occurs; or if clinical response is inadequate after 3 months of therapy.

Overdose and treatment
Overdose of cholestyramine has not been reported. Chief potential risk is intestinal obstruction; treatment would depend on location and degree of obstruction and on amount of gut motility.

▶ Special considerations
● To mix, sprinkle powder on surface of preferred beverage or wet food, let stand a few minutes, and stir to obtain uniform suspension; avoid excess foaming by using large glass and mixing slowly. Use at least 90 ml of water or other fluid (if carbonated fluid is used, minimize excess foaming by mixing the powder slowly in a large glass), soups, milk, or pulpy fruit; rinse container and have patient drink this to be sure he ingests entire dose.
● Cholestyramine has been used to treat cardiac glycoside overdose because it binds these agents and prevents enterohepatic recycling. When used as an adjunct to hyperlipidemia, monitor levels of cardiac glycosides and other drugs to ensure appropriate dosage during and after therapy with cholestyramine.
● Determine serum cholesterol level frequently during first few months of therapy and periodically thereafter.
● Monitor bowel function. Treat constipation promptly by decreasing dosage, adding a stool softener, or discontinuing drug.
● Monitor for signs of vitamin A, D, or K deficiency.
● Questran-Light contains aspartame and provides 1.6 calories per packet or scoop.

Information for the patient
● Explain disease process and rationale for therapy, and encourage patient to comply with continued blood testing and special diet; although therapy is not curative, it helps control serum cholesterol level.
● Attempt to increase patient awareness of other cardiac risk factors; encourage patient to control weight and not to smoke.
● Tell patient not to take the powder in dry form; teach him to mix drug with fluids or pulpy fruits.

Geriatric use
Patients over age 60 are more likely to experience adverse GI effects, as well as adverse nutritional effects.

Pediatric use
Children may be at greater risk of hyperchloremic acidosis during cholestyramine therapy.

Breast-feeding
Safety in breast-feeding women has not been established.

choline magnesium trisalicylates
Trilisate

choline salicylate
Arthropan

- Pharmacologic classification: salicylate
- Therapeutic classification: nonnarcotic analgesic, antipyretic, anti-inflammatory
- Pregnancy risk category C

How supplied
Available by prescription only
Tablets: 500 mg, 750 mg, 1,000 mg of salicylate (as choline and magnesium salicylate)
Solution: 500 mg of salicylate/5 ml (as choline and magnesium salicylate); 870 mg/5 ml (as choline salicylate)

Indications, route, and dosage
Arthritis, mild
Adults: 1 to 2 teaspoonfuls (5 to 10 ml) or 1 to 2 tablets b.i.d. Total daily dose can also be given at one time.
Rheumatoid arthritis and osteoarthritis
Adults: 3 to 4 teaspoonfuls (10 to 15 ml) or 2 to 3 tablets b.i.d. Total daily dose can also be given at one time.

Each 500-mg tablet or 5 ml of liquid choline and magnesium salicylate or 870 mg of choline salicylate is equal in salicylate content to 650 mg of aspirin.
Juvenile rheumatoid arthritis
Children: 107 to 133 mg/kg/day of choline salicylate in divided doses.
Mild-to-moderate pain and fever
Adults: 2.5 to 5 ml P.O. q 4 hours p.r.n.
Children: 2 g/m²/day in four to six divided doses or as shown below.
Children age 2 to 4: 217.5 mg q 4 hours p.r.n.
Children age 4 to 6: 326.5 mg q 4 hours p.r.n.
Children age 6 to 9: 435 mg q 4 hours p.r.n.
Children age 9 to 11: 543.8 mg q 4 hours p.r.n.
Children age 11 to 12: 652.5 mg q 4 hours p.r.n.

Pharmacodynamics
- *Analgesic action:* Choline salicylates produce analgesia by an ill-defined effect on the hypothalamus (central action) and by blocking generation of pain impulses (peripheral action). The peripheral action may involve inhibition of prostaglandin synthesis.
- *Anti-inflammatory action:* These drugs exert their anti-inflammatory effect by inhibiting prostaglandin synthesis; they may also inhibit the synthesis or action of other inflammation mediators.
- *Antipyretic action:* Choline salicylates relieve fever by acting on the hypothalamic heat-regulating center to produce peripheral vasodilation. This increases peripheral blood supply and promotes sweating, which leads to loss of heat and to cooling by evaporation. These drugs do not affect platelet aggregation and should not be used to prevent thrombosis.

Pharmacokinetics
- *Absorption:* These salicylate salts are absorbed rapidly and completely from the GI tract. Peak therapeutic effect occurs in 2 hours.
- *Distribution:* Protein binding depends on concentration and ranges from 75% to 90%, decreasing as serum concentration increases. Severe toxic side effects may occur at serum concentrations greater than 400 mcg/ml.
- *Metabolism:* Drugs are hydrolyzed to salicylate in the liver.
- *Excretion:* Metabolites are excreted in urine.

Contraindications and precautions
These drugs are contraindicated in patients with known hypersensitivity to salicylates or other nonsteroidal anti-inflammatory drugs (NSAIDs) and when GI ulcer or GI bleeding are present.

Choline salicylates should be used cautiously in patients with a history of GI disease and increased risk of GI bleeding because the drug may worsen these conditions; and in patients with decreased renal or hepatic function because of potential for drug accumulation (especially magnesium salicylate).

Patients with known "triad" symptoms (aspirin hypersensitivity, rhinitis/nasal polyps, and asthma) are at high risk of cross-sensitivity to salicylates and NSAIDs with precipitation of bronchospasm. Salicylates may mask the signs and symptoms of acute infection (fever, myalgia, erythema); carefully evaluate patients with high risk (for example, those with diabetes).

Interactions
Concomitant use of choline salicylates with drugs that are highly protein-bound (phenytoin, sulfonylureas, warfarin) may cause displacement of either drug, and adverse effects. Monitor therapy closely for both drugs. The adverse GI effects of choline salicylates may be potentiated by concomitant use of other GI-irritant drugs (such as steroids, antibiotics, and other NSAIDs). Use together with caution. Choline salicylates decrease renal clearance of lithium carbonate, thus increasing serum lithium levels and the risk of adverse effects. Ammonium chloride and other urine acidifiers increase choline salicylate blood levels; monitor for choline salicylate blood levels and thus toxicity. Antacids in high doses, and other urine alkalizers, decrease choline salicylate blood levels; monitor for decreased salicylate effect. Corticosteroids enhance salicylate elimination; monitor for decreased effect. Food and antacids delay and decrease absorption of choline salicylates.

Effects on diagnostic tests
Choline salicylates may interfere with urinary glucose analysis performed via Clinistix, Tes-Tape, Clinitest, and Benedict's solution. These drugs also interfere with urinary 5-hydroxyindole acetic acid (5-HIAA) and vanillymandelic acid (VMA).

Adverse reactions
- DERM: rash, bruising.
- EENT: tinnitus, hearing loss.
- GI: nausea, vomiting, GI distress, occult bleeding.
- Other: hypersensitivity manifested by *anaphylaxis* or asthma, abnormal liver function tests, hepatitis.
  Note: Drug should be discontinued if the following occur: hypersensitivity (aspirin-induced bronchospasm) reaction, severe hepatic dysfunction, or signs and symptoms of salicylism.

Overdose and treatment
Clinical manifestations of overdose include metabolic acidosis with respiratory alkalosis, hyperpnea, and tachypnea from increased CO_2 production and direct stimulation of the respiratory center.

To treat overdose of choline salicylates, empty stomach immediately by inducing emesis with ipecac syrup, if patient is conscious, or by gastric lavage. Administer activated charcoal via nasogastric tube. Provide symptomatic and supportive measures (respiratory support and correction of fluid and electrolyte imbalances). Monitor laboratory parameters and vital signs closely. Hemodialysis is effective in removing choline salicylates, but is used only in severe poisoning.

▶ **Special considerations**
Besides those relevant to all *salicylates*, consider the following recommendations.
● Do not mix choline salicylates with antacids.
● Administer oral solution of choline salicylate mixed with fruit juice. Follow with a full 8-oz glass of water to ensure passage into stomach.
● Monitor serum magnesium levels to prevent possible magnesium toxicity.
● Use of choline salicylates should be avoided in the third trimester of pregnancy.

Geriatric use
Patients over age 60 may be more susceptible to the toxic effects of these drugs.

Pediatric use
● The safety of long-term choline salicylate use in children under age 14 has not been established.
● Because of epidemiologic association with Reye's syndrome, the Centers for Disease Control recommend that children with chicken pox or flulike symptoms should not be given salicylates.
● Febrile, dehydrated children can develop toxicity rapidly. Ordinarily, they should not receive more than five doses in 24 hours.

Breast-feeding
Salicylates are distributed into breast milk. Avoid use in breast-feeding women.

PHARMACOLOGIC CLASS

cholinergics

acetylcholine chloride
bethanechol chloride
carbachol chloride

The basic components of cholinergic drugs were first synthesized in the 1860s; by the 1930s, physicians were using them and some of their synthetic analogues therapeutically.

Pharmacology
These agents are used to simulate the actions of acetylcholine at postganglionic (muscarinic) neuroeffector sites.
Acetylcholine is of little use clinically because of its susceptibility to acetylcholinesterase and butyrylcholinesterase and its relatively nonspecific action at both sympathetic and parasympathetic ganglia.

Clinical indications and actions
GI and urinary tract atony
Bethanechol is used to treat paralytic ileus, postoperative abdominal distention, and gastric atony or stasis. Bethanechol enhances gastric tone, contractions, and GI peristaltic activity, increasing gastric acid secretions.

It also relieves gastric atony and retention after bilateral vagotomy for peptic ulcer. In some patients, bethanechol has proven effective in treating congenital megacolon. Bethanechol is used to treat postoperative or postpartum urinary retention and, in certain cases, neurogenic bladder; it increases ureteral peristalsis and induces contraction of the urinary bladder's detrusor muscle.

Glaucoma
Topical carbachol is used to treat glaucoma. In narrow-angle glaucoma, it causes the iris sphincter to contract; that allows aqueous humor to flow out through the trabecular space at Schlemm's canal. In open-angle glaucoma, physostigmine enhances trabecular network tone and alignment, permitting aqueous humor to flow through the Schlemm's canal, thereby reducing intraocular pressure.
Because of its short duration of action, acetylcholine is used only for perioperative miosis.

Overview of adverse reactions
Cholinergics may cause dizziness, confusion, hallucinations, muscle weakness, nervousness, miosis, blurred vision, tearing, bronchospasm, bronchial constriction, nausea, vomiting, and belching. They may also precipitate asthma attacks in susceptible patients.
Clinical effects of overdose primarily involve muscarinic symptoms, such as nausea, vomiting, diarrhea, abdominal discomfort, involuntary defecation, urinary urgency, increased bronchial and salivary secretions, respiratory depression, skin flushing or heat sensation, and bradycardia; cardiac arrest has also occurred.

▶ **Special considerations**
● Regularly monitor patient's vital signs, especially heart rate and respirations, and fluid intake and output; evaluate for changes in muscle strength and observe closely for adverse drug effects or signs of acute toxicity.
● Impose safety precautions. Patient may become restless or have hallucinations and may need assistance with ambulation.
● All cholinergics are contraindicated in pregnant women.

Information for the patient
● Instruct patient to take medication exactly as ordered; advise patient to take with food and milk to reduce gastric irritation, if appropriate.
● Advise patient to report dyspnea, irregular pulse, increased salivation, nausea, vomiting, diarrhea, severe abdominal pain, muscle weakness, or sweating.

Geriatric use
Use cautiously when administering cholinergics to elderly patients, because they may be more sensitive to drug effects. Lower doses may be indicated.

Pediatric use
Safety and effectiveness in children not established.

Breast-feeding
Some cholinergics may be excreted in breast milk, possibly resulting in infant toxicity. Breast-feeding women should avoid these drugs.

Representative combinations
Physostigmine salicylate with atropine: Atrophysine; with 1-hyoscyamine hydrobromide: Phyatromine-H; with

pilocarpine and methylcellulose: Isopto P-ES, Miocel, Sol.

cholinesterase inhibitors

Amine or quaternary ammonium compounds
ambenonium chloride
demecarium bromide
edrophonium chloride
neostigmine bromide
neostigmine methylsulfate
physostigmine salicylate
physostigmine sulfate
pyridostigmine bromide

Organophosphates
echothiophate iodide

Cholinesterase inhibitors are divided into two main categories: amine or quaternary ammonium compounds and organophosphates. The inhibition of cholinesterases has varied effects based on where the enzymes are inhibited, with the most significant effects occurring at sites of cholinergic neuroeffector transmission. Anticholinesterases are used both systemically and topically, and should be used under careful medical supervision as the therapeutic/toxic margin is quite small. Also, wide variations in response may occur even in the same patient; therefore, caution should be exercised because the first sign of adverse reactions may be subtle. Note that adverse systemic effects may occur even after topical application due to systemic absorption of agent.

Pharmacology
Amine or quaternary ammonium compounds interact reversibly with the anionic site of the cholinesterase (ionic bonding) as well as with the esteratic site (reversible acylation). They are more selective for acetylcholinesterase and may enhance neuromuscular function with only a few autonomic side effects; however, some agents, like physostigmine, may cross the blood-brain barrier and cause central effects. The quaternary ammonium compounds have nicotinic agonist activity as well, which indirectly enhances neuromuscular function. Their confinement to the periphery makes them useful for peripheral action.

The organophosphates form irreversible bonds at the esteratic site and are moderately selective for butyrocholinesterase. When neuromuscular transmission is enhanced by these agents, excessive effects on glands and smooth muscle also occur due to the presense of the enzyme in those sites. Because they are non-ionized, they readily penetrate the blood-brain barrier, causing central effects. As with the amine or quaternary ammonium agents, the organoposphates can be absorbed from the skin.

Clinical indications and actions
Muscle atony or paralysis; atropine or tricyclic antidepressant poisoning
Systemically, anticholinesterase agents are used to abolish muscle paralysis due to neuromuscular blocking agents, to improve muscle function in myasthenia gravis, to treat intestinal distention, and to restore GI

tonicity postpartum and postoperatively. They also are used to treat atropine or tricyclic antidepressant poisoning.
Glaucoma and other ocular disorders
Topically, anticholinesterase agents are applied to the eye to treat wide-angle glaucoma, marginal corneal ulcers, accommodative convergent strabismus, accommodative esotropia, and to improve the function of extraocular muscles and eyelids in myasthenia gravis. They also may be used in the emergency treatment of acute congestive glaucoma. When alternated with mydriatics, reversibly acting anticholinesterases may be used to break adhesions between lens and iris.

Overview of adverse reactions
Adverse systemic effects may result from systemic administration or systemic absorption following topical application. The most frequent of these include excessive salivation, sweating, lacrimation, bronchoconstriction, tracheobronchial secretion, marked miosis, blurred vision, nausea, vomiting, diarrhea, abdominal cramps, involuntary defecation, pallor, *hypertension or hypotension, bradycardia,* urinary frequency and urgency, and enuresis. Administration of atropine can antagonize these effects.

Topical application may result in stinging, lacrimation, ocular pain, browache, blurred vision, conjunctival and intraocular hyperemia, blepharospasm, transient rise in intraocular pressure, pigment cysts of the iris, anterior and posterior synechia, fibrinous iritis, cataracts (especially in elderly patients), and allergies. Atropine can antagonize these effects as well.

▶ Special considerations
● Administer oral forms with food or milk to reduce the muscarinic side effects by slowing down absorption and reducing peak serum levels.
● Observe patients closely for cholinergic reactions, especially with parenteral forms.
● Have atropine available to reduce or reverse hypersensitivity reactions.
● Administer atropine prior to or concurrently with large doses of parenteral anticholinesterases to counteract muscarinic side effects.
● Dosage must be individualized according to severity of disease and patient response.
● Myasthenic patients may become refractory to these medications after prolonged use; however, responsiveness may be restored by reducing the dose or discontinuing the drug for a few days.

Information for the patient
● Tell patient to take with food or milk to reduce adverse effects.
● Advise patient to keep daily record of dose and effects during initial phase of therapy to help identify an optimum therapeutic regimen.
● Warn patient to take drug exactly as prescribed, and to take missed dose as soon as possible. If almost time for next dose, patient should skip the missed dose and return to prescribed schedule. Patient should not double the dose.
● Advise patient to store drug away from children, heat, and light.

Geriatric use
No specific recommendations available.

Pediatric use
No specific recommendations available.

Breast-feeding
Excretion of anticholinesterase agents into breast milk is unknown. Use with caution.

Representative combinations
None.

---

chorionic gonadotropin, human (HCG)
A.P.L., Chorex 5, Chorex-10, Chorigon, Choron 10, Corgonject-5, Follutein Gonic, Pregnyl, Profasi HP

● Pharmacologic classification: gonadotropin
● Therapeutic classification: ovulation stimulant, spermatogenesis stimulant
● Pregnancy risk category X

How supplied
Available by prescription only
Injection: 200 USP units/ml, 500 USP units/ml, 1,000 USP units/ml, 2,000 USP units/ml

Indications, route, and dosage
To induce ovulation and pregnancy
Adults: 5,000 to 10,000 USP units I.M. 1 day after last dose of menotropins.
Hypogonadotropic hypogonadism
Adults: 500 to 1,000 USP units I.M. three times weekly for 3 weeks, then twice weekly for 3 weeks; or 4,000 USP units I.M. three times weekly for 6 to 9 months, then 2,000 USP units three times weekly for 3 more months.
Nonobstructive prepubertal cryptorchidism
Children age 4 to 9: 5,000 USP units I.M. every other day for 4 doses or 4,000 USP units I.M. three times a week for 3 weeks or 15 doses of 500 to 1,000 USP units I.M. given over 6 weeks.
Diagnosis of errors in testosterone biosynthesis (especially 5-alpha reductase deficiency); diagnosis of bilateral cryptorchidism
Children: Dosage varies considerably; 3,000 to 5,000 USP units I.M. per dose may be given for one to four doses.

Pharmacodynamics
● *Ovulation stimulant action:* HCG mimics the action of luteinizing hormone in stimulating the ovulation of a mature ovarian follicle.
● *Spermatogenesis stimulant action:* HCG stimulates androgen production in Leydig's cells of the testis and causes maturation of the cells lining the seminiferous tubules of the testes.

Pharmacokinetics
● *Absorption:* HCG must be administered I.M. Peak blood concentrations occur within 6 hours.
● *Distribution:* HCG is distributed primarily into the testes and the ovaries.
● *Metabolism:* Unknown.
● *Excretion:* HCG is excreted in urine.

Contraindications and precautions
HCG is contraindicated in patients with precocious puberty or androgen-responsive cancer (prostatic, testicular, male breast) because it stimulates androgen production, and in patients with known hypersensitivity to HCG.
HCG should be used only by clinicians experienced in treating infertility disorders.
HCG should be used cautiously in patients with asthma, seizure disorders, migraines, or cardiac or renal diseases, because it may exacerbate these conditions.

Interactions
None reported.

Effects on diagnostic tests
None reported.

Adverse reactions
● CNS: headache, fatigue, irritability, restlessness, depression.
● GU: early puberty (growth of testes, penis, pubic and axillary hair; voice change, down on upper lip; growth of body hair), hyperstimulation (ovarian enlargement), rupture of ovarian cysts (after use of gonadotropins).
● Local: pain at injection site.
● Other: gynecomastia, edema.

▶ **Special considerations**
● Young male patients receiving HCG must be observed carefully for the development of precocious puberty.
● Carefully monitor patients with disorders that may be aggravated by fluid retention.
● Pregnancies that occur after stimulation of ovulation with gonadotropins show a relatively high incidence of multiple births.
● HCG is usually used only after failure of clomiphene in anovulatory patients.
● In infertility, encourage daily intercourse from day before chorionic gonadotropin is given until ovulation occurs.
● Be alert to symptoms of ectopic pregnancy, usually evident between 8 to 12 weeks' gestation.

Information for the patient
● Teach patient and family how to assess for edema and to report it promptly.
● Advise patient and family to report signs of precocious puberty promptly.
● Advise patient receiving HCG for infertility that multiple births are possible.

Geriatric use
Not indicated for geriatric use.

Pediatric use
Treating prepubertal cryptorchidism with HCG can help predict future need for orchidopexy. Induction of androgen secretion may induce precocious puberty in patient treated for cryptorchidism. Instruct parent to report the following: axillary, facial, or pubic hair; penile growth; acne; and deepening of voice.

---

chymopapain
Chymodiactin

- Pharmacologic classification: proteolytic enzyme
- Therapeutic classification: chemonucleolytic agent
- Pregnancy risk category C

How supplied
Available by prescription only
Powder for injection: 4,000 or 10,000 pKat unit vials

Indications, route, and dosage
Herniated lumbar intervertebral disk
Adults: 2,000 to 4,000 pKat units per disk injected intradiskally. Maximum dose in a patient with multiple disk herniation is 8,000 pKat units.

Pharmacodynamics
Chemonucleolytic action: Mechanism of action has not been clearly established in humans; in animals, chymopapain hydrolyzes the noncollagenous polypeptides or proteins that maintain the chondromucoprotein structure of the nucleus pulposis. Hydrolysis of chondromucoprotein decreases intradiskal osmotic pressure and fluid accumulation, thereby reducing symptoms of compression. Drug has no effect on collagen.

Pharmacokinetics
- *Absorption:* Chymopapain is available only for intradiskal administration. It acts directly at the site of injection.
- *Distribution:* After intradiskal injection, chymopapain and its immunologically reactive fragments (CIP) are detectable in serum.
- *Metabolism:* Chymopapain serum levels are low, and drug is inactivated rapidly by plasma alpha-2 macroglobulin; extradiskal activity is unlikely.
- *Excretion:* Chymopapain and CIP serum levels remain steady for 24 hours and then decline. Only small amounts of CIP occur in urine.

Contraindications and precautions
Chymopapain is contraindicated in patients with known hypersensitivity to the drug or to papaya or its derivatives (for example, meat tenderizers); in patients previously treated with the drug, because of the increased risk of alergic reaction; in patients with severe spondylolisthesis, paralysis with rapidly progressing neurologic dysfunction, or evidence of cauda equina lesion or spinal cord tumor; for injection into the subarachnoid space (extreme toxicity will result) or outside the lumbar region, because no data exists on drug safety or efficacy in other body sites; and in combination with radio contrast media, such use in animals has produced increased neurotoxicity, including paralysis and death. Chymopapain should be used only by clinicians experienced in the diagnosis and medical and surgical treatment of lumbar disk disease, in the use of chymopapain, and in the management of potential complications.

Care must be taken to ensure that chymopapain and radiocontrast media are not injected into the subarachnoid space through the dural canal; if any doubt about needle tip location or extravasation into the subarach-

noid or intrathecal spaces exists, treatment should be discontinued immediately.

Interactions
Concomitant use with radiocontrast media increases risk of neurotoxicity.

Effects on diagnostic tests
None reported.

Adverse reactions
- CNS: acute transverse myelitis, paraplegia, headache, dizziness.
- CV: *cerebral hemorrhage,* hypotension, *cardiovascular collapse.*
- DERM: pruritic urticaria, rash, pruritus, pilomotor erection, erythema.
- GI: abdominal pain or cramps, constipation, vomiting.
- GU: decreased or uncontrolled urination.
- Other: hypersensitivity (hypotension, *bronchospasm, anaphylaxis*), sacral burning, leg pain, hypalgesia, numbness, tingling, weakness or paresthesia of legs or toes, lumbar pain, soreness or spasm.

Note: Drug should be discontinued if injection into other than disk space is known or suspected or if patient shows signs of hypersensitivity.

Overdose and treatment
Doses of over 100 times the recommended amount have been given *without* toxic effects; toxic effects after overdosage would probably be extreme manifestations of adverse reactions. Treat symptomatically.

▶ Special considerations
- Drug should be administered in the hospital by clinicians experienced and trained in diagnosis of lumbar disk disease.
- Before treatment, question patient about allergy to papaya or its derivatives.
- Monitor patient for at least 1 hour after injection for hypersensitivity reaction; hypotension and bronchospasm can rapidly lead to anaphylaxis and death. Maintain an open I.V. line to permit rapid management of anaphylaxis, and keep resuscitative measures available.
- Anaphylaxis occurs in 0.4% to 1% of patients and may occur immediately or up to 1 hour after injection; risk of anaphylaxis is greater in women with elevated erythrocyte sedimentation rate and in patients undergoing general anesthesia.
- One in 18,000 patients develops acute transverse myelitis/myelopathy, manifested by acute onset of severe back pain, weakness, and sensory changes at the thoracic level that progress to paraplegia or paraparesis over 4 to 48 hours; patients with injection of two or more disks after diskography have an increased risk.
- A skin test (ChymoFAST) may detect hypersensitivity.
- Pretreatment of the patient with histamine-receptor antagonists (H_1 and H_2) is recommended to decrease the severity of chymopapain-induced allergic reactions.
- The patient should be well hydrated before the procedure because of the abrupt decrease in intravascular volume during anaphylaxis.

Information for the patient
- Warn patient to call at once if he develops delayed allergic reaction of rash, itching, or urticaria (up to 15 days postinjection) or if he develops sudden, severe pain, muscle weakness, or sensory changes in the back.

• Up to 50% of patients will experience back pain, stiffness, and soreness and up to 30% will have back spasm after treatment. Reassure patient this is temporary but may last for several days.

Geriatric use
Drug should be used with caution in elderly patients.

chymotrypsin
Catarase, Zolyse

• Pharmacologic classification: proteolytic enzyme
• Therapeutic classification: zonulolytic agent, anti-inflammatory
• Pregnancy risk category C

How supplied
Available by prescription only
Ophthalmic solution: 150 USP units, 300 USP units, 750 USP units

Indications, route, and dosage
Adjunct in cataract surgery
Adults: After corneoscleral or corneoscleral-conjunctival incision, the posterior chamber of the eye is irrigated with 0.25 to 2 ml of a chymotrypsin solution containing 150 units/ml (1:5,000) or 75 units/ml (1:10,000). After iridectomy or iridotomy and placement of sutures, and a waiting period of 2 to 4 minutes, the posterior chamber is then irrigated with at least 2 ml of diluent or 0.9% sodium chloride injection. If the zonules are still intact, another irrigation with 1 to 2 ml of chymotrypsin solution may be made through the iridectomy opening; after another waiting period of 2 to 4 minutes, the chamber is irrigated again with at least 2 ml of diluent or 0.9% sodium chloride injection.

Pharmacodynamics
Zonulolytic action: When used as an adjunct to cataract surgery, chymotrypsin facilitates lens extraction by dissolving the zonules (supporting filaments), which hold the lens.

Pharmacokinetics
Absorption, distribution, metabolism, and excretion are unknown.

Contraindications and precautions
Chymotrypsin is contraindicated in patients with known hypersensitivity to chymotrypsin or trypsin. The ophthalmic solution should not be used in patients with high vitreous pressure and a gaping incisional wound or in patients with congenital cataracts. Ophthalmic solution should be used with caution during cataract surgery in patients under age 20 because of risk of excessive loss of vitreous humor.

Interactions
Topical instillation of epinephrine 1:100 into the eye will inactivate chymotrypsin in about 1 hour; isoflurophate, chloramphenicol, serum, blood, detergents, alkalies, acids, and antiseptics also will inactivate the ophthalmic solution of chymotrypsin.

Effects on diagnostic tests
None reported.

Adverse reactions
• EENT: transient increases in intraocular pressure, corneal edema, uveitis.

Overdose and treatment
No information available.

▶ Special considerations
• Ophthalmic chymotrypsin is instilled into the posterior chamber of the eye after incision. The patient is under local or general anesthesia, and the pupil is dilated with a mydriatic.
• Instruments and syringes must be free of enzyme-inactivating alcohol and other antispetic solutions before using ophthalmic solution.
• Reconstitute immediately before use.

ciclopirox olamine
Loprox

• Pharmacologic classification: N-hydrox-ypyridinone derivative
• Therapeutic classification: topical anti-fungal
• Pregnancy risk category B

How supplied
Available by prescription only
Cream: 1%
Lotion: 1%

Indications, route, and dosage
Tinea pedis, tinea cruris, and tinea corporis; cutaneous candidiasis; tinea versicolor
Adults and children over age 10: Massage gently into the affected and surrounding areas b.i.d., in the morning and evening.

Pharmacodynamics
Antifungal and antibacterial activity: Although the exact mechanism of action is unknown, ciclopirox appears to act by causing intracellular depletion of essential cellular components or ions. The drug is active against many fungi, including dermatophytes and yeast, as well as against some gram-positive and gram-negative bacteria.

Pharmacokinetics
• *Absorption:* Rapid but minimal percutaneous absorption.
• *Distribution:* Minimal.
• *Metabolism:* After percutaneous absorption, ciclopirox has an elimination half-life of about 2 hours.
• *Excretion:* After percutaneous absorption, ciclopirox and its metabolites are excreted rapidly in the urine.

Contraindications and precautions
Ciclopirox is contraindicated in patients who have shown hypersensitivity to the drug.

Effects on diagnostic tests
None reported.

Interactions
None reported.

Adverse reactions
● DERM: pruritus or burning around the area of application.

Note: Drug should be discontinued if hypersensitivity occurs.

Overdose and treatment
No information available.

▶ Special considerations
● Drug is for topical use only; avoid contact with eyes.
● Do not apply occlusive dressings.

Information for the patient
● Advise patient to use drug for full treatment period even if symptoms have improved. Patient should call if no improvement occurs in 4 weeks.
● Tell patient to avoid occlusive wrapping or dressing.
● Advise patient to wash hands thoroughly after applying drug, to avoid contacting eyes with the medication.
● If sensitivity or chemical irritation occurs, advise patient to discontinue treatment and call promptly.
● Inform patient with tinea versicolor that hypopigmentation from the disease will not resolve immediately.

Pediatric use
Safety and efficacy in children under age 10 have not been established.

Breast-feeding
It is unknown if the medication is excreted in breast milk; therefore, ciclopirox should be used with caution in breast-feeding women.

cimetidine
Tagamet

● Pharmacologic classification: histamine₂-receptor antagonist
● Therapeutic classification: antiulcer agent
● Pregnancy risk category B

How supplied
Available by prescription only
Tablets: 200 mg, 300 mg, 400 mg, 800 mg
Injection: 150 mg/ml
Liquid: 300 mg/5 ml

Indications, route, and dosage
Duodenal ulcer (short-term treatment)
Adults: 800 mg h.s. for maximum of 8 weeks. Alternatively, give 400 mg P.O. b.i.d. or 300 mg P.O. q.i.d. with meals and h.s. When healing occurs, stop treatment or give bedtime dose only to control nocturnal hypersecretion.
Parenteral: 300 mg diluted to 20 ml with normal saline solution or other compatible I.V. solution by I.V. push over 1 to 2 minutes q 6 hours. Or 300 mg diluted in 100 ml dextrose 5% solution or other compatible I.V. solution by I.V. infusion over 15 to 20 minutes q 6 hours. Or 300 mg I.M. q 6 hours (no dilution necessary). To

increase dose, give 300-mg doses more frequently to maximum daily dose of 2,400 mg.
Duodenal ulcer prophylaxis
Adults: 400 mg P.O. h.s.
Active benign gastric ulcer
Adults: 300 mg q.i.d. with meals and h.s. for up to 8 weeks.
Pathologic hypersecretory conditions (such as Zollinger-Ellison syndrome, systemic mastocytosis, and multiple endocrine adenomas); †short-bowel syndrome
Adults: 300 mg P.O. q.i.d. with meals and h.s.; adjust to individual needs. Maximum daily dose is 2,400 mg. Parenteral: 300 mg diluted to 20 ml with 0.9% normal saline solution or other compatible I.V. solution by I.V. push over 1 to 2 minutes q 6 hours. Or 300-mg diluted in 100 ml dextrose 5% solution or other compatible I.V. solution by I.V. infusion over 15 to 20 minutes q 6 hours. To increase dose, give 300 mg doses more frequently to maximum daily dose of 2,400 mg.
Symptomatic relief of gastroesophageal reflux
Adults: 800 mg P.O. b.i.d. or 400 mg q.i.d., before meals and h.s.
Upper GI bleeding, peptic esophagitis, stress ulcer
Adults: 1 to 2 g I.V. or P.O. daily, in four divided doses.
Children: 20 to 40 mg/kg daily in divided doses.
Continuous infusion for patients unable to tolerate oral medication
Adults: 37.5 mg/hour (900 mg/day) by continuous I.V. infusion. Use an infusion pump if total volume is below 250 ml/day.

Pharmacodynamics
Antiulcer action: Cimetidine competitively inhibits histamine's action at histamine₂ (H₂) receptors in gastric parietal cells, inhibiting basal and nocturnal gastric acid secretion (such as from stimulation by food, caffeine, insulin, histamine, betazole, or pentagastrin). Cimetidine may also enhance gastromucosal defense and healing.
  A 300-mg oral or parenteral dose inhibits about 80% of gastric acid secretion for 4 to 5 hours.

Pharmacokinetics
● Absorption: Approximately 60% to 75% of oral dose is absorbed. Absorption rate (but not extent) may be affected by food.
● Distribution: Cimetidine is distributed to many body tissues. About 15% to 20% of drug is protein-bound. Cimetidine apparently crosses the placenta and is distributed in breast milk.
● Metabolism: Approximately 30% to 40% of dose is metabolized in the liver. Drug has a half-life of 2 hours in patients with normal renal function; half-life increases with decreasing renal function.
● Excretion: Cimetidine is excreted primarily in urine (48% of oral dose, 75% of parenteral dose); 10% of oral dose is excreted in feces. Some drug also is excreted in breast milk.

Contraindications and precautions
Cimetidine is contraindicated in patients with cimetidine allergy or cross-sensitivity to other H₂-receptor antagonists.
  Use caution when administering large parenteral doses to patients with asthma because the drug may exacerbate the symptoms of the disease.
  Use caution when administering cimetidine to pa-

tients with cirrhosis, severely impaired hepatic function, and moderately to severely impaired renal function, because drug accumulation may occur.

Interactions

Cimetidine decreases the metabolism of the following drugs, thus increasing potential toxicity and possibly necessitating dosage reduction: beta-adrenergic blockers (such as propranolol), phenytoin, lidocaine, procainamide, quinidine, benzodiazepines, disulfiram, metronidazole, xanthines, tricyclic antidepressants, oral contraceptives, isoniazid, warfarin, and carmustine.

Effects on diagnostic tests

Cimetidine may antagonize pentagastrin's effect during gastric acid secretion tests; it may cause false-negative results in skin tests using allergen extracts.

Cimetidine therapy increases prolactin levels, serum alkaline phosphatase levels, and serum creatinine levels.

FD and C blue dye #2 used in Tagamet tablets may impair interpretation of Hemoccult and Gastroccult tests on gastric content aspirate. Be sure to wait at least 15 minutes after tablet administration before drawing the sample, and follow test manufacturer's instructions closely.

Adverse reactions

● CNS: dizziness, confusion (particularly in elderly or critically ill patients), headache, depression.
● CV: bradycardia.
● GI: jaundice, diarrhea.
● GU: interstitial nephritis, reversible impotence, urinary retention, mild gynecomastia with prolonged use.
● HEMA: *agranulocytosis (rare)*, neutropenia (rare), *thrombocytopenia, aplastic anemia.*
● Other: rash, allergic reaction, pain at I.M. injection site, fever (rare), urticaria.

Overdose and treatment

Clinical effects of overdose include respiratory failure and tachycardia. Overdose is rare; intake of up to 10 g has caused no untoward effects.

Support respiration and maintain a patent airway. Induce emesis or use gastric lavage; follow with activated charcoal to prevent further absorption. Treat tachycardia with propranolol if necessary.

▶ Special considerations

Besides those relevant to all H_2-receptor antagonists, consider the following recommendations.
● For I.V. use, cimetidine must be diluted prior to administration. Do not dilute drug with sterile water for injection; use normal saline solution, dextrose 5% or 10% injection, lactated Ringer's solution, or 5% sodium bicarbonate injection to a total volume of 20 ml. I.M. administration may be painful.
● After administration of the liquid via nasogastric tube, tube should be flushed to clear it and ensure drug's passage to stomach.
● Hemodialysis removes cimetidine; schedule dose after dialysis session.
● Dosage adjustments may be necessary in patients with renal impairment.
● Other unlabeled uses include pancreatic insufficiency, hives, and hirsutism.

Information for the patient

Warn patient to take drug as directed and to continue taking it even after pain subsides, to allow for adequate healing. Urge patient to avoid smoking, because it may increase gastric acid secretion and worsen disease.

Geriatric use

Use caution when administering cimetidine to elderly patients because of the potential for adverse reactions affecting the CNS.

Breast-feeding

Cimetidine is excreted in breast milk. Breast-feeding women should avoid this drug.

---

cinoxacin
Cinobac

● Pharmacologic classification: quinolone antibiotic
● Therapeutic classification: urinary tract antiseptic
● Pregnancy risk category B

How supplied

Available by prescription only
Capsules: 250 mg, 500 mg

Indications, route, and dosage
Initial and recurrent urinary tract infections caused by susceptible organisms

Adults and children age 12 or older: 1 g daily, in two to four divided doses for 7 to 14 days. Not recommended for children under age 12.

Dosage in renal failure

Patients with renal disease require dosage reduction, as follows: If creatinine clearance is 50 to 80 ml/minute, give 500 mg P.O., followed by 250 mg t.i.d.; if creatinine clearance is 20 to 50 ml/minute, 250 mg b.i.d.; if creatinine clearance is below 20 ml/minute, 250 mg daily.

Pharmacodynamics

Antibacterial action: Cinoxacin inhibits microbial synthesis of deoxyribonucleic acid (DNA). It acts against most strains of *Escherichia coli, Klebsiella, Enterobacter, Proteus mirabilis, P. vulgaris, Morganella morganii, Serratia,* and *Citrobacter* and certain other organisms. It usually is not effective against *Pseudomonas,* enterococci, or staphylococci.

Pharmacokinetics

● *Absorption:* Cinoxacin is well absorbed from the GI tract. Peak plasma concentrations occur 1 to 2 hours after administration. Food decreases peak concentrations but not the total absorption.
● *Distribution:* Cinoxacin concentrates in renal tissue; it is 60% to 80% protein-bound and has only fair prostatic penetration (30% to 60% of plasma levels).
● *Metabolism:* Approximately 30% to 40% of cinoxacin dose is metabolized in the liver to inactive compounds.
● *Excretion:* Inactive metabolites and unchanged drug are excreted in the urine. Peak urine concentrations occur within 2 to 4 hours and usually exceed the minimum inhibitory concentration of susceptible organisms for 12 hours. In patients with normal renal function, plasma half-life is 1 to 1½ hours.

Contraindications and precautions
Cinoxacin is contraindicated in patients with known hypersensitivity to the drug or to nalidixic acid.

Cinoxacin should be administered cautiously to patients with a history of hepatic or renal dysfunction, because drug accumulation may occur.

Interactions
Concomitant use with probenecid reduces renal tubular secretion of cinoxacin, leading to a twofold increase in serum cinoxacin concentrations, prolonged half-life, reduced elimination rate, and approximately a 20% decrease in urine drug concentration. Decreased urine concentration may result in reduced antibacterial effectiveness; increased serum concentration may lead to increased risk of toxicity.

Concomitant use with antacids may result in urine alkalinization and reduction of serum concentration of cinoxacin by up to 50%.

Effects on diagnostic tests
Blood urea nitrogen levels may increase slightly during cinoxacin therapy.

Adverse reactions
● CNS: dizziness, headache, drowsiness, insomnia, convulsions.
● DERM: rash, urticaria, pruritus, photosensitivity.
● EENT: photophobia, tinnitus.
● GI: nausea, vomiting, abdominal pain, diarrhea.
   Note: Drug should be discontinued if patient develops hypersensitivity reaction.

Overdose and treatment
No information available.

▶ Special considerations
● Obtain clean-catch urine specimen for culture and sensitivity testing before starting therapy; repeat as needed.
● Drug should be taken with food.
● Avoid overuse of antacids and sodium bicarbonate during cinoxacin therapy.

Information for the patient
● Advise patient to take drug with meals to help reduce adverse GI effects.
● Warn patient that drug may cause photophobia in bright sunlight.
● Advise patient that drug may cause dizziness. The patient should avoid driving and other activities that require alertness until adverse CNS effects of the drug are known.

Pediatric use
Do not administer drug to prepubertal children because it may prove toxic to cartilage in weight-bearing joints.

Breast-feeding
Data regarding drug excretion in breast milk are not available. However, alternative feeding method is recommended.

---

ciprofloxacin hydrochloride (ophthalmic)
Ciloxan

● Pharmacologic classification: fluoroquinolone
● Therapeutic classification: antibacterial agent
● Pregnancy risk category C

How supplied
Available by prescription only
Ophthalmic solution: 0.3% in 2.5- and 5-ml containers

Indications, route, and dosage
Corneal ulcers caused by Pseudomonas aeruginosa, Staphylococcus aureus, S. epidermidis, Streptococcus pneumoniae, *and possibly* Serratia marcescens *and* Streptococcus viridans
Adults and children over age 12: 2 drops in the affected eye q 15 minutes for the first 6 hours, then 2 drops q 30 minutes for the remainder of the first day. On day 2, administer 2 drops hourly. On days 3 to 14, administer 2 drops q 4 hours.
Bacterial conjunctivitis caused by Staphylococcus aureus *and* S. epidermidis *and possibly* Streptococcus pneumoniae
Adults and children over age 12: 1 or 2 drops into the conjunctival sac of the affected eye q 2 hours while awake, for the first 2 days. Then 1 or 2 drops q 4 hours while awake, for the next 5 days.

Pharmacodynamics
Antibacterial action: Inhibits bacterial DNA gyrase, an enzyme necessary for bacterial replication. Bacteriostatic or bactericidal, depending on concentration.

Pharmacokinetics
● *Absorption:* Systemic absorption is limited. One study in which the drug was administered in each eye every 2 hours while awake for 2 days, followed by every 4 hours while awake for an additional 5 days, showed that the maximum plasma concentration was below 5 ng/ml, and the mean plasma concentration was usually below 2.5 ng/ml.
● *Distribution:* Unknown.
● *Metabolism:* Unknown.
● *Excretion:* Unknown.

Contraindications and precautions
Ophthalmic ciprofloxacin is contraindicated in patients with hypersensitivity to ciprofloxacin or other quinolone antibiotics. Drug should not be injected into the eye.

Serious hypersensitivity reactions, including anaphylaxis, have occurred in patients receiving systemic quinolone therapy. Discontinue drug at the first sign of hypersensitivity, such as skin rash.

Prolonged use may result in overgrowth of nonsusceptible organisms, including fungi. Institute appropriate therapy if superinfection occurs.

Interactions
None reported.

Effects on diagnostic tests
None reported.

Adverse reactions
● EENT: local burning or discomfort, white crystalline precipitate (in the superficial portion of the corneal defect in patients with corneal ulcers), margin crusting, crystals or scales, foreign body sensation, itching, conjunctival hyperemia, bad taste in mouth.

Overdose and treatment
A topical overdose of the drug may be flushed from the eye with warm tap water.

▶ Special considerations
If corneal epithelium is still compromised after 14 days of treatment, continue therapy.

Information for the patient
● Teach patient how to instill drug correctly. Remind him not to touch the tip of the bottle with his hands and to avoid contact of the tip with the eye or surrounding tissue.
● Remind patient not to share washcloths or towels with other family members to avoid spreading infection.
● Advise patient to wash hands before and after instilling solution.

Pediatric use
Safety and efficacy in children under age 12 have not been established.

Breast-feeding
It is unknown if drug is excreted in breast milk after application to the eye; however, systemically administered ciprofloxacin has been detected in human milk. Use caution.

---

ciprofloxacin (systemic)
Cipro

● Pharmacologic classification: quinolone antibiotic
● Therapeutic classification: antibiotic
● Pregnancy risk category C

How supplied
Available by prescription only
Tablets: 250 mg, 500 mg, 750 mg
Injection: 200 mg per 20-ml vial; 400 mg per 40-ml vial; 200 mg in 100 ml 5% dextrose in water; 400 mg in 200 ml 5% dextrose of water

Indications, route, and dosage
Mild to moderate urinary tract infection caused by susceptible bacteria
Adults: 250 mg P.O. or I.V. q 12 hours.
Infectious diarrhea, mild to moderate respiratory tract infections, bone and joint infections, and severe or complicated urinary tract infections
Adults: 500 mg P.O. q 12 hours or 400 mg I.V. q 12 hours.

Severe or complicated infections of the respiratory tract, bones, joints, skin, or skin structures
Adults: 750 mg P.O. q 12 hours.

Dosage adjustments for patients in renal failure

ORAL CIPROFLOXACIN

Creatinine clearance (ml/min)	Dose
>50	No adjustment
30 to 50	250 to 500 mg q 12 hr
5 to 29	250 to 500 mg q 18 hr
Patients on hemodialysis or peritoneal dialysis	250 to 500 mg q 24 hr (after dialysis)

I.V. CIPROFLOXACIN

Creatinine clearance (ml/min)	Dose
>30	No adjustment
5 to 29	200 to 400 mg. I.V. q 18 to 24 hr

Pharmacodynamics
Ciprofloxacin inhibits DNA gyrase, preventing bacterial DNA replication. The following organisms have been reported to be susceptible to ciprofloxacin: *Campylobacter jejuni, Citrobacter diversus, Citrobacter freundii, Enterobacter cloacae, Escherichia coli* (including enterotoxigenic strains), *Haemophilus parainfluenzae, Klebsiella pneumoniae, Morganella morganii, Proteus mirabilis, Proteus vulgaris, Providencia stuartii, Providencia rettgeri, Pseudomonas aeruginosa, Serratia marcescens, Shigella flexneri, Shigella sonnei, Staphylococcus aureus* (penicillinase- and nonpenicillinase-producing strains), *Staphylococcus epidermidis, Streptococcus faecalis,* and *Streptococcus pyogenes.*

Pharmacokinetics
● *Absorption:* About 70% of ciprofloxacin is absorbed after oral administration. Food delays rate of absorption but not extent.
● *Distribution:* Peak serum levels occur within 1 to 2 hours after oral dosing. Ciprofloxacin is 20% to 40% protein-bound. Cerebrospinal fluid levels are only about 10% of plasma levels.
● *Metabolism:* Probably hepatic. Four metabolites have been identified; each has less antimicrobial activity than the parent compound.
● *Excretion:* Primarily renal. Serum half-life is about 4 hours in adults with normal renal function.

Contraindications and precautions
Ciprofloxacin is contraindicated in patients allergic to the drug or to other quinolone antibiotics. This drug should not be used in children because animal studies have shown that it can induce arthropathy in immature animals. Patients should be well hydrated to prevent crystalluria. Avoid urine alkalinization. Because drug may cause CNS stimulation, use with caution in patients with suspected or known CNS disturbances, epi-

---

lepsy, severe cerebral arterosclerosis, or other conditions that may induce seizures.

Interactions
Aluminum- and magnesium-containing antacids may interfere with ciprofloxacin absorption. Separate administration by at least 2 hours. Concomitant use with probenecid interferes with renal tubular secretion and results in higher plasma levels of ciprofloxacin; use with sucralfate reduces absorption of ciprofloxacin by 50%. Ciprofloxacin may attenuate elimination of theophylline, increasing the risk of theophylline toxicity.

Effects on diagnostic tests
None reported.

Adverse reactions
● CNS: headache, restlessness, dizziness, light-headedness, insomnia, nightmares, hallucinations, manic reaction, irritability, tremor, ataxia, seizures, lethargy, drowsiness, weakness, malaise, anorexia, phobia, depersonalization, depression, paresthesia.
● CV: palpitations, atrial flutter, ventricular ectopy, syncope, hypertension, angina pectoris, *myocardial infarction, cardiopulmonary arrest, cerebral thrombosis.*
● DERM: rash, pruritus, urticaria, photosensitivity, flushing, cutaneous candidiasis, hyperpigmentation, erythema nodosum.
● GI: nausea, diarrhea, vomiting, abdominal discomfort, painful oral mucosa, oral candidiasis, dysphagia, *intestinal perforation,* gastrointestinal bleeding
● Musculoskeletal: joint pain or stiffness, back pain.
● Respiratory: epistaxis, pulmonary or laryngeal edema, dyspnea.
● Other: blurred or disturbed vision, diplopia, tinnitus, unpleasant taste.

Overdose and treatment
To treat ciprofloxacin overdose, empty the stomach by induced vomiting or lavage. Provide general supportive measures and maintain hydration. Peritoneal dialysis or hemodialysis may be helpful, particularly if patient's renal function is compromised.

▶ Special considerations
● Duration of therapy depends upon type and severity of infection. Therapy should continue for 2 days after symptoms have abated. Most infections are well controlled in 1 to 2 weeks, but bone or joint infections may require therapy for 4 weeks or longer.
● Closer monitoring of theophylline levels may be necessary because of increased risk of theophylline toxicity in patient receiving ciprofloxacin.

Information for the patient
● Ciprofloxacin may be taken with or without meals. The preferred time is 2 hours after a meal.
● Tell patient to avoid taking with antacids and to drink plenty of fluids during drug therapy.
● Tell patient drug may cause dizziness, light-headedness, or drowsiness. Patient should avoid hazardous activities that require mental alertness until CNS reaction to drug is determined.

Pediatric use
Avoid use in children.

Breast-feeding
Ciprofloxacin may be secreted in milk. Consider discontinuing breast-feeding or drug therapy to avoid serious toxicity in the infant.

---

cisplatin (cis-platinum)
Platinol, Platinol AQ

● Pharmacologic classification: alkylating agent (cell cycle-phase nonspecific)
● Therapeutic classification: antineoplastic
● Pregnancy risk category D

How supplied
Available by prescription only
Injection: 10-mg and 50-mg vials (lyophilized); 50-mg and 100-mg vials (aqueous)

Indications, route, and dosage
Dosage and indications may vary. Check current literature for recommended protocol.
Adjunctive therapy in metastatic testicular cancer
Adults: 20 mg/m² I.V. daily for 5 days. Repeat q 3 weeks for three cycles or more. Usually used in therapeutic regimen with bleomycin and vinblastine.
Adjunctive therapy in metastatic ovarian cancer, head and neck cancers, lung cancer, and esophageal cancer
Adults: 100 mg/m² I.V. Repeat q 4 weeks or 50 mg/m² I.V. q 3 weeks with concurrent doxorubicin hydrochloride therapy (ovarian cancer only). Give as I.V. infusion in 1 liter of solution with 37.5 g mannitol over 6 to 8 hours.
Treatment of advanced bladder cancer
Adults: 50 to 70 mg/m² I.V. once q 3 to 4 weeks. Patients who have received other antineoplastics or radiation therapy should receive 50 mg/m² q 4 weeks.
Note: Prehydration and mannitol diuresis may significantly reduce renal toxicity and ototoxicity.

Pharmacodynamics
Antineoplastic action: Cisplatin exerts its cytotoxic effects by binding with DNA and inhibiting DNA synthesis and, to a lesser extent, by inhibition of protein and RNA synthesis. Cisplatin also acts as a bifunctional alkylating agent, causing intrastrand and interstrand cross-links of DNA. Interstrand cross-linking appears to correlate well with the cytotoxicity of the drug.

Pharmacokinetics
● *Absorption:* Cisplatin is not administered orally or intramuscularly.
● *Distribution:* Cisplatin distributes widely into tissues, with the highest concentrations found in the kidneys, liver, and prostate. Cisplatin can accumulate in body tissues, with drug being detected up to 6 months after the last dose. Cisplatin does not readily cross the blood-brain barrier. The drug is extensively and irreversibly bound to plasma proteins and tissue proteins.
● *Metabolism:* The metabolic fate of cisplatin is unclear.
● *Excretion:* Cisplatin is excreted primarily unchanged in urine. In patients with normal renal function, the half-life of the initial elimination phase is 25 to 79 minutes and the terminal phase 58 to 78 hours. The terminal half-life of total cisplatin is up to 10 days.

Contraindications and precautions

Cisplatin is contraindicated in patients with a history of hypersensitivity to cisplatin or other platinum-containing compounds. Patients who have been previously exposed to these agents should undergo skin testing before cisplatin therapy because of potential for allergic reaction. The drug is also contraindicated in patients with myelosuppression or hearing impairment because drug may worsen these conditions.

Cisplatin should be used with caution or dosage adjusted in patients with impaired renal function because of the drug's nephrotoxic effects. It is usually not used in patients with a creatinine clearance below 50 ml/minute. Perform baseline audiometry before therapy begins. Cisplatin can impair fertility. Aspermia has been reported after cisplatin therapy.

Interactions

Concomitant use with aminoglycosides potentiates the cumulative nephrotoxicity caused by cisplatin; additive toxicity is the mechanism for this interaction. Therefore, aminoglycosides should not be used within 2 weeks of cisplatin therapy. Concomitant use with loop diuretics increases the risk of ototoxicity; closely monitor the patient's audiologic status. Concomitant use with phenytoin may decrease serum concentration of phenytoin.

Effects on diagnostic tests

Cisplatin therapy may increase BUN, serum creatinine, and serum uric acid levels. It may decrease creatinine clearance, serum calcium, magnesium, phosphate, and potassium levels, indicating nephrotoxicity.

Adverse reactions

- CNS: peripheral neuritis, loss of taste, *seizures*, headache.
- EENT: tinnitus, high-frequency hearing loss may occur in both ears.
- GI: nausea and vomiting, beginning 1 to 4 hours after dose and lasting 24 hours; diarrhea; metallic taste; stomatitis.
- GU: more prolonged and severe renal toxicity with repeated courses of therapy (dose-limiting).
- HEMA: mild myelosuppression in 25% to 30% of patients; *leukopenia; thrombocytopenia;* anemia; nadirs in circulating platelets and leukocytes on days 18 to 23, with recovery by day 39.
- Other: anaphylactoid reaction, hyperuricemia, hypomagnesemia.

Note: Drug should be discontinued if signs of neurotoxicity appear.

Overdose and treatment

Clinical manifestations of overdose include leukopenia, thrombocytopenia, nausea, and vomiting.

Treatment is generally supportive and includes transfusion of blood components, antibiotics for possible infections, and antiemetics. Cisplatin can be removed by dialysis, but only within 3 hours after administration.

▶ **Special considerations**

Besides those relevant to all *alkylating agents*, consider the following recommendations.

- Review hematologic status and creatinine clearance before therapy.
- Reconstitute 10-mg vial with 10 ml and 50-mg vial with 50 ml of sterile water for injection to yield a concentration of 1 mg/ml. The drug may be diluted further in a saline-containing solution for I.V. infusion.

- Do not use aluminum needles for reconstitution or administration of cisplatin; a black precipitate may form. Use stainless steel needles.
- Drug is stable for 24 hours in normal saline solutions at room temperature. Do not refrigerate because precipitation may occur. Discard any solution containing precipitate.
- Infusions are most stable in chloride-containing solutions, such as normal saline, 0.5 normal saline, or 0.25 normal saline.
- Mannitol may be given as a 12.5-g I.V. bolus before starting cisplatin infusion. Follow by infusion of mannitol at rate up to 10 g/hour, as necessary, to maintain urine output during cisplatin infusion and for 6 to 24 hours after infusion.
- I.V. sodium thiosulfate may be administered with cisplatin infusion to decrease risk of nephrotoxicity.
- Hydrate patient with normal saline solution before giving drug. Maintain urine output of 100 ml/hour for 4 consecutive hours before and for 24 hours after infusion.
- Hydrate patient by encouraging oral fluid intake when possible.
- Avoid all I.M. injections when platelets are low.
- Nausea and vomiting may be severe and protracted (up to 24 hours). Antiemetics can be started 24 hours before therapy. Monitor fluid intake and output. Continue I.V. hydration until patient can tolerate adequate oral intake.
- High-dose metoclopramide (2 mg/kg I.V.) has been used to prevent and treat nausea and vomiting. Dexamethasone 10 to 20 mg has been given intravenously with metoclopramide to help alleviate nausea and vomiting. Many patients respond favorably to treatment with ondansetron (Zofran). Pretreatment with this 5-HT$_3$ antagonist should begin 30 minutes before cisplatin therapy.
- Treat extravasation with local injections of a ⅙ M sodium thiosulfate solution (prepared by mixing 4 ml of sodium thiosulfate 10% and 6 ml of sterile water for injection).
- Monitor CBC, platelet count, and renal function studies before initial and subsequent doses. Do not repeat dose unless platelet count is over 100,000/mm^3, WBC count is over 4,000/mm^3, serum creatinine level is under 1.5 mg/dl, or BUN level is under 25 mg/dl.
- Renal toxicity becomes more severe with repeated doses. Renal function must return to normal before next dose can be given.
- Monitor electrolytes extensively; aggressive supplementation is often required after a course of therapy.
- Anaphylactoid reaction usually responds to immediate treatment with epinephrine, corticosteroids, or antihistamines.
- Drug is given with bleomycin and vinblastine for testicular cancer and with doxorubicin for ovarian cancer.
- Avoid contact with skin. If contact occurs, wash drug off immediately with soap and water.

Information for the patient

- Stress importance of adequate fluid intake and increase in urine output, to facilitate uric acid excretion.
- Tell patient to report tinnitus immediately, to prevent permanent hearing loss. Patient should have audiometric tests before initial and subsequent courses.
- Advise patient to avoid exposure to people with infections.
- Tell patient to promptly report any unusual bleeding or bruising.

Pediatric use
● Pediatric dosage of cisplatin has not been fully established. Unlabeled uses of cisplatin include osteogenic sarcoma and neuroblastoma.
● Ototoxicity appears to be more severe in children.

Breast-feeding
It is unknown if cisplatin distributes into breast milk. However, because of the risk to the infant of serious adverse reactions, mutagenicity, and carcinogenicity, breast-feeding is not recommended.

clarithromycin
Biaxin Filmtabs

● Pharmacologic classification: macrolide
● Therapeutic classification: antibiotic
● Pregnancy risk category C

How supplied
Available by prescription only
Tablets: 250 mg, 500 mg

Indications, route, and dosage
Pharyngitis or tonsillitis caused by Streptococcus pyogenes
Adults: 250 mg P.O. q 12 hours for 10 days.
Acute maxillary sinusitis caused by S. pneumoniae
Adults: 500 mg P.O. q 12 hours for 14 days.
Acute exacerbations of chronic bronchitis caused by Moraxella (Branhamella) catarrhalis *or* S. pneumoniae; *pneumonia caused by* S. pneumoniae *or* Mycoplasma pneumoniae
Adults: 250 mg P.O. q 12 hours for 7 to 14 days.
Acute exacerbations of chronic bronchitis caused by Haemophilus influenzae
Adults: 500 mg P.O. q 12 hours for 7 to 14 days.
Uncomplicated skin and skin structure infections caused by Staphylococcus aureus *or* Streptococcus pyogenes
Adults: 250 mg P.O. q 12 hours for 7 to 14 days.

Pharmacodynamics
Antibiotic action: Clarithromycin, a macrolide antibiotic that is a derivative of erythromycin, binds to the 50S subunit of bacterial ribosomes, blocking protein synthesis. It is bacteriostatic or bactericidal, depending on the concentration.

Pharmacokinetics
● *Absorption:* Clarithromycin is rapidly absorbed from the GI tract; absolute bioavailability is about 50%. Peak serum levels are acheived within 2 hours of dosing. Although food slightly delays onset of absorption and formation of the active metabolite, clarithromycin may be taken without regard to meals because food doesn't alter the total amount of drug absorbed.
● *Distribution:* Drug is widely distributed; because it readily penetrates cells, tissue concentrations are higher than plasma levels. Plasma half-life is dose-dependent; half-life is 3 to 4 hours at doses of 250 mg q 12 hours and increases to 5 to 7 hours at doses of 500 mg q 12 hours.
● *Metabolism:* Clarithromycin's major metabolite, 14-hydroxy clarithromycin, has significant antimicrobial activity. It is about twice as active against *H. influenzae* as the parent drug.
● *Excretion:* In patients taking 250 mg of the drug q 12 hours, about 20% is eliminated in the urine unchanged; this increases to 30% in patients taking 500 mg q 12 hours. The major metabolite accounts for about 15% of drug in the urine. Elimination half-life of the active metabolite is dose-dependent: 5 to 6 hours with 250 mg q 12 hours; 7 hours with 500 mg q 12 hours.

Contraindications and precautions
Clarithromycin is contraindicated in patients with hypersensitivity to the drug, erythromycin, or other macrolides. Do not use during pregnancy unless no alternative therapy is available. Drug has exhibited adverse effects on fetal development and pregnancy outcome in animal studies at 2 to 17 times the serum levels achieved in humans who were treated at the maximum recommended dosage.

Because drug is excreted by the liver and kidney, use cautiously in patients with hepatic or renal impairment. Dosage adjustments are not necessary in patients with liver dysfunction but are recommended in patients with severe renal impairment.

Pseudomembranous colitis has been reported with nearly all antibacterial agents. Consider this diagnosis in patients who develop diarrhea secondary to antibiotic therapy. Although most patients respond to withdrawal of drug therapy alone, it may be necessary to institute treatment with an antibacterial agent effective against *Clostridium difficile*, an organism linked to this disorder.

Interactions
Preliminary studies indicate that clarithromycin may increase serum levels of theophylline and carbamazepine. Monitor plasma levels of these agents carefully. Other macrolides have been associated with various drug interactions, including increased prothrombin time in patients taking warfarin; increased digoxin levels in patients receiving digoxin; acute ergot toxicity in patients recieving ergotamine or dihydroergotamine; and decreased metabolism of cyclosporine, hexobarbital, triazolam, or phenytoin. The effect of clarithromycin is unknown.

Effects on diagnostic tests
None reported.

Adverse reactions
● CNS: headache.
● GI: diarrhea, nausea, abnormal taste, dyspepsia, abdominal pain or discomfort.
● Other: overgrowth of nonsusceptible organisms, pseudomembranous colitis.

Overdose and treatment
No information available.

▶ Special considerations
● Obtain specimen for culture and sensitivity tests before first dose. Therapy may begin pending test results.
● Clarithromycin may be taken without regard to meals.
● Drug may cause overgrowth of nonsusceptible bacteria or fungi. Monitor for signs and symptoms of superinfection.

Information for the patient
● Tell patient to take all of the medication prescribed, even if he feels better.
● Tell patient that he may take drug without regard to meals.

Pediatric use
Safety and efficacy in children under age 12 have not been established.

Breast-feeding
It is unknown if the drug is excreted in breast milk; however, other macrolides have been found in breast milk. Use with caution.

clemastine fumarate
Tavist, Tavist-1

● Pharmacologic classification: ethanol-amine-derivative antihistamine
● Therapeutic classification: antihistamine (H$_1$-receptor antagonist)
● Pregnancy risk category C

How supplied
Available without prescription
Tablets: 1.34 mg (Tavist-1), 2.68 mg (Tavist)
Syrup: 0.67 mg/5 ml (equivalent to 0.5 mg base/5 ml)

Indications, route, and dosage
Rhinitis, allergy symptoms
Adults and children age 12 or older: 1.34 to 2.68 mg P.O. b.i.d. or t.i.d. Maximum recommended daily dosage is 8.04 mg.
Children age 6 to 11: 0.67 mg b.i.d.; not to exceed 4.02 mg/day.
Allergic skin manifestation of urticaria and angioedema
Adults and children age 12 or older: 2.68 mg up to t.i.d. maximum.
Children age 6 to 11: 1.34 mg b.i.d.; not to exceed 4.02 mg/day.

Pharmacodynamics
Antihistamine action: Antihistamines compete with histamine for histamine H$_1$-receptor sites on the smooth muscle of the bronchi, GI tract, uterus, and large blood vessels; by binding to cellular receptors, they prevent access of histamine and suppress histamine-induced allergic symptoms, even though they do not prevent its release.

Pharmacokinetics
● *Absorption:* Clemastine is absorbed readily from the GI tract; action begins in 15 to 30 minutes and peaks in 2 to 7 hours.
● *Distribution:* Unknown.
● *Metabolism:* Unknown.
● *Excretion:* Clemastine is excreted in urine.

Contraindications and precautions
Clemastine is contraindicated in patients with known hypersensitivity to this drug or other antihistamines with similar chemical structures (carbinoxamine and diphenhydramine); during an acute asthmatic attack, because it thickens bronchial secretions; and in patients

who have taken monoamine oxidase (MAO) inhibitors within the preceding 2 weeks.
Clemastine should be used with caution in patients with narrow-angle glaucoma; in those with pyloroduodenal obstruction or urinary bladder obstruction from prostatic hypertrophy or narrowing of the bladder neck, because of their marked anticholinergic effects; in patients with cardiovascular disease, hypertension, or hyperthyroidism, because of the risk of palpitations and tachycardia; and in patients with renal disease, diabetes, bronchial asthma, urinary retention, or stenosing peptic ulcers.
Clemastine should not be used during pregnancy (especially in the third trimester) or during breast-feeding. Antihistamines have caused convulsions and other severe reactions, especially in premature infants.

Interactions
MAO inhibitors interfere with the detoxification of clemastine and thus prolong and intensify their central depressant and anticholinergic effects. Additive CNS depression may occur when clemastine is given concomitantly with other CNS depressants, such as alcohol, barbiturates, tranquilizers, sleeping aids, or antianxiety agents.
Clemastine may diminish the effects of sulfonylureas and may partially counteract the anticoagulant effects of heparin.

Effects on diagnostic tests
Discontinue clemastine 4 days before diagnostic skin tests; antihistamines can prevent, reduce, or mask positive skin test response.

Adverse reactions
● CNS: sedation, drowsiness.
● CV: hypotension, palpitations, tachycardia.
● DERM: rash, urticaria.
● GI: epigastric distress, anorexia, nausea, vomiting, constipation, dry mouth.
● GU: urinary retention.
● HEMA: hemolytic anemia, thrombocytopenia, agranulocytosis.
● Respiratory: thick bronchial secretions.

Overdose and treatment
Clinical manifestations of overdose may include either CNS depression, sedation, reduced mental alertness, apnea, and cardiovascular collapse) or CNS stimulation (insomnia, hallucinations, tremors, or convulsions). Anticholinergic symptoms, such as dry mouth, flushed skin, fixed and dilated pupils, and GI symptoms, are common, especially in children.
Treat overdose by inducing emesis with ipecac syrup (in conscious patient), followed by activated charcoal to reduce further drug absorption. Use gastric lavage if patient is unconscious or ipecac fails. Treat hypotension with vasopressors, and control seizures with diazepam or phenytoin. *Do not give stimulants.*

▶ Special considerations
Besides those relevant to all *antihistamines,* consider the following recommendation.
● Clemastine is indicated for treatment of urticaria only at dosages of 2.68 mg up to t.i.d.

Geriatric use
Elderly patients are more susceptible to the sedative effect of drug. Instruct the geriatric patient to change

---

positions slowly and gradually. Elderly people may experience dizziness or hypotension more readily than younger people.

Pediatric use
Clemastine is not indicated for use in premature infants or neonates. Children, especially those under age 6, may experience paradoxical hyperexcitability.

Breast-feeding
Antihistamines such as clemastine should not be used during breast-feeding. Many of these drugs are secreted in breast milk, exposing the infant to risks of unusual excitability; premature infants are at particular risk for seizures.

clidinium bromide
Quarzan

- Pharmacologic classification: anticholinergic
- Therapeutic classification: antimuscarinic, gastrointestinal antispasmodic
- Pregnancy risk category C

How supplied
Available by prescription only
Capsules: 2.5 mg, 5 mg

Indications, route, and dosage
Adjunctive therapy for peptic ulcers
Dosage should be individualized according to severity of symptoms and occurrence of adverse effects.
Adults: 2.5 to 5 mg P.O. t.i.d. or q.i.d. before meals and h.s.
Elderly or debilitated patients: 2.5 mg P.O. t.i.d. before meals.

Pharmacodynamics
Anticholinergic action: Clidinium competitively blocks acetylcholine at cholinergic neuroeffector sites, decreasing gastric motility and inhibiting gastric acid secretion.

Pharmacokinetics
- *Absorption:* Clidinium is poorly absorbed from the GI tract. Effects usually appear about 1 hour after the dose is administered.
- *Distribution:* Clidinium does not cross the blood-brain barrier; little else is known about its distribution.
- *Metabolism:* Clidinium is metabolized mainly in the liver. Its duration of effect is about 3 hours.
- *Excretion:* Approximately 36% of a dose is excreted in urine over a 7-day period.

Contraindications and precautions
Clidinium is contraindicated in patients with narrow-angle glaucoma, because drug-induced cycloplegia and mydriasis may increase intraocular pressure; in patients with obstructive uropathy, obstructive GI tract disease, severe ulcerative colitis, myasthenia gravis, paralytic ileus, intestinal atony, or toxic megacolon, because the drug may exacerbate these conditions; and in patients with known hypersensitivity to anticholinergics.
Administer clidinium cautiously to patients with au-

tonomic neuropathy, hyperthyroidism, coronary artery disease, cardiac arrhythmias, congestive heart failure, or ulcerative colitis, because the drug may exacerbate symptoms of these disorders; to patients with hepatic or renal disease, because toxic accumulation can occur; to patients over age 40, because the drug increases the glaucoma risk; to patients with hiatal hernia associated with reflux esophagitis, because the drug may decrease lower esophageal sphincter tone; and in hot or humid environments, because the drug may predispose the patient to heatstroke.

Interactions
Concurrent administration of antacids decreases oral absorption of anticholinergics. Administer clidinium at least 1 hour before antacids.
Concomitant administration of drugs with anticholinergic effects may cause additive toxicity.
Decreased GI absorption of many drugs has been reported after the use of anticholinergics (for example, levodopa and ketoconazole). Conversely, slowly dissolving digoxin tablets may yield higher serum digoxin levels when administered with anticholinergics.
Use cautiously with oral potassium supplements (especially wax-matrix formulations) because the incidence of potassium-induced GI ulcerations may be increased.

Effects on diagnostic tests
None reported.

Adverse reactions
- CNS: headache, insomnia, drowsiness, dizziness, confusion or excitement (in elderly patients), nervousness, weakness.
- CV: palpitations, tachycardia, orthostatic hypotension.
- DERM: urticaria, decreased sweating or anhidrosis, other dermal manifestations.
- EENT: blurred vision, mydriasis, increased intraocular pressure, cycloplegia, photophobia.
- GI: dry mouth, dysphagia, heartburn, taste loss, nausea, vomiting, paralytic ileus, abdominal distention, constipation.
- GU: urinary hesitancy and retention, impotence.
- Other: fever, allergic reaction.
  Note: Drug should be discontinued if hypersensitivity, urinary retention, confusion or excitement, skin rash, or curare-like symptoms develop.

Overdose and treatment
Clinical signs of overdose include curare-like symptoms and peripheral effects such as dilated, nonreactive pupils; blurred vision; hot, flushed, dry skin; dryness of mucous membranes; dysphagia; decreased or absent bowel sounds; urinary retention; hyperthermia; tachycardia; hypertension; and increased respiration.
Treatment is primarily symptomatic. Monitor vital signs closely. If patient is alert, induce emesis (or use gastric lavage) and follow with a saline cathartic and activated charcoal to prevent further absorption of orally administered drug. In severe cases, physostigmine may be administered to block clidinium's antimuscarinic effects. Give fluids, as needed, to treat shock. If urinary retention occurs, catheterization may be necessary.

▶ Special considerations
Recommendations for use of clidinium, for care and teaching of the patient during therapy, and for use in

children and during breast-feeding are the same as those for all *anticholinergics.*

Geriatric use
Clidinium should be administered cautiously to elderly patients. Lower doses are indicated.

Breast-feeding
Clidinium may be excreted in breast milk, possibly resulting in infant toxicity. Clidinium may decrease milk production; advise patient to avoid breast-feeding while taking this drug.

---

clindamycin hydrochloride
Cleocin HCl

clindamycin palmitate hydrochloride
Cleocin Pediatric

clindamycin phosphate
Cleocin Phosphate, Cleocin T

- Pharmacologic classification: lincomycin derivative
- Therapeutic classification: antibiotic
- Pregnancy risk category C

How supplied
Available by prescription only
Capsules: 75 mg, 150 mg, 300 mg
Solution: 75 mg/5 ml
Injection: 150 mg, 300 mg, 600 mg
Topical solution: 10 mg/ml

Indications, route, and dosage
Infections caused by sensitive organisms
Adults: 150 to 450 mg P.O. q 6 hours; or 300 mg I.M. or I.V. q 6, 8, or 12 hours. Up to 2,700 mg I.M. or I.V. daily, divided q 6, 8, or 12 hours. May be used for severe infections.
Children over age 1 month: 20 to 30 mg/kg/day P.O. in divided doses q 6 hours; or 25 to 40 mg/kg/day I.M. or I.V. in divided doses q 6 or 8 hours.
Acne vulgaris
Adults: Apply thin film of topical solution to affected areas b.i.d.

Pharmacodynamics
Antibacterial action: Clindamycin inhibits bacterial protein synthesis by binding to ribosome's 50S subunit. Clindamycin may produce bacteriostatic or bactericidal effects on susceptible bacteria, including most aerobic gram-positive cocci and several anaerobic gram-negative and gram-positive organisms. It is considered a first-line drug in the treatment of *Bacteroides fragilis* and most other gram-positive and gram-negative anerobes. It is also effective against *Mycloplasma pneumoniae, Leptotrichia buccalis,* and some gram-positive cocci and bacilli.

Pharmacokinetics
- *Absorption:* When administered orally, clindamycin is absorbed rapidly and almost completely from the GI tract, regardless of formulation. Peak concentrations of 1.9 to 3.9 mcg/ml occur in 45 to 60 minutes. Drug may

also be given I.M. with good absorption. Peak concentrations occur in about 3 hours. With 300-mg dose, peak concentrations are about 6 mcg/ml; with 600-mg dose, about 10 mcg/ml.
- *Distribution:* Clindamycin is distributed widely to most body tissues and fluids (except CSF) and crosses the placenta. Approximately 93% of drug is bound to plasma proteins.
- *Metabolism:* Clindamycin is metabolized partially to inactive metabolites.
- *Excretion:* About 10% of clindamycin dose is excreted unchanged in urine; the remainder is excreted as inactive metabolites (with some drug excreted in breast milk). Plasma half-life is 2½ to 3 hours in patients with normal renal function; 3½ to 5 hours in anephric patients; and 7 to 14 hours in patients with hepatic disease. Peritoneal dialysis and hemodialysis do not remove drug.

Contraindications and precautions
Clindamycin is contraindicated in patients hypersensitive to the drug or to lincomycin, and those with a history of inflammatory bowel disease or antibiotic-induced colitis.

Clindamycin should be administered cautiously to patients with renal or hepatic dysfunction because it may exacerbate these conditions; to patients with asthma or significant allergies; to newborns; and to patients with tartrazine sensitivity. Topical solution should be administered cautiously to atopic patients because of potential for contact dermatitis.

Interactions
When used concomitantly, clindamycin may potentiate the action of neuromuscular blocking agents (such as tubocurarine and pancuronium). Concomitant use with kaolin products may reduce GI absorption of clindamycin. Concomitant use with such antidiarrheals as diphenoxylate and opiates may prolong or worsen clindamycin-induced diarrhea by reducing excretion of bacterial toxins. When used concomitantly, erythromycin may act as an antagonist, blocking clindamycin from reaching its site of action. When used concurrently with other acne preparations (such as benzoyl peroxide or tretinoin), topical clindamycin may cause a cumulative irritant or drying effect. Reportedly, clindamycin inactivates aminoglycosides in vitro.

Effects on diagnostic tests
Liver function test results may become abnormal in some patients during clindamycin therapy.

Adverse reactions
- DERM: maculopapular rash, urticaria, *erythema multiforme,* contact dermatitis and dryness (with topical solution).
- EENT: stinging in eyes (with topical solution).
- GI: nausea; vomiting; abdominal pain; diarrhea; *pseudomembranous enterocolitis* (usually from *Clostridium difficile*); esophagitis; flatulence; anorexia; bloody or tarry stools; dysphagia; elevated serum glutamic-oxaloacetic transaminase (SGOT), alkaline phosphatase, and bilirubin levels.
- HEMA: transient leukopenia, eosinophilia, thrombocytopenia.
- Local: pain, induration, sterile abscess (with I.M. injection); thrombophlebitis, pain (with I.V. administration).
- Other: unpleasant or bitter taste, *anaphylaxis,* sen-

---

sitization and systemic adverse effects (with topical solution).

Note: Drug should be discontinued if patient develops persistent diarrhea or hypersensitivity reaction.

Overdose and treatment
No information available.

▶ **Special considerations**
● Culture and sensitivity tests should be done before treatment starts and should be repeated as needed.
● Do not refrigerate reconstituted oral solution, because it will thicken. Drug remains stable for 2 weeks at room temperature.
● I.M. preparation should be given deep I.M. Rotate sites. Doses exceeding 600 mg are not recommended.
● I.M. injection may increase creatinine phosphokinase levels because of muscle irritation.
● For I.V. infusion, dilute each 300 mg in 50 ml of dextrose 5%, normal saline, or lactated Ringer's solution and give no faster than 30 mg/minute. Do not administer more than 1.2 g/hour.
● Topical form may produce adverse systemic effects.
● Monitor renal, hepatic, and hematopoietic functions during prolonged therapy.
● Do not administer diphenoxylate compound (Lomotil) to treat drug-induced diarrhea because this may worsen and prolong diarrhea.

Information for the patient
● Warn patient that I.M. injection may be painful.
● Instruct patient to report adverse effects – especially diarrhea. Warn patient not to treat diarrhea himself.
● Advise patient to take capsules with full glass of water to prevent dysphagia.
● Instruct patient using topical solution to wash, rinse, and dry affected areas before application. Warn him not to use topical solution near eyes, nose, mouth, or other mucous membranes, and caution him to avoid sharing washcloths and towels with family members.

Geriatric use
Elderly patients may tolerate drug-induced diarrhea poorly. Monitor closely for change in bowel frequency.

Pediatric use
Administer drug cautiously, if at all, to neonates and infants. Monitor closely, especially for diarrhea.

Breast-feeding
Clindamycin is excreted in breast milk. Alternative feeding method is recommended during clindamycin therapy.

clobetasol propionate
Dermovate*, Temovate

● Pharmacologic classification: topical adrenocorticoid
● Therapeutic classification: anti-inflammatory
● Pregnancy risk category C

How supplied
Available by prescription only
Cream: 0.05%

Lotion: 0.05%
Ointment: 0.05%

Indications, route, and dosage
Inflammation of corticosteroid-responsive dermatoses
Adults: Apply a thin layer to affected skin areas b.i.d., once in the morning and once at night. Limit treatment to 14 days, with no more than 50 g of the cream or ointment per week.

Pharmacodynamics
Anti-inflammatory action: Clobetasol stimulates the synthesis of enzymes needed to decrease the inflammatory response. Clobetasol is a high-potency group I fluorinated corticosteroid that is usually reserved for the management of severe dermatoses that have not responded satisfactorily to a less potent formulation.

Pharmacokinetics
● *Absorption:* The amount of clobetasol absorbed depends on the potency of the preparation, the amount applied, and the nature of the skin at the application site. It ranges from about 1% in areas with a thick stratum corneum (such as the palms, soles, elbows, and knees) to as high as 36% in areas with a thin stratum corneum (face, eyelids, and genitals). Absorption increases in areas of skin damage, inflammation, or occlusion. Some systemic absorption of topical steroids occurs, especially through the oral mucosa.
● *Distribution:* After topical application, clobetasol is distributed throughout the local skin. Any drug absorbed into the circulation is rapidly removed from the blood and distributed into muscle, liver, skin, intestines, and kidneys.
● *Metabolism:* After topical administration, clobetasol is metabolized primarily in the skin. The small amount absorbed into systemic circulation is metabolized primarily in the liver to inactive compounds.
● *Excretion:* Inactive metabolites are excreted by the kidneys, primarily as glucuronides and sulfates, but also as unconjugated products. Small amounts of the metabolites are also excreted in feces.

Contraindications and precautions
Clobetasol is contraindicated in patients who are hypersensitive to any component of the preparation and in patients with viral, fungal, or tubercular skin lesions.
Clobetasol should be used with extreme caution in patients with impaired circulation, because the drug may increase the risk of skin ulceration.

Interactions
None reported.

Effects on diagnostic tests
None significant.

Adverse reactions
● Local: burning, itching, irritation, dryness, folliculitis, hypertrichosis, acneiform eruptions, hypopigmentation, perioral dermatitis, allergic contact dermatitis, maceration, secondary infection, atrophy, striae, miliaria.
Significant systemic absorption may produce the following effects.
● CNS: euphoria, insomnia, headache, psychotic behavior, pseudotumor cerebri, mental changes, nervousness, restlessness.
● CV: congestive heart failure, hypertension, edema.

- EENT: cataracts, glaucoma, thrush.
- GI: peptic ulcer, irritation, increased appetite.
- Immune: immunosuppression, increased susceptibility to infection.
- Metabolic: hypokalemia, sodium retention, fluid retention, weight gain, hyperglycemia, osteoporosis, growth suppression in children.
- Musculoskeletal: muscle atrophy.
- Other: withdrawal syndrome (nausea, fatigue, anorexia, dyspnea, hypotension, hypoglycemia, myalgia, arthralgia, fever, dizziness, and fainting).

Note: Drug should be discontinued if local irritation, infection, systemic absorption, or hypersensitivity reaction occurs.

Overdose and treatment
No information available.

▶ Special considerations
Besides those relevant to all *topical adrenocorticoids,* consider the following recommendations.
- Clobetasol should not be used with occlusive dressings. Advise patient not to cover affected area or use occlusive dressings.
- "Pulse" therapy is sometimes used with topical steroids of this potency – that is, b.i.d. for 3 days, then none for 3 days. Intermittent use prevents cumulative effects.

Pediatric use
Clobetasol treatment is not recommended in patients under age 12.

clocortolone pivalate
Cloderm

- Pharmacologic classification: topical adrenocorticoid
- Therapeutic classification: anti-inflammatory
- Pregnancy risk category C

How supplied
Available by prescription only
Cream: 0.1%

Indications, route, and dosage
Inflammation of corticosteroid-responsive dermatoses
Adults and children: Apply cream sparingly and gently rub into the affected area daily to q.i.d.

Pharmacodynamics
Anti-inflammatory action: Clocortolone stimulates the synthesis of enzymes needed to decrease the inflammatory response. Clocortolone cream is a group IV fluorinated glucocorticoid with a potency similar to that of betamethasone valerate cream 0.01%, flurandrenolide cream 0.025%, and hydrocortisone valerate cream and ointment 0.2%.

Pharmacokinetics
- *Absorption:* The amount of clocortolone absorbed depends on the amount applied and on the nature of the skin at the application site. It ranges from about 1% in areas with a thick stratum corneum (such as the palms, soles, knees, and elbows) to as much as 36% in areas of the thinnest stratum corneum (face, eyelids, and genitals). Absorption increases in areas of skin damage, inflammation, or occlusion. Some systemic absorption of topical steroids occurs, especially through the oral mucosa.
- *Distribution:* After topical application, clocortolone is distributed throughout the local skin. Any drug that is absorbed into circulation is removed rapidly from the blood and distributed into muscle, liver, skin, intestines, and kidneys.
- *Metabolism:* After topical administration, clocortolone is metabolized primarily in the skin. The small amount that is absorbed into systemic circulation is metabolized primarily in the liver to inactive compounds.
- *Excretion:* Inactive metabolites are excreted by the kidneys, primarily as glucuronides and sulfates, but also as unconjugated products. Small amounts of the metabolites are also excreted in feces.

Contraindications and precautions
Clocortolone is contraindicated in patients who are hypersensitive to any component of the preparation and in patients with viral, fungal, or tubercular skin lesions. It should be used with extreme caution in patients with impaired circulation because the drug may increase the risk of skin ulceration. Avoid using on the face or genital areas because increased absorption may result in striae.

Interactions
None significant.

Effects on diagnostic tests
None reported.

Adverse reactions
- Local: burning, itching, irritation, dryness, folliculitis, hypertrichosis, acneiform eruptions, hypopigmentation, perioral dermatitis, allergic contact dermatitis, maceration, secondary infection, atrophy, striae, miliaria.

Significant systemic absorption may produce the following reactions.
- CNS: euphoria, insomnia, headache, psychotic behavior, pseudotumor cerebri, mental changes, nervousness, restlessness.
- CV: congestive heart failure, hypertension, edema.
- DERM: delayed healing, acne, skin eruptions, striae.
- EENT: cataracts, glaucoma, thrush.
- GI: peptic ulcer, irritation, increased appetite.
- Immune: immunosuppression, increased susceptibility to infection.
- Metabolic: hypokalemia, sodium retention, fluid retention, weight gain, hyperglycemia, osteoporosis, growth suppression in children.
- Musculoskeletal: muscle atrophy.
- Other: withdrawal syndrome (nausea, fatigue, anorexia, dyspnea, hypotension, hypoglycemia, myalgia, arthralgia, fever, dizziness, and fainting).

Note: Drug should be discontinued if local irritation, infection, systemic absorption, or hypersensitivity reaction occurs.

Overdose and treatment
No information available.

▶ **Special considerations**

Recommendations for use of clocortolone, for care and teaching of patients during therapy, and for use in elderly patients, children, and breast-feeding women are the same as those for all *topical adrenocorticoids*.

clofazimine
Lamprene

- Pharmacologic classification: substituted iminophenazine dye
- Therapeutic classification: leprostatic
- Pregnancy risk category C

How supplied
Available by prescription only
Capsules: 50 mg, 100 mg

Indications, route, and dosage
Dapsone-resistant leprosy
Adults: 50 to 100 mg P.O. once daily; usually given with rifampin 600 mg once daily or once monthly for at least 2 years.
Erythema nodosum leprosum
Adults: 100 to 200 mg P.O. daily for up to 3 months. Taper dosage to 100 mg daily as soon as possible. Dosages above 200 mg daily are not recommended.
†*Atypical mycobacterial infections*
Adults: 100 mg P.O. q 8 hours. Usually given with several other antitubercular agents.

Pharmacodynamics
Leprostatic action: Clofazimine is a bright red iminophenazine dye, a relative of aniline dyes. It exerts a slow bactericidal effect on *Mycobacterium leprae* (Hansen's bacillus). Clinical benefit is usually noted in 1 to 3 months, with clearing observed by 6 months. Administration with dapsone produces a more rapid effect on leprosy lesions. No cross-resistance with dapsone or rifampin has been reported. Clofazimine inhibits mycobacterial growth and preferentially binds to mycobacterial DNA. Although the precise mechanism is unknown, the drug also exhibits anti-inflammatory properties in controlling erythema nodosum leprosum reactions.

Clofazimine also appears to have an important role in the treatment of atypical mycobacterial infections, such as *M. avium* infections, which have become prominent recently in AIDS patients. Some efficacy has been demonstrated when used in combination with ansamycin, ethionamide, or ethambutol. Further clinical information is required.

Pharmacokinetics
- *Absorption:* Absorption is variable (45% to 62%) after oral administration.
- *Distribution:* Highly lipophilic, the drug is distributed widely into fatty tissues and is taken up by macrophages into the reticuloendothelial system. Little, if any, crosses the blood-brain barrier or enters the CNS.
- *Metabolism:* The drug's metabolism has not been completely defined; however, some evidence exists of enterohepatic cycling. Serum half-lives of up to 70 days have been noted.
- *Excretion:* Most is excreted in feces; some in sputum,

sebum, and sweat; very little in urine. The drug is excreted in breast milk.

Contraindications and precautions
Use cautiously in a patient with abdominal pain or diarrhea; discontinue if patient becomes colicky or if pain and other symptoms worsen.

Interactions
Dapsone may inhibit the anti-inflammatory activity of clofazimine, but this is unconfirmed; continued treatment with both drugs is still advisable.

Effects on diagnostic tests
Clofazimine therapy can elevate blood sugar, albumin, serum bilirubin, and AST (SGOT) and can cause hypokalemia and eosinophilia.

Adverse reactions
- CNS: dizziness, drowsiness, fatigue, headache, giddiness, neuralgia, taste disorder.
- CV: thromboembolism, anemia, vascular pain.
- DERM: pink to brownish black pigmentation, ichthyosis, dryness, rash, pruritus, phototoxicity, erythroderma, acneiform eruptions, monilial cheilosis.
- EENT: conjunctival and corneal pigmentation; dryness, burning, itching, and irritation of eye.
- GI: abdominal pain, epigastric pain, diarrhea, nausea, vomiting, GI intolerance, bowel obstruction, GI bleeding, anorexia, constipation, weight loss, hepatitis, jaundice, eosinophilic enteritis, enlarged liver.
- Other: depression secondary to skin pigmentation.

Overdose and treatment
No information available.

▶ **Special considerations**
- Administer with meals. Use clofazimine in combination with other antileprosy drugs.
- Severe GI symptoms may necessitate withdrawal of drug if dosage reduction does not relieve symptoms.
- Pink to brownish black pigmentation of skin occurs in 75% to 100% of patients.
- Observe patient for signs of depression.

Information for the patient
- Tell patient to take drug with meals to minimize GI problems.
- Advise patient to store drug away from heat and light and out of children's reach.
- Explain that pink to brownish-black pigmentation of skin may occur. Although reversible, it may take several months or years to disappear after drug is stopped. Also explain that discoloration of eyes, urine, feces, sputum, sweat, and tears also may occur.
- Tell patient not to expect benefits for 1 to 3 months; observable benefits may take up to 6 months.
- Suggest using skin oil or cream to help relieve dryness or ichthyosis.

Breast-feeding
Clofazimine is excreted in breast milk; it should not be administered to breast-feeding women unless potential benefit to mother exceeds risk to infant.

---

clofibrate
Atromid-S

- Pharmacologic classification: fibric acid derivative
- Therapeutic classification: antilipemic
- Pregnancy risk category C

How supplied
Available by prescription only
Capsules: 500 mg

Indications, route, and dosage
Hyperlipidemia and xanthoma tuberosum; Type III hyperlipidemia that does not respond adequately to diet
Adults: 2 g P.O. daily in two to four divided doses. Some patients may respond to lower doses as assessed by serum lipid monitoring.
Clofibrate should not be used in children.

Pharmacodynamics
Antilipemic action: Clofibrate may lower serum triglyceride levels by accelerating catabolism of very low-density lipoproteins; drug lowers serum cholesterol levels (to a lesser degree) by inhibiting cholesterol biosynthesis. Both mechanisms are unknown. Drug is closely related to gemfibrozil.

Pharmacokinetics
- *Absorption:* Clofibrate is absorbed slowly but completely from the GI tract. Peak plasma concentration occurs 2 to 6 hours after a single dose. Serum triglyceride levels decrease in 2 to 5 days, with peak clinical effect at 21 days.
- *Distribution:* Clofibrate is distributed into extracellular space as its active form, clofibric acid, which is up to 98% protein-bound. Animal studies suggest that fetal concentration levels may exceed maternal concentration levels.
- *Metabolism:* Clofibrate is hydrolyzed by serum enzymes to clofibric acid, which is metabolized by the liver.
- *Excretion:* 20% of clofibric acid is excreted unchanged in urine; 70% is eliminated in urine as conjugated metabolite. Plasma half-life after a single dose ranges from 6 to 25 hours; in patients with renal impairment and cirrhosis, half-life can be as long as 113 hours.

Contraindications and precautions
Clofibrate is contraindicated in patients with renal or hepatic dysfunction because drug accumulation increases the incidence of adverse reactions; in patients with primary biliary cirrhosis because cholesterol levels may be raised rather than lowered in such patients; and in pregnant or lactating patients because fetal drug concentrations may exceed those in the mother and because it is believed that the fetus' immature liver cannot metabolize clofibrate.
Use cautiously in patients with a history of liver disease or peptic ulcer disease.

Interactions
Clofibrate potentiates the effects of oral anticoagulants, which may cause fatal hemorrhage; if such a combination is necessary, reduce oral anticoagulant dosage by 50%, and evaluate prothrombin time frequently.
Clofibrate may also enhance the effects of sulfonylureas, causing hypoglycemia; a dosage adjustment may be needed.
Concomitant use with furosemide may cause increased diuresis as both drugs compete for albumin binding sites; use cautiously.
Concomitant administration with chlolestyramine decreases absorption rate of clofibrate.

Effects on diagnostic tests
Clofibrate therapy may increase serum levels of creatine phosphokinase, serum transaminase, serum amylase, alanine aminotransferase, and serum aspartate aminotransferase. Drug may decrease plasma beta-lipoprotein and plasma fibrinogen concentrations.

Adverse reactions
- CNS: drowsiness, headache, fatigue, weakness.
- CV: increased risk of angina, cardiac arrhythmias, intermittent claudication, increased incidence of thrombophlebitis and pulmonary emboli.
- DERM: rash, dry skin, dry brittle hair, alopecia, pruritus, urticaria.
- GI: nausea, diarrhea, hepatomegaly, gastritis, two-fold increase in risk of gallstones during long-term therapy, increased risk of liver cancer.
- GU: decreased libido, sexual ability; renal dysfunction (hematuria, proteinuria, dysuria, and anuria).
- HEMA: leukopenia, eosinophilia, anemia.
- Other: flulike syndrome with weakness and muscle aches, weight gain, polyphagia.
Note: Drug should be discontinued if liver function tests show significant abnormalities; if serum amylase level increases; if a paradoxical increase in cholesterol or low-density lipoprotein levels occur; or if no therapeutic response occurs after 3 months of therapy, except in treating xanthoma tuberosum, which may require up to 12 months of treatment.

Overdose and treatment
No information available.

▶ Special considerations
- Warn patient to report flulike symptoms immediately.
- Clofibrate should not be used indiscriminately; it may pose an increased risk of gallstones, heart disease, and cancer.
- Monitor serum cholesterol and triglyceride levels regularly during clofibrate therapy.
- Use cautiously in patients with a history of gallbladder disease.
- Observe patient for serious adverse reactions: thrombophlebitis, pulmonary embolism, angina, and dysrhythmias; monitor renal and hepatic function, blood counts, and serum electrolyte and blood glucose levels.
- Studies suggest clofibrate may increase the risk of death from cancer, postcholecystectomy complications, and pancreatitis.

Information for the patient
- Stress importance of close medical supervision and of reporting any adverse reactions; encourage patient to comply with prescribed regimen and diet.
- Warn patient not to exceed prescribed dose.
- Recommend taking with food to minimize GI discomfort.
- Emphasize that drug therapy will not replace diet,

---

exercise, and weight reduction for the control of hyperlipidemia.

Pediatric use
Safety and efficacy have not been established in children younger than age 14.

Breast-feeding
Available data suggest clofibrate may enter breast milk; alternative feeding method is recommended during therapy.

---

clomiphene citrate
Clomid, Milophene, Serophene

- Pharmacologic classification: chlorotrianisene derivative
- Therapeutic classification: ovulation stimulant
- Pregnancy risk category C

How supplied
Available by prescription only
Tablets: 50 mg

Indications, route, and dosage
To induce ovulation
Adults: 50 mg P.O. daily for 5 days, starting any time; or 50 mg P.O. daily starting on day 5 of menstrual cycle (first day of menstrual flow is day 1). Dose may be increased to 100 mg to 250 mg if ovulation does not occur. Repeat the 5-day course each ovulatory cycle until conception occurs or until 3 courses of therapy are completed.
†Male infertility
Adults: 25 mg P.O. daily for 25 days, then with 5 days rest; or 100 mg P.O. every Monday, Wednesday, and Friday.

Pharmacodynamics
Ovulation stimulant action: The precise mechanism of action for inducing ovulation in anovulatory females has not been determined. The drug appears to stimulate the release of the pituitary gonadotropin, follicle-stimulating hormone (FSH), and luteinizing hormone (LH), which results in development and maturation of the ovarian follicle, ovulation, and subsequent development and function of the corpus luteum.

Pharmacokinetics
- *Absorption:* Clomiphene citrate is absorbed readily from the GI tract.
- *Distribution:* The drug may undergo enterohepatic recirculation or may be stored in body fat.
- *Metabolism:* Clomiphene citrate is metabolized by the liver.
- *Excretion:* The half-life is approximately 5 days. Drug is excreted principally in the feces via biliary elimination.

Contraindications and precautions
Clomiphene citrate is contraindicated in patients with liver disease or a history of liver dysfunction because of potential hepatotoxic effects; in patients with abnormal bleeding of undetermined origin; during pregnancy or suspected pregnancy, because of its fetal effects;

and in patients with fibroids or abnormal uterine bleeding.

Do not use clomiphene in the presence of an ovarian cyst or in patients with polycystic ovary syndrome because drug may enlarge or promote cyst formation. Use cautiously in patients with visual disturbances, mental depression, or thrombophlebitis because drug may exacerbate these disorders.

Interactions
None reported.

Effects on diagnostic tests
Clomiphene therapy may increase levels of serum thyronine, thyroxine-binding globulin, and sex hormone-binding globulin. It may also increase sulfobromophthalein retention and FSH and LH secretion.

Adverse reactions
- CNS: headache, restlessness, insomnia, dizziness, light-headedness, depression, fatigue, tension.
- CV: vasomotor flushes resembling menopausal "hot flashes," hypertension.
- DERM: urticaria, rash or allergic dermatitis.
- EENT: blurred vision, diplopia, light flashes, photophobia (signs of impending visual toxicity).
- GI: nausea, vomiting, bloating, distention, abdominal discomfort or pain, increased appetite, weight gain, yellowing of skin and eyes (indicating hepatotoxicity).
- GU: urinary frequency and polyuria, ovarian enlargement and cyst that regress spontaneously when the drug is stopped, heavier menses, multiple pregnancies.
- Other: reversible alopecia, breast discomfort.
Note: Drug should be discontinued if any adverse visual symptoms occur during treatment. If ovarian enlargement or cyst development occurs, therapy should be interrupted until the ovaries have returned to pretreatment size; thereafter, treatment should be reinstated at decreased dosage for a shorter period.

Overdose and treatment
No information available.

▶ Special considerations
- Human chorionic gonadotropin (5,000 to 10,000 units) may be administered 5 to 7 days after the last dose of drug to stimulate ovulation.
- Instruct patient on all aspects of infertility testing and therapy.

Information for the patient
- Patients with visual disturbances should report these symptoms immediately.
- Advise patient of the possibility of multiple births. The risk increases with higher doses.
- Teach patient to take basal body temperature every morning (starting on day 1 of menstrual period) and chart on a graph to detect ovulation.
- Instruct patient on importance of properly timed coitus.
- Advise patient to discontinue drug immediately if abdominal symptoms, weight gain, edema, or bloating occur, because these may indicate ovarian enlargement or ovarian cysts.
- Since the drug may cause dizziness or visual disturbances, warn patient to avoid hazardous tasks until her response to the drug is known.
- Advise patient to discontinue the drug and call im-

---

mediately if she suspects she is pregnant, because drug may have teratogenic effects.

clomipramine hydrochloride
Anafranil

- Pharmacologic classification: tricyclic antidepressant (TCA)
- Therapeutic classification: antiobsessional agent
- Pregnancy risk category C

How supplied
Available by prescription only
Capsules: 25 mg, 50 mg, 75 mg

Indications, route, and dosage
Treatment of obsessive-compulsive disorder (OCD)
Adults: Initially, 25 mg P.O. daily, gradually increasing to 100 mg P.O. daily (in divided doses, with meals) during the first 2 weeks. Maximum dosage is 250 mg daily. After titration, entire daily dose may be given h.s.
Children and adolescents: Initially, 25 mg P.O. daily, gradually increased to a maximum of 3 mg/kg or 100 mg P.O. daily, whichever is smaller (in divided doses, with meals) over the first 2 weeks. Maximum daily dosage is 3 mg/kg or 200 mg, whichever is smaller. After titration, entire daily dose may be given h.s.

Pharmacodynamics
Antiobsessional action: A selective inhibitor of serotonin (5-HT) reuptake into neurons within the CNS. It may also have some blocking activity at postsynaptic dopamine receptors. The exact mechanism by which clomipramine treats OCD is unknown.

Pharmacokinetics
- *Absorption:* Clomipramine is well absorbed from the GI tract, but extensive first-pass metabolism limits bioavailablity to about 50%.
- *Distribution:* Clomipramine distributes well into lipophilic tissues; the volume of distribution is about 12 liters/kg. It is about 98% bound to plasma proteins.
- *Metabolism:* Primarily hepatic. Several metabolites have been identified; desmethylclomipramine is the primary active metabolite.
- *Excretion:* About 66% is excreted in the urine and the remainder in the feces. Mean elimination half-life of the parent compound is about 36 hours; the elimination half-life of desmethylclomipramine may be from 4.4 to 233 days.

Contraindications and precautions
Clomipramine is contraindicated in patients with a history of hypersensitivity to clomipramine or other TCAs. It is also contraindicated in combination with an MAO inhibitor, in patients who have received an MAO inhibitor within the previous 2 weeks, and during the acute recovery period after a myocardial infarction.

Use with caution in patients with a history of seizure disorders, in patients with brain damage of various etiologies, or in patients receiving other seizure threshold-lowering drugs. Use cautiously in patients who are at 0risk for suicide; in patients who are hyperthyroid or are receiving thyroid medication; in urine retention; in patients with narrow-angle glaucoma or increased intraocular pressure; in patients with cardiovascular disease, impaired hepatic function, or tumors of the adrenal medulla; or in patients who are receiving electroshock therapy or electrocautery.

Interactions
Concomitant administration of MAO inhibitors with TCAs may cause hyperpyretic crisis, seizures, coma, and death.

Concurrent use of barbiturates increases the activity of hepatic microsomal enzymes with repeated doses and may decrease TCA blood levels. Monitor for decreased effectiveness. Barbiturates, alcohol, and other CNS depressants may cause an exaggerated depressant effect when used concomitantly with TCAs.

Methylphenidate may increase TCA blood levels. Epinephrine and norepinephrine may produce an increased hypertensive effect in patients taking TCAs.

Effects on diagnostic tests
None reported.

Adverse reactions
- CNS: somnolence, tremor, dizziness, headache, insomnia, libido change, nervousness, myoclonus, increased appetite, fatigue.
- CV: postural hypotension, palpitations, tachycardia.
- DERM: increased sweating, rash, pruritus.
- EENT: otitis media (children), abnormal vision, pharyngitis, rhinitis.
- GI: dry mouth, constipation, nausea, dyspepsia, diarrhea, anorexia, nausea, abdominal pain.
- GU: micturition disorder, urinary tract infection, dysmenorrhea, impotence, ejaculation failure.
- Other: myalgia.

Overdose and treatment
Signs and symptoms of clomipramine overdose are similar to those of other TCAs and have included sinus tachycardia, intraventricular block, hypotension, irritability, fixed and dilated pupils, drowsiness, delerium, stupor, hyperreflexia, and hyperpyrexia.

Treatment should include gastric lavage with large quantities of fluid. Lavage should be continued for 12 hours because the anticholinergic effects of the drug slow gastric emptying. Hemodialysis, peritoneal dialysis, and forced diuresis are ineffective because of the high degree of plasma protein binding. Support respirations and monitor cardiac function. Treat shock with plasma expanders or corticosteroids; treat seizures with diazepam.

▶ Special considerations
- To minimize the risk of overdose, dispense this drug in small quantities.
- Monitor for urine retention and constipation. Suggest stool softener or high-fiber diet, as needed, and encourage adequate fluid intake.
- Do not withdraw drug abruptly.

Information for the patient
- Warn patient to avoid hazardous activities that require alertness or good psychomotor coordination until adverse CNS effects are known. This is especially important during initial titration period when daytime sedation and dizziness may occur.
- Tell patient to avoid alcohol and other depressants.

- Suggest to patient that dry mouth may be relieved with saliva substitutes or sugarless candy or gum.
- Tell patient adverse GI effects can be minimized by taking the drug with meals during the titration period. Later, the entire daily dose may be taken at bedtime to limit daytime drowsiness.
- Tell patient to avoid using nonprescription medications, particularly antihistamines and decongestants, unless recommended by physician or pharmacist.
- Encourage patient to continue therapy, even if adverse reactions are troublesome.

Breast-feeding
It is not known if the drug is excreted in breast milk. Use with caution in breast-feeding women.

clonazepam
Klonopin, Rivotril

- Pharmacologic classification: benzodiazepine
- Therapeutic classification: anticonvulsant
- Controlled substance schedule IV
- Pregnancy risk category C

How supplied
Available by prescription only
Tablets: 0.5 mg, 1 mg, 2 mg

Indications, route, and dosage
Absence and atypical absence seizures; akinetic and myoclonic seizures
Adults: Initial dosage should not exceed 1.5 mg P.O. daily, divided into three doses. May be increased by 0.5 to 1 mg q 3 days until seizures are controlled. Maximum recommended daily dosage is 20 mg.
Children up to age 10 or weighing 30 kg or less: 0.01 to 0.03 mg/kg P.O. daily (not to exceed 0.05 mg/kg daily), divided q 8 hours. Increase dosage by 0.25 to 0.5 mg q 3rd day to a maximum maintenance dosage of 0.1 to 0.2 mg/kg daily.
Nocturnal myoclonus; †bipolar disorder
Adults: 0.5 mg t.i.d. or 1.5 mg at bedtime.

Pharmacodynamics
Anticonvulsant action: Mechanism of anticonvulsant activity is unknown; clonazepam appears to act in the limbic system, thalamus, and hypothalamus.

Clonazepam is used to treat myoclonic, atonic, and absence seizures resistant to other anticonvulsants and to suppress or eliminate attacks of sleep-related nocturnal myoclonus (restless legs syndrome).

Pharmacokinetics
- *Absorption:* Clonazepam is well absorbed from the GI tract; action begins in 20 to 60 minutes and persists for 6 to 8 hours in infants and children and up to 12 hours in adults.
- *Distribution:* Clonazepam is distributed widely throughout the body; it is approximately 47% protein-bound.
- *Metabolism:* Clonazepam is metabolized by the liver to several metabolites.
- *Excretion:* Clonazepam is excreted in urine.

Contraindications and precautions
Clonazepam is contraindicated in patients with known hypersensitivity to clonazepam and other benzodiazepines and in patients with significant hepatic disease, chronic respiratory disease, and untreated open-angle glaucoma or narrow-angle glaucoma. It should be used with caution (and at lower doses) in patients with decreased renal function and in patients for whom excessive salivation may be dangerous.

Interactions
Concomitant use of clonazepam with other CNS depressants (alcohol, narcotics, tranquilizers, anxiolytics, barbiturates) and other anticonvulsants will produce additive CNS depressant effects. Concomitant use with valproic acid may induce absence seizures.

Effects on diagnostic tests
Clonazepam may elevate liver function test values.

Adverse reactions
- CNS: drowsiness, ataxia, behavioral disturbances (especially in children), slurred speech, tremor, confusion, headache.
- CV: thrombophlebitis, *arrhythmias* (deaths have occurred).
- DERM: rash.
- EENT: increased salivation, diplopia, nystagmus, abnormal eye movements, rhinorrhea.
- GI: constipation, gastritis, change in appetite, nausea, abnormal thirst, sore gums.
- GU: dysuria, enuresis, nocturia, urinary retention.
- HEMA: leukopenia, thrombocytopenia, eosinophilia.
- Metabolic: hypocalcemia.
- Respiratory: *respiratory depression,* chest congestion, shortness of breath.

Note: Drug should be discontinued if signs of hypersensitivity occur or if liver function or hematologic tests show significant abnormalities.

Overdose and treatment
Symptoms of overdose may include ataxia, confusion, coma, decreased reflexes, and hypotension. Treat overdose with gastric lavage and supportive therapy. Flumazenil, a specific benzodiazepine antagonist, may be useful. Vasopressors should be used to treat hypotension. Carefully monitor vital signs, ECG, and fluid and electrolyte balance. Clonazepam is not dialyzable.

▶ Special considerations
- Abrupt withdrawal may precipitate status epilepticus; after long-term use, lower dosage gradually.
- Concomitant use with barbiturates or other CNS depressants may impair ability to perform tasks requiring mental alertness, such as driving a car. Warn patient to avoid such combined use.
- Monitor complete blood counts and liver function tests periodically.
- Monitor for oversedation, especially in elderly patients.

Information for the patient
- Explain rationale for therapy and risks and benefits that may be anticipated.
- Teach patient signs and symptoms of adverse reactions and need to report them promptly.
- Tell patient to avoid alcohol and other sedatives to prevent added CNS depression.

● Warn patient not to discontinue drug or change dosage unless prescribed.
● Advise patient to avoid tasks that require mental alertness until degree of sedative effect is determined.

Geriatric use
Elderly patients may require lower doses because of diminished renal function; such patients also are at greater risk for oversedation from CNS depressants.

Pediatric use
Long-term safety in children has not been established.

Breast-feeding
Alternative feeding method is recommended during clonazepam therapy.

---

clonidine hydrochloride
Catapres, Catapres-TTS, Dixarit*

● Pharmacologic classification: centrally acting antiadrenergic agent
● Therapeutic classification: antihypertensive
● Pregnancy risk category C

How supplied
Available by prescription only
Tablets: 0.1 mg, 0.2 mg, 0.3 mg
Transdermal: TTS-1 (releases 0.1 mg/24 hours), TTS-2 (releases 0.2 mg/24 hours), TTS-3 (releases 0.3 mg/24 hours)

Indications, route, and dosage
Hypertension
Adults: Initially, 0.1 mg P.O. b.i.d.; then increased by 0.1 to 0.2 mg daily or every few days until desired response is achieved. Usual dosage range is 0.2 to 1.2 mg daily in divided doses. Maximum effective dosage is 2.4 mg/day. If transdermal patch is used, apply to area of intact skin once every 7 days.
Children: No dosing recommendations for children.
†Adjunctive therapy in nicotine withdrawal
Adults: Initially, 0.05 mg P.O. daily, gradually increased to 0.2 mg P.O. daily as tolerated. Alternatively, apply transdermal patch (0.1 mg) and replace weekly for the first 2 or 3 weeks after smoking cessation.
†Prophylaxis for vascular headache
Adults: 0.05 mg P.O. t.i.d.
†Adjunctive treatment of menopausal symptoms
Adults: 0.025 to 0.075 mg P.O. b.i.d.
†Adjunctive therapy in opiate withdrawal
Adults: 5 to 17 mcg/kg P.O. daily in divided doses for up to 10 days. Adjust dosage to avoid hypotension and excessive sedation, and slowly withdraw drug.

Pharmacodynamics
Antihypertensive action: Clonidine decreases peripheral vascular resistance by stimulating central alpha-adrenergic receptors, thus decreasing cerebral sympathetic outflow; drug may also inhibit renin release. Initially, clonidine may stimulate peripheral alpha-adrenergic receptors, producing transient vasoconstriction.

Pharmacokinetics
● Absorption: Clonidine is absorbed well from the GI tract when administered orally; after oral administration, blood pressure begins to decline in 30 to 60 minutes, with maximal effect occurring in 2 to 4 hours. Clonidine is absorbed well percutaneously after transdermal topical administration; transdermal therapeutic plasma levels are achieved 2 to 3 days after initial application.
● Distribution: Clonidine is distributed widely into the body.
● Metabolism: Clonidine is metabolized in the liver, where nearly 50% is transformed to inactive metabolites.
● Excretion: Approximately 65% of a given dose is excreted in urine; 20% is excreted in feces. Half-life of clonidine ranges from 6 to 20 hours in patients with normal renal function. After oral administration, the antihypertensive effect lasts up to 8 hours; after transdermal application, the antihypertensive effect persists for up to 7 days.

Contraindications and precautions
Clonidine is contraindicated in patients with known hypersensitivity to the drug.
Clonidine should be used cautiously in patients with severe coronary insufficiency, diabetes mellitus, myocardial infarction, cerebrovascular disease, chronic renal failure, a history of depression, or those taking other antihypertensives.

Interactions
Clonidine may increase CNS depressant effects of alcohol, barbiturates, and other sedatives.
Tricyclic antidepressants, monoamine oxidase inhibitors, and tolazoline may inhibit the antihypertensive effects of clonidine; use with propranolol or other beta blockers may cause a paradoxical hypertensive response.

Effects on diagnostic tests
Clonidine may decrease urinary excretion of vanillylmandelic acid and catecholamines; it may slightly increase blood or serum glucose levels and may cause a weakly positive Coombs' test.

Adverse reactions
● CNS: drowsiness, dizziness, fatigue, sedation, nervousness, headache.
● CV: orthostatic hypotension, bradycardia, severe rebound hypertension.
● DERM: pruritus, contact dermatitis from transdermal patch.
● EENT: dry mouth.
● GI: constipation.
● GU: impotence, urinary retention.
● Metabolic: glucose intolerance.

Overdose and treatment
Clinical signs of overdose include bradycardia, CNS depression, respiratory depression, hypothermia, apnea, seizures, lethargy, agitation, irritability, diarrhea, and hypotension; hypertension has also been reported. After overdose with oral clonidine, do not induce emesis, because rapid onset of CNS depression can lead to aspiration. After adequate airway is assured, empty stomach by gastric lavage followed by administration of activated charcoal. If overdose occurs in patients receiving transdermal therapy, remove transdermal

---

patch. Further treatment is usually symptomatic and supportive.

▶ **Special considerations**
● Monitor pulse and blood pressure frequently; dosage is usually adjusted to patient's response and tolerance.
● Do not discontinue abruptly; reduce dosage gradually over 2 to 4 days to prevent severe rebound hypertension.
● Patients with renal impairment may respond to smaller doses of the drug.
● Give 4 to 6 hours before scheduled surgery.
● Clonidine may be used to lower blood pressure quickly in some hypertensive emergencies.
● Monitor weight daily during initiation of therapy, to monitor fluid retention.
● Clonidine has been used investigationally to prevent migraine, to treat severe dysmenorrhea and menopausal flushing, as an adjunct to smoking cessation therapy, and to aid rapid detoxification in the management of opiate withdrawal in opiate-dependent patients.
● Therapeutic plasma levels are achieved 2 or 3 days after applying transdermal form. Patient may need oral antihypertensive therapy during this interim period.

Information for the patient
● Explain disease and rationale for therapy; emphasize importance of follow-up visits in establishing therapeutic regimen.
● Teach patient signs and symptoms of adverse effects and need to report them; patient should also report excessive weight gain (more than 5 lb [2.25 kg] per week).
● Warn patient to avoid hazardous activities that require mental alertness until tolerance develops to sedation, drowsiness, and other CNS effects.
● Advise patient to avoid sudden position changes to minimize orthostatic hypotension.
● Advise patient that ice chips, hard candy, or gum will relieve dry mouth.
● Warn patient to call for specific instructions before taking nonprescription cold preparations.
● Advise taking last dose at bedtime to ensure nighttime blood pressure control.
● Advise patient not to discontinue drug suddenly; rebound hypertension may develop.

Geriatric use
Elderly patients may require lower doses because they may be more sensitive to clonidine's hypotensive effects.

Pediatric use
Efficacy and safety in children have not been established; use drug only if potential benefit outweighs risk.

Breast-feeding
Clonidine is distributed into breast milk. An alternate feeding method is recommended during treatment.

clorazepate dipotassium
Novoclopate*, Tranxene*, Tranxene-SD Half Strength, Tranxene-SD

● Pharmacologic classification: benzodiazepine
● Therapeutic classification: antianxiety agent; anticonvulsant; sedative-hypnotic
● Controlled substance schedule IV
● Pregnancy risk category D

How supplied
Available by prescription only
Capsules: 3.75 mg, 7.5 mg, 15 mg
Tablets: 3.75 mg, 7.5 mg, 11.25 mg, 15 mg, 22.5 mg

Indications, route, and dosage
Acute alcohol withdrawal
Adults: Day 1 – initially, 30 mg P.O., followed by 30 to 60 mg P.O. in divided doses; Day 2 – 45 to 90 mg P.O. in divided doses; Day 3 – 22.5 to 45 mg P.O. in divided doses; Day 4 – 15 to 30 mg P.O. in divided doses; gradually reduce daily dose to 7.5 to 15 mg.
Anxiety
Adults: 15 to 60 mg P.O. daily.
As an adjunct in epilepsy
Adults and children over age 12: Maximum recommended initial dosage is 7.5 mg P.O. t.i.d. Dosage increases should be no greater than 7.5 mg/week. Maximum daily dosage should not exceed 90 mg.
Children between age 9 and 12: Maximum recommended initial dosage is 7.5 mg P.O. b.i.d. Dosage increases should be no greater than 7.5 mg/week. Maximum daily dosage should not exceed 60 mg/day.

Pharmacodynamics
● *Anxiolytic and sedative actions:* Clorazepate depresses the CNS at the limbic and subcortical levels of the brain. It produces an antianxiety effect by enhancing the effect of the neurotransmitter gamma-aminobutyric acid (GABA) on its receptor in the ascending reticular activating system, which increases inhibition and blocks both cortical and limbic arousal.
● *Anticonvulsant action:* Clorazepate suppresses the spread of seizure activity produced by epileptogenic foci in the cortex, thalamus, and limbic structures by enhancing presynaptic inhibition.

Pharmacokinetics
● *Absorption:* After oral administration, clorazepate is hydrolyzed in the stomach to desmethyldiazepam, which is absorbed completely and rapidly. Peak serum levels occur at 1 to 2 hours.
● *Distribution:* Clorazepate is distributed widely throughout the body. Approximately 80% to 95% of an administered dose is bound to plasma protein.
● *Metabolism:* Desmethyldiazepam is metabolized in the liver to oxazepam.
● *Excretion:* Inactive glucuronide metabolites are excreted in urine. The half-life of desmethyldiazepam ranges from 30 to 200 hours.

Contraindications and precautions
Clorazepate is contraindicated in patients with known hypersensitivity to the drug; in patients with acute narrow-angle glaucoma or untreated open-angle glau-

coma, because of the drug's possible anticholinergic effect; in patients in shock or coma, because the drug's hypnotic or hypotensive effect may be prolonged or intensified; in patients with acute alcohol intoxication who have depressed vital signs, because the drug will worsen CNS depression; and in infants younger than age 30 days, in whom slow metabolism of the drug causes it to accumulate.

Clorazepate should be used cautiously in patients with psychoses, because the drug is rarely beneficial in such patients and may induce paradoxical reactions; in patients with myasthenia gravis or Parkinson's disease, because it may exacerbate the disorder; in patients with impaired renal or hepatic function, which prolongs elimination of the drug; in elderly or debilitated patients, who are usually more sensitive to the drug's CNS effects; and in individuals prone to addiction or drug abuse.

Interactions
Clorazepate potentiates the CNS depressant effects of phenothiazines, narcotics, barbiturates, alcohol, antihistamines, monoamine oxidase inhibitors, general anesthetics, and antidepressants. Concomitant use with cimetidine and possibly disulfiram causes diminished hepatic metabolism of clorazepate, which increases its plasma concentration.

Heavy smoking accelerates clorazepate's metabolism, thus lowering clinical effectiveness. Antacids delay the drug's absorption and reduce the total amount absorbed.

Benzodiazepines may reduce serum levels of haloperidol. Clorazepate may decrease the therapeutic effectiveness of levodopa.

Effects on diagnostic tests
Clorazepate therapy may elevate liver function test results. Minor changes in EEG patterns, usually low-voltage, fast activity, may occur during and after clorazepate therapy.

Adverse reactions
● CNS: confusion, depression, drowsiness, lethargy, hangover effect, ataxia, dizziness, syncope, nightmares, fatigue, slurred speech, tremors, vertigo, headache, paradoxical reactions.
● CV: bradycardia, palpitations, *cardiovascular collapse,* transient hypotension.
● DERM: rash, urticaria.
● EENT: diplopia, blurred vision, nystagmus.
● GI: constipation, dry mouth, nausea, vomiting, anorexia, dysphagia, abdominal discomfort.
● GU: urinary incontinence or retention.
● Other: *respiratory depression,* dysarthria, behavior problems, hepatic dysfunction, changes in libido.
  Note: Drug should be discontinued if hypersensitivity or the following paradoxical reactions occur: acute hyperexcited state, anxiety, hallucinations, increased muscle spasticity, insomnia, or rage.

Overdose and treatment
Clinical manifestations of overdose include somnolence, confusion, coma, hypoactive reflexes, dyspnea, labored breathing, hypotension, bradycardia, slurred speech, and unsteady gait or impaired coordination.

Support blood pressure and respiration until drug effects subside; monitor vital signs. Flumazenil, a specific benzodiazepine antagonist, may be useful. Mechanical ventilatory assistance via endotracheal tube may be required to maintain a patent airway and support adequate oxygenation. Treat hypotension with I.V. fluids and vasopressors such as dopamine and phenylephrine as needed. Induce emesis if patient is conscious. Use gastric lavage if ingestion was recent, but only if an endotracheal tube is present to prevent aspiration. After emesis or lavage, administer activated charcoal with a cathartic as a single dose. Dialysis is of limited value. Do not use barbiturates because they may worsen CNS adverse effects.

▶ Special considerations
Besides those relevant to all *benzodiazepines,* consider the following recommendations.
● Lower doses are effective in elderly patients and patients with renal or hepatic dysfunction.
● Store in a cool, dry place away from direct light.

Information for the patient
● Advise patient of potential for physical and psychological dependence with chronic use of clorazepate.
● Instruct patient not to alter drug regimen in any way without medical approval.
● Warn patient that sudden position changes may cause dizziness. Advise patient to dangle legs for a few minutes before getting out of bed to prevent falls and injury.
● Advise patient to take antacids 1 hour before or after clorazepate.
● Tell patient not to suddenly discontinue the drug.

Geriatric use
● Lower doses are usually effective in elderly patients because of decreased elimination. Use with caution.
● Elderly patients who receive this drug require supervision with ambulation and activities of daily living during initiation of therapy or after an increase in dose.

Pediatric use
Safety has not been established in children under age 9.

Breast-feeding
The breast-fed infant of a mother who uses clorazepate may become sedated, have feeding difficulties, or lose weight. Avoid use in breast-feeding women.

clotrimazole
Gyne-Lotrimin, Lotrimin, Mycelex, Mycelex-G

● Pharmacologic classification: synthetic imidazole derivative
● Therapeutic classification: topical antifungal
● Pregnancy risk category B

How supplied
Available by prescription only
Vaginal tablets: 500 mg
Topical cream: 1%
Topical lotion: 1%
Topical solution: 1%
Lozenges: 1%

Available without prescription
Vaginal tablets: 100 mg
Vaginal cream: 1%

Indications, route, and dosage
Tinea pedis, tinea cruris, tinea versicolor, tinea corporis, cutaneous candidiasis
Adults and children: Apply thinly and massage into cleansed affected and surrounding area, morning and evening, for prescribed period (usually 1 to 4 weeks; however, therapy may take up to 8 weeks).
Vulvovaginal candidiasis
Adults: Insert one 100-mg tablet intravaginally daily at bedtime for 7 consecutive days. Alternatively, non-pregnant women may insert two 100-mg tablets once daily for 3 consecutive days or one 500-mg tablet one time only at bedtime. If vaginal cream is used, insert one applicatorful intravaginally, once daily at bedtime for 7 to 14 consecutive days.
Oropharyngeal candidiasis
Adults and children: Administer orally and dissolve slowly (15 to 30 minutes) in mouth; usual dosage is one lozenge 5 times daily for 14 consecutive days.

Pharmacodynamics
Antifungal action: Clotrimazole alters cell membrane permeability by binding with phospholipids in the fungal cell membrane. Clotrimazole inhibits or kills many fungi, including yeast and dermatophytes, and also is active against some gram-positive bacteria.

Pharmacokinetics
● *Absorption:* Absorption is limited with topical administration.
● *Distribution:* Minimal with local application.
● *Metabolism:* Unknown.
● *Excretion:* Unknown.

Contraindications and precautions
Clotrimazole is contraindicated in patients with hypersensitivity to the drug. Clotrimazole lozenges should be used cautiously in patients with hepatic impairment because abnormal liver function test results have been reported. It should be used with caution intravaginally during first trimester of pregnancy because of possible adverse effects to the fetus.

Interactions
None reported.

Effects on diagnostic tests
Abnormal liver function test results have been reported in patients receiving clotrimazole lozenges.

Adverse reactions
● GI: lower abdominal cramps.
● GU: vaginal soreness during intercourse, dyspareunia, vaginal burning, urinary frequency.
● Local: blistering, erythema, pruritus, burning, stinging, irritation.
Note: Drug should be discontinued if hypersensitivity occurs.

Overdose and treatment
Discontinue therapy.

▶ Special considerations
Patients treated with clotrimazole lozenges, especially those who have preexisting liver dysfunction, should have periodic liver function tests.

Information for the patient
● Advise patient that clotrimazole lozenges must dissolve slowly in the mouth to achieve maximum effect. Tell patient not to chew lozenges.
● Advise patient using intravaginal application to insert the medication high into the vagina and to refrain from sexual contact during treatment period to avoid reinfection. Also tell patient to use a sanitary napkin to prevent staining of clothing and to absorb discharge.
● Tell patient to complete the full course of therapy. Improvement usually will be noted within a week. Patient should call if no improvement occurs in 4 weeks or if condition worsens.
● Advise patient to watch for and report irritation or sensitivity and, if this occurs, to discontinue use.

Pediatric use
Not recommended for use in children under age 3.

Breast-feeding
It is unknown whether clotrimazole is excreted in breast milk. Drug should be used with caution in breast-feeding women.

cloxacillin sodium
Cloxapen, Tegopen

● Pharmacologic classification: penicillinase-resistant penicillin
● Therapeutic classification: antibiotic
● Pregnancy risk category B

How supplied
Available by prescription only
Capsules: 250 mg, 500 mg
Oral solution: 125 mg/5 ml (after reconstitution)

Indications, route, and dosage
Systemic infections caused by susceptible organisms
Adults: 2 to 4 g P.O. daily, divided into doses given q 6 hours.
Children: 50 to 100 mg/kg P.O. daily, divided into doses given q 6 hours.

Pharmacodynamics
Antibiotic action: Cloxacillin is bactericidal; it adheres to bacterial penicillin-binding proteins, thereby inhibiting bacterial cell wall synthesis.
  Cloxacillin resists the effects of penicillinases—enzymes that inactivate penicillin—and therefore is active against many strains of penicillinase-producing bacteria; this activity is most pronounced against penicillinase-producing staphylococci; some strains may remain resistant. Cloxacillin is also active against gram-positive aerobic and anaerobic bacilli but has no significant effect on gram-negative bacilli.

Pharmacokinetics
● *Absorption:* Cloxacillin is absorbed rapidly but incompletely (37% to 60%) from the GI tract; it is relatively acid stable. Peak plasma concentrations occur ½ to 2 hours after an oral dose. Food may decrease both rate and extent of absorption.
● *Distribution:* Cloxacillin is distributed widely. CSF penetration is poor but enhanced in meningeal inflam-

mation. Cloxacillin crosses the placenta; it is 90% to 96% protein-bound.

● *Metabolism:* Cloxacillin is only partially metabolized.
● *Excretion:* Cloxacillin and metabolites are excreted in urine by renal tubular secretion and glomerular filtration; they are also excreted in breast milk. Elimination half-life in adults is ½ to 1 hour, extended minimally to 2½ hours in patients with renal impairment.

Contraindications and precautions
Cloxacillin is contraindicated in patients with known hypersensitivity to any other penicillin or to cephalosporins.

Cloxacillin should be administered with caution to patients with renal impairment, because it is excreted in urine; decreased dosage is required in moderate to severe renal failure.

Interactions
Concomitant use with aminoglycosides produces synergistic bactericidal effects against *Staphylococcus aureus.* However, the drugs are physically and chemically incompatible and are inactivated when mixed or given together. In vivo inactivation has been reported when aminoglycosides and penicillins are used concomitantly.

Probenecid blocks renal tubular secretion of carbenicillin, raising its serum concentrations.

Effects on diagnostic tests
Cloxacillin alters test results for urine and serum proteins; it produces false-positive or elevated results in turbidimetric urine and serum protein tests using sulfosalicylic acid or trichloroacetic acid; it also reportedly produces false results on the Bradshaw screening test for Bence Jones protein.

Cloxacillin may cause transient elevations in liver function study results and transient reductions in red blood cell, white blood cell, and platelet counts.

Elevated liver function test results may indicate drug-induced cholestasis or hepatitis.

Cloxacillin may falsely decrease serum aninoglycoside concentrations.

Adverse reactions
● GI: nausea, vomiting, epigastric distress, diarrhea, *pseudomembranous colitis, intrahepatic cholestasis.*
● GU: *acute interstitial nephritis.*
● HEMA: eosinophilia, leukopenia, granulocytopenia, thrombocytopenia, *agranulocytosis.*
● Other: *hypersensitivity* (rash, urticaria, chills, fever, sneezing, wheezing, *anaphylaxis*), bacterial and fungal superinfection.
   Note: Drug should be discontinued if immediate hypersensitivity reactions occur or if signs of acute interstitial nephritis or pseudomembranous colitis occur. Alternate therapy should be considered if any of the following occurs: drug fever, eosinophilia, hematuria, neutropenia, or unexplained elevations in serum creatinine or BUN levels, or in liver function studies.

Overdose and treatment
Clinical signs of overdose include neuromuscular irritability or seizures. No specific recommendation is available. Treatment is symptomatic. After recent ingestion (within 4 hours), empty the stomach by induced emesis or gastric lavage; follow with activated charcoal to reduce absorption. Cloxacillin is not appreciably removed by hemodialysis or peritoneal dialysis.

▶ Special considerations
Besides those relevant to all *penicillins,* consider the following recommendations.
● Give drug with water only; acid in fruit juice or carbonated beverage may inactivate drug.
● Give dose on empty stomach; food decreases absorption.

Pediatric use
Elimination of cloxacillin is reduced in neonates; safe use of drug in neonates has not been established.

Breast-feeding
Cloxacillin is excreted into breast milk; drug should be used with caution in breast-feeding women.

clozapine
Clozaril

● Pharmacologic classification: tricyclic dibenzodiazepine derivative
● Therapeutic classification: antipsychotic
● Pregnancy risk category B

How supplied
Available by prescription only
Tablets: 25 mg, 100 mg

Indications, route, and dosage
Treatment of schizophrenia in severely ill patients unresponsive to other therapies
Adults: Initially, 25 mg P.O. once or twice daily, titrated upward at 25 to 50 mg daily (if tolerated) to a daily dosage of 300 to 450 mg daily by the end of 2 weeks. Individual dosage is based on clinical response, patient tolerance, and adverse reactions. Subsequent increases of dosage should occur no more than once or twice weekly and should not exceed 100 mg. Many patients respond to doses of 300 to 600 mg daily, but some patients require as much as 900 mg daily. Do not exceed 900 mg/day.

Pharmacodynamics
Antipsychotic action: Clozapine binds to dopamine receptors (both D-1 and D-2) within the limbic system of the CNS. It also may interfere with adrenergic, cholinergic, histaminergic, and serotoninergic receptors.

Pharmacokinetics
● *Absorption:* Peak levels occur about 2.5 hours after oral administration. Food does not appear to interfere with bioavailability.
● *Distribution:* The drug is about 95% bound to serum proteins.
● *Metabolism:* Nearly complete; very little unchanged drug appears in the urine.
● *Excretion:* Approximately 50% of the drug appears in the urine and 30% in the feces, mostly as metabolites. Elimination half-life appears proportional to dose and may range from 8 to 12 hours.

Contraindications and precautions
Contraindicated in patients with a history of clozapine-induced agranulocytosis or severe granulocytopenia and in patients with severe CNS depression or coma. It is also contraindicated in patients currently taking

---

other drugs that suppress bone marrow function and in patients with myelosuppressive disorders.

Because clozapine has potent anticholinergic effects, use cautiously in patients with prostatic hypertrophy or glaucoma.

Seizures may occur, especially in patients receiving high doses of the drug. Patients should avoid hazardous activities, such as driving, swimming, or climbing, while taking the drug.

Clozapine therapy carries a significant risk of agranulocytosis (early trials estimate the incidence at 1.3%). If possible, patients should receive at least two trials of a standard antipsychotic drug therapy before clozapine therapy is initiated. Baseline white blood cell (WBC) and differential counts are required before therapy; WBC counts must be monitored weekly and for at least 4 weeks after therapy is discontinued.

If WBC count drops below 3,500/mm³ after initiating therapy or drops substantially from baseline, monitor patient closely for signs of infection. If WBC count is 3,000 to 3,500/mm³ and granulocyte count is above 1,500/mm³, perform twice weekly WBC and differential counts. If WBC count drops below 3,000/mm³ and granulocyte count drops below 1,500/mm³, therapy should be interrupted and the patient monitored for signs of infection. Therapy may be cautiously restarted if WBC count returns above 3,000/mm³ and granulocyte count returns above 1,500/mm³, but twice weekly monitoring of WBC and differential counts should continue until the WBC count exceeds 3,500/mm³.

If the WBC count drops below 2,000/mm³ and granulocyte count drops below 1,000/mm³, the patient may require protective isolation. If the patient develops an infection, prepare cultures according to policy and administer antibiotics as appropriate. Some clinicians may perform bone marrow aspiration to assess bone marrow function. Subsequent clozapine therapy is contraindicated.

Interactions
Clozapine may potentiate the hypotensive effects of antihypertensives. Anticholinergics may potentiate the anticholinergic effects of clozapine.

Administration of clozapine to a patient taking a benzodiazepine may pose a risk of respiratory arrest. Avoid concomitant use.

Increased serum levels of warfarin, digoxin, and other highly protein-bound drugs may occur. Monitor closely for adverse reactions.

Potentially increased bone marrow toxicity may follow concomitant use with drugs that suppress bone marrow function.

Use together with other CNS-active drugs cautiously because of the potential for additive effects.

Effects on diagnostic tests
Toxic effects of the drug may be evidenced by depressed blood counts.

Adverse reactions
● CNS: drowsiness, sedation, *seizures*, dizziness, syncope, vertigo, headache, tremor, disturbed sleep or nightmares, restlessness, hypokinesia or akinesia, agitation, rigidity, akathisia, confusion, fatigue, insomnia, hyperkinesia, weakness, lethargy, ataxia, slurred speech, depression, myoclonia, anxiety.
● CV: tachycardia, hypotension, hypertension, chest pain, ECG changes.
● DERM: rash.

● GI: constipation, nausea, vomiting, salivation, dry mouth.
● GU: urinary abnormalities, incontinence, abnormal ejaculation, urinary frequency or urgency, urinary retention.
● HEMA: *leukopenia, granulocytopenia, agranulocytosis.*
● Other: fever, muscle pain or spasm, muscle weakness, weight gain.

Overdose and treatment
Fatalities have occurred at doses exceeding 2.5 g. Symptoms include drowsiness, delerium, coma, hypotension, hypersalivation, tachycardia, respiratory depression, and, rarely, seizures.

Treat symptomatically. Establish an airway and ensure adequate ventilation. Gastric lavage with activated charcoal and sorbitol may be effective. Monitor vital signs. Avoid epinephrine (and derivatives), quinidine, and procainamide when treating hypotension and cardiac arrhythmias.

▶ Special considerations
● Clozapine therapy must be given with a monitoring program that ensures weekly testing of WBC counts. Blood tests must be performed weekly, and no more than a 1-week supply of drug can be distributed.
● To discontinue clozapine therapy, withdraw drug gradually (over a 1- to 2-week period). However, changes in the patient's clinical status (including the development of leukopenia) may require abrupt discontinuation of the drug. If so, monitor closely for recurrence of psychotic symptoms.
● To reinstate therapy in patients withdrawn from the drug, follow usual guidelines for dosage buildup. However, reexposure of the patient may increase the risk and severity of adverse reactions. If therapy was terminated for WBC counts below 2,000/mm³ or granulocyte counts below 1,000/mm³, the drug should not be continued.
● Some patients experience transient fevers (temperature above 100.4° F. [38° C.]), especially in the first 3 weeks of therapy. Monitor patients closely.
● Assess patient periodically for abnormal body movement.

Information for the patient
● Warn patient about the risk of developing agranulocytosis. He should know that safe use of the drug requires weekly blood tests to monitor for agranulocytosis. Advise patient to promptly report flu-like symptoms, fever, sore throat, lethargy, malaise, or other signs of infection.
● Advise patient to check with physician before taking any OTC drugs or alcohol.
● Tell patient that ice chips or sugarless candy or gum may help to relieve dry mouth.
● Warn patient to rise slowly to upright position to avoid orthostatic hypotension.

Pediatric use
Safe use in children has not been established.

Breast-feeding
Animal studies have shown that the drug is excreted in breast milk. Women taking clozapine should not breast-feed.

coccidioidin
Spherulin

- Pharmacologic classification: *Coccidioides immitis* antigen
- Therapeutic classification: skin test antigen
- Pregnancy risk category C

How supplied
Available by prescription only
Injection: 1:10 dilution (0.5 ml), 1:100 dilution (1 ml)

Indications, route, and dosage
Diagnostic aid in coccidioidomycosis
Adults and children: 0.1 ml of a 1:100 dilution intradermally into the volar surface of the forearm. Use the 1:10 dilution skin test on persons nonreactive to the 1:100 dilution.
To assess cell-mediated immunity
Adults and children: Given in a battery of at least four different antigens to which the patient probably has been exposed in the past. The antigens are administered intradermally 5 to 10 cm apart on the forearm. The usual coccidioidin dose is 0.1 ml of the 1:100 dilution.

Pharmacodynamics
Antigenic action: Intradermal administration of coccidioidin evokes a delayed hypersensitivity reaction in a patient who has become sensitive to *Coccidioides immitis.*

Pharmacokinetics
- *Absorption:* When coccidioidin is injected intradermally, a delayed hypersensitivity reaction appears in 5 to 6 hours and peaks in 24 to 48 hours.
- *Distribution:* Injection must be given intradermally; S.C. injection invalidates the test.
- *Metabolism:* Not applicable.
- *Excretion:* Not applicable.

Contraindications and precautions
Use of coccidioidin is contraindicated in patients with hypersensitivity to thimerosal or other mercuric compounds, a component of this preparation; and in patients with erythema nodosum, because these patients have a high incidence of severe reactions.

Interactions
None significant.

Effects on diagnostic tests
None significant.

Adverse reactions
- *Systemic:* reaction consisting of fever or erythema nodosum.
- *Local:* immediate wheal reaction; occasionally large reaction resulting in vesiculation, local tissue necrosis, and scar formation.
- *Other: anaphylaxis,* Arthus reaction.

Overdose and treatment
No information available.

▶ Special considerations
- A positive reaction may cause a transitory rise in titer of complement fixation antibody to histoplasma antigen, but not to coccidioidin.
- Coccidioidin may cause a skin test cross reaction with other fungi (*Histoplasma, Blastomyces*).
- Coccidioidin may boost level of skin sensitivity to coccidioidin in already sensitive patients.
- The skin test may be negative in anergic patients or after a long time has elapsed since infection.
- Interpretation of results is as follows:
Positive reaction: Induration of 5 mm or more. Erythema without induration is considered negative. Read the test at 24 and 48 hours, since some reactions may not be noticeable after 36 hours. A positive reaction indicates present or past infection with *Coccidioides immitis.*
Negative reaction: A negative test means the individual has not been sensitized to coccidioidin or has lost sensitivity.
- After injection of coccidioidin, observe patient for 15 minutes for immediate-type reaction. Keep epinephrine 1:1,000 available to treat possible anaphylaxis.
- Accurate dilution, dosage, and administration are essential with the use of coccidioidin. Normal saline solution may be used for dilutions.
- Erythema is not considered indicative of a delayed hypersensitivity reaction or positive response.
- Obtain history of allergies and reactions to skin tests. Patients allergic to mercury (merthiolate and thimerosal) should not receive this test.
- Reactivity to this test may be depressed or suppressed for as long as 6 weeks in individuals who have received concurrent virus vaccines, who are receiving a corticosteroid or immunosuppressive agents, and who have had viral infections.
- Take history of patient's travel to endemic areas (such as California, Arizona, New Mexico, and western Texas).
- Patients with coccidioidal erythema nodosum may have a severe reaction; use a dilution of 1:10,000 for the initial skin test. If this is negative, use a 1:1,000 dilution.

Information for the patient
- Have patient report any unusual side effects.
- Tell patient that the induration will subside in a few days.

Geriatric use
Elderly patients who are anergic may not react to the test.

Breast-feeding
Benefit of the test to the breast-feeding woman should be weighed against possible risk to the infant.

---

codeine phosphate
codeine sulfate

- Pharmacologic classification: opioid
- Therapeutic classification: analgesic, antitussive
- Controlled substance schedule II
- Pregnancy risk category C

How supplied
Available by prescription only
Tablets: 15 mg, 30 mg, 60 mg; 15 mg, 30 mg, 60 mg (soluble)
Oral solution: 15 mg/5 ml codeine phosphate
Injection: 25 mg/5 ml, 30 mg/ml, 60 mg/ml codeine phosphate

Indications, route, and dosage
Mild to moderate pain
Adults: 15 to 60 mg P.O. or 15 to 60 mg (phosphate) S.C. or I.M. q 4 hours, p.r.n., or around the clock.
Children: 0.5 mg/kg (or 15 mg/m²) q 4 to 6 hours.
Nonproductive cough
Adults: 10 to 20 mg P.O. q 4 to 6 hours. Maximum dosage: 120 mg/24 hours.
Children age 6 to 11: 5 to 10 mg q 4 to 6 hours, not to exceed 60 mg daily.
Children age 2 to 6: 1 mg/kg daily divided into four equal doses, administered q 4 to 6 hours.

Pharmacodynamics
- *Analgesic action:* Codeine (methylmorphine) has analgesic properties that result from its agonist activity at the opiate receptors.
- *Antitussive action:* Codeine has a direct suppressant action on the cough reflex center.

Pharmacokinetics
- *Absorption:* Codeine is well absorbed after oral or parenteral administration. It is about two thirds as potent orally as parenterally. After oral or subcutaneous administration, action occurs in less than 30 minutes. Peak analgesic effect is seen at ½ to 1 hour, and the duration of action is 4 to 6 hours.
- *Distribution:* Codeine is distributed widely throughout the body; it crosses the placenta and enters breast milk.
- *Metabolism:* Codeine is metabolized mainly in the liver, by demethylation, or conjugation with glucuronic acid.
- *Excretion:* Codeine is excreted mainly in the urine as norcodeine and free and conjugated morphine.

Contraindications and precautions
Codeine is contraindicated in patients with known hypersensitivity to the drug or phenanthrene opioids (hydrocodone, hydromorphone, morphine, oxycodone, or oxymorphone).

Administer codeine with extreme caution to patients with supraventricular arrhythmias. It is about two thirds as potent avoid, or administer drug with extreme caution to patients with head injury or increased intracranial pressure, because drug obscures neurologic parameters; and during pregnancy and labor, because drug readily crosses placenta (premature infants are especially sensitive to respiratory and CNS depressant effects of opioids).

Administer codeine cautiously to patients with renal or hepatic dysfunction, because drug accumulation or prolonged duration of action may occur; to patients with pulmonary disease (asthma, chronic obstructive pulmonary disease), because drug depresses respiration and suppresses cough reflex; to patients undergoing biliary tract surgery, because drug may cause biliary spasm; to patients with convulsive disorders, because drug may precipitate seizures; to elderly or debilitated patients, who are more sensitive to both therapeutic and adverse drug effects; and to patients prone to physical or psychic addiction, because of the high risk of addiction to this drug.

Interactions
Concomitant use with other CNS depressants (narcotic analgesics, general anesthetics, antihistamines, phenothiazines, barbiturates, benzodiazepines, sedative-hypnotics tricyclic antidepressants, monoamine oxidase inhibitors, alcohol, and muscle relaxants) potentiates drug's respiratory and CNS depression, sedation, and hypotensive effects. Concomitant use with cimetidine may also increase respiratory and CNS depression, causing confusion, disorientation, apnea, or seizures.

Drug accumulation and enhanced effects may result from concomitant use with other drugs that are extensively metabolized in the liver (rifampin, phenytoin, digitoxin); combined use with anticholinergics may cause paralytic ileus.

Patients who become physically dependent on this drug may experience acute withdrawal syndrome if given a narcotic antagonist.

Severe cardiovascular depression may result from concomitant use with general anesthetics.

Effects on diagnostic tests
Codeine may increase plasma amylase and lipase levels, delay gastric emptying, increase biliary tract pressure resulting from contraction of the sphincter of Oddi, and may interfere with hepatobiliary imaging studies.

Adverse reactions
- CNS: sedation, drowsiness, dysphoria, dizziness, euphoria, insomnia, agitation, confusion, headache, tremor, miosis, *seizures,* psychic dependence.
- CV: tachycardia, bradycardia, palpitations, chest wall rigidity, hypertension, hypotension, syncope, edema, *shock, cardiopulmonary arrest.*
- DERM: flushing, rashes, pruritus, pain at injection site.
- GI: dry mouth, anorexia, biliary spasms (colic), ileus, nausea, vomiting, constipation.
- GU: urinary retention or hesitancy, decreased libido.
- Other: apnea, *respiratory depression.*
Note: Drug should be discontinued if hypersensitivity, seizures, or life-threatening cardiac arrhythmias occur.

Overdose and treatment
The most common signs and symptoms of overdose are CNS depression, respiratory depression, and miosis (pinpoint pupils). Other acute toxic effects include hypotension, bradycardia, hypothermia, shock, apnea, cardiopulmonary arrest, circulatory collapse, pulmonary edema, and convulsions.

To treat acute overdose, first establish adequate respiratory exchange via a patent airway and ventilation as needed; administer narcotic antagonist (naloxone) to reverse respiratory depression. (Because the duration of action of codeine is longer than that of naloxone, repeated naloxone dosing is necessary.) Naloxone should not be given unless the patient has clinically significant respiratory or cardiovascular depression. Monitor vital signs closely.

If the patient presents within 2 hours of ingestion of an oral overdose, empty the stomach immediately by inducing emesis (ipecac syrup) or using gastric lavage. Use caution to avoid any risk of aspiration. Administer activated charcoal via nasogastric tube for further removal of the drug in an oral overdose.

Provide symptomatic and supportive treatment (continued respiratory support, correction of fluid or electrolyte imbalance). Monitor laboratory parameters, vital signs, and neurologic status closely.

▶ **Special considerations**
Besides those relevant to all *opioids*, consider the following recommendations.
● Codeine and aspirin have additive analgesic effects. Give together for maximum pain relief.
● Codeine has much less abuse potential than morphine.

Geriatric use
Lower doses are usually indicated for elderly patients, who may be more sensitive to the therapeutic and adverse effects of the drug.

Pediatric use
Administer cautiously to children. Codeine-containing cough preparations may be hazardous in young children. Use a calibrated measuring device and do not exceed the recommended daily dose:
Age 6 to 11: 60 mg/day.
Age 5 (average 18 kg): 18 mg/day
Age 4 (average 16 kg): 16 mg/day
Age 3 (average 14 kg): 14 mg/day
Age 2 (average 12 kg): 12 mg/day

Breast-feeding
Drug is excreted in breast milk; assess risk to benefit ratio before administering.

colchicine

● Pharmacologic classification: *Colchicum autumnale* alkaloid
● Therapeutic classification: antigout
● Pregnancy risk category C (oral), D (parenteral)

How supplied
Available by prescription only
Injection: 1 mg (1/60 grain)/2 ml ampule
Tablets: 0.6 mg (1/100 grain), 0.5 mg (1/120 grain) as sugar-coated granules

Indications, route, and dosage
To prevent acute attacks of gout as prophylactic or maintenance therapy
Adults: 0.5 or 0.6 mg P.O. daily; 1 to 1.8 mg P.O. daily for more severe cases.

To prevent attacks of gout in patients undergoing surgery
Adults: 0.5 to 0.6 mg P.O. t.i.d. 3 days before and 3 days after surgery.
Acute gout, acute gouty arthritis
Adults: Initially, 1 to 1.2 mg P.O., then 0.5 or 0.6 mg hourly, or 1 to 1.2 mg q 2 hours until pain is relieved or until nausea, vomiting, or diarrhea ensues. Or 2 mg I.V. followed by 2 mg I.V. in 12 hours if necessary. Total I.V. dose over 24 hours (one course of treatment) not to exceed 4 mg.
†*Familial Mediterranean fever*
Colchicine has been used effectively to treat familial Mediterranean fever (hereditary disorder characterized by acute episodes of fever, peritonitis, and pleuritis).
Adults: 1 to 2 mg/day in divided doses.
†*Amyloidosis suppressant*
Adults: 500 to 600 mcg P.O. b.i.d. or t.i.d.
†*Dermatitis herpetiformis suppressant*
Adults: 600 mcg P.O. t.i.d. or q.i.d.
†*Antiosteolytic in Paget's disease*
Adults: 600 mcg P.O. t.i.d.
†*Hepatic cirrhosis*
Adults: 1 mg 5 days weekly.
†*Primary biliary cirrhosis*
Adults: 0.6 mg twice daily.

Pharmacodynamics
● *Antigout action:* Colchicine's exact mechanism of action is unknown, but it is involved in leukocyte migration inhibition; reduction of lactic acid production by leukocytes, resulting in decreased deposits of uric acid; and interference with kinin formation.
● *Anti-inflammatory action:* Colchicine reduces the inflammatory response to deposited uric acid crystals and diminishes phagocytosis.

Pharmacokinetics
● *Absorption:* When administered P.O., colchicine is rapidly absorbed from the GI tract. Unchanged drug may be reabsorbed from the intestine by biliary processes.
● *Distribution:* Colchicine is distributed rapidly into various tissues after reabsorption from the intestine. It is concentrated in leukocytes and distributed into the kidneys, liver, spleen, and intestinal tract, but is absent in the heart, skeletal muscle, and brain.
● *Metabolism:* Colchicine is metabolized partially in the liver and also slowly metabolized in other tissues.
● *Excretion:* Colchicine and its metabolites are excreted primarily in the feces, with lesser amounts excreted in urine.

Contraindications and precautions
Colchicine is contraindicated in patients with serious GI, renal, or cardiac disorders and should be used cautiously in patients who may have early signs of these disorders, because the drug may exacerbate these conditions. Colchicine is also contraindicated in patients with blood dyscrasias or hypersensitivity to colchicine. Use with caution in elderly or debilitated patients.

Interactions
When used concomitantly, colchicine and sulfinpyrazone may lead to leukemia in some patients. However, a cause-and-effect relationship has not been established. Colchicine induces reversible malabsorption of vitamin B_{12}, may increase sensitivity to CNS depressants, and may enhance the response to sympatho-

mimetic agents. Colchicine is inhibited by acidifying agents and by alcohol consumption; its actions are increased by alkalinizing agents.

Effects on diagnostic tests

Colchicine therapy may increase alkaline phosphatase, AST (SGOT), and ALT (SGPT) levels and may decrease serum carotene, cholesterol, and thrombocyte values.

Colchicine may cause false-positive results of urine tests for red blood cells or hemoglobin.

Adverse reactions

● CNS: peripheral neuritis, purpura, myopathy, mental confusion, loss of deep tendon reflexes.
● GI: vomiting, diarrhea, abdominal pain, nausea.
● GU: dysuria, urinary frequency, reversible azoospermia, nephrotoxicity (with toxic doses).
● HEMA: bone marrow depression with *aplastic anemia, agranulocytosis, thrombocytopenia.*
● Other: alopecia, dermatosis, hypersensitivity, pain and erythema at I.V. infusion site.

Overdose and treatment

Clinical manifestations of overdose include nausea, vomiting, abdominal pain, and diarrhea. Diarrhea may be severe and bloody from hemorrhagic gastroenteritis. Burning sensations in the throat, stomach, and skin also may occur. Extensive vascular damage may result in shock, hematuria, and oliguria, indicating kidney damage. Patient develops severe dehydration, hypotension, and muscle weakness with an ascending paralysis of the CNS. Patient usually remains conscious, but delirium and convulsions may occur. Death may result from respiratory depression.

There is no known specific antidote. Treatment begins with gastric lavage and preventive measures for shock. Recent studies support the use of hemodialysis and peritoneal dialysis; atropine and morphine may relieve abdominal pain; paregoric usually is administered to control diarrhea and cramps. Respiratory assistance may be needed.

▶ Special considerations

● To avoid cumulative toxicity, a course of oral colchicine should not be repeated for at least 3 days; a course of I.V. colchicine should not be repeated for several weeks.
● Do not administer I.M. or subcutaneously; severe local irritation occurs.
● Obtain baseline laboratory studies, including CBC, before initiating therapy and periodically thereafter.
● Give I.V. by slow I.V. push over 2 to 5 minutes by direct I.V. injection or into tubing of a free-flowing I.V. with compatible I.V. fluid. Avoid extravasation. Do not dilute colchicine injection with 0.9% sodium chloride, dextrose 5% injection, or any other fluid that might change pH of colchicine solution. If lower concentration of colchicine injection is needed, dilute with sterile water for injection. However, if diluted solution becomes turbid, do not inject.
● Discontinue drug if weakness, anorexia, nausea, vomiting, or diarrhea appears. First sign of acute overdosage may be GI symptoms, followed by vascular damage, muscle weakness, and ascending paralysis. Delirium and convulsions may occur without loss of consciousness.
● Store the drug in a tightly closed, light-resistant container, away from moisture and high temperatures.

Information for the patient

● Advise patient to report rash, sore throat, fever, unusual bleeding, bruising, tiredness, weakness, numbness, or tingling.
● Tell patient to discontinue colchicine as soon as gout pain is relieved or at the first sign of nausea, vomiting, stomach pain, or diarrhea. Advise patient to report persistent symptoms.
● Instruct patient to avoid alcohol during colchicine therapy, because alcohol may inhibit drug action.

Geriatric use

Administer with caution to elderly or debilitated patients, especially those with renal, GI, or heart disease or hematologic disorders. Reduce dosage if weakness, anorexia, nausea, vomiting, or diarrhea appears.

Pediatric use

Safety and efficacy for use in children have not been established.

Breast-feeding

Safe use has not been established. It is not known whether this drug is excreted in breast milk.

---

colestipol hydrochloride
Colestid

● Pharmacologic classification: anion exchange resin
● Therapeutic classification: antilipemic
● Pregnancy risk category C

How supplied

Available by prescription only
Granules: 500-mg bottles, 5-g packets

Indications, route, and dosage

Primary hypercholesterolemia and xanthomas
Adults: 15 to 30 g P.O. daily in two to four divided doses.
Children: 10 to 20 g or 500 mg/kg daily in two to four divided doses (lower dosages of 125 to 250 mg/kg used when serum cholesterol levels were 15% to 20% above normal after only dietary management).

Pharmacodynamics

Antilipemic action: Bile is normally excreted into the intestine to facilitate absorption of fat and other lipid materials. Colestipol binds with bile acid, forming an insoluble compound that is excreted in feces. With less bile available in the digestive system, less fat and lipid materials in food are absorbed, more cholesterol is used by the liver to replace its supply of bile acids, and the serum cholesterol level decreases.

Pharmacokinetics

● *Absorption:* Colestipol is not absorbed. Cholesterol levels may decrease in 24 to 48 hours, with peak effect occurring at 1 month. In some patients, the initial decrease is followed by a return to or above baseline cholesterol levels on continued therapy.
● *Distribution:* None.
● *Metabolism:* None.
● *Excretion:* Colestipol is excreted in feces; cholesterol levels return to baseline within 1 month after therapy stops.

Contraindications and precautions

Colestipol is contraindicated in patients with complete biliary obstruction or complete atresia because bile is not secreted into the intestine; in patients with primary biliary cirrhosis because cholesterol levels may be further increased in these cases; and in patients with known hypersensitivity to the drug.

Use colestipol cautiously in patients with constipation because of the risk of fecal impaction; in patients with malabsorption, because the condition may deteriorate from further decreased absorption of fats and fat-soluble vitamins E, A, D, and K; and in pregnant women, because impaired maternal absorption of vitamins and other nutrients is a potential threat to the fetus.

Interactions

Colestipol impairs absorption of digitalis glycosides (including digoxin and digitoxin), tetracycline, penicillin G, chenodril, and thiazide diuretics, thus decreasing their therapeutic effect.

Dosage of any oral medication may require adjustment to compensate for possible binding with colestipol; give other drugs at least 1 hour before or 4 to 6 hours after colestipol (longer if possible); readjustment must also be made when colestipol is withdrawn, to prevent high-dose toxicity.

Effects on diagnostic tests

Colestipol alters serum levels of alkaline phosphatase, aspartate aminotransferase, chloride, phosphorus, potassium, and sodium.

Adverse reactions

● DERM: rashes, sore skin, tongue, and perianal skin.
● GI: constipation, fecal impaction, aggravation of hemorrhoids, abdominal discomfort, flatulence, nausea, vomiting, steatorrhea.
● Other: vitamin A, D, and K deficiency from decreased absorption; hyperchloremic acidosis with long-term use or very high dosage.

Note: Drug should be discontinued if constipation worsens even after reduction in dosage; if a paradoxical increase in serum cholesterol level occurs; or if inadequate clinical response occurs after 1 to 3 months of treatment except when treating xanthoma tuberosum, which may require up to 12 months of treatment.

Overdose and treatment

Overdose of colestipol has not been reported. Chief potential risk is intestinal obstruction; treatment would depend on location and degree of obstruction and on amount of gut motility.

▶ Special considerations

● To mix, sprinkle granules on surface of preferred beverage or wet food, let stand a few minutes, and stir to obtain uniform suspension; avoid excess foaming by using large glass and mixing slowly. Use at least 90 ml of water or other fluid, soups, milk, or pulpy fruit; rinse container and have patient drink this to be sure he ingests entire dose.
● Monitor levels of cardiac glycosides and other drugs to ensure appropriate dosage during and after therapy with colestipol.
● Determine serum cholesterol level frequently during first few months of therapy and periodically thereafter.
● Monitor bowel habits; treat constipation promptly by decreasing dosage, increasing fluid intake, adding a stool softener, or discontinuing drug.

● Monitor for signs of vitamin A, D, or K deficiency.

Information for the patient

● Explain disease process and rationale for therapy and encourage patient to comply with continued blood testing and special diet; although therapy is not curative, it helps control serum cholesterol level.
● Teach patient how to administer drug.

Geriatric use

Elderly patients are more likely to experience adverse GI effects, as well as adverse nutritional effects.

Pediatric use

Safety in children has not been established; drug is not usually recommended; however, it has been used in a limited number of children with hypercholesteremia.

Breast-feeding

Safety in breast-feeding women has not been established.

---

colfosceril palmitate
Exosurf Neonatal

● Pharmacologic classification: phospholipid
● Therapeutic classification: lung surfactant

How supplied

Available by prescription only
Intratracheal suspension: 108 mg/10-ml vial (13.5 mg/ml when reconstituted with 8 ml sterile water for injection provided)

Indications, route, and dosage
Prevention and treatment (rescue) of respiratory distress syndrome (RDS) in premature infants
Prophylaxis: 67.5 mg/kg of body weight intratracheally for the first dose, administered as soon as possible after birth; second and third doses should be administered approximately 12 and 24 hours later to all infants remaining on mechanical ventilation at those times.
Rescue: Initially, 67.5 mg/kg of body weight intratracheally, administered as soon as possible after diagnosis of RDS is confirmed; second dose, approximately 12 hours after the first, provided the infant remains on mechanical ventilation.

Administer using endotracheal tube adapter supplied by manufacturer.

Infant should be suctioned before administration; however, suction should not be performed for 2 hours after administration except when necessary.

Pharmacodynamics
Surfactant action: Endogenous pulmonary surfactant lowers surface tension on alveolar surfaces during respiration and stabilizes alveoli against collapse at rest in transpulmonary pressures. Colfosceril replenishes surfactant and restores surface activity to the lungs.

Pharmacokinetics
Absorption: Colfosceril is administered directly to the target organ, where biophysical effects occur at the

---

alveolar surface. Most of the dose becomes lung-as-sociated within hours of administration.

Contraindications and precautions

Colfosceril should be used only by medical personnel familiar with endotracheal intubation and respiratory management of critically ill neonates. Because the drug can rapidly alter lung compliance and oxygenation, close monitoring of the neonate is necessary before, during, and after drug administration. If chest expansion improves dramatically after administration, peak ventilator pressures should be reduced immediately to avoid potentially fatal pulmonary air leak. Be prepared to rapidly reduce FIO_2 in infants who become pink and display transcutaneous O_2 saturations in excess of 95% to avoid hyperoxia. Marked hypocapnea and subsequent decreases in brain blood flow can occur in infants with arterial or transcutaneous CO_2 measurements less than 30 mm Hg.

At least one study of colfosceril in infants weighing less than 700 grams revealed increased incidence of pulmonary hemorrhage after treatment. Generally, the risk of pulmonary hemorrhage is higher in younger, smaller, male infants and those with a patent ductus arteriosus.

Mucus plugging of the endotracheal tube can occur. If respiration becomes markedly impaired during or shortly after dosing, attempt to suction the airway. If suctioning is not immediately successful, replace the blocked tube immediately.

Effects on diagnostic tests

Abnormal laboratory values are common in critically ill, mechanically ventilated patients. No higher incidence was seen in colfosceril-treated patients.

Adverse reactions

● Respiratory: *pulmonary hemorrhage, apnea.*

Overdose and treatment

Overdose may result in acute airway obstruction. Treatment should be symptomatic and supportive.

▶ Special considerations

● Five different-sized endotracheal tube adapters are supplied; select size based on inside diameter of endotracheal tube.
● To prepare, reconstitute immediately before use with 8 ml of sterile water for injection (supplied). Fill a 10- or 12-ml syringe with 8 ml of sterile water using an 18G or 19G needle. Allow vacuum to draw water into vial. Aspirate as much as possible of the 8 ml out of the vial into the syringe while maintaining the vacuum; then, suddenly release the syringe plunger. The last step should be repeated 3 or 4 times to ensure adequate mixing. If vacuum is not present, do not use vial.
● The appropriate volume for the entire dose should be drawn into the syringe from below the froth of the vial. The reconstituted suspension will be milky white. Each ml contains 13.5 mg colfosceril, 1.5 mg cetyl alcohol, 1 mg tyloxapol, and sodium chloride to provide a 0.1 normal concentration.
● Continuous ECG and transcutaneous oxygen saturation monitoring is recommended. During dosing, heart rate, color, chest expansion, facial expressions, oximeter, and endotracheal tube patency and position should be monitored.
● A videotape is available from the manufacturer demonstrating techniques for safe administration and should

be viewed by the health care professional who will administer the drug.

---

colistimethate sodium (polymyxin E)
Coly-Mycin M Parenteral

colistin sulfate
Coly-Mycin S

● Pharmacologic classification: polymyxin antibiotic
● Therapeutic classification: antibiotic
● Pregnancy risk category C

How supplied

Available by prescription only
Oral suspension: 25 mg colistin (as sulfate) per 5 ml when reconstituted
Injection: 150-mg vial Coly-Mycin M powder for reconstitution

Indications, route, and dosage

Severe infections caused by susceptible strains of gram-negative bacteria when other agents (such as aminoglycosides) are contraindicated or ineffective

Colistimethate sodium
Adults and children: 2.5 to 5 mg/kg I.M. or I.V. daily in two to four divided doses. The maximum daily dose is 7 mg/kg.

Colistin sulfate
Adults and children: 5 to 15 mg/kg P.O. daily in three divided doses.

Pharmacodynamics

Antibacterial action: The bactericidal action of colistin and colistimethate resembles that of cationic detergent, damaging bacterial membranes and causing leakage of cell contents. Drug is effective against many gram-negative organisms, including many strains of *Acinetobacter, Citrobacter, Escherichia coli, Enterobacter, Haemophilus influenzae, Klebsiella pneumoniae, Pseudomonas aeruginosa, Salmonella, Shigella,* and some strains of *Bordetella* and *Vibrio.* Gram-positive organisms and most strains of *Proteus, Neisseria, Serratia,* and *Bacteroides fragilis* organisms resist treatment with colistin.

Pharmacokinetics

● *Absorption:* With oral colistin administration, systemic absorption is negligible. With I.M. colistimethate administration, peak concentrations occur in approximately 2 hours.
● *Distribution:* Colistimethate is distributed widely; however, it does not enter synovial, cerebrospinal, pleural, or pericardial fluid. Approximately 50% of colistimethate binds to plasma proteins.
● *Metabolism:* Parenterally administered colistimethate is hydrolyzed to colistin.
● *Excretion:* Colistin is excreted in the feces. Parenteral colistimethate is excreted in the urine by filtration. In patients with normal renal function, plasma half-life is 1½ to 8 hours; in patients lacking functioning kidneys, plasma half-life may be prolonged up to 3 days.

Contraindications and precautions
Colistin and colistimethate are contraindicated in patients with known hypersensitivity to colistin or colistimethate.

Colistimethate should be administered cautiously to patients undergoing anesthesia because it may potentiate neuromuscular blockade induced by neuromuscular blocking agents.

Interactions
When used concomitantly, colistimethate may potentiate renal toxicity of other nephrotoxic drugs, such as aminoglycosides, amphotericin B, capreomycin, methoxyflurane, polymyxin B, and vancomycin. Colistimethate may cause additive neuromuscular effects when used with other neuromuscular blocking agents, such as tubocurarine, succinylcholine, gallamine, and decamethonium.

Effects on diagnostic tests
None reported.

Adverse reactions
● CNS: circumoral and lingual paresthesias; paresthesias of extremities; *neuromuscular blockade with respiratory arrest*, especially in patients with impaired renal function; dizziness; slurring of speech; vertigo.
● DERM: pruritus, urticaria.
● GI: nausea, vomiting, discomfort.
● GU: *nephrotoxicity* (decreased urine output, increased BUN and serum creatinine levels).
● Local: pain at I.M. injection site.
● Other: drug fever, overgrowth of nonsusceptible organisms.
  Note: These effects occur with parenteral colistimethate administration, not with oral colistin sulfate administration. Drug should be discontinued if BUN and serum creatinine levels increase or if urine output decreases.

Overdose and treatment
No information available.

▶ **Special considerations**
● Systemic polymyxin therapy should only be considered in life-threatening gram-negative infections such as *Pseudomonas* when other drugs cannot be used.
● Culture and sensitivity tests should be done before starting therapy. This drug should be reserved for patients unresponsive to or intolerant of other agents.
● Reconstitute 150-mg vial with 2 ml of sterile water for injection. When mixing, swirl gently to avoid frothing. Reconstituted solution will provide 75 mg/ml.
● I.M. preparations should be given deep I.M. and sites rotated.
● For direct I.V. injection, administer half of daily dose over 3 to 5 minutes at 12-hour intervals.
● For continuous I.V. infusion, directly inject half of daily dose over 3 to 5 minutes and follow in 2 hours with infusion containing other half, at rate of 5 mg/hour. Continuous infusion may be prepared in any commercially available crystalloid solution containing dextrose or sodium chloride or in lactated Ringer's solution.
● I.V. infusion solution remains stable for 24 hours.
● Colistin is available in combination with neomycin and hydrocortisone for otic use.

Information for the patient
● Warn patient that injection may be painful.
● Caution patient to continue taking oral form as directed, even if he feels better. Inform him that oral suspension remains stable for 14 days when stored in refrigerator.

collagenase
Biozyme-C, Santyl

● Pharmacologic classification: enzyme concentrate derived from *Clostridium histolytica*
● Therapeutic classification: topical proteolytic enzyme preparation

How supplied
Available by prescription only
Ointment: 250 units/g

Indications, route, and dosage
To promote debridement of necrotic tissue in dermal ulcers and severe burns
Adults and children: Apply ointment to lesion daily or every other day.

Pharmacodynamics
Enzymatic debriding agent: Collagenase liquefies necrotic tissue without damaging granulation tissue. It hydrolyzes peptide bonds of undenatured and denatured collagen.

Pharmacokinetics
● *Absorption:* Limited with topical use.
● *Distribution:* None.
● *Metabolism:* None.
● *Excretion:* None.

Contraindications and precautions
Collagenase is contraindicated in patients with hypersensitivity to the drug. It should be used with caution near the eyes.

Interactions
When used concomitantly, the enzyme activity of collagenase is adversely affected by detergents, benzalkonium chloride, hexachlorophene, nitrofurazone, tincture of iodine, and any medication or material containing heavy metal ions.

Effects on diagnostic tests
None reported.

Adverse reactions
● Local: pain, burning, erythema.
  Note: Drug should be discontinued if sensitization occurs.

Overdose and treatment
Action of enzyme can be stopped by applying aluminum acetate solution to the lesion as soon as possible.

▶ **Special considerations**
● Store drug at temperatures not exceeding 98.6° F. (37° C.).

- Avoid local skin irritation by covering the skin surrounding the lesion with a protectant.
- Observe patient for sensitivity reaction with prolonged use.
- Monitor debilitated patients for systemic infections; debriding enzymes may increase risk of bacteremia.
- Use strict aseptic technique when applying collagenase. Cleanse lesion with hydrogen peroxide or 0.9% sodium chloride buffer solution.
- Discontinue therapy when debridement of tissue has been achieved and granulation tissue has developed.

Information for the patient
Teach patient to cover surrounding area with a protectant (zinc oxide paste) to decrease possibility of irritation, to cleanse lesion with hydrogen peroxide or 0.9% sodium chloride buffer solution, and to maintain strict aseptic conditions when changing dressings.

Breast-feeding
Women should avoid breast-feeding if product is used in breast area.

coral snake, North American (Micrurus fulvius), antivenin

- Pharmacologic classification: antivenin
- Therapeutic classification: snake antivenin
- Pregnancy risk category D

How supplied
Available by prescription only
Injection: combination package – 1 vial antivenin and 1 vial diluent (10 ml bacteriostatic water for injection)

Indications, route, and dosage
Eastern and Texas coral snake bite
Adults and children: 3 to 5 vials slow I.V. through running I.V. of 0.9% normal saline solution. Give first 1 to 2 ml over 3 to 5 minutes, and watch for signs of allergic reaction. If no signs develop, continue injection. Up to 10 vials may be needed. Not effective for Sonoran or Arizona coral snake bites.

Pharmacodynamics
Antivenin action: This product neutralizes and binds venom.

Pharmacokinetics
No information available.

Contraindications and precautions
Use with caution in persons with sensitivity to horse serum derived preparations.

Interactions
None reported.

Effects on diagnostic tests
None reported.

Adverse reactions
- Systemic: *hypersensitivity, anaphylaxis.*
  Note: Drug should be discontinued if severe systemic reactions occur.

Overdose and treatment
No information available.

▶ Special considerations
- If possible, hospitalize patient for observation.
- Splint bitten limb to prevent spread of venom.
- Obtain a thorough patient history of allergies, especially to horses and horse immune serum, and of previous reactions to immunizations.
- Before administering antivenin, a skin test for sensitivity to equine serum should be performed, because this product is derived from horses immunized with Eastern coral snake venom. For an intradermal test, use a 1:10 dilution of the antivenin serum in normal saline solution.
- Epinephrine solution 1:1,000 should be available to treat allergic reactions.
- Ask patient when he received his last tetanus immunization; a booster may be appropriate at this time.
- Venom is neurotoxic and may rapidly cause respiratory paralysis and death. Monitor patient carefully for 24 hours. Be ready to take supportive measures, such as mechanical ventilation.
- Avoid use of narcotic analgesics and other drugs that produce sedation or respiratory depression.
- Monitor patient closely over the next 24 hours for reactions to both the snake bite and the antivenin.
- Refrigerate antivenin at 2° to 8° C. (36° to 46° F.).

Information for the patient
Tell patient that this product is derived from an animal source (that is, horses) and that he may experience allergic reactions, such as rash, joint swelling or pain, or difficulty breathing.

Pediatric use
The amount of antivenin given to a child is not based on weight. Children receive the same dosage as adults.

Breast-feeding
Patient should discontinue breast-feeding until the venom's effects have subsided and if symptoms of serum sickness develop.

corn oil
Lipomul

- Pharmacologic classification: modular supplement
- Therapeutic classification: enteral nutritional therapy

How supplied
Available without a prescription
Liquid: 473-ml container with 10 g corn oil/15 ml (sugar-free)

Indications, route, and dosage
To increase caloric intake
Adults: 45 ml P.O. b.i.d. to q.i.d. after or between meals, alone or with proteins, milk, or other energy sources.
Children: 30 ml P.O. daily to q.i.d. after or between meals, alone or with proteins, milk, or other energy sources.

Pharmacodynamics
Nutritional action: Corn oil is a nutritional supplement that provides a source of fat and increases caloric intake. Enteral nutrition products may be administered orally by nasogastric tube, feeding gastrostomy, or needle-catheter jejunostomy. Defined formula diets may be monomeric, oligomeric (containing amino acids or short peptides and simple carbohydrates) or polymeric (containing more complex protein and carbohydrate sources). Individual modular supplements of protein, carbohydrate, or fat are used when formulas do not offer sufficient flexibility. Except for patients with lactose or other allergies (for example, to corn or gluten), the protein or carbohydrate source is not critical. The formulations contain varying amounts of vitamins, electrolytes, and minerals.

Pharmacokinetics
No information is available regarding systemic absorption, distribution, metabolism, or excretion.

Contraindications and precautions
Corn oil is contraindicated in patients with GI obstruction and in those with gallbladder disease or diabetes. Use cautiously in patients with steatorrhea, partial GI obstruction, or enterostomies.

Interactions
Corn oil may increase the absorption of griseofulvin.

Effects on diagnostic tests
None reported.

Adverse reactions
None reported.

Overdose and treatment
No information available.

▶ Special considerations
● Give frequent small doses with meals or mix with milk to reduce nausea and diarrhea.
● Increase administration rate gradually when beginning therapy.
● Observe patient closely for abdominal distention or signs of intestinal obstruction.
● Consider sodium and potassium content of formulas in patients with renal or hepatic disease.

corticotropin (adrenocortico-tropic hormone, ACTH)
ACTH, Acthar, ACTHGel, Cortigel-40, Cortigel-80, Cortrophin Gel, Cortrophin-Zinc, HP Acthar Gel

● Pharmacologic classification: anterior pituitary hormone
● Therapeutic classification: diagnostic aid, replacement hormone, multiple sclerosis and nonsuppurative thyroiditis treatment
● Pregnancy risk category C

How supplied
Available by prescription only
Injection: 25 units/vial, 40 units/vial

Repository injection: 40 units/ml, 80 units/ml

Indications, route, and dosage
Diagnostic test of adrenocortical function
Adults: Up to 80 units I.M. or S.C. in divided doses; or a single dose of repository form; or 10 to 25 units (aqueous form) in 500 ml of dextrose 5% in water I.V. over 8 hours, between blood samplings.

Individual dosages vary with adrenal glands' sensitivity to stimulation and with the specific disease. Infants and younger children require larger doses per kilogram than do older children and adults.
Replacement hormone
Adults: 40 units S.C. or I.M. in four divided doses (aqueous); 40 units q 12 to 24 hours (gel or repository injection).
Exacerbations of multiple sclerosis
Adults: 80 to 120 units I.M. daily for 2 to 3 weeks.
Severe allergic reactions, collagen disorders, dermatologic disorders, inflammation
Adults: 40 to 80 units/day I.M. or S.C. Adjust dosage based upon patient response.
Infantile spasms
Infants: 40 to 120 units I.M. (of repository injection) daily or 80 to 240 units I.M. every other day.

Pharmacodynamics
● *Diagnostic action:* Corticotropin is used to test adrenocortical function. Corticotropin binds with a specific receptor in the adrenal cell plasma membrane, stimulating the synthesis of the entire spectrum of adrenal steroids, one of which is cortisol. The effect of corticotropin is measured by analyzing plasma cortisol before and after drug administration. In patients with primary adrenocortical insufficiency, corticotropin does not increase plasma cortisol concentrations significantly.
● *Anti-inflammatory action:* In nonsuppurative thyroiditis and acute exacerbations of multiple sclerosis, corticotropin stimulates release of adrenal cortex hormones, which combat tissue responses to inflammatory processes.

Pharmacokinetics
● *Absorption:* Corticotropin is absorbed rapidly after I.M. administration; absorption occurs over 8 to 16 hours after I.M. administration of zinc or repository form. Maximum stimulation occurs after infusing 1 to 6 units of corticotropin over 8 hours. Peak cortisol levels are achieved within 1 hour of I.M. or rapid I.V. administration of corticotropin. Peak 17-hydroxycorticosteroid levels are achieved within 7 to 24 hours with zinc and 3 to 12 hours with the repository form.
● *Distribution:* The exact distribution of corticotropin is unknown, but it is removed rapidly from plasma by many tissues.
● *Metabolism:* Unknown.
● *Excretion:* Corticotropin probably is excreted by the kidneys. Its duration of action is about 2 hours with zinc form and up to 3 days with the repository form. Half-life is about 15 minutes.

Contraindications and precautions
Corticotropin is contraindicated in patients with known hypersensitivity to corticotropin, primary adrenocortical insufficiency, or congenital adrenogenital syndrome (because corticotropin will be ineffective) and in any condition associated with adrenocortical hyperfunction (which may become exacerbated). Corticotropin also may exacerbate congestive heart failure (CHF) or hy-

pertension (because of sodium and fluid retention), ocular herpes simplex (because of the risk of corneal perforation), sensitivity to proteins of porcine origin (because corticotropin often is obtained from pigs), osteoporosis, and scleroderma.

Corticotropin should be used cautiously in patients with acquired immune deficiency syndrome (AIDS) or a predisposition to AIDS because of an increased risk of uncontrollable infection or neoplasms; in patients with diabetes mellitus, which may become exacerbated; in patients with ulcerative colitis, diverticulitis, peptic ulcer, or gastritis because symptoms of disease progression may be masked or perforation may occur without warning; and in patients with systemic fungal or tuberculosis infection, which may become exacerbated.

Use in hypothyroidism and cirrhosis may result in an enhanced corticotropin effect. Use in gouty arthritis should be limited to a few days because rebound attacks may follow withdrawal after prolonged use. Corticotropin may aggravate existing emotional instability or psychotic tendencies. Corticotropin should be used cautiously in patients with myasthenia gravis because it *may* cause muscle weakness.

Interactions
Concomitant use of corticotropin with diuretics may accentuate the electrolyte loss associated with diuretic therapy; use with amphotericin B or carbonic anhydrase inhibitors may cause severe hypokalemia. Amphotericin B also decreases adrenal responsiveness to corticotropin. Concurrent use with insulin or oral antidiabetic agents may require increased dosage of the hypoglycemic agent; use with hepatic enzyme-inducing agents may increase corticotropin metabolism resulting from induction of hepatic microsomal enzymes; use with digitalis glycosides may increase the risk of dysrhythmias or digitalis toxicity associated with hypokalemia; and use with cortisone, hydrocortisone, or estrogens may elevate plasma cortisol levels abnormally.

Effects on diagnostic tests
Corticotropin therapy alters blood and urinary glucose levels; sodium and potassium levels; protein-bound iodine levels; radioactive iodine (^{131}I) uptake and liothyronine (T_3) uptake; total protein values; serum amylase, urine amino acid, serotonin, uric acid, calcium, and 17-ketosteroid levels; and leukocyte counts.

High plasma cortisol concentrations may be reported erroneously in patients receiving spironolactone, cortisone, or hydrocortisone when fluorometric analysis is used. This does not occur with the radioimmunoassay or competitive protein-binding method. However, therapy can be maintained with prednisone, dexamethasone, or betamethasone because they are not detectable by the fluorometric method.

Adverse reactions
Uncontrollable adverse reactions may be associated with chronic use of more than 40 units/day.
● CNS: *convulsions*, dizziness, papilledema, headache, euphoria, insomnia, mood swings, personality changes, depression, psychosis, vertigo.
● CV: hypertension, CHF, necrotizing angiitis.
● DERM: impaired wound healing; thin, fragile skin; petechiae; ecchymoses; facial erythema; increased sweating; acne; hyperpigmentation; allergic skin reactions; hirsutism.
● EENT: cataracts, glaucoma, exophthalmos.

● GI: peptic ulcer with *perforation* and *hemorrhage; pancreatitis;* abdominal distention; ulcerative esophagitis; nausea; vomiting.
● GU: menstrual irregularities.
● Metabolic: sodium and fluid retention, calcium and potassium loss, hypokalemic alkalosis, negative nitrogen balance.
● Other: muscle weakness, steroid myopathy, loss of muscle mass, osteoporosis, vertebral compression fractures, cushingoid state, suppression of growth in children, activation of latent diabetes mellitus, progressive increase in antibodies, loss of corticotropin stimulatory effect, *hypersensitivity*.

Overdose and treatment
Specific information unavailable. Treatment is supportive, as appropriate.

▶ Special considerations
● Cosyntropin is less antigenic and less likely to cause allergic reactions than corticotropin. However, allergic reactions occur rarely with corticotropin.
● In patient with suspected sensitivity to porcine proteins, skin testing should be performed. To decrease the risk of anaphylactic reaction in patient with limited adrenal reserves, 1 mg of dexamethasone may be given at midnight before the corticotropin test and 0.5 mg at start of test.
● Use with caution if surgery or emergency treatment is required.
● Observe neonates of corticotropin-treated women for signs of hypoadrenalism.
● Counteract edema by low-sodium, high-potassium intake; nitrogen loss by high-protein diet; and psychotic symptoms by reducing corticotropin dosage or administering sedatives.
● Corticotropin may mask signs of chronic disease and decrease host resistance and ability to localize infection.
● Insulin or oral hypoglycemic dosages may need to be increased during corticotropin therapy.
● Monitor weight, fluid exchange, and resting blood pressure levels until minimal effective dosage is achieved.
● Refrigerate reconstituted product and use within 24 hours.
● If administering gel, warm it to room temperature, draw into large needle, and give slowly, deep I.M. with a 22G needle.
● Corticotropin must not be discontinued abruptly, especially after prolonged therapy. An addisonian crisis may occur.

Information for the patient
● Warn patient that injection is painful.
● Tell patient to report marked fluid retention, muscle weakness, abdominal pain, seizures, or headache.
● Tell patient not to be vaccinated during corticotropin therapy.
● Show patient how to monitor for edema, and teach him about the need for fluid and salt restriction as appropriate.
● Warn patient not to discontinue medication except as prescribed. Tell patient that abrupt discontinuation may provoke severe adverse reactions.

Geriatric use
Use with caution in elderly patients because they are more likely to develop osteoporosis.

Pediatric use
Use with caution because prolonged use of corticotropin will inhibit skeletal growth. Intermittent administration is recommended.

Breast-feeding
Safety has not been established. Because the potential for severe adverse reactions exists, benefits and risks must be weighed.

cortisone acetate
Cortelan*, Cortistab*, Cortone

- Pharmacologic classification: glucocorticoid, mineralocorticoid
- Therapeutic classification: anti-inflammatory, replacement therapy
- Pregnancy risk category C

How supplied
Available by prescription only
Tablets: 5 mg, 10 mg, 25 mg
Injection: 25 mg/ml, 50 mg/ml suspension

Indications, route, and dosage
Adrenal insufficiency, allergy, inflammation
Adults: 25 to 300 mg P.O. or I.M. daily or on alternate days. Doses highly individualized, depending on severity of disease.
Children: 20 to 300 mg/m² P.O. or 7 to 37.5 mg/m² I.M. daily. Dosage must be highly individualized.

Pharmacodynamics
Adrenocorticoid replacement: Cortisone acetate is an adrenocorticoid with both glucocorticoid and mineralocorticoid properties. A weak anti-inflammatory agent, cortisone acetate has only about 80% of the anti-inflammatory activity of an equal weight of hydrocortisone. It is a potent mineralocorticoid, however, having twice the potency of prednisone. Cortisone (or hydrocortisone) is usually the drug of choice for replacement therapy in patients with adrenal insufficiency. It is usually not used for inflammatory or immunosuppressant activity because of the extremely large doses that must be used and because of the unwanted mineralocorticoid effects. The injectable form has a slow onset but a long duration of action. It is usually used only when the oral dosage form cannot be used.

Pharmacokinetics
- *Absorption:* Cortisone is absorbed readily after oral administration, with peak effects in about 1 to 2 hours. The suspension for injection has a variable onset of 24 to 48 hours.
- *Distribution:* Cortisone is distributed rapidly to muscle, liver, skin, intestines, and kidneys. Cortisone is extensively bound to plasma proteins (transcortin and albumin). Only the unbound portion is active. Cortisone is distributed into breast milk and through the placenta.
- *Metabolism:* Cortisone is metabolized in the liver to the active metabolite hydrocortisone, which in turn is metabolized to inactive glucuronide and sulfate metabolites.
- *Excretion:* The inactive metabolites and small amounts of unmetabolized drug are excreted by the kidneys. Insignificant quantities of the drug are also

excreted in feces. The biological half-life of cortisone is 8 to 12 hours.

Contraindications and precautions
Cortisone is contraindicated in patients with systemic fungal infections (except in adrenal insufficiency) or a hypersensitivity to ingredients of adrenocorticoid preparations. Patients who are receiving cortisone should not be given live virus vaccines because cortisone suppresses the immune response.

Cortisone should be used with extreme caution in patients with GI ulceration, renal disease, hypertension, osteoporosis, diabetes mellitus, thromboembolic disorders, seizures, myasthenia gravis, congestive heart failure (CHF), tuberculosis, hypoalbuminemia, hypothyroidism, cirrhosis of the liver, emotional instability, psychotic tendencies, hyperlipidemias, glaucoma, or cataracts, because the drug may exacerbate these conditions.

Because adrenocorticoids increase the susceptibility to and mask symptoms of infection, cortisone should not be used (except in life-threatening situations) in patients with viral or bacterial infections not controlled by anti-infective agents.

Interactions
When used concomitantly, cortisone may decrease the effects of oral anticoagulants by unknown mechanisms (rarely); increase the metabolism of isoniazid and salicylates; and cause hyperglycemia, requiring dosage adjustment of insulin or oral hypoglycemic agents in diabetic patients.

Use with barbiturates, phenytoin, or rifampin may cause decreased corticosteroid effects because of increased hepatic metabolism. Use with cholestyramine, colestipol, or antacids decreases cortisone's effect by adsorbing the corticosteroid, decreasing the amount absorbed.

Cortisone may enhance hypokalemia associated with diuretic or amphotericin B therapy. The hypokalemia may increase the risk of toxicity in patients concurrently receiving digitalis glycosides.

Concomitant use with estrogens may reduce the metabolism of cortisone by increasing the concentration of transcortin. The half-life of cortisone is then prolonged because of increased protein binding. Concomitant administration of ulcerogenic drugs, such as the nonsteroidal anti-inflammatory agents, may increase the risk of GI ulceration.

Effects on diagnostic tests
Cortisone therapy suppresses reactions to skin tests; causes false-negative results in the nitroblue tetrazolium test for systemic bacterial infections; and decreases ^{131}I uptake and protein-bound iodine concentrations in thyroid function tests.

It may increase glucose and cholesterol levels; decrease serum potassium, calcium, thyroxine, and triiodothyronine levels; and increase urine glucose and calcium levels.

Adverse reactions
When administered in high doses or for prolonged therapy, cortisone suppresses release of adrenocorticotropic hormone (ACTH) from the pituitary gland; in turn, the adrenal cortex stops secreting endogenous corticosteroids. The degree and duration of hypothalamic-pituitary-adrenal (HPA) axis suppression produced by the drug is highly variable among patients and depends

on the dose, frequency and time of administration, and duration of cortisone therapy.

- CNS: euphoria, insomnia, headache, psychotic behavior, pseudotumor cerebri, mental changes, nervousness, restlessness.
- CV: CHF, hypertension, edema.
- DERM: delayed healing, acne, skin eruptions, striae.
- EENT: cataracts, glaucoma, thrush.
- GI: peptic ulcer, irritation, increased appetite.
- Immune: immunosuppression, increased susceptibility to infection.
- Metabolic: hypokalemia, sodium retention, fluid retention, weight gain, hyperglycemia, osteoporosis, growth suppression in children.
- Musculoskeletal: muscle atrophy, weakness.
- Local: atrophy at I.M. injection sites.
- Other: *pancreatitis,* hirsutism, cushingoid symptoms, withdrawal syndrome (nausea, fatigue, anorexia, dyspnea, hypotension, hypoglycemia, myalgia, arthralgia, fever, dizziness and fainting). *Sudden withdrawal may be fatal or may exacerbate the underlying disease.* Acute adrenal insufficiency may follow increased stress (infection, surgery, trauma) or abrupt withdrawal after long-term therapy.

Overdose and treatment
Acute ingestion, even in massive doses, is rarely a clinical problem. Toxic signs and symptoms rarely occur if the drug is used for less than 3 weeks, even at large dosage ranges. However, chronic use causes adverse physiologic effects, including suppression of the HPA axis, cushingoid appearance, muscle weakness, and osteoporosis.

▶ Special considerations
Recommendations for use of cortisone and for care and teaching of patients during therapy are the same as those for all *systemic adrenocorticoids.*

Pediatric use
Chronic use of cortisone in children and adolescents may delay growth and maturation.

---

cosyntropin
Cortrosyn

- Pharmacologic classification: anterior pituitary hormone
- Therapeutic classification: diagnostic agent
- Pregnancy risk category C

How supplied
Available by prescription only
Injection: 0.25 mg/vial

Indications, route, and dosage
Diagnostic test of adrenocortical function
Adults and children: 0.25 to 1 mg I.M. or I.V. (unless label prohibits I.V. administration) between blood samplings. To administer as I.V. infusion, dilute 0.25 mg in dextrose 5% in water or normal saline solution, and infuse over 6 to 8 hours (40 mcg/hour).
Children under age 2: 0.125 mg I.M. or I.V.

Pharmacodynamics
Diagnostic action: Cosyntropin is used to test adrenal function. The drug binds with a specific receptor in the adrenal cell plasma membrane to initiate synthesis of its entire spectrum of hormones, one of which is cortisol. In patients with primary adrenocortical insufficiency, cosyntropin does not increase plasma cortisol levels significantly.

Pharmacokinetics
- *Absorption:* Cosyntropin is inactivated by the proteolytic enzymes in the GI tract. After I.M. administration, cosyntropin is absorbed rapidly. After rapid I.V. administration, plasma cortisol levels begin to rise within 5 minutes and double within 15 to 30 minutes. Peak levels occur within 1 hour after I.M. or rapid I.V. administration.
- *Distribution:* Distribution of cosyntropin is not fully understood, but the drug is removed rapidly from plasma by many tissues.
- *Metabolism:* Unknown.
- *Excretion:* Cosyntropin probably is excreted by the kidneys.

Contraindications and precautions
Cosyntropin is contraindicated in patients with known hypersensitivity to the drug; however, it is less antigenic than corticotropin and less likely to produce allergic reactions.

Cosyntropin should be used cautiously in patients with preexisting allergic disease or a history of allergic reactions to corticotropin, because hypersensitivity reactions are possible.

Interactions
Concomitant use of cosyntropin with cortisone, hydrocortisone, or estrogens may cause abnormally elevated plasma cortisol levels. High plasma cortisol levels may be reported erroneously in patients receiving spironolactone, cortisone, or hydrocortisone when fluorometric analysis is used. This does not occur with the radioimmunoassay or competitive protein-binding method. However, therapy can be maintained with prednisone, dexamethasone, or betamethasone because these are not detectable by the fluorometric method.

Effects on diagnostic tests
Cosyntropin therapy alters blood glucose levels.

Adverse reactions
Except for hypersensitivity reactions, short-term administration of cosyntropin is unlikely to produce adverse reactions. Discontinue if hypersensitivity reaction occurs.

Overdose and treatment
Acute overdose probably requires no therapy other than symptomatic treatment and supportive care, as appropriate.

▶ Special considerations
- More cortisol is secreted if dosage is given slowly, not rapidly I.V.
- Cosyntropin is less antigenic than corticotropin and less likely to produce allergic reactions.
- Some clinicians prefer plasma cortisol concentration determinations at 60 minutes after injection of cosyntropin.

• Determine if patient is taking medications containing spironolactone, cortisone, hydrocortisone, or estrogen.
• Reconstitute powder by adding 1 ml of normal saline solution to 0.25-mg vial to yield a solution containing 0.25 mg/ml.
• Reconstituted solution remains stable at room temperature for 24 hours or for 21 days at 2° to 8° C. (36° to 46° F.).
• A normal response to cosyntropin includes morning control plasma cortisol level exceeding 5 mcg/100 ml plasma; 30 minutes after the injection, cortisol levels rise by 7 mcg/100 ml above control; 30 minute cortisol levels exceed 18 mcg/100 ml.

Information for the patient
Find out if the patient is taking spironolactone, cortisone, hydrocortisone, or estrogen. These medications may interfere with test results.

━━━━━━━━━━━━━━━━

co-trimoxazole (trimethoprim-sulfamethoxazole)
Apo-Sulfatrim*, Bactrim, Bactrim DS, Bactrim I.V. Infusion, Bethaprim SS, Cotrim, Novotrimel*, Protrin*, Roubac*, Septra, Septra DS, Septra I.V. Infusion, SMZ-TMP, Sulfatrim, Sulmeprim

• Pharmacologic classification: sulfonamide and folate antagonist
• Therapeutic classification: antibiotic
• Pregnancy risk category B (D at term)

How supplied
Available by prescription only
Tablets: trimethoprim 80 mg and sulfamethoxazole 400 mg; trimethoprim 160 mg and sulfamethoxazole 800 mg
Suspension: trimethoprim 40 mg and sulfamethoxazole 200 mg/5 ml
Injectable: trimethoprim 16 mg and sulfamethoxazole 80 mg/ml (5 ml/ampule)

Indications, route, and dosage
Urinary tract infections and shigellosis
Adults: 160 mg trimethoprim and 800 mg sulfa-methoxazole (double-strength tablet) q 12 hours for 10 to 14 days in urinary tract infections and for 5 days in shigellosis. For simple cystitis or acute urethral syndrome, may give one to three double-strength tablets as a single dose.
Children: 8 mg/kg trimethoprim and 40 mg/kg sulfamethoxazole daily in two divided doses q 12 hours (10 days for urinary tract infections; 5 days for shigellosis).
Otitis media
Children: 8 mg/kg trimethoprim and 40 mg/kg sulfamethoxazole daily, in two divided doses q 12 hours for 10 days.
Pneumocystis carinii *pneumonitis*
Adults and children: 20 mg/kg trimethoprim and 100 mg/kg sulfamethoxazole daily, in equally divided doses q 6 hours for 14 days.
Chronic bronchitis
Adults: 160 mg trimethoprim and 800 mg sulfamethoxazole q 12 hours for 10 to 14 days. Not recommended for infants less than age 2 months.

Dosage in renal failure (parenteral form)
In patients with impaired renal function, dose or frequency of administration must be modified according to degree of renal impairment, severity of infection, and susceptibility of organism.

Creatinine clearance (ml/min/1.73 m^2)	Dosage in adults
> 30	Usual adult dose
15 to 30	One-half the usual adult dose
< 15	Use is not recommended

Creatinine clearance (ml/min/1.73 m^2)	Dosage in children
> 30	Usual pediatric dose
20 to 30	One-half the usual pediatric dose
< 20	Use is contraindicated

Pharmacodynamics
Antibacterial action: Co-trimoxazole is generally bactericidal; it acts by sequential blockade of folic acid enzymes in the synthesis pathway. The sulfamethoxazole component inhibits formation of dihydrofolic acid from para-aminobenzoic acid (PABA), whereas trimethoprim inhibits dihydrofolate reductase. Both drugs block folic acid synthesis, preventing bacterial cell synthesis of essential nucleic acids.

Co-trimoxazole is effective against *Escherichia coli, Klebsiella, Enterobacter, Proteus mirabilis, Haemophilus influenzae, Streptococcus pneumoniae, Staphylococcus aureus, Acinetobacter, Salmonella, Shigella,* and *Pneumocystis carinii.*

Pharmacokinetics
• *Absorption:* Co-trimoxazole is well absorbed from the GI tract after oral administration; peak serum levels occur at 1 to 4 hours.
• *Distribution:* Co-trimoxazole is distributed widely into body tissues and fluids, including middle ear fluid, prostatic fluid, bile, aqueous humor, and CSF. Protein binding is 44% for trimethoprim, 70% for sulfamethoxazole. Co-trimoxazole crosses the placenta.
• *Metabolism:* Co-trimoxazole is metabolized by the liver.
• *Excretion:* Both components of co-trimoxazole are excreted primarily in urine by glomerular filtration and renal tubular secretion; some drug is excreted in breast milk. Trimethoprim's plasma half-life in patients with normal renal function is 8 to 11 hours, extended to 26 hours in severe renal dysfunction; sulfamethoxazole's plasma half-life is normally 10 to 13 hours, extended to 30 to 40 hours in severe renal dysfunction. Hemodialysis removes some co-trimoxazole.

Contraindications and precautions
Do not give co-trimoxazole to patients with known hypersensitivity to sulfonamides (or any other drug containing sulfur, such as thiazides, furosemide, and oral sulfonylureas) or to patients with known hypersensitivity to trimethoprim. Sulfonamides also are contraindicated in patients with severe renal or hepatic dysfunction or porphyria; during pregnancy at term; and during lactation.

━━━━━━━━━━━━━━━━

Co-trimoxazole should be used cautiously in patients with acquired immunodeficiency syndrome (AIDS), because of the increased incidence of adverse reactions; and in patients with mild to moderate renal or hepatic impairment, urinary obstruction because of the hazard of drug accumulation, severe allergies, asthma, blood dyscrasias, and folate or glucose-6-phosphate dehydrogenase deficiency.

Interactions
Co-trimoxazole may inhibit hepatic metabolism of oral anticoagulants, displacing them from binding sites and enhancing anticoagulant effects. Concomitant use of co-trimoxazole with PABA antagonizes sulfonamide effects. Concomitant use with oral sulfonylureas enhances their hypoglycemic effects, probably by displacement of sulfonylureas from protein-binding sites.

Concomitant use of urinary acidifying agents (ammonium chloride or ascorbic acid) decreases urinary pH and sulfonamide solubility, thereby increasing the risk of crystalluria.

Effects on diagnostic tests
Co-trimoxazole alters urine glucose test results utilizing cupric sulfate (Benedict's reagent or Clinitest).

Co-trimoxazole may elevate liver function test results; it may decrease serum concentration levels of erythrocytes, platelets, or leukocytes.

Adverse reactions
● CNS: headache, mental depression, seizures, hallucinations.
● DERM: *erythema multiforme (Stevens-Johnson syndrome),* generalized skin eruption, epidermal necrolysis, *exfoliative dermatitis,* photosensitivity, urticaria, pruritus, petechiae.
● GI: nausea, vomiting, diarrhea, abdominal pain, anorexia, stomatitis.
● GU: toxic nephrosis with oliguria and anuria, crystalluria, hematuria.
● HEMA: *agranulocytosis, aplastic anemia,* megaloblastic anemia, thrombocytopenia, leukopenia, hemolytic anemia.
● Hepatic: jaundice.
● Other: hypersensitivity, serum sickness, drug fever, *anaphylaxis.*
Note: Patients with AIDS have a much higher incidence of all adverse reactions, especially hypersensitivity, rash, fever, hematologic toxicity, and liver function test abnormalities.

Drug should be discontinued if signs of toxicity or hypersensitivity occur; if hematologic abnormalities are accompanied by sore throat, pallor, fever, jaundice, purpura, or weakness; if crystalluria is accompanied by renal colic, hematuria, oliguria, proteinuria, urinary obstruction, urolithiasis, increased blood urea nitrogen levels, or anuria; or if severe diarrhea indicates pseudomembranous colitis. If signs of megaloblastic anemia develop, drug should be discontinued and folinic acid administered to rescue the bone marrow.

Overdose and treatment
Clinical signs of overdose include mental depression, confusion, headache, nausea, vomiting, diarrhea, facial swelling, slight elevations in liver function test results, and bone marrow depression.

Treat by emesis or gastric lavage, followed by supportive care (correction of acidosis, forced fluids, and/or urinary alkalinization to enhance solubility and ex-

cretion). Treatment of renal failure may be required; transfuse appropriate blood products in severe hematologic toxicity; use folinic acid to rescue bone marrow. Hemodialysis has limited ability to remove co-trimoxazole.

▶ Special considerations
Besides those relevant to all *sulfonamides,* consider the following recommendations.
● Co-trimoxazole has been used effectively to treat chronic bacterial prostatitis and as prophylaxis against recurrent urinary tract infection in women and "traveler's" diarrhea.
● For I.V. use, dilute infusion in dextrose 5% in water. Do not mix with other drugs. Do not administer by rapid infusion or bolus injection. Infuse slowly over 60 to 90 minutes. Change infusion site every 48 to 72 hours.
● I.V. infusion must be diluted before use. Each 5 ml should be added to 125 ml dextrose 5% in water (D_5W). Do not refrigerate solution; diluted solutions must be used within 6 hours. A dilution of 5 ml per 100 ml may be prepared for patients requiring fluid restriction, but these solutions should be used within 4 hours.
● Check solution carefully for precipitate before starting infusion. Do not use solution containing a precipitate.
● Assess I.V. site for signs of phlebitis or infiltration.
● Shake oral suspension thoroughly before administering.
● Note that DS means double-strength.

Geriatric use
In elderly patients, diminished renal function may prolong half-life. Such patients also have an increased risk of adverse reactions.

Breast-feeding
Use with caution in breast-feeding women.

PHARMACOLOGIC CLASS

coumarin derivatives

dicumarol
warfarin sodium

Oral anticoagulants were discovered in 1924, when some cows developed a bleeding disorder after eating spoiled sweet clover. Since 1954, when human clinical trials established their safety and effectiveness in clotting disorders, oral anticoagulants have significantly reduced morbidity and mortality in patients with various disorders.

Pharmacology
Dicumarol and warfarin are coumarin derivatives. They interfere with the hepatic synthesis of vitamin K-dependent clotting factors II, VII, IX, and X, decreasing the blood's coagulation potential; they have no direct effect on established thrombi and cannot reverse ischemic tissue damage. However, oral anticoagulant therapy may prevent additional clot formation or extension of formed clots, as well as other complications of thrombosis.

Clinical indications and actions
Treatment or prevention of thrombosis or embolism

Interference with clotting factor synthesis by oral anticoagulants is used to prevent or treat deep vein thrombosis or pulmonary embolism and to prevent coronary occlusion, myocardial infarction, or other thrombotic events in selected patients.

Overview of adverse reactions

Adverse reactions to oral anticoagulants are usually an extension of their therapeutic actions. Bleeding is the primary complication: it ranges from mild gum bleeding to major hemorrhage.

▶ Special considerations

● Obtain prothrombin time (PT) before initiation of drug and daily during initial therapy for dosage adjustment; follow hospital policy for anticoagulant administration.
● Dosage is determined by PT; therapy usually aims to maintain PT at 1.5 to 2 times normal. Numerical PT values depend on procedure and reagents used in the individual laboratory.
● During maintenance therapy, check PT as often as twice a week or as infrequently as every 6 weeks, depending on consistency of PT and patient's reliability and clinical status.
● Because of delayed onset of action, heparin is commonly given during the first few days of treatment. Do not check PT within 5 hours of intermittent heparin use; however, PT may be checked at any time during continuous heparinization.
● Use caution when adding or stopping any drug in patients taking anticoagulants; some drugs alter clotting time or interact with coumarin derivatives and the combination may cause either hemorrhage or rethrombosis.
● Check patient regularly for bleeding gums, bruises on arms or legs, petechiae, nosebleeds, hemoptysis, melena, tarry stools, hematuria, or hematemesis, which indicate increased bleeding; for sudden onset of lumbar pain, which may signal retroperitoneal hemorrhage; and for fever and skin rash, which may signal other severe complications.
● Prescribe administration at same time daily to ensure compliance and daily laboratory result availability.
● After cardiac valve replacement, a coumarin anticoagulant may be given concomitantly with dipyridamole to help prevent postoperative thromboembolic complications.

Information for the patient

● Explain disease process and rationale for drug therapy; stress importance of complying with recommended amount and timing of dosage, and of keeping follow-up appointments.
● Stress importance of taking a missed dose as soon as possible. If the missed dose is not remembered until the next day, the patient should not take it; doubling the dose can cause bleeding. Tell the patient to report any missed doses.
● Tell patient to carry a card that identifies him as a potential bleeder, and to inform any other physicians or dentists who may be treating him.
● Tell patient and family to watch for bruising and other signs of increased bleeding, and to call immediately if these or other severe complications occur; heavier-than-usual menses may also necessitate dosage adjustment.

● Warn patient to avoid nonprescription products containing aspirin, other salicylates, or drugs that may interact with the anticoagulant, causing an increase or decrease in its action. Advise patient to seek medical approval before stopping or starting any medication.
● Explain that PT is increased by fever, long periods of hot weather, malnutrition, and diarrhea.
● Tell patient that drugs may turn alkaline urine red-orange.
● Advise patient not to substantially alter daily intake of leafy green vegetables (asparagus, broccoli, cabbage, lettuce, turnip greens, spinach, watercress) or of fish, pork or beef liver, green tea, or tomatoes; these foods contain vitamin K, and widely varying daily intake may alter anticoagulant effect.
● Explain that smoking may also increase dosage requirement, because of changes in metabolism; light to moderate alcohol intake does not significantly alter PT.
● Advise patient to take special precautions against cutting or bruising his skin; for example, by using an electric razor when shaving and a soft toothbrush to prevent gum irritation.

Geriatric use

Elderly patients are more susceptible to effects of anticoagulants and are at greater risk of hemorrhage. That may be caused by altered hemostatic mechanisms or age-related deterioration of hepatic and renal functions.

Pediatric use

Infants, especially neonates, may be more susceptible to anticoagulants because of vitamin K deficiency.

Breast-feeding

Women should avoid breast-feeding during therapy with anticoagulants if possible; these drugs appear in breast milk, and may cause coagulation problems in the infant. Recent evidence suggests that these quantities may be insufficient to cause clinical problems; however, more data are needed to establish safety.

Representative combinations

None.

---

cromolyn sodium
Intal Aerosol Spray, Intal Nebulizer Solution, Nasalcrom, Opticrom

● Pharmacologic classification: chromone derivative
● Therapeutic classification: mast cell stabilizer, antiasthmatic
● Pregnancy risk category B

How supplied

Available by prescription only
Aerosol: 800 mcg/metered spray
Solution: 20 mg/2 ml for nebulization
Ophthalmic solution: 4% (with benzalkonium chloride 0.01%, EDTA 0.01%, and phenylethyl alcohol 0.4%)
Nasal solution: 5.2 mg/metered spray (40 mg/ml)

Indications, route, and dosage

Adjunct in treatment of severe perennial bronchial asthma

Adults and children over age 5: 2 q.i.d. at regular intervals. Also available as an aqueous solution administered through a nebulizer.

Prevention and treatment of allergic rhinitis

Adults and children over age 5: 1 spray (5.2 mg) of the nasal solution in each nostril t.i.d or q.i.d. May give up to 6 times daily.

Prevention of exercise-induced bronchospasm

Adults and children over age 5: 2 metered sprays using inhaler no more than 1 hour before anticipated exercise.

Inhalation of 20 mg of the oral inhalation solution may be used in adults or children age 2 and over. Repeat inhalation as required for protection during long exercise.

Allergic ocular disorders (giant papillary conjunctivitis, vernal keratoconjunctivitis, vernal keratitis, and allergic keratoconjunctivitis)

Adults and children over age 4: Instill 1 to 2 drops in each eye 4 to 6 times daily at regular intervals. One drop contains approximately 1.6 mg cromolyn sodium.

Pharmacodynamics

● Antiasthmatic action: Cromolyn prevents release of the mediators of Type I allergic reactions, including histamine and slow-reacting substance of anaphylaxis (SRS-A), from sensitized mast cells after the antigen-antibody union has taken place. Cromolyn does not inhibit the binding of the IgE to the mast cell nor the interaction between the cell-bound IgE and the specific antigen. It does inhibit the release of substances (such as histamine and SRS-A) in response to the IgE binding to the mast cell. The main site of action occurs locally on the lung mucosa, nasal mucosa, and eyes.

● Bronchodilating action: Besides the mast cell stabilization, recent evidence suggests that the drug may have a bronchodilating effect by an unknown mechanism. Comparative studies have shown cromolyn and theophylline to be equally efficacious but less effective than orally inhaled B$_2$-adrenergic agonists in preventing this bronchospasm.

● Ocular antiallergy action: Cromolyn inhibits the degranulation of sensitized mast cells that occurs after exposure to specific antigens, preventing the release of histamine and SRS-A.

Cromolyn has no direct anti-inflammatory, vasoconstrictor, antihistamine, antiserotonin, or corticosteroid-like properties.

Cromolyn dissolved in water and given orally has been found to be effective in managing food allergy, inflammatory bowel disease (Crohn's disease, ulcerative colitis), and systemic mastocytosis.

Pharmacokinetics

● Absorption: Only 0.5% to 2% of an oral dose is absorbed. The amount reaching the lungs depends on the patient's ability to use the inhaler correctly, the amount of bronchoconstriction, and the size or presence of mucous plugs. The degree of absorption depends on the method of administration; the most absorption occurs with the aerosol via metered-dose inhaler, and the least occurs with the administration of the solution via power-operated nebulizer. Less than 7% of an intranasal dose of cromolyn as a solution is absorbed systemically. Only minimal absorption (0.03%) of an ophthalmic dose occurs after instillation into the eye. The absorption half-life from the lung is 1 hour. A plasma concentration of 9 mcg/ml can be achieved 15 minutes after following a 20-mg dose.

● Distribution: Cromolyn does not cross most biological membranes because it is ionized and lipid-insoluble at the body's pH. Less than 0.1% of a cromolyn dose crosses to the placenta; it is not known if the drug is distributed into breast milk.

● Metabolism: None significant.

● Excretion: Cromolyn is excreted unchanged in urine (50%) and bile (approximately 50%). Small amounts may be excreted in the feces or exhaled. The elimination half-life is 81 minutes.

Contraindications and precautions

Cromolyn is contraindicated in patients with a hypersensitivity to cromolyn or any ingredient in these products. It should be not be used to treat acute asthma, especially status asthmaticus, because it is a prophylactic drug with no benefit in acute situations.

Cromolyn's safety in pregnancy has not been established. It should be used only when benefit clearly outweighs the risk to the fetus.

Interactions

None reported.

Effects on diagnostic tests

None reported.

Adverse reactions

● CNS: dizziness, headache, vertigo, neuritis.
● DERM: rash, urticaria, dermatitis.
● EENT: lacrimation, swollen parotid gland, irritation of the throat and trachea, cough, bronchospasm after inhalation of dry powder; esophagitis; nasal congestion; pharyngeal irritation; wheezing.
● GI: nausea, dry mouth, vomiting, esophagitis.
● GU: dysuria, urinary frequency, nephrosis.
● Other: joint swelling and pain, angioedema, myalgia.

Overdose and treatment

No information available.

▶ Special considerations

● Pulmonary status should be monitored before and immediately after therapy.
● Bronchospasm or cough occasionally occur after inhalation and may require stopping the therapy. Prior bronchodilation may help but it may still be necessary to stop the cromolyn therapy.
● Asthma symptoms may recur if cromolyn dosage is reduced below the recommended dosage.
● Patients with impaired renal or hepatic function should receive reduced dosage.
● Eosinophilic pneumonia or pulmonary infiltrates with eosinophilia requires stopping the drug.
● Nasal solution may cause nasal stinging or sneezing immediately after instillation of the drug but this reaction rarely requires discontinuation of the drug.
● Watch for recurrence of asthmatic symptoms when corticosteroids are also used. Use only when acute episode has been controlled, airway is cleared, and patient is able to inhale.
● Patients considered for cromolyn therapy should have pulmonary function tests to confirm significant bronchodilator-reversible component of airway obstruction.
● Protect oral solution and ophthalmic solution from direct sunlight.

● Therapeutic effects may not be seen for 2 to 4 weeks after initiating therapy.

Information for the patient
● Teach correct use of metered-dose inhaler: exhale completely before placing mouthpiece between lips, then inhale deeply and slowly with steady, even breath; remove inhaler from mouth, hold breath for 5 to 10 seconds, and exhale.
● Teach patient how to instill eye drops correctly. Because ophthalmic solution contains benzalkonium chloride as a preservative, advise patient not to wear soft contact lenses during treatment.
● Urge patient to call if drug causes wheezing or coughing.
● Instruct patients with asthma or seasonal or perennial allergic rhinitis to administer the drug at regular intervals to ensure clinical effectiveness.
● Advise patient that gargling and rinsing mouth after administration can help reduce mouth dryness.
● The patient who is taking prescribed adrenocorticoids should continue taking them during cromolyn therapy, if appropriate.
● Tell a patient who uses a bronchodilator inhaler to administer a dose about 5 minutes before taking cromolyn (unless otherwise indicated); explain that this step helps reduce adverse reactions.

Pediatric use
Cromolyn use in children under age 5 is limited to the inhalation route of administration. The safety of the nebulizer solution in children under age 2 has not been established. Safety of the nasal solution in children under age 6 has not been established.

crotaline (Crotalidae) antivenin, polyvalent

● Pharmacologic classification: antivenin
● Therapeutic classification: snake anti-venin
● Pregnancy risk category C

How supplied
Available by prescription only
Injection: combination package – one vial of lyophilized serum, one vial of diluent (10 ml bacteriostatic water for injection), and one 1-ml vial of normal horse serum (diluted 1:10) for sensitivity testing

Indications, route, and dosage
Crotalid (pit viper) bites, including those from rattlesnakes, copperheads, and cotton-mouth moccasins
Adults and children: The following initial doses (given I.M., S.C., or I.V.) are recommended (based on level of envenomation): minimal – 2 to 4 vials; moderate – 5 to 9 vials; severe – 10 to 15 or more vials.
  Subsequent dosages are based on the patient's response; 10 ml q 30 minutes to 2 hours, as needed, may be given. If bite is in an extremity, inject part of the initial dose at various sites around the limb above the swelling; do not inject in finger or toe.
  The smaller the patient, the larger the initial dose. The amount of antivenin given to a child is not based on weight. Children may require a larger dose than adults.
  Note: I.V. route is preferred and is mandatory if shock is present.

Pharmacodynamics
Antivenin action: Crotaline antivenin neutralizes and binds venom.

Pharmacokinetics
When given I.M., crotaline antivenin may not reach maximum blood levels until about 8 hours after administration.

Contraindications and precautions
Crotaline antivenin is contraindicated in patients with a history of allergy or a positive sensitivity test to horse serum. However, the risk of administering antivenin must be weighed against the risk of withholding it, because severe envenomation can be fatal.

Interactions
Concomitant use of crotaline antivenin with corticosteroids may mask the severity of hypovolemia in moderate to severe envenomation and may have little, if any, effect on the local tissue response to snake venoms. However, corticosteroids may be administered, if necessary, to treat immediate or delayed allergic reactions to antivenin.

Effects on diagnostic tests
None reported.

Adverse reactions
● Systemic: *hypersensitivity,* shock, *anaphylaxis, serum sickness* (marked by malaise, fever, nausea, vomiting, urticaria, lymphadenopathy, edema, arthralgia, muscle weakness, and peripheral neuritis occurring 5 to 24 days after administration).

Overdose and treatment
No information available.

▶ Special considerations
● Immobilize patient immediately. Splint the bitten extremity.
● Obtain a thorough patient history of allergies, especially to horses and horse immune serum, and previous reactions to immunizations.
● Early use of antivenin (within 4 hours of the bite) is recommended for best results.
● This product is derived from horses immunized with *Crotalidae* venom. Therefore, test patient for sensitivity (against a control of normal saline solution in opposing extremity) before giving it. Give 0.02 to 0.03 ml of the 1:10 dilution of horse serum (provided) intradermally. Read results after 5 to 30 minutes.
Positive reaction: wheal with or without pseudopodia and surrounding erythema. If sensitivity test is positive, follow desensitization schedule.
● Epinephrine solution 1:1,000 should be available to treat allergic reactions.
● Pregnancy is not a contraindication to the use of crotaline antivenin when indicated.
● Monitor circumference of bitten area before and after antivenin administration.
● Find out when the patient received last tetanus immunization; a booster may be indicated at this time.
● Type and cross-match as soon as possible because

---

hemolysis from venom prevents accurate cross matching.
● Monitor fluid intake and urine output.
● Watch patient carefully for delayed allergic reactions or relapse.
● This painful snakebite characteristically requires supportive, symptomatic, and pharmacologic management.
● Monitor vital signs at frequent intervals (that is, every 30 minutes) until symptoms subside (usually in 1 to 3 hours). Also monitor hemoglobin and hematocrit levels, CBC with differential, platelets, coagulation studies (prothrombin time and partial thromboplastin time), bleeding time, chemistry panel, and urinalysis.
● Antibiotic therapy may be necessary for wound infection.

Information for the patient
● Tell patient that he may experience allergic reactions (such as rash, joint swelling or pain, fever, or difficulty breathing) because this product is derived from an animal source, namely horses. Explain that he will be monitored closely and given medication, as needed, to ease such effects.
● Warn patient that delayed reactions to antivenin may occur up to 24 days after its administration. Have patient call if he experiences such symptoms as fever, general malaise, swollen lymph nodes, edema, nausea and vomiting, and joint and muscle pain.

Breast-feeding
Patient should discontinue breast-feeding until the effects of the venom have subsided and if symptoms of serum sickness develop.

---

crotamiton
Eurax

- Pharmacologic classification: synthetic chloroformate salt
- Therapeutic classification: scabicide and antipruritic
- Pregnancy risk category C

How supplied
Available by prescription only
Cream: 10%
Lotion: 10% (emollient base)

Indications, route, and dosage
Scabicide
Adults and children: Wash thoroughly and scrub away loose scales, then towel dry; massage drug onto skin of the entire body from the neck to the toes (with special attention to skin folds, creases, and interdigital spaces). Repeat application in 24 hours. Take a cleansing bath 48 hours after the final application. Repeat if necessary.
Antipruritic
Adults and children: Apply locally b.i.d. or t.i.d.

Pharmacodynamics
The mechanisms of crotamiton's scabicidal and antipruritic actions are unknown. Crotamiton is toxic to the parasitic mite *Sarcoptes scabiei.*

Pharmacokinetics
Absorption, distribution, metabolism, and excretion of crotamiton have not been reported.

Contraindications and precautions
Do not apply crotamiton to acutely inflamed or raw skin.
Crotamiton is contraindicated in patients with a history of hypersensitivity to the drug and in those who exhibit primary irritation after application of the drug.

Interactions
None reported.

Effects on diagnostic tests
None reported.

Adverse reactions
● Local: irritation, contact dermatitis.
Note: Drug should be discontinued if sensitization develops.

Overdose and treatment
Discontinue therapy.

▶ Special considerations
● Avoid applying crotamiton to the face, eyes, mucous membranes, or urethral meatus.
● Patients may require isolation and special care of linens until treatment is complete.
● If primary irritation or hypersensitivity occurs, discontinue treatment and remove drug with soap and water.

Information for the patient
● All clothing and bed linen used by the patient should be machine-washed in hot water and dried in hot dryer or dry-cleaned.
● Patient should reapply drug if accidentally washed off but should avoid overuse.
● Advise patient that pruritus may persist after treatment.

---

cyanocobalamin (vitamin B₁₂)
Bay Bee-12, Berubigen, Betalin 12, Cabadon-M, Cobex, Crystimin-1000, Cyanoject, Cyomin, Kaybovite-1000, Pernavit, Redisol, Rubesol-1000, Rubramin PC, Sytobex, Vibal

hydroxocobalamin (vitamin B₁₂ₐ)
Alphamin, AlphaRedisol, Codroxomin, Droxomin, Hybalamin, Hydrobexan, Hydro-Cobex, Hydroxo-12, Hydroxocobalamin, LA-12, Vibal L.A.

- Pharmacologic classification: water-soluble vitamin
- Therapeutic classification: vitamin, nutrition supplement
- Pregnancy risk category A (C if > recommended daily allowance [RDA])

How supplied
Available by prescription only
Injection: 30-ml vials (30 mcg/ml, 100 mcg/ml, 120 mcg/ml with benzyl alcohol, 1,000 mcg/ml, 1,000 mcg/ml

---

with benzyl alcohol), 10-ml vials (100 mcg/ml, 100 mcg/ml with benzyl alcohol, 1,000 mcg/ml, 1,000 mcg/ml with benzyl alcohol, 1,000 mcg/ml with methyl and propyl parabens), 5-ml vials (1,000 mcg/ml with benzyl alcohol), 1-ml vials (1,000 mcg/ml with benzyl alcohol), 1-ml unimatic (1,000 mcg/ml with benzyl alcohol)
Tablets: 25 mcg, 50 mcg, 100 mcg, 250 mcg, 500 mcg, 1,000 mcg

Indications, route, and dosage

Vitamin B_{12} deficiency from any cause except malabsorption related to pernicious anemia or other GI disease
Adults: 25 mcg P.O. daily as dietary supplement, or 30 to 100 mcg S.C. or I.M. daily for 5 to 10 days, depending on severity of deficiency.
Maintenance dose: 100 to 200 mcg I.M. monthly. For subsequent prophylaxis, advise adequate nutrition and daily RDA vitamin B_{12} supplements.
Children: 1 mcg P.O. daily as dietary supplement, or 1 to 30 mcg S.C. or I.M. daily for 5 to 10 days, depending on severity of deficiency.
Maintenance dose: At least 60 mcg I.M. or S.C. monthly. For subsequent prophylaxis, advise adequate nutrition and daily RDA vitamin B_{12} supplements.
Pernicious anemia or vitamin B_{12} malabsorption
Adults: Initially, 100 to 1,000 mcg I.M. daily for 2 weeks, then 100 to 1,000 mcg I.M. monthly for life. If neurologic complications are present, follow initial therapy with 100 to 1,000 mcg I.M. once every 2 weeks before starting monthly regimen.
Children: 1,000 to 5,000 mcg I.M. or S.C. given over 2 or more weeks in 100-mcg increments; then 60 mcg I.M. or S.C. monthly for life.
Methylmalonic aciduria
Neonates: 1,000 mcg I.M. daily for 11 days with a protein-restricted diet.
Diagnostic test for vitamin B_{12} deficiency without concealing folate deficiency in patients with megaloblastic anemias
Adults and children: 1 mcg I.M. daily for 10 days with diet low in vitamin B_{12} and folate. Reticulocytosis between days 3 and 10 confirms diagnosis of vitamin B_{12} deficiency.
Schilling test flushing dose
Adults and children: 1,000 mcg I.M. in a single dose.

Pharmacodynamics

Nutritional action: Vitamin B_{12} can be converted to coenzyme B_{12} in tissues and, as such, is essential for conversion of methyl-malonate to succinate and synthesis of methionine from homocystine, a reaction that also requires folate. Without coenzyme B_{12}, folate deficiency occurs. Vitamin B_{12} is also associated with fat and carbohydrate metabolism and protein synthesis. Cells characterized by rapid division (epithelial cells, bone marrow, and myeloid cells) appear to have the greatest requirement for vitamin B_{12}.
Vitamin B_{12} deficiency may cause megaloblastic anemia, GI lesions, and neurologic damage; it begins with an inability to produce myelin followed by gradual degeneration of the axon and nerve. Parenteral administration of vitamin B_{12} completely reverses the megaloblastic anemia and GI symptoms of vitamin B_{12} deficiency.

Pharmacokinetics

● *Absorption:* After oral administration, vitamin B_{12} is absorbed irregularly from the distal small intestine. Vitamin B_{12} is protein-bound, and this bond must be split by proteolysis and gastric acid before absorption. Absorption depends on sufficient intrinsic factor and calcium. Vitamin B_{12} is inadequate in malabsorptive states and in pernicious anemia. Vitamin B_{12} is absorbed rapidly from I.M. and S.C. injection sites; the plasma level peaks within 1 hour. After oral administration of doses below 3 mcg, peak plasma levels are not reached for 8 to 12 hours.
● *Distribution:* Vitamin B_{12} is distributed into the liver, bone marrow, and other tissues, including the placenta. At birth, the vitamin B concentration in neonates is three to five times that in the mother. Vitamin B_{12} is distributed into breast milk in concentrations approximately equal to the maternal vitamin B_{12} concentration. Unlike cyanocobalamin, hydroxocobalamin is absorbed more slowly parenterally and may be taken up by the liver in larger quantities; it also produces a greater increase in serum cobalamin levels and less urinary excretion.
● *Metabolism:* Cyanocobalamin and hydroxocobalamin are metabolized in the liver.
● *Excretion:* In healthy persons receiving only dietary vitamin B_{12}, approximately 3 to 8 mcg of the vitamin is secreted into the GI tract daily, mainly from bile, and all but about 1 mcg is reabsorbed; less than 0.25 mcg is usually excreted in the urine daily. When vitamin B_{12} is administered in amounts that exceed the binding capacity of plasma, the liver, and other tissues, it is free in the blood for urinary excretion.

Contraindications and precautions

Vitamin B_{12} is contraindicated in patients with known hypersensitivity to cobalt, vitamin B_{12}, or any component of these medications. An intradermal test dose is recommended. After starting vitamin B_{12} therapy, serum potassium concentrations should be monitored to avoid fatal hypokalemia. Vitamin B_{12} should be administered cautiously to persons who are susceptible to gout (because of the potential for increased nucleic acid degeneration) and to those with heart disease (because of the potential for increased blood volume).
Vitamin B_{12} should not be used in patients with hereditary optic nerve atrophy (Leber's disease) because rapid optic nerve atrophy has been reported as an adverse effect.

Interactions

Concomitant use of the following drugs decreases vitamin B_{12} absorption from the GI tract: aminoglycosides, colchicine, extended-release potassium preparations, aminosalicylic acid and its salts, anticonvulsants, cobalt irradiation of the small bowel, and excessive alcohol intake. Concurrent administration of colchicine may increase neomycin-induced malabsorption of vitamin B_{12}. Large amounts of ascorbic acid should not be administered within 1 hour of taking vitamin B_{12} because ascorbic acid may destroy vitamin B_{12}. In patients with pernicious anemia, vitamin B_{12} absorption and intrinsic factor secretion may be increased. Vitamin B_{12} and chloramphenicol should not be given concurrently because of an antagonized hematopoietic response. Careful monitoring of the hematologic response and alternate therapy is necessary.

Effects on diagnostic tests

Vitamin B_{12} therapy may cause false-positive results for intrinsic factor antibodies, which are present in the blood of half of all patients with pernicious anemia.

Methotrexate, pyrimethamine, and most anti-infectives invalidate diagnostic blood assays for vitamin B_{12}.

Adverse reactions

● CV: *pulmonary edema, congestive heart failure (early in treatment)*, peripheral vascular thrombosis.
● DERM: itching, transitory exanthema, urticaria.
● EENT: severe optic nerve atrophy in patients with 2Leber's disease.
● GI: mild, transient diarrhea.
● HEMA: polycythemia vera.
● Local: pain at injection site.
● Other: *anaphylactic shock* and death, feeling that entire body is swelling, hypokalemia.

Overdose and treatment

Not applicable. Even in large doses, vitamin B_{12} is usually nontoxic.

▶ Special considerations

● The recommended RDA for vitamin B_{12} is 0.3 mcg in infants to 2 mcg in adults, as follows:
Infants age 0 to 6 months: 0.3 mcg
Children age 6 months to 1 year: 0.5 mcg
Children age 1 to 3 years: 0.7 mcg
Children age 4 to 6 years: 1.0 mcg
Children age 7 to 10 years: 1.4 mcg
Children age 11 to adult: 2.0 mcg
Pregnant women: 2.2 mcg
Lactating women: 2.6 mcg
● Determine patient's diet and drug history, including patterns of alcohol use, to identify poor nutritional habits.
● Oral solution should be administered promptly after mixing with fruit juice. Ascorbic acid causes instability of vitamin B_{12}.
● Administer oral vitamin B_{12} with meals to increase absorption.
● Monitor bowel function because regularity is essential for consistent absorption of oral preparations.
● Do not mix the parenteral form with dextrose solutions, alkaline or strongly acidic solutions, or oxidizing and reducing agents, because anaphylactic reactions may occur with I.V. use. Check compatibility with pharmacist.
● Parenteral therapy is preferred for patients with pernicious anemia because oral administration may be unreliable. In patients with neurologic complications, prolonged inadequate oral therapy may lead to permanent spinal cord damage. Oral therapy is appropriate for mild conditions without neurologic signs and for those patients who refuse or are sensitive to the parenteral form.
● Monitor vital signs in patients with cardiac disease and those receiving parenteral vitamin B_{12}. Watch for symptoms of pulmonary edema, which tend to develop early in therapy.
● Patients with a history of sensitivities and those suspected of being sensitive to vitamin B_{12} should receive an intradermal test dose before therapy begins. Sensitization to vitamin B_{12} may develop after as many as 8 years of treatment.
● Expect therapeutic response to occur within 48 hours; it is measured by laboratory values and effect on fa-

tigue, GI symptoms, anorexia, pallid or yellow complexion, glossitis, distaste for meat, dyspnea on exertion, palpitation, neurologic degeneration (paresthesias, loss of vibratory and position sense and deep reflexes, incoordination), psychotic behavior, anosmia, and visual disturbances.
● Therapeutic response to vitamin B_{12} may be impaired by concurrent infection, uremia, folic acid or iron deficiency, or drugs having bone marrow suppressant effects. Large doses of vitamin B_{12} or B_{12a} may improve folate-deficient megaloblastic anemia.
● Expect reticulocyte concentration to rise in 3 to 4 days, peak in 5 to 8 days, and then gradually decline as erythrocyte count and hemoglobin rise to normal levels (in 4 to 6 weeks).
● Monitor potassium levels during the first 48 hours, especially in patients with pernicious anemia or megaloblastic anemia. Potassium supplements may be required. Conversion to normal erythropoiesis increases erythrocyte potassium requirement and can result in fatal hypokalemia in these patients.
● Patients with mild peripheral neurologic defects may respond to concomitant physical therapy. Usually, neurologic damage that does not improve after 12 to 18 months of therapy is considered irreversible. Severe vitamin B_{12} deficiency that persists for 3 months or longer may cause permanent spinal cord degeneration.
● Continue periodic hematologic evaluations throughout the patient's lifetime.

Information for the patient

● Emphasize the importance of a well-balanced diet. To prevent progression of subacute combined degeneration, do not use folic acid instead of vitamin B_{12} to prevent anemia.
● Tell the patient to avoid smoking, which appears to increase requirement for vitamin B_{12}.
● Tell patient to report infection or disease in case his condition requires increased dosage of vitamin B_{12}.
● Tell patient with pernicious anemia that he must have lifelong treatment with vitamin B_{12} to prevent recurring symptoms and the risk of incapacitating and irreversible spinal cord damage.

Pediatric use

● Safety and efficacy of vitamin B_{12} for use in children have not been established. Intake for children should be 0.5 to 2 mcg daily, as recommended by the Food and Nutrition Board of the National Academy of Sciences – National Research Council.
● Some of these products contain benzyl alcohol, which has been associated with a fatal "gasping syndrome" in premature infants.

Breast-feeding

Vitamin B_{12} is excreted in breast milk in concentrations that approximate the maternal vitamin B_{12} level. The Food and Nutrition Board of the National Academy of Sciences – National Research Council recommends that breast-feeding women consume 2.6 mcg/day of vitamin B_{12}.

---

cyclandelate
Cyclospasmol

- Pharmacologic classification: mandelic acid derivative
- Therapeutic classification: antispasmodic, vasodilator
- Pregnancy risk category C

How supplied
Available by prescription only
Tablets: 100 mg
Capsules: 200 mg, 400 mg

Indications, route, and dosage
Adjunct in vascular ischemic states
Drug is possibly effective in intermittent claudication, arteriosclerosis obliterans, vasospasm and muscular ischemia associated with thrombophlebitis, nocturnal leg cramps, Raynaud's phenomenon, selected cases of ischemic cerebral vascular disease.
Adults: Initially, 1.2 to 1.6 g daily in divided doses before meals and h.s. When clinical response is noted, decrease dosage by 200 mg decrements until maintenance dosage is reached. Maintenance dose is 400 to 800 mg daily in two to four divided doses.

Pharmacodynamics
Cyclandelate relaxes smooth muscle directly via inhibition of phosphodiesterase, increasing concentration of cyclic adenosine monophosphate (cAMP).

Pharmacokinetics
- *Absorption:* Cyclandelate is absorbed completely and rapidly from the GI tract; maximum effect of a single dose occurs in 1½ hours. Clinical improvement may require several weeks.
- *Distribution:* Not available.
- *Metabolism:* Metabolic fate of cyclandelate is not fully understood; animal studies indicate metabolism to mandelic acid, presumably by serum and hepatic enzymes.
- *Excretion:* Cyclandelate is excreted in urine.

Contraindications and precautions
Cyclandelate is contraindicated in patients with known hypersensitivity to the drug. Use cyclandelate with extreme caution in patients with severe obliterative coronary artery disease, since blood flow to diseased areas may be compromised by drug's vasodilating effects elsewhere. Although prolonged bleeding time has not been reported with human therapeutic use, it has occurred in animals at very high doses; keep this possibility in mind when giving drug to patients with active bleeding. Use drug cautiously in patients with glaucoma.

The efficacy of cyclandelate in the treatment of peripheral vascular disease has not been established, and the drug should not be used as a substitute for appropriate medical or surgical therapy for the treatment of peripheral or cerebral vascular disease.

Interactions
None reported.

Effects on diagnostic tests
None reported.

Adverse reactions
- CNS: headache, tingling of extremities, dizziness.
- CV: mild flushing, tachycardia.
- GI: eructation, nausea, heartburn, pain.
- Other: sweating.

Overdose and treatment
Clinical signs of overdose include nausea, vomiting, flushing, severe hypotension, tachycardia, and cardiac arrhythmias.

To reduce absorption, induce emesis and give activated charcoal followed by a cathartic. Thereafter treat symptomatically and supportively. Treat hypotension with I.V. fluids and dopamine.

▶ Special considerations
Minimize GI distress by administering drug with meals or antacids.

Information for the patient
- Explain that drug is an adjunct and not a substitute for appropriate medical or surgical therapy.
- Explain that clinical improvement may require several weeks; encourage patient to comply with long-term therapy.

Breast-feeding
Safety in breast-feeding women has not been established.

cyclizine hydrochloride
Marezine

cyclizine lactate
Marezine, Marzine*

- Pharmacologic classification: piperazine-derivative antihistamine
- Therapeutic classification: antiemetic and antivertigo agent
- Pregnancy risk category B

How supplied
Available with or without prescription

hydrochloride
Tablets: 50 mg

lactate
Injection: 50 mg/ml

Indications, route, and dosage
Motion sickness (prophylaxis and treatment)
Adults: 50 mg P.O. (hydrochloride) ½ hour before travel, then q 4 to 6 hours, p.r.n., to maximum of 200 mg daily; or 50 mg I.M. (lactate) q 4 to 6 hours, p.r.n.

Pharmacodynamics
- *Antiemetic action:* Cyclizine probably inhibits nausea and vomiting by centrally depressing sensitivity of the labyrinth apparatus that relays stimuli to the chemoreceptor trigger zone and thus stimulates the vomiting center in the brain.

• *Antivertigo action:* Cyclizine depresses conduction in vestibular-cerebellar pathways and reduces labyrinth excitability.

Pharmacokinetics
• *Absorption:* Not well characterized; onset of action is between 30 and 60 minutes.
• *Distribution:* Drug is well distributed throughout the body.
• *Metabolism:* Cyclizine is metabolized in the liver.
• *Excretion:* Unknown: drug effect lasts 4 to 6 hours.

Contraindications and precautions
Cyclizine is contraindicated in patients with known hypersensitivity to drug or other antiemetic antihistamines with a similar chemical structure, such as buclizine, meclizine, or dimenhydrinate.

Cyclizine should be used with caution in patients with narrow-angle glaucoma, asthma, prostatic hypertrophy, severe heart failure, or GU or GI obstruction, because of its anticholinergic effects. Drug may mask signs of intestinal obstruction or brain tumor.

Interactions
Additive sedative and CNS depressant effects may occur when cyclizine is used concomitantly with other CNS depressants, such as alcohol, barbiturates, tranquilizers, sleeping agents, or antianxiety agents; drug should not be given to patients taking ototoxic medications, such as aminoglycosides, salicylates, vancomycin, loop diuretics, and cisplatin, because it may mask signs of ototoxicity.

Effects on diagnostic tests
Discontinue cyclizine 4 days before diagnostic skin testing, to avoid preventing, reducing, or masking test response.

Adverse reactions
• CNS: drowsiness, dizziness, vertigo, auditory and visual hallucinations, restlessness, nervousness, insomnia, euphoria.
• CV: hypotension, tachycardia, palpitations.
• EENT: blurred vision, tinnitus, dry nose and throat.
• GI: anorexia, nausea, vomiting, diarrhea, constipation, dry mouth, cholestatic jaundice.
• GU: urinary retention and frequency, dysuria.

Overdose and treatment
Overdose and treatment for cyclizine is not documented; however, symptoms may be anticipated to approximate those of other antihistamine H₁-receptor antagonists. Clinical manifestations of overdose may include either CNS depression (sedation, reduced mental alertness, apnea, and cardiovascular collapse) or CNS stimulation (insomnia, hallucinations, tremors, or convulsions). Anticholinergic symptoms, such as dry mouth, flushed skin, fixed and dilated pupils, and GI symptoms, are common, especially in children.

Treat overdose with gastric lavage to empty stomach contents; inducing emesis with ipecac syrup may be ineffective. Treat hypotension with vasopressors, and control seizures with diazepam or phenytoin. *Do not give stimulants.*

▶ **Special considerations**
Besides those relevant to all *antihistamines,* consider the following recommendations.
• Injectable cyclizine is for I.M. use only. When giving

I.M., aspirate and check carefully for blood return; inadvertent I.V. administration can cause anaphylactic reaction.
• Injectable solution is incompatible with many drugs; check compatibility before mixing in same syringe.
• Store in a cool place; at room temperature, injection may turn slightly yellow but does not indicate loss of potency.

Information for the patient
• Instruct patients to position themselves in places of minimal motion (such as in the middle, not front or back, of ship), to avoid excessive intake of food or drink, and not to read while in motion.
• Tell patient to avoid hazardous activities requiring mental alertness until CNS reaction is determined.

Geriatric use
Elderly patients are usually more sensitive to adverse effects of antihistamines and are especially likely to experience a greater degree of dizziness, sedation, hyperexcitability, dry mouth, and urinary retention than younger patients.

Pediatric use
Not indicated for use in children under age 6; they may experience paradoxical hyperexcitability.

Breast-feeding
Antihistamines such as cyclizine should not be used during breast-feeding. Many of these drugs are secreted in breast milk, exposing the infant to risks of unusual excitability; premature infants are at particular risk for convulsions. Cyclizine also may inhibit lactation.

---

cyclobenzaprine
Flexeril

• Pharmacologic classification: tricyclic antidepressant derivative
• Therapeutic classification: skeletal muscle relaxant
• Pregnancy risk category B

How supplied
Available by prescription only
Tablets: 10 mg

Indications, route, and dosage
Adjunct in acute, painful musculoskeletal conditions
Adults: 20 to 40 mg P.O. divided b.i.d. to q.i.d.; maximum dosage, 60 mg daily. Drug should not be administered for more than 2 to 3 weeks.

Pharmacodynamics
Skeletal muscle relaxant action: Cyclobenzaprine relaxes skeletal muscles through an unknown mechanism of action. Cyclobenzaprine is a CNS depressant.

Cyclobenzaprine also potentiates the effects of norepinephrine and exhibits anticholinergic effects similar to those of tricyclic antidepressants, including central and peripheral antimuscarinic actions, sedation, and an increase in heart rate.

Pharmacokinetics

● *Absorption:* Cyclobenzaprine is almost completely absorbed during first pass through GI tract. Onset of action occurs within 1 hour, with peak concentrations in 3 to 8 hours. Duration of action is 12 to 24 hours.
● *Distribution:* Cyclobenzaprine is 93% plasma protein-bound.
● *Metabolism:* During first pass through GI tract and liver, drug and metabolites undergo enterohepatic recycling.
● *Excretion:* Cyclobenzaprine is excreted primarily in urine as conjugated metabolites; also in feces via bile as unchanged drug.

Contraindications and precautions

Cyclobenzaprine is contraindicated in patients with hyperthyroidism, congestive heart failure, arrhythmias, heart block, or conduction disorders, because of its cardiovascular effects, in those in acute recovery stage after myocardial infarction, in known hypersensitivity to the drug, and in patients who have received monoamine oxidase (MAO) inhibitors within 14 days.

Administer cautiously to patients with urinary retention, narrow-angle glaucoma, increased intraocular pressure, impaired hepatic or renal function, and those receiving anticholinergic drugs because of its adverse anticholinergic effects.

Interactions

Concomitant use with CNS depressant drugs, including alcohol, narcotics, anxiolytics, antipsychotics, tricyclic antidepressants, and parenteral magnesium salts, may potentiate the CNS depressant's effects.

Antimuscarinic effects may be potentiated when cyclobenzaprine is used with antidyskinetics or antimuscarinics (especially atropine and related compounds).

Cyclobenzaprine may decrease or block the antihypertensive effects of guanadrel or guanethidine. Concurrent use with MAO inhibitors is not recommended for outpatients.

Hyperpyretic crisis, severe seizures, and death have resulted from the tricyclic antidepressant-like effect of cyclobenzaprine. Allow 14 days to elapse after discontinuance of MAO inhibitor therapy before starting cyclobenzaprine, and 5 to 7 days after discontinuance of cyclobenzaprine therapy and start of MAO inhibitor.

Effects on diagnostic tests

None significant.

Adverse reactions

● CNS: drowsiness, dizziness, fatigue, headache, nervousness, confusion, ataxia, vertigo, tremors, hypertonia, paresthesia, disorientation, insomnia, depressed mood, anxiety, agitation, abnormal thinking and dreaming, excitement, hallucinations.
● CV: *tachycardia*, hypotension, syncope, palpitations, vasodilation, *arrhythmia.*
● GI: dyspepsia, nausea, constipation, unpleasant taste, vomiting, anorexia, diarrhea, GI pain, gastritis, flatulence, dry mouth.
● Other: blurred vision, rash, urinary frequency or retention, decreased libido, impotence, tinnitus, jaundice, thirst.
    Note: Drug should be discontinued if the patient develops signs of hypersensitivity or shows no therapeutic benefit after 14 days of therapy.

Overdose and treatment

Clinical manifestations of overdose include severe drowsiness, troubled breathing, syncope, seizures, tachycardia, arrhythmias, hallucinations, increase or decrease in body temperature, and vomiting.

To treat overdose, induce emesis or perform gastric lavage. As ordered, give 20 to 30 g activated charcoal every 4 to 6 hours for 24 to 48 hours. Take ECG and monitor cardiac functions for arrhythmias. Monitor vital signs, especially body temperature and ECG. Maintain adequate airway and fluid intake. If needed, 1 to 3 mg I.V. physostigmine may be given to combat severe life-threatening antimuscarinic effects. Provide supportive therapy for arrhythmias, cardiac failure, circulatory shock, seizures, and metabolic acidosis as necessary.

▶ **Special considerations**
● Drug may cause effects and adverse reactions similar to those of tricyclic antidepressants.
● Note that drug's antimuscarinic effect may inhibit salivary flow, resulting in development of dental caries, periodontal disease, oral candidiasis, and mouth discomfort.
● Allow 14 days to elapse after discontinuance of MAO inhibitors before starting cyclobenzaprine; 5 to 7 days after discontinuing cyclobenzaprine before starting MAO inhibitors.
● Monitor for GI problems.
● Cyclobenzaprine is intended for short-term (2 or 3 weeks) treatment, because risk-benefit ratio associated with prolonged use is not known. Additionally, muscle spasm accompanying acute musculoskeletal conditions is usually transient.
● Spasmolytic effect usually begins within 1 or 2 days and may be manifested by lessening of pain and tenderness and an increase in range of motion and ability to perform activities of daily living.

Information for the patient

● Warn patient about possible drowsiness and dizziness. Tell patient to avoid hazardous activities that require alertness until reaction to drug is known.
● Advise patient to avoid alcohol and other CNS depressants (unless prescribed), because combined use with cyclobenzaprine will cause additive effects.
● Advise patient to relieve dry mouth (anticholinergic effect) with frequent clear water rinses, extra fluid intake, or with sugarless gum or candy.
● Tell patient to report discomfort immediately.
● Patient should use cough and cold preparations cautiously, as some may contain alcohol.
● If treatment lasts longer than 2 weeks, patient should check with dentist to minimize risk of dental disease (tooth decay, fungal infections, or gum disease).

Geriatric use

Elderly patients are more sensitive to drug's effects.

Pediatric use

Not recommended for children under age 15.

cyclopentolate hydrochloride
AK-Pentolate, Cyclogyl, I-Pentolate, Minims Cyclopentolate*, Pentolair

- Pharmacologic classification: anticholinergic agent
- Therapeutic classification: cyloplegic, mydriatic
- Pregnancy risk category C

How supplied
Available by prescription only
Ophthalmic solution: 0.5%, 1%, 2%

Indications, route, and dosage
Diagnostic procedures requiring mydriasis and cycloplegia
Adults: Instill 1 drop of 1% solution in eye, followed by another drop in 5 minutes. Use 2% solution in heavily pigmented irises.
Children: Instill 1 drop of 0.5%, 1%, or 2% solution in each eye, followed by 1 drop of 0.5% or 1% solution in 5 minutes, if necessary.

Pharmacodynamics
Cycloplegic and mydriatic action: Anticholinergic action prevents the sphincter muscle of the iris and the muscle of the ciliary body from responding to cholinergic stimulation. This results in unopposed adrenergic influence, producing pupillary dilation (mydriasis) and paralysis of accommodation (cycloplegia).

Pharmacokinetics
- *Absorption:* Peak mydriatic effect occurs within 30 to 60 minutes and cycloplegic effect within 25 to 75 minutes.
- *Distribution:* Unknown.
- *Metabolism:* Unknown.
- *Excretion:* Recovery from mydriasis usually occurs in about 24 hours; recovery from cycloplegia may occur in 6 to 24 hours.

Contraindications and precautions
Cyclopentolate is contraindicated in patients with narrow-angle glaucoma and in patients with hypersensitivity to any component of the preparation. It should be used with caution in patients in whom increased intraocular pressure may occur; and in children because of increased risk of cardiovascular and CNS effects. Do not use solutions more concentrated than 0.5% in neonates.

Interactions
Cyclopentolate may increase the bioavailability of nitrofurantoin from the anticholinergic effect of delayed gastric emptying. It also may interfere with the antiglaucoma action of pilocarpine, carbachol, or cholinesterase inhibitors.

Effects on diagnostic tests
None reported.

Adverse reactions
- CNS: ataxia, irritability, confusion (failure to identify people), somnolence, hallucinations, *seizures*, and behavioral disturbances in children.
- CV: flushing, tachycardia.
- Eye: burning sensation on instillation, increased intraocular pressure, blurred vision, exudate, photophobia, ocular congestion, contact dermatitis, conjunctivitis.
- Other: dry skin and mouth, fever, urinary retention.
  Note: Drug should be discontinued if behavioral disturbances occur.

Overdose and treatment
Clinical manifestations of overdose include flushing, warm dry skin, dry mouth, dilated pupils, delirium, hallucinations, tachycardia, bladder distention, ataxia, hypotension, respiratory depression, coma, and death. Induce emesis or give activated charcoal. Use physostigmine to antagonize cyclopentolate's anticholinergic activity, and in severe toxicity; propranolol may be used to treat symptomatic tachyarrhythmias unresponsive to physostigmine.

▶ Special considerations
Superior to homatropine hydrobromide, cyclopentolate has a shorter duration of action.

Information for the patient
- Warn patient that drug will cause burning sensation when instilled.
- Advise patient to protect eyes from bright illumination; dark glasses may reduce sensitivity.

Geriatric use
Drug should be used with caution in elderly patients because undiagnosed narrow-angle glaucoma may be present.

Pediatric use
- Avoid getting the preparation in a child's mouth while administering.
- Infants and young children may experience an increased sensitivity to the cardiopulmonary and CNS effects of cyclopentolate.
- Young infants should not be given any solution more concentrated than 0.5%.

Breast-feeding
No data available; however, use cyclopentolate with extreme caution in breast-feeding women because of potential for CNS and cardiopulmonary effects in infants.

cyclophosphamide
Cytoxan, Neosar

- Pharmacologic classification: alkylating agent (cell cycle-phase nonspecific)
- Therapeutic classification: antineoplastic
- Pregnancy risk category D

How supplied
Available by prescription only
Tablets: 25 mg, 50 mg
Injection: 100-mg, 200-mg, 500-mg, 1-g, 2-g vials

Indications, route, and dosage
Dosage and indications may vary. Check literature for recommended protocols.

Breast, head, neck, lung, and ovarian carcinoma; Hodgkin's disease; chronic lymphocytic or myelocytic and acute lymphoblastic leukemia; neuroblastoma; retinoblastoma; non-Hodgkin's lymphomas; multiple myeloma; mycosis fungoides; sarcomas; severe rheumatoid disorders; glomerular and nephrotic syndrome (in children); immunosuppression after transplants

Adults: 40 to 50 mg/kg P.O. or I.V. in single dose or in two to five doses, then adjust for maintenance; or 2 to 4 mg/kg P.O. daily for 10 days, then adjust for maintenance. Maintenance dosage, 1 to 5 mg/kg P.O. daily; 10 to 15 mg/kg I.V. q 7 to 10 days; or 3 to 5 mg/kg I.V. twice weekly.

Children: 2 to 8 mg/kg or 60 to 250 mg/m² P.O. or I.V. daily for 6 days (dosage depends on susceptibility of neoplasm); divide oral dosages; give I.V. dosages once weekly. Maintenance dosage is 2 to 5 mg/kg or 50 to 150 mg/m² P.O. twice weekly.

†*Polymyositis*
Adults: 1 to 2 mg/kg P.O. daily.
†*Rheumatoid arthritis*
Adults: 1.5 to 3 mg/kg P.O. daily.
†*Wegener's granulomatosis*
Adults: 1 to 2 mg/kg P.O. daily (usually administered with prednisone).

Pharmacodynamics
Antineoplastic action: The cytotoxic action of cyclophosphamide is mediated by its two active metabolites. These metabolites function as alkylating agents, preventing cell division by cross-linking DNA strands. This results in an imbalance of growth within the cell, leading to cell death. Cyclophosphamide also has significant immunosuppressive activity.

Pharmacokinetics
• *Absorption:* Cyclophosphamide is almost completely absorbed from the GI tract at doses of 100 mg or less. Higher doses (300 mg) are approximately 75% absorbed.
• *Distribution:* Cyclophosphamide is distributed throughout the body, although only minimal amounts have been found in saliva, sweat, and synovial fluid. The concentration in the cerebrospinal fluid is too low for treatment of meningeal leukemia. The active metabolites are approximately 50% bound to plasma proteins.
• *Metabolism:* Cyclophosphamide is metabolized to its active form by hepatic microsomal enzymes. The activity of these metabolites is terminated by metabolism to inactive forms.
• *Excretion:* Cyclophosphamide and its metabolites are eliminated primarily in urine, with 15% to 30% excreted as unchanged drug. The plasma half-life ranges from 4 to 6½ hours.

Contraindications and precautions
Use cyclophosphamide with caution in young men and women of childbearing age because it may impair fertility; in pregnant women because it may be fetotoxic; in lactating women because of potential harm to the neonate; and in patients with myelosuppression or infections because of potentially severe immunosuppression.

Interactions
Concomitant use of cyclophosphamide with barbiturates, phenytoin, or chloral hydrate increases the rate of metabolism of cyclophosphamide to toxic metabolites. These agents are known to be inducers of hepatic microsomal enzymes. These drugs should be discontinued before cyclophosphamide therapy.

Corticosteroids are known to initially inhibit the metabolism of cyclophosphamide, reducing its effect. Eventual reduction of dose or discontinuation of steroids may increase metabolism of cyclophosphamide to a toxic level. Other drugs that may inhibit cyclophosphamide metabolism include allopurinol, chloramphenicol, chloroquine, imipramine, phenothiazines, potassium iodide, and vitamin A.

Patients on cyclophosphamide therapy who receive succinylcholine as an adjunct to anesthesia may experience prolonged respiratory distress and apnea. This may occur up to several days after the discontinuation of cyclophosphamide. The mechanism of this interaction is that cyclophosphamide depresses the activity of pseudocholinesterases, the enzyme responsible for the inactivation of succinylcholine. Use succinylcholine with caution or not at all.

Concomitant use of cyclophosphamide may potentiate the cardiotoxic effects of doxorubicin.

Effects on diagnostic tests
Cyclophosphamide may suppress positive reaction to *Candida,* mumps, tricophyton, and tuberculin TB skin tests. A false-positive result for the Papanicolaou test may occur. Cyclophosphamide therapy may also increase serum uric acid concentrations and decrease serum pseudocholinesterase concentrations.

Adverse reactions
• CV: *cardiotoxicity* (with very high doses and in combination with doxorubicin), thrombophlebitis.
• GI: anorexia; nausea and vomiting beginning within 6 hours, lasting 4 hours; stomatitis; mucositis; diarrhea.
• GU: gonadal suppression (may be irreversible), *hemorrhagic cystitis* (may develop in approximately 10% of patients because of poor hydration), bladder fibrosis, *nephrotoxicity.*
• HEMA: *bone marrow depression* (dose-limiting); *leukopenia* (nadir between days 8 and 15, recovery in 17 to 28 days); *thrombocytopenia;* anemia.
• Metabolic: hyperuricemia syndrome of inappropriate ADH secretion (with high doses).
• Other: reversible alopecia in 50% of patients, especially with high doses; secondary malignancies; *pulmonary fibrosis* (with high doses); fever; *anaphylaxis;* dermatitis.
Note: Drug should be discontinued if hemorrhagic cystitis develops.

Overdose and treatment
Clinical manifestations of overdose include myelosuppression, alopecia, nausea, vomiting, and anorexia. Treatment is generally supportive and includes transfusion of blood components and antiemetics. Cyclophosphamide is dialyzable.

▶ **Special considerations**
Besides those relevant to all *alkylating agents,* consider the following recommendations.
• Follow institutional guidelines for the safe preparation, administration, and disposal of chemotherapeutic drugs.

• Reconstitute vials with appropriate volume of bacteriostatic or sterile water for injection to give a concentration of 20 mg/ml.
• Reconstituted solution is stable 6 days if refrigerated or 24 hours at room temperature.
• Cyclophosphamide can be given by direct I.V. push into a running I.V. line or by infusion in normal saline solution or dextrose 5% in water.
• Avoid all I.M. injections when platelet counts are low.
• Oral medication should be taken with or after a meal. Higher oral doses (400 mg) may be tolerated better if divided into smaller doses.
• Administration with cold foods such as ice cream may improve toleration of oral dose.
• Push fluid (3 liters daily) to prevent hemorrhagic cystitis. Some clinicians use uroprotectant agents such as mesna. Drug should not be given at bedtime, because voiding afterward is too infrequent to avoid cystitis. If hemorrhagic cystitis occurs, discontinue drug. Cystitis can occur months after therapy has been discontinued.
• Reduce dosage of cyclophosphamide if patient is concomitantly receiving corticosteroid therapy and develops viral or bacterial infections.
• Monitor for cyclophosphamide toxicity if patient's corticosteroid therapy is discontinued.
• Monitor uric acid, CBC, and renal and hepatic functions.
• Observe for hematuria and ask patient if he has dysuria.
• Nausea and vomiting are most common with high doses of I.V. cyclophosphamide.
• Use cautiously in severe leukopenia, thrombocytopenia, malignant cell infiltration of bone marrow, after recent radiation therapy or chemotherapy, and in hepatic or renal disease.
• The dosage of cyclophosphamide should be adjusted for renal impairment.
• Has been used successfully to treat many nonmalignant conditions, for example, multiple sclerosis, because of its immunosuppressive activity.

Information for the patient
• Advise both male and female patients to practice contraception while taking this drug and for 4 months after; drug is potentially teratogenic.
• Emphasize importance of continuing medication despite nausea and vomiting.
• Advise patient to report vomiting that occurs shortly after an oral dose.
• Warn patient that alopecia is likely to occur, but that it is reversible.
• Encourage adequate fluid intake to prevent hemorrhagic cystitis and to facilitate uric acid excretion.

Breast-feeding
Cyclophosphamide is excreted into breast milk; therefore, breast-feeding should be discontinued because of the risk of serious adverse reactions, mutagenicity, and carcinogenicity in the infant.

cycloserine
Seromycin

• Pharmacologic classification: isoxizolidone, d-alanine analog
• Therapeutic classification: antitubercular agent
• Pregnancy risk category C

How supplied
Available by prescription only
Capsules: 250 mg

Indications, route, and dosage
Adjunctive treatment in pulmonary or extrapulmonary tuberculosis
Adults: Initially, 250 mg P.O. q 12 hours for 2 weeks; then, if blood levels are below 25 to 30 mcg/ml and there are no clinical signs of toxicity, dosage is increased to 250 mg P.O. q 8 hours for 2 weeks. If optimum blood levels are still not achieved, and there are no signs of clinical toxicity, then dosage is increased to 250 mg P.O. q 6 hours. Maximum dosage is 1 g/day. If CNS toxicity occurs, drug is discontinued for 1 week, then resumed at 250 mg/day for 2 weeks. If no serious toxic effects occur, dose is increased by 250-mg increments every 10 days until blood levels reach 25 to 30 mcg/ml.

Pharmacodynamics
Antibiotic action: Cycloserine inhibits bacterial cell utilization of amino acids, thereby inhibiting cell wall synthesis. Its action is bacteriostatic or bactericidal, depending on organism susceptibility and drug concentration at infection site. Cycloserine is active against Mycobacterium tuberculosis, M. bovis, and some strains of M. kansasii, M. marinum, M. ulcerans, M. avium, M. smegmatis, and M. intracellulare. It is also active against some gram-negative and gram-positive bacteria, including Staphylococcus aureus, Enterobacter, and Escherichia coli. Cycloserine is considered adjunctive therapy in tuberculosis and is combined with other antituberculosis agents to prevent or delay development of drug resistance by M. tuberculosis.

Pharmacokinetics
• Absorption: About 80% of an oral dose of cycloserine is absorbed from the GI tract; peak serum concentrations occur 3 to 4 hours after ingestion.
• Distribution: Cycloserine is distributed widely into body tissues and fluids, including CSF. Cycloserine crosses the placenta; it does not bind to plasma proteins.
• Metabolism: Cycloserine may be metabolized partially.
• Excretion: Cycloserine is excreted primarily in urine by glomerular filtration. Small amounts of drug are excreted in feces and breast milk. Elimination plasma half-life in adults is 10 hours. Cycloserine is hemodialyzable.

Contraindications and precautions
Cycloserine is contraindicated in patients with known hypersensitivity to cycloserine; in patients with mental depression, epilepsy, severe anxiety, or psychosis because drug may exacerbate symptoms of these disorders; in patients with severe renal impairment be-

cause of potential for drug accumulation; and in frequent users of alcohol because of increased potential for seizures.

Use cautiously in patients taking isoniazid, ethionamide, or phenytoin.

Interactions
Concomitant use with isoniazid or ethionamide increases hazard of CNS toxicity, drowsiness, and dizziness; concomitant use with alcohol may increase incidence of seizures.

Cycloserine may inhibit metabolism of phenytoin, producing toxic blood levels of phenytoin. Dosage adjustment may be required.

Effects on diagnostic tests
Cycloserine may elevate serum transaminase levels, especially in patients with preexisting hepatic disease.

Adverse reactions
● CNS: drowsiness, headache, tremor, dysarthria, vertigo, confusion, loss of memory, *possible suicidal tendencies* and other psychotic symptoms, nervousness, hallucinations, depression, hyperirritability, paresthesias, paresis, hyperreflexia.
● Other: hypersensitivity (allergic dermatitis).
Note: Drug should be discontinued if patient shows signs of hypersensitivity reaction, CNS toxicity, or severe personality changes.

Overdose and treatment
Signs of overdose include CNS depression accompanied by dizziness, hyperreflexia, confusion, or convulsions.

Treat with gastric lavage and supportive care, including oxygen, I.V. fluids, pressor agents (for circulatory shock), and body temperature stabilization. Treat seizures with anticonvulsants and pyridoxine.

▶ Special considerations
● Give drug after meals to avoid gastric irritation.
● Obtain specimens for culture and sensitivity testing before first dose, but therapy can begin before test results are complete; repeat periodically to detect drug resistance.
● Monitor hematologic, renal, and liver function studies before and periodically during therapy to minimize toxicity; toxic reactions may occur at blood levels in excess of 30 mcg/ml.
● Assess level of consciousness and neurologic function; monitor for personality changes and other early signs of CNS toxicity.
● Pyridoxine, anticonvulsants, tranquilizers, or sedatives may be prescribed to relieve adverse reactions.

Information for the patient
● Explain disease process and rationale for long-term therapy.
● Teach signs and symptoms of hypersensitivity and other adverse reactions, and emphasize need to report *any* unusual effects and skin rash promptly.
● Warn patient to avoid hazardous tasks that require mental alertness because drug may cause patient to become drowsy or dizzy.
● Warn patient not to use alcohol; explain hazard of serious CNS toxicity.
● Advise patient to take drug after meals to avoid gastric irritation.
● Urge patient to complete entire prescribed regimen,

to comply with instructions for around-the-clock dosage, and not to discontinue drug without medical approval.
● Explain importance of follow-up appointments.

Geriatric use
Because elderly patients commonly have renal impairment, which decreases excretion of drugs, cycloserine should be used with caution.

Breast-feeding
Cycloserine is excreted in breast milk; use with caution in breast-feeding women.

---

cyclosporine
Sandimmune

● Pharmacologic classification: polypeptide antibiotic
● Therapeutic classification: immunosuppressant
● Pregnancy risk category C

How supplied
Available by prescription only
Capsules: 25 mg, 100 mg
Oral solution: 100 mg/ml
Injection: 50 mg/ml

Indications, route, and dosage
Prophylaxis of organ rejection in kidney, liver, and heart transplants
Adults and children: 15 mg/kg P.O. daily 4 to 12 hours before transplantation. Continue this daily dose postoperatively for 1 to 2 weeks. Then, gradually reduce dosage by 5% per week to maintenance level of 5 to 10 mg/kg/day. Alternatively, administer an I.V. concentrate of 5 to 6 mg/kg 4 to 12 hours before transplantation. Postoperatively, administer this dose daily as an I.V. dilute solution infusion (50 mg per 20 to 100 ml infused over 2 to 6 hours) until patient can tolerate oral forms.

Pharmacodynamics
Immunosuppressant action: The exact mechanism is unknown; purportedly, its action is related to the inhibition of induction of interleukin II, which plays a role in both cellular and humoral immune responses.

Pharmacokinetics
● *Absorption:* Absorption after oral administration varies widely between patients and in the same individual. Only 30% of an oral dose reaches systemic circulation; peak levels occur at 3 to 4 hours.
● *Distribution:* Cyclosporine is distributed widely outside the blood volume. About 33% to 47% is found in plasma; 4% to 9%, in leukocytes; 5% to 12%, in granulocytes; and 41% to 58%, in erythrocytes. In plasma, approximately 90% is bound to proteins, primarily lipoproteins. Cyclosporine crosses the placenta; cord blood levels are about 60% those of maternal blood. Cyclosporine enters breast milk.
● *Metabolism:* Cyclosporine is metabolized extensively in the liver.
● *Excretion:* Elimination is primarily in the feces (biliary excretion) with only 6% of the drug found in urine.

Contraindications and precautions

Cyclosporine is contraindicated in patients with known hypersensitivity to the drug or to polyoxyethylated castor oil. It should be used cautiously in patients with renal or hepatic toxicity or hypertension because drug may exacerbate the signs and symptoms of these conditions.

Interactions

Concomitant use with amphotericin B is likely to increase nephrotoxicity because both drugs are nephrotoxic, and amphotericin may increase cyclosporine blood levels.

Except for corticosteroids, cyclosporine should not be used concomitantly with immunosuppressive agents because of the increased risk of malignancy (lymphoma) and susceptibility to infection.

Erythromycin, ketoconazole, diltiazem, verapamil, and possibly corticosteroids impair hepatic enzyme metabolism and increase plasma cyclosporine levels; reduced dosage of cyclosporine may be necessary. Phenytoin, rifampin, phenobarbital, and co-trimoxazole increase hepatic metabolism and may lower plasma levels of cyclosporine.

Effects on diagnostic tests

Cyclosporine therapy may alter CBC and differential blood tests and may increase serum lipid levels; drug elevation of serum BUN and creatinine and liver function tests may signal nephrotoxicity or hepatotoxicity.

Adverse reactions

● CNS: tremor, *seizures,* headache, paresthesia, ataxia, depression.
● CV: hypertension, chest pain.
● DERM: acne, hirsutism, oily skin, brittle nails.
● EENT: gum hyperplasia, oral thrush, mouth ulcers, visual disturbances, sore throat.
● GI: nausea, vomiting, diarrhea, anorexia, difficulty swallowing, constipation.
● GU: nephrotoxicity, increased BUN and serum creatinine levels, *acute or chronic renal failure.*
● HEMA: leukopenia, thrombocytopenia, anemia.
● Hepatic: hepatotoxicity.
● Other: *anaphylaxis* (with I.V. only), flushing, night sweats, gynecomastia, joint pains.
    Note: Drug should be discontinued if hypersensitivity occurs.

Overdose and treatment

Clinical manifestations of overdose include extensions of common adverse effects. Hepatotoxicity and nephrotoxicity often accompany nausea and vomiting; tremor and seizures may occur. Up to 2 hours after ingestion, empty stomach by induced emesis or lavage; thereafter, treat supportively. Monitor vital signs and fluid and electrolyte levels closely. Cyclosporine is not removed by hemodialysis or charcoal hemoperfusion.

▶ Special considerations

● Cyclosporine usually is prescribed with corticosteroids.
● Possible kidney rejection should be considered before discontinuation of drug for suspected nephrotoxicity.
● Monitor hepatic and renal function tests routinely; hepatotoxicity may occur in the first month after transplantation, but renal toxicity may be delayed for 2 to 3 months.

● Dose should be given at same time each day. Oral solution should be measured carefully in oral syringe and mixed with plain or chocolate milk or fruit juice to increase palatability; it should be served in a glass to minimize drug adherence to container walls. Drug can be taken with food to minimize nausea.

Information for the patient

● Teach patient about rationale for therapy; explain possible side effects and importance of reporting them, especially fever, sore throat, mouth sores, abdominal pain, unusual bleeding or bruising, pale stools, or dark urine.
● Encourage compliance with therapy and follow-up visits.
● Teach patient how and when to take medication for optimal benefit and minimal discomfort; caution against discontinuing drug without medical approval.
● Advise patient to make oral solution more palatable by diluting with room-temperature milk, chocolate milk, or orange juice.

Pediatric use

Safety and efficacy have not been established; however, drug has been used in children as young as 6 months. Use with caution.

Breast-feeding

Safety during breast-feeding has not been established; breast-feeding women should avoid drug.

---

cyproheptadine hydrochloride
Periactin

● Pharmacologic classification: piperidine-derivative antihistamine
● Therapeutic classification: antihistamine (H₁-receptor antagonist), antipruritic agent
● Pregnancy risk category B

How supplied

Available by prescription only
Tablets: 4 mg
Syrup: 2 mg/5 ml

Indications, route, and dosage
Allergy symptoms, pruritus, cold urticaria, allergic conjunctivitis, †appetite stimulant, †vascular cluster headaches

Adults: 4 mg P.O. t.i.d. or q.i.d. Maximum dosage is 0.5 mg/kg daily.
Children age 7 to 14: 4 mg P.O. b.i.d. or t.i.d. Maximum dosage is 16 mg daily.
Children age 2 to 6: 2 mg P.O. b.i.d. or t.i.d. Maximum dosage is 12 mg daily.

Drug also has been used experimentally to stimulate appetite and increase weight gain in children.

Pharmacodynamics
Antihistamine action: Antihistamines compete with histamine for histamine H₁-receptor sites on smooth muscle of the bronchi, GI tract, uterus, and large blood vessels; they bind to cellular receptors, preventing access of histamine, thereby suppressing histamine-

---

induced allergic symptoms. They do not directly alter histamine or its release.

Cyproheptadine also displays significant anticholinergic and antiserotonin activity.

Pharmacokinetics
• *Absorption:* Cyproheptadine is well absorbed from the GI tract; peak action occurs in 6 to 9 hours.
• *Distribution:* Unknown.
• *Metabolism:* Cyproheptadine appears to be almost completely metabolized in the liver.
• *Excretion:* Cyproheptadine's metabolites are excreted primarily in urine; unchanged drug is not excreted in urine. Small amounts of unchanged cyproheptadine and metabolites are excreted in feces.

Contraindications and precautions
Cyproheptadine is contraindicated in patients with known hypersensitivity to this drug or other antihistamines with similar chemical structures, such as azatadine; in patients experiencing asthmatic attacks, because cyproheptadine thickens bronchial secretions; and in patients who have taken monoamine oxidase (MAO) inhibitors within the preceding 2 weeks.

Cyproheptadine should be used with caution in patients with narrow-angle glaucoma; in those with pyloroduodenal obstruction or urinary bladder obstruction from prostatic hyperthrophy or narrowing of the bladder neck, because of their marked anticholinergic effects; in patients with cardiovascular disease, hypertension, or hyperthyroidism, because of the risk of palpitations and tachycardia; and in patients with renal disease, diabetes, bronchial asthma, urinary retention, or stenosing peptic ulcers.

Antihistamines should not be used during pregnancy (especially in the third trimester) or during breast-feeding. Antihistamines have caused convulsions and other severe reactions, especially in premature infants.

Interactions
MAO inhibitors interfere with the detoxification of antihistamines and thus prolong and intensify their central depressant and anticholinergic effects; additive sedative effects result when cyproheptadine is used concomitantly with alcohol or other CNS depressants, such as barbiturates, tranquilizers, sleeping aids, and antianxiety agents.

Serum amylase and prolactin concentrations may be increased when these drugs are administered with thyrotropin-releasing hormone.

Effects on diagnostic tests
Cyproheptadine should be discontinued 4 days before diagnostic skin tests. Antihistamines can prevent, reduce, or mask positive skin test response.

Adverse reactions
• CNS: stimulation, sedation, drowsiness, headache, fatigue, excitability, appetite stimulation, agitation, confusion, visual hallucinations, ataxia, tremors, disturbed coordination.
• CV: hypotension, palpitations, tachycardia.
• DERM: urticaria, photosensitivity.
• EENT: dry nose and throat, blurred vision, tinnitus.
• GI: dry mouth, constipation, jaundice.
• GU: urinary frequency and retention.
• HEMA: hemolytic anemia, leukopenia, thrombocytopenia, appetite stimulation, *agranulocytosis.*
• Metabolic: weight gain.

Overdose and treatment
Clinical manifestations of overdose may include either CNS depression (sedation, reduced mental alertness, apnea, and cardiovascular collapse) or CNS stimulation (insomnia, hallucinations, tremors, or convulsions). Anticholinergic symptoms, such as dry mouth, flushed skin, fixed and dilated pupils, and GI symptoms, are common, especially in children.

Treat overdose by inducing emesis with ipecac syrup (in conscious patient), followed by activated charcoal to reduce further drug absorption. Use gastric lavage if patient is unconscious or ipecac fails. Treat hypotension with vasopressors, and control seizures with diazepam or phenytoin. *Do not give stimulants.*

▶ **Special considerations**
Besides those relevant to all *antihistamines*, consider the following recommendations.
• Cyproheptadine can cause weight gain. Monitor weight.
• In some patients, sedative effect disappears within 3 or 4 days.

Geriatric use
Elderly patients are more susceptible to the sedative effect of drug. Instruct patient to change positions slowly and gradually. Elderly patients may experience dizziness or hypotension more readily than younger patients.

Pediatric use
CNS stimulation (agitation, confusion, tremors, hallucinations) is more common in children and may require dosage reduction. Drug is not indicated for use in newborn or premature infants.

Breast-feeding
Antihistamines such as cyproheptadine should not be used during breast-feeding. Many of these drugs are secreted in breast milk, exposing the infant to risks of unusual excitability; premature infants are at particular risk for convulsions.

cytarabine (ARA-C, cytosine arabinoside)
Cytosar-U

• Pharmacologic classification: antimetabolite (cell cycle-phase specific, S phase)
• Therapeutic classification: antineoplastic
• Pregnancy risk category D

How supplied
Available by prescription only
Injection: 100-mg, 500-mg, 1-g, 2-g vials

Indications, route, and dosage
Dosage and indications may vary. Check literature for recommended protocols.
Acute myelocytic and other acute leukemias
Adults and children: 100 to 200 mg/m² or 3 mg/kg daily by continuous I.V. infusion or rapid I.V. injection in divided doses for 5 days at 2-week intervals for remission induction; or 30 mg/m² intrathecally (range: 5 to 75 mg/m²) q 4 days until cerebrospinal fluid findings are nor-

---

mal. Doses up to 3 g/m² q 12 hours for 12 doses have been given by continuous infusion for refractory acute leukemias.

Pharmacodynamics

Antineoplastic action: Cytarabine requires conversion to its active metabolite within the cell. This metabolite acts as a competitive inhibitor of the enzyme DNA polymerase, disrupting the normal synthesis of DNA.

Pharmacokinetics

● *Absorption:* Cytarabine is poorly absorbed (less than 20%) across the GI tract because of rapid deactivation in the gut lumen. After I.M. or subcutaneous administration, peak plasma levels are less than after I.V. administration.
● *Distribution:* Cytarabine rapidly distributes widely through the body. Approximately 13% of the drug is bound to plasma proteins. The drug penetrates the blood-brain barrier only slightly after a rapid I.V. dose; however, when the drug is administered by a continuous I.V. infusion, cerebrospinal fluid levels achieve a concentration 40% to 60% of that of plasma levels.
● *Metabolism:* Cytarabine is metabolized primarily in the liver but also in the kidneys, GI mucosa, and granulocytes.
● *Excretion:* The elimination of cytarabine has been described as biphasic, with an initial half-life of 8 minutes and a terminal phase half-life of 1 to 3 hours. Cytarabine and its metabolites are excreted in urine. Less than 10% of a dose is excreted as unchanged drug in urine.

Contraindications and precautions

Cytarabine is contraindicated in patients with a history of hypersensitivity to the drug.

Interactions

When used concomitantly, cytarabine decreases the cellular uptake of methotrexate, reducing its effectiveness.

Temporary damage to GI mucosa by cytarabine may impair oral absorption of digoxin.

Effects on diagnostic tests

Cytarabine therapy may increase blood and urine levels of uric acid. It may also increase serum alkaline phosphatase, AST (SGOT), and bilirubin concentrations, which indicate drug-induced hepatotoxicity.

Adverse reactions

● CNS: neurotoxicity; neuritis and peripheral neuropathy (with high-doses).
● DERM: rash, alopecia.
● EENT: *keratitis.*
● GI: nausea; vomiting; diarrhea; dysphagia; reddened area at juncture of lips, followed by sore mouth, oral ulcers in 5 to 10 days; high dose given via rapid I.V. may cause projectile vomiting.
● HEMA: *leukopenia* (nadir 7 to 9 days after drug stopped), anemia, *thrombocytopenia,* reticulocytopenia (platelet nadir occurring on day 10), *megaloblastosis, bone marrow depression* (dose-limiting).
● Hepatic: hepatotoxicity (usually mild and reversible).
● Metabolic: hyperuricemia.
● Other: flulike syndrome.
  Note: Drug should be discontinued if the polymorphonuclear granulocyte count falls below 1,000/mm³; if the platelet count falls below 50,000/mm³ during main-

tenance therapy (not during remission induction therapy).

Overdose and treatment

Clinical manifestations of overdose include myelosuppression, nausea, vomiting, and megaloblastosis.

Treatment is usually supportive and includes transfusion of blood components and antiemetics.

▶ Special considerations

● To reconstitute the 100-mg vial for I.V. administration use 5 ml bacteriostatic water for injection (20 mg/ml) and for the 500-mg vial with 10 ml bacteriostatic water for injection (50 mg/ml).
● Drug may be further diluted with dextrose 5% in water or normal saline solution for continuous I.V. infusion.
● For intrathecal injection, dilute the drug in 5 to 15 ml of lactated Ringer's solution, Elliot's B solution, or normal saline solution with no preservative, and administer after withdrawing an equivalent volume of cerebrospinal fluid.
● Do not reconstitute the drug with bacteriostatic diluent for intrathecal administration because the preservative, benzyl alcohol, has been associated with a higher incidence of neurologic toxicity.
● Reconstituted solutions are stable for 48 hours at room temperature. Infusion solutions up to a concentration of 5 mg/ml are stable for 7 days at room temperature. Discard cloudy reconstituted solution.
● Dose modification may be required in thrombocytopenia, leukopenia, renal or hepatic disease, and after other chemotherapy or radiation therapy.
● Watch for signs of infection (cough, fever, sore throat). Monitor CBC.
● Excellent mouth care can help prevent oral adverse reactions.
● Nausea and vomiting are more frequent when large doses are administered rapidly by I.V. push. These reactions are less frequent with infusion. To reduce nausea, give antiemetic before administering.
● Monitor intake and output carefully. Maintain high fluid intake and give allopurinol, if ordered, to avoid urate nephropathy in leukemia induction therapy. Monitor uric acid levels.
● Monitor hepatic function.
● Monitor patients receiving high doses for cerebellar dysfunction.
● Prescribe steroid eye drops (dexamethasone) to prevent drug-induced keratitis.
● Avoid I.M. injections of any drugs in patients with severely depressed platelet count (thrombocytopenia) to prevent bleeding.
● Pyridoxine supplements may be administered to prevent neuropathies; reportedly, however, prophylactic use of pyridoxine does not prevent cytarabine neurotoxicity.

Information for the patient

● Encourage adequate fluid intake to increase urine output and facilitate excretion of uric acid.
● Advise patient to avoid exposure to people with infections.

Breast-feeding

It is not known whether cytarabine distributes into breast milk. However, because of the risk of serious adverse reactions, mutagenicity, and carcinogenicity in the infant, breast-feeding is not recommended.

---

cytomegalovirus immune globulin (CMV-IGIV, cytomegalovirus immune serum intravenous [human], CytoMune-IV)
CytoGam

- Pharmacologic classification: immune globulin
- Therapeutic classification: immune serum
- Pregnancy risk category C

How supplied
Available by prescription only
Injection: 2.5 g as lyophilized powder with 50 ml sterile water (diluent supplied)

Indications, route, and dosage
To attenuate primary cytomegalovirus (CMV) disease in seronegative kidney transplant recipients who receive a kidney from a CMV seropositive donor
Adults: The maximum total dosage per infusion is 150 mg/kg I.V. administered as follows:
- within 72 hours of transplant: 150 mg/kg
- 2 weeks post-transplant: 100 mg/kg
- 4 weeks post-transplant: 100 mg/kg
- 6 weeks post-transplant: 100 mg/kg
- 8 weeks post-transplant: 100 mg/kg
- 12 weeks post-transplant: 50 mg/kg
- 16 weeks post-transplant: 50 mg/kg

Administer initial dose at 15 mg/kg/hour. Increase to 30 mg/kg/hour after 30 minutes if no untoward reactions occur, then increase to 60 mg/kg/hour after a subsequent 30 minutes if no untoward reactions occur. Volume is not to exceed 75 ml/hour. Subsequent doses may be administered at 15 mg/kg/hour for 15 minutes, increasing as with initial dose at 15-minute intervals.

Pharmacodynamics
Immune action: CMV immune globulin contains a relatively high concentration of immunoglobulin G (IgG) antibodies against CMV and can raise relevant antibodies in CMV-exposed patients to levels sufficient to attenuate or reduce the incidence of serious CMV disease.

Pharmacokinetics
- *Absorption:* CMV immune globulin is administered intravenously.
- *Distribution:* Unknown; other immune globulins distribute between the intravascular and extravascular spaces.
- *Metabolism:* Unknown.
- *Excretion:* Unknown.

Contraindications and precautions
CMV immune globulin is contraindicated in patients with history of sensitivity to other human immune globulin preparations and in patients with selective IgA deficiency.

Interactions
Vaccination with live-virus vaccines should be deferred for at least 3 months after CMV immune globulin administration because of the potential for interference with the immune response to live virus vaccines.

Adverse reactions
- GI: nausea, vomiting.
- Other: flushing, chills, muscle cramps, back pain, fever, wheezing.

Overdose and treatment
Little data is available. Presumed major manifestations would be related to volume overload.

If anaphylaxis or drop in blood pressure occurs, discontinue infusion and administer supportive therapy, including drugs such as diphenhydramine and epinephrine.

▶ Special considerations
- Monitor patient closely during each change or infusion rate.
- Infusion should begin within 6 hours and finish within 12 hours of reconstitution.
- Administer through a separate I.V. line using a constant infusion pump. Filters are not necessary.
- If unable to administer through separate line, piggyback into preexisting line of sodium chloride injection or one of the following dextrose solutions with or without sodium chloride: dextrose 2.5% in water, dextrose 5% in water, dextrose 10% in water, dextrose 20% in water. Do not dilute more than 1:2 with any of the above solutions.
- Monitor vital signs before infusion, midway through infusion, after the infusion, and before any increase in infusion rate.
- Reconstitute as follows. Remove tab portion of vial cap and clean rubber stopper with 70% alcohol or equivalent. Add 50 ml sterile water for injection. *Do not shake vial; avoid foaming.* After adding water, release residual vacuum in vial to hasten the dissolving process. Rotate vial gently to wet all undissolved powder. Allow 30 minutes for powder to dissolve before administration. Inspect vial for clarity and particles.
- Store in refrigerator at 35.6° to 46.4° F. (2° to 8° C.).
- CMV immune globulin provides passive immunity.
- Off-label uses include liver transplants and allergenic bone marrow transplants.

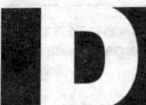

dacarbazine (DTIC)
DTIC-Dome

- Pharmacologic classification: alkylating agent (cell cycle-phase nonspecific)
- Therapeutic classification: antineoplastic
- Pregnancy risk category C

How supplied
Available by prescription only
Injection: 100-mg, 200-mg

Indications, route, and dosage
Dosage and indications may vary. Check current literature for recommended protocols.
Metastatic malignant melanoma
Adults: 2 to 4.5 mg/kg or 70 to 160 mg/m² I.V. daily for 10 days, then repeat q 4 weeks as tolerated; or 250 mg/m² I.V. daily for 5 days, repeated at 3-week intervals.
Hodgkin's disease
Adults: 150 mg/m² for 5 days, repeated q 4 weeks; or 375 mg/m² on day 1, repeated q 15 days (usually used in combination with other drugs).

Pharmacodynamics
Antineoplastic action: Three mechanisms have been proposed to explain the cytotoxicity of dacarbazine: alkylation, in which DNA and RNA synthesis are inhibited; antimetabolite activity as a false precursor for purine synthesis; and binding with protein sulfhydryl groups.

Pharmacokinetics
- *Absorption:* Because of poor absorption from the GI tract, dacarbazine is not administered orally.
- *Distribution:* Dacarbazine is thought to localize in body tissues, especially the liver. The drug crosses the blood-brain barrier to a limited extent. It is minimally bound to plasma proteins.
- *Metabolism:* Dacarbazine is rapidly metabolized in the liver to several compounds, some of which may be active.
- *Excretion:* The elimination of dacarbazine occurs in a biphasic manner, with an initial phase half-life of 19 minutes and terminal phase of 5 hours in patients with normal renal and hepatic function. Approximately 30% to 45% of a dose is excreted in urine.

Contraindications and precautions
Dacarbazine is contraindicated in patients with a history of hypersensitivity to the drug.

Interactions
None reported.

Effects on diagnostic tests
Dacarbazine therapy causes transient increases in serum BUN, ALT (SGPT), AST (SGOT), and alkaline phosphatase levels.

Adverse reactions
- CNS: confusion, headache, paresthesia.
- DERM: phototoxicity, urticaria.
- EENT: blurred vision.
- GI: severe nausea and vomiting begin within 1 to 3 hours in 90% of patients, last 1 to 12 hours; anorexia.
- HEMA: *bone marrow depression* (dose-limiting), *leukopenia and thrombocytopenia* (nadir between 3 and 4 weeks), anemia.
- Local: severe pain if I.V. infiltrates or if solution is too concentrated; tissue damage.
- Other: flulike syndrome (fever, malaise, myalgia beginning 7 days after treatment is stopped and possibly lasting 7 to 21 days), alopecia, facial flushing.
   Note: Drug should be discontinued if hematopoietic toxicity is evident.

Overdose and treatment
Clinical manifestations of overdose include myelosuppression and diarrhea.
   Treatment is usually supportive and includes transfusion of blood components and monitoring of hematologic parameters.

▶ Special considerations
Besides those relevant to all *alkylating agents*, consider the following recommendations.
- To reconstitute the drug for I.V. administration, use a volume of sterile water for injection that gives a concentration of 10 mg/ml (9.9 ml for 100-mg vial, 19.7 ml for 200-mg vial).
- Drug may be diluted further with dextrose 5% in water to a volume of 100 to 200 ml for I.V. infusion over 30 minutes. Increase volume or slow the rate of infusion to decrease pain at infusion site.
- Drug may be administered I.V. push over 1 to 2 minutes.
- A change in solution color from ivory to pink indicates *some* drug degradation. During infusion, protect the solution from light to avoid possible drug breakdown.
- Treatment of extravasation with application of hot packs may relieve burning sensation, local pain, and irritation.
- Discard refrigerated solution after 72 hours; room temperature solution after 8 hours.
- Nausea and vomiting may be minimized by administering dacarbazine by I.V. infusion and by hydrating patient 4 to 6 hours before therapy.
- Monitor uric acid levels.
- Reduce dosage when giving repeated doses to a patient with severely impaired renal function.
- Use lower dose if renal function or bone marrow is impaired. Stop drug if WBC count falls to 3,000/mm³ or platelet count drops to 100,000/mm³. Monitor CBC.
- Monitor daily temperature. Observe for signs of infection.
- Avoid all I.M. injections when platelet count is below 100,000/mm³.
- Anticoagulants and aspirin products should be used cautiously. Watch closely for signs of bleeding.

Information for the patient
● Advise patient to avoid sunlight and sunlamps for first 2 days after treatment.
● Tell patient to avoid contact with people who have infections.
● Reassure patient that growth of hair should return after treatment has ended.
● Reassure patient that flulike syndrome may be treated with mild antipyretics such as acetaminophen.
● Tell patient to avoid aspirin and aspirin-containing products. Teach him the signs and symptoms of bleeding, and urge him to report them promptly.

Breast-feeding
It is not known whether dacarbazine distributes into breast milk. However, because of the risk of serious adverse reactions, mutagenicity, and carcinogenicity in the infant, breast-feeding is not recommended.

dactinomycin (actinomycin D)
Cosmegen

● Pharmacologic classification: antibiotic antineoplastic (cell cycle–phase non-specific)
● Therapeutic classification: antineoplastic
● Pregnancy risk category C

How supplied
Available by prescription only
Injectable: 500-mcg vial

Indications, route, and dosage
Dosage and indications may vary. Check current literature for recommended protocols.
Melanomas, sarcomas, trophoblastic tumors in women, testicular cancer
Adults: 10 to 15 mcg/kg I.V. for a maximum of 5 days every 4 to 6 weeks; or 500 mcg/m² I.V. once a week (maximum 2 mg per week) for 3 weeks.
Wilms' tumor, rhabdomyosarcoma, Ewing's sarcoma
Children: 10 to 15 mcg/kg/day or 450 mcg/m²/day I.V. (maximum dose: 500 mcg/day for 5 days or 2.4 mg/m² in divided doses over 7 days). If all signs of toxicity have disappeared, may be repeated in 4 to 6 weeks.
    Note: Use body surface area calculation in obese or edematous patients.
    For isolation-perfusion, use 50 mcg/kg for lower extremity or pelvis; 35 mcg/kg for upper extremity.

Pharmacodynamics
Antineoplastic action: Dactinomycin exerts its cytotoxic activity by intercalating between DNA base pairs and uncoiling the DNA helix. The result is inhibition of DNA synthesis and DNA-dependent RNA synthesis.

Pharmacokinetics
● *Absorption:* Due to its vesicant properties, dactinomycin must be administered intravenously.
● *Distribution:* Dactinomycin is widely distributed into body tissues, with the highest levels found in the bone marrow and nucleated cells. The drug does not cross the blood-brain barrier to any significant extent.
● *Metabolism:* Dactinomycin is only minimally metabolized in the liver.

● *Excretion:* Dactinomycin and its metabolites are excreted in the urine and bile. The plasma elimination half-life of the drug is 36 hours.

Contraindications and precautions
Dactinomycin is contraindicated in patients who are infected with chicken pox or herpes zoster because of risk of serious generalized disease and death. Drug should be used during pregnancy only when potential benefits to the mother outweigh risks to the fetus.
    Use with extreme caution in patients with renal, hepatic, or bone marrow impairment and viral infections. Use cautiously in metastatic testicular tumors, in combination with chlorambucil and methotrexate therapy. Extreme bone marrow and GI toxicity can occur with this combined therapy.
    Also use cautiously in patients who have received cytotoxic drugs or radiation therapy within 6 weeks, or in patients with a history of gout, infection, or hematologic compromise because of increased potential for adverse effects.

Interactions
None reported.

Effects on diagnostic tests
Dactinomycin therapy may increase blood and urine concentrations of uric acid.

Adverse reactions
Bone marrow depression and GI reactions are the dose-limiting toxicity factors.
● DERM: erythema; desquamation; hyperpigmentation of skin, especially in previously irradiated areas; acnelike eruptions (reversible).
● GI: anorexia, nausea, vomiting, abdominal pain, diarrhea, stomatitis, esophagitis, pharyngitis.
● HEMA: anemia, *leukopenia, thrombocytopenia, pancytopenia,* agranulocytosis.
● Local: phlebitis, severe damage to soft tissue.
● Other: reversible alopecia, hepatotoxicity.
    Note: Drug should be discontinued if diarrhea and stomatitis develop. Therapy may be resumed when these conditions subside.

Overdose and treatment
Clinical manifestations of overdose include myelosuppression, nausea, vomiting, glossitis, and oral ulceration.
    Treatment is generally supportive and includes antiemetics and transfusion of blood components.

▶ ## Special considerations
● To reconstitute for I.V. administration, add 1.1 ml of sterile water for injection to drug to give a concentration of 0.5 mg/ml. Do not use a preserved diluent, as precipitation may occur.
● Use gloves when preparing and administering this drug.
● May dilute further with dextrose 5% in water or normal saline for administration by I.V. infusion.
● Discard any unused solution because it doesn't contain any preservatives.
● May administer by I.V. push injection into the tubing of a freely flowing I.V. infusion. Do *not* administer through an in-line I.V. filter.
● Treatment of extravasation includes topical administration of dimethylsulfoxide and cold compresses.
● To reduce nausea, give antiemetic before adminis-

tering. Nausea usually occurs within 30 minutes of a dose.
● Monitor CBC daily and platelet counts every third day. Observe for signs of bleeding.
● Monitor renal and hepatic functions.
● Patients who have received other cytotoxic drugs or radiation within 6 weeks of dactinomycin may exhibit erythema, followed by hyperpigmentation or edema, or both; desquamation; vesiculation; and, rarely, necrosis.

Information for the patient
● Advise patient to avoid exposure to people with infections.
● Warn patient that alopecia may occur but is usually reversible.
● Tell patient to promptly report sore throat, fever, or any signs of bleeding.

Pediatric use
Restrict use of dactinomycin in infants to those age 6 months or older; adverse reactions are more frequent in infants under age 6 months.

Breast-feeding
The distribution of dactinomycin into breast milk is unknown. However, due to risks of serious adverse reactions, mutagenicity, and carcinogenicity in infants, breast-feeding is not recommended.

danazol
Cyclomen*, Danocrine

● Pharmacologic classification: androgen
● Therapeutic classification: antiestrogen, androgen
● Pregnancy risk category X

How supplied
Available by prescription only
Capsules: 50 mg, 100 mg, 200 mg

Indications, route, and dosage
Endometriosis
Adults: 200 to 400 mg P.O. daily in divided doses b.i.d. In moderate to severe cases, increase to 800 mg daily in divided doses b.i.d. Therapy is continued for 3 to 6 months; may continue for 9 months.
Fibrocystic breast disease
Adults: 100 to 400 mg P.O. daily in two divided doses uninterrupted for 2 to 6 months.
Prevention of hereditary angioedema
Adults: 200 mg P.O. b.i.d. or t.i.d., continued until favorable response is achieved. Then, dosage should be decreased by half at 1- to 3-month intervals.

Pharmacodynamics
● *Antiestrogenic action:* Danazol's antiestrogenic actions cause regression and atrophy of normal and ectopic endometrial tissue. Danazol also decreases the rate of growth and nodularity of abnormal breast tissue in fibrocystic breast disease.
● *Androgenic action:* Danazol's androgenic effects increase levels of the C4 component of complement, which reduces the frequency and severity of attacks associated with hereditary angioedema.

Pharmacokinetics
● *Absorption:* The amount of danazol absorbed by the body is not proportional to the administered dose; doubling the dose of danazol produces an increase of only 35% to 40% in drug absorption.
● *Distribution:* Unknown.
● *Metabolism:* Danazol is metabolized to 2-hydroxymethylethisterone.
● *Excretion:* Unknown.

Contraindications and precautions
Danazol is contraindicated in patients with severe renal or cardiac disease because these conditions may be worsened by the fluid and electrolyte retention this drug may cause; in patients with hepatic disease because impaired elimination may cause toxic accumulation of the drug; in patients with undiagnosed abnormal genital bleeding because danazol can stimulate the growth of cancerous breast or prostate tissue in males; and in pregnant and breast-feeding patients because animal studies have shown that administration of androgens during pregnancy causes masculinization of the fetus.
    Rule out the possibility of breast cancer before beginning therapy with danazol for fibrocystic breast disease. Carefully evaluate breast nodules or masses that may appear or enlarge with danazol therapy.
    Observe female patients carefully for signs of excessive virilization. If possible, discontinue therapy at the first sign of virilization because some adverse effects (deepening of the voice, clitoral enlargement) are not reversible.

Interactions
In patients with diabetes, danazol may cause decreases in blood glucose levels, which may require adjustment of insulin or oral hypoglycemic drugs. Danazol may potentiate the action of warfarin-type anticoagulants, prolonging prothrombin time. It may increase the plasma concentrations of cyclosporine.

Effects on diagnostic tests
Glucose tolerance test results may be abnormal. Total serum thyroxine (T_4) may be decreased; triiodothyronine (T_3) may be increased. Prothrombin time (especially in patients on anticoagulant therapy) may be prolonged.

Adverse reactions
● CNS: dizziness, headache, sleep disorders, fatigue, nervousness, tremor, irritability, anxiety, mental depression, paresthesia, emotional lability.
● CV: elevated blood pressure.
● DERM: acne, hirsutism, oily skin or hair.
● EENT: visual disturbances.
● GI: gastroenteritis, change in appetite.
● Hepatic: reversible jaundice.
● Other: muscle cramps or spasms, flushing, sweating, vaginitis, vaginal bleeding, menstrual irregularities, edema, weight gain, deepening of voice, clitoral enlargement, testicular atrophy, decrease in breast size, change in libido, altered serum lipid profiles.

Overdose and treatment
No specific recommendations are available. Empty stomach by induced emesis or gastric lavage; follow with activated charcoal to reduce absorption. Treatment is supportive.

▶ **Special considerations**
Besides those relevant to all *androgens*, consider the following recommendations.
● Because drug may cause hepatic dysfunction, periodic liver function studies should be performed.
● To treat endometriosis and fibrocystic breast disease, danazol therapy should begin during menstruation.
● Tests should rule out pregnancy before therapy with danazol. Urge female patients to use effective barrier methods of contraception during danazol therapy.

Information for the patient
● Tell patients desiring birth control to use a nonhormonal contraceptive; during danazol treatment, ovulation may not be suppressed by hormonal contraceptives.
● Advise patient to report voice changes or other signs of virilization promptly. Some androgenic effects, such as deepening of the voice, may not be reversible upon discontinuation of drug.
● Tell patient to immediately report nausea, vomiting, headache, and visual disturbances, which may suggest pseudotumor cerebri.
● Advise patient who is taking danazol for fibrocystic disease to examine breasts regularly. If breast nodule enlarges during treatment, patient should call immediately.
● Advise female patients that amenorrhea usually occurs after 6 to 8 weeks of therapy.
● Advise male patients that periodic evaluation of semen may be indicated.

Pediatric use
Use with caution because of possible androgenic effects. Use danazol with extreme caution in children to avoid precocious puberty and premature closure of the epiphyses. Conduct X-ray examinations every 6 months to assess skeletal maturation.

Geriatric use
Use with caution. Observe elderly male patients for the development of prostatic hypertrophy; symptomatic prostatic hypertrophy or prostatic carcinoma mandates discontinuation of danazol.

Breast-feeding
Because of the potential for serious adverse reactions to the infant, a decision should be made to discontinue breast-feeding or the drug, depending on the drug's importance to the woman.

dantrolene sodium
Dantrium

● Pharmacologic classification: hydantoin derivative
● Therapeutic classification: skeletal muscle relaxant
● Pregnancy risk category C

How supplied
Available by prescription only
Capsules: 25 mg, 50 mg, 100 mg
Injection: 20 mg parenteral (contains 3 g mannitol)

Indications, route, and dosage
Spasticity resulting from upper motor neuron disorders
Adults: 25 mg P.O. daily, increased gradually in increments of 25 mg at 4- to 7-day intervals, up to 100 mg b.i.d. to q.i.d., to maximum of 400 mg daily.
Children: 0.5 mg/kg daily P.O. b.i.d., increased gradually as needed by 0.5 mg/kg b.i.d. to q.i.d. to maximum of 100 mg q.i.d.
Prevention of malignant hyperthermia in susceptible patients who require surgery
Adults: 4 to 8 mg/kg/day P.O. given in three to four divided doses for 1 to 2 days before procedure; administer last dose 3 to 4 hours before procedure. Alternatively, give 2.5 mg/kg I.V. over 1 hour approximately 75 minutes before procedure.
Management of malignant hyperthermia crisis
Adults and children: 1 mg/kg I.V. initially; may repeat dose up to cumulative dose of 10 mg/kg.
Prevention of recurrence of malignant hyperthermia after crisis
Adults: 4 to 8 mg/kg/day P.O. given in four divided doses for up to 3 days after crisis. Alternatively, give 1 mg/kg I.V. initially, then individualize dose up to maximum of 10 mg/kg based on clinical response.
† *To reduce succinylcholine-induced muscle fasciculations and postoperative muscle pain*
Adults over 45 kg: 100 mg P.O. 2 hours before succinylcholine.
Adults under 45 kg: 150 mg P.O. 2 hours before succinylcholine.

Pharmacodynamics
Skeletal muscle relaxant action: A hydantoin derivative, dantrolene is chemically and pharmacologically unrelated to other skeletal muscle relaxants. It directly affects skeletal muscle, reducing muscle tension. It interferes with the release of calcium ion from the sarcoplasmic reticulum, resulting in decreased muscle contraction. This mechanism is of particular importance in malignant hyperthermia when increased myoplasmic calcium ion concentrations activate acute catabolism in the skeletal muscle cell. Dantrolene prevents or reduces the increase in myoplasmic calcium concentrations associated with malignant hyperthermia crises.

Pharmacokinetics
● *Absorption:* 35% of oral dose is absorbed through GI tract, with peak concentrations reached within 5 hours. Therapeutic effect in patients with upper motor neuron disorders may take 1 week or more.
● *Distribution:* Dantrolene is substantially plasma protein-bound, mainly to albumin.
● *Metabolism:* Dantrolene is metabolized in the liver to its less active 5-hydroxy derivatives, and to its amino derivative by reductive pathways.
● *Excretion:* Dantrolene is excreted in urine as metabolites.

Contraindications and precautions
Dantrolene is contraindicated in patients with active hepatic disease (hepatitis, cirrhosis), upper motor neuron disorders, and those in whom spasticity helps maintain upright posture and balance.
Administer cautiously to patients with cardiac function impairment (may cause pleural effusion), pulmonary function impairment (especially chronic obstructive pulmonary disease), or preexisting hepatic disease.

Also administer cautiously to patients over age 35, especially women, and in patients receiving other drugs (especially estrogens) concomitantly, because of increased risk of hepatotoxicity.

There are no contraindications to the use of I.V. dantrolene in management of malignant hyperthermia crisis.

Interactions

Concomitant use with other CNS depressant drugs, including alcohol, narcotics, anxiolytics, antipsychotics, and tricyclic antidepressants, may increase CNS depression. Reduce dosage of one or both if used concurrently. Use of dantrolene in women over age 35 who are also receiving estrogen therapy may increase incidence of hepatotoxicity.

Effects on diagnostic tests

Dantrolene therapy alters liver function test results (increased ALT [SGPT], AST [SGOT], alkaline phosphatase, and lactic dehydrogenase), blood urea nitrogen levels, and total serum bilirubin.

Adverse reactions

● CNS: skeletal muscle weakness, drowsiness, dizziness, light-headedness, mental depression, confusion, fatigue, malaise, speech disturbance, headache, increased nervousness, hallucinations.
● CV: tachycardia, erratic blood pressure, phlebitis, pleural effusion with pericarditis.
● DERM: pruritus, urticaria, acneiform rash, eczematoid eruption, photosensitivity reactions.
● EENT: excessive tearing, visual and auditory disturbances.
● GI: nausea, severe diarrhea, anorexia, vomiting, gastric irritation, abdominal cramps, constipation, difficulty swallowing, GI bleeding, alteration of taste.
● GU: urinary frequency, incontinence, nocturia, crystalluria, hematuria, difficulty achieving erection.
● Hepatic: *hepatitis.*
● Other: sweating, backache, myalgia, chills, fever, drooling.
Note: Drug should be discontinued if hypersensitivity or liver function test abnormality occurs, or if improvement does not occur after 45 days of oral therapy.

Overdose and treatment

Clinical manifestations of overdose include exaggeration of adverse reactions, particularly CNS depression, and nausea and vomiting.

Treatment includes supportive measures, gastric lavage, and observation of symptoms. Maintain adequate airway, have emergency ventilation equipment on hand, monitor ECG, and administer large quantities of I.V. solutions to prevent crystalluria. Monitor vital signs closely. The benefit of dialysis is not known.

▶ Special considerations

● To prepare suspension for single oral dose, dissolve contents of appropriate number of capsules in fruit juice or other suitable liquid.
● Before therapy begins, check patient's baseline neuromuscular functions—posture, gait, coordination, range of motion, muscle strength and tone, presence of abnormal muscle movements, and reflexes—for later comparisons.
● May cause muscle weakness and impaired walking ability. Use with caution and carefully supervise patients receiving this drug for prophylactic treatment for malignant hyperthermia.

● Walking should be supervised until patient's reaction to drug is known. With relief of spasticity, patient may lose ability to maintain balance.
● Improvement may require a week or more of drug therapy.
● Because of the risk of hepatic injury, drug should be discontinued if improvement is not evident within 45 days.
● Perform baseline and regularly scheduled liver function tests (alkaline phosphatase, ALT [SGPT], AST [SGOT], and total bilirubin), blood cell counts, and renal function tests.
● Risk of hepatotoxicity may be greater in women, patients over age 35, patients taking other medications, and patients taking high dantrolene doses (400 mg or more daily) for prolonged periods.
● Clinical signs of malignant hyperthermia include skeletal muscle rigidity (often the first sign), sudden tachycardia, cardiac arrhythmias, cyanosis, tachypnea, severe hypercarbia, unstable blood pressure, rapidly rising temperature, acidosis, and shock.
● In malignant hyperthermia crisis, drug should be given by rapid I.V. injection as soon as reaction is recognized.
● To reconstitute, add 60 ml sterile water for injection to 20-mg vial. Do not use bacteriostatic water for injection. Reconstituted solution is stable for only 6 hours.
● Treating malignant hyperthermia requires continual monitoring of body temperature, management of fever, correction of acidosis, maintenance of fluid and electrolyte balance, monitoring of intake and output, adequate oxygenation, and seizure precautions.

Information for the patient

● Instruct patient to report promptly the onset of jaundice: yellow skin or sclerae, dark urine, clay-colored stools, itching, and abdominal discomfort. Hepatotoxicity occurs more frequently between the third and twelfth month of therapy.
● Advise patients susceptible to malignant hyperthermia to wear medical identification (for example, Medic Alert) indicating diagnosis, physician's name and telephone number, drug causing reaction, and treatment used.
● Because hepatotoxicity occurs more commonly after concurrent use of other drugs with dantrolene, warn patient to avoid nonprescription medications, alcoholic beverages, and other CNS depressants except as prescribed.
● Photosensitivity reactions are possible. Advise patient to avoid excessive or unnecessary exposure to sunlight and to use protective clothing and a sunscreen agent.
● Drug may cause drowsiness. Warn patient to avoid hazardous activities that require alertness until CNS depressant effects are determined.
● Advise patient to report any adverse reactions immediately.
● Tell patient to store drug away from heat and direct light (not in bathroom medicine cabinet). Keep out of reach of children.
● If patient misses a dose, tell him to take it within 1 hour; otherwise, he should omit the dose and return to regular dosing schedule. Tell him not to double doses.

Geriatric use

Administer with extreme caution to elderly patients.

Pediatric use
Not recommended for long-term use in children under age 5.

Breast-feeding
Dantrolene is not recommended for use by breast-feeding women.

dapiprazole hydrochloride
Rev-Eyes

- Pharmacologic classification: alpha-adrenergic blocking agent
- Therapeutic classification: mydriatic reversal agent
- Pregnancy risk category B

How supplied
Available by prescription only
Ophthalmic powder: lyophilized, 25 mg dapiprazole/vial; 5 ml diluent; 0.5% solution when reconstituted

Indications, route, and dosage
Treatment of iatrogenically induced mydriasis produced by adrenergic or parasympatholytic agents
Adults: Instill 2 drops, followed in 5 minutes by another 2 drops.

Pharmacodynamics
Miotic action: Dapiprazole blocks alpha-adrenergic receptors in smooth muscle, producing miosis through an effect on the dilator muscle of the iris. It has no significant activity on ciliary muscle contraction nor does it significantly alter intraocular pressure in normotensive eyes or in eyes with increased intraocular pressure. Eye color can affect the rate of pupillary constriction but not the final pupil size.

Pharmacokinetics
Information not available.

Contraindications and precautions
Dapiprazole is contraindicated in patients with hypersensitivity to any ingredient and when constriction is undesirable; for example, in acute iritis.

Interactions
None reported.

Adverse reactions
- CNS: headache, browache.
- Eye: conjunctival injection lasting 20 minutes, burning on instillation, ptosis, lid erythema, lid edema, chemosis, itching, punctate keratitis, corneal edema, photophobia, dry eyes, tearing, blurry vision.

▶ Special considerations
- Dapiprazole is not indicated for the reduction of intraocular pressure or treatment of open-angle glaucoma.
- Do not touch dropper to any surface to avoid contamination.
- Do not use in same patient more than once per week.
- Apply topically to conjunctiva of each eye after ophthalmic examination to reverse diagnostic mydriasis.

- To prepare, remove and discard aluminum seals and rubber stoppers from both drug and diluent vials. Pour diluent into drug vial and attach dropper assembly. Shake container to ensure mixing. Store at room temperature for 21 days. Discard any solution that is discolored.

Pediatric use
Safety and efficacy have not been established.

Breast-feeding
It is unknown if the drug is excreted in breast milk.

dapsone
Avlosulfon*

- Pharmacologic classification: synthetic sulfone
- Therapeutic classification: antileprotic, antimalarial agent
- Pregnancy risk category C

How supplied
Available by prescription only
Tablets: 25 mg, 100 mg

Indications, route, and dosage
All forms of leprosy (Hansen's disease)
Adults: 50 to 100 mg P.O. daily for indefinite period, plus rifampin 600 mg daily for 6 months.
Children: 1 to 1.5 mg/kg P.O. daily.
Prophylaxis for leprosy patient's close contacts
Adults: 50 mg P.O. daily.
Children age 6 to 12: 25 mg P.O. daily.
Children age 2 to 5: 25 mg P.O. three times weekly.
Infants age 6 to 23 months: 12 mg P.O. three times weekly.
Infants under age 6 months: 6 mg P.O. three times weekly.
Dermatitis herpetiformis
Adults: Initially, 50 mg P.O. daily; may increase up to 400 mg/day.
Malaria suppression or prophylaxis
Adults: 100 mg P.O. weekly, with pyrimethamine 12.5 mg P.O. weekly.
Children: 2 mg/kg P.O. weekly, with pyrimethamine 0.25 mg/kg weekly.
Continue prophylaxis throughout exposure and 6 months postexposure.
†*Pneumocystis carinii* pneumonia
Adults: 100 mg P.O. daily. Usually administered with trimethoprim, 20 mg/kg daily divided q.i.d.

Pharmacodynamics
Antibiotic action: Dapsone is bacteriostatic and bactericidal; like sulfonamides, it is thought to act principally by inhibition of folic acid. It acts against *Mycobacterium leprae* and *M. tuberculosis,* and has some activity against *Pneumocystis carinii* and *Plasmodium.*

Pharmacokinetics
- *Absorption:* Dapsone is absorbed completely, but rather slowly, from the GI tract after oral administration; peak serum levels occur 2 to 8 hours after ingestion.
- *Distribution:* Dapsone is distributed widely into most

body tissues and fluids. Dapsone is 50% to 80% protein-bound.

● *Metabolism:* Dapsone undergoes acetylation by liver enzymes; rate varies and is genetically determined. Almost 50% of blacks and whites are slow acetylators, whereas over 80% of Chinese, Japanese, and Eskimos are fast acetylators. Dosage adjustment may be required.

● *Excretion:* Dapsone and metabolites are excreted primarily in urine; small amounts of drug are excreted in feces and possibly in breast milk. Dapsone undergoes enterohepatic circulation; half-life in adults ranges between 10 and 50 hours (average 28 hours). Orally administered charcoal may enhance excretion. Dapsone is dialyzable.

Contraindications and precautions
Dapsone is contraindicated in patients with known hypersensitivity to dapsone or its derivatives and in patients with severe anemia.

Dapsone should be used cautiously in patients with glucose-6-phosphate dehydrogenase (G6PD) deficiency, methemoglobin reductase deficiency, or hemoglobin M; in patients predisposed to hemolysis induced by other drugs or conditions (certain infections or diabetic ketosis) because of potential adverse hematologic effects; and in patients taking probenecid because of decreased excretion and drug accumulation. Special care must be taken to recognize leprosy reactional states.

Interactions
Concomitant use of dapsone with nitrite, phenylhydrazine, nitrofurantoin, or primaquine increases hazard of hemolysis in patients with G6PD deficiency; with probenecid may increase dapsone serum levels by blocking renal tubular secretion; with para-aminobenzoic acid (PABA) antagonizes dapsone's antibacterial effect.

Rifampin-induced hepatic enzymes increase metabolic rate and reduce dapsone serum levels.

Effects on diagnostic tests
None reported.

Adverse reactions
● CNS: psychosis, headache, dizziness, lethargy, severe malaise, paresthesias.
● DERM: *allergic dermatitis* (generalized or fixed maculopapular rash).
● EENT: tinnitus, allergic rhinitis.
● GI: anorexia, abdominal pain, *nausea, vomiting.*
● HEMA: *aplastic anemia, agranulocytosis, hemolytic anemia, methemoglobinemia,* possible leukopenia.
● Hepatic: *hepatitis,* cholestatic jaundice.
● Other: fever, phototoxicity.

Note: Drug should be discontinued if patient shows signs of hypersensitivity reaction, dermatologic toxicity, muscle weakness, hepatotoxicity, or marked hematologic abnormalities (leukopenia, thrombocytopenia, anemia); reduce dosage or temporarily discontinue dapsone if hemoglobin level falls below 9 g/dl, if leukocyte level falls below 5,000/mm³, or if erythrocyte count falls below 2.5 million/mm³ or remains low.

Leprosy reactional states
When treating leprosy with dapsone, it is essential to recognize two types of leprosy reactional states that are related to effectiveness of dapsone therapy.

Type I, reversal reaction, includes erythema, followed by swelling of skin and nerve lesions in tuberculoid patients; skin lesions may ulcerate and multiply, and acute neuritis may cause neural dysfunction. Severe cases require hospitalization, analgesics, corticosteroids, and nerve trunk decompression while dapsone therapy is continued.

Type II, erythema nodosum leprosum (ENL), occurs primarily in lepromatous leprosy, with an incidence of about 50% during the first year of therapy. Signs and symptoms include tender erythematous skin nodules, fever, malaise, orchitis, neuritis, albuminuria, iritis, joint swelling, epistaxis, and depression; skin lesions may ulcerate. Treatment includes corticosteroids and analgesics.

Additional treatment guidelines are available from National Hansen's Disease Center, (504) 642-7771.

Overdose and treatment
Signs of overdose include nausea, vomiting, and hyperexcitability, occurring within minutes or up to 24 hours after ingestion; methemoglobin-induced depression, cyanosis, and convulsions may occur. Hemolysis is a late complication (up to 14 days after ingestion).

Treat by gastric lavage, followed by activated charcoal; treat dapsone-induced methemoglobinemia in G-6-PD patients with methylene blue. Hemodialysis may also be used to enhance elimination.

▶ Special considerations
● Give drug with or after meals to avoid gastric irritation.
● Obtain specimens for culture and sensitivity testing before first dose, but therapy may begin before test results are complete; repeat periodically to detect drug resistance.
● Observe patient for adverse effects and monitor hematologic and liver function studies to minimize toxicity.
● Monitor dapsone serum concentrations periodically to maintain effective levels. Levels of 0.1 to 7 are usually effective and safe.
● Observe skin and mucous membranes for early signs of allergic reactions or leprosy reactional states.
● Isolation of patient with inactive leprosy is not required; however, surfaces in contact with discharge from nose or skin lesions should be disinfected.
● Therapeutic effect on leprosy may not be evident until 3 to 6 months after start of therapy.
● Monitor vital signs frequently during early weeks of drug therapy. Frequent or high fever may require reduced dosage or discontinuation of drug.
● Because dapsone is dialyzable, patients undergoing hemodialysis may require dosage adjustments.

Information for the patient
● Explain disease process and rationale for long-term therapy to patient and family; emphasize that improvement may not occur for 3 to 6 months.
● Teach signs and symptoms of hypersensitivity and other adverse reactions, and emphasize need to report these promptly; explain possibility of cumulative effects; urge patient to report *any* unusual effects or reactions and to report loss of appetite, nausea, or vomiting promptly.
● Teach patient how to take drug and the need to comply with prescribed regimen. Encourage patient to report no improvement or worsening of symptoms after 3 months of drug treatment. Urge patient not to discontinue drug without medical approval.
● Explain importance of follow-up visits and need to

monitor close contacts at 6- to 12-month intervals for 10 years.
• Teach sanitary disposal of secretions from nose or skin lesions.
• Assure patient and family that inactive leprosy is no barrier to employment or school attendance.
• New mothers need not be separated from infant during therapy; teach signs of cyanosis and methemoglobinemia.

Geriatric use
Elderly patients often have decreased renal function, which decreases drug excretion. Use with caution in elderly patients.

Pediatric use
Use with caution in children.

Breast-feeding
Dapsone is excreted in breast milk and is tumorigenic in animals. An alternative feeding method is recommended during therapy with dapsone.

---

daunorubicin hydrochloride
Cerubidine

• Pharmacologic classification: antibiotic antineoplastic (cell cycle-phase nonspecific)
• Therapeutic classification: antineoplastic
• Pregnancy risk category D

How supplied
Available by prescription only
Injection: 20-mg vials

Indications, route, and dosage
Dosage and indications may vary. Check current literature for recommended protocols.
Remission induction in acute nonlymphocytic leukemia (myelogenous, monocytic, erythroid)
Adults: As a single agent – 30 to 60 mg/m² I.V. daily on days 1, 2, and 3 q 3 to 4 weeks; or 800 mcg to 1 mg/kg for 3 to 6 days, repeated q 3 to 4 weeks. Maximum dosage is 550 mg/m² (450 mg/m² for patients who have received chest irradiation). In combination – 25 to 45 mg/m² I.V. daily on days 1, 2, and 3 of the first course and on days 1 and 2 of subsequent courses with cytosine arabinoside infusions.
Adults age 60 and over: Initially, 30 mg/m² I.V. daily for 3 days. Repeat courses q 3 to 4 weeks with 30 mg/m² daily for 2 days.
Children: 25 mg/m² weekly, usually combined with vincristine and prednisone.
Note: Dose should be reduced if hepatic function is impaired.

Pharmacodynamics
Antineoplastic action: Daunorubicin exerts its cytotoxic activity by intercalating between DNA base pairs and uncoiling the DNA helix. The result is inhibition of DNA synthesis and DNA-dependent RNA synthesis. The drug may also inhibit polymerase activity.

Pharmacokinetics
• *Absorption:* Because of its vesicant nature, daunorubicin must be given intravenously.
• *Distribution:* Daunorubicin is widely distributed into body tissues, with the highest concentrations found in the spleen, kidneys, liver, lungs, and heart. The drug does not cross the blood-brain barrier.
• *Metabolism:* The drug is extensively metabolized in the liver by microsomal enzymes. One of the metabolites has cytotoxic activity.
• *Excretion:* Daunorubicin and its metabolites are primarily excreted in bile, with a small portion excreted in urine. Plasma elimination has been described as biphasic, with an initial phase half-life of 45 minutes and a terminal phase half-life of 18½ hours.

Contraindications and precautions
Daunorubicin is contraindicated in patients with life-threatening myelosuppression, preexisting cardiac disease, severe infections, or hepatic or renal dysfunction because drug may worsen these conditions. Drug should not be used in pregnant patients because of significant risk to the fetus. Use cautiously in patients with moderate hepatic, renal, cardiac, or bone marrow dysfunction.

Interactions
When used concomitantly, other hepatotoxic drugs may increase the risk of hepatotoxicity with daunorubicin. Do not mix daunorubicin with either heparin sodium or dexamethasone phosphate. Admixture of these agents results in the formation of a precipitate.

Effects on diagnostic tests
Daunorubicin therapy may increase blood and urine concentrations of uric acid.
Daunorubicin therapy may also cause an increase in serum alkaline phosphatase, AST (SGOT), and bilirubin levels, indicating drug-induced hepatotoxicity.

Adverse reactions
• CV: *irreversible cardiomyopathy* (dose-related), ECG changes, arrhythmias, *pericarditis, myocarditis.*
• DERM: rash.
• GI: nausea, vomiting, stomatitis, esophagitis, anorexia, diarrhea.
• GU: nephrotoxicity, transient red urine.
• HEMA: *bone marrow depression* (dose-limiting), anemia, *pancytopenia* (nadir between 10 and 14 days), *leukopenia, thrombocytopenia.*
• Hepatic: hepatotoxicity.
• Local: severe cellulitis or tissue slough if drug extravasates.
• Metabolic: hyperuricemia.
• Other: generalized alopecia, fever, chills.
Note: Drug should be discontinued if patient develops signs of congestive heart failure or cardiomyopathy.

Overdose and treatment
Clinical manifestations of overdose include myelosuppression, nausea, vomiting, and stomatitis.
Treatment is usually supportive and includes transfusion of blood components and antiemetics.

▶ Special considerations
• To reconstitute the drug for I.V. administration, add 4 ml of sterile water for injection to a 20-mg vial to give a concentration of 5 mg/ml.
• Drug may be diluted further into 100 ml of dextrose

5% in water or normal saline solution and infused over 30 to 45 minutes.
• For I.V. push administration, withdraw reconstituted drug into syringe containing 10 to 15 ml of normal saline solution, and inject over 2 to 3 minutes into the tubing of a freely flowing I.V. infusion. Reconstituted solution is stable for 24 hours at room temperature.
• Reddish color of drug looks similar to that of doxorubicin (Adriamycin). Do not confuse the two drugs.
• Erythematous streaking along the vein or flushing in the face indicate that the drug is being administered too rapidly.
• Extravasation may be treated with topical application of dimethyl sulfoxide and ice packs to the site.
• Antiemetics may be used to prevent or treat nausea and vomiting.
• Darkening or redness of the skin may occur in prior radiation fields.
• To prevent cardiomyopathy, cumulative dose should be limited to 550 mg/m² (450 mg/m² when patient has been receiving any other cardiotoxic agent, such as cyclophosphamide, or radiation therapy that encompasses the heart).
• Dosage should be reduced in patients with hepatic or renal impairment; in patients with serum bilirubin of 1.2 to 3 mg/dl, reduce dose by 25%; with serum bilirubin or creatinine levels over 3 mg/dl, reduce dose by 50%.
• Monitor ECG before treatment and monthly during treatment.
• Monitor CBC and hepatic function.
• Note if resting pulse rate is high (a sign of cardiac adverse reactions).
• Do not use a scalp tourniquet or apply ice to prevent alopecia, because this may compromise effectiveness of drug.
• Nausea and vomiting may be very severe and last 24 to 48 hours.

Information for the patient
• Warn patient that urine may be red for 1 to 2 days and that this is a drug effect, not bleeding.
• Advise patient that alopecia may occur, but that it is usually reversible.
• Tell patient to avoid exposure to people with infections.
• Encourage adequate fluid intake to increase urine output and facilitate excretion of uric acid.
• Warn patient that nausea and vomiting may be severe and may last for 24 to 48 hours.
• Tell patient to call if he develops a sore throat, fever, or any signs of bleeding.

Geriatric use
• Elderly patients have an increased incidence of drug-induced cardiotoxicity.
• Be sure to monitor for hematologic toxicity because some elderly patients have poor bone marrow reserve.

Pediatric use
Children have an increased incidence of drug-induced cardiotoxicity, which may occur at lower doses in children. The total lifetime dosage for children over age 2 is 300 mg/m²; for children under age 2, 10 mg/kg.

Breast-feeding
It is not known whether daunorubicin distributes into breast milk. However, because of the potential for serious adverse reactions, mutagenicity, and carcinogenicity in the infant, breast-feeding is not recommended.

deferoxamine mesylate
Desferal Mesylate

• Pharmacologic classification: chelating agent
• Therapeutic classification: heavy metal antagonist
• Pregnancy risk category C

How supplied
Available by prescription only
Injectable powder for injection: 500-mg vial

Indications, route, and dosage
Acute iron intoxication
Adults and children: 1 g I.M. or I.V. followed by 500 mg I.M. or I.V. every 4 hours for two doses; then 500 mg I.M. or I.V. every 4 to 12 hours if needed. I.V. infusion rate should not exceed 15 mg/kg hourly. Do not exceed 6 g in 24 hours.
Chronic iron overload resulting from multiple transfusions
Adults and children: 500 mg to 1 g I.M. daily and 2 g slow I.V. infusion in separate solution along with each unit of blood transfused. I.V. infusion rate should not exceed 15 mg/kg hourly. Alternatively, give 1 to 2 g via a subcutaneous infusion over 8 to 24 hours.

Pharmacodynamics
Chelating action: Deferoxamine chelates iron by binding ferric ions to the 3 hydroxamino groups of the molecule. It also chelates aluminum to a lesser extent.

Pharmacokinetics
• *Absorption:* Deferoxamine is absorbed poorly after oral administration; however, absorption of the drug may occur in patients with acute iron toxicity.
• *Distribution:* Deferoxamine distributes widely into the body after parenteral administration.
• *Metabolism:* Small amounts of deferoxamine are metabolized by plasma enzymes.
• *Excretion:* Deferoxamine is excreted in urine as unchanged drug or as ferrioxamine, the deferoxamine-iron complex.

Contraindications and precautions
Deferoxamine is contraindicated in patients with severe renal failure or anuria, because the drug and ferrioxamine are excreted primarily by the kidneys *except* for management of iron or aluminum intoxication in dialysis patients. The drug also is contraindicated in pregnant women or in women who may become pregnant.

Deferoxamine should be used cautiously in patients with pyelonephritis and in patients with hearing or vision deficits, because drug may exacerbate these conditions.

Interactions
None reported.

Effects on diagnostic tests
None reported.

Adverse reactions
• CV: hypotension, tachycardia.
• DERM: cutaneous wheal formation, rash, pruritus.

- EENT: blurred vision, decreased visual acuity, visual field changes, night blindness, optic neuropathy, retinal pigmentation, cataracts, audiographic hearing loss with or without clinical loss.
- GI: diarrhea, abdominal discomfort.
- Local: pain, erythema, and swelling at injection site.
- Other: *anaphylactoid reactions,* fever.
    Note: Drug should be discontinued if hypersensitivity reaction develops, if hearing or vision changes occur, or if renal function deteriorates significantly.

Overdose and treatment
Acute intoxication is anticipated to include extension and exacerbation of adverse reactions. Treat symptomatically. Ferrioxamine can be removed by hemodialysis.

▶ Special considerations
- Observe closely and be prepared to treat hypersensitivity reactions; monitor renal, vision, and hearing function throughout therapy.
- Use I.M. route for acute iron intoxication, if patient is not in shock. If patient is in shock, administer I.V. *slowly;* avoid subcutaneous route.
- Deferoxamine has been used to treat iron overload from congenital anemias and in the diagnosis and treatment of primary hemochromatosis. The drug also has been applied topically to remove corneal rust rings and has been used I.V. or intraperitoneally to promote aluminum excretion or removal.

Information for the patient
- Advise patient that ophthalmic and, possibly, audiometric examinations are needed every 3 to 6 months during continuous therapy; stress importance of reporting any changes in vision or hearing.
- Explain that drug may turn urine red.

Geriatric use
Drug should be used with caution, because elderly patients are more likely to have visual or hearing impairment and renal dysfunction than younger patients.

Pediatric use
Deferoxamine is safe and effective in children over age 3.

dehydrocholic acid
Antrocholin, Cholan-DH, Decholin, Hepahydrin

- Pharmacologic classification: bile acid
- Therapeutic classification: laxative
- Pregnancy risk category C

How supplied
Available with and without prescription
Tablets: 130 mg, 244 mg, 250 mg

Indications, route, and dosage
Constipation, biliary tract conditions
Adults and children age 12 and over: 250 to 500 mg P.O. b.i.d. or t.i.d. after meals. Do not exceed 1.5 g/day.

Pharmacodynamics
- *Hydrocholeretic action:* Dehydrocholic acid increases the water content of bile, producing larger volumes of low-viscosity bile. Bile acid production remains the same.
- *Laxative action:* Dehydrocholic acid is a stimulant cathartic.

Pharmacokinetics
- *Absorption:* Absorbed readily from the GI tract.
- *Distribution:* Dehydrocholic acid is concentrated in the liver.
- *Metabolism:* Unknown.
- *Excretion:* Drug is excreted in bile.

Contraindications and precautions
Drug is contraindicated in patients with cholelithiasis, jaundice, marked hepatic insufficiency, complete obstruction of the hepatic or common bile ducts, or complete GI or GU tract obstruction, because of increased risk of adverse effects. Do not use when abdominal pain, vomiting, or nausea is present.

Interactions
None reported.

Effects on diagnostic tests
None reported.

Adverse reactions
- GI: loose stools, cramping.
- Metabolic: fluid and electrolyte imbalance.

Overdose and treatment
No information available.

▶ Special considerations
- Monitor fluid and electrolyte balance.
- Patients with biliary fistula may require concomitant bile salts.
- Drug is also useful in preventing bacterial accumulation after biliary tract surgery.
- Frequent use may lead to laxative dependence.

Information for the patient
Instruct patient on the importance of exercise, adequate fluid intake, and a high-fiber diet to prevent constipation.

Geriatric use
Use cautiously because elderly patients are more likely to have partial obstruction of the GI or GU tracts.

Pediatric use
Drug is not recommended in children under age 6.

---

demecarium bromide
Humorsol

- Pharmacologic classification: cholinesterase inhibitor
- Therapeutic classification: miotic
- Pregnancy risk category C

How supplied
Available by prescription only
Ophthalmic solution: 0.125% and 0.25% in 5-ml ocumeter

Indications, route, and dosage
Glaucoma, postiridectomy
Adults: Instill 1 drop of 0.125% or 0.25% solution in eyes twice weekly up to b.i.d., depending on intraocular pressure.
Convergent strabismus
Children: Instill 1 drop of 0.125% solution in each eye daily for 2 to 3 weeks, taper to 1 drop q 2 days for 3 to 4 weeks, then 1 drop once or twice weekly. Reevaluate q 4 to 12 weeks, adjusting dose as needed. Therapy should be discontinued after 4 months if control of condition still requires every-other-day therapy or if patient shows no response.

Drug is antidote for atropine in glaucoma or preglaucoma patients and is used to control postoperative rise in intraocular pressure.

Pharmacodynamics
Miotic action: Demecarium inhibits the enzymatic destruction of acetylcholine by inactivating cholinesterase. This leaves acetylcholine free to act on the effector cells of the iridic sphincter and ciliary muscles, causing pupillary constriction and accommodation spasm.

Pharmacokinetics
- *Absorption:* Unknown.
- *Distribution:* Unknown.
- *Metabolism:* Unknown.
- *Excretion:* Although demecarium is a reversible inhibitor of cholinesterase, its duration of action is similar to that of irreversible cholinesterase inhibitors. Maximal decrease in intraocular pressure occurs in 24 hours and may persist for over a week.

Contraindications and precautions
Demecarium is contraindicated in patients with active uveal inflammation, narrow-angle glaucoma, secondary glaucoma resulting from iridocyclitis, ocular hypertension, vasomotor instability, bronchial instability, bronchial asthma, spastic GI conditions, peptic ulcer, severe bradycardia, hypotension, recent myocardial infarction, epilepsy, Parkinson's disease, or history of retinal detachment, because the drug may aggravate the signs or symptoms of these disorders. It should be used with caution in patients with myasthenia gravis who are also receiving systemic anticholinesterase therapy and in patients exposed to organophosphorus insecticides.

Interactions
When used concomitantly, demecarium may increase neuromuscular blocking effects of succinylcholine, antagonize antiglaucoma effect of cyclopentolate and belladonna alkaloids, interfere with pilocarpine-induced

miosis, increase the toxicity of carbamate organophosphate insecticides, add to effects of systemic anticholinesterase agents used for myasthenia gravis, and decrease duration of echothiophate-induced miosis; echothiophate usually is tried first.

Effects on diagnostic tests
None reported.

Adverse reactions
- CNS: muscle weakness, headache
- CV: bradycardia, *arrhythmias*.
- DERM: contact dermatitis.
- Eye: iris cysts (reversible with discontinuation), lens opacity, blurred vision, eye or brow pain, retinal detachment, vitreous hemorrhage, eyelid twitching, iritis, conjunctival and intraocular hyperemia, ocular pain, paradoxical increased intraocular pressure.
- GI: nausea, vomiting, abdominal pain, diarrhea, salivation.
- GU: urinary incontinence.
- Respiratory: dyspnea.

Note: Drug should be discontinued immediately if excessive salivation, sweating, urinary incontinence, diarrhea, or muscle weakness occurs.

Overdose and treatment
Clinical manifestations of overdose include nausea, vomiting, abdominal pain, diarrhea, increased salivation, headache, syncope, tremor, urinary incontinence, dyspnea, hypotension, bradycardia, and arrhythmias. When swallowed accidentally, vomiting is usually spontaneous; if not, induce emesis and follow with activated charcoal or a cathartic. Treat cardiovascular or blood pressure responses with epinephrine; treat accidental dermal exposure by washing the area twice with water. Atropine sulfate, given S.C. or I.V., is the antidote of choice.

▶ Special considerations
- Demecarium is a potent, long-acting drug capable of producing cumulative systemic side effects. Follow prescribed concentration and dosage schedule closely; monitor patient.
- Wash hands immediately before and after administering; if solution contacts skin, wash promptly with large amount of water.
- Check patient for lenticular opacities every 6 months.
- Store in tightly closed original container.

Information for the patient
- Teach patient correct way to use and store medication and adequate safety measures; stress compliance with schedule and importance of close, constant medical supervision. Warn patient never to exceed recommended dosage.
- Warn patient to stop drug at least 2 weeks before scheduled ophthalmic surgery or other surgery involving general anesthesia.
- Instruct patient to use at bedtime because drug blurs vision.
- Reassure patient that blurred vision usually diminishes with prolonged use.

Geriatric use
Use with regard to the potential for cumulative side effects and toxicity.

Pediatric use
Use with regard to potential for cumulative side effects and toxicity.

Breast-feeding
No data available; however, patients using demecarium probably should avoid breast-feeding.

demeclocycline hydrochloride
Declomycin, Ledermycin

- Pharmacologic classification: tetracycline antibiotic
- Therapeutic classification: antibiotic
- Pregnancy risk category D

How supplied
Available by prescription only
Capsules: 150 mg
Tablets: 150 mg, 300 mg

Indications, route, and dosage
Infections caused by susceptible organisms
Adults: 150 mg P.O. q 6 hours, or 300 mg P.O. q 12 hours.
Children over age 8: 6 to 12 mg/kg P.O. daily, divided q 6 to 12 hours.
Gonorrhea
Adults: 600 mg P.O. initially, then 300 mg P.O. q 12 hours for 4 days (total 3 g).
Uncomplicated urethral, endocervical, or rectal infection
Adults: 300 mg P.O. q.i.d. for at least 7 days.
†*Syndrome of inappropriate antidiuretic hormone (a hyposmolar state)*
Adults: 600 to 1,200 mg P.O. daily in divided doses.

Pharmacodynamics
Antibacterial action: Demeclocycline is bacteriostatic. Tetracyclines bind reversibly to ribosomal subunits, thereby inhibiting bacterial protein synthesis. Demeclocycline is active against many gram-negative and gram-positive organisms, *Mycoplasma, Rickettsia, Chlamydia,* and spirochetes.

Pharmacokinetics
- *Absorption:* Demeclocycline is 60% to 80% absorbed from the GI tract after oral administration; peak serum levels occur at 3 to 4 hours. Food or milk reduces absorption by 50%; antacids chelate with tetracyclines and further reduce absorption.
Demeclocycline has the greatest affinity of all tetracyclines for calcium ions.
- *Distribution:* Demeclocycline is distributed widely into body tissues and fluids, including synovial, pleural, prostatic, and seminal fluids; bronchial secretions; saliva; and aqueous humor; CSF penetration is poor. Demeclocycline crosses the placenta; it is 36% to 91% protein-bound.
- *Metabolism:* Demeclocycline is not metabolized.
- *Excretion:* Demeclocycline is excreted primarily unchanged in urine by glomerular filtration; some drug may be excreted in breast milk. Plasma half-life is 10 to 17 hours in adults with normal renal function. Hemodialysis and peritoneal dialysis remove only minimal amounts of demeclocycline.

Contraindications and precautions
Demeclocycline is contraindicated in patients with known hypersensitivity to any tetracycline. It also is contraindicated during the second half of pregnancy because it may cause fatty infiltration of the liver in the mother and may cause permanent discoloration or hypoplasia of tooth enamel or impaired skeletal growth in the fetus. It is contraindicated in children under age 8 because it may cause permanent discoloration of teeth, enamel defects, and retardation of bone growth.
Use demeclocycline with caution in patients with decreased renal function, because it may elevate BUN levels and exacerbate renal dysfunction, and in patients likely to be exposed to direct sunlight or ultraviolet light because of the risk of photosensitivity reactions.

Interactions
Oral absorption of tetracycline is impaired by concomitant use with antacids containing aluminum, calcium, or magnesium or laxatives containing magnesium because of chelation; absorption of tetracycline is also impaired by food, milk and other dairy products, iron products, and sodium bicarbonate.
Tetracyclines may antagonize bactericidal effects of penicillin, inhibiting cell growth because of bacteriostatic action; administer penicillin 2 to 3 hours before tetracycline.
Concomitant use of tetracycline increases the risk of nephrotoxicity from methoxyflurane. When used concomitantly with oral anticoagulants, it necessitates lowered dosages of oral anticoagulants because of enhanced effects; and when used with digoxin, lowered dosages of digoxin because of increased bioavailability.

Effects on diagnostic tests
Demeclocycline causes false-negative results in urine tests using glucose oxidase reagent (Clinistix or Tes-Tape). It also causes false elevations in fluorometric tests for urinary catecholamines.
Demeclocycline may elevate serum BUN levels in patients with decreased renal function.

Adverse reactions
- CV: pericarditis.
- DERM: maculopapular and erythematous rashes, photosensitivity, increased pigmentation, urticaria, discolored nails and teeth.
- EENT: dysphagia, glossitis.
- GI: anorexia, nausea, vomiting, diarrhea, enterocolitis, anogenital inflammation.
- GU: reversible nephrotoxicity (Fanconi's syndrome) with outdated tetracyclines, progressive renal dysfunction in patients with preexisting renal impairment.
- HEMA: neutropenia, eosinophilia.
- Metabolic: increased BUN levels, diabetes insipidus syndrome (polyuria, polydipsia and weakness).
- Other: hypersensitivity, bacterial and fungal superinfection.
Note: Drug should be discontinued if signs of toxicity, hypersensitivity, progressive renal dysfunction, or superinfection occur; if erythema follows exposure to sunlight or ultraviolet light; or if severe diarrhea indicates pseudomembranous colitis.

Overdose and treatment
Clinical signs of overdose are usually limited to the GI tract. Treatment may include antacids or gastric lavage if ingestion occurred within the preceding 4 hours.

▶ **Special considerations**
Besides those relevant to all *tetracyclines,* consider the following recommendations.
● As an anti-infective, demeclocycline is usually reserved for patients intolerant of other antibiotics.
● A reversible diabetes insipidus syndrome has been reported with long-term use of demeclocycline; monitor patient for this disorder (weakness, polyuria, polydipsia).

Pediatric use
Drug should not be used in children younger than age 9.

Breast-feeding
Avoid use in breast-feeding women.

---

deserpidine
Harmonyl

● Pharmacologic classification: rauwolfia alkaloid, peripherally acting adrenergic-blocking agent
● Therapeutic classification: antihypertensive, antipsychotic
● Pregnancy risk category C

How supplied
Available by prescription only
Tablets: 0.25 mg

Indications, route, and dosage
Hypertension
Adults: Initially, 0.75 to 1 mg P.O. daily; maximum maintenance dosage is 0.25 mg P.O. daily. However, some clinicians avoid the initial loading dose and recommend treatment with 0.25 mg P.O. daily.
Psychosis
Adults: 0.1 to 1 mg P.O. daily.

Pharmacodynamics
● *Antihypertensive action:* The exact mechanism of deserpidine's antihypertensive action is unknown. Hypotension is thought to result from depletion of catecholamine and serotonin stores in many organs and from decreased catecholamine uptake by adrenergic neurons. Continuous therapy causes venous dilation, decreasing venous return and thus decreasing cardiac output.
● *Antipsychotic action:* Deserpidine depletes brain stores of serotonin and catecholamines, producing a tranquilizing effect.

Pharmacokinetics
● *Absorption:* Deserpidine is believed to be absorbed rapidly; however, onset of antihypertensive activity is delayed for 3 to 6 days. Maximum antihypertensive effect usually does not occur for at least 2 to 3 weeks.
● *Distribution:* Deserpidine appears to be distributed widely into the body; high concentrations are found in adipose tissue.
● *Metabolism:* Deserpidine is metabolized extensively in the liver.
● *Excretion:* Deserpidine is excreted as unchanged drug and metabolites in urine and feces. Antihypertensive effect may persist for several days to weeks after chronic therapy is discontinued.

Contraindications and precautions
Deserpidine is contraindicated in patients with known hypersensitivity to the drug; in patients receiving electroconvulsive therapy, because cerebral depletion of serotonin and catecholamines may predispose patient to convulsions and extrapyramidal reactions; and in patients with mental depression, ulcerative colitis, or peptic ulcer disease, because the drug may exacerbate these conditions.

Interactions
Deserpidine may potentiate antihypertensive effects of other antihypertensive agents and depressant effects of alcohol and CNS depressants.
Concomitant use with quinidine or cardiac glycosides may increase risk of cardiac arrhythmia in some patients.
Concomitant use with monoamine oxidase inhibitors may cause excitability and hypertension.

Effects on diagnostic tests
Rauwolfia therapy alters detection of urinary corticosteroids by colorimetric assay and may interfere with excretion of urine catecholamines and vanillylmandelic acid.

Adverse reactions
● CNS: mental confusion, depression, drowsiness, nervousness, paradoxical anxiety, nightmares, extrapyramidal symptoms, sedation.
● CV: orthostatic hypotension, bradycardia, dyspnea, syncope, edema.
● DERM: pruritus, rash.
● EENT: dry mouth, nasal stuffiness, glaucoma, uveitis, optic atrophy, conjunctival injection.
● GI: hyperacidity, nausea, vomiting, diarrhea, GI bleeding.
● Other: impotence, weight gain, dysuria.
Note: Drug should be discontinued if patient shows signs of mental depression.

Overdose and treatment
Signs of overdose include hypotension, bradycardia, CNS depression, coma, respiratory depression, hypothermia, diarrhea, vomiting, skin flushing, miosis, leg pain, and tremors.
After acute ingestion, empty stomach by induced emesis or gastric lavage; follow with a saline cathartic. Subsequent treatment is usually symptomatic and supportive.

▶ **Special considerations**
Besides those relevant to all *rauwolfia alkaloids,* consider the following recommendations.
● Hypotensive effect may be accompanied by bradycardia.
● Drowsiness, dizziness, and sedation are common adverse effects; therefore, patient may need assistance during walking.
● Use of deserpidine has decreased because of the availability of newer drugs with milder CNS effects.

Information for the patient
Warn patient to avoid hazardous activities that require mental alertness until tolerance develops to drowsiness, dizziness, or other CNS effects.

Geriatric use
Lower dose may be necessary because of decreased drug clearance in elderly.

Pediatric use
The safety and efficacy of deserpidine in children have not been established; use only if potential benefit outweighs risk.

Breast-feeding
Deserpidine is distributed into breast milk; an alternative feeding method is recommended during therapy.

desipramine hydrochloride
Norpramin, Pertofrane

- Pharmacologic classification: dibenzazepine tricyclic antidepressant
- Therapeutic classification: antidepressant, antianxiety agent
- Pregnancy risk category C

How supplied
Available by prescription only
Tablets: 10 mg, 25 mg, 50 mg, 75 mg, 100 mg, 150 mg
Pertofrane
Capsules: 25 mg, 50 mg

Indications, route, and dosage
Depression
Adults: 75 to 150 mg P.O. daily in divided doses, increasing to a maximum of 300 mg daily. Alternatively, the entire dosage can be given at bedtime.
Elderly patients and adolescents: 25 to 50 mg P.O. daily, increasing gradually to a maximum of 100 mg daily.

Pharmacodynamics
Antidepressant action: Desipramine is thought to exert its antidepressant effects by inhibiting reuptake of norepinephrine and serotonin in CNS nerve terminals (presynaptic neurons), which results in increased concentrations and enhanced activity of these neurotransmitters in the synaptic cleft. Desipramine more strongly inhibits reuptake of norepinephrine than serotonin; it has a lesser incidence of sedative effects and less anticholinergic and hypotensive activity than its parent compound, imipramine.

Pharmacokinetics
- *Absorption:* Desipramine is absorbed rapidly from the GI tract after oral administration.
- *Distribution:* Desipramine is distributed widely into the body, including the CNS and breast milk. Drug is 90% protein-bound. Peak effect occurs in 4 to 6 hours; steady state, within 2 to 11 days, with full therapeutic effect in 2 to 4 weeks. Proposed therapeutic plasma levels (parent drug and metabolite) range from 125 ng/ml to 300 ng/ml.
- *Metabolism:* Desipramine is metabolized by the liver; a significant first-pass effect may explain variability of serum concentrations in different patients taking the same dosage.
- *Excretion:* Drug is excreted primarily in urine.

Contraindications and precautions
Desipramine is contraindicated in patients with known hypersensitivity to tricyclic antidepressants, trazodone, and related compounds; in the acute recovery phase of myocardial infarction (MI) because of its potential arrhythmogenic effects and ECG changes; in patients in coma or severe respiratory depression because of added CNS depressant effects; and during or within 14 days of therapy with monoamine oxidase inhibitors.

Desipramine should be used cautiously in patients with other cardiac disease (arrhythmias, congestive heart failure [CHF], angina pectoris, valvular disease, or heart block); respiratory disorders; epilepsy and other seizure disorders; scheduled electroconvulsive therapy; bipolar disease; glaucoma, hyperthyroidism, or patients taking thyroid replacement; Type I and Type II diabetes; prostatic hypertrophy, paralytic ileus, or urinary retention; hepatic or renal dysfunction; or Parkinson's disease; and in those undergoing surgery using general anesthesia.

If product contains tartrazine, drug may precipitate asthma in patients with aspirin allergy.

Interactions
Concomitant use of desipramine with sympathomimetics, including epinephrine, phenylephrine, phenylpropanolamine, and ephedrine (often found in nasal sprays) may increase blood pressure; use with warfarin may increase prothrombin time and cause bleeding.

Concomitant use with thyroid medication, pimozide, or antiarrhythmic agents (quinidine, disopyramide, procainamide) may increase incidence of cardiac arrhythmias and conduction defects.

Desipramine may decrease hypotensive effects of centrally acting antihypertensive drugs, such as guanethidine, guanabenz, guanadrel, clonidine, methyldopa, and reserpine. Concomitant use with disulfiram or ethchlorvynol may cause delirium and tachycardia. Additive effects are likely after concomitant use of desipramine and CNS depressants, including alcohol, analgesics, barbiturates, narcotics, tranquilizers, and anesthetics (oversedation); atropine and other anticholinergic drugs, including phenothiazines, antihistamines, meperidine, and antiparkinsonian agents (oversedation, paralytic ileus, visual changes, and severe constipation); and metrizamide (increased risk of seizures).

Barbiturates and heavy smoking induce desipramine metabolism and decrease therapeutic efficacy; phenothiazines and haloperidol decrease its metabolism, decreasing therapeutic efficacy. Methylphenidate, cimetidine, oral contraceptives, propoxyphene, and beta blockers may inhibit desipramine metabolism, increasing plasma levels and toxicity.

Effects on diagnostic tests
Desipramine may prolong conduction time (elongation of Q-T and PR intervals, flattened T waves on ECG); it also may elevate liver function test results, decrease white blood cell counts, and decrease or increase serum glucose levels.

Adverse reactions
- CNS: drowsiness, dizziness, sedation, excitation, tremor, weakness, headache, nervousness, *seizures,* peripheral neuropathy, extrapyramidal symptoms, anxiety, vivid dreams, confusion (more marked in elderly patients).
- CV: orthostatic hypotension, tachycardia, *arrhyth-*

mias, *MI, stroke, heart block, CHF,* palpitations, hypertension (including some surgical patients), ECG changes.
● EENT: blurred vision, tinnitus, mydriasis, increased intraocular pressure.
● GI: dry mouth, constipation, nausea, vomiting, anorexia, diarrhea, paralytic ileus, jaundice.
● GU: urine retention.
● Other: sweating, photosensitivity, hypersensitivity (rash, urticaria, drug fever, edema).

After abrupt withdrawal of long-term therapy, nausea, headache, and malaise (does not indicate addiction) may occur.

Note: Drug should be discontinued (not abruptly) if signs of hypersensitivity occur. Monitor carefully for the following: urine retention, extreme dry mouth, rash, excessive sedation, seizures, tachycardia, sore throat, fever, or jaundice. Dizziness, fatigue, or orthostatic hypotension may indicate need for reduced dosage.

Overdose and treatment
The first 12 hours after acute ingestion are a stimulatory phase characterized by excessive anticholinergic activity (agitation, irritation, confusion, hallucinations, parkinsonian symptoms, hyperthermia, seizures, urine retention, dry mucous membranes, pupillary dilatation, constipation, and ileus). This is followed by CNS depressant effects, including hypothermia, decreased or absent reflexes, sedation, hypotension, cyanosis, and cardiac irregularities, including tachycardia, conduction disturbances, and quinidine-like effects on the ECG.

Severity of overdose is best indicated by widening of the QRS complex, which usually represents a serum level in excess of 1,000 ng/ml; serum levels are generally not helpful. Metabolic acidosis may follow hypotension, hypoventilation, and convulsions.

Treatment is symptomatic and supportive, including maintaining airway, stable body temperature, and fluid and electrolyte balance. Induce emesis with ipecac if patient is conscious; follow with gastric lavage and activated charcoal to prevent further absorption. Dialysis is of little use. Treat seizures with parenteral diazepam or phenytoin; arrhythmias, with parenteral phenytoin or lidocaine; and acidosis, with sodium bicarbonate. *Do not give barbiturates;* these may enhance CNS and respiratory depressant effects.

▶ **Special considerations**
Besides those relevant to all *tricyclic antidepressants,* consider the following recommendations.
● Check standing and sitting blood pressure to assess orthostasis before administering desipramine.
● Desipramine has a lesser incidence of sedative effects. It has less anticholinergic and hypotensive effects than its parent compound imipramine.
● The full dose may be given at bedtime to help offset daytime sedation.
● Tolerance usually develops to the sedative effects of the drug during the initial weeks of therapy.
● The drug should not be withdrawn abruptly, but tapered gradually over time.
● The drug should be discontinued at least 48 hours before surgical procedures.

Information for the patient
● The full dose may be taken at bedtime to alleviate daytime sedation.
● Explain that the full effects of the drug may not become apparent for 4 weeks or more after initiation of therapy.
● Tell patient to take the medication exactly as prescribed and not to double dose for missed ones.
● To prevent dizziness, advise patient to lie down for about 30 minutes after each dose at start of therapy and to avoid sudden postural changes, especially when rising to upright position.
● Warn patient not to stop taking drug suddenly.
● Encourage patient to report any unusual or troublesome effects, especially confusion, movement disorders, rapid heartbeat, dizziness, fainting, or difficulty urinating.
● Tell patient chewing gum, sugarless hard candy, or ice may alleviate dry mouth.
● Stress importance of regular dental hygiene to avoid caries.
● Warn patient to avoid alcohol while taking this medicaiton.
● Tell patient to store drug safely away from children.

Geriatric use
Elderly patients may be more susceptible to adverse cardiac reactions.

Pediatric use
Drug is not recommended for patients under age 12.

Breast-feeding
Desipramine is excreted in breast milk in concentrations equal to those in maternal serum. The potential benefit to the mother should outweigh the possible adverse reactions in the infant.

---

deslanoside
Cedilanid-D Injection

● Pharmacologic classification: digitalis glycoside
● Therapeutic classification: antiarrhythmic, inotropic
● Pregnancy risk category C

How supplied
Available by prescription only
Injection: 0.2 mg/ml

Indications, route, and dosage
Congestive heart failure, paroxysmal atrial tachycardia, atrial fibrillation and flutter
Adults: Loading dosage is 1.2 to 1.6 mg I.M. or I.V. in 2 divided doses over 24 hours; for maintenance, use another cardiac glycoside.
†*Premature and full-term neonates:* 22 mcg/kg I.M. or I.V. divided into two or three doses at 3- or 4-hour intervals.
†*Children age 2 weeks to 3 years:* 25 mcg/kg I.M. or I.V. divided into two or three doses at 3- or 4-hour intervals.
†*Children age 3 and older:* 22.5 mcg/kg I.M. or I.V. divided into two or three doses at 3- or 4-hour intervals.

Pharmacodynamics
Deslanoside has effects similar to those of digoxin but may have a slightly faster onset of action. Its clinical usefulness is somewhat limited because its therapeutic

---

serum level profile has not yet been defined and because an oral dosage form is unavailable.

Deslanoside's effects on the myocardium are dose-related and involve both direct and indirect mechanisms. The drug directly increases the force and velocity of myocardial contraction, AV node refractory period, and total peripheral resistance. At higher doses, increased sympathetic outflow occurs. The drug indirectly depresses the SA node and prolongs conduction to the AV node.

• *Inotropic action:* In patients with heart failure, increased contractile force boosts cardiac output, improves systolic emptying, and decreases diastolic heart size. It also increases ventricular end-diastolic pressure and consequently decreases pulmonary and systemic venous pressures. Increased myocardial contractility and cardiac output reflexively reduce sympathetic tone in patients with congestive heart failure. This compensates for the drug's direct vasoconstrictive action and thereby reduces total peripheral resistance; it also slows the heart rate and causes diuresis in edematous patients.

• *Antiarrhythmic action:* Deslanoside-induced heart rate slowing in patients without congestive heart failure is negligible and stems mainly from vagal (cholinergic) and sympatholytic effects on the SA node; however, with toxic doses, heart-rate slowing results from direct depression of SA node automaticity. Although therapeutic doses produce little effect on the action potential, toxic doses increase automaticity (increased spontaneous diastolic depolarization) in all heart regions except the SA node.

Pharmacokinetics

• *Absorption:* Deslanoside is inconsistently and incompletely absorbed from the GI tract. After I.V. administration, effects occur in about 10 minutes; peak effects occur in about 20 minutes.

• *Distribution:* Deslanoside is widely distributed in body tissues; highest concentrations occur in the heart, kidneys, intestine, stomach, liver, and skeletal muscle; lowest concentrations are in the plasma and brain. Deslanoside crosses both the blood-brain barrier and the placenta; consequently, fetal and maternal serum drug levels are presumably similar. About 25% of drug is bound to plasma proteins.

• *Metabolism:* Drug's metabolism is minimal.

• *Excretion:* Deslanoside is excreted initially unchanged in the urine; elimination half-life is about 33 hours.

Contraindications and precautions

Deslanoside is contraindicated in patients with ventricular fibrillation, because it may cause ventricular asystole; in patients with digitalis toxicity, because of potential for additive toxicity; and in patients with hypersensitivity to the drug.

Deslanoside should be used with extreme caution, if at all, in patients with idiopathic hypertrophic subaortic stenosis, because the drug may increase obstruction of left ventricular outflow; in patients with incomplete AV block who do not have an artificial pacemaker (especially those with Stokes-Adams syndrome), because the drug may induce advanced or complete AV block; in patients with hypersensitive carotid sinus syndrome, because the drug increases vagal tone (carotid sinus massage has induced ventricular fibrillation in patients receiving cardiac glycosides); in patients with Wolff-Parkinson-White syndrome, because the drug may in-

crease conduction through accessory pathways; in patients with sinus node disease (for example, sick sinus syndrome), because the drug may worsen sinus bradycardia or SA block; and in patients with acute glomerulonephritis and congestive heart failure, because the drug may accumulate rapidly to toxic levels.

Deslanoside should be used with caution in patients with severe pulmonary disease, hypoxia, myxedema, acute myocardial infarction, severe heart failure, acute myocarditis, or an otherwise damaged myocardium, because of the increased risk of drug-induced arrhythmias in these patients; in patients with chronic constrictive pericarditis, because such patients may respond unfavorably to the drug; in patients with frequent premature ventricular contractions or ventricular tachycardia (especially if these arrhythmias are not caused by heart failure), because the drug may induce additional arrhythmias; in patients with low cardiac output states caused by valvular stenosis, chronic pericarditis, or chronic cor pulmonale, because the drug may decrease heart rate and subsequently further reduce cardiac output; in patients with conditions that increase cardiac sensitivity to cardiac glycosides, including hypokalemia, chronic pulmonary disease, and acute hypoxemia; and in patients with hypertension, because I.V. administration may transiently increase blood pressure.

Interactions

Concomitant use of deslanoside with other drugs that affect AV conduction (such as procainamide, propranolol, and verapamil) may have additive cardiac effects. Concomitant use with sympathomimetics (such as ephedrine, epinephrine, and isoproterenol), rauwolfia, or succinylcholine may increase the risk of cardiac arrhythmias.

Concomitant use with I.V. calcium preparations may cause synergistic cardiac effects, precipitating arrhythmias; use with electrolyte-altering agents may increase or decrease serum electrolyte levels, in turn predisposing the patient to deslanoside toxicity. For example, concomitant use with diuretics (such as ethacrynic acid, furosemide, and bumetanide) may cause hypokalemia and hypomagnesemia; thiazides may cause hypercalcemia. Fatal cardiac arrhythmias may result. Concomitant use with amphotericin B, corticosteroids, corticotropin, edetate disodium, laxatives, or sodium polystyrene sulfonate may deplete total body potassium levels. Concomitant use with glucagon, high-dose dextrose, or dextrose-insulin infusions reduces extracellular potassium. Patients receiving these drugs may be predisposed to digitalis toxicity.

Effects on diagnostic tests

None reported.

Adverse reactions

• CNS: fatigue, generalized weakness, agitation, hallucinations, headache, malaise, dizziness, vertigo, stupor, paresthesia.

• CV: *increased severity of congestive heart failure, arrhythmias* (most commonly conduction disturbances with or without AV block, premature ventricular contractions, and supraventricular arrhythmias), hypotension. (These effects may be life-threatening and require immediate attention.)

• EENT: yellow-green halos around visual images, blurred vision, light flashes, photophobia, diplopia.

• GI: anorexia, nausea, vomiting, diarrhea.

Note: Drug should be discontinued if signs of digitalis toxicity are present (nausea, vomiting, arrhythmias).

Overdose and treatment
Clinical effects of overdose mainly involve the gastrointestinal, CNS, and cardiovascular systems.

Hyperkalemia may occur with severe intoxication and may develop rapidly, possibly resulting in life-threatening cardiac effects. Signs of cardiac toxicity may occur with or without other toxicity signs and commonly precede other toxic manifestations. Because most toxic cardiac effects also may be manifestations of heart disease, it may be difficult to determine whether these result from underlying heart disease or from drug therapy. Patients with chronic drug toxicity commonly have ventricular arrhythmias and/or AV conduction disturbances. In patients with digoxin-induced ventricular tachycardia, mortality is high; this condition may progress to ventricular fibrillation or asystole.

If toxicity is suspected, the drug should be discontinued immediately and the serum drug concentration measured. (Usually, the drug requires at least 6 hours to equilibrate between plasma and tissue; therefore, plasma levels drawn earlier may show higher levels than those present after the drug is distributed to the tissues.)

Any interacting drugs probably also should be discontinued. Ventricular arrhythmias may be treated with I.V. potassium, I.V. phenytoin, I.V. lidocaine, or I.V. propranolol. Refractory ventricular tachyarrhythmias may be controlled with overdrive pacing. Procainamide may be used for ventricular arrhythmias that do not respond to the above treatments. In severe AV block, asystole, and hemodynamically significant sinus bradycardia, atropine may restore normal heart rate.

▶ **Special considerations**
● Do not administer calcium salts to patient receiving deslanoside because this may cause serious arrhythmias. Because deslanoside predisposes to postcardioversion arrhythmias, it is commonly withheld 1 to 2 days before elective cardioversion in patients with atrial fibrillation. (However, consider consequences of increased ventricular response to atrial fibrillation while deslanoside is withheld.)
● Elective cardioversion should be postponed in patients with signs of drug toxicity.
● Hypothyroid patients are sensitive to drug; hyperthyroid patients may need larger doses.
● Obtain baseline heart rate and rhythm, blood pressure, and serum electrolyte levels before giving first dose.
● Ask patient about use of cardiac glycosides within previous 2 to 3 weeks before administering loading dose.
● Always divide loading dose over first 24 hours unless clinical situation indicates otherwise. Use only for rapid digitalization, not maintenance therapy.
● Dosage must be adjusted to patient's clinical condition; ECG and serum levels of drug, calcium, potassium, and magnesium must be monitored. Serum potassium should be maintained at 4 to 5 mEq/liter to prevent ventricular irritability.
● Monitor clinical status. Take apical and radial pulses for full minute. Watch for significant changes (sudden rate increase or decrease, pulse deficit, irregular beats, and especially regularization of a previously irregular rhythm). Check blood pressure and obtain 12-lead ECG if these changes occur.

● Excessive slowing of pulse rate (to 60 beats/minute or less) may be a sign of drug toxicity. Withhold drug and reevaluate therapy if this occurs.
● Observe patient's eating patterns. Ask him if he has experienced nausea, vomiting, anorexia, visual disturbances, or other toxicity symptoms.
● I.M. injection is painful; give I.V. if possible.
● Monitor serum potassium levels. Take corrective action before hypokalemia occurs.

Geriatric use
Use deslanoside with extreme caution in elderly patients; dosage should be adjusted to avoid systemic accumulation.

Pediatric use
Pediatric patients have poorly defined serum drug level ranges; however, toxicity apparently does not occur at same concentrations considered toxic in adults. Divided daily dosing is recommended for infants and children under age 10. Children over age 10 require adult doses proportional to body weight.

Breast-feeding
Safety and effectiveness has not been established.

desmopressin acetate
DDAVP, Stimate

● Pharmacologic classification: posterior pituitary hormone
● Therapeutic classification: antidiuretic; hemostatic agent
● Pregnancy risk category B

How supplied
Available by prescription only
Nasal solution: 2.5-ml vials, 0.1 mg/ml
Injection: 10-ml vials, 4 mcg/ml

Indications, route, and dosage
Nonnephrogenic diabetes insipidus, temporary polyuria, and polydipsia associated with pituitary trauma
Adults: 0.1 to 0.4 ml intranasally daily in one to three doses. Adjust morning and evening doses separately for adequate diurnal rhythm of water turnover. Alternatively, may administer injectable form in dosage of 0.5 to 1 ml I.V. or S.C. daily, usually in two divided doses.
Children age 3 months to 12 years: 0.05 to 0.3 ml intranasally daily in one or two doses; or 2 to 4 mcg I.V. daily in divided doses.
Hemophilia A and von Willebrand's disease
Adults and children: 0.3 mcg/kg diluted in normal saline solution and infused I.V. slowly over 15 to 30 minutes. May repeat dosage, if necessary, as indicated by laboratory response and the patient's clinical condition.

Pharmacodynamics
● *Antidiuretic action:* Desmopressin is used to control or prevent signs and complications of neurogenic diabetes insipidus. The site of action is primarily at the renal tubular level. Desmopressin increases cyclic 3′,5′-adenosine monophosphate, which increases water permeability at the renal tubule and collecting duct, re-

sulting in increased urine osmolality and decreased urinary flow rate.
● *Hemostatic action:* Desmopressin increases Factor VIII activity by releasing endogenous Factor VIII from plasma storage sites.

Pharmacokinetics
● *Absorption:* Desmopressin is destroyed in the GI tract. After intranasal administration, 10% to 20% of the dose is absorbed through nasal mucosa; antidiuretic action occurs within 1 hour and peaks in 1 to 5 hours. After I.V. infusion, plasma Factor VIII activity increases within 15 to 30 minutes and peaks between 1½ and 3 hours.
● *Distribution:* Distribution is not fully understood.
● *Metabolism:* Unknown.
● *Excretion:* Plasma levels decline in two phases: the half-life of the fast phase is about 8 minutes; the slow phase, 75½ minutes. Duration of action after intranasal administration is 8 to 20 hours; after I.V. administration, it is 12 to 24 hours for mild hemophilia and approximately 3 hours for von Willebrand's disease.

Contraindications and precautions
Desmopressin is contraindicated in patients with known hypersensitivity to the drug and in those with type IIB or platelet-type von Willebrand's disease (pseudomophilia). It should be used cautiously in patients with allergic rhinitis, nasal congestion, or upper respiratory infection because these states may interfere with the drug's absorption. Large doses of desmopressin may produce a slight rise in blood pressure when used in patients with coronary artery disease or hypertension.

Interactions
Concomitant use of desmopressin with carbamazepine, chlorpropamide, or clofibrate may potentiate desmopressin's antidiuretic action. Concomitant use with lithium, epinephrine, norepinephrine, demeclocycline, heparin, or alcohol may decrease the antidiuretic effect.

Effects on diagnostic tests
None reported.

Adverse reactions
● CNS: headache, *seizures,* confusion, drowsiness, *coma.*
● CV: slight rise in blood pressure at high doses, hypotension with rapid I.V. injection.
● EENT: nasal congestion, rhinitis.
● GI: nausea, abdominal cramps.
● GU: anuria, vulval pain, problems with urination.
● Local: pain, redness at injection site.
● Other: weight gain, flushing, *anaphylaxis.*
   Note: Drug should be discontinued if signs or symptoms of anaphylaxis, hypersensitivity, or water intoxication occur.

Overdose and treatment
Clinical manifestations of overdose include drowsiness, listlessness, headache, confusion, anuria, and weight gain (water intoxication). Treatment requires water restriction and temporary withdrawal of desmopressin until polyuria occurs. Severe water intoxication may require osmotic diuresis with mannitol, hypertonic dextrose, or urea – alone or with furosemide.

▶ Special considerations
Besides those relevant to all *posterior pituitary hormones,* consider the following recommendations.

● Desmopressin is administered intranasally through a flexible catheter called a rhinyle. A measured quantity is drawn up into the catheter, one end is inserted into the patient's nose, and the patient blows on the other end to deposit drug into nasal cavity.
● Patients may be switched from intranasal to subcutaneous desmopressin (for example, during episodes of rhinorrhea). They should receive one tenth of their usual dosage parenterally.
● Observe for early signs of water intoxication – drowsiness, listlessness, headache, confusion, anuria, and weight gain – to prevent seizures, coma, and death.
● Adjust patient's fluid intake to reduce risk of water intoxication and of sodium depletion, especially in young or elderly patients.
● Patient should be weighed daily and observed for edema.
● Desmopressin is not indicated for hemophilia A patients with Factor VIII levels up to 5% or in patients with severe von Willebrand's disease.
● Desmopressin therapy may enable some patients to avoid the hazards of contaminated blood products.
● Check expiration date.

Information for the patient
● Some patients may have difficulty measuring and inhaling drug into nostrils. Teach them correct administration technique, then evaluate their proficiency at drug administration and accurate measurement on return visits.
● Emphasize that patient should not increase or decrease dosage unless it is prescribed.
● Review with patient fluid intake measurement and methods for measuring fluid output.
● Tell patient to call if signs of water intoxication (drowsiness, listlessness, headache, or shortness of breath) develop.
● Tell patient to store drug away from heat and direct light, not in bathroom, where heat and moisture can cause drug to deteriorate.

Geriatric use
● Elderly patients have an increased risk of hyponatremia and water intoxication; therefore, restriction of their fluid intake is recommended.
● Because elderly patients are more sensitive to this drug's effects, they may need a lower dosage.

Pediatric use
● Use of desmopressin in infants under age 3 months is not recommended because of infants' increased tendency to develop fluid imbalance.
● Use with caution in infants because of risk of hyponatremia and water intoxication.
● Safety and efficacy of parenteral desmopressin have not been established for management of diabetes insipidus in children under age 12.

desonide
DesOwen, Tridesilon

- Pharmacologic classification: topical adrenocorticoid
- Therapeutic classification: anti-inflammatory
- Pregnancy risk category C

How supplied
Available by prescription only
Cream, ointment: 0.05%

Indications, route, and dosage
Adjunctive therapy for inflammation in acute and chronic corticosteroid-responsive dermatoses
Adults and children: Apply sparingly to affected area b.i.d. to q.i.d.

Pharmacodynamics
Anti-inflammatory action: Desonide stimulates the synthesis of enzymes needed to decrease the inflammatory response. Desonide is a group IV nonfluorinated glucocorticoid with a potency similar to that of alclometasone dipropionate 0.05% and fluocinolone acetonide 0.01%.

Pharmacokinetics
- *Absorption:* The amount of desonide absorbed depends on the amount applied and on the nature of the skin at the application site. It ranges from about 1% in areas with a thick stratum corneum (such as the palms, soles, elbows, and knees) to as much as 36% in areas of the thinnest stratum corneum (face, eyelids, and genitals). Absorption increases in areas of skin damage, inflammation, or occlusion. Some systemic absorption of topical steroids occurs, especially through the oral mucosa.
- *Distribution:* After topical application, desonide is distributed throughout the local skin layer. Any drug that is absorbed into circulation is removed rapidly from the blood and distributed into muscle, liver, skin, intestines, and kidneys.
- *Metabolism:* After topical administration, desonide is metabolized primarily in the skin. The small amount that is absorbed into systemic circulation is metabolized primarily in the liver to inactive compounds.
- *Excretion:* Inactive metabolites are excreted by the kidneys, primarily as glucuronides and sulfates, but also as unconjugated products. Small amounts of the metabolites are also excreted in feces.

Contraindications and precautions
Desonide is contraindicated in patients who are hypersensitive to any component of the preparation and in patients with viral, fungal, or tubercular skin lesions.

Desonide should be used with extreme caution in patients with impaired circulation, because the drug may increase the risk of skin ulceration.

Interactions
None significant.

Effects on diagnostic tests
None reported.

Adverse reactions
- Local: burning, itching, irritation, dryness, folliculitis, hypertrichosis, acneiform eruptions, hypopigmentation, perioral dermatitis, allergic contact dermatitis, maceration, secondary infection, atrophy, striae, miliaria.

Significant systemic absorption may produce the following effects.
- CNS: euphoria, insomnia, headache, psychotic behavior, pseudotumor cerebri, mental changes, nervousness, restlessness.
- CV: congestive heart failure, hypertension, edema.
- EENT: cataracts, glaucoma, thrush.
- GI: peptic ulcer, irritation, increased appetite.
- Immune: increased susceptibility to infection.
- Metabolic: hypokalemia, sodium retention, fluid retention, weight gain, hyperglycemia, osteoporosis, growth suppression in children.
- Musculoskeletal: muscle atrophy.
- Other: withdrawal syndrome (nausea, fatigue, anorexia, dyspnea, hypotension, hypoglycemia, myalgia, arthralgia, fever, dizziness, and fainting).

Note: Drug should be discontinued if local irritation, infection, systemic absorption, or hypersensitivity reaction occurs.

Overdose and treatment
No information available.

▶ Special considerations
Recommendations for use of desonide, for care and teaching of patients during therapy, and for use in elderly patients, children, and breast-feeding women are the same as those for all *topical adrenocorticoids.*

desoximetasone
Topicort

- Pharmacologic classification: topical adrenocorticoid
- Therapeutic classification: anti-inflammatory
- Pregnancy risk category C

How supplied
Available by prescription only
Cream: 0.05%, 0.25%
Gel: 0.05%
Ointment: 0.25%

Indications, route, and dosage
Inflammation of corticosteroid-responsive dermatoses
Adults and children: Apply sparingly in a very thin film and rub in gently to the affected area once daily to t.i.d.

Pharmacodynamics
Anti-inflammatory action: Desoximetasone stimulates the synthesis of enzymes needed to decrease the inflammatory response. Desoximetasone is a synthetic fluorinated corticosteroid. The 0.05% gel and cream have a potency of group III; the 0.25% cream and ointment have a potency of group II.

Pharmacokinetics
- *Absorption:* The amount of desoximetasone absorbed depends on the strength of the preparation, the

amount applied, and the nature of the skin at the application site. It ranges from about 1% in areas with a thick stratum corneum (such as the palms, soles, elbows, and knees) to as much as 36% in areas of the thinnest stratum corneum (face, eyelids, and genitals). Absorption increases in areas of skin damage, inflammation, or occlusion. Some systemic absorption of topical steroids, especially through the oral mucosa, may occur.

• *Distribution:* After topical application, desoximetasone is distributed throughout the local skin. Any drug that is absorbed into circulation is removed rapidly from the blood and distributed into muscle, liver, skin, intestines, and kidneys.

• *Metabolism:* After topical administration, desoximetasone is metabolized primarily in the skin. The small amount that is absorbed into systemic circulation is metabolized primarily in the liver to inactive compounds.

• *Excretion:* Inactive metabolites are excreted by the kidneys, primarily as glucuronides and sulfates, but also as unconjugated products. Small amounts of the metabolites are also excreted in feces.

Contraindications and precautions
Desoximetasone is contraindicated in patients who are hypersensitive to any component of the preparation and in patients with viral, fungal, or tubercular skin lesions.

Desoximetasone should be used with extreme caution in patients with impaired circulation, because the drug may increase the risk of skin ulceration. Avoid using on the face and genital areas because increased absorption may result in striae.

Interactions
None significant.

Effects on diagnostic tests
None reported.

Adverse reactions
• Local: burning, itching, irritation, dryness, folliculitis, hypertrichosis, acneiform eruptions, hypopigmentation, perioral dermatitis, allergic contact dermatitis, maceration, secondary infection, atrophy, striae, miliaria.

Significant systemic absorption may produce the following reactions.
• CNS: euphoria, insomnia, headache, psychotic behavior, pseudotumor cerebri, mental changes, nervousness, restlessness.
• CV: *congestive heart failure*, hypertension, edema.
• DERM: delayed healing, acne, skin eruptions, striae.
• EENT: cataracts, glaucoma, thrush.
• GI: peptic ulcer, GI irritation, increased appetite.
• Immune: immunosuppression, increased susceptibility to infection.
• Metabolic: hypokalemia, sodium retention, fluid retention, weight gain, hyperglycemia, osteoporosis, growth suppression in children.
• Musculoskeletal: muscle atrophy.
• Other: withdrawal syndrome (nausea, fatigue, anorexia, dyspnea, hypotension, hypoglycemia, myalgia, arthralgia, fever, dizziness, and fainting).
Note: Drug should be discontinued if local irritation, infection, systemic absorption, or hypersensitivity reaction occurs.

Overdose and treatment
No information available.

▶ Special considerations
Recommendations for use of desoximetasone, for care and teaching of patients during therapy, and for use in elderly patients, children, and breast-feeding women are the same as those for all *topical adrenocorticoids.*

---

desoxycorticosterone acetate
Doca Acetate, Percorten Acetate

desoxycorticosterone pivalate
Percorten Pivalate

• Pharmacologic classification: mineralocorticoid
• Therapeutic classification: mineralocorticoid replacement therapy
• Pregnancy risk category C

How supplied
Available by prescription only
Desoxycorticosterone acetate
Injection: 5 mg/ml
Pellets: 125 mg
Desoxycorticosterone pivalate
Repository injection: 25 mg/ml suspension

Indications, route, and dosage
Adrenal insufficiency (partial replacement), salt-losing adrenogenital syndrome
Desoxycorticosterone acetate
Adults: 1 to 5 mg I.M. daily. Alternatively, give 1 to 6 mg I.M. for 3 or 4 days, then adjust dosage based upon clinical and serum electrolyte response. Or implant one pellet (125 mg) for each 0.5 mg of the daily injected maintenance dose. Repeat at 8- to 12-month intervals.
Desoxycorticosterone pivalate
Adults: 25 mg I.M. for each 1 mg of the daily maintenance dose of acetate. Repeat at 4-week intervals.

Pharmacodynamics
Adrenal hormone replacement: Desoxycorticosterone regulates electrolyte homeostasis by acting renally at the distal tubules to enhance the reabsorption of sodium ions (and thus water) from the tubular fluid into the plasma and enhance the excretion of both potassium and hydrogen ions.

Desoxycorticosterone is an adrenal cortical steroid with potent mineralocorticoid activity, but essentially no glucocorticoid properties. It is used for partial steroid hormone replacement in adrenal insufficiency and in patients with salt-losing forms of congenital adrenogenital syndrome. When treating adrenocortical insufficiency with desoxycorticosterone, an exogenous glucocorticoid is also needed for adequate control. (Cortisone or hydrocortisone are usually the drugs of choice for replacement because they have both mineralocorticoid and glucocorticoid activity.)

Pharmacokinetics
• *Absorption:* Desoxycorticosterone is not administered orally because it is destroyed in the GI tract. When administered I.M., the acetate salt is absorbed readily and must be replaced daily. Absorption from the subcutaneously implanted acetate pellets is much slower. The pellets must be replaced every 8 to 12 months. The pivalate suspension is absorbed gradually after

I.M. injection. It must be reinjected approximately every 4 weeks to maintain therapy.

● *Distribution:* Once absorbed, desoxycorticosterone is rapidly removed from the blood and distributed to muscle, liver, skin, intestines, and kidneys. It has a plasma half-life of about 70 minutes. It is extensively bound to plasma proteins (transcortin and albumin). Only the unbound portion is active. Adrenocorticoids are distributed into breast milk and through the placenta.

● *Metabolism:* Desoxycorticosterone is metabolized in the liver to inactive glucuronide and sulfate metabolites.

● *Excretion:* The inactive metabolites and small amounts of unmetabolized drug are excreted by the kidneys. Insignificant quantities of drug are excreted in feces.

Contraindications and precautions

Desoxycorticosterone is contraindicated in patients who are hypersensitive to desoxycorticosterone acetate or pivalate. It should be used with extreme caution in patients with hypertension, congestive heart failure (CHF), or cardiac disease, because the drug may exacerbate these conditions. Treatment should be stopped if weight or blood pressure increases significantly or if edema or cardiac enlargement develops.

The use of mineralocorticoids should be accompanied by adequate glucocorticoid therapy in adrenal insufficiency or the salt-losing form of adrenogenital syndrome.

Patients with Addison's disease are more sensitive to the action of desoxycorticosterone and may develop severe adverse reactions. Treatment should be discontinued if weight or blood pressure increases significantly or if edema or cardiac enlargement develops.

Interactions

Concomitant use of desoxycorticosterone with barbiturates, phenytoin, or rifampin may cause decreased corticosteroid effects due to increased hepatic metabolism. Desoxycorticosterone may increase the metabolism of isoniazid and salicylates. It may increase hypokalemia associated with diuretic or amphotericin B therapy. The hypokalemia may increase the risk of toxicity in patients concurrently receiving digitalis glycosides.

Effects on diagnostic tests

Desoxycorticosterone therapy increases serum sodium levels and decreases serum potassium levels. In addisonian patients, it causes a tendency to react with severe hypoglycemia within 3 hours of receiving desoxycorticosterone; therefore, perform glucose tolerance tests only if necessary.

Adverse reactions

● CNS: frontal and occipital headaches, dizziness.
● CV: sodium and water retention, leading to increased blood volume, edema, hypertension, CHF, cardiac arrhythmias, cardiomegaly.
● Metabolic: hypokalemia, unusual weight gain.
● Musculoskeletal: arthralgias and tendon contractures, extreme weakness of extremities with ascending paralysis secondary to low potassium.
Note: Drug should not be discontinued without medical supervision; rapid withdrawal may cause an addisonian crisis.

Overdose and treatment

Acute toxicity is manifested as an extension of the therapeutic effect, such as disturbances in fluid and electrolyte balance, hypokalemia, edema, hypertension, and cardiac insufficiency. In acute poisoning, treat symptomatically and take measures to correct fluid and electrolyte imbalances.

▶ Special considerations

Besides those relevant to all *systemic adrenocorticoids,* consider the following recommendations.

● Plasma renin activity is usually the most sensitive laboratory test used to evaluate the adequacy of drug therapy. It is profoundly abnormal before clinical signs and symptoms become apparent.
● Drug should be used only with other supplemental measures, such as glucocorticoids, control of electrolytes, and control of infection.
● Supplemental dosages may be required in times of great stress such as infection, trauma, or surgery.
● I.M. injections should be given in the upper outer quadrant of the buttocks. It is important to alternate injection sites. The upper extremities are not recommended as injection sites.
● To identify the proper dosage for replacement therapy by pellet implantation, administer desoxycorticosterone acetate by I.M. injection daily.
● If I.M. administration is impossible, administer drug subcutaneously.
● Once a maintenance dose has been identified, sterile pellets of desoxycorticosterone acetate may be implanted below the skin over the scapula. After implantation, the mineralocorticoid effects usually last 8 to 12 months. Signs that additional mineralocorticoid is needed include anorexia, weight loss, fatigue, and a gradual decrease in blood pressure. Before more pellets are implanted, the daily maintenance requirement of desoxycorticosterone acetate injection should again be determined over a 4- to 6-week period, because hormone requirements may have changed.
● Desoxycorticosterone pivalate suspension may also be used for maintenance therapy. After the dosage requirement has been determined by daily injections of the acetate salt, 25 mg of desoxycorticosterone pivalate may be substituted for every 1 mg of desoxycorticosterone acetate. The pivalate salt is injected into the upper outer quadrant of the buttocks, using a 20G needle, approximately every 4 weeks. High sodium intake accelerates sodium retention and potassium loss. If edema develops, restrict dietary sodium. Give potassium supplements as necessary.
● Monitor for significant patient weight gain, edema, hypertension, or severe headaches.

Information for the patient

● Teach patients to recognize signs of electrolyte imbalance: muscle weakness, paresthesias, numbness, fatigue, anorexia, nausea, altered mental status, increased urination, altered heart rhythm, severe or continuing headaches, unusual weight gain, or swelling of the feet.
● Advise patient to inject missed doses as soon as possible, unless it is almost time for the next dose, but not to double the next dose.

Pediatric use

Chronic use of desoxycorticosterone in children and adolescents may delay growth and maturation.

---

dexamethasone (systemic)
Decadron, Deronil*, Dexasone*, Dexone, Hexadrol, SK-Dexamethasone

dexamethasone acetate
Dalalone D.P., Decadron L.A., Decaject L.A., Decameth L.A., Dexacen, Dexasone L.A., Dexon L.A., Solurex L.A.

dexamethasone sodium phosphate
AK-Dex, Dalalone, Decadrol, Decadron, Decaject, Decameth, Dexacen, Dexasone, Dexon, Dexone, Hexadrol Phosphate, Oradexon*, Solurex

- Pharmacologic classification: glucocorticoid
- Therapeutic classification: anti-inflammatory, immunosuppressant
- Pregnancy risk category C

How supplied
Available by prescription only
Dexamethasone
Tablets: 0.25 mg, 0.5 mg, 0.75 mg, 1 mg, 1.5 mg, 2 mg, 4 mg, 6 mg
Elixir: 0.5 mg/5 ml
Oral solution: 0.5 mg/5 ml, 0.5 mg/0.5 ml
Dexamethasone acetate
Injection: 8 mg/ml, 16 mg/ml suspension
Dexamethasone sodium phosphate
Injection: 4 mg/ml, 10 mg/ml, 20 mg/ml, 24 mg/ml

Indications, route, and dosage
Cerebral edema
Children: 0.2 mg/kg P.O., I.M., or I.V. daily in divided doses.
Dexamethasone sodium phosphate
Adults: Initially, 10 mg I.V., then 4 to 6 mg I.M. q 6 hours for 2 to 4 days, then taper over 5 to 7 days.
Inflammatory conditions, allergic reactions, neoplasias
Adults: 0.5 to 9 mg P.O. b.i.d., t.i.d., or q.i.d.
Children: 0.0833 to 0.333 mg/kg daily in three divided doses.
Dexamethasone sodium phosphate
Adults: 0.2 to 6 mg intra-articularly, intralesional, or into soft tissue; or 0.5 to 9 mg I.M.
Children: 0.02776 to 0.16665 mg/kg I.M.
Dexamethasone acetate
Adults: 0.8 to 1.6 mg I.M. or into lesions q 1 to 3 weeks; or 4 to 16 mg intra-articularly or into tissue q 1 to 3 weeks.
Shock (other than adrenal crisis)
Dexamethasone sodium phosphate
Adults: 1 to 6 mg/kg I.V. daily as a single dose; or 40 mg I.V. q 2 to 6 hours, p.r.n.
Dexamethasone suppression test
Adults: 0.5 mg P.O. q 6 hours for 48 hours.
Adrenal insufficiency
Dexamethasone sodium phosphate
Children: 0.0233 mg/kg I.M. in three divided doses; or 0.00776 to 0.01165 mg/kg I.M. daily.

Pharmacodynamics
Anti-inflammatory action: Dexamethasone stimulates the synthesis of enzymes needed to decrease the inflammatory response. It causes suppression of the immune system by reducing activity and volume of the lymphatic system, producing lymphocytopenia (primarily T-lymphocytes), decreasing passage of immune complexes through basement membranes, and possibly by depressing reactivity of tissue to antigen-antibody interactions.

Dexamethasone is a long-acting synthetic adrenocorticoid with strong anti-inflammatory activity and minimal mineralocorticoid properties. It is 25 to 30 times more potent than an equal weight of hydrocortisone.

The acetate salt is a suspension and should not be used I.V. It is particularly useful as an anti-inflammatory agent in intra-articular, intradermal, and intralesional injections.

The sodium phosphate salt is highly soluble and has a more rapid onset and a shorter duration of action than does the acetate salt. It is most commonly used for cerebral edema and unresponsive shock. It can also be used in intra-articular, intralesional, or soft tissue inflammation. Other uses for dexamethasone are symptomatic treatment of bronchial asthma, chemotherapy-induced nausea, and as a diagnostic test for Cushing's syndrome.

Pharmacokinetics
- *Absorption:* After oral administration, dexamethasone is absorbed readily, and peak effects occur in about 1 to 2 hours. The suspension for injection has a variable onset and duration of action (ranging from 2 days to 3 weeks), depending on whether it is injected into an intra-articular space, a muscle, or the blood supply to the muscle.
- *Distribution:* Dexamethasone is removed rapidly from the blood and distributed to muscle, liver, skin, intestines, and kidneys. Dexamethasone is bound weakly to plasma proteins (transcortin and albumin). Only the unbound portion is active. Adrenocorticoids are distributed into breast milk and through the placenta.
- *Metabolism:* Dexamethasone is metabolized in the liver to inactive glucuronide and sulfate metabolites.
- *Excretion:* The inactive metabolites and small amounts of unmetabolized drug are excreted by the kidneys. Insignificant quantities of drug are also excreted in feces. The biological half-life of dexamethasone is 36 to 54 hours.

Contraindications and precautions
Dexamethasone is contraindicated in patients who are hypersensitive to ingredients of adrenocorticoid preparations and in those with systemic fungal infections (except in adrenal insufficiency). Patients who are receiving dexamethasone should not be given live virus vaccines because dexamethasone suppresses the immune response.

Dexamethasone should be used with extreme caution in patients with GI ulceration, renal disease, hypertension, osteoporosis, diabetes mellitus, thromboembolytic disorders, seizures, myasthenia gravis, congestive heart failure (CHF), tuberculosis, hypoalbuminemia, hypothyroidism, cirrhosis of the liver, emotional instability, psychotic tendencies, hyperlipidemias, glaucoma, or cataracts, because the drug may exacerbate these conditions.

Because adrenocorticoids increase susceptibility to and mask symptoms of infection, dexamethasone should not be used (except in life-threatening situations) in patients with viral or bacterial infections not controlled by anti-infective agents.

Interactions

When used concomitantly, dexamethasone may in rare cases decrease the effects of oral anticoagulants by unknown mechanisms.

Dexamethasone increases the metabolism of isoniazid and salicylates; causes hyperglycemia, requiring dosage adjustment of insulin or oral hypoglycemic agents in diabetic patients; and may enhance hypokalemia associated with diuretic or amphotericin B therapy. The hypokalemia may increase the risk of toxicity in patients concurrently receiving digitalis glycosides.

Concomitant use of barbiturates, phenytoin, and rifampin may cause decreased corticosteroid effects because of increased hepatic metabolism. Cholestyramine, colestipol, and antacids decrease the corticosteroid effect by adsorbing the corticosteroid, decreasing the amount absorbed.

Concomitant use with estrogens may reduce the metabolism of dexamethasone by increasing the concentration of transcortin. The half-life of the corticosteroid is then prolonged because of increased protein-binding. Concomitant administration of ulcerogenic drugs, such as the nonsteroidal anti-inflammatory agents, may increase the risk of GI ulceration.

Effects on diagnostic tests

Dexamethasone suppresses reactions to skin tests; causes false-negative results in the nitroblue tetrazolium test for systemic bacterial infections; and decreases ^{131}I uptake and protein-bound iodine concentrations in thyroid function tests.

Dexamethasone may increase glucose and cholesterol levels; may decrease levels of serum potassium, calcium, thyroxine, and triiodothyronine; and may increase urine glucose and calcium levels.

Adverse reactions

When administered in high doses or for prolonged periods, dexamethasone suppresses the release of adrenocorticotropic hormone (ACTH) from the pituitary gland, stopping secretion of endogenous corticosteroids from the adrenal cortex. The degree and duration of hypothalamic-pituitary-adrenal (HPA) axis suppression produced by glucocorticoids is highly variable among patients and depends on the dose, frequency and time of administration, and duration of glucocorticoid therapy.

● CNS: euphoria, insomnia, headache, psychotic behavior, pseudotumor cerebri, mental changes, nervousness, restlessness.
● CV: CHF, hypertension, edema.
● DERM: delayed healing, acne, skin eruptions, striae.
● EENT: cataracts, glaucoma, thrush.
● GI: peptic ulcer, irritation, increased appetite.
● Immune: immunosuppression, increased susceptibility to infection.
● Metabolic: hypokalemia, sodium retention, fluid retention, weight gain, hyperglycemia, osteoporosis, growth suppression in children.
● Musculoskeletal: muscle atrophy, weakness.
● Local: atrophy at I.M. injection sites.
● Other: pancreatitis, hirsutism, cushingoid symptoms, withdrawal syndrome (nausea, fatigue, anorexia, dyspnea, hypotension, hypoglycemia, myalgia, arthralgia, fever, dizziness, and fainting). *Sudden discontinuation*

may be fatal or may exacerbate the underlying disease. Acute adrenal insufficiency may follow increased stress (infection, surgery, trauma) or abrupt withdrawal after long-term therapy.

Overdose and treatment

Acute ingestion, even in massive doses, rarely poses a clinical problem. Toxic signs and symptoms rarely occur if drug is used for less than 3 weeks, even at large dosage ranges. However, chronic use causes adverse physiologic effects, including suppression of the HPA axis, cushingoid appearance, muscle weakness, and osteoporosis.

▶ Special considerations

Recommendations for use of dexamethasone, for care and teaching of patients during therapy, and for use in elderly patients and breast-feeding women are the same as those for all *systemic adrenocorticoids*.
● This drug is being used investigationally to prevent hyaline membrane disease (respiratory distress syndrome) in premature infants. The suspension (acetate salt) is administered I.M. to the mother two or three times daily for 2 days before delivery.

Pediatric use

Chronic use of dexamethasone in children and adolescents may delay growth and maturation.

---

dexamethasone (topical)
Aeroseb-Dex, Decaderm, Decaspray

dexamethasone sodium phosphate
Decadron Cream

● Pharmacologic classification: glucocorticoid
● Therapeutic classification: anti-inflammatory
● Pregnancy risk category C

How supplied

Available by prescription only
Dexamethasone
Aerosol: 0.01%, 0.04%
Gel: 0.1%
Dexamethasone sodium phosphate
Cream: 0.1%

Indications, route, and dosage
Inflammation of corticosteroid-responsive dermatoses

Adults and children: Apply gel or aerosol sparingly once daily to q.i.d.

For aerosol use on scalp, shake can well and apply to dry scalp after shampooing. Hold can upright. Slide applicator tube under hair so that it touches scalp. Spray while moving tube to all affected areas, keeping tube under hair and in contact with scalp throughout spraying, which should take about 2 seconds. Inadequately covered areas may be spot sprayed. Slide applicator tube through hair to touch scalp, press and immediately release spray button. Do not massage medication into scalp or spray forehead or eyes.

---

326 **DEXAMETHASONE (OPHTHALMIC)**

Pharmacodynamics
Anti-inflammatory action: Dexamethasone stimulates the synthesis of enzymes needed to decrease the inflammatory response. Dexamethasone is a synthetic fluorinated corticosteroid. It is usually classed as a group V or group VI potency anti-inflammatory agent. Occlusive dressings may be used in severe cases. The aerosol spray is usually used for dermatologic conditions of the scalp.

Pharmacokinetics
• *Absorption:* Drug absorption depends on the potency of the preparation, the amount applied, and the nature of the skin at the application site. It ranges from about 1% in areas with a thick stratum corneum (such as the palms, soles, elbows, and knees) to as high as 36% in areas of the thinnest stratum corneum (face, eyelids, and genitals). Absorption increases in areas of skin damage, inflammation, or occlusion. Some systemic absorption occurs, especially through the oral mucosa.
• *Distribution:* After topical applications, dexamethasone is distributed throughout the local skin layer. If absorbed into circulation, the drug is distributed rapidly into muscle, liver, skin, intestines, and kidneys.
• *Metabolism:* After topical administration, dexamethasone is metabolized primarily in the skin. The small amount that is absorbed into systemic circulation is primarily metabolized in the liver to inactive compounds.
• *Excretion:* Inactive metabolites are excreted by the kidneys, primarily as glucuronides and sulfates, but also as unconjugated products. Small amounts of the metabolites are also excreted in feces.

Contraindications and precautions
Dexamethasone is contraindicated in patients who are hypersensitive to any component of the preparation and in patients with viral, fungal, or tubercular skin lesions. It should be used with extreme caution in patients with impaired circulation, because the drug may increase the risk of skin ulceration.

Interactions
None significant.

Effects on diagnostic tests
None reported.

Adverse reactions
• Local: burning, itching, irritation, dryness, folliculitis, hypertrichosis, acneiform eruptions, hypopigmentation, perioral dermatitis, and allergic contact dermatitis. Use of occlusive dressings may result in maceration, secondary infection, skin atrophy, striae, and miliaria.
The following effects may occur from systemic absorption.
• CNS: euphoria, insomnia, headache, psychotic behavior, pseudotumor cerebri, mental changes, nervousness, restlessness.
• CV: congestive heart failure, hypertension, edema.
• DERM: delayed healing, acne, skin eruptions, striae.
• EENT: cataracts, glaucoma, thrush.
• GI: peptic ulcer, irritation, increased appetite.
• Immune: immunosuppression, increased susceptibility to infection.
• Metabolic: hypokalemia, sodium retention, fluid retention, weight gain, hyperglycemia, osteoporosis, growth suppression in children.
• Musculoskeletal: muscle atrophy.

• Other: withdrawal syndrome (nausea, fatigue, anorexia, dyspnea, hypotension, hypoglycemia, myalgia, arthralgia, fever, dizziness, and fainting).
Note: Drug should be discontinued if local irritation, infection, systemic absorption, or hypersensitivity reaction occurs.

Overdose and treatment
No information available.

▶ Special considerations
Recommendations for use of dexamethasone, for care and teaching of patients during therapy, and for use in elderly patients, children, and breast-feeding women are the same as those for all *topical adrenocorticoids.*

dexamethasone (ophthalmic suspension)
Maxidex

dexamethasone sodium phosphate
AK-Dex, Decadron, Dexair, I-Methasone, Maxidex, Ocu-Dex

• Pharmacologic classification: corticosteroid
• Therapeutic classification: ophthalmic anti-inflammatory
• Pregnancy risk category C

How supplied
Available by prescription only
Dexamethasone
Ophthalmic suspension: 0.1%
Dexamethasone sodium phosphate
Ophthalmic ointment: 0.05%
Ophthalmic solution: 0.1%

Indications, route, and dosage
Uveitis; iridocyclitis; inflammation of eyelids, conjunctiva, cornea, anterior segment of globe; corneal injury from burns or penetration by foreign bodies
Adults and children: Instill 1 to 2 drops into conjunctival sac. For initial therapy of severe cases, instill the solution or suspension into the conjunctival sac every hour during the day and every 2 hours during the night. Instill the ointment into the conjunctival sac three or four times daily initially and once or twice daily thereafter. The ointment may also be used at night with daytime use of the suspension or solution. The duration of treatment depends on the type and severity of the disease.

Pharmacodynamics
Anti-inflammatory action: Corticosteroids stimulate the synthesis of enzymes needed to decrease the inflammatory response. Dexamethasone, a long-acting fluorinated synthetic adrenocorticoid with strong anti-inflammatory activity and minimal mineralocorticoid activity, is 25 to 30 times more potent than an equal weight of hydrocortisone. Dexamethasone is poorly soluble and therefore has a slower onset of action but a longer duration of action when applied in a liquid suspension. The sodium phosphate salt is highly soluble and has a rapid onset but short duration of action.

Pharmacokinetics
• *Absorption:* After ophthalmic administration, dexamethasone is absorbed through the aqueous humor. Because only low doses are administered, little if any systemic absorption occurs.
• *Distribution:* Drug is distributed throughout the local tissue layers. Any drug absorbed into circulation is rapidly removed from the blood and distributed into muscle, liver, skin, intestines, and kidneys.
• *Metabolism:* Dexamethasone is primarily metabolized locally. The small amount that is absorbed into systemic circulation is metabolized primarily in the liver to inactive compounds.
• *Excretion:* Inactive metabolites are excreted by the kidneys, primarily as glucuronides and sulfates, but also as unconjugated products. Small amounts of the metabolites are also excreted in feces.

Contraindications and precautions
Dexamethasone is contraindicated in patients who are hypersensitive to any component of the preparation; in patients with fungal infections of the eye; and in patients with acute, untreated purulent bacterial, viral, or fungal ocular infections. It should be used cautiously in patients with corneal abrasions. If a bacterial infection does not respond promptly to appropriate anti-infective therapy, dexamethasone should be discontinued and other therapy applied.

Intraocular pressure should be measured every 2 to 4 weeks for the first 2 months of ophthalmic corticosteroid therapy and then, if no increase in intraocular pressure has occurred, every 1 to 2 months thereafter. Dexamethasone is more likely than other ophthalmic products to increase intraocular pressure in susceptible patients.

Interactions
None reported.

Effects on diagnostic tests
None reported.

Adverse reactions
• Eye: transient burning or stinging on administration; mydriasis, ptosis, epithelial punctate keratitis, and possible corneal or scleral malacia; increased intraocular pressure, thinning of the cornea, interference with corneal wound healing, increased susceptibility to viral or fungal corneal infection, and corneal ulceration; glaucoma, cataracts, defects in visual acuity and visual field with long-term use.
• Systemic: edema, sodium retention, hypothalamic-pituitary-adrenal (HPA) axis suppression (rare, but may occur with excessive doses or long-term use).
Note: Drug should be discontinued if topical application results in local irritation, infection, significant systemic absorption, or hypersensitivity reaction; if visual acuity decreases or visual field is diminished; or if burning, stinging, or watering of eyes does not quickly resolve after administration.

Overdose and treatment
No information available.

▶ Special considerations
Recommendations for administration of dexamethasone and for care and teaching of patients during therapy are the same as those for all *ophthalmic adrenocorticoids.*

dexamethasone sodium phosphate (inhalant)

Nasal inhalants
Decadron Phosphate Turbinaire

Oral inhalants
Decadron Phosphate Respihaler

• Pharmacologic classification: glucocorticoid
• Therapeutic classification: anti-inflammatory, antiasthmatic
• Pregnancy risk category C

How supplied
Available by prescription only
Nasal aerosol: 84 mcg/metered spray; 170 doses/canister
Oral inhalation aerosol: 84 mcg/metered spray; 170 doses/canister

Indications, route, and dosage
Control of bronchial asthma in patients with steroid-dependent asthma
Oral inhaler
Adults: 3 inhalations t.i.d. or q.i.d., to a maximum dosage of 12 inhalations daily.
Children: 2 inhalations t.i.d. or q.i.d., to a maximum dosage of 8 inhalations daily.
Relief of symptoms of perennial or seasonal rhinitis; prevention of recurrence of nasal polyps after surgical removal
Nasal inhaler
Adults: 2 sprays (168 mcg) into each nostril b.i.d. or t.i.d. Maximum dosage of 12 sprays daily (1,008 mcg).
Children age 6 to 12: 1 or 2 sprays (84 to 168 mcg) into each nostril b.i.d. Maximum dosage is 8 sprays daily (672 mcg).

Pharmacodynamics
• *Anti-inflammatory action:* Dexamethasone stimulates the synthesis of enzymes needed to decrease the inflammatory response.
• *Antiasthmatic action:* Dexamethasone is used as a nasal inhalant for the symptomatic treatment of seasonal or perennial rhinitis and nasal polyposis. It is used as an oral inhalant to treat bronchial asthma in patients who require corticosteroids to control symptoms.

Pharmacokinetics
• *Absorption:* Approximately 30% to 50% of an orally inhaled dose is systemically absorbed. Onset of action usually occurs within a few days, but may take as long as 7 days in some patients.
• *Distribution:* Distribution following intranasal aerosol administration has not been described. After oral aerosol administration, most of the drug is distributed into the mouth and throat. The remainder is distributed through the trachea and bronchial tissue. When absorbed systemically, dexamethasone is distributed rapidly to muscle, liver, skin, intestines, and kidneys. Dexamethasone is bound weakly to plasma proteins (transcortin and albumin). Only the unbound portion is active. Dexamethasone transfers across the placenta and is distributed into breast milk.

● *Metabolism:* Dexamethasone is metabolized primarily in the liver to inactive glucuronide and sulfate metabolites. Some drug may be metabolized locally in the lung tissue.
● *Excretion:* The inactive metabolites and small amounts of unmetabolized drug are excreted by the kidneys. Insignificant quantities of drug are excreted in feces. The biological half-life of dexamethasone is 36 to 54 hours.

Contraindications and precautions
Dexamethasone inhalant is contraindicated in patients with acute status asthmaticus, hypersensitivity to any component of the preparation, or nasal infections.

Use cautiously in patients with diabetes mellitus, peptic ulcer, or tuberculosis because systemic absorption of drug can aggravate these diseases. Also use cautiously in patients receiving systemic corticosteroids because of increased risk of hypothalamic-pituitary-adrenal axis suppression; when switching inhalant for oral systemic administration because withdrawal symptoms may occur; and in patients with healing nasal septal ulcers, oral or nasal surgery, or trauma.

Prolonged use of dexamethasone may produce posterior subcapsular cataracts or glaucoma with possible damage to the optic nerves, and may enhance the establishment of secondary ocular infections from fungi or viruses.

Interactions
None reported.

Effects on diagnostic tests
None reported.

Adverse reactions
● EENT: (after oral inhalation) flushing, rash, dry mouth, hoarseness, irritation of the tongue or throat, and impaired sense of taste; (after nasal inhalation) itchy nose, dryness, burning, irritation and sneezing, infrequent epistaxis, bloody mucus.
● Immune: suppression of immune response; fungal overgrowth and infections of the nose, mouth, or throat.
● Other: headache, nausea, GI upset.
    Note: Drug should be discontinued if no improvement is evident after 7 to 10 days, or if nasal or oral infections develop.

Overdose and treatment
No information available.

▶ Special considerations
Recommendations for use of inhalant dexamethasone and for care and teaching of the patient during therapy are the same as those for all *inhalant adrenocorticoids.*

Breast-feeding
Breast-feeding is not recommended because systemically absorbed drug may be excreted in breast milk.

dexchlorpheniramine maleate
Polaramine, Polaramine Repetabs

● Pharmacologic classification: propylamine-derivative antihistamine
● Therapeutic classification: antihistamine (H_1-receptor antagonist), antipruritic
● Pregnancy risk category B

How supplied
Available by prescription only
Tablets: 2 mg
Tablets (repeat-action): 4 mg, 6 mg
Syrup: 2 mg/5 ml

Indications, route, and dosage
Rhinitis, allergy symptoms, contact dermatitis, pruritus, allergic conjunctivitis, adjunct to epinephrine for anaphylaxis after control of acute manifestations
Adults and children age 12 or older: 1 to 2 mg P.O. (tablets or syrup) t.i.d. or q.i.d.; or 4 to 6 mg (timed-release) b.i.d. or t.i.d.
Children age 6 to 11: 1 mg every 4 to 6 hours or 4 mg repeat-action tablet at bedtime.
Children age 2 to 5: 0.5 mg every 4 to 6 hours; do not use repeat-action form.

Pharmacodynamics
Antihistamine action: Antihistamines compete with histamine for histamine H_1-receptor sites on smooth muscle of the bronchi, GI tract, uterus, and large blood vessels; they bind to cellular receptors, preventing access of histamine, thereby suppressing histamine-induced allergic symptoms. They do not directly alter histamine or its release.

Pharmacokinetics
● *Absorption:* Dexchlorpheniramine is well absorbed from the GI tract. Action begins within 30 to 60 minutes.
● *Distribution:* Dexchlorpheniramine is distributed extensively throughout the body and is 70% protein-bound. Plasma half-life ranges from 20 to 24 hours.
● *Metabolism:* Dexchlorpheniramine is metabolized by the liver.
● *Excretion:* Drug and metabolites are excreted in urine.

Contraindications and precautions
Dexchlorpheniramine is contraindicated in patients with known hypersensitivity to this drug or other antihistamines with similar chemical structures (brompheniramine, chlorpheniramine, and triprolidine); during an acute asthmatic attack, because dexchlorpheniramine thickens bronchial secretions; and in patients who have taken monoamine oxidase (MAO) inhibitors within the preceding 2 weeks, because these drugs prolong and intensify the effects of antihistamines.

Dexchlorpheniramine should be used with caution in patients with narrow-angle glaucoma; in those with pyloroduodenal obstruction or urinary bladder obstruction from prostatic hypertrophy or narrowing of the bladder neck, because of their marked anticholinergic effects; in patients with cardiovascular disease, hypertension, or hyperthyroidism, because of the risk of palpitations and tachycardia; and in patients with renal disease,

---

diabetes, bronchial asthma, urinary retention, or stenosing peptic ulcers.

Dexchlorpheniramine should not be used during pregnancy (especially in the third trimester) or during breast-feeding. Antihistamines have caused convulsions, and other severe reactions have occurred, especially in premature infants.

Interactions
MAO inhibitors interfere with detoxification of antihistamines and thus prolong and intensify their central depressant and anticholinergic effects; additive CNS depression may occur when dexchlorpheniramine is given concomitantly with other CNS depressants, such as alcohol, barbiturates, tranquilizers, sleeping aids, and antianxiety agents.

Dexchlorpheniramine may diminish the effects of sulfonylureas, enhance the effects of epinephrine, and may partially counteract the anticoagulant effects of heparin.

Effects on diagnostic tests
Dexchlorpheniramine should be discontinued 4 days before diagnostic skin tests; antihistamines can prevent, reduce, or mask positive skin test response.

Adverse reactions
● CNS: (especially in the elderly) drowsiness, dizziness, stimulation, weakness.
● CV: palpitations, tachycardia, hypotension.
● DERM: eruptions, urticaria, photosensitivity.
● EENT: blurred vision, tinnitus.
● GI: dry mouth, nausea, vomiting, diarrhea, constipation, anorexia.
● GU: polyuria, dysuria, urinary retention.

Overdose and treatment
Clinical manifestations of overdose may include either CNS depression (sedation, reduced mental alertness, apnea, and cardiovascular collapse) or CNS stimulation (insomnia, hallucinations, tremors, or convulsions). Anticholinergic symptoms, such as dry mouth, flushed skin, fixed and dilated pupils, and GI symptoms, are common, especially in children.

Treat overdose by inducing emesis with ipecac syrup (in conscious patient), followed by activated charcoal to reduce further drug absorption. Use gastric lavage if patient is unconscious or ipecac fails. Treat hypotension with vasopressors, and control seizures with diazepam or phenytoin. *Do not give stimulants.*

▶ **Special considerations**
Besides those relevant to all *antihistamines,* consider the following recommendation.
● Repeat-action dexchlorpheniramine tablets must be swallowed whole. Do not crush or permit patient to chew tablet. Regular tablets may be crushed or mixed with food.

Geriatric use
Elderly patients are usually more sensitive to adverse effects of antihistamines and are especially likely to experience a greater degree of dizziness, sedation, hyperexcitability, dry mouth, and urinary retention than younger patients. Symptoms usually respond to a decrease in medication dosage.

Pediatric use
Repeat-action tablets are not recommended for use in children under age 6; drug is not indicated for use in newborns or premature infants. Infants and children under age 6 may experience paradoxical hyperexcitability.

Breast-feeding
Small quantities of drug are excreted in breast milk; drug should not be used during breast-feeding because it exposes the infant to risks of unusual excitability; premature infants are at particular risk for convulsions.

dexpanthenol
Ilopan, Intrapan, Panthoderm (topical), Tonestat

● Pharmacologic classification: vitamin B complex analog
● Therapeutic classification: GI stimulant, emollient
● Pregnancy risk category C

How supplied
Available by prescription only
Injection: 250 mg/ml in vials, ampules, and prefilled syringes
Topical cream: 2% cream

Indications, route, and dosage
Emollient and protectant: colostomy area or other surgical sites
Adults and children: Apply p.r.n.
Itching, wounds, insect bites, poison ivy, poison oak, diaper rash, chafing, mild eczema, decubitus ulcers, dry lesions
Adults and children: Apply topically p.r.n.
Prevention of postoperative adynamic ileus
Adults: 250 to 500 mg I.M.; repeat in 2 hours. Then give q 6 hours, as needed.
Treatment of adynamic ileus
Adults: 500 mg I.M., repeat in 2 hours. Then give q 6 hours, as needed.

Pharmacodynamics
● *Emollient action:* By stimulating granulation and epithelialization, dexpanthenol promotes healing and relieves itching.
● *GI stimulant action:* Dexpanthenol stimulates the acetylation of choline to acetylcholine, which increases peristalsis. The exact mechanism of this action is unknown.

Pharmacokinetics
● *Absorption:* Dexpanthenol is absorbed from I.M. sites.
● *Distribution:* After conversion to pantothenic acid, drug is distributed widely, mainly as coenzyme A. Some concentration occurs in the liver, adrenal glands, heart, and kidneys.
● *Metabolism:* Conversion to pantothenic acid occurs readily.
● *Excretion:* Most metabolites are excreted in urine; remainder in feces.

Contraindications and precautions
Dexpanthenol is contraindicated in patients with ileus due to obstruction, because of potential for severe cramping and worsening of condition; and on wounds in patients with hemophilia, because of potential for severe bleeding.

Interactions
When used concomitantly, antibiotics, barbiturates, and narcotics have stimulated an allergic response to dexpanthenol. Succinylcholine's actions are prolonged in the presence of dexpanthenol; therefore, give these drugs at least 1 hour apart.

Effects on diagnostic tests
None reported.

Adverse reactions
- CV: slight decreases in blood pressure.
- DERM: itching, red patches, dermatitis, tingling.
- GI: intestinal colic, vomiting, diarrhea.
  Note: Drug should be discontinued if hypersensitivity reactions occur.

Overdose and treatment
No information available.

▶ Special considerations
- For I.V. administration, dilute in glucose or lactate Ringer's solutions and infuse slowly.
- Be sure to monitor fluid and electrolytes (especially potassium) in patients with adynamic ileus. Anemia, hypoproteinemia, and infection may contribute to the condition.
- Avoid concomitant use with drugs that decrease GI motility.

Information for the patient
Advise patient of the adverse reactions.

Pediatric use
Safety of parenteral form has not been established.

---

dextran 1
Promit

dextran, low molecular weight (dextran 40)
Gentran 40, 10% LMD Rheomacrodex

dextran, high molecular weight (dextran 70, dextran 75)
Gentran 75, Macrodex

- Pharmacologic classification: glucose polymer
- Therapeutic classification: plasma volume expander
- Pregnancy risk category C

How supplied
Available by prescription only
Dextran 1
Injection: 150 mg/ml, in 20-ml vials

Low molecular weight
Injection: 10% dextran 40 in dextrose 5% or 0.9% sodium chloride
High molecular weight
Injection: 6% dextran 70 in 0.9% sodium chloride or dextrose 5%; 6% dextran 75 in 0.9% sodium chloride or dextrose 5%

Indications, route, and dosage
Prevention of severe anaphylactic reaction caused by low or high molecular weight dextran
Adults: 20 ml of dextran 1 by rapid I.V. push 1 to 2 minutes before dextran infusion.
Children: 0.3 ml/kg by rapid I.V. push 1 to 2 minutes before dextran infusion.
Plasma volume expansion
Dosage depends on amount of fluid loss.
Adults: Initially, 500 ml of dextran 40 with central venous pressure monitoring. Infuse remaining dose slowly. Total daily dose should not exceed 2 g/kg (20 ml/kg) body weight. If therapy continues past 24 hours, do not exceed 1 g/kg daily. Continue for no longer than 5 days. The usual dose of dextran 70 or 75 solution is 30 g (500 ml of 6% solution) I.V. In emergency situations, may be administered at a rate of 1.2 to 2.4 g/minute (20 to 40 ml/minute). Total dose during the first 24 hours is not to exceed 1.2 g/kg; actual dose depends on the amount of fluid loss and resultant hemoconcentration and must be determined individually. In normovolemic patients, the rate of administration should not exceed 240 mg/minute (4 ml/minute).
Children: The total dosage of dextran 70 or 75 should not exceed 1.2 g/kg (20 ml/kg), with the dose based on the body weight or surface area. If therapy is continued, dosage should not exceed 0.6 g/kg (10 ml/kg) daily.
Priming pump oxygenators
Adults: Dextran 40 can be used as the only priming fluid or as an additive to other primers in pump oxygenators. Dextran 40 is added to the perfusion circuit as the 10% solution in a dose of 1 to 2 g/kg (10 to 20 ml/kg); total dose should not exceed 2 g/kg (20 ml/kg).
Prophylaxis of venous thrombosis and pulmonary embolism
Adults: Dextran 40 therapy should usually be given during the surgical procedure. On the day of surgery, dextran 40 (10% solution) is given at the dose of 50 to 100 g (500 to 1,000 ml or approximately 10 ml/kg). Treatment is continued for 2 to 3 days at a dose of 50 g (500 ml) daily. Then, if needed, 50 g (500 ml) may be given q 2 or 3 days for up to 2 weeks to reduce the risk of thromboembolism (deep venous thrombosis [DVT]) or pulmonary embolism.
Reduction of blood sludging
Adults: 500 ml of 10% solution by I.V. infusion.

Pharmacodynamics
- *Plasma-expanding action:* Dextran 40 (10%) has an average molecular weight of 40,000, the osmotic equivalent of twice the volume of plasma. Dextran 40 has a duration of action of 2 to 4 hours. Dextran 70 has an average molecular weight of 70,000; the I.V. infusion results in an expansion of the plasma volume slightly in excess of the volume infused. This effect, useful in treating shock, lasts for approximately 12 hours.
  Dextran 40, 70, and 75 enhance the blood flow, particularly in the microcirculation. Dextran 40 can be used

---

to prime oxygenator pumps, as the only fluid or in combination with other fluids.
• *Prophylaxis of venous thrombosis and pulmonary embolism:* Dextran 40 inhibits vascular stasis and platelet adhesiveness and alters the structure and lysability of fibrin clots. Dextran 40 increases cardiac output, arterial, venous, and microcirculatory flow, and reduces mean transit time, mainly by expanding plasma volume and by reducing blood viscosity through hemodilution and reducing red cell aggregation.

Pharmacokinetics
• *Absorption:* Dextran 40 and 70 are given by I.V. infusion. The plasma concentration depends on the rate of infusion and the rate of disappearance of the drug from the plasma.
• *Distribution:* Dextran is distributed throughout the vascular system.
• *Metabolism:* Dextran molecules with molecular weights above 50,000 are enzymatically degraded by dextranase to glucose at a rate of about 70 to 90 mg/kg/day. This is a variable process.
• *Excretion:* Dextran molecules with molecular weights below 50,000 are eliminated by renal excretion, with 40% of dextran 70 appearing in the urine within 24 hours. Approximately 50% of dextran 40 is excreted in the urine within 3 hours, 60% within 6 hours, and 75% within 24 hours. The remaining 25% is hydrolyzed partially and excreted in urine, excreted partially in feces, and partially oxidized.

Contraindications and precautions
Dextran 40 and 70 are contraindicated in patients with a known hypersensitivity to dextran; in patients with marked hemostatic defects of all types (such as thrombocytopenia and hypofibrinogenemia), including those caused by drugs (such as heparin and warfarin); in patients with marked cardiac decompensation; and in patients with renal disease with severe oliguria or anuria.

Interactions
None reported.

Effects on diagnostic tests
Falsely elevated blood glucose levels may occur in patients receiving dextran 40 or 70 if the test uses high concentrations of acid. Dextran may cause turbidity, which interferes with bilirubin assays that use alcohol, total protein levels using biuret reagent, and blood glucose levels using the orthotoluidine method. Blood typing and cross-matching using enzyme techniques may give unreliable readings if the samples are taken after the dextran infusion.

Dextran 40 administration has been associated with abnormal renal and hepatic function test results.

Adverse reactions
• DERM: hypersensitivity reaction (rash, pruritus, nasal congestion, mild hypotension, dyspnea) occurs rarely (dextran 40 has less antigenic potential than dextran 70); urticaria.
• GI: nausea, vomiting.
• GU: tubular stasis and blocking, increased viscosity and specific gravity of urine in patients having diminished urine flow, which may lead to acute tubular failure that is usually associated with dehydration or shock.
• HEMA: decreased level of hemoglobin and hematocrit; increased bleeding times caused by interference

with platelet function can occur, especially when the higher-molecular-weight product is used in doses exceeding 1.5 liters.
• Hepatic: increased serum transaminase levels with dextran 40.
• Other: *anaphylactic reaction,* fever, infection at injection site, venous thrombosis or phlebitis extending from injection site, extravasation, hypervolemia.

Overdose and treatment
No information available.

▶ Special considerations
• Patients with dehydration should be well hydrated before dextran infusions.
• Dextran in sodium chloride solution is hazardous when given to patients with heart failure, severe renal failure, and clinical states in which edema exists with sodium restriction. (Dextrose 5% solution should be used.)
• Dextran works as a plasma expander via colloidal osmotic effect, thereby drawing fluid from interstitial to intravascular space. It provides plasma expansion slightly greater than volume infused. Observe for circulatory overload or a rise in central venous pressure readings.
• Dextran 1 should be given just before infusing low- or high-molecular weight dextran. Repeat dosage of dextran 1 if more than 15 minutes elapses during infusion.
• Avoid doses that exceed the recommendations because dose-related increases in the incidence of wound hematoma, wound seroma, wound bleeding, distant bleeding (such as hematuria and melena), and pulmonary edema have been observed.
• Monitor urine flow rate during administration. If oliguria or anuria occurs or is not reversed by the initial infusion (500 ml), administration should be discontinued.
• Monitor urine or serum osmolarity; urine specific gravity will be increased by urine dextran concentration.
• Monitor central venous pressure (CVP) when dextran is given by rapid I.V. infusion. A precipitous rise in CVP or other signs of fluid overload indicate the need to stop the infusion.
• Check hemoglobin and hematocrit; do not allow to fall below 30% by volume.
• Observe patient closely during early phase of infusion; check for infiltration, phlebitis, and anaphylactic reactions.
• Dextran may interfere with analysis of blood grouping, cross-matching, bilirubin, blood glucose, and protein.
• Store at constant 77° F. (25° C.). Solution may precipitate in storage. Discard any solution that is not clear.
• Dextran does not contain a preservative. Discard any partially used containers.

Geriatric use
Use dextran with caution in elderly patients because they may be at increased risk of fluid overload.

Breast-feeding
It is unknown whether dextran crosses into human milk. A decision should be made to discontinue breast-feeding or the drug.

---

dextranomer
Debrisan, Envisan

- Pharmacologic classification: synthetic polysaccharide
- Therapeutic classification: topical debriding agent
- Pregnancy risk category C

How supplied
Available by prescription only
Beads: 4 g, 25 g, 60 g, 120 g
Dressing pad: 3 g
Paste: 10 g

Indications, route, and dosage
To clean exudative wounds
Adults and children: Apply to affected area daily or more often if area becomes wet. Apply to ⅛" or ¼" thickness, and cover with sterile gauze.

Pharmacodynamics
Debriding action: Dextranomer cleanses wound surfaces by capillary action, drawing wound exudate, bacteria, and contaminants into the beads and therefore enhancing formation of granulative tissue and promoting wound healing.

Pharmacokinetics
- *Absorption:* Limited with topical use.
- *Distribution:* None.
- *Metabolism:* None.
- *Excretion:* None.

Contraindications and precautions
Dextranomer is contraindicated in deep fistulas, sinus tracts, or any area where complete removal is not assured; and in dry wounds because it is ineffective in cleaning dry wounds.

Interactions
Dextranomer should not be used concomitantly with topical antibiotics or debriding enzymes.

Effects on diagnostic tests
None reported.

Adverse reactions
- Local: transient pain at site, bleeding, erythema, contact dermatitis.
  Note: Drug should be discontinued if sensitization develops.

Overdose and treatment
No information available.

▶ Special considerations
- Use strict aseptic technique when applying dextranomer.
- Dextranomer is not an enzyme and cannot be used for dry wounds.
- Clean wound before applying, leaving area moist; cover wound to a thickness of at least ¼"; then bandage lightly to hold beads in place. Be sure to leave room for expansion (1 g of beads absorbs 4 ml of exudate).
- When product is saturated and grayish yellow, irrigate

wound and remove beads or paste; beads must be removed thoroughly, especially before any surgical treatment, and vigorous irrigation or soaking may be necessary.
- If dressing becomes dry, do not remove it without prior wetting to loosen bandage and beads.
- Stop treatment when area is free of exudate.
- Do not use in areas where complete removal cannot be ensured – for example, in fistulas or sinus tracts.

Information for the patient
- Teach patient how to perform dressing changes before discharge.
- Advise patient to avoid drug contact with eyes and to wash hands well after application.

Breast-feeding
Women should avoid breast-feeding if drug is used in breast area.

---

dextroamphetamine sulfate
Dexampex, Dexedrine, Ferndex, Oxydess II, Robese, Spancap #1

- Pharmacologic classification: amphetamine
- Therapeutic classification: CNS stimulant, short-term adjunctive anorexigenic agent, sympathomimetic amine
- Controlled substance schedule II
- Pregnancy risk category C

How supplied
Available by prescription only
Tablets: 5 mg, 10 mg
Elixir: 5 mg/5 ml
Capsules (sustained-release): 5 mg, 10 mg, 15 mg

Indications, route, and dosage
Narcolepsy
Adults: 5 to 60 mg P.O. daily in divided doses. Long-acting dosage forms allow once-daily dosing.
Children over age 12: 10 mg P.O. daily, with 10-mg increments weekly, p.r.n.
Children age 6 to 12: 5 mg P.O. daily, with 5-mg increments weekly, p.r.n.
†*Short-term adjunct in exogenous obesity*
Adults: Single 10- to 15-mg sustained-release capsule, up to 30 mg daily; or in divided doses, 5 to 10 mg ½ hour before meals.
Attention deficit disorders with hyperactivity
Children age 6 and older: 5 mg once daily or b.i.d., with 5-mg increments weekly, p.r.n.
Children age 3 to 5: 2.5 mg P.O. daily, with 2.5-mg increments weekly, p.r.n.; not recommended for children under age 3.

Pharmacodynamics
- *CNS stimulant action:* Amphetamines are sympathomimetic amines with CNS stimulant activity; in hyperactive children, they have a paradoxical calming effect.
- *Anorexigenic action:* Anorexigenic effects are thought to occur in the hypothalamus, where decreased smell and taste acuity decreases appetite. They may be tried for short-term control of refractory obesity, with caloric restriction and behavior modification.

The cerebral cortex and reticular activating system appear to be the primary sites of activity; amphetamines release nerve terminal stores of norepinephrine, promoting nerve impulse transmission. At high dosages, effects are mediated by dopamine.

Amphetamines are used to treat narcolepsy and as adjuncts to psychosocial measures in attention deficit disorder in children. Their precise mechanism of action in these conditions is unknown.

Pharmacokinetics

● *Absorption:* Dextroamphetamine sulfate is rapidly absorbed from the GI tract; peak serum concentrations occur 2 to 4 hours after oral administration; long-acting capsules are absorbed more slowly and have a longer duration of action.

● *Distribution:* Dextroamphetamine sulfate is distributed widely throughout the body.

● *Metabolism:* Unknown.

● *Excretion:* Excreted in urine.

Contraindications and precautions

Dextroamphetamine is contraindicated in patients with hypersensitivity or idiosyncratic reaction to amphetamines; in patients with hyperthyroidism, angina pectoris, glaucoma, any degree of hypertension, or other severe cardiovascular disease; and in patients with a history of substance abuse. It also is contraindicated for concomitant use with monoamine oxidase (MAO) inhibitors or within 14 days of discontinuing MAO inhibitors.

It should be used with caution in patients with diabetes mellitus; in elderly, debilitated, or hyperexcitable patients; and in children with Gilles de la Tourette's syndrome. Amphetamine-induced CNS stimulation superimposed on CNS depression can cause seizures. Some formulations (Dexedrine) contain tartrazine, which may induce allergic reactions in hypersensitive individuals.

Interactions

Concomitant use with MAO inhibitors (or drugs with MAO-inhibiting activity, such as furazolidone) or within 14 days of such therapy may cause hypertensive crisis; use with antihypertensives may antagonize antihypertensive effects.

Concomitant use with antacids, sodium bicarbonate, or acetazolamide enhances reabsorption of dextroamphetamine and prolongs duration of action; use with ascorbic acid enhances dextroamphetamine excretion and shortens duration of action.

Concomitant use with phenothiazines or haloperidol decreases dextroamphetamine effects; barbiturates antagonize dextroamphetamine by CNS depression; use with theophylline, caffeine, or other CNS stimulants produces additive effects.

Dextroamphetamine may alter insulin requirements.

Effects on diagnostic tests

Dextroamphetamine may elevate plasma corticosteroid levels and may interefere with urinary steroid determinations.

Adverse reactions

● CNS: restlessness, tremor, hyperactivity, talkativeness, insomnia, irritability, dizziness, headache, chills, overstimulation, dysphoria, psychosis.

● CV: tachycardia, palpitations, hypertension, hypotension.

● DERM: urticaria.

● GI: nausea, vomiting, cramps, dry mouth, diarrhea, constipation, metallic taste, anorexia, weight loss.

● Other: impotence, changes in libido.

Note: Drug should be discontinued if signs of hypersensitivity or idiosyncrasy occur.

Overdose and treatment

Individual responses to overdose vary widely. Toxic symptoms may occur at 15 mg and 30 mg and can cause severe reactions; however, doses of 400 mg or more have not always proved fatal.

Symptoms of overdose include restlessness, tremor, hyperreflexia, tachypnea, confusion, aggressiveness, hallucinations, and panic; fatigue and depression usually follow excitement stage. Other symptoms may include arrhythmias, shock, alterations in blood pressure, nausea, vomiting, diarrhea, and abdominal cramps; death is usually preceded by convulsions and coma.

Treat overdose symptomatically and supportively: if ingestion is recent (within 4 hours), use gastric lavage or emesis and sedate with a barbiturate; monitor vital signs and fluid and electrolyte balance. Urinary acidification may enhance excretion. Saline catharsis (magnesium citrate) may hasten GI evacuation of unabsorbed sustained-release drug.

▶ Special considerations

Besides those relevant to all *amphetamines,* consider the following recommendations.

● Administer dextroamphetamine 30 to 60 minutes before meals when using as an anorexigenic agent. To minimize insomnia, avoid giving within 6 hours of bedtime.

● Check vital signs regularly. Observe patient for signs of excessive stimulation.

● When tolerance to anorexigenic effect develops, dosage should be discontinued, not increased.

● Monitor blood and urine glucose levels. Drug may alter daily insulin requirement in patients with diabetes.

● For narcolepsy, patient should take first dose on awakening.

Information for the patient

● Tell patient to avoid drinks containing caffeine, which increases stimulant effects of the drug.

● Warn patient to avoid hazardous activities that require alertness until CNS response to drug is determined.

● Patient should take drug early in the day to minimize insomnia.

● Tell patient not to crush sustained-release forms or to increase dosage.

● Tell patient to take dose 60 minutes before next meal when drug is used as an appetite suppressant.

Geriatric use

Lower doses are recommended for use in elderly patients.

Pediatric use

Dextroamphetamine is not recommended for treatment of obesity in children under age 12.

Breast-feeding

Safety has not been established. Alternative feeding method is recommended during therapy with dextroamphetamine sulfate.

---

dextromethorphan hydrobromide
Balminil D.M.*, Benylin DM Cough,
Broncho-Grippol-DM*, Congespirin,
Cremacoat 1, Delsym, Demo-Cineol*,
DM Cough, DM Syrup*, Hold, Koffex*,
Mediquell, Neo-DM*, PediaCare 1,
Pertussin 8 Hour Cough Formula,
Robidex*, St. Joseph for Children,
Sedatuss*, Sucrets Cough Control

- Pharmacologic classification: levorphanol derivative (dextrorotatory methyl ether)
- Therapeutic classification: antitussive (nonnarcotic)
- Pregnancy risk category C

How supplied
Available without a prescription
Syrup: 5 mg/5 ml, 7.5 mg/5 ml, 10 mg/5 ml, 15 mg/5 ml
Liquid (sustained-action): 30 mg/5 ml
Lozenges: 5 mg
Chewable pieces: 15 mg

Indications, route, and dosage
Nonproductive cough (chronic)
Adults and children age 12 and older: 10 to 20 mg q 4 hours, or 30 mg q 6 to 8 hours. Or the controlled-release liquid twice daily (60 mg b.i.d.). Maximum dosage is 120 mg daily.
Children age 6 to 11: 5 to 10 mg q 4 hours, or 15 mg q 6 to 8 hours. Or the controlled-release liquid twice daily (30 mg b.i.d.). Maximum dosage is 60 mg daily.
Children age 2 to 5: 2.5 to 5 mg q 4 hours, or 7.5 mg q 6 to 8 hours b.i.d.; or the sustained-action liquid 15 mg b.i.d. Maximum dosage is 30 mg daily.

Pharmacodynamics
Antitussive action: Dextromethorphan suppresses the cough reflex by direct action on the cough center in the medulla. Dextromethorphan is almost equal in antitussive potency to codeine, but causes no analgesia or addiction and little or no CNS depression and has no expectorant action; it also produces fewer subjective and GI side effects than codeine. Treatment is intended to relieve cough frequency without abolishing protective cough reflex. In therapeutic doses, drug does not inhibit ciliary activity.

Pharmacokinetics
- *Absorption:* Dextromethorphan is absorbed readily from the GI tract; action begins within 15 to 30 minutes.
- *Distribution:* Unknown.
- *Metabolism:* Dextromethorphan is metabolized extensively by the liver. Plasma half-life is approximately 11 hours.
- *Excretion:* Little drug is excreted unchanged: metabolites are excreted primarily in urine; about 7% to 10% is excreted in feces. Antitussive effect persists for 5 to 6 hours.

Contraindications and precautions
Dextromethorphan is contraindicated in patients with known hypersensitivity to this drug; and in patients who have taken MAO inhibitors within the preceding 2 weeks.
Dextromethorphan should be used with caution in patients with asthma and other respiratory conditions in which thick secretions are present, because this drug may impair mobilization of secretions.

Interactions
Concomitant use with monoamine oxidase (MAO) inhibitors may cause nausea, hypotension, excitation, hyperpyrexia, and coma; do not give dextromethorphan to patients at any interval less than 2 weeks after MAO inhibitors are discontinued.

Effects on diagnostic tests
None reported.

Adverse reactions
- CNS: drowsiness, dizziness.
- GI: nausea.

Overdose and treatment
Clinical manifestations of overdose may include nausea, vomiting, drowsiness, dizziness, blurred vision, nystagmus, shallow respirations, urinary retention, toxic psychosis, stupor, and coma.
Treatment of overdose involves administering activated charcoal to reduce drug absorption and I.V. naloxone to support respiration. Other symptoms are treated supportively.

▶ Special considerations
- Treatment is intended to relieve cough intensity and frequency, without completely abolishing the protective cough reflex.
- Use with percussion and chest vibration.
- Monitor nature and frequency of coughing.

Information for the patient
- Tell patient to call if cough persists more than 7 days.
- Suggest sugarless throat lozenges to decrease throat irritation and resulting cough.
- Suggest a humidifier to filter out dust, smoke, and air pollutants.

Pediatric use
Syrup, tablets, and lozenges are not recommended for children under age 2. Sustained-action liquid may be used in children under age 2, but dosage must be individualized.

Breast-feeding
Safety has not been established.

dextrose (D-glucose)
$D_{2.5}W$, D_5W, $D_{10}W$, $D_{20}W$, $D_{25}W$, $D_{30}W$, $D_{38.5}W$, $D_{40}W$, $D_{50}W$, $D_{60}W$, $D_{70}W$

- Pharmacologic classification: carbohydrate
- Therapeutic classification: I.V. hyperalimentation (IVH) component, caloric agent, fluid volume replacement
- Pregnancy risk category C

How supplied
Available by prescription only
Injection: 1,000 ml (2.5%, 5%, 10%, 20%, 30%, 40%, 50%, 60%, 70%); 650 ml (38.5%); 500 ml (5%, 10%,

20%, 30%, 40%, 50%, 60%, 70%); 400 ml (5%); 250 ml (5%, 10%); 100 ml (5%); 70-ml pin-top vial (70% for additive use only); 50 ml (5% and 50% available in vial, ampule, and Bristoject); 10 ml (25%); 5-ml ampule (10%); 3-ml ampule (10%)

Indications, route, and dosage
Fluid replacement and caloric supplementation in patient who cannot maintain adequate oral intake or who is restricted from doing so
Adults and children: Dosage depends on fluid and caloric requirements. Use peripheral I.V. infusion of 2.5%, 5%, or 10% solution, or central I.V. infusion of 20% solution for minimal fluid needs. Use 50% solution to treat insulin-induced hypoglycemia. Solutions from 40% to 70% are used diluted in admixtures, normally with amino acid solutions, because IVH should be given through a central vein.

Pharmacodynamics
Metabolic action: Dextrose is a rapidly metabolized source of calories and fluids in patients with inadequate oral intake. While increasing blood glucose concentrations, dextrose may decrease body protein and nitrogen losses, promote glycogen deposition, and decrease or prevent ketosis if sufficient doses are given. Dextrose also may induce diuresis. Parenterally injected doses of dextrose undergo oxidation to carbon dioxide and water. A 5% solution is isotonic and is administered peripherally. Concentrated dextrose infusions provide increased caloric intake with less fluid volume; they may be irritating if given by peripheral infusions. Concentrated solutions (greater than 12.5%) should be administered only by central venous catheters.

Pharmacokinetics
• *Absorption:* After oral administration, dextrose (a monosaccharide) is absorbed rapidly by the small intestine, principally by an active mechanism. In patients with hypoglycemia, blood glucose concentrations increase within 10 to 20 minutes after oral administration. Peak blood concentrations may occur 40 minutes after oral administration.
• *Distribution:* As a source of calories and water for hydration, dextrose solutions expand plasma volume.
• *Metabolism:* Dextrose is metabolized to carbon dioxide and water.
• *Excretion:* In some patients, dextrose solutions may produce diuresis.

Contraindications and precautions
Dextrose is contraindicated in patients with diabetic coma while blood glucose levels are excessively high. Concentrated solutions should not be used in the presence of intracranial or intraspinal hemorrhage. Dextrose is contraindicated in patients with delirium tremens and in dehydrated patients with glucose-galactose malabsorption syndrome and in patients with blood glucose levels of 250 mg/dl for 3 days. Hypertonic solutions also are contraindicated in patients with a known corn allergy. Dextrose solutions must be used cautiously in patients with diabetes mellitus or carbohydrate intolerance. I.V. administration may cause fluid or solute overload and resultant congestive conditions with peripheral or pulmonary edema; risk is directly proportional to the electrolyte concentration. Hypomagnesemia, hypokalemia, and hypophosphatemia may result from I.V. dextrose administration. Rapid administration of hypertonic dextrose solutions may lead to hyperglycemia and hyperosmolar syndrome.

Interactions
Dextrose should be administered cautiously, especially if it contains sodium ions, to patients receiving corticosteroids or corticotropin. Dextrose administration may cause vitamin B_6 deficiency. Additives must be introduced aseptically, mixed thoroughly, and not stored; incompatibility is possible. Dextrose must not be administered with blood through the same infusion set because of possible pseudoagglutination of red blood cells.

Effects on diagnostic tests
None reported.

Adverse reactions
• CNS: confusion, unconsciousness, hyperosmolar syndrome (with concentrated solutions).
• CV: (with fluid overload) *pulmonary edema,* exacerbated hypertension, and congestive heart failure in susceptible patients. Prolonged or concentrated infusions may cause phlebitis and sclerosis of vein, especially with peripheral route of administration.
• DERM: sloughing and tissue necrosis if extravasation occurs with concentrated solutions.
• GU: glycosuria, osmotic diuresis.
• Metabolic: (with rapid infusion of concentrated solution or prolonged infusion) hyperglycemia, hypervolemia, hyperosmolarity. Rapid termination of long-term infusions may cause hypoglycemia from rebound hyperinsulinemia.

Overdose and treatment
If fluid or solute overload occurs during I.V. therapy, reevaluate the patient's condition and institute appropriate corrective treatment. Decrease infusion rate or adjust insulin dosage as needed.

▶ Special considerations
• Monitor infusion rate for maximum dextrose infusion of 0.5 g/kg/hour, using the largest available peripheral vein and a well-placed needle or catheter.
• Avoid rapid administration, which may cause hyperglycemia, hyperosmolar syndrome, or glycosuria.
• Infuse concentrated solutions slowly; rapid infusion can cause hyperglycemia and fluid shifts.
• Hypertonic solutions are more likely than isotonic or hypotonic solutions to cause irritation; they should be administered into larger central veins.
• Injection site should be checked frequently during the day to prevent irritation, tissue sloughing, necrosis, and phlebitis.
• Carefully monitor patient's intake, output, and body weight, especially in patients with renal dysfunction.
• Monitor serum glucose levels during long-term treatment.
• Monitor vital signs for significant changes.
• Depletion of pancreatic insulin production and secretion can occur. To avoid an adverse effect on insulin production, patient may need to have insulin added to infusions.
• Fluid imbalance or changes in electrolyte concentrations and acid-base balance should be evaluated clinically by periodic laboratory determinations during prolonged therapy. Additional electrolyte supplementation may be required.
• Excessive administration of potassium-free solutions

may result in hypokalemia. Potassium should be added to dextrose solutions and administered to fasting patients with good renal function; special precautions should be taken with patients receiving digitalis.

• To avoid rebound hypoglycemia, dextrose 5% or 10% solution is advisable upon discontinuation of concentrated dextrose infusions.

Pediatric use
Use with caution in infants of diabetic women, except as may be indicated in newborn infants who are hypoglycemic.

dextrothyroxine sodium
Choloxin

• Pharmacologic classification: thyroid hormone
• Therapeutic classification: antilipemic
• Pregnancy risk category C

How supplied
Available by prescription only
Tablets: 1 mg, 2 mg, 4 mg, 6 mg

Indications, route, and dosage
Primary type II hyperlipoproteinemia
Adults: Initial dose 1 to 2 mg daily, increased gradually by 1 to 2 mg daily at monthly intervals to a maximum of 4 to 8 mg daily.
Children: Initial dose 0.05 mg/kg daily, increased slowly by 0.05 mg/kg daily at monthly intervals to a maximum of 4 mg daily.

Pharmacodynamics
Antilipemic action: Dextrothyroxine accelerates hepatic catabolism of low-density lipoprotein (LDL) and increases bile secretion to lower cholesterol and LDL levels.

Pharmacokinetics
• *Absorption:* Dextrothyroxine is 25% absorbed from the GI tract.
• *Distribution:* Drug is almost completely protein-bound.
• *Metabolism:* Not completely understood; some drug is deiodinated in peripheral tissues, and a small amount is metabolized by the liver.
• *Excretion:* Drug is excreted in urine and feces; half-life is 18 hours. Serum lipids return to pretreatment levels 6 weeks to 3 months after discontinuing therapy.

Contraindications and precautions
Dextrothyroxine is contraindicated in patients with heart disease or a history of hypertension or rheumatic heart disease because drug increases myocardial oxygen demand and such patients are at increased risk of angina or myocardial infarction; in patients with advanced liver or kidney disease or a history of iodism because the drug may exacerbate these conditions; and in pregnant or lactating women because thyroid hormones cross the placenta and enter breast milk.

Dextrothyroxine 2-mg and 6-mg tablets contain tartrazine dye (FD&C Yellow No. 5), which may cause allergic reactions in some individuals, usually patients sensitive to aspirin.

Interactions
Dextrothyroxine may potentiate effects of oral anticoagulants (warfarin); if concomitant use is unavoidable, reduce anticoagulant dose by one third and monitor prothrombin time frequently, readjusting dose as needed. Dextrothyroxine can also increase blood glucose levels, necessitating increased insulin or oral hypoglycemic dosage in patients with diabetes mellitus. Dextrothyroxine may enhance effects of other thyroid preparations; it may increase myocardial stimulant effects of cardiac glycosides. Patients with coronary artery disease receiving dextrothyroxine may be more susceptible to arrhythmias after administration of catecholamines. Cholestyramine and colestipol may decrease absorption of dextrothyroxine.

Effects on diagnostic tests
Dextrothyroxine therapy alters serum levels of thyroxine (T_4), alkaline phosphatase, aspartate aminotransferase, and bilirubin; it may also decrease radioactive iodine uptake and alter urinary and blood glucose levels.

Adverse reactions
Adverse reactions are most common in patients with hypothyroidism, with heart disease, and at dosages greater than 8 mg/day; they may not occur until 1 to 6 weeks after initiation of therapy.
• CNS: headache, tinnitus, dizziness, psychic changes, paresthesia.
• CV: palpitations, tachycardia, peripheral edmea, angina pectoris, arrhythmias, ischemic ECG changes, myocardial infarction.
• EENT: visual disturbances, ptosis, hoarseness.
• GI: dyspepsia, nausea, vomiting, diarrhea, constipation, bitter taste, decreased appetite.
• Metabolic: insomnia, weight loss, sweating, flushing, hyperthermia, hair loss, menstrual irregularities.
• Other: malaise, tiredness, muscle pain.
Note: Drug should be discontinued if signs or symptoms of heart disease develop.

Overdose and treatment
Clinical signs of overdose include signs and symptoms of hyperthyroidism—palpitations, diarrhea, abdominal cramps, nervousness, sweating, heat intolerance, fever, increased pulse and blood pressure, arrhythmias, and congestive heart failure.

Empty stomach by induced emesis or gastric lavage. Give oxygen and treat fever, fluid loss, and congestive heart failure. Propranolol is useful to treat increased sympathetic activity.

▶ Special considerations
• Observe patient for signs of hyperthyroidism.
• Some preparations contain tartrazine, which may precipitate allergic reactions, especially in persons allergic to aspirin.
• Dextrothyroxine therapy is an adjunct to adequate dietary management and patients receiving the drug should continue to reduce total saturated fat and cholesterol intake.
• Because it may cause adverse hormonal and cardiac effects, the use of dextrothyroxine is limited to euthyroid patients with no history of cardiovascular disease.

Information for the patient
• Explain disease process and rationale for therapy; stress importance of close monitoring and of reporting any adverse reactions.

- Encourage patient to comply with prescribed regimen and adhere to diet; dextrothyroxine is not curative.
- Warn patient not to exceed prescribed dosage.
- Recommend taking with food to minimize GI discomfort.

Geriatric use
Elderly patients may be more sensitive to the effects of dextrothyroxine.

Pediatric use
Children with familial hypercholesterolemia have been treated for 1 year or longer without adverse effects on growth. However, continue the drug in children only if it has lowered serum cholesterol level significantly.

Breast-feeding
Dextrothyroxine may be excreted in breast milk; alternative feeding method is recommended during therapy.

---

dezocine
Dalgan

- Pharmacologic classification: opiate (narcotic) agonist-antagonist
- Therapeutic classification: analgesic
- Pregnancy risk category C

How supplied
Available by prescription only
Injection: 5 mg/ml, 10 mg/ml, 15 mg/ml

Indications, route, and dosage
Management of moderate to severe pain
Adults: 5 to 20 mg I.M. q 3 to 6 hours or 2.5 to 10 mg I.V. q 2 to 4 hours. Maximum recommended single I.M. dose is 20 mg, with a maximum daily dosage of 120 mg. Maximum dosage for I.V. use has not been determined.
Dosage in renal and hepatic failure
Limited studies suggest that the drug should be used with caution and in lower doses. The half-life increases in the presence of hepatic failure. The primary means of drug elimination is renal excretion of the metabolite.

Pharmacodynamics
Analgesic action: A synthetic opioid agonist-antagonist, dezocine produces postoperative analgesia qualitatively similar to morphine.

Pharmacokinetics
- *Absorption:* The drug is rapidly and completely absorbed after I.M. administration. Peak levels appear 10 to 90 minutes after I.M. administration, and peak analgesic effects appear to lag blood levels by 20 to 60 minutes.
- *Distribution:* After a 10-mg I.M. injection, peak serum levels average 19 ng/ml. The average volume of distribution is 10.1 liters/kg and is increased by hepatic disease. The degree of serum protein binding is not known.
- *Metabolism:* Probably hepatic. A glucuronide conjugate has been identified.
- *Excretion:* Approximately 66% of a dose appears in the urine: about 1% is unchanged drug; the remainder is the metabolite. The half-life of the drug is about 2.4

hours and is prolonged in the presence of hepatic disease.

Contraindications and precautions
Dezocine is contraindicated in patients hypersensitive to the drug.

Dezocine produces a dose-dependent respiratory depression similar to that of morphine, usually peaking within 15 minutes of administration. The drug should be used only in clinical settings where adequate respiratory support and an opiate antagonist (naloxone hydrochloride [Narcan]) is available. Use with caution and in lower doses in patients with chronic respiratory disease.

Use with extreme caution in patients with head injury. Dezocine can obscure clinical signs in such patients. Related drugs have exhibited enhanced respiratory-depressant effects and elevations of CSF pressure (caused by cerebral vasodilation as a response to elevated CO_2 levels).

Use of dezocine is not recommended in patients who are opioid-dependent because it may precipitate a withdrawal syndrome. In animal studies, dezocine had greater antagonist activity than pentazocine but less than nalorphine.

Note that the injection contains sulfite preservatives, which may cause allergic reactions in certain hypersensitive patients.

Use cautiously in patients undergoing biliary surgery. Related drugs have caused significant increases in pressure within the common bile duct.

Plasma concentrations higher than 45 ng/ml are associated with an increased incidence of adverse effects.

Interactions
Patients receiving chronic opioid therapy (opioid-dependent patients) may experience withdrawal symptoms after dezocine.

Concurrent use with alcohol or other CNS depressants may increase the risk of CNS depression.

Effects on diagnostic tests
In clinical trials, less than 1% of the patients experienced increased alkaline phosphatase and AST (SGOT).

Adverse reactions
- CNS: dizziness, vertigo, anxiety, mood disorders, sleep disturbances, headache, slurred speech, chills.
- CV: edema, hypotension, irregular heartbeat, hypertension, chest pain.
- DERM: rash, pruritus, local irritation at the injection site.
- GI: nausea, vomiting, dry mouth, constipation, diarrhea, abdominal distress.
- HEMA: low hemoglobin.
- Other: sweating, flushing, pallor, thrombophlebitis.

Overdose and treatment
Dezocine overdose has not been reported. However, based on animal studies, it may be expected to cause respiratory depression, delirium, and cardiovascular dysfunction.

Treat overdosage with naloxone hydrochloride to reverse the respiratory depressant effects. Continuous cardiovascular monitoring is recommended, with measures to maintain a patent airway. Vasopressors, I.V. fluids, oxygen, and controlled ventilation may be required.

▶ **Special considerations**

● Although currently not a controlled substance, dezocine will replace morphine in animal drug-dependence studies. Drugs of this type (mixed opioid agonist-antagonists) tend to elicit less potential for abuse as compared with agonists. However, in persons with a history of opiate use or dependence, abuse of this drug is a potential risk.

● Animal tests reveal that dezocine has limited ability to produce physical dependence. Tolerance or physical dependence has not been reported in humans.

● Currently, the drug is not recommended for patients with chronic pain because of limited experience and because the drug can precipitate an abstinence syndrome in patients with substantial tolerance to opiates.

Information for the patient
Warn the patient to move about cautiously because the drug may cause dizziness.

Geriatric use
Like other potent analgesics, dezocine should be administered with caution to elderly patients.

Pediatric use
Safety and efficacy in children under age 18 have not been established.

Breast-feeding
Because it is not known if the drug is excreted in breast milk, breast-feeding is not recommended during therapy with dezocine.

diazepam
Apo-Diazepam*, E-Pam*, Meval*, Neo-Calme*, Novodipam*, Rival*, Valium, Valrelease, Vivol*

● Pharmacologic classification: benzodiazepine
● Therapeutic classification: antianxiety agent; skeletal muscle relaxant; amnesic agent; anticonvulsant; sedative-hypnotic
● Controlled substance schedule IV
● Pregnancy risk category D

How supplied
Available by prescription only
Tablets: 2 mg, 5 mg, 10 mg
Capsules (extended-release): 15 mg
Oral solution: 5 mg/ml; 5 mg/5 ml
Oral suspension: 5 mg/5 ml
Injection: 5 mg/ml in 2-ml ampules or 10-ml vials
Disposable syringe: 2-ml Tel-E-Ject

Indications, route, and dosage
Anxiety and tension
Adults: 2 to 10 mg P.O. b.i.d. to q.i.d.; or 2 to 5 mg I.M. or I.V., repeated in 3 to 4 hours as needed.
Acute alcohol withdrawal
Adults: 10 mg P.O. t.i.d. or q.i.d. for the first 24 hours; reduce to 5 mg t.i.d. or q.i.d., if needed; or 10 mg I.M. or I.V. initially, followed by 5 to 10 mg in 3 to 4 hours, if needed.

Adjunct to skeletal muscle spasm
Adults: 2 to 10 mg t.i.d. to q.i.d.; or 5 to 10 mg I.M. or I.V., repeated in 3 to 4 hours, if needed.
Tetanus
Infants age 1 month to children age 5: 1 to 2 mg I.M. or I.V., repeated q 3 to 4 hours.
Children age 5 and older: 5 to 10 mg q 3 to 4 hours, as needed.
Adjunct to convulsive disorders
Adults: 2 to 10 mg b.i.d. to q.i.d.
Children over age 6 months: 1 to 2.5 mg P.O. t.i.d. or q.i.d.
Adjunct to anesthesia; endoscopic procedures
Adults: 5 to 10 mg I.M. before surgery; or administer slowly I.V. just before procedure, titrating dose to effect. Usually, less than 10 mg is used, but up to 20 mg may be given.
Status epilepticus
Adults: 5 to 10 mg I.V., repeated at 10- to 15-minute intervals to a maximum dose of 30 mg. Repeat q 3 to 4 hours, if needed.
Infants age 1 month to children age 5: 0.2 to 0.5 mg/kg I.V. q 2 to 5 minutes to a maximum dose of 5 mg.
Children age 5 and over: 1 mg I.V. q 2 to 5 minutes to a maximum of 10 mg; repeat in 2 to 4 hours, as needed.
Note: One sustained-release capsule can be substituted for oral diazepam; 5 mg t.i.d. of oral solution may be substituted for oral tablets.

Pharmacodynamics
● *Anxiolytic and sedative-hypnotic actions:* Diazepam depresses the CNS at the limbic and subcortical levels of the brain. It produces an anti-anxiety effect by influencing the effect of the neurotransmitter gamma-aminobutyric acid (GABA) on its receptor in the ascending reticular activating system, which increases inhibition and blocks cortical and limbic arousal.
● *Anticonvulsant action:* Diazepam suppresses the spread of seizure activity produced by epileptogenic foci in the cortex, thalamus, and limbic structures by enhancing presynaptic inhibition.
● *Amnesic action:* The exact mechanism of action is unknown.
● *Skeletal muscle relaxant action:* The exact mechanism is unknown, but it is believed to involve inhibiting polysynaptic afferent pathways.

Pharmacokinetics
● *Absorption:* When administered orally, diazepam is absorbed through the GI tract. Onset of action occurs within 30 to 60 minutes, with peak action in 1 to 2 hours. I.M. administration results in erratic absorption of the drug; onset of action usually occurs in 15 to 30 minutes. After I.V. administration, rapid onset of action occurs 1 to 5 minutes after injection.
● *Distribution:* Diazepam is distributed widely throughout the body. Approximately 85% to 95% of an administered dose is bound to plasma protein.
● *Metabolism:* Diazepam is metabolized in the liver to the active metabolite desmethyldiazepam.
● *Excretion:* Most metabolites of diazepam are excreted in urine, with only small amounts excreted in feces. Half-life of desmethyldiazepam is 30 to 200 hours. Duration of effect is 3 hours; this may be prolonged up to 90 hours in elderly patients and in patients with hepatic or renal dysfunction.

Contraindications and precautions

Diazepam is contraindicated in patients with known hypersensitivity to the drug; in patients with acute narrow-angle glaucoma or untreated open-angle glaucoma, because of the drug's possible anticholinergic effect; in patients in shock or coma, because the drug's hypnotic or hypotensive effect may be prolonged or intensified; in patients with acute alcohol intoxication who have depressed vital signs, because the drug will worsen CNS depression; and in infants younger than age 30 days, in whom slow metabolism of the drug causes it to accumulate.

Diazepam should be used cautiously in patients with psychoses, because the drug is rarely beneficial in such patients and may induce paradoxical reactions; in patients with myasthenia gravis or Parkinson's disease, because it may exacerbate the disorder; in patients with impaired renal or hepatic function, which prolongs elimination of the drug; in elderly or debilitated patients, who are usually more sensitive to the drug's CNS effects; and in individuals prone to addiction or drug abuse. Abrupt withdrawal of diazepam may precipitate seizures in patients with seizure disorders. Use of I.V. diazepam in patients with petit mal or Lennox-Gastaut syndrome may precipitate tonic status epilepticus.

Interactions

Diazepam potentiates the CNS depressant effects of phenothiazines, narcotics, barbiturates, alcohol, antihistamines, monoamine oxidase inhibitors, general anesthetics, and antidepressants. Concomitant use with cimetidine and possibly disulfiram causes diminished hepatic metabolism of diazepam, which increases its plasma concentration.

Antacids may decrease the rate of absorption of diazepam.

Haloperidol may change the seizure patterns of patients treated with diazepam; benzodiazepines also may reduce the serum levels of haloperidol.

Diazepam reportedly can decrease digoxin clearance; monitor patients for digoxin toxicity.

Patients receiving diazepam and nondepolarizing neuromuscular blocking agents such as pancuronium and succinylcholine have intensified and prolonged respiratory depression.

Heavy smoking accelerates diazepam's metabolism, thus lowering clinical effectiveness.

Oral contraceptives may impair the metabolism of diazepam.

Diazepam may inhibit the therapeutic effect of levodopa.

Effects on diagnostic tests

Diazepam therapy may elevate liver function test results. Minor changes in EEG patterns, usually low-voltage, fast activity, may occur during and after diazepam therapy.

Adverse reactions

● CNS: confusion, depression, drowsiness, lethargy, hangover effect, ataxia, dizziness, syncope, nightmares, fatigue, slurred speech, tremors, vertigo, headache, muscle cramps, paresthesia, nervousness, euphoria.
● CV: *cardiovascular collapse*, transient hypotension, bradycardia, arrhythmias (with I.V.).
● DERM: rash, urticaria.
● EENT: diplopia, blurred vision, photosensitivity, nystagmus.

● GI: constipation, salivation changes, anorexia, metallic taste, depressed gag reflex (with I.V.), nausea, vomiting, abdominal discomfort.
● GU: urinary incontinence or retention.
● Local: pain, phlebitis at the injection site, desquamation of the skin at the I.V. site.
● Other: blood dyscrasias, *respiratory depression*, dysarthria, hepatic dysfunction, changes in libido, tissue necrosis (with intra-arterial administration), lactic acidosis (high-dose I.V. use).

Note: Drug should be discontinued if hypersensitivity and the following paradoxical reactions occur: acute hyperexcited state, anxiety, hallucinations, increased muscle spasticity, insomnia, or rage.

Overdose and treatment

Clinical manifestations of overdose include somnolence, confusion, coma, hypoactive reflexes, dyspnea, labored breathing, hypotension, bradycardia, slurred speech, and unsteady gait or impaired coordination.

Support blood pressure and respiration until drug effects subside; monitor vital signs. Mechanical ventilatory assistance via endotracheal tube may be required to maintain a patent airway and support adequate oxygenation. Flumazenil, a specific benzodiazepine antagonist, may be useful. Use I.V. fluids and vasopressors such as dopamine and phenylephrine to treat hypotension as needed. If the patient is conscious, induce emesis; use gastric lavage if ingestion was recent, but only if an endotracheal tube is present to prevent aspiration. After emesis or lavage, administer activated charcoal with a cathartic as a single dose. Dialysis is of limited value.

▶ Special considerations

Besides those relevant to all *benzodiazepines*, consider the following recommendations.
● Do not discontinue the drug suddenly; decrease dosage slowly over 8 to 12 weeks after long-term therapy.
● To enhance taste, oral solution can be mixed with liquids or semisolid foods, such as applesauce or puddings, immediately before administration.
● Patient should not crush or chew extended-release capsule but should swallow the capsule whole.
● Shake oral suspension well before administering.
● When prescribing with opiates for endoscopic procedures, reduce opiate dose by at least one third.
● Parenteral forms of diazepam may be diluted in normal saline solution; a slight precipitate may form, but the solution can still be used.
● Diazepam interacts with plastic. Do not store diazepam in plastic syringes or administer it in plastic administration sets, which will decrease availability of the infused drug.
● I.V. route is preferred because of rapid and more uniform absorption.
● For I.V. administration, drug should be infused slowly, directly into a large vein, at a rate not exceeding 5 mg/minute for adults or 0.25 mg/kg of body weight over 3 minutes for children. Do not inject diazepam into small veins to avoid extravasation into subcutaneous tissue. Observe the infusion site for phlebitis. If direct I.V. administration is not possible, inject diazepam directly into I.V. tubing at point closest to vein insertion site to prevent extravasation.
● Administration by continuous I.V. infusion is not recommended.
● Inject I.M. dose deep into deltoid muscle. Aspirate for backflow to prevent inadvertent intra-arterial ad-

ministration. Use I.M. route only if I.V. or oral routes are unavailable.

• Patients should remain in bed under observation for at least 3 hours after parenteral administration of diazepam to prevent potential hazards; keep resuscitation equipment nearby.

• During prolonged therapy, periodically monitor blood counts and liver function studies.

• Lower doses are effective in patients with renal or hepatic dysfunction.

• Assess gag reflex postendoscopy and before resuming oral intake to prevent aspiration.

• Anticipate possible transient increase in frequency or severity of seizures when diazepam is used as adjunctive treatment of convulsive disorders. Impose seizure precautions.

• Do not mix diazepam with any other drug in a syringe or infusion container.

Information for the patient
• Advise patient of the potential for physical and psychological dependence with chronic use.

• Warn patient that sudden changes of position can cause dizziness. Advise patient to dangle legs for a few minutes before getting out of bed to prevent falls and injury.

• Encourage patient to avoid or limit smoking to prevent increased diazepam metabolism.

• Warn female patient to call immediately if she becomes pregnant.

• Warn patient to avoid alcohol while taking diazepam.

• Advise patient not to suddenly discontinue the drug.

Geriatric use
• Elderly patients are more sensitive to the CNS depressant effects of diazepam. Use with caution.

• Lower doses are usually effective in elderly patients because of decreased elimination.

• Elderly patients who receive this drug require assistance with walking and activities of daily living during initiation of therapy or after an increase in dose.

• Parenteral administration of this drug is more likely to cause apnea, hypotension, and bradycardia in elderly patients.

Pediatric use
• Safe use of oral diazepam in infants less than age 6 months has not been established. Safe use of parenteral diazepam in infants younger than age 30 days has not been established.

• Closely observe neonates of mothers who took diazepam for a prolonged period during pregnancy; the infants may show withdrawal symptoms. Use of diazepam during labor may cause neonatal flaccidity.

Breast-feeding
Diazepam is distributed into breast milk. The breast-fed infant of a mother who uses diazepam may become sedated, have feeding difficulties, or lose weight. Avoid use in breast-feeding women.

diazoxide
Hyperstat I.V., Proglycem

• Pharmacologic classification: peripheral vasodilator
• Therapeutic classification: antihypertensive, antihypoglycemic
• Pregnancy risk category C

How supplied
Available by prescription only
Injection: 300 mg/20 ml
Capsule: 50 mg
Oral suspension: 50 mg/ml in 30-ml bottle

Indications, route, and dosage
Hypertensive crisis
Adults and children: 1 to 3 mg/kg I.V. (up to a maximum of 150 mg) every 5 to 15 minutes until an adequate reduction in blood pressure is achieved.

Note: The use of 300-mg I.V. bolus push is no longer recommended. Switch to therapy with oral antihypertensives as soon as possible.
Hypoglycemia from hyperinsulinism
Adults and children: Usual daily dosage is 3 to 8 mg/kg/day P.O. divided in two or three equal doses.

Infants and newborns: Usual daily dosage is 8 to 15 mg/kg/day P.O. divided in two or three equal doses.

Pharmacodynamics
• *Antihypertensive action:* Diazoxide directly relaxes arteriolar smooth muscle, causing vasodilation and reducing peripheral vascular resistance, thus reducing blood pressure.

• *Antihypoglycemic action:* Diazoxide increases blood glucose levels by inhibiting pancreatic secretion of insulin, by stimulating catecholamine release, or by increasing hepatic release of glucose.

Diazoxide is a nondiuretic congener of thiazide diuretics.

Pharmacokinetics
• *Absorption:* After I.V. administration, blood pressure should decrease promptly, with maximum decrease in less than 5 minutes. After oral administration, hyperglycemic effect begins in 1 hour.

• *Distribution:* Diazoxide is distributed throughout the body; highest concentration is found in kidneys, liver, and adrenal glands; diazoxide crosses placenta and blood-brain barrier. Drug is approximately 90% protein-bound.

• *Metabolism:* Diazoxide is metabolized partially in the liver.

• *Excretion:* Diazoxide and its metabolites are excreted slowly by the kidneys. Duration of antihypertensive effect varies widely, ranging from 30 minutes to 72 hours (average 3 to 12 hours) after I.V. administration; after oral administration, antihypoglycemic effect persists for about 8 hours. Antihypertensive and antihypoglycemic effects may be prolonged in patients with renal dysfunction.

Contraindications and precautions
Diazoxide is contraindicated in patients with known hypersensitivity to the drug or to other thiazide derivatives. I.V. diazoxide is contraindicated in patients with coarc-

---

tation of the aorta or an atrioventricular shunt; oral diazoxide is contraindicated in patients with functional hypoglycemia.

Diazoxide should be used cautiously in patients who may be harmed by sodium and water retention and in patients with impaired cerebral, cardiac, or renal function, because the drug may reduce blood pressure abruptly, resulting in decreased perfusion.

Interactions
Diazoxide may potentiate antihypertensive effects of other antihypertensive agents, especially if I.V. diazoxide is administered within 6 hours after patient has received another antihypertensive agent.

Concomitant use of diazoxide with phenytoin may increase metabolism and decrease the plasma protein binding of phenytoin.

Concomitant use of diazoxide with diuretics may potentiate antihypoglycemic, hyperuricemic, or antihypertensive effects of diazoxide.

Diazoxide may displace warfarin, bilirubin, or other highly protein-bound substances from protein-binding sites.

Concomitant use with other thiazides may enhance effects of diazoxide. Diazoxide may alter insulin and oral hypoglycemic requirements in previously stable diabetic patients.

Effects on diagnostic tests
Diazoxide inhibits glucose-stimulated insulin release and may cause false-negative insulin response to glucagon. Prolonged use of oral diazoxide may decrease hemoglobin and hematocrit levels.

Adverse reactions
● CNS: headache, dizziness, light-headedness, euphoria.
● CV: sodium and water retention, orthostatic hypotension, sweating, flushing, warmth, angina, *myocardial ischemia, arrhythmias,* ECG changes.
● GI: nausea, vomiting, abdominal discomfort.
● Metabolic: hyperglycemia, hyperuricemia.
● Other: hypertrichosis (ceases when treatment stops).

Overdose and treatment
Overdose is manifested primarily by hyperglycemia; ketoacidosis and hypotension may occur.

Treat acute overdose supportively and symptomatically. If hyperglycemia develops, give insulin and replace fluid and electrolyte losses; use vasopressors if hypotension fails to respond to conservative treatment. Prolonged monitoring may be necessary because of diazoxide's long half-life.

▶ Special considerations
Diazoxide is used to treat only hypoglycemia resulting from hyperinsulinism; it is not used to treat functional hypoglycemia. It may be used temporarily to control preoperative or postoperative hypoglycemia in patients with hyperinsulinism.
● I.V. use of diazoxide is seldom necessary for more than 4 or 5 days.
● After I.V. injection, monitor blood pressure every 5 minutes for 15 to 30 minutes, then every hour when patient is stable. Discontinue if severe hypotension develops or if blood pressure continues to fall 30 minutes after drug infusion; keep patient recumbent during this time and have norepinephrine available. Monitor I.V. site for infiltration or extravasation.

● Monitor patient's intake and output carefully. If fluid or sodium retention develops, diuretics may be given 30 to 60 minutes after diazoxide. Keep patient recumbent for 8 to 10 hours after diuretic administration.
● Monitor daily blood glucose and electrolyte levels, watching diabetic patients closely for severe hyperglycemia or hyperglycemic hyperosmolar nonketotic coma; also monitor daily urine glucose and ketone levels, intake and output, and weight. Check serum uric acid levels frequently.
● Protect solutions from light, heat, or freezing; do not administer solutions that have darkened or that contain particulate matter.
● Significant hypotension does not occur after oral administration in doses used to treat hypoglycemia.
● Drug may be given by constant I.V. infusion (7.5 to 30 mg/minute) until adequate blood pressure reduction occurs.

Information for the patient
● Explain that orthostatic hypotension can be minimized by rising slowly and avoiding sudden position changes.
● Tell patient to report any adverse effect immediately, including pain and redness at injection site, which may indicate infiltration.
● Have patient check weight daily and report gains of over 5 lb/week, because diazoxide causes sodium and water retention.
● Reassure patient that excessive hair growth is a common reaction that subsides when drug treatment is completed.

Geriatric use
Elderly patients may have a more pronounced hypotensive response.

Pediatric use
Use with caution in children.

Breast-feeding
It is not known whether diazoxide is distributed into breast milk; an alternative feeding method is recommended during therapy.

dibucaine
Nupercainal

● Pharmacologic classification: local anesthetic (amine)
● Therapeutic classification: local anesthestic
● Pregnancy risk category C

How supplied
Available without a prescription
Ointment: 1%
Cream: 0.5%

Indications, route, and dosage
Topical for temporary relief of pain and itching associated with abrasions, sunburn, minor burns, hemorrhoids, and other minor skin conditions
Adults and children: Apply to affected areas as needed. For hemorrhoids, insert ointment into rectum using a

---

rectal applicator in the morning, evening, and after each bowel movement.

Pharmacodynamics
Anesthetic action: Dibucaine inhibits conduction of nerve impulses and decreases cell membrane permeability to ions, anesthetizing local nerve endings.

Pharmacokinetics
- *Absorption:* Dibucaine has limited absorption.
- *Distribution:* None.
- *Metabolism:* None.
- *Excretion:* None.

Contraindications and precautions
Dibucaine is contraindicated in patients with known hypersensitivity. It is also contraindicated for use on large skin areas, on broken skin or mucous membranes, and in eyes.

Interactions
None reported.

Effects on diagnostic tests
None reported.

Adverse reactions
- Hypersensitivity: urticaria, edema, burning or stinging, tenderness.
- Local: irritation, inflammation, contact dermatitis, cutaneous lesions.
  Note: Drug should be discontinued if sensitization occurs or if condition worsens.

Overdose and treatment
Cleanse area thoroughly with mild soap and water.

▶ Special considerations
Use dibucaine topically only, for short periods.

Information for the patient
- Advise patient to call if condition worsens or if symptoms persist for more than 7 days after use.
- Explain correct use of drug.
- Emphasize need to wash hands thoroughly after use.
- Caution patient to apply drug sparingly to minimize untoward effects.
- Advise keeping drug out of reach of children.

Geriatric use
Dosage should be adjusted to patient's age, size, and physical condition.

Pediatric use
Dosage should be adjusted to patient's age, size, and physical condition.

Breast-feeding
Drug should not be used in breast-feeding women.

dichlorphenamide
Daranide, Oratrol

- Pharmacologic classification: carbonic anhydrase inhibitor
- Therapeutic classification: adjunctive treatment for open-angle glaucoma and perioperative treatment for acute angle-closure glaucoma
- Pregnancy risk category C

How supplied
Available by prescription only
Tablets: 50 mg

Indications, route, and dosage
Adjunct in glaucoma
Adults: Initially, 100 to 200 mg P.O., followed by 100 mg q 12 hours until desired response is obtained. Maintenance dosage is 25 to 50 mg P.O. daily b.i.d. or t.i.d. Give miotics concomitantly.

Pharmacodynamics
Antiglaucoma action: In open-angle glaucoma and perioperatively for acute angle-closure glaucoma, dichlorphenamide decreases the formation of aqueous humor, lowering intraocular pressure.

Pharmacokinetics
There is no suitable assay for determining dichlorphenamide in plasma or urine; pharmacokinetics are not fully understood.

Contraindications and precautions
Dichlorphenamide is contraindicated in patients with hepatic insufficiency, low potassium or sodium levels, hyperchloremic acidosis, or severe renal impairment.
  Dichlorphenamide should be used with caution in patients with respiratory acidosis or other severe respiratory problems because drug may produce acidosis; in patients with diabetes because drug may cause hyperglycemia and glycosuria; in patients taking cardiac glycosides because they are more susceptible to digitalis toxicity from dichlorphenamide-induced hypokalemia; and in patients taking other diuretics.

Interactions
Dichlorphenamide alkalizes urine, thereby decreasing excretion of amphetamines, procainamide, quinidine, and flecainide; dichlorphenamide increases excretion of salicylates, phenobarbital, and lithium, lowering plasma levels of these drugs and necessitating dosage adjustments.

Effects on diagnostic tests
Because it alkalizes urine, dichlorphenamide may cause false-positive results for proteinuria when Albustix or Albutest tests are performed; dichlorphenamide also may decrease iodine uptake by the thyroid.

Adverse reactions
- CNS: drowsiness, paresthesia.
- DERM: rash.
- EENT: transient myopia.
- GI: nausea, vomiting, anorexia.
- GU: crystalluria, renal calculi.

• HEMA: *aplastic anemia,* hemolytic anemia, leukopenia.
• Metabolic: *hyperchloremic acidosis,* hypokalemia, asymptomatic hyperuricemia.
Note: Drug should be discontinued if blood pH level is below 7.2 or Pco_2 level is markedly elevated.

Overdose and treatment
Specific recommendations are unavailable. Treatment is supportive and symptomatic. Carbonic anhydrase inhibitors increase bicarbonate excretion and may cause hypokalemia and hyperchloremic acidosis. Induce emesis or perform gastric lavage. Do not induce catharsis because this may exacerbate electrolyte imbalance. Monitor fluid and electrolyte levels.

▶ Special considerations
Besides those relevant to all *carbonic anhydrase inhibitors,* consider the following recommendations.
• Drug should be given daily for glaucoma.
• Monitor patients with glaucoma for eye pain, to ensure drug efficacy.

Geriatric use
Elderly and debilitated patients require close observation because they are more susceptible to drug-induced diuresis. Excessive diuresis promotes rapid dehydration, leading to hypovolemia, hypokalemia, and hyponatremia, and may cause circulatory collapse. Reduced dosages may be indicated.

Breast-feeding
Safety of dichlorphenamide in breast-feeding women has not been established.

---

diclofenac sodium
Voltaren

• Pharmacologic classification: nonsteroidal anti-inflammatory
• Therapeutic classification: antiarthritic agent, anti-inflammatory
• Pregnancy risk category B

How supplied
Available by prescription only
Tablets (enteric-coated): 25 mg, 50 mg, 75 mg

Indications, route, and dosage
Osteoarthritis
Adults: 100 to 150 mg P.O. daily in divided doses.
Ankylosing spondylitis
Adults: 25 mg P.O. q.i.d. An additional 25 mg dose may be needed at bedtime.
Rheumatoid arthritis
Adults: 150 to 200 mg P.O. daily in divided doses.

Pharmacodynamics
Anti-inflammatory action: Diclofenac exerts its anti-inflammatory and antipyretic actions through an unknown mechanism that may involve inhibition of prostaglandin synthesis.

Pharmacokinetics
• *Absorption:* After oral, rectal, or I.M. administration, diclofenac is rapidly and almost completely absorbed, with peak plasma concentrations occurring in 10 to 30 minutes. Absorption is delayed by food, with peak plasma concentrations occurring in 2½ to 12 hours; however, bioavailability is unchanged.
• *Distribution:* Diclofenac is highly (nearly 100%) protein-bound.
• *Metabolism:* Diclofenac undergoes first-pass metabolism, with 60% of unchanged drug reaching systemic circulation. The principal and only active metabolite, 4′-hydroxydiclofenac, has approximately 3% the activity of the parent compound. The mean terminal half-life is approximately 1.2 to 1.8 hours after an oral dose.
• *Excretion:* Approximately 40% to 60% of diclofenac is excreted in the urine; the balance is excreted in the bile. The 4′-hydroxy metabolite accounts for 20% to 30% of the dose excreted in the urine; the other metabolites account for 10% to 20%; 5% to 10% excreted unchanged in the urine. More than 90% is excreted within 72 hours. Moderate renal impairment does not alter the elimination rate of unchanged diclofenac but may reduce the elimination rate of the metabolites. Hepatic impairment does not appear to affect the pharmacokinetics of diclofenac.

Contraindications and precautions
Diclofenac is contraindicated in patients with hypersensitivity to it and those in whom diclofenac, aspirin, or other nonsteroidal anti-inflammatory drugs (NSAIDs) induce asthma, urticaria, or other allergic reactions. Allergic reactions, including anaphylaxis, have been reported. Diclofenac should not be used in patients with hepatic porphyria because it may exacerbate this condition.

Serious GI toxicity, including ulceration and hemorrhage, can occur at any time in patients on chronic NSAID therapy. Peptic ulceration and gastrointestinal bleeding have been reported. Monitor for ulceration and bleeding in all patients who receive prolonged treatment with diclofenac sodium, even those without previous GI tract symptoms. Maintain therapy with the lowest effective dosage.

Periodically monitor serum transaminase levels (particularly ALT [SGPT]) and other indicators of liver function because mild to moderate hepatic dysfunction has been reported during therapy with diclofenac.

Because this drug is excreted by the kidneys, its use in patients with impaired renal function requires close monitoring. Fluid retention and edema have occurred in some patients.

Interactions
Concomitant administration of diclofenac and aspirin lowers plasma levels of diclofenac and is not recommended. Concomitant use with warfarin requires close monitoring of anticoagulant dosage because diclofenac, like other NSAIDs, affects platelet function. Concurrent use with digoxin, methotrexate, and cyclosporine may increase the toxicity of these drugs; with lithium decreases renal clearance of lithium and therefore increases its plasma levels and may lead to lithium toxicity; with insulin or oral hypoglycemics may alter the patient's response to these agents. Concurrent use of diclofenac may inhibit the action of diuretics; use with potassium-sparing diuretics may increase serum potassium levels.

Effects on diagnostic tests

Diclofenac increases platelet aggregation time but does not affect bleeding time, plasma thrombin clotting time, plasma fibrinogen, or Factors V and VII to XII.

Adverse reactions

● CNS: headache, dizziness, paresthesia, seizures, memory disturbance, nightmares, tic, psychotic reaction, disorientation.
● CV: congestive heart failure, hypertension, myocardial infarction, palpitations, chest pain, premature ventricular contractions, tachycardia.
● DERM: urticaria, eczema, dermatitis, alopecia, photosensitivity, bullous eruption, Stevens-Johnson syndrome, erythema multiforme major, allergic purpura, rash, pruritus, exfoliative dermatitis (rare).
● Endocrine: hypoglycemia, flushing (rare).
● GI: abdominal pain or cramps, constipation, diarrhea, indigestion, nausea, abdominal distention, flatulence, liver test abnormalities, bleeding, peptic ulcer (possibly with bleeding or perforation), esophageal lesions.
● GU: azotemia, proteinuria, acute renal failure, oliguria, interstitial nephritis, nephrotic syndrome, papillary necrosis.
● HEMA: leukopenia, thrombocytopenia, decreased hemoglobin levels, epistaxis, purpura, *agranulocytosis* (rare), *aplastic anemia* (rare).
● Metabolic: fluid retention.
● Respiratory: asthma, dyspnea, hyperventilation.
● Special senses: blurred vision, scotoma, diplopia, taste disorder, reversible hearing loss, amblyopia, night blindness, vitreous floaters.
● Other: hypersensitivity (swelling of lips and tongue, laryngeal edema, anaphylactoid reaction, angioedema, *anaphylaxis* [rare], edema of the pharynx), malaise, excess perspiration, bruising, weight loss.
Note: Drug should be discontinued if abnormal liver function test results persist or worsen or if patient develops clinical signs of liver disease.

Overdose and treatment

None reported. There is no special antidote. Supportive and symptomatic treatment may include induction of vomiting or gastric lavage. Treatment with activated charcoal or dialysis may also be appropriate.

▶ Special considerations

● Concurrent administration with other drugs, such as glucocorticoids, that produce adverse gastrointestinal effects may aggravate such effects.
● Periodic evaluation of hematopoietic function is recommended because bone marrow abnormalities have occurred. Regular check of hemoglobin level is important to detect toxic effects on the GI tract.
● Because the anti-inflammatory, antipyretic, and analgesic effects of diclofenac may mask the usual signs of infection, monitor carefully for infection.
● Monitor renal function during treatment. Use with caution and at reduced dosage in patients with renal impairment.
● Periodic ophthalmologic examinations are recommended during prolonged therapy.
● Monitor liver function during therapy. Abnormal liver function test results and severe hepatic reactions may occur.

Geriatric use

Use with caution in elderly patients. Elderly patients may be more susceptible to adverse reactions, especially GI toxicity. Reduce dosage to lowest level that controls symptoms.

Pediatric use

Not recommended for use in children.

Breast-feeding

Low levels of diclofenac have been measured in human breast milk. Risk-to-benefit ratio must be considered.

dicloxacillin sodium
Dycill, Dynapen, Pathocil

● Pharmacologic classification: penicillinase-resistant penicillin
● Therapeutic classification: antibiotic
● Pregnancy risk category B

How supplied

Available by prescription only
Capsules: 125 mg, 250 mg, 500 mg
Oral suspension: 62.5 mg/5 ml (after reconstitution)

Indications, route, and dosage
Systemic infections caused by susceptible organisms

Adults: 1 to 4 g P.O. daily, divided into doses given q 6 hours.
Children: 25 to 50 mg/kg P.O. daily, divided into doses given q 6 hours. Serious infection may require higher dosage (75 to 100 mg/kg/day in divided doses q 6 hours).

Pharmacodynamics

Antibiotic action: Dicloxacillin is bactericidal; it adheres to bacterial penicillin-binding proteins, thus inhibiting bacterial cell wall synthesis. Dicloxacillin resists the effects of penicillinases—enzymes that inactivate penicillin—and is thus active against many strains of penicillinase-producing bacteria; this activity is most important against penicillinase-producing staphylococci; some strains may remain resistant. Dicloxacillin is also active against a few gram-positive aerobic and anaerobic bacilli but has no significant effect on gram-negative bacilli.

Pharmacokinetics

● *Absorption:* Dicloxacillin is absorbed rapidly but incompletely (35% to 76%) from the GI tract; it is relatively acid stable. Peak plasma levels occur ½ to 2 hours after an oral dose. Food may decrease both rate and extent of absorption.
● *Distribution:* Dicloxacillin is distributed widely into bone, bile, and pleural and synovial fluids. CSF penetration is poor but is enhanced by meningeal inflammation. Dicloxacillin crosses the placenta; it is 95% to 99% protein-bound.
● *Metabolism:* Dicloxacillin is metabolized only partially.
● *Excretion:* Dicloxacillin and metabolites are excreted in urine by renal tubular secretion and glomerular filtration; they are also excreted in breast milk. Elimination half-life in adults is ½ to 1 hour, extended minimally to 2½ hours in patients with renal impairment.

Contraindications and precautions
Dicloxacillin is contraindicated in patients with known hypersensitivity to any other penicillin or to cephalosporins.

Dicloxacillin should be used cautiously in patients with renal impairment because it is excreted in urine; decreased dosage is required in moderate to severe renal failure.

Interactions
Concomitant use with aminoglycosides produces synergistic bactericidal effects against *Staphylococcus aureus*. However, the drugs are physically and chemically incompatible and are inactivated when mixed or given together.

Probenecid blocks renal tubular secretion of dicloxacillin, raising its serum levels.

Effects on diagnostic tests
Dicloxacillin alters test results for urine and serum proteins; it produces false-positive or elevated results in turbidimetric urine and serum protein tests using sulfosalicylic acid or trichloroacetic acid; it also reportedly produces false results on the Bradshaw screening test for Bence Jones protein.

Dicloxacillin may cause transient elevations in liver function study results and transient reductions in red blood cell, white blood cell, and platelet counts. Elevated liver function test results may indicate drug-induced cholestasis or hepatitis.

Dicloxacillin may falsely decrease serum aminoglycoside concentrations.

Adverse reactions
● CNS: neuromuscular irritability, seizures.
● GI: nausea, vomiting, epigastric distress, flatulence, *diarrhea, pseudomembranous colitis, intrahepatic cholestasis*.
● GU: acute interstitial nephritis.
● HEMA: eosinophilia, leukopenia, granulocytopenia, thrombocytopenia, agranulocytosis.
● Other: *hypersensitivity reaction* (pruritus, urticaria, rash, *anaphylaxis*), bacterial or fungal superinfection.
   Note: Drug should be discontinued if immediate hypersensitivity reactions occur or if signs of interstitial nephritis or pseudomembranous colitis occur. Patient may require alternate therapy if any of the following occurs: drug fever, eosinophilia, hematuria, neutropenia, or unexplained elevations in serum creatinine levels, BUN levels, or liver function studies.

Overdose and treatment
Clinical signs of overdose include neuromuscular irritability or seizures. No specific recommendations. Treatment is supportive. After recent ingestion (4 hours or less), empty the stomach by induced emesis or gastric lavage; follow with activated charcoal to reduce absorption. Dicloxacillin is not appreciably dialyzable.

▶ Special considerations
Besides those relevant to all *penicillins*, consider the following recommendations.
● Give drug with water only; acid in fruit juice or carbonated beverage may inactivate drug.
● Give dose on empty stomach; food decreases absorption.
● Regularly assess renal, hepatic, and hematopoietic function during prolonged therapy.

Information for the patient
Tell patient to report severe diarrhea promptly. He should also report any rash or itching.

Geriatric use
Half-life may be prolonged in elderly patients because of impaired renal function.

Pediatric use
Elimination of dicloxacillin is reduced in neonates; safe use of drug in neonates has not been established.

Breast-feeding
Dicloxacillin is excreted into breast milk; drug should be used with caution in breast-feeding women.

dicumarol

● Pharmacologic classification: coumarin derivative
● Therapeutic classification: oral anticoagulant
● Pregnancy risk category D

How supplied
Available by prescription only
Tablets: 25 mg, 50 mg

Indications, route, and dosage
Treatment of pulmonary emboli; prevention and treatment of deep vein thrombosis, myocardial infarction, rheumatic heart disease with heart valve damage, atrial arrhythmias
Adults: 25 to 200 mg P.O. daily, based on prothrombin times (PT).

Pharmacodynamics
Anticoagulant action: Dicumarol inhibits vitamin K-dependent activation of clotting factors II, VII, IX, and X, which are formed in the liver; it has no direct effect on established thrombi and cannot reverse ischemic tissue damage. However, dicumarol may prevent additional clot formation, extension of formed clots, and secondary complications of thrombosis.

Pharmacokinetics
● *Absorption:* Dicumarol is absorbed slowly and incompletely from the GI tract, causing erratic bioavailability.
● *Distribution:* Dicumarol is highly bound to plasma proteins, primarily albumin; it crosses the placenta.
● *Metabolism:* Dicumarol is hydroxylated by the liver to inactive metabolites.
● *Excretion:* Metabolites are reabsorbed from bile and excreted in urine and breast milk. Unabsorbed drug is excreted in feces. Half-life of parent drug is 1 to 2 days and is dose-dependent. Therapeutic effect is relatively more dependent on clotting factor depletion (Factor X has a half-life of 40 hours), and PT will not peak for 1 to 3 days. Duration of action more closely reflects drug's half-life, ranging from 2 to 10 days.

Contraindications and precautions
Dicumarol is contraindicated in patients with hemophilia, thrombocytopenic purpura, leukemia with pronounced bleeding tendency, open wounds or ulcers,

impaired hepatic or renal function, severe hypertension (diastolic pressure over 110 mm Hg), acute nephritis, or subacute bacterial endocarditis, because of the potential for excessive bleeding.

Administer dicumarol with extreme caution (avoid when possible) to psychiatric patients or to debilitated or cachectic patients; administer it cautiously during menses or when any drainage tube is being used, and to any patient in whom slight bleeding is dangerous.

Interactions
Oral anticoagulants interact with many drugs; thus, any change in drug regimen, including use of nonprescription compounds, requires careful monitoring.

Concomitant use with amiodarone, anabolic steroids, chloramphenicol, metronidazole, cimetidine, clofibrate, dextrothyroxine and other thyroid preparations, salicylates, streptokinase, urokinase, disulfiram, or sulfonamides will markedly increase dicumarol's anticoagulant effect. Avoid concomitant use.

Concomitant use with ethacrynic acid, indomethacin, mefenamic acid, phenylbutazone, salicylates, or sulfinpyrazone will increase dicumarol's anticoagulant effect and cause severe irritation of GI tract (may be ulcerogenic). Avoid concomitant use when possible.

Concomitant use with allopurinol, moxalactam, cefoperazone, cefamandole, cefotetan, danazol, diflunisal, erythromycin, glucagon, heparin, miconazole, quinidine, sulindac, or vitamin E can increase dicumarol's anticoagulant effect. Monitor carefully.

Concomitant use with glutethimide and rifampin will decrease dicumarol's anticoagulant effect significantly; avoid concomitant use.

Concomitant use with carbamazepine, griseofulvin, corticosteroids, etchlorvynol, oral contraceptives, and vitamin K can decrease dicumarol's anticoagulant effect. Monitor carefully.

Concomitant use with chloral hydrate may increase or decrease anticoagulant effect; monitor therapy carefully and avoid when possible. Acute alcohol intoxication increases anticoagulant effect, and chronic alcohol abuse decreases anticoagulant effect but may predispose patient to bleeding problems.

Effects on diagnostic tests
Dicumarol prolongs both PT and partial thromboplastin time (PTT) and may cause false decreases in serum theophylline levels (as determined by the Schack and Waxler ultraviolet method).

Adverse reactions
● DERM: dermatitis, urticaria, alopecia, rash, petechiae, ecchymoses.
● GI: anorexia, nausea, vomiting, cramps, diarrhea, bleeding gums, mouth ulcers, hematemesis, melena.
● GU: hematuria.
● HEMA: *hemorrhage with excessive dosage*, leukopenia, *agranulocytosis*.
● Other: fever, hemoptysis.
Note: Drug should be discontinued if patient shows any signs of internal or external bleeding, or develops necrosis of skin or other tissues or signs of allergy.

Overdose and treatment
Clinical manifestations of overdose vary with severity and may include internal or external bleeding, or skin necrosis of fat-rich areas, but most common sign is hematuria. Excessive prolongation of PT or minor bleeding mandates withdrawal of therapy. Treatment to

control bleeding may include oral or I.V. phytonadione (vitamin K₁) and if necessary in severe hemorrhage, fresh frozen plasma or whole blood. Use of phytonadione may interfere with subsequent oral anticoagulant therapy.

▶ Special considerations
Besides those relevant to all *coumarin derivatives*, consider the following recommendations.

Geriatric use
Elderly patients are more susceptible to effects of anticoagulants and are at increased risk of hemorrhage; that may be from altered hemostatic mechanisms or age-related deterioration of hepatic and renal functions.

Pediatric use
Infants, especially neonates, may be more susceptible to anticoagulants because of vitamin K deficiency.

Breast-feeding
Women should avoid breast-feeding during anticoagulant therapy if possible; oral anticoagulants appear in breast milk, and may cause coagulation problems in the infant. Some recent evidence suggests that these quantities may be insufficient to cause clinical problems; however, more data are needed.

dicyclomine hydrochloride
Antispas, A-Spas, Bentyl, Bentylol★, Byclomine, Cyclocen, Dibent, Dicen, Di-Cyclonex, Dilomine, Di-Spaz, Formulex★, Lomine★, Neoquess, Or-Tyl, Protylol★, Spasmoban★, Spasmoject, Viscerol★

● Pharmacologic classification: anticholinergic
● Therapeutic classification: antimuscarinic, gastrointestinal antispasmodic
● Pregnancy risk category C

How supplied
Tablets: 20 mg
Capsules: 10 mg, 20 mg
Syrup: 10 mg/5 ml
Injection: 10 mg/ml in 2-ml vials, 10-ml vials, 2-ml ampules, or 2-ml prefilled syringe

Indications, route, and dosage
Adjunctive therapy for peptic ulcers and treatment of functional bowel and irritable bowel syndrome
Adults: 10 to 20 mg P.O. t.i.d. or q.i.d.; 20 mg I.M. q 4 to 6 hours.
Children over 6 months: 5 to 10 mg P.O. t.i.d. or q.i.d.
Infant colic
Infants over 6 months: 5 to 10 mg P.O. t.i.d. or q.i.d. Adjust dosage according to patient's needs and response.

Pharmacodynamics
Antispasmodic action: Dicyclomine exerts a nonspecific, direct spasmolytic action on smooth muscle. It also has some local anesthetic properties that may contribute to spasmolysis in the GI and biliary tracts.

Pharmacokinetics
• *Absorption:* About 67% of an oral dose is absorbed from the GI tract.
• *Distribution:* Largely unknown.
• *Metabolism:* Unknown.
• *Excretion:* After oral administration, 80% of a dose is excreted in urine and 10% in feces.

Contraindications and precautions
Dicyclomine is contraindicated in patients with obstructive uropathy, obstructive GI tract disease, severe ulcerative colitis, myasthenia gravis, paralytic ileus, intestinal atony, or toxic megacolon, because the drug may exacerbate these conditions; and in patients with known hypersensitivity to anticholinergics. The drug is also contraindicated in infants under age 6 months.

Administer dicyclomine cautiously to patients with narrow-angle glaucoma, because drug-induced cycloplegia and mydriasis may increase intraocular pressure; to in patients with autonomic neuropathy, hyperthyroidism, coronary artery disease, cardiac arrhythmias, congestive heart failure, or ulcerative colitis, because the drug may exacerbate the symptoms associated with these disorders; to patients with hepatic or renal disease, because toxic accumulation can occur; to patients over age 40, because the drug increases the glaucoma risk; to patients with hiatal hernia associated with reflux esophagitis, because the drug may decrease lower esophageal sphincter tone; and in hot or humid environments, because the drug may predispose the patient to heatstroke.

Interactions
Concurrent administration of antacids decreases oral absorption of anticholinergics. Administer dicyclomine at least 1 hour before antacids.

Concomitant administration of drugs with anticholinergic effects may cause additive toxicity.

Decreased GI absorption of many drugs has been reported after the use of anticholinergics (for example, levodopa and ketoconazole). Conversely, slowly dissolving digoxin tablets may yield higher serum digoxin levels when administered with anticholinergics.

Use cautiously with oral potassium supplements (especially wax-matrix formulations) because the incidence of potassium-induced GI ulcerations may be increased.

Effects on diagnostic tests
None reported.

Adverse reactions
• CNS: headache, insomnia, drowsiness, dizziness, nervousness, insomnia, weakness, confusion or excitement (in elderly).
• CV: palpitations, tachycardia.
• DERM: urticaria, decreased sweating or anhidrosis, other dermal manifestations.
• EENT: blurred vision, mydriasis, cycloplegia, increased intraocular pressure.
• GI: dry mouth, dysphagia, loss of taste, nausea, constipation, vomiting, paralytic ileus, abdominal distention, heartburn.
• GU: urinary hesitancy and retention, impotence.
• Other: fever, allergic reaction.
Note: Drug should be discontinued if hypersensitivity, urinary retention, or curare-like symptoms develop.

Overdose and treatment
Clinical signs of overdose include curare-like symptoms, of CNS stimulation followed by depression, and such psychotic symptoms as disorientation, confusion, hallucinations, delusions, anxiety, agitation, and restlessness. Peripheral effects may include dilated, nonreactive pupils; hot, flushed, dry skin; tachycardia; hypertension; and increased respiration.

Treatment is primarily symptomatic and supportive, as necessary. Maintain patent airway. If the patient is alert, induce emesis (or use gastric lavage) and follow with a saline cathartic and activated charcoal to prevent further drug absorption. In severe cases, physostigmine may be administered to block dicyclomine's antimuscarinic effects. Give fluids, as needed, to treat shock; diazepam to control psychotic symptoms; and pilocarpine (instilled into the eyes) to relieve mydriasis. If urinary retention occurs, catheterization may be necessary.

▶ **Special considerations**
Besides those relevant to all *anticholinergics,* consider the following recommendation.
• Never give dicyclomine I.V. or S.C.

Information for the patient
Tell patient syrup formulation may be diluted with water.

Geriatric use
Dicyclomine should be administered cautiously to elderly patients. Lower doses are indicated.

Pediatric use
Drug's safety and effectiveness in children has not been established. Administer cautiously to infants; seizures have been reported.

Breast-feeding
Dicyclomine may be excreted in breast milk; it may also decrease milk production. Breast-feeding women should avoid this drug.

---

didanosine (ddI)
Videx

• Pharmacologic classification: purine analog
• Therapeutic classification: antiviral agent
• Pregnancy risk category B

How supplied
Available by prescription only
Chewable tablets: 25 mg, 50 mg, 100 mg, 150 mg
Powder for solution (buffered): 100 mg/packet, 167 mg/packet, 250 mg/packet, 375 mg/packet
Powder for oral solution (pediatric): 10 mg/ml, in 2-g and 4-g bottles

Indications, route, and dosage
Advanced human immunodeficiency virus (HIV) infection in patients who can't tolerate or no longer respond to zidovudine therapy
Adults 75 kg and over: 300 mg (2 150-mg tablets) P.O. q 12 hours, or 375 mg buffered powder P.O. q 12 hours.

Adults 50 to 74 kg: 200 mg (2 100-mg tablets) P.O. q 12 hours, or 250 mg buffered powder P.O. q 12 hours.
Adults 35 to 49 kg: 125 mg (1 25-mg tablet and 1 100-mg tablet) P.O. q 12 hours, or 167 mg buffered powder P.O. q 12 hours.
Children: 200 mg/m² daily in divided doses q 12 hours. Children over age 1 should receive a 2-tablet dose, and children under age 1 should receive a 1-tablet dose. Pediatric oral solution (10 mg/ml).
Children with body surface area of 1.1 to 1.4 m²: 100 mg (tablets) P.O. q 12 hours, or 125 mg (12.5 ml) pediatric solution q 12 hours.
Children with body surface area of 0.8 to 1 m²: 75 mg P.O. q 12 hours, or 94 mg (about 9.5 ml) pediatric solution q 12 hours.
Children with body surface area of 0.5 to 0.7 m²: 50 mg P.O. q 12 hours, or 62 mg (about 6 ml) of pediatric solution q 12 hours.
Children with body surface area of less than 0.5 m²: 25 mg P.O. q 12 hours, or 31 mg (3 ml) pediatric solution q 12 hours.

Pharmacodynamics
Antiviral actions: Didanosine is a synthetic purine analog of deoxyadenosine. After didanosine enters the cell, it is converted to its active form dideoxyadenosine triphosphate (ddATP), which inhibits replication of HIV by preventing DNA replication. In addition, ddATP inhibits the enzyme HIV-RNA dependent DNA polymerase (reverse transcriptase).

Pharmacokinetics
● *Absorption:* Didanosine degrades rapidly in gastric acid. Commercially available preparations contain buffers to raise stomach pH. Bioavailability averages about 33%; tablets may exhibit better bioavailability than buffered powder for oral solution. Food can decrease absorption by 50%.
● *Distribution:* Didanosine is widely distributed; drug penetration into the CNS varies, but CSF levels average 46% of concurrent plasma levels.
● *Metabolism:* Didanosine's metabolism is not fully understood, but is probably similar to that of endogenous purines.
● *Excretion:* Didanosine is excreted in urine as allantoin, hypoxanthine, xanthine, and uric acid. Serum half-life averages 0.8 hours.

Contraindications and precautions
Didanosine is contraindicated in patients with hypersensitivity to any component of the formulation.
Because several controlled clinical trials have demonstrated that zidovudine prolongs survival and decreases incidence of opportunistic infections in patients with advanced HIV infection, zidovudine should be considered the preferred drug for initial therapy. Didanosine should be reserved for adults and children age 6 months and over who can't tolerate or do not respond to zidovudine therapy.
Drug should be discontinued if patient develops abdominal pain, nausea, vomiting, or elevated biochemical markers for pancreatitis, a potentially fatal complication. Restart drug only after pancreatitis is ruled out. About 9% of patients developed pancreatitis in phase I clinical trials; dosage levels were at or below the current recommended treatment dose. The development of pancreatitis appears to be dose related, and patients with conditions that predispose them to higher plasma levels of drug (such as renal impairment) or those with a history of pancreatitis may be at higher risk for this complication.

Digital numbness, tingling, or pain in the feet or hands may signal peripheral neuropathy, which occurred in 34% of patients in phase I clinical trials at doses at or below the currently recommended dose. Incidence of neuropathy appears higher in patients with a history of neuropathy or prior neurotoxic drug therapy and lower in children.

Use cautiously in patients who need sodium restriction because each buffered tablet contains 264.5 mg sodium and each effervescent packet contains 1,380 mg sodium. When treating a patient with phenylketonuria, know that tablets contain phenylalanine (22.5 mg for each 100-mg tablet; 33.7 mg for each 150-mg tablet). When treating a patient with renal impairment, note that the magnesium hydroxide content of each tablet is 15.7 mEq, to prevent magnesium toxicity.

Interactions
Ketoconazole, dapsone, and other drugs that require gastric acid for adequate absorption may be rendered ineffective because of the buffering action of didanosine formulations on gastric acid. Administer such drugs 2 hours before didanosine. Tetracyclines and fluoroquinolones may show decreased absorption because of buffering agents in didanosine tablets or antacids in pediatric suspension. Concurrently used antacids containing magnesium or aluminum hydroxides may produce enhanced adverse effects, such as diarrhea or constipation.

Effects on diagnostic tests
None reported.

Adverse reactions
● CNS: headache, insomnia, dizziness, *seizures*, confusion, anxiety, nervousness, hypertonia, abnormal thinking.
● CV: hypertension.
● DERM: rash, pruritus.
● EENT: retinal depigmentation.
● GI: diarrhea, nausea, vomiting, abdominal pain, *pancreatitis*, dry mouth, dyspepsia, liver abnormalities, flatulence.
● HEMA: leukopenia, granulocytopenia, thrombocytopenia, anemia.
● Other: peripheral neuropathy, asthenia, pain, myalgia, arthritis, pneumonia, infection, cough, myopathy.

Overdose and treatment
There is no specific information regarding the treatment of overdose; however, experience with patients in phase I clinical trials suggest possible effects of overdose. Patients who received doses 10 times greater than the currently recommended dosage developed diarrhea, pancreatitis, peripheral neuropathy, hyperuricemia, and hepatic dysfunction. Treatment is supportive. No specific antidote is known, and it is unknown if drug is dialyzable.

▶ Special considerations
● Administer didanosine on an empty stomach, regardless of dosage form used. Studies have shown that administering drug with meals can result in a 50% decrease in absorption.
● Most patients over age 1 should receive two tablets per dose. Tablets contain buffers that raise stomach pH to levels that prevent degradation of the active drug.

Tablets should be thoroughly chewed before swallowing, and the patient should drink at least 1 oz water with each dose. If tablets are manually crushed, mix drug in 1 oz water; stir to disperse uniformly, then have patient drink it immediately. Know that single-dose packets containing buffered powder for oral solution are available.

• To administer buffered powder for oral solution, carefully open the packet and pour the contents into 4 oz water. Do not use fruit juice or other acidic beverages. Stir for 2 or 3 minutes until the powder dissolves completely. Administer immediately.

• In early clinical trials, about one-third of patients taking buffered powder for oral solution developed diarrhea. Although there is no evidence that other formulations have a lower incidence of diarrhea, consider substituting the chewable tablets if diarrhea occurs.

• When preparing powder or crushing tablets, take care to avoid excessive dispersal of drug particles into the air.

• The pediatric powder for oral solution must be prepared by a pharmacist before dispensing. It must be constituted with Purified Water, USP, then diluted with antacid (manufacturer recommends either Mylanta Double Strength Liquid or Maalox TC) to a final concentration of 10 mg/ml. The admixture is stable for 30 days if refrigerated (36° to 46° F [2° to 8° C]). Be sure to shake well before measuring the dose.

Information for the patient
Tell patient to take didanosine on an empty stomach to ensure adequate absorption, to chew tablets thoroughly before swallowing, and to drink at least 1 oz water with each dose. Remind patient who is using buffered powder for oral solution not to use fruit juice or other acidic beverages. Be sure he understands how to mix the solution.

Pediatric use
Retinal depigmentation occurred in some children receiving this drug. Children should receive dilated retinal examinations at least every 6 months or if a change in vision occurs.

Breast-feeding
It is unknown if drug is excreted in breast milk. Because of the risk of serious adverse effects in the infant, breast-feeding is not recommended.

dienestrol
DV, Estraguard, Ortho Dienestrol

• Pharmacologic classification: estrogen
• Therapeutic classification: topical estrogen
• Pregnancy risk category X

How supplied
Available by prescription only
Cream: 0.01% dienestrol

Indications, route, and dosage
Atrophic vaginitis and kraurosis vulvae
Postmenopausal adults: One to two applications of cream daily for 1 to 2 weeks. If therapy is continued,

one half of the initial dose is given one to three times weekly for 1 or 2 weeks.

Pharmacodynamics
Estrogenic action: Dienestrol causes development, cornification, and secretion in atrophic vaginal tissue.

Pharmacokinetics
Topically applied dienestrol can be absorbed in significant quantities, particularly when used in large doses. Its pharmacokinetics are not well known.

Contraindications and precautions
Dienestrol is contraindicated in patients with estrogen-responsive carcinoma (breast or genital tract cancer) or undiagnosed abnormal genital bleeding because it may worsen these conditions; in pregnant patients because it may be fetotoxic; and in breast-feeding women because it may adversely affect the infant.

Carefully monitor patients who have breast nodules, fibrocystic breast disease, or a family history of breast cancer. Because of the risk of thromboembolism, therapy with this drug should be discontinued at least 1 week before elective surgical procedures associated with an increased incidence of thromboembolism.

Interactions
None reported.

Effects on diagnostic tests
Dienestrol increases sulfobromophthalein retention, prothrombin time and clotting Factors VII to X, and norepinephrine-induced platelet aggregability. It decreases antithrombin III concentration.

Dienestrol also increases thyroid-binding globulin concentration; as a result, total thyroid concentration (measured by protein-bound iodine or total thyroxine) increases, and free triiodothyronine resin uptake decreases. Serum folate and pyridoxine concentrations may decrease; triglyceride, glucose, and phospholipid levels may increase. Glucose tolerance may be impaired. Pregnanediol excretion may decrease.

Adverse reactions
• GU: vaginal discharge; with excessive use, uterine bleeding.
• Local: increased discomfort, burning sensation. Systemic effects possible.
• Other: breast tenderness.

Overdose and treatment
Serious toxicity after dienestrol overdose has not been reported.

▶ **Special considerations**
Besides those relevant to all *estrogens,* consider the following recommendations.
• Systemic absorption of drug may occur with intravaginal use, causing systemic reactions.
• After vaginal mucosa has been restored, a maintenance dose of one applicatorful of cream one to three times weekly may be used. Attempts to reduce dosage or discontinue therapy should be made at 3- to 6-month intervals.

Information for the patient
• Instruct patient to wash vaginal area with soap and water before application and to apply drug at bedtime to increase its absorption and effectiveness. Patient

shouldn't wear tampon while receiving vaginal therapy. She may need to wear sanitary pad to protect clothing.
● Tell patient to remain recumbent for 30 minutes after drug application to prevent drug loss.
● Warn patient not to exceed prescribed dose.
● Withdrawal bleeding may occur if estrogen is stopped suddenly.

Breast-feeding
Dienestrol is contraindicated in breast-feeding women.

diethylpropion hydrochloride
Nobesine, Nu-Dispoz, Regibon, Ro-Diet, Tenuate, Tepanil

● Pharmacologic classification: amphetamine
● Therapeutic classification: short-term adjunctive anorexigenic agent, sympathomimetic amine
● Controlled substance schedule IV
● Pregnancy risk category C

How supplied
Available by prescription only
Tablets: 25 mg
Tablets (controlled-release): 75 mg

Indications, route, and dosage
Short-term adjunct in exogenous obesity
Adults: 25 mg P.O. t.i.d. before meals or 75 mg controlled-release tablet P.O. at midmorning. An additional 25-mg dose may be added in the evening to control night hunger.

Pharmacodynamics
Anorexigenic action: The precise mechanism of action for appetite control is unknown; anorexigenic effects are thought to occur in the hypothalamus, where decreased smell and taste acuity decreases appetite. The cerebral cortex and reticular activating system appear to be the primary sites of activity; amphetamines release nerve terminal stores of norepinephrine, promoting nerve impulse transmission.

Diethylpropion is used adjunctively with caloric restriction and behavior modification to control appetite in exogenous obesity. Diethylpropion is a sympathomimetic amine and is considered the safest of its class for potential use in patients with mild to moderate hypertension.

Pharmacokinetics
● *Absorption:* Diethylpropion is readily absorbed after oral administration; therapeutic effects persist for 4 hours with regular tablets, longer with controlled-release preparation.
● *Distribution:* Widely distributed throughout the body.
● *Metabolism:* Metabolized in the liver.
● *Excretion:* Excreted in urine.

Contraindications and precautions
Diethylpropion is contraindicated in patients with hypersensitivity or idiosyncratic reaction to sympathomimetic amines; in patients with severe cardiovascular disease, hyperthyroidism, moderate to severe hyper-

tension, or advanced arteriosclerosis; and in patients with a history of substance abuse.

Diethylpropion also is contraindicated for use with monoamine oxidase (MAO) inhibitors or within 14 days of such use. It should be used with caution in patients with epilepsy because it may increase seizures, and in patients with diabetes mellitus or hyperexcitability states. Habituation or psychic dependence may occur.

Interactions
Concomitant use with MAO inhibitors (or drugs with MAO-inhibiting effects, such as furazolidone) or within 14 days of such therapy may cause hypertensive crisis. Diethylpropion may decrease antihypertensive effects of guanethidine; it may also decrease insulin requirements in diabetic patients as a result of weight loss. Diethylpropion may increase the effects of antidepressants; excessive concomitant use of caffeine produces additive CNS stimulation. Barbiturates antagonize diethylpropion by CNS depression and may decrease its effects.

Effects on diagnostic tests
None reported.

Adverse reactions
● CNS: headache, nervousness, dizziness.
● CV: tachycardia, palpitations, rise in blood pressure.
● DERM: urticaria.
● EENT: blurred vision.
● GI: nausea, abdominal cramps, dry mouth, diarrhea, constipation.
● Other: impotence, libidinal changes, menstrual upset.
Note: Drug should be discontinued if signs of hypersensitivity or idiosyncrasy occur.

Overdose and treatment
Symptoms of acute overdose include restlessness, tremor, hyperreflexia, tachypnea, confusion, aggressive behavior, hallucinations, blood pressure changes, arrhythmias, nausea, vomiting, diarrhea, and cramps. Fatigue and depression usually follow initial stimulation; convulsions and coma may follow.

Treat overdose symptomatically and supportively: if ingestion is recent (within 4 hours) use gastric lavage or emesis. Treatment may require administration of a sedative and, if acute hypertension develops, I.V. phentolamine. Monitor vital signs and fluid and electrolyte balance.

▶ Special considerations
Besides those relevant to all *amphetamines,* consider the following recommendations.
● Diethylpropion can be used to stop nighttime overeating. Drug rarely causes insomnia.
● Do not crush 75-mg controlled-release tablets.

Information for the patient
● Tell patient to avoid drinks containing caffeine to prevent overstimulation.
● Tell patient to swallow controlled-release tablet whole and not to chew or crush it.
● Warn patient against exceeding prescribed dosage.
● Tell patient drug may color urine pink to brown. This is not harmful.

Geriatric use
In elderly patients, lower dosages may be effective because of diminished renal function.

Pediatric use
Diethylpropion is not recommended for weight reduction in children under age 12.

Breast-feeding
Diethylpropion is excreted in breast milk; alternative feeding method is recommended during therapy with this drug.

---

diethylstilbestrol
Stilboestrol*

diethylstilbestrol diphosphate
Honvol*, Stilphostrol

- Pharmacologic classification: estrogen
- Therapeutic classification: estrogen replacement, antineoplastic, †contraceptive (postcoital)
- Pregnancy risk category X

How supplied
Available by prescription only
Diethylstilbestrol
Tablets: 1 mg, 5 mg
Tablets (enteric-coated): 0.1 mg, 0.25 mg, 1 mg, 5 mg
Diethystilbestrol diphosphate
Tablets: 50 mg
Injection: 50 mg/ml

Indications, route, and dosage
Female hypogonadism, ovariectomy, primary ovarian failure
Adults: 0.2 to 0.5 mg P.O. daily in cycles of 3 weeks on and 1 week off.
Moderate to severe vasomotor symptoms of menopause; atrophic vaginitis or kraurosis vulvae
Adults: 0.2 to 0.5 mg P.O. daily in cycles of 3 weeks on and 1 week off. However, doses up to 2 mg P.O. daily may be required.
†Postcoital contraception ("morning-after pill")
Adults: 25 mg P.O. b.i.d. for 5 days, starting within 72 hours after coitus.
Prostatic cancer
Adults: 1 to 3 mg P.O. daily or 50 to 200 mg (diphosphate) P.O. t.i.d. Alternatively, 0.5 g (diphosphate) I.V. followed by 1 g daily for 5 or more days. Maintenance dosage is 0.25 to 0.5 g I.V. once or twice weekly.
Breast cancer
Men and postmenopausal women: 15 mg P.O. daily.

Pharmacodynamics
- *Estrogen replacement action:* Diethylstilbestrol mimics the action of endogenous estrogen in treating female hypogonadism, menopausal symptoms, and atrophic vaginitis.
- *Antineoplastic action:* Drug inhibits growth of hormone-sensitive tissue in advanced, inoperable prostatic cancer and in certain carefully selected cases of breast cancer in men and postmenopausal women.
- *Topical estrogenic action:* Drug causes development, cornification, and secretion in atrophic vaginal tissue.

Pharmacokinetics
- *Absorption:* Diethylstilbestrol is well absorbed from the GI tract when administered orally.
- *Distribution:* Very little information is available; drug probably distributes extensively into most body tissues.
- *Metabolism:* Drug undergoes conjugation with glucuronic acid in the liver.
- *Excretion:* Drug appears in both urine and feces, primarily as the glucuronide conjugate.

Contraindications and precautions
Diethylstilbestrol is contraindicated in patients with thrombophlebitis, thromboembolism or history of thromboembolism associated with estrogen use, estrogen-responsive carcinoma (breast or genital tract cancer), or undiagnosed abnormal genital bleeding; and in pregnant and breast-feeding women.

Administer drug cautiously to patients with disorders that may be aggravated by fluid and electrolyte accumulation, such as asthma, seizure disorders, migraine, or cardiac, renal, or hepatic dysfunction. Carefully monitor female patients who have breast nodules, fibrocystic breast disease, or a family history of breast cancer. Because of the risk of thromboembolism, therapy with this drug should be discontinued at least 1 week before elective surgical procedures associated with an increased incidence of thromboembolism.

Interactions
Concomitant administration of diethylstilbestrol with drugs that induce hepatic metabolism, such as rifampin, barbiturates, primidone, carbamazepine, and phenytoin, may result in decreased estrogenic effects from a given dose. These drugs are known to accelerate the rate of metabolism of certain other agents. Concomitant use with anticoagulants may decrease the effects of warfarin-type anticoagulants.

Concomitant use with adrenocorticosteroids increases the risk of fluid and electrolyte accumulation.

Effects on diagnostic tests
Diethylstilbestrol may cause increases in blood glucose levels, necessitating dosage adjustment of insulin or oral hypoglycemic drugs. Diethylstilbestrol increases sulfobromophthalein retention, prothrombin and clotting Factors VII to X, and norepinephrine-induced platelet aggregability. Increases in thyroid-binding globulin concentration may occur, resulting in increased total thyroid concentrations (measured by protein-bound iodine or total thyroxine) and decreased uptake of free triiodothyronine resin. Antithrombin III concentrations decrease; serum folate and pyridoxine concentrations and pregnanediol excretion may decrease; triglyceride, glucose, and phospholipid levels may increase. Glucose tolerance may be impaired.

Adverse reactions
- CNS: headache, dizziness, chorea, depression, lethargy.
- CV: *thrombophlebitis; thromboembolism;* hypertension; edema; *increased risk of stroke, pulmonary embolism, and myocardial infarction.*
- DERM: melasma, urticaria, acne, seborrhea, oily skin, hirsutism or hair loss.
- EENT: worsening of myopia or astigmatism, intolerance to contact lenses.

- GI: nausea, vomiting, abdominal cramps, bloating, diarrhea, constipation, anorexia, increased appetite, excessive thirst, weight changes.
- GU: breakthrough bleeding, altered menstrual flow, dysmenorrhea, amenorrhea, cervical erosion, altered cervical secretions, enlargement of uterine fibromas, vaginal candidiasis, loss of libido, cystitis-like syndrome; *in males:* gynecomastia, testicular atrophy, impotence.
- Hepatic: cholestatic jaundice.
- Metabolic: hyperglycemia, hypercalcemia, folic acid deficiency.
- Other: leg cramps, breast tenderness or enlargement.

Note: Drug should be discontinued if severe depression occurs during use or signs and symptoms of thrombotic disorders are noted.

Overdose and treatment
Serious toxicity after overdose of this drug has not been reported. Nausea may be expected to occur. Appropriate supportive care should be provided.

▶ Special considerations
Besides those relevant to all *estrogens,* diethylstilbestrol requires the following special considerations.
- Administer diethylstilbestrol diphosphate injection as an I.V. infusion. Dilute the dose in 300 ml of normal saline solution or dextrose 5% in water, and administer no faster than 1 to 2 ml/minute for the first 15 minutes. The flow rate may then be adjusted so that the remainder of the dose is administered over 1 hour.
- To be effective as a postcoital contraceptive ("morning-after pill"), diethylstilbestrol must be taken within 72 hours (preferably within 24 hours) after coitus. Nausea and vomiting are common with this large dose.
- A pregnancy test is advised before starting diethylstilbestrol therapy.
- A higher incidence of cardiovascular death has been reported in men taking diethylstilbestrol tablets (5 mg daily) for prostatic cancer over a long time. This effect is not associated with a daily dosage of 1 mg three times daily.
- According to the U.S. Department of Health and Human Services 1985 DES Task Force, women who used diethylstilbestrol during pregnancy may have a greater risk of breast cancer, but limited data available do not confirm a causal relationship to the drug.
- For women who received diethylstilbestrol during pregnancy, the DES Task Force recommends regular breast examinations according to general National Cancer Institute guidelines, and annual gynecologic examinations.

Information for the patient
Warn patient to stop taking drug immediately if she becomes pregnant, because it can affect the fetus adversely.

Geriatric use
Use with caution in elderly patients. Administering estrogens to postmenopausal women may be associated with increased incidence of endometrial or breast cancer.

Breast-feeding
Drug is not recommended for use in breast-feeding women.

---

difenoxin hydrochloride (with atropine sulfate)
Motofen

- Pharmacologic classification: opioid agonist
- Therapeutic classification: antidiarrheal
- Controlled substance schedule IV
- Pregnancy risk category C

How supplied
Available by prescription only
Tablets: 1 mg (with atropine sulfate 0.025 mg)

Indications, route, and dosage
Adjunctive treatment of acute nonspecific diarrhea, and acute exacerbations of chronic functional diarrhea
Adults: Initially 2 mg P.O., then 1 mg P.O. after each loose bowel movement. Total dosage should not exceed 8 mg daily. Not recommended for use longer than 2 days.

Pharmacodynamics
Antidiarrheal action: Difenoxin exerts a direct effect on the intestinal wall to slow motility. Atropine sulfate has been added to the formulation to minimize the potential for drug abuse.

Pharmacokinetics
- *Absorption:* Rapidly absorbed after oral administration.
- *Distribution:* Peak levels occur about 1 hour after a dose.
- *Metabolism:* Metabolized to an inactive hydroxylated metabolite and conjugates.
- *Excretion:* In urine and feces, as parent drug and metabolites. Over 90% of the drug is excreted within 24 hours of a single dose.

Contraindications and precautions
Difenoxin is contraindicated in patients allergic to difenoxin or atropine, in children under age 2, and in patients with diarrhea from pseudomembranous colitis associated with antibiotic administration. Also contraindicated in patients with jaundice or diarrhea from organisms that may penetrate the intestinal mucosa (including toxigenic *Escherichia coli, Salmonella,* or *Shigella*). Difenoxin is the principal metabolite of diphenoxylate (Lomotil) and is chemically related to meperidine. Use cautiously in patients with a history of drug abuse or in those currently receiving drugs with a high abuse potential.

Atropine has been added to the medication to prevent abuse. The small amount of atropine in the medication is unlikely to cause clinical problems, but patients may experience dry mouth, tachycardia, urine retention, and flushing. The atropine may exacerbate preexisting glaucoma.

Interactions
Concomitant use with monoamine oxidase inhibitors may cause hypertensive crisis. Avoid concomitant use. Use with alcohol, CNS depressants, tranquilizers, narcotics, or barbiturates may enhance CNS depression. Closely monitor patients.

Effects on diagnostic tests
None reported.

Adverse reactions
● CNS: dizziness and light-headedness, drowsiness, headache, tiredness, nervousness, insomnia, and confusion.
● EENT: burning eyes, blurred vision.
● GI: nausea, vomiting, dry mouth, epigastric distress, constipation.
● GU: urinary retention.

Overdose and treatment
Overdose can result in respiratory depression, coma, and death. Patients who overdose with difenoxin should be observed for at least 48 hours. Respiratory depression may occur up to 30 hours after ingestion. Gastric lavage, establishment of a patent airway, and mechanically assisted ventilation are advised. Naloxone will reverse the respiratory depression; however, because difenoxin has a longer duration of action than naloxone, supplemental naloxone injections will be necessary.

▶ **Special considerations**
Besides those relevant to all *opioids*, consider the following recommendations.
● Monitor patients closely for fluid and electrolyte imbalance. Difenoxin-induced decreases in peristalsis may result in fluid retention in the colon, with subsequent dehydration and, possibly, delayed difenoxin intoxication.

Information for the patient
● Advise patient to avoid hazardous activities that require mental alertness until the CNS effects of the drug are known.
● Advise patient to adhere to dosing schedule. Overdose with difenoxin may result in respiratory depression and coma.
● Encourage proper storage to keep drug out of the reach of children.

Geriatric use
Use cautiously in elderly patients. The drug may aggravate pre-existing glaucoma, exacerbate blurred vision, or contribute to urinary retention.

Pediatric use
Safety in children under age 12 has not been established. The drug is contraindicated in children under age 2.

Breast-feeding
Because of the potential for serious adverse effects on neonates, consider discontinuing the drug or recommend discontinuing breast-feeding during therapy.

diflorasone diacetate
Florone, Flutone*, Maxiflor, Psorcon

● Pharmacologic classification: topical adrenocorticoid
● Therapeutic classification: anti-inflammatory
● Pregnancy risk category C

How supplied
Available by prescription only
Cream, ointment: 0.05%

Indications, route, and dosage
Inflammation of corticosteroid-responsive dermatoses
Adults and children: Apply ointment sparingly in a thin film once daily to t.i.d.; apply cream b.i.d. to q.i.d.

Pharmacodynamics
Anti-inflammatory action: Diflorasone stimulates the synthesis of enzymes needed to decrease the inflammatory response. Diflorasone is a high-potency (group II) anti-inflammatory agent similar in potency to triamcinolone acetonide 0.5%.

Pharmacokinetics
● *Absorption:* The amount of diflorasone absorbed depends on the amount applied and on the nature of the skin at the application site. It ranges from about 1% in areas with a thick stratum corneum (such as the palms, soles, elbows, and knees) to as high as 36% in areas of the thinnest stratum corneum (face, eyelids, and genitals). Absorption increases in areas of skin damage, inflammation, or occlusion. Some systemic absorption of topical steroids occurs, especially through the oral mucosa.
● *Distribution:* After topical application, diflorasone is distributed throughout the local skin. Any drug absorbed into the circulation is distributed rapidly into muscle, liver, skin, intestines, and kidneys.
● *Metabolism:* After topical administration, diflorasone is metabolized primarily in the skin. The small amount absorbed into the systemic circulation is metabolized primarily in the liver to inactive compounds.
● *Excretion:* Inactive metabolites are excreted by the kidneys, primarily as glucuronides and sulfates, but also as unconjugated products. Small amounts of the metabolites are also excreted in feces.

Contraindications and precautions
Diflorasone is contraindicated in patients who are hypersensitive to any component of the preparation and in patients with viral, fungal, or tubercular skin lesions.
Diflorasone should be used with extreme caution in patients with impaired circulation, because its use may increase the risk of skin ulceration. Avoid using on the face and genital areas because increased absorption may result in striae.

Interactions
None significant.

Effects on diagnostic tests
None reported.

Adverse reactions
● *Local:* burning, itching, irritation, dryness, folliculitis, hypertrichosis, acneiform eruptions, hypopigmentation, perioral dermatitis, allergic contact dermatitis, maceration, secondary infection, atrophy, striae, miliaria.

Significant systemic absorption may produce the following reactions.

● *CNS:* euphoria, insomnia, headache, psychotic behavior, pseudotumor cerebri, mental changes, nervousness, restlessness.
● *CV:* congestive heart failure, hypertension, edema.
● *EENT:* cataracts, glaucoma, thrush.
● *GI:* peptic ulcer, irritation, increased appetite.
● *Immune:* immunosuppression, increased susceptibility to infection.
● *Musculoskeletal:* muscle atrophy.
● *Other:* withdrawal syndrome (nausea, fatigue, anorexia, dyspnea, hypotension, hypoglycemia, myalgia, arthralgia, fever, dizziness, and fainting).

Note: Drug should be discontinued if local irritation, infection, systemic absorption, or hypersensitivity reaction occurs.

Overdose and treatment
No information available.

▶ Special considerations
Recommendations for use of diflorasone, for care and teaching of patients during therapy, and for use in elderly patients, children, and breast-feeding women are the same as those for all *topical adrenocorticoids.*

diflunisal
Dolobid

● Pharmacologic classification: nonsteroidal anti-inflammatory, salicylic acid derivative
● Therapeutic classification: nonnarcotic analgesic, antipyretic, anti-inflammatory
● Pregnancy risk category C

How supplied
Available by prescription only
Tablets: 250 mg, 500 mg

Indications, route, and dosage
Mild to moderate pain and osteoarthritis
Adults: 500 to 1,000 mg daily in two divided doses, usually q 12 hours. Maximum dosage is 1,500 mg daily.
Adults over age 70: Start with one-half the usual adult dose.

Pharmacodynamics
Analgesic, antipyretic, and anti-inflammatory actions: Mechanisms of action are unknown, but are probably related to inhibition of prostaglandin synthesis. Diflunisal is a salicylic acid derivative, but is not hydrolyzed to free salicylate in vivo.

Pharmacokinetics
● *Absorption:* Diflunisal is absorbed rapidly and completely via the GI tract. Peak plasma concentrations occur in 2 to 3 hours. Analgesia is achieved within 1 hour and peaks within 2 to 3 hours.
● *Distribution:* The drug is highly protein-bound.

● *Metabolism:* The drug is metabolized in the liver. Diflunisal is not metabolized to salicylic acid.
● *Excretion:* The drug is excreted in urine. Half-life is 8 to 12 hours.

Contraindications and precautions
Diflunisal is contraindicated in patients with known hypersensitivity to the drug or other nonsteroidal anti-inflammatory drugs (NSAIDs), and in patients in whom aspirin or other salicylates provoke asthma, urticaria, and rhinitis.

Serious GI toxicity, particularly ulceration or hemorrhage, can occur at any time in patients on chronic NSAID therapy. Diflunisal should be administered cautiously to patients with active GI bleeding or history of peptic ulcer disease because the drug may exacerbate these conditions; and in patients with renal impairment or compromised cardiac function because peripheral edema has been seen in some patients.

Patients with known "triad" symptoms (aspirin hypersensitivity, rhinitis/nasal polyps, and asthma) are at high risk of bronchospasm. Diflunisal may mask the signs and symptoms of acute infection (fever, myalgia, erythema); carefully evaluate patients with high risk (such as those with diabetes).

Interactions
Concomitant use of diflunisal with anticoagulants and thrombolytic drugs may potentiate their anticoagulant effects by the platelet-inhibiting effect of diflunisal. Concomitant use of diflunisal with other highly protein-bound drugs (phenytoin, sulfonylureas, warfarin) may cause displacement of either drug, and adverse effects. Monitor therapy closely for both drugs. Concomitant use of diflunisal with other GI-irritating drugs such as alcohol, steroids, antibiotics, and other NSAIDs may potentiate the adverse GI effects of diflunisal; use together with caution.

Antacids and food delay and decrease the absorption of diflunisal.

Concurrent use of diflunisal with hydrochlorothiazide may increase the plasma concentration of hydrochlorothiazide, but decrease its hyperuricemic, diuretic, antihypertensive, and natriuretic effects. Concomitant use with furosemide may decrease furosemide's hyperuricemic effect. Concurrent use with antihypertensives may decrease their effect on blood pressure; concurrent use with diuretics may increase nephrotoxic potential. Concurrent use with gold compounds may increase nephrotoxicity. Concurrent use of diflunisal and indomethacin has been associated with decreased renal clearance of indomethacin. Fatal GI hemorrhage has also been reported. Concurrent use with acetaminophen may increase serum acetaminophen levels by as much as 50%, leading to potential hepatotoxicity. This interaction may also be nephrotoxic.

Concurrent use with lithium may result in increased lithium serum levels. Diflunisal may decrease the renal excretion of methotrexate, verapamil, and nifedipine. Probenecid may decrease the renal clearance of diflunisal. Aspirin may decrease the bioavailibity of diflunisal.

Effects on diagnostic tests
The physiologic effects of the drug may prolong bleeding time; increase serum BUN, creatinine, and potassium levels; decrease serum uric acid; and increase liver function tests (serum transaminase, alkaline phosphatase, and lactic dehydrogenase).

Adverse reactions
- CNS: dizziness, somnolence, insomnia, headache, fatigue.
- CV: palpitations, syncope.
- DERM: rash, pruritus, sweating.
- EENT: tinnitus, stomatitis, dry mucous membranes.
- GI: nausea, dyspepsia, GI pain, diarrhea, vomiting, constipation, flatulence.
- GU: dysuria, renal impairment, hematuria.
- Other: chest pain, dyspnea, muscle cramps, elevated liver enzymes, peripheral edema.

Note: Drug should be discontinued if hypersensitivity, hepatic toxicity, or salicylism occurs.

Overdose and treatment
Clinical manifestations of overdose include drowsiness, nausea, vomiting, hyperventilation, tachycardia, sweating, tinnitus, disorientation, stupor, and coma.

To treat overdose of diflunisal, empty stomach immediately by inducing emesis with ipecac syrup if patient is conscious, or by gastric lavage. Administer activated charcoal via nasogastric tube. Provide symptomatic and supportive measures (respiratory support and correction of fluid and electrolyte imbalances). Monitor laboratory parameters and vital signs closely. Hemodialysis has little effect.

▶ Special considerations
Besides those relevant to all *NSAIDs,* consider the following recommendations.
- Similar to aspirin, diflunisal is a salicylic acid derivative but is metabolized differently.
- Diflunisal is recommended for twice-daily dosing for added patient convenience and compliance.
- Do not break, crush, or allow patient to chew diflunisal. He should swallow medication whole.
- Administer diflunisal with water, milk, or meals to minimize GI upset.
- Do not administer concurrently with aspirin or acetaminophen.
- Monitor results of laboratory tests, especially renal and liver function studies. Assess presence and amount of peripheral edema. Monitor weight frequently.
- Evaluate patient's response to diflunisal therapy as evidenced by a reduction in pain or inflammation. Monitor vital signs frequently, especially temperature.
- Assess patient for signs and symptoms of potential hemorrhage, such as bruising, petechiae, coffee ground emesis, and black, tarry stools.
- Institute safety measures to prevent injury if patient experiences CNS effects.

Information for the patient
- Instruct patient in diflunisal regimen and need for compliance. Advise him to report any adverse reactions.
- Tell patient to take diflunisal with foods to minimize GI upset and to swallow capsule whole.
- Caution patient to avoid activities requiring alertness or concentration, such as driving, until CNS effects are known.
- Instruct patient in safety measures to prevent injury.

Geriatric use
- Patients over age 60 may be more susceptible to the toxic effects (particularly GI toxicity) of these drugs.
- The effects of these drugs on renal prostaglandins may cause fluid retention and edema, a significant drawback for elderly patients, especially those with congestive heart failure.

Pediatric use
Do not use long-term diflunisal therapy in children under age 14; safe use has not been established.

Breast-feeding
Because diflunisal is distributed into breast milk, breast-feeding is not recommended.

---

digitoxin
Crystodigin, Purodigin

- Pharmacologic classification: digitalis glycoside
- Therapeutic classification: antiarrhythmic agent, inotropic agent
- Pregnancy risk category C

How supplied
Available by prescription only
Tablets: 0.05 mg, 0.1 mg, 0.15 mg, 0.2 mg
Injection: 0.2 mg/ml

Indications, route, and dosage
Congestive heart failure, paroxysmal atrial tachycardia, atrial fibrillation and flutter
Adults: Loading dosage is 1.2 to 1.6 mg I.V. or P.O. in divided doses over 24 hours; maintenance dosage is 0.1 mg daily but can range from 0.05 to 0.3 mg daily.
Children age 2 to 12: Loading dosage is 0.03 mg/kg or 0.75 mg/m² I.M., I.V., or P.O. in divided doses over 24 hours; maintenance ¹⁄₁₀ loading dose or 0.003 mg/kg or 0.075 mg/m² daily. Monitor closely for toxicity.
Children age 1 to 2: Loading dosage is 0.04 mg/kg over 24 hours in divided doses; maintenance dosage is 0.004 mg/kg daily. Monitor closely for toxicity.
Children age 2 weeks to 1 year: Loading dosage is 0.045 mg/kg I.M., I.V., or P.O. in divided doses over 24 hours; maintenance dosage is 0.0045 mg/kg daily. Monitor closely for toxicity.
Premature infants, neonates, and severely ill older infants: Loading dosage is 0.022 mg/kg I.M., I.V., or P.O. in divided doses over 24 hours; maintenance dosage is 0.0022 mg/kg daily. Monitor closely for toxicity.

Pharmacodynamics
- *Inotropic action:* Digitoxin's effect on the myocardium is dose-related and involves both direct and indirect mechanisms. It directly increases the force and velocity of myocardial contraction, AV node refractory period, and total peripheral resistance; at higher doses, it also increases sympathetic outflow. It indirectly depresses the SA node and prolongs conduction to the AV node. In patients with heart failure, increased contractile force boosts cardiac output, improves systolic emptying, and decreases diastolic heart size. Digitoxin also reduces ventricular end diastolic pressure and, consequently, pulmonary and systemic venous pressures. Increased myocardial contractility and cardiac output reflexively reduce sympathetic tone in patients with congestive heart failure. This compensates for the drug's direct vasoconstrictive action, thereby reducing total peripheral resistance. It also slows increased heart rate and causes diuresis in edematous patients.

• *Antiarrhythmic action:* Digitoxin-induced heart-rate slowing in patients without congestive heart failure is negligible and stems mainly from vagal (cholinergic) and sympatholytic effects on the SA node; however, with toxic doses, heart-rate slowing results from direct depression of SA node automaticity. Therapeutic doses produce little effect on the action potential, but toxic doses increase the automaticity (spontaneous diastolic depolarization) of all cardiac regions except the SA node.

Pharmacokinetics
• *Absorption:* Digitoxin is absorbed rapidly and completely from the GI tract. After oral administration, therapeutic effects appear in 1 to 2 hours, with peak effects occurring in 8 to 12 hours. After I.V. administration, clinical effects appear in 30 minutes to 2 hours, with peak effects occurring in 4 to 12 hours.
• *Distribution:* Digitoxin is distributed widely in body tissues; highest concentrations appear in the heart, kidneys, intestine, stomach, liver, and skeletal muscle; lowest concentrations appear in the plasma and brain. Little of the drug crosses the blood-brain barrier. About 97% is bound to plasma proteins. Usual therapeutic steady-state serum levels range from 20 to 35 ng/ml.
• *Metabolism:* Digitoxin is metabolized extensively, apparently in the liver, to active metabolites (one of which is digoxin) and inactive metabolites. Dosage reduction may be necessary in patients with hepatic impairment.
• *Excretion:* After it is metabolized and enters the enterohepatic recirculation, digitoxin is eventually excreted in urine. Elimination half-life ranges from 5 to 14 days.

Contraindications and precautions
Digitoxin is contraindicated in patients with ventricular fibrillation, because the drug may induce arrhythmias; in patients with digitoxin toxicity; and in patients with hypersensitivity to the drug.

Digitoxin should be used with extreme caution, if at all, in patients with idiopathic hypertrophic subaortic stenosis, because the drug may cause increased obstruction of left ventricular outflow; in patients with incomplete AV block who do not have an artificial pacemaker (especially those with Stokes-Adams syndrome), because the drug may induce advanced or complete AV block; in patients with hypersensitive carotid sinus syndrome, because the drug increases vagal tone (carotid sinus massage has induced ventricular fibrillation in patients receiving cardiac glycosides); in patients with Wolff-Parkinson-White syndrome, because the drug may cause fatal ventricular arrhythmias; in patients with sinus node disease (such as sick sinus syndrome), because the drug may worsen sinus bradycardia or SA block; in patients with severe pulmonary disease, hypoxia, myxedema, acute myocardial infarction, severe heart failure, acute myocarditis, or an otherwise damaged myocardium, because the drug increases the risk of arrhythmias in these patients; in patients with chronic constrictive pericarditis, because such patients may respond unfavorably to the drug; in patients with frequent premature ventricular contractions or ventricular tachycardia (especially if these arrhythmias do not result from heart failure), because the drug may induce arrhythmias; in patients with low cardiac output states caused by valvular stenosis, chronic pericarditis, or chronic cor pulmonale, because the drug may decrease heart rate, which, in turn, may reduce cardiac output; and in patients with conditions that increase cardiac sensitivity to digitalis, including hypokalemia, chronic pulmonary disease, and acute hypoxemia.

Interactions
Concomitant use of digitoxin with antacids containing aluminum and/or magnesium hydroxide, magnesium trisilicate, kaolin-pectin, aminosalicylic acid, and sulfasalazine interferes with absorption of orally administered digitoxin. Cholestyramine and colestipol may bind digitoxin in the GI tract and impair absorption.

Concomitant use with other cardiac drugs that may affect AV conduction (such as procainamide, propranolol, and verapamil) may have additive cardiac effects. Concomitant use with sympathomimetics (such as ephedrine, epinephrine, and isoproterenol), rauwolfia alkaloids, or succinylcholine may increase the risk of arrhythmias. Concomitant use with I.V. calcium preparations may cause synergistic effects that precipitate arrhythmias.

Concomitant use with electrolyte-altering agents may increase or decrease serum electrolyte concentrations, predisposing the patient to digitoxin toxicity. For example, such diuretics as ethacrynic acid, furosemide, and bumetanide may cause hypokalemia and hypomagnesemia; thiazides may cause hypercalcemia. Fatal cardiac arrhythmias may result. Amphotericin B, corticosteroids, corticotropin, edetate disodium, laxatives, and sodium polystyrene sulfonate deplete total body potassium levels, possibly leading to drug toxicity. Glucagon, large dextrose doses, and dextrose-insulin infusions reduce extracellular potassium levels, possibly causing digitoxin toxicity.

Concomitant use with barbiturates, hydantoins, rifampin, and phenylbutazone may stimulate microsomal enzymes that metabolize digitoxin in the liver, possibly causing decreased serum digitoxin levels.

Effects on diagnostic tests
Digitoxin may interfere with the Zimmerman reaction, causing falsely elevated urinary 17-ketogenic steroid levels.

Adverse reactions
• CNS: fatigue, generalized weakness, agitation, hallucinations, headache, malaise, dizziness, vertigo, stupor, paresthesias.
• CV: *increased severity of congestive heart failure, arrhythmias* (most commonly, conduction disturbances with or without AV block, premature ventricular contractions, and supraventricular arrhythmias), hypotension. (Toxic cardiac effects may be life-threatening and require immediate attention.)
• EENT: yellow-green halos around visual images, blurred vision, light flashes, photophobia, diplopia.
• GI: anorexia, nausea, vomiting, diarrhea.
   Note: Drug should be discontinued if signs of digitalis toxicity are present (nausea, vomiting, arrhythmias).

Overdose and treatment
Clinical effects of overdose are primarily gastrointestinal, CNS, and cardiac reactions. Severe intoxication may cause hyperkalemia, which may develop rapidly and result in life-threatening cardiac manifestations. Cardiac signs of digitoxin toxicity may occur with or without other toxicity signs and commonly precede other toxic effects. Because toxic cardiac effects also may occur as manifestations of heart disease, determining whether these effects result from underlying heart dis-

ease or digitoxin toxicity may be difficult. Digitoxin has caused almost every kind of arrhythmia; various combinations of arrhythmias may occur in the same patient. Patients with chronic digitoxin toxicity commonly have ventricular arrhythmias and/or AV conduction disturbances. Patients with digitoxin-induced ventricular tachycardia have a high mortality because ventricular fibrillation or asystole may result.

Treatment requires immediate discontinuation of the drug and measurement of serum drug levels. Usually, drug takes at least 6 hours to equilibriate between plasma and tissue; plasma levels drawn earlier may show higher digitoxin levels than those present after the drug distributes into the tissues.

Other treatment measures include immediate emesis induction, gastric lavage, and administration of activated charcoal to reduce absorption of drug remaining in the gut. Cholestyramine or colestipol may be given to bind digitoxin in the gut, since the drug undergoes extensive enterohepatic recycling. Multiple doses of activated charcoal (such as 50 g q 6 hours) may help reduce further absorption, especially of any drug undergoing enterohepatic recirculation. Any interacting drugs should probably be discontinued. Ventricular arrhythmias may be treated with I.V. potassium (replacement doses; but not in patients with significant AV block), I.V. phenytoin, I.V. lidocaine, or I.V. propranolol. Refractory ventricular tachyarrhythmias may be controlled with overdrive pacing. Procainamide may be used for ventricular arrhythmias that do not respond to the above treatments. In severe AV block, asystole, and hemodynamically significant sinus bradycardia, atropine restores a normal rate.

Administration of specific antibody fragments (digoxin immune Fab [Digibind]) is a promising new treatment for life-threatening digitoxin toxicity. These fragments bind digitoxin in the bloodstream and are excreted in the urine, rapidly decreasing serum levels and therefore cardiac drug concentrations. Each 40 mg of Fab fragments will bind about 0.6 mg of digoxin or digitoxin.

▶ **Special considerations**
● Obtain baseline heart rate and rhythm, blood pressure, and serum electrolyte levels before giving first dose.
● Question patient about use of cardiac glycosides within previous 2 to 3 weeks before administering loading dose. Always divide loading dose over first 24 hours unless clinical situation indicates otherwise.
● Adjust dose to patient's clinical condition; monitor ECG and serum levels of digitoxin, calcium, potassium, and magnesium. Therapeutic blood digitoxin levels range from 25 to 35 ng/ml.
● I.M. injection is painful and dose is poorly absorbed; give I.V. if parenteral route is necessary.
● Monitor clinical status. Take apical-radial pulse for a full minute. Watch for significant changes (sudden rate increase, pulse deficit, irregular beats, and especially regularization of a previously irregular rhythm). Check blood pressure and obtain 12-lead ECG if these changes occur.
● Because digitoxin predisposes patient to postcardioversion arrhythmias, most clinicians withhold drug 1 to 2 days before elective cardioversion in patients with atrial fibrillation. (However, consider the consequences of increased ventricular response to atrial fibrillation if digitoxin is withheld.)

● Elective cardioversion should be postponed in patients with signs of digitoxin toxicity.
● Do not administer calcium salts to patient receiving digitoxin. Calcium affects cardiac contractility and excitability in much the same way that digitoxin does and may lead to serious arrhythmias.
● Thyroid function inversely affects plasma levels of digitalis glycosides. Patients with myxedema require lower doses, while thyrotoxic patients may be relatively insensitive to digitalis glycosides.
● Monitor patient's eating patterns. Ask about nausea, vomiting, anorexia, visual disturbances, and other symptoms of toxicity. Watch closely for toxicity signs in children and elderly patients.
● Monitor serum potassium levels. Take corrective action before hypokalemia occurs.
● Digitoxin is a long-acting drug; watch for cumulative effects.
● Protect solution from light.
● Consider that different brands may not be therapeutically interchangeable.

Information for the patient
Instruct patient and responsible family member about drug action, medication regimen, how to take pulse, reportable signs, and follow-up plans.

Geriatric use
Digitoxin should be used with caution in elderly patients; adjust dosage to prevent systemic accumulation.

Pediatric use
Pediatric patients have a poorly defined serum concentration level range; however, toxicity apparently does not occur at the same concentration levels considered toxic in adults. Divided daily dosing is recommended for infants and children under age 10; older children require adult doses proportional to body weight.

digoxin
Lanoxicaps, Lanoxin, Novodigoxin⋆

● Pharmacologic classification: digitalis glycoside
● Therapeutic classification: antiarrhythmic, inotropic
● Pregnancy risk category A

How supplied
Available by prescription only
Tablets: 0.125 mg, 0.25 mg, 0.5 mg
Capsules: 0.05 mg, 0.10 mg, 0.20 mg
Elixir: 0.05 mg/ml
Injection: 0.05⋆ mg/ml, 0.1 mg/ml (pediatric), 0.25 mg/ml

Indications, route, and dosage
Congestive heart failure, atrial fibrillation and flutter, paroxysmal atrial tachycardia
Tablets, elixir
Adults: For rapid digitalization, give 0.75 to 1.25 mg P.O. over 24 hours in two or more divided doses q 6 to 8 hours. For slow digitalization, give 0.125 to 0.5 mg daily for 5 to 7 days. Maintenance dose is 0.125 to 0.5 mg daily.
Children: 17 mcg/kg P.O. daily. Alternatively, administer according to age as follows:

Children age 10 and over: For rapid digitalization, give 0.75 to 1.25 mg P.O. over 24 hours in two or more divided doses q 6 to 8 hours. For slow digitalization, give 0.125 to 0.5 mg daily for 5 to 7 days. Maintenance dose is 20% to 33% of the total digitalizing dose.

Children age 5 to 10: 20 to 35 mcg/kg P.O. over 24 hours in two or more divided doses q 6 to 8 hours. Maintenance dose is 20% to 33% of the total digitalizing dose.

Children age 2 to 5: 30 to 40 mcg/kg P.O. over 24 hours in two or more divided doses q 6 to 8 hours. Maintenance dose is 20% to 33% of the total digitalizing dose.

Infants age 1 month to 2 years: 35 to 60 mcg/kg P.O. over 24 hours in two or more divided doses q 6 to 8 hours. Maintenance dose is 20% to 33% of the total digitalizing dose.

Premature infants and neonates: 20 to 35 mcg/kg P.O. over 24 hours in two or more divided doses q 6 to 8 hours. Maintenance dose is 20% to 33% of the total digitalizing dose.

Capsules

Adults: For rapid digitalization, give 0.4 to 0.6 mg P.O. initially, followed by 100 to 300 mcg q 6 to 8 hours, as needed and tolerated, for 24 hours. For slow digitalization, give 0.05 to 0.35 mg daily in one or two divided doses for 7 to 22 days as needed until therapeutic serum levels are reached. Maintenance dose is 0.05 to 0.35 mg daily in one or two divided doses.

Children: Digitalizing dose is based on child's age and is administered in three or more divided doses over the first 24 hours. Initial dose should be 50% of the total dose; subsequent doses are given q 4 to 8 hours as needed and tolerated.

Children age 10 and over: For rapid digitalization, give 8 to 12 mcg/kg P.O. over 24 hours, divided as above. Maintenance dose is 25% to 35% of the total digitalizing dose, given daily as a single dose.

Children age 5 to 10: For rapid digitalization, give 15 to 30 mcg/kg P.O. over 24 hours, divided as above. Maintenance dose is 25% to 35% of the total digitalizing dose, divided and given in two or three equal portions daily.

Children age 2 to 5: For rapid digitalization, give 25 to 35 mcg/kg P.O. over 24 hours, divided as above. Maintenance dose is 25% to 35% of the total digitalizing dose, divided and given in two or three equal portions daily.

Infants age 1 month to 2 years: For rapid digitalization, give 30 to 50 mcg/kg P.O. over 24 hours, divided as above. Maintenance dose is 25% to 35% of the total digitalizing dose, divided and given in two or three equal portions daily.

Neonates: For rapid digitalization, give 20 to 30 mcg/kg P.O. over 24 hours, divided as above. Maintenance dose is 25% to 35% of the total digitalizing dose, divided and given in two or three equal portions daily.

Premature infants: For rapid digitalization, give 15 to 25 mcg/kg P.O. over 24 hours, divided as above. Maintenance dose is 20% to 30% of the total digitalizing dose, divided and given in two or three equal portions daily.

Injection

Adults: For rapid digitalization, give 0.4 to 0.6 mg I.V. initially, followed by 100 to 300 mcg I.V. q 6 to 8 hours, as needed and tolerated, for 24 hours. For slow digitalization, give 0.05 to 0.35 mg I.V. daily in one or two divided doses, for 7 to 22 days as needed until therapeutic serum levels are reached. Maintenance dose is 0.05 to 0.35 mg I.V. daily in one or two divided doses.

Children: Digitalizing dose is based on child's age and is administered in three or more divided doses over the first 24 hours. Initial dose should be 50% of the total dose; subsequent doses are given q 4 to 8 hours as needed and tolerated.

Children age 10 and over: For rapid digitalization, give 8 to 12 mcg/kg I.V. over 24 hours, divided as above. Maintenance dose is 25% to 35% of the total digitalizing dose, given daily as a single dose.

Children age 5 to 10: For rapid digitalization, give 15 to 30 mcg/kg I.V. over 24 hours, divided as above. Maintenance dose is 25% to 35% of the total digitalizing dose, divided and given in two or three equal portions daily.

Children age 2 to 5: For rapid digitalization, give 25 to 35 mcg/kg I.V. over 24 hours, divided as above. Maintenance dose is 25% to 35% of the total digitalizing dose, divided and given in two or three equal portions daily.

Infants age 1 month to 2 years: For rapid digitalization, give 30 to 50 mcg/kg I.V. over 24 hours, divided as above. Maintenance dose is 25% to 35% of the total digitalizing dose, divided and given in two or three equal portions daily.

Neonates: For rapid digitalization, give 20 to 30 mcg/kg I.V. over 24 hours, divided as above. Maintenance dose is 25% to 35% of the total digitalizing dose, divided and given in two or three equal portions daily.

Premature infants: For rapid digitalization, give 15 to 25 mcg/kg I.V. over 24 hours, divided as above. Maintenance dose is 20% to 30% of the total digitalizing dose, divided and given in two or three equal portions daily.

Pharmacodynamics

Digoxin is the most widely used cardiac glycoside. Multiple oral forms and a parenteral form are available, facilitating the drug's use in both acute and chronic clinical settings.

● *Inotropic action:* Digoxin's effect on the myocardium is dose-related and involves both direct and indirect mechanisms. It directly increases the force and velocity of myocardial contraction, AV node refractory period, and total peripheral resistance; at higher doses, it also increases sympathetic outflow. It indirectly depresses the SA node and prolongs conduction to the AV node. In patients with heart failure, increased contractile force boosts cardiac output, improves systolic emptying, and decreases diastolic heart size. It also reduces ventricular end-diastolic pressure and, consequently, pulmonary and systemic venous pressures. Increased myocardial contractility and cardiac output reflexively reduce sympathetic tone in patients with congestive heart failure. This compensates for the drug's direct vasoconstrictive action, thereby reducing total peripheral resistance. It also slows increased heart rate and causes diuresis in edematous patients.

● *Antiarrhythmic action:* Digoxin-induced heart-rate slowing in patients without congestive heart failure is negligible and stems mainly from vagal (cholinergic) and sympatholytic effects on the SA node; however, with toxic doses, heart-rate slowing results from direct depression of SA node automaticity. Therapeutic doses produce little effect on the action potential, but toxic doses increase the automaticity (spontaneous diastolic depolarization) of all cardiac regions except the SA node.

Pharmacokinetics

• *Absorption:* With tablet or elixir administration, 60% to 85% of dose is absorbed. With capsule form, bioavailability increases. About 90% to 100% of a dose is absorbed. With I.M. administration, about 80% of dose is absorbed. With oral administration, onset of action occurs in 30 minutes to 2 hours, with peak effects occurring in 6 to 8 hours. With I.M. administration, onset of action occurs in 30 minutes, with peak effects in 4 to 6 hours. With I.V. administration, action occurs in 5 to 30 minutes, with peak effects in 1 to 5 hours.

• *Distribution:* Digoxin is distributed widely in body tissues; highest concentrations occur in the heart, kidneys, intestine, stomach, liver, and skeletal muscle; lowest concentrations are in the plasma and brain. Digoxin crosses both the blood-brain barrier and the placenta; fetal and maternal digoxin levels are equivalent at birth. About 20% to 30% of drug is bound to plasma proteins. Usual therapeutic range for steady-state serum levels is 0.5 to 2 ng/ml. In treatment of atrial tachyarrhythmias, higher serum levels (such as 2 to 4 ng/ml) may be needed. Because of drug's long half-life, achievement of steady-state levels may take 7 days or longer, depending on patient's renal function. Toxic symptoms may appear within the usual therapeutic range; however, these are more frequent and serious with levels above 2.5 ng/ml.

• *Metabolism:* In most patients, a small amount of digoxin apparently is metabolized in the liver and gut by bacteria. This metabolism varies and may be substantial in some patients. Drug undergoes some enterohepatic recirculation (also variable). Metabolites have minimal cardiac activity.

• *Excretion:* Most of dose is excreted by the kidneys as unchanged drug. Some patients excrete a substantial amount of metabolized or reduced drug. In patients with renal failure, biliary excretion is a more important excretion route. In healthy patients, terminal half-life is 30 to 40 hours. In patients lacking functioning kidneys, half-life increases to at least 4 days.

Contraindications and precautions

Digoxin is contraindicated in patients with ventricular fibrillation, because the drug may induce arrhythmias; in patients with digoxin toxicity; and in patients with hypersensitivity to digoxin.

Digoxin should be used with extreme caution, if at all, in patients with idiopathic hypertrophic subaortic stenosis, because the drug may cause increased obstruction of left ventricular outflow; in patients with incomplete AV block who do not have an artificial pacemaker (especially those with Stokes-Adams syndrome), because the drug may induce advanced or complete AV block; in patients with hypersensitive carotid sinus syndrome, because the drug increases vagal tone (carotid sinus massage has induced ventricular fibrillation in patients receiving cardiac glycosides); in patients with Wolff-Parkinson-White syndrome, because the drug may cause fatal ventricular arrhythmias; in patients with sinus node disease (such as sick sinus syndrome), because the drug may worsen sinus bradycardia or SA block; in patients with severe pulmonary disease, hypoxia, myxedema, acute myocardial infarction, severe heart failure, acute myocarditis, or an otherwise damaged myocardium, because the drug increases the risk of arrhythmias in these patients; in patients with chronic constrictive pericarditis, because such patients may respond unfavorably to the drug; in patients with frequent premature ventricular contrac-

tions or ventricular tachycardia (especially if these arrhythmias do not result from heart failure), because the drug may induce arrhythmias; in patients with low cardiac output states caused by valvular stenosis, chronic pericarditis, or chronic cor pulmonale, because the drug may decrease heart rate, which, in turn, may reduce cardiac output; and in patients with conditions that increase cardiac sensitivity to digitalis, including hypokalemia, chronic pulmonary disease, and acute hypoxemia.

I.V. digoxin should be used with caution in patients with hypertension, because I.V. administration may increase blood pressure transiently.

Interactions

Concomitant use of digoxin with antacids containing aluminum and/or magnesium hydroxide, magnesium trisilicate, kaolin-pectin, aminosalicylic acid, and sulfasalazine decreases absorption of orally administered digoxin. Cholestyramine and colestipol may bind digoxin in the GI tract and impair absorption.

Concomitant use with cytotoxic agents or radiation therapy may decrease digoxin absorption if the intestinal mucosa is damaged. (Use of digoxin elixir or capsules is recommended in this situation.) Concomitant use with amiodarone, diltiazem, flecainide, nifedipine, verapamil, or quinidine may cause increased serum digoxin levels, predisposing the patient to toxicity. Concomitant use with cardiac drugs affecting AV conduction (such as procainamide, propranolol, and verapamil) may cause additive cardiac effects. Concomitant use with sympathomimetics (such as ephedrine, epinephrine, and isoproterenol) or rauwolfia alkaloids may increase the risk of arrhythmia.

When used concomitantly, erythromycin and tetracycline may interfere with bacterial flora that allow formation of inactive reduction products in the GI tract, possibly causing a significant increase in digoxin bioavailability and, consequently, increased serum digoxin levels.

Concomitant use with I.V. calcium preparations may cause synergistic effects that precipitate arrhythmias. Concomitant use with electrolyte-altering agents may increase or decrease serum electrolyte concentrations, predisposing the patient to digoxin toxicity. For example, such diuretics as ethacrynic acid, furosemide, bumetanide, and thiazides may cause hypokalemia and hypomagnesemia; thiazides may cause hypercalcemia. Fatal cardiac arrhythmias may result. Amphotericin B, corticosteroids, corticotropin, edetate disodium, laxatives, and sodium polystyrene sulfonate deplete total body potassium, possibly causing digoxin toxicity. Glucagon, large dextrose doses, and dextrose-insulin infusions reduce extracellular potassium, possibly leading to digitalis toxicity. Concomitant use with succinylcholine may precipitate cardiac arrhythmias by potentiating digoxin's effects.

Effects on diagnostic tests

None reported.

Adverse reactions

• CNS: fatigue, generalized weakness, agitation, hallucinations, headache, malaise, dizziness, vertigo, stupor, paresthesias.

• CV: *increased severity of congestive heart failure, arrhythmias* (most commonly, conduction disturbances with or without AV block, premature ventricular contractions, and supraventricular arrhythmias), hypoten-

sion. (Toxic cardiac effects may be life-threatening and require immediate attention.)
● EENT: yellow-green halos around visual images, blurred vision, light flashes, photophobia, diplopia.
● GI: anorexia, nausea, vomiting, diarrhea.
Note: Drug should be discontinued if signs of digitalis toxicity are present (nausea, vomiting, arrhythmias).

Overdose and treatment

Clinical effects of overdose are primarily gastrointestinal, CNS, and cardiac reactions.

Severe intoxication may cause hyperkalemia, which may develop rapidly and result in life-threatening cardiac manifestations. Cardiac signs of digoxin toxicity may occur with or without other toxicity signs and commonly precede other toxic effects. Because toxic cardiac effects also can occur as manifestations of heart disease, determining whether these effects result from underlying heart disease or digoxin toxicity may be difficult. Digoxin has caused almost every kind of arrhythmia; various combinations of arrhythmias may occur in the same patient. Patients with chronic digoxin toxicity commonly have ventricular arrhythmias and/or AV conduction disturbances. Patients with digoxin-induced ventricular tachycardia have a high mortality, because ventricular fibrillation or asystole may result.

If toxicity is suspected, the drug should be discontinued and serum drug level measurements obtained. Usually, the drug takes at least 6 hours to distribute between plasma and tissue and reach equilibrium; plasma levels drawn earlier may show higher digoxin levels than those present after the drug distributes into the tissues.

Other treatment measures include immediate emesis induction, gastric lavage, and administration of activated charcoal to reduce absorption of drug remaining in the gut. Multiple doses of activated charcoal (such as 50 g q 6 hours) may help reduce further absorption, especially of any drug undergoing enterohepatic recirculation. Some clinicians advocate cholestyramine administration if digoxin was recently ingested; however, it may not be useful if the ingestion is life-threatening. Any interacting drugs probably should be discontinued. Ventricular arrhythmias may be treated with I.V. potassium (replacement doses; but not in patients with significant AV block), I.V. phenytoin, I.V. lidocaine, or I.V. propranolol. Refractory ventricular tachyarrhythmias may be controlled with overdrive pacing. Procainamide may be used for ventricular arrhythmias that do not respond to the above treatments. In severe AV block, asystole, and hemodynamically significant sinus bradycardia, atropine restores a normal rate.

Administration of digoxin-specific antibody fragments (digoxin immune Fab [Digibind]) is a promising new treatment for life-threatening digoxin toxicity. Each 40 mg of digoxin immune Fab binds about 0.6 mg of digoxin in the bloodstream. The complex is then excreted in the urine, rapidly decreasing serum levels and therefore cardiac drug concentrations.

▶ Special considerations

● Obtain baseline heart rate and rhythm, blood pressure, and serum electrolyte levels before giving first dose.
● Question patient about use of cardiac glycosides within the previous 2 to 3 weeks before administering a loading dose. Always divide loading dose over first 24 hours unless clinical situation indicates otherwise.
● Adjust dose to patient's clinical condition; monitor

ECG and serum levels of digoxin, calcium, potassium, and magnesium. Therapeutic serum digoxin levels range from 0.5 to 2 ng/ml. Take corrective action before hypokalemia occurs.
● Monitor clinical status. Take apical-radial pulse for a full minute. Watch for significant changes (sudden rate increase or decrease, pulse deficit, irregular beats, and especially regularization of a previously irregular rhythm). Check blood pressure and obtain 12-lead ECG if these changes occur.
● GI absorption may be reduced in patients with congestive heart failure, especially right heart failure.
● Digoxin dosage generally should be reduced and serum level monitoring performed if patient is receiving digoxin concomitantly with amiodarone, diltiazem, flecainide, nifedipine, verapamil, or quinidine. Also monitor patient closely for signs and symptoms of digoxin toxicity. Obtain serum digoxin levels if you suspect toxicity.
● Because digoxin may predispose patients to postcardioversion asystole, most clinicians withhold digoxin 1 or 2 days before elective cardioversion in patients with atrial fibrillation. (However, consider consequences of increased ventricular response to atrial fibrillation if drug is withheld.)
● Elective cardioversion should be postponed in patients with signs of digoxin toxicity.
● Do not administer calcium salts to patient receiving digoxin. Calcium affects cardiac contractility and excitability in much the same way that digoxin does and may lead to serious arrhythmias.
● Hypothyroid patients are highly sensitive to glycosides; hyperthyroid patients may need larger doses.
● Monitor patient's eating patterns. Ask him about nausea, vomiting, anorexia, visual disturbances, and other evidence of toxicity.
● Consider that different brands may not be therapeutically interchangeable.
● Digoxin solution is enclosed in newly available soft capsule (Lanoxicaps). Because these capsules are better absorbed than tablets, dose is usually slightly smaller.

Information for the patient

Instruct patient and responsible family member about drug action, medication regimen, how to take pulse, reportable signs, and follow-up plans.

Geriatric use

Digoxin should be used with caution in elderly patients; adjust dosage to prevent systemic accumulation.

Pediatric use

Pediatric patients have a poorly defined serum concentration range; however, toxicity apparently does not occur at same concentrations considered toxic in adults. Divided daily dosing is recommended for infants and children under age 10; older children require adult doses proportional to body weight.

---

digoxin immune Fab (ovine)
Digibind

● Pharmacologic classification: antibody fragment
● Therapeutic classification: digitalis glycoside antidote
● Pregnancy risk category C

How supplied
Available by prescription only
Injection: 40-mg vial

Indications, route, and dosage
Potentially life-threatening digoxin or digitoxin intoxication

Adults and children: Administered I.V. over 30 minutes or as a bolus if cardiac arrest is imminent. Dosage varies according to the amount of drug to be neutralized; average dose is 10 vials (400 mg). However, if toxicity resulted from acute digoxin ingestion, and neither a serum digoxin level nor an estimated ingestion amount is known, 20 vials (800 mg) should be administered. See package insert for complete, specific dosage instructions.

Pharmacodynamics
Digitalis antidote: Specific antigen-binding fragments bind to free digoxin in extracellular fluid and intravascularly to prevent and reverse pharmacologic and toxic effects of the digitalis glycoside. This binding is preferential for digoxin and digitoxin; preliminary evidence suggests some binding to other digoxin derivatives and cardioactive metabolites.

Once free digoxin is bound and removed from serum, tissue-bound digoxin is released into the serum to maintain efflux-influx balance. As digoxin is released, it, too, is bound and removed by digoxin immune Fab, resulting in a reduction of serum and tissue digoxin. Cardiac glycoside toxicity begins to subside within 30 minutes after completion of a 15-to-30-minute I.V. infusion of digoxin immune Fab. The onset of action and response is variable and appears to depend on rate of infusion, dose administered relative to body load of glycoside, and possibly other, as yet unidentified factors. Reversal of toxicity, including hyperkalemia, is usually complete within 2 to 6 hours after administration of digoxin immune Fab.

Pharmacokinetics
● *Absorption:* Peak serum concentrations occur at the completion of I.V. infusion. Digoxin immune Fab has a serum half-life of 15 to 20 hours. The association reaction between Fab fragments and glycoside molecules appears to occur rapidly; data is limited.
● *Distribution:* The drug's distribution is not fully characterized. After I.V. administration, it appears to distribute rapidly throughout extracellular space, into both plasma and interstitial fluid. It is not known if digoxin immune Fab crosses the placental barrier or is distributed into breast milk.
● *Metabolism:* Unknown.
● *Excretion:* It is excreted in urine via glomerular filtration.

Contraindications and precautions
There are no known contraindications. No systemic allergic reactions have been reported; however, patients sensitive to or intolerant of sheep or other products of ovine origin may be intolerant of digoxin immune Fab. In these high-risk patients, skin testing is recommended. This drug should be used cautiously in patients with low cardiac output and congestive heart failure (CHF), because the condition may worsen from the subsequent decrease in effective inotropic concentrations of digoxin. A causal relationship has not been established.

Ventricular tachycardia may develop in patients with preexisting atrial fibrillation because of the reversal of the glycoside effects on the AV node.

Renal impairment may delay elimination of Fab-digoxin complex.

Interactions
When used concomitantly, digoxin immune Fab will bind cardiac glycosides, including digoxin, digitoxin, and lanatoside C. This will also occur if redigitalization is attempted before elimination of digoxin immune Fab is complete (several days with normal renal function; 1 week or longer with renal impairment).

Effects on diagnostic tests
Digoxin immune Fab therapy alters standard cardiac glycoside determinations by radioimmunoassay procedures. Results may be falsely increased or decreased, depending on separation method used. Serum potassium levels may decrease rapidly.

Adverse reactions
● CV: CHF, *ventricular tachycardia.*
● Metabolic: hypokalemia.
● Other: *hypersensitivity.*

Note: Adverse reactions are related more to the withdrawal of digitalis than to a direct effect of the antibody fragment; these may include exacerbation of CHF, low cardiac output, increased ventricular rate in the presence of pre-existing atrial fibrillation, and hypokalemia as serum potassium levels rapidly decrease.

Overdose and treatment
Limited information is available; however, administration of doses larger than needed for neutralizing the cardiac glycoside may subject the patient to increased risk of allergic or febrile reaction or delayed serum sickness. Large doses may also prolong the time span required before redigitalization.

▶ Special considerations
● Give I.V. using a 0.22-micron filter needle over 30 minutes or as a bolus injection when cardiac arrest is imminent. Dose depends on amount of digoxin to be neutralized. Each 40-mg vial binds approximately 0.6 mg of digoxin or digitoxin. Reconstitute vial with 4 ml of sterile water for injection, mix gently, and use immediately. May be stored in refrigerator up to 4 hours.
● Skin testing may be appropriate for high-risk patients. One of two methods may be used:
Intradermal test–Dilute 0.1 ml of reconstituted solution in 9.9 ml of sterile saline for injection; then withdraw and inject 0.1 ml of this solution intradermally. Inspect site after 20 minutes for signs of erythema or urticaria.
Scratch test–Dilute as for intradermal test. Place one drop of diluted solution on skin and make a ¼ " scratch through the drop with a sterile needle. Inspect site after

20 minutes for signs of erythema or urticaria. If results are positive, avoid use of digoxin immune Fab unless necessary. If systemic reaction occurs, treat symptomatically.

● Pretreat patients with sensitivity or allergy to sheep or ovine products, or when skin test results are positive, with an antihistamine such as diphenhydramine and a corticosteroid before administering digoxin immune Fab.
● Keep medications and equipment for cardiopulmonary resuscitation readily available during administration of digoxin immune Fab for patients who respond poorly to withdrawal of digoxin's inotropic effects. Dopamine or dobutamine, or other cardiac load-reducing agents, may be used. Catecholamines may aggravate arrhythmias induced by digitalis toxicity and should be used with caution.
● Measure serum digoxin or digitoxin levels before giving antidote, because serum concentrations may be difficult to interpret after therapy with antidote.
● Closely monitor temperature, blood pressure, ECG, and potassium concentration before, during, and after administration of antidote.
● Potassium levels must be checked repeatedly, because severe digitalis intoxication can cause life-threatening hyperkalemia, and reversal by digoxin immune Fab may lead to rapid hypokalemia.
● Suicidal ingestion often involves more than one medication. Be alert for possible toxic manifestations secondary to these other medications.
● Delay redigitalization until elimination of Fab fragments is complete; may take several days with normal renal function, a week or longer with impaired renal function.

Pediatric use
● Risk-to-benefit ratio must be considered. Use in infants and small children has not produced adverse effects.
● Monitor for volume overload in small children.
● Very small doses may require diluting the reconstituted solution with 36 ml of sterile saline for injection to produce a 1 mg/ml solution.
● Infants may require smaller doses; the manufacturer recommends reconstituting as directed and administering with a tuberculin syringe.

Breast-feeding
It is unknown whether digoxin immune Fab is distributed into breast milk. It should be used with caution in breast-feeding women.

---

dihydroergotamine mesylate
D.H.E. 45

● Pharmacologic classification: ergot alkaloid
● Therapeutic classification: vasoconstrictor
● Pregnancy risk category X

How supplied
Available by prescription only
Injection: 1 mg/ml parenteral

Indications, route, and dosage
To prevent or abort vascular headaches, including migraine and cluster headaches
Adults: 1 mg I.M. or I.V., repeated at 1-hour intervals, up to total of 3 mg I.M. The total I.V. dose should not exceed 2 mg. Maximum weekly dose is 6 mg.

Pharmacodynamics
Vasoconstrictor action: By stimulating alpha-adrenergic receptors, dihydroergotamine causes peripheral vasoconstriction (if vascular tone is low). However, the drug causes vasodilation in hypertonic blood vessels. At high doses, it is a competitive alpha-adrenergic blocker. In therapeutic doses, dihydroergotamine inhibits the reuptake of norepinephrine, which increases its vasoconstricting activity. A weak antagonist of serotonin, the drug reduces the increased rate of platelet aggregation caused by serotonin.

In the treatment of vascular headaches, dihydroergotamine probably causes direct vasoconstriction of the dilated carotid artery bed while decreasing the amplitude of pulsations. Its serotoninergic and catecholamine effects also appear to be involved.

Effects on blood pressure are unpredictable but usually minimal. The vasoconstrictor effect is more pronounced on veins and venules than on arteries and arterioles.

Pharmacokinetics
● *Absorption:* Dihydroergotamine is incompletely and irregularly absorbed from the GI tract. Onset of action is probably dependent on how promptly after onset of headache the drug is given. After I.M. injection, the onset of action occurs within 15 to 30 minutes, and after I.V. injection, within a few minutes. Duration of action persists 3 to 4 hours after I.M. injection.
● *Distribution:* 90% of a dose is plasma protein-bound.
● *Metabolism:* Dihydroergotamine is extensively metabolized, probably in the liver (extensive first-pass metabolism).
● *Excretion:* 10% of a dose is excreted in urine within 72 hours as metabolites; the rest in feces by biliary elimination.

Contraindications and precautions
Dihydroergotamine is contraindicated in patients with peripheral vascular disease, coronary artery disease, hypertension, or sepsis because of the cardiovascular effects of the drug; in patients with impaired hepatic or renal function, because of the potential for accumulation and toxicity; in patients with known hypersensitivity to the drug; and during pregnancy.

Interactions
Concomitant use with antihypertensive drugs may antagonize their antihypertensive effects. Concomitant use with erythromycin may cause ergot toxicity.

Effects on diagnostic tests
None reported.

Adverse reactions
● CV: transient bradycardia or tachycardia, severe vasospasm, numbness, tingling in fingers and toes, precordial distress and pain, increased arterial pressure.
● GI: nausea, vomiting.
● Other: localized edema, itching, weakness in legs, dizziness, muscle pain in extremities.

Note: Drug should be discontinued if severe vaso-spasm or hypersensitivity occurs.

Overdose and treatment
Clinical manifestations of overdose include symptoms of ergot toxicity, including peripheral ischemia, pares-thesia, headache, nausea, and vomiting.

Treatment requires prolonged and careful monitoring. Provide respiratory support, treat convulsions if nec-essary, and apply warmth (not direct heat) to ischemic extremities if vasospasm occurs. Administer vasodilator (nitroprusside, prazosin, or tolazoline) if needed.

▶ Special considerations
Besides those relevant to all *ergot alkaloids,* consider the following recommendations.
● Dihydroergotamine is most effective when used at first sign of migraine, or as soon after onset as possible.
● If severe vasospasm occurs, keep extremities warm. Provide supportive treatment to prevent tissue damage. Administer vasodilators (nitroprusside, prazosin, or to-lazoline) if needed.
● Protect ampules from heat and light. Do not use if discolored.
● For short-term use only. Do not exceed recom-mended dose.
● Ergotamine rebound or an increase in frequency or duration of headaches may occur when drug is stopped.
● Dihydroergotamine has also been used to treat pos-tural hypotension.

Information for the patient
● Advise patient to lie down and relax in a quiet, dark-ened room after dose is administered.
● Urge patient to report immediately any feelings of numbness or tingling in fingers and toes, or red or violet blisters on hands or feet.
● Warn patient to avoid alcoholic beverages, because alcohol may worsen headaches.
● Smoking may increase the adverse effects of dihy-droergotamine. Patient should avoid smoking while tak-ing this drug.
● Tell patient to avoid prolonged exposure to very cold temperatures while taking this medication. Cold may increase adverse reactions.
● Advise patient to report illness or infection, which may increase sensitivity to drug reactions.

Geriatric use
Administer cautiously, because elderly patients are more sensitive to drug's reactions.

Breast-feeding
Breast-feeding should be avoided during therapy with dihydroergotamine.

dihydrotachysterol
DHT, DHT Intensol, Hytakerol

● Pharmacologic classification: vitamin D analog
● Therapeutic classification: antihypocal-cemic
● Pregnancy risk category C (diffused in doses greater than RDA)

How supplied
Available by prescription only
Tablets: 0.125 mg, 0.2 mg, 0.4 mg
Capsules: 0.125 mg
Solution: 0.2 mg/ml (Intensol), 0.2 mg/5 ml (in 4% al-cohol), 0.25 mg/ml (in sesame oil)

Indications, route, and dosage
Familial hypophosphatemia
Adults and children: 0.5 to 2 mg P.O. daily. Maintenance dose is 0.3 to 1.5 mg daily.
Hypocalcemia associated with hypoparathy-roidism and pseudohypoparathyroidism
Adults: Initially, 0.8 to 2.4 mg P.O. daily for several days. Maintenance dose is 0.2 to 2 mg daily, as required for normal serum calcium levels. Average dose is 0.6 mg daily.
Children: Initially, 1 to 5 mg P.O. for several days. Main-tenance dose is 0.2 to 1 mg daily, as required for normal serum calcium levels.
Renal osteodystrophy in chronic uremia
Adults: 0.1 to 0.6 mg P.O. daily.

Pharmacodynamics
Antihypocalcemic action: Once activated to its 25-hy-droxy form, dihydrotachysterol works with parathyroid hormone to regulate levels of calcium. It appears to have little activity as the parent compound.

Pharmacokinetics
● *Absorption:* Absorbed readily from the small intes-tine.
● *Distribution:* Drug is distributed widely; it is largely protein-bound.
● *Metabolism:* Drug is metabolized in the liver, and has a duration of action up to 9 weeks.
● *Excretion:* Dihydrotachysterol is excreted in urine and bile.

Contraindications and precautions
Dihydrotachysterol is contraindicated in patients with hypercalcemia or sensitivity to vitamin D.

Interactions
Antacids may alter absorption of dihydrotachysterol. Barbiturates, phenytoin, and primidone may increase metabolism and therefore reduce activity of dihydro-tachysterol. The resulting increases in calcium may po-tentiate the effects of digitalis glycosides. Excessive use of mineral oil may interfere with intestinal absorption of vitamin D analogs. Concurrent use with cholestyr-amine and colestipol may result in decreased intestinal absorption of vitamin D analogs.

Effects on diagnostic tests
Drug alters serum alkaline phosphatase concentrations and cholesterol levels and may alter electrolytes, such as magnesium, phosphate, and calcium, in serum and urine.

Adverse reactions
Signs and symptoms of hypercalcemia:
● CNS: headache, lethargy, depression, amnesia, disorientation, hallucinations, syncope and coma.
● EENT: vertigo, tinnitus.
● GI: nausea, vomiting, abdominal cramps, constipation, anorexia.
● Other: weakness, polyuria and polydipsia (with impairment of renal function).
   Note: Drug should be discontinued if patient develops signs or symptoms of hypercalcemia.

Overdose and treatment
Hypercalcemia is the only clinical manifestation of overdose. Treatment involves discontinuing therapy, instituting a low-calcium diet, increasing fluid intake, and providing supportive measures. In severe cases, death from cardiac and renal failure has occurred. Calcitonin administration may help reverse hypercalcemia.

▶ Special considerations
● Monitor serum and urine calcium levels. Observe patient for signs and symptoms of hypercalcemia.
● There is some evidence that monitoring urine calcium and urine creatinine is very helpful in screening for hypercalciuria. The ratio of urine calcium to urine creatinine should be less than or equal to 0.18. A value > 0.2 suggests hypercalciuria, and the dose should be decreased regardless of serum calcium.
● Adequate dietary calcium intake is necessary; usually supplemented with 10 to 15 g oral calcium lactate or gluconate daily.
● 1 mg is equal to 120,000 units ergocalciferol (vitamin D_2).
● Store in tightly closed, light-resistant containers. Do not refrigerate.

Information for the patient
Explain the importance of a calcium-rich diet.

Pediatric use
Some infants may be hyperreactive to drug.

Breast-feeding
Do not use in breast-feeding women.

---

dihydroxyaluminum sodium carbonate (DSC)
Rolaids

● Pharmacologic classification: aluminum salt
● Therapeutic classification: antacid
● Pregnancy risk category C

How supplied
Available without prescription
Tablets: 324 mg

Indications, route, and dosage
Antacid
Adults: Chew 1 to 2 tablets, p.r.n.

Pharmacodynamics
Antiulcer action: DSC neutralizes gastric acid, decreasing the direct acid irritant effect. This increases pH, thereby inactivating pepsin. DSC also enhances mucosal barrier integrity and increases gastroesophageal sphincter tone.

Pharmacokinetics
● *Absorption:* Unknown.
● *Distribution:* Primarily local.
● *Metabolism:* None.
● *Excretion:* DSC is excreted in feces; some aluminum may be excreted in breast milk.

Contraindications and precautions
DSC is contraindicated in patients with renal failure, hypophosphatemia, appendicitis, undiagnosed rectal or GI bleeding, constipation, fecal impaction, chronic diarrhea, or intestinal obstruction because drug may exacerbate the symptoms associated with these conditions.
   DSC should be used cautiously in patients with restricted sodium intake or congestive heart failure because of high sodium content (53 mg sodium/tablet); in patients with hemorrhoids because the drug may exacerbate this condition; and in patients with decreased GI motility, such as elderly patients and those receiving such drugs as anticholinergics or antidiarrheals, because these patients may be predisposed to intestinal obstruction.

Interactions
DSC may decrease absorption of tetracycline, coumarin anticoagulants, antimuscarinics, chenodiol, diazepam, chlordiazepoxide, ciprofloxacin, isoniazid, digoxin, iron salts, and potassium salts, thereby decreasing their effectiveness.
   Drug also may cause premature release of enterically coated drugs; separate DSC from all oral medications by 1 hour.

Effects on diagnostic tests
DSC may interfere with evaluation of Meckel's diverticulum, reticuloendothelial imaging, and other tests using radiopaque media.
   DSC may increase serum gastrin levels.

Adverse reactions
● GI: constipation, anorexia, obstruction, decreased bowel motility.
● Other: aluminum toxicity, dehydration.

Overdose and treatment
No information available.

▶ Special considerations
● Closely monitor dehydrated patients and those with restricted fluid intake or suspected intestinal obstruction.
● Monitor bowel function. If patient is constipated, you may need to prescribe a laxative or alternate DSC with a magnesium-containing antacid (unless contraindicated).
● DSC has a high sodium content. Monitor sodium lev-

---

els if administering drug in high doses or for prolonged periods to patient who must limit sodium intake.

Information for the patient
● Caution patient to use drug only as directed and to chew tablets thoroughly.
● Tell patient to take drug 1 to 2 hours apart from other medications.

Pediatric use
Use with caution in children under age 6.

Breast-feeding
Although some aluminum may be excreted in breast milk, no problems have been associated with use by breast-feeding women.

---

diltiazem hydrochloride
Cardizem, Cardizem CD, Cardizem SR, Dilacor SR

● Pharmacologic classification: calcium channel blocker
● Therapeutic classification: antianginal
● Pregnancy risk category C

How supplied
Available by prescription only
Tablets: 30 mg, 60 mg, 90 mg, 120 mg
Capsules (sustained-release): 60 mg, 90 mg, 120 mg (Cardizem SR); 180 mg, 240 mg, 300 mg (Cardizem CD); 180 mg, 240 mg (Dilacor SR)
Injection: 5 mg/ml

Indications, route, and dosage
Management of Prinzmetal's or variant angina or chronic stable angina pectoris
Adults: 30 mg P.O. q.i.d. before meals and h.s. Dosage may be increased gradually to 240 mg/day, in divided doses three to four times a day.
Hypertension
Adults: 60 to 120 mg P.O. b.i.d. (Cardizem SR); or 180 to 240 mg (Cardizem CD or Dilacor SR) once a day. Adjust dosage according to patient response. Maximum hypotensive effect is usually evident after 14 days. Usual dosage range is 240 to 360 mg daily for Cardizem CD, 180 mg to 480 mg once daily for Dilacor SR.
Atrial fibrillation or flutter
Adults: 0. 25 mg/kg I.V. as a bolus injection over 2 minutes. Repeat after 15 minutes if response is not adequate.

Pharmacodynamics
Antianginal action: By dilating systemic arteries, diltiazem decreases total peripheral resistance and afterload, slightly reduces blood pressure, and increases cardiac index, when given in high doses (over 200 mg). Afterload reduction, which occurs at rest and with exercise, and the resulting decrease in myocardial oxygen consumption account for diltiazem's effectiveness in controlling chronic stable angina.

Diltiazem also decreases myocardial oxygen demand and cardiac work by reducing heart rate, relieving coronary artery spasm (through coronary artery vasodilation), and dilating peripheral vessels. These effects relieve ischemia and pain. In patients with Prinz-

metal's angina, diltiazem inhibits coronary artery spasm, increasing myocardial oxygen delivery.

Pharmacokinetics
● *Absorption:* Approximately 80% of a dose of diltiazem is absorbed rapidly from the GI tract. However, only about 40% of the drug enters systemic circulation because of a significant first-pass effect in the liver. Peak serum levels occur in about 2 to 3 hours.
● *Distribution:* About 70% to 85% of circulating diltiazem is bound to plasma proteins.
● *Metabolism:* Diltiazem is metabolized in the liver.
● *Excretion:* About 35% of the drug is excreted in the urine and about 65% in the bile as unchanged drug and inactive and active metabolites. Elimination half-life is 3 to 9 hours. Half-life may increase in elderly patients; however, renal dysfunction does not appear to affect half-life.

Contraindications and precautions
Diltiazem is contraindicated in patients with severe hypotension (systolic blood pressure below 90 mm Hg), because of the drug's hypotensive effect; in patients with second- or third-degree AV block or sick sinus syndrome (unless a functioning artificial ventricular pacemaker is in place), because of the drug's effect on the cardiac conduction system; and in patients with known hypersensitivity to the drug.

Diltiazem should be used with caution in patients with congestive heart failure; in patients with impaired ventricular function or conduction abnormalities, because the drug may worsen this condition; in patients receiving beta blockers or digoxin; because this may result in excessive bradycardia or conduction abnormalities; in patients with impaired liver or kidney function; and in elderly patients, because plasma half-life may be prolonged.

Interactions
When used concomitantly, beta blockers may cause combined effects that result in congestive heart failure, conduction disturbances, dysrhythmia, and hypotension. Concomitant use with digoxin may cause serum digoxin levels to increase by 20% to 50%. Concomitant use with cyclosporine may cause increased serum cyclosporine levels and subsequent cyclosporine-induced nephrotoxicity.

Effects on diagnostic tests
None reported.

Adverse reactions
● CNS: headache, fatigue, drowsiness, dizziness, nervousness, depression, insomnia, confusion.
● CV: edema, *arrhythmia*, flushing, bradycardia, hypotension, conduction abnormalities.
● DERM: rash, pruritus.
● GI: nausea, vomiting, diarrhea.
● GU: nocturia, polyuria.
● Hepatic: transient elevation of liver enzymes.
● Other: photosensitivity, akathisia.

Overdose and treatment
Clinical effects of overdose primarily are extensions of the drug's adverse reactions. Heart block, asystole, and hypotension are the most serious effects and require immediate attention.

Treatment may involve I.V. isoproterenol, norepinephrine, epinephrine, atropine, or calcium gluconate

---

*Canada only   †Unlabeled clinical use   Italicized adverse reactions are life-threatening.

administered in usual doses. Adequate hydration must be ensured. Inotropic agents, including dobutamine and dopamine, may be used, if necessary. If the patient develops severe conduction disturbances (such as heart block and asystole) with hypotension that does not respond to drug therapy, cardiac pacing should be initiated immediately with cardiopulmonary resuscitation measures, as indicated.

▶ **Special considerations**
Besides those relevant to all *calcium channel blockers*, consider the following recommendations.
● If diltiazem is added to therapy of a patient receiving digoxin, monitor serum digoxin levels and observe patient closely for signs of toxicity, especially elderly patients, those with unstable renal function, and those with serum digoxin levels in the upper therapeutic range.
● Sublingual nitroglycerin may be administered concomitantly, as needed, if patient has acute angina symptoms.
● Diltiazem has been used investigationally to prevent reinfarction after non Q wave myocardial infarction; as an adjunct in the treatment of peripheral vascular disorders; and in the treatment of a variety of spastic smooth muscle disorders, including esophageal spasm.

Information for the patient
Nitrate therapy prescribed during titration of diltiazem dosage may cause dizziness. Urge patient to continue compliance.

Geriatric use
Diltiazem should be used with caution in elderly patients because drug's half-life may be prolonged.

Breast-feeding
Diltiazem is excreted in breast milk; therefore, women should discontinue breast-feeding during diltiazem therapy.

---

dimenhydrinate
Apo-Dimenhydrinate★, Calm X, Dimentabs, Dinate, Dommanate, Dramamine, Dramilin, Dramocen, Dramoject, Dymenate, Gravol★, Hydrate, Marmine, Motion-Aid, Nauseatol★, Novodimenate★, PMS-Dimenhydrinate★, Reidamine, Travamine★, Wehamine

● Pharmacologic classification: ethanol-amine-derivative antihistamine
● Therapeutic classification: antihistamine (H₁-receptor antagonist), antiemetic and antivertigo agent
● Pregnancy risk category B

How supplied
Available with or without prescription
Tablets: 50 mg
Liquid: 12.5 mg/4 ml
Injection: 50 mg/ml
Rectal: 50 mg, 100 mg

Indications, route, and dosage
Nausea, vomiting, dizziness of motion sickness (prophylaxis and treatment)
Adults and children age 12 and older: 50 to 100 mg q 4 to 6 hours P.O., I.V., or I.M. (and rectally where available). For I.V. administration, dilute each 50-mg dose in 10 ml of normal saline solution and inject slowly over 2 minutes.
Children: 5 mg/kg/day P.O. in four divided doses; or 150 mg/m²/day P.O. in four divided doses, not to exceed 300 mg/day, or according to the following schedule:
Children age 6 to 12: 25 to 50 mg P.O. q 6 to 8 hours; maximum dosage is 150 mg/day.
Children age 2 to 6: 12.5 to 25 mg P.O. q 6 to 8 hours maximum dosage is 75 mg/day.
Children under age 2: 1.25 mg/kg I.M. or I.V.; or 37.5 mg/m² I.M. or I.V. Do not use in neonates and premature infants.

Drug has been used to treat Meniere's disease. Dosage is 50 mg I.M. for acute attack, 25 to 50 mg t.i.d. for maintenance.

Pharmacodynamics
Antiemetic and antivertigo action: Dimenhydrinate probably inhibits nausea and vomiting by centrally depressing sensitivity of the labyrinth apparatus that relays stimuli to the chemoreceptor trigger zone and stimulates the vomiting center in the brain.

Pharmacokinetics
● *Absorption:* Dimenhydrinate is well absorbed. Action begins within 15 to 30 minutes after oral administration, 20 to 30 minutes after I.M. administration, and almost immediately after I.V. administration.
● *Distribution:* Dimenhydrinate is well distributed throughout the body and crosses the placenta.
● *Metabolism:* Dimenhydrinate is metabolized in the liver.
● *Excretion:* Metabolites are excreted in urine.

Contraindications and precautions
Dimenhydrinate is contraindicated in patients with known hypersensitivity to this drug or to other antiemetic antihistamines with a similar chemical structure, such as diphenhydramine; and in those sensitive to theophylline, because dimenhydrinate is the 8-chlorotheophylline salt of diphenhydramine.

Dimenhydrinate should be used with caution in patients with narrow-angle glaucoma, asthma, prostatic hypertrophy, or GU or GI obstruction, because of the drug's anticholinergic effects; and in patients with seizure disorders. Drug may mask signs of brain tumor or intestinal obstruction.

Interactions
Additive CNS sedation and depression may occur when drug is used concomitantly with other CNS depressants, such as alcohol, barbiturates, tranquilizers, sleeping agents, and antianxiety agents.

Dimenhydrinate may mask the signs of ototoxicity caused by known ototoxic agents, including the aminoglycosides, salicylates, vancomycin, loop diuretics, and cisplatin.

Effects on diagnostic tests
Dimenhydrinate may alter or confuse test results for xanthines (caffeine, aminophylline) because of its 8-chlorotheophylline content; discontinue dimenhydri-

---

nate 4 days before diagnostic skin tests, to avoid preventing, reducing, or masking test response.

Adverse reactions
• CNS: drowsiness, dizziness, headache, incoordination, convulsions.
• CV: palpitations, hypotension.
• EENT: blurred vision, tinnitus, dry mouth and respiratory passages.
• GI: constipation, diarrhea, anorexia.
• GU: urinary frequency, dysuria.

Overdose and treatment
Clinical manifestations of overdose may include either CNS depression (sedation, reduced mental alertness, apnea, and cardiovascular collapse) or CNS stimulation (insomnia, hallucinations, tremors, or convulsions). Anticholinergic symptoms, such as dry mouth, flushed skin, fixed and dilated pupils, and GI symptoms, are likely to occur, especially in children.

Use gastric lavage to empty stomach contents; emetics may be ineffective. Diazepam or phenytoin may be used to control seizures. Treat supportively.

▶ **Special considerations**
Besides those relevant to all *antihistamines,* consider the following recommendations.
• Incorrectly administered or undiluted I.V. solution is irritating to veins and may cause sclerosis.
• Parenteral solution is incompatible with many drugs; do not mix other drugs in the same syringe.
• Advise safety measures for all patients; dimenhydrinate has a high incidence of drowsiness. Tolerance to CNS depressant effects usually develops within a few days.
• To prevent motion sickness, patient should take medication ½ hour before traveling and again before meals and at bedtime.
• Antiemetic effect may diminish with prolonged use.

Information for the patient
Tell patient to avoid hazardous activities, such as driving or operating heavy machinery, until the adverse CNS effects of the drug are known.

Geriatric use
Elderly patients are usually more sensitive to adverse effects of antihistamines and are especially likely to experience a greater degree of dizziness, sedation, hyperexcitability, dry mouth, and urinary retention than younger patients.

Pediatric use
Safety in neonates has not been established. Infants and children under age 6 may experience paradoxical hyperexcitability. I.V. dosage for children has not been established.

Breast-feeding
Antihistamines should not be used during breast-feeding. Many of these drugs, including dimenhydrinate, are secreted in breast milk, exposing the infant to risks of unusual excitability; premature infants are at particular risk for convulsions.

dimercaprol
BAL in Oil

• Pharmacologic classification: chelating agent
• Therapeutic classification: heavy metal antagonist
• Pregnancy risk category C

How supplied
Available by prescription only
Injection: 100 mg/ml

Indications, route, and dosage
Severe arsenic or gold poisoning
Adults and children: 3 mg/kg deep I.M. every 4 hours for 2 days, then q.i.d. on 3rd day; then b.i.d. for 10 days.
Mild arsenic or gold poisoning
Adults and children: 2.5 mg/kg deep I.M. q.i.d. for 2 days, then b.i.d. on 3rd day; then once daily for 10 days.
Severe gold dermatitis
Adults and children: 2.5 mg/kg deep I.M. every 4 hours for 2 days, then b.i.d. for 7 days.
Gold-induced thrombocytopenia
Adults and children: 100 mg deep I.M. b.i.d. for 15 days.
Mercury poisoning
Adults and children: Initially, 5 mg/kg deep I.M., then 2.5 mg/kg daily or b.i.d. for 10 days.
Acute lead encephalopathy or blood lead level greater than 100 mcg/dl
Adults and children: 4 mg/kg deep I.M. injection, then give simultaneously with edetate calcium disodium (250 mg/m^2) every 4 hours for 5 days. Use separate injection sites.

Pharmacodynamics
Chelating action: The sulfhydryl groups of dimercaprol form heterocyclic ring complexes with heavy metals, particularly arsenic, mercury, and gold, preventing or reversing their binding to body ligands.

Pharmacokinetics
• *Absorption:* Dimercaprol is absorbed slowly through the skin. After I.M. injection, peak serum levels occur in 30 to 60 minutes.
• *Distribution:* Dimercaprol is distributed to all tissues, mainly the intracellular space, with the highest concentrations of dimercaprol occurring in the liver and kidneys.
• *Metabolism:* Uncomplexed dimercaprol is metabolized rapidly to inactive products.
• *Excretion:* Most dimercaprol-metal complexes and inactive metabolites are excreted in urine and feces.

Contraindications and precautions
Dimercaprol is contraindicated in patients with iron, cadmium, selenium, or uranium poisoning, because the complexes formed are more toxic than the metals themselves; and in patients with impaired hepatic function except those with postarsenical jaundice.

Dimercaprol should be used cautiously in patients with impaired renal function, because toxic levels may result; and in patients with hypertension because drug may worsen the hypertension.

Interactions

Iron, cadmium, selenium, and uranium form toxic complexes with dimercaprol. Delay iron therapy for 24 hours after stopping dimercaprol.

Effects on diagnostic tests

Dimercaprol therapy blocks thyroid uptake of ^{131}I, causing decreased values.

Adverse reactions

● CNS: seizures, stupor, and/or coma with doses over 5 mg/kg; headache; anxiety; restlessness; paresthesia.
● CV: transient hypertension, tachycardia.
● DERM: contact edema and erythema.
● EENT: burning sensation of lips, throat, and eyes; pain in teeth; blepharospasm; lacrimation; rhinorrhea; excessive salivation.
● GI: nausea, vomiting, abdominal pain.
● Local: pain, sterile abscess after I.M. injection.
● Other: fever, muscle aches, pain, spasms, sweating.
   Note: Drug should be discontinued if renal failure or hypersensitivity develops.

Overdose and treatment

Clinical signs of overdose include vomiting, seizures, stupor, coma, hypertension, and tachycardia; effects subside in 1 to 6 hours. Support cardiovascular and respiratory status; control seizures with diazepam.

▶ Special considerations

● Treat patient as soon as possible after poisoning, for optimal therapeutic effect; administer drug by deep I.M. injection only.
● Monitor vital signs and intake and output during therapy, and keep urine alkaline to prevent renal failure.
● Adverse effects of dimercaprol are usually mild and transitory and occur in about one half of patients who receive an I.M. dose of 5 mg/kg. In patients who receive doses in excess of 5 mg/kg, adverse effects usually occur within 30 minutes after injection and subside in 1 to 6 hours.
● Drug has strong garlic odor.

Information for the patient

Advise patient that drug may cause a bad taste in the mouth and/or bad breath. It also may cause a burning sensation of the lips, mouth, throat, eyes, and penis and pain in the teeth.

Geriatric use

Drug should be used with caution.

Pediatric use

Fever is common, usually appearing after the second or third dose, and may persist throughout therapy. Acrodynia in infants and children has been treated with 3 mg/kg of dimercaprol I.M. every 4 hours for 2 days, then every 6 hours for 1 day, followed by every 12 hours for 7 to 8 days.

dinoprostone (prostaglandin E₂)
Prostin E₂

● Pharmacologic classification: prostaglandin
● Therapeutic classification: oxytocic

How supplied

Available by prescription only
Vaginal suppositories: 20 mg

Indications, route, and dosage

Abort second-trimester pregnancy, evacuate uterus in cases of missed abortion, intrauterine fetal deaths up to 28 weeks of gestation, benign hydatidiform mole
Adults: Insert 20-mg suppository high into posterior vaginal fornix. Repeat q 3 to 5 hours until abortion is complete. Do not exceed 240 mg.
†*To ripen cervix before induction of labor*
Adults: Insert ¼ suppository into vagina.

Pharmacodynamics

Oxytocic action: Dinoprostone stimulates myometrial contractions in the gravid uterus similar to the contractions of term labor. The exact mechanism of action is unknown, but it may result from one or more of the following: direct stimulation, regulation of cellular calcium transport, or regulation of intracellular concentrations of cyclic 3', 5'-adenosine monophosphate. Reductions in plasma estrogen and progesterone levels play a role in the drug's uterine action, but this effect does not occur consistently. Dinoprostone facilitates cervical dilations by directly softening the cervix.

Pharmacokinetics

● *Absorption:* Following vaginal insertion, dinoprostone is diffused slowly into the maternal blood. There is also some local absorption into the uterus through the cervix or local vascular and lymphatic channels, but this accounts for only a small portion of the dose. Contractions appear within 10 minutes of dosing, with a peak effect in 17 hours. There is no correlation of activity with plasma concentrations.
● *Distribution:* Drug is distributed widely in the mother.
● *Metabolism:* Drug is metabolized in the lungs, liver, kidneys, spleen, and other maternal tissues. There are at least nine inactive metabolites.
● *Excretion:* Drug and metabolites are excreted primarily in urine, with small amounts in feces.

Contraindications and precautions

Dinoprostone is contraindicated in patients sensitive to the drug; in patients with acute pelvic inflammatory disease, because drug may worsen fever and associated symptoms; in pregnant women when membranes have ruptured; and in patients with history of pelvic surgery, uterine fibroid disease, or cervical stenosis, because of risk of retention of placenta and hemorrhage. Use cautiously in patients with epilepsy, diabetes, and hypotension or hypertension, because drug may exacerbate symptoms of these disorders.

Interactions

Used concomitantly, dinoprostone enhances the effects of oxytocin and other oxytocics. Cervical laceration and

---

*Canada only   †Unlabeled clinical use   Italicized adverse reactions are life-threatening.

trauma have been reported when oxytocin is used concurrently.

Effects on diagnostic tests
None reported.

Adverse reactions
● CV: hypotension, syncope, flushing, hot flashes, fainting.
● GI: nausea, vomiting, diarrhea.
● Respiratory: *bronchospasm*, wheezing, dyspnea.
● Other: chest pain, chest tightness, fever, headache, chills, abdominal pain, uterine bleeding, and uterine rupture have been reported less frequently.
   Note: Drug should be discontinued if wheezing, troubled breathing, or tightness in chest occurs.

Overdose and treatment
Clinical manifestations of overdose are extensions of adverse reactions. Because the drug is rapidly metabolized, treatment involves discontinuing the drug and providing supportive treatment.

▶ Special considerations
● Store the suppositories in the freezer at −4° F. (−20° C.) and warm to room temperature (in foil) just before use.
● To prevent absorption through the skin, use gloves and keep handling of drug to a minimum.
● Administer the drug only in medical facilities where intensive care and surgical facilities are accessible.
● Confirmation of fetal death is imperative before administration when used for missed abortion or intrauterine fetal death.
● Premedicate with antiemetic and antidiarrheal agents to minimize the GI effects.
● Not for rectal administration.
● Abortion should be complete within 30 hours.
● Dinoprostone-induced fever is transient and self-limiting. Sponge baths or increased fluid intake usually corrects this problem.
● After administration, patient should remain supine for 10 minutes.

Information for the patient
● Advise the patient of the expected adverse reactions, especially fever, which is self-limiting.
● Instruct patient to remain in prone position for 10 minutes after insertion.

diphenhydramine hydrochloride
Beldin, Benadryl, Benadryl Children's Allergy, Benadryl Complete Allergy, Bendylate, Benylin, Compoz, Diahist, Diphen, Diphenadril, Fenylhist, Fynex, Hydramine, Hydril, Insomnal∗, Nervine Nighttime Sleep-Aid, Noradryl, Nordryl, Nytol with DPH, Robalyn, Sleep-Eze 3, Sominex Formula 2, Twilite, Tusstat, Valdrene

● Pharmacologic classification: ethanol-amine-derivative antihistamine
● Therapeutic classification: antihistamine (H_1-receptor antagonist), antiemetic and antivertigo agent, antitussive, sedative-hypnotic, topical anesthetic, antidyskinetic (anticholinergic) agent
● Pregnancy risk category C

How supplied
Available with or without prescription
Tablets: 25 mg, 50 mg
Capsules: 25 mg, 50 mg
Elixir: 12.5 mg/5 ml (14% alcohol)
Syrup: 12.5 mg/5 ml, 13.3 mg/5 ml (5% alcohol)
Injection: 10 mg/ml, 50 mg/ml
Cream: 1%, 2%
Lotion: 2%

Indications, route, and dosage
Allergic rhinitis, urticaria, allergic reactions to blood or plasma (antihistamine)
Adults: 25 to 50 mg P.O. q 4 to 6 hours p.r.n.; or 10 to 50 mg I.V. or deep I.M.
Children: 1.25 mg/kg P.O. q 4 to 6 hours; or 37.5 mg/m² P.O. q 4 to 6 hours, not to exceed 300 mg/day. (For children weighing less than 9.1 kg, 6.25 to 12.5 mg P.O. q 4 to 6 hours. For children weighing 9.1 kg and over, 12.5 to 25 mg P.O. q 4 to 6 hours.) Or 1.25 mg/kg or 37.5 mg/m² I.M. q.i.d., not to exceed 300 mg/day.
Motion sickness or vertigo
Adults: 25 to 50 mg P.O. q 4 to 6 hours p.r.n.; or 10 mg I.M. or I.V. initially, then 20 to 50 mg I.M. or I.V. q 2 to 3 hours p.r.n.
Children: 1 to 1.5 mg/kg P.O. q 4 to 6 hours p.r.n.; or 1 to 1.5 mg/kg I.M. q 6 hours, not to exceed 300 mg/day.
Cough
Adults: 25 mg P.O. q 4 to 6 hours.
Children age 6 to 12: 12.5 mg P.O. q 4 to 6 hours; maximum dosage is 50 mg/day.
Children age 2 to 5: 6.25 mg P.O. q 4 to 6 hours; maximum dosage is 25 mg/day.
Insomnia
Adults: 50 mg P.O. h.s.
Control of dyskinetic movement
Adults: Initially, 25 mg t.i.d., increased to 50 mg q.i.d.; or 10 to 50 mg I.M. or I.V.
†Local anesthesia
Adults: 2 ml of a 1% solution injected locally (as in dental procedures). Particularly useful in patients who are allergic to amide or ester local anesthetics.

Pharmacodynamics

● *Antihistamine action:* Antihistamines compete for histamine H_1-receptor sites on the smooth muscle of the bronchi, GI tract, uterus, and large blood vessels; by binding to cellular receptors, they prevent access of histamine and suppress histamine-induced allergic symptoms, even though they do not prevent its release.
● *Antivertigo, antiemetic, and antidyskinetic action:* Central antimuscarinic actions of antihistamines probably are responsible for these effects of diphenhydramine.
● *Antitussive action:* Diphenhydramine suppresses the cough reflex by a direct effect on the cough center.
● *Sedative action:* Mechanism of the CNS depressant effects of diphenhydramine is unknown.
● *Anesthetic action:* Diphenhydramine is structurally related to local anesthetics, which prevent initiation and transmission of nerve impulses; this is the probable source of its topical and local anesthetic effects.

Pharmacokinetics

● *Absorption:* Diphenhydramine is well absorbed from the GI tract. Action begins within 15 to 30 minutes and peaks in 1 to 4 hours.
● *Distribution:* Diphenhydramine is distributed widely throughout the body, including the CNS; drug crosses the placenta and is excreted in breast milk. Diphenhydramine is approximately 82% protein-bound.
● *Metabolism:* About 50% to 60% of an oral dose of diphenhydramine is metabolized by the liver before reaching the systemic circulation (first-pass effect); virtually all available drug is metabolized by the liver within 24 to 48 hours.
● *Excretion:* Plasma elimination half-life of diphenhydramine is about 3½ hours; drug and metabolites are excreted primarily in urine.

Contraindications and precautions

Diphenhydramine is contraindicated in patients with known hypersensitivity to this drug or antihistamines with similar chemical structures (carbinoxamine and clemastine); during an acute asthma attack, because diphenhydramine thickens bronchial secretions; and in patients who have taken monoamine oxidase (MAO) inhibitors within the past 2 weeks. (See Interactions.)

Diphenhydramine should be used with caution in patients with narrow-angle glaucoma; in those with pyloroduodenal obstruction or urinary bladder obstruction from prostatic hypertrophy or narrowing of the bladder neck, because of their marked anticholinergic effects; in patients with cardiovascular disease, hypertension, or hyperthyroidism, because of the risk of palpitations and tachycardia; and in patients with renal disease, diabetes, bronchial asthma, urinary retention, or stenosing peptic ulcers.

Diphenhydramine should not be used during pregnancy, especially in the third trimester, or during breastfeeding. Antihistamines have caused convulsions and other severe reactions, especially in premature infants.

Benadryl 25 contains bisulfites, which can cause severe reactions in individuals allergic to these chemicals.

Interactions

MAO inhibitors interfere with the detoxification of diphenhydramine and thus prolong their central depressant and anticholinergic effects; additive CNS depression may occur when diphenhydramine is given concomitantly with other CNS depressants, such as alcohol, barbiturates, tranquilizers, sleeping aids, and antianxiety agents.

Diphenhydramine may diminish the effects of sulfonylureas, enhance the effects of epinephrine, and partially counteract the anticoagulant effects of heparin.

Effects on diagnostic tests

Discontinue diphenhydramine 4 days before diagnostic skin tests; antihistamines can prevent, reduce, or mask positive skin test response.

Adverse reactions

● CNS: drowsiness, sedation, dizziness, disturbed coordination, confusion, headache, insomnia, restlessness, vertigo; (in children) fever, ataxia, excitement, convulsions, hallucinations.
● CV: hypotension, palpitations, tachycardia, extrasystoles.
● DERM: photosensitivity, urticaria.
● EENT: blurred vision, diplopia, dry nose and throat.
● GI: dry mouth, nausea, vomiting, diarrhea, constipation, epigastric distress, anorexia.
● GU: urinary frequency, dysuria, urinary retention.
● HEMA: leukopenia, agranulocytosis, hemolytic anemia.
● Respiratory: chest tightness, wheezing, thickened bronchial secretions, *anaphylaxis*.

Overdose and treatment

Drowsiness is the usual clinical manifestation of overdose. Seizures, coma, and respiratory depression may occur with profound overdose. Anticholinergic symptoms, such as dry mouth, flushed skin, fixed and dilated pupils, and GI symptoms, are common, especially in children.

Treat overdose by inducing emesis with ipecac syrup (in conscious patient), followed by activated charcoal to reduce further drug absorption. Use gastric lavage if patient is unconscious or ipecac fails. Treat hypotension with vasopressors, and control seizures with diazepam or phenytoin. *Do not give stimulants.*

▶ Special considerations

Besides those relevant to all *antihistamines,* consider the following recommendations.
● Diphenhydramine injection is compatible with most I.V. solutions but is *incompatible* with some drugs; check compatibility before mixing in the same I.V. line.
● Alternate injection sites to prevent irritation. Administer deep I.M. into large muscle.
● Drowsiness is the most common side effect during initial therapy but usually disappears with continued use of the drug.
● Injectable and elixir solutions are light-sensitive; protect from light.

Geriatric use

Elderly patients are usually more sensitive to adverse effects of antihistamines and are especially likely to experience a greater degree of dizziness, sedation, hyperexcitability, dry mouth, and urinary retention than younger patients. Symptoms usually respond to a decrease in medication dosage.

Pediatric use

Diphenhydramine should not be used in premature infants or neonates. Infants and children, especially those under age 6, may experience paradoxical hyperexcitability.

Breast-feeding
Antihistamines should not be used during breast-feeding. Many of these drugs are secreted in breast milk, exposing the infant to risks of unusual excitability; premature infants are at particular risk for convulsions.

diphenoxylate hydrochloride (with atropine sulfate)
Diphenatol, Latropine, Lofene, Lomanate, Lomotil, Lonox, Lo-Quel, Lo-Trol, Nor-Mil

- Pharmacologic classification: opiate
- Therapeutic classification: antidiarrheal
- Controlled substance schedule V
- Pregnancy risk category C

How supplied
Available by prescription only
Tablets: 2.5 mg diphenoxylate hydrochloride and 0.025 mg atropine sulfate per tablet
Liquid: 2.5 mg diphenoxylate hydrochloride and 0.025 mg atropine sulfate/5 ml

Indications, route, and dosage
Acute, nonspecific diarrhea
Adults: 1 to 2 tablets or tsp t.i.d. or q.i.d. initially; decrease dose to 1 tablet or tsp b.i.d. or t.i.d.
Children age 2 and over: 0.3 to 0.4 mg/kg/day diphenoxylate component in divided doses; or administer according to diphenoxylate component, as follows:
Children over age 12: Give usual adult dose.
Children age 9 to 12 (23 to 55 kg): 1.75 to 2.5 mg q.i.d.
Children age 6 to 9 (17 to 32 kg): 1.25 to 2.5 mg q.i.d.
Children age 5 to 6 (16 to 23 kg): 1.25 to 2.25 mg q.i.d.
Children age 4 to 5 (14 to 20 kg): 1 to 2 mg q.i.d.
Children age 3 to 4 (12 to 16 kg): 1 to 1.5 mg q.i.d.
Children age 2 to 3 (11 to 14 kg): 0.75 to 1.5 mg q.i.d.

Pharmacodynamics
Antidiarrheal action: Diphenoxylate is a meperidine analogue that inhibits GI motility locally and centrally. In high doses, it may produce an opiate effect. Atropine is added in subtherapeutic doses to prevent abuse by deliberate overdose.

Pharmacokinetics
- *Absorption:* About 90% of an oral dose is absorbed. Action begins in 45 to 60 minutes.
- *Distribution:* Diphenoxylate is distributed in breast milk.
- *Metabolism:* Diphenoxylate is metabolized extensively by the liver.
- *Excretion:* Metabolites are excreted mainly in feces via the biliary tract, with lesser amounts excreted in urine. Duration of effect is 3 to 4 hours.

Contraindications and precautions
Diphenoxylate is contraindicated in patients with known hypersensitivity to this drug, atropine, or meperidine; in patients with obstructive jaundice because of potential for hepatic coma; in patients with diarrhea caused by pseudomembranous colitis because of potential for toxic megacolon. Use cautiously in patients with diarrhea caused by poisoning or by infection by *Shigella, Salmonella,* and some strains of *Escherichia coli,* be-

cause expulsion of intestinal contents may be a protective mechanism.

Diphenoxylate should be used with extreme caution in patients with impaired hepatic function, cirrhosis, advanced hepatorenal disease, or abnormal liver function test results, because the drug may precipitate hepatic coma. The atropine component may exacerbate pre-existing glaucoma.

Interactions
Diphenoxylate may precipitate hypertensive crisis in patients receiving monoamine oxidase inhibitors. Concomitant use with such CNS depressants as barbiturates, tranquilizers, and alcohol may result in an increased depressant effect.

Effects on diagnostic tests
Diphenoxylate may decrease urinary excretion of phenolsulfonphthalein (PSP) during the PSP excretion test; drug may increase serum amylase levels.

Adverse reactions
- CNS: sedation, dizziness, headache, drowsiness, lethargy, restlessness, depression, euphoria.
- CV: tachycardia.
- DERM: pruritus, giant urticaria, rash, dryness.
- EENT: mydriasis.
- GI: dry mouth, nausea, vomiting, abdominal discomfort or distention, paralytic ileus, anorexia, fluid retention in bowel (may mask depletion of extracellular fluid and electrolytes, especially in young children treated for acute gastroenteritis), abdominal cramps, toxic megacolon, constipation.
- GU: urinary retention.
- Other: possible physical dependence in long-term use, angioedema, respiratory depression, flushing, fever, dry mucous membranes.
Note: Drug should be discontinued if signs of CNS depression develop, or if response does not occur within 48 hours.

Overdose and treatment
Clinical effects of overdose include drowsiness, low blood pressure, marked seizures, apnea, blurred vision, miosis, flushing, dry mouth and mucous membranes, and psychotic episodes.

Treatment is supportive; maintain airway and support vital functions. A narcotic antagonist, such as naloxone, may be given. Gastric lavage may be performed. Monitor patient for 48 to 72 hours.

▶ Special considerations
- Monitor vital signs and intake and output; observe patient for adverse reactions, especially CNS reactions.
- Monitor bowel function.
- Drug is usually ineffective in treating antibiotic-induced diarrhea.
- Reduce dosage as soon as symptoms are controlled.

Information for the patient
- Warn patient to take drug exactly as ordered and not to exceed recommended dose.
- Advise patient to maintain adequate fluid intake during course of diarrhea and teach him about diet and fluid replacement.
- Caution patient to avoid driving while taking this drug because it may cause drowsiness and dizziness; warn patient to avoid alcohol while taking this drug because additive depressant effect may occur.

• Advise patient to call if drug is not effective within 48 hours.
• Warn patient that prolonged use may result in tolerance and that use of larger-than-recommended doses may result in drug dependence.

Geriatric use
Elderly patients may be more susceptible to respiratory depression and to exacerbation of preexisting glaucoma.

Pediatric use
Drug is contraindicated in children younger than age 2; some children may experience respiratory depression. Children, especially those with Down's syndrome, appear to be particularly sensitive to atropine content of this medication.

Breast-feeding
Diphenoxylate is excreted in breast milk; drug effects have been noted in nursing infants of women taking the drug.

---

diphtheria and tetanus toxoids, adsorbed, combined (Td)

• Pharmacologic classification: toxoid
• Therapeutic classification: diphtheria and tetanus prophylaxis agent
• Pregnancy risk category C

How supplied
Available by prescription only
Available in pediatric (DT) and adult (Td) strengths
Injection: pediatric – 6.6 to 15 Lf units of inactivated diphtheria and 5 to 10 Lf units of inactivated tetanus per 0.5 ml, in 5-ml vials; adult – 1.4 to 2 Lf units of inactivated diphtheria and 5 to 10 Lf units of inactivated tetanus per 0.5 ml, in 5-ml vials

Indications, route, and dosage
Primary immunization
Adults and children over age 6: Use adult strength. Give 0.5 ml I.M. 4 to 8 weeks apart for two doses and a third dose 1 year later.
Children age 1 to 6: Use pediatric strength. Give two 0.5-ml doses I.M. at least 8 weeks apart. Give a third dose 6 to 12 months after the second injection. If the final immunizing dose is given after the 7th birthday, use the adult strength.
Infants age 6 weeks to 1 year: Use pediatric strength. Give three 0.5-ml doses I.M. at least 8 weeks apart. Give a fourth dose 6 to 12 months after third injection.
Booster dose
Adults and children over age 6: After primary immunization, give booster dose of 0.5 ml Td (adult strength) q 10 years.
Children age 4 to 6: If primary immunization with DT occurs before 4th birthday, give booster dose of 0.5 ml.

Pharmacodynamics
Diphtheria and tetanus prophylaxis: Diphtheria and tetanus toxoids promote active immunization to diphtheria and tetanus by inducing production of antitoxins.

Pharmacokinetics
No information available.

Contraindications and precautions
Contraindicated in patients with a history of systemic or anaphylactic reactions to the use of this product.
Some clinicians recommend deferring (if possible) elective immunization under the following conditions: poliomyelitis outbreaks, acute respiratory or other active infection, or febrile illness. Patients receiving immunosuppressive agents (corticosteroids, antimetabolites, alkylating agents, or radiation therapy), immunosuppressed patients, or patients who have recently received an injection of immune globulin may not respond optimally.

Interactions
Concomitant use with corticosteroids or immunosuppressants may impair the immune response to diphtheria and tetanus toxoids. Avoid elective immunization under these circumstances.

Effects on diagnostic tests
None reported.

Adverse reactions
• Local: stinging, edema, erythema, pain, induration; a nodule may develop and last several weeks.
• Systemic: fretfulness, drowsiness, anorexia, vomiting, chills, fever, flushing, malaise, arthralgia, myalgia, *anaphylaxis.*

Overdose and treatment
No information available.

▶ Special considerations
• Obtain a thorough history of allergies and reactions to immunizations.
• Epinephrine solution 1:1,000 should be available to treat allergic reactions.
• Diphtheria and tetanus toxoids are used primarily when pertussis vaccine is contraindicated or used separately.
• These toxoids are not used to treat active tetanus or diphtheria infections.
• Teratogenicity has not been reported. Immunization during pregnancy is recommended when needed.
• To prevent sciatic nerve damage, avoid administration in gluteal muscle. During primary immunization, do not inject same site more than once.
• Store toxoids between 2° and 8° C (36° to 46° F). Do not freeze. Shake well before withdrawing each dose.

Information for the patient
• Inform patient that he may experience discomfort at the injection site and that a nodule may develop there and persist for several weeks after immunization. He also may develop fever, headache, upset stomach, general malaise, or body aches and pains. Tell patient to relieve such effects with acetaminophen.
• Tell patient to report any distressing adverse reactions.
• Stress the importance of keeping all scheduled appointments for subsequent doses because full immunization requires a series of injections.

---

diphtheria and tetanus toxoids and pertussis vaccine, adsorbed (DTP)
Tri-Immunol

- Pharmacologic classification: combination toxoid and vaccine
- Therapeutic classification: diphtheria, tetanus, and pertussis prophylaxis agent

How supplied
Available by prescription only
Injection: 12.5 Lf units inactivated diphtheria, 5 Lf units inactivated tetanus, and 4 protective units pertussis per 0.5 ml, in 7.5-ml vials

Indications, route, and dosage
Primary immunization
Children age 6 weeks to 6 years: 0.5 ml I.M. 2 months apart for three doses and a fourth dose 1 year later.
Booster immunization
Booster dosage is 0.5 ml I.M. when starting school, at age 4 to 6. Not advised for adults or for children over age 6.

Pharmacodynamics
Diphtheria, tetanus, and pertussis (whooping cough) prophylaxis: DTP promotes active immunity to diphtheria, tetanus, and pertussis by inducing production of antitoxin and antibodies.

Pharmacokinetics
No information available.

Contraindications and precautions
Not recommended for use in adults or children age 7 and over (use diphtheria and tetanus toxoids). Defer immunization during acute illness, or if the patient has a history of seizures after use of this product.
    Children with a history of neurologic disorders (including seizures) should not receive the pertussis component.
    A history of any of the following effects from a previous administration of pertussis vaccine precludes further use of this component (use diphtheria and tetanus toxoids instead): fever greater than 103° F. (39.4° C.), focal neurologic signs, screaming episodes, shock, collapse, somnolence, or encephalopathy. This preparation also is contraindicated in patients with known hypersensitivity to thimerosal, which is a component of this vaccine.

Interactions
Concomitant use of DTP with corticosteroids or immunosuppressants may impair the immune response to the toxoids and vaccine. Avoid elective immunization under these circumstances.

Effects on diagnostic tests
None reported.

Adverse reactions
- Local: soreness, redness, and induration at injection site; a nodule may develop and last several weeks.
- Systemic: slight fever, chills, malaise, drowsiness, fretfulness, anorexia, vomiting, *convulsions, encephalopathy, anaphylaxis.*

Overdose and treatment
No information available.

▶ Special considerations
- Obtain thorough history of allergies and reactions to immunizations, especially to pertussis vaccine.
- Epinephrine solution 1:1,000 should be available to treat allergic reactions.
- DTP may be given at same time as trivalent oral polio vaccine and, if indicated, when the patient receives vaccines against *Haemophilus influenzae* type b, measles, mumps, and rubella.
- Do not use DTP to treat active tetanus, diphtheria, or pertussis infections.
- Store between 2° and 8° C. (36° to 46° F.). Do not freeze.

Information for the patient
- Explain to parents that their child may experience discomfort at the injection site after immunization and that a nodule may develop there and persist for several weeks. The child also may develop fever, upset stomach, or general malaise. Recommend acetaminophen liquid to relieve such discomfort.
- Tell parents to report any worrisome or intolerable reactions promptly.
- Stress the importance of keeping scheduled appointments for subsequent doses. Full immunization requires a series of injections.

diphtheria antitoxin, equine

- Pharmacologic classification: antitoxin
- Therapeutic classification: diphtheria antitoxin
- Pregnancy risk category D

How supplied
Available by prescription only
Injection: not less than 500 units/ml in 10,000-unit and 20,000-unit vials

Indications, route, and dosage
Diphtheria prevention
Adults and children: 1,000 to 10,000 units I.M. (dose dependent on length of time since exposure, extent of exposure, and individual's medical condition).
Diphtheria treatment
Adults and children: 20,000 to 120,000 units slow I.V. infusion in normal saline solution (dose based on extent of disease). A 1:20 dilution of the antitoxin is infused at 1 ml/minute. Additional doses may be given in 24 hours. I.M. route may be used in mild cases. Begin antibiotic therapy.

Pharmacodynamics
Antitoxin action: Diphtheria antitoxin neutralizes and binds toxin.

Pharmacokinetics
Absorption, distribution, metabolism, and excretion have not been described.

Contraindications and precautions
Because this product is derived from horses immunized with diphtheria toxin, an intradermal or scratch skin test and a conjunctival test for sensitivity to equine serum (against a control of normal saline solution) should be performed before administering diphtheria antitoxin. If the sensitivity test is positive, check desensitization schedule.

Interactions
None reported.

Effects on diagnostic tests
None reported.

Adverse reactions
● Local: erythema, tenderness, and induration at injection site.
● Systemic: hypersensitivity, *anaphylaxis;* serum sickness (urticaria, pruritus, fever, malaise, and arthralgia) may occur within 7 to 12 days. Discontinue if severe systemic reactions occur.

Overdose and treatment
No information available.

▶ Special considerations
● Obtain a thorough patient history of allergies, especially to horses and horse immune serum; of asthma; and of previous reactions to immunizations.
● Epinephrine solution 1:1,000 should be available to treat allergic reactions.
● All asymptomatic nonimmunized contacts of patients with diphtheria should receive prompt prophylaxis with antibiotic therapy and have cultures taken before and after treatment. The patient should receive diphtheria toxoid and be monitored for 7 days thereafter.
● Therapy should begin immediately, without waiting for culture and sensitivity test results, if patient has clinical symptoms of diphtheria (sore throat, fever, and tonsillar membrane involvement).
● Refrigerate the antitoxin at 2° to 8° C. (36° to 46° F.). It may also be warmed to 32° to 34° C. (90° to 93° F.); higher temperatures will diminish potency.

Information for the patient
● Tell patient that he may experience allergic reactions (such as rash, joint swelling or pain, or difficulty breathing) but that he will be monitored closely and will receive medication, as needed, to relieve such effects.
● Delayed effects associated with this antitoxin may occur in 7 to 12 days after treatment. Encourage patient to report any and all unusual symptoms.

Breast-feeding
Patient should discontinue breast-feeding until the toxin's effects subside or if symptoms of serum sickness develop.

diphtheria toxoid, adsorbed
(for pediatric use)

● Pharmacologic classification: toxoid
● Therapeutic classification: diphtheria prophylaxis agent

How supplied
Available by prescription only
Injection: suspension of 15 Lf units inactivated diphtheria per 0.5 ml, in 5-ml vials

Indications, route, and dosage
Diphtheria immunization
Children under age 6: 0.5 ml I.M. 6 to 8 weeks apart for two doses and a third dose 1 year later. Booster dosage is 0.5 ml I.M. at 5- to 10-year intervals. Not advised for adults or for children over age 6; instead, use adult strength of diphtheria toxoid (usually available as diphtheria and tetanus toxoids, adsorbed combined).

Pharmacodynamics
Diphtheria prophylaxis: Diphtheria toxoid promotes active immunity to diphtheria by inducing production of antitoxin. Protection thought to last 10 years or more.

Pharmacokinetics
Absorption, distribution, metabolism, and excretion have not been described.

Contraindications and precautions
Diphtheria toxoid is contraindicated in patients with any febrile illness other than a mild upper respiratory infection or any other active infection. Defer elective immunization during these situations and during outbreaks of poliomyelitis.

Defer immunization until the 2nd year of life in infants with a history of seizures or CNS damage. (Alternatively, one tenth the recommended initial dosage may be used, followed by standard doses if no untoward effect occurs.)

Diphtheria toxoid is not recommended for adults or for children older than age 6. This preparation also is contraindicated in patients with known hypersensitivity to thimerosal, a component of the toxoid, and in immunosuppressed patients (those with congenital immunodeficiencies, cancer, or acquired immune deficiency syndrome and those undergoing treatment with corticosteroids, antineoplastic agents, or radiation).

Interactions
Concomitant use of diphtheria toxoid with corticosteroids or immunosuppressants may impair the immune response to the toxoid. Avoid elective immunization under these circumstances.

Effects on diagnostic tests
None reported.

Adverse reactions
● Local: erythema, pain, and sterile abscess induration at injection site; a nodule may develop and persist for several weeks.
● Systemic: fever, malaise, urticaria, tachycardia, flushing, pruritus, hypotension, myalgia, arthralgia, *anaphylaxis,* drowsiness.

Overdose and treatment
No information available.

▶ Special considerations
• Obtain a thorough history of allergies and reactions to immunizations.
• Epinephrine solution 1:1,000 should be available to treat allergic reactions.
• This preparation is used primarily when products containing tetanus toxoid or pertussis vaccine would not be advisable.
• Shake well before using.
• Do not use diphtheria toxoid to treat active diphtheria infections.
• Store between 2° to 8° C. (36° to 46° F.). Do not freeze.

Information for the patient
• Explain to parents that their child may experience discomfort at the injection site after immunization and may develop a nodule there that can persist for several weeks. The child also may develop fever, general malaise, or body aches and pains. Recommend acetaminophen liquid to relieve minor discomfort.
• Tell parents to report any worrisome or intolerable adverse reactions promptly.
• Emphasize the importance of keeping scheduled appointments for subsequent doses. Full immunization requires a series of injections.

---

dipivefrin hydrochloride
Propine Sterile Ophthalmic Solution

• Pharmacologic classification: sympathomimetic agent
• Therapeutic classification: antiglaucoma agent
• Pregnancy risk category B

How supplied
Available by prescription only
Ophthalmic solution: 0.1%

Indications, route, and dosage
To reduce intraocular pressure in chronic open-angle glaucoma
Adults: For initial glaucoma therapy, 1 drop in eye q 12 hours.

Pharmacodynamics
Antiglaucoma action: Dipivefrin is a prodrug converted to epinephrine in the eye. It decreases aqueous humor production and enhances outflow. It is often used with a miotic agent.

Pharmacokinetics
• *Absorption:* Action begins in about 30 minutes, with peak effect in 1 hour.
• *Distribution:* Unknown.
• *Metabolism:* Unknown.
• *Excretion:* Unknown.

Contraindications and precautions
Dipivefrin is contraindicated in patients with hypersensitivity to any component of the preparation and in narrow-angle glaucoma. It should be used with caution in aphakic patients, because macular edema may occur.

Interactions
When used concomitantly, dipivefrin may enhance the lowering of intraocular pressure caused by miotic agents and carbonic anhydrase inhibitors. Depending on the extent of systemic absorption and the amount present, there may be additive toxic effects with sympathomimetics, and an increased risk of cardiac arrhythmias with digoxin, anesthetics, or tricyclic antidepressants.

Effects on diagnostic tests
None reported.

Adverse reactions
• Eye: burning, stinging, ocular congestion, conjunctival hyperemia, photophobia, mydriasis, blurred vision, ocular pain.

Overdose and treatment
Overdose is quite rare with ophthalmic use but may cause the following effects after accidental ingestion: hypertension with tachycardia or bradycardia, cardiac arrhythmias, precordial pain, anxiety, nervousness, insomnia, muscle tremor, cerebral hemorrhage, seizures, altered mental status, anorexia, nausea and vomiting, and acute renal failure. To treat oral overdose, dilute immediately then initiate emesis followed by activated charcoal and a cathartic, unless the patient is comatose or obtunded. Monitor urinary output. As ordered, treat seizures with I.V. diazepam, and hypertension with nitroprusside; treat arrhythmias appropriately, depending on the type of arrhythmia. Preparations containing sulfites may cause GI or cardiac toxicities and hypotension.

▶ Special considerations
• Drug may cause fewer adverse reactions than with conventional epinephrine therapy; it often is used concomitantly with other antiglaucoma agents.
• Store away from heat and light.

Information for the patient
• Teach patient correct way to instill drops and warn him not to touch eye with dropper.
• Teach patient that if also using other eye drops, he should instill dipivefrin first, then wait at least 5 minutes before using the other drops.
• Instruct patient not to blink more than usual and not to close his eyes tightly after instillation.
• Tell patient instillation of drug may cause transient burning or stinging.

Geriatric use
Drug should be used with caution in elderly patients, to avoid precipitating narrow-angle glaucoma.

---

dipyridamole
Persantine, Pyridamole

- Pharmacologic classification: pyrimidine analogue
- Therapeutic classification: coronary vasodilator, platelet aggregation inhibitor
- Pregnancy risk category C

How supplied
Available by prescription only
Tablets: 25 mg, 50 mg, 75 mg
Injection: 10 mg/ampule

Indications, route, and dosage
Chronic angina pectoris
Adults: 50 mg P.O. t.i.d. at least 1 hour before meals, to a maximum of 400 mg daily. Two to three months of therapy may be required to achieve a clinical response.
Inhibition of platelet adhesion in patients with prosthetic heart valves, in combination with warfarin or aspirin
Adults: 100 to 400 mg P.O. daily.
As an alternative to exercise in thallium myocardial perfusion imaging
Adults: 0.142 mg/kg/minute infused over 4 minutes (0.57 mg/kg total).

Pharmacodynamics
Coronary vasodilating action: Dipyridamole increases coronary blood flow by selectively dilating the coronary arteries. Coronary vasodilator effect follows inhibition of serum adenosine deaminase, which allows accumulation of adenosine, a potent vasodilator. Dipyridamole inhibits platelet adhesion by increasing effects of prostacyclin or by inhibiting phosphodiesterase.

Pharmacokinetics
- *Absorption:* Absorption is variable and slow; bioavailability ranges from 27% to 59%. Serum concentrations of dipyridamole peak 2 to 2½ hours after oral administration.
- *Distribution:* Animal studies indicate wide distribution in body tissues; small amounts cross the placenta. Protein binding ranges from 91% to 97%.
- *Metabolism:* Dipyridamole is metabolized by the liver.
- *Excretion:* Elimination occurs via biliary excretion of glucuronide conjugates. Some dipyridamole and conjugates may undergo enterohepatic circulation and fecal excretion; a small amount is excreted in urine. Half-life varies from 1 to 12 hours.

Contraindications and precautions
Drug is ineffective in acute angina; do not substitute for other appropriate treatment such as nitroglycerin.
Dipyridamole is contraindicated in patients with known hypersensitivity to the drug.
Use drug cautiously in patients with hypotension and in patients taking anticoagulants.

Interactions
Aminophylline inhibits the action of dipyridamole.

Effects on diagnostic tests
Dipyridamole's physiologic effects on platelet aggregation will cause an increase in bleeding time.

Adverse reactions
- CNS: headache, dizziness, syncope.
- CV: flushing, chest pain.
- GI: nausea, vomiting, diarrhea.
- Other: sweating, rash, weakness.
Note: Drug should be discontinued if excessive hypotension occurs.

Overdose and treatment
Clinical signs of overdose include peripheral vasodilation and hypotension. Maintain blood pressure and treat symptomatically.

▶ Special considerations
- Be alert for adverse reactions, including signs of bleeding and prolonged bleeding time, especially at high doses and during long-term therapy.
- Monitor blood pressure.
- Give drug at least 1 hour before meals.
- When used as a pharmacologic "stress test," total doses beyond 60 mg appear to be unnecessary.
- Dilute I.V. form to at least a 1:2 ratio with 0.45% sodium chloride injection, 0.9% sodium chloride injection, or 5% dextrose in water to a total volume of 20 to 50 ml. Inject thallium within 5 minutes of dipyridamole.

Information for the patient
- Explain that clinical response may require 2 to 3 months of continuous therapy; encourage patient compliance.
- Discuss adverse reactions and how to manage therapy.

Pediatric use
Dosage has not been established in children.

Breast-feeding
Safety in breast-feeding women has not been established.

disopyramide phosphate
Napamide, Norpace, Norpace CR, Rythmodon*, Rythmodon-LA*

- Pharmacologic classification: pyridine derivative antiarrhythmic
- Therapeutic classification: ventricular antiarrhythmic, supraventricular antiarrhythmic, atrial antitachyarrhythmic
- Pregnancy risk category C

How supplied
Available by prescription only
Capsules: 100 mg, 150 mg
Capsules (extended-release): 100 mg, 150 mg

Indications, route, and dosage
Premature ventricular contractions (unifocal, multifocal, or coupled); ventricular tachycardia not severe enough to require electrocardioversion
Adults: Usual maintenance dosage is 150 to 200 mg P.O. q 6 hours; for patients who weigh less than 50 kg or those with renal, hepatic, or cardiac impairment, dosage is 100 mg P.O. q 6 hours. May give sustained-release capsule q 12 hours.

Children age 12 to 18: 6 to 15 mg/kg/day.
Children age 4 to 12: 10 to 15 mg/kg/day.
Children age 1 to 4: 10 to 20 mg/kg/day.
Children under age 1: 10 to 30 mg/kg/day.

All children's doses should be divided into equal amounts and given every 6 hours. Extended-release capsules not recommended for use in children.

Dosage adjustment for patients with renal failure

Adults: Patients with hepatic insufficiency or moderately impaired renal function should receive 100 mg P.O. q 6 hours or 200 mg (extended-release) q 12 hours. Patients with severe impaired renal function should receive only 100 mg (regular-release) at the following intervals:

Creatinine clearance (ml/minute)	Dosage interval
30 to 40	q 8 hours
15 to 30	q 12 hours
< 15	q 24 hours

Pharmacodynamics

Antiarrhythmic action: A Class IA antiarrhythmic agent, disopyramide depresses phase O of the action potential. It is considered a myocardial depressant because it decreases myocardial excitability and conduction velocity and may depress myocardial contractility. It also possesses anticholinergic activity that may modify the drug's direct myocardial effects. In therapeutic doses, disopyramide reduces conduction velocity in the atria, ventricles, and His-Purkinje system. By prolonging the effective refractory period (ERP), it helps control atrial tachyarrhythmias (however, this indication is unapproved in the United States). Its anticholinergic action, which is much greater than quinidine's, may increase AV node conductivity.

Disopyramide also has a greater myocardial depressant (negative inotropic) effect than quinidine. It helps manage premature ventricular beats by suppressing automaticity in the His-Purkinje system and ectopic pacemakers. At therapeutic doses, it usually does not prolong the QRS segment duration and PR interval but may prolong the QT interval.

Pharmacokinetics

• *Absorption:* Disopyramide is rapidly and well absorbed from the GI tract; about 60% to 80% of the drug reaches systemic circulation. Onset of action usually occurs in 30 minutes; peak blood levels occur approximately 2 hours after administration of conventional capsules and 5 hours after administration of extended-release capsules.
• *Distribution:* Disopyramide is well distributed throughout extracellular fluid but is not extensively bound to tissues. Plasma protein binding varies, depending on drug concentration levels, but generally ranges from about 50% to 65%. Usual therapeutic serum level ranges from 2 to 4 mcg/ml, although some patients may require up to 7 mcg/ml. Levels above 9 mcg/ml generally are considered toxic.
• *Metabolism:* Disopyramide is metabolized in the liver to one major metabolite that possesses little antiarrhythmic activity but greater anticholinergic activity than the parent compound.

• *Excretion:* About 90% of an orally administered dose is excreted in the urine as unchanged drug and metabolites; 40% to 60% is excreted as unchanged drug. Usual elimination half-life is about 7 hours but lengthens in patients with renal and/or hepatic insufficiency. Duration of effect is usually 6 to 7 hours.

Contraindications and precautions

Disopyramide is contraindicated in patients with second- or third-degree heart block (unless a pacemaker is in place), because of the drug's effects on AV conduction; in patients with myasthenia gravis, because the drug's anticholinergic effect may precipitate a myasthenic crisis; in patients with untreated glaucoma or urinary retention (particularly from prostatic hypertrophy), because of the drug's anticholinergic effect (however, disopyramide may be used with caution in such patients if they are treated appropriately and monitored carefully); in patients with uncompensated congestive heart failure and cardiogenic shock, because of the drug's negative inotropic effect; and in patients with known hypersensitivity to the drug.

Disopyramide should be used with caution in patients with sick sinus syndrome, Wolff-Parkinson-White syndrome, or bundle branch block, because of the drug's unpredictable effects on AV conduction; and in patients with renal or hepatic insufficiency, because decreased drug elimination may cause toxicity.

Interactions

When used concomitantly, other antiarrhythmic agents may cause additive or antagonistic cardiac effects and additive toxicity. Concomitant use with enzyme inducers, such as rifampin, may impair disopyramide's antiarrhythmic activity. Concomitant use with anticholinergic agents may cause additive anticholinergic effects. Concomitant use with warfarin may potentiate anticoagulant effects. Oral antidiabetic agents or insulin may cause additive hypoglycemia.

Effects on diagnostic tests

The physiologic effects of disopyramide may cause a decrease in blood glucose concentrations.

Adverse reactions

• CNS: dizziness, agitation, depression, fatigue, muscle weakness, *syncope.*
• CV: *hypotension, congestive heart failure, heart block,* edema, chest pain.
• DERM: rash (1% to 3%).
• EENT: blurred vision, dry eyes and nose.
• GI: nausea, vomiting, anorexia, bloating, abdominal pain, constipation, dry mouth.
• GU: urinary retention and hesitancy (particularly in males).
• Hepatic: cholestatic jaundice.
• Metabolic: hypoglycemia.
Note: Drug should be discontinued if hypotension, progressive heart failure, or heart block occurs; if the QRS complex widens by 25% to 50% over baseline; or if the QT interval lengthens.

Overdose and treatment

Clinical manifestations of overdose include anticholinergic effects, severe hypotension, widening of QRS complex and QT interval, ventricular arrhythmias, cardiac conduction disturbances, bradycardia, congestive heart failure, asystole, loss of consciousness, seizures, apnea episodes, and respiratory arrest.

Treatment involves general supportive measures (including respiratory and cardiovascular support) and hemodynamic and ECG monitoring. If ingestion was recent, gastric lavage, emesis induction, and administration of activated charcoal may decrease absorption. Isoproterenol or dopamine may be administered to correct hypotension, after adequate hydration has been ensured. Digoxin and diuretics may be administered to treat heart failure. Hemodialysis and charcoal hemoperfusion may effectively remove disopyramide. Some patients may require intraaortic balloon counterpulsation, mechanically assisted respiration, and/or endocardial pacing.

▶ **Special considerations**
● Correct any underlying electrolyte abnormalities, especially hypokalemia, before administering drug, because disopyramide may be ineffective in patients with these problems.
● Do not give sustained-release capsules for rapid control of ventricular arrhythmias if therapeutic blood drug levels must be attained rapidly, or if patient has cardiomyopathy, possible cardiac decompensation, or severe renal impairment.
● Watch for signs of developing heart block, such as QRS complex widening by more than 25% or QT interval lengthening by more than 25% above baseline.
● Disopyramide may cause hypoglycemia in some patients; monitor serum glucose levels in patients with altered serum glucose regulatory mechanisms.
● If drug causes constipation, administer laxatives and ensure proper diet.
● Disopyramide is commonly prescribed for patients with heart failure who cannot tolerate quinidine or procainamide.
● Pharmacist may prepare disopyramide suspension; 100-mg capsules are used with cherry syrup to prepare suspension (this may be best form for young children).
● Disopyramide is removed by hemodialysis. Dosage adjustments may be necessary in patients undergoing dialysis.

Information for the patient
● When changing from immediate-release to sustained-release capsules, advise patient to begin taking sustained-release capsule 6 hours after last immediate-release capsule.
● Teach patient importance of taking drug on time, exactly as prescribed. To do this, he may have to use an alarm clock for night doses.
● Advise patient to use sugarless gum or hard candy to relieve dry mouth.

Geriatric use
Elderly patients may need dosage reduction. Monitor closely for toxicity signs; also monitor serum electrolyte and drug levels.

Pediatric use
Although drug's safety and effectiveness in children has not been established, current recommendations call for total daily dosage given in equally divided doses every 6 hours or at intervals based on individual requirements.

Monitor pediatric patients during initial titration period; dose titration should begin at lower end of recommended ranges. Monitor serum drug levels and therapeutic response carefully.

Breast-feeding
Disopyramide is distributed into breast milk. Alternate infant feeding methods are recommended during disopyramide therapy.

disulfiram
Antabuse

● Pharmacologic classification: aldehyde dehydrogenase inhibitor
● Therapeutic classification: alcoholic deterrent
● Pregnancy risk category C

How supplied
Available by prescription only
Tablets: 250 mg, 500 mg

Indications, route, and dosage
Adjunct in management of chronic alcoholism
Adults: Maximum of 500 mg q morning for 1 to 2 weeks. Can be taken in evening if drowsiness occurs. Maintenance dosage is 125 to 500 mg daily (average dose 250 mg) until permanent self-control is established. Treatment may continue for months or years.

Pharmacodynamics
Antialcoholic action: Disulfiram irreversibly inhibits aldehyde dehydrogenase, which prevents the oxidation of alcohol after the acetaldehyde stage. It interacts with ingested alcohol to produce acetaldehyde levels five to ten times higher than are produced by normal alcohol metabolism. Excess acetaldehyde produces a highly unpleasant reaction (nausea and vomiting) to even a small quantity of alcohol. Tolerance to disulfiram does not occur; rather, sensitivity to alcohol increases with longer duration of therapy.

Pharmacokinetics
● *Absorption:* Disulfiram is absorbed completely after oral administration, but 3 to 12 hours may be required before effects occur. Toxic reactions to alcohol may occur up to 2 weeks after the last dose of disulfiram.
● *Distribution:* Disulfiram is highly lipid-soluble and is initially localized in adipose tissue.
● *Metabolism:* Mostly oxidized in the liver and excreted in urine as free drug and metabolites (for example, diethyldithiocarbamate, diethylamine, and carbon disulfide).
● *Excretion:* 5% to 20% is unabsorbed and is eliminated in feces. A small amount is eliminated through the lungs, but most is excreted in the urine. Several days may be required for total elimination of the drug.

Contraindications and precautions
Disulfiram is contraindicated in patients with severe myocardial disease or coronary occlusion because of the potential for adverse cardiac effects; in patients with psychosis; in patients with a hypersensitivity to disulfiram or to other thiuram derivatives; in patients with chronic intoxication; and in pregnant women.

Disulfiram should be given cautiously to patients with a history of rubber contact dermatitis or hypersensitivity to thiuram derivatives. Patients who have received metronidazole, paraldehyde, alcohol, or alcohol-containing preparations (such as vitamin tonics and cough syrups) may experience a disulfiram reaction.

Disulfiram should be given cautiously or not at all to patients with diabetes mellitus, chronic or acute nephritis, hepatitis cirrhosis or insufficiency, seizure disorders, cerebral damage, abnormal EEG results, or drug dependence.

Interactions

Disulfiram interferes with the metabolism of alcohol, diazepam, chlordiazepoxide, barbiturates, coumarin anticoagulants, paraldehyde, and phenytoin; therefore, it may increase the blood concentration of these drugs.

Disulfiram inhibits the metabolism of caffeine, greatly increasing its half-life. Exaggerated or prolonged effects of caffeine may occur.

Concomitant use of disulfiram with metronidazole can produce psychosis or confusion and should be avoided. Use with isoniazid may produce ataxia, unsteady gait, or marked behavioral changes and should be avoided.

Disulfiram has been reported to produce a synergistic CNS stimulation when used with marijuana.

Effects on diagnostic tests

Disulfiram may decrease urinary vanilmandelic acid excretion and increase urinary concentrations of homovanillic acid. Decrease of radioactive iodine (^{131}I); uptake or protein-bound iodine levels may occur rarely. Serum cholesterol levels may be elevated.

Adverse reactions

- CNS: drowsiness, headache, fatigue, delirium, depression, neuritis.
- DERM: acneiform or allergic dermatitis.
- EENT: optic neuritis.
- GI: metallic or garlic-like aftertaste.
- GU: impotence.
- Hepatic: toxicity.
- Other: "disulfiram reaction" (throbbing headache, dyspnea, nausea, copious vomiting, sweating, thirst, chest pain, palpitations, hyperventilation, hypotension, syncope, anxiety, weakness, blurred vision, confusion). Severe reactions may cause respiratory depression, *cardiovascular collapse*, arrhythmias, *myocardial infarction, acute congestive heart failure, convulsions,* unconsciousness, and death.

Overdose and treatment

Overdose symptoms include GI upset and vomiting, abnormal EEG findings, drowsiness, altered consciousness, hallucinations, speech impairment, incoordination, and coma. Treat overdose or accidental overingestion by gastric aspiration or lavage along with supportive therapy.

Treatment of alcohol-induced disulfiram reaction is supportive and symptomatic. These reactions are not usually life-threatening. Emergency equipment and drugs should be available, because arrhythmias and severe hypotension may occur. Treat severe reactions like shock by administering plasma or electrolyte solutions as needed. Large I.V. doses of ascorbic acid, iron, and antihistamines have been used but are of questionable value. Hypokalemia has been reported; it requires careful monitoring and potassium supplements.

▶ Special considerations

- Drug use requires close medical supervision. Patients should clearly understand consequences of disulfiram therapy and give informed consent before use.
- Use drug only in patients who are cooperative and well motivated, and are receiving supportive psychiatric therapy.
- Complete physical examination and laboratory studies (CBC, SMA-12, transaminases) should precede therapy and be repeated regularly.
- Disulfiram should *not* be administered for at least 12 hours after the last alcohol ingestion.

Information for the patient

- Explain to the patient that although disulfiram can help discourage use of alcohol, it is not a cure for alcoholism.
- Inform patient of the seriousness of the disulfiram-alcohol reaction and the consequences of alcohol use.
- Warn patient to avoid all sources of alcohol: sauces or soups made with sherry or other wines or alcohol (even "cooking alcohol") and cough syrups. External applications of after-shave lotion, liniments, or other topical preparations may cause disulfiram reaction (because of the products' alcohol content).
- Tell patient that alcohol reaction may occur for up to 2 weeks after a single dose of disulfiram. The longer the disulfiram therapy, the more sensitive patient will be to alcohol.
- Warn patient that drug may cause drowsiness.
- Instruct patient to carry identification card stating that disulfiram is being used and including the phone number of the physician or clinic to contact if a reaction occurs.

PHARMACOLOGIC CLASS

diuretics, loop

**bumetanide
ethacrynate sodium
ethacrynic acid
furosemide**

Loop diuretics are sometimes referred to as high-ceiling diuretics because they produce a peak diuresis greater than that produced by other agents. Loop diuretics are particularly useful in edema associated with compromised renal function. Ethacrynic acid was synthesized during the search for compounds that might interact with renal sulfhydryl groups like mercurial diuretics. Unfortunately, ethacrynic acid is associated with ototoxicity and a higher incidence of GI reactions and is therefore used less frequently. Structurally similar to furosemide, bumetanide is approximately 40 times more potent.

Pharmacology

Loop diuretics inhibit sodium and chloride reabsorption in the ascending loop of Henle, thus increasing renal excretion of sodium, chloride, and water; like thiazide diuretics, loop diuretics increase excretion of potassium. Loop diuretics produce greater maximum diuresis and electrolyte loss than thiazide diuretics.

Furosemide and bumetanide, but not ethacrynic acid, have some renal vasodilatory effect, which may temporarily increase glomerular filtration rate (GFR), and

COMPARING LOOP DIURETICS

DRUG AND ROUTE	ONSET	PEAK	DURATION	USUAL DOSAGE
bumetanide				
I.V.	≤5 min	15 to 45 min	4 to 6 hr	0.5 to 1 mg ≤ t.i.d
P.O.	30 to 60 min	1 to 2 hr	4 to 6 hr	0.5 to 2 mg/day
ethacrynic acid				
I.V.	≤5 min	¼ to ½ hr	2 hr	50 mg/day
P.O.	≤30 min	2 hr	6 to 8 hr	50 to 100 mg/day
furosemide				
I.V.	≤5 min	⅓ to 1 hr	2 hr	20 to 40 mg q 2 hr, p.r.n.
P.O.	30 to 60 min	1 to 2 hr	6 to 8 hr	20 to 80 mg ≤b.i.d.

peripheral vasodilatory effect, which may decrease peripheral vascular resistance.

Clinical indications and actions
Edema
Loop diuretics effectively relieve edema associated with congestive heart failure (CHF). They may be useful in patients refractory to other diuretics; because furosemide and bumetanide may increase GFR, they are useful in patients with renal impairment. I.V. loop diuretics are used adjunctively in acute pulmonary edema to decrease peripheral vascular resistance. Loop diuretics also are used to treat edema associated with hepatic cirrhosis and nephrotic syndrome.

Hypertension
Loop diuretics are used in patients with mild to moderate hypertension, although thiazides are the initial diuretics of choice in most patients. Loop diuretics are preferred in patients with CHF or renal impairment; used I.V., they are a helpful adjunct in managing hypertensive crises.

Overview of adverse reactions
The most common adverse effects associated with therapeutic doses of loop diuretics are metabolic and electrolyte disturbances, particularly potassium depletion, which may require replacement by other diuretic therapy. Loop diuretics may also cause hypochloremic alkalosis, hyperglycemia, hyperuricemia, and hypomagnesemia. Rapid parenteral administration of loop diuretics may cause hearing loss (including deafness) and tinnitus. Toxic doses produce profound diuresis, leading to hypovolemia and cardiovascular collapse.

▶ Special considerations
● Monitor blood pressure and pulse rate (especially during rapid diuresis), establish baseline values before therapy, and watch for significant changes.
● Advise safety measures for all ambulatory patients until response to the diuretic is known.
● Establish baseline and periodically review CBC, including white blood cell count; serum electrolytes; CO_2; BUN and creatinine levels; and results of liver function tests.
● Administer diuretics in the morning so major diuresis

occurs before bedtime. To prevent nocturia, do not prescribe diuretics for use after 6 p.m.
● Consider possible dosage adjustment in the following circumstances: reduced dosage for patients with hepatic dysfunction; increased dosage in patients with renal impairment, oliguria, or decreased diuresis (inadequate urine output may result in circulatory overload, causing water intoxication, pulmonary edema, and CHF); increased doses of insulin or oral hypoglycemics in diabetic patients; and reduced dosages of other antihypertensive agents.
● Monitor patient for edema and ascites. Observe lower extremities of ambulatory patients and the sacral area of patients on bed rest.
● Patient should be weighed each morning immediately after voiding and before breakfast – in same type of clothing and on the same scale. Weight provides guide for clinical response to diuretic therapy.
● Consult dietitian on possible need for dietary potassium supplementation.
● Patients taking digitalis are at increased risk of digitalis toxicity from potassium depletion.
● Ototoxicity may follow prolonged use or administration of large doses.
● Patients with liver disease are especially susceptible to diuretic-induced electrolyte imbalance; in extreme cases, stupor, coma, and death can result.
● Patient should have urinal or commode readily available.

Information for the patient
● Explain to the patient the rationale for therapy and the diuretic effect of these drugs (increased volume and frequency of urination).
● Teach patient signs of adverse effects, especially hypokalemia (weakness, fatigue, muscle cramps, paresthesias, confusion, nausea, vomiting, diarrhea, headache, dizziness, or palpitations), and importance of reporting such symptoms promptly.
● Advise patient to eat potassium-rich foods, such as citrus fruits, potatoes, dates, raisins, and bananas; to avoid high-sodium foods such as lunch meat, smoked meats, and processed cheeses; and not to add salt to other foods. Recommend salt substitutes.

● Emphasize importance of keeping follow-up appointments to monitor effectiveness of diuretic therapy.
● Tell patient to report increased edema or weight or excess diuresis (more than 2-lb weight loss/day).
● With initial doses, caution patient to change position slowly, especially when rising to upright position, to prevent dizziness from orthostatic hypotension.
● Instruct patient to call at once if chest, back, or leg pain; shortness of breath; or dyspnea occurs.

Geriatric use
Elderly and debilitated patients require close observation, because they are more susceptible to drug-induced diuresis. In elderly patients, excessive diuresis can quickly lead to dehydration, hypovolemia, hypokalemia, and hyponatremia and may cause circulatory collapse. Reduced dosages may be indicated.

Pediatric use
Use loop diuretics with caution in neonates. The usual pediatric dose can be used, but dosage intervals should be extended.

Breast-feeding
Loop diuretics should not be used by breast-feeding women.

Representative combinations
None.

PHARMACOLOGIC CLASS

diuretics, osmotic

mannitol
urea

Osmotic diuretics are used to reduce intraocular and intracranial pressure. Most clinicians prefer mannitol because it is relatively less toxic and more stable in solution. Mannitol, but not urea, is approved for prevention and, adjunctively, for treatment of acute renal failure or oliguria.

$$\text{Males:} \quad \frac{\text{Creatinine}}{\text{clearance}} = \frac{\text{weight (kg)} \times (140 - \text{age})}{72 \times \text{serum creatinine (mg/dl)}}$$

Females: $0.85 \times$ male value

Pharmacology
Osmotic diuretics elevate osmotic pressure of the glomerular filtrate, thereby hindering tubular reabsorption of solutes and water and promoting renal excretion of water, sodium, potassium, chloride, calcium, phosphorus, magnesium, and uric acid. Osmotic diuretics also elevate osmotic pressure in blood and promote the shift of intracellular water into the blood.

Clinical indications and actions
Acute renal failure or oliguria
Mannitol is used to prevent and treat the oliguric phase of acute renal failure. It enhances renal blood flow by its osmotic diuretic effect and by vasodilating effects.
Reduction of intracranial pressure
Osmotic diuretics reduce intracranial pressure and control cerebral edema caused by trauma or disease and during surgery by drawing water from cells (including those in the brain and CSF) into the blood. A rebound

effect may occur 12 hours after the administration of urea.
Reduction of intraocular pressure
Osmotic diuretics are used to reduce intraocular pressure when it cannot be reduced by other means; these drugs are especially useful in acute angle-closure glaucoma, in absolute or secondary glaucoma, and before surgery. Their osmotic effect draws fluid from the anterior chamber of the eye, reducing intraocular pressure. Urea, unlike mannitol, penetrates the eye and may cause a rebound increase in intraocular pressure if plasma urea levels fall below that in the vitreous humor. Because urea penetrates the eye, it should not be used when irritation is present.
Drug intoxication
Mannitol is used alone or with other diuretics to enhance urinary excretion of toxins, including aspirin, some barbiturates, bromides, imipramine, and lithium. Besides promoting diuresis, mannitol maintains renal blood flow.

Overview of adverse reactions
The most severe adverse effects associated with mannitol are fluid and electrolyte imbalance. Circulatory overload may follow administration of mannitol to patients with inadequate urine output. The most common adverse reactions associated with urea are headache, nausea, and vomiting; a rebound increase in intraocular pressure also may occur.

▶ Special considerations
● Maintain adequate hydration. Monitor fluid and electrolyte balance.
● Monitor I.V. infusion carefully for inflammation at the infusion site.
● Patient should have frequent mouth care or fluids as appropriate to relieve thirst.
● In patients with urethral catheter, an hourly urometer collection bag should be used to facilitate accurate measurement of urine output.

Information for the patient
● Tell patient he may feel thirsty or experience mouth dryness, and emphasize importance of drinking only the amount of fluids provided, as ordered.
● With initial doses, warn patient to change position slowly, especially when rising to an upright position, to prevent dizziness from orthostatic hypotension.
● Instruct patient to call immediately if he experiences chest, back, or leg pain; shortness of breath; or apnea.

Geriatric use
Elderly or debilitated patients will require close observation and may require lower dosages. In elderly patients, excessive diuresis can quickly lead to dehydration, hypovolemia, hypokalemia, and hyponatremia.

Pediatric use
No specific recommendations available.

Breast-feeding
Safety has not been established.

Representative combinations
None.

PHARMACOLOGIC CLASS

diuretics, potassium-sparing

amiloride hydrochloride
spironolactone
triamterene

Potassium-sparing diuretics are less potent than many others; in particular, amiloride and triamterene have little clinical effect when used alone. However, because they protect against potassium loss, they are used with other more potent diuretic agents. Spironolactone, an aldosterone antagonist, is particularly useful in patients with edema and hypertension associated with hyperaldosteronism.

Pharmacology
Amiloride and triamterene act directly on the distal renal tubules, inhibiting sodium reabsorption and potassium excretion, thereby reducing the potassium loss associated with other diuretic therapy. Spironolactone competitively inhibits aldosterone at the distal renal tubules, also promoting sodium excretion and potassium retention.

Clinical indications and actions
Edema
All potassium-sparing diuretics are used to manage edema associated with hepatic cirrhosis, nephrotic syndrome, and congestive heart failure.
Hypertension
Amiloride and spironolactone are used to treat mild and moderate hypertension; the exact mechanism is unknown. Spironolactone may block the effect of aldosterone on arteriolar smooth muscle.
Diagnosis of primary hyperaldosteronism
Because spironolactone inhibits aldosterone, correction of hypokalemia and hypertension is presumptive evidence of primary hyperaldosteronism.

Overview of adverse reactions
Hyperkalemia is the most important adverse reaction; it occurs with all drugs in this class and may lead to cardiac arrhythmias. Other adverse reactions include nausea, vomiting, headache, weakness, fatigue, bowel disturbances, cough, and dyspnea.

Potassium-sparing diuretics are contraindicated in patients with serum potassium levels above 5.5 mEq/liter, in those receiving other potassium-sparing diuretics or potassium supplements, and in patients with anuria, acute or chronic renal insufficiency, diabetic nephropathy, or known hypersensitivity to the drug. They should be used cautiously in patients with severe hepatic insufficiency because electrolyte imbalance may precipitate hepatic encephalopathy, and in patients with diabetes, who are at increased risk of hyperkalemia.

▶ Special considerations
• Monitor for hyperkalemia and cardiac arrhythmias; measure serum potassium and other electrolyte levels frequently, and check for significant changes. Monitor the following at baseline and periodic intervals: CBC including white blood cell count, CO_2, BUN, and creatinine levels and, especially, liver function studies.
• Monitor vital signs, intake and output, weight, and blood pressure daily; check patient for edema, oliguria, or lack of diuresis, which may indicate drug tolerance.

• Patient should be weighed each morning immediately after voiding and before breakfast—in the same type of clothing and on the same scale; the patient's weight provides an index for therapeutic response.
• Monitor patient with hepatic disease in whom mild drug-induced acidosis may be hazardous; watch for mental confusion, lethargy, or stupor. Patients with hepatic disease are especially susceptible to diuretic-induced electrolyte imbalance; in extreme cases, coma and death can result.
• Administer diuretics in morning to ensure that major diuresis occurs before bedtime. To prevent nocturia, do not prescribe diuretics for use after 6 p.m.
• Establish safety measures for all ambulatory patients until response to diuretic is known; diuretic therapy may cause orthostatic hypotension, weakness, ataxia, and confusion.
• Consider possible dosage adjustments in the following circumstances: reduced dosage for patients with hepatic dysfunction and for those taking other antihypertensive agents; increased dosage in patients with renal impairment; and changes in insulin requirements in diabetic patients.
• Monitor for other signs of toxicity: lethargy, confusion, stupor, muscle twitching, increased reflexes, and convulsions (water intoxication); severe weakness, headache, abdominal pain, malaise, nausea, and vomiting (metabolic acidosis); sore throat, rash, or jaundice (blood dyscrasia from hypersensitivity); joint swelling, redness, and pain (hyperuricemia); hypotension (in patients taking other antihypertensive drugs); and hyperglycemia (in diabetic patients).
• Patient should have urinal or commode readily available.

Information for the patient
• Explain signs and symptoms of possible adverse effects and the importance of reporting any unusual effect, especially weakness, fatigue, shortness of breath, chest or back pain, heaviness in the legs, muscle cramps, headache, dizziness, palpitations, mental confusion, nausea, vomiting, or diarrhea.
• Tell patient to report increased edema or weight or excess diuresis (more than 2-lb weight loss per day) and to record weight each morning after voiding and before dressing and breakfast, using same scale.
• Teach patient how to minimize dizziness from orthostatic hypotension by avoiding sudden postural changes.
• Advise patient to avoid potassium-rich food and potassium-containing salt substitutes or supplements, which increase the hazard of hyperkalemia.
• Advise patient to take drug at the same time each morning to avoid interrupted sleep from nighttime diuresis.
• Advise patient to take drug with or after meals to minimize GI distress.
• Caution patient to avoid hazardous activities, such as driving or operating machinery, until response to drug is known.
• Tell patient to seek medical approval before taking unprescribed drugs; many contain sodium and potassium and can cause electrolyte imbalance.
• Emphasize importance of keeping follow-up appointments to monitor effectiveness of diuretic therapy.

Geriatric use
Elderly and debilitated patients require close observation because they are more susceptible to drug-in-

---

duced diuresis and hyperkalemia. Reduced dosages may be indicated.

Pediatric use
Use drugs with caution; children are more susceptible to hyperkalemia.

Breast-feeding
Safety has not been established; drug may be excreted in breast milk.

Representative combinations
Amiloride with hydrochlorothiazide: Moduretic.
  Spironolactone with hydrochlorothiazide: Aldactazide, Spiranazide.
  Triamterene with hydrochlorothiazide: Dyazide, Maxzide.

PHARMACOLOGIC CLASS

diuretics, thiazide

bendroflumethiazide
benzthiazide
chlorothiazide
hydrochlorothiazide
hydroflumethiazide
methyclothiazide
polythiazide
trichlormethiazide

diuretics, thiazide-like

chlorthalidone
indapamide
metolazone
quinethazone

Thiazide diuretics were discovered and synthesized as an outgrowth of studies on carbonic anhydrase inhibitors. Until the 1950s, organic mercurials were the only effective diuretics available; though potent, they were also toxic. Introduction of the thiazides in 1957 proved a major advance because these were the first potent – and safe – diuretics.

Pharmacology
Thiazide diuretics interfere with sodium transport across tubules of the cortical diluting segment of the nephron, thereby increasing renal excretion of sodium, chloride, water, potassium, and calcium.

The exact mechanism of thiazides' antihypertensive effect is unknown; however, it is thought to be partially caused by direct arteriolar dilatation. Thiazides initially decrease extracellular fluid volume, plasma volume, and cardiac output; extracellular fluid volume and plasma volume revert to near baseline levels in several weeks but remain slightly below normal. Cardiac output returns to normal or slightly above. Total body sodium remains slightly below pretreatment levels. Peripheral vascular resistance is initially elevated but falls below pretreatment levels with chronic diuretic therapy.

In diabetes insipidus, thiazides cause a paradoxical decrease in urine volume and increase in renal concentration of urine, possibly because of sodium depletion and decreased plasma volume, which leads to an increase in renal water and sodium reabsorption.

Clinical indications and actions
Edema
Thiazide diuretics are used to treat edema associated with right-sided heart failure, mild to moderate left-sided heart failure, and nephrotic syndrome and, with spironolactone, to treat edema and ascites secondary to hepatic cirrhosis.

Efficacy and toxicity profiles of thiazide and thiazide-like diuretics are equivalent at comparable dosages; the single exception is metolazone, which may be more effective in patients with impaired renal function. Usually, thiazide diuretics are less effective than loop diuretics in patients with renal insufficiency.

Hypertension
Thiazide diuretics are commonly used for initial management of all degrees of hypertension. Used alone, they reduce mean blood pressure by only 10 to 15 mm Hg; in mild hypertension, thiazide diuresis alone will usually reduce blood pressure to desired levels. However, in moderate to severe hypertension that does not respond to thiazides alone, combination therapy with another antihypertensive agent is necessary.

Diabetes insipidus
In diabetes insipidus, thiazides cause a paradoxical decrease in urine volume; urine becomes more concentrated, possibly because of sodium depletion and decreased plasma volume. Thiazides are particularly effective in nephrogenic diabetes insipidus.

Overview of adverse reactions
Therapeutic doses of thiazide diuretics cause electrolyte and metabolic disturbances, the most common being potassium depletion; patients may require dietary supplementation. Other abnormalities include hypochloremic alkalosis, hyponatremia, hypercalcemia, hyperuricemia, elevated cholesterol levels, and hyperglycemia. Overdose of thiazides may produce lethargy that can progress to coma within a few hours.

▶ Special considerations
● Thiazides and thiazide-like diuretics (except metolazone) are ineffective in patients with a glomerular filtration rate below 25 ml/min.
● Because thiazides may cause adverse lipid effects, consider an alternative agent in patients with significant hyperlipidemia.
● Monitor intake and output, weight, and serum electrolyte levels regularly.
● Monitor serum potassium levels; consult dietitian to provide high-potassium diet. Foods rich in potassium include citrus fruits, tomatoes, bananas, dates, and apricots. Watch for signs of hypokalemia (for example, muscle weakness or cramps). Patients also taking digitalis have an increased risk of digitalis toxicity from the potassium-depleting effect of these diuretics.
● Thiazides may be used with potassium-sparing diuretics to prevent potassium loss.
● Check insulin requirements in patients with diabetes. Severe hyperglycemia may be treated with oral hyperglycemic agents.
● Monitor serum creatinine and BUN levels regularly. Drug is not as effective if these levels are more than twice normal.
● Monitor blood uric acid levels, especially in patients with a history of gout.
● Prescribe drug for use in morning to prevent nocturia.
● Antihypertensive effects persist for approximately week after discontinuation of the drug.

COMPARING THIAZIDES
Under most conditions, thiazide diuretics differ mainly in duration of action.

DRUG	EQUIVALENT DOSE	ONSET	PEAK	DURATION
bendroflumethiazide	5 mg	Within 2 hr	4 hr	6 to 12 hr
benzthiazide	50 mg	Within 2 hr	4 to 6 hr	6 to 12 hr
chlorothiazide	500 mg	Within 2 hr	4 hr	6 to 12 hr
cyclothiazide	2 mg	Within 6 hr	7 to 12 hr	18 to 24 hr
hydrochlorothiazide	50 mg	Within 2 hr	4 to 6 hr	6 to 12 hr
hydroflumethiazide	50 mg	Within 2 hr	4 hr	6 to 12 hr
methyclothiazide	5 mg	Within 2 hr	4 to 6 hr	24 hr
polythiazide	2 mg	Within 2 hr	6 hr	24 to 48 hr
trichlormethiazide	2 mg	Within 2 hr	6 hr	24 hr

● Instruct patient to report any joint swelling, pain, or redness; these signs may indicate hyperuricemia.

Information for the patient
● Explain rationale of therapy and diuretic effects of these drugs (increased volume and frequency of urination).
● Warn patient to call immediately if signs of electrolyte imbalance occur; these include weakness, fatigue, muscle cramps, paresthesias, confusion, nausea, vomiting, diarrhea, headache, dizziness, and palpitations.
● Tell patient to report any increased edema or weight or excess diuresis (more than a 2-lb weight loss per day); advise patient to record weight each morning after voiding and before dressing and breakfast, using the same scale.
● Advise patient to take drug with food to minimize gastric irritation; to eat potassium-rich foods, such as citrus fruits, potatoes, dates, raisins, and bananas; to avoid high-sodium foods, such as lunch meat, smoked meats, and processed cheeses; and not to add salt to other foods. Recommend salt substitutes.
● Counsel patient to avoid smoking because nicotine increases blood pressure.
● Tell patient to seek medical approval before taking nonprescription drugs; many contain sodium and potassium and can cause electrolyte imbalances; many diet aids and cold preparations contain drugs that may raise blood pressure.
● Warn patient about photosensitivity reactions. Explain that thiazide-related photosensitivity is a photoallergy in which ultraviolet radiation alters drug structure, causing allergic reactions in some persons; reaction occurs 10 days to 2 weeks after initial sun exposure.
● Emphasize importance of keeping follow-up appointments to monitor effectiveness of diuretic therapy.

With initial doses
● Caution patient to change position slowly, especially when rising to upright position, to prevent dizziness from orthostatic hypotension.
● Instruct patient to call immediately if chest, back, or leg pain; shortness of breath; or dyspnea occurs.
● Tell patient to take drug only as prescribed and at the same time each day, to prevent nighttime diuresis and interrupted sleep.

Geriatric use
Elderly and debilitated patients require close observation and may require reduced dosages. They are more sensitive to excess diuresis because of age-related changes in cardiovascular and renal function. In elderly patients, excess diuresis can quickly lead to dehydration, hypovolemia, hyponatremia, hypomagnesemia, and hypokalemia.

Pediatric use
Safety and effectiveness have not been established for all thiazide diuretics.

Breast-feeding
Thiazides are distributed in breast milk; safety and effectiveness in breast-feeding women have not been established.

Representative combinations
Bendroflumethiazide with nadolol: Corzide; with potassium chloride: Naturetin W/K; with rauwolfia serpentina: Rauzide; with raudixin and potassium chloride: Rautrax; with rauwolfia serpentina and potassium chloride: Rautrax-N; with raudixin and potassium chloride: Rautrax-N, modified; with reserpine: Exna-R.
Chlorthalidone with atenolol: Tenoretic; with reserpine: Regroton; *Chlorothiazide* with methyldopa: Aldochlor; with reserpine: Diupres.
Hydrochlorothiazide with deserpidine: Oreticyl; with guanethidine monosulfate: Esimil; with hydralazine: Apresazide, Apresoline-Esidrix, Hydralazide; with methyldopa: Aldoril; with pindolol: Viskazide*; with propranolol: Inderide; with reserpine: Hydropine, Hydropres, Hydroserp, Hydroserpine, Hydrotensin, Mallopress, Serpasil-Esidrex, Thia-Serp; with hydralazine and reserpine: Harbolin, Ser-Ap-Es, Serapine, Serpahyde, Thia-Serpa-Zine, Unipres; with spironolactone: Aldactazide; with timolol maleate: Timolide; with triamterene: Dyazide, Maxide; with amiloride: Moduretic.
Hydroflumethiazide with reserpine: Salutensin.
Methyclothiazide with cryptenamine: Diutensin; with reserpine: Diutensin-R; with deserpidine: Enduronyl; with pargyline: Eutron.
Polythiazide with prazosin: Minizide; with reserpine: Renese-R.

*Canada only   †Unlabeled clinical use   Italicized adverse reactions are life-threatening.

Quinethazone with reserpine: Hydromox R.
Trichlormethiazide with reserpine: Metatensin, Naqui-val.

dobutamine hydrochloride
Dobutrex

- Pharmacologic classification: adrenergic, beta₁ agonist
- Therapeutic classification: inotropic agent
- Pregnancy risk category C

How supplied
Available by prescription only
Injection: 12.5 mg/ml in 20-ml vials (parenteral)

Indications, route, and dosage
To increase cardiac output in short-term treatment of cardiac decompensation caused by depressed contractility
Adults: 2.5 to 10 mcg/kg/minute as an I.V. infusion. Rarely, infusion rates up to 40 mcg/kg/minute may be needed. Titrate dosage carefully to patient response.

Pharmacodynamics
Inotropic action: Dobutamine selectively stimulates beta₁-adrenergic receptors to increase myocardial contractility and stroke volume, resulting in increased cardiac output (a positive inotropic effect in patients with normal hearts or in congestive heart failure). At therapeutic doses, dobutamine decreases peripheral resistance (afterload), reduces ventricular filling pressure (preload), and may facilitate AV node conduction. Systolic blood pressure and pulse pressure may remain unchanged or increased from increased cardiac output. Increased myocardial contractility results in increased coronary blood flow and myocardial oxygen consumption. Heart rate usually remains unchanged; however, excessive doses do have chronotropic effects. Dobutamine does not appear to affect dopaminergic receptors, nor does it cause renal or mesenteric vasodilation; however, urine flow may increase because of increased cardiac output.

Pharmacokinetics
- *Absorption:* After I.V. administration, onset of action occurs within 2 minutes, with peak concentrations achieved within 10 minutes. Effects persist a few minutes after I.V. is discontinued.
- *Distribution:* Dobutamine is widely distributed throughout the body.
- *Metabolism:* Dobutamine is metabolized by the liver and by conjugation to inactive metabolites.
- *Excretion:* Dobutamine is excreted mainly in urine, with minor amounts in feces, as its metabolites and conjugates.

Contraindications and precautions
Dobutamine is contraindicated in patients with idiopathic hypertrophic subaortic stenosis or known hypersensitivity to the drug or its ingredients. Use with extreme caution after myocardial infarction (may intensify or extend myocardial ischemia). Dobutamine increases AV conduction; therefore, patients with atrial fibrillation should have therapeutic levels of a cardiac glycoside before administration of dobutamine.

Drug contains sodium bisulfite and may trigger allergic reaction in patients with sulfite sensitivity.

Interactions
Concomitant use with inhalation hydrocarbon anesthetics, especially halothane and cyclopropane, may trigger ventricular arrhythmias. Beta-adrenergic blockers may antagonize the cardiac effects of dobutamine, resulting in increased peripheral resistance and predominance of alpha-adrenergic effects.

Dobutamine may decrease the hypotensive effects of guanadrel and guanethidine; however, these agents may potentiate the pressor effects of dobutamine, possibly resulting in hypertension and cardiac arrhythmias. Concomitant use with nitroprusside may cause higher cardiac output and lower pulmonary wedge pressure. Theoretically, rauwolfia alkaloids may prolong the actions of dobutamine (a denervation supersensitivity response).

Effects on diagnostic tests
None reported.

Adverse reactions
- CV: ectopic heart beats, increased heart rate, angina, chest pain, palpitation, hypertension.
- GI: nausea, vomiting.
- Other: tingling sensation, paresthesias, dyspnea, headache, mild leg cramps.
  Note: Drug should be discontinued if hypersensitivity reaction to drug or sulfites or if cardiac arrhythmia occurs.

Overdose and treatment
Clinical manifestations of overdose include nervousness and fatigue. No treatment is necessary beyond dosage reduction or withdrawal of drug.

▶ **Special considerations**
Besides those relevant to all *adrenergics*, consider the following recommendations.
- Before administration of dobutamine, correct hypovolemia with appropriate plasma volume expanders.
- Monitor ECG, blood pressure, cardiac output, and pulmonary wedge pressure via central venous pressure line or Swan-Ganz catheter.
- Before giving dobutamine, administer digitalis if patient has atrial fibrillation (dobutamine increases AV conduction).
- Most patients experience an increase of 10 to 20 mm Hg in systolic blood pressure; some show an increase of 50 mm Hg or more. Most also experience an increase in heart rate of 5 to 15/beats minute; some show increases of 30 or more beats/minute. Premature ventricular arrhythmias may also occur in about 5% of patients. Dosage reduction may be necessary when these occur.
- Dose should be adjusted to meet individual needs and achieve desired clinical response. Drug must be administered by I.V. infusion using an infusion pump or other device to control flow rate.
- Concentration of infusion solution should not exceed 5,000 mcg/ml; the solution should be used within 24 hours. Rate and duration of infusion depend on patient response.
- Pink discoloration of solution indicates slight oxidation but no significant loss of potency.
- Dobutamine is incompatible with alkaline solution (sodium bicarbonate). Also, do not mix with or give through same I.V. line as heparin, hydrocortisone sodium succinate, cefazolin, cefamandole, neutral cephalothin, penicillin, or ethacrynate sodium.

Information for the patient
● Advise patient to report any adverse reactions.
● Inform patient that he'll need frequent monitoring of vital signs.

Geriatric use
Lower doses are indicated, because elderly patients may be more sensitive to the drug's effects.

Pediatric use
Not recommended for use in children. Safety and efficacy not established.

Breast-feeding
It is unknown if dobutamine is excreted in breast milk. Administer cautiously to breast-feeding women.

---

docusate calcium
D-C-S, Pro-Cal-Sof, Surfak

docusate potassium
Dialose, Diocto-K, Kasof

docusate sodium
Afko-Lube, Colace, Diocto, Dioeze, Diosuccin, Disonate, Di-Sosul, Doss, Doxinate, D.S.S., Duosol, Modane Soft, Molatoc, Pro-Sof, Regulax SS, Regulex*, Regutol, Stulex, Theravac Plus, Theravac-SB

● Pharmacologic classification: surfactant
● Therapeutic classification: emollient laxative
● Pregnancy risk category C

How supplied
Available without prescription
Tablets: 50 mg, 100 mg
Capsules: 50 mg, 60 mg, 100 mg, 120 mg, 240 mg, 250 mg, 300 mg
Syrup: 50 mg/15 ml, 60 mg/15 ml
Liquid: 150 mg/15 ml
Solution: 50 mg/ml

Indications, route, and dosage
Stool softener
Docusate sodium
Adults and older children: 50 to 300 mg P.O. daily until bowel movements are normal. Alternatively, add 50 to 100 mg to saline or oil retention enema to treat fecal impaction.
Children age 6 to 12: 40 to 120 mg P.O. daily.
Children age 3 to 6: 20 to 60 mg P.O. daily.
Children under age 3: 10 to 40 mg P.O. daily.
Docusate calcium or docusate potassium
Adults and older children: 240 mg P.O. daily until bowel movements are normal.
   Higher doses are for initial therapy. Adjust dose to individual response. Usual dosage in children and adults with minimal needs is 50 to 150 mg (docusate calcium) P.O. daily.

Pharmacodynamics
Laxative action: Docusate salts act as detergents in the intestine, reducing surface tension of interfacing liquids;

this promotes incorporation of fat and additional liquid, softening the stool.

Pharmacokinetics
● *Absorption:* Docusate salts are absorbed minimally in the duodenum and jejunum; drug acts in 1 to 3 days.
● *Distribution:* Docusate salts are distributed primarily locally, in the gut.
● *Metabolism:* None.
● *Excretion:* Docusate salts are excreted in feces.

Contraindications and precautions
Docusate salts are contraindicated in patients receiving mineral oil because they may increase absorption to dangerous levels.

Interactions
Docusate salts may increase absorption of mineral oil.

Effects on diagnostic tests
None reported.

Adverse reactions
● EENT: throat irritation.
● GI: bitter taste, mild abdominal cramping, diarrhea.
Note: Drug should be discontinued if severe cramping occurs.

Overdose and treatment
No information available.

▶ Special considerations
● Liquid (but not syrup) may be diluted in juice or other flavored liquid to improve taste.
● After administration of liquid through nasogastric tube, tube should be flushed afterward to clear it and ensure dispersion into stomach.
● Avoid using docusate sodium in sodium-restricted patients.
● Docusate salts are available in combination with casanthranol (Peri-Colace), senna (Senokot, Gentlax), and phenolphthalein (Ex-Lax, Feen-a-Mint, Correctol).
● Docusate salts are the preferred laxative for most patients who must avoid straining at stool, such as those recovering from myocardial infarction or rectal surgery. They also are used commonly to treat patients with postpartum constipation.
● Docusate salts are less likely than other laxatives to cause laxative dependence; however, their effectiveness may decrease with long-term use.

Information for the patient
Docusate salts lose their effectiveness over time; advise patient to report failure of medication.

Geriatric use
Docusate salts are good choices for elderly patients because they rarely cause laxative dependence and cause fewer adverse effects and are gentler than some other laxatives.

Breast-feeding
Because absorption of docusate salts is minimal, they presumably pose no risk to breast-feeding infants.

---

dopamine hydrochloride
Dopastat, Intropin

- Pharmacologic classification: adrenergic
- Therapeutic classification: inotropic, vasopressor
- Pregnancy risk category C

How supplied
Available by prescription only
Injection: 40 mg/ml, 80 mg/ml, and 160 mg/ml parenteral concentrate for injection for I.V. infusion; 0.8 mg/ml (200 or 400 mg) in dextrose 5%; 1.6 mg/ml (400 or 800 mg) in dextrose 5%, and 3.2 mg/ml (800 mg) in dextrose 5% parenteral injection for I.V. infusion.

Indications, route, and dosage
Adjunct in shock to increase cardiac output, blood pressure, and urine flow
Adults: 1 to 5 mcg/kg/minute I.V. infusion, up to 50 mcg/kg/minute. Infusion rate may be increased by 1 to 4 mcg/kg/minute at 10- to 30-minute intervals until optimum response is achieved. In severely ill patient, infusion may begin at 5 mcg/kg/minute and gradually increase by increments of 5 to 10 mcg/kg/minute until optimum response is achieved.
Short-term treatment of severe, refractory, chronic congestive heart failure
Adults: Initially, 0.5 to 2 mcg/kg/minute I.V. infusion. Dosage may be increased until desired renal response occurs. Average dosage, 1 to 3 mcg/kg/minute.

Pharmacodynamics
Vasopressor action: An immediate precursor of norepinephrine, dopamine stimulates dopaminergic, beta-adrenergic, and alpha-adrenergic receptors of the sympathetic nervous system. The main effects produced are dose-dependent. It has a direct stimulating effect on beta$_1$ receptors (in I.V. doses of 2 to 10 mcg/kg/minute) and little or no effect on beta$_2$ receptors. In I.V. doses of 0.5 to 2 mcg/kg/minute it acts on dopaminergic receptors, causing vasodilation in the renal, mesenteric, coronary, and intracerebral vascular beds; in I.V. doses above 10 mcg/kg/minute, it stimulates alpha receptors.

Low to moderate doses result in cardiac stimulation (positive inotropic effects) and renal and mesenteric vasodilation (dopaminergic response). High doses result in increased peripheral resistance and renal vasoconstriction.

Pharmacokinetics
- *Absorption:* Onset of action after I.V. administration occurs within 5 minutes and persists for less than 10 minutes.
- *Distribution:* Dopamine is widely distributed throughout the body; however, it does not cross the blood-brain barrier.
- *Metabolism:* Dopamine is metabolized to inactive compounds in the liver, kidneys, and plasma by monoamine oxidase and catechol-O-methyltransferase (COMT). About 25% is metabolized to norepinephrine within adrenergic nerve terminals.
- *Excretion:* Dopamine is excreted in urine, mainly as its metabolites.

Contraindications and precautions
Dopamine is contraindicated in patients with pheochromocytoma and in those with uncorrected tachyarrhythmias or ventricular fibrillation because of potential for severe cardiovascular effects.

Commercially available dopamine solutions containing sulfites should be administered cautiously to patients with asthma and other patients with known hypersensitivity to them. Administer cautiously to patients with ischemic heart disease. Monitor patients with a history of occlusive vascular disease for decreased circulation to extremities.

Interactions
Concomitant use with monoamine oxidase inhibitors may prolong and intensify the effects of dopamine. Use with beta-adrenergic blockers antagonizes the cardiac effects of dopamine; use with alpha-adrenergic blockers may antagonize the peripheral vasoconstriction caused by high doses of dopamine.

Combined use with general anesthetics, especially halothane and cyclopropane, may cause ventricular arrhythmias and hypertension. Use with I.V. phenytoin may cause hypotension and bradycardia; use with diuretics increases diuretic effects of both agents. Use with oxytocics may cause advanced vasoconstriction. Dosage adjustments may be needed.

Dopamine decreases hypotensive effects of guanadrel, guanethidine, methyldopa, and trimethaphan through potentiated pressor effects of dopamine. Use with digitalis glycosides, levodopa, and sympathomimetics increases risk of cardiac arrhythmias.

Effects on diagnostic tests
Dopamine may cause elevated urinary catecholamine levels. Drug may also cause increased serum glucose levels although level usually doesn't rise above normal limits.

Adverse reactions
- CV: ectopic heartbeats, tachycardia, angina, palpitation, vasoconstriction, hypotension, cardiac conduction abnormalities, widened QRS complex, bradycardia, hypertension, *ventricular arrhythmias* (high doses).
- GI: nausea, vomiting.
- Other: dyspnea, headache, azotemia, anxiety, and piloerection. Extravasation can cause local necrosis and sloughing of tissue.
   Note: Drug should be discontinued if patient develops signs of hypersensitivity to drug or sulfite preservative, cardiac arrhythmias, or tachyphylaxis.

Overdose and treatment
Clinical manifestations of overdose include excessive, severe hypertension. No treatment is necessary beyond dosage reduction or withdrawal of drug. If that fails to lower blood pressure, a short-acting alpha-adrenergic blocking agent may be helpful.

▶ Special considerations
Besides those relevant to all *adrenergics*, consider the following recommendations.
- Hypovolemia should be corrected with appropriate plasma volume expanders before administration of dopamine.
- Dopamine is administered by I.V. infusion using an infusion device to control rate of flow.
- Administer dopamine into a large vein to prevent the possibility of extravasation. If necessary to administer

---

in hand or ankle veins, change injection site to larger vein as soon as possible. Monitor continuously for free flow. Central venous access is recommended.

● Adjust dose to meet individual needs of patient and to achieve desired clinical response. If dose required to obtain desired systolic blood pressure exceeds optimum rate of renal response, reduce dose as soon as hemodynamic condition is stabilized.

● Significant hypokalemia may result with excessive administration of potassium-free solutions. Monitor electrolyte levels.

● Severe hypotension may result with abrupt withdrawal of infusion; therefore, reduce dose gradually.

● If extravasation occurs, stop infusion and infiltrate site promptly with 10 to 15 ml of sodium chloride injection containing 5 to 10 mg of phentolamine. Use syringe with a fine needle, and infiltrate area liberally with phentolamine solution.

● Do not mix other drugs in dopamine solutions. Discard solutions after 24 hours.

● Monitor blood pressure, cardiac output, ECG, and intake and output during infusion, especially if dose exceeds 50 mcg/kg/minute. Watch for cold extremities.

Information for the patient
● Advise patient to report any adverse reactions.
● Inform patient of need for frequent monitoring of his vital signs and condition.

Geriatric use
Lower doses are indicated, because elderly patients may be more sensitive to drug's effects.

---

doxapram hydrochloride
Dopram

● Pharmacologic classification: analeptic
● Therapeutic classification: CNS and respiratory stimulant
● Pregnancy risk category C

How supplied
Available by prescription only
Injection: 20 mg/ml (benzyl alcohol 0.9%)

Indications, route, and dosage
Postanesthesia respiratory stimulation, drug-induced CNS depression, acute hypercapnia associated with chronic obstructive pulmonary disease
Adults: 0.5 to 1 mg/kg of body weight (up to 2 mg/kg in CNS depression) I.V. injection or infusion. Maximum dosage is 4 mg/kg, up to 3 g in 1 day. Infusion rate is 1 to 3 mg/minute (initial dose is 5 mg/minute for postanesthesia).
Chronic obstructive pulmonary disease (COPD)
Adults: Infusion of 1 to 2 mg/minute. Maximum dosage is 3 mg/minute for a maximum duration of 2 hours. *Do not use drug with mechanical ventilation.*

Start flow rate at 1 mg/minute until satisfactory respiratory response is achieved, using infusion pump to regulate rate. Patient can be maintained with 1 to 3 mg/minute; however, dosage is usually titrated to respiratory response.

Pharmacodynamics
Respiratory stimulant action: Doxapram increases respiratory rate by direct stimulation of the medullary respiratory center and possibly by indirect action on chemoreceptors in the carotid artery and aortic arch. Doxapram causes increased release of catecholamines.

Pharmacokinetics
● *Absorption:* After I.V. administration, action begins within 20 to 40 seconds; peak effect occurs in 1 to 2 minutes. Plasma half-life ranges from about 2½ to 4 hours; pharmacologic action persists for 5 to 12 minutes.
● *Distribution:* Doxapram is distributed throughout the body.
● *Metabolism:* Drug is 99% metabolized by the liver.
● *Excretion:* Metabolites are excreted in urine.

Contraindications and precautions
Doxapram is contraindicated in patients with head trauma and epilepsy or other seizure disorders because of the risk of drug-induced convulsions; in patients with acute bronchial asthma, pulmonary embolism, pneumothorax, pulmonary fibrosis, airway obstruction, severe dyspnea and respiratory failure from muscle paresis, because of risk of hypoxia and subsequent arrhythmias; and in patients with coronary artery disease, severe hypertension, frank uncompensated heart failure, or cerebrovascular accident, because of drug's vasopressor effects.

Doxapram should be used with caution in patients with a history of severe tachycardia or cardiac arrhythmia, because of the risk of hypoxia and subsequent arrhythmia; and in patients with increased cerebrospinal fluid pressure or cerebral edema, pheochromocytoma, or hyperthyroidism, because of drug's vasopressor effects.

Interactions
Concomitant use with MAO inhibitors or sympathomimetic drugs may produce added pressor effects.

Discontinue anesthetics, such as halothane, cyclopropane, and enflurane, at least 10 minutes before giving doxapram; these agents sensitize the myocardium to catecholamines.

Doxapram temporarily may mask residual effects of neuromuscular blockers used after anesthesia.

Effects on diagnostic tests
Doxapram may cause T-wave depression on ECG, decreased erythrocyte and leukocyte counts, reduced hemoglobin and hematocrit levels, increased BUN levels, and albuminuria.

Adverse reactions
● CNS: *seizures*, headache, dizziness, apprehension, disorientation, pupillary dilatation, bilateral Babinski's signs, flushing, sweating, paresthesias.
● CV: chest pain and tightness, arrhythmias, hypertension, phlebitis.
● DERM: pruritus.
● GI: nausea, vomiting, diarrhea, urge to defecate.
● GU: urinary retention, stimulation of bladder with incontinence.
● Respiratory: cough, sneezing, hiccups, *bronchospasm*, rebound hypoventilation.
Note: Drug should be discontinued if hypotension or dyspnea occurs.

Adverse reactions associated with doxapram and nikethamide are the same: clinical experience to date indicates that doxapram has greater margin of safety and lower incidence of adverse effects.

Overdose and treatment
Signs of overdose include hypertension, tachycardia, arrhythmias, skeletal muscle hyperactivity, and dyspnea.

Treatment is supportive. Keep oxygen and resuscitative equipment available, but use oxygen with caution, because rapid increase in PO_2 can suppress carotid chemoreceptor activity. Keep I.V. anticonvulsants available to treat seizures.

▶ Special considerations
● Doxapram's use as an analeptic is strongly discouraged; drug should be used only in surgery or emergency room.
● Establish adequate airway before administering drug; prevent aspiration of vomitus by placing patient on his side.
● Monitor blood pressure, heart rate, deep tendon reflexes, and arterial blood gas (ABG) levels before giving drug and every 30 minutes afterward; in patients with COPD, draw ABG levels before infusion and every ½ hour during infusion. Discontinue drug if ABG levels deteriorate or mechanical ventilation is started.
● For I.V. infusion, dilute to 1 mg/ml. Do not infuse doxapram faster than recommended rate because hemolysis may occur. Drug should be used only on an intermittent basis; maximum infusion period is 2 hours.
● Avoid repeated injections in the site for long periods, because of risk of thrombophlebitis or local skin irritation.
● Do not combine doxapram, which is acidic, with alkaline solutions, such as thiopental sodium; solution is compatible with dextrose 5% or 10% and 0.9% NaCl.
● Give concomitant oxygen cautiously to patients with COPD who are narcotized or those who have just undergone surgery; doxapram-stimulated respiration increases oxygen demand.
● Monitor patient for signs of toxicity—tachycardia, muscle tremor, spasticity, and hyperactive reflexes—and blood pressure changes, especially hypertensive patients.

Geriatric use
No specific recommendations exist for use of doxapram in elderly patients. However, elderly patients may be predisposed to one of several illnesses that preclude its use.

Pediatric use
Safety in children under age 12 has not been established.

Breast-feeding
Safe use in breast-feeding has not been established. Distribution into breast milk is unknown.

doxazosin mesylate
Cardura

● Pharmacologic classification: alpha-adrenergic blocking agent
● Therapeutic classification: antihypertensive
● Pregnancy risk category B

How supplied
Available by prescription only
Tablets: 1 mg, 2 mg, 4 mg, 8 mg

Indications, route, and dosage
Essential hypertension
Adult: Dosage must be individualized. Initially, administer 1 mg P.O. daily. Increase dosage as necessary and tolerated. Maintenance dosage ranges from 2 to 16 mg daily.

Pharmacodynamics
Hypotensive action: Doxazosin selectively blocks postsynaptic alpha$_1$-adrenergic receptors, dilating both resistance (arterioles) and capacitance (veins) vessels. It lowers both supine and standing blood pressure, producing more pronounced effects on diastolic pressure. Maximum reductions occur 2 to 6 hours after dosing and are associated with a small increase in standing heart rate. Doxazosin has a greater effect on blood pressure and heart rate in the standing position.

Pharmacokinetics
● *Absorption:* Doxazosin is readily absorbed from the GI tract after oral administration. Peak plasma levels are obtained in 2 to 3 hours.
● *Distribution:* Doxazosin is 98% protein-bound. It is distributed in breast milk in concentrations about 20 times greater than in maternal plasma.
● *Metabolism:* Extensively metabolized in the liver by O-demethylation or hydroxylation. Secondary peaking of plasma levels suggests enterohepatic recycling.
● *Excretion:* 63% is excreted in bile and feces (4.8% as unchanged drug); 9% is excreted in urine.

Contraindications and precautions
Doxazosin is contraindicated in patients with known hypersensitivity to quinazolines. Use with caution in patients with impaired hepatic function or those receiving drugs known to influence hepatic metabolism. Concurrent administration with other antihypertensives may result in marked hypotension, especially postural hypotension, and syncope with sudden loss of consciousness, particularly with the first few doses. Use with caution.

Interactions
None reported.

Effects on diagnostic tests
Mean WBC and neutrophil counts may be decreased.

Adverse reactions
● CNS: depression, dizziness, nervousness, paresthesia, somnolence, anxiety, insomnia, asthenia, drowsiness, ataxia, hypertonia, weakness, fatigue, lassitude, headache.

● CV: palpitations, *orthostatic hypotension,* hypotension, tachycardia, *arrhythmias,* chest pain.
● DERM: pruritus, rash, sweating, alopecia, lichen planus.
● EENT: abnormal vision, conjunctivitis, reddened sclera, tinnitus, vertigo.
● GI: nausea, vomiting, diarrhea, constipation, dry mouth, abdominal discomfort and pain, flatulence.
● GU: incontinence, polyuria, decreased libido, sexual dysfunction.
● Respiratory: dyspnea, sinusitis, bronchitis, cold symptoms, bronchospasm, epistaxis, flulike symptoms, pharyngitis, rhinitis.
● Other: edema, weight gain, facial edema, fever, flushing, arthritis, joint pain, arthralgia, and muscle pain in neck, back, shoulder, and extremities.

Overdose and treatment
Keep patient supine to restore blood pressure and heart rate. If necessary, treat shock with volume expanders. Administer vasopressors and monitor and support renal function.

▶ Special considerations
● Postural effects are most likely to occur 2 to 6 hours after dose. Monitor blood pressure during this time after the first dose and after subsequent increases in dosage. Daily doses greater than 4 mg increase the potential for excessive postural effects.
● Tolerance to doxazosin's antihypertensive effects has not been observed.
● No apparent differences exist in the hypotensive response of whites and blacks or of elderly patients.
● First-dose effect (orthostatic hypotension) occurs with doxazosin but is less pronounced than with prazosin or terazosin.

Information for the patient
● Tell patient that orthostatic hypotension and syncope are possible especially after first few doses and with dosage changes. Patient should arise slowly to prevent postural hypertension.
● Caution patient that drug may cause drowsiness and somnolence. Patient should avoid driving and other hazardous tasks that require alertness for 12 to 24 hours after first dose, after dosage increases, and after resumption of interrupted therapy.
● Tell patient to report bothersome palpitations or dizziness to physician.

Pediatric use
Safety and efficacy have not been established.

Breast-feeding
Doxazosin accumulates in breast milk in concentrations about 20 times greater than in maternal plasma concentrations.

doxepin hydrochloride
Adapin, Sinequan, Triadapin*

● Pharmacologic classification: tricyclic antidepressant
● Therapeutic classification: antidepressant
● Pregnancy risk category C

How supplied
Available by prescription only
Capsules: 10 mg, 25 mg, 50 mg, 75 mg, 100 mg, 150 mg
Oral concentrate: 10 mg/ml

Indications, route, and dosage
Depression
Adults: Initially, 50 to 75 mg P.O. daily in divided doses, to a maximum of 300 mg daily. Alternatively, entire dosage may be given at bedtime.

Pharmacodynamics
Antidepressant action: Doxepin is thought to exert its antidepressant effects by inhibiting reuptake of norepinephrine and serotonin in CNS nerve terminals (presynaptic neurons), which results in increased levels and enhanced activity of these neurotransmitters in the synaptic cleft. Doxepin more actively inhibits reuptake of serotonin than norepinephrine. Anxiolytic effects of this drug usually precede antidepressant effects. Doxepin also may be used as an anxiolytic. Doxepin has the greatest sedative effect of all tricyclic antidepressants; tolerance to this effect usually develops in a few weeks.

Pharmacokinetics
● *Absorption:* Doxepin is absorbed rapidly from the GI tract after oral administration.
● *Distribution:* Doxepin is distributed widely into the body, including the CNS and breast milk. Drug is 90% protein-bound. Peak effect occurs in 2 to 4 hours; steady state is achieved within 7 days. Therapeutic concentrations (parent drug and metabolite) are thought to range from 150 to 250 ng/ml.
● *Metabolism:* Doxepin is metabolized by the liver to the active metabolite desmethyldoxepin. A significant first-pass effect may explain variability of serum concentrations in different patients taking the same dosage.
● *Excretion:* Most of drug is excreted in urine.

Contraindications and precautions
Doxepin is contraindicated in patients with known hypersensitivity to tricyclic antidepressants, trazodone, and related compounds; in the acute recovery phase of myocardial infarction (MI) because of its potential arrhythmogenic effects and ECG changes; in patients in coma or severe respiratory depression because of additive CNS depression; and during or within 14 days of therapy with monoamine oxidase inhibitors. Doxepin is also contraindicated in breast-feeding women because of the hazard of respiratory depression in the infant.

Doxepin should be used cautiously in patients with other cardiac disease (arrhythmias, congestive heart failure [CHF], angina pectoris, valvular disease, or heart block); respiratory disorders; alcoholism, epilepsy, and

---

other seizure disorders; scheduled electroconvulsive therapy; bipolar disease; glaucoma; hyperthyroidism, or in those taking thyroid replacement; Type I and Type II diabetes; prostatic hypertrophy, paralytic ileus, or urinary retention; hepatic or renal dysfunction; or Parkinson's disease; and in those undergoing surgery with general anesthesia.

Interactions
Concomitant use of doxepin with sympathomimetics, including epinephrine, phenylephrine, phenylpropanolamine, and ephedrine (often found in nasal sprays) may increase blood pressure; use with warfarin may increase prothrombin time and cause bleeding.

Concomitant use with thyroid medication, pimozide, and antiarrhythmic agents (quinidine, disopyramide, procainamide) may increase incidence of cardiac dysrhythmias and conduction defects.

Doxepin may decrease hypotensive effects of centrally acting antihypertensive drugs, such as guanethidine, guanabenz, guanadrel, clonidine, methyldopa, and reserpine. Concomitant use with disulfiram or ethchlorvynol may cause delirium and tachycardia. Additive effects are likely after concomitant use of doxepin with CNS depressants, including alcohol, analgesics, barbiturates, narcotics, tranquilizers, and anesthetics (oversedation); atropine and other anticholinergic drugs, including phenothiazines, antihistamines, meperidine, and antiparkinsonian agents (oversedation, paralytic ileus, visual changes, and severe constipation); and metrizamide (increased risk of convulsions).

Barbiturates and heavy smoking induce doxepin metabolism and decrease therapeutic efficacy; phenothiazines and haloperidol decrease its metabolism, decreasing therapeutic efficacy; methylphenidate, cimetidine, oral contraceptives, propoxyphene, and beta blockers may inhibit doxepin metabolism, increasing plasma levels and toxicity.

Effects on diagnostic tests
Doxepin may prolong conduction time (elongation of Q-T and PR intervals, flattened T waves on ECG); it also may elevate liver function test results, decrease white blood cell counts, and decrease or increase serum glucose levels.

Adverse reactions
● CNS: drowsiness, dizziness, sedation, excitation, tremors, weakness, headache, nervousness, *seizures*, peripheral neuropathy, extrapyramidal symptoms, anxiety, vivid dreams, decreased libido, confusion (more marked in elderly patients).
● CV: orthostatic hypotension, tachycardia, arrhythmias, *MI, stroke, heart block, CHF*, palpitations, hypertension, ECG changes.
● EENT: blurred vision, tinnitus, mydriasis, increased intraocular pressure.
● GI: dry mouth, constipation, nausea, vomiting, anorexia, diarrhea, paralytic ileus, jaundice.
● GU: urinary retention.
● Other: sweating, photosensitivity, hypersensitivity (rash, urticaria, drug fever, edema).

After abrupt withdrawal of long-term therapy, nausea, headache, and malaise (does not indicate addiction) may occur.

Note: Drug should be discontinued (not abruptly) if signs of hypersensitivity occur, and the following reactions reported: urinary retention, extreme dry mouth, rash, excessive sedation, seizures, tachycardia, sore throat, fever, or jaundice.

Overdose and treatment
The first 12 hours after acute ingestion are a stimulatory phase characterized by excessive anticholinergic activity (agitation, irritation, confusion, hallucinations, hyperthermia, parkinsonian symptoms, seizure, urinary retention, dry mucous membranes, pupillary dilatation, constipation, and ileus). This is followed by CNS depressant effects, including hypothermia, decreased or absent reflexes, sedation, hypotension, cyanosis, and cardiac irregularities, including tachycardia, conduction disturbances, and quinidine-like effects on the ECG.

Severity of overdose is best indicated by widening of QRS complex. Usually, this represents a serum concentration in excess of 1,000 ng/ml. Serum concentrations are usually not helpful. Metabolic acidosis may follow hypotension, hypoventilation, and convulsions.

Treatment is symptomatic and supportive, including maintaining airway, stable body temperature, and fluid and electrolyte balance. Induce emesis with ipecac if patient is conscious; follow with gastric lavage and activated charcoal to prevent further absorption. Dialysis is of little use. Physostigmine may be cautiously used to reverse central anticholinergic effects. Treat seizures with parenteral diazepam or phenytoin; arrhythmias, with parenteral phenytoin or lidocaine; and acidosis, with sodium bicarbonate. *Do not give barbiturates:* these may enhance CNS and respiratory depressant effects.

▶ Special considerations
Recommendations for administration of doxepin, for the care of the patient during therapy, and for use in pediatric patients are the same as those for all *tricyclic antidepressants*.

Information for the patient
● Teach patient to dilute oral concentrate with 120 ml water, milk, or juice (grapefruit, orange, pineapple, prune, or tomato). Drug is incompatible with carbonated beverages.
● Tell patient to use ice chips, sugarless gum or hard candy, or saliva substitutes to treat dry mouth.
● Advise patient to avoid alcohol or other sedative drugs while taking doxepin. Drug has a strong sedative effect and such combinations can cause excessive sedation.
● Warn patient to avoid taking any other drugs while taking doxepin unless they have been prescribed.
● Instruct patient to take full dose at bedtime.
● Tell patient to store drug safely away from children.

Geriatric use
Elderly patients are more likely to develop adverse CNS reactions.

Breast-feeding
Patient should not breast-feed while taking doxepin; doxepin is excreted in breast milk, especially if the mother is taking high doses.

---

doxorubicin hydrochloride
Adriamycin

- Pharmacologic classification: antineoplastic antibiotic (cell cycle-phase nonspecific)
- Therapeutic classification: antineoplastic
- Pregnancy risk category D

How supplied
Available by prescription only
Injection: 10-mg, 20-mg, 50-mg, 100-mg, 150-mg vials
Injection (preservative-free): 2 mg/ml

Indications, route, and dosage
Dosage and indications may vary. Check current literature for recommended protocol.
Cancer of bladder, kidney, breast, cervix, head, neck, liver, lungs, ovary, prostate, stomach, testes, brain, or blood and lymph system; sarcomas
Adults: 60 to 75 mg/m² I.V. as a single dose q 3 weeks; or 25 to 30 mg/m² I.V. as a single daily dose on days 1 to 3 of 4-week cycle. Alternatively, 20 mg/m² I.V. once weekly. Maximum cumulative dosage is 550 mg/m² (450 mg/m² in patients who have received chest irradiation).

Pharmacodynamics
Antineoplastic action: Doxorubicin exerts its cytotoxic activity by intercalating between DNA base pairs and uncoiling the DNA helix. The result is inhibition of DNA synthesis and DNA-dependent RNA synthesis. Doxorubicin also inhibits protein synthesis.

Pharmacokinetics
- *Absorption:* Because of its vesicant effects, doxorubicin must be administered intravenously.
- *Distribution:* Doxorubicin distributes widely into body tissues, with the highest concentrations found in the liver, heart, and kidneys. The drug does not cross the blood-brain barrier.
- *Metabolism:* Doxorubicin is extensively metabolized by hepatic microsomal enzymes to several metabolites, one of which possesses cytotoxic activity.
- *Excretion:* Doxorubicin and its metabolites are excreted primarily in bile. A minute amount is eliminated in urine. The plasma elimination of doxorubicin is described as biphasic with a half-life of about ½ hour in the initial phase and 16½ hours in the terminal phase.

Contraindications and precautions
Doxorubicin is contraindicated in patients with hepatic dysfunction, depressed bone marrow function or impaired cardiac function and in patients who have previously received lifetime cumulative doses of doxorubicin or daunorubicin because of increased potential for cardiac or hematopoietic toxicity.

Interactions
Concomitant use with streptozocin may increase the plasma half-life of doxorubicin by an unknown mechanism, increasing the activity of doxorubicin. Concomitant use of daunorubicin or cyclophosphamide may potentiate the cardiotoxicity of doxorubicin through additive effects on the heart. Doxorubicin should not be mixed with heparin sodium, fluorouracil, aminophylline, cephalosporins, dexamethasone phosphate, or hydrocortisone sodium phosphate because it will result in a precipitate. Serum digoxin levels may be decreased if used concomitantly with doxorubicin.

Effects on diagnostic tests
Doxorubicin therapy may increase blood and urine concentrations of uric acid.

Adverse reactions
- CV: *cardiotoxicity,* seen in such ECG changes as sinus tachycardia, T-wave flattening, ST segment depression, and voltage reduction; *arrhythmias; irreversible cardiomyopathy,* sometimes with pulmonary edema.
- DERM: hyperpigmentation, especially in previously irradiated areas.
- GI: nausea, vomiting, diarrhea, stomatitis, esophagitis.
- GU: transient red urine.
- HEMA: *leukopenia,* especially agranulocytosis, during days 10 to 15, with recovery by day 21; *thrombocytopenia; bone marrow depression* (dose-limiting).
- Local: severe cellulitis.
- Other: hyperpigmentation of nails and dermal creases, complete alopecia.
  Note: Drug should be discontinued if hematopoietic toxicity becomes severe.

Overdose and treatment
Clinical manifestations of overdose include myelosuppression, nausea, vomiting, mucositis, and irreversible myocardial toxicity.
Treatment is usually supportive and includes transfusion of blood components, antiemetics, antibiotics for infections which may develop, symptomatic treatment of mucositis, and digitalis preparations.

▶ Special considerations
- To reconstitute, add 5 ml of normal saline solution to the 10-mg vial, 10 ml to the 20-mg vial, and 25 ml to the 50-mg vial, to yield a concentration of 2 mg/ml.
- Drug may be further diluted with normal saline solution or dextrose 5% in water and administered by I.V. infusion.
- Drug may be administered by I.V. push injection over 5 to 10 minutes into the tubing of a freely flowing I.V. infusion.
- The alternative dosage schedule (once-weekly dosing) has been found to cause a lower incidence of cardiomyopathy.
- If cumulative dose exceeds 550 mg/m² body surface area, 30% of patients develop cardiac adverse reactions, which begin 2 weeks to 6 months after stopping drug.
- The occurrence of streaking along a vein or facial flushing indicates that the drug is being administered too rapidly.
- Applying a scalp tourniquet or ice may decrease alopecia. However, *do not* use these if treating leukemias or other neoplasms where tumor stem cells may be present in scalp.
- Drug should be discontinued or rate of infusion slowed if tachycardia develops. Treat extravasation with topical application of dimethyl sulfoxide and ice packs.
- Monitor CBC and hepatic function.
- Decrease dosage as follows if serum bilirubin level increases: 50% of dose when bilirubin level is 1.2 to 3

mg/100 ml; 25% of dose when bilirubin level exceeds 3 mg/100 ml.

• Esophagitis is very common in patients who have also received radiation therapy.

Information for the patient

• Encourage adequate fluid intake to increase urine output and facilitate excretion of uric acid.
• Advise patient to avoid exposure to people with infections.
• Warn patient that alopecia will occur. Explain that hair growth should resume 2 to 5 months after drug is stopped.
• Advise that urine will become reddish for 1 to 2 days after the dose and does not indicate bleeding. The urine may stain clothes.
• Tell patient not to receive any immunizations during therapy and for several weeks after. Other members of the patient's household should also not receive immunizations during the same period.
• Tell patient to call if he notices unusual bruising or bleeding.

Geriatric use

Patients over age 70 have an increased incidence of drug-induced cardiotoxicity. Caution should be taken in elderly patients with low bone marrow reserve to prevent serious hematologic toxicity.

Pediatric use

Children under age 2 have a higher incidence of drug-induced cardiotoxicity.

Breast-feeding

It is not known whether doxorubicin distributes into breast milk. However, because of the risk of serious adverse reactions, mutagenicity, and carcinogenicity in the infant, breast-feeding is not recommended.

---

doxycycline hyclate
Doryx, Doxy-100, Doxy-200, Doxy-Caps, Doxychel, Doxy-Lemmon, Doxy-Tabs, Vibramycin, Vibra-Tabs, Vivox

• Pharmacologic classification: tetracycline
• Therapeutic classification: antibiotic
• Pregnancy risk category D

How supplied

Available by prescription only
Capsules: 50 mg, 100 mg
Tablets: 50 mg, 100 mg
Injection: 100 mg, 200 mg
Syrup: 50 mg/5 ml
Suspension: 25 mg/5 ml

Indications, route, and dosage
Infections caused by sensitive organisms
Adults: 100 mg P.O. q 12 hours on 1st day, then 100 mg P.O. daily; or 200 mg I.V. on 1st day in one or two infusions, then 100 to 200 mg I.V. daily.
Children over age 8 weighing less than 45 kg: 4.4 mg/kg P.O. or I.V. daily, divided q 12 hours 1st day, then 2.2 to 4.4 mg/kg daily. For children weighing more than 45 kg, dosage is same as adults.

Give I.V. infusion slowly (minimum 1 hour). Infusion must be completed within 12 hours (within 6 hours in lactated Ringer's solution or dextrose 5% in lactated Ringer's solution).
Gonorrhea in patients allergic to penicillin
Adults: 200 mg P.O. initially, followed by 100 mg P.O. at bedtime, then 100 mg P.O. b.i.d. for 3 days; or 300 mg P.O. initially and repeat dose in 1 hour.
†**Late latent syphilis of more than 1 year's duration, gummas, and cardiovascular syphilis (alternate therapy) in nonpregnant patients allergic to penicillin**
Adults: 100 mg P.O. b.i.d. for 2 weeks.
Chlamydia trachomatis, nongonococcal urethritis, and uncomplicated urethral, endocervical, or rectal infections and prophylaxis for rape victims
Adults: 100 mg P.O. b.i.d. for at least 7 days.
†**To prevent "traveler's diarrhea" commonly caused by enterotoxigenic Escherichia coli**
Adults: 100 mg P.O. b.i.d.
Lymphogranuloma venereum
Adults: 100 mg P.O. b.i.d. for 21 days.
Chemoprophylaxis for malaria in travelers to areas where chloroquine-resistant Plasmodium falciparum is endemic and mefloquine is contraindicated
Adults: 100 mg P.O. once daily. Begin prophylaxis 1 to 2 days before travel to malarious areas, continue daily while in affected area, and continue for 4 weeks after return from malarious area.
Children over age 8: 2 mg/kg P.O. daily as a single dose, not to exceed 100 mg daily. Employ the same dosage schedule as for adults.

Pharmacodynamics
Antibacterial action: Doxycycline is bacteriostatic; it binds reversibly to ribosomal units, thereby inhibiting bacterial protein synthesis.

Doxycycline's spectrum of activity includes many gram-negative and gram-positive organisms, *Mycoplasma, Rickettsia, Chlamydia,* and spirochetes.

Pharmacokinetics
• *Absorption:* Doxycycline is 90% to 100% absorbed after oral administration; peak serum levels occur at 1½ to 4 hours. Doxycycline has the least affinity for calcium of all tetracyclines; its absorption is insignificantly altered by milk or other dairy products.
• *Distribution:* Doxycycline is distributed widely into body tissues and fluids, including synovial, pleural, prostatic, and seminal fluids; bronchial secretions; saliva; and aqueous humor. CSF penetration is poor. Doxycycline readily crosses the placenta; it is 25% to 93% protein-bound.
• *Metabolism:* Doxycycline is insignificantly metabolized; some hepatic degradation occurs.
• *Excretion:* Doxycycline is excreted primarily unchanged in urine by glomerular filtration; some drug may be excreted in breast milk. Plasma half-life is 22 to 24 hours after multiple dosing in adults with normal renal function; 20 to 30 hours in patients with severe renal impairment. Some drug is excreted in feces.

Contraindications and precautions
Doxycycline is contraindicated in patients with known hypersensitivity to any tetracycline; during the second half of pregnancy; and in children under age 8 because

---

of the risk of permanent discoloration of teeth, enamel defects, and retardation of bone growth.

Use doxycycline with caution in patients with impaired renal function, as serum half-life is prolonged; and in patients likely to be exposed to direct sunlight or ultraviolet light because of the risk of photosensitivity reactions.

Interactions

Concomitant use of doxycycline with antacids containing aluminum, calcium, or magnesium or laxatives containing magnesium decreases oral absorption of doxycycline because of chelation; oral iron products and sodium bicarbonate also impair absorption of tetracyclines.

Doxycycline may antagonize bactericidal effects of penicillin, inhibiting cell growth because of bacteriostatic action; administer penicillin 2 to 3 hours before tetracycline.

Concomitant use of doxycycline with oral anticoagulants necessitates lowered dosage of oral anticoagulants because of enhanced effects; when used with digoxin, lowered dosages of digoxin because of increased bioavailability.

Effects on diagnostic tests

Doxycycline causes false-negative results in urine tests using glucose oxidase reagent (Clinistix or TesTape); parenteral dosage form may cause false-negative Clinitest results.

Doxycycline also causes false elevations in fluorometric tests for urinary catecholamines.

Adverse reactions

● CNS: *intracranial hypertension.*
● CV: pericarditis.
● DERM: maculopapular and erythematous rashes, photosensitivity, increased pigmentation, urticaria, discolored nails.
● EENT: sore throat, glossitis, dysphagia.
● GI: anorexia, epigastric distress, nausea, vomiting, diarrhea, enterocolitis, anogenital inflammation.
● GU: reversible nephrotoxicity (Fanconi's syndrome) with outdated tetracyclines.
● HEMA: neutropenia, eosinophilia.
● Local: thrombophlebitis.
● Other: hypersensitivity, bacterial and fungal superinfection, discolored teeth.

Note: Drug should be discontinued if signs of toxicity or hypersensitivity or superinfection occur; if erythema follows exposure to sunlight or ultraviolet light; or if severe diarrhea indicates pseudomembranous colitis.

Overdose and treatment

Clinical signs of overdose are usually limited to the GI tract; give antacids or empty stomach by gastric lavage if ingestion occurred within the preceding 4 hours.

▶ Special considerations

Besides those relevant to all *tetracyclines,* consider the following recommendations.
● Reconstitute powder for injection with sterile water for injection. Use 10 ml in a 100-mg vial and 20 ml in a 200-mg vial. Dilute solution to 100 to 1,000 ml for I.V. infusion. Do not infuse solutions more concentrated than 1 mg/ml.
● Reconstituted solution is stable for 72 hours if refrigerated and protected from light.
● Do not inject S.C. or I.M.

● Doxycycline may be used in patients with impaired renal function; it does not accumulate or cause a significant rise in BUN levels.

Pediatric use
Drug should not be used in children younger than age 9.

Breast-feeding
Avoid use in breast-feeding women.

dronabinol (THC)
Marinol

● Pharmacologic classification: cannabinoid
● Therapeutic classification: antiemetic
● Controlled substance schedule II
● Pregnancy risk category B

How supplied
Available by prescription only
Capsules: 2.5 mg, 10 mg

Indications, route, and dosage
Nausea and vomiting associated with cancer chemotherapy
Adults and children: 5 mg/m^2 P.O. 1 to 3 hours before administration of chemotherapy; then same dose q 2 to 4 hours after chemotherapy for a total of 4 to 6 doses daily. Dose may be increased in increments of 2.5 mg/m^2 to a maximum of 15 mg/m^2 per dose.

Pharmacodynamics
Antiemetic action: Dronabinol is a synthetic cannabinoid that inhibits vomiting centers in the brain and possibly in the chemoreceptor trigger zone and other sites.

Pharmacokinetics
● *Absorption:* About 10% to 20% of dose is absorbed; action begins in 30 to 60 minutes, with peak action in 1 to 3 hours.
● *Distribution:* Dronabinol is distributed rapidly into many tissue sites. Drug is 97% to 99% protein-bound.
● *Metabolism:* Dronabinol undergoes extensive metabolism in the liver. Metabolite activity is unknown.
● *Excretion:* Dronabinol is excreted primarily in feces, via the biliary tract. Drug effect may persist for several days after treatment ends; duration varies considerably among patients.

Contraindications and precautions
Dronabinol is contraindicated in patients with nausea and vomiting not secondary to cancer chemotherapy or not refractory to conventional antiemetics; and in patients with hypersensitivity to sesame oil or dronabinol.

Dronabinol should be used cautiously in elderly patients and patients with hypertension, cardiac disease, or psychiatric illness, because of possible CNS and cardiovascular adverse effects. In particular, drug may exacerbate underlying psychiatric illness.

Interactions
When used concomitantly with alcohol or other sedatives or psychotomimetic drugs, dronabinol may have an additive sedative effect. Dronabinol may alter ethanol

---

*Canada only   †Unlabeled clinical use   Italicized adverse reactions are life-threatening.

elimination, increasing it in some patients and decreasing it in others. Concomitant use with anticholinergics may cause tachycardia.

Effects on diagnostic tests
None reported.

Adverse reactions
• CNS: drowsiness, dizziness, euphoria, altered thinking, mood changes, psychosis, hallucinations, impaired coordination, irritability, anxiety, ataxia, visual distortions, confusion, depression, weakness, paresthesias.
• CV: orthostatic hypotension, tachycardia.
• GI: dry mouth, diarrhea.
• Other: muscle pain.
   Note: Drug should be discontinued if blood pressure drops.

Overdose and treatment
Treat overdose with symptomatic and supportive therapy. Observe patient in a quiet environment and provide supportive measures, including reassurance.

▶ **Special considerations**
• Dronabinol is used only in patients with nausea and vomiting resulting from cancer chemotherapy who do not respond to other treatment; drug should be given before chemotherapy infusion.
• Monitor frequency and degree of vomiting.
• Monitor pulse, blood pressure, and fluid intake and output to help prevent dehydration; observe for signs of confusion.
• Dronabinol is the major active ingredient of *Cannabis sativa* (marijuana) and therefore has a potential for abuse.

Information for the patient
• Warn patient to avoid driving and other activities requiring sound judgment until extent of CNS depressant effects are known.
• Urge family to ensure that patient is supervised by a responsible person during and immediately after treatment.
• Caution patient and family to anticipate drug's mood-altering effects.

Geriatric use
Elderly patients may be more susceptible to adverse reactions.

Breast-feeding
Dronabinol is concentrated and excreted in breast milk and is absorbed by breast-feeding infants.

droperidol
Inapsine

• Pharmacologic classification: butyrophenone derivative
• Therapeutic classification: tranquilizer
• Pregnancy risk category C

How supplied
Available by prescription only
Injection: 2.5 mg/ml

Indications, route, and dosage
Anesthestic premedication
Adults: 2.5 to 10 mg I.M. or I.V. 30 to 60 minutes before induction of general anesthesia.
Children age 2 to 12: 0.088 to 0.165 mg/kg I.V. or I.M.
Adjunct for induction of general anesthesia
Adults: 0.22 to 0.275 mg/kg I.V. (preferably) or I.M. concomitantly with an analgesic and/or general anesthetic.
Children: 0.088 to 0.165 mg/kg I.V. or I.M.
Adjunct for maintenance of general anesthesia
Adults: 1.25 to 2.5 mg I.V.
For use without a general anesthetic during diagnostic procedures
Adults: 2.5 to 10 mg I.M. 30 to 60 minutes before the procedure. Additional doses of 1.25 to 2.5 mg I.V. are given as needed.
Adjunct to regional anesthesia
Adult: 2.5 to 5 mg I.M. or slow I.V. injection.
†*Antiemetic*
Adults: 6.25 mg I.M. or by slow I.V. injection

Pharmacodynamics
Tranquilizer action: Droperidol produces marked sedation by directly blocking subcortical receptors. Droperidol also blocks CNS receptors at the chemoreceptor trigger zone, producing an antiemetic effect.

Pharmacokinetics
• *Absorption:* Droperidol is well absorbed after I.M. injection. Sedation begins in 3 to 10 minutes, peaks at 30 minutes, and lasts for 2 to 4 hours; some alteration of consciousness may persist for 12 hours.
• *Distribution:* Distribution of droperidol is not well understood; drug crosses the blood-brain barrier and is distributed in the CSF. It also crosses the placenta.
• *Metabolism:* Droperidol is metabolized by the liver to p-fluoro-phenylacetic acid and p-hydroxypiperidine.
• *Excretion:* Droperidol and its metabolites are excreted in urine and feces.

Contraindications and precautions
Droperidol is contraindicated in patients with known hypersensitivity or intolerance to the drug. It should be used cautiously in patients with hypotension and other cardiovascular disease, because of its vasodilatory effects; in patients with hepatic or renal disease, in whom drug clearance may be impaired; and in patients taking other CNS depressants, including alcohol, opiates, and sedatives, because droperidol may potentiate the effects of these drugs.

Interactions
Droperidol potentiates the CNS depressant effects of opiate or other analgesics and has an additive or potentiating effect when used concomitantly with other CNS depressants, such as alcohol, barbiturates, tranquilizers, and sedative-hypnotics. When used concurrently, the dosage of both drugs should be reduced.

Effects on diagnostic tests
Droperidol temporarily alters the EEG pattern, which returns slowly to normal after administration of the drug. Droperidol may decrease pulmonary artery pressure.

Adverse reactions
• CNS: sedation, altered consciousness, respiratory depression, postoperative hallucinations, extrapyramidal reactions (dystonia [extended tongue, stiff rotated

---

*Canada only   †Unlabeled clinical use   Italicized adverse reactions are life-threatening.

neck, upward rotation of eyes], akathesia [restlessness], fine tremors of limbs).
• CV: hypotension with rebound tachycardia, bradycardia (occasional), hypertension when combined with fentanyl or other parenteral analgesics (rare).
Note: Drug should be discontinued if patient shows signs of hypersensitivity, severe persistent hypotension, respiratory depression, paradoxical hypertension, or dystonia.

Overdose and treatment
Clinical signs of overdose include extension of the drug's pharmacologic actions. Treat overdose symptomatically and supportively.

▶ **Special considerations**
• Monitor vital signs and watch carefully for extrapyramidal reactions. Droperidol is related to haloperidol and is more likely than other antipsychotics to cause extrapyramidal symptoms.
• If opiates are required during recovery from anesthesia to prevent potentiation of respiratory depression, they should be used initially in reduced dosages (as low as ¼ to ⅓ of the usual recommended dosage).
• Droperidol has been used for its antiemetic effects in preventing or treating cancer chemotherapy-induced nausea and vomiting, especially that produced by cisplatin.
• Observe for postoperative hallucinations or emergence delirium and drowsiness.
• Be prepared to treat severe hypotension.

Information for the patient
Advise patient of possible postoperative effects.

Geriatric use
Drug should be used with caution.

Pediatric use
Safety and efficacy in children younger than age 2 have not been established.

Breast-feeding
It is unknown whether droperidol distributes into breast milk.

---

dyclonine hydrochloride
Dyclone

• Pharmacologic classification: topical local anesthetic (unclassified)
• Therapeutic classification: local anesthetic
• Pregnancy risk category C

How supplied
Available by prescription only
Solution: 0.5%, 1%

Available without a prescription
Lozenges: 1.2 mg, 3 mg

Indications, route, and dosage
Relief of pain and itching from minor burns, insect bites, or irritations, or episiotomy or anogenital lesions; to anesthetize mucous membranes before endoscopic procedures
Adults and children: Dosage varies with area to be anesthetized and technique used. Generally, apply to affected area as needed. If used before urologic endoscopy, instill 6 to 30 ml of the solution into the urethra before the procedure. Have patient retain the solution for 5 to 10 minutes.
Local anesthesia before laryngoscopy, bronchoscopy, esophagoscopy, or endotracheal procedures
Adults: Before bronchoscopy, 2 ml of the 1% dyclonine hydrochloride solution (20 mg) may be sprayed into the larynx and trachea every 5 minutes until the laryngeal reflex is abolished; 2 or 3 applications usually are required. Five minutes should elapse before bronchoscopy is performed. For esophagoscopy after pharyngeal anesthesia, 10 to 15 ml of the 0.5% solution (50 to 75 mg) is swallowed. To produce local analgesia in the throat and oral cavity, 5 to 10 ml of the 0.5% or 1% solution (25 to 100 mg) may be swabbed, gargled, or sprayed and then expectorated. For relief of esophageal pain, 5 to 15 ml of the 0.5% solution (25 to 75 mg) may be swallowed.
For temporary relief of minor sore throat pain or mouth irritation
Adults and children over age 12: Dissolve one lozenge slowly in the mouth; may be repeated q 2 hours if needed.

Pharmacodynamics
Anesthetic action: Dyclonine blocks conduction of nerve impulses at the sensory nerve endings by altering cell membrane permeability to ionic transfer.

Pharmacokinetics
• *Absorption:* Limited with short-term topical use. Topical application produces local anesthesia within 2 to 10 minutes, lasting for about 30 minutes.
• *Distribution:* None.
• *Metabolism:* None.
• *Excretion:* None.

Contraindications and precautions
Dyclonine hydrochloride is contraindicated in patients with hypersensitivity to the drug or in patients undergoing cystoscopic procedures after excretion urography, because visualization may be impaired. It should be used with caution on ulcerated or inflamed areas or for prolonged periods, as increased absorption nonselectively increases drug effectiveness, untoward effects, and systemic toxicity.

Interactions
None reported.

Effects on diagnostic tests
None reported.

Adverse reactions
• CNS: stimulation or depression.
• Local: irritation or stinging.
Note: Drug should be discontinued if sensitization occurs.

Overdose and treatment
No information available.

▶ **Special considerations**
If used as an oral topical anesthetic, dyclonine may impair patient's swallowing ability. Watch for aspiration.

Information for the patient
● Explain correct use of drug, and stress avoidance of contact with eyes; emphasize need to wash hands thoroughly after use.
● Caution patient to apply drug sparingly, to minimize systemic effects.
● Advise keeping drug out of reach of children.

Pediatric use
Lozenges are not recommended for children under age 12.

Breast-feeding
Drug should not be used in breast-feeding women.

---

dyphylline
Dilor, Dyflex, Dy-Phyl-Lin, Lufyllin, Neothylline, Oxystat, Protophylline*

● Pharmacologic classification: xanthine derivative
● Therapeutic classification: bronchodilator
● Pregnancy risk category C

How supplied
Available by prescription only
Tablets: 200 mg, 400 mg
Elixir: 100 mg/15 ml, 160 mg/15 ml
Injection: 250 mg/ml in vials and ampules

Indications, route, and dosage
For relief of acute and chronic bronchial asthma and reversible bronchospasm associated with chronic bronchitis and emphysema
Adults: 200 to 800 mg P.O. q 6 hours; or 500 mg initially, followed by 250 to 500 mg I.M. at 6-hour intervals. It should be given very slowly.

Pharmacodynamics
Bronchodilating action: The exact mechanism is not known, but the action of dyphylline is similar to that of theophylline. Unlike other theophylline derivatives, dyphylline is not metabolized to theophylline *in vivo;* therefore, serum theophylline concentrations cannot be used to determine dosage adjustments. Use dyphilline serum levels, which are available.

Pharmacokinetics
● *Absorption:* Approximately 75% of an oral dose is absorbed rapidly; peak concentration occurs in 1 hour.
● *Distribution:* Drug is distributed rapidly and widely in body fluids and tissues.
● *Metabolism:* Metabolism of dyphylline is unknown; however, dyphylline is not metabolized to theophylline. Half-life is approximately 2 hours; it increases in patients with decreased renal function.
● *Excretion:* About 88% of the drug is excreted unchanged in urine.

Contraindications and precautions
Dyphylline is contraindicated in patients with hypersensitivity to xanthines. Use cautiously in patients with compromised cardiac or circulatory function, diabetes, glaucoma, hypertension, hyperthyroidism, peptic ulcer, or gastroesophageal reflux, because drug may worsen these symptoms or conditions.

Interactions
Concomitant use of dyphylline and xanthines, sympathomimetics, or ephedrine produces synergistic effects. Probenecid increases the half-life of dyphylline by blocking renal tubular secretion.
Alkali-sensitive drugs: reduced activity. Do not add to I.V. fluids containing aminophylline.
Beta-adrenergic blockers: antagonism. Propanolol and nadolol, especially, may cause bronchospasm in sensitive patients. Use together cautiously.
Troleandomycin, erythromycin, and cimetidine: decreased hepatic clearance of theophylline; elevated theophylline levels. Monitor for signs of toxicity.
Barbiturates, phenytoin: enhanced metabolism and decreased theophylline blood levels. Monitor for decreased theophylline effect.

Effects on diagnostic tests
None reported.

Adverse reactions
● CNS: irritability, restlessness, headache, insomnia, dizziness, convulsions, depression, light-headedness, muscle twitching.
● CV: palpitations, marked hypotension, flushing, sinus tachycardia, *ventricular tachycardia* and other life-threatening dysrhythmias, extrasystoles, *circulatory failure.*
● DERM: urticaria.
● GI: nausea, vomiting, epigastric pain, loss of appetite, diarrhea, bitter aftertaste, dyspepsia.
● Respiratory: tachypnea, *respiratory arrest.*
● Other: fever, urinary retention, hyperglycemia.
Note: Drug should be discontinued if an adverse reaction intensifies; this signals impending overdose.

Overdose and treatment
Clinical manifestations of overdose include nausea, vomiting, insomnia, irritability, tachycardia, extrasystoles, tachypnea, and tonic/clonic seizures. The onset of toxicity may be sudden and severe, with dysrhythmias and seizures as the first signs. Induce emesis, except in convulsing patients, then give activated charcoal and cathartics. Treat arrhythmias with lidocaine and seizures with I.V. benzodiazepine; support respiratory and cardiovascular function.

▶ **Special considerations**
● I.V. use of injectable form is not recommended.
● Dose should be decreased in renal insufficiency.
● Gastric irritation may be relieved by taking oral drug after meals; no evidence that antacids reduce this adverse reaction. May produce less gastric discomfort than theophylline.
● Monitor vital signs and intake and output. Expected clinical effects include improvement in quality of pulse and respiration.
● Dyphylline is metabolized faster than theophylline; dosage intervals may have to be decreased to ensure continual therapeutic effect. Higher daily doses may be

---

needed. Dyphilline may be less effective than theophylline.

• Discard dyphylline ampule if precipitate is present. Protect from light.

Information for the patient

• Instruct patient about dosage schedule. Explain why dosage must be maintained. If a dose is missed, take as soon as possible; do not double up on doses.
• Advise the patient of the adverse reactions and possible signs of toxicity.
• Warn that nonprescription remedies may contain ephedrine in combination with theophylline salts; excessive CNS stimulation may result. Patient should not take *any* other medications unless prescribed.
• Tell patient to avoid consuming large quantities of xanthine-containing foods and beverages.

Geriatric use

• Use reduced doses and monitor patient closely.
• Warn patients to take safety precautions, because dizziness may occur.

Pediatric use

Pediatric dosage has not been established.

Breast-feeding

Drug is excreted in breast milk and may cause irritability, insomnia, or fretfulness in the breast-fed infant.

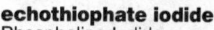

echothiophate iodide
Phospholine Iodide

- Pharmacologic classification: cholines-terase inhibitor
- Therapeutic classification: miotic
- Pregnancy risk category C

How supplied
Available by prescription only
Ophthalmic: powder for reconstitution to make 0.03%, 0.06%, 0.125%, and 0.25% solutions

Indications, route, and dosage
Open-angle glaucoma, conditions obstructing aqueous outflow
Adults and children: Instill 1 drop of 0.03% to 0.125% solution into conjunctival sac daily. Maximum dosage is 1 drop b.i.d. Use lowest possible dosage to continuously control intraocular pressure.
Diagnosis of convergent strabismus
Adults: Instill 1 drop of 0.125% solution daily h.s. for 2 to 3 weeks.
Treatment of convergent strabismus
Adults: Instill 1 drop of 0.03% to 0.125% solution daily or every other day h.s.

Pharmacodynamics
Miotic action: Echothiophate inhibits the enzymatic destruction of acetylcholine by inactivating cholinesterase. Acetylcholine acts on the effector cells of the iridic sphincter and ciliary muscles, causing pupillary constriction and accommodation spasm.

Pharmacokinetics
- *Absorption:* Unknown.
- *Distribution:* Unknown.
- *Metabolism:* Unknown.
- *Excretion:* Duration of effect can be up to 1 week or longer.

Contraindications and precautions
Echothiophate is contraindicated in patients with hypersensitivity to cholinesterase inhibitors, active uveal inflammation or inflammatory diseases of the iris or ciliary body, narrow-angle or angle-closure glaucoma (most cases) or epilepsy, vasomotor instability, parkinsonism, iodide hypersensitivity, bronchial asthma, spastic GI conditions, urinary tract obstruction, peptic ulcer, severe bradycardia or hypotension, vascular hypertension, myocardial infarction, or history of retinal detachment because the drug can worsen these symptoms or disorders.

Drug should be used with caution in patients routinely exposed to organophosphate insecticides, because of potential for additive toxicity; it may cause nausea, vomiting, and diarrhea, progressing to muscle weakness and respiratory difficulty. It should be used cautiously in patients with myasthenia gravis who are receiving anticholinesterase therapy.

Interactions
When used concomitantly, echothiophate may increase the neuromuscular-blocking effects of succinylcholine, antagonize the antiglaucoma effect of cyclopentolate and the belladonna alkaloids, increase the toxicity of carbonate organophosphate insecticides and cholinesterase inhibitors, and add to effects of systemic anticholinesterase agents used for myasthenia gravis.

Effects on diagnostic tests
Echothiophate therapy decreases plasma cholinesterase activity.

Adverse reactions
- CNS: muscle weakness, headache.
- CV: bradycardia, hypotension, *arrhythmias.*
- Eye: reversible iris cysts, blurred or dimmed vision, eye or brow pain, lid twitching, conjunctival and intraocular hyperemia, lens opacities, lacrimation, retinal detachment, excessive vitreous hemorrhage; paradoxical, increased intraocular pressure.
- GI: diarrhea, nausea, vomiting, abdominal pain, intestinal cramps, salivation.
- GU: frequent urination, urinary incontinence.
- Respiratory: dyspnea.
  Note: Drug should be discontinued if the following occur: salivation, diarrhea, profuse sweating, urinary incontinence, or muscle weakness.

Overdose and treatment
Clinical manifestations of overdose include tremor, syncope, headache, bradycardia, hypotension, arrhythmias, diarrhea, nausea, vomiting, abdominal pain, excessive salivation, urinary incontinence, and dyspnea. Toxicity can be cumulative, with symptoms appearing weeks to months after initiating therapy.

To treat accidental overdose after ingestion, employ general measures, such as emesis, cathartics, or lavage to remove the drug from the GI tract. Treat dermal exposure by washing the area twice with soap and water. The extent of echothiophates' potential toxicity is not well known; observe patient closely for signs and symptoms, and treat symptomatically and supportively. Atropine sulfate (S.C., I.M., or I.V.) has been suggested as the antidote of choice.

▶ Special considerations
- Reconstitute powder carefully to avoid contamination; use only diluent provided. Discard refrigerated, reconstituted solution after 6 months; discard solution at room temperature after 1 month.
- Drug should be discontinued at least 2 weeks preoperatively if succinylcholine is to be used in surgery. Inform anesthesiologist.
- Echothiophate iodide is a potent, long-acting, irreversible drug.

Information for the patient
● Warn patient that transient brow ache or dimmed or blurred vision is common at first but usually disappears within 5 to 10 days; advise instillation at bedtime to minimize effects of blurred vision.
● Patient or family must inform physician or anesthesiologist about use of this drug before undergoing any general anesthesia.
● Teach patient correct use, storage, and reconstitution of product.

Geriatric use
Elderly patients may be at increased risk for adverse reactions.

Pediatric use
Safety and efficacy have not been established; iris cysts have been reported, but these generally resolve spontaneously when drug is discontinued. Many ophthalmologists avoid using drug in children because of reports of lens opacities in adults.

econazole nitrate
Spectazole

● Pharmacologic classification: synthetic imidazole derivative
● Therapeutic classification: antifungal
● Pregnancy risk category C

How supplied
Available by prescription only
Cream: 1% (water-soluble base)

Indications, route, and dosage
Tinea pedis, tinea cruris, and tinea corporis; cutaneous candidiasis
Adults and children: Gently rub sufficient quantity into affected areas b.i.d. in the morning and evening.
Tinea versicolor
Adults and children: Gently rub into affected area once daily.

Pharmacodynamics
Antifungal action: Although exact mechanism of action is unknown, econazole is thought to exert its effects by altering cellular membranes and interfering with intracellular enzymes. Econazole is active against many fungi, including dermatophytes and yeasts, as well as some gram-positive bacteria.

Pharmacokinetics
● *Absorption:* Minimal but rapid percutaneous absorption.
● *Distribution:* Minimal.
● *Metabolism:* Unknown.
● *Excretion:* Unknown.

Contraindications and precautions
Econazole nitrate is contraindicated in patients with known hypersensitivity and during the first trimester of pregnancy. It should be used in second and third trimesters only if deemed essential to patient's welfare.

Interactions
None reported.

Effects on diagnostic tests
None reported.

Adverse reactions
● Local: chemical irritation, burning, itching, stinging, erythema.
  Note: Drug should be discontinued if sensitization develops, condition persists or worsens, or irritation occurs.

Overdose and treatment
Discontinue therapy.

▶ Special considerations
● Wash affected area with soap and water, and dry thoroughly before applying drug.
● Do not apply econazole to the eye or administer intravaginally.

Information for the patient
● Instruct patient to wash hands well after application.
● Advise patient to use medication for entire treatment period, even though symptoms lessen. Relief of symptoms usually occurs within the first week or two of therapy.
● Advise patient with tinea pedis (athlete's foot) to wear well-fitting, well-ventilated shoes. Shoes and all-cotton socks should be changed daily.

Breast-feeding
Drug should be used with caution in breast-feeding women, as it is unknown whether econazole is distributed into breast milk.

edetate calcium disodium (calcium EDTA)
Calcium Disodium Versenate

● Pharmacologic classification: chelating agent
● Therapeutic classification: heavy metal antagonist
● Pregnancy risk category C

How supplied
Available by prescription only
Injection: 200 mg/ml

Indications, route, and dosage
Symptomatic lead poisoning without encephalopathy and blood lead concentrations less than 100 mcg/dl
Adults and children: 1 g/m^2 I.V. or I.M. daily for 3 to 5 days.
Severe lead poisoning with symptoms of encephalopathy and/or blood lead concentrations greater than 100 mcg/dl
Adults and children: 250 mg/m^2 per dose (1.5 g/m^2 daily) deep I.M. injection or continuous I.V. infusion 4 hours after initial dimercaprol injection and at 4-hour intervals thereafter usually for 5 days.

Pharmacodynamics
Chelating action: Calcium in edetate calcium disodium is displaced by divalent and trivalent heavy metals,

forming a soluble complex, which is then excreted in urine, removing the heavy metal.

Pharmacokinetics
• *Absorption:* Edetate calcium disodium is well absorbed after I.M. or S.C. injection. After I.V. administration, chelated lead appears in urine within 1 hour; peak excretion of lead occurs in 24 to 48 hours.
• *Distribution:* Edetate calcium disodium is distributed primarily in extracellular fluid.
• *Metabolism:* None.
• *Excretion:* Edetate calcium disodium is excreted rapidly in urine. After I.V. administration, 50% of drug is excreted in urine unchanged or as a metal chelate in 1 hour; 95% of drug is excreted in 24 hours.

Contraindications and precautions
Edetate calcium disodium is contraindicated in patients with severe renal disease and anuria because of its possible nephrotoxic effects. Avoid rapid I.V. infusion in patients with lead encephalopathy because it may increase intracranial pressure to lethal levels.

Edetate calcium disodium should be used cautiously in patients with renal insufficiency or dehydration, who are at increased risk of renal failure because of its potential for nephrotoxicity.

Interactions
None reported.

Effects on diagnostic tests
None reported.

Adverse reactions
• CNS: headache, malaise, fatigue, paresthesia, numbness, tingling.
• CV: thrombophlebitis, hypotension.
• DERM: skin and mucous membrane lesions, including cheilosis with long-term use.
• GI: anorexia, nausea, and vomiting.
• GU: proteinuria, microscopic hematuria, *renal tubular necrosis.*
• Other: excessive thirst, hypercalcemia, myalgia, arthralgia, bone marrow suppression with long-term use, sudden fever and chills.
    Note: Drug should be discontinued if any of the following occur: hypersensitivity; increases in proteinuria, urinary erythrocytes, or large renal epithelial cells; T-wave inversion on ECG; anuria.

Overdose and treatment
Clinical signs of overdose include acute renal failure with anuria, and altered consciousness consistent with increased intracranial pressure, in patients with lead encephalopathy. Reduce intracranial pressure with hyperventilation and furosemide or mannitol; monitor vital signs and ECG closely. Barbiturate infusion may be needed in severe cases; hemodialysis may be needed in acute renal failure.

▶ Special considerations
• Add 1% procaine before I.M. injection to decrease pain at site.
• Avoid rapid I.V. infusion and infusions of large fluid volumes in patients with lead encephalopathy.
• Hydrate patient before giving drug, to ensure adequate urine flow; monitor renal status frequently.
• Monitor intake and output, urinalysis, BUN levels and ECG throughout therapy.

• Parenterally administered edetate calcium disodium has been used in poisoning by radioactive and nuclear fusion products and other heavy metals except mercury, gold, or arsenic poisoning. It has also been used to aid diagnosis of lead poisoning.
• For I.V. infusion, dilute drug with dextrose 5% solution or 0.9% sodium chloride; administer one half the daily dose over at least a 1-hour period in asymptomatic patients; 2 hours in symptomatic patients. The second daily infusion should be given 6 or more hours after the first infusion. If administered as a single dose, infuse over 12 to 24 hours.
• If drug is administered as a continuous I.V. infusion, interrupt infusion for at least 1 hour before a blood lead concentration to avoid a falsely elevated value.

Information for the patient
As appropriate, explain measures to avoid future heavy metal poisoning.

Pediatric use
I.M. route is recommended for children.

---

edetate disodium (EDTA)
Chealamide, Disotate, Endrate

• Pharmacologic classification: chelating agent
• Therapeutic classification: heavy metal antagonist
• Pregnancy risk category C

How supplied
Available by prescription only
Injection: 150 mg/ml

Indications, route, and dosage
Hypercalcemia
Adults: 50 mg/kg daily by slow I.V. infusion to a maximum of 3 g in 24 hours. Dilute in 500 ml of dextrose 5% in water (D_5W) or 0.9% sodium chloride. Give over 3 or more hours.
Children: 40 to 70 mg/kg daily by slow I.V. infusion administered over 3 to 4 hours.
Digitalis-induced cardiac arrhythmias
Adults and children: I.V. infusion of 15 mg/kg/hour; maximum dosage is 60 mg/kg daily. Dilute in D_5W.

Pharmacodynamics
Chelating agent: Edetate disodium binds many divalent and trivalent ions but has the strongest affinity for calcium, with which it forms a stable complex readily excreted by the kidney. Edetate disodium also chelates magnesium, zinc, and other trace metals, increasing their urinary excretion; it does not decrease CSF calcium concentrations.

Pharmacokinetics
• *Absorption:* Edetate disodium is absorbed poorly from the GI tract.
• *Distribution:* Edetate disodium does not enter the CSF in significant amounts but distributes widely throughout the rest of the body.
• *Metabolism:* None.
• *Excretion:* After I.V. administration, edetate disodium

---

is excreted rapidly in urine; 95% of the dose is excreted within 24 hours.

Contraindications and precautions

Edetate disodium is contraindicated in patients with severe renal failure or anuria; in patients with suspected or known hypocalcemia, active or healed tuberculosis, or severe heart, renal, or coronary artery disease; in elderly patients with generalized arteriosclerosis; and in patients with a history of seizures, because drug may exacerbate the signs and symptoms of these conditions.

Edetate disodium should be used cautiously in patients with renal impairment; in patients with incipient congestive heart failure, because its effect on calcium concentration depresses cardiac function and because large sodium and fluid loads are delivered during therapy; and in patients with hypokalemia or hypomagnesemia, because drug may lower total body stores via increased renal excretion.

Drug should not be used to treat lead poisoning; edetate calcium disodium should be used instead.

Interactions

Edetate disodium interferes with the cardiac effects of digitalis glycosides indirectly by decreasing intracellular calcium by both chelation and urinary excretion of extracellular calcium.

Drug may decrease insulin requirements in diabetic patients by chelation of zinc in exogenous insulin.

Effects on diagnostic tests

Edetate disodium lowers serum calcium concentrations when measured by oxalate or other precipitation methods and by colorimetry. The drug also lowers blood glucose concentration in diabetic patients. Edetate disodium-induced hypomagnesemia decreases serum alkaline phosphatase levels.

Adverse reactions

● CNS: *seizures*, headache, circumoral paresthesia, numbness.
● CV: *severe cardiac arrhythmias*, hypotension.
● DERM: erythema, *exfoliative dermatitis*.
● GI: nausea, diarrhea, vomiting, abdominal cramps, anorexia.
● GU: urinary urgency, nocturia, polyuria, proteinuria, acute tubular necrosis.
● Metabolic: severe hypocalcemia, hypomagnesemia.
● Local: pain at infusion site, erythema, dermatitis.
● Other: fever, chills, back pain, muscle pain and weakness.

Note: Drug should be discontinued if hypocalcemia, cardiac arrhythmias, tetany, or seizures occur.

Overdose and treatment

Clinical signs of overdose may include hypotension, cardiac arrhythmias, and cardiac arrest. Treat hypotension with fluids, if necessary. Treat arrhythmias with lidocaine, and seizures and tetany with calcium replacement; use I.V. diazepam for refractory seizures. Replace magnesium and potassium, as needed.

▶ Special considerations

● Monitor infusion site closely. Extravasation severely irritates tissue; rotate infusion sites with multiple doses or chronic therapy.
● Do not exceed recommended rate of infusion or dosage; rapid infusion and/or high concentrations of ed-

etate disodium may precipitously decrease serum calcium levels, causing seizures and death. Therefore, have I.V. calcium replacement readily available whenever drug is administered.
● Monitor calcium levels, and observe patient for seizures or altered vital signs and ECG during infusion. Administer infusion over at least 3 hours; have patient remain supine for 20 to 30 minutes after infusion, because of possible postural hypotension. Drug also exerts a negative inotropic effect on the heart.
● Edetate disodium also has been used topically or by iontophoresis to treat corneal calcium deposits.
● Although once considered useful in treating digitalis-induced arrhythmias, edetate disodium has been replaced by digoxin immune Fab as the drug of choice for digoxin toxicity.

Information for the patient

● Explain possible adverse reactions; stress importance of reporting signs and symptoms of adverse reactions promptly.
● Tell diabetic patients that insulin dosage may need adjustment.

Geriatric use

Elderly patients with renal or cardiac failure are at increased risk; lower doses are recommended.

Pediatric use

Safety and efficacy in pediatric patients have not been established; give recommended dose slowly, over at least 3 hours.

edrophonium chloride

Enlon, Tensilon

● Pharmacologic classification: cholinesterase inhibitor
● Therapeutic classification: cholinergic agonist, diagnostic agent
● Pregnancy risk category C

How supplied

Available by prescription only
Injection: 10 mg/ml in 1-ml ampule or 10-ml vial

Indications, route, and dosage

Curare antagonist (to reverse neuromuscular blocking action)
Adults: 10 mg I.V. given over 30 to 45 seconds, repeated as necessary to 40 mg maximum dose. Larger doses may potentiate rather than antagonize effect of curare.
Diagnostic aid in myasthenia gravis
Adults: 1 to 2 mg I.V. within 15 to 30 seconds, then 8 mg if no response (increase in muscular strength).
Children weighing more than 75 pounds (34 kg): 2 mg I.V. If no response within 45 seconds, give 1 mg q 45 seconds to maximum of 10 mg.
Children weighing up to 75 pounds (34 kg): 1 mg I.V. If no response within 45 seconds, give 1 mg q 45 seconds to maximum of 5 mg.
Infants: 0.5 mg I.V.
To differentiate myasthenic crisis from cholinergic crisis
Adults: 1 mg I.V. If no response in 1 minute, repeat dose once. Increased muscular strength confirms myas-

EFLORNITHINE HYDROCHLORIDE 403

thenic crisis; no increase or exaggerated weakness confirms cholinergic crisis.

†*Paroxysmal supraventricular tachycardia*
Adults: 10 mg I.V. given over 1 minute or less.

Pharmacodynamics
Cholinergic action: Edrophonium blocks acetylcholine's hydrolysis by cholinesterase, resulting in acetylcholine accumulation at cholinergic synapses. That leads to increased cholinergic receptor stimulation at the neuromuscular junction and vagal sites. Edrophonium is a short-acting agent which makes it particularly useful for the diagnosis of myasthenia gravis.

Pharmacokinetics
● *Absorption:* Action begins 30 to 60 seconds after I.V. administration and 2 to 10 minutes after I.M. administration.
● *Distribution:* Edrophonium may cross the placenta; little else is known.
● *Metabolism:* Exact metabolic fate is unknown; drug is not hydrolyzed by cholinesterases. Duration of effect ranges from 5 to 10 minutes after I.V. administration and 5 to 30 minutes after I.M. administration.
● *Excretion:* Exact excretion mode is unknown.

Contraindications and precautions
Edrophonium is contraindicated in patients with mechanical obstruction of the GI or urinary tract because of its stimulatory effect on smooth muscle and in patients with bradycardia, hyperthyroidism, or hypotension, because it may exacerbate these conditions.

Administer edrophonium cautiously to patients with cardiac disease because of stimulating effects on cardiovascular system; to patients with peptic ulcer disease, because it may increase gastric acid secretion; and to patients with bronchial asthma, because it may precipitate asthma attacks.

Interactions
Concomitant use with procainamide or quinidine may reverse edrophonium's cholinergic effect on muscle. Use with corticosteroids may decrease edrophonium's cholinergic effects; when corticosteroids are stopped, however, cholinergic effects may increase, possibly affecting muscle strength.

Concomitant use with succinylcholine may cause prolonged respiratory depression from plasma esterase inhibition, leading to delayed succinylcholine hydrolysis. Concomitant use with ganglionic blockers, such as mecamylamine, may lead to a critical blood pressure decrease, usually preceded by abdominal symptoms. Magnesium administration has a direct depressant effect on skeletal muscle and concomitant administration may antagonize edrophonium's anticholinesterase effect. Concomitant use with other cholinergic drugs may lead to additive toxicity.

Effects on diagnostic tests
None reported.

Adverse reactions
● CNS: weakness, *respiratory paralysis,* sweating.
● CV: hypotension, bradycardia, palpitations.
● EENT: miosis, blurred vision.
● GI: nausea, vomiting, diarrhea, abdominal cramps, excessive salivation.
● Other: increased bronchial secretions, *bronchospasm,* muscle cramps, muscle fasciculation.

Note: Drug should be discontinued if hypersensitivity, difficulty breathing, or paralysis develops.

Overdose and treatment
Clinical signs of overdose include muscle weakness, nausea, vomiting, diarrhea, blurred vision, miosis, excessive tearing, bronchospasm, increased bronchial secretions, hypotension, incoordination, excessive sweating, cramps, fasciculations, paralysis, bradycardia or tachycardia, excessive salivation, and restlessness or agitation. Muscles first weakened by overdose include neck, jaw, and pharyngeal muscles, followed by muscle weakening of the shoulder, upper extremities, pelvis, outer eye, and legs.

Discontinue drug immediately. Support respiration; bronchial suctioning may be performed. Atropine may be given to block edrophonium's muscarinic effects but will not counter the drug's paralytic effects on skeletal muscle. Avoid atropine overdose, because it may lead to bronchial plug formation.

▶ **Special considerations**
Besides those relevant to all *cholinesterase inhibitors,* consider the following recommendations.
● Of all cholinergics, edrophonium has the most rapid onset of action but the shortest duration of effect; consequently, it is not used to treat myasthenia gravis.
● When giving edrophonium to differentiate myasthenic crisis from cholinergic crisis, evaluate patient's muscle strength closely.
● For easier administration, use a tuberculin syringe with an I.V. needle.

Information for the patient
Tell patient drug's adverse effects will be transient because of its short duration of effect.

Geriatric use
Elderly patients may be more sensitive to effects of this drug. Use with caution.

Pediatric use
Children may require I.M. administration; with this route, drug effects may be delayed for 2 to 10 minutes.

Breast-feeding
Safety not established. Breast-feeding women should avoid edrophonium.

eflornithine hydrochloride (DFMO)
Ornidyl

● Pharmacologic classification: ornithine decarboxylase inhibitor
● Therapeutic classification: antiprotozoal
● Pregnancy risk category C

How supplied
Available by prescription only
Injection: 200 mg/ml in 100-ml vials (concentrated)

Indications, route, and dosage
Treatment of meningoencephalitic stage of Trypanosoma brucei gambiense *infection (sleeping sickness); treatment of* Pneumocystis carinii *pneumonia in acquired immunodeficiency syndrome patients*
Adults: 100 mg/kg (46 mg/lb) q 6 hours administered by I.V. infusion over a minimum of 45 minutes daily for 14 days.
Dosage in renal failure
Excretion of the drug parallels creatinine clearance. Estimate creatinine clearance from serum creatinine as follows:

$$\text{Males: } \frac{\text{Creatinine}}{\text{clearance}} = \frac{\text{weight (kg)} \times (140\text{-age})}{72 \times \text{serum creatinine (mg/dl)}}$$

Females: 0.85 x male value.

Pharmacodynamics
Antiprotozoal action: Eflornithine is a selective, enzyme-activated, irreversible inhibitor of ornithine decarboxylase, blocking the conversion of ornithine to putrescine – the first and rate-limiting step in the biosynthesis of polyamine – which is thought to play an important role in cell differentiation and division.

Pharmacokinetics
● *Absorption:* Not applicable; administered by I.V. infusion.
● *Distribution:* Eflornithine is not significantly bound to plasma proteins. It does cross the blood-brain barrier, diffusing into the CNS in CSF at levels up to 51% of corresponding serum concentrations.
● *Metabolism:* Not significant.
● *Excretion:* 80% of the I.V. dose is excreted unchanged in the urine within 24 hours. The terminal plasma elimination half-life is 3 to 4 hours.

Contraindications and precautions
Use with caution in patients with renal impairment. In clinical trials, anemia was common among patients receiving the drug; however, many of these patients were anemic before therapy. Leukopenia usually occurs within 8 days after the start of treatment. This drug has also been associated with thrombocytopenia, seizures, and hearing impairment. Consider these potential complications during therapy.

Interactions
Other drugs should not be administered I.V. simultaneously during eflornithine administration.

Effects on diagnostic tests
None reported.

Adverse reactions
● CNS: seizures.
● HEMA: *myelosuppression,* anemia, leukopenia, thrombocytopenia.
● Other: hearing impairment (rare).

▶ **Special considerations**
● Because the drug is a myelosuppressant, careful monitoring of hematologic status is necessary for safe and effective use. Some degree of myelosuppression may be unavoidable; in most patients, problems resolve after discontinuation of the drug.
● Eflornithine concentrate is hypertonic and must be diluted with sterile water for injection before use. Diluted

drug must be used within 24 hours of preparation and stored at 39 F. (4 C.) to minimize risk of microbial proliferation.
● Perform CBC and platelet counts before therapy, twice weekly during therapy, and weekly after completion of therapy until hematologic values return to baseline.
● Patients should be monitored for at least 24 months to ensure further therapy in the event of relapse.
● To prepare solutions within 10% of plasma tonicity, use strict aseptic technique; withdraw the entire contents of each 100-ml vial of eflornithine and inject 25 ml into each of four diluent bags (100 ml of sterile water for injection per bag). Concentration will be 40 mg/ml (5,000 mg of eflornithine in 125 ml final volume).
● Serial audiograms are recommended to monitor degree of hearing impairment.

Geriatric use
Use cautiously because elderly patients may develop some degree of renal impairment.

Pediatric use
Safety and efficacy have not been established.

Breast-feeding
It is unknown if eflornithine is excreted in breast milk. Consider potential for serious adverse reactions in breast-fed infants against importance of drug to mother.

emetine hydrochloride

● Pharmacologic classification: ipecac alkaloid
● Therapeutic classification: amebicide
● Pregnancy risk category X

How supplied
Available by prescription only
Injection: 65 mg/ml

Indications, route, and dosage
Acute fulminating amebic dysentery
Adults: 1 mg/kg daily, up to 60 mg daily (one or two doses), deep S.C. or I.M. for 3 to 5 days to control symptoms. Give another antiamebic drug simultaneously.
Children: 1 mg/kg daily in two doses I.M. or S.C. for up to 5 days; maximum dosage 10 mg/day in children younger than age 8, and 20 mg/day in children older than age 8.
Amebic hepatitis and abscess
Adults: 60 mg daily (one or two doses) deep S.C. or I.M. for 10 days.
Dosage should be decreased by 50% in elderly and debilitated patients.

Pharmacodynamics
Amebicidal action: Emetine is amebicidal against protozoa, especially *Entamoeba histolytica;* it causes degeneration of the nucleus and reticulum of amebic cytoplasm.

Pharmacokinetics
● *Absorption:* Emetine causes nausea and vomiting and is absorbed erratically after oral administration; therefore, it is administered I.M. or S.C.

• *Distribution:* Emetine is distributed into the liver, lungs, kidneys, and spleen; it crosses the placenta.
• *Metabolism:* Largely unknown.
• *Excretion:* Emetine is excreted slowly by the kidneys over 2 months or longer. It is unknown if emetine is excreted in breast milk.

Contraindications and precautions

Emetine is contraindicated in patients with organic heart disease because it may cause cardiac abnormalities; in patients with kidney disease because of its slow renal elimination; in patients with recent polyneuropathy or muscle disease because it can exacerbate these conditions; and during pregnancy because of possible hazard to the fetus. Intravenous administration of emetine is dangerous and contraindicated.

Because it accumulates over time, emetine should not be used in patients who have received it during the preceding 6 weeks. Such vulnerable patients should receive emetine only if safer agents have failed.

Emetine also is contraindicated in children, except those with severe dysentery uncontrolled by other amebicides, and should be used with caution in patients about to undergo surgery and with extreme caution in elderly patients.

Interactions

None reported. However, emetine's GI effects may decrease absorption of orally administered drugs.

Effects on diagnostic tests

Emetine may alter ECG tracings for 6 weeks: it may widen the QRS complex, prolong the PR or QT interval, or cause inversion or flattening of the T wave, increased amplitude of the P wave, ST deformation, premature beats, AV junctional rhythm, or transient atrial fibrillation.

Decreased serum potassium levels, increased serum transaminase levels, and thrombocytopenia have also been reported.

Adverse reactions

• CNS: dizziness, headache, mild sensory disturbances, central or peripheral nerve function changes, neuromuscular symptoms (weakness, aching, stiffness, tenderness, pain, tremor).
• CV: *acute toxicity* (hypotension, tachycardia, precordial pain, dyspnea, palpitations, *ECG abnormalities*, gallop rhythm, cardiac dilatation, severe acute degenerative myocarditis, pericarditis, congestive heart failure and death).
• DERM: eczematous, urticarial purpuric lesions.
• GI: nausea, vomiting, diarrhea, abdominal cramps, loss of sense of taste, epigastric burning or pain, constipation.
• Metabolic: decreased serum potassium levels.
• Local: skeletal muscle stiffness, aching, tenderness, muscle weakness at injection site, cellulitis, tissue necrosis.
• Other: edema.
Note: Acute toxicity can occur at any dosage. Drug should be discontinued if signs of hypersensitivity or toxicity occur.

Overdose and treatment

Overdose is characterized by tremor, weakness, and muscle pain. Nausea, vomiting, and diarrhea are common. Purpura, dermatitis, hemoptysis, or arrhythmias and heart failure may occur.

Treatment of emetine overdose is supportive: fluid management and blood pressure stabilization are important.

▶ Special considerations

• ECG should be taken preceding therapy, after the fifth dose, at completion of therapy, and 1 week after discontinuation.
• Emetine should not be administered I.V. The I.M. route is acceptable, but deep S.C. is preferred. Rotate injection sites and apply warm soaks to relieve local discomfort.
• Patients should be confined to bed during treatment and for several days thereafter.
• Monitor vital signs and record pulse rate and blood pressure two or three times daily.
• Assess cardiac and pulmonary status closely; be alert for shortness of breath, dyspnea on exertion, chest pain, or signs of congestive heart failure.
• Also monitor neuromuscular function, especially neck and extremities; fatigue, listlessness, and muscle stiffness usually precede more serious signs of toxicity.
• Monitor intake and output, odor and consistency of stools, and presence of mucus, blood, or other foreign matter in stools.
• Send fecal specimens to laboratory promptly; infection is detectable only in warm specimens. Repeat fecal examinations at 3-month intervals to assure elimination of amebae.
• Also check family members and suspected contacts for infestation. Patients with acute amebic dysentery often become asymptomatic carriers.
• Isolation of patient is not required.
• This drug is irritating; avoid contact with eyes or mucous membranes.
• Suspect an emetine-induced reaction if diarrhea recurs after initial relief.
• Do not exceed recommended dose or extend therapy beyond 10 days.

Information for the patient

• Counsel patient on need for medical follow-up after discharge.
• Advise patient to report any adverse effects.
• Instruct patient about limiting activities during treatment.
• To help prevent reinfection, instruct patient and family members in proper hygiene, including disposal of feces and hand washing after defecation and before handling, preparing, or eating food, and about the risks of eating raw food and the control of contamination by flies.
• Advise use of liquid soap or reserved bar of soap to prevent cross contamination.
• Encourage other household members and suspected contacts to be tested and, if necessary, treated.
• Isolation is not required, but patient must refrain from preparing, processing, or serving food until treatment is complete.

Geriatric use

Emetine should be used with extreme caution in elderly patients; dosage should be decreased by 50% of the recommended adult dosage.

Pediatric use

Emetine is contraindicated in children, except those with severe dysentery uncontrolled by other amebicides.

Breast-feeding
Safety has not been established.

enalaprilat
Vasotec I.V.

enalapril maleate
Vasotec

- Pharmacologic classification: angiotensin-converting enzyme (ACE) inhibitor
- Therapeutic classification: antihypertensive
- Pregnancy risk category C

How supplied
Available by prescription only
Tablets: 2.5 mg, 5 mg, 10 mg, 20 mg
Injection: 1.25 mg/ml in 2-ml vials

Indications, route, and dosage
Mild to severe hypertension, heart failure
Adults: Initially, 5 mg P.O. once daily; then adjust according to response. Usual dosage range is 10 to 40 mg daily as a single dose or as two divided doses. Alternatively, patients temporarily unable to take P.O. medications may receive enalaprilat 1.25 mg every 6 hours. Administer over a 5-minute period.
Dosage in renal failure
In patients with a creatinine clearance below 30 ml/minute, begin therapy at 2.5 mg/day. Gradually titrate dosage according to response. Patients undergoing hemodialysis should receive a supplemental dose of 2.5 mg on dialysis days.

Pharmacodynamics
Antihypertensive action: Enalapril inhibits ACE, preventing conversion of angiotensin I to angiotensin II, a potent vasoconstrictor. Reduced angiotensin II levels decrease peripheral arterial resistance, lowering blood pressure, and decrease aldosterone secretion, thus reducing sodium and water retention.

Pharmacokinetics
- *Absorption:* Approximately 60% of a given dose of enalapril is absorbed from the GI tract; blood pressure decreases within 1 hour, with peak antihypertensive effect at 4 to 6 hours.
- *Distribution:* Full distribution pattern of enalapril is unknown; drug does not appear to cross the blood-brain barrier.
- *Metabolism:* Enalapril is metabolized extensively to the active metabolite enalaprilat.
- *Excretion:* About 94% of a dose of enalapril is excreted in urine and feces as enalaprilat and enalapril.

Contraindications and precautions
Enalapril is contraindicated in patients with known hypersensitivity to the drug.

Enalapril should be used cautiously in patients with collagen vascular disease or immune disease and in patients taking drugs that may depress immune function or cause decreased white blood cell (WBC) count: such patients are at increased risk of developing enalapril-induced neutropenia, especially if they also have renal impairment. Enalapril also should be used cau-

tiously in patients with renal dysfunction because the drug may worsen this condition.

Interactions
Indomethacin and aspirin may decrease enalapril's antihypertensive effect; enalapril may increase antihypertensive effects of diuretics or other antihypertensive drugs.

Enalapril may enhance effects of potassium-sparing diuretics, potassium supplements, and salt substitutes, thereby causing hyperkalemia; such products should be used cautiously.

Enalapril may decrease the renal clearance of lithium.

Effects on diagnostic tests
Enalapril may elevate BUN and serum creatinine levels and, less commonly, liver enzyme and bilirubin levels; it may slightly decrease hemoglobin and hematocrit levels. Rare cases of neutropenia, thrombocytopenia, and bone marrow depression have been reported.

Adverse reactions
- CNS: headache, dizziness, fatigue, insomnia.
- CV: hypotension, orthostasis.
- DERM: rash.
- GI: diarrhea, nausea.
- GU: renal function impairment.
- HEMA: neutropenia, *thrombocytopenia, agranulocytosis, bone marrow depression.*
- Other: cough, angioedema.
  Note: Drug should be discontinued if neutropenia or renal failure occurs.

Overdose and treatment
Little clinical data is available. The most likely manifestation would be hypotension. After acute ingestion, empty stomach by induced emesis or gastric lavage. Follow with activated charcoal to reduce absorption. Consider hemodialysis in severe cases. Subsequent treatment is usually symptomatic and supportive.

▶ Special considerations
- Discontinue diuretic therapy 2 to 3 days before beginning enalapril therapy, to reduce risk of hypotension; if drug does not adequately control blood pressure, diuretics should be reinstated.
- Perform WBC and differential counts before treatment, every 2 weeks for 3 months, and periodically thereafter.
- Proteinuria and nephrotic syndrome may occur in patients who are on enalapril therapy.
- Enalapril may be given before, during, or after meals because food does not appear to affect absorption.

Information for the patient
- Tell patient to report feelings of light-headedness, especially in first few days, so dosage can be adjusted; signs of infection, such as sore throat and fever, because drug may decrease WBC count; facial swelling or difficulty breathing, because drug may cause angioedema; and loss of taste, which may necessitate discontinuing drug.
- Advise patient to avoid sudden position changes, to minimize orthostatic hypotension.
- Warn patient to seek medical approval before taking nonprescription cold preparations.
- Advise patient to take drug 1 hour before meals.

Geriatric use
Elderly patients may need lower doses because of impaired drug clearance.

Pediatric use
Safety and efficacy of enalapril in children have not been established; use only if potential benefit outweighs risk.

Breast-feeding
It is unknown whether enalapril is distributed into breast milk; an alternative feeding method is recommended during therapy.

ephedrine
Bofedrol

ephedrine hydrochloride
Efedron

ephedrine sulfate
Ectasule Minus, Ephed II, Slo-Fedrin, Vicks Va-tro-nol

- Pharmacologic classification: adrenergic
- Therapeutic classification: bronchodilator, vasopressor (parenteral form), nasal decongestant
- Pregnancy risk category C

How supplied
Available without prescription as appropriate
Capsules: 25 mg, 50 mg
Capsules (extended-release): 15 mg, 30 mg, 60 mg
Solution: 11 mg/5 ml, 20 mg/5 ml
Nasal solution: 0.6% jelly; 0.5% and 1%
Injection: 5 mg/ml, 20 mg/ml, 25 mg/ml, 50 mg/ml (parenteral)

Indications, route, and dosage
To correct hypotensive states
Adults: 25 to 50 mg I.M. or S.C., or 10 to 25 mg slow I.V. bolus. If necessary, a second I.M. dose of 50 mg or I.V. dose of 25 mg may be administered. Additional I.V. doses may be given in 5 to 10 minutes. Maximum dosage, 150 mg daily.
Children: 3 mg/kg S.C. or 100 mg/m² I.V. daily, divided into four to six doses.
Orthostatic hypotension
Adults: 25 mg P.O. once daily to q.i.d.
Children: 3 mg/kg P.O. daily, divided into four to six doses.
Bronchodilator or nasal decongestant
Adults: 25 to 50 mg q 3 to 4 hours as needed; 12.5 to 25 mg I.M., I.V., or S.C. repeated as determined by patient response; or 15 to 60 mg extended-release capsules P.O. q 8 to 12 hours. As nasal decongestant, 0.5% to 1% solution applied topically to nasal mucosa as drops, or on a nasal pack. Instill no more often than q 4 hours.
Children: 2 to 3 mg/kg or 100 mg/m² P.O. daily in four to six divided doses.
Severe, acute bronchospasm
Adults: 12.5 to 25 mg I.M., S.C., or I.V.
Enuresis
Adults: 25 to 50 mg P.O. h.s.

Myasthenia gravis
Adults: 25 mg t.i.d. to q.i.d.

Pharmacodynamics
Ephedrine is both a direct- and indirect-acting sympathomimetic that stimulates alpha- and beta-adrenergic receptors. Release of norepinephrine from its storage sites is one of its indirect effects. In therapeutic doses, ephedrine relaxes bronchial smooth muscle and produces cardiac stimulation with increased systolic and diastolic blood pressure when norepinephrine stores are not depleted.
- *Bronchodilator action:* Ephedrine relaxes bronchial smooth muscle by stimulating beta₂-adrenergic receptors, resulting in increased vital capacity, relief of mild bronchospasm, improved air exchange, and decreased residual volume.
- *Vasopressor action:* Ephedrine produces positive inotropic effects with low doses by action on beta₁ receptors in the heart. Vasodilation results from its effect on beta₂-adrenergic receptors; vasoconstriction from its alpha-adrenergic effects. Pressor effects may result from vasoconstriction or cardiac stimulation; however, when peripheral vascular resistance is decreased, blood pressure elevation results from increased cardiac output.
- *Nasal decongestant action:* Ephedrine stimulates alpha-adrenergic receptors in blood vessels of nasal mucosa, producing vasoconstriction and nasal decongestion.

Pharmacokinetics
- *Absorption:* Ephedrine is rapidly and completely absorbed after oral, S.C., or I.M. administration. After oral administration, onset of action occurs within 15 to 60 minutes and persists 2 to 4 hours. Pressor and cardiac effects last 1 hour after I.V. dose of 10 to 25 mg or I.M. or S.C. dose of 25 to 50 mg; they last up to 4 hours after oral dose of 15 to 50 mg.
- *Distribution:* Ephedrine is widely distributed throughout the body.
- *Metabolism:* Ephedrine is slowly metabolized in the liver by oxidative deamination, demethylation, aromatic hydroxylation, and conjugation.
- *Excretion:* Most of a dose is excreted unchanged in urine. Rate of excretion depends on urine pH.

Contraindications and precautions
Ephedrine is contraindicated in patients with narrow-angle glaucoma or psychoneurosis, because the drug may exacerbate these conditions. The injectable form is contraindicated during general anesthesia with cyclopropane or halothane, because the patient may experience cardiac arrhythmias.
   Administer with extreme caution to hypertensive or hyperthyroid patients (increased incidence of adverse reactions), elderly patients (especially men with enlarged prostate), diabetic patients, and those with cardiovascular disease or a history of sensitivity to ephedrine or other sympathomimetics.

Interactions
Concomitant use of other sympathomimetic agents may add to their effects and toxicity. Use with alpha-adrenergic blocking agents may decrease vasopressor effects of ephedrine. Concomitant beta-adrenergic blocking agents may block cardiovascular and bronchodilating effects of ephedrine. Use with general anesthetics (especially cyclopropane or halothane) and dig-

---

italis glycosides may sensitize myocardium to effects of ephedrine, causing cardiac arrhythmias.

Monoamine oxidase (MAO) inhibitors may potentiate the pressor effects of ephedrine, possibly resulting in hypertensive crisis. Allow 14 days to lapse after withdrawal of MAO inhibitor before using ephedrine. Reserpine, guanethidine, methyldopa, and diuretics may decrease ephedrine's pressor effects.

Concomitant use with atropine blocks reflex bradycardia and enhances pressor effects. Administration with a theophylline derivative such as aminophylline reportedly produces a greater incidence of adverse reactions than either drug when used alone.

Effects on diagnostic tests
None reported.

Adverse reactions
● CNS: nervousness, anxiety, apprehension, fear, tension, agitation, excitation, restlessness, insomnia, weakness, irritability, talkativeness, dizziness, lightheadedness, vertigo, tremor, hyperactive reflexes, confusion, delirium, hallucinations, euphoria.
● CV: hypertension, palpitations, tachycardia, arrhythmias, precordial pain.
● GI: nausea, vomiting, mild epigastric distress, anorexia.
● GU: urinary retention, difficult urination, priapism.
● Other: fever; pallor; dryness of mouth, throat, and nose; respiratory difficulty; sweating; rebound congestion; and tachyphylaxis.

Overdose and treatment
Clinical manifestations of overdose include exaggeration of common adverse reactions, especially cardiac arrhythmias, extreme tremor or seizures, nausea and vomiting, fever, and CNS and respiratory depression.

Treatment requires supportive and symptomatic measures. If patient is conscious, induce emesis with ipecac followed by activated charcoal. If patient is depressed or hyperactive, perform gastric lavage. Maintain airway and blood pressure. Do not administer vasopressors. Monitor vital signs closely.

A beta blocker (such as propranolol) may be used to treat cardiac arrhythmias. A cardioselective beta blocker is recommended in asthmatic patients. Phentolamine may be used for hypertension; paraldehyde or diazepam for seizures; dexamethasone for pyrexia.

▶ Special considerations
Besides those relevant to all *adrenergics,* consider the following recommendations.
● As a pressor agent, ephedrine is not a substitute for blood, plasma, fluids, or electrolytes. Correct fluid volume depletion before administration.
● Tolerance may develop after prolonged or excessive use. Increased dose may be needed. Also, if drug is discontinued for a few days and readministered, effectiveness may be restored.
● To prevent insomnia, last dose should be taken at least 2 hours before bedtime.
● With parenteral dosing, monitor vital signs closely during infusion. Tachycardia is common.

Information for the patient
● Tell patient using nonprescription product to follow directions on label, to take last dose a few hours before bedtime to reduce possibility of insomnia, to take only as directed, and not to increase dose or frequency.

● Warn patient not to crush, break, or chew extended-release capsules. If capsule is too large to swallow, patient may open it and mix contents with applesauce, jelly, honey, or syrup and swallow without chewing.
● Advise patient to store drug away from heat and light (not in bathroom medicine cabinet) and to keep out of reach of children.
● Instruct patient who misses a dose to take it as soon as remembered if within 1 hour. If beyond 1 hour, patient should skip dose and return to regular schedule.
● Teach patient to be aware of palpitations and significant pulse rate changes.
● Instruct patient to clear nose before instillation of nasal solutions.

Geriatric use
Administer cautiously, because elderly patients may be more sensitive to drug's effects. Lower dose may be recommended.

Pediatric use
Administer cautiously to children.

Breast-feeding
Breast-feeding should be avoided during treatment with ephedrine.

---

epinephrine
Bronkaid Mist, Bronkaid Mistometer*, Dysne-Inhal*, EpiPen, EpiPen Jr., Primatene Mist Solution, Sus-Phrine

epinephrine bitartrate
AsthmaHaler, Bronitin Mist, Bronkaid Mist Suspension, Epitrate, Medihaler-Epi, Primatene Mist Suspension

epinephrine hydrochloride
Adrenalin Chloride, AsthmaNefrin, Epifrin, Glaucon, microNefrin, S-2 Inhalant, Vaponefrin

epinephryl borate
Epinal, Eppy/N

● Pharmacologic classification: adrenergic
● Therapeutic classification: bronchodilator, vasopressor, cardiac stimulant, local anesthetic (adjunct), topical antihemorrhagic, antiglaucoma agent
● Pregnancy risk category C

How supplied
Available by prescription only
Injection: 0.01 mg/ml (1:100,000), 0.1 mg/ml (1:10,000), 0.5 mg/ml (1:2,000), 1 mg/ml (1:1,000) parenteral; 5 mg/ml (1:200) parenteral suspension
Ophthalmic: 0.1%, 0.25%, 0.5%, 1%, 2% solution

Available without prescription
Nebulizer inhaler: 1% (1:100), 1.25%, 2.25%
Aerosol inhaler: 160 mcg, 200 mcg, 250 mcg/metered spray

Indications, route, and dosage

Severe anaphylaxis or asthma

Adults: Initially, 0.1 to 0.5 mg (0.1 to 0.5 mg of a 1:1000 solution) S.C. or I.M.; may be repeated at 10- to 15-minute intervals if needed. Alternatively, 0.1 to 0.25 mg (1 to 2.5 ml of a 1:10,000 solution) I.V. slowly over 5 to 10 minutes. May be repeated every 5 to 15 minutes if needed or followed by a 1 to 4 mcg/minute I.V. infusion.

Children: 0.01 mg/kg (0.01 ml/kg of a 1:1000 solution) or 0.3 mg/m^2 (0.3 ml/m^2 of a 1:1000 solution) S.C. Dosage not to exceed 0.5 mg. May be repeated at 20-minute to 4-hour intervals as needed. Alternatively, 0.02 to 0.025 mg/kg (0.004 to 0.005 ml/kg) or 0.625 mg/m^2 (0.125 ml/m^2) of a 1:200 solution. May be repeated but not more often than q 6 hours. Alternatively, 0.1 mg (10 ml of a 1:100,000 dilution) I.V. slowly over 5 to 10 minutes followed by a 0.1 to 1.5 mcg/kg/minute I.V. infusion.

Bronchodilator

Adults and children: One inhalation via metered aerosol, repeated once if needed after 1 minute; subsequent doses should not be repeated for at least 3 hours. Alternatively, one or two deep inhalations via hand-bulb nebulizer of a 1% (1:100) solution; may be repeated at 1-to 2-minute intervals. Alternatively, 0.03 ml (0.3 mg) of a 1% solution via IPPB.

To restore cardiac rhythm in cardiac arrest

Adults: Initially, 0.5 to 1 mg (range: 0.1 to 1 mg [1 to 10 ml of a 1:10,000 solution]) I.V. bolus; may be repeated q 5 minutes if needed. Alternatively, initial dose followed by 0.3 mg S.C. or 1 to 4 mcg/minute I.V. infusion. Alternatively, 1 mg (10 ml of a 1:10,000 solution) intratracheally, or 0.1 to 1 mg (1 to 10 ml of a 1:10,000 solution) intracardiac.

Children: Initially, 0.01 mg/kg (0.1 ml/kg of a 1:10,000 solution) I.V. bolus or intratracheally; may be repeated q 5 minutes if needed.

Alternatively, initially, 0.1 mcg/kg/minute; may increase in increments of 0.1 mcg/kg/minute to a maximum of 1 mcg/kg/minute. Alternatively, 0.005 to 0.01 mg/kg (0.05 to 0.1 ml/kg of a 1:10,000 solution) by intracardiac injection.

Infants: Initially, 0.01 to 0.03 mg/kg (0.1 to 0.3 ml/kg of a 1:10,000 solution) I.V. bolus or by intratracheal injection. May be repeated q 5 minutes if needed.

Hemostatic use

Adults: 1:50,000 to 1:1,000, applied topically.

To prolong local anesthetic effect

Adults and children: 1:500,000 to 1:50,000 mixed with local anesthetic.

Open-angle glaucoma

Adults: 1 or 2 drops of 1% to 2% solution instilled daily or b.i.d.

Pharmacodynamics

Epinephrine acts directly by stimulating alpha- and beta-adrenergic receptors in the sympathetic nervous system. Its main therapeutic effects include relaxation of bronchial smooth muscle, cardiac stimulation, and dilation of skeletal muscle vasculature.

● *Bronchodilator action:* Epinephrine relaxes bronchial smooth muscle by stimulating beta$_2$-adrenergic receptors. Epinephrine constricts bronchial arterioles by stimulating alpha-adrenergic receptors, resulting in relief of bronchospasm, reduced congestion and edema, and increased tidal volume and vital capacity. By inhibiting histamine release, it may reverse bronchiolar constriction, vasodilation, and edema.

● *Cardiovascular and vasopressor actions:* As a cardiac stimulant, epinephrine produces positive chronotropic and inotropic effects by action on beta$_1$ receptors in the heart, increasing cardiac output, myocardial oxygen consumption, and force of contraction, and decreasing cardiac efficiency. Vasodilation results from its effect on beta$_2$ receptors; vasoconstriction results from alpha-adrenergic effects.

● *Local anesthetic (adjunct) action:* Epinephrine acts on alpha receptors in skin, mucous membranes, and viscera; it produces vasoconstriction, which reduces absorption of local anesthetic, thus prolonging its duration of action, localizing anesthesia, and decreasing risk of anesthetic's toxicity.

● *Local vasoconstriction action:* Epinephrine's effect results from action on alpha receptors in skin, mucous membranes, and viscera, which produces vasoconstriction and hemostasis in small vessels.

● *Antiglaucoma action:* Epinephrine's exact mechanism of lowering intraocular pressure is unknown. When applied topically to the conjunctiva or injected into the interior chamber of the eye, epinephrine constricts conjunctival blood vessels, contracts the dilator muscle of the pupil, and may dilate the pupil.

Pharmacokinetics

● *Absorption:* Well absorbed after S.C. or I.M. injection, epinephrine has a rapid onset of action and short duration of action. Bronchodilation occurs within 5 to 10 minutes and peaks in 20 minutes after S.C. injection; onset after oral inhalation is within 1 minute.

Topical administration or intraocular injection usually produces local vasoconstriction within 5 minutes and lasts less than 1 hour. After topical application to the conjunctiva, reduction of intraocular pressure occurs within 1 hour, peaks in 4 to 8 hours, and persists up to 24 hours.

● *Distribution:* Epinephrine is distributed widely throughout the body.

● *Metabolism:* Drug is metabolized at sympathetic nerve endings, liver, and other tissues to inactive metabolites.

● *Excretion:* Epinephrine is excreted in urine, mainly as its metabolites and conjugates.

Contraindications and precautions

Epinephrine is contraindicated in patients with shock (except anaphylactic shock), organic heart disease, cardiac dilatation, and arrhythmias, because it increases myocardial oxygen demand; in patients with organic brain damage or cerebral arteriosclerosis, because of potential adverse CNS effects; in patients with narrow-angle glaucoma, because the drug may worsen the condition; and in patients with known sensitivity to the drug. Epinephrine is contraindicated in conjunction with local anesthetics in fingers, toes, ears, nose, or genitalia, because vasoconstriction in these extremities may induce tissue necrosis.

Administer with extreme caution to patients with hypertension or hyperthyroidism; and to elderly patients, diabetic patients, and those with cardiovascular diseases, history of sensitivity to sympathomimetics, Parkinson's disease (temporary increase in tremor or rigidity), bronchial asthma, or psychoneurotic disorders. Use with extreme caution in patients receiving inhalational anesthetics because of the potential for cardiac arrhythmias. Use cautiously in patients with sulfite hypersensitivity; some epinephrine preparations contain sulfites. Epinephrine may delay the second stage of labor in pregnant women because the drug inhibits spontaneous or oxytocin-induced uterine contractions. It may also cause anoxia in the fetus. However, there is some evidence that epinephrine added to lidocaine to prolong epidural anesthesia is safe.

Interactions

Concomitant use with other sympathomimetics may produce additive effects and toxicity. Beta-adrenergic blockers antagonize cardiac and bronchodilating effects of epinephrine; alpha-adrenergic blockers antagonize vasoconstriction and hypertension. Use with general anesthetics (especially cyclopropane and halothane) and digitalis glycosides may sensitize the myocardium to epinephrine's effects, causing arrhythmias. Use with tricyclic antidepressants, antihistamines, and thyroid hormones may potentiate adverse cardiac effects of epinephrine. Concomitant use with oxytocics or ergot alkaloids may cause severe hypertension.

Because phenothiazines may cause reversal of its pressor effects, epinephrine should not be used to treat circulatory collapse or hypotension caused by phenothiazines; such use may cause further lowering of blood pressure.

Use with guanethidine may decrease its hypotensive effects while potentiating epinephrine's effects, resulting in hypertension and cardiac arrhythmias.

Concomitant use with hypoglycemic agents may decrease their effects; dosage adjustments may be necessary.

Concomitant use of ophthalmic epinephrine with topical miotics, topical beta-adrenergic blocking agents, osmotic diuretics, and carbonic anhydrase inhibitors may cause additive lowering of intraocular pressure. Concomitant use with miotics offers the advantage of reducing the ciliary spasm, mydriasis, blurred vision, and increased IOP that may occur with miotics or epinephrine alone.

Effects on diagnostic tests

Epinephrine therapy alters blood glucose and serum lactic acid levels (both may be increased), increases blood urea nitrogen levels, and interferes with tests for urinary catecholamines.

Adverse reactions

● CNS: fear, anxiety, tenseness, restlessness, headache, tremor, dizziness, light-headedness, nervousness, sleeplessness, excitability, weakness, psychomotor agitation, disorientation, impaired memory, panic, hallucinations, *suicidal tendencies*.
● CV: ECG changes, (decreased T-wave amplitude), disturbances in cardiac rhythm and rate (palpitations, tachycardia), angina, arrhythmias, syncope, hypertension.
● EENT: ocular discomfort, conjunctival irritation, lacrimation, blurred vision, mydriasis, localized melanin-like pigmentary deposits in the conjunctiva or eyelids (prolonged ophthalmic use).
● GI: nausea, vomiting.
● Other: sweating, pallor, respiratory difficulty, rebound nasal congestion, respiratory weakness, apnea, contact dermatitis. Extravasation can cause local necrosis and bleeding at injection site.
Note: Drug should be discontinued if hypersensitivity occurs.

Overdose and treatment

Clinical manifestations of overdose may include a sharp increase in systolic and diastolic blood pressure, rise in venous pressure, severe anxiety, irregular heartbeat, severe nausea or vomiting, severe respiratory distress, unusually large pupils, unusual paleness and coldness of skin, pulmonary edema, renal failure, and metabolic acidosis.

Treatment includes symptomatic and supportive measures, because epinephrine is rapidly inactivated in the body. Monitor vital signs closely. Trimethaphan or phentolamine may be needed for hypotension; beta blockers (such as propranolol) for arrhythmias.

▶ Special considerations

Besides those relevant to all *adrenergics*, consider the following recommendations.
● After S.C. or I.M. injection, massaging the site may hasten absorption.
● Epinephrine is destroyed by oxidizing agents, alkalies (including sodium bicarbonate), halogens, permanganates, chromates, nitrates, and salts of easily reducible metals such as iron, copper, and zinc.
● A tuberculin syringe may assure greater accuracy in measurement of parenteral doses.
● To avoid hazardous medication errors, check carefully type of solution prescribed, concentration, dosage, and route before administration. Do not mix with alkali.
● Before withdrawing epinephrine suspension into syringe, shake vial or ampule thoroughly to disperse particles; then inject promptly. Do not use if preparation is discolored or contains a precipitate.
● Repeated injections may cause tissue necrosis from vascular constriction. Rotate injection sites, and observe for signs of blanching.
● Avoid I.M. injection into buttocks. Epinephrine-induced vasoconstriction favors growth of the anaerobe *Clostridium perfringens*.
● Monitor blood pressure, pulse, respirations, and urine output, and observe patient closely. Epinephrine may widen pulse pressure. If arrhythmias occur, discontinue epinephrine immediately. Watch for changes in intake/output ratio.
● Patients receiving I.V. epinephrine should be on cardiac monitor. Keep resuscitation equipment available.
● When drug is administered I.V., check patient's blood pressure repeatedly during first 5 minutes, then every 3 to 5 minutes until patient is stable.
● Intracardiac administration requires external cardiac massage to move drug into coronary circulation.
● Drying effect on bronchial secretions may make mucus plugs more difficult to dislodge. Bronchial hygiene program, including postural drainage, breathing exercises, and adequate hydration, may be necessary.
● Epinephrine may increase blood glucose levels. Closely observe patients with diabetes for loss of diabetes control.
● Monitor amount, consistency, and color of sputum.

Inhalation

● Treatment should start with first symptoms of bronchospasm. Patient should use the fewest number of inhalations that provide relief. To prevent excessive dosage, at least 1 or 2 minutes should elapse before taking additional inhalations of epinephrine. Dosage requirements vary. Warn patient that overuse or too-frequent use can cause severe adverse reactions.

Nasal

● Instill nose drops with patient's head in lateral, head-low position to prevent entry of drug into throat.

Ophthalmic
● Ophthalmic preparation may cause mydriasis with blurred vision and sensitivity to light in some patients being treated for glaucoma. Drug is usually administered at bedtime or after prescribed miotic to minimize these symptoms.
● Patients should have regular tonometer readings during continuous therapy, especially elderly patients.
● When using separate solutions of epinephrine and a topical miotic, instill the miotic 2 to 10 minutes before epinephrine.

Information for the patient
Urge patient to report diminishing effect. Repeated or prolonged use of epinephrine can cause tolerance to the drug's effects. Continuing to take epinephrine despite tolerance can be hazardous. Interrupting drug therapy for 12 hours to several days may restore responsiveness to drug.

Inhalation
● Instruct patient in correct use of inhaler.
● Tell patient to avoid contact with eyes, and to take no more than two inhalations at a time with 1- to 2-minute intervals between.
● Instruct patient to rinse mouth and throat with water immediately after inhalation to avoid swallowing residual drug (the propellant in the aerosol preparation may cause epigastric pain and systemic effects) and to prevent dryness of oropharyngeal membranes.
● Tell patient to save applicator; refills may be available.
● Tell patient to call immediately if he receives no relief within 20 minutes or if condition worsens.

Nasal
● Tell patient to call if symptoms are not relieved in 20 minutes or if they become worse, and to report bronchial irritation, nervousness, or sleeplessness, which require reduction of dosage.
● Warn patient that intranasal applications may sting slightly and cause rebound congestion or drug-induced rhinitis after prolonged use. Nose drops should be used for 3 or 4 days only. Encourage patient to use drug exactly as prescribed.
● Tell patient to rinse nose dropper or spray tip with hot water after each use to avoid contaminating the solution.
● To avoid excessive systemic absorption, instruct patient to gently press finger against nasolacrimal duct for at least 1 or 2 minutes immediately after drug instillation.

Ophthalmic
● To minimize systemic absorption, tell patient to press finger to lacrimal sac during and for 1 to 2 minutes after instillation of eye drops.
● To prevent contamination, tell patient not to touch applicator tip to any surface; keep container tightly closed.
● Tell patient not to use if epinephrine solution is discolored or contains a precipitate.
● Advise patient to remove soft contact lenses before instilling eye drops to avoid staining or damaging them.
● Tell patient to apply a missed dose as soon as possible. If too close to time for next dose, the patient should wait and apply at regularly scheduled time.
● Tell patient to store drug away from heat and light (not in bathroom medicine cabinet where heat and moisture can cause drug to deteriorate) and out of children's reach.

Geriatric use
Elderly patients may be more sensitive to effects of epinephrine, so lower doses are indicated.

Pediatric use
Safety and efficacy of ophthalmic epinephrine in children have not been established. Use with caution.

Breast-feeding
Epinephrine is excreted in breast milk. Patient should avoid breast-feeding during therapy with epinephrine.

---

epoetin alfa (erythropoietin)
Epogen, Procrit

● Pharmacologic classification: glycoprotein
● Therapeutic classification: antianemic agent
● Pregnancy risk category C

How supplied
Available by prescription only
Injection: 2,000 units, 3,000 units, 4,000 units, 10,000 units

Indications, route, and dosage
Anemia associated with chronic renal failure
Adults: Initiate therapy at 50 to 100 units/kg three times weekly. Patients receiving dialysis should receive the drug I.V.; chronic renal failure patients not on dialysis may receive the drug S.C. or I.V.

Reduce dosage when the target hematocrit is reached, or if the hematocrit rises more than four points within any 2-week period. Increase the dosage if the hematocrit doesn't rise by five to six points after 8 weeks of therapy and the target range of 30% to 33% has not been reached.

Individualize dosage for maintenance range. Usually, dosage is changed by 25 units/kg three times weekly.
Anemia related to zidovudine therapy in patients infected with human immunodeficiency virus (HIV)
Adults: Before therapy, determine endogenous serum epoetin alfa levels. Patients with levels ≥ 500 milliunits/ml are unlikely to respond to therapy.

Initial dose for patients with levels ≤ 500 milliunits/ml who are receiving zidovudine ≤ 4,200 mg weekly is 100 units/kg I.V. or S.C. three times weekly for 8 weeks. If response is inadequate after 8 weeks, increase dose by increments of 50 to 100 units/kg three times weekly and reevaluate response q 4 to 8 weeks. Individualize maintenance dose to maintain response, which may be influenced by zidovudine dose or infection or inflammation.

Pharmacodynamics
Antianemic action: Epoetin alfa is a glycoprotein consisting of 165 amino acids synthesized using recombinant DNA technology. It mimics naturally occurring erythropoietin, which is produced by the kidney. It stimulates the division and differentiation of cells within bone marrow to produce red blood cells.

Pharmacokinetics

● *Absorption:* Epoetin alfa may be given S.C. or I.V. After S.C. administration, peak serum levels occur within 5 to 24 hours.
● *Distribution:* Information not available.
● *Metabolism:* Information not available.
● *Excretion:* Information not available.

Contraindications and precautions

Epoetin alfa is contraindicated in patients hypersensitive to mammalian cell-derived products, or to human albumin. It is also contraindicated in patients with uncontrolled hypertension.

The rapid rise in the hematocrit can cause loss of control of blood pressure. Reduce dosage so that the hematocrit doesn't increase by more than four points within any 2-week period. The drug may have to be temporarily withheld until blood pressure is controlled.

During the initiation of therapy, patients should avoid hazardous activities, such as driving or operating heavy machinery. There appears to be a higher potential for seizures during the initiation of therapy, but their relationship to the drug is uncertain.

Patients who are receiving dialysis may require increased anticoagulation with heparin.

Interactions

None reported.

Effects on diagnostic tests

Moderate increases in BUN, uric acid, creatinine, phosphorus, and potassium levels have been reported.

Adverse reactions

● CNS: headache.
● CV: hypertension, clots at I.V. infusion site.
● GI: nausea, diarrhea, vomiting.
● Other: arthralgia, seizures.
   Note: Discontinue drug if hematocrit rises beyond target range of 30% to 33%.

Overdose and treatment

Maximum safe dose has not been established. Doses up to 1,500 units/kg have been administered three times weekly for 3 weeks without direct toxic effects.

The drug can cause polycythemia; phlebotomy may be used to bring hematocrit within appropriate levels.

▶ Special considerations

● Hematocrit should be monitored at least twice weekly during the initiation of therapy and during any dosage adjustment. Close monitoring of blood pressure is also recommended.
● For HIV-infected patients treated with zidovudine, measure hematocrit once weekly until stabilized and then periodically.
● If a patient fails to respond to epoetin alfa therapy, consider the following possible causes: vitamin deficiency, iron deficiency, underlying infection, occult blood loss, underlying hematologic disease, hemolysis, aluminum intoxication, osteitis fibrosa cystica, or increased dosage of zidovudine.
● Most patients eventually require supplemental iron therapy. Before and during therapy, monitor patient's iron stores, including serum ferritin and transferrin saturation.
● Hematocrit should be measured twice weekly until it has stabilized and during adjustment to a maintenance dosage in patients with chronic renal failure. An interval

of 2 to 6 weeks may elapse before a dosage change is reflected in the hematocrit.
● Routine monitoring of complete blood count with differential and platelet counts is recommended.

Information for the patient

● Explain the importance of regularly monitoring blood pressure in light of the potential drug effects.
● Patients should adhere to dietary restrictions during therapy. They should understand that epoetin alfa will not influence the disease process.

Pediatric use

Safety and efficacy in children have not been established.

Breast-feeding

It is unknown whether epoetin alfa is excreted in breast milk. Use with caution in breast-feeding women.

---

ergocalciferol (vitamin D₂)

Calciferol, Deltalin Gelseals, Drisdol, Vitamin D capsules

● Pharmacologic classification: vitamin
● Therapeutic classification: antihypocalcemic
● Pregnancy risk category C (D if > recommended daily allowance [RDA])

How supplied

Available by prescription only
Capsules: 0.625 mg (25,000 units), 1.25 mg (50,000 units)
Tablets: 1.25 mg (50,000 units)
Injection: 12.5 mg (500,000 units)/ml

Available without prescription
Liquid: 8,000 units/ml in 60-ml dropper bottle

Indications, route, and dosage
Nutritional rickets or osteomalacia

Adults: 25 to 125 mcg P.O. daily if patient has normal GI absorption. With severe malabsorption, 250 mcg to 7.5 mg P.O. or 250 mcg I.M. daily.
Children: 25 to 125 mcg P.O. daily if patient has normal GI absorption. With malabsorption, 250 to 625 mcg.

Familial hypophosphatemia

Adults: 250 mcg to 1.5 mg P.O. daily with phosphate supplements.
Children: 1 to 2 mg P.O. daily with phosphate supplements. Increase daily dosage in 250- to 500-mg increments at 3- to 4-month intervals until adequate response is obtained.

Vitamin D-dependent rickets

Adults: 250 mcg to 1.5 mg P.O. daily.
Children: 75 to 125 mcg P.O. daily.

Anticonvulsant-induced rickets and osteomalacia

Adults: 50 mcg to 1.25 mg P.O. daily.

Hypoparathyroidism and pseudohypoparathyroidism

Adults: 625 mcg to 5 mg P.O. daily with calcium supplements.
Children: 1.25 to 5 mg P.O. daily with calcium supplements.

Pharmacodynamics
Antihypocalcemic action: Once activated, ergocalciferol acts to regulate the serum concentrations of calcium by regulating absorption from the GI tract and resorption stored in bone.

Pharmacokinetics
• *Absorption:* Drug is absorbed readily from the small intestine. Onset of action is 10 to 24 hours.
• *Distribution:* Drug is distributed widely and bound to proteins stored in the liver.
• *Metabolism:* Ergocalciferol is metabolized in the liver and kidney. It has an average half-life of 24 hours and a duration of up to 6 months.
• *Excretion:* Bile (feces) is the primary excretion route. A small percentage is excreted in urine.

Contraindications and precautions
Ergocalciferol is contraindicated in patients with hypercalcemia or vitamin D toxicity, malabsorption syndrome, or abnormal sensitivity to vitamin D effects.

Use with extreme caution in patients with impaired renal function, heart disease, renal stones, arteriosclerosis; and in patients receiving cardiac glycosides.

Interactions
Concomitant use of ergocalciferol and cardiac glycosides may result in cardiac arrhythmias. Concomitant use with thiazide diuretics may cause hypercalcemia in patients with hypoparathyroidism; with magnesium-containing antacids may lead to hypermagnesemia; with verapamil may induce recurrence of atrial fibrillation when supplemental calcium and calciferol have induced hypercalcemia. Corticosteroids counteract the drug's effects. Administration of phenobarbital and phenytoin may increase the drug's metabolism to inactive metabolites. Cholestyramine, colestipol, and excessive use of mineral oil may interfere with the absorption of ergocalciferol.

Effects on diagnostic tests
Ergocalciferol may falsely increase serum cholesterol levels and may elevate AST (SGOT) and ALT (SGPT) levels.

Adverse reactions
Adverse reactions listed are usually seen in vitamin D toxicity only.
• CNS: headache, dizziness, ataxia, irritability, weakness, somnolence, decreased libido, overt psychosis, *convulsions.*
• CV: calcifications of soft tissues, including the heart; hypertension, arrhythmias.
• DERM: pruritus.
• EENT: dry mouth, metallic taste, rhinorrhea, conjunctivitis (calcific), photophobia, tinnitus.
• GI: anorexia, nausea, vomiting, constipation, diarrhea.
• GU: polyuria, albuminuria, hypercalciuria, nocturia, impaired renal function, renal calculi.
• Metabolic: hypercalcemia, hyperphosphatemia.
• Other: bone and muscle pain, bone demineralization, weight loss, weakness, fever, overt psychosis, polydipsia.
Note: Drug should be discontinued if adverse reactions become severe.

Overdose and treatment
Clinical manifestations of overdose include hypercalcemia, hypercalciuria, and hyperphosphatemia, which may be treated by stopping therapy, starting a low calcium diet, and increasing fluid intake. A loop diuretic, such as furosemide, may be given with saline I.V. infusion to increase calcium excretion. Supportive measures should be provided. In severe cases, death from cardiac or renal failure may occur. Calcitonin may decrease hypercalcemia.

▶ Special considerations
• I.M. injection of ergocalciferol dispersed in oil is preferable in patients who are unable to absorb the oral form.
• If I.V. route is necessary, use only water-miscible solutions intended for dilution in large-volume parenterals. Use cautiously in cardiac patients, especially if they are receiving cardiotonic glycosides. In such patients, hypercalcemia may precipitate arrhythmias.
• Monitor eating and bowel habits; dry mouth, nausea, vomiting, metallic taste, and constipation can be early signs of toxicity.
• Patients with hyperphosphatemia require dietary phosphate restrictions and binding agents to avoid metastatic calcifications and renal calculi.
• When high therapeutic doses are used, frequent serum and urine calcium, potassium, and urea determinations should be made.
• Malabsorption caused by inadequate bile or hepatic dysfunction may require addition of exogenous bile salts.
• Doses of 60,000 IU daily can cause hypercalcemia.
• Patients taking ergocalciferol should restrict their intake of magnesium-containing antacids.

Information for the patient
• Explain the importance of a diet rich in calcium.
• Caution patient not to increase daily dose on his own initiative. Vitamin D is a fat-soluble vitamin; vitamin D toxicity is thus more likely to occur.
• Tell patient to avoid magnesium-containing antacids and mineral oil.
• Tell patient to swallow tablets whole without crushing or chewing.

Pediatric use
Some infants may be hyperreactive to this drug.

Breast-feeding
Very little appears in the breast milk; however, the effect on infants of amounts greater than RDA levels of vitamin D is not known.

---

ergonovine maleate
Ergotrate Maleate

• Pharmacologic classification: ergot alkaloid
• Therapeutic classification: oxytocic

How supplied
Available by prescription only
Tablets: 0.2 mg
Injection: 0.2-mg ampules

Indications, route, and dosage
Prevent or treat postpartum and postabortion hemorrhage due to uterine atony or subinvolution
Adults: 0.2 mg I.M. q 2 to 4 hours, maximum five doses; or 0.2 mg I.V. (only for severe uterine bleeding or other life-threatening emergency) over 1 minute while blood pressure and uterine contractions are monitored. I.V. dose may be diluted to 5 ml with 0.9% sodium chloride injection. After initial I.M. or I.V. dose, may give 0.2 to 0.4 mg P.O. q 6 to 12 hours for 2 to 7 days. Decrease dose if severe uterine cramping occurs.
To diagnose coronary artery spasm (Prinzmetal's angina)
Adults: 0.05 to 0.40 mg I.V.

Pharmacodynamics
Oxytocic action: Ergonovine maleate stimulates contractions of uterine and vascular smooth muscle. This produces intense uterine contractions, followed by periods of relaxation. The drug produces vasoconstriction of primarily capacitance blood vessels, causing an increased central venous pressure and elevated blood pressure. The clinical effect is secondary to contraction of the uterine wall around bleeding vessels, producing hemostasis.

Pharmacokinetics
● *Absorption:* Absorption is rapid following oral and I.M. administration. Onset of action is immediate for I.V., 2 to 5 minutes for I.M., and 6 to 15 minutes for oral doses.
● *Distribution:* Not fully known.
● *Metabolism:* Drug is metabolized in the liver.
● *Excretion:* Primarily nonrenal elimination in feces has been suggested.

Contraindications and precautions
Drug is contraindicated in patients sensitive to ergot preparations; in threatened spontaneous abortion, induction of labor, or before delivery of placenta, because captivation of placenta may occur; and in patients with a history of allergic or idiosyncratic reactions to this drug. Because of the potential for adverse cardiovascular effects, use cautiously in patients with hypertension; toxemia; sepsis; occlusive vascular disease; and hepatic, renal, and cardiac disease.

Interactions
Ergonovine maleate will enhance the vasoconstrictor potential of other ergot alkaloids and sympathomimetic amines. Combined use of local anesthetics with vasoconstrictors (lidocaine with epinephrine) or smoking (nicotine) will enhance vasoconstriction. If patient is not also taking digitalis, cautious administration of calcium gluconate I.V. may produce desired oxytocic action in calcium-deficient patients.

Effects on diagnostic tests
The concentration of serum prolactin may appear decreased.

Adverse reactions
● CNS: headache, confusion, dizziness, ringing in ears.
● CV: chest pain, weakness in legs (peripheral vasospasm), hypertension, thrombophlebitis.
● GI: nausea, vomiting, diarrhea, cramping.
● Respiratory: shortness of breath.
● Other: itching; sweating; pain in arms, legs, or lower back; hypersensitivity, signs of *shock*.

Note: Drug should be discontinued if hypertension or allergic reactions occur.

Overdose and treatment
Clinical manifestations of overdose include seizures, with nausea, vomiting, diarrhea, dizziness, fluctuations in blood pressure, weak pulse, chest pain, tingling, and numbness and coldness in the extremities. Rarely, gangrene has occurred. Treatment after oral overdose requires immediate gastric lavage and emesis, followed with activated charcoal and cathartics. Treat seizures with anticonvulsants and hypercoagulability with heparin; give vasodilators to improve blood flow. Gangrene may require amputation.

▶ Special considerations
● Contractions begin 5 to 15 minutes after P.O. administration, immediately after I.V. injection. May continue 3 hours or more after P.O. or I.M. administration, 45 minutes after I.V. injection.
● Monitor blood pressure, pulse rate, uterine response, and character and amount of vaginal bleeding. Watch for sudden changes in vital signs, and frequent periods of uterine relaxation.
● Hypocalcemia may decrease patient response; I.V. administration of calcium salts is necessary.
● High doses during delivery may cause uterine tetany and possible infant hypoxia or intracranial hemorrhage.
● Store tablets in tightly closed, light-resistant container. Discard if discolored.
● Store I.V. solutions below 46.4 F. (8 C.). Daily stock may be kept at cool room temperature for 60 days.
● Ergonovine has been used as a diagnostic agent for angina pectoris.

Information for the patient
● Tell patient not to smoke while taking this medication.
● Advise the patient of adverse reactions.

Breast-feeding
Ergot alkaloids inhibit lactation. This drug is excreted in breast milk, and ergotism has been reported in breast-fed infants of mothers treated with other ergot alkaloids. Use with caution.

ergotamine tartrate
Ergomar, Ergostat, Medihaler-Ergotamine, Wigrettes

● Pharmacologic classification: ergot alkaloid
● Therapeutic classification: vasoconstrictor
● Pregnancy risk category X

How supplied
Available without prescription, as appropriate
Tablets (sublingual): 2 mg
Aerosal inhaler: 360 mcg/metered spray

Indications, route, and dosage
To prevent or abort vascular headache, including migraine and cluster headaches
Adults: Initially, 2 mg S.L., then 1 to 2 mg S.L. q ½ hour, to maximum 6 mg daily and 10 mg weekly. Alternatively, initially, inhalation; if not relieved in 5 minutes, repeat

inhalation. May repeat inhalations at least 5 minutes apart up to maximum of 6 inhalations per 24 hours or 15 inhalations weekly.

Pharmacodynamics

Vasoconstricting action: By stimulating alpha-adrenergic receptors, ergotamine in therapeutic doses causes peripheral vasoconstriction (if vascular tone is low); however, if vascular tone is high, it produces vasodilation. In high doses, it is a competitive alpha-adrenergic blocker. In therapeutic doses, it inhibits the reuptake of norepinephrine, which increases the vasoconstricting activity of ergotamine. A weaker serotonin antagonist, it reduces the increased rate of platelet aggregation caused by serotonin.

In the treatment of vascular headaches, ergotamine probably causes direct vasoconstriction of dilated carotid artery beds while decreasing the amplitude of pulsations. Its serotoninergic and catecholamine effects also seem to be involved.

Pharmacokinetics

● *Absorption:* Ergotamine is rapidly absorbed after inhalation and variably absorbed after oral administration. Peak concentrations are reached within ½ to 3 hours. Caffeine may increase rate and extent of absorption. Drug undergoes first-pass metabolism after oral administration.
● *Distribution:* Ergotamine is widely distributed throughout the body.
● *Metabolism:* Ergotamine is extensively metabolized in the liver.
● *Excretion:* 4% of a dose is excreted in urine within 96 hours; remainder of a dose presumed to be excreted in feces. Ergotamine is dialyzable. Onset of action depends on how promptly drug is given after onset of headache.

Contraindications and precautions

Ergotamine is contraindicated in patients with sepsis or peripheral vascular disease, because of adverse vascular effects; in patients with impaired renal or hepatic function because of the potential for accumulation and toxicity; and in patients with malnutrition, severe pruritus, severe hypertension, or known hypersensitivity to drug or ergot alkaloids. Ergotamine is also contraindicated in women who are or who may become pregnant.

Interactions

Concomitant use with propranolol or other beta blockers may intensify ergotamine's vasoconstrictor effects. Use with troleandomycin appears to interfere with the detoxification of ergotamine in the liver; use concurrently with caution.

Effects on diagnostic tests

None reported.

Adverse reactions

● CV: numbness or tingling in fingers and toes, transient sinus tachycardia or bradycardia, arterial spasm, symptoms of impaired peripheral circulation (cold, numb, painful extremities with or without paresthesia; diminished or absent pulse in affected extremity; claudication of legs), coronary insufficiency, precipitation or aggravation of angina pectoris.
● GI: nausea, vomiting, abdominal pain, diarrhea, epigastric pain, ischemic colitis.

● Other: weakness in legs, localized edema, muscle pain or stiffness, fatigue, polydipsia, itching.
Note: Drug should be discontinued if patient develops hypersensitivity, signs and symptoms of impaired circulation, severe headaches, or worsening of migraine.

Overdose and treatment

Clinical manifestations of overdose include adverse vasospastic effects, nausea, vomiting, lassitude, impaired mental function, delirium, severe dyspnea, hypotension, hypertension, rapid and weak pulse, unconsciousness, spasms of the limbs, seizures, and shock.

Treatment requires supportive and symptomatic measures, with prolonged and careful monitoring. If patient is conscious and ingestion is recent, empty stomach by emesis or gastric lavage; if comatose, perform gastric lavage after placement of endotracheal tube with cuff inflated. Activated charcoal and a saline (magnesium sulfate) cathartic may be used. Provide respiratory support. Apply warmth (not direct heat) to ischemic extremities if vasospasm occurs. As needed, administer vasodilators (nitroprusside, prazosin, or tolazoline) and if necessary, I.V. diazepam to treat convulsions. Dialysis may be helpful.

▶ Special considerations

Besides those relevant to all *alpha-adrenergic blocking agents,* consider the following recommendations.
● Ergotamine is most effective when used in prodromal stage of headache or as soon as possible after onset. Provide quiet, low-light environment to relax patient after dose is administered.
● Store drug in light-resistant container.
● Sublingual tablet is preferred during early stage of attack because of its rapid absorption.
● Obtain an accurate dietary history to determine possible relationship between certain foods and onset of headache.
● Rebound headache or an increase in duration or frequency of headache may occur when drug is stopped.
● If patient experiences severe vasoconstriction with tissue necrosis, administer I.V. sodium nitroprusside or intra-arterial tolazoline. I.V. heparin and 10% dextran 40 in 5% dextrose injection also may be administered to prevent vascular stasis and thrombosis.

Information for the patient

● Instruct patient in correct use of inhaler.
● Urge patient to report immediately any feelings of numbness or tingling in fingers or toes, or red or violet blisters on hands or feet.
● Tell patient to avoid alcoholic beverages, because alcohol may worsen headache; and to avoid smoking, because it may increase adverse effects of drug.
● Warn patient to avoid prolonged exposure to very cold temperatures, which may increase adverse effects of drug.
● Tell patient to promptly report illness or infection, which may increase sensitivity to drug effects.
● Tell the patient that the body may need time to adjust, depending on the amount used and length of time involved, after discontinuing the medication.
● Patients who use inhaler should call promptly if mouth, throat, or lung infection occurs, or if condition worsens. Cough, hoarseness, or throat irritation may occur. Patient should gargle and rinse mouth after each dose to help prevent hoarseness and irritation.

- Advise patient to call promptly if persistent numbness or tingling and chest, muscle, or abdominal pain occur.
- Advise patient not to exceed recommended dosage.
- Tell patient not to eat, drink, or smoke while sublingual tablet is dissolving.

Geriatric use
Administer cautiously to elderly patients.

Pediatric use
Safety and efficacy of ergotamine in children has not been established. However, some clinicians recommend 1 mg sublingually in older children and adolescents; if no improvement, additional 1 mg dose may be given in 30 minutes.

Breast-feeding
Ergotamine is distributed into breast milk; therefore, it should be used with caution in breast-feeding women. Excessive dosage or prolonged administration of the drug may inhibit lactation.

---

erythrityl tetranitrate
Cardilate

- Pharmacologic classification: nitrate
- Therapeutic classification: antianginal, vasodilator
- Pregnancy risk category C

How supplied
Available by prescription only
Tablets: 10 mg (chewable); 5 mg, 10 mg (oral, sublingual, intrabuccal)

Indications, route, and dosage
Prophylaxis and long-term management of frequent or recurrent angina pain, reduced exercise tolerance associated with angina pectoris
Adults: 5 mg sublingually or buccally t.i.d. or 10 mg P.O., before meals, chewed t.i.d., increasing in 2 to 3 days if needed.

Pharmacodynamics
Antianginal action: Erythrityl tetranitrate shares the antianginal and vasodilating actions of other nitrates, although it does not relieve acute angina.

Pharmacokinetics
- *Absorption:* Erythrityl tetranitrate is absorbed when administered orally, sublingually, and intrabuccally. Onset of action occurs within 5 to 10 minutes after administration of sublingual, intrabuccal, and chewable tablets; within 30 minutes with other oral forms.
- *Distribution:* Little is known about drug's distribution; however, it is probably similar to that of nitroglycerin and other nitrates.
- *Metabolism:* Drug is metabolized in the liver and serum similarly to other nitrates. Metabolites are unknown.
- *Excretion:* Drug is excreted in the urine. Duration of effect for sublingual, intrabuccal, and chewable tablets is 30 minutes to 3 hours; for other oral forms, 60 to 90 minutes to maximal effect, lasting up to 6 hours.

Contraindications and precautions
Erythrityl tetranitrate is contraindicated in patients with head trauma or cerebral hemorrhage, because it may increase intracranial pressure, or in patients with a history of hypersensitivity or idiosyncratic reaction to nitrates; and in patients with severe anemia, because nitrate ions readily oxidize hemoglobin to methemoglobin.

Use caution when administering erythrityl tetranitrate to patients with increased intracranial pressure, because the drug dilates meningeal vessels; in patients with open or closed-angle glaucoma, although intraocular pressure is increased only briefly and aqueous humor drainage from the eye is unimpeded; in patients with diuretic-induced fluid depletion or low systolic blood pressure (below 90 mm Hg), because of the drug's hypotensive effect; and in patients in the initial days after acute myocardial infarction, because the drug may cause excessive hypotension and tachycardia.

Interactions
Concomitant use of erythrityl tetranitrate with alcohol, antihypertensive drugs, beta blockers, phenothiazines, or other nitrates may cause additive hypotensive effects. Concomitant use of oral erythrityl tetranitrate forms with ergot alkaloids may increase ergot alkaloid bioavailability and precipitate angina.

Effects on diagnostic tests
Erythrityl tetranitrate may interfere with serum cholesterol determination tests using the Zlatkis-Zak color reaction, resulting in a falsely decreased value.

Adverse reactions
- CNS: headache, dizziness, blurred vision.
- CV: orthostatic hypotension, tachycardia, palpitations, ankle edema, syncope, fainting.
- DERM: cutaneous vasodilation with flushing, rash, dermatitis.
- GI: dry mouth, nausea, vomiting.
- Local: sublingual burning, skin irritation.
- Other: hypersensitivity.
  Note: Drug should be discontinued if rash, dermatitis, blurred vision, or dry mouth occurs.

Overdose and treatment
Clinical effects of overdose result primarily from vasodilation and methemoglobinemia and include hypotension; persistent throbbing headache; palpitations; visual disturbance; flushing of the skin and sweating (with skin later becoming cold and cyanotic); nausea and vomiting; colic and bloody diarrhea; orthostasis; initial hyperpnea, dyspnea and slow respiratory rate; bradycardia; heart block; increased intracranial pressure with confusion, fever, paralysis, and tissue hypoxia from methemoglobinemia, possibly leading to cyanosis, metabolic acidosis, circulatory collapse, coma, and clonic convulsions. Death may follow circulatory collapse or asphyxia.

Treatment includes gastric lavage; administration of activated charcoal may help remove remaining gastric contents. Blood gas measurements and methemoglobin levels should be monitored, as indicated. Supportive care includes respiratory support and oxygen, passive movement of extremities to aid venous return, recumbent positioning (Trendelenburg position, if necessary), maintenance of adequate body temperature, and administration of I.V. fluids. An I.V. alpha-adrenergic agonist (such as phenylephrine) may be considered if patient requires further treatment. For methemoglobinemia, methylene blue (1 to 2 mg/kg I.V.) may be given. Epinephrine and related compounds are contraindicated in nitrate overdose.

▶ **Special considerations**
● If drug causes headache (most likely with initial doses), administer aspirin or acetaminophen. Dose may need to be reduced temporarily, but tolerance usually develops.
● Additional dose may be administered before anticipated stress or at bedtime if angina is nocturnal.
● Monitor blood pressure and intensity and duration of response to drug.
● Drug may cause orthostatic hypotension. To minimize this, have patient change to upright position slowly, go up and down stairs carefully, and lie down at the first sign of dizziness.
● Do not discontinue drug abruptly, because coronary vasospasm may occur. To avoid withdrawal symptoms, dosage should be reduced gradually after long-term use.
● Store medication in cool place, in tightly closed container away from light. To ensure freshness, replace supply every 3 months. Remove cotton from container because it absorbs drug.
● Erythrityl tetranitrate has proven effective in some patients with diffuse esophageal spasm without gastroesophageal reflux.

Information for the patient
● Warn patient that drug may cause headache initially but that this symptom usually responds to common headache remedies.
● Instruct patient to take medication regularly, even long-term, as prescribed, and to keep it easily accessible at all times. Tell patient drug is physiologically necessary, not addictive.
● Teach patient to take oral tablets on empty stomach, either 30 minutes before or 1 to 2 hours after meals; to swallow oral tablets whole; and to chew chewable tablets thoroughly before swallowing.
● Instruct patient to wet sublingual tablet with saliva, place it under tongue until completely absorbed, and sit down and rest. Burning sensation indicates potency. If patient complains of tingling sensation with drug placed sublingually, he may try holding tablet in buccal pouch.
● Instruct patient to avoid alcohol while taking this drug because severe hypotension and cardiovascular collapse may occur.
● Advise patient to change positions gradually to avoid excessive dizziness.
● Tell patient to call promptly if blurred vision, dry mouth, or persistent headache occurs.

erythromycin base
E-Mycin, Eryc, Eryc Sprinkle*, Eryfed, Ethril 500, Erythrocin, Erythromycin Base Filmtabs, Robimycin

erythromycin estolate
Ilosone

erythromycin ethylsuccinate
E.E.S., E-Mycin E, EryPed, Pediamycin, Pediazole, Wyamycin E

erythromycin glucceptate
Ilotycin Glucceptate

erythromycin lactobionate
Erythrocin Lactobionate

erythromycin stearate
Apo-Erythro-S*, Erypar Filmseal, Erythrocin Stearate, Ethril, Novorythro*, Wyamycin S

erythromycin (topical)
Akne-Mycin, A/T/S, EryDerm, Erymax, Eryvette, Sansac*, Staticin, T-Stat

● Pharmacologic classification: erythromycin
● Therapeutic classification: antibiotic
● Pregnancy risk category C

How supplied
Available by prescription only
Oral suspension: 200 mg/5 ml, 125 mg/5 ml, 400 mg/5 ml
Erythromycin base
Tablets (enteric-coated): 250 mg, 330 mg, 500 mg
Pellets (enteric-coated): 125 mg, 250 mg
Erythromycin estolate
Tablets: 250 mg, 500 mg
Tablets (chewable): 125 mg, 250 mg
Capsules: 125 mg, 250 mg
Drops: 100 mg/ml
Suspension: 125 mg/5 ml, 250 mg/5 ml
Erythromycin ethylsuccinate
Tablets (chewable): 200 mg, 400 mg
Topical solution: 1.5%, 2%
Oral suspension: 400 mg/5 ml
Powder for oral suspension: 200 mg/5 ml (after reconstitution)
Granules for oral suspension: 400 mg/5 ml (after reconstitution)
Ophthalmic ointment: 5 mg/g
Erythromycin glucceptate
Injection: 500-mg and 1-g vials
Erythromycin lactobionate
Injection: 500-mg and 1-g vials
Erythromycin stearate
Tablets (film-coated): 250 mg, 500 mg

Indications, route, and dosage
Acute pelvic inflammatory disease caused by Neisseria gonorrhoeae
Adults: 500 mg I.V. (erythromycin glucceptate, lactobionate) q 6 hours for 3 days, then 250 mg (erythromycin base, estolate, stearate) or 400 mg (erythromycin ethylsuccinate) P.O. q 6 hours for 7 days.
Endocarditis prophylaxis for dental procedures in patients allergic to penicillin
Erythromycin base, estolate, stearate
Adults: 1 g P.O. 1 hour before procedure, then 500 mg P.O. 6 hours later.
Treatment of intestinal amebiasis in patients who cannot receive metronidazole
Erythromycin base, estolate, stearate
Adults: 250 mg P.O. q 6 hours for 10 to 14 days.
Children: 30 to 50 mg/kg P.O. daily, divided q 6 hours for 10 to 14 days.

Mild to moderately severe respiratory tract, skin, and soft-tissue infections caused by susceptible organisms
Erythromycin base, estolate, stearate
Adults: 250 to 500 mg P.O. q 6 hours.
Erythromycin ethylsuccinate
Adults: 400 to 800 mg P.O. q 6 hours; or 15 to 20 mg/kg I.V. daily, as continuous infusion or divided q 6 hours.
Oral erythromycin salts
Children: 30 to 50 mg/kg P.O. daily, divided q 6 hours; or 15 to 20 mg/kg I.V. daily, divided q 4 to 6 hours.
Syphilis
Erythromycin base, estolate, stearate
Adults: 500 mg P.O. q.i.d. for 15 days.
Legionnaire's disease
Adults: 500 mg to 1 g I.V. or P.O. q 6 hours for 21 days.
Uncomplicated urethral, endocervical, or rectal infections when tetracyclines are contraindicated
Adults: 500 mg P.O. q.i.d. for at least 7 days.
Urogenital Chlamydia trachomatis infections during pregnancy
Adults: 500 mg P.O. q.i.d. for at least 7 days or 250 mg P.O. q.i.d. for at least 14 days.
Conjunctivitis caused by C. trachomatis in neonates
Neonates: 50 mg/kg/day in four divided doses for at least 2 weeks.
Pneumonia of infancy caused by C. trachomatis
Infants: 50 mg/kg/day in four divided doses for at least 3 weeks.
Topical treatment of acne vulgaris
Adults and children: Apply to the affected area b.i.d.
Prophylaxis of ophthalmia neonatorum
Neonates: Apply ointment no later than 1 hour after birth. Use new tube for each infant and do not flush after instillation. Infants born to women with gonorrhea should also be given I.M. or I.V. penicillin G 50,000 units (for term) or 20,000 units (for low birth weight).

Pharmacodynamics
Antibacterial action: Erythromycin inhibits bacterial protein synthesis by binding to the ribosomal 50S subunit. It is used in the treatment of *Haemophilus influenzae, Entamoeba histolytica, Mycoplasma pneumoniae, Corynebacterium diphtheriae* and *C. minutissimum, Legionella pneumophila,* and *Bordetella pertussis.* It may be used as an alternative to penicillins or tetracycline in the treatment of *Streptococcus pneumoniae, S. viridans, Listeria monocytogenes, Staphylococcus aureus, Chlamydia trachomatis, Neisseria gonorrhoeae,* and *Ureponema pallidium.*

Pharmacokinetics
● *Absorption:* Because base salt is acid-sensitive, it must be buffered or have enteric coating to prevent destruction by gastric acids. Acid salts and esters (estolate, ethylsuccinate, and stearate) are not affected by gastric acidity and therefore are well absorbed. Base and stearate preparations should be given on empty stomach. Absorption of estolate and ethylsuccinate preparations is unaffected or possibly even enhanced by presence of food. When administered topically, drug is absorbed minimally.
● *Distribution:* Erythromycin is distributed widely to most body tissues and fluids except CSF, where it appears only in low concentrations. Drug crosses the placenta. About 80% of erythromycin base and 96% of erythromycin estolate are protein-bound.
● *Metabolism:* Erythromycin is metabolized partially in the liver to inactive metabolites.
● *Excretion:* Erythromycin is excreted mainly unchanged in bile. Only small drug amounts (less than 5%) are excreted in urine; some drug is excreted in breast milk. In patients with normal renal function, plasma half-life is about 1½ hours. Peritoneal hemodialysis does not remove drug.

Contraindications and precautions
Erythromycin is contraindicated in patients with known hypersensitivity to drug. Erythromycin estolate is contraindicated in patients with hepatic disease because drug may be hepatotoxic.

Other erythromycin forms should be administered cautiously to patients with preexisting hepatic disease because drug may exacerbate hepatic dysfunction.

Interactions
Concomitant use of erythromycin may inhibit metabolism of theophylline (possibly leading to elevated serum theophylline levels), warfarin (causing excessive anticoagulant effect), carbamazepine (possibly causing toxicity), and cyclosporine (resulting in elevation of serum cyclosporine levels to nearly nephrotoxic ranges).

When used concomitantly with topical desquamating or abrasive acne preparations, topical erythromycin has a cumulative irritant effect.

Effects on diagnostic tests
Erythromycin may interfere with fluorometric determination of urinary catecholamines. Liver function test results may become abnormal during erythromycin therapy (rare).

Adverse reactions
● DERM: urticaria; rashes; erythema, burning, dryness, pruritus (with topical application).
● EENT: eye irritation (with topical application), hearing loss (with high I.V. doses, especially in patients with renal failure).
● GI: abdominal pain and cramps, nausea, vomiting, diarrhea.
● Hepatic: cholestatic jaundice (with estolate).
● Local: venous irritation, thrombophlebitis (both after I.V. injection).
● Other: overgrowth of nonsusceptible bacteria or fungi, *anaphylaxis*, fever, sensitivity reaction (with topical application).
Note: Drug should be discontinued if patient develops hypersensitivity reaction.

Overdose and treatment
No information available.

▶ Special considerations
● Culture and sensitivity tests should be performed before treatment starts and then as needed.
● Base and stearate preparations should be given on empty stomach. Absorption of estolate and ethylsuccinate preparations is unaffected or possibly even enhanced by presence of food. When administered topically, drug is minimally absorbed.
● Erythromycin estolate may cause serious hepatotoxicity (reversible cholestatic jaundice) in adults. Monitor liver function tests for increased serum bilirubin, AST (SGOT), and alkaline phosphatase levels. Other

erythromycin salts can cause less severe hepatotoxicity. (Patients who develop hepatotoxicity from erythromycin estolate may react similarly to any erythromycin preparation.)

• If patient is receiving erythromycin concomitantly with theophylline, monitor serum theophylline levels.

• If patient is receiving erythromycin concomitantly with warfarin, monitor for prolonged prothrombin time and abnormal bleeding.

• Reconstitute injectable form (lactobionate) according to manufacturer's instructions and dilute every 250 mg in at least 100 ml of normal saline solution. Continuous infusions are preferred, but drug may be given by intermittent infusion at a maximum concentration of 5 mg/ml infused over 20 to 60 minutes.

• Do not administer erythromycin lactobionate with other drugs because of chemical instability. Reconstituted solutions are acidic and should be completely administered within 8 hours of preparation.

• Drug may cause overgrowth of nonsusceptible bacteria or fungi.

• Although drug is bacteriostatic, it may be bactericidal in high concentrations or against highly susceptible organisms.

Information for the patient

• For best absorption, instruct patient to take oral form with full glass of water 1 hour before or 2 hours after meals. (However, patient receiving enteric-coated tablets may take them with meals). Advise patient not to take drug with fruit juice. If patient is taking chewable tablets, instruct him not to swallow them whole.

• If patient is using topical solution, instruct him to wash, rinse, and dry affected areas before applying it. Warn patient not to apply solution near eyes, nose, mouth, or other mucous membranes. Caution patient to avoid sharing washcloths and towels with family members.

• Instruct patient applying ophthalmic ointment to wash hands before and after applying ointment. Instruct him to cleanse eye area of excess exudate before applying ointment. Warn him not to allow tube to touch the eye or surrounding tissue. Instruct him to promptly report signs of sensitivity, such as itching eyelids and constant burning.

• Instruct patient to take drug exactly as directed and to continue taking it for prescribed period, even after he feels better.

• Instruct patient to report adverse reactions promptly.

Breast-feeding

Although drug is excreted in breast milk, no adverse reactions have been reported. Administer cautiously to breast-feeding women.

---

esmolol
Brevibloc

• Pharmacologic classification: beta₁-adrenergic blocking agent
• Therapeutic classification: antiarrhythmic
• Pregnancy risk category C

How supplied
Available by prescription only
Injection: 250 mg/ml, in 10-ml ampules

Indications, route, and dosage
Supraventricular tachycardia

Adults: Dosage range is 50 to 200 mcg/kg/min; average dose is 100 mcg/kg/min. Individual dosage adjustment requires step-wise titration in which each step consists of a loading dose followed by a maintenance dose.

To begin treatment, administer a loading infusion of 500 mcg/kg/min for 1 minute followed by a 4-minute maintenance infusion of 50 mcg/kg/min. If tachycardia does not subside within 5 minutes, repeat the loading dose and follow with a maintenance infusion increased to 100 mcg/kg/min. Continue titration, repeating loading infusion and increasing each maintenance infusion by 50 mcg/kg/min. As the patient's heart rate or blood pressure reaches a safety end-point, omit the loading infusion and reduce the increase in maintenance infusion from 50 mcg/kg/min to 25 mcg/kg/min or less; also, increase the interval between titration steps from 5 to 10 minutes.

Pharmacodynamics
Antiarrhythmic action: Esmolol, a beta₁ blocker with rapid onset and very short duration of action, decreases blood pressure and heart rate in a dose-related, titratable manner. Its hemodynamic effects are similar to those of propranolol, but it does not increase vascular resistance.

Pharmacokinetics
• *Absorption:* Absorption is immediate after I.V. infusion.
• *Distribution:* Esmolol is distributed rapidly throughout the plasma. Distribution half-life is about 2 minutes. Esmolol is 55% protein-bound.
• *Metabolism:* Drug is hydrolyzed rapidly by plasma esterases.
• *Excretion:* Esmolol is excreted by the kidneys as metabolites. Elimination half-life is about 9 minutes.

Contraindications and precautions
Esmolol is contraindicated in patients hypersensitive to the drug; and should not be used in patients with cardiac failure, cardiogenic shock, second- or third-degree atrioventricular block, or sinus bradycardia (less than 45 beats/minute) because the drug may worsen cardiac depression. Esmolol is not for use on a long-term basis when transfer to another agent is anticipated.

Esmolol should be used with caution in atopic patients, and in patients with bronchial asthma, emphysema, or bronchitis because it may precipitate bronchospasm. In patients with diabetes, esmolol may mask tachycardia associated with hypoglycemia.

Interactions
Because of esmolol's short duration of action and the short periods of time over which it is used, many of the drug interactions associated with other beta blockers do not apply. Concurrent use of esmolol with insulin or oral antidiabetic agents may mask symptoms of developing hypoglycemia, such as rising pulse rate and blood pressure. Use with nondepolarizing neuromuscular blocking agents such as gallamine, metocurine, pancuronium, or tubocurarine may potentiate and prolonge their action; careful postoperative monitoring of the patient may be necessary after concurrent or sequential use, especially if there is a possibility of incomplete reversal of neuromuscular blockade.

Use with antihypertensives may potentiate their hypotensive effects and requires dosage adjustments based on blood pressure measurements.

Use with monoamine oxidase (MAO) inhibitors, including pargyline, furazolidone, and procarbazine, may cause significant hypertension—theoretically as long as 14 days after discontinuation of the MAO inhibitor. Concurrent use of esmolol with MAO inhibitors is not recommended.

Concurrent use of esmolol with intravenous phenytoin may produce additive cardiac depressant effects. Concurrent use with reserpine may result in additive and possibly excessive beta-adrenergic blockade with bradycardia and hypotension. Close observation is recommended.

Concurrent use of esmolol with sympathomimetic amines having beta-adrenergic stimulant activity may cause mutual but transient inhibition of therapeutic effects. Use with xanthines, especially aminophylline or theophylline, may cause mutual inhibition of therapeutic effects and (except for dyphylline) may decrease theophylline clearance, especially in patients with increased theophylline clearance induced by smoking; concurrent use requires careful monitoring to prevent toxic accumulation of theophylline. Concomitant I.V. administration with digoxin may increase digoxin blood levels 10% to 20%; I.V. administration of morphine increases esmolol steady-state levels by 46%.

Effects on diagnostic tests
None reported.

Adverse reactions
● CV: hypotension.
● DERM: induration or inflammation at infusion site, edema, erythema.
● Other: breathing difficulty, urinary retention, speech disorders, pain, fever, pallor, flushing, diaphoresis, drowsiness, dizziness, confusion, paresthesias.

Overdose and treatment
Limited information available. Hypotension would be the most likely symptom.

Symptoms of esmolol overdose usually disappear quickly after esmolol is withdrawn. In addition to immediate discontinuation of esmolol infusion, treatment is supportive and symptomatic.

Some clinicians report the effective use of glucagon to combat the cardiovascular effects (bradycardia, hypotension) of overdose with beta blockers. An I.V. dose of 2 to 3 mg is administered over 30 seconds and repeated if necessary, followed by infusion at 5 mg/hour until the patient's condition has stabilized.

▶ **Special considerations**
● Esmolol hydrochloride injection must be diluted and administered by intravenous infusion. Concentrations that exceed 10 mg of esmolol hydrochloride per ml may produce irritation.
● To prepare esmolol hydrochloride injection for administration by intravenous infusion, aseptically remove 20 ml from a 500 ml bottle of intravenous fluid (5% dextrose injection USP, 5% dextrose in Ringer's injection, 5% dextrose and 0.45% sodium chloride injection USP, 5% dextrose and 0.9% sodium chloride injection USP, lactated Ringer's injection USP, 0.45% sodium chloride injection USP, or 0.9% sodium chloride injection USP) and then add 5 g esmolol hydrochloride injection to the bottle to produce a solution containing 10 mg of esmolol hydrochloride per ml.

● Not compatible with 5% sodium bicarbonate injection USP.
● Diluted solutions of esmolol hydrochloride are stable for at least 24 hours at room temperature.
● If irritation occurs at the infusion site, the infusion should be stopped and resumed at another site. Use of butterfly needles for I.V. administration of esmolol is not recommended.
● To convert to other antiarrhythmic therapy after control has been achieved with esmolol, reduce the infusion rate of esmolol by one-half 30 minutes after administration of the first dose of the alternative agent. If after the second dose of the alternative agent a satisfactory response is maintained for 1 hour, then discontinue esmolol.
● Monitor patient's pulse and blood pressure.

Geriatric use
Although adequate and well-controlled studies have not been done in the geriatric population, the elderly may be less sensitive to some of the effects of beta blockers. However, reduced metabolic and excretory capabilities in many elderly patients may lead to increased myocardial depression and require dosage reduction of beta blockers. Dosage adjustment should be based on clinical response.

Pediatric use
Adequate and well-controlled studies have not been done. Safety and efficacy in children have not been established.

Breast-feeding
It is not known whether esmolol is excreted in human breast milk; no problems associated with breast-feeding have been reported.

estazolam
ProSom

● Pharmacologic classification: benzodiazepine
● Therapeutic classification: hypnotic
● Pregnancy risk category X

How supplied
Available by prescription only
Tablets: 1 mg, 2 mg

Indications, route, and dosage
Short-term management of insomnia characterized by difficulty in falling asleep, frequent nocturnal awakenings, or early-morning awakenings
Adults: Initially, 1 mg P.O. h.s.; may increase to 2 mg as needed and tolerated.
Older adults: 1 mg P.O. h.s.
Small or debilitated older adults: Initially, 0.5 mg P.O. h.s.; may increase with care to 1 mg if needed.

Pharmacodynamics
Hypnotic action: Estazolam depresses the CNS at the limbic and subcortical levels of the brain. It produces a sedative-hypnotic effect by potentiating the effect of the neurotransmitter gamma-aminobutyric acid on its receptor in the ascending reticular activating system,

---

which increases inhibition and blocks both cortical and limbic arousal.

Pharmacokinetics
● *Absorption:* Estazolam is rapidly and completely absorbed through the GI tract in 1 to 3 hours. Peak levels occur within 2 hours (range is 0.5 to 6 hours).
● *Distribution:* Estazolam is 93% protein-bound.
● *Metabolism:* Extensively metabolized in the liver.
● *Excretion:* Metabolites are excreted primarily in the urine. Less than 5% is excreted in urine as unchanged drug; 4% of a 2-mg dose is excreted in feces. Elimination half-life ranges from 10 to 24 hours; clearance is accelerated in smokers.

Contraindications and precautions
Estazolam is contraindicated in patients with a history of hypersensitivity to benzodiazepines, and during pregnancy because of the risk of fetal damage. Use with caution in elderly and debilitated patients and in those with hepatic impairment, compromised respiratory function, depression, impaired renal function, or sleep apnea.

Interactions
Estazolam potentiates CNS depressant effects of phenothiazines, narcotics, antihistamines, MAO inhibitors, barbiturates, alcohol, general anesthetics, and tricyclic antidepressants. Concurrent use with cimetidine, disulfiram, oral contraceptives, and isoniazid may diminish hepatic metabolism, resulting in increased plasma concentrations of estazolam and increased CNS depressant effects. Heavy smoking accelerates estazolam's metabolism, resulting in diminished clinical efficacy. Like other benzodiazepines, estazolam increases phenytoin and digoxin levels, possibly resulting in toxicity. Use with probenecid results in more rapid onset and more prolonged benzodiazepine effect. Theophylline antagonizes estazolam's pharmacologic effects. Rifampin increases clearance and decreases half-life of estazolam.

Effects on diagnostic tests
AST (SGOT) levels may be increased.

Adverse reactions
● CNS: headache, abnormal coordination, nervousness, apprehension, malaise, confusion, somnolence, irritability, drowsiness, hypokinesia, amnesia, lethargy, hangover effect, ataxia, dizziness, euphoria, talkativeness, apathy, hostility, weakness, tremor, depression, syncope, nightmares, slurred speech, daytime sedation, restlessness, possible hallucinations and paradoxical reactions in elderly patients.
● CV: palpitations, chest pain, hypotension (rare), tachycardia.
● GI: nausea, vomiting, diarrhea, constipation, dry mouth, taste aberrations, anorexia, abdominal discomfort, heartburn, dyspepsia, flatulence.
● DERM: rash, urticaria, sweating, flushes, acne (rare), dry skin (rare).
● EENT: abnormal vision, ear pain, eye irritation, eye pain, eye swelling, photophobia, tinnitus, sinusitis, epistaxis, diplopia (rare), decreased hearing (rare).
● GU: urinary frequency and urgency, urinary hesitancy, menstrual cramps, decreased libido, vaginal discharge and itching, penile discharge, nocturia.
● Respiratory: cold, flulike symptoms, pharyngitis, asthma, cough, dyspnea, hyperventilation.
● Other: leg pain, back pain, body pain, muscle stiffness, myalgia, allergic reaction, swollen lymph nodes, edema, weight gain.

Overdose and treatment
Somnolence, confusion with reduced or absent reflexes, respiratory depression, apnea, hypotension, impaired coordination, slurred speech, seizures, or coma can occur from benzodiazepine overdose. If excitation occurs, do not use barbiturates. Remember that multiple agents may have been ingested. Gastric evacuation and lavage should be performed immediately. Monitor respiration, pulse rate, and blood pressure. Use symptomatic and supportive measures. Maintain airway and administer fluids.

▶ Special considerations
Besides those relevant to all *benzodiazepines*, consider the following recommendations.
● Remove all potential safety hazards, such as cigarettes, from patient's reach.
● Regularly perform blood counts, urinalysis, and blood chemistry analyses.
● Withdraw drug slowly after prolonged use.
● Encourage good sleep habits and regular exercise. Advise the avoidance of caffeine or other stimulants, especially late in the day.

Information for the patient
● Tell patient to avoid alcohol and other CNS depressants while taking this medication. After taking the drug in the evening, patient should avoid alcohol the following day.
● Tell patient to inform physician of medications he is taking and of usual alcohol consumption.
● Warn that drug may cause drowsiness. Advise special caution and avoidance of driving or operating hazardous machinery until adverse CNS effects of the drug are known.
● Nocturnal sleep may be disturbed for 1 or 2 nights after stopping the drug.
● Tell patient to inform physician of pregnancy or the plan to become pregnant while taking this drug.
● Warn patient not to discontinue drug abruptly after taking it daily for prolonged period, not to vary dosage or increase dose unless directed by physician, and not to use if breast-feeding (estazolam is excreted in breast milk).

Geriatric use
Elderly patients may be more susceptible to CNS depressant effects of estazolam. Use with caution. Lower dosage may be required. To prevent injury from dizziness and falls, elderly patients should be supervised during daily living activities, especially at the start of treatment and after any increase in dosage.

Pediatric use
Safety and efficacy have not been established.

Breast-feeding
Estazolam is excreted in breast milk and should not be used by patients who are breast-feeding.

---

esterified estrogens
Estratab, Menest

- Pharmacologic classification: estrogen
- Therapeutic classification: estrogen replacement, antineoplastic
- Pregnancy risk category X

How supplied
Tablets: 0.3 mg, 0.625 mg, 1.25 mg, 2.5 mg

Indications, route, and dosage
Prostatic cancer
Adults: 1.25 to 2.5 mg P.O. t.i.d.
Breast cancer
Men and postmenopausal women: 10 mg P.O. t.i.d. for 3 or more months.
Female hypogonadism, ovariectomy, primary ovarian failure
Adults: 2.5 mg daily to t.i.d. in cycles of 3 weeks on, 1 week off.
Menopausal symptoms
Adults: 0.625 to 1.25 mg P.O. daily in cycles of 3 weeks on, 1 week off.

Pharmacodynamics
Estrogenic action: Esterified estrogen mimics the action of endogenous estrogen in treating female hypogonadism, menopausal symptoms, and atrophic vaginitis. It inhibits growth of hormone-sensitive tissue in advanced, inoperable prostatic cancer, and in certain carefully selected cases of breast cancer in men and postmenopausal women.

Pharmacokinetics
- *Absorption:* After oral administration, esterified estrogens are well absorbed but substantially inactivated by the liver. Therefore, esterified estrogens are usually administered parenterally.
- *Distribution:* Esterified estrogens are approximately 50% to 80% plasma protein-bound, particularly the estradiol-binding globulin. Distribution occurs throughout the body with highest concentrations appearing in fat.
- *Metabolism:* Esterified estrogens are metabolized primarily in the liver, where they are conjugated with sulfate and glucuronide.
- *Excretion:* Most esterified estrogens are eliminated through the kidneys, in the form of sulfate or glucuronide conjugates.

Contraindications and precautions
Esterified estrogens are contraindicated in patients with thrombophlebitis or thromboembolism because of their association with thromboembolic disorders; in patients with estrogen-responsive carcinoma (breast or genital tract cancer); and in patients with undiagnosed abnormal genital bleeding. The drugs are also contraindicated in pregnant women because they may be fetotoxic and in breast-feeding women because they may adversely affect the infant.

Esterified estrogens should be administered cautiously to patients with disorders that may be aggravated by fluid and electrolyte accumulation, such as asthma, seizure disorders, migraine, or cardiac, renal, or hepatic dysfunction. Carefully monitor female patients who have breast nodules, fibrocystic breast disease, or a family history of breast cancer. Because of the risk of thromboembolism, therapy with esterified estrogens should be discontinued at least 1 week before elective surgical procedures associated with an increased incidence of thromboembolism.

Interactions
Concomitant administration of drugs that induce hepatic metabolism, such as rifampin, barbiturates, primidone, carbamazepine, and phenytoin, may result in decreased estrogenic effects from a given dose. These drugs are known to accelerate the rate of metabolism of certain other agents.

In patients with diabetes, esterified estrogens may increase blood glucose levels, necessitating dosage adjustment of insulin or oral hypoglycemic drugs.

Concomitant use with anticoagulants may decrease the effects of warfarin-type anticoagulants. Concomitant use with adrenocorticosteroids or adrenocorticotropic hormone may cause greater risk of fluid and electrolyte accumulation.

Effects on diagnostic tests
Therapy with esterified estrogens increases sulfobromophthalein retention, prothrombin time and clotting Factors VII to X, and norepinephrine-induced platelet aggregability. Increases in the thyroid-binding globulin concentration may occur, resulting in increased total thyroid concentrations (measured by protein-bound iodine or total thyroxine) and decreased uptake of free triiodothyronine resin. Serum folate, pyridoxine, and antithrombin III concentrations may decrease; triglyceride, glucose, and phospholipid levels may increase. Glucose tolerance may be impaired. Pregnanediol excretion may decrease.

Adverse reactions
- CNS: headache, dizziness, chorea, depression, libido changes, lethargy.
- CV: thrombophlebitis; *thromboembolism;* hypertension; edema; *increased risk of stroke, pulmonary embolism, and myocardial infarction.*
- DERM: melasma, rash, acne, hirsutism or hair loss, seborrhea, oily skin.
- EENT: worsening of myopia or astigmatism, intolerance to contact lenses.
- GI: nausea, vomiting, abdominal cramps, bloating, diarrhea, constipation, anorexia, increased appetite, weight changes.
- GU: breakthrough bleeding, altered menstrual flow, dysmenorrhea, amenorrhea, cervical erosion, altered cervical secretions, enlargement of uterine fibromas, vaginal candidiasis; *in males:* gynecomastia, testicular atrophy, impotence.
- Hepatic: cholestatic jaundice.
- Metabolic: hyperglycemia, hypercalcemia, folic acid deficiency.
- Other: breast changes (tenderness, enlargement, secretion).

Overdose and treatment
Serious toxicity after overdose of these drugs has not been reported. Nausea may be expected to occur. Appropriate supportive care should be provided.

▶ Special considerations
Recommendations for administration of esterified estrogens and for care and teaching of the patient during therapy are the same as those for all *estrogens.*

Breast-feeding
Esterified estrogens are contraindicated in breast-feeding women.

---

estradiol
Estrace, Estrace Vaginal Cream, Estraderm

estradiol cypionate
Depestro, depGynogen, Depo-Estradiol Cypionate, Depogen, Dura-Estrin, Estra-D, Estro-Cyp, Estrofem, Estroject-LA, Estronol-LA, Hormogen Depot

estradiol valerate
Delestrogen*, Dioval, Dioval XX, Dioval 40, Duragen, Estradiol L.A., Estradiol L.A. 20, Estradiol L.A. 40, Estraval, Gynogen L.A. 10, Gynogen L.A. 20, L.A.E. 20, Valergen-10, Valergen-20, Valergen-40

polyestradiol phosphate
Estradurin

- Pharmacologic classification: estrogen
- Therapeutic classification: estrogen replacement, antineoplastic
- Pregnancy risk category X

How supplied
Available by prescription only
Estradiol
Tablets: 1 mg, 2 mg
Vaginal: 0.1 mg/g cream (in nonliquefying base)
Transdermal: 4 mg/10 cm² (delivers 0.05 mg/24 hours); 8 mg/20 cm² (delivers 0.1 mg/24 hours)
Estradiol cypionate
Injection: 1 mg/ml, 5 mg/ml (in oil)
Estradiol valerate
Injection: 10 mg/ml, 20 mg/ml, 40 mg/ml (in oil)
Polyestradiol phosphate
Injection: 40 mg/2 ml

Indications, route, and dosage
Atrophic vaginitis, atrophic dystrophy of the vulva, menopausal symptoms, hypogonadism, ovariectomy, primary ovarian failure
Estradiol tablets: 1 to 2 mg P.O. daily, in cycles of 21 days on and 7 days off or cycles of 5 days on and 2 days off; or 0.2 to 1 mg I.M. weekly.
Estradiol valerate injection: 10 to 20 mg I.M. once a month.
Estradiol transdermal: Place one Estraderm transdermal patch on trunk of the body twice weekly. Administer on an intermittent cyclic schedule (3 weeks on and 1 week off).
Atrophic vaginitis
Estradiol vaginal cream: 2 to 4 g daily for 1 to 2 weeks. When vaginal mucosa is restored, begin maintenance dosage of 1 g one to three times weekly.
Postpartum breast engorgement
Estradiol valerate injection: 10 to 25 mg I.M. at end of first stage of labor.

Female hypogonadism
Estradiol cypionate injection: 1.5 to 2 mg I.M. at monthly intervals.
Inoperable breast cancer
Estradiol tablets: 10 mg t.i.d. for 3 months.
Inoperable prostatic cancer
Estradiol valerate injection: 30 mg I.M. q 1 to 2 weeks
Estradiol tablets: 1 to 2 mg t.i.d.
Inoperable prostatic carcinoma, advancing
Polyestradiol phosphate injection: 40 mg I.M. q 2 to 4 weeks.

Pharmacodynamics
Estrogenic action: Estradiol mimics the action of endogenous estrogen in treating female hypogonadism, menopausal symptoms, and atrophic vaginitis. It inhibits growth of hormone-sensitive tissue in advanced, inoperable prostatic cancer and in certain carefully selected cases of breast cancer in men and postmenopausal women.

Pharmacokinetics
- *Absorption:* After oral administration, estradiol and the other natural unconjugated estrogens are well absorbed but substantially inactivated by the liver. Therefore, unconjugated estrogens are usually administered parenterally.
  After I.M. administration, absorption begins rapidly and continues for days. The cypionate and valerate esters administered in oil have prolonged durations of action because of their slow absorption characteristics.
  Topically applied estradiol is absorbed readily into the systemic circulation.
- *Distribution:* Estradiol and the other natural estrogens are approximately 50% to 80% plasma protein-bound, particularly the estradiol-binding globulin. Distribution occurs throughout the body, with highest concentrations appearing in fat.
- *Metabolism:* The steroidal estrogens, including estradiol, are metabolized primarily in the liver, where they are conjugated with sulfate and glucuronide. Because of the rapid rate of metabolism, nonesterified forms of estrogen, including estradiol, must usually be administered daily.
- *Excretion:* The majority of estrogen elimination occurs through the kidneys in the form of sulfate and/or glucuronide conjugates.

Contraindications and precautions
Estradiol is contraindicated in patients with thrombophlebitis or thromboembolism, estrogen-responsive carcinoma (breast or genital tract cancer), or undiagnosed abnormal genital bleeding; and in pregnant or breast-feeding women.
  This drug should be administered cautiously to patients with disorders that may be aggravated by fluid and electrolyte accumulation, such as asthma, seizure disorders, migraine, or cardiac, renal, or hepatic dysfunction. Carefully monitor female patients who have breast nodules, fibrocystic breast disease, or a family history of breast cancer. Because of the risk of thromboembolism, therapy with this drug should be discontinued at least 1 week before elective surgical procedures associated with an increased incidence of thromboembolism.
  The 2-mg tablet of Estrace contains the dye tartrazine, which may cause hypersensitivity reactions (bronchial asthma, anaphylaxis) in rare individuals. In many

---

cases, these individuals are also sensitive to aspirin and have nasal polyps.

Interactions

Concomitant administration of drugs that induce hepatic metabolism (such as rifampin, barbiturates, primidone, carbamazepine, and phenytoin) may decrease estrogenic effects from a given dose. These drugs are known to accelerate the rate of metabolism of certain other agents.

In patients with diabetes, estradiol may increase blood glucose levels, necessitating dosage adjustment of insulin or oral hypoglycemic drugs.

Concomitant use with anticoagulants may decrease the effects of warfarin-type anticoagulants.

Use with adrenocorticosteroids or adrenocorticotropic hormone increases the risk of fluid and electrolyte accumulation.

Use with hepatotoxic medications (especially dantrolene) increases risk of liver damage.

Effects on diagnostic tests

Estradiol increases sulfobromophthalein retention, prothrombin and clotting Factors VII to X, and norepinephrine-induced platelet aggregability. Increases in thyroid-binding globulin concentrations may occur, resulting in increased total thyroid concentrations (measured by protein-bound iodine or total thyroxine) and decreased uptake of free triiodothyronine resin. Serum folate, pyridoxine, and antithrombin III concentrations may decrease; triglyceride, glucose, and phospholipid levels may increase. Glucose tolerance may be impaired. Pregnanediol excretion may decrease.

Adverse reactions

● CNS: headache, dizziness, chorea, depression, libido changes, lethargy, premenstrual-like syndrome.
● CV: thrombophlebitis, *thromboembolism*, hypertension, *edema*.
● DERM: melasma, urticaria, acne, seborrhea, oily skin, hirsutism or hair loss.
● EENT: worsening of myopia or astigmatism, intolerance to contact lenses.
● GI: nausea, vomiting, abdominal cramps, bloating, diarrhea, constipation, anorexia, increased appetite, weight changes.
● GU: breakthrough bleeding, altered menstrual flow, dysmenorrhea, amenorrhea, cervical erosion, altered cervical secretions, enlargement of uterine fibromas, vaginal candidiasis; *in males:* gynecomastia, testicular atrophy, impotence.
● Hepatic: cholestatic jaundice.
● Metabolic: hyperglycemia, hypercalcemia, folic acid deficiency.
● Other: breast changes (tenderness, enlargement, secretions), leg cramps, exacerbation of porphyria.

Overdose and treatment

Serious toxicity after overdose of this drug has not been reported. Nausea may be expected to occur. Appropriate supportive care should be provided.

▶ Special considerations

Besides those relevant to all *estrogens,* consider the following recommendations.
● Before injection, make sure drug is well dispersed in solution by rolling the reconstituted vial between the palms.
● Administer by deep I.M. injection into large muscles.

Information for the patient
● Tell patient not to apply patch to her breast areas.
● Remind the patient not to use the same skin site for at least 1 week after removal of the transdermal system.

Geriatric use
Frequent physical examinations are recommended in postmenopausal women taking estrogen.

Breast-feeding
Estradiol is contraindicated in breast-feeding women.

---

estramustine phosphate sodium
Emcyt

● Pharmacologic classification: estrogen, alkylating agent
● Therapeutic classification: antineoplastic
● Pregnancy risk category C

How supplied
Available by prescription only
Capsules: 140 mg

Indications, route, and dosage
Dosage and indications may vary. Check literature for recommended protocols.
Palliative treatment of metastatic or progressive cancer of the prostate
Adults: 10 to 16 mg/kg P.O. in three to four divided doses. Usual dosage is 14 mg/kg daily. Therapy should continue for up to 3 months and, if successful, be maintained as long as the patient responds.

Pharmacodynamics
Antineoplastic action: The exact mechanism of action is unclear. However, the estrogenic portion of the molecule may act as a carrier of the drug to facilitate selective uptake by tumor cells with estradiol hormone receptors, such as those in the prostate gland. At that point, the nitrogen mustard portion of the drug acts as an alkylating agent.

Pharmacokinetics
● *Absorption:* After oral administration, about 75% of a dose is absorbed across the GI tract.
● *Distribution:* Estramustine distributes widely into body tissues.
● *Metabolism:* Estramustine is extensively metabolized in the liver.
● *Excretion:* Estramustine and its metabolites are eliminated primarily in feces, with a small amount excreted in urine. The terminal phase of plasma elimination has a half-life of 20 hours.

Contraindications and precautions
Estramustine is contraindicated in patients with a history of hypersensitivity to the drug or to estradiol or mechlorethamine; cross-sensitivity may occur. The drug is also contraindicated in patients with peptic ulcers, severe liver disease, cardiac disease, or impaired bone marrow function because it may worsen these conditions.

Because of the drug's cardiovascular toxicity, it should be used cautiously in patients with thromboembolic

---

disorders, cerebrovascular disorders, or coronary artery disease.

Interactions
Concomitant use of estramustine with anticoagulants may decrease the anticoagulant effect by an unknown mechanism and requires increased dosage of anticoagulants.

Effects on diagnostic tests
Estramustine therapy may increase norepinephrine-induced platelet aggregability. A reduced response to the metyrapone test may occur during therapy with estramustine. Glucose tolerance may be decreased.

Adverse reactions
- CNS: anxiety, headache, emotional liability.
- CV: *myocardial infarction*, *cerebrovascular accident*, edema, *pulmonary emboli*, thrombophlebitis, *congestive heart failure*, hypertension.
- DERM: rash, pruritus.
- GI: nausea and vomiting (dose-limiting), diarrhea, anorexia.
- HEMA: *leukopenia*, *thrombocytopenia*, hypercalcemia.
- Other: painful gynecomastia and breast tenderness, thinning of hair, hyperglycemia, infertility, azoospermia.
  Note: Drug should be discontinued if intractable GI toxicity occurs.

Overdose and treatment
Clinical manifestations of overdose include headache, nausea, vomiting, and myelosuppression.

Treatment is usually supportive and includes induction of emesis, gastric lavage, transfusion of blood components, and appropriate symptomatic therapy. Hematologic monitoring should continue for at least 6 weeks after the ingestion.

▶ Special considerations
Besides those relevant to all *alkylating agents*, consider the following recommendations.
- Drug may be administered with meals or antacids to reduce the incidence of GI upset. However, calcium-rich foods may impair absorption.
- Store capsules in refrigerator.
- Phenothiazines can be used to treat nausea and vomiting.
- Monitor blood pressure at baseline and routinely during therapy. Estramustine may cause hypertension.
- Estramustine may exaggerate preexisting peripheral edema or congestive heart failure. Weight gain should be monitored regularly in these patients.
- Monitor glucose tolerance periodically throughout therapy.
- Patient may continue estramustine as long as he's responding favorably. Some patients have taken the drug for more than 3 years.

Information for the patient
- Emphasize importance of continuing medication despite nausea and vomiting.
- Advise patient to call immediately if vomiting occurs shortly after a dose is taken.
- Because of the possibility of mutagenic effects, advise couples of childbearing age to use contraceptive measures.

Geriatric use
Use with caution in elderly patients, who are more likely to have vascular disorders, because the use of estrogen is associated with vascular complications.

estrogen and progestin
Brevicon 21-Day, Brevicon 28-Day, Demulen 1/35-21, Demulen 1/35-28, Enovid 5 mg, Enovid-E21, Loestrin 21 1/20, Loestrin 21 1.5/30, Loestrin Fe 1/20, Loestrin Fe 1.5/30, Lo/Ovral, Lo/Ovral-28, Modicon 21, Modicon 28, Nordette-21, Nordette-28, Norinyl 1 + 35 21-Day, Norinyl 1 + 35 28-Day, Norinyl 1 + 50 21-Day, Norinyl 1 + 50 28-Day, Norinyl 1 + 80 21-Day, Norinyl 1 + 80 28-Day, Norinyl 2 mg, Norlestrin 21 1/50, Norlestrin 21 2.5/50, Norlestrin 28 1/50, Norlestrin Fe 1/50, Norlestrin Fe 2.5/50, Ortho-Novum 1/35 21, Ortho-Novum 1/35 28, Ortho-Novum 1/50 21, Ortho-Novum 1/50 28, Ortho-Novum 1/80 21, Ortho-Novum 1/80 28, Ortho-Novum 2 mg 21, Ortho-Novum 7/7/7-21, Ortho-Novum 7/7/7-28, Ortho-Novum 10/11-21, Ortho-Novum 10/11-28, Ovcon-35, Ovcon-50, Ovral, Ovral-28, Ovulen-21, Ovulen-28, Tri-Norinyl-21, Tri-Norinyl-28, Triphasil-21, Triphasil-28

- Pharmacologic classification: estrogen with progestin
- Therapeutic classification: contraceptive (hormonal)
- Pregnancy risk category X

How supplied
Available by prescription only
Tablets – monophasic type
Mestranol 0.1 mg and norethynodrel 2.5 mg
Mestranol 0.1 mg and norethindrone 2 mg
Mestranol 0.1 mg and ethynodiol diacetate 1 mg
Mestranol 0.08 mg and norethindrone 1 mg
Mestranol 0.075 mg and norethynodrel 5 mg
Mestranol 0.05 mg and norethindrone 1 mg
Ethinyl estradiol 0.05 mg and norethindrone 1 mg
Ethinyl estradiol 0.05 mg and norethindrone acetate 1 mg
Ethinyl estradiol 0.05 mg and ethynodiol diacetate 1 mg
Ethinyl estradiol 0.05 mg and norethindrone acetate 2.5 mg
Ethinyl estradiol 0.05 mg and norgestrel 0.5 mg
Ethinyl estradiol 0.035 mg and norethindrone 1 mg
Ethinyl estradiol 0.035 mg and norethindrone 0.5 mg
Ethinyl estradiol 0.035 mg and norethindrone 0.4 mg
Ethinyl estradiol 0.035 mg and ethynodiol diacetate 1 mg
Ethinyl estradiol 0.03 mg and norethindrone acetate 1.5 mg
Ethinyl estradiol 0.03 mg and norgestrel 0.3 mg
Ethinyl estradiol 0.03 mg and levonorgestrel 0.15 mg
Ethinyl estradiol 0.02 mg and norethindrone 1 mg
Tablets – biphasic type
10 tablets ethinyl estradiol 0.035 mg and norethindrone 0.5 mg; 11 tablets ethinyl estradiol 0.035 mg and norethindrone 1 mg

---

Tablets – triphasic type

● 7 tablets ethinyl estradiol 0.035 mg and norethindrone 0.5 mg; 9 tablets ethinyl estradiol 0.035 mg and norethindrone 1 mg; 5 tablets ethinyl estradiol 0.035 mg and norethindrone 0.5 mg

● 7 tablets ethinyl estradiol 0.035 mg and norethindrone 0.5 mg; 7 tablets ethinyl estradiol 0.035 mg and norethindrone 0.75 mg; 7 tablets ethinyl estradiol 0.035 mg and norethindrone 1 mg

● 6 tablets ethinyl estradiol 0.03 and levonorgestrel 0.05 mg; 5 tablets ethinyl estradiol 0.04 mg and levonorgestrel 0.075 mg; 10 tablets ethinyl estradiol 0.03 mg and levonorgestrel 0.125 mg

Indications, route, and dosage
Contraception

1 tablet P.O. daily, beginning on day 5 of menstrual cycle (first day of menstrual flow is day 1). With 20- and 21-tablet packages, new dosing cycle begins 7 days after last tablet taken. With 28-tablet packages, dosage is 1 tablet daily without interruption; extra tablets are placebos or contain iron. If next menstrual period doesn't begin on schedule, rule out pregnancy before starting new dosing cycle. If menstrual period begins, start new dosing cycle 7 days after last tablet was taken. If all doses have been taken on schedule and one menstrual period is missed, continue dosing cycle. If two consecutive menstrual periods are missed, pregnancy test is required before new dosing cycle is started.

Biphasic oral contraceptives
Ortho-Novum 10/11

1 color tablet daily for 10 days, then next color tablet for 11 days.

Triphasic oral contraceptives
Ortho-Novum 7/7/7, Tri-Norinyl, Triphasil

1 tablet daily in the sequence specified by the manufacturer.

Hypermenorrhea

Use high-dose combinations only. Dosage is same as for contraception.

Endometriosis

Cyclic therapy: 1 tablet Ortho-Novum 10 mg P.O. daily for 20 days from day 5 to day 24 of menstrual cycle. *Suppressive therapy:* 1 tablet Enovid 5 mg or 10 mg P.O. daily for 2 weeks, starting on day 5 of menstrual cycle. Continue without interruption for 6 to 9 months, increasing dose by 5 to 10 mg every 2 weeks, up to 20 mg daily. Up to 40 mg daily may be needed if breakthrough bleeding occurs.

Pharmacodynamics

Contraceptive action: Estrogen components of oral contraceptives inhibit the release of follicle-stimulating hormone, thereby stopping follicular development and suppressing ovulation.

Progestin components of oral contraceptives inhibit the release of luteinizing hormone, preventing ovulation even in the event of incomplete suppression of follicular development. Progestins also change the endometrial environment to inhibit nidation (implantation of the fertilized egg into the endometrium) and cause thickening of the cervical mucus, blocking the upward migration of sperm.

Pharmacokinetics

● *Absorption:* Most components of oral contraceptives are absorbed relatively well from the GI tract. Bioavailabilities range from 40% to 70%; considerable individual variation exists in extent of absorption. Peak concentrations occur from ½ to 4 hours (usually about 2) after dosing.

● *Distribution:* Protein binding of the various drugs used in oral contraceptives is high, ranging from 80% to 98%. These agents are distributed extensively into virtually all body tissues.

● *Metabolism:* All of these drugs undergo metabolic transformation before excretion; their rates of metabolism may thus be affected by agents that induce or inhibit metabolism.

● *Excretion:* Very little, if any, of these drugs is excreted unchanged in urine or feces. They appear primarily as sulfate and glucuronide conjugates.

Contraindications and precautions

Oral contraceptives are contraindicated in patients with thromboembolic disorders, cerebrovascular or coronary artery disease, or myocardial infarction because of their association with thromboembolic disease; in patients with known or suspected cancer of the breast or reproductive organs or with benign or malignant liver tumors because of their association with tumorigenesis; in patients with undiagnosed abnormal vaginal bleeding; in women known or believed to be pregnant or breast-feeding; in adolescents with incomplete epiphyseal closure; in women smokers over age 35; and in all women over age 40.

Oral contraceptives should be used cautiously in patients with systemic lupus erythematosus, hypertension, mental depression, migraine, epilepsy, asthma, diabetes mellitus, amenorrhea, scanty or irregular periods, fibrocystic breast disease, family history (mother, grandmother, sister) of breast or genital tract cancer, or renal or gallbladder disease. Development or worsening of any of these conditions should be reported. Prolonged therapy may be inadvisable in women who plan to become pregnant.

Interactions

Concomitant use of certain drugs increases the metabolism of oral contraceptives, resulting in reduced efficacy, breakthrough bleeding, and occasionally contraceptive failure. Such drugs include rifampin, barbiturates, phenylbutazone, phenytoin, primidone, carbamazepine, and isoniazid. Similar effects may occur with concomitant use of neomycin, penicillin V, tetracycline, griseofulvin, chloramphenicol, nitrofurantoin, sulfonamides, and antihistamines.

Oral contraceptive use may require adjustment of dosage of insulin or oral hypoglycemic agents. Oral contraceptives may counteract the effectiveness of oral warfarin-type anticoagulants and of anticonvulsants, antihypertensives, and tricyclic antidepressants.

Effects on diagnostic tests

The following test results may be elevated in users of oral contraceptives: sulfobromophthalein retention, prothrombin and clotting Factors VII to X, plasminogen, norepinephrine-induced platelet aggregation, fibrinogen, thyroid-binding globulin, triglycerides, phospholipids, transcortin and corticosteroids, transferrin, prolactin, renin, and vitamin A.

The following test results may be decreased in users of oral contraceptives: antithrombin III, metyrapone, pregnanediol excretion, free triiodothyronine resin uptake, glucose tolerance, zinc, and vitamin B_{12}.

Adverse reactions
● CNS: headache, dizziness, depression, libido changes, lethargy, migraine.
● CV: *thromboembolism,* hypertension, edema.
● DERM: rash, acne, seborrhea, oily skin, erythema multiforme, hyperpigmentation.
● EENT: worsening of myopia or astigmatism, intolerance of contact lenses, unexplained loss of vision, optic neuritis, diplopia, retinal thrombosis, papilledema.
● GI: nausea, vomiting, abdominal cramps, bloating, diarrhea, constipation, changes in appetite, weight gain, bowel ischemia.
● GU: breakthrough bleeding, granulomatous colitis, dysmenorrhea, amenorrhea, cervical erosion or abnormal secretions, enlargement of uterine fibromas, vaginal candidiasis, urinary track infections.
● Hepatic: gallbladder disease, cholestatic jaundice, liver tumors.
● Metabolic: hyperglycemia, hypercalcemia, folic acid deficiency.
● Other: breast tenderness, enlargement, or secretion; increase in varicosities; possible increased risk of congenital anomalies.
   Adverse effects may be more serious, frequent, and rapid in onset with high-dose than with low-dose combinations.
   Note: Drug should be discontinued if patient becomes hypertensive during therapy.

Overdose and treatment
Serious toxicity after overdose of this drug has not been reported. Nausea and vomiting may be expected to occur. Withdrawal bleeding may occur.

▶ Special considerations
Besides those relevant to all *estrogens and progestins,* oral contraceptives require the following special considerations.
● Astigmatic error and myopic refractive error may be increased twofold to threefold, usually after 6 months of oral contraceptive therapy. Changes in ocular contour and lubricant quality of tears may necessitate change in size and shape of contact lenses.

Information for the patient
● Warn patient that headache, nausea, dizziness, breast tenderness, spotting, and breakthrough bleeding are common at first. These should diminish after 3 to 6 dosing cycles (months). However, breakthrough bleeding in patients taking high-dose estrogen-progestin combinations for menstrual disorders may necessitate dosage adjustment.
● Advise patient to use an additional method of birth control for the first week of administration in the initial cycle.
● Tell patient to take tablets at same time each day for efficacy of medication; nighttime dosing may reduce incidence of nausea and headaches.
● If one menstrual period is missed and tablets have been taken on schedule, tell patient to continue taking them. If two consecutive menstrual periods are missed, tell patient to stop drug and have pregnancy test. Progestogens may cause birth defects if taken early in pregnancy.
● Teach patient to take drug at the same time each day at 24-hour intervals; to keep tablets in original container, and to take them in correct (color-coded) sequence.
● Suggest taking the drug with or immediately after food to reduce nausea.

● Stress importance of annual Papanicolaou smears and gynecologic examinations while taking estrogen-progestin combinations.
● Warn patient of possible delay in achieving pregnancy when drug is discontinued.
● Advise patient of increased risks associated with simultaneous use of cigarettes and oral contraceptives.
● Instruct patient to weigh herself at least twice a week and to report any sudden weight gain or edema.
● Warn patient to avoid exposure to ultraviolet light or prolonged exposure to sunlight; chloasma seems to be aggravated by sunlight. With anticipated exposure (as in summer), taking pill at bedtime will reduce daytime levels of circulating hormone.
● Many clinicians recommend that pregnancy should be avoided for 2 months after stopping drug. Patient should seek medical advice about how soon pregnancy may be safely attempted after hormonal therapy is stopped.
● Inform patient that oral contraceptives decrease viscosity of the cervical mucus and increase susceptibility to vaginal infections. Good hygienic practices are essential.
● Instruct patient to use another form of contraception if she is receiving ampicillin, antiepileptics, phenylbutazone, rifampin, or tetracycline, because intermittent bleeding and unwanted pregnancy might result from effect of drug interactions.
● Instruct patient as follows regarding missed doses.

Monophasic or biphasic cycles
For 20-, 21-, or 24-day dosing schedule:
● If one regular dose, take tablet as soon as possible; if remembered on the next day, take 2 tablets, then continue regular dosing schedule.
● If two consecutive days are missed, take 2 tablets a day for next 2 days, then resume regular dosing schedule.
● If 3 consecutive days are missed, discontinue drug and substitute other contraceptive method until period begins or pregnancy is ruled out. Then start new cycle of tablets.
   For 28-day dosing schedule:
Follow instructions for 21-day dosing schedule; if one of the last seven tablets is missed, be sure to take first tablet of next month's cycle on regularly scheduled day.

Triphasic cycle
For 21-day dosing schedule:
● If 1 day is missed, take dose as soon as possible; if remembered on the next day, take 2 tablets, then continue regular dosing schedule while using additional method of contraception for remainder of cycle.
● If 2 consecutive days are missed, take 2 tablets/day for next 2 days, then continue regular schedule while using additional contraceptive method for remainder of cycle.
● If 3 consecutive days are missed, discontinue drug and use other contraceptive method until period begins or pregnancy is ruled out. Then start new cycle of tablets.
   For 28-day dosing schedule:
Follow instructions for 21-day dosing schedule; if one of the last seven tablets was missed, be sure to take first tablet of next month's cycle on regularly scheduled day.

Pediatric use
● To avoid later fertility and menstrual problems, hormonal contraception is not advised for the adolescent

---

until after at least 2 years of well-established menstrual cycles and completion of physiologic maturation.

• An estrogen-dominant agent is the best choice for the adolescent with scanty menses, moderate or severe acne, or candidiasis. A progestin-dominant agent is the best choice for the adolescent with dysmenorrhea, hypermenorrhea, fibrocystic breast disease, or cyclic premenstrual weight gain.

Breast-feeding
Oral contraceptives are contraindicated in breast-feeding women.

estrogenic substances, conjugated
Estracon, Premarin, Progens Tabs

• Pharmacologic classification: estrogen
• Therapeutic classification: estrogen replacement, antineoplastic, antiosteoporotic
• Pregnancy risk category X

How supplied
Available by prescription only
Tablets: 0.3 mg, 0.625 mg, 0.9 mg, 1.25 mg, 2.5 mg
Injection: 25 mg/5 ml
Vaginal cream: 0.0625%

Indications, route, and dosage
Abnormal uterine bleeding (hormonal imbalance)
Adults: 25 mg I.V. or I.M. Repeat in 6 to 12 hours.
Castration, primary ovarian failure, and osteoporosis
Adults: 0.625 mg to 1.25 mg P.O. daily in cycles of 3 weeks on, 1 week off.
Female hypogonadism
Adults: 2.5 to 7.5 mg P.O. daily in divided doses for 20 consecutive days followed by 10 days without the drug.
Menopausal symptoms; atrophic vaginitis or kraurosis vulvae
Adults: 0.3 mg to 1.25 mg P.O. daily in cycles of 3 weeks on, 1 week off. Alternatively, 2 to 4 g intravaginally or topically once daily in cycles of 3 weeks on, 1 week off.
Postpartum breast engorgement
Adults: 3.75 mg P.O. q 4 hours for five doses or 1.25 mg q 4 hours for 5 days.
Prostatic cancer
Adults: 1.25 to 2.5 mg P.O. t.i.d.
Breast cancer
Adults: 10 mg P.O. t.i.d. for 3 months or more.

Pharmacodynamics
Estrogenic action: Conjugated estrogenic substances mimic the action of endogenous estrogen in treating female hypogonadism, menopausal symptoms, and atrophic vaginitis. They inhibit growth of hormone-sensitive tissue in advanced, inoperable prostatic cancer and in certain carefully selected cases of breast cancer in men and postmenopausal women; they also retard progression of osteoporosis by enhancing calcium and phosphate retention and limiting bone decalcification.

Pharmacokinetics
• *Absorption:* Not well characterized. After I.M. administration, absorption begins rapidly and continues for days.
• *Distribution:* Conjugated estrogens are approximately 50% to 80% plasma protein-bound, particularly the estradiol-binding globulin. Distribution occurs throughout the body, with highest concentrations appearing in fat.
• *Metabolism:* Conjugated estrogens are metabolized primarily in the liver, where they are conjugated with sulfate and glucuronide. Because of the rapid rate of metabolism, nonesterified forms of estrogen, including estradiol, must usually be administered daily.
• *Excretion:* The majority of estrogen elimination occurs through the kidneys, in the form of sulfate or glucuronide conjugates, or both.

Contraindications and precautions
Conjugated estrogens are contraindicated in patients with thrombophlebitis or thromboembolism because of the potential for increased clotting abnormalities; in patients with estrogen-responsive carcinoma (breast or genital tract cancer) because they may stimulate tumor growth; and in patients with undiagnosed abnormal genital bleeding. The drugs are also contraindicated in pregnant women because they may be fetotoxic and in breast-feeding women because they may have adverse effects upon the infant.

Administer these drugs cautiously in patients with disorders that may be aggravated by fluid and electrolyte accumulation, such as asthma, seizure disorders, migraine, or cardiac, renal, or hepatic dysfunction. Carefully monitor female patients who have breast nodules, fibrocystic breast disease, or a family history of breast cancer. Because of the risk of thromboembolism, therapy with this drug should be discontinued at least 1 week before elective surgical procedures associated with an increased incidence of thromboembolism.

Interactions
Concomitant administration of drugs that induce hepatic metabolism (such as rifampin, barbiturates, primidone, carbamazepine, and phenytoin) may decrease estrogenic effects from a given dose. These drugs are known to accelerate the rate of metabolism of certain other agents.

In patients with diabetes, estrogens may cause increases in blood glucose levels, necessitating dosage adjustment of insulin or oral hypoglycemic drugs.

Use with anticoagulants may decrease the effects of warfarin-type anticoagulants. Use with adrenocorticosteroids or adrenocorticotropic hormone increases the risk of fluid and electrolyte accumulation.

Effects on diagnostic tests
Therapy with estrogens increases sulfobromophthalein retention, prothrombin and clotting Factors VII to X, and norepinephrine-induced platelet aggregability. Increases in thyroid-binding globulin concentration may occur, resulting in increased total thyroid concentration (measured by protein-bound iodine or total thyroxine) and decreased uptake of free triiodothyronine resin. Serum folate, pyridoxine, and antithrombin III concentrations may decrease; triglyceride, glucose, and phospholipid levels may increase. Glucose tolerance may be impaired. Pregnanediol excretion may decrease.

Adverse reactions
• CNS: headache, dizziness, chorea, depression, libido changes, lethargy.
• CV: thrombophlebitis; *thromboembolism;* hypertension; edema; *increased risk of stroke, pulmonary embolism, and myocardial infarction.*
• DERM: melasma, urticaria, acne, seborrhea, oily skin, flushing (when given rapidly I.V.), hirsutism or hair loss.
• EENT: worsening of myopia or astigmatism, intolerance to contact lenses.
• GI: nausea, vomiting, abdominal cramps, bloating, diarrhea, constipation, anorexia, increased appetite, weight changes.
• GU: breakthrough bleeding, altered menstrual flow, dysmenorrhea, amenorrhea, cervical erosion, altered cervical secretions, enlargement of uterine fibromas, vaginal candidiasis; *in males:* gynecomastia, testicular atrophy, impotence.
• Hepatic: cholestatic jaundice.
• Metabolic: hyperglycemia, hypercalcemia, folic acid deficiency.
• Other: breast changes (tenderness, enlargement, secretions), leg cramps.

Overdose and treatment
Serious toxicity after overdose of this drug has not been reported. Nausea may be expected to occur. Provide appropriate supportive care.

▶ Special considerations
Besides those relevant to all *estrogens,* consider the following recommendations.
• For the rapid treatment of dysfunctional uterine bleeding or reduction of surgical bleeding, parenteral administration is preferred.
• Refrigerate before reconstitution. After adding diluent, agitate gently until drug is in solution.

Geriatric use
Chronic use for menopausal symptoms may be associated with increased risk of certain types of cancer. Frequent physical examinations are recommended.

Breast-feeding
Estrogens are contraindicated in breast-feeding women.

PHARMACOLOGIC CLASS

estrogens

chlorotrianisene
dienestrol
diethylstilbestrol
diethylstilbestrol diphosphate
esterified estrogens
estradiol
estradiol cypionate
estradiol valerate
estrogen and progestin
estrogenic substances, conjugated
estrone
estropipate
ethinyl estradiol
polyestradiol phosphate
quinestrol

Estrogens were first discovered in the urine of humans and animals in 1930. Since that time, numerous synthetic modifications of the naturally occurring estrogen molecules and completely synthetic estrogenic compounds have been developed. Estrogens have many uses: in treating the symptoms of menopause, atrophic vaginitis, breast cancer, and other diseases; in the prophylaxis of osteoporosis, and when combined with progestins, as contraceptives.

Pharmacology
Conjugated estrogens and estrogenic substances are normally obtained from the urine of pregnant mares. Other estrogens are manufactured synthetically. Of the six naturally occurring estrogens in humans, three (estradiol, estrone, and estriol) are present in significant quantities. The estrogens promote the development and maintenance of the female reproductive system and secondary sexual characteristics. Estrogens inhibit the release of pituitary gonadotropins and also have various metabolic effects, including retention of fluid and electrolytes, retention and deposition in bone of calcium and phosphorous, and mild anabolic activity. Estrogens and estrogenic substances administered as drugs have effects related to endogenous estrogen's mechanism of action. They can mimic the action of endogenous estrogen when used as replacement therapy or produce such useful effects as inhibiting ovulation or inhibiting growth of certain hormone-sensitive cancers.

Use of estrogens is not without risk. Long-term use is associated with an increased incidence of endometrial cancer, gall bladder disease, and thromboembolic disease. Elevations in blood pressure often occur as well.

Clinical indications and actions
Moderate to severe vasomotor symptoms of menopause
Endogenous estrogens are markedly reduced in concentration after menopause. This commonly results in vasomotor symptoms, such as hot flashes and dizziness. Chlorotrianisene, diethylstilbestrol, estradiol cypionate, and ethinyl estradiol serve to mimic the action of endogenous estrogens in preventing these symptoms.
Atrophic vaginitis/kraurosis vulvae
Chlorotrianisene and diethylstilbestrol stimulate development, cornification, and secretory activity in vaginal tissues.
Carcinoma of the breast
Conjugated estrogens, diethylstilbestrol, esterified estrogens, estradiol, and ethinyl estradiol inhibit the growth of hormone-sensitive cancers in certain carefully selected male and post-menopausal female patients.
Carcinoma of the prostate
Chlorotrianisene, conjugated estrogens, diethylstilbestrol, esterified estrogens, estradiol, estradiol valerate, estrone, and ethinyl estradiol inhibit growth of hormone-sensitive cancer tissue in males with advanced disease.
Prophylaxis of postmenopausal osteoporosis
Conjugated estrogens serve to replace or augment the activity of endogenous estrogen in causing calcium and phosphate retention and preventing bone decalcification.
Contraception
Estrogens are also used in combination with progestins for ovulation control to prevent conception.

Overview of adverse reactions

Acute reactions: changes in menstrual bleeding patterns (spotting, prolongation or absence of bleeding), abdominal cramps, swollen feet or ankles, bloated sensation (fluid and electrolyte retention), breast swelling and tenderness, weight gain, nausea, loss of appetite, headache, photosensitivity, loss of libido.

With chronic administration: increased blood pressure (sometimes into the hypertensive range), thromboembolic disease, cholestatic jaundice, benign hepatomas, endometrial carcinoma (rare). Risk of thromboembolic disease increases markedly with cigarette smoking, especially in women over age 35.

▶ **Special considerations**
● Estrogens are contraindicated in patients with thrombophlebitis or thromboembolic disorders; cancer of the breast, reproductive organs, or genitals; or undiagnosed abnormal genital bleeding. They should be used cautiously in patients with hypertension, asthma, mental depression, bone disease, blood dyscrasias, gallbladder disease, migraine, seizures, diabetes mellitus, amenorrhea, heart failure, hepatic or renal dysfunction, or a family history (mother, grandmother, or sister) of breast or genital tract cancer. Development or worsening of these conditions may require discontinuation of the drug.
● Give patient the package insert describing estrogen adverse reactions, and also provide verbal explanation.
● Pathologist should be advised of estrogen therapy when specimen is sent.
● Patients with diabetes mellitus should be monitored more closely for loss of diabetes control.
● If patient is receiving a warfarin-type anticoagulant, monitor prothrombin time for possible anticoagulant dosage adjustment.
● Patients who become pregnant while on estrogen therapy should stop taking the drug immediately, because it may adversely affect the fetus.
● Estrogen therapy is usually administered cyclically. The drugs are usually given once daily for 3 weeks, followed by 1 week without the drugs, and then this regimen is repeated as necessary.

Information for the patient

● Warn patient to report immediately abdominal pain; pain, numbness, or stiffness in legs or buttocks; pressure or pain in chest; shortness of breath; severe headaches; visual disturbances, such as blind spots, flashing lights, or blurriness; vaginal bleeding or discharge; breast lumps; swelling of hands or feet; yellow skin and sclera; dark urine; and light-colored stools.
● Tell male patients on long-term therapy about possible gynecomastia and impotence, which will disappear when therapy is terminated.
● Explain to patients on cyclic therapy for postmenopausal symptoms that, although withdrawal bleeding may occur in week off drug, fertility has not been restored; ovulation does not occur.
● Teach female patients how to perform routine breast self-examination.
● Teach patient that medical supervision is essential during prolonged estrogen therapy.
● Inform patient that nausea, when present, usually disappears with continued therapy. Nausea can be relieved by taking medication at mealtimes or bedtime (if only one daily dose is required).
● Diabetic patients should report symptoms of hyperglycemia or glycosuria.

● Teach patient how to apply estrogen ointments or transdermal estrogen locally. Explain what symptoms may occur in a systemic reaction to estrogen ointment.
● Teach patient how to insert intravaginal estrogen suppository. Advise use of perineal pads instead of tampons when using intravaginal suppositories.
● Tell women who are planning to breast-feed not to take estrogens.

Geriatric use

Postmenopausal women with long-term estrogen use have an increased risk of endometrial cancer.

Pediatric use

Because of the effects of estrogen on epiphyseal closure, estrogens should be used with caution in adolescents whose bone growth is not complete.

Breast-feeding

Estrogens are contraindicated in breast-feeding women.

Representative combinations

Ethynodiol diacetate with ethinyl estradiol: Demulen; with mestranol: Ovulen.
  Estradiol with testosterone: Testrolix; with testosterone and chlorobutanol: Depo-Testadiol.
  Estradiol cypionate with testosterone: D-Diol, Dep-Tesestro, Dep-Testradiol, Duo-Cyp, Duo-Ionate, Duracrine, Estran-C, Menoject, T.E. Ionate.
  Estradiol valerate with testosterone enanthate: Bi-Nate, Deladumone, Delatestadiol, Duoval-P.A., Estran E.V., Estra-Testrin, Teev, Tesogen, Testanate, Valertest.
  Estrogenic substances (conjugated) with meprobamate: Milprem, PMB 200, PMB 400; with methyltestosterone: Menotab-M, Premarin with Methyltestosterone.
  Estrone with hydrocortisone acetate: Estro-V HC; with estradiol: Tri-Orapin; with estradiol and vitamin B_{12}: Ovest, Ovulin; with estriol and estradiol: Estro Plus, Hormonin; with potassium estrone sulfate: Dura-Keelin, Estro-Plus, Gynlin, Mer-Estrone, Sodestrin, Spanestrin; with testosterone: Andesterone, Anestro, Di-Hormone, Di-Met, Diorapin, Di-Steroid, Estratest; with testosterone and vitamins: Android-G, Geratic Forte, Geriamic, Geritag; with testosterone, vitamins and minerals: Geramine.

---

estrone
Bestrone, Estrone-A, Estronol, Kestrone-5, Theelin Aqueous

estropipate
Ogen

● Pharmacologic classification: estrogen
● Therapeutic classification: estrogen replacement
● Pregnancy risk category X

How supplied

Available by prescription only
Estrone
Injection: 2 mg/ml, 5 mg/ml (aqueous suspension)
Estropipate as estrone sodium sulfate
Tablets: 0.625 mg, 1.25 mg, 2.5 mg, 5 mg

Indications, route, and dosage
Atrophic vaginitis and menopausal symptoms
Estrone
Adults: 0.1 to 0.5 mg I.M. two or three times weekly.
Estropipate
Adults: 0.625 to 5 mg P.O. daily for 21 days, followed by 7 days of no medication.
Female hypogonadism, primary ovarian failure, or after castration
Estrone
Adults: 0.1 to 2 mg weekly in single or divided doses.
Estropipate
Adults: 1.25 to 7.5 mg P.O. daily for 3 weeks, followed by 8 to 10 days off therapy. The cycle may be repeated if no withdrawal bleeding occurs within 10 days of discontinuing therapy.
Prostatic cancer
Estrone
Adults: 2 to 4 mg I.M. two to three times weekly.

Pharmacodynamics
Estrogenic action: Estrone mimics the action of endogenous estrogen in treating female hypogonadism, menopausal symptoms, and atrophic vaginitis.

Pharmacokinetics
● *Absorption:* After oral administration, estradiol and the other natural unconjugated estrogens are well absorbed but substantially inactivated by the liver. Therefore, unconjugated estrogens are usually administered parenterally.

After I.M. administration, absorption begins rapidly and continues for days. The cypionate and valerate esters administered in oil have prolonged durations of action because of their slow absorption characteristics.

Topically applied estradiol is absorbed readily into the systemic circulation.
● *Distribution:* Estradiol and the other natural estrogens are approximately 50% to 80% plasma protein-bound, particularly the estradiol-binding globulin. Distribution occurs throughout the body, with highest concentrations appearing in fat.
● *Metabolism:* The steroidal estrogens, including estradiol, are metabolized primarily in the liver, where they are conjugated with sulfate and glucuronide. Because of the rapid rate of metabolism, nonesterified forms of estrogen, including estradiol, must usually be administered daily.
● *Excretion:* The majority of estrogen elimination occurs through the kidneys in the form of sulfate and/or glucuronide conjugates.

Contraindications and precautions
Estrone is contraindicated in patients with thrombophlebitis or thromboembolism because of its association with thromboembolic disorders; estrogen-responsive carcinoma (breast or genital tract cancer); and undiagnosed abnormal genital bleeding. The drug is also contraindicated in pregnant or breast-feeding women.

This drug should be administered cautiously to patients with disorders that may be aggravated by fluid and electrolyte accumulation, such as asthma, seizure disorders, migraine, or cardiac, renal, or hepatic dysfunction. Carefully monitor female patients who have breast nodules, fibrocystic breast disease, or a family history of breast cancer. Because of the risk of thromboembolism, therapy with this drug should be discontinued at least 4 weeks before elective surgical procedures associated with an increased incidence of thromboembolism.

Interactions
Concomitant administration of drugs that induce hepatic metabolism (such as rifampin, barbiturates, primidone, carbamazepine, and phenytoin) may decrease estrogenic effects from a given dose. These drugs are known to accelerate the rate of metabolism of certain other agents.

Estrogens may decrease elimination rate of corticosteroids.

In patients with diabetes, estrone may cause increases in blood glucose levels, necessitating dosage adjustment of insulin or oral hypoglycemic drugs.

Use with anticoagulants may decrease the effects of warfarin-type anticoagulants. Use with adrenocorticosteroids or adrenocorticotropic hormone increases the risk of fluid and electrolyte accumulation.

Effects on diagnostic tests
Therapy with estrogens increases sulfobromophthalein retention, prothrombin and clotting Factors VII to X, and norepinephrine-induced platelet aggregability. Increases in thyroid-binding globulin concentration may occur, resulting in increased total thyroid concentration (measured by protein-bound iodine or total thyroxine) and decreased uptake of free triiodothyronine resin. Serum folate, pyridoxine, and antithrombin III concentrations may decrease; triglyceride, glucose, and phospholipid levels may increase. Glucose tolerance may be impaired. Pregnanediol excretion may decrease.

Adverse reactions
● CNS: headache, dizziness, chorea, depression, libido changes, lethargy.
● CV: thrombophlebitis, *thromboembolism*, hypertension, edema.
● DERM: melasma, urticaria, acne, seborrhea, oily skin, hirsutism or hair loss.
● EENT: worsening of myopia or astigmatism, intolerance to contact lenses.
● GI: nausea, vomiting, abdominal cramps, bloating, diarrhea, constipation, anorexia, increased appetite, weight changes.
● GU: breakthrough bleeding, altered menstrual flow, dysmenorrhea, amenorrhea, cervical erosion, altered cervical secretion, enlargement of uterine fibromas, vaginal candidiasis; *in males:* gynecomastia, testicular atrophy, impotence.
● Hepatic: cholestatic jaundice.
● Metabolic: hyperglycemia, hypercalcemia, folic acid deficiency.
● Other: breast changes (tenderness, enlargement, secretions), leg cramps.

Overdose and treatment
Serious toxicity after overdose of this drug has not been reported. Nausea may be expected to occur. Provide appropriate supportive care.

▶ Special considerations
Besides those relevant to all *estrogens,* consider the following recommendations.
● Administer estrone I.M. only.
● When used for progressive, inoperable prostate cancer, remission should be apparent within 3 weeks of therapy.

---

*Canada only   †Unlabeled clinical use   Italicized adverse reactions are life-threatening.

• When submitting specimens to pathologist for evaluation, be sure to note that patient is taking estrogens.

Geriatric use
Frequent physical examinations are recommended for postmenopausal women taking estrogens.

Breast-feeding
Estrone is contraindicated in breast-feeding women.

ethacrynate sodium
ethacrynic acid
Edecrin

• Pharmacologic classification: loop diuretic
• Therapeutic classification: diuretic
• Pregnancy risk category B

How supplied
Available by prescription only
Tablets: 25 mg, 50 mg
Injectable: 50 mg (with 62.5 mg of mannitol and 0.1 mg of thimerosal)

Indications, route, and dosage
Acute pulmonary edema
Adults: 50 to 100 mg of ethacrynate sodium I.V. slowly over several minutes.
Edema
Adults: 50 to 200 mg P.O. daily. Refractory cases may require up to 200 mg b.i.d.
Children: Initially, 25 mg P.O., given cautiously and increased in 25-mg increments daily until desired effect is achieved.

Pharmacodynamics
Diuretic action: Ethacrynic acid inhibits sodium and chloride reabsorption in the proximal part of the ascending loop of Henle, promoting the excretion of sodium, water, chloride, and potassium.

Pharmacokinetics
• *Absorption:* Ethacrynic acid is absorbed rapidly from the GI tract; diuresis occurs in 30 minutes and peaks in 2 hours. After I.V. administration of ethacrynate sodium, diuresis occurs in 5 minutes and peaks in 15 to 30 minutes.
• *Distribution:* In animal studies, ethacrynic acid was found to accumulate in the liver. Ethacrynic acid does not enter the cerebrospinal fluid, and its distribution into breast milk or the placenta is unknown.
• *Metabolism:* In animals, ethacrynic acid is metabolized by the liver to a potentially active metabolite.
• *Excretion:* Animal studies show that 30% to 65% of ethacrynate sodium is excreted in urine and 35% to 40% is excreted in bile, as the metabolite. Duration of action is 6 to 8 hours after oral administration and about 2 hours after I.V. administration.

Contraindications and precautions
Ethacrynic acid is contraindicated in patients with known hypersensitivity, anuria, hypotension, dehydration with low serum sodium levels, or metabolic alkalosis with hypokalemia, because the drug may exacerbate these conditions.

Ethacrynic acid should be used with caution in patients with hearing impairment or cirrhosis, especially those with a history of electrolyte imbalance or hepatic encephalopathy; in patients with diabetes because it may alter carbohydrate metabolism; in patients with increasing azotemia or oliguria; and in patients receiving cardiac glycosides (digoxin, digitoxin), because ethacrynic acid–induced hypokalemia may predispose such patients to digitalis toxicity.

Interactions
Concomitant use of ethacrynic acid with other diuretics may enhance the diuretic effect of the other drugs; reduce dosage when adding ethacrynic acid to a diuretic regimen. Concomitant use of potassium-sparing diuretics (spironolactone, triamterene, amiloride) may decrease the potassium loss induced by ethacrynic acid and may be a therapeutic advantage; severe potassium loss may occur if ethacrynic acid is administered with other potassium-depleting drugs, such as steroids and amphotericin B. Ethacrynic acid may reduce renal clearance of lithium, elevating serum lithium levels; monitor lithium levels and adjust dosage.

Diabetic patients may need increased dosages of insulin or oral hypoglycemics when taking ethacrynic acid. Ethacrynic acid may potentiate the hypotensive effect of antihypertensive agents; patients may require dosage reduction.

Concomitant administration of ethacrynic acid and aminoglycosides or other ototoxic drugs may increase the incidence of deafness; avoid use of such combinations.

Effects on diagnostic tests
Ethacrynic acid therapy alters electrolyte balance and liver and renal function tests.

Adverse reactions
• CV: volume depletion and dehydration, orthostatic hypotension.
• DERM: dermatitis.
• EENT: transient deafness with too-rapid I.V. injection.
• GI: abdominal discomfort and pain, diarrhea.
• HEMA: *agranulocytosis,* neutropenia, thrombocytopenia.
• Metabolic: hypochloremic alkalosis; asymptomatic hyperuricemia; fluid and electrolyte imbalances, including hypokalemia, hypocalcemia, hypomagnesemia, and hyponatremia; hyperglycemia and impairment of glucose tolerance.
Note: Drug should be discontinued if excessive diuresis, electrolyte abnormalities, increasing azotemia, oliguria, hematuria, bloody stools, or severe or watery diarrhea occurs.

Overdose and treatment
Clinical manifestations of overdose include profound electrolyte and volume depletion, which may precipitate circulatory collapse.

Treatment of ethacrynic acid overdose is primarily supportive; replace fluid and electrolytes as needed.

▶ Special considerations
Besides those relevant to all *loop diuretics,* consider the following recommendations.
• Do not give ethacrynate sodium either I.M. or S.C. because it may cause severe local pain and irritation. When giving I.V., check infusion site frequently for infiltration (edema or skin blanching).
• Infuse ethacrynate sodium slowly over 20 to 30 min-

utes, by I.V. infusion or by direct I.V. injection over a period of several minutes; rapid injection may cause hypotension.

● Do not administer ethacrynate sodium simultaneously with whole blood or blood products; hemolysis may occur.

● I.V. ethacrynate sodium has been used to treat hypercalcemia and to manage ethylene glycol poisoning and bromide intoxication.

● Periodically assess hearing function in patients receiving high-dose therapy.

Geriatric use
Elderly and debilitated patients require close observation because they are more susceptible to drug-induced diuresis. Excessive diuresis promotes rapid dehydration, leading to hypovolemia, hypokalemia, hyponatremia, and circulatory collapse. Reduced dosages may be indicated.

Pediatric use
● Use ethacrynate sodium or ethacrynic acid with caution in neonates. The usual pediatric dosage can be used, but dosage intervals should be extended.
● Safety for use in children has not been established.

Breast-feeding
Ethacrynic acid should not be used by breast-feeding women.

---

ethambutol hydrochloride
Myambutol

● Pharmacologic classification: semisynthetic antitubercular
● Therapeutic classification: antitubercular agent
● Pregnancy risk category B

How supplied
Available by prescription only
Tablets: 100 mg, 400 mg

Indications, route, and dosage
Adjunctive treatment in pulmonary tuberculosis
Adults and children age 13 and older: Initial treatment for patients who have not received previous antitubercular therapy, 15 mg/kg P.O. daily single dose. Retreatment: 25 mg/kg P.O. daily single dose for 60 days with at least one other antitubercular drug; then decrease to 15 mg/kg P.O. daily single dose.

Pharmacodynamics
Antitubercular action: Ethambutol is bacteriostatic; it interferes with mycolic acid incorporation into the mycobacterial cell wall. Ethambutol is active against *Mycobacterium tuberculosis, M. bovis,* and *M. marinum,* and some strains of *M. kansasii, M. avium, M. fortuitum,* and *M. intracellulare.* Ethambutol is considered adjunctive therapy in tuberculosis and is combined with other antituberculosis agents to prevent or delay development of drug resistance by *Mycobacterium tuberculosis.*

Pharmacokinetics
● *Absorption:* Ethambutol is absorbed rapidly from the GI tract; peak serum levels occur 2 to 4 hours after ingestion.
● *Distribution:* Ethambutol is distributed widely into body tissues and fluids, especially into lungs, erythrocytes, saliva, and kidneys; lesser amounts distribute into brain, ascitic, pleural, and cerebrospinal fluids. Ethambutol is 8% to 22% protein-bound.
● *Metabolism:* Ethambutol undergoes partial hepatic metabolism.
● *Excretion:* After 24 hours, about 50% of an oral dose of ethambutol and 8% to 15% of its metabolites are excreted in urine; 20% to 25% is excreted in feces. Small amounts of drug may be excreted in breast milk. Plasma half-life in adults is about 3½ hours; half-life is prolonged in decreased renal or hepatic function. Ethambutol can be removed by peritoneal dialysis and to a lesser extent by hemodialysis.

Contraindications and precautions
Ethambutol is contraindicated in patients with known hypersensitivity to ethambutol.

Ethambutol should be used cautiously in patients with preexisting visual disturbances, in whom ethambutol-induced visual changes are difficult to identify; monthly vision tests are mandatory at high dosage levels. Use drug with caution in patients with gout and in patients with decreased renal or hepatic function.

Interactions
Ethambutol may potentiate adverse effects of agents that produce neurotoxicity.

Effects on diagnostic tests
Ethambutol may elevate serum urate levels and liver function test results.

Adverse reactions
● CNS: headache, dizziness, mental confusion, possible hallucinations, peripheral neuritis (numbness and tingling of extremities).
● EENT: optic neuritis (vision loss and loss of color discrimination, especially red and green).
● GI: anorexia, nausea, vomiting, abdominal pain, impaired liver function.
● Metabolic: *elevated uric acid levels.*
● Other: *anaphylactoid reactions,* fever, malaise, bloody sputum, joint pain.
  Note: Drug should be discontinued if patient shows signs of hypersensitivity reaction or substantive visual changes.

Overdose and treatment
No specific recommendation is available. Treatment is supportive. After recent ingestion (4 hours or less), empty stomach by induced emesis or gastric lavage. Follow with activated charcoal to decrease absorption.

▶ Special considerations
● Give drug with food if necessary to prevent gastric irritation; food does not interfere with absorption.
● Obtain specimens for culture and sensitivity testing before first dose, but therapy can begin before test results are complete; repeat periodically to detect drug resistance.
● Assess visual status before therapy; test visual acuity and color discrimination monthly in patients taking more

---

than 15 mg/kg/day. Visual disturbances are dose related and reversible if detected in time.
● Monitor blood (including serum uric acid), renal, and liver function studies before and periodically during therapy to minimize toxicity.
● Monitor for change in renal function. Dosage reduction may be necessary.

Information for the patient
● Explain disease process and rationale for long-term therapy.
● Teach signs and symptoms of hypersensitivity and other adverse reactions, and emphasize need to notify you if these occur; urge patient to report *any* unusual effects, especially blurred vision, or red-green color blindness, or changes in urinary elimination.
● Assure patient that visual alterations will disappear within several weeks or months after drug is discontinued.
● Urge patient to complete entire prescribed regimen, to comply with instructions for around-the-clock dosage, to avoid missing doses, and not to discontinue drug without medical approval. Explain importance of keeping follow-up appointments.

Pediatric use
Not recommended for use in children under age 13.

Breast-feeding
Ethambutol is excreted in breast milk; use with caution in breast-feeding women.

---

ethanolamine oleate
Ethamolin

● Pharmacologic classification: oleic acid/ 2-aminoethanol combination
● Therapeutic classification: sclerosing agent
● Pregnancy risk category C

How supplied
Available by prescription only
Injection: 5% solution in 2-ml ampules

Indications, route, and dosage
Treatment of bleeding esophageal varices and prevention of recurrent bleeding
Adults: Local injection of 1.5 to 5 ml per varix. Maximum total dose per treatment should not exceed 20 ml or about 0.4 ml/kg. Injections should be performed by physicians familiar with sclerotherapy.

Pharmacodynamics
Sclerosing action: Ethanolamine oleate is a mild sclerosing agent that initiates a local inflammatory response that leads to scarring which prevents bleeding. The oleic acid component is responsible for the inflammatory response, and it may also promote local clot formation by initiating the release of tissue factor and activate Hageman factor. However, the ethanolamine component may chelate calcium and inhibit fibrin clot formation *in situ.*

Pharmacokinetics
● *Absorption:* When injected locally, ethanolamine oleate is cleared via the portal vein within 5 minutes.
● *Distribution:* Information not available.
● *Metabolism:* Information not available.
● *Excretion:* Information not available.

Contraindications and precautions
Contraindicated in patients hypersensitive to ethanolamine, oleic acid, or ethanolamine oleate.
Sclerotherapy is not indicated for patients with esophageal varices that have not bled. It is also not indicated for varicosities of the leg.
Be prepared to treat anaphylaxis in patients undergoing sclerotherapy with ethanolamine oleate. Although rare, it has been fatal. Have epinephrine 1:1,000 available, and control allergic reactions with antihistamines.
Severe injection necrosis may occur. Assess respiratory status.

Interactions
None reported.

Effects on diagnostic tests
None reported.

Adverse reactions
● GI: esophageal ulcer, esophageal stricture, esophagitis, esophageal tearing, local mucosal sloughing or necrosis, *periesophageal abscess and perforation.*
● GU: acute renal failure.
● Respiratory: *pleural effusion or infiltration,* pneumonia, *aspiration pneumonia.*
● Other: pyrexia, retrosternal pain, *anaphylaxis.*

Overdose and treatment
Overdosage can result in severe esophageal intramural necrosis. Death has resulted from such overdosage. Specific antidotes are not known.

▶ Special considerations
● Ethanolamine oleate will not correct portal hypertension, the cause of esophageal varices. Vascular recanalization and collateral formation may occur, and patients may need further treatment.
● Patients with concomitant cardiopulmonary disease should receive smaller volumes of sclerosing agents to minimize adverse reactions. Submucosal injections are not recommended because they are more likely to cause mucosal ulceration.
● Timing of therapy is quite variable with no clear consensus. However, therapy may be initiated at the first bleeding episode, with follow-up sclerotherapy at 1 week, 6 weeks, 3 months, and 6 months, if needed.

Information for the patient
● Explain the technique to the patient, and that several follow-up visits will be necessary for successful sclerotherapy.
● Tell patient to report chest pain, shortness of breath, or bleeding immediately.

Pediatric use
Safe use in children has not been established.

Breast-feeding
It is not known whether ethanolamine is excreted in breast milk. Use with caution in breast-feeding women.

---

ethaverine hydrochloride
Circubid, Ethaquin, Ethatab, Ethavex-100, Isovex, Pavaspan

- Pharmacologic classification: isoquinoline derivative
- Therapeutic classification: peripheral vasodilator
- Pregnancy risk category C

How supplied
Available by prescription only
Tablets: 100 mg
Capsules: 100 mg
Capsules (timed-release): 150 mg

Indications, route, and dosage
Peripheral and cerebrovascular insufficiency associated with arterial spasm; spastic conditions of gastrointestinal and genitourinary tracts
Adults: 100 to 200 mg P.O. t.i.d. or 150-mg sustained-release capsule P.O. q 12 hours.

Pharmacodynamics
Vasodilating action: Ethaverine directly relaxes smooth muscle via inhibition of phosphodiesterase, increasing concentration levels of cyclic adenosine monophosphate.

Pharmacokinetics
Pharmacokinetic parameters of ethaverine are not available; however, it may be assumed that they are similar to those of papaverine because the two drugs are closely related.

Contraindications and precautions
Ethaverine is contraindicated in patients with complete atrioventricular dissociation because the drug is a myocardial depressant.
 Use cautiously in patients with glaucoma.

Interactions
Ethaverine may decrease the antiparkinsonian effects of levodopa, exacerbating such symptoms as rigidity and tremors. Alcohol may intensify ethaverine-induced dizziness and drowsiness.

Effects on diagnostic tests
None reported.

Adverse reactions
- CNS: drowsiness, dizziness, headache.
- CV: hypotension, flushing, sweating, myocardial depression, arrhythmias.
- DERM: rash.
- GI: nausea, anorexia, abdominal distress, dryness of throat, constipation, diarrhea.
- Hepatic: jaundice, altered liver function test.
- Other: respiratory depression, malaise, lassitude.
 Note: Drug should be discontinued if patient becomes markedly jaundiced or if there are signs of hepatotoxicity (abnormal liver function tests, GI symptoms, or eosinophilia).

Overdose and treatment
Clinical signs of overdose include nausea, vomiting, flushing, severe hypotension, tachycardia, and cardiac arrhythmias.
 To reduce absorption, induce emesis and give activated charcoal followed by a cathartic. Treat symptomatically and supportively. Treat hypotension with I.V. fluids and dopamine.

▶ Special considerations
Monitor and record vital signs during therapy.

Information for the patient
- Warn patient of importance of reporting pronounced adverse reactions, especially signs of hepatic dysfunction.
- Warn patient not to drive or perform other tasks requiring alertness during therapy.

Breast-feeding
Safety in breast-feeding women has not been established.

ethchlorvynol
Placidyl

- Pharmacologic classification: chlorinated tertiary acetylenic carbinol
- Therapeutic classification: sedative-hypnotic
- Controlled substance schedule IV
- Pregnancy risk category C

How supplied
Available by prescription only
Capsules: 200 mg, 500 mg, 750 mg (contains tartrazine)

Indications, route, and dosage
Sedation
Adults: 200 mg P.O. b.i.d. or t.i.d.
Insomnia
Adults: 500 mg to 1 g P.O. h.s. May repeat 100 to 200 mg if awakened in early morning.

Pharmacodynamics
Sedative-hypnotic action: The activity of ethchlorvynol is similar to that of the barbiturates. It causes nonspecific depression of the CNS, particularly the reticular activating system. Low doses do not significantly depress respiration. The cellular mechanism is unknown.

Pharmacokinetics
- *Absorption:* Ethchlorvynol is absorbed completely and rapidly after oral administration. Peak serum concentrations occur within 2 hours. Action begins in 15 to 60 minutes.
- *Distribution:* Drug distributes throughout the body, including the CNS, and is extensively stored in fatty tissue.
- *Metabolism:* Ethchlorvynol is metabolized primarily in the liver; however, significant metabolism occurs in the kidney as well. In overdose, the metabolic pathways can be saturated.
- *Excretion:* Inactive metabolites of the drug are ex-

creted in urine. Half-life is 10 to 20 hours, but the duration of sleep is about 5 hours.

Contraindications and precautions

Ethchlorvynol is contraindicated in patients with known hypersensitivity to the drug; in patients with porphyria; and in patients with persistent pain and insomnia unless the insomnia persists after the pain is controlled, because the drug increases sensitivity to pain. The 750-mg dosage form is contraindicated in individuals allergic to aspirin, because it contains tartrazine and because significant cross-reactivity has been demonstrated.

Because drug depresses the CNS, administer ethchlorvynol cautiously to patients who are depressed or who have suicidal tendencies, and those with a history of drug abuse or addiction.

Ethchlorvynol should be used cautiously in patients with hepatic or renal dysfunction, because decreased elimination of the drug may lead to accumulation and toxicity; and in patients who have shown unpredictable or paradoxical reactions to barbiturates or chloral hydrate, because drug may cause a similar reaction.

Interactions

When used concomitantly, ethchlorvynol will decrease the effect of oral anticoagulants (warfarin) by increasing hepatic metabolism. Ethchlorvynol will add to or potentiate the CNS depressant effects of barbiturates, benzodiazepines, alcohol, antihistamines, narcotics, tranquilizers, and other CNS depressants. Concomitant use with MAO inhibitors may cause increased sedation. Concomitant use with amitriptyline may cause delirium.

Effects on diagnostic tests

Ethchlorvynol may cause a false-positive phentolamine test.

Adverse reactions

● CNS: hangover, dizziness, facial numbness, ataxia, fatigue, nightmares, prolonged hypnosis, excitement, hysteria.
● CV: hypotension.
● DERM: rash, urticaria.
● GI: nausea, vomiting, gastric upset, unpleasant aftertaste.
● HEMA: thrombocytopenia.
● Hepatic: cholestatic jaundice.
● Other: muscle weakness, blurred vision, syncope without hypotension, hypersensitivity.

Note: Drug should be discontinued if profound weakness, excitement, hysteria, hypotension, or hypersensitivity occurs.

Overdose and treatment

Clinical manifestations of overdose include stupor, coma, and severe respiratory depression. Hypotension, hypothermia, areflexia, and bradycardia may occur.

Treatment is supportive, with emphasis on improving respiratory function and preventing possible pulmonary edema. Empty stomach by emesis or lavage. Hemoperfusion is the most effective means of increasing elimination; hemodialysis and peritoneal dialysis, especially with aqueous solutions, are of limited value.

▶ **Special considerations**
● Monitor level of consciousness and vital signs to prevent possible adverse effects.
● Administer with food to reduce ataxia, giddiness, or stomach upset.

● Patients who are suicidal or depressed or who have a history of drug abuse should be observed to prevent hoarding or self-dosing. Overdose is difficult to treat and carries a high mortality rate.
● Discontinue drug after 1 week; drug is effective only for short-term use.
● Monitor prothrombin times of patient on an oral anticoagulant to determine effectiveness of drug.
● Slight darkening of liquid in the capsules from exposure to air and light does not affect safety or potency. Store in tight, light-resistant container to avoid possible deterioration.

Information for the patient
● Advise patient to take the medication with food to avoid or lessen giddiness, ataxia, or GI upset.
● Warn patient not to attempt tasks that require mental alertness or physical coordination before the CNS effects of the drug are known, and to avoid alcohol and the use of other CNS depressants or antidepressants unless prescribed.
● Tell patient not to change the dose or frequency or discontinue the drug without medical approval.
● Tell patient to promptly report muscle weakness, excitability, or syncope.
● Advise patient of potential for physical and psychological dependence with chronic use.
● Emphasize the dangers of combining this drug with alcohol. An excessive depressant effect is possible even if the drug is taken the evening before ingestion of alcohol.

Geriatric use
Elderly patients, especially those with hepatic dysfunction, will show an increased response and sensitivity. Use lowest dose possible.

Pediatric use
Not recommended for use in children; safety has not been established.

Breast-feeding
Safety of ethchlorvynol in breast-feeding women has not been established.

ethinyl estradiol
Estinyl, Feminone

● Pharmacologic classification: estrogen
● Therapeutic classification: estrogen replacement, antineoplastic
● Pregnancy risk category X

How supplied
Available by prescription only
Tablets: 0.02 mg, 0.05 mg, 0.5 mg

Indications, route, and dosage
Breast cancer (at least 5 years after menopause)
Adults: 1 mg P.O. t.i.d.
Female hypogonadism
Adults: 0.05 mg daily to t.i.d. for 2 weeks a month, followed by 2 weeks progesterone therapy; continue for 3 to 6 monthly dosing cycles, followed by 2 months off.

Menopausal symptoms
Adults: 0.02 to 0.05 mg P.O. daily for cycles of 3 weeks on, 1 week off.
Postpartum breast engorgement
Adults: 0.5 to 1 mg P.O. daily for 3 days, then taper over 7 days to 0.1 mg and discontinue.
Prostatic cancer
Adults: 0.15 to 2 mg P.O. daily.

Pharmacodynamics
Estrogenic action: Ethinyl estradiol mimics the action of endogenous estrogen in treating female hypogonadism, menopausal symptoms, and atrophic vaginitis. It inhibits growth of hormone-sensitive tissue in advanced, inoperable prostatic cancer and in certain carefully selected cases of breast cancer in men and postmenopausal women.

Pharmacokinetics
• *Absorption:* After oral administration, estradiol and the other natural unconjugated estrogens are well absorbed but substantially inactivated by the liver. Therefore, unconjugated estrogens are usually administered parenterally.

After I.M. administration, absorption begins rapidly and continues for days. The cypionate and valerate esters administered in oil have prolonged durations of action because of their slow absorption characteristics.

Topically applied estradiol is absorbed readily into the systemic circulation.
• *Distribution:* Estradiol and the other natural estrogens are approximately 50% to 80% plasma protein-bound, particularly the estradiol-binding globulin. Distribution occurs throughout the body, with highest concentrations appearing in fat.
• *Metabolism:* The steroidal estrogens, including estradiol, are metabolized primarily in the liver, where they are conjugated with sulfate and glucuronide. Because of the rapid rate of metabolism, nonesterified forms of estrogen, including estradiol, must usually be administered daily.
• *Excretion:* The majority of estrogen elimination occurs through the kidneys in the form of sulfate and/or glucuronide conjugates.

Contraindications and precautions
Ethinyl estradiol is contraindicated in patients with thrombophlebitis or thromboembolism because of its association with thromboembolic disorders; in patients with estrogen-responsive carcinoma (breast or genital tract cancer) because the drug may induce tumor growth; in patients with undiagnosed abnormal genital bleeding; in pregnant women because it may be fetotoxic; and in breast-feeding women because of the potential for adverse effects on the infant.

This drug should be administered cautiously in patients with disorders that may be aggravated by fluid and electrolyte accumulation, such as asthma, seizure disorders, migraine, or cardiac, renal, or hepatic dysfunction. Carefully monitor female patients who have breast nodules, fibrocystic breast disease, or a family history of breast cancer. Because of the risk of thromboembolism, therapy with this drug should be discontinued at least 1 week before elective surgical procedures associated with an increased incidence of thromboembolism.

Interactions
Concomitant administration of drugs that induce hepatic metabolism (such as rifampin, barbiturates, primidone, carbamazepine, and phenytoin) may decrease estrogenic effects from a given dose. These drugs are known to accelerate the rate of metabolism of certain other agents. Concomitant use of estrogens with corticosteroids may decrease corticosteroid elimination.

In patients with diabetes, ethinyl estradiol may increase blood glucose levels, necessitating dosage adjustment of insulin or oral hypoglycemic drugs.

Use with anticoagulants may decrease the effects of warfarin-type anticoagulants. Use with adrenocorticosteroids or adrenocorticotropic hormone increases the risk of fluid and electrolyte accumulation.

Effects on diagnostic tests
Therapy with ethinyl estradiol increases sulfobromophthalein retention, prothrombin and clotting Factors VII to X, and norepinephrine-induced platelet aggregability. Increases in thyroid-binding globulin concentration may occur, resulting in increased total thyroid concentration (measured by protein-bound iodine or total thyroxine) and decreased uptake of free triiodothyronine resin. Serum folate, pyridoxine, and antithrombin III concentrations may decrease; triglyceride, glucose, and phospholipid levels may increase. Glucose tolerance may be impaired. Pregnanediol excretion may decrease.

Adverse reactions
• CNS: headache, dizziness, chorea, depression, libido changes, lethargy.
• CV: thrombophlebitis, *thromboembolism,* hypertension, edema.
• DERM: melasma, urticaria, acne, seborrhea, oily skin, hirsutism or hair loss.
• EENT: worsening of myopia or astigmatism, intolerance to contact lenses.
• GI: nausea, vomiting, abdominal cramps, bloating, diarrhea, constipation, anorexia, increased appetite, weight changes.
• GU: breakthrough bleeding, altered menstrual flow, dysmenorrhea, amenorrhea, cervical erosion, altered cervical secretion, enlargement of uterine fibromas, vaginal candidiasis; *in males:* gynecomastia, testicular atrophy, impotence.
• Hepatic: cholestatic jaundice.
• Metabolic: hyperglycemia, hypercalcemia, folic acid deficiency.
• Other: breast changes (tenderness, enlargement, secretions), leg cramps.

Overdose and treatment
Serious toxicity after overdose of this drug has not been reported. Nausea may be expected to occur. Provide appropriate supportive care.

▶ Special considerations
Recommendations for administration of ethinyl estradiol and for care and teaching of patient during therapy are the same as those for all *estrogens.*

Geriatric use
Use with caution in patients whose condition may be aggravated by fluid retention.

Breast-feeding
Ethinyl estradiol is contraindicated in breast-feeding women.

ethionamide
Trecator-SC

- Pharmacologic classification: isonicotinic acid derivative
- Therapeutic classification: antitubercular agent
- Pregnancy risk category C

How supplied
Available by prescription only
Tablets: 250 mg

Indications, route, and dosage
Adjunctive treatment in pulmonary or extrapulmonary tuberculosis (when first-line agents cannot be used or have failed)
Adults: 500 mg to 1 g P.O. in one to three divided doses. Concomitant administration of other effective antitubercular drugs and pyridoxine is recommended.
Children: Optimum dosage has not been established.

Pharmacodynamics
Antitubercular action: Ethionamide appears to disrupt bacterial peptide synthesis. It may inhibit incorporation of mycolic acid into the mycobacterial cell wall; its exact mechanism of antibacterial action is unknown. It is either bacteriostatic or bactericidal, depending on organism susceptibility and drug concentration at infection site. Ethionamide is active against *Mycobacterium tuberculosis, M. bovis, M. kansasii,* and some strains of *M. avium* and *M. intracellulare.* Ethionamide is considered adjunctive therapy in tuberculosis and is given with another antitubercular agent to prevent or delay development of drug resistance by *M. tuberculosis.*

Pharmacokinetics
- *Absorption:* About 80% of an oral dose of ethionamide is absorbed from the GI tract; peak serum levels occur 3 hours after ingestion.
- *Distribution:* Ethionamide is distributed widely into body tissues and fluids, and has good CSF penetration. Ethionamide crosses the placenta; it is 10% protein-bound.
- *Metabolism:* Ethionamide is metabolized extensively, probably in the liver.
- *Excretion:* Ethionamide is excreted primarily in urine; 1% to 5% is excreted unchanged in 24 hours; the rest is excreted as metabolites. Plasma half-life is about 3 hours. It is not known if ethionamide is excreted in breast milk.

Contraindications and precautions
Ethionamide is contraindicated in patients with severe hepatic impairment and in patients with known hypersensitivity to drug.

Ethionamide should be used cautiously in patients with known hypersensitivity to chemically related drugs such as isoniazid or pyrazinamide to avoid cross-hypersensitivity; and in patients with diabetes because drug may hinder stabilization of serum glucose. Incidence of ethionamide-induced hepatic dysfunction is higher in diabetic patients.

Interactions
Ethionamide may intensify adverse reactions of concomitantly used antitubercular drugs.

Concomitant use with cycloserine or alcohol increases hazard of neurotoxicity.

Effects on diagnostic tests
Ethionamide may cause transient elevations of liver function test results; it may decrease serum protein-bound iodine and thyroxine (T_4) values.

Adverse reactions
- CNS: peripheral neuritis, psychic disturbances (especially mental depression), tremor, paresthesia, seizures, dizziness, olfactory disturbances, blurred vision.
- CV: postural hypotension, ganglionic blockade.
- DERM: rash, photosensitivity, acne.
- GI: anorexia, metallic taste in mouth, nausea, vomiting, sialorrhea, epigastric distress, diarrhea, stomatitis, weight loss.
- HEMA: thrombocytopenia.
- Hepatic: jaundice, hepatitis, elevated AST (SGOT) and ALT (SGPT) levels.
- Other: hypoglycemia, goiter, gynecomastia, impotence, acute rheumatic symptoms.
Note: Drug should be discontinued if patient shows signs of hypersensitivity reaction, hepatic dysfunction, or acute bleeding disorder.

Overdose and treatment
No specific recommendation is available. Treatment is supportive. After recent ingestion (within 4 hours), empty stomach by induced emesis or gastric lavage. Follow with activated charcoal to decrease absorption.

▶ Special considerations
- Give drug with or after meals to avoid gastric irritation. Severe irritation requires adjustment.
- Obtain specimens for culture and sensitivity testing before first dose, but therapy may begin before test results are complete; repeat periodically to detect drug resistance.
- Monitor renal and liver function studies before and every 2 to 4 weeks during therapy to detect and minimize toxicity.
- Observe patient for adverse effects, especially hepatic dysfunction and CNS toxicity; vitamin B_6 may be prescribed to prevent or relieve peripheral neuritis or neurotoxicity.
- Closely monitor the diabetic patient for hyperglycemia.
- Establish safety measures in case postural hypotention occurs.

Information for the patient
- Explain disease process and rationale for long-term therapy.
- Teach signs and symptoms of hypersensitivity and other adverse reactions, and emphasize need to report *any* unusual effects.
- Encourage patient to call if GI distress persists or becomes severe, if rash develops, or if patient develops symptoms or signs of hepatic dysfunction: loss of appetite, fatigue, malaise, jaundice, or dark urine.
- Advise patient to take drug with food to minimize gastric irritation.
- Advise patient to avoid alcohol.

• Be sure patient understands how and when to take drug; urge patient to complete entire prescribed regimen, to comply with instructions for around-the-clock dosage, and to keep follow-up appointments.

Pediatric use
When necessary, drug may be used in children even though optimal dose has not been established.

Breast-feeding
Safe use has not been established. An alternative feeding method is recommended during therapy.

ethosuximide
Zarontin

- Pharmacologic classification: succinimide derivative
- Therapeutic classification: anticonvulsant
- Pregnancy risk category C

How supplied
Available by prescription only
Capsules: 250 mg
Syrup: 250 mg/5 ml

Indications, route, and dosage
Absence seizures
Adults and children over age 6: Initially, 250 mg P.O. b.i.d. May increase by 250 mg q 4 to 7 days up to 1.5 g daily.
Children age 3 to 6: 20 mg/kg or 1.2 g/m² P.O. daily in a single dose or divided b.i.d. up to 1.5 g daily.

Pharmacodynamics
Anticonvulsant action: Ethosuximide raises the seizure threshold; it suppresses characteristic spike-and-wave pattern by depressing neuronal transmission in the motor cortex and basal ganglia. It is indicated for absence seizures refractory to other drugs.

Pharmacokinetics
• *Absorption:* Ethosuximide is absorbed from the GI tract; steady-state plasma levels occur in 4 to 7 days.
• *Distribution:* Ethosuximide is distributed widely throughout the body; protein binding is minimal.
• *Metabolism:* Ethosuximide is metabolized extensively in the liver to several inactive metabolites.
• *Excretion:* Ethosuximide is excreted in urine, with small amounts excreted in bile and feces.

Contraindications and precautions
Ethosuximide is contraindicated in patients with known hypersensitivity to succinimides. It should be used with extreme caution in patients with hepatic or renal disease and in those taking other CNS depressants or anticonvulsants. Ethosuximide may increase the incidence of generalized tonic-clonic seizures if used alone to treat patient with mixed seizures; abrupt withdrawal may precipitate petit mal seizures. Anticonvulsants have been associated with an increased incidence of birth defects.

Interactions
Concomitant use of ethosuximide and other CNS depressants (alcohol, narcotics, anxiolytics, antidepressants, antipsychotics, and other anticonvulsants) causes additive CNS depression and sedation.

Effects on diagnostic tests
Ethosuximide may elevate liver enzyme levels and may cause false-positive Coombs' test results. It may also cause abnormal results of renal function tests.

Adverse reactions
• CNS: drowsiness, headache, fatigue, dizziness, ataxia, irritability, hiccups, euphoria, lethargy, psychotic behavior.
• DERM: urticaria, pruritic and erythematous rashes, hirsutism, *Stevens-Johnson syndrome,* lupus-like syndromes.
• EENT: myopia.
• GI: nausea, vomiting, diarrhea, gum hypertrophy, weight loss, cramps, tongue swelling, anorexia, epigastric and abdominal pain.
• GU: vaginal bleeding.
• HEMA: leukopenia, eosinophilia, *agranulocytosis, pancytopenia, aplastic anemia.*
  Note: Drug should be discontinued if signs of hypersensitivity, rash, or unusual skin lesions or any of the following signs of blood dyscrasia occur: joint pain, fever, sore throat, or unusual bleeding or bruising.

Overdose and treatment
Symptoms of ethosuximide overdose, when used alone or with other anticonvulsants, include CNS depression, ataxia, stupor, and coma. Treatment is symptomatic and supportive. Carefully monitor vital signs and fluid and electrolyte balance.

▶ Special considerations
Besides those relevant to all *succinimide derivatives,* consider the following recommendations.
• Administer ethosuximide with food to minimize GI distress.
• Avoid abrupt discontinuation of drug. This may precipitate petit mal seizures.
• Observe patient for dermatologic reactions, joint pain, unexplained fever, or unusual bruising or bleeding (which may signal hematologic or other severe adverse reactions).

Information for the patient
• Tell patient to take drug with food or milk to prevent GI distress, to avoid use with alcoholic beverages, and to avoid hazardous tasks that require alertness if drug causes drowsiness, dizziness, or blurred vision.
• Warn patient not to discontinue drug abruptly; this may cause seizures.
• Encourage patient to wear a Medic Alert bracelet or necklace.
• Tell patient to report the following effects: skin rash, joint pain, fever, sore throat, or unusual bleeding or bruising.
• If pregnancy occurs, patient should call promptly.
• Tell patient to protect pediatric syrup from freezing.

Geriatric use
Use with caution in elderly patients.

Pediatric use
Ethosuximide is not recommended for children under age 3.

Breast-feeding
Safe use has not been established. Alternative feeding method is recommended during therapy with ethosuximide.

ethotoin
Peganone

- Pharmacologic classification: hydantoin derivative
- Therapeutic classification: anticonvulsant
- Pregnancy risk category D

How supplied
Available by prescription only
Tablets: 250 mg, 500 mg

Indications, route, and dosage
Generalized tonic-clonic or complex-partial seizures
Adults: Initially, 250 mg P.O. q.i.d. after meals; may increase slowly over several days to 3 g daily divided q.i.d.
Children: 80 mg/kg or 2.5 mg/m² P.O. daily or divided b.i.d.

Pharmacodynamics
Anticonvulsant action: Like other hydantoin derivatives, ethotoin stabilizes neuronal membranes and limits seizure activity by increasing efflux of sodium ions across cell membranes in the motor cortex during generation of nerve impulses. However, ethotoin lacks the antiarrhythmic effects of phenytoin.

Ethotoin is indicated for tonic-clonic (grand mal) and partial seizures. It is less toxic and less effective than phenytoin and usually is given with other anticonvulsants.

Pharmacokinetics
- *Absorption:* Ethotoin is absorbed rapidly from the GI tract.
- *Distribution:* Ethotoin is distributed widely throughout the body; its therapeutic range is believed to be 15 to 50 mcg/ml.
- *Metabolism:* Ethotoin is metabolized by the liver, probably by a saturable mechanism (at high doses, a small increase in dosage may produce a large increase in plasma levels).
- *Excretion:* Ethotoin is excreted in urine and feces; small amounts appear in saliva and breast milk.

Contraindications and precautions
Ethotoin is contraindicated in patients with hepatic dysfunction or hematologic disorders. It should be used with caution in patients taking other hydantoin derivatives; concomitant use with phenacemide has caused extreme paranoid symptoms.

Interactions
Concomitant use of ethotoin with phenacemide may cause extreme paranoia. Use of ethotoin with oral contraceptives may decrease the efficacy of oral contraceptives.

The use of anticonvulsants during pregnancy has been associated with an increased incidence of birth defects.

Effects on diagnostic tests
Ethotoin may raise liver enzyme levels.

Adverse reactions
- CNS: fatigue, insomnia, dizziness, headache, numbness.
- CV: chest pain.
- DERM: rash.
- EENT: diplopia, nystagmus.
- GI: nausea, vomiting, diarrhea, gingival hyperplasia (rare).
- HEMA: thrombocytopenia, leukopenia, *agranulocytosis,* pancytopenia, megaloblastic anemia.
- Other: fever, lymphadenopathy.
  Note: Drug should be discontinued if signs of hypersensitivity occur, if a lymphoma-like syndrome develops, or if laboratory tests show hepatic or hematologic changes.

Overdose and treatment
Symptoms of overdose may include drowsiness, nausea, nystagmus, ataxia, and dysarthria; hypotension, respiratory depression, and coma may follow.

Treat overdose with gastric lavage or emesis and follow with supportive treatment. Carefully monitor vital signs and fluid and electrolyte balance. Hemodialysis or total exchange transfusion has been used for managing severe overdose, especially in children.

▶ Special considerations
Besides those relevant to all *hydantoin derivatives,* consider the following recommendations.
- Obtain complete blood count and urinalysis at start of therapy and monthly thereafter.
- Administer ethotoin after meals. Schedule doses as evenly as possible over 24 hours.
- Ethotoin generally produces milder adverse effects than phenytoin; however, larger doses needed to maintain therapeutic effect frequently cause GI distress.
- Use cautiously in patients receiving phenacemide.
- Ethotoin may be removed by hemodialysis. Dosage adjustments may be necessary in patients undergoing dialysis.

Information for the patient
- Warn patient to avoid hazardous activities that require alertness until CNS response to drug has been determined.
- Tell patient to avoid alcohol while taking this drug, to take drug with food or milk to prevent GI distress, and never to discontinue drug abruptly.
- Patient should call at once if adverse reactions, especially rash, swollen glands, bleeding or bruising, yellow skin or eyes, fever, sore throat, or infection, occur.
- Warn patient that pregnancy should be avoided during therapy. Patient should call promptly if pregnancy occurs.

Geriatric use
Use with caution in elderly patients.

Pediatric use
Pediatric dosage form unavailable.

Breast-feeding
Ethotoin is distributed into breast milk. Alternative feeding method is recommended during therapy with ethotoin.

---

ethyl chloride
Ethyl Chloride Spray

- Pharmacologic classification: halogenated hydrocarbon
- Therapeutic classification: local anesthetic, counterirritant
- Pregnancy risk category C

How supplied
Available by prescription only
Liquid spray

Indications, route, and dosage
As a local anesthetic in minor operative procedures and to relieve pain caused by insect stings and burns
Adults and children: Dosage varies with different procedures. Use smallest dosage needed to produce desired effect. For local anesthesia, use the fine-spray nozzle; hold container about 12″ (30 cm) from area and spray downward until a light frosting appears.
For infants: Hold a cotton ball saturated with ethyl chloride to area for a few seconds.
As a counterirritant to relieve myofascial and visceral pain syndromes
Adults, children, and infants: Dosage varies with use. Use smallest dosage needed to produce desired effect. Use the large-sized nozzle; hold container 24″ from skin and spray at an acute angle in one direction in a sweeping motion until area has been covered.

Pharmacodynamics
Anesthetic action: Rapid vaporization of ethyl chloride freezes superficial tissues, producing insensitivity of peripheral nerve endings and local anesthesia. Anesthesia lasts for up to 1 minute.

Pharmacokinetics
- *Absorption:* Limited with topical use.
- *Distribution:* None.
- *Metabolism:* None.
- *Excretion:* None.

Contraindications and precautions
Ethyl chloride is contraindicated for use near eyes or on broken skin or mucous membranes; it should not be inhaled.

Freezing and thawing process may damage epithelial cells; avoid repeated use over long periods.

Ethyl chloride is highly flammable and explosive; it should not be used near open fire and should be stored away from heat or open flame.

Interactions
None reported.

Effects on diagnostic tests
None reported.

Adverse reactions
- Local: skin lesions, rash, urticaria, burning, stinging, tenderness, inflammation, frostbite, tissue necrosis with prolonged use, pain and muscle spasm from excessive cooling.
  Note: Drug should be discontinued if sensitization develops.

Overdose and treatment
Discontinue use and clean area thoroughly.

▶ **Special considerations**
- Do not apply to broken skin or mucous membranes.
- Protect adjacent skin with petrolatum to prevent tissue damage.
- When using ethyl chloride as a counterirritant, avoid frosting the skin, as excessive cooling may increase spasms and pain.

Information for the patient
Advise patient that drug will produce a temporary numbness.

Pediatric use
Use smaller amounts of drug.

Breast-feeding
Cleanse breast area of drug before breast-feeding.

---

etidronate disodium
Didronel

- Pharmacologic classification: pyrophosphate analog
- Therapeutic classification: antihypercalcemic
- Pregnancy risk category B

How supplied
Available by prescription only
Tablets: 200 mg, 400 mg
Injection: 50 mg/ml

Indications, route, and dosage
Symptomatic Paget's disease
Adults: 5 mg/kg P.O. daily as a single dose 2 hours before a meal with water or juice. Patient should not eat or take antacids or vitamins with mineral supplements for 2 hours after dose. May give up to 10 mg/kg/day in severe cases not to exceed 6 months. Maximum dosage is 20 mg/kg/day, not to exceed 3 months.
Heterotopic ossification in spinal cord injuries
Adults: 20 mg/kg/day for 2 weeks, then 10 mg/kg/day for 10 weeks. Total treatment period 12 weeks.
Heterotopic ossification after total hip replacement
Adults: 20 mg/kg/day for 1 month before total hip replacement and for 3 months afterward.
Hypercalcemia associated with malignancy
Adults: 7.5 mg/kg I.V. daily for 3 days. May repeat up to 7 days. Then wait 7 days before beginning a second course of treatment.

Pharmacodynamics
Bone-metabolism inhibitor action: Although the exact mechanism is not known, etidronate acts on bone by

---

adsorbing to hydroxyapatite crystals in the bone, thereby inhibiting their growth and dissolution. It also decreases the number of osteoclasts in bone, thereby slowing excessive remodeling of pagetic or heterotopic bone.

Pharmacokinetics
● *Absorption:* Absorption following an oral dose is variable and is decreased in the presence of food. Absorption may also be dose related.
● *Distribution:* Approximately half of the dose is distributed to bone.
● *Metabolism:* Etidronate is not metabolized.
● *Excretion:* About 50% of the drug is excreted within 24 hours in urine.

Contraindications and precautions
No known contraindications. Use cautiously in patients with restricted calcium and vitamin D intake. Because of potential for intestinal irritation, use cautiously in patients with enterocolitis. Patients with impaired renal function should be monitored closely because the drug may accumulate.

Interactions
None reported.

Effects on diagnostic tests
Drug may elevate serum phosphate.

Adverse reactions
● GI: (seen most frequently at 20 mg/kg/day) diarrhea, increased frequency of bowel movements, nausea.
● Other: increased or recurrent bone pain at pagetic sites, pain at previously asymptomatic sites, increased risk of fracture, elevated serum phosphate.

Overdose and treatment
Clinical manifestations of overdose include diarrhea, nausea, and hypocalcemia. Treat with gastric lavage and emesis. Administer calcium if required.

▶ Special considerations
● Drug should be taken in a single dose. However, if nausea occurs, dosage may be divided.
● Monitor drug effect by serum alkaline phosphate and urinary hydroxyproline excretion; both are lowered by effective therapy.

Information for the patient
● Instruct patient to take drug on an empty stomach with water or juice and to avoid food, antacids, and vitamins with mineral supplements for 2 hours.
● Remind patient that improvement may take at least 3 months and may continue even after the drug is stopped.

etodolac (ultradol)
Lodine

● Pharmacologic classification: nonsteroidal anti-inflammatory
● Therapeutic classification: antiarthritic
● Pregnancy risk category C

How supplied
Available by prescription only
Capsules: 200 mg, 300 mg

Indications, route, and dosage
Acute and chronic management of osteoarthritis and pain
Adults: For acute pain, give 200 to 400 mg P.O. q 6 to 8 hours p.r.n., not to exceed 1,200 mg daily. For patients weighing 60 kg (132 lb) or less, total daily dose should not exceed 20 mg/kg.

For osteoarthritis, give 800 to 1,200 mg P.O. daily in divided doses initially, followed by adjustments of 600 to 1,200 mg in divided doses: 200 mg P.O. t.i.d. or q.i.d.; 300 mg P.O. b.i.d., t.i.d., or q.i.d.; 400 mg P.O. b.i.d. or t.i.d. Total daily dosage is not to exceed 1,200 mg. For patients weighing 60 kg or less, total daily dosage should not exceed 20 mg/kg.

Pharmacodynamics
Antiarthritic action: The mechanism of action of etodolac is unknown but presumed to be associated with inhibition of prostaglandin biosynthesis.

Pharmacokinetics
● *Absorption:* Etodolac is well-absorbed from GI tract, with peak concentrations reached in 1 to 1.5 hours. Onset of analgesic activity occurs within 30 minutes, lasting 4 to 6 hours. Antacids do not appear to affect absorption of etodolac; however, they can decrease peak concentrations reached by 15% to 20% but have no effect when peak levels are reached.
● *Distribution:* Found in liver, lungs, heart, and kidneys.
● *Metabolism:* Extensively metabolized in the liver.
● *Excretion:* Excreted in urine primarily as metabolites; 16% is excreted in feces.

Contraindications and precautions
Etodolac is contraindicated for use in patients with a history of hypersenstivity to the drug and in those patients in whom etodolac or other NSAIDs induced asthma, rhinitis, urticaria, or other allergic reactions. Use with caution in patients with a history of GI bleeding, ulceration, and perforation, or renal or hepatic impairment.

GI ulceration or bleeding can occur with any NSAID, sometimes without warning. Patients receiving chronic therapy should be closely watched for signs and symptoms of GI bleeding.

Interactions
Like other NSAIDs, etodolac may cause changes in elimination of cyclosporine, digoxin, lithium, and methotrexate, resulting in increased levels of these drugs. It may enhance nephrotoxicity associated with cyclosporine. Although the clinical significance is unknown, concurrent use with aspirin reduces etodolac's protein-binding without altering its clearance. Use with warfarin

results in decreased protein-binding of warfarin but does not change its clearance. No dosage adjustment is necessary.

Effects on diagnostic tests
A false-positive test for urinary bilirubin may be caused by phenolic metabolites. Decreased serum uric acid levels and borderline elevations of one or more liver test results may occur.

Adverse reactions
● CNS: asthenia, malaise, dizziness, depression, nervousness.
● CV: anemia, hypertension, *CHF*, flushing, palpitations.
● GI: dyspepsia, flatulence, abdominal pain, diarrhea, nausea, constipation, gastritis, melena, vomiting, anorexia, peptic ulcer with or without bleeding and *perforation.*
● GU: dysuria, urinary frequency.
● EENT: blurred vision, tinnitus, photophobia.
● DERM: pruritus, rash.
● Hepatic: hepatitis.
● Respiratory: asthma.
● Other: ulcerative stomatitis, thirst, dry mouth, chills, fever, edema.

▶ Special considerations
● Minimal GI blood loss has been reported at doses up to 1,200 mg daily; endoscopy scores are comparable to placebo at doses up to 1,000 mg daily.
● No apparent interaction occurs when administered with diuretics, phenytoin, or glyburide. Use caution with concurrent use of diuretics in patients with cardiac, renal, or hepatic failure.
● Monitor for signs and symptoms of GI ulceration and bleeding.
● Etodolac 1,200 mg was shown to cause less GI bleeding than ibuprofen 2,400 mg daily, indomethacin 200 mg daily, naproxen 750 mg daily, or piroxicam 20 mg daily.
● Etodolac is not recommended to treat rheumatoid arthritis.

Information for the patient
● Tell patient to inform physician of any GI complaints.
● Caution patient to avoid use during pregnancy.
● Tell patient that etodolac may be taken with food.

Geriatric use
Etodolac is well-tolerated in older and younger adults and generally does not require age-related dosage adjustments. No age-related differences have been reported.

Pediatric use
Safety and efficacy have not been established.

Breast-feeding
It is unknown if etodolac is excreted in breast milk. Use with caution.

---

etomidate
Amidate

● Pharmacologic classification: nonbarbiturate hypnotic
● Therapeutic classification: I.V. anesthetic, sedative
● Pregnancy risk category C

How supplied
Available by prescription only
Injection: 2 mg/ml

Indications, route, and dosage
Induction of general anesthesia
Adults and children over age 10: 0.2 to 0.6 mg/kg I.V. over a period of 30 to 60 seconds.

Pharmacodynamics
Anesthetic and sedative actions: Etomidate, like naturally occurring gamma-aminobutyric acid, decreases the firing rate of neurons within the ascending reticular activating system.

Pharmacokinetics
● *Absorption:* Etomidate is only given I.V. Onset of action is rapid, usually beginning in 60 seconds; duration of action is usually 3 to 5 minutes.
● *Distribution:* Etomidate distributes widely into body tissue and is highly protein-bound (76%).
● *Metabolism:* Etomidate is metabolized rapidly in the liver.
● *Excretion:* About 75% of a given dose is excreted in urine as an active metabolite; 10% of drug is excreted in bile and 13% in feces.

Contraindications and precautions
Etomidate is contraindicated in patients allergic to the drug. It should be used cautiously in elderly or debilitated patients with underlying pulmonary disease, because of increased respiratory depression. Monitor patients on prolonged use for signs of adrenal insufficiency, because etomidate may block adrenal steroid production. It is not recommended for use during labor and delivery because safety has not been established.

Interactions
None significant.

Effects on diagnostic tests
Reduced plasma cortisol levels have been reported, lasting for 6 to 8 hours after induction.

Adverse reactions
● CNS: transient skeletal muscle movements (chiefly myoclonic, some tonic), averting movements.
● CV: hypertension, hypotension, tachycardia, bradycardia, *arrhythmias.*
● GI: postoperative nausea or vomiting after induction of anesthesia.
● Local: transient venous pain on injection.
● Other: hiccups, snoring, transient apnea.
Note: Drug should be discontinued if patient shows signs of hypersensitivity or adrenal insufficiency or if prolonged apnea occurs.

Overdose and treatment
Clinical signs include CNS depression and respiratory arrest. Treat patient supportively, using mechanical ventilation if necessary, until drug effects subside.

▶ **Special considerations**
● Etomidate is compatible with commonly used pre-anesthetic agents.
● During short procedures in adults, smaller increments of I.V. etomidate may be used to supplement subpotent anesthetics, such as nitrous oxide.
● Transient muscle movements may be reduced by injection of 0.1 mg of fentanyl before giving etomidate, probably by reducing total dose of etomidate.
● Muscle movements are more common in patients with transient venous irritation and pain.
● Etomidate has a much lower incidence of cardiovascular and respiratory effects than thiopental sodium and is therefore used to advantage in high-risk surgical patients.

Geriatric use
Drug should be used with caution in elderly patients.

Pediatric use
Use is not recommended in patients younger than age 10.

Breast-feeding
It is unknown whether etomidate enters breast milk; therefore, it should be used with caution in breast-feeding women.

---

etoposide (VP-16)
VePesid

● Pharmacologic classification: podophyllotoxin (cell cycle-phase specific, G2 and late S phases)
● Therapeutic classification: antineoplastic
● Pregnancy risk category D

How supplied
Available by prescription only
Injection: 100 mg/5 ml multiple-dose vials
Capsules: 50 mg

Indications, route, and dosage
Dosage and indications may vary. Check literature for current protocol.
Small-cell carcinoma of the lung
Adults: 70 mg/m²/day P.O. (rounded to the nearest 50 mg) for 4 days; or 100 mg/m² P.O. (rounded to the nearest 50 mg) daily for 5 days. Repeat q 3 to 4 weeks. Alternatively, 35 mg/m² I.V. daily for 4 days or 50 mg/m² I.V. daily for 5 days. Repeat q 3 to 4 weeks.
Testicular carcinoma
Adults: 50 to 100 mg/m² I.V. daily on days 1 to 5; or 100 mg/m²/day on days 1, 3, and 5 of a regimen repeated q 3 or 4 weeks.

Pharmacodynamics
Antineoplastic action: Etoposide exerts its cytotoxic action by arresting cells in the metaphase portion of cell division. The drug also inhibits cells from entering mitosis and depresses DNA and RNA synthesis.

Pharmacokinetics
● *Absorption:* Etoposide is only moderately absorbed across the GI tract after oral administration. The bioavailability ranges from 25% to 75%, with an average of 50% of the dose being absorbed.
● *Distribution:* Etoposide distributes widely into body tissues; the highest concentrations are found in the liver, spleen, kidney, healthy brain tissue, and brain tumor tissue. The drug crosses the blood-brain barrier to a limited and variable extent. Etoposide is approximately 94% bound to serum albumin.
● *Metabolism:* Only a small portion of a dose of etoposide is metabolized. Metabolism occurs in the liver.
● *Excretion:* Etoposide is excreted primarily in the urine as unchanged drug. A smaller portion of a dose is excreted in the feces. The plasma elimination of etoposide is described as biphasic, with an initial phase half-life of about ½ to 2 hours and a terminal phase of about 5½ to 11 hours.

Contraindications and precautions
Etoposide is contraindicated in patients with a history of hypersensitivity to the drug.

Interactions
Concomitant use of etoposide increases the cytotoxicity of cisplatin against certain tumors. The mechanism of this synergistic cytotoxic activity is unknown.

Effects on diagnostic tests
None reported.

Adverse reactions
● CNS: headache, weakness, visual disturbances, peripheral neuropathy (especially if administered with other neurotoxic medications).
● CV: hypotension from rapid infusion, palpitation, tachycardia.
● GI: nausea and vomiting (in 30%), anorexia, stomatitis.
● HEMA: *bone marrow depression* (dose-limiting), *leukopenia, thrombocytopenia.*
● Local: infrequent phlebitis; pain at I.V. site.
● Other: occasional fever, reversible alopecia, *anaphylaxis* (rare), generalized pain, chills, diaphoresis.
Note: Drug should be discontinued if severe hematopoietic toxicity results.

Overdose and treatment
Clinical manifestations of overdose include myelosuppression, nausea, and vomiting.
Treatment is usually supportive and includes transfusion of blood components, antiemetics, and appropriate symptomatic therapy.

▶ **Special considerations**
● To prepare solution, dilute prescribed dose to a concentration of 0.2 to 0.4 mg/ml with normal saline solution or dextrose 5% in water. Higher concentrations may crystallize. Discard solution if cloudy.
● Solutions diluted to 0.2 mg/ml are stable for 96 hours at room temperature in plastic or glass unprotected from light; solutions diluted to 0.4 mg/ml are stable for 48 hours under the same conditions.
● Administer infusion over 30 to 60 minutes to avoid hypotensive reactions.
● Treatment of extravasation includes local injections of hyaluronidase, which aids in systemic reabsorption of etoposide.

Canada only   †Unlabeled clinical use   Italicized adverse reactions are life-threatening.

- Pretreatment with antiemetics may reduce frequency and duration of nausea and vomiting.
- GI toxicity occurs more frequently after oral administration.
- At doses below 200 mg, extent of absorption after oral administration is not affected by food.
- Intrapleural and intrathecal administration of this drug is contraindicated due to severe toxicity.
- Dosage reduction may be required for patients with impaired renal function.
- Capsules must be stored under refrigeration.
- Have diphenhydramine, hydrocortisone, epinephrine, and airway available in case of an anaphylactic reaction.
- Monitor blood pressure before infusion and at 30-minute intervals during infusion. If systolic blood pressure falls below 90 mm Hg, stop infusion.
- Monitor CBC. Observe patient for signs of bone marrow depression.
- Etoposide has produced complete remissions in small-cell lung cancer and testicular cancer.

Information for the patient
- Emphasize importance of continuing medication despite nausea and vomiting.
- Tell patient to call immediately if vomiting occurs shortly after dose is taken.
- Advise patient to avoid exposure to people with infections.
- Tell patient not to receive immunizations during therapy with etoposide. Other members of the patient's household should also receive no immunizations during the same period of time.
- Tell patient to promptly report a sore throat or fever or unusual bruising or bleeding.
- Reassure patient that hair should grow back after treatment has ended.

Geriatric use
Elderly patients may be particularly susceptible to the hypotensive effects of etoposide.

Pediatric use
Safety and effectiveness in children have not been established.

Breast-feeding
Etoposide is excreted into breast milk. Therefore, because of the risk of serious adverse reactions, mutagenicity, and carcinogenicity in the infant, breast-feeding is not recommended.

Factor IX complex
Konyne-HT, Profilnine Heat-Treated,
Proplex SX-T, Proplex T

- Pharmacologic classification: blood derivative
- Therapeutic classification: systemic hemostatic
- Pregnancy risk category C

How supplied
Available by prescription only
Injection: Vials, with diluents. Units specified on label.

Indications, route, and dosage
Factor IX deficiency (hemophilia B or Christmas disease), anticoagulant overdose
Adults and children: Determine units required by multiplying 0.8 to 1 by body weight (in kg), then by percent of desired Factor IX level increase; administer by slow I.V. infusion or I.V. push. Dosage is highly individualized, depending on degree of deficiency, desired level of Factor IX, body weight, and severity of bleeding.

Factor IX complex can also be used to reverse coumarin anticoagulation when emergency situations such as surgery preclude less hazardous therapy.

One unit of Factor IX complex (Factor IX units) equals the average of Factor II, VII, IX, and X activity in 1 ml of normal fresh pooled plasma less than 1 hour old.
Hemostasis in patients with Factor VIII inhibitors
Adults and children: Usual dose is > 5 IU/kg I.V. Repeat q 12 hours p.r.n.
Hemostasis in Factor VII deficiency (Proplex T only)
Adults and children: Determine units required by multiplying 0.5 by body weight (kg) multiplied by percent of Factor VII increase desired. Administer I.V., and repeat q 6 to 8 hours.

Pharmacodynamics
Hemostatic action: Factor IX complex directly replaces deficient clotting factor.

Pharmacokinetics
- *Absorption:* Factor IX complex must be given parenterally for systemic effect.
- *Distribution:* Equilibration within extravascular space takes 4 to 6 hours.
- *Metabolism:* Factor IX complex is rapidly cleared by plasma.
- *Excretion:* Half-life is approximately 24 hours.

Contraindications and precautions
Factor IX complex is contraindicated in hepatic disease, intravascular coagulation, or fibrinolysis.

Administer Factor IX complex cautiously to neonates and infants susceptible to hepatitis, which Factor IX

complex may transmit; presently available heat-treated products lessen this risk.

Only Proplex T may be used to treat Factor VII deficiency.

Interactions
Concurrent administration with aminocaproic acid increases the risk of thrombosis.

Effects on diagnostic tests
None reported.

Adverse reactions
- CNS: headache, tingling sensation.
- CV: thromboembolic reactions, hypotension, tachycardia, possible *intravascular hemolysis* in patients with blood types A, B, and AB.
- Other: transient fever, chills, flushing, hypersensitivity, viral hepatitis, *disseminated intravascular coagulation (DIC)*.
  Note: Drug should be discontinued if signs of allergic reaction appear.

Overdose and treatment
Clinical manifestations of overdose include a risk of DIC on repeated use because of increased levels of Factors II, IX, and X.

▶ Special considerations
- Refrigerate vials until needed; before reconstituting, warm to room temperature. Use 20 ml sterile water for injection of each vial of lyophilized drug. To mix, gently roll vial between hands; do not shake or mix with other I.V. solutions. Keep product away from heat (but do not refrigerate, because this may cause precipitation of active ingredient), and use within 3 hours.
- Adverse reactions are usually related to too-rapid infusion. Take baseline pulse rate before I.V. administration; if pulse rate increases significantly during infusion, reduce flow rate or stop drug. If patient complains of tingling sensation, fever, chills, or headache, decrease flow rate. A rate of 100 units/minute is usually well-tolerated; do not give drug faster than 3 ml/minute.
- Monitor coagulation studies before and during therapy; monitor vital signs regularly, and be alert for allergic reactions.
- Patient should be immunized with hepatitis B vaccine to decrease the risk of transmission of hepatitis.

Information for the patient
Teach or review proper storage, preparation, and injection technique for the specific product which the patient uses.

Pediatric use
Administer cautiously to neonates and other infants because of increased risk of hepatitis; only heat-treated products are now available, thus decreasing the risk.

---

*Canada only   †Unlabeled clinical use   Italicized adverse reactions are life-threatening.

famotidine
Pepcid

- Pharmacologic classification: histamine₂-receptor antagonist
- Therapeutic classification: antiulcer agent
- Pregnancy risk category B

How supplied
Available by prescription only
Tablets: 20 mg, 40 mg
Injection: 10 mg/ml
Suspension: 40 mg/5 ml

Indications, route, and dosage
Duodenal and gastric ulcer
Adults: For acute therapy, 40 mg P.O. h.s. for 4 to 8 weeks; for maintenance therapy, 20 mg P.O. h.s.
Pathologic hypersecretory conditions (such as Zollinger-Ellison syndrome), †short bowel syndrome
Adults: 20 mg P.O. q 6 hours. As much as 160 mg q 6 hours may be administered.
Hospitalized patients with intractable ulcers or hypersecretory conditions, or patients who can't take oral medication
Adults: 20 mg I.V. q 12 hours.

Pharmacodynamics
Antiulcer action: Famotidine competitively inhibits histamine's action at H₂-receptors in gastric parietal cells. This inhibits basal and nocturnal gastric acid secretion resulting from stimulation by such factors as caffeine, food, and pentagastrin.

Pharmacokinetics
- *Absorption:* When administered orally, approximately 40% to 45% of dose is absorbed; onset of action occurs in 1 hour, with peak action in 1 to 3 hours. After parenteral administration, peak action occurs in 30 minutes.
- *Distribution:* Famotidine is distributed widely to many body tissues.
- *Metabolism:* About 30% to 35% of an administered dose is metabolized by the liver (minimal first-pass metabolism).
- *Excretion:* Most drug is excreted unchanged in urine. Famotidine has a longer duration of effect than its 2½ to 3½ hour half-life suggests.

Contraindications and precautions
Famotidine is contraindicated in patients with famotidine allergy.

Famotidine should be used cautiously in patients with severely impaired hepatic function because inadequate hepatic metabolism may cause accumulation of the drug and toxic effects.

Dosage increase may be necessary in patients with creatinine clearance less than 10 ml/minute.

Interactions
Famotidine may cause enteric coatings to dissolve too rapidly because of increased gastric pH. It may decrease ketoconazole's absorption, requiring an increased dose of ketoconazole.

Effects on diagnostic tests
Famotidine may antagonize pentagastrin during gastric acid secretion tests. Famotidine may elevate hepatic enzyme levels.

In skin tests using allergen extracts, the drug may cause false-negative results.

Adverse reactions
- CNS: headache, malaise, dizziness, drowsiness, anxiety, depression.
- DERM: dryness, flushing, alopecia, acne, pruritus.
- EENT: tinnitus.
- GI: dry mouth, diarrhea, constipation, nausea, vomiting, anorexia, stomach pain, unusual taste, flatulence.
- HEMA: *thrombocytopenia.*
- Hepatic: increased liver enzyme levels.
- Local: transient irritation at I.V. site.
- Other: decreased libido, joint or muscle pain, allergic reaction.

Overdose and treatment
Overdose has not been reported. Treatment should include gastric lavage or induced emesis, followed by activated charcoal to prevent further absorption and by necessary supportive and symptomatic therapy. Hemodialysis does not remove famotidine.

▶ Special considerations
Besides those relevant to all *H₂-receptor antagonists,* consider the following recommendations.
- Famotidine is not recommended for use longer than 8 weeks in patients with uncomplicated duodenal ulcer.
- After administration via nasogastric tube, tube should be flushed to clear it and ensure drug's passage to stomach.
- For I.V. push administration, dilute with normal saline solution to total volume of 5 to 10 ml; administer over period exceeding 2 minutes. For I.V. infusion, dilute in 100 ml of dextrose 5% solution; administer over 15 to 30 minutes. Drug is stable at room temperature for 48 hours. Do not use drug if it is discolored or contains precipitate.
- Antacids may be administered concurrently.
- Drug appears to cause fewer adverse reactions and drug interactions than cimetidine.

Information for the patient
- Caution patient to take drug only as directed and to continue taking doses even after pain subsides, to ensure adequate healing.
- Instruct patient to take dose at bedtime.

Geriatric use
Use caution when administering famotidine to elderly patients because of the increased risk of adverse reactions, particularly those affecting the CNS.

Breast-feeding
Famotidine may be excreted in breast milk. Use with caution in breast-feeding women.

---

fat emulsions
Intralipid 10%, Intralipid 20%, Liposyn 10%, Liposyn 20%, Liposyn II 10%, Liposyn II 20%, Soyacal 10%, Soyacal 20%, Travamulsion 10%, Travamulsion 20%

- Pharmacologic classification: lipid
- Therapeutic classification: I.V. hyperalimentation (IVH)
- Pregnancy risk category C (except Soyacal 10%, category B)

How supplied
Available by prescription only
Injection: 50 ml (10%, 20%), 100 ml (10%, 20%), 200 ml (10%, 20%), 250 ml (10%, 20%), 500 ml (10%, 20%)

Indications, route, and dosage
Source of calories adjunctive to IVH
Intralipid
Adults: 1 ml/minute I.V. for 15 to 30 minutes (10% emulsion); or 0.5 ml/minute I.V. for 15 to 30 minutes (20% emulsion). If no adverse reactions occur, increase rate to deliver 500 ml over 4 to 8 hours. Total daily dose should not exceed 2.5 g/kg.
Children: 0.1 ml/minute for 10 to 15 minutes (10% emulsion); or 0.05 ml/minute I.V. for 10 to 15 minutes (20% emulsion). If no adverse reactions occur, increase rate to deliver 1 g/kg over 4 hours. Daily dose should not exceed 4 g/kg, which equals 60% of daily caloric intake. Protein-carbohydrate IVH should supply remaining 40%.
Fatty acid deficiency
Intralipid
Adults and children: 8% to 10% of total caloric intake I.V.
Prevention of fatty acid deficiency
Liposyn
Adults: 500 ml (10% emulsion) I.V. twice weekly. Infuse initially at a rate of 1 ml/minute for 30 minutes. Rate may be increased but should not exceed 500 ml over 4 to 6 hours.
Children: 5 to 10 ml/kg (10% emulsion) I.V. daily. Infuse initially at a rate of 0.1 ml/minute for 30 minutes. Rate may be increased but should not exceed 100 ml/hour.

Pharmacodynamics
Metabolic action: I.V. fat emulsions are prepared from either soybean or safflower oil and provide a mixture of neutral triglycerides, predominantly fatty acids. Besides the major component, fatty acids (linoleic, oleic, palmitic, stearic, and linolenic), these preparations also contain 1.2% egg yolk (an emulsifier) and glycerol (to adjust tonicity). I.V. fat emulsions are isotonic and may be given centrally or peripherally.
   Linoleic, linolenic, and arachidonic acids are essential in humans. Clinical manifestations of essential fatty acid deficiency (EFAD) include scaly dermatitis, alopecia, growth retardation, poor wound healing, thrombocytopenia, and fatty liver. I.V. fat emulsions prevent or reverse the biochemical and clinical manifestations of EFAD and provide 1.1 kcal/ml (10%) or 2.2 kcal/ml (20%).

Pharmacokinetics
- *Absorption:* These products are administered as an I.V. infusion, through either a peripheral or a central vein.
- *Distribution:* Fat emulsions distribute through the plasma compartment.
- *Metabolism:* Fat emulsions are metabolized and used as an energy source, causing increased heat production, decreased respiratory quotient, and increased oxygen consumption.
- *Excretion:* The infused fat particles are cleared from the bloodstream in a manner similar to chylomicrons.

Contraindications and precautions
I.V. fat emulsions are contraindicated in patients with impaired fat metabolism, such as pathologic hyperlipidemia, lipoid nephrosis, or acute pancreatitis, if accompanied by hyperlipidemia. Because I.V. fat emulsions contain egg yolk phospholipids, they should not be administered to patients with severe egg allergies. Safety during pregnancy has not been established.
   Fat emulsions must be used cautiously in patients with severe liver damage, pulmonary disease, anemia, or blood coagulation disorders; they also must be used cautiously when danger of fat embolism exists. All patients must have their capacity to eliminate I.V. fat emulsions monitored to ensure clearance of the lipemia between daily infusions. Discontinue use if abnormal parameters result.

Interactions
None reported.

Effects on diagnostic tests
Abnormally high mean corpuscular hemoglobin and mean corpuscular hemoglobin concentration values may be found in blood samples drawn during or shortly after fat emulsion infusion. Fat emulsions may cause transient abnormalities in liver function tests and may alter results of serum bilirubin tests (especially in infants).

Adverse reactions
Early reactions to fat overload:
- CNS: headache, sleepiness, dizziness, insomnia.
- DERM: flushing, diaphoresis, urticaria, pruritus.
- EENT: pressure over eyes.
- GI: nausea, vomiting.
- HEMA: hyperlipemia, hypercoagulability, thrombocytopenia in neonates (rare).
- Local: irritation at infusion site, sepsis, thrombophlebitis.
- Other: fever, dyspnea, chest and back pains, cyanosis, deposition of I.V. fat, *sepsis.*
Delayed reactions:
- CNS: focal seizures.
- CV: *shock.*
- HEMA: thrombocytopenia, leukopenia, leukocytosis, splenomegaly, shock.
- Hepatic: transient increased liver function test, hepatomegaly, jaundice.
- Other: fever, splenomegaly, fat accumulation in lungs.

Overdose and treatment
Clinical manifestations of overdose or "overloading syndrome" include focal seizures, splenomegaly, leukocytosis, fever, and shock. The infusion should be discontinued until visual inspection of the plasma, determination of triglyceride concentrations, or nephelometric

measurement of plasma light-scattering activity confirms clearance of the lipid. Reevaluate the patient and institute appropriate corrective measures.

▶ **Special considerations**
● Only the intralipid brand of fat emulsion can be mixed with amino acid solution, dextrose, electrolytes, and vitamins in the same I.V. container. Do not mix other lipid solutions with other substances.
● Do not use an in-line filter when administering this drug because the fat particles (0.5 mcg) are larger than the 0.22 mcg cellulose filter.
● Fat emulsions may extract small amounts of plasticizers from I.V. administration sets made of polyvinylchloride. Nonphthalate administration sets are available; however, phthalate extraction can be minimized from regular I.V. tubing by not storing primed administration sets.
● Discard the fat emulsion if it separates or becomes oily.
● Change all I.V. tubing at each infusion because lipids support bacterial growth.
● Avoid rapid infusion by using an infusion pump to regulate the rate.
● Check injection site daily for signs of inflammation or infection.
● Watch closely for adverse effects, especially during the first half hour of infusion.
● Monitor serum lipid levels closely when patient is receiving fat emulsion therapy. Lipemia must clear between dosing.
● Monitor hepatic function carefully in long-term use.
● Do not store contents of partly used containers for later use.
● Store Intralipid 10% and Liposyn 10% at room temperature (77° F [25° C]) or below. Do not freeze.

Pediatric use
● Premature and small-for-gestational-age infants have poor clearance of I.V. fat emulsions, so lower doses are necessary to decrease the likelihood of fat overload.
● Because free fatty acids displace bilirubin bound to albumin, caution must be observed when administering fat emulsions to jaundiced or premature infants. Deaths in preterm infants have been reported from intravascular fat accumulation in the lungs.
● Monitor the infant's ability to eliminate the infused fat (triglycerides or plasma free fatty acids) daily.
● Check platelet count frequently in neonates receiving fat emulsions I.V. because they tend to develop thrombocytopenia.

---

felodipine
Plendil

● Pharmacologic classification: calcium channel blocker
● Therapeutic classification: antihypertensive
● Pregnancy risk category C

How supplied
Tablets (extended-release): 5 mg, 10 mg

Indications, route, and dosage
Hypertension
Adults: 5 mg P.O. daily. Adjust dosage according to patient response, generally at intervals not less than 2 weeks. Usual dose is 5 to 10 mg daily; maximum recommended dose is 20 mg daily in most patients. Elderly patients or patients with impaired hepatic function should not receive more than 10 mg daily.

Pharmacodynamics
Antihypertensive action: A dihydropyridine-derivative calcium channel blocker, felodipine blocks the entry of calcium ions into vascular smooth muscle and cardiac cells. This type of calcium channel blocker shows some selectivity for smooth muscle as compared to cardiac muscle.

Pharmacokinetics
● *Absorption:* Felodipine is almost completely absorbed, but extensive first-pass metabolism reduces absolute bioavailability to about 20%. Plasma levels peak within 2.5 to 5 hours after a dose.
● *Distribution:* Felodipine is over 99% bound to plasma proteins.
● *Metabolism:* Metabolism of felodipine is probably hepatic; at least six inactive metabolites have been identified.
● *Excretion:* Over 70% of a dose appears in urine, and 10% appears in feces as metabolites.

Contraindications and precautions
Felodipine is contraindicated in patients with hypersensitivity to the drug. Use cautiously in patients with heart failure, particularly those receiving beta-adrenergic blockers. Also use cautiously in patients with impaired hepatic function because clearance of drug from the blood depends on the liver. Although felodipine metabolites accumulate in the plasma of patients with renal disease, these metabolites are inactive.

Also use cautiously in patients with angina. A reflex increase in heart rate is common during the first week of therapy and may precipitate chest pain in certain patients. The increased heart rate usually diminishes gradually over time, but increases of 5 to 10 beats/minute may persist with chronic dosing. Administration of beta-adrenergic blockers will attenuate this effect.

Interactions
Felodipine may alter the pharmacokinetics of metoprolol. No dosage adjustment appears necessary; however, monitor for adverse effects. Cimetidine decreases the clearance of felodipine. Lower doses of felodipine should be used. In clinical trials, felodipine decreased peak serum levels of digoxin, but total absorbed drug was unchanged. Clinical significance is unknown.

Effects on diagnostic tests
None reported.

Adverse reactions
● CNS: headache, dizziness, paresthesia.
● CV: peripheral edema, chest pain, palpitations, increased heart rate.
● DERM: rash.
● EENT: pharyngitis, rhinorrhea.
● GI: dyspepsia, abdominal pain, nausea, constipation, diarrhea.
● Respiratory: upper respiratory infection, cough.

• Other: flushing, asthenia, muscle cramps, back pain, gingival hyperplasia.

Overdose and treatment
Expected symptoms would be peripheral vasodilation, bradycardia, and hypotension. Provide supportive care. Intravenous fluids or sympathomimetics may be useful in treating hypotension, and atropine (0.5 to 1 mg I.V.) may treat bradycardia. It is not known if the drug may be removed by dialysis.

▶ **Special considerations**
Besides those relevant to all *calcium channel blockers,* consider the following recommendations.
• Peripheral edema appears to be both dose- and age-dependent. It's more common in patients taking higher doses, especially those who are age 60 or over.
• Felodipine may be administered without regard to meals. However, a small study reported a more than twofold increase of bioavailability when drug was taken with doubly concentrated grape juice as compared with water or orange juice.

Information for the patient
• Tell patient to observe good oral hygiene and to see a dentist regularly because drug has been associated with mild gingival hyperplasia.
• Remind patient to swallow tablet whole and not to crush or chew it.
• Be sure patient understands that he should continue taking drug, even when feeing better. He should watch his diet and check with the physician or pharmacist before taking any other medications, including OTC drugs.

Geriatric use
Higher blood levels of drug are seen in elderly patients. Mean clearance of drug from elderly hypertensive patients (average age 74) was less than half of that observed in young patients (average age 26). Check blood pressures closely during dosage adjustment. Maximum daily dose is 10 mg.

Pediatric use
Safety and efficacy in children have not been established.

Breast-feeding
It is unknown if drug is excreted in breast milk. Because of the risk of serious adverse effects to the infant, breast-feeding is not recommended.

---

fenfluramine hydrochloride
Pondimin

• Pharmacologic classification: amphet-amine congener
• Therapeutic classification: short-term adjunctive anorexigenic agent, indirect-acting sympathomimetic amine
• Controlled substance schedule IV
• Pregnancy risk category C

How supplied
Available by prescription only
Tablets: 20 mg

Indications, route, and dosage
Short-term adjunct in exogenous obesity
Adults: Initially, 20 mg P.O. t.i.d. before meals; maximum of 40 mg t.i.d. Adjust dosage according to patient's response.
†*Autism*
Children: 1.5 mg/kg/day P.O.

Pharmacodynamics
Anorexigenic action: The mechanism of fenfluramine's anorexigenic effects is incompletely understood; it appears to involve stimulation of the hypothalamus and may be related to brain serotonin levels or to increased glucose use.

Fenfluramine differs from other sympathomimetics in that it usually depresses the CNS. As an anorexigenic, it is considered a second-line drug. However, because of its depressant effects, it may be especially useful for tense, nervous patients and others who should avoid CNS stimulation; it can also be used to help prevent nighttime snacking if taken before the evening meal.

Fenfluramine may *improve* glucose tolerance and is considered the anorexigenic agent of choice in patients with type II (non-insulin-dependent) diabetes; it also has a slightly hypotensive effect.

Fenfluramine is used adjunctively with caloric restriction and behavior modification to control appetite in patients with exogenous obesity.

Fenfluramine is being investigated as a means to improve intellectual functioning in patients with autism. It reduces excessive serotoninergic activity in these patients, but has variable effects on social behavior and attention span.

Pharmacokinetics
• *Absorption:* Fenfluramine is well absorbed after oral administration; maximal anorexia occurs at 2 to 4 hours.
• *Distribution:* Fenfluramine is distributed widely throughout the body, including the CNS.
• *Metabolism:* Fenfluramine is metabolized in the liver.
• *Excretion:* Most drug and metabolites are excreted in urine; rate of elimination is pH-dependent.

Contraindications and precautions
Fenfluramine is contraindicated in patients with hypersensitivity or idiosyncratic reaction to sympathomimetic amines; in depressed or alcoholic patients; in patients with symptomatic cardiovascular disease; and in patients with a history of substance abuse. Fenfluramine also is contraindicated for use with monoamine oxidase (MAO) inhibitors or within 14 days of such use.

Fenfluramine should be used with caution in patients with hypertension, diabetes mellitus, or a history of depressive disorder. Habituation or psychological dependence may occur with prolonged use.

Fenfluramine should be used with caution in patients undergoing general anesthesia; fatal cardiac arrest has been reported. Therefore, when possible, fenfluramine should be discontinued for 1 week before surgery; if surgery cannot be postponed, full cardiac monitoring and resuscitative equipment must be available.

Fenfluramine is not recommended for intermittent courses of therapy in weight control.

Interactions
Concomitant use with MAO inhibitors (or drugs with MAO-inhibiting activity) and use within 14 days of such therapy may cause hypertensive crisis. Fenfluramine may increase hypotensive effects of other drugs, es-

---

pecially guanethidine, methyldopa, and reserpine; concomitant use with other CNS depressants will produce additive effects.

Effects on diagnostic tests
None reported.

Adverse reactions
● CNS: drowsiness, dizziness, incoordination, headache, euphoria or depression, anxiety, insomnia, weakness or fatigue, agitation, hallucinations.
● CV: palpitations, hypotension, hypertension, chest pain.
● DERM: rashes, urticaria, burning sensation.
● EENT: eye irritation, blurred vision.
● GI: diarrhea, dry mouth, nausea, vomiting, abdominal pain, constipation.
● GU: changes in libido, dysuria, increased urinary frequency, impotence.
● Other: sweating, chills, fever.
   Note: Drug should be discontinued if signs of hypersensitivity or idiosyncrasy occur or if pulmonary hypertension develops.

Overdose and treatment
Symptoms of acute overdose include nystagmus, jaw tremor, confusion, sweating, abdominal pain, hyperventilation, and dilated, nonreactive pupils. Higher doses may cause convulsions, coma, and arrhythmias leading to cardiac arrest.
   Treat overdose symptomatically and supportively. If ingestion is recent (within 4 hours), use gastric lavage or emesis; avoid drug-induced emesis, as subsequent development of coma may cause aspiration. Treatment may include use of I.V. beta blockers for tachycardia and other arrhythmias, and diazepam or phenobarbital for convulsions. Monitor vital signs and fluid and electrolyte balance.

▶ Special considerations
Besides those relevant to all *amphetamines,* consider the following recommendations.
● Because of possible hypoglycemia, patients with diabetes may have altered insulin or sulfonylurea requirements. Monitor glucose levels.
● Fenfluramine should not be discontinued abruptly; severe mental depression may result.
● If tolerance to drug effect occurs, do not increase the dose. Discontinue drug.

Information for the patient
● Tell patient to avoid use of alcohol, caffeine, or other stimulants.
● Warn patient not to discontinue drug abruptly.
● Encourage patient to report palpitations, nervousness, or dizziness.

Geriatric use
Lower doses are recommended for elderly patients.

Pediatric use
Fenfluramine is not recommended for weight reduction in children under age 12.

---

fenoprofen calcium
Nalfon

● Pharmacologic classification: nonsteroidal anti-inflammatory
● Therapeutic classification: nonnarcotic analgesic, antipyretic, anti-inflammatory
● Pregnancy risk category B (D in third trimester)

How supplied
Available by prescription only
Tablets: 600 mg
Capsules: 200 mg, 300 mg

Indications, route, and dosage
Rheumatoid arthritis and osteoarthritis
Adults: 300 to 600 mg P.O. t.i.d. to q.i.d. Maximum dosage is 3.2 g daily.
Mild to moderate pain
Adults: 200 mg P.O. q 4 to 6 hours, p.r.n.

Pharmacodynamics
Analgesic, anti-inflammatory, and antipyretic actions: Mechanisms of action unknown, but fenoprofen is thought to inhibit prostaglandin synthesis. Fenoprofen decreases platelet aggregation and may prolong bleeding time.

Pharmacokinetics
● *Absorption:* Fenoprofen is absorbed rapidly and completely from the GI tract. The onset of analgesic activity occurs within 15 to 30 minutes, with peak plasma levels achieved in 2 hours. The duration of action is approximately 4 to 6 hours.
● *Distribution:* The drug is 99% protein-bound.
● *Metabolism:* Fenoprofen is metabolized in the liver.
● *Excretion:* The drug is excreted chiefly in urine with a serum half-life of 2½ to 3 hours. A small amount is excreted in feces.

Contraindications and precautions
Fenoprofen is contraindicated in patients with known hypersensitivity to the drug; in patients in whom aspirin or other nonsteroidal anti-inflammatory drugs (NSAIDs) induce symptoms of asthma, urticaria, or rhinitis; and in patients with renal impairment, because it may induce renal failure.
   Serious GI toxicity, including ulceration or hemorrhage, can occur at any time in patients on chronic NSAID therapy. Fenoprofen should be administered cautiously to patients with a history of GI disease because it can irritate the GI tract, and to patients with impaired cardiac function and bleeding abnormalities.
   Patients with known "triad" symptoms (aspirin hypersensitivity, rhinitis/nasal polyps, and asthma) are at high risk of bronchospasm. NSAIDs may mask the signs and symptoms of acute infection (fever, myalgia, erythema); carefully evaluate patients with high risk (such as those with diabetes).

Interactions
Concomitant use of fenoprofen with anticoagulants and thrombolytic drugs (coumarin derivatives, heparin, streptokinase, and urokinase) may potentiate anticoagulant effects. Bleeding problems may occur if feno-

---

profen is used with other drugs that inhibit platelet aggregation, such as azlocillin, parenteral carbenicillin, dextran, dipyridamole, mezlocillin, piperacillin, sulfinpyrazone, ticarcillin, valproic acid, or with cefamandole, cefoperazone, moxalactam, plicamycin, aspirin, salicylates, or other anti-inflammatory agents. Concomitant use with salicylates, anti-inflammatory agents, alcohol, corticotropin, or steroids may cause increased GI adverse reactions, including ulceration and hemorrhage. Aspirin may decrease the bioavailability of fenoprofen.

Because of the influence of prostaglandins on glucose metabolism, concomitant use with insulin or oral hypoglycemic agents may potentiate hypoglycemic effects. Fenoprofen may displace highly protein-bound drugs from binding sites. Toxicity may occur with coumarin derivatives, phenytoin, verapamil, or nifedipine. Increased nephrotoxicity may occur with gold compounds, other anti-inflammatory agents, or acetaminophen. Fenoprofen may decrease the renal clearance of methotrexate and lithium.

Fenoprofen may decrease the effectiveness of antihypertensives or diuretics. Concomitant use with diuretics may increase nephrotoxic potential.

Effects on diagnostic tests
The physiologic effects of the drug may increase bleeding time, BUN, serum creatinine, potassium, alkaline phosphatase, lactic dehydrogenase, and transaminase concentrations. Drug may also cause false elevations in both free and total serum triiodothyronine, but thyroid-stimulating hormone and thyroxine are unaffected.

Adverse reactions
- CNS: headache, drowsiness, dizziness, somnolence.
- CV: peripheral edema, tachycardia, congestive heart failure (CHF), palpitations, fluid retention.
- DERM: pruritus, rash, urticaria.
- EENT: visual disturbances, tinnitus, hearing loss.
- GI: epigastric distress, nausea, vomiting, diarrhea, bleeding, constipation, anorexia, change in taste.
- GU: reversible renal failure, hematuria, nocturia, dysuria, urinary frequency, oliguria.
- Other: prolonged bleeding time, anemia, elevated liver enzymes, jaundice, cholestatic hepatitis, dyspnea, pyrexia.
   Note: Drug should be discontinued if hypersensitivity or renal or hepatic toxicity occurs.

Overdose and treatment
Little is known about the acute toxicity of fenoprofen. Nonoliguric renal failure, tachycardia, and hypotension have been observed. Other symptoms include drowsiness, dizziness, confusion and lethargy, nausea, vomiting, headache, tinnitus, and blurred vision. Elevations in serum creatinine and BUN levels have been reported. To treat an overdose of fenoprofen, empty stomach immediately by inducing emesis with ipecac syrup or by gastric lavage. Administer activated charcoal via nasogastric tube. Provide symptomatic and supportive measures (respiratory support and correction of fluid and electrolyte imbalances). Monitor laboratory parameters and vital signs closely. Dialysis is of little value.

▶ Special considerations
Besides those relevant to all *NSAIDs*, consider the following recommendations.
- Fenoprofen has been used to treat fever, acute gouty arthritis, and juvenile arthritis.

- Monitor for potential CNS effects. Institute safety measures to prevent injury.
- Monitor renal, hepatic, and auditory function in patients on long-term therapy. Stop drug if abnormalities occur.

Information for the patient
- Tell patient to avoid activities that require alertness or concentration until CNS effects of the drug are known.
- Instruct patient in safety measures to prevent injury.
- Advise patient to call for specific instruction before taking any nonprescription analgesic.

Geriatric use
- Patients over age 60 may be more susceptible to the toxic effects of fenoprofen, especially adverse GI reactions. Use with caution.
- The effects of this drug on renal prostaglandins may cause fluid retention and edema, a significant drawback for elderly patients and those with CHF.

Pediatric use
Safe use of fenoprofen in children has not been established.

Breast-feeding
Because fenoprofen is distributed into breast milk, avoid use in breast-feeding women.

---

fentanyl citrate
Sublimaze

- Pharmacologic classification: opioid agonist
- Therapeutic classification: analgesic, adjunct to anesthesia, anesthetic
- Controlled substance schedule II
- Pregnancy risk category C

How supplied
Available by prescription only
Injection: 50 mcg/ml

Indications, route, and dosage
Preoperatively
Adults: 0.05 to 0.1 mg I.M. 30 to 60 minutes before surgery.
Adjunct to general anesthetic
Adults: 0.005 to 0.1 mg I.V. q 2 to 3 minutes, p.r.n. Dose should be reduced in elderly and poor-risk patients.
Postoperative analgesic
Adults: 0.05 to 0.1 mg I.M. q 1 to 2 hours, p.r.n.
Children age 2 to 12: 1 to 2 mcg/kg I.M. q 1 to 2 hours p.r.n.

Pharmacodynamics
Analgesic action: Fentanyl binds to the opiate receptors as an agonist to alter the patient's perception of painful stimuli, thus providing analgesia for moderate to severe pain. Its CNS and respiratory depressant effects are similar to those of morphine. The drug has little hypnotic activity and rarely causes histamine release.

Pharmacokinetics
- *Absorption:* Onset of action after I.V. administration is rapid; peak levels occur within 5 to 15 minutes, with

---

*Canada only   †Unlabeled clinical use   Italicized adverse reactions are life-threatening.

peak analgesia within 30 minutes. Duration of action is 1 to 2 hours.
- *Distribution:* Redistribution has been suggested as the main cause of the brief analgesic effect of fentanyl.
- *Metabolism:* Fentanyl is metabolized in the liver.
- *Excretion:* Fentanyl is excreted in the urine as metabolites and unchanged drug.

Contraindications and precautions
Fentanyl is contraindicated in patients with known hypersensitivity to the drug.

Administer fentanyl with extreme caution to patients with supraventricular arrhythmias or bradycardia; avoid, or administer drug with extreme caution to patients with head injury or increased intracranial pressure, because drug obscures neurologic parameters; and during pregnancy and labor, because drug readily crosses placenta (premature infants are especially sensitive to respiratory and CNS depressant effects of fentanyl). Administer fentanyl cautiously to patients with renal or hepatic dysfunction, because drug accumulation or prolonged duration of action may occur; to patients with pulmonary disease (asthma, chronic obstructive pulmonary disease), because drug depresses respiration and suppresses cough reflex; to patients undergoing biliary tract surgery, because drug may cause biliary spasm; to patients with convulsive disorders, because drug may precipitate seizures; in elderly or debilitated patients, who are more sensitive to both therapeutic and adverse drug effects; and to patients prone to physical or psychic addiction, because of the high abuse potential for this drug.

Muscular rigidity that may be associated with reduced pulmonary compliance or apnea, laryngospasm, and bronchoconstriction may occur and may be treated by use of assisted ventilation or I.V. neuromuscular blocking drugs.

The manufacturer states that use of fentanyl is not recommended in patients who have received monoamine oxidase (MAO) inhibitors within the preceding 14 days.

Interactions
Concomitant use with other CNS depressants (narcotic analgesics, general anesthetics, antihistamines, phenothiazines, barbiturates, benzodiazepines, sedative-hypnotics, tricyclic antidepressants, alcohol, and muscle relaxants) potentiates drug's respiratory and CNS depression, sedation, and hypotensive effects. Concomitant use with cimetidine may also increase respiratory and CNS depression, causing confusion, disorientation, apnea, or seizures; such use requires that dosage of fentanyl be reduced by one quarter to one third.

Drug accumulation and enhanced effects may result from concomitant use with drugs that are extensively metabolized in the liver (rifampin, phenytoin, digitoxin); combined use with anticholinergics may cause paralytic ileus.

Patients who become physically dependent on this drug may experience acute withdrawal syndrome if given a narcotic antagonist.

Severe cardiovascular depression may result from concomitant use with general anesthetics; diazepam may produce cardiovascular depression when given with high doses of fentanyl.

When used to supplement conduction anesthesia, such as spinal anesthesia and some peridural anesthetics, fentanyl can alter respiration by blocking intercostal nerves.

When used with fentanyl, droperidol may cause hypotension and a decrease in pulmonary artery pressure. (*Note:* A droperidol-fentanyl combination, Innovar, is available.) The manufacturer warns that fentanyl should not be given to a patient who has received MAO inhibitors within the past 14 days.

Effects on diagnostic tests
Fentanyl increases plasma amylase and lipase levels.

Adverse reactions
- CNS: sedation, somnolence, clouded sensorium, euphoria, insomnia, agitation, confusion, headache, tremor, seizures, dysphoria, miosis, *seizures*, dizziness.
- CV: tachycardia, bradycardia, palpitations, chest wall rigidity, hypertension, hypotension, syncope, edema, *shock, cardiopulmonary arrest.*
- DERM: flushing, rash, pruritus, pain at injection site, diaphoresis.
- GI: dry mouth, anorexia, biliary spasms (colic), ileus, nausea, vomiting, constipation.
- GU: urine retention, urinary hesitancy, decreased libido.
- Other: *apnea, respiratory depression,* skeletal muscle (particularly chest wall) rigidity, blurred vision.

Note: Drug should be discontinued if hypersensitivity, seizures, or life-threatening cardiac arrhythmias occur.

Overdose and treatment
The most common signs and symptoms of fentanyl overdose are an extension of its actions. They include CNS depression, respiratory depression, and miosis (pinpoint pupils). Other acute toxic effects include hypotension, bradycardia, hypothermia, shock, apnea, cardiopulmonary arrest, circulatory collapse, pulmonary edema, and seizures.

To treat acute overdose, first establish adequate respiratory exchange via a patent airway and ventilation as needed; administer a narcotic antagonist (naloxone) to reverse respiratory depression. (Because the duration of action of fentanyl is longer than that of naloxone, repeated dosing is necessary.) Naloxone should not be given unless the patient has clinically significant respiratory or cardiovascular depression. Monitor vital signs closely.

Provide symptomatic and supportive treatment (continued respiratory support, correction of fluid or electrolyte imbalance). Monitor laboratory parameters, vital signs, and neurologic status closely.

▶ Special considerations
Besides those relevant to all *opioid agonists,* consider the following recommendations.
- Observe patient for delayed onset of respiratory depression. The high lipid solubility of fentanyl may contribute to this potential adverse effect.
- Monitor patient's heart rate. Fentanyl may cause bradycardia. Pretreatment with an anticholinergic (such as atropine or glycopyrrolate) may minimize this effect.
- High doses can produce muscle rigidity. This effect can be reversed by naloxone.
- Many anesthesiologists employ epidural and intrathecal fentanyl as a potent adjunct to epidural anesthesia.

---

*Canada only   †Unlabeled clinical use   Italicized adverse reactions are life-threatening.

Geriatric use
Lower doses are usually indicated for elderly patients, because they may be more sensitive to the therapeutic and adverse effects of the drug.

Pediatric use
Safe use in children under age 2 has not been established.

Breast-feeding
Fentanyl is excreted into breast milk. Administer cautiously to breast-feeding women.

---

ferrous fumarate
Femiron, Feostat, Fumasorb, Fumerin, Hemocyte, Ircon-FA, Neo-Fer★, Novofumar★, Palafer★, Palmiron, Span-FF

- Pharmacologic classification: oral iron supplement
- Therapeutic classification: hematinic
- Pregnancy risk category A

How supplied
Ferrous fumarate is 33% elemental iron. All products are available without prescription.
Tablets: 63 mg, 195 mg, 200 mg, 325 mg
Tablets (chewable): 100 mg
Tablets (extended-release): 325 mg
Suspension: 100 mg/5 ml, 45 mg/0.6 ml

Indications, route, and dosage
Iron-deficiency states
Adults: 200 mg P.O. t.i.d. or q.i.d. Dosage is adjusted gradually, as needed and as tolerated. For extended-release tablet, 300 mg P.O. b.i.d.

Pharmacodynamics
Hematinic action: Ferrous fumarate replaces iron, an essential component in the formation of hemoglobin.

Pharmacokinetics
- *Absorption:* Iron is absorbed from the entire length of the GI tract, but primary absorption sites are the duodenum and proximal jejunum. Up to 10% of iron is absorbed by healthy individuals; patients with iron-deficiency anemia may absorb up to 60%. Enteric coating and some extended-release formulas have decreased absorption, because they are designed to release iron past the points of highest absorption; food may decrease absorption by 33% to 50%.
- *Distribution:* Iron is transported through GI mucosal cells directly into the blood, where it is immediately bound to a carrier protein, transferrin, and transported to the bone marrow for incorporation into hemoglobin. Iron is highly protein-bound.
- *Metabolism:* Iron is liberated by the destruction of hemoglobin, but is conserved and reused by the body.
- *Excretion:* Healthy individuals lose only small amounts of iron each day. Men and postmenopausal women lose about 1 mg/day, and premenopausal women about 1.5 mg/day. The loss usually occurs in nails, hair, feces, and urine; trace amounts are lost in bile and sweat.

Contraindications and precautions
Ferrous fumarate is contraindicated in patients with hemochromatosis, hemosiderosis, hemolytic anemia, or known hypersensitivity to any components of the product.

Ferrous fumarate should be administered with extreme caution to patients with peptic ulcer, regional enteritis, ulcerative colitis, or hepatitis, because iron has irritant effects on the GI mucosa; and with reasonable caution to patients requiring prolonged therapy.

Interactions
Ascorbic acid (vitamin C) increases ferrous fumarate absorption.

Antacids, cholestyramine, pancreatic extracts, and vitamin E decrease ferrous fumarate absorption (separate doses by 1- to 2-hour intervals); doxycycline may interfere with ferrous fumarate absorption even when doses are separated; chloramphenicol delays response to iron therapy. Concomitant use of ferrous fumarate and tetracycline inhibits absorption of both drugs; give tetracycline 3 hours after or 2 hours before iron supplement.

Ferrous fumarate decreases penicillamine absorption; separate doses by at least 2 hours.

Effects on diagnostic tests
Ferrous fumarate blackens feces and may interfere with tests for occult blood in the stool; the guaiac test and orthotoluidine test may yield false-positive results, but benzidine test is usually not affected.

Iron overload may decrease uptake of technetium 99m and thus interfere with skeletal imaging.

Adverse reactions
- GI: nausea, vomiting, anorexia, constipation, dark stools.
- HEMA: hemosiderosis (long-term use).
- Other: liquid preparations may stain teeth.
  Note: GI symptoms are exacerbated with long-term use.

Overdose and treatment
The lethal dose of iron is between 200 to 250 mg/kg; fatalities have occurred with lower doses. Symptoms may follow ingestion of 20 to 60 mg/kg. Clinical signs of acute overdose may occur as follows.

Between ½ hour and 8 hours after ingestion, patient may experience lethargy, nausea and vomiting, green then tarry stools, weak and rapid pulse, hypotension, dehydration, acidosis, and coma. If death does not immediately ensue, symptoms may clear for about 24 hours.

At 12 to 48 hours, symptoms may return, accompanied by diffuse vascular congestion, pulmonary edema, shock, convulsions, anuria, and hyperthermia. Death may follow.

Treatment requires immediate support of airway, respiration, and circulation. In conscious patient with intact gag reflex, induce emesis with ipecac; if not, empty stomach by gastric lavage. Follow emesis with lavage, using a 1% sodium bicarbonate solution, to convert iron to less irritating, poorly absorbed form. (Phosphate solutions have been used, but carry hazard of other adverse effects.) X-ray abdomen to determine continued presence of excess iron; if serum iron levels exceed 350 mg/dl, deferoxamine may be used for systemic chelation.

Survivors are likely to sustain organ damage, in-

---

cluding pyloric or antral stenosis, hepatic cirrhosis, CNS damage, and intestinal obstruction.

▶ **Special considerations**
Besides those relevant to all *oral iron supplements*, consider the following recommendations.

Geriatric use
Iron-induced constipation is common in elderly patients; stress proper diet to minimize this adverse effect. Elderly patients may need higher doses, because reduced gastric secretions and achlorhydria may lower capacity for iron absorption.

Pediatric use
Overdose of iron may be fatal; treat *immediately*.

Breast-feeding
Iron supplements are often recommended for breast-feeding women; no adverse effects of such use have been documented.

---

ferrous gluconate
Apo-Ferrous Gluconate*, Fergon, Ferralet, Fertinic*, Novoferrogluc*, Simron

- Pharmacologic classification: oral iron supplement
- Therapeutic classification: hematinic
- Pregnancy risk category A

How supplied
Ferrous gluconate is 11.6% elemental iron. All products are available without prescription.
Tablets: 300 mg, 320 mg, 325 mg (320-mg tablet contains 37 mg Fe$^+$)
Capsules: 86 mg, 325 mg, 435 mg
Elixir: 300 mg/5 ml (contains 35 mg Fe$^+$)

Indications, route, and dosage
Iron deficiency
Adults: 325 mg P.O. q.i.d., dosage increased as needed and tolerated, up to 650 mg q.i.d.
Children age 2 and older: 16 mg/kg P.O. t.i.d.
Children under age 2: Dosage must be individualized; 5 ml of elixir contains 300 mg ferrous gluconate (35 mg elemental iron).

Pharmacodynamics
Hematinic action: Ferrous gluconate replaces iron, an essential component in the formation of hemoglobin.

Pharmacokinetics
- *Absorption:* Iron is absorbed from the entire length of the GI tract, but primary absorption sites are the duodenum and proximal jejunum. Up to 10% of iron is absorbed by healthy individuals; patients with iron-deficiency anemia may absorb up to 60%. Food may decrease absorption by 33% to 50%.
- *Distribution:* Iron is transported through GI mucosal cells directly into the blood, where it is immediately bound to a carrier protein, transferrin, and transported to the bone marrow for incorporation into hemoglobin. Iron is highly protein-bound.

- *Metabolism:* Iron is liberated by the destruction of hemoglobin, but is conserved and reused by the body.
- *Excretion:* Healthy individuals lose only small amounts of iron each day. Men and postmenopausal women lose about 1 mg/day, premenopausal women about 1.5 mg/day. Loss usually occurs in nails, hair, feces, and urine; trace amounts are lost in bile and sweat.

Contraindications and precautions
Ferrous gluconate is contraindicated in patients with hemochromatosis, hemosiderosis, hemolytic anemia, or known hypersensitivity to any components of the product.

Ferrous gluconate should be administered with extreme caution to patients with peptic ulcer, regional enteritis, ulcerative colitis, or hepatitis because of iron's irritant effects on the GI mucosa; it should be administered with reasonable caution to patients on long-term therapy.

Interactions
Ascorbic acid (vitamin C) increases ferrous gluconate absorption.

Antacids, cholestyramine, pancreatic extracts, and vitamin E decrease ferrous gluconate absorption (separate doses by 1- to 2-hour intervals); doxycycline may interfere with ferrous gluconate absorption even when doses are separated; chloramphenicol delays response to iron therapy. Concomitant use of ferrous gluconate and tetracycline inhibits absorption of both drugs; give tetracycline 3 hours after or 2 hours before iron supplement.

Ferrous gluconate decreases penicillamine absorption; separate doses by at least 2 hours.

Effects on diagnostic tests
Ferrous gluconate blackens feces and may interfere with test for occult blood in the stools; the guaiac test and orthotoluidine test may yield false-positive results, but benzidine test is usually not affected.

Iron overload may decrease uptake of technetium 99m and thus interfere with skeletal imaging.

Adverse reactions
- GI: nausea, vomiting, anorexia, constipation, dark stools.
- HEMA: hemosiderosis (long-term use).
- Other: liquid preparations may stain teeth.
Note: GI symptoms are exacerbated with long-term use.

Overdose and treatment
The lethal dose of iron is between 200 to 250 mg/kg; fatalities have occurred with lower doses. Symptoms may follow ingestion of 20 to 60 mg/kg. Clinical signs of acute overdose may occur as follows.

Between ½ hour and 8 hours after ingestion, patient may experience lethargy, nausea and vomiting, green then tarry stools, weak and rapid pulse, hypotension, dehydration, acidosis, and coma. If death does not immediately ensue, symptoms may clear for about 24 hours.

At 12 to 48 hours, symptoms may return, accompanied by diffuse vascular congestion, pulmonary edema, shock, convulsions, anuria, and hyperthermia. Death may follow.

Treatment requires immediate support of airway, respiration, and circulation. In conscious patient with intact gag reflex, induce emesis with ipecac; if not, empty

---

*Canada only   †Unlabeled clinical use   Italicized adverse reactions are life-threatening.

stomach by gastric lavage. Follow emesis with lavage, using a 1% sodium bicarbonate solution, to convert iron to less irritating, poorly absorbed form. (Phosphate solutions have been used, but carry hazard of other adverse effects.) Take abdominal X-ray to determine continued presence of excess iron; if serum iron levels exceed 350 mg/dl, deferoxamine may be used for systemic chelation.

Survivors are likely to sustain organ damage, including pyloric or antral stenosis, hepatic cirrhosis, CNS damage, and intestinal obstruction.

▶ **Special considerations**
Besides those relevant to all *iron supplements*, consider the following recommendations.

Geriatric use
Iron-induced constipation is common in elderly patients; stress proper diet to minimize this adverse effect. Elderly patients may need higher doses, because of reduced gastric secretions and achlorhydria may lower capacity for iron absorption.

Pediatric use
Overdose may be fatal; treat *immediately.*

Breast-feeding
Iron supplements are often recommended for breast-feeding women; no adverse effects of such use have been documented.

---

ferrous sulfate
Apo-Ferrous Sulfate*, Feosol, Fer-In-Sol, Fer-Iron, Fero-Grad*, Fero-Gradumet, Ferospace, Ferralyn, Ferra-TD, Fesofor*, Mol-Iron, Novoferrosulfa*, PMS Ferrous Sulfate*, Slow Fe

- Pharmacologic classification: oral iron supplement
- Therapeutic classification: hematinic
- Pregnancy risk category A

How supplied
Ferrous sulfate is 20% elemental iron; dried and powdered (exsiccated), it is about 32% elemental iron. All products are available without a prescription.
Tablets: 195 mg, 300 mg, 325 mg; 200 mg (exsiccated); 160 mg (exsiccated, extended-release)
Capsules: 150 mg, 225 mg, 250 mg, 390 mg, 525 mg (extended-release); 190 mg (exsiccated); 150 mg, 167 mg (exsiccated, extended-release)
Syrup: 90 mg/5 ml
Elixir: 220 mg/5 ml
Liquid: 75 mg/0.6 ml, 125 mg/ml

Indications, route, and dosage
Iron deficiency
Adults: 300 mg P.O. b.i.d.; dosage gradually increased to 300 mg q.i.d. as needed and tolerated. For extended-release capsule, 150 to 250 mg P.O. one or two times daily; for extended-release tablets, 160 to 525 mg one or two times daily.
Children: 10 mg/kg P.O. t.i.d.

Prophylaxis for iron-deficiency anemia
Adults: 300 mg P.O. daily.
Children: 5 mg/kg P.O. daily in divided doses.

Pharmacodynamics
Hematinic action: Ferrous sulfate replaces iron, an essential component in the formation of hemoglobin.

Pharmacokinetics
- *Absorption:* Iron is absorbed from the entire length of the GI tract, but primary absorption sites are the duodenum and proximal jejunum. Up to 10% of iron is absorbed by healthy individuals; patients with iron-deficiency anemia may absorb up to 60%. Enteric coating and some extended-release formulas have decreased absorption, because they are designed to release iron past the points of highest absorption; food may decrease absorption by 33% to 50%.
- *Distribution:* Iron is transported through GI mucosal cells directly into the blood, where it is immediately bound to a carrier protein, transferrin, and transported to the bone marrow for incorporation into hemoglobin. Iron is highly protein-bound.
- *Metabolism:* Iron is liberated by the destruction of hemoglobin, but is conserved and reused by the body.
- *Excretion:* Healthy individuals lose very little iron each day. Men and postmenopausal women lose about 1 mg/day, and premenopausal women about 1.5 mg/day. The loss usually occurs in nails, hair, feces, and urine; trace amounts are lost in bile and sweat.

Contraindications and precautions
Ferrous sulfate is contraindicated in patients with hemochromatosis, hemosiderosis, hemolytic anemia, or known hypersensitivity to components of the product.

Ferrous sulfate should be administered with extreme caution to patients with peptic ulcer, regional enteritis, ulcerative colitis, or hepatitis because of iron's irritant effects on the GI mucosa; it should be administered with caution to patients on long-term therapy.

Interactions
Ascorbic acid (vitamin C) increases ferrous sulfate absorption.

Antacids, cholestyramine, pancreatic extracts, and vitamin E decrease ferrous sulfate absorption (separate doses by 1- to 2-hour intervals); doxycycline may interfere with ferrous sulfate absorption even when doses are separated; chloramphenicol delays response to iron therapy. Concomitant use of ferrous sulfate and tetracycline inhibits absorption of both drugs; give tetracycline 3 hours after or 2 hours before iron supplement.

Ferrous sulfate decreases penicillamine absorption; separate doses by at least 2 hours.

Effects on diagnostic tests
Ferrous sulfate blackens feces and may interfere with tests for occult blood in the stool; the guaiac test and orthotoluidine test may yield false-positive results, but benzidine test is usually not affected.

Iron overload may decrease uptake of technetium 99m and thus interfere with skeletal imaging.

Adverse reactions
- GI: nausea, vomiting, anorexia, constipation, dark stools.
- HEMA: hemosiderosis (with long-term use).
- Other: liquid preparations may stain teeth.

Note: GI symptoms are exacerbated with long-term use.

Overdose and treatment

The lethal dose of iron is between 200 to 250 mg/kg; fatalities have occurred with lower doses. Symptoms may follow ingestion of 20 to 60 mg/kg. Clinical signs of acute overdose may occur as follows.

Between ½ hours to 8 hours after ingestion, patient may experience lethargy, nausea and vomiting, green then tarry stools, weak and rapid pulse, hypotension, dehydration, acidosis, and coma. If death does not immediately ensue, symptoms may clear for about 24 hours.

At 12 to 48 hours, symptoms may return, accompanied by diffuse vascular congestion, pulmonary edema, shock, convulsions, anuria, and hyperthermia. Death may follow.

Treatment requires immediate support of airway, respiration, and circulation. In conscious patient with intact gag reflex, induce emesis with ipecac; if not, empty stomach by gastric lavage. Follow emesis with lavage, using a 1% sodium bicarbonate solution, to convert iron to less irritating, poorly absorbed form. (Phosphate solutions have been used, but carry hazard of other adverse effects.) Take abdominal X-ray to determine continued presence of excess iron; if serum iron levels exceed 350 mg/dl, deferoxamine may be used for systemic chelation.

Survivors are likely to sustain organ damage, including pyloric or antral stenosis, hepatic cirrhosis, CNS damage, and intestinal obstruction.

▶ **Special considerations**

Besides those relevant to all *iron supplements,* consider the following recommendations.

Geriatric use

Iron-induced constipation is common in elderly patients; stress proper diet to minimize this adverse effect. Elderly patients may need higher doses, because reduced gastric secretions and achlorhydria may lower capacity for iron absorption.

Pediatric use

Iron extended-release capsules or tablets are usually not recommended for children. Overdose may be fatal; treat immediately.

Breast-feeding

Iron supplements often are recommended for breast-feeding women; no adverse effects have been documented.

fibrinolysin and deoxyribonuclease, combined (bovine)
Elase

- Pharmacologic classification: proteolytic enzyme
- Therapeutic classification: topical debriding agent
- Pregnancy risk category C

How supplied

Available by prescription only

Dry powder: 25 units fibrinolysin and 15,000 units deoxyribonuclease in a 30-ml vial

Ointment: 30 units fibrinolysin and 20,000 units deoxyribonuclease in 30-g tube

Indications, route, and dosage
Topical debridement of inflamed and infected skin lesions and wounds

Adults and children: Apply ointment or solution as a spray at intervals for as long as enzyme action is desired, usually at least once daily, but 2 or 3 times daily may be preferred; apply solution as a wet dressing 3 or 4 times daily.

Intravaginal treatment of cervicitis and vaginitis

Adults: Using applicator, insert 5 ml of ointment (or 10 ml in severe cases) high into the vagina once daily at bedtime for 5 days, or as prescribed. After 1 or 2 minutes, insert tampon. Remove tampon before next treatment.

Irrigating agent for the treatment of abscesses, empyema cavities, fistulae, sinus tracts, or subcutaneous hematomas

Irrigate and replace solution every 6 to 10 hours.

Pharmacodynamics

Debriding action: Digests necrotic tissues by proteolytic action; fibrinolysis is directed toward denatured proteins in devitalized tissues. Produces clear surfaces and facilitates wound healing.

Pharmacokinetics

- *Absorption:* Limited with topical use.
- *Distribution:* None.
- *Metabolism:* None.
- *Excretion:* None.

Contraindications and precautions

Fibrinolysin is contraindicated in patients with hypersensitivity to bovine products or mercury compounds.

Interactions

None reported.

Effects on diagnostic tests

None reported.

Adverse reactions

- Local: hyperemia, irritation, itching, burning.
  Note: Drug should be discontinued if hypersensitivity reaction occurs.

Overdose and treatment

No specific recommendations available.

▶ **Special considerations**

● Use solution promptly after preparation; do not use after 24 hours.

● Enzyme must be in constant contact with substrate surface for optimal activity. Therefore, remove dense, dry skin before applying drug.

● To apply ointment, clean wound and skin area carefully with normal saline solution, hydrogen peroxide, or water; moisten thoroughly, then gently dry area. Apply a thin layer of ointment to the affected area, and cover with loose-fitting, nonadhering or pertrolatum gauze dressing.

● Change dressing at least once daily; flush away enzyme and debris before reapplication.

● Solution may be applied topically as a spray or as a wet dressing. As a spray, apply using an atomizer; as a wet dressing, saturate gauze dressing with solution and pack affected area.

● Avoid using spray near eyes or mucous membranes.

Information for the patient

Be sure patient understands how to use product; teach correct application.

Breast-feeding

Cleanse breast area thoroughly before breast-feeding.

---

filgrastim (granulocyte colony stimulating factor, G-CSF)
Neupogen

● Pharmacologic classification: biologic response modifier
● Therapeutic classification: colony stimulating factor
● Pregnancy risk category C

How supplied

Available by prescription only
Injection: 300 mcg/ml in 1-ml and 1.6-ml single-dose vials

Indications, route, and dosage
To decrease incidence of infection after cancer chemotherapy for nonmyeloid malignancies

Adults: Initially, 5 mcg/kg S.C. or I.V. as a single daily dose; may increase dose incrementally by 5 mcg/kg for each course of chemotherapy according to duration and severity of absolute neutrophil count (ANC) nadir.

Do not administer earlier than 24 hours after or within 24 hours before chemotherapy.

Filgrastim should be given daily for up to 2 weeks until ANC nadir reaches 10,000/mm³ after the anticipated chemoinduced ANC nadir. Duration of treatment depends on the myelosuppressive potential of the chemotherapy used. Discontinue if ANC nadir surpasses 10,000/mm³.

Pharmacodynamics

Immunostimulant action: Filgrastim is a naturally occurring cytokine glycoprotein that stimulates proliferation, differentiation, and functional activity of neutro-phils, causing a rapid rise in WBC counts within 2 to 3 days in patients with normal bone marrow function or 7 to 14 days in patients with bone marrow suppression. Blood counts return to pretreatment levels, usually within 1 week after therapy ends.

Pharmacokinetics

● *Absorption:* After S.C. bolus dose, blood levels suggest rapid absorption with peak levels in 4 to 5 hours.
● *Distribution:* Unknown.
● *Metabolism:* Unknown.
● *Excretion:* Unknown.

Contraindications and precautions

Filgrastim is contraindicated in patients with hypersensitivity to products derived from *Escherichia coli.* Avoid use in patients with malignancies with myeloid characteristics because filgrastim may act as a growth factor for any tumor.

Interactions

No evidence of drug interactions exists.

Effects on diagnostic tests

WBC counts may be increased to 100,000/mm³ or more. Transient increases in neutrophils, as well as reversible elevations in uric acid, lactate dehydrogenase, and alkaline phosphatase levels, have been reported. Transient decreases in blood pressure and increases in serum creatinine and aminotransferase levels were also reported.

Adverse reactions

● CNS: skeletal pain, fatigue, headache, generalized weakness.
● CV: chest pain, *arrhythmia,* MI.
● DERM: alopecia, skin rash.
● GI: nausea, vomiting, diarrhea, anorexia, constipation.
● Respiratory: dyspnea, cough.
● Other: stomatitis, neutropenic fever, mucositis, fever, sore throat, unspecified pain, splenomegaly.

Overdose and treatment

Maximum tolerated dose has not been determined. There have been no reports of overdose.

▶ **Special considerations**

● Store in refrigerator; do not freeze. Avoid shaking. Before injection, allow to reach room temperature for a maximum of 6 hours. Discard after 6 hours. Use only one dose per vial; do not reenter vial.

● Obtain CBC and platelet counts before and twice weekly during therapy.

● Filgrastim is not compatible with 0.9% sodium chloride.

● Regular monitoring of hematocrit and platelet counts is recommended.

● Adult respiratory distress syndrome may occur in septic patients because of the influx of neutrophils at the site of inflammation.

● MI and arrhythmias have occurred; closely monitor patients with preexisting cardiac conditions.

● Bone pain is the most frequent adverse reaction and may be controlled with nonnarcotic analgesics if mild to moderate or may require narcotic analgesics if severe.

Information for the patient
● Review "Information for Patients" section of package insert with patient. Thorough instruction is essential if home use is prescribed.
● When drug can be safely and effectively self-administered, instruct patient in proper dosage and administration techniques.
● Manufacturer has reimbursement hotline to answer questions about insurance reimbursement procedures. Hotline operates from Monday through Friday 9 a.m. to 5 p.m. Eastern Standard Time: 1-800-272-9376; in Washington, D.C., 1-202-637-6698.

Geriatric use
No age-related problems have been reported.

Pediatric use
Efficacy is not established but there is no evidence of greater toxicity in children than in adults.

Breast-feeding
It is unknown if filgrastim is distributed into breast milk. Risk-to-benefit ratio must be assessed.

---

finasteride
Proscar

● Pharmacologic classification: steroid (synthetic 4-azasteroid) derivative
● Therapeutic classification: androgen synthesis inhibitor
● Pregnancy risk category X

How supplied
Available by prescription only
Tablets: 5 mg

Indications, route and dosage
Symptomatic benign prostatic hyperplasia (BPH)
Men: 5 mg P.O. daily.

Pharmacodynamics
Androgen synthesis inhibition: Finasteride competitively inhibits steroid 5α-reductase, an enzyme responsible for formation of the potent androgen 5α-dihydrotestosterone (DHT) from testosterone. Because DHT influences development of the prostate gland, decreasing levels of this hormone in adult males should relieve the symptoms associated with BPH.

Pharmacokinetics
● *Absorption:* Average bioavailability was 63% in one study. Maximum plasma concentrations are reached within 2 hours of a dose.
● *Distribution:* Finasteride is about 90% bound to plasma proteins. Drug crosses the blood-brain barrier.
● *Metabolism:* Finasteride is extensively metabolized by the liver; at least 2 metabolites have been identified. Metabolites are responsible for less than 20% of the drug's total activity.
● *Excretion:* 39% of an oral dose is excreted in urine as metabolites; 57%, in feces. No unchanged drug is found in urine.

Contraindications and precautions
Finasteride is contraindicated in patients with hypersensitivity to the drug; in pregnant and breast-feeding women; and in children. Because drug is metabolized extensively in the liver, use cautiously in patients with hepatic dysfunction.
  Baseline and periodic digital rectal examinations are recommended. Remember that this drug will decrease serum prostate specific antigen (PSA) levels even in prostate cancer. However, in clinical trials, drug did not appear to decrease the rate of prostate cancer detection.

Interactions
Small, clinically insignificant increases in theophylline clearance and decreased half-life (10%) have been observed.

Effects on diagnostic tests
Finasteride will decrease levels of PSA even in prostate cancer. This does not indicate a beneficial effect.

Adverse reactions
● GU: impotence, decreased volume of ejaculate.
● Other: decreased libido.

Overdose and treatment
Experience with overdose is limited. Patients have received single doses of 400 mg and multiple doses of up to 80 mg daily for 3 months without adverse effects.

▶ Special considerations
● Closely evaluate patient for conditions that might mimic BPH before therapy, including hypotonic bladder, prostate cancer, infection, stricture, or other neurologic conditions.
● Because it is not possible to identify prospectively which patients will respond to finasteride, a minimum of 6 months of therapy may be necessary.
● Patients who have large residual urine volumes or severely diminished urine flows should be monitored carefully. Not all patients respond to this drug, and these patients may not be candidates for finasteride therapy.
● Long-term effects of this drug on the complications of BPH, including acute urinary obstruction, or the incidence of surgery are not known.
● No dosage adjustments are necessary in patients with renal impairment. Decreased urinary excretion of metabolites is associated with an increased excretion of metabolites in the feces.
● Sustained increases in serum PSA should be carefully evaluated. In patients receiving finasteride therapy, this could indicate noncompliance to therapy.
● Current investigations aim to determine drug's effectiveness as adjuvant therapy after radical prostatectomy; as adjunctive treatment of prostate cancer; and as treatment of male pattern baldness, acne, and hirsutism.

Information for the patient
● Crushed tablets should not be handled by women who are or may become pregnant because of the risk of adverse effects on a male fetus.
● A patient whose sexual partner is or may become pregnant should avoid exposing her to his semen or should discontinue the drug.
● Patients should understand that finasteride may decrease the volume of ejaculate but does not appear to impair normal sexual function. However, impotence and

---

*Canada only   †Unlabeled clinical use   Italicized adverse reactions are life-threatening.

decreased libido have occurred in less than 4% of the patients treated with this drug.

Geriatric use
Although drug's elimination rate is decreased in elderly patients, dosage adjustments are not necessary.

Pediatric use
This drug is not indicated for use in children.

Breast-feeding
It is unknown if drug is excreted in breast milk; however, this drug is not indicated for use in women.

flavoxate hydrochloride
Urispas

- Pharmacologic classification: flavone derivative
- Therapeutic classification: urinary tract spasmolytic
- Pregnancy risk category B

How supplied
Available by prescription only
Tablets: 100 mg

Indications, route, and dosage
Symptomatic relief of dysuria, frequency, urgency, nocturia, incontinence, and suprapubic pain associated with urologic disorders
Adults and children over age 12: 100 to 200 mg P.O. t.i.d. or q.i.d.

Pharmacodynamics
Spasmolytic action: Flavoxate exerts a direct spasmolytic effect on smooth muscle, primarily in the urinary tract. Acting on the detrusor muscle, this agent increases bladder capacity in patients with bladder spasticity; drug also has antihistaminic, antimuscarinic, local anesthetic, and analgesic effects.

Pharmacokinetics
- *Absorption:* Flavoxate is absorbed well from the GI tract; peak levels occur in approximately 2 hours.
- *Distribution:* Unknown.
- *Metabolism:* Unknown.
- *Excretion:* Flavoxate is excreted in the urine; 10% to 30% appears in the urine within 6 hours.

Contraindications and precautions
Flavoxate is contraindicated in patients with pyloric or duodenal obstruction, GI hemorrhage, obstructive uropathies of the lower urinary tract, and obstructive lesions of the intestine or ileus, because it may exacerbate of these symptoms of illnesses. Exercise caution when using drug in patients with glaucoma and in those performing hazardous tasks because drug causes drowsiness, vertigo, and ocular disturbances.

Interactions
Flavoxate enhances the antimuscarinic effects of atropine and related compounds. It may also potentiate the effects of CNS depressants.

Effects on diagnostic tests
None reported.

Adverse reactions
- CNS: nervousness, vertigo, confusion, headache, dizziness, drowsiness, mental confusion (especially in elderly patients).
- CV: tachycardia, palpitations.
- DERM: urticaria, dermatoses.
- GI: nausea, vomiting, abdominal pain, constipation (at high doses).
- Ocular: blurred vision, increased intraocular tension, disturbed accommodation.
- Other: dysuria, hyperpyrexia, eosinophilia, dry mouth and throat.

Overdose and treatment
Clinical manifestations of overdose include clumsiness, dizziness, drowsiness, fever, flushing, hallucinations, shortness of breath, nervousness, restlessness, or irritability. Treatment begins with gastric lavage or emesis and may include slow I.V. physostigmine 0.4 to 2 mg up to 5 mg total dose. As appropriate, excitement may be controlled with 2% thiopental I.V. drip or a rectal infusion of 2% chloral hydrate 100 to 200 ml. Treat fever symptomatically. Respiratory depression may require artificial respiration.

▶ Special considerations
Dosage may be reduced with improvement of symptoms.

Information for the patient
- Tell patient that flavoxate may be taken on an empty stomach or with food or milk if gastric irritation occurs.
- Because of potential for drowsiness, blurred vision, and confusion, warn patient to avoid driving or other hazardous activities that require alertness.

Geriatric use
Warn family members that elderly patients are more likely to become confused.

Pediatric use
Safety has not been established in children under age 12.

Breast-feeding
It is unknown if drug is distributed into breast milk. Use cautiously in breast-feeding women.

flecainide acetate
Tambocor

- Pharmacologic classification: benza-mide derivative local anesthetic (amide)
- Therapeutic classification: ventricular antiarrhythmic
- Pregnancy risk category C

How supplied
Available by prescription only
Tablets: 50 mg, 100 mg, 150 mg

Indications, route, and dosage
Life-threatening ventricular tachycardia and premature ventricular contractions
Adults: 100 mg P.O. q 12 hours; may be increased in increments of 50 mg b.i.d. every 4 days until efficacy is achieved. Maximum dosage is 400 mg daily for most patients.
Dosage in renal failure
Dosage should be reduced in renal impairment (creatinine clearance < 35 ml/min) beginning at 100 mg/day (50 mg b.i.d.); increase dosage cautiously at intervals longer than 4 days.

Pharmacodynamics
Antiarrhythmic action: A Class IC antiarrhythmic agent, flecainide suppresses SA node automaticity and prolongs conduction in the atria, AV node, ventricles, accessory pathways, and His-Purkinje system. It has the most pronounced effect on the His-Purkinje system, as shown by QRS complex widening; this leads to a prolonged QT interval. The drug has relatively little effect on action potential duration except in Purkinje's fibers, where it shortens it. A proarrhythmic (arrhythmogenic) effect may result from the drug's potent effects on the conduction system. Effects on the sinus node are strongest in patients with sinus node disease (sick sinus syndrome). Flecainide also exerts a moderate negative inotropic effect.

Pharmacokinetics
● *Absorption:* Flecainide is rapidly and almost completely absorbed from the GI tract; bioavailability of commercially available tablets is 85% to 90%. Peak plasma levels usually occur within 2 to 3 hours.
● *Distribution:* Flecainide is apparently well distributed throughout the body. Only about 40% binds to plasma proteins. Trough serum levels ranging from 0.2 to 1 mcg/ml provide the greatest therapeutic benefit. Trough serum levels higher than 0.7 mcg/ml have been associated with increased adverse effects.
● *Metabolism:* Flecainide is metabolized in the liver to inactive metabolites. About 30% of an orally administered dose escapes metabolism and is excreted in the urine unchanged.
● *Excretion:* Elimination half-life averages about 20 hours. Plasma half-life may be prolonged in patients with congestive heart failure and renal disease.

Contraindications and precautions
Flecainide is contraindicated in patients with a history of hypersensitivity to this drug; and in patients with significant conduction delay, including second- or third-degree heart block, sick sinus syndrome, and right bundle branch block with bifascicular block (unless an artificial pacemaker is in place), because it may further depress cardiac conduction. Because of its mild negative inotropic and arrhythmogenic effects, flecainide also is contraindicated in patients with cardiogenic shock.

Use flecainide only in patients with life-threatening arrhythmias. Data from the Cardiac Arrhythmia Suppression Trial (CAST) showed that the drug may increase the risk of sudden death in patients who have had a myocardial infarction and who have asymptomatic nonsustained ventricular tachycardia. Use flecainide with caution in patients with preexisting left ventricular dysfunction, because it may worsen cardiac function; in patients with atrial flutter, because it may accelerate the ventricular rate; in patients with preexisting sinus node dysfunction, because it may cause marked effects on the sinus node; in patients with permanent artificial pacemakers or temporary pacing electrodes, because the drug may increase pacing thresholds and may suppress ventricular escape rhythms; in patients with preexisting left ventricular dysfunction or sustained ventricular tachycardia, because the drug may cause proarrhythmic effects; and in patients with renal or hepatic dysfunction, because these conditions can cause increased drug levels and subsequent toxicity.

Interactions
Concomitant use with digoxin may cause increased serum digoxin levels; concomitant use with beta-adrenergic blockers (such as propranolol) may cause additive negative inotropic effects.

When used concomitantly, other antiarrhythmic drugs may cause additive, synergistic, or antagonistic cardiac effects and may cause additive adverse effects. For example, amiodarone may increase serum flecainide levels; disopyramide may cause an additive negative inotropic effect; verapamil also may have an additive negative inotropic effect and may exacerbate AV nodal dysfunction.

Concomitant use with acidifying and alkalizing agents changes urinary pH, which in turn alters flecainide elimination; alkalization decreases renal flecainide excretion, and acidification increases it. When drugs that can markedly affect urine acidity (such as ammonium chloride) or alkalinity (such as high-dose antacids, carbonic anhydrase inhibitors, sodium bicarbonate) are given, monitor for possible subtherapeutic or toxic levels and effects. Cimetidine may decrease both the renal and nonrenal clearance of flecainide.

Effects on diagnostic tests
None reported.

Adverse reactions
● CNS: dizziness, headache, fatigue, tremor.
● CV: *arrhythmias*, chest pain, *congestive heart failure*, bradycardia, torsades de pointes.
● EENT: blurred vision and other visual disturbances.
● GI: nausea, constipation, abdominal pain.
● Other: dyspnea, edema.
Note: Drug should be discontinued if congestive heart failure worsens despite optimum therapy and reduced dosage; if second- or third-degree AV block or bifascicular block occurs (unless an artificial pacemaker is in place); or if unexplained jaundice, signs of hepatic dysfunction, or blood dyscrasias develop.

Overdose and treatment
Clinical effects of overdose include increased PR and QT intervals, increased QRS complex duration, decreased myocardial contractility, conduction disturbances, and hypotension.

Treatment generally involves symptomatic and supportive measures along with ECG, blood pressure, and respiratory monitoring. Inotropic agents, including dopamine and dobutamine, may be used. Hemodynamic support, including use of an intra-aortic balloon pump and transvenous pacing, may be needed. Because of drug's long half-life, supportive measures may need to be continued for extended periods. Hemodialysis is ineffective in reducing serum drug levels.

▶ **Special considerations**

• Hypokalemia or hyperkalemia may alter drug effects and should be corrected before drug therapy begins.

• Initiation of therapy should be done in the hospital with careful monitoring of patients with symptomatic congestive heart failure, sinus node dysfunction, sustained ventricular tachycardia, or underlying structural heart disease and in patients changing from another antiarrhythmic in whom discontinuation of current antiarrhythmic is likely to cause life-threatening arrhythmias.

• Loading doses may exacerbate arrhythmias and therefore are not recommended. Dosage adjustments should be made at intervals of at least 4 days because of this drug's long half-life.

• Most patients can be adequately maintained on an every-12-hour dosage schedule, but some need to receive drug every 8 hours.

• Twice-daily dosing improves patient compliance.

• Drug's full therapeutic effect may take 3 to 5 days. I.V. lidocaine may be administered while awaiting full effect.

• Flecainide is the first class IC antiarrhythmic. This drug class appears to be highly effective and has a relatively low incidence of adverse effects. Incidence of adverse effects increases when trough serum drug levels exceed 0.7 mcg/ml. Periodically monitor blood levels, especially in patients with renal failure or congestive heart failure.

• Drug may increase acute and chronic endocardial pacing thresholds and may suppress ventricular escape rhythms. Pacing threshold should be determined before drug is administered, after 1 week of therapy, and regularly thereafter. It should not be given to patients with preexisting poor thresholds or nonprogrammable artificial pacemakers unless pacing rescue is available.

• In CHF and myocardial dysfunction, initial dosage should not exceed 100 mg q 12 hours; common initial dosage is 50 mg q 12 hours.

• Use in hepatic impairment has not been fully evaluated; however, because flecainide is metabolized extensively (probably in the liver) it should be used in patients with significant hepatic impairment only when benefits clearly outweigh risks. Dosage reduction may be necessary and patients should be monitored carefully for signs of toxicity. Serum levels also must be monitored.

Geriatric use
Elderly patients are more susceptible to adverse effects. Careful monitoring is recommended.

Pediatric use
Safety and efficacy have not been established in children younger than age 18. Limited data suggest usefulness in management of paroxysmal reentrant supraventricular tachycardia.

Breast-feeding
Limited data indicate that this drug is excreted in breast milk. Breast-feeding is not recommended during flecainide therapy because of the risk of adverse effects on the infant.

floxuridine
FUDR

• Pharmacologic classification: antimetabolite (cell cycle-phase specific, S phase)
• Therapeutic classification: antineoplastic
• Pregnancy risk category C

How supplied
Available by prescription only
Injection: 500-mg vials

Indications, route, and dosage
Dosage and indications may vary. Check current literature for recommended protocol.
Brain, breast, head, neck, liver, gallbladder, and bile duct cancer
Adults: 0.1 to 0.6 mg/kg daily by intra-arterial infusion; or 0.4 to 0.6 mg/kg daily into hepatic artery.

Pharmacodynamics
Antineoplastic action: Floxuridine exerts its cytotoxic activity after conversion to its active form, by competitively inhibiting the enzyme thymidylate synthetase; this halts DNA synthesis and leads to cell death.

Pharmacokinetics
• *Absorption:* Floxuridine is not administered orally.
• *Distribution:* Floxuridine crosses the blood-brain barrier to a limited extent.
• *Metabolism:* Floxuridine is metabolized to fluorouracil in the liver after intraarterial infusions and rapid I.V. injections.
• *Excretion:* Approximately 60% of a dose of floxuridine is excreted through the lungs as carbon dioxide. A small amount is excreted by the kidneys as unchanged drug and metabolites.

Contraindications and precautions
Floxuridine is contraindicated in patients with poor nutritional status, depressed bone marrow function, or serious infections because these patients are at high risk for serious drug-related toxicity. Floxuridine should be discontinued immediately if myocardial ischemia occurs.

Interactions
None significant.

Effects on diagnostic tests
Floxuridine therapy may increase serum concentrations of ALT (SGPT), alkaline phosphatase, AST (SGOT), bilirubin, and LDH; these increases indicate drug-induced hepatotoxicity.

Adverse reactions
• CNS: cerebellar ataxia, vertigo, nystagmus, *seizures*, depression, hemiplegia, hiccups, lethargy.
• DERM: erythema, dermatitis, pruritus, rash.
• EENT: blurred vision.
• GI: stomatitis, cramps, nausea, vomiting, diarrhea, bleeding, enteritis.
• HEMA: *bone marrow depression* (dose-limiting), *leukopenia*, anemia, *thrombocytopenia*.
• Hepatic: cholangitis, jaundice, elevated liver enzymes.

Note: Drug should be discontinued if stomatitis, GI bleeding, esophagopharyngitis, or thromboembolic events occur; if the leukocyte count falls below 3,500/mm³; or if the platelet count falls below 100,000/mm³.

Overdose and treatment
Clinical manifestations of overdose include myelosuppression, diarrhea, alopecia, dermatitis, and hyperpigmentation.

Treatment is usually supportive and includes transfusion of blood components and antidiarrheal agents.

▶ Special considerations
• To reconstitute, use 5 ml sterile water for injection to give a concentration of 100 mg/ml.
• Dilute to appropriate volume for infusion device with dextrose 5% in water or normal saline solution.
• Administration by infusion pump maintains a continuous, uniform rate. Reconstituted floxuridine solutions are stable for 14 days when refrigerated.
• Observe arterial perfused area. Check line for bleeding, blockage, displacement, or leakage.
• Floxuridine is often administered via hepatic arterial infusion in treating hepatic metastases.
• Severe skin and GI adverse reactions require stopping drug.
• Excellent mouth care can help prevent oral adverse reactions.
• Monitor intake and output, CBC, and renal and hepatic function.
• Therapeutic effect may be delayed 1 to 6 weeks. Make sure patient is aware of time required for improvement.
• To prevent bleeding, avoid I.M. injections of any drugs in patients with thrombocytopenia.
• Floxuridine may be given concurrently with doxorubicin in the same infusion.

Information for the patient
Advise patient to report nausea, vomiting, stomach pain, or any unusual bruising or bleeding.

Breast-feeding
It is not known whether floxuridine distributes into breast milk. However, because of the risk of serious adverse reactions, mutagenicity, and carcinogenicity in the infant, breast-feeding is not recommended.

fluconazole
Diflucan

• Pharmacologic classification: bis-triazole derivative
• Therapeutic classification: antifungal
• Pregnancy risk category C

How supplied
Available by prescription only
Tablets: 50 mg, 100 mg, 200 mg
Injection: 200 mg/100 ml, 400 mg/200 ml

Indications, route, and dosage
Oropharyngeal and esophageal candidiasis
Adults: 200 mg P.O. or I.V. on the first day followed by 100 mg P.O. or I.V. once daily. As much as 400 mg daily has been used for esophageal disease. Treatment should continue for at least 2 weeks after resolution of symptoms.
Systemic candidiasis
Adults: 400 mg P.O. or I.V. on the first day, followed by 200 mg P.O. or I.V. once daily. Treatment should continue for at least 2 weeks after resolution of symptoms.
Cryptococcal meningitis
Adults: 400 mg P.O. or I.V. on the first day, followed by 200 mg P.O. or I.V. once daily. Some patients require a dosage of 400 mg once daily depending on their clinical response. The duration of therapy for initial treatment is 10 to 12 weeks after the CSF culture becomes negative.
Dosage in renal failure
Patient receiving hemodialysis should receive one full dose after each session.

Creatinine clearance (ml/min/1.73 m²)	Percentage of usual adult dose
>50	100
21 to 49	50
11 to 20	25

Pharmacodynamics
Antifungal action: Fluconazole exerts its fungistatic effects by inhibiting fungal cytochrome P-450 and interfering with sterols in the fungal cell. The spectrum of activity includes *Cryptococcus neoformans, Candida sp.* (including systemic *C. albicans), Aspergillus flavus, A. fumigatus, Coccidioides immitis,* and *Histoplasma capsulatum.*

Pharmacokinetics
• *Absorption:* After oral administration, absorption is rapid and complete. Peak plasma concentration after an oral dose occurs in 1 to 2 hours.
• *Distribution:* Fluconazole is well distributed to various sites, including CNS, saliva, sputum, blister fluid, urine, normal skin, nails, and blister skin. CNS concentrations approach 50% to 90% of that of serum. Fluconazole is 12% protein-bound.
• *Metabolism:* Fluconazole is partially metabolized.
• *Elimination:* Fluconazole is primarily excreted via the kidneys. Over 80% of an administered dose is excreted unchanged in the urine. The excretion rate diminishes as renal function decreases.

Contraindications and precautions
Fluconazole is contraindicated in patients with known hypersensitivity to the drug.

Interactions
Concomitant use with cimetidine may reduce fluconazole's serum concentrations; use with phenytoin may significantly increase phenytoin serum levels. Fluconazole has been shown to increase the hypoglycemic effects of the sulfonylureas tolbutamide, glyburide, and glipizide. Fluconazole therapy may reduce cyclosporine levels and may enhance the hypoprothrombinemic effects of warfarin. Rifampin can lower fluconazole levels; hydrochlorothiazide has decreased fluconazole's clearance, raising the drug's serum levels. The incidence of elevated hepatic transaminase levels is higher in patients taking rifampin, isoniazid, and sulfonylureas, phenytoin, or valproic acid.

Effects on diagnostic tests
Increased liver transaminase serum levels may occur with fluconazole.

Adverse reactions
● CNS: dizziness, headache.
● DERM: itching, rash.
● GI: nausea, vomiting, abdominal pain, diarrhea.
● HEMA: thrombocytopenia.
● Hepatic: elevated transaminase levels.
● Metabolic: hypokalemia.

Overdose and treatment
Treatment is largely supportive.

▶ Special considerations
● Fluconazole dose should be adjusted in patients with renal dysfunction.
● Fluconazole is not compatible with other I.V. medications.
● Adverse reactions (including transaminase elevations) are more frequent and more severe in patients with severe underlying illness (including acquired immunodeficiency syndrome [AIDS] and malignancies).

Breast-feeding
Safety has not been established.

---

flucytosine (5FC)
Ancobon

● Pharmacologic classification: fluorinated pyrimidine
● Therapeutic classification: antifungal
● Pregnancy risk category C

How supplied
Available by prescription only
Capsules: 250 mg, 500 mg

Indications, route, and dosage
Severe fungal infections caused by susceptible strains of Candida and Cryptococcus
Adults and children weighing more than 50 kg: 50 to 150 mg/kg daily q 6 hours P.O.
Adults and children weighing less than 50 kg: 1.5 to 4.5 g/m²/day in four divided doses P.O.
Severe infections, such as meningitis, may require doses up to 250 mg/kg.
Dosage in renal failure
In patients with a creatinine clearance of 10 to 50 ml/min/1.73 m² reduce dosage by 50% to 70%, or increase dosage interval to every 12 to 24 hours. In patients with a creatinine clearance <10 ml/min/1.73 m² reduce dosage by 20% to 80%, or increase dosage interval to 24 to 48 hours. If possible, serum levels should be monitored. Flucytosine is removed by hemodialysis and peritoneal dialysis.
Dosage of 20 to 50 mg/kg P.O. immediately after hemodialysis every 2 to 3 days ensures therapeutic blood levels.

Pharmacodynamics
Antifungal action: Flucytosine penetrates fungal cells, where it is converted to fluorouracil, which interferes with pyrimidine metabolism; it also may be converted to fluorodeoxyuredylic acid, which interferes with DNA synthesis. Because human cells lack the enzymes needed to convert the drug to these toxic metabolites, flucytosine is selectively toxic to fungal, not host cells. It is active against some strains of *Cryptococcus* and *Candida*.

Pharmacokinetics
● *Absorption:* About 75% to 90% of an oral dose of flucytosine is absorbed. Peak serum concentrations occur at 2 to 6 hours after a dose. Food decreases the rate of absorption.
● *Distribution:* Flucytosine is distributed widely into the liver, kidneys, spleen, heart, bronchial secretions, joints, peritoneal fluid, and aqueous humor. CSF levels vary from 60% to 100% of serum levels. Drug is 2% to 4% bound to plasma proteins.
● *Metabolism:* Only small amounts of flucytosine are metabolized.
● *Excretion:* About 75% to 95% of a dose is excreted unchanged in urine; less than 10% is excreted unchanged in feces. Serum half-life is 2½ to 6 hours with normal renal function; as long as 1,160 hours with creatinine clearance below 2 ml/minute.

Contraindications and precautions
Flucytosine is contraindicated in patients with known hypersensitivity to the drug. It should be used with caution in patients with bone marrow depression (regardless of origin), as it may exacerbate this condition; and in patients with impaired renal function, to prevent toxic drug accumulation. In patients with impaired renal function, serum concentrations should be determined to maintain therapeutic range (25 to 120 mcg/ml).

Interactions
Flucytosine potentiates the efficacy and toxicity of amphotericin B.

Effects on diagnostic tests
Flucytosine causes falsely elevated creatinine values on iminohydrolase enzymatic assay.
Flucytosine may increase alkaline phosphatase, AST (SGOT), ALT (SGPT), BUN, and serum creatinine levels and may decrease white blood cell, red blood cell, and platelet counts.

Adverse reactions
● CNS: dizziness, drowsiness, confusion, headache, vertigo, hallucinations.
● DERM: occasional rash.
● GI: *nausea, vomiting, diarrhea,* abdominal bloating.
● HEMA: anemia, leukopenia, bone marrow depression, thrombocytopenia.
● Hepatic: elevated AST (SGOT) and ALT (SGPT) levels.
● Metabolic: elevated serum alkaline phosphatase, BUN, and serum creatinine levels.

Overdose and treatment
Flucytosine overdose may affect cardiovascular and pulmonary function. Treatment is largely supportive. Induced emesis or lavage may be useful within 4 hours after ingestion. Activated charcoal and osmotic cathartics also may be helpful. Flucytosine is readily removed by either hemodialysis or peritoneal dialysis.

▶ Special considerations
● Hematologic studies and renal and hepatic function studies should also precede therapy and should be

---

repeated frequently thereafter, to evaluate dosage and monitor for adverse effects.
• Give capsules over a 15-minute period to reduce nausea, vomiting, and GI distress.
• Monitor intake/output to ensure adequate renal function.
• Flucytosine is usually given concomitantly with amphotericin B because they are synergistic.
• Protect drug from light.
• Because flucytosine is removed by hemodialysis, dosage adjustments should be made in patients undergoing hemodialysis.

Information for the patient
• Teach patient the signs and symptoms of adverse reactions and the need to report them.
• Tell patient to call promptly if urine output decreases or signs of bleeding or bruising occur.
• Explain that adequate response may require several weeks or months of therapy. Advise patient to adhere to medical regimen and to return as instructed for follow-up visits.

Breast-feeding
Safety has not been established.

fludarabine phosphate
Fludara

• Pharmacologic classification: antimetabolite
• Therapeutic classification: antineoplastic
• Pregnancy risk category D

How supplied
Available by prescription only
Injection: 50 mg as lyophilized powder

Indications, route, and dosage
Treatment of B-cell chronic lymphocytic leukemia (CLL) in patients who have not responded or responded inadequately to at least one standard alkylating agent regimen
Adults: Usually, 25 mg/m² I.V. over 30 minutes for 5 consecutive days q 28 days. Therapy based on patient response and tolerance.

Pharmacodynamics
Antineoplastic action: After rapid conversion of fludarabine to its active metabolite, the metabolite appears to inhibit DNA synthesis by inhibiting DNA polymerase alpha, ribonucleotide reductase, and DNA primase. The exact mechanism of action is not fully established.

Pharmacokinetics
• *Absorption:* Fludarabine is administered I.V.
• *Metabolism:* Rapidly dephosphorylated and then phosphorylated intracellularly to its active metabolite.
• *Distribution:* Unknown.
• *Excretion:* 23% is excreted in urine as unchanged active metabolite.

Contraindications and precautions
Fludarabine is contraindicated in patients with hypersensitivity to the drug or its components. Administer with caution to patients with renal insufficiency, hematologic impairment, or myelosuppression.

Interactions
Concomitant use with other myelosuppressive agents may cause additive toxicity.

Effects on diagnostic tests
None reported.

Adverse reactions
• CNS: fatigue, malaise, weakness, paresthesia, headache, sleep disorder, depression, cerebellar syndrome, agitation, confusion, peripheral neuropathy.
• CV: edema, angina, phlebitis, arrhythmias, *CHF*, deep venous thrombosis, transient ischemic attack, aneurysm, *CVA*, hemorrhage.
• DERM: rash, pruritus, seborrhea.
• EENT: visual disturbances, hearing loss, sinusitis, epistaxis.
• GI: nausea, vomiting, diarrhea, constipation, anorexia, stomatitis, bleeding, esophagitis, mucositis.
• GU: dysuria, urinary infection, urinary hesitancy, proteinuria, hematuria, renal failure.
• HEMA: thrombocytopenia, neutropenia, anemia.
• Respiratory: cough, pneumonia, dyspnea, pharyngitis, allergic pneumonitis, hemoptysis, bronchitis.
• Other: fever, chills, infection, pain, myalgia, tumor lysis syndrome, alopecia, anaphylaxis, diaphoresis, hyperglycemia, dehydration, liver failure, cholelithiasis.

Overdose and treatment
Irreversible CNS toxicity characterized by delayed blindness, coma, and death is associated with high doses. Severe thrombocytopenia and neutropenia secondary to bone marrow suppression also occur. There is no specific antidote, and treatment consists of discontinuing therapy and taking supportive measures.

▶ Special considerations
• Used investigationally in the treatment of non-Hodgkin's lymphoma, macroglobulinemic lymphoma, prolymphocytic leukemia or prolymphocytoid variant of CLL, mycosis fungoides, hairy cell leukemia, and Hodgkin's disease.
• Fludarabine should be administered under the direct supervision of a physician experienced in antineoplastic therapy.
• Careful hematologic monitoring is required, especially of neutrophil and platelet counts.
• Tumor lysis syndrome (hyperuricemia, hyperphosphatemia, hypocalcemia, metabolic acidosis, hyperkalemia, hematuria, urate crystalluria, and renal failure) has occurred in CLL patients with large tumors.
• Severe neurologic effects are seen when high doses are used to treat acute leukemia.
• Advanced age, renal insufficiency, and bone marrow impairment may predispose patient to severe toxicity; toxic effects are dose-dependent.
• Optimal duration of therapy has not been established; three additional cycles after achieving maximal response are recommended before discontinuing drug.
• To prepare, add 2 ml of sterile water for injection to the solid cake of fludarabine. Dissolution should occur within 15 seconds and each ml will contain 25 mg of drug, 25 mg of mannitol, and sodium hydroxide. Use within 8 hours of reconstitution. Fludarabine has been further diluted in 100 ml or 125 ml of dextrose 5% in water or normal saline.

● Follow institutional protocol and guidelines for proper handling and disposal of chemotherapeutic agents.
● Store drug in refrigerator at 35.6° to 46.4° F (2° to 8° C).

Geriatric use
Advanced age may increase toxicity potential.

Pediatric use
Safety and efficacy have not been established.

Breast-feeding
It is unknown if fludarabine is excreted in breast milk. Risk-benefit ratio must be determined.

fludarabine phosphate
Fludara

● Pharmacologic classification: antimetabolite
● Therapeutic classification: antineoplastic
● Pregnancy risk category D

How supplied
Available by prescription only
Injection: 50 mg as lyophilized powder

Indications, route, and dosage
Treatment of B-cell chronic lymphocytic leukemia (CLL) in patients who have not responded or responded inadequately to at least one standard alkylating agent regimen
Adults: Usually, 25 mg/m² I.V. over 30 minutes for 5 consecutive days q 28 days. Therapy based on patient response and tolerance.

Pharmacodynamics
Antineoplastic action: After rapid conversion of fludarabine to its active metabolite, the metabolite appears to inhibit DNA synthesis by inhibiting DNA polymerase alpha, ribonucleotide reductase, and DNA primase. The exact mechanism of action is not fully established.

Pharmacokinetics
● *Absorption:* Fludarabine is administered I.V.
● *Metabolism:* Rapidly dephosphorylated and then phosphorylated intracellularly to its active metabolite.
● *Distribution:* Unknown.
● *Excretion:* 23% is excreted in urine as unchanged active metabolite.

Contraindications and precautions
Fludarabine is contraindicated in patients with hypersensitivity to the drug or its components. Administer with caution to patients with renal insufficiency, hematologic impairment, or myelosuppression.

Interactions
Concomitant use with other myelosuppressive agents may cause additive toxicity.

Effects on diagnostic tests
None reported.

Adverse reactions
● CNS: fatigue, malaise, weakness, paresthesia, headache, sleep disorder, depression, cerebellar syndrome, agitation, confusion, peripheral neuropathy.
● CV: edema, angina, phlebitis, arrhythmias, *CHF,* deep venous thrombosis, transient ischemic attack, aneurysm, *CVA,* hemorrhage.
● DERM: rash, pruritus, seborrhea.
● EENT: visual disturbances, hearing loss, sinusitis, epistaxis.
● GI: nausea, vomiting, diarrhea, constipation, anorexia, stomatitis, bleeding, esophagitis, mucositis.
● GU: dysuria, urinary infection, urinary hesitancy, proteinuria, hematuria, renal failure.
● HEMA: thrombocytopenia, neutropenia, anemia.
● Respiratory: cough, pneumonia, dyspnea, pharyngitis, allergic pneumonitis, hemoptysis, bronchitis.
● Other: fever, chills, infection, pain, myalgia, tumor lysis syndrome, alopecia, anaphylaxis, diaphoresis, hyperglycemia, dehydration, liver failure, cholelithiasis.

Overdose and treatment
Irreversible CNS toxicity characterized by delayed blindness, coma, and death is associated with high doses. Severe thrombocytopenia and neutropenia secondary to bone marrow suppression also occur. There is no specific antidote, and treatment consists of discontinuing therapy and taking supportive measures.

▶ Special considerations
● Used investigationally in the treatment of non-Hodgkin's lymphoma, macroglobulinemic lymphoma, prolymphocytic leukemia or prolymphocytoid variant of CLL, mycosis fungoides, hairy cell leukemia, and Hodgkin's disease.
● Fludarabine should be administered under the direct supervision of a physician experienced in antineoplastic therapy.
● Careful hematologic monitoring is required, especially of neutrophil and platelet counts.
● Tumor lysis syndrome (hyperuricemia, hyperphosphatemia, hypocalcemia, metabolic acidosis, hyperkalemia, hematuria, urate crystalluria, and renal failure) has occurred in CLL patients with large tumors.
● Severe neurologic effects are seen when high doses are used to treat acute leukemia.
● Advanced age, renal insufficiency, and bone marrow impairment may predispose patient to severe toxicity; toxic effects are dose-dependent.
● Optimal duration of therapy has not been established; three additional cycles after achieving maximal response are recommended before discontinuing drug.
● To prepare, add 2 ml of sterile water for injection to the solid cake of fludarabine. Dissolution should occur within 15 seconds and each ml will contain 25 mg of drug, 25 mg of mannitol, and sodium hydroxide. Use within 8 hours of reconstitution. Fludarabine has been further diluted in 100 ml or 125 ml of dextrose 5% in water or normal saline.
● Follow institutional protocol and guidelines for proper handling and disposal of chemotherapeutic agents.
● Store drug in refrigerator at 35.6° to 46.4° F (2° to 8° C).

Geriatric use
Advanced age may increase toxicity potential.

Pediatric use
Safety and efficacy have not been established.

Breast-feeding
It is unknown if fludarabine is excreted in breast milk. Risk-benefit ratio must be determined.

---

fludrocortisone acetate
Florinef

- Pharmacologic classification: mineralocorticoid, glucocorticoid
- Therapeutic classification: mineralocorticoid replacement therapy
- Pregnancy risk category C

How supplied
Available by prescription only
Tablets: 0.1 mg

Indications, route, and dosage
Adrenal insufficiency (partial replacement), salt-losing adrenogenital syndrome
Adults: 0.1 to 0.2 mg P.O. daily.
Children: 0.05 to 0.1 mg P.O. daily.

Pharmacodynamics
Adrenal hormone replacement: Fludrocortisone, a synthetic glucocorticoid with potent mineralocorticoid activity, is used for partial replacement of steroid hormones in adrenocortical insufficiency and in salt-losing forms of congenital adrenogenital syndrome. In treating adrenocortical insufficiency, an exogenous glucocorticoid must also be administered for adequate control. (Cortisone or hydrocortisone are usually the drugs of choice for replacement because they produce both mineralocorticoid and glucocorticoid activity.) Fludrocortisone is administered on a variable schedule ranging from three times weekly to twice daily, depending on individual requirements.

Pharmacokinetics
- *Absorption:* Fludrocortisone is absorbed readily from the GI tract, reaching peak concentrations in about 1½ hours.
- *Distribution:* Fludrocortisone is removed rapidly from the blood and distributed to muscle, liver, skin, intestines, and kidneys. It has a plasma half-life of about 30 minutes. It is extensively bound to plasma proteins (transcortin and albumin). Only the unbound portion is active. Adrenocorticoids are distributed into breast milk and through the placenta.
- *Metabolism:* Fludrocortisone is metabolized in the liver to inactive glucuronide and sulfate metabolites.
- *Excretion:* The inactive metabolites and small amounts of unmetabolized drug are excreted by the kidneys. Insignificant quantities of drug are also excreted in feces. The biological half-life is 18 to 36 hours.

Contraindications and precautions
Fludrocortisone is contraindicated in patients with hypersensitivity to fludrocortisone acetate. It should be used with extreme caution in patients with hypertension, congestive heart failure (CHF), or cardiac disease and should be discontinued if a significant increase in weight or blood pressure, edema, or cardiac enlargement occurs.

The use of fludrocortisone should be accompanied by adequate glucocorticoid therapy in adrenal insufficiency or the salt-losing form of adrenogenital syndrome.

Patients with Addison's disease are more sensitive to the action of fludrocortisone and may develop adverse reactions to an exaggerated degree. Stop treatment in the event of a significant increase in weight or blood pressure, or the development of edema or cardiac enlargement.

Sodium retention and potassium loss are accelerated by a high sodium intake. If edema develops, restriction of dietary sodium and administration of potassium supplements may be necessary.

Interactions.
Concomitant use with barbiturates, phenytoin, or rifampin may cause decreased corticosteroid effects because of increased hepatic metabolism. Fludrocortisone may enhance hypokalemia associated with diuretic or amphotericin B therapy. The hypokalemia may increase the risk of toxicity in patients concurrently receiving digitalis glycosides. Fludrocortisone may increase the metabolism of isoniazid and salicylates.

Effects on diagnostic tests
Fludrocortisone therapy increases serum sodium levels and decreases serum potassium levels. Glucose tolerance tests should be performed only if necessary, because addisonian patients tend to develop severe hypoglycemia within 3 hours of the test.

Adverse reactions
- CNS: frontal and occipital headaches, dizziness.
- CV: sodium and water retention, leading to increased blood volume, edema, hypertension, CHF, cardiac arrhythmias, and cardiomegaly.
- Metabolic: hypokalemia, unusual weight gain.
- Musculoskeletal: arthralgias and tendon contractures, extreme weakness of extremities with ascending paralysis secondary to low potassium.
   Note: Drug should not be discontinued without direct medical supervision; rapid discontinuation may cause an addisonian crisis.

Overdose and treatment
Acute toxicity is manifested as an extension of the therapeutic effect, such as disturbances in fluid and electrolyte balance, hypokalemia, edema, hypertension, and cardiac insufficiency. In acute toxicity, administer symptomatic treatment and correct fluid and electrolyte imbalance.

▶ Special considerations
Besides those relevant to all *systemic adrenocorticoids,* consider the following recommendations.
- Plasma renin activity is usually the most sensitive laboratory test used to evaluate the adequacy of drug therapy. It is profoundly abnormal before clinical signs and symptoms become apparent.
- Use only with other supplemental measures, such as glucocorticoids, control of electrolytes, and control of infection.
- Supplemental dosages may be required in times of physiologic stress from serious illness, trauma, or surgery.
- Monitor for significant patient weight gain, edema, hypertension, or severe headaches.

Information for the patient

● Teach patient to recognize signs of electrolyte imbalance: muscle weakness, paresthesia, numbness, fatigue, anorexia, nausea, altered mental status, increased urination, altered heart rhythm, severe or continuing headaches, unusual weight gain, or swelling of the feet.
● Tell patient to take missed doses as soon as possible, unless it is almost time for the next dose, and not to double doses.

Pediatric use

Chronic use of fludrocortisone in children and adolescents may delay growth and maturation.

flumazenil
Mazicon

● Pharmacologic classification: benzodiazepine antagonist
● Therapeutic classification: antidote
● Pregnancy risk category C

How supplied

Available by prescription only
Injection: 0.1 mg/ml in 5-ml and 10-ml multiple-dose vials

Indications, route, and dosage

Complete or partial reversal of the sedative effects of benzodiazepines after anesthesia or short diagnostic procedures (conscious sedation)
Adults: Initially, 0.2 mg I.V. over 15 seconds. If patient does not reach the desired level of consciousness after 45 seconds, repeat dose. Repeat at 1-minute intervals until a cumulative dose of 1 mg has been given (initial dose plus four additional doses). Most patients respond after 0.6 to 1 mg of drug. If resedation occurs, dosage may be repeated after 20 minutes, but no more than 1 mg should be given at one time, and patient should not receive more than 3 mg/hour.
Management of suspected benzodiazepine overdose
Adults: Initially, 0.2 mg I.V. over 15 seconds. If patient does not reach the desired level of consciousness after 30 seconds, administer 0.3 mg over 30 seconds. If patient still does not respond adequately, give 0.5 mg over 30 seconds; then repeat 0.5-mg doses at 1-minute intervals until a cumulative dose of 3 mg has been given. Most patients with benzodiazepine overdose respond to cumulative doses between 1 and 3 mg; rarely, patients who respond partially after 3 mg may require additional doses. Do not give more than 5 mg over 5 minutes initially; sedation that persists after this dosage is unlikely to be caused by benzodiazepines. If resedation occurs, dosage may be repeated after 20 minutes, but no more than 1 mg should be given at one time, and patient should not receive more than 3 mg/hour.

Pharmacodynamics

Antidote action: Flumazenil competitively inhibits the actions of benzodiazepines on the gamma-aminobutyric acid (GABA)-benzodiazepine receptor complex.

Pharmacokinetics

● *Distribution:* After administration, flumazenil redistributes rapidly (initial distribution half-life is 7 to 15 minutes). Drug is about 50% bound to plasma proteins.
● *Metabolism:* Flumazenil is rapidly extracted from the blood and metabolized by the liver. Metabolites that have been identified are inactive. Ingestion of food during an I.V. infusion enhances extraction of drug from plasma, probably by increasing hepatic blood flow.
● *Excretion:* About 90% to 95% of drug appears in the urine as metabolites; the remainder is excreted in the feces. Plasma half-life is about 54 minutes.

Contraindications and precautions

Flumazenil is contraindicated in patients with hypersensitivity to the drug or benzodiazepines; in patients who show evidence of serious tricyclic or tetracyclic antidepressant overdose; and in those who received the benzodiazepine to treat a potentially life-threatening condition (such as status epilepticus). Drug is also contraindicated in benzodiazepine-dependent patients because it may precipitate seizures.

Use cautiously in patients at high risk for seizures (including those undergoing concurrent sedative-hypnotic drug withdrawal, patients who have recently received multiple doses of a parenteral benzodiazepine, and patients who show some signs of seizure activity, such as myoclonic jerking). Also use cautiously in patients who may be at risk for unrecognized benzodiazepine dependence (such as those in intensive care units), patients with head injury (because of the risk of precipitating seizures), patients who have received neuromuscular blockers, and psychiatric patients (because the drug has precipitated panic attacks in patients with panic disorder).

Interactions

Use flumazenil with caution in mixed overdose because it can obscure symptoms of poisoning by drugs that can cause seizures or arrhythmias, such as antidepressants. Seizures or arrhythmias can develop after flumazenil removes the effects of the benzodiazepine overdose.

Effects on diagnostic tests

None reported.

Adverse reactions

● CNS: dizziness, abnormal or blurred vision, headache, *seizures,* fatigue, agitation, emotional lability.
● CV: *arrhythmias,* cutaneous vasodilation.
● GI: nausea, vomiting.
● Local: pain at injection site.
● Other: increased sweating.

Overdose and treatment

In clinical trials, large doses of flumazenil were administered I.V. to volunteers in the absence of a benzodiazepine agonist. No serious adverse reactions, clinical signs or symptoms, or altered laboratory tests were noted.

In patients with benzodiazepine overdosage, large doses of flumazenil may produce agitation or anxiety, hyperesthesia, increased muscle tone, or seizures. Seizures may be treated with barbiturates, phenytoin, or benzodiazepines.

▶ Special considerations

● Onset of action is usually evident within 1 to 2 minutes of injection, and peak effect occurs within 6 to 10 minutes. Because duration of action of flumazenil is shorter than that of benzodiazepines, monitor patient carefully and administer additional drug as needed. Duration and degree of effect depend on plasma levels of the sedating benzodiazepine and the dose of flumazenil.

● To minimize pain at the injection site, drug should be given through a freely flowing I.V. solution running into a large vein. Compatible solutions include dextrose 5% in water, lactated Ringer's injection, or 0.9% sodium chloride solution.

● Resedation may occur after reversal of benzodiazepine effect because flumazenil has a shorter duration of action than that of benzodiazepines. Patients should be monitored for resedation according to duration of drug being reversed: monitor closely after long-acting benzodiazepines (such as diazepam) or after high doses of shorter-acting benzodiazepines (such as 10 mg of midazolam). Usually, serious resedation is unlikely in patients who fail to show signs of resedation 2 hours after a 1-mg dose of flumazenil.

● Do not expect patients to recall information from the postprocedure period because drug does not reverse the amnesiac effects of benzodiazepines. Therefore, important instructions should be given to family caregivers or in writing to patient.

● Because of the risk of resedation, patients should avoid hazardous activities, such as driving a car, and alcohol, CNS depressants, and OTC drugs within 24 hours of the procedure.

● Flumazenil can be administered by direct injection or diluted with a compatible solution. Unused drug that has been drawn into a syringe or diluted should be discarded within 24 hours.

Geriatric use

No dosage adjustments appear necessary in elderly patients.

Pediatric use

Because clinical trials have not been performed to identify flumazenil's clinical risks, benefits, or dosage range, the manufacturer does not recommend its use in children.

Breast-feeding

It is unknown if drug is excreted in breast milk. Use with caution.

flunisolide

Nasal inhalant
Nasalide

Oral inhalant
AeroBid

● Pharmacologic classification: glucocorticoid
● Therapeutic classification: anti-inflammatory, antiasthmatic
● Pregnancy risk category C

How supplied

Available by prescription only
Nasal inhalant: 25 mcg/metered spray; 200 doses/bottle
Oral inhalant: 250 mcg/metered spray; 50 doses/inhaler

Indications, route, and dosage
Steroid-dependent asthma

Adults: Two inhalations b.i.d. Do not exceed 8 inhalations a day.
Children age 6 and older: One inhalation t.i.d. Do not exceed four inhalations a day.

Pharmacodynamics

● *Anti-inflammatory action:* Flunisolide stimulates the synthesis of enzymes needed to decrease the inflammatory response. The anti-inflammatory and vasoconstrictor potency of topically applied flunisolide is several hundred times greater than that of hydrocortisone and about equal to that of an equal weight of triamcinolone; the metabolite, 6-beta-hydroxyflunisdolide, has about three times the activity of hydrocortisone.

● *Antiasthmatic action:* The nasal inhalant form of flunisolide is used in the symptomatic treatment of seasonal or perennial rhinitis. In patients who require corticosteroids to control symptoms, the oral inhalant form is used to treat bronchial asthma.

Pharmacokinetics

● *Absorption:* Approximately 50% of a nasally inhaled dose is absorbed systemically. Peak plasma concentrations occur within 10 to 30 minutes. After oral inhalation, about 70% of the dose is absorbed from the lungs and GI tract. Only about 20% of an orally inhaled dose of flunisolide reaches systemic circulation unmetabolized because of extensive metabolism in the liver. Onset of action usually occurs in a few days but may take as long as 4 weeks in some patients.

● *Distribution:* Distribution following intranasal administration has not been described. After oral inhalation, 10% to 25% of the drug is distributed to the lungs; the remainder is deposited in the mouth and swallowed. No evidence exists of tissue storage of flunisolide or its metabolites. When absorbed, it is 50% bound to plasma proteins.

● *Metabolism:* Flunisolide that is swallowed undergoes rapid metabolism in the liver or GI tract to a variety of metabolites, one of which has glucocorticoid activity. Flunisolide and its 6-beta-hydroxy metabolite are eventually conjugated in the liver, by glucuronic acid or surface sulfate, to inactive metabolites.

● *Excretion:* Excretion of flunisolide administered by inhalation has not been described; however, when the drug is administered systemically, the metabolites are excreted in approximately equal portions in feces and urine. The biological half-life of flunisolide averages about 2 hours.

Contraindications and precautions
Flunisolide is contraindicated in patients with acute status asthmaticus; in patients with tuberculosis or viral, fungal, or bacterial respiratory infections; and in patients who are hypersensitive to any component of the preparation.

It should be used cautiously in patients receiving systemic corticosteroids because of increased risk of hypothalamic-pituitary-adrenal axis suppression; when substituting inhalant for oral systemic administration (because withdrawal symptoms may occur); and in patients with healing nasal septal ulcers, oral or nasal surgery, or trauma.

Interactions
None reported.

Effects on diagnostic tests
None reported.

Adverse reactions
● EENT: (after oral inhalation) flushing, rash, dry mouth, hoarseness, irritation of the tongue or throat, and impaired sense of taste; (after nasal inhalation) itchy nose, dryness, burning, irritation and sneezing, infrequent epistaxis, bloody mucus.
● Immune: suppression of immune response; fungal overgrowth and infections of the nose, mouth, or throat.
● Other: restlessness, anxiety, altered taste.
Note: Drug should be discontinued if no improvement is evident after 4 weeks, or if nasal or oral infections develop.

Overdose and treatment
No information available.

▶ Special considerations
Recommendations for use of flunisolide and for care and teaching of the patient during therapy are the same as those for all *inhalant adrenocorticoids.*

fluocinolone acetonide
Fluoderm*, Fluolar*, Fluonid, Fluonide*, Flurosyn, Neo-Synalar, Synalar, Synalar-HP, Synamol*, Synandone*, Synemol

● Pharmacologic classification: topical adrenocorticoid
● Therapeutic classification: anti-inflammatory
● Pregnancy risk category C

How supplied
Available by prescription only
Cream: 0.01%, 0.025%, 0.2%
Ointment: 0.025%
Solution: 0.01%

Indications, route, and dosage
Inflammation of corticosteroid-responsive dermatoses
Adults and children over age 2: Apply cream, ointment, or solution sparingly daily to q.i.d. Treat multiple or extensive lesions sequentially, applying to only small areas at any one time. Occlusive dressings may be used for severe or resistant dermatoses.

Pharmacodynamics
Anti-inflammatory action: Fluocinolone stimulates the synthesis of enzymes needed to decrease the inflammatory response. It is a high-potency fluorinated glucocorticoid. Preparations of 0.01% potency are in group V; 0.025% potency in group III or IV; and 0.2% potency in group II.

Pharmacokinetics
● Absorption: The amount absorbed depends on the strength of the preparation, the amount applied, and the nature of the skin at the application site. It ranges from about 1% in areas with a thick stratum corneum (such as the palms, soles, elbows, and heels) to as high as 36% in areas of the thinnest stratum corneum (face, eyelids, and genitals). Absorption increases in areas of skin damage, inflammation, or occlusion. Some systemic absorption of topical steroids occurs, especially through the oral mucosa.
● Distribution: After topical application, fluocinolone is distributed throughout the local skin. Any drug absorbed into the circulation is distributed rapidly into muscle, liver, skin, intestines, and kidneys.
● Metabolism: After topical administration, fluocinolone is metabolized primarily in the skin. The small amount absorbed into systemic circulation is metabolized primarily in the liver to inactive compounds.
● Excretion: Inactive metabolites are excreted by the kidneys, primarily as glucuronides and sulfates, but also as unconjugated products. Small amounts of the metabolites are also excreted in feces.

Contraindications and precautions
Fluocinolone is contraindicated in patients who are hypersensitive to any component of the preparation and in patients with viral, fungal, or tubercular skin lesions.

Fluocinolone should be used with extreme caution in patients with impaired circulation because the drug may increase the risk of skin ulceration.

Avoid using on the face or genital areas because increased absorption may result in striae.

Interactions
None significant.

Effects on diagnostic tests
None significant.

Adverse reactions
● Local: burning, itching, irritation, dryness, folliculitis, hypertrichosis, acneiform eruptions, hypopigmentation, perioral dermatitis, allergic contact dermatitis, maceration, secondary infection, atrophy, striae, miliaria.
Significant systemic absorption can produce the following reactions.
● CNS: euphoria, insomnia, headache, psychotic behavior, pseudotumor cerebri, mental changes, nervousness, restlessness.
● CV: *congestive heart failure,* hypertension, edema.
● EENT: cataracts, glaucoma, thrush.

● GI: peptic ulcer, irritation, increased appetite.
● Immune: immunosuppression, increased susceptibility to infection.
● Metabolic: hypokalemia, sodium retention, fluid retention, weight gain, hyperglycemia, osteoporosis, growth suppression in children.
● Musculoskeletal: muscle atrophy.
● Other: withdrawal syndrome (nausea, fatigue, anorexia, dyspnea, hypotension, hypoglycemia, myalgia, arthralgia, fever, dizziness, and fainting).

Note: Drug should be discontinued if local irritation, infection, systemic absorption, or hypersensitivity reaction occurs.

Overdose and treatment
No information available.

▶ Special considerations
Recommendations for use of fluocinolone, for care and teaching of patients during therapy, and for use in elderly patients, children, and breast-feeding women are the same as those for all *topical adrenocorticoids*.

---

fluocinonide
FAPG, Lidex, Lidex-E, Lidemol*,
Lyderm*, Metosyn*

● Pharmacologic classification: topical adrenocorticoid
● Therapeutic classification: anti-inflammatory
● Pregnancy risk category C

How supplied
Available by prescription only
Cream, gel, ointment, solution: 0.05%

Indications, route, and dosage
Inflammation of corticosteroid-responsive dermatoses
Adults and children: Apply sparingly once daily to q.i.d. Occlusive dressings may be used for severe or resistant dermatoses.

Pharmacodynamics
Anti-inflammatory action: Fluocinonide stimulates the synthesis of enzymes needed to decrease the inflammatory response. Fluocinonide is a high-potency fluorinated glucocorticoid categorized as a group II topical steroid.

Pharmacokinetics
● *Absorption:* The amount absorbed depends on the amount applied and on the nature of the skin at the application site. It ranges from about 1% in areas of thick stratum corneum (such as the palms, soles, elbows, and knees) to as high as 36% in areas of thin stratum corneum (face, eyelids, and genitals). Absorption increases in areas of skin damage, inflammation, or occlusion. Some systemic absorption of steroids occurs, especially through the oral mucosa.
● *Distribution:* After topical application, fluocinonide is distributed throughout the local skin. Any drug absorbed into circulation is removed rapidly from the blood and distributed into muscle, liver, skin, intestines, and kidneys.

● *Metabolism:* After topical administration, fluocinonide is metabolized primarily in the skin. The small amount absorbed into systemic circulation is metabolized primarily in the liver to inactive compounds.
● *Excretion:* Inactive metabolites are excreted by the kidneys, primarily as glucuronides and sulfates, but also as unconjugated products. Small amounts of the metabolites are excreted in feces.

Contraindications and precautions
Fluocinonide is contraindicated in patients who are hypersensitive to any component of the preparation and in patients with viral, fungal, or tubercular skin lesions.

Fluocinonide should be used with extreme caution in patients with impaired circulation because the drug may increase the risk of skin ulceration.

Avoid using on the face or genital areas because increased absorption may result in striae.

Interactions
None significant.

Effects on diagnostic tests
None reported.

Adverse reactions
● Local: burning, itching, irritation, dryness, folliculitis, hypertrichosis, acneiform eruptions, hypopigmentation, perioral dermatitis, allergic contact dermatitis, maceration, secondary infection, atrophy, striae, miliaria.

Significant systemic absorption may cause the following reactions.
● CNS: euphoria, insomnia, headache, psychotic behavior, pseudotumor cerebri, mental changes, nervousness, restlessness.
● CV: *congestive heart failure,* hypertension, edema.
● DERM: delayed healing, acne, skin eruptions, striae.
● EENT: cataracts, glaucoma, thrush.
● GI: peptic ulcer, irritation, increased appetite.
● Immune: immunosuppression, increased susceptibility to infection.
● Metabolic: hypokalemia, sodium retention, fluid retention, weight gain, hyperglycemia, osteoporosis, growth suppression in children.
● Musculoskeletal: muscle atrophy.
● Other: withdrawal syndrome (nausea, fatigue, anorexia, dyspnea, hypotension, hypoglycemia, myalgia, arthralgia, fever, dizziness, and fainting).

Note: Drug should be discontinued if local irritation, infection, systemic absorption, or hypersensitivity reaction occurs.

Overdose and treatment
No information available.

▶ Special considerations
Recommendations for use of fluocinonide, for care and teaching of patients during therapy, and for use in elderly patients, children, and breast-feeding women are the same as those for all *topical adrenocorticoids*.

---

fluorescein sodium
Fluorescite, Fluor-I-Strip, Fluor-I-Strip
A.T., Ful-Glo, Funduscein

- Pharmacologic classification: dye
- Therapeutic classification: diagnostic aid
- Pregnancy risk category C

How supplied
Available by prescription only
Parenteral injection: 10%, 25%
Ophthalmic solution: 2%
Ophthalmic strips: 0.6 mg, 1 mg, 9 mg

Indications, route, and dosage
Diagnostic aid in corneal abrasions and foreign bodies; fitting hard contact lenses; lacrimal patency; fundus photography; applanation tonometry
Adults and children: For topical solution, instill 1 drop of 2% solution followed by irrigation, or moisten strip with sterile water. Touch conjunctiva or fornix with moistened tip. Flush eye with irrigating solution. Patient should blink several times after application.
Retinal angiography
Adults: 5 ml of 10% solution (500 mg) or 3 ml of 25% solution (750 mg) injected rapidly into antecubital vein by physician or a specially trained nurse.
Children: 0.077 ml of 10% solution (7.7 mg/kg of body weight) or 0.044 ml of 25% solution (11 mg/kg of body weight) injected rapidly into antecubital vein by physician.

Pharmacodynamics
Diagnostic adjunct: Fluorescein stains abraded or ulcerated areas of the cornea fluorescent green under normal light and bright yellow if viewed under cobalt blue light. Foreign bodies appear surrounded by a green fluorescent ring, and lesions of the conjunctiva appear orange-yellow.

Pharmacokinetics
- *Absorption:* Unknown.
- *Distribution:* Unknown.
- *Metabolism:* Unknown.
- *Excretion:* Drug is excreted in urine. Urine attains a bright yellow color that fades in 24 to 36 hours.

Contraindications and precautions
Fluorescein sodium is contraindicated in patients with hypersensitivity to any component of the preparation. Injectable preparation should be used cautiously in patients with a history of allergy or bronchial asthma. It should not be used in patients wearing soft contact lenses; the lenses may become discolored.

Interactions
None reported.

Effects on diagnostic tests
Bright yellow discoloration of urine may interfere with routine urinalysis.

Adverse reactions
The following reactions may follow use of the injected drug.

- CNS: headache, dizziness, syncope, *seizures.*
- CV: basilar artery ischemia, hypotension, *shock, cardiac arrest.*
- DERM: yellow discoloration (fades in 6 to 12 hours), urticaria, pruritus, angioedema.
- GI: nausea, vomiting, GI distress, strong taste with high dosages.
- GU: bright yellow urine (persists for 24 to 36 hours).
- Respiratory: transient dyspnea, *anaphylaxis, bronchospasm.*
- Other: extravasation and thrombophlebitis at injection site.
   Note: Drug should be discontinued if symptoms of hypersensitivity occur.

Overdose and treatment
The 2% solution of fluorescein sodium alone is considered nontoxic; however, some preparations may contain boric acid: 10 to 20 g of boric acid have been tolerated by children, and 80 to 297 g by adults. In other cases, as little as 5 g in infants or 20 g in adults has been fatal. Clinical manifestations of overdose include hypotension, shock, restlessness, weakness, seizures, nausea, vomiting, diarrhea, oliguria, hypothermia, hyperthermia, and erythematous rash.
   Use emesis followed by a cathartic for substantial accidental ingestion unless the patient is comatose or obtunded. Treat hypotension with fluids and Trendelenburg positioning. Treat seizures with I.V. diazepam.

▶ Special considerations
- Never instill drug in eye of patient wearing soft contact lens; this will cause permanent discoloration of lens.
- Topical anesthetic may be used before instillation to partially relieve burning and irritation.
- Use strict aseptic technique; preparation is contaminated easily by *Pseudomonas.*
- Fluorescein is water-soluble. Do not freeze; store below 80° F. (26.7° C.).
- After I.V. injection, yellow skin discoloration may last 6 to 12 hours; urine will be bright yellow for 24 to 36 hours, and routine urinalysis of sample taken within 1 hour will be abnormal.
- Keep emergency supplies and medications on hand to manage or treat respiratory and/or cardiac arrest.
- Intermittent nausea lasting 1 to 4 minutes follows I.V. injection in 5% to 10% of patients; assist patient as necessary.

Information for the patient
- Explain that fluorescein may discolor soft contact lenses; contact lenses should be removed before use. After using fluorescein, eyes should be flushed with normal saline solution; allow at least 1 hour before replacing lenses.
- Explain that yellow skin discoloration may persist for 6 to 12 hours and that urine will be bright yellow for 24 to 36 hours after I.V. injection; reassure patient that this is not harmful.
- Explain that, although uncommon, mild nausea may occur; reassure patient that it will subside in a few minutes.

---

fluorometholone
Fluor-Op Ophthalmic, FML Liquifilm Ophthalmic, FML Ointment

- Pharmacological classification: corticosteroid
- Therapeutic classification: ophthalmic anti-inflammatory
- Pregnancy risk category C

How supplied
Available by prescription only
Ophthalmic ointment: 0.1%
Ophthalmic suspension: 0.1%, 0.25%

Indications, route, and dosage
Inflammatory and allergic conditions of cornea, conjunctiva, sclera, anterior uvea
Adults and children: In severe cases, instill 2 drops of suspension in conjunctival sac every hour or ½" ointment q 4 hours during the first 1 to 2 days of therapy. In mild to moderate cases, 1 to 2 drops of suspension may be used b.i.d. to q.i.d. or ½" ointment daily to t.i.d.

Pharmacodynamics
Anti-inflammatory action: Fluorometholone stimulates the synthesis of enzymes needed to decrease the inflammatory response. Fluorometholone is a synthetic fluorinated corticosteroid that is less likely than hydrocortisone, prednisolone, or dexamethasone to cause intraocular hypertension.

Pharmacokinetics
- *Absorption:* After ophthalmic administration, fluorometholone is absorbed mainly into the aqueous humor. Slight systemic absorption typically occurs.
- *Distribution:* Fluorometholone is distributed throughout the local tissue layers. Any drug absorbed into circulation is removed rapidly from the blood and distributed into muscle, liver, skin, intestines, and kidneys.
- *Metabolism:* Fluorometholone is primarily metabolized locally. The small amount absorbed into systemic circulation is metabolized primarily in liver to inactive compounds.
- *Excretion:* Inactive metabolites are excreted by the kidneys, primarily as glucuronides and sulfates, but also as unconjugated products. Small amounts of the metabolites are also excreted in the feces.

Contraindications and precautions
Fluorometholone is contraindicated in patients who are hypersensitive to any component of the preparation; in patients with fungal infections of the eye; and in patients with acute, untreated purulent bacterial, viral, or fungal ocular infections. If a bacterial infection does not respond promptly to appropriate anti-infective therapy, fluorometholone should be discontinued and another therapy applied.

Intraocular pressure should be measured every 2 to 4 weeks for the first 2 months of ophthalmic corticosteroid therapy; then, if no increase in intraocular pressure has occurred, every 1 to 2 months thereafter.

Interactions
None reported.

Effects on diagnostic tests
None reported.

Adverse reactions
- Eye: transient burning or stinging on administration; mydriasis, ptosis, epithelial punctate keratitis, and corneal or scleral malacia (rare); increased intraocular pressure, thinning of the cornea, interference with corneal wound healing, increased susceptibility to viral or fungal corneal infection, corneal ulceration; glaucoma, cataracts, and defects in visual acuity and visual field (with long-term use).
- Systemic: HPA axis suppression, fluid retention; rare, but may occur with excessive doses or long-term use.
Note: Drug should be discontinued if topical application results in local irritation, infection, significant systemic absorption, or hypersensitivity reaction; if visual acuity decreases or visual field diminishes; or if burning, stinging, or watering of eyes does not quickly resolve after administration.

Overdose and treatment
No information available.

▶ Special considerations
Recommendations for administration of fluorometholone and for care and teaching of patients during therapy are the same as those for all *ophthalmic adrenocorticoids.*

Pediatric use
Safety and efficacy in children under age 2 have not been established.

fluorouracil (5-FU)
Adrucil, Efudex, Fluroplex

- Pharmacologic classification: antimetabolite (cell cycle-phase specific, S phase)
- Therapeutic classification: antineoplastic
- Pregnancy risk category D

How supplied
Available by prescription only
Injection: 50 mg/ml in 10-ml and 20-ml vials and 1,000 mg/20 ml vials
Cream: 1%, 5%
Topical solution: 1%, 2%, 5%

Indications, route, and dosage
Dosage and indications may vary. Check current literature for recommended protocol.
Colon, rectal, breast, ovarian, cervical, gastric, esophageal, bladder, liver, pancreatic, and unknown primary cancers
Adults and children: 7 to 12 mg/kg I.V. for 4 days, then (after 3 days) 7 to 10 mg/kg q 3 to 4 days for 2 weeks. Alternatively, 12 mg/kg I.V. for 5 days, followed (after 1 day) by 6 mg/kg I.V. every other day for 4 or 5 doses, for a total course of 2 weeks. Maintenance infusion is 7 to 12 mg/kg I.V. q 7 to 10 days or 300 to 500 mg/m² every 4 to 5 days, repeated monthly. Do not exceed 800 mg/day (400 mg/day in severely ill patients).

Actinic or solar keratoses
Adults: Sufficient cream or lotion to cover lesions twice a day. Usually, 1% preparations are used on head, neck, and chest, 2% and 5% on hands.

Superficial basal cell carcinomas
Adults: 5% solution or cream in a sufficient amount to cover lesion twice a day.

Pharmacodynamics
Antineoplastic action: Fluorouracil exerts its cytotoxic activity by acting as an antimetabolite, competing for the enzyme that is important in the synthesis of thymidine, an essential substrate for DNA synthesis. Therefore, DNA synthesis is inhibited. The drug also inhibits RNA synthesis to a lesser extent.

Pharmacokinetics
● *Absorption:* Because fluorouracil is absorbed poorly after oral administration, it is given parenterally.
● *Distribution:* Fluorouracil distributes widely into all areas of body water and tissues, including tumors, bone marrow, liver, and intestinal mucosa. Fluorouracil crosses the blood-brain barrier to a significant extent.
● *Metabolism:* A small amount of fluorouracil is converted in the tissues to the active metabolite, with a majority of the drug degraded in the liver.
● *Excretion:* Metabolites of fluorouracil are primarily excreted through the lungs as carbon dioxide. A small portion of a dose is excreted in urine as unchanged drug.

Contraindications and precautions
Fluorouracil is contraindicated in patients with poor nutritional status, depressed bone marrow function, recent major surgery, or serious infections because of the increased potential for toxicity; and in pregnant patients because the drug may be fetotoxic.

Interactions
When used concomitantly, leucovorin calcium given as a continuous infusion causes increased binding of fluorouracil to substrate, increased fluorouracil cell uptake, and increased inhibition of thymidine synthetase. Significance is unknown.

Effects on diagnostic tests
Fluorouracil may decrease plasma albumin concentration because of drug-induced protein malabsorption.

Adverse reactions
● CNS: acute cerebellar syndrome, drowsiness, euphoria.
● CV: mild angina, ECG changes.
● DERM: maculopapular rash, dryness, erythema, hyperpigmentation (especially in blacks), nail changes, pigmented palmar creases, pruritus, suppuration, burning, swelling, scarring.
● GI: anorexia, proctitis, paralytic ileus, stomatitis, diarrhea (GI ulcer may precede leukopenia), nausea, vomiting, GI toxicity (dose-limiting).
● HEMA: *bone marrow depression* (dose-limiting), *leukopenia* (nadir in 7 to 14 days), anemia, thrombocytopenia.
● Other: photosensitivity, lacrimation, reversible alopecia, weakness, malaise.
   Note: Drug should be discontinued if intractable vomiting, stomatitis, diarrhea, GI ulceration, or GI bleeding occurs; if the leukocyte count falls below 3,000/mm³; or if the platelet count falls below 100,000/mm³.

Overdose and treatment
Clinical manifestations of overdose include myelosuppression, diarrhea, alopecia, dermatitis, hyperpigmentation, nausea, and vomiting.

Treatment is usually supportive and includes transfusion of blood components, antiemetics, and antidiarrheals.

▶ Special considerations
● To reconstitute, withdraw solution through a 5-micron filter and add to vial.
● Drug may be administered I.V. push over 1 to 2 minutes.
● Drug may be further diluted in dextrose 5% in water or normal saline solution for infusions up to 24 hours in duration.
● Use plastic I.V. containers for administering continuous infusions. Solution is more stable in plastic I.V. bags than in glass bottles.
● Do not use cloudy solution. If crystals form, redissolve by warming at a temperature of 140° F (60° C). Allow solution to cool to body temperature before using.
● Use new vein site for each dose.
● Give antiemetic before administering to decrease nausea.
● If extravasation occurs, treat as a chemical phlebitis with warm compresses.
● Do not refrigerate fluorouracil.
● Drug can be diluted in 120 ml of a 0.2 M sodium bicarbonate solution and administered orally.
● General photosensitivity occurs for 2 to 3 months after a dose.
● Ingestion and systemic absorption may cause leukopenia, thrombocytopenia, stomatitis, diarrhea or GI ulceration, bleeding, and hemorrhage. A topical local anesthetic may be used to soothe mouth lesions. Encourage good and frequent mouth care.
● Monitor intake and output, CBC, and renal and hepatic function.
● Avoid I.M. injections in patients with low platelet counts.
● Apply topical drug while using plastic gloves. Wash hands immediately after handling medication. Avoid topical use with occlusive dressings.
● Apply topical solution with caution near eyes, nose, and mouth.
● Topical application to larger ulcerated areas may cause systemic toxicity.
● For superficial basal cell carcinoma confirmed by biopsy, use 5% strength. Apply 1% concentration on the face. Reserve higher concentrations for thicker-skinned areas or resistant lesions. Occlusion may be required.
● Do not continue to treat lesions resistant to fluorouracil; they should be biopsied.

Information for the patient
● Warn patient to avoid strong sunlight or ultraviolet light because it will intensify the skin reaction. Encourage use of sunscreens.
● Tell patient to avoid exposure to people with infections.
● Reassure patient that hair should grow back after treatment is discontinued.
● Tell patient to apply topical fluorouracil with gloves and wash hands thoroughly after application.
● Warn patient that treated area may be unsightly during therapy and for several weeks after therapy is stopped. Complete healing may not occur until 1 or 2 months after treatment is stopped.

Breast-feeding
It is not known whether fluorouracil distributes into breast milk. However, because of the potential for serious adverse reactions, mutagenicity, and carcinogenicity in the infant, breast-feeding is not recommended.

---

fluoxetine
Prozac

- Pharmacologic classification: serotonin uptake inhibitor
- Therapeutic classification: antidepressant
- Pregnancy risk category B

How supplied
Available by prescription only
Pulvules: 20 mg
Oral suspension: 20 mg/5 ml

Indications, route, and dosage
Depression, †panic disorder
Adults: 20 mg P.O. daily in the morning. Increase dosage as needed after several weeks to 40 mg daily with a dose in the morning and at noon. Do not exceed 80 mg daily.

†Obsessive-compulsive disorder
Adults: Initially, 20 mg P.O. daily. Gradually increase dosage as needed and tolerated to 60 to 80 mg daily.

Pharmacodynamics
Antidepressant action: The antidepressant action of fluoxetine is purportedly related to its inhibition of CNS neuronal uptake of serotonin. Fluoxetine blocks uptake of serotonin, but not of norepinephrine, into human platelets. Animal studies suggest it is a much more potent uptake inhibitor of serotonin than of norepinephrine.

Pharmacokinetics
- *Absorption:* Fluoxetine is well absorbed after oral administration. Its absorption is not altered by food.
- *Distribution:* Fluoxetine is apparently highly protein-bound (about 95%).
- *Metabolism:* Fluoxetine is metabolized primarily in the liver to active metabolites.
- *Excretion:* Drug is excreted by the kidneys. Elimination half-life is 2 to 3 days. Norfluoxetine (the primary active metabolite) has an elimination half-life of 7 to 9 days.

Contraindications and precautions
There are no known contraindications to fluoxetine. In early trials, about 4% of all patients taking the drug developed a rash or urticaria, and all recovered after the drug was discontinued. Because a substantial percentage of patients taking fluoxetine may experience anxiety, nervousness, and insomnia, administering this drug early in the day may avoid sleep disturbance. Monitor changes in weight during therapy because significant weight loss may occur, especially in underweight patients.

Interactions
Concomitant use with diazepam may prolong the half-life of diazepam. Concomitant use with tryptophan may lead to increased adverse CNS effects (agitation, restlessness) and GI distress. Avoid concomitant administration with other highly protein-bound drugs (such as warfarin). Avoid concomitant administration with other psychoactive drugs (MAO inhibitors, antipsychotics).

Effects on diagnostic tests
None reported.

Adverse reactions
- CNS: headache, nervousness, insomnia, drowsiness, sedation, anxiety, tremor, dizziness, fatigue, diminished concentration, abnormal dreams, agitation, suicidal ideation.
- CV: hot flushes, palpitations.
- DERM: sweating, rash, pruritus.
- GI: nausea, diarrhea, dry mouth, anorexia, dyspepsia, constipation, abdominal pain, vomiting, taste change, flatulence, gastroenteritis.
- GU: sexual dysfunction, urinary tract infection, frequent micturition, painful menstruation.
- Musculoskeletal: back, joint, or muscle pain.
- Respiratory: flulike syndrome, upper respiratory infection, pharyngitis, nasal congestion, sinusitis, cough, dyspnea, bronchitis, rhinitis.
- Other: asthenia, fever, chest pain, allergy, viral infection, limb pain, weight loss.

Overdose and treatment
Symptoms of overdose include agitation, restlessness, hypomania, and other signs of CNS excitation; and, in patients who took higher doses of fluoxetine, nausea and vomiting. Among approximately 38 reports of acute overdose with fluoxetine, two fatalities involved plasma concentrations of 4.57 mg/liter and 1.93 mg/liter. One involved 1.8 g of fluoxetine with an undetermined amount of maprotiline; another death involved combined ingestion of fluoxetine, codeine, and temazepam. One other patient developed two tonic-clonic seizures after taking 3 g of fluoxetine; these seizures remitted spontaneously and did not require treatment with anticonvulsants.

To treat fluoxetine overdose, establish and maintain an airway; ensure adequate oxygenation and ventilation. Activated charcoal, which may be used with sorbitol, may be as effective as emesis or lavage.

Monitor cardiac and vital signs, and provide usual supportive measures. Fluoxetine-induced seizures that do not subside spontaneously may respond to diazepam. Forced diuresis, dialysis, hemoperfusion, and exchange transfusion are unlikely to be of benefit.

▶ Special considerations
- Consider the inherent risk of suicide until significant improvement of depressive state occurs. High-risk patients should have close supervision during initial drug therapy. To reduce risk of suicidal overdose, prescribe the smallest quantity of pulvules consistent with good management.
- Full antidepressant effect may be delayed until 4 weeks of treatment or longer.
- Treatment of acute depression usually requires at least several months of continuous drug therapy; optimal duration of therapy has not been established.
- Because of its long elimination half-life, changes in fluoxetine dosage will not be reflected in plasma for several weeks, affecting titration to final dose and withdrawal from treatment.
- Impaired hepatic function can delay the elimination of fluoxetine and its metabolite norfluoxetine, prolong-

---

ing the drug's elimination half-life. Therefore, use fluoxetine with caution in patients with liver disease.
● In patients with severely impaired renal function, chronic administration of fluoxetine is associated with significant accumulation of this drug or its metabolites.
● Prescribe lower or less frequent dosage in patients with renal or hepatic impairment. Also consider lower or less frequent dosage in elderly patients and others with concurrent disease or multiple drug therapy.

Information for the patient
● Tell patient drug may cause dizziness or drowsiness. Patient should avoid hazardous tasks that require alertness until CNS response to drug is established.
● Tell patient to avoid ingestion of alcohol and to seek medical approval before taking other drugs.
● Tell patient to promptly report rash or hives, anxiety or nervousness, anorexia (especially in underweight patients), suspicion of pregnancy, or intent to become pregnant.

---

fluoxymesterone
Android-F, Halotestin, Hysterone, Oratestryl

● Pharmacologic classification: androgen
● Therapeutic classification: androgen replacement, antineoplastic
● Controlled substance schedule III
● Pregnancy risk category X

How supplied
Available by prescription only
Tablets: 2 mg, 5 mg, 10 mg

Indications, route, and dosage
Male hypogonadism
Adults: 5 to 20 mg P.O. daily, in a single dose or in three or four divided doses.
Palliation of breast cancer in women
Adults: 10 to 40 mg P.O. daily in three or four divided doses.
Postpartum breast engorgement
Adults: 2.5 mg P.O. shortly after parturition followed by 5 to 10 mg daily for 4 to 5 days in divided doses.
†Stimulation of erythropoiesis
Adults: 10 mg P.O. b.i.d. Doses up to 40 mg daily have been used.

Pharmacodynamics
● *Androgenic action:* Fluoxymesterone mimics the action of the endogenous androgen testosterone by stimulating receptors in androgen-responsive organs and tissues. It exerts inhibitory, anti-estrogenic effects on hormone-responsive breast tumors and metastases.
● *Antianemic action:* Fluoxymesterone enhances the production of erythropoietic stimulating factors, thereby increasing the production of red blood cells.

Pharmacokinetics
Fluoxymesterone is eliminated primarily by hepatic metabolism. Its pharmacokinetics are otherwise described poorly.

Contraindications and precautions
Fluoxymesterone is contraindicated in patients with severe renal or cardiac disease (fluid and sodium retention caused by fluoxymesterone may aggravate renal and cardiac disease); in patients with hepatic disease, because impaired elimination of the drug may cause this accumulation; in male patients with prostate or breast cancer or benign prostatic hypertrophy with obstruction; in patients with undiagnosed abnormal genital bleeding, because drug can stimulate the growth of cancerous breast or prostate tissue; in pregnant and breast-feeding women, because animal studies have shown that administration of androgens during pregnancy causes masculinization of the fetus; and in patients with known hypersensitivity to the drug.
The brands Halotestin and Oratestryl contain the dye tartrazine. Rare individuals, particularly those who are known to be sensitive to aspirin and who have nasal polyps, may suffer severe hypersensitivity reactions (for example, anaphylaxis) after ingesting tartrazine.

Interactions
In patients with diabetes, decreased blood glucose levels may require adjustment of insulin or oral hypoglycemic drug dosage.
Fluoxymesterone may potentiate the action of anticoagulants, resulting in increased prothrombin time. Concurrent administration with oxyphenbutazone may increase serum oxyphenbutazone concentrations.

Effects on diagnostic tests
Fluoxymesterone may cause abnormal results of the glucose tolerance test. Thyroid function test results (protein-bound iodine, radioactive iodine uptake, thyroid-binding capacity) may decrease. Prothrombin time (especially in patients on anticoagulant therapy) may be prolonged. Abnormal liver function test may occur. Because of this agent's anabolic activity, serum sodium, potassium, calcium, phosphate, and cholesterol levels may all rise.

Adverse reactions
● Androgenic: *in females:* deepening of voice, clitoral enlargement, changes in libido; *in males:* prepubertal – premature epiphyseal closure, priapism, phallic enlargement; postpubertal – testicular atrophy, oligospermia, decreased ejaculatory volume, impotence, gynecomastia, epididymitis.
● CNS: headache, anxiety, mental depression, generalized paresthesia.
● CV: edema.
● DERM: acne, oily skin, hirsutism, flushing, sweating, male pattern baldness.
● GI: gastroenteritis, nausea, vomiting, diarrhea, constipation, change in appetite, weight gain.
● GU: bladder irritability, priapism, virilization in females, vaginitis, menstrual irregularities.
● HEMA: polycythemia; *suppression of clotting factors II, V, VII, and X.*
● Hepatic: cholestatic hepatitis, *jaundice.*
● Other: hypercalcemia, *hepatocellular cancer* (with long-term use).
Note: Drug should be discontinued if hypercalcemia, edema, hypersensitivity reaction, priapism, or excessive sexual stimulation develops; or if virilization occurs in females.

Overdose and treatment
No information available.

▶ Special considerations
Besides those relevant to all *androgens*, consider the following recommendations.
● Observe female patients carefully for signs of excessive virilization. If possible, therapy should be discontinued at the first sign of virilization because some adverse effects (deepening of the voice, clitoral enlargement) are not reversible.
● Patients with metastatic breast cancer should have regular determinations of serum calcium levels to identify potential for serious hypercalcemia.
● When drug is used in breast cancer, subjective effects may not appear for about 1 month; objective improvement not for 3 months.
● Watch for symptoms of hypoglycemia in patients with diabetes. Dosage of antidiabetic drug may need adjustment.
● If patient is receiving anticoagulants concurrently with fluoxymesterone, monitor for ecchymoses, petechiae, and other signs of bleeding.
● Halotestin and Oratestryl contain tartrazine. Observe for signs of allergic reactions in patients sensitive to aspirin or tartrazine.

Information for the patient
● Explain to patient on drug for palliation of breast cancer that virilization usually occurs at dosage used. Tell patient to report androgenic effects immediately. Stopping drug will prevent further androgenic changes but probably will not reverse those already present.
● Tell female patient to report menstrual irregularities; discontinue therapy pending etiologic determination.
● Advise male patient to report overly frequent or persistent penile erections.
● Advise patient to report persistent GI distress, diarrhea, or the onset of jaundice.

Geriatric use
Use with caution. Observe elderly male patients for the development of prostatic hypertrophy. Development of symptomatic prostatic hypertrophy or prostatic cancer mandates discontinuing the drug.

Pediatric use
Fluoxymesterone should be used with extreme caution in pediatric patients to avoid precocious puberty and premature closure of the epiphyses. X-ray examinations every 6 months are recommended to assess skeletal maturation.

Breast-feeding
Because of potential adverse effects on the infant, a decision should be made to discontinue breast-feeding or to discontinue the drug, depending on the woman's need for the drug.

---

fluphenazine decanoate
Modecate Decanoate*, Prolixin Decanoate

fluphenazine enanthate
Moditen Enanthate*, Prolixin Enanthate

fluphenazine hydrochloride
Permitil Hydrochloride, Prolixin Hydrochloride

● Pharmacologic classification: phenothiazine (piperazine derivative)
● Therapeutic classification: antipsychotic
● Pregnancy risk category C

How supplied
Available by prescription only
Fluphenazine hydrochloride
Tablets: 1 mg, 2.5 mg, 5 mg, 10 mg
Oral concentrate: 5 mg/ml (contains 14% alcohol)
Elixir: 2.5 mg/5 ml (with 14% alcohol)
I.M. injection: 2.5 mg/ml
Fluphenazine enanthate
Depot injection: 25 mg/ml
Fluphenazine decanoate
Depot injection: 25 mg/ml

Indications, route, and dosage
Psychotic disorders
Adults: Initially, 0.5 to 10 mg fluphenazine hydrochloride P.O. daily in divided doses q 6 to 8 hours; may increase cautiously to 20 mg. Maintenance dosage is 1 to 5 mg P.O. daily. I.M. doses are one third to one half that of oral doses. Lower doses for geriatric patients (1 to 2.5 mg daily).
Adults and children over age 12: 12.5 to 25 mg of long-acting esters (fluphenazine decanoate and enanthate) I.M. or S.C. q 1 to 6 weeks. Maintenance dosage is 25 to 100 mg, p.r.n.
Children age 12 and under: 0.25 to 3.5 mg fluphenazine hydrochloride P.O. daily in divided doses q 4 to 6 hours; or one third to one half of oral dose I.M.; maximum dosage is 10 mg daily.

Pharmacodynamics
Antipsychotic action: Fluphenazine is thought to exert its antipsychotic effects by postsynaptic blockade of CNS dopamine receptors, thereby inhibiting dopamine-mediated effects.
  Fluphenazine has many other central and peripheral effects; it produces both alpha and ganglionic blockade and counteracts histamine- and serotonin-mediated activity. Its most prominent adverse reactions are extrapyramidal.

Pharmacokinetics
● *Absorption:* Rate and extent of absorption vary with route of administration; oral tablet absorption is erratic and variable. Oral and I.M. dosages have an onset of action within ½ to 1 hour. Long-acting decanoate and enanthate salts act within 24 to 72 hours.
● *Distribution:* Fluphenazine is distributed widely into the body, including breast milk. CNS concentrations are usually higher than those in plasma. Drug is 91% to

---

99% protein-bound. Peak effects of oral dose usually occur at 2 hours; steady-state serum levels are achieved within 4 to 7 days.
- *Metabolism:* Fluphenazine is metabolized extensively by the liver, but no active metabolites are formed; duration of action is about 6 to 8 hours after oral administration; 1 to 6 weeks (average, 2 weeks) after I.M. depot administration.
- *Excretion:* Most of drug is excreted in urine via the kidneys; some is excreted in feces via the biliary tract.

Contraindications and precautions
Fluphenazine is contraindicated in patients with known hypersensitivity to phenothiazines and related compounds, including allergic reactions involving hepatic function; in patients with blood dyscrasias and bone marrow depression because of possible agranulocytosis; in patients with disorders accompanied by coma, brain damage, or CNS depression because of additive CNS depression; in patients with circulatory collapse or cerebrovascular disease because of its hypotensive effect; and for use with adrenergic blocking agents or spinal or epidural anesthetics because of potential hypotension and alpha blockade.

Fluphenazine should be used cautiously in patients with cardiac disease (arrhythmias, congestive heart failure, angina pectoris, valvular disease, or heart block), encephalitis, Reye's syndrome, head injury, respiratory disease, epilepsy and other seizure disorders, glaucoma, prostatic hypertrophy, urinary retention, hepatic or renal dysfunction, Parkinson's disease, pheochromocytoma, or hypocalcemia. Some oral preparations of fluphenazine contain tartrazine; use of such products may cause allergic reaction in patients with aspirin allergy.

Interactions
Concomitant use of fluphenazine with sympathomimetics, including epinephrine, phenylephrine, phenylpropanolamine, and ephedrine (often found in nasal sprays), and appetite suppressants may decrease their stimulatory and pressor effects.

Fluphenazine may inhibit blood pressure response to centrally acting antihypertensive drugs such as guanethidine, guanabenz, guanadrel, clonidine, methyldopa, and reserpine. Additive effects are likely after concomitant use of fluphenazine with CNS depressants, including alcohol, analgesics, barbiturates, narcotics, tranquilizers, and general, spinal, or epidural anesthetics, or parenteral magnesium sulfate (oversedation, respiratory depression, and hypotension); antiarrhythmic agents, quinidine, disopyramide, and procainamide (increased incidence of cardiac arrhythmias and conduction defects); atropine or other anticholinergic drugs, including antidepressants, monoamine oxidase inhibitors, phenothiazines, antihistamines, meperidine, and antiparkinsonian agents (oversedation, paralytic ileus, visual changes, and severe constipation); nitrates (hypotension); and metrizamide (increased risk of convulsions).

Beta-blocking agents may inhibit fluphenazine metabolism, increasing plasma levels and toxicity.

Concomitant use with propylthiouracil increases risk of agranulocytosis; concomitant use with lithium may result in severe neurologic toxicity with an encephalitis-like syndrome, and a decreased therapeutic response to fluphenazine.

Pharmacokinetic alterations and subsequent decreased therapeutic response to fluphenazine may follow concomitant use with phenobarbital (enhanced renal excretion), aluminum- and magnesium-containing antacids and antidiarrheals (decreased absorption), or caffeine, and with heavy smoking (increased metabolism).

Fluphenazine may antagonize therapeutic effect of bromocriptine on prolactin secretion; it also may decrease the vasoconstricting effects of high-dose dopamine, and may decrease effectiveness and increase toxicity of levodopa (by dopamine blockade). Fluphenazine may inhibit metabolism and increase toxicity of phenytoin and tricyclic antidepressants.

Effects on diagnostic tests
Fluphenazine causes false-positive test results for urinary porphyrins, urobilinogen, amylase, and 5-hydroxyindoleacetic acid (5-HIAA), because of darkening of urine by metabolites; it also causes false-positive urine pregnancy test results using human chorionic gonadotropin.

Fluphenazine elevates test results for liver enzymes and protein-bound iodine, and causes quinidine-like ECG effects.

Adverse reactions
- CNS: extrapyramidal symptoms—dystonia, akathisia, torticollis, tardive dyskinesia, sedation (low incidence), pseudoparkinsonism, drowsiness (frequent), *neuroleptic malignant syndrome* (dose-related; *fatal respiratory failure* in over 10% of patients if untreated), dizziness, headache, insomnia, exacerbation of psychotic symptoms.
- CV: *asystole,* orthostatic hypotension, tachycardia, dizziness and fainting, arrhythmias, ECG changes, increased anginal pain after I.M. injection.
- EENT: blurred vision, tinnitus, mydriasis, increased intraocular pressure, ocular changes (retinal pigmentary change with long-term use).
- GI: dry mouth, constipation, nausea, vomiting, anorexia, diarrhea.
- GU: urine retention, gynecomastia, hypermenorrhea, inhibited ejaculation.
- HEMA: transient leukopenia, *agranulocytosis,* thrombocytopenia, anemia (within 30 to 90 days).
- Local: contact dermatitis from concentrate or injectable form, muscle necrosis from I.M. injection.
- Other: hyperprolactinemia, photosensitivity, increased appetite or weight gain, hypersensitivity (rash, urticaria, drug fever, edema, cholestatic jaundice [in 0.1% to 4% of patients within first 30 days]), decreased libido.

After abrupt withdrawal of long-term therapy, patient may develop gastritis, nausea, vomiting, dizziness, tremors, feeling of heat or cold, sweating, tachycardia, headache or insomnia.

Note: Drug should be discontinued immediately if any of the following occurs: hypersensitivity, jaundice, agranulocytosis, neuroleptic malignant syndrome (marked hyperthermia, extrapyramidal effects, autonomic dysfunction), or if severe extrapyramidal symptoms occur even after dosage is lowered. Drug should be discontinued 48 hours before and 24 hours after myelography utilizing metrizamide because of the risk of convulsions. When feasible, drug should be withdrawn slowly and gradually; many drug effects persist after withdrawal.

---

*Canada only   †Unlabeled clinical use   Italicized adverse reactions are life-threatening.

Overdose and treatment

CNS depression is characterized by deep, unarousable sleep and possible coma, hypotension or hypertension, extrapyramidal symptoms, dystonia, abnormal involuntary muscle movements, agitation, seizures, arrhythmias, ECG changes, hypothermia or hyperthermia, and autonomic nervous system dysfunction.

Treatment is symptomatic and supportive, including maintaining vital signs, airway, stable body temperature, and fluid and electrolyte balance.

Do not induce vomiting: drug inhibits cough reflex, and aspiration may occur. Use gastric lavage, then activated charcoal and saline cathartics; dialysis does not help. Regulate body temperature as needed. Treat hypotension with I.V. fluids: *do not give epinephrine.* Treat seizures with parenteral diazepam or barbiturates; arrhythmias with parenteral phenytoin (1 mg/kg with rate titrated to blood pressure); extrapyramidal reactions with benztropine or parenteral diphenhydramine at 2 mg/kg/minute.

▶ **Special considerations**
Besides those relevant to all *phenothiazines,* consider the following recommendations.
● Note that depot injection (25 mg/ml) and I.M. injection (2.5 mg/ml) are not interchangeable.
● The depot injection form is not recommended for patients who are not stabilized on a phenothiazine. This form has a prolonged elimination; its action could not be terminated in case of adverse reactions.

Information for the patient
● Tell patient drug may cause dizziness or drowsiness. Patient should avoid hazardous tasks that require alertness until CNS response to drug is established.
● Tell patient to avoid ingestion of alcohol and to seek medical approval before taking other drugs.
● Tell patient to promptly report rash or hives, anxiety or nervousness, anorexia (especially in underweight patients), suspicion of pregnancy, or intent to become pregnant.

Pediatric use
Fluphenazine may be used in children over age 6.

Breast-feeding
Fluphenazine enters breast milk. Caution should be observed, and the potential benefits to the mother should outweigh the potential harm to the infant.

flurandrenolide
Cordran, Cordran SP, Drenison*

● Pharmacologic classification: topical adrenocorticoid
● Therapeutic classification: anti-inflammatory
● Pregnancy risk category C

How supplied
Available by prescription only
Cream: 0.025%, 0.05%
Lotion: 0.05%
Ointment: 0.025%, 0.05%
Tape: 4 mcg/cm²

Indications, route, and dosage
Inflammation of corticosteroid-responsive dermatoses
Adults and children: Apply cream, lotion, or ointment sparingly b.i.d. or t.i.d. Apply tape q 12 hours.

Occlusive dressings may be used for severe or resistant dermatoses. The tape is usually applied as an occlusive dressing to clean, dry affected areas.

Pharmacodynamics
Anti-inflammatory action: Flurandrenolide stimulates the synthesis of enzymes needed to decrease the inflammatory response. Depending on strength, flurandrenolide is either a group III (0.05%) or group IV (0.025%) fluorinated glucocorticoid.

Pharmacokinetics
● *Absorption:* The amount absorbed depends on the strength of the preparation, the amount applied, and the nature of the skin at the application site. It ranges from about 1% in areas with a thick stratum corneum (such as the palms, soles, elbows, and knees) to as high as 36% in areas of the thinnest stratum corneum (face, eyelids, and genitals). Absorption increases in areas of skin damage, inflammation, or occlusion. Some systemic absorption may occur, especially through the oral mucosa.
● *Distribution:* After topical application, drug is distributed throughout the local skin. Any drug that is absorbed into circulation is removed rapidly from the blood and distributed into muscle, liver, skin, intestines, and kidneys.
● *Metabolism:* After topical administration, flurandrenolide is metabolized primarily in the skin. The small amount that is absorbed into systemic circulation is metabolized primarily in the liver to inactive compounds.
● *Excretion:* Inactive metabolites are excreted by the kidneys, primarily as glucuronides and sulfates, but also as unconjugated products. Small amounts of the metabolites are also excreted in feces.

Contraindications and precautions
Flurandrenolide is contraindicated in patients who are hypersensitive to any component of the preparation and in patients with viral, fungal, or tubercular skin lesions.

Flurandrenolide should be used with extreme caution in patients with impaired circulation because it may increase the risk of skin ulceration.

Avoid using on the face or genital areas because increased absorption may result in striae.

Interactions
None significant.

Effects on diagnostic tests
None significant.

Adverse reactions
● Local: burning, itching, irritation, dryness, folliculitis, hypertrichosis, acneiform eruptions, hypopigmentation, perioral dermatitis, allergic contact dermatitis, maceration, secondary infection, atrophy, striae, miliaria.

Significant systemic absorption can produce the following reactions.
● CNS: euphoria, insomnia, headache, psychotic behavior, pseudotumor cerebri, mental changes, nervousness, restlessness.
● CV: *congestive heart failure,* hypertension, edema.

- EENT: cataracts, glaucoma, thrush.
- GI: peptic ulcer, irritation, increased appetite.
- Immune: immunosuppression, increased susceptibility to infection.
- Metabolic: hypokalemia, sodium retention, fluid retention, weight gain, hyperglycemia, osteoporosis, growth suppression in children.
- Musculoskeletal: muscle atrophy.
- Other: withdrawal syndrome (nausea, fatigue, anorexia, dyspnea, hypotension, hypoglycemia, myalgia, arthralgia, fever, dizziness, and fainting).

Note: Drug should be discontinued if local irritation, infection, systemic absorption, or hypersensitivity reaction occurs.

Overdose and treatment
No information available.

▶ Special considerations
Recommendations for use of flurandrenolide, for care and teaching of patients during therapy, and for use in elderly patients, children, and breast-feeding women are the same as those for all *topical adrenocorticoids*.

---

flurazepam hydrochloride
Apo-Flurazepam*, Dalmane, Durapam, Novoflupam*, Som-Pam*, Somnol*

- Pharmacologic classification: benzodiazepine
- Therapeutic classification: sedative-hypnotic
- Controlled substance schedule IV
- Pregnancy risk category D

How supplied
Available by prescription only
Capsules: 15 mg, 30 mg

Indications, route, and dosage
Insomnia
Adults: 15 to 30 mg P.O. h.s. May repeat dose once after 1 hour (but after 2 a.m.)
Adults over age 65: 15 mg P.O. h.s.

Pharmacodynamics
Sedative action: Flurazepam depresses the CNS at the limbic and subcortical levels of the brain. It produces a sedative effect by potentiating the effect of the neurotransmitter gamma-aminobutyric acid (GABA) on its receptor in the ascending reticular activating system, which increases inhibition and blocks both cortical and limbic arousal.

Pharmacokinetics
- *Absorption:* When administered orally, flurazepam is absorbed rapidly through the GI tract. Onset of action occurs within 20 minutes, with peak action in 1 to 2 hours. The duration of action is 7 to 10 hours.
- *Distribution:* Flurazepam is distributed widely throughout the body. Approximately 97% of an administered dose is bound to plasma protein.
- *Metabolism:* Flurazepam is metabolized in the liver to the active metabolite desalkylflurazepam.
- *Excretion:* Desalkylflurazepam is excreted in urine. It has a half-life of 50 to 100 hours.

Contraindications and precautions
Flurazepam is contraindicated in patients with known hypersensitivity to the drug; in patients with acute narrow-angle glaucoma or untreated open-angle glaucoma, because of the drug's possible anticholinergic effect; in patients in shock or coma, because the drug's hypnotic or hypotensive effect may be prolonged or intensified; and in patients with acute alcohol intoxication who have depressed vital signs, because the drug will worsen CNS depression.

Flurazepam should be used cautiously in patients with psychoses, because the drug is rarely beneficial in such patients and may induce paradoxical reactions; in patients with myasthenia gravis or Parkinson's disease, because it may exacerbate the disorder; in patients with impaired renal or hepatic function, which prolongs elimination of the drug; in elderly or debilitated patients, who are usually more sensitive to the drug's CNS effects; and in individuals prone to addiction or drug abuse.

Interactions
Flurazepam potentiates the CNS depressant effects of phenothiazines, narcotics, barbiturates, alcohol, antihistamines, monoamine oxidase inhibitors, general anesthetics, and antidepressants.

Concomitant use with cimetidine and possibly disulfiram causes diminished hepatic metabolism of flurazepam, which increases its plasma concentration.

Heavy smoking accelerates flurazepam's metabolism, thus lowering clinical effectiveness.

Benzodiazepines may decrease plasma levels of haloperidol.

Flurazepam may decrease the therapeutic effects of levodopa.

Effects on diagnostic tests
Flurazepam therapy may elevate liver function test results. Minor changes in EEG patterns, usually low-voltage, fast activity, may occur during and after flurazepam therapy.

Adverse reactions
- CNS: confusion, depression, drowsiness, lethargy, daytime sedation, disturbed coordination, hangover effect, ataxia, dizziness, syncope, nightmares, fatigue, slurred speech, tremors, vertigo, headache.
- CV: palpitations, chest pains, tachycardia, hypotension (rare).
- DERM: rash (rare), flushing, sweating, urticaria.
- EENT: diplopia, blurred vision, nystagmus.
- GI: constipation, dry mouth, taste alterations, anorexia, nausea, vomiting, abdominal discomfort.
- GU: urinary incontinence or retention.
- HEMA: leukopenia, granulocytopenia (rare).
- Hepatic: hepatic dysfunction.
- Other: *respiratory depression,* dysarthria, changes in libido.

Note: Drug should be discontinued if hypersensitivity or the following paradoxical reactions occur: acute hyperexcited state, anxiety, hallucinations, increased muscle spasticity, insomnia, or rage.

Overdose and treatment
Clinical manifestations of overdose include somnolence, confusion, hypoactive reflexes, dyspnea, labored breathing, hypotension, bradycardia, slurred speech, unsteady gait or impaired coordination and, eventually, coma.

Support blood pressure and respiration until drug effects subside; monitor vital signs. Mechanical ventilatory assistance via endotracheal tube may be required to maintain a patent airway and support adequate oxygenation. Use I.V. fluids to promote diuresis and vasopressors such as dopamine and phenylephrine to treat hypotension, as needed.

If the patient is conscious, induce emesis. Use gastric lavage if ingestion was recent, but only if an endotracheal tube is present to prevent aspiration. After emesis or lavage, administer activated charcoal with a cathartic as a single dose. Dialysis is of limited value. Do not use barbiturates if excitation occurs to avoid exacerbation of excitatory state or potentiation of CNS depressant effects.

▶ **Special considerations**
Besides those relevant to all *benzodiazepines*, consider the following recommendations.
● Studies have demonstrated a "carryover effect." The drug is most effective after 3 or 4 nights of use because of the long half-life. Do not increase dose more frequently than every 5 days.
● Monitor hepatic function, and AST (SGOT), ALT (SGPT), bilirubin, and alkaline phosphatase levels for changes.
● Flurazepam is useful for patients who have trouble falling asleep and who awaken frequently at night and early in the morning.
● Although prolonged use is not recommended, this drug has proven effective for up to 4 weeks of continuous use.
● Rapid withdrawal after prolonged use can cause withdrawal symptoms.
● Lower doses are effective in patients with renal or hepatic dysfunction.
● Store in a cool, dry place, away from light.

Information for the patient
● Advise patients to avoid alcohol while taking flurazepam.
● Advise female patient not to take the drug if she is pregnant. If she suspects pregnancy, she should contact her physician immediately.
● Emphasize the potential for excessive CNS depression if this drug is taken with alcohol, even if the drug is taken the evening before ingestion of alcohol.

Geriatric use
● Elderly patients are more susceptible to the CNS depressant effects of flurazepam. They may require assistance and supervision with walking and daily activities during initiation of therapy or after an increase in dose.
● Lower doses usually are effective in elderly patients because of decreased elimination.

Pediatric use
● Closely observe a neonate for withdrawal symptoms if the mother took flurazepam during pregnancy. Use of flurazepam during labor may cause neonatal flaccidity.
● Not for use in children under age 15.
● Neonates are more sensitive to flurazepam because of slower metabolism. The possibility of toxicity is greatly increased.

Breast-feeding
Flurazepam is excreted in breast milk. A breast-fed infant may become sedated, have feeding difficulties, or lose weight. Avoid use in breast-feeding women.

flurbiprofen
Ansaid

● Pharmacologic classification: nonsteroidal anti-inflammatory, phenylalkanoic acid derivative
● Therapeutic classification: antiarthritic agent
● Pregnancy risk category B

How supplied
Available by prescription only
Tablets: 50 mg, 100 mg

Indications, route, and dosage
Rheumatoid arthritis and osteoarthritis
Adults: 200 to 300 mg P.O. daily, divided b.i.d. or t.i.d.
Dosage in renal failure
Patients with end-stage renal disease may exhibit accumulation of flurbiprofen metabolites, but the half-life of the parent compound is unchanged. Monitor patients closely and adjust dosage accordingly.

Pharmacodynamics
Anti-inflammatory action: A nonsteroidal anti-inflammatory drug (NSAID), flurbiprofen interferes with the synthesis of prostaglandins.

Pharmacokinetics
● *Absorption:* Well absorbed after oral administration, with peak levels occurring in about 1.5 hours. Administering with food alters the rate, but not extent, of absorption.
● *Distribution:* Flurbiprofen is highly bound (> 99%) to plasma proteins.
● *Metabolism:* Primarily in the liver. The major metabolite shows little anti-inflammatory activity.
● *Excretion:* Primarily in the urine. Average elimination half-life is 6.5 hours.

Contraindications and precautions
Contraindicated in patients with a history of an allergic response (including asthma or urticaria) to aspirin or NSAIDs.
Serious GI toxicity, including ulceration and hemorrhage, can occur at any time in patients receiving chronic NSAID therapy.

Interactions
Patients taking oral anticoagulants may exhibit increased bleeding tendencies. Monitor patients closely.
Aspirin may decrease flurbiprofen levels. Concomitant use is not recommended.
Flurbiprofen may decrease the effectiveness of diuretics. Monitor patients closely.
Antacids and food may decrease the rate, but not the extent, of absorption.

Effects on diagnostic tests
None reported.

Adverse reactions
● CNS: headache, anxiety, insomnia, increased reflexes, tremor, amnesia, asthenia, somnolence, malaise, depression, dizziness.
● CV: edema.
● DERM: rash.
● EENT: rhinitis, tinnitus, visual changes.
● GI: dyspepsia, diarrhea, abdominal pain, nausea, constipation, *GI bleeding*, flatulence, vomiting.
● GU: urinary tract infection.
● Hepatic: elevated liver enzymes.
● Other: weight changes.

Overdose and treatment
Overdosage has resulted in lethargy, coma, respiratory depression, epigastric pain and distress.
   Treatment should be supportive. Emptying the stomach by emesis or lavage would be of little use if the ingestion took place more than an hour before treatment, but is still recommended.

▶ Special considerations
Besides those relevant to all *NSAIDs,* consider the following recommendations.
● Patients with impaired hepatic or renal function and elderly or debilitated patients should be closely monitored and probably should receive lower doses. These patients may be at risk for renal toxicity. Periodically monitor renal function.
● Patients receiving long-term therapy should have periodic liver function studies, ophthalmologic examinations, and hematocrit determinations.

Information for the patient
● Teach patient the signs and symptoms of GI bleeding, and tell him to discontinue the drug and call promptly if these symptoms appear.
● Tell patient to take drug with food, milk, or antacid to minimize GI upset.
● Advise the patient to avoid hazardous activities that require alertness until the adverse CNS effects of the drug are known.
● Tell the patient to call immediately if edema, substantial weight gain, black stools, skin rash, itching, or visual disturbances occur.

Pediatric use
Safe use in children has not been established.

Breast-feeding
A breast-feeding woman taking 200 mg of flurbiprofen daily could deliver as much as 0.1 mg to the infant daily. Breast-feeding is not recommended during therapy with flurbiprofen.

flurbiprofen sodium
Ocufen Liquifilm

● Pharmacologic classification: nonsteroidal anti-inflammatory
● Therapeutic classification: ophthalmic anti-inflammatory, antimiotic
● Pregnancy risk category C

How supplied
Available by prescription only
Ophthalmic solution: 0.03%

Indications, route, and dosage
Inhibition of intraoperative miosis
Adults: Instill 1 drop into the eye(s) undergoing surgery approximately every ½ hour, beginning 2 hours before surgery. Give a total of 4 drops.

Pharmacodynamics
● *Anti-inflammatory action:* Flurbiprofen acts by inhibiting the cyclo-oxygenase enzyme that is essential in converting arachidonic acid to prostaglandin. When applied topically, it inhibits prostaglandin synthesis in the iris, ciliary body, and conjunctiva. It does not affect intraocular pressure or tonographic aqueous outflow resistance.
● *Antimiotic action:* Flurbiprofen inhibits or reduces miosis and possibly some manifestations of ocular inflammation induced by ocular trauma. When administered prophylactically, topical flurbiprofen inhibits intraoperative trauma-induced miosis. However, the drug has little, if any, effect, if administered after trauma-induced miosis is present. Flurbiprofen does not inhibit or reduce light-induced miosis.

Pharmacokinetics
● *Absorption:* No information is available concerning absorption after ophthalmic administration.
● *Distribution:* Flurbiprofen is at least 99% bound to plasma proteins. Whether flurbiprofen crosses the placenta or is distributed into breast milk is unknown.
● *Metabolism:* After ophthalmic administration, flurbiprofen is absorbed systemically and is metabolized primarily in the liver where it is converted mainly to inactive glucuronide and sulfate compounds.
● *Excretion:* Inactive metabolites are excreted by the kidneys, primarily as glucuronides and sulfates. The biological half-life of orally administered flurbiprofen is 6 to 10 hours.

Contraindications and precautions
Flurbiprofen is contraindicated in patients who are hypersensitive to any component of the preparation. Ophthalmic flurbiprofen is contraindicated in patients with active epithelial herpes simplex keratitis and should be used with extreme caution in patients with a history of this disorder, because it *may worsen* this condition and may delay wound healing. It should be used with caution in patients who may be affected adversely by a prolonged bleeding time, because flurbiprofen can inhibit platelet aggregation.
   Because of a potential for cross-sensitivity between flurbiprofen and aspirin or other nonsteroidal anti-inflammatory drugs (NSAIDs), flurbiprofen should be used

with particular caution in patients in whom aspirin or other NSAIDs may trigger asthma, rhinitis, or urticaria.

Interactions
None reported.

Effects on diagnostic tests
None reported.

Adverse reactions
● Eye: transient burning and/or stinging on administration.
Note: Drug should be discontinued if ophthalmic application causes excessive local irritation, prolonged bleeding time, or signs of hypersensitivity reaction.

Overdose and treatment
Overdosage ordinarily will not cause acute complications. After accidental ingestion, fluids are recommended to dilute the drug.

▶ **Special considerations**
Store away from heat in a dark, tightly closed container; protect drug from freezing.

Information for the patient
● Teach patient not to touch eye dropper to eye.
● Remind patient to keep drug container closed tightly.
● Advise patient not to use more drug than the amount prescribed or to use flurbiprofen for other eye problems unless prescribed.
● Instruct patient to discard drug when outdated or no longer needed.

Pediatric use
Safety and efficacy in children have not been established.

---

flutamide
Eulexin

● Pharmacologic classification: nonsteroidal antiandrogen
● Therapeutic classification: antineoplastic agent
● Pregnancy risk category D

How supplied
Available by prescription only
Capsules: 125 mg

Indication, route, and dosage
Treatment of metastatic prostatic carcinoma (stage D2) in combination with LHRH analogs, such as leuprolide acetate
Adults: 250 mg P.O. q 8 hours.

Pharmacodynamics
Antitumor action: Flutamide inhibits androgen uptake or prevents binding of androgens in nucleus of cells within target tissues. Prostatic carcinoma is known to be androgen-sensitive.

Pharmacokinetics
● *Absorption:* Rapid and complete absorption occurs after oral administration.

● *Distribution:* Studies in animals show that the drug concentrates in the prostate. The drug and its active metabolite is about 95% protein bound.
● *Metabolism:* rapid, with at least six metabolites identified. Over 97% of the drug is metabolized within 1 hour of administration.
● *Excretion:* Over 95% in the urine.

Contraindications and precautions
Flutamide is contraindicated in patients allergic to the drug.
Periodic liver tests should be performed in patients receiving prolonged therapy with flutamide. Animal studies indicate that flutamide may harm the fetus if administered to a pregnant woman.

Interactions
None reported.

Effects on diagnostic tests
Elevation of plasma testosterone and estradiol levels has been reported. Serum ALT (SGPT), AST (SGOT), bilirubin, and creatinine levels may be increased.

Adverse reactions
● CNS: loss of libido, drowsiness, confusion, nervousness.
● CV: edema, hypertension.
● DERM: rash, photosensitivity.
● GI: diarrhea, nausea, vomiting.
● GU: impotence.
● Metabolic: gynecomastia, elevation of hepatic enzymes, hepatitis.
● Other: hot flashes.

Overdose and treatment
No experience with overdose in humans has been reported. Dosage as high as 1,500 mg daily for 36 weeks has been reported without serious adverse effects.

▶ **Special considerations**
Explain to the patient that flutamide must be taken continuously with the agent used for medical castration (such as leuprolide acetate) to produce full benefit of therapy. Leuprolide suppresses testosterone production, while flutamide inhibits testosterone action at the cellular level. Together they can impair the growth of androgen-responsive tumors.

Information for the patient
● Tell patient not to discontinue either leuprolide or flutamide without medical approval.
● Explain to patient that some symptoms may worsen initially before they improve.

Pediatric use
Safe use in children has not been established.

Breast-feeding
It is unknown whether flutamide is excreted in breast milk. This drug is not indicated for breast-feeding women.

---

fluticasone propionate
Cutivate

- Pharmacologic classification: corticosteroid
- Therapeutic classification: topical anti-inflammatory
- Pregnancy risk category C

How supplied
Available by prescription only
Cream: 0.05%
Ointment: 0.005%

Indications, route, dosage
Relief of inflammation and pruritus of corticosteroid-responsive dermatoses
Adults: Apply sparingly to affected area b.i.d. and rub in gently and completely. Treatment beyond 2 consecutive weeks is not recommended; total dose should not exceed 50 g/week.

Pharmacodynamics
Anti-inflammatory action: Fluticasone stimulates synthesis of enzymes needed to decrease inflammation.

Pharmacokinetics
- *Absorption:* The amount of fluticasone absorbed depends on the the amount applied, application site, vehicle used, use of occlusive dressing, and integrity of epidermal barrier. Some systemic absorption does occur.
- *Distribution:* Fluticasone is distributed throughout the local skin.
- *Metabolism:* Fluticasone is metabolized primarily by the skin.
- *Excretion:* Information not available.

Contraindications and precautions
Fluticasone is contraindicated in patients with a history of hypersensitivity to it or any of its components, and in patients with viral, fungal, herpetic, or tubercular skin lesions. Use with caution in pediatric patients because of increased susceptibility for systemic absorption and toxicity.

Interactions
No significant interactions reported.

Effects on diagnostic tests
None significant.

Adverse reactions
- DERM: stinging, burning, itching, irritation, dryness, folliculitis, erythema, skin atrophy, leukoderma, vesicles, rash, hypertrichosis, acneiform eruptions, hypopigmentation, perioral dermatitis, allergic contact dermatitis, secondary infection, striae, milaria.
  Significant systemic absorption can produce the following reactions:
- CNS: euphoria, insomnia, headache, psychotic behavior, pseudotumor cerebri, mental changes, nervousness, restlessness.
- CV: CHF, hypertension, edema.
- EENT: cataracts, glaucoma, thrush.
- GI: peptic ulcer, irritation, increased appetite.

- Other: immunosuppression, increased susceptibility to infection, hypokalemia, sodium retention, fluid retention, weight gain, hyperglycemia, osteoporosis, muscular atrophy, growth suppression in children, withdrawal syndrome.
  Note: Drug should be discontinued if local irritation, systemic infection, systemic absorption, or hypersenstivity reactions occur.

▶ Special considerations
- Do not use for treatment of rosacea, perioral dermatitis, or acne.
- Mixing with other bases or vehicles may affect potency far beyond expectations.
- The risk of adverse reactions may be minimized by changing to a less potent agent.
- To cover the adult body one time requires 12 to 26 g.
- Use of more than 50 g weekly is not recommended.

Information for the patient
- Tell patient to apply agent sparingly and rub in lightly. Washing the area before application may increase drug penetration.
- Tell patient that if condition persists or worsens, or if burning or irritation develops, to notify physician.
- Tell patient to avoid prolonged use, contact with eyes or use around genital area, rectal area, on face and in skin creases.

Pediatric use
Children may be more susceptible to topical steroid-induced hypothalamic-pituitary-adrenal axis suppression as they may absorb proportionally larger amounts and be more susceptible to systemic toxicity. Do not exceed 15 g weekly.

Breast-feeding
Use with caution in women who are breast-feeding as it is unknown whether topical corticosteroids undergo sufficient absorption to produce systemic effects in the infant.

folic acid (vitamin B₉)
Folvite

- Pharmacologic classification: folic acid derivative
- Therapeutic classification: vitamin supplement
- Pregnancy risk category A (C if > recommended daily allowance [RDA])

How supplied
Available by prescription only
Injection: 10-ml vials (5 mg/ml with 1.5% benzyl alcohol or 10 mg/ml with 1.5% benzyl alcohol and 0.2% EDTA)
Tablets: 0.1 mg, 0.4 mg, 0.8 mg, 1 mg

Indications, route, and dosage
Megaloblastic or macrocytic anemia secondary to folic acid deficiency, hepatic disease, alcoholism, intestinal obstruction, excessive hemolysis
Pregnant and lactating women: 0.8 mg P.O., S.C., or I.M. daily.

Adults and children age 4 and older: 1 mg P.O., S.C., or I.M. daily for 4 to 5 days. After anemia secondary to folic acid deficiency is corrected, proper diet and RDA supplements are necessary to prevent recurrence.
Children under age 4: Up to 0.3 mg P.O., S.C., or I.M. daily.

Prevention of megaloblastic anemia of pregnancy and fetal damage
Adults: 1 mg P.O., S.C., or I.M. daily throughout pregnancy.

Nutritional supplement
Adults: 0.1 mg P.O., S.C., or I.M. daily.
Children: 0.05 mg P.O. daily.

Tropical sprue
Adults: 3 to 15 mg P.O. daily.

Test of megaloblastic anemia patients to detect folic acid deficiency without masking pernicious anemia
Adults and children: 0.1 to 0.2 mg P.O. or I.M. for 10 days while maintaining a diet low in folate and vitamin B_{12}. (Reticulosis, reversion to normoblastic hematopoiesis, and return to normal hemoglobin levels indicate folic acid deficiency.)

Pharmacodynamics
Nutritional action: Exogenous folate is required to maintain normal erythropoiesis and to perform nucleoprotein synthesis. Folic acid stimulates production of red and white blood cells and platelets in certain megaloblastic anemias.

Dietary folic acid is present in foods, primarily as reduced folate polyglutamate. This vitamin may be absorbed only after hydrolysis, reduction, and methylation occur in the GI tract. Conversion to active tetrahydrofolate may require vitamin B_{12}.

The oral synthetic form of folic acid is a monoglutamate and is absorbed completely after administration, even in malabsorption syndromes.

Pharmacokinetics
• Absorption: Folic acid is absorbed rapidly from the GI tract, mainly from the proximal part of the small intestine. Peak folate activity in blood occurs within 30 to 60 minutes after oral administration. Normal serum folate concentrations range from 0.005 to 0.015 mcg/ml. Usually, serum levels below 0.005 mcg/ml indicate folate deficiency; those below 0.002 mcg/ml usually result in megaloblastic anemia.
• Distribution: The active tetrahydrofolic acid and its derivatives are distributed into all body tissues; the liver contains about half of the total body folate stores. Folate is actively concentrated in the CSF. Folic acid is distributed into breast milk.
• Metabolism: Folic acid is metabolized in the liver to N^5-methyltetrahydrofolic acid, the main form of folate storage and transport.
• Excretion: A single 0.1-mg to 0.2-mg dose of folic acid usually results in only a trace amount of the drug in the urine. After administering large doses, excessive folate is excreted unchanged in urine. Small amounts of folic acid have been recovered in feces. About 0.05 mg/day of normal body folate stores is lost by a combination of urinary and fecal excretion and oxidative cleavage of the molecule.

Contraindications and precautions
Folic acid is contraindicated in patients with pernicious, aplastic, or normocytic anemias. Folic acid may ob-

scure the diagnosis of pernicious anemia, which can cause disabling neurologic complications.

Interactions
Concomitant use of folic acid (15 to 20 mg/day) decreases serum phenytoin levels to subtherapeutic concentrations, possibly with increased frequency of seizures. Folic acid appears to increase the metabolic clearance of phenytoin and cause redistribution of phenytoin in the CSF and brain.

Conversely, phenytoin and primidone may decrease serum folate levels and produce symptoms of folic acid deficiency in long-term therapy. Para-aminosalicylic acid and sulfasalazine may cause a similar deficiency. Although oral contraceptives may also impair folate metabolism and produce folate depletion, they are unlikely to induce anemia or megaloblastic changes.

Folic acid may interfere with the antimicrobial actions of pyrimethamine against toxoplasmosis.

Folic acid antagonists, pyrimethamine, trimethoprim, or triamterene may cause dihydrofolate reductase deficiency, which may interfere with folic acid utilization.

Effects on diagnostic tests
Folic acid therapy alters serum and erythrocyte folate concentrations; falsely low serum and erythrocyte folate levels may occur with the Lactobacillus casei assay in patients receiving anti-infectives, such as tetracycline, which suppress the growth of this organism.

Adverse reactions
• DERM: rash, pruritus, erythema.
• Other: allergic bronchospasm, general malaise, anaphylaxis.

Overdose and treatment
Folic acid is relatively nontoxic. Adverse GI and CNS effects have been reported rarely in patients receiving 15 mg of folic acid daily for 1 month.

▶ Special considerations
• The RDA for folic acid is 25 to 200 mcg in children and 180 to 200 mcg in adults; 100 mcg/day is considered an adequate oral supplement. Pregnant women require 400 mcg daily. During the first 6 months of lactation, women require 280 mcg daily; during the second 6 months, this requirement decreases to 260 mcg daily.
• Many drugs, such as oral contraceptives and alcohol, can cause folate deficiencies.
• Ensure that patients do not also have vitamin B_{12} deficiency; folic acid can improve hematologic measurements while allowing progression of neurologic damage. Do not use as sole treatment of pernicious anemia.
• Patients undergoing renal dialysis are at risk for folate deficiency.
• Monitor complete blood counts to measure effectiveness of drug treatment.
• Protect folic acid injections from light.

Information for the patient
• Teach patient about dietary sources of folic acid, such as yeast, whole grains, leafy vegetables, beans, nuts, and fruit.
• Tell patient that folate is destroyed by overcooking and canning.
• Stress the importance of administering folic acid only under medical supervision.

Breast-feeding
Folic acid is excreted in breast milk. Daily doses of 0.8 mg are sufficient to maintain a normo-blastic bone marrow after clinical symptoms have subsided and blood components have returned to normal.

---

foscarnet sodium (phosphonoformic acid)
Foscavir

- Pharmacologic classification: pyrophosphate analog
- Therapeutic classification: antiviral agent
- Pregnancy risk category C

How supplied
Injection: 24 mg/ml in 250-ml and 500-ml vials

Indications, route, and dosage
Cytomegalovirus (CMV) retinitis in patients with acquired immunodeficiency syndrome (AIDS)
Adults: Initially, 60 mg/kg I.V. as an induction treatment in patients with normal renal function. Administer as an I.V. infusion over 1 hour q 8 hours for 2 or 3 weeks, depending on clinical response. Follow with a maintenance infusion of 90 mg/kg daily administered over 2 hours; increase as needed and tolerated to 120 mg/kg daily if disease shows signs of progression.
Dosage adjustment in patients with renal failure
Adults: First, calculate patient's creatinine clearance from this equation:
for male patients: creatinine clearance = (140 − age)/(serum creatinine × 72).
for female patients: multiply the above value by 0.85
Administer according to the following table.
Induction dose

Creatinine clearance (ml/minute/kg)	Dose to be administered q 8 hours (mg/kg)
1.6	60
1.5	57
1.4	53
1.3	49
1.2	46
1.1	42
1	39
0.9	35
0.8	32
0.7	28
0.6	25
0.5	21
0.4	18

Maintenance dose

Creatinine clearance (ml/min/kg)	Equivalent to 90 mg/kg daily	Equivalent to 120 mg/kg daily
1.4	90	120
1.2 to 1.4	78	104
1 to 1.2	75	100
0.8 to 1	71	94
0.6 to 0.8	63	84
0.4 to 0.6	57	76

Pharmacodynamics
Antiviral action: An organic analog of pyrophosphate, a compound used in many enzymatic reactions, foscarnet inhibits all known herpesviruses in vitro by blocking the pyrophosphate binding site on DNA polymerases and reverse transcriptases.

Pharmacokinetics
- *Distribution:* Foscarnet is about 14% to 17% bound to plasma proteins. Animal studies indicate that the drug is deposited in bone.
- *Metabolism:* Unknown.
- *Excretion:* About 80% to 90% of drug appears in the urine unchanged. Drug clearance is dependent on renal function. Plasma half-life is about 3 hours.

Contraindications and precautions
Foscarnet is contraindicated in patients with hypersensitivity to the drug.

Use cautiously in patients with abnormal renal function because decreased renal function will result in accumulation of drug and enhanced toxicity. Because foscarnet is nephrotoxic, it has the potential to further worsen a patient's renal impairment. Some degree of nephrotoxicity occurs in most patients treated with drug. To minimize nephrotoxicity, patient must be adequately hydrated before and during the infusion.

Because drug is highly toxic and toxicity is probably dose related, the lowest effective maintenance dose should be used throughout therapy.

Administration of drug is associated with a transient decrease in ionized serum calcium. This decrease may not always be reflected in the patient's laboratory values, and it is caused by a direct chemical effect of the drug on serum calcium. This effect is dose related. Advise patients to report perioral tingling, numbness in the extremities, and paresthesia.

Creatinine clearance should be determined before therapy and frequently thereafter because of the drug's adverse effects on renal function. A baseline 24-hour creatinine clearance is recommended, followed by regular determinations. Recommended intervals are two to three times weekly during induction and at least every 1 to 2 weeks during maintenance therapy. If creatinine clearance drops to below 0.4 ml/minute/kg, discontinue drug.

Because drug can adversely affect important serum electrolytes, such as potassium, calcium, magnesium, and phosphorus, regular determinations of these electrolytes are recommended using a schedule similar to that established for creatinine clearance.

Interactions
Nephrotoxic drugs, such as amphotericin B and aminoglycosides, may increase risk of nephrotoxicity. Avoid concomitant use.

Pentamidine may increase the risk of nephrotoxicity; severe hypocalcemia has also been reported. Don't use together.

Zidovudine may increase the incidence or severity of anemia. Monitor blood counts.

Adverse reactions
● CNS: headache, *seizures*, fatigue, visual disturbances, rigors, malaise, asthenia, paresthesia, dizziness, hypesthesia, neuropathy, tremor, ataxia, generalized spasms, dementia, stupor, sensory disturbances, meningitis, aphagia, abnormal coordination, leg cramps, EEG abnormalities, vertigo, *coma*, encephalopathy, abnormal gait, hypertonia, visual field defects, dyskinesias, extrapyramidal reactions, speech disorders, paralysis, peripheral neuropathy, nystagmus, cerebral edema.
● CV: hypertension, palpitations, ECG abnormalities, sinus tachycardia, first-degree AV block, hypotension, flushing.
● DERM: rash, increased sweating, pruritus, skin ulceration, erythematous rash, seborrhea, skin discoloration.
● GI: nausea, diarrhea, vomiting, abdominal pain, anorexia, constipation, dysphagia, rectal hemorrhage, dry mouth, melena, flatulence, ulcerative stomatitis, pancreatitis.
● GU: *abnormal renal function*, decreased creatinine clearance and increased serum creatinine, albuminuria, dysuria, polyuria, urethral disorder, urine retention, urinary tract infections, *acute renal failure*.
● HEMA: anemia, granulocytopenia, leukopenia, *bone marrow suppression*, thrombocytopenia, platelet abnormalities, thrombocytosis, WBC abnormalities, lymphadenopathy.
● Respiratory: cough, dyspnea, pneumonitis, sinusitis, pharyngitis, rhinitis, respiratory insufficiency, pulmonary infiltration, stridor, pneumothorax, *bronchospasm*, hemoptysis.
● Other: fever, pain, infection, sepsis, hypokalemia, hypomagnesemia, hypophosphatemia or hyperphosphatemia, hypocalcemia.

▶ **Special considerations**
● Anemia is common (up to 33% of patients treated with drug) and may be severe enough to require transfusions.
● Do not exceed the recommended dosage, infusion rate, or frequency of administration. Know that all doses must be individualized according to patient's renal function.
● An infusion pump must be used to administer foscarnet.
● Unlike ganciclovir, foscarnet does not require cellular activation by thymidine kinase or other kinases. Foscarnet may be active against certain CMV strains resistant to ganciclovir.

Information for the patient
● Make sure patient understands that adverse reactions to drug are common and that he should report for all laboratory studies and follow-up appointments to check his progress.
● Advise patient to report perioral tingling, numbness in the extremities, and paresthesia.

Geriatric use
It is unknown if age alters drug response. However, elderly patients are likely to have preexisting renal function impairment, which requires alterations in dosage.

Pediatric use
Safety and efficacy in children have not been established. Postmortem studies in animals show that up to 40% of a dose is deposited in the teeth and bones. It is likely that similar deposition may be seen in growing children.

Breast-feeding
It is unknown if drug is excreted in human breast milk; however, animal studies indicate that drug may concentrate in breast milk when administered at high doses. Use with caution.

fosinopril sodium
Monopril

● Pharmacologic classification: angiotensin-converting enzyme inhibitor
● Therapeutic classification: antihypertensive
● Pregnancy risk category D

How supplied
Available by prescription only
Tablets: 10 mg, 20 mg

Indications, route, and dosage
Treatment of hypertension
Adults: Initially, 10 mg P.O. daily; adjust dose based on blood pressure response at peak and trough levels. Usual dose: 20 to 40 mg; maximum up to 80 mg. Dose may be divided.

Pharmacodynamics
Antihypertensive action: Fosinopril is believed to lower blood pressure primarily by suppressing the renin-angiotensin-aldosterone system, although it has also been effective in patients with low-renin hypertension.

Pharmacokinetics
● *Absorption:* Absorbed slowly through GI tract, primarily via proximal small intestine.
● *Distribution:* Greater than 95% protein-bound; peak concentrations are achieved in about 3 hours.
● *Metabolism:* Hydrolyzed primarily in the liver and gut wall by esterases.
● *Excretion:* 50% of the drug is excreted in urine; the remainder, in feces.

Contraindications and precautions
Fosinopril is contraindicated in patients hypersensitive to the drug or other angiotensin-converting enzyme (ACE) inhibitors. Use with caution in patients taking potassium-containing salts or sodium substitutes, in those with impaired liver function, and in those undergoing surgery.

Interactions
Excessive hypotension may occur with concurrent use of diuretics, especially if patient is volume depleted. Effect may be minimized by stopping diuretic or in-

creasing sodium intake before starting fosinopril. Concurrent use of potassium supplements or potassium-sparing diuretics may result in hyperkalemia; monitor potassium levels. When used with lithium, increased serum lithium levels and symptoms of lithium toxicity may occur; monitor lithium levels frequently. Risk is increased if diuretic is also used. Antacids may impair absorption of fosinopril; separate administration by at least 2 hours.

Effects on diagnostic tests

False low measurements of digoxin levels may result with the DIGI TAB radioimmunoassay kit for digoxin; other kits may be used. Transient elevations of BUN and serum creatinine levels and liver function tests and decreases in hematocrit or hemoglobin may also occur.

Adverse reactions

● CNS: headache, dizziness, fatigue, light-headedness, syncope, memory disturbances, mood change, paresthesia, sleep disturbance, drowsiness, weakness, *CVA.*
● CV: chest pain, angina, *MI,* hypertensive crisis, rhythm disturbances, palpitations, hypotension, flushing, claudication, orthostatic hypotension, *cardiac arrest.*
● DERM: urticaria, rash, photosensitivity, pruritus.
● EENT: tinnitus, vision disturbances, eye irritation.
● GI: nausea, vomiting, diarrhea, pancreatitis, hepatitis, dysphagia, abdominal distention, abdominal pain, flatulence, constipation, heartburn, appetite change, weight change, dry mouth.
● GU: sexual dysfunction, decreased libido, urinary frequency, renal insufficiency, *acute renal failure.*
● HEMA: *neutropenia, agranulocytosis, pancytopenia,* anemia, *thrombocytopenia.*
● Respiratory: cough, bronchospasm, pharyngitis, sinusitis, rhinitis, laryngitis, hoarseness, epistaxis.
● Other: angioedema, fever, arthralgia, musculoskeletal pain, myalgia, jaundice, gout.

Overdose and treatment

Human overdose has never been reported; however, the most common manifestation of overdose is likely to be hypotension. Treat with infusion of 0.9% sodium chloride. Hemodialysis and peritoneal dialysis are not effective in removing the drug.

▶ Special considerations

● Diuretic therapy is usually discontinued 2 to 3 days before the start of ACE inhibitor therapy to reduce the risk of hypotension. If fosinopril does not adequately control blood pressure, diuretic may be reinstituted with care. Monitor potassium levels.
● Perform CBC with differential counts before therapy, then every 2 weeks for 3 months and periodically thereafter.
● Food in the GI tract may slow absorption.
● Incidence of postural hypotension is low.
● Blood pressure is lowered within 1 hour of a single dose of 10 to 40 mg, with peak reductions occurring 2 to 6 hours after dose. The antihypertensive effect lasts 24 hours.
● Effectiveness of fosinopril is unaffected by age, sex, or weight.

Information for the patient

● Tell patient to take antacids 2 hours after dose.
● Recommend taking drug on an empty stomach – 1 hour before and 2 hours after meals.
● Tell patient to inform physician of any light-headedness in the first few days of therapy and of any signs of infection such as fever or sore throat. Patient should call physician and discontinue therapy immediately if any of the following effects occurs: swelling of tongue, lips, face, mucous membranes, eyes, lips, or extremities; difficulty swallowing or breathing; or hoarseness.
● Warn patient to avoid sudden position changes until effect of drug is known; however, postural hypotension is infrequent.

Geriatric use

No age-related differences have been observed.

Pediatric use

Safety and efficacy have not been established.

Breast-feeding

Avoid use; significant levels have been detected in breast milk.

---

fructose (levulose)

● Pharmacologic classification: carbohydrate
● Therapeutic classification: parenteral nutritional therapy, caloric agent
● Pregnancy risk category C

How supplied

Available by prescription only
Injection: 1,000 ml (10%)

Indications, route, and dosage

Source of carbohydrate calories primarily when fluid replacement is also indicated and as a dextrose substitute for patients with diabetes

Adults and children: Dosage depends on caloric needs. I.V. infusion rate should not exceed 1 g/kg/hour. Single liter of 10% solution yields 375 calories.

Pharmacodynamics

Metabolic action: Like dextrose, fructose is a monosaccharide that is metabolized rapidly; it is converted to glycogen more quickly than is dextrose. Insulin is not required for phosphorylation and conversion to glucose. Fructose is a source of carbohydrates that restores blood glucose levels, minimizes liver glycogen depletion, and exerts a protein-sparing action. Fructose undergoes oxidation to carbon dioxide and water, and this antiketogenic characteristic offers a valuable alternative to dextrose as a carbohydrate source in diabetic patients. I.V. infusion of fructose offers low serum glucose levels and less glycosuria than does dextrose. However, fructose may not be used to treat hypoglycemia because it tends to deplete hepatic adenosine triphosphate levels.

Fructose is metabolized mainly in the liver to fructose-1-phosphate. This then splits into D-glyceraldehyde and dihydroxyacetone phosphate by aldolase B.

The absence of this enzyme results in hereditary fructose intolerance.

Pharmacokinetics
• *Absorption:* Fructose is administered intravenously.
• *Distribution:* As a source of calories and water for hydration, fructose solutions expand plasma volume.
• *Metabolism:* Fructose is metabolized mainly in the liver.
• *Excretion:* Fructose may produce diuresis in some patients.

Contraindications and precautions
Fructose is contraindicated in patients with hereditary fructose intolerance. This may precipitate the reversible renal dysfunctions of Fanconi's syndrome. Clinical evaluation and periodic laboratory tests must be performed routinely while patients receive fructose therapy. Fluid balance, electrolyte concentrations, and acid-base balance must be monitored.

Use cautiously in patients with diabetes mellitus. When administered at a rate greater than 1 g/kg/hour, lactic acidosis may result from very rapid lactic acid production. Lactic acidosis also may occur with administration to patients with hepatic disease. Do not administer to patients with gout because of a possible increase in uric acid levels. Fluid or solute overload, resulting in dilution of serum electrolyte levels, overhydration, congestion, or pulmonary edema, may occur. Excessive administration of potassium-free solutions may result in hypokalemic states.

Interactions
Many drugs added to I.V. solutions may be incompatible. Consult appropriate tables or pharmacist before preparing admixtures. Administration of fructose without simultaneous administration of electrolytes and blood in the same infusion set may cause pseudoagglutination of red blood cells.

Effects on diagnostic tests
None reported.

Adverse reactions
• CV: increased pulse rate, precipitation or exacerbation of congestive heart failure (CHF) in susceptible patients, *pulmonary edema.*
• Hepatic: hepatomegaly.
• Metabolic: metabolic acidosis, hypervolemia.
• Local: extravasation at infusion site may cause sloughing of skin, thrombophlebitis.
• Other: increased respiratory rate.

Overdose and treatment
In case of overhydration or solute overload, reevaluate and correct therapy as appropriate.

▶ Special considerations
• Do not use in patients with hereditary fructose intolerance, hypoglycemia, or gout.
• Infusion rate should not exceed 1 g/kg/hour.
• Infusion sites should be checked frequently to avoid irritation and extravasation during long-term treatment, for redness, swelling, or irritation.
• Monitor patient for signs of fluid overload, pulmonary edema, and CHF. Watch for shortness of breath, increased pulse rate, or edema in the extremities.

Pediatric use
• Safety and efficacy of this solution have not been demonstrated in patients under age 12.
• Rapid administration may cause increased pulse and respiration rates and increased liver size in infants. Blood pH and carbon dioxide levels may decrease.

furazolidone
Furoxone

• Pharmacologic classification: nitrofuran derivative
• Therapeutic classification: antibacterial, antiprotozoal agent
• Pregnancy risk category C

How supplied
Available by prescription only
Tablets: 100 mg
Liquid: 50 mg/15 ml

Indications, route, and dosage
Gastroenteritis, adjunctive therapy in cholera
Adults: 100 mg P.O. q.i.d.
Children age 5 to 12: 25 to 50 mg P.O. q.i.d.
Treatment of bacterial or protozoal diarrhea and enteritis caused by susceptible organisms
Adults: 100 mg P.O. q.i.d.
Children age 5 and over: 25 to 50 mg P.O. q.i.d.
Children age 1 to 4: 17 to 25 mg P.O. q.i.d.
Infants age 1 month to 11 months: 8 to 17 mg P.O. q.i.d. Dosage based on 5 mg/kg daily; maximum dosage is 8.8 mg/kg/day. Duration of therapy should not exceed 7 days.

Pharmacodynamics
Antibacterial and antiprotozoal action: Furazolidone presumably works by inhibiting several vital enzymatic reactions; its activity includes monoamine oxidase (MAO) inhibition. Spectrum of activity includes many gram-positive and gram-negative enteric organisms, including *Vibrio cholerae.* It is also effective against protozoa, including *Giardia lamblia* and *Trichomonas.*

Pharmacokinetics
• *Absorption:* Furazolidone is absorbed poorly after oral administration and is inactivated in the intestine.
• *Distribution:* Distribution is unknown.
• *Metabolism:* Furazolidone is metabolized via intestinal degradation.
• *Excretion:* Furazolidone is excreted mainly in feces, with approximately 5% excreted in urine.

Contraindications and precautions
Furazolidone is contraindicated in infants under age 1 month because of the possibility of inducing hemolytic anemia, and in patients with known hypersensitivity to the drug.

Furazolidone should be administered cautiously to patients with glucose-6-phosphate dehydrogenase (G6PD) deficiency because it may cause hemolytic anemia.

Interactions
When used concomitantly with alcohol, furazolidone may lead to a disulfiram-type reaction, possibly causing

---

*Canada only   †Unlabeled clinical use   Italicized adverse reactions are life-threatening.

flushing, nausea, vomiting, hypotension, sweating, and tachycardia. Concomitant use with sympathomimetic drugs and tyramine-containing foods or beverages may lead to hypertensive crisis (from furazolidone's MAO-inhibiting properties). Concomitant use with tricyclic antidepressants may cause toxic psychosis.

Effects on diagnostic tests
Furazolidone therapy may cause false-positive results on some urine glucose tests using Benedict's reagent (for example, Clinitest).

Adverse reactions
- CNS: headache, malaise.
- GI: nausea and vomiting, colitis, pruritus ani.
- HEMA: hemolysis (with G6PD deficiency).
- Other: disulfiram-type reaction (with alcohol).
  Note: Drug should be discontinued if signs or symptoms of hemolytic anemia occur or if adverse effects become intolerable. Dosage reduction may alleviate nausea and vomiting.

Overdose and treatment
No information available.

▶ Special considerations
- Culture and sensitivity tests should be done before initiating therapy.
- Diarrhea usually resolves within 2 to 5 days after therapy begins.
- Monitor blood and urine tests in patients with G6PD deficiency.
- Store drug in dark place at 35.6° to 59° F. (2° to 15° C.).
- Drug may turn urine brown.

Information for the patient
- Instruct patient to continue taking drug exactly as directed, even if he feels better.
- Instruct patient to avoid beverages and medications containing alcohol during therapy and for 4 days afterward to avoid disulfiram-type reactions (nausea, sweating, flushing, tachycardia).
- If patient is taking high doses (more than 400 mg/day) or is on long-term therapy, advise him to avoid all drugs containing stimulants or decongestants and tyramine-rich foods and beverages.

Pediatric use
Furazolidone is contraindicated in infants under age 1 month because it increases the risk of drug-induced hemolytic anemia.

---

furosemide
Lasix, Novosemide*, SK-Furosemide, Uritol*

- Pharmacologic classification: loop diuretic
- Therapeutic classification: diuretic, antihypertensive
- Pregnancy risk category C

How supplied
Available by prescription only
Tablets: 20 mg, 40 mg, 80 mg
Solution: 10 mg/ml, 40 mg/5 ml

Injection: 10 mg/ml

Indications, route, and dosage
Acute pulmonary edema
Adults: 40 mg I.V. injected slowly; then 80 mg I.V. within 1 hour if needed.
Infants and children: 1 mg/kg I.M. or I.V. q 2 hours until response is achieved; maximum dosage is 6 mg/kg/day.
Edema
Adults: 20 to 80 mg P.O. daily in morning, with second dose given in 6 to 8 hours, carefully titrated up to 600 mg daily if needed; or 20 to 40 mg I.M. or I.V. Increase by 20 mg q 2 hours until desired response is achieved. I.V. dosage should be given slowly over 1 to 2 minutes.
Infants and children: 2 mg/kg/day, increased by 1 to 2 mg/kg in 6 to 8 hours if needed, carefully titrated not to exceed 6 mg/kg/day.
Hypertension
Adults: 40 mg P.O. b.i.d. Adjust dosage according to response.
Hypertensive crisis, acute renal failure
Adults: 100 to 200 mg I.V. over 1 to 2 minutes.
Chronic renal failure
Adults: Initially, 80 mg P.O. daily; increase by 80 to 120 mg daily until desired response is achieved.

Pharmacodynamics
- *Diuretic action:* Loop diuretics inhibit sodium and chloride reabsorption in the proximal part of the ascending loop of Henle, promoting the excretion of sodium, water, chloride, and potassium.
- *Antihypertensive action:* This drug effect may be the result of renal and peripheral vasodilatation and a temporary increase in glomerular filtration rate and a decrease in peripheral vascular resistance.

Pharmacokinetics
- *Absorption:* About 60% of a given furosemide dose is absorbed from the GI tract after oral administration. Food delays oral absorption but does not alter diuretic response. Diuresis begins in 30 to 60 minutes; peak diuresis occurs 1 to 2 hours after oral administration. Diuresis follows I.V. administration within 5 minutes and peaks in 20 to 60 minutes.
- *Distribution:* Furosemide is about 95% plasma protein-bound. It crosses the placenta and distributes into breast milk.
- *Metabolism:* Furosemide is metabolized minimally by the liver.
- *Excretion:* About 50% to 80% of a furosemide dose is excreted in urine; plasma half-life is about 30 minutes. Duration of action is 6 to 8 hours after oral administration and about 2 hours after I.V. administration.

Contraindications and precautions
Furosemide is contraindicated in patients with known hypersensitivity, anuria, hepatic coma, or electrolyte depletion and in the presence of rising BUN and serum creatinine levels or oliguria, even though it is used to produce diuresis in patients with renal impairment, because rapid fluid and electrolyte changes can exacerbate these conditions.

Furosemide should be used with caution in patients hypersensitive to sulfonamides; in patients with hepatic cirrhosis and ascites because changes in electrolyte balance may precipitate hepatic encephalopathy; and in patients receiving cardiac glycosides (digoxin, digitoxin) because furosemide-induced hypokalemia may

---

predispose them to digitalis toxicity. Rapid I.V. administration of furosemide increases risk of ototoxicity.

Interactions

Furosemide potentiates the hypotensive effect of most other antihypertensive agents and of other diuretics; both actions are used to therapeutic advantage.

Concomitant use with potassium-sparing diuretics (spironolactone, triamterene, amiloride) may decrease furosemide-induced potassium loss; use with other potassium-depleting drugs, such as steroids and amphotericin B, may cause severe potassium loss.

Furosemide may reduce renal clearance of lithium and increase lithium levels; lithium dosage may require adjustment.

Indomethacin and probenecid may reduce furosemide's diuretic effect; their combined use is not recommended. However, if there is no therapeutic alternative, an increased furosemide dosage may be required.

Concomitant administration of furosemide with ototoxic or nephrotoxic drugs may result in enhanced toxicity.

Furosemide could prolong neuromuscular blockade by muscle relaxants.

Patients receiving I.V. furosemide within 24 hours of a dose of chloral hydrate have experienced sweating, flushing, and blood pressure fluctuations; if possible, use an alternative sedative in patients receiving I.V. furosemide.

Effects on diagnostic tests

Furosemide therapy alters electrolyte balance and liver and renal function tests.

Adverse reactions

● CV: volume depletion and dehydration, orthostatic hypotension.
● DERM: dermatitis, photosensitivity.
● EENT: transient deafness with too-rapid I.V. injection.
● GI: abdominal discomfort and pain, diarrhea (with oral solution).
● HEMA: *agranulocytosis,* transient leukopenia, thrombocytopenia.
● Metabolic: hypochloremic alkalosis; asymptomatic hyperuricemia; fluid and electrolyte imbalances, including hypocalcemia, hypokalemia, hypomagnesemia, and hyponatremia; hyperglycemia; and impairment of glucose tolerance.
Note: Drug should be discontinued if dehydration or hypotension occurs or if BUN and creatinine levels rise.

Overdose and treatment

Clinical manifestations of overdose include profound electrolyte and volume depletion, which may precipitate circulatory collapse.

Treatment is chiefly supportive; replace fluids and electrolytes.

▶ Special considerations

Besides those relevant to all *loop diuretics,* consider the following recommendations.
● Give I.V. furosemide slowly, over 1 to 2 minutes, at a rate not to exceed 4 mg/minute; for I.V. infusion, dilute furosemide in dextrose 5% in water, normal saline solution, or lactated Ringer's solution, and use within 24 hours.
● Furosemide has been used to treat hypercalcemia

at dosages of 80 to 100 mg I.V., given every 1 to 2 hours.

Information for the patient

● Warn patient about photosensitivity reaction. Explain that this reaction is a photoallergy in which ultraviolet radiation alters drug structure, causing allergic reactions in some persons.
● Tell patient that photosensitivity reactions occur 10 days to 2 weeks after initial sun exposure.

Geriatric use

Elderly and debilitated patients require close observation because they are more susceptible to drug-induced diuresis. Excessive diuresis promotes rapid dehydration, leading to hypovolemia, hypokalemia, hyponatremia, and circulatory collapse. Reduced dosages may be indicated.

Pediatric use

Use furosemide with caution in neonates. The usual pediatric dosage can be used, but dosing intervals should be extended.

Sorbitol content of oral preparations may cause diarrhea, especially at high dosages.

Breast-feeding

Furosemide should not be used by breast-feeding women.

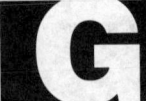

gallamine triethiodide
Flaxedil

- Pharmacologic classification: nondepolarizing neuromuscular blocking agent
- Therapeutic classification: skeletal muscle relaxant
- Pregnancy risk category C

How supplied
Available by prescription only
Injection: 20 mg/ml parenteral – for I.V. use only

Indications, route, and dosage
Adjunct to anesthesia to induce skeletal muscle relaxation, facilitate intubation and mechanical ventilation, reduce fractures and dislocations, weaken muscle contractions in pharmacologically or electrically induced convulsions
Dose depends on anesthetic used, individual needs, and response. Doses are representative and must be adjusted.
Adults and children over age 1 month: Initially, 1 mg/kg I.V. to maximum of 100 mg, regardless of patient's weight. Additional doses of 0.5 to 1 mg/kg q 30 to 40 minutes may be administered if necessary.
Infants under age 1 month but over 11 pounds (5 kg): Initially, 0.25 to 0.75 mg/kg I.V., with additional doses of 0.1 to 0.5 mg/kg q 30 to 40 minutes if necessary.

Pharmacodynamics
Skeletal muscle relaxant action: Gallamine produces skeletal muscle paralysis by causing a decreased response to acetylcholine (ACh) at the myoneural junction. Because of its high affinity for ACh receptor sites, gallamine competitively blocks access of ACh to the motor end-plate, thus blocking depolarization.

Pharmacokinetics
- *Absorption:* After I.V. administration, muscle relaxation occurs rapidly and reaches a maximum in about 3 minutes. The duration is related to total dosage, number of doses, anesthetic used, and depth of anesthesia. After usual doses, the duration of action averages 15 to 20 minutes.
- *Distribution:* After I.V. administration, gallamine is distributed in the extracellular fluid and rapidly reaches its site of action. It is substantially bound to serum albumin; the extent of binding is pH dependent.
- *Metabolism:* Unknown.
- *Excretion:* Gallamine is excreted unchanged in urine.

Contraindications and precautions
Gallamine is contraindicated in patients with myasthenia gravis because of potential for prolonged neuromuscular blockade; in patients with impaired renal function because of decreased elimination of drug and potential for accumulation and toxicity; and in patients with shock or hypersensitivity to gallamine or iodides, in whom tachycardia may be hazardous. Administer cautiously to elderly or debilitated patients; to those with cardiac, hepatic, or pulmonary impairment, respiratory depression, myasthenic syndrome of lung cancer, dehydration, thyroid disorders, collagen diseases, porphyria, familial periodic paralysis, or electrolyte disturbances; and in those undergoing cesarean section. Commercially available formulations containing sulfites should be administered cautiously to patients with known sensitivity to sulfites.

Neonates are particularly sensitive to the effects of gallamine and respond to usual doses with prolonged neuromuscular blockade.

Gallamine may increase blood pressure. Hyperthermia may increase the duration and intensity of drug's effects; hypothermia may decrease its duration and intensity.

Administer gallamine cautiously at reduced dose to pregnant women receiving magnesium sulfate.

Interactions
Concomitant use with many general anesthetics, particularly ether, methoxyflurane, enflurane, halothane, and cyclopropane, potentiates gallamine's effects. Use with aminoglycoside antibiotics (amikacin, gentamicin, kanamycin, neomycin, netilmycin, or streptomycin), polymyxin antibiotics (polymyxin B sulfate, colistin, or colistimethate sodium), capreomycin sulfate, clindamycin, and lincomycin reportedly potentiates neuromuscular blockade, leading to increased skeletal muscle relaxation and possibly respiratory paralysis. Concomitant use with I.V. diazepam may increase the intensity and duration of neuromuscular blockade; with opiate analgesics may cause additive respiratory depressant effects. Potassium-depleting agents – thiazide diuretics, furosemide, ethacrynic acid, chlorthalidone, carbonic anhydrase inhibitors, amphotericin B, corticosteroids, and cotropin – may prolong neuromuscular blockade; so may quinine, quinidine, beta-adrenergic blocking agents, and high doses of lidocaine.

Effects on diagnostic tests
None reported.

Adverse reactions
- CV: *tachycardia.*
- Other: *respiratory paralysis, dose-related prolonged apnea,* residual muscle weakness, increased oropharyngeal secretions, allergic or idiosyncratic hypersensitivity reactions.

  Note: Drug should be discontinued if the patient develops hypersensitivity or cardiovascular collapse.

Overdose and treatment
Clinical manifestations of overdose include apnea or prolonged paralysis, which should be treated by maintaining an adequate airway and manual or mechanical ventilation until complete recovery of normal respiration is assured. Anticholinesterase agents (edrophonium, neostigmine, or pyridostigmine) may antagonize gallamine. Administration of atropine before or along with

---

the antagonist will counteract its muscarinic effects. Fluids and vasopressors may be necessary to combat shock or severe hypotension.

A peripheral nerve stimulator may be used to determine the degree of neuromuscular blockade as well as the nature of the blockade.

▶ **Special considerations**
● Administration of this drug requires direct medical supervision.
● Determine baseline electrolyte levels and monitor regularly.
● Vital signs should be checked every 15 minutes, especially for developing tachycardia. Gallamine appears to induce substantial tachycardia, even at low doses.
● Measure intake and output for signs of renal dysfunction.
● Keep airway clear. Have emergency respiratory support (endotracheal equipment, ventilator, oxygen, atropine, and neostigmine) on hand.
● Determine whether patient has iodide allergy or sulfite sensitivity.
● Protect drug from light or excessive heat; use only fresh solutions.
● Do not mix with meperidine or barbiturate solutions.
● Give slowly by I.V. injection (over 30 to 90 seconds).
● May be preferred muscle relaxant in patients with bradycardia.
● Use of a peripheral nerve stimulator is recommended to monitor the degree of neuromuscular blockade and of muscle relaxation, to minimize the possibility of overdose, and to assess recovery in patients undergoing general anesthesia.
● Patients with hypoalbuminemia usually require lower doses.
● Drug does not relieve pain or affect consciousness; therefore, if indicated, assess need for pain medication.

Geriatric use
Elderly patients are more sensitive to the drug's effects.

Pediatric use
Not recommended for use in children weighing less than 11 pounds (5 kg).

Breast-feeding
It is unknown whether drug is excreted in breast milk. Use with caution.

gallium nitrate
Ganite

● Pharmacologic classification: heavy metal
● Therapeutic classification: antihypercalcemic agent
● Pregnancy risk category C

How supplied
Available by prescription only
Injection: 500 mg in 20-ml single-dose vial (25 mg/ml)

Indications, route, and dosage
Treatment of cancer-related hypercalcemia after hydration
Adults: Usually, 200 mg/m² I.V. daily for 5 consecutive days. In patients who are hypercalcemic with few symptoms, 100 mg/m² I.V. for 5 days may be used. Dilute in 1,000 ml of normal saline solution or dextrose 5% in water and administer by I.V. infusion over 24 hours. Maintain adequate hydration throughout treatment. If serum calcium levels return to within normal limits in less than 5 days, discontinue therapy.

Pharmacodynamics
Hypocalcemic action: Gallium inhibits calcium resorption from bone by reducing increased bone turnover, but the precise mechanism for inhibiting calcium resorption is unknown.

Pharmacokinteics
● *Absorption:* Plasma half-life is dependent on dosage.
● *Distribution:* Steady-state levels are achieved in 24 to 48 hours.
● *Metabolism:* Drug is *not* metabolized by liver or kidneys.
● *Excretion:* Excreted by the kidneys; hydration and diuresis do not affect renal clearance of gallium.

Contraindications and precautions
Gallium is contraindicated in patients hypersensitive to the drug and in those with severe renal impairment.

Interactions
Concurrent use with other potentially nephrotoxic drugs, such as aminoglycosides and amphotericin B, may increase risk of renal insufficiency.

Adverse reactions
● CNS: lethargy, confusion, paresthesia.
● CV: anemia, asymptomatic hypotension, tachycardia, leukopenia.
● GI: nausea, vomiting, diarrhea, constipation.
● DERM: skin rash.
● EENT: acute optic neuritis, tinnitus (rare), partial loss of auditory acuity (rare).
● Respiratory: rhonchi, pleural effusion, pulmonary infiltrates, dyspnea, mild respiratory alkalosis.
● Other: hypocalcemia, decreased sodium bicarbonate, lower extremity edema, hypothermia, fever.

Overdose and treatment
Nausea, vomiting, and renal insufficiency may follow rapid I.V. infusion of gallium or use of doses higher than 200 mg/m². Treat by discontinuing drug and by vigorous hydration with or without diuretics. Monitor serum calcium levels, renal function, and urine output. Balance intake and output levels.

▶ **Special considerations**
● Store undiluted solution at room temperature. After further dilution, solution may be stored at room temperature for 48 hours or in refrigerator for 7 days. Discard unused portion because product contains no preservatives.
● Gallium is nontoxic to bone cells and its use does not interfere with subsequent chemotherapy.
● Gallium is significantly more effective than calcitonin in reaching normocalcemia (75% vs. 27%) and superior in maintaining normocalcemia. Median duration of normocalcemia and hypocalcemia after therapy is 7.5 days.

• Monitor serum creatinine levels; elevated BUN and serum creatinine levels have been observed.
• Adequate hydration of patient is essential. Use extreme care to avoid fluid overload in cardiac-compromised patients.

Geriatric use
No age-specific data available.

Pediatric use
Safety and efficacy have not been established.

Breast-feeding
It is unknown if gallium is excreted in breast milk; risk-benefit ratio must be assessed.

ganciclovir (DHPG)
Cytovene

• Pharmacologic classification: synthetic nucleoside
• Therapeutic classification: antiviral agent
• Pregnancy risk category C

How supplied
Available by prescription only
Injection: 500-mg vial

Indications, route, and dosage
Treatment of cytomegalovirus (CMV) retinitis
Adults: 5 mg/kg I.V. q 12 hours for 14 to 21 days, followed by a maintenance dose of 5 mg/kg once daily for 5 days per week.
Dosage in adult patients with renal failure

Creatinine clearance (ml/min/1.73 m²)	Dosage
>80	5 mg/kg I.V. q 12 hours
50 to 79	2.5 mg/kg I.V. q 12 hours
25 to 49	2.5 mg/kg I.V. q 24 hours
<25	1.25 mg/kg I.V. q 24 hours

Pharmacodynamics
Antiviral action: Ganciclovir is a synthetic nucleoside analog of 2'-deoxyguanosine. It competitively inhibits viral DNA polymerase, and may be incorporated within viral DNA to cause early termination of DNA replication. It has shown activity against CMV, herpes simplex virus type 1 and type 2 (HSV-1 and HSV-2), varicella-zoster virus, and Epstein-Barr virus.

Pharmacokinetics
• *Absorption:* Ganciclovir is administered I.V. because less than 7% is absorbed after oral administration.
• *Distribution:* The drug is only 2% to 3% protein-bound. It preferentially concentrates within CMV-infected cells because of the action of cellular kinases that convert it to ganciclovir triphosphate.

• *Metabolism:* Most (>90%) of the drug is excreted unchanged.
• *Excretion:* The elimination half-life is about 3 hours in patients with normal renal function; it can be as long as 30 hours in patients with severe renal failure. The primary route of excretion is through the kidneys by glomerular filtration and some renal tubular secretion.

Contraindications and precautions
Ganciclovir is contraindicated in patients who are hypersensitive to ganciclovir or acyclovir.
About 40% of the patients who receive the drug experience some form of hematologic toxicity, including granulocytopenia or thrombocytopenia. Granulocytopenia usually occurs during the first week, but may occur anytime during therapy. Patients with drug-induced immunosuppression seem more likely to develop thrombocytopenia than patients with acquired immunodeficiency syndrome (AIDS). Cell counts usually recover within 3 to 7 days after discontinuing the drug.
In animal studies, the drug has shown carcinogenic and mutagenic activity and has also caused aspermatogenesis. It should be used only to treat immunocompromised patients with CMV retinitis.

Interactions
There may be a higher incidence of neutropenia in patients also receiving zidovudine. Use with cytotoxic drugs may result in additive toxicity (bone marrow depression, stomatitis, alopecia). Use with probenecid may decrease the renal clearance of ganciclovir. Concomitant use of imipenem-cilastatin may increase the risk of seizures.

Effects on diagnostic tests
None reported.

Adverse reactions
• CNS: disorientation, confusion, seizures, dizziness, headaches.
• CV: arrhythmias, hypotension, hypertension.
• DERM: rash, alopecia, pruritus.
• GI: nausea, vomiting, diarrhea.
• GU: hematuria.
• HEMA: *neutropenia, thrombocytopenia, anemia.*
• Other: hepatotoxicity, fever.

Overdose and treatment
Overdose may result in emesis, neutropenia, or GI disturbances. Treatment should be symptomatic and supportive. Hemodialysis may be useful. Hydrate the patient to reduce plasma levels.

▶ Special considerations
• Administer the drug over 1 hour; do not administer as a rapid I.V. bolus. Ganciclovir should not be given I.M.
• Reconstitute with sterile water for injection. Do not reconstitute with bacteriostatic water for injection because this may lead to the formation of a precipitate.
• Reconstituted solutions are stable for 12 hours. Do not refrigerate.
• Monitor complete blood count to detect neutropenia, which may occur in as many as 40% of patients who take the drug. It usually appears after about 10 days of therapy, and may be associated with a higher dosage (15 mg/kg/day). Neutropenia is reversible, but may necessitate discontinuation of therapy. Patients may re-

sume therapy with the drug when blood counts return to normal.
• Patients with renal failure will probably need dosage adjustments to prevent toxicity.

Information for the patient
• Tell the patient that maintenance infusions are necessary to prevent recurrence of the disease.
• Advise the patient to immediately report any signs or symptoms of infection (fever, sore throat) or easy bruising or bleeding.

Geriatric use
Because the major route of excretion is by glomerular filtration, use in elderly patients with compromised renal function requires caution.

Pediatric use
There has been very little experience with the drug in children under age 12. Use with extreme caution, keeping in mind the possible potential for carcinogenic and reproductive toxicity.

Breast-feeding
Breast-feeding is not recommended during treatment with ganciclovir. Patients should be instructed to discontinue breast-feeding until at least 72 hours after the last treatment.

---

gemfibrozil
Lopid

• Pharmacologic classification: fibric acid derivative
• Therapeutic classification: antilipemic
• Pregnancy risk category B

How supplied
Available by prescription only
Tablets: 600 mg
Capsules: 300 mg

Indications, route, and dosage
Type IV hyperlipidemia (hypertriglyceridemia) and severe hypercholesterolemia unresponsive to diet and other drugs
Adults: 1,200 mg P.O. administered in two divided doses 30 minutes before the morning and evening meals.

Pharmacodynamics
Antilipemic action: Gemfibrozil increases serum high-density lipoprotein cholesterol, inhibits lipolysis in adipose tissue, and reduces hepatic triglyceride synthesis; drug is closely related to clofibrate pharmacologically.

Pharmacokinetics
• *Absorption:* Gemfibrozil is well absorbed from the GI tract; peak plasma concentrations occur 1 to 2 hours after an oral dose. Plasma levels of very low-density lipoprotein (VLDL) decrease in 2 to 5 days; peak clinical effect occurs in 4 weeks. Further decreases in plasma VLDL levels occur over several months.
• *Distribution:* Gemfibrozil is 95% protein-bound.
• *Metabolism:* Gemfibrozil is metabolized by the liver.
• *Excretion:* Elimination of gemfibrozil is mostly in urine but some is excreted in feces. After a single dose, half-

life is 1½ hours; after multiple doses, half-life decreases to about 1¼ hours.

Contraindications and precautions
Gemfibrozil is contraindicated in patients with hypersensitivity to the drug; in patients with gallbladder disease because it may increase cholesterol excretion through the bile and cause cholelithiasis; and in patients with hepatic dysfunction (including primary biliary cirrhosis) or severe renal dysfunction. Drug may cause paradoxical increase in serum cholesterol levels in patients with primary biliary cirrhosis. Hepatic or severe renal disease may increase drug's adverse reactions.

Interactions
Gemfibrozil enhances effect of oral anticoagulants, increasing risk of hemorrhage; adjust anticoagulant dose to maintain the desired prothrombin time, and monitor frequently. Myopathy with rhabdomyolysis can occur with use of gemfibrozil and lovastatin, as well as with similar cholesterol-lowering drugs (such as simvastatin and pravastatin). Avoid concomitant use.

Effects on diagnostic tests
Gemfibrozil therapy may elevate serum levels of creatine phosphokinase, alanine aminotransferase, alkaline phosphatase, aspartate aminotransferase, and lactate dehydrogenase; and it may decrease serum potassium, hematocrit, hemoglobin, and leukocyte counts.

Adverse reactions
• CNS: blurred vision, headache, dizziness.
• DERM: rash, dermatitis, pruritus.
• GI: abdominal and epigastric pain, dry mouth, dyspepsia, anorexia, diarrhea, nausea, vomiting, flatulence.
• HEMA: anemia, leukopenia.
• Hepatic: elevated enzyme levels.
• Other: pain in extremities.
  Note: Drug should be discontinued if liver function test results rise significantly or show worsening abnormalities; if gallstones are found; or if clinical response is inadequate after 3 months of treatment.

Overdose and treatment
No information available.

▶ Special considerations
Because gemfibrozil is pharmacologically related to clofibrate, adverse reactions associated with clofibrate may also occur with gemfibrozil. Some studies suggest clofibrate increases risk of death from cancer, postcholecystectomy complications, and pancreatitis. These hazards have not been studied in gemfibrozil but should be kept in mind.

Information for the patient
• Stress importance of close medical supervision and of reporting any adverse reactions; encourage patient to comply with prescribed regimen and diet.
• Warn patient not to exceed prescribed dose.
• Recommend taking drug with food to minimize GI discomfort.

Pediatric use
Safety and efficacy in children under age 18 have not been established.

Breast-feeding
Safety in breast-feeding women has not been established.

---

gentamicin sulfate
Cidomycin*, Garamycin, Gentacidin

- Pharmacologic classification: aminoglycoside
- Therapeutic classification: antibiotic
- Pregnancy risk category C

How supplied
Available by prescription only
Injection: 40 mg/ml (adult), 10 mg/ml (pediatric), 2 mg/ml (intrathecal)
Ophthalmic ointment: 3 mg/g
Ophthalmic solution: 3 mg/ml
Topical: 0.1% ointment, 0.1% cream

Indications, route, and dosage
Serious infections caused by susceptible organisms
Adults with normal renal function: 3 mg/kg I.M. or I.V. infusion (in 50 to 200 ml of normal saline solution or dextrose 5% in water infused over 30 minutes to 2 hours) daily in divided doses q 8 hours. May be given by direct I.V. push if necessary. For life-threatening infections, patient may receive up to 5 mg/kg/day in three to four divided doses.
Children with normal renal function: 2 to 2.5 mg/kg I.M. or I.V. infusion q 8 hours.
Infants and neonates over age 1 week with normal renal function: 2.5 mg/kg I.M. or I.V. infusion q 8 hours.
Neonates under age 1 week: 2.5 mg/kg I.V. q 12 hours. For I.V. infusion, dilute in normal saline solution or dextrose 5% in water and infuse over 30 minutes to 2 hours.
Meningitis
Adults: Systemic therapy as above; may also use 4 to 8 mg intrathecally daily.
Children: Systemic therapy as above; may also use 1 to 2 mg intrathecally daily.
Endocarditis prophylaxis for GI or GU procedure or surgery
Adults: 1.5 mg/kg I.M. or I.V. 30 to 60 minutes before procedure or surgery and q 8 hours after, for two doses. Given separately with aqueous penicillin G or ampicillin.
Children: 2.5 mg/kg I.M. or I.V. 30 to 60 minutes before procedure or surgery and q 8 hours after, for two doses. Given separately with aqueous penicillin G or ampicillin.
External ocular infections caused by susceptible organisms
Adults and children: Instill 1 to 2 drops in eye q 4 hours. In severe infections, may use up to 2 drops q 1 hour. Apply ointment to lower conjunctival sac b.i.d. or t.i.d.
Primary and secondary bacterial infections; superficial burns; skin ulcers; and infected lacerations, abrasions, insect bites, or minor surgical wounds
Adults and children over age 1: Rub in small amount gently t.i.d. or q.i.d., with or without gauze dressing.
Dosage in renal failure
Initial dose is same as for those with normal renal function. Subsequent doses and frequency determined by renal function studies and blood concentrations; keep peak serum concentrations between 4 and 10 mcg/ml,

and trough serum concentrations between 1 and 2 mcg/ml. One method is to administer 1 mg/kg doses and adjust the dosing interval based upon steady-state serum creatinine:

$$\frac{\text{creatinine}}{(\text{mg/100 ml})} \times 8 = \frac{\text{dosing interval}}{(\text{in hours})}$$

Posthemodialysis to maintain therapeutic blood levels
Adults: 1 to 1.7 mg/kg I.M. or I.V. infusion after each dialysis.
Children: 2 mg/kg I.M. or I.V. infusion after each dialysis.

Pharmacodynamics
Antibiotic action: Gentamicin is bactericidal; it binds directly to the 30S ribosomal subunit, thus inhibiting bacterial protein synthesis. Its spectrum of activity includes many aerobic gram-negative organisms (including most strains of *Pseudomonas aeruginosa*) and some aerobic gram-positive organisms. Gentamicin may act against some bacterial strains resistant to other aminoglycosides; bacterial strains resistant to gentamicin may be susceptible to tobramycin, netilmicin, or amikacin.

Pharmacokinetics
- *Absorption:* Gentamicin is absorbed poorly after oral administration and is given parenterally; after I.M. administration, peak serum concentrations occur at 30 to 90 minutes.
- *Distribution:* Gentamicin is distributed widely after parenteral administration; intraocular penetration is poor. CSF penetration is low even in patients with inflamed meninges. Intraventricular administration produces high concentrations throughout the CNS. Protein-binding is minimal. Gentamicin crosses the placenta.
- *Metabolism:* Not metabolized.
- *Excretion:* Gentamicin is excreted primarily in urine by glomerular filtration; small amounts may be excreted in bile and breast milk. Elimination half-life in adults is 2 to 3 hours. In patients with severe renal damage, half-life may extend to 24 to 60 hours.

Contraindications and precautions
Gentamicin is contraindicated in patients with known hypersensitivity to gentamicin or any other aminoglycoside.

Gentamicin should be used cautiously in patients with decreased renal function because of potential for decreased drug clearance; in patients with tinnitus, vertigo, or high-frequency hearing loss, who are susceptible to ototoxicity; in patients with dehydration because of increased risk of ototoxicity and nephrotoxicity; in patients with myasthenia gravis, parkinsonism, or hypocalcemia because it may aggravate muscle weakness; in neonates and other infants; and in elderly patients because of decreased renal clearance.

Interactions
Concomitant use with the following drugs may increase the hazard of nephrotoxicity, ototoxicity, or neurotoxicity: methoxyflurane, polymyxin B, vancomycin, capreomycin, cisplatin, cephalosporins, amphotericin B, and other aminoglycosides; hazard of ototoxicity is also increased during use with ethacrynic acid, furosemide, bumetanide, urea, or mannitol. Dimenhydrinate and

---

other antiemetic and antivertigo drugs may mask gentamicin-induced ototoxicity.

Concomitant use with a penicillin results in synergistic bactericidal effect against *Pseudomonas aeruginosa, Escherichia coli, Klebsiella, Citrobacter, Enterobacter, Serratia,* and *Proteus mirabilis*; however, the drugs are physically and chemically incompatible and are inactivated when mixed or given together.

Gentamicin may potentiate neuromuscular blockade produced by general anesthetics or neuromuscular blocking agents such as succinylcholine and tubocurarine.

Effects on diagnostic tests
Gentamicin-induced nephrotoxicity may elevate levels of blood urea nitrogen (BUN), nonprotein nitrogen, or serum creatinine, and increase urinary excretion of casts.

Adverse reactions
● CNS: headache, lethargy, neuromuscular blockade with respiratory depression.
● DERM: small percentage of minor skin irritation; possible photosensitivity; allergic contact dermatitis.
● EENT: ototoxicity (tinnitus, vertigo, hearing loss), burning, stinging, transient irritation from ophthalmic ointment or solution.
● GI: diarrhea.
● GU: *nephrotoxicity (cells or casts in the urine; oliguria; proteinuria; decreased creatinine clearance; increased BUN, nonprotein nitrogen, and serum creatinine levels).*
● Other: hypersensitivity reactions (eosinophilia, fever, rash, urticaria, pruritus), bacterial and fungal superinfections
  Note: Drug should be discontinued if signs of ototoxicity, nephrotoxicity, or hypersensitivity occur.

Overdose and treatment
Clinical signs of overdose include ototoxicity, nephrotoxicity, and neuromuscular toxicity. Drug can be removed by hemodialysis or peritoneal dialysis. Treatment with calcium salts or anticholinesterases reverses neuromuscular blockade.

▶ Special considerations
Besides those relevant to all *aminoglycosides,* consider the following recommendations.
● Increased risk of toxicity is associated with prolonged peak serum concentration greater than 10 mcg/ml and/or trough serum concentration greater than 2 mcg/ml.
● For local application to skin infections, remove crusts by gently soaking with warm water and soap or wet compresses before applying ointment or cream; cover with protective gauze.
● Because gentamicin is dialyzable, patients undergoing hemodialysis may need dosage adjustments.

Information for the patient
Teach patient proper topical application of drug; emphasize need to call promptly if lesions worsen or skin irritation develops.

gentian violet
Genapax

● Pharmacologic classification: triphenylmethane (rosaniline) dye
● Therapeutic classification: topical antibacterial, antifungal
● Pregnancy risk category C

How supplied
Available by prescription only
Tampons: 5 mg

Available without a prescription
Solution: 1%, 2%

Indications, route, and dosage
Cutaneous or mucocutaneous infections caused by Candida albicans **and other superficial skin infections**
Adults and children: Apply solution to lesion with cotton b.i.d. or t.i.d. for 3 days. To treat vulvovaginal candidiasis, insert one tampon high into vagina and retain 3 to 4 hours once or twice daily for 12 consecutive days. Additional tampon may be used overnight in resistant cases.

Pharmacodynamics
Antifungal action: The mechanism of antifungal action is unknown; however, its antibacterial action is thought to be related to the bacterial cell characteristics that underlie the Gram stain. Gentian violet inhibits the growth of many fungi, including yeasts and dermatophytes, and is effective against some gram-positive bacteria. It has largely been replaced by more specific agents that don't stain the skin.

Pharmacokinetics
Absorption, distribution, metabolism, and excretion of gentian violet base have not been reported.

Contraindications and precautions
Gentian violet is contraindicated in patients with known hypersensitivity to the drug and for use on ulcerated areas.

Drug turns skin and clothing purple; if applied to granulation tissue, tattooing (permanent discoloration) may result.

Interactions
None reported.

Effects on diagnostic tests
None reported.

Adverse reactions
● Local: vulvovaginal burning, irritation, vesicle formation.
  Note: Drug should be discontinued if sensitization develops.

Overdose and treatment
Laryngeal obstruction may develop after prolonged or frequent use of drug. Specific treatment information is not available.

▶ Special considerations
● Store gentian violet solution in a tight container at temperature less than 104° F. (40° C.); tampons at 59° to 86° F. (15° to 30° C.).
● Tattooing of the skin may occur if drug is applied to granulation tissue.
● Pregnant patients may require longer treatment periods. Treatment may be repeated if infection persists.

Information for the patient
● Advise patient how to administer drug. Be sure patient understands how to use drug and to report adverse reactions.
● If patient is using the vaginal tampon form of the drug, advise her to remove the tampon after 3 to 4 hours and to continue therapy for its full course, even through menstruation.
● Advise patient to refrain from sexual intercourse or have partner use condom during course of therapy to prevent reinfection.
● Tell patient that drug may stain skin and clothing.
● When used in infants for oral candidiasis, advise parent to hold infant's face downward after application to minimize swallowing of medication.
● Advise patients with candidiasis to avoid use of occlusive dressings and to apply enough solution to cover only the affected area.

Breast-feeding
Safety has not been established.

---

glipizide
Glucotrol

● Pharmacologic classification: sulfonyl-urea
● Therapeutic classification: antidiabetic agent
● Pregnancy risk category C

How supplied
Available by prescription only
Tablets: 5 mg, 10 mg

Indications, route, and dosage
Adjunct to diet to lower blood glucose levels in patients with non-insulin-dependent diabetes mellitus (type II)
Adults: Initially, 5 mg P.O. daily before breakfast. Elderly patients or those with liver disease may be started on 2.5 mg. Usual maintenance dosage is 10 to 15 mg. Maximum recommended daily dose is 40 mg.
To replace insulin therapy
If insulin dosage is more than 20 units daily, patient may be started at usual dosage besides 50% of the insulin dosage. If insulin dosage is less than 20 units, insulin may be discontinued.

Pharmacodynamics
Antidiabetic action: Glipizide lowers blood glucose levels by stimulating insulin release from functioning beta cells in the pancreas. After prolonged administration, the drug's hypoglycemic effects appear to reflect extrapancreatic effects, possibly including reduction of basal hepatic glucose production and enhanced peripheral sensitivity to insulin. The latter may result either

from an increase in the number of insulin receptors or from changes in events subsequent to insulin binding.

Pharmacokinetics
● *Absorption:* Glipizide is absorbed rapidly and completely from the GI tract. Onset of action occurs within 1½ hours, with maximum hypoglycemic effects within 2 to 3 hours.
● *Distribution:* Glipizide probably is distributed within the extracellular fluid. It is approximately 92% to 99% protein-bound.
● *Metabolism:* Glipizide is metabolized almost completely by the liver to inactive metabolites.
● *Excretion:* Glipizide and its metabolites are excreted primarily in urine; small amounts are excreted in feces. Renal clearance of unchanged glipizide increases with increasing urinary pH. The duration of action is 10 to 24 hours; half-life is 2 to 4 hours.

Contraindications and precautions
Glipizide is contraindicated in patients with known hypersensitivity to sulfonylureas or thiazides; in those with nonfunctioning beta cells; and in those with impaired adrenal, pituitary, or thyroid function. It should not be used in patients with burns, acidosis, diabetic coma, severe infection, ketosis, or severe trauma or in those requiring major surgery because such conditions of severe physiologic stress require insulin for adequate control of serum glucose levels.
Glipizide should be used cautiously in patients with hepatic or renal insufficiency because of the important roles of the liver in metabolism and the kidneys in elimination.

Interactions
Concomitant use of glipizide with alcohol may produce a disulfiram-like reaction consisting of nausea, vomiting, abdominal cramps, and headaches. Use with anticoagulants may increase plasma levels of both drugs and, after continued therapy, may reduce plasma levels and effectiveness of the anticoagulant. Concomitant use with chloramphenicol, guanethidine, insulin, monoamine oxidase inhibitors, probenecid, salicylates, or sulfonamides may enhance the hypoglycemic effect by displacing glipizide from its protein-binding sites. Cimetidine may poentiate the hypoglycemic effects by preventing hepatic metabolism.
Concomitant use with beta-adrenergic blocking agents (including ophthalmics) may mask symptoms of hypoglycemia, such as rising pulse rate and blood pressure, and may prolong hypoglycemia by blocking gluconeogenesis. Use with drugs that may increase blood glucose levels (adrenocorticoids, glucocorticoids, amphetamines, baclofen, corticotropin, epinephrine, estrogens, ethacrynic acid, furosemide, oral contraceptives, phenytoin, thiazide diuretics, triamterene, and thyroid hormones) may require dosage adjustments.
Because smoking increases corticosteroid release, patients who smoke may require higher dosages of glipizide.

Effects on diagnostic tests
Glipizide therapy alters cholesterol, alkaline phosphatase, AST (SGOT), lactic dehydrogenase, and blood urea nitrogen levels.

Adverse reactions
- CNS: weakness, paresthesia, dizziness.
- DERM: eczema, pruritus, erythema, urticaria, facial flushing, morbilliform or maculopapular eruptions.
- GI: *cholestatic jaundice,* nausea, vomiting, epigastric fullness, heartburn, constipation.
- HEMA: leukopenia, thrombocytopenia, mild anemia, *agranulocytosis.*
- Metabolic: hypoglycemia, dilutional hyponatremia.
- Other: *hypersensitivity reactions.*

    Note: Drug should be discontinued if signs or symptoms of hypersensitivity, including jaundice, skin eruptions, blood dyscrasias, or severe diarrhea, occur, or if progressive increases in serum alkaline phosphatase levels occur.

Overdose and treatment
Clinical manifestations of overdose include low blood glucose levels, tingling of lips and tongue, hunger, nausea, decreased cerebral function (lethargy, yawning, confusion, agitation, and nervousness), increased sympathetic activity (tachycardia, sweating, and tremor), and ultimately convulsions, stupor, and coma.

    Mild hypoglycemia (without loss of consciousness or neurologic findings) responds to treatment with oral glucose and dosage adjustments. If the patient loses consciousness or experiences other neurologic changes, he should receive a rapid injection of dextrose 50%, followed by continuous infusion of dextrose 10% at a rate to maintain blood glucose levels more than 100 mg/dl. Monitor for 24 to 48 hours.

▶ Special considerations
Besides those relevant to all *sulfonylureas,* consider the following recommendations.
- To improve glucose control in patients who receive 15 mg/day or more, divided doses, usually given before the morning and evening meals, are recommended.
- Some patients taking glipizide can be controlled effectively on a once-daily regimen; others show better response with divided dosing.
- Glipizide is a second-generation sulfonylurea oral hypoglycemic. It appears to cause fewer adverse reactions than first-generation sulfonylureas.
- Glipizide has a mild diuretic effect that may be useful in patients with congestive heart failure or cirrhosis.
- When substituting glipizide for chlorpropamide, monitor patient carefully during the 1st week because of the prolonged retention of chlorpropamide.
- Patients who may be more sensitive to this drug, such as elderly, debilitated, or malnourished individuals, should begin therapy with lower dosage (2.5 mg once daily).
- Use in pregnancy is usually not recommended. If glipizide must be used, the manufacturer recommends that the drug be discontinued at least 1 month before expected delivery to prevent neonatal hypoglycemia.
- Oral hypoglycemic agents have been associated with an increased risk of cardiovascular mortality as compared to diet or diet and insulin therapy.

Information for the patient
- Emphasize to patient the importance of following prescribed diet, exercise, and medical regimen.
- Instruct patient to take the medication at the same time each day.
- Tell patient that, if a dose is missed, it should be taken immediately, unless it's almost time to take the next dose. Patient should not take double doses.

- Tell patient to avoid alcohol when taking glipizide. Remind him that many foods and nonprescription medications contain alcohol.
- Encourage patient to wear a Medic-Alert bracelet or necklace.
- If glipizide causes GI upset, suggest that the drug be taken with food.
- Teach patient how to monitor blood glucose, urine glucose, and ketone levels, as prescribed.
- Teach patient how to recognize the signs and symptoms of hyperglycemia and hypoglycemia and what to do if they occur.

Geriatric use
- Elderly patients may be more sensitive to the effects of this drug because of reduced metabolism and elimination.
- Hypoglycemia causes more neurologic symptoms in elderly patients.
- Elderly patients should begin with a lower dosage (2.5 mg once daily).

Pediatric use
Glipizide is ineffective in insulin-dependent (type I, juvenile-onset) diabetes.

---

glucagon

- Pharmacologic classification: antihypoglycemic agent
- Therapeutic classification: antihypoglycemic, diagnostic agent
- Pregnancy risk category B

How supplied
Available by prescription only
Powder for injection: 1 mg (1 unit)/vial, 10 mg (10 units)/vial

Indications, route, and dosage
Coma of insulin-shock therapy
Adults: 0.5 to 1 mg S.C., I.M., or I.V. 1 hour after coma develops; may repeat within 25 minutes, if necessary. In deep coma, also give glucose 10% to 50% I.V. for faster response. When patient responds, give additional carbohydrate immediately.
Severe insulin-induced hypoglycemia during diabetic therapy
Adults and children: 0.5 to 1 mg S.C., I.M., or I.V.; may repeat q 20 minutes for 2 doses, if necessary. If coma persists, give glucose 10% to 50% I.V.
Diagnostic aid for radiologic examination
Adults: 0.25 to 2 mg I.V. or I.M. before initiation of radiologic procedure.

Pharmacodynamics
- *Antihypoglycemic action:* Glucagon increases plasma glucose levels and causes smooth muscle relaxation and an inotropic myocardial effect because of the stimulation of adenylate cyclase to produce cyclic 3',5'-adenosine monophosphate (AMP). Cyclic AMP initiates a series of reactions that leads to the degradation of glycogen to glucose. Hepatic stores of glycogen are necessary for glucagon to exert an antihypoglycemic effect.
- *Diagnostic action:* The mechanism by which gluca-

---

gon relaxes the smooth muscles of the stomach, esophagus, duodenum, small bowel, and colon has not been fully defined.

Pharmacokinetics
● *Absorption:* Glucagon is destroyed in the GI tract; therefore, it must be given parenterally. After I.V. administration, hyperglycemic activity peaks within 30 minutes; relaxation of the GI smooth muscle occurs within 1 minute. After I.M. administration, relaxation of the GI smooth muscle occurs within 10 minutes. Administration to comatose hypoglycemic patients with normal liver glycogen stores) usually produces a return to consciousness within 20 minutes.
● *Distribution:* Distribution is not fully understood.
● *Metabolism:* Glucagon is degraded extensively by the liver, in the kidneys and plasma, and at its tissue receptor sites in plasma membranes.
● *Excretion:* Metabolic products are excreted by the kidneys. Half-life is about 3 to 10 minutes. Duration after I.M. administration is up to 32 minutes; after I.V. administration, up to 25 minutes.

Contraindications and precautions
Glucagon is contraindicated in patients with hypersensitivity to the drug, often a result of its protein nature.

Glucagon should be used cautiously in patients with a history of insulinoma because, although it initially raises blood glucose levels in patients with insulinoma, its insulin-releasing effect subsequently may cause hypoglycemia. The drug also should be used with caution in patients with pheochromocytoma because the drug stimulates release of catecholamines.

Interactions
Concomitant use of glucagon with epinephrine increases and prolongs the hyperglycemic effect. Phenytoin appears to inhibit glucagon-induced insulin release. Use with caution as a diagnostic agent in patients with diabetes mellitus.

Effects on diagnostic tests
Glucagon lowers serum potassium levels.

Adverse reactions
● CNS: dizziness, light-headedness.
● DERM: *Stevens-Johnson syndrome* (one case reported).
● GI: nausea, vomiting.
● Other: hypersensitivity.
  Note: Drug should be discontinued if signs or symptoms of hypersensitivity, including dizziness, rash, or difficulty breathing, occur.

Overdose and treatment
Clinical manifestations of overdose include nausea, vomiting, and hypokalemia. Treat symptomatically.

▶ Special considerations
● Glucagon should be used only under direct medical supervision.
● If patient experiences nausea and vomiting from glucagon administration and cannot retain some form of sugar for 1 hour, consider administration of I.V. dextrose.
● For I.V. drip infusion, glucagon is compatible with dextrose solution but forms a precipitate in chloride solutions.
● Glucagon has a positive inotropic and chronotropic

action on the heart and may be used to treat overdose of beta-adrenergic blockers.
● Glucagon may be used as a diagnostic aid in radiologic examination of the stomach, duodenum, small intestine, and colon when a hypotonic state is desirable.

Information for the patient
● Teach patient how to mix and inject the medication properly, using an appropriate-sized syringe and injecting at a 90-degree angle. *Instructions for mixing injection:* For 2 mg or less, must use manufacturer's diluent; for doses over 2 mg, use sterile water for injection rather than manufacturer's diluent.
● Recommend that patient use medication within 3 months after mixing and store the mixed solution in refrigerator. Patient should store unmixed medication at room temperature and not in the bathroom, where heat and humidity can cause it to deteriorate.
● Instruct patient and family members how to administer glucagon and how to recognize hypoglycemia. Urge them to call immediately in emergencies.
● Tell patient to expect response usually within 20 minutes after injection and that injection may be repeated if no response occurs. Patient should seek medical assistance if second injection is needed.

Pediatric use
Glucagon should not be used to treat newborn asphyxia or hypoglycemia in premature infants or in infants who have had intrauterine growth retardation.

Breast-feeding
No information is available about excretion of glucagon into breast milk. However, because glucagon is destroyed in the GI tract and because of its short-term use, it is unlikely to cause problems in the breast-feeding infant.

---

glutamic acid hydrochloride
Acidulin

● Pharmacologic classification: amino acid
● Therapeutic classification: digestive aid
● Pregnancy risk category C

How supplied
Available without prescription
Capsules: 340 mg
Tablets: 500 mg

Indications, route, and dosage
Hypoacidity
Adults: 340 mg to 1.02 g P.O. t.i.d. before meals.

Pharmacodynamics
Digestive action: Glutamic acid hydrochloride reacts with the stomach contents to release hydrochloric acid.

Pharmacokinetics
Absorption, distribution, metabolism, and excretion have not been described.

Contraindications and precautions
Drug is contraindicated in patients with hyperacidity and peptic ulcers.

Interactions
None significant.

Effects on diagnostic tests
None reported.

Adverse reactions
None reported.

Overdose and treatment
Clinical manifestations of massive overdose include systemic acidosis, which may be treated symptomatically with sodium bicarbonate.

▶ **Special considerations**
Drug is used instead of hydrochloric acid to avoid damaging tooth enamel; however, glutamic acid hydrochloride is not as effective in decreasing gastric pH.

Information for the patient
Tell patient this agent should be taken immediately before or during a meal with water.

Breast-feeding
No problems reported. Patient should consult physician before using.

---

glutethimide
Doriden, Doriglute

- Pharmacologic classification: piperidine-dione
- Therapeutic classification: sedative-hypnotic
- Controlled substance schedule II
- Pregnancy risk category C

How supplied
Available by prescription only
Tablets: 250 mg, 500 mg

Indications, route, and dosage
Insomnia
Adults: 250 to 500 mg P.O. h.s. May be repeated, but not less than 4 hours before intended awakening. Total daily dose should not exceed 1 g.

Pharmacodynamics
Sedative-hypnotic action: Glutethimide's cellular mechanism of action is not known. Like the barbiturates, glutethimide produces a nonspecific depression of the CNS. The mesencephalic activating system is particularly affected, decreasing arousal.

Pharmacokinetics
- *Absorption:* Glutethimide is absorbed erratically after oral administration. Peak serum levels may occur at any point from 1 to 6 hours. Action may begin in 30 minutes and lasts for 4 to 8 hours.
- *Distribution:* Glutethimide distributes throughout the body, with large concentrations found in fat tissue. Slightly more than 50% of the drug is protein-bound.
- *Metabolism:* Glutethimide is metabolized in the liver to inactive metabolites.
- *Excretion:* Inactive metabolites are excreted primarily in urine, with minor excretion in feces. Less than 2%

of the drug is excreted unchanged. Half-life of glutethimide is 10 to 12 hours; duration of action is 4 to 8 hours.

Contraindications and precautions
Glutethimide is contraindicated in patients with known hypersensitivity to the drug and in those with porphyria, severe renal failure, or uncontrolled pain.

Glutethimide should be used cautiously in patients with conditions such as prostatic hypertrophy, bladder neck obstruction, narrow-angle glaucoma, or stenosing peptic ulcer that may be worsened by the drug's anticholinergic effects.

Because this drug depresses the CNS, avoid use in depressed patients or those with suicidal tendencies, and in patients with a history of drug abuse or addiction. The abuse potential, persistence of side effects, and potential lethality of glutethimide overdose mandates the use of other agents in these patients.

Interactions
Glutethimide increases the metabolism of warfarin, decreasing the hypothrombic effect. Glutethimide will add to or potentiate the effects of alcohol, barbiturates, benzodiazepines, narcotics, antihistamines, tranquilizers, and other CNS depressants. Use of glutethimide with tricyclic antidepressants increases anticholinergic effects.

Effects on diagnostic tests
Glutethimide may cause a false-positive phentolamine test. It may interfere with urinary 17-hydroxycorticosteroids (as determined by the Glenn-Nelson technique).

Adverse reactions
- CNS: residual sedation, hangover, headache, vertigo, paradoxical excitation, dizziness, ataxia, confusion.
- DERM: purpuric or urticarial rash, *exfoliative dermatitis* (rarely).
- EENT: dry mouth, blurred vision.
- GI: gastric irritation, nausea, diarrhea, hiccups, dry mouth.
- GU: urinary retention, bladder atony.
- Other: hypersensitivity (thrombocytopenic purpura, leukopenia, *aplastic anemia,* jaundice), nocturnal diaphoresis.

Note: Drug should be discontinued if hypersensitivity, paradoxical excitation, or skin rash occurs.

Overdose and treatment
Clinical manifestations of overdose include prolonged coma, hypotension, hypothermia followed by fever, and inadequate ventilation even without significant respiratory depression. Absence of pupillary reflexes, dilated pupils, loss of deep tendon reflexes, tonic muscle spasms, and apnea may occur.

Treatment of overdose involves support of respiration and cardiovascular function; mechanical ventilation may be necessary. Maintain adequate urine output with adequate hydration while avoiding pulmonary edema. Empty gastric contents by emesis or by lavage with a 1:1 mixture of water and castor oil. Charcoal and resin hemoperfusion are effective in removing the drug; hemodialysis and peritoneal dialysis are of minimal value. Because of the significant storage of glutethimide in fat tissue, blood levels can often show large fluctuations with worsening of symptoms.

▶ **Special considerations**
● Assess level of consciousness and vital signs frequently to prevent possible adverse reactions.
● Monitor prothrombin time in patients taking anticoagulants; anticoagulant dosage may need adjusting.
● Tell patient to store medicine in a cool, dry, dark place out of the reach of children.
● Drug is effective for short-term use only.
● Abrupt discontinuation may cause withdrawal symptoms. Discontinue gradually.

Information for the patient
● Advise patient to avoid alcohol, barbiturates, benzodiazepines, and other CNS depressants unless prescribed by the physician. Tell patient to call physician before taking any nonprescription cold or allergy preparations to prevent possibility of increased CNS depressant activity.
● Warn patient not to increase the dose or frequency unless prescribed.
● Tell patient not to attempt tasks requiring mental alertness or physical coordination until the drug's CNS effects are known.
● Advise patient that abrupt discontinuation of the drug may cause withdrawal symptoms.
● Tell patient to report skin rash or increased excitability.
● Advise patient of potential for physical and psychological dependence with chronic use.
● Advise safety precaution measures (for example, supervised walking and raised bed rails), especially for elderly patients.
● Emphasize the dangers of combining this drug with alcohol. An excessive depressant effect is possible even if the drug is taken the evening before ingestion of alcohol.

Geriatric use
Elderly patients, especially those with decreased renal function, will have increased effects. Use with caution in lowest possible effective dose.

Pediatric use
Drug is not recommended for use in children.

Breast-feeding
Glutethimide is excreted in breast milk. It may cause sedation in the infants of breast-feeding women, and should be used only when benefits far outweigh the risks.

---

glyburide
DiaBeta, Micronase

● Pharmacologic classification: sulfonylurea
● Therapeutic classification: antidiabetic agent
● Pregnancy risk category B

How supplied
Available by prescription only
Tablets: 1.25 mg, 2.5 mg, 5 mg

Indications, route, and dosage
Adjunct to diet to lower blood glucose levels in patients with non-insulin-dependent diabetes mellitus (type II)
Adults: Initially, 2.5 to 5 mg P.O. daily with breakfast. Patients who are more sensitive to hypoglycemic drugs should be started at 1.25 mg daily. Usual maintenance dosage is 1.25 to 20 mg daily, either as a single dose or in divided doses.
To replace insulin therapy
Adults: If insulin dosage is more than 40 units/day, patient may be started on 5 mg of glyburide daily besides 50% of the insulin dose. Patients maintained on less than 20 units/day should receive 2.5 to 5 mg/day; those maintained on 20 to 40 units/day should receive 5 mg/day. In all patients, glyburide is substituted and insulin discontinued abruptly.

Pharmacodynamics
Antidiabetic action: Glyburide lowers blood glucose levels by stimulating insulin release from functioning beta cells in the pancreas. After prolonged administration, the drug's hypoglycemic effects appear to be related to extrapancreatic effects, possibly including reduction of basal hepatic glucose production and enhanced peripheral sensitivity to insulin. The latter may result either from an increase in the number of insulin receptors or from changes in events subsequent to insulin binding.

Pharmacokinetics
● *Absorption:* Glyburide is absorbed almost completely from the GI tract. Onset of action occurs within 2 hours; hypoglycemic effects peak within 3 to 4 hours.
● *Distribution:* Glyburide is 99% protein-bound. Its distribution is not fully understood.
● *Metabolism:* Glyburide is metabolized completely by the liver to inactive metabolites.
● *Excretion:* Glyburide is excreted as metabolites in urine and feces in equal proportions. Its duration of action is 24 hours; its half-life is 10 hours.

Contraindications and precautions
Glyburide is contraindicated in patients with known hypersensitivity to sulfonylureas or thiazides and in patients with nonfunctioning pancreatic beta cells. It should not be used in patients with burns, acidosis, diabetic coma, severe infection, ketosis, or severe trauma or in patients requiring major surgery because such conditions of severe physiologic stress require insulin for adequate control of blood glucose.

Glyburide should be used cautiously in patients with hepatic or renal insufficiency because of the important roles of the liver in metabolism and the kidneys in elimination; and in patients with impaired adrenal, pituitary, or thyroid function.

Interactions
Concomitant use of glyburide with alcohol may produce a disulfiram-like reaction consisting of nausea, vomiting, abdominal cramps, and headaches. Use with anticoagulants may increase plasma levels of both drugs and, after continued therapy, may reduce plasma levels and anticoagulant effect. Use with chloramphenicol, guanethidine, insulin, monoamine oxidase inhibitors, probenecid, salicylates, or sulfonamides may enhance the hypoglycemic effect by displacing glyburide from its protein-binding sites.

Concomitant use of glyburide with beta-adrenergic blocking agents (including ophthalmics) may increase the risk of hypoglycemia, mask its symptoms (increased pulse rate and blood pressure), and prolong its effects by blocking gluconeogenesis. Use with drugs that may increase blood glucose levels (adrenocorticoids, diazoxide, glucocorticoids, amphetamines, baclofen, corticotropin, epinephrine, ethacrynic acid, furosemide, phenytoin, thiazide diuretics, triamterene, and thyroid hormones) may require dosage adjustments.

Because smoking increases corticosteroid release, smokers may require higher dosages of glyburide.

Effects on diagnostic tests
Glyburide therapy alters cholesterol, alkaline phosphatase, and blood urea nitrogen levels.

Adverse reactions
● CNS: weakness, paresthesias, dizziness.
● DERM: eczema, pruritus, erythema, urticaria, facial flushing, morbilliform or maculopapular eruptions.
● GI: *cholestatic jaundice,* nausea, vomiting, epigastric fullness, heartburn, constipation.
● HEMA: leukopenia, thrombocytopenia, mild anemia, *agranulocytosis.*
● Metabolic: *hypoglycemia,* dilutional hyponatremia.
● Other: *hypersensitivity reactions.*
Note: Drug should be discontinued if signs or symptoms of hypersensitivity, including jaundice, skin eruptions, blood dyscrasias, and severe diarrhea, occur, or if serial and progressive increases in serum alkaline phosphatase levels occur.

Overdose and treatment
Clinical manifestations of overdose include low blood glucose levels, tingling of lips and tongue, hunger, nausea, decreased cerebral function (lethargy, yawning, confusion, agitation, and nervousness), increased sympathetic activity (tachycardia, sweating, and tremor) and ultimately convulsions, stupor, and coma.

Mild hypoglycemia, without loss of consciousness or neurologic findings, responds to treatment with oral glucose and dosage adjustments. The patient with severe hypoglycemia should be hospitalized immediately. If hypoglycemic coma is suspected, the patient should receive rapid injection of dextrose 50%, followed by a continuous infusion of dextrose 10% at a rate to maintain blood glucose levels greater than 100 mg/dl. Monitor for 24 to 48 hours.

▶ **Special considerations**
Besides those relevant to all *sulfonylureas,* consider the following recommendations.
● To improve control in patients receiving 10 mg/day or more, divided doses, usually given before the morning and evening meals, are recommended.
● Some patients taking glyburide may be controlled effectively on a once-daily regimen, whereas others show better response with divided dosing.
● Glyburide is a second-generation sulfonylurea oral hypoglycemic agent. It appears to cause fewer adverse reactions than first-generation drugs.
● Glyburide has a mild diuretic effect that may be useful in patients who have chronic heart failure or cirrhosis.
● When substituting glyburide for chlorpropamide, monitor patient closely during the 1st week because of the prolonged retention of chlorpropamide in the body.
● In elderly, debilitated, or malnourished patients or those with renal or liver dysfunction, glyburide therapy should start with 1.25 mg once a day.
● Oral hypoglycemic agents have been associated with

an increased risk of cardiovascular mortality as compared to diet or diet and insulin therapy.

Information for the patient
● Emphasize to patient the importance of following prescribed diet, exercise, and medical regimen.
● Tell patient to take the medication at the same time each day. If a dose is missed, it should be taken immediately, unless it's almost time to take the next dose. Instruct patient not to take double doses.
● Advise patient to avoid alcohol while taking glyburide. Remind him that many foods and nonprescription medications contain alcohol.
● Encourage patient to wear a Medic Alert bracelet or necklace.
● If drug causes GI upset, suggest that it be taken with food.
● Teach patient how to monitor blood glucose and urine glucose and ketone levels as prescribed.
● Teach patient how to recognize the signs and symptoms of hyperglycemia and hypoglycemia and what to do if they occur.

Geriatric use
● Elderly patients may be more sensitive to the effects of this medication because of reduced metabolism and elimination.
● Hypoglycemia causes more neurologic symptoms in elderly patients.

Pediatric use
Glyburide is ineffective in insulin-dependent (type I, juvenile-onset) diabetes. Safety and effectiveness in children have not been established.

---

glycerin (glycerol)
Glyrol, Osmoglyn, Ophthalgan

glycerin, anhydrous
Fleet Babylax, Sani-Supp

● Pharmacologic classification: trihydric alcohol, ophthalmic osmotic vehicle
● Therapeutic classification: laxative (osmotic), ophthalmic osmotic agent, adjunctive agent in treating glaucoma, lubricant
● Pregnancy risk category C

How supplied
Available by prescription only
Ophthalmic solution: 7.5 ml containers
Oral solution: 50% (0.6 g/ml), 75% (0.94 g/ml)

Available without prescription
Suppository: 4 ml/applicator
Adult/infant rectal solution: 4 ml/applicator

Indications, route, and dosage
Constipation
Adults and children age 6 and older: 3 g as a suppository or 5 to 15 ml as an enema.
Children under age 6: 1 to 1.5 g as a suppository or 2 to 5 ml as an enema.

Reduction of intraocular pressure
Adults: 1 to 1.8 g/kg P.O. 60 to 90 minutes preoperatively; additional doses at 5-hour intervals.

Drug is useful in acute angle-closure glaucoma; before iridectomy (with carbonic anhydrase inhibitors or topical miotics); in trauma or disease, such as congenital glaucoma and some secondary glaucoma forms; and before or after surgery, such as retinal detachment surgery, cataract extraction, or keratoplasty.

Reduction of corneal edema
Adults: 1 to 2 drops of ophthalmic solution topically before eye examination; 1 to 2 drops q 3 to 4 hours for corneal edema.

Drug is used to facilitate ophthalmoscopic and gonioscopic examination and to differentiate superficial edema and deep corneal edema.

Pharmacodynamics
● *Laxative action:* Glycerin suppositories produce laxative action by causing rectal distention, thereby stimulating the urge to defecate; by causing local rectal irritation; and by triggering a hyperosmolar mechanism that draws water into the colon.

● *Antiglaucoma action:* Orally administered glycerin helps reduce intraocular pressure by increasing plasma osmotic pressure, thereby drawing water into the blood from extravascular spaces. It also reduces intraocular fluid volume independently of routine flow mechanisms, decreasing intraocular pressure; it may cause tissue dehydration and decreased CSF pressure.

Topically applied glycerin produces a hygroscopic (moisture-retaining) effect that reduces edema and improves visualization in ophthalmoscopy or gonioscopy. Glycerin reduces fluid in the cornea via its osmotic action and clears corneal haze.

Pharmacokinetics
For rectal form
● *Absorption:* Glycerin suppositories are absorbed poorly; after rectal administration, laxative effect occurs in 15 to 30 minutes.
● *Distribution:* When administered by suppository, glycerin is distributed locally.
● *Metabolism:* Not reported.
● *Excretion:* Glycerin is excreted in the feces.

For oral form
● *Absorption:* With oral administration, glycerin is absorbed rapidly from the GI tract, with peak serum levels occurring in 60 to 90 minutes; intraocular pressure decreases in 10 to 30 minutes. Peak action occurs in 30 minutes to 2 hours, with effects persisting for 4 to 8 hours. Intracranial pressure decreases in 10 to 60 minutes; this effect persists for 2 to 3 hours.
● *Distribution:* Glycerin is distributed throughout the blood but does not enter ocular fluid; drug may enter breast milk.
● *Metabolism:* After oral administration, about 80% of dose is metabolized in the liver, 10% to 20% in the kidneys.
● *Excretion:* Glycerin is excreted in feces and urine.

Contraindications and precautions
Glycerin is contraindicated in patients with known glycerin hypersensitivity. Glycerin suppositories are contraindicated in patients who are recovering from rectal surgery.

Orally administered glycerin should be used cautiously in patients with cardiac, renal, or hepatic disease, because it may cause a fluid shift precipitating pulmonary edema or congestive heart failure; in elderly and dehydrated patients because it may cause seizures and disorientation; and in diabetic patients because it may lead to diabetic ketoacidosis and coma.

Interactions
Concomitant use with diuretics may result in additive effects.

Effects on diagnostic tests
None reported.

Adverse reactions
● CNS: mild headache, dizziness (with oral administration).
● Eye: pain, irritation.
● GI: thirst, nausea, vomiting, diarrhea and cramping pain (with oral administration); rectal discomfort or local hyperemia (after rectal administration).
● Metabolic: mild hyperglycemia, mild glycosuria.
Note: Drug should be discontinued if symptoms of hypersensitivity occur.

Overdose and treatment
If excess glycerin is administered into eye, irrigate conjunctiva with sterile normal saline solution or water. Systemic effects are not expected.

▶ Special considerations
● When administering glycerin orally, do not give hypotonic fluids to relieve thirst and headache from glycerin-induced dehydration because these will counteract drug's osmotic effects.
● Use topical tetracaine hydrochloride or proparacaine before ophthalmic instillation to prevent discomfort.
● Don't touch tip of dropper to eye, surrounding tissues, or tear-film; glycerin will absorb moisture.
● To prevent or relieve headache, have patient remain supine during and after oral administration.
● Monitor diabetic patients for possible alteration of serum and urine glucose levels; dosage adjustment may be necessary.
● Commercially available solutions may be poured over ice and sipped through a straw.
● Hyperosmolar laxatives are used most commonly to help laxative-dependent patients reestablish normal bowel habits.
● Other uses include reducing intracranial pressure in patients with cerebrovascular accident, meningitis, encephalitis, Reye's syndrome, or CNS trauma or tumors and reducing brain volume during neurosurgical procedures through oral or intravenous administration, or both.
● Store drug in tightly closed original container.

Information for the patient
● Tell patient to call if he experiences severe headache from oral dose.
● Teach patient correct way to instill drops and warn him not to touch eye with the dropper.
● Tell patient to lie down during and after administration of glycerin to prevent or relieve headache.

Geriatric use
Dehydrated elderly patients may experience seizures and disorientation.

Pediatric use
Safety and effectiveness of ophthalmic glycerin solutions in children has not been established.

Breast-feeding
Glycerin's safety in breast-feeding women has not been established; possible risks must be weighed against benefits.

---

glycopyrrolate
Robinul, Robinul Forte

- Pharmacologic classification: anticholinergic
- Therapeutic classification: antimuscarinic, gastrointestinal antispasmodic
- Pregnancy risk category B

How supplied
Available by prescription only
Tablets: 1 mg, 2 mg
Injection: 0.2 mg/ml in 1-ml, 2-ml, 5-ml, and 20-ml vials

Indications, route, and dosage
Blockade of cholinergic effects of anticholinesterase drugs used to reverse neuromuscular blockade
Adults and children: 0.2 mg I.V. for each 1 mg neostigmine or equivalent dose of pyridostigmine. May be given I.V. without dilution or may be added to dextrose injection and given by infusion.

Preoperatively to diminish secretions and block cardiac vagal reflexes
Adults: 4.4 mcg/kg I.M. 30 to 60 minutes before anesthesia.
Children: 4.4 to 8.8 mcg/kg I.M. 30 to 60 minutes before anesthesia.

Arrhythmias (intraoperative)
Adults: 100 mcg I.V.; repeat at 2- to 3-minute intervals as needed.
Children: 4.4 mcg/kg (up to a maximum of 100 mcg) I.V.; repeat at 2- to 3-minute intervals as needed.

Adjunctive therapy in peptic ulcers and other GI disorders
Adults: 1 to 2 mg P.O. t.i.d. or 0.1 mg I.M. t.i.d. or q.i.d. Dosage should be individualized.

Pharmacodynamics
Anticholinergic action: Glycopyrrolate inhibits acetylcholine's muscarinic actions on autonomic effectors innervated by postganglionic cholinergic nerves. That action blocks adverse muscarinic effects associated with anticholinesterase agents used to reverse curariform-induced neuromuscular blockade. Glycopyrrolate decreases secretions and GI motility by the same mechanism. Glycopyrrolate blocks cardiac vagal reflexes by blocking vagal inhibition of the sinoatrial node.

Pharmacokinetics
- *Absorption:* Glycopyrrolate is poorly absorbed from the GI tract (10% to 25%) after oral administration. Glycopyrrolate is rapidly absorbed when given I.M.; serum concentrations peak in 30 to 45 minutes. Action begins in 1 minute after I.V. and 15 to 30 minutes after I.M. or S.C. administration.
- *Distribution:* Glycopyrrolate is rapidly distributed. Because it is a quaternary amine, it does not cross the blood-brain barrier or enter the CNS.
- *Metabolism:* Glycopyrrolate's exact metabolic fate is unknown. Duration of effect is up to 7 hours when given parenterally and up to 12 hours when given orally.
- *Excretion:* Small drug amounts are eliminated in the urine as unchanged drug and metabolites. Most of the drug is excreted unchanged in feces or bile.

Contraindications and precautions
Glycopyrrolate is contraindicated in patients with narrow-angle glaucoma, because drug-induced cycloplegia and mydriasis may increase intraocular pressure; in patients with obstructive uropathy, because the drug may exacerbate urinary retention; and in patients with myasthenia gravis, paralytic ileus, intestinal atony, or toxic megacolon, because the drug may worsen these conditions.

Administer glycopyrrolate cautiously to patients with hyperthyroidism, ulcerative colitis, coronary artery disease, congestive heart failure, cardiac arrhythmias, or hypertension, because it may exacerbate these conditions; to patients with hiatal hernia associated with reflux esophagitis, because the drug may decrease lower esophageal sphincter tone, thus worsening the condition; to patients over age 40, because it increases the glaucoma risk; and in hot or humid environments, because it may predispose the patient to heatstroke.

Interactions
Concurrent administration of antacids decreases oral absorption of anticholinergics. Administer glycopyrrolate at least 1 hour before antacids.

Concomitant administration of drugs with anticholinergic effects may cause additive toxicity.

Decreased GI absorption of many drugs has been reported after the use of anticholinergics (for example, levodopa and ketoconazole). Conversely, slowly dissolving digoxin tablets may yield higher serum digoxin levels when administered with anticholinergics.

Use cautiously with oral potassium supplements (especially wax-matrix formulations) because the incidence of potassium-induced GI ulcerations may be increased.

Effects on diagnostic tests
None reported.

Adverse reactions
- CNS: weakness, nervousness, drowsiness, dizziness, confusion or excitement (in elderly), headache.
- CV: palpitations, tachycardia, *paradoxical bradycardia*, orthostatic hypotension.
- DERM: urticaria, decreased sweating or anhidrosis, other dermal manifestations.
- EENT: dilated pupils, blurred vision, photophobia, cycloplegia, increased intraocular pressure.
- GI: constipation, dry mouth, nausea, vomiting, epigastric distress, dysphagia, loss of taste, abdominal distention.
- GU: urinary hesitancy, urine retention.
- Other: burning at injection site, bronchial plug formation, fever.

Note: Drug should be discontinued if hypersensitivity; urine retention; confusion; hallucinations; dilated, nonreactive pupils; or hot, dry, flushed skin occurs.

Overdose and treatment

Clinical effects of overdose include such peripheral effects as dilated, nonreactive pupils; blurred vision; flushed, hot, dry skin; dryness of mucous membranes; dysphagia; decreased or absent bowel sounds; urine retention; hyperthermia; tachycardia; hypertension; and increased respiration.

Treatment is primarily symptomatic and supportive, as needed. If patient is alert, induce emesis (or use gastric lavage) and follow with a saline cathartic and activated charcoal to prevent further drug absorption. In severe cases, physostigmine may be administered to block glycopyrrolate's antimuscarinic effects. Give fluids, as needed, to treat shock. If urine retention occurs, catheterization may be necessary.

▶ Special considerations

Besides those relevant to all *anticholinergics,* consider the following recommendations.
● Check all dosages carefully. Even slight overdose could lead to toxic effects.
● For immediate treatment of bradycardia, some clinicians prefer atropine over glycopyrrolate.
● Do not mix glycopyrrolate with I.V. solutions containing sodium chloride or bicarbonate.
● May be administered with neostigmine or physostigmine in same syringe.
● Drug is incompatible with thiopental, methohexital, secobarbital, pentobarbital, chloramphenicol, dimenhydrinate, and diazepam.

Geriatric use

Administer glycopyrrolate cautiously to elderly patients. However, glycopyrrolate may be the preferred anticholinergic in elderly patients.

Breast-feeding

Drug may be excreted in breast milk, possibly resulting in infant toxicity. Breast-feeding women should avoid this drug. Glycopyrrolate may decrease milk production.

PHARMACOLOGIC CLASS

gold salts

auranofin
aurothioglucose
gold sodium thiomalate

Gold compounds suppress or prevent the progression of active adult and juvenile rheumatoid arthritis and synovitis through an unknown mechanism. They do not produce analgesia or antipyresis. They should be considered in treating rheumatoid arthritis that progresses despite several months of treatment with salicylates or other nonsteroidal anti-inflammatory drugs (NSAIDs), rest, and physical therapy. Gold compounds can induce remission of arthritis but are more toxic than the NSAIDs alone. Treatment with gold compounds should begin before irreversible joint damage occurs and should include concomitant NSAIDs until complete remission of arthritis has been achieved. Improvement occurs slowly and may require 2 to 6 months before onset of disease control.

Pharmacology

Aurothioglucose and gold sodium thiomalate are aurous salts in which the gold is attached to sulfur; they contain about 50% gold. Auranofin contains about 29% gold and differs chemically and in some pharmacologic actions. It has the advantage of being effective for rheumatoid arthritis when administered orally.

These compounds exhibit anti-inflammatory, antiarthritic, and immunomodulating effects. They can decrease the rheumatoid factor and immunoglobulin concentrations. The exact mechanism in rheumatoid arthritis is still unclear; some data suggest that activity comes from nonprotein-bound gold. These drugs affect numerous cellular processes involved with inflammation, modulate various humoral and cellular immune responses, and achieve clinical responses in patients with rheumatoid arthritis.

Therapeutic effects occur gradually. After 6 to 8 weeks, benefits typically are limited to some reduction in morning stiffness; 3 to 6 months may be required to gain full therapeutic benefit.

Clinical indications and actions
Rheumatoid arthritis

The injectable gold compounds (aurothioglucose and gold sodium thiomalate) are used to treat both adult and juvenile types of rheumatoid arthritis. They should not be used until adequate trials of salicylates or other anti-inflammatory agents, rest, and physical therapy have failed to produce improvement. Gold compounds are of little value after advanced disease has damaged cartilage and bone; they will not reverse extensive deformities.

Gold compounds may halt progression of the disease, improve grip strength, and decrease erythrocyte sedimentation rate (ESR), rheumatoid factor (RF), and elevated serum protein and immunoglobulin concentrations.

Gold therapy may be useful in treating psoriatic arthritis.

Auranofin, given orally, is similarly effective in treating rheumatoid arthritis. Patients who received oral auranofin after 6 months of parenteral therapy maintained equal disease control.

Overview of adverse reactions

The incidence of adverse drug reactions is high but most reactions respond favorably to discontinuation of therapy. Adverse drug reactions may occur at any time during treatment or many months after the gold is stopped. However, most reactions occur during the second or third month of therapy, after a cumulative dose of 300 to 500 mg of aurothioglucose or 400 to 800 mg of gold sodium thiomalate.

Skin reactions include dermatitis, erythema, and chrysiasis (gray-blue pigmentation). Lung injury may occur as gold bronchitis, interstitial pneumonitis, and fibrosis, with shortness of breath and cough. Granulocytopenia, thrombocytopenia with or without purpura, leukopenia, eosinophilia, and hypoplastic and aplastic anemia have all been rare. Hepatic toxicity may cause hepatitis with jaundice or intrahepatic cholestatic hepatitis with elevated liver enzyme levels. Proteinuria and albuminuria may occur.

GI disturbances (loose stools, diarrhea, or other bowel habit changes) are the most frequently reported adverse drug reactions, particularly with auranofin. Ulcerative colitis, although rare, may be life-threatening. Other reactions may include conjunctivitis, iritis, corneal ulcers, headache, EEG abnormalities, peripheral neuritis, and sensory-motor polyradiculoneuropathy (including Guillain-Barrè syndrome); stomatitis, vaginitis, proctitis, metallic taste, diffuse glossitis or gingivitis; and sensitivity reaction – anaphylactoid or "nitroid type" (flushing, syncope, dizziness, sweating and nausea, vomiting, and weakness). Adverse reactions to thiomalate preparation are probably caused by the vehicle rather than the gold. Using one of the other gold products may help eliminate this problem.

▶ **Special considerations**
● Carefully monitor for toxic reactions (pruritus, rash, metallic taste, sore mouth, or GI reactions).
● Gold therapy is contraindicated in patients with history of necrotizing enterocolitis, pulmonary fibrosis, exfoliative dermatitis, bone marrow aplasia, or severe hematologic disorders; and in patients receiving other drugs that have the potential to cause blood dyscrasias.
● Use cautiously, if at all, in patients who have preexisting renal disease, liver disease, inflammatory bowel disease, skin rash, marked hypertension, compromised cerebral or cardiovascular circulation, or allergy or hypersensitivity to gold or other heavy metals.
● Complete blood count and platelet count should be monitored at least monthly.
● Moderately severe skin reactions and mucous membrane reactions often benefit from a topical steroid cream, oral antihistamine, and soothing lotions.
● Before each injection, urinalysis should be done for protein and sediment changes.
● Do not restart gold therapy in patients who have had severe reaction to gold.
● Gold therapy may alter liver function tests.
● Administer all injectable gold salts I.M. intragluteally.

Information for the patient
● Encourage patient compliance by reinforcing that 2 to 6 months' treatment may be required before therapeutic benefit is seen.
● Explain to the patient the importance of taking gold therapy according to the prescribed dosage and of having monthly follow-up blood test.
● Tell patient to continue taking other prescribed antiarthritic drug therapy, such as NSAIDs.
● Tell patient joint pain may increase after a gold injection and last for 1 to 2 days, but this usually subsides after the first few injections.
● Advise patient to minimize exposure to sunlight or artificial ultraviolet light, because skin rash may develop or be aggravated by such exposure.
● Tell patient good oral hygiene is important.

Pediatric use
Auranofin is not recommended for use in children. No age-related problems have been documented for aurothioglucose and gold sodium thiomalate.

Breast-feeding
Gold salts are not recommended for use by breast-feeding women because of the potential for adverse reactions in the infant.

Representative combinations
None.

gold sodium thiomalate
Myochrysine

● Pharmacologic classification: gold salt
● Therapeutic classification: antiarthritic
● Pregnancy risk category C

How supplied
Available by prescription only
Injection: 25 mg/ml, 50 mg/ml with benzyl alcohol

Indications, route, and dosage
Rheumatoid arthritis
Adults: Initially, 10 mg I.M., followed by 25 mg in 1 week and continued for second and third doses at weekly intervals. Then, 50 mg weekly until 14 to 20 doses have been given. If improvement occurs without toxicity, continue 50 mg q 2 weeks for 4 doses; then, 50 mg q 3 weeks for 4 doses; then, 50 mg/month indefinitely as maintenance therapy to cumulative dose of 800 mg to 1 g. If relapse occurs during maintenance therapy, resume injections at weekly intervals.
Children: Initiate therapy with 10-mg test dose, then give 1 mg/kg/week or one-quarter the adult dose I.M. for 20 weeks. If response is good, may be given q 3 to 4 weeks indefinitely. Maximum single dose for children under age 12 is 50 mg.

Pharmacodynamics
Antiarthritic action: Gold sodium thiomalate is thought to be effective against rheumatoid arthritis by altering the immune system to reduce inflammation. Although the exact mechanism of action remains unknown, these compounds have reduced serum concentrations of immunoglobulins and rheumatoid factors in patients with arthritis.

Pharmacokinetics
● *Absorption:* Absorption of gold sodium thiomalate is rapid, with peak levels occurring within 3 to 6 hours.
● *Distribution:* Higher tissue concentrations occur with parenteral gold salts, with a mean steady-state plasma level of 1 to 5 mcg/ml. Drug is distributed widely throughout the body in lymph nodes, bone marrow, kidneys, liver, spleen, and tissues. About 85% to 90% is protein-bound.
● *Metabolism:* Gold sodium thiomalate is not broken down into its elemental form. The half-life with cumulative dosing is 14 to 40 days.
● *Excretion:* About 70% of the drug is excreted in the urine, 30% in the feces.

Contraindications and precautions
Gold compounds are contraindicated in patients with uncontrolled diabetes mellitus, systemic lupus erythematosus, Sjögren's syndrome, agranulocytosis, or blood dyscrasias; in patients who recently received radiation therapy; in breast-feeding patients, because the drug distributes into breast milk; and in patients with a history of sensitivity to gold compounds. They should be administered cautiously to patients with marked hypertension, compromised cerebral or cardiovascular function, or renal or hepatic dysfunction, because gold may exacerbate these conditions; and to women of child-bearing age, because gold compounds are teratogenic in high doses in animals.

Interactions
Concomitant use with other drugs known to cause blood dyscrasias causes an additive risk of hematologic toxicity.

Effects on diagnostic tests
Serum protein-bound iodine test, especially when done by the chloric acid digestion method, gives false readings during and for several weeks after gold therapy.

Adverse reactions
Adverse reactions to gold are considered severe and potentially life-threatening.
● CNS: dizziness, syncope, sweating.
● CV: bradycardia.
● DERM: rash, pruritus, dermatitis, *exfoliative dermatitis*.
● EENT: corneal gold deposition, corneal ulcers.
● GI: diarrhea, abdominal pain, nausea, vomiting, stomatitis, enterocolitis, anorexia, metallic taste, dyspepsia, flatulence.
● GU: albuminuria, proteinuria, nephrotic syndrome, nephritis, acute tubular necrosis.
● HEMA: thrombocytopenia (with or without purpura), *aplastic anemia, agranulocytosis*, leukopenia, eosinophilia.
● Hepatic: jaundice, elevated liver enzymes.
● Other: gold bronchitis and interstitial pneumonitis, partial or complete loss of hair, fever, *anaphylaxis*, angioneurotic edema.

Overdose and treatment
When severe reactions to gold occur, corticosteroids, dimercaprol (a chelating agent), or penicillamine may be given to aid in the recovery. Prednisone 40 to 100 mg/day in divided doses is recommended to manage severe renal, hematologic, pulmonary, or enterocolitic reactions to gold. Dimercaprol may be used concurrently with steroids to facilitate the removal of the gold when the steroid treatment alone is ineffective.

▶ Special considerations
Besides those relevant to all *gold salts*, consider the following recommendations.
● Gold salts should be administered only under close medical supervision.
● Most adverse reactions are readily reversible if drug is discontinued immediately.
● Vasomotor adverse effects are more common with gold sodium thiomalate than with other gold salts.
● Administer all gold salts I.M., preferably intragluteally. Normal color of drug is pale yellow; do not use if it darkens.
● Observe patient for 30 minutes after administration because of possible anaphylactic reaction.
● When giving gold sodium thiomalate, advise patient to lie down and to remain recumbent for 10 to 20 minutes after injection.
● Patient's urine should be analyzed for protein and sediment changes before each injection.
● Complete blood count and platelet count should be monitored monthly.
● If adverse reactions are mild, some rheumatologists order resumption of gold therapy after 2 to 3 weeks' rest.

Information for the patient
● Urge patients to have scheduled monthly platelet counts. Drug should be stopped if the platelet count falls below 100,000/mm³.
● Reassure patient that beneficial drug effect may be delayed for 3 months. However, if response is inadequate after 6 months, auranofin will probably be discontinued.
● Explain that vasomotor adverse reactions – faintness, weakness, dizziness, flushing, nausea, vomiting, diaphoresis – may occur immediately after injection. Advise patient to lie down until symptoms subside.
● Tell patient to continue taking the drug if he experiences mild diarrhea; however, if diarrhea persists, or if he notes blood in his stool, he should call physician immediately.
● Tell patient that stomatitis is often preceded by a metallic taste. Advise him to report this symptom immediately.
● Advise patient to report any rashes or other skin problems immediately.
● Encourage patient to take the drug exactly as prescribed.
● Tell patient to continue taking concomitant drug therapy, such as nonsteroidal anti-inflammatory drugs, as prescribed.
● Tell patient that drug may increase sensitivity to sunlight and tanning beds. He should avoid exposure to excessive sunlight, wear protective clothing, and use a sunscreen.

Geriatric use
Administer usual adult dose. Use cautiously in patients with decreased renal function.

Pediatric use
Use in children younger than age 6 is not recommended. Children age 6 to 12 may receive one-fourth the usual adult dose.

Breast-feeding
Gold sodium thiomalate is not recommended for use in breast-feeding women.

---

gonadorelin acetate
Lutrepulse

● Pharmacologic classification: gonadotropin-releasing hormone (GnRH)
● Therapeutic classification: fertility agent
● Pregnancy risk category B

How supplied
Available by prescription only
Injection: 0.8 mg/10 ml, 3.2 mg/10 ml, in 10-ml vials
Supplied as a kit with I.V. supplies and portable infusion pump.

Indications, route, and dosage
To induce ovulation in women with primary hypothalamic amenorrhea
Adults: 5 mcg I.V. q 90 minutes for 21 days. If no response after three treatment intervals, dosage may be increased.

Pharmacodynamics

Ovulation-stimulating action: Mimics the action of GnRH, which results in the synthesis and release of luteinizing hormone (LH) from the anterior pituitary. LH subsequently acts upon the reproductive organs to regulate hormone synthesis.

Pharmacokinetics

● *Absorption:* Gonadorelin is administered I.V. using a portable pump designed to administer the drug in a pulsatile fashion to mimic the endogenous hormone.
● *Distribution:* The drug has a low plasma volume of distribution (10 to 15 liters) and a high rate of clearance from plasma.
● *Metabolism:* The drug is rapidly metabolized. Several biologically inactive peptide fragments have been identified.
● *Excretion:* The drug is excreted primarily in the urine. The high initial clearance rate (half-life of 2 to 10 minutes) is followed by a somewhat slower terminal half-life of 10 to 40 minutes.

Contraindications and precautions

Gonadorelin is contraindicated in patients hypersensitive to the drug, with conditions that could be complicated by pregnancy (such as a pituitary prolactinoma), who are anovulatory from any cause other than a hypothalamic disorder, and with ovarian cysts.

Interactions

Concomitant use of ovarian-stimulating drugs should be avoided to decrease the risk of ovarian hyperstimulation.

Effects on diagnostic tests

None reported.

Adverse reactions

● GU: ovarian hyperstimulation.
● Local: hematoma, infection, inflammation, mild phlebitis.
● Other: multiple pregnancy.

Overdose and treatment

No harmful effects are expected if the pump were to malfunction and deliver the entire contents of the highest concentration vial (3.2 mg). Bolus doses of up to 3,000 mcg have not proven harmful in clinical trials. However, continuous exposure (nonpulsatile administration) to gonadorelin might temporarily reduce pituitary responsiveness.

▶ Special considerations

● Patients usually require pelvic ultrasound on days 7 and 14 after establishment of a baseline scan. Some clinicians prefer shorter intervals between scans.
● To mimic the action of the naturally occurring hormone, gonadorelin requires a pulsatile administration with the special portable infusion pump. The pulse period is set at 1 minute (drug is infused over 1 minute); pulse interval is set at 90 minutes.
● To administer 2.5 mcg/pulse, reconstitute the 0.8-mg vial with 8 ml of supplied diluent, and set the pump to deliver 25 microliters/pulse. To administer 5 mcg/pulse, use the same dosage strength and dilution but set the pump to deliver 50 microliters/pulse.
● Some patients may require higher doses. To administer 10 mcg/pulse, reconstitute the 3.2-mg vial with 8 ml of supplied diluent, and set the pump to deliver 25 microliters/pulse. To administer 20 mcg/pulse, use this dosage strength and dilution but set the pump to deliver 50 microliters/pulse.

Information for the patient

● Because similar drugs have caused anaphylaxis, teach the patient about the signs and symptoms of hypersensitivity reactions (hives, wheezing, difficulty breathing) and instruct her to report these immediately.
● Patients should understand that a multiple pregnancy is possible (incidence about 12%). Close monitoring of dosage and ultrasonography of the ovaries are necessary to monitor drug response.
● Encourage patients to adhere to the close monitoring schedule required by the therapy. Regular pelvic examinations, midluteal phase serum progesterone determinations, and multiple ovarian ultrasound scans are necessary. Inspect the I.V. site at each visit.
● Instruct the patient about proper aseptic technique and I.V. site care. Provide available written instructions. Cannula and I.V. site should be changed every 48 hours.

Pediatric use

Safety and efficacy in children under age 18 have not been established.

Breast-feeding

It is not known if the drug is excreted in breast milk; however, there is no reason to administer the drug to a breast-feeding woman.

---

gonadorelin hydrochloride
Factrel

● Pharmacologic classification: luteinizing hormone releasing hormone
● Therapeutic classification: diagnostic agent
● Pregnancy risk category B

How supplied

Available by prescription only
Injection: 100 mcg, 500 mcg

Indications, route, and dosage
Diagnosis of hypogonadism

Adults and children age 12 and older: 100 mcg S.C. or I.V. In women for whom the phase of the menstrual cycle can be established, perform the test between day 1 and day 7.

Pharmacodynamics

Gonadotropic action: Gonadorelin stimulates the release of luteinizing hormone and follicle-stimulating hormone from the anterior pituitary. Serial measurement of luteinizing hormone levels in blood after gonadorelin injection allows assessment of pituitary gonadotropic function.

Pharmacokinetics

● *Absorption:* Limited information is available. Gonadorelin has a duration of action of 3 to 5 hours and a half-life of a few minutes.
● *Distribution:* This drug has a low plasma volume of distribution (10 to 15 liters) and a high rate of clearance from plasma.

---

*Canada only   †Unlabeled clinical use   Italicized adverse reactions are life-threatening.

• *Metabolism:* The drug is rapidly metabolized. Several biologically inactive peptide fragments have been identified.

• *Excretion:* The drug is excreted primarily in the urine. The high initial clearance rate (half-life of 2 to 10 minutes) is followed by a somewhat slower terminal half-life of 10 to 40 minutes.

Contraindications and precautions
Gonadorelin is contraindicated in patients who have demonstrated hypersensitivity to it.

Interactions
Perform diagnostic testing with gonadorelin in the absence of drugs that affect the pituitary secretion of gonadotropins, such as androgens, estrogens, progestins, adrenocorticoids, or glucocorticosteroids. Levodopa and spironolactone may elevate gonadotropin levels. Digoxin and oral contraceptives may decrease gonadotropin levels. Metoclopramide or phenothiazines also may affect test results.

Effects on diagnostic tests
Therapy with gonadorelin elevates luteinizing hormone levels.

Adverse reactions
• CNS: headache, flushing, nausea, light-headedness.
• Local: occasional pain and pruritus when administered S.C.

Overdose and treatment
Specific information unavailable. Treatment is supportive.

▶ **Special considerations**
• As a single injection, gonadorelin can aid in evaluating the functional capacity and response of the gonadotropins of the anterior pituitary. Prolonged or repeated administration may be necessary to measure pituitary gonadotropic reserve.
• Although no hypersensitivity reactions have been reported to date, use cautiously in patients who are allergic to other drugs.
• The gonadorelin test can be performed concomitantly with other post-treatment evaluation.
• For specific test methodology and interpretation of test results, refer to the manufacturer's full product information available from pharmacist.
• Reconstitute vial with 1 ml of accompanying sterile diluent. Prepare solution immediately before use. After reconstitution, store at room temperature and use within 1 day. Discard unused reconstituted solution and diluent.

Breast-feeding
Problems in humans have not been reported. However, caution is advised.

goserelin acetate
Zoladex

• Pharmacologic classification: synthetic decapeptide
• Therapeutic classification: luteinizing hormone-releasing hormone (LHRH; GnRH) analog
• Pregnancy risk category X

How supplied
Available by prescription only
Implant: 3.6 mg

Indications, route, and dosage
Palliative treatment of advanced carcinoma of the prostate
Adults: 1 implant S.C. q 28 days into the upper abdominal wall.

Pharmacodynamics
Hormonal action: Chronic administration of goserelin, an LHRH, acts on the pituitary to decrease the release of follicle-stimulating hormone (FSH) and luteinizing hormone (LH). In males, the result is dramatically lowered serum levels of testosterone.

Pharmacokinetics
• *Absorption:* Goserelin is slowly absorbed from implant site. Drug levels peak in 12 to 15 days.
• *Distribution:* No information available.
• *Metabolism:* No information available.
• *Excretion:* Elimination half-life is about 4.2 hours in patients with normal renal function. Substantial renal impairment prolongs half-life, but this does not appear to increase the incidence of adverse effects.

Contraindications and precautions
The manufacturer states that goserelin is contraindicated during pregnancy.

Initially, LHRH analogs such as goserelin may cause a worsening of the symptoms of prostatic cancer because the drug initially increases testosterone serum levels. A few patients may experience increased bone pain. Rarely, disease exacerbation (spinal cord compression or ureteral obstruction) has occurred.

Interactions
None reported.

Effects on diagnostic tests
Serum testosterone levels increase during the first week of therapy and then decrease. Serum acid phosphatase may increase initially and will decrease by week 4.

Adverse reactions
• CNS: lethargy, pain (worsened in the first 30 days), dizziness, insomnia, anxiety, depression, headache, chills, fever.
• CV: edema, *CHF, arrhythmias, cerebrovascular accident,* hypertension, *myocardial infarction,* peripheral vascular disorder, chest pain.
• DERM: rash, sweating.
• EENT: upper respiratory infection.
• GI: nausea, vomiting, diarrhea, constipation, ulcer.
• GU: decreased erections, lower urinary tract symp-

toms, renal insufficiency, urinary obstruction, urinary tract infection.
● HEMA: anemia.
● Other: hot flashes, sexual dysfunction, gout, hyperglycemia, weight increase, breast swelling and tenderness.

Overdose and treatment
No information is available regarding accidental or intentional overdosage in humans. In animal studies, doses up to 1 mg/kg/day did not produce nonendocrine-related symptoms.

▶ Special considerations
● The implant comes in a preloaded syringe. If the package is damaged, do not use the syringe. Make sure that the drug is visible in the translucent chamber of the syringe.
● Drug should be given every 28 days, always under direct supervision of a physician. Local anesthesia may be used before injection.
● Administer the drug in the upper abdominal wall using aseptic technique. After cleaning the area with an alcohol swab (and injecting a local anesthetic), stretch the patient's skin with one hand while grasping the barrel of the syringe with the other. Insert the needle into the S.C. fat, then change the needle direction to parallel the abdominal wall. Push the needle in until the hub touches the patient's skin, then withdraw it about 1 cm (this creates a gap for the drug to be injected) before depressing the plunger completely.
● After inserting the needle, do not aspirate since blood will be seen instantly in the chamber if a large vessel is penetrated (a new syringe and injection site will be needed).
● Store the drug at room temperature, not to exceed 77° F (25° C).

Information for the patient
Advise the patient to report every 28 days for a new implant. However, a delay of a couple of days is permissible.

Pediatric use
Safety and efficacy in children under age 18 have not been established.

Breast-feeding
It is not known if the drug is excreted in breast milk. However, this drug is not indicated for use in women.

griseofulvin microsize
Fulvicin-U/F, Grifulvin V, Grisactin

griseofulvin ultramicrosize
Fulvicin P/G, Gris-PEG, Grisactin Ultra

● Pharmacologic classification: *Penicillium* antibiotic
● Therapeutic classification: antifungal
● Pregnancy risk category C

How supplied
Available by prescription only

Microsize
Capsules: 125 mg, 250 mg
Tablets: 250 mg, 500 mg
Oral suspension: 125 mg/5 ml
Ultramicrosize
Tablets: 125 mg, 165 mg, 250 mg, 330 mg
Tablets, film-coated: 125 mg, 250 mg

Indications, route, and dosage
Tinea corporis, tinea capitis, or tinea cruris infections
Adults: 330 to 375 mg ultramicrosize P.O. daily, or 500 mg microsize P.O. daily.
Children over age 2: 7.3 mg/kg ultramicrosize P.O. daily or 10 to 11 mg/kg or 300 mg/m² microsize P.O. daily.
Tinea pedis or tinea unguium infections
Adults: 660 to 750 mg ultramicrosize P.O. daily or 1 g microsize P.O. daily.
Children over age 2: 7.3 mg/kg ultramicrosize P.O. daily or 10 to 11 mg/kg or 300 mg/m² microsize P.O. daily.

Pharmacodynamics
Antifungal action: Griseofulvin disrupts the fungal cell's mitotic spindle, interfering with cell division; it also may inhibit DNA replication. Drug is also deposited in keratin precursor cells, inhibiting fungal invasion. It is active against *Trichophyton, Microsporum,* and *Epidermophyton.*

Pharmacokinetics
● *Absorption:* Griseofulvin is absorbed primarily in the duodenum and varies among individuals. Ultramicrosize preparations are absorbed almost completely; microsize absorption ranges from 25% to 70% and may be increased by giving with a high-fat meal. Peak concentrations occur at 4 to 8 hours.
● *Distribution:* Griseofulvin concentrates in skin, hair, nails, fat, liver, and skeletal muscle; it is tightly bound to new keratin.
● *Metabolism:* Griseofulvin is oxidatively demethylated and conjugated with glucuronic acid to inactive metabolites in the liver.
● *Excretion:* About 50% of griseofulvin and its metabolites is excreted in urine and 33% in feces within 5 days. Less than 1% of a dose appears unchanged in urine. Griseofulvin is also excreted in perspiration. Elimination half-life is 9 to 24 hours.

Contraindications and precautions
Griseofulvin is contraindicated in patients with known hypersensitivity to the drug; it is also contraindicated in patients with hepatocellular failure and in patients with porphyria because it interferes with porphyrin metabolism. Griseofulvin should be used with caution in patients with penicillin hypersensitivity because both drugs are produced by *Penicillium.* It should be reserved for mycotic disease unresponsive to other topical treatment.

Interactions
Griseofulvin may potentiate the effects of alcohol, producing tachycardia and flushing; it may decrease prothrombin time in patients taking warfarin, by enzyme induction; and it may decrease the efficacy of oral contraceptives.
Concomitant use of barbiturates may impair absorption of griseofulvin and increase dosage requirements.

Effects on diagnostic tests
Griseofulvin can cause proteinuria; it also may decrease granulocyte counts.

Adverse reactions
● CNS: headaches (in early stages of treatment), transient decrease in hearing, fatigue with large doses, occasional mental confusion, impaired performance of routine activities, psychotic symptoms, dizziness, insomnia.
● DERM: rash, urticaria, photosensitivity reactions (may aggravate lupus erythematosus).
● GI: nausea, vomiting, excessive thirst, flatulence, diarrhea.
● HEMA: leukopenia, *granulocytopenia*.
● Metabolic: porphyria.
● Other: estrogen-like effects in children, oral thrush.
  Note: Drug should be discontinued if granulocytopenia occurs.

Overdose and treatment
Symptoms of overdose include headache, lethargy, confusion, vertigo, blurred vision, nausea, vomiting, and diarrhea. Treatment is supportive. After recent ingestion (within 4 hours), empty stomach by induced emesis or gastric lavage. Follow with activated charcoal to decrease absorption. A cathartic may also be helpful.

▶ Special considerations
● Commercial formulation of this drug has changed, decreasing the dosage required for an equivalent therapeutic effect. Dosages equivalent to the original formulation (before 1971) for 1 g of griseofulvin are 250 mg ultramicrosize or 500 mg microsize. Dosages may vary slightly depending on your manufacturer.
● Identification of organism should be confirmed before therapy begins.
● Give drug with or after meals consisting of a high-fat content (if allowed), to minimize GI distress.
● Assess nutrition and monitor food intake; drug may alter taste sensation, suppressing appetite.
● Check complete blood counts regularly for possible adverse effects; monitor renal and liver function studies periodically.
● Treatment of tinea pedis may require combined oral and topical therapy.
● Ultramicrosize griseofulvin is absorbed more rapidly and completely than microsize and is effective at one-half to two-thirds the usual dose.

Information for the patient
● Encourage patient to maintain adequate nutritional intake; offer suggestions to improve taste of food.
● Stress importance of completing prescribed regimen to prevent relapse even though symptoms may abate quickly.
● Teach signs and symptoms of adverse effects and hypersensitivity, and tell patient to report them immediately.
● Advise patient to avoid exposure to intense indoor light and sunlight to reduce the risk of photosensitivity reactions.
● Explain that drug may potentiate alcohol effects, and advise patient to avoid alcohol during therapy.
● Teach correct personal hygiene and skin care.

Pediatric use
Safety in children under age 2 has not been established.

Breast-feeding
Safety has not been established.

---

guaifenesin
Anti-Tuss, Balminil Expectorant*, Baytussin, Breonesin, Colrex Expectorant, Cremacoat 2, Gee-Gee, GG-CEN, Glyate, Glycotuss, Glytuss, Guiatuss, Halotussin, Humibid L.A., Hytuss, Hytuss-2X, Malotuss, Neo-Spec*, Nortussin, Resyl*, Robafen, Robitussin, S-T Expectorant

● Pharmacologic classification: propanediol derivative
● Therapeutic classification: expectorant
● Pregnancy risk category C

How supplied
Available without prescription
Tablets: 100 mg, 200 mg
Capsules: 200 mg
Syrup: 67 mg/5 ml, 100 mg/5 ml

Indications, route, and dosage
As expectorant
Adults and children age 12 and older: 200 to 400 mg q 4 hours; maximum dosage is 2.4 g/day.
Children age 6 to 11: 100 to 200 mg q 4 hours; maximum dosage is 1.2 g/day.
Children age 2 to 5: 50 to 100 mg q 4 hours; maximum dosage is 600 mg/day.
Children under age 2: Individualize dosage.
  For self-medication, the recommended dosage is half the usual dosage.

Pharmacodynamics
Expectorant action: Guaifenesin increases respiratory tract fluid by reducing adhesiveness and surface tension, decreasing viscosity of the secretions and thereby facilitating their removal.

Pharmacokinetics
Unknown.

Contraindications and precautions
Guaifenesin is contraindicated in patients with known hypersensitivity to this medication.

Interactions
None significant.

Effects on diagnostic tests
Guaifenesin may cause color interference with tests for 5-hydroxyindoleacetic acid and vanillylmandelic acid.

Adverse reactions
● CNS: drowsiness.
● GI: diarrhea, vomiting, and nausea occur with excessive doses.

Overdose and treatment
No information available.

▶ **Special considerations**
● The efficacy of guaifenesin as an expectorant has not been clearly established because of conflicting results of clinical studies.
● Drug should be taken with a glass of water to help loosen mucus in lungs.

Information for the patient
● Instruct patient to call if cough persists for more than 1 week, if cough recurs, or if cough is accompanied by fever, skin rash, or persistent headache.
● Advise patient to use sugarless throat lozenges to decrease throat irritation and associated cough and to report cough that persists longer than 7 days.
● Recommend humidifier to filter out dust, smoke, and air pollutants.
● Encourage deep-breathing exercises.

Geriatric use
No specific recommendations are available. Note that most liquid preparations contain alcohol (3.5% to 10%).

Pediatric use
Individualize dosage for children under age 2.

Breast-feeding
Distribution into breast milk is unknown. Safe use in breast-feeding has not been established.

guanabenz acetate
Wytensin

● Pharmacologic classification: centrally acting antiadrenergic agent
● Therapeutic classification: antihypertensive
● Pregnancy risk category C

How supplied
Available by prescription only
Tablets: 4 mg, 8 mg

Indications, route, and dosage
Hypertension (generally considered a Step 2 agent)
Adults: Initially, 4 mg P.O. b.i.d. Dosage may be increased in increments of 4 to 8 mg/day every 1 to 2 weeks. The usual maintenance dosage ranges from 8 to 16 mg daily. Maximum dosage is 32 mg b.i.d.
Children age 12 and older: Initially, 0.5 to 4 mg daily; maintenance dosage ranges from 4 to 24 mg daily, administered in two divided doses.
†*Management of opiate withdrawal*
Adults: 4 mg P.O. b.i.d. to q.i.d.

Pharmacodynamics
Antihypertensive action: Guanabenz lowers blood pressure by stimulating central alpha₂-adrenergic receptors, decreasing cerebral sympathetic outflow and thus decreasing peripheral vascular resistance. Guanabenz may also antagonize antidiuretic hormone (ADH) secretion and ADH activity in the kidney.

Pharmacokinetics
● *Absorption:* After oral administration, 70% to 80% of guanabenz is absorbed from the GI tract; antihyper-

tensive effect occurs within 60 minutes, peaking at 2 to 4 hours.
● *Distribution:* Guanabenz appears to be distributed widely into the body; drug is about 90% protein-bound.
● *Metabolism:* Guanabenz is metabolized extensively in the liver; several metabolites are formed.
● *Excretion:* Guanabenz and its metabolites are excreted primarily in urine; remaining drug is excreted in feces. Duration of antihypertensive effect varies from 6 to 12 hours.

Contraindications and precautions
Guanabenz is contraindicated in patients with known hypersensitivity to the drug. It should be used cautiously in patients with vascular insufficiency, severe coronary insufficiency, recent myocardial infarction, cerebrovascular disease, or severe hepatic or renal failure.

Interactions
Guanabenz may increase CNS depressant effects of alcohol, phenothiazines, benzodiazepines, barbiturates, and other sedatives; tricyclic antidepressants may inhibit antihypertensive effects of guanabenz.

Effects on diagnostic tests
Guanabenz may reduce serum cholesterol and total triglyceride levels slightly, but it does not alter high-density lipoprotein fraction; drug may cause nonprogressive elevations in liver enzyme levels.
Chronic use of guanabenz decreases plasma norepinephrine, dopamine, beta-hydroxylase, and plasma renin activity.

Adverse reactions
● CNS: drowsiness, sedation, dizziness, weakness, headache, ataxia, depression.
● CV: *severe rebound hypertension.*
● EENT: dry mouth.
● GU: sexual dysfunction.
Note: Drug should be discontinued if intolerable adverse reactions, such as sedation and dry mouth, do not subside.

Overdose and treatment
Clinical signs of overdose include bradycardia, CNS depression, respiratory depression, hypothermia, apnea, seizures, lethargy, agitation, irritability, diarrhea, and hypotension.
Do not induce emesis; CNS depression occurs rapidly. After adequate respiration is assured, empty stomach by gastric lavage; then give activated charcoal and a saline cathartic to decrease absorption. Follow with symptomatic and supportive care.

▶ **Special considerations**
● To ensure overnight blood pressure control and minimize daytime drowsiness, give last dose at bedtime.
● Investigational uses include managing opiate withdrawal and adjunctive therapy in patients with chronic pain.
● Abrupt discontinuation of guanabenz will cause severe rebound hypertension; reduce dosage gradually over 2 to 4 days.
● Reduced dosages may be required in patients with hepatic impairment.

Information for the patient
● Explain signs and symptoms of adverse effects and importance of reporting them.

• Warn patient to avoid hazardous activities that require mental alertness and to avoid alcohol and other CNS depressants.

• Suggest taking drug at bedtime until tolerance develops to sedation, drowsiness, and other CNS effects.

• Advise patient to avoid sudden position changes to minimize orthostatic hypotension, and to relieve dry mouth with ice chips or sugarless gum.

• Warn patient to seek medical approval before taking nonprescription cold preparations.

• Advise patient not to discontinue this drug suddenly; severe rebound hypertension may occur.

Geriatric use
Elderly patients may be more sensitive to the antihypertensive and sedative effects of guanabenz.

Pediatric use
Guanabenz has been used to treat hypertension in a limited number of children over age 12; its safety and efficacy in younger children have not been established.

Breast-feeding
It is not known if guanabenz is distributed into breast milk; an alternative feeding method is recommended during therapy.

---

guanadrel sulfate
Hylorel

• Pharmacologic classification: adrenergic neuron blocking agent
• Therapeutic classification: antihypertensive
• Pregnancy risk category B

How supplied
Available by prescription only
Tablets: 10 mg, 25 mg

Indications, route, and dosage
Hypertension
Adults: Initially, 5 mg P.O. b.i.d.; adjust dosage until blood pressure is controlled. Most patients require 20 to 75 mg daily, usually given b.i.d.

Pharmacodynamics
Antihypertensive action: Guanadrel reduces blood pressure by peripheral inhibition of norepinephrine release in adrenergic nerve endings, thus decreasing arteriolar vasoconstriction.

Pharmacokinetics
• *Absorption:* Guanadrel is absorbed rapidly and almost completely from the GI tract. Antihypertensive effect usually occurs at ½ to 2 hours; peak effect occurs at 4 to 6 hours.
• *Distribution:* Guanadrel is distributed widely into the body; drug is about 20% protein-bound; it does not enter the CNS.
• *Metabolism:* Approximately 40% to 50% of a given dose is metabolized by the liver.
• *Excretion:* Guanadrel and its metabolites are eliminated primarily in urine. Antihypertensive activity persists for 4 to 14 hours. Plasma half-life is about 10 hours but varies considerably with each individual.

Contraindications and precautions
Guanadrel is contraindicated in patients with known hypersensitivity to the drug; in patients with known or suspected pheochromocytoma, because guanadrel may increase sensitivity to circulating catecholamines; and in patients with congestive heart failure, because the drug may interfere with normal sympathetic compensation.

Guanadrel should be used cautiously in patients with bronchial asthma, peptic ulcer disease, or regional vascular disease, because the drug may worsen these conditions.

Interactions
Guanadrel may potentiate antihypertensive effects of other antihypertensive agents and pressor effects of such agents as norepinephrine and metaraminol. Monoamine oxidase (MAO) inhibitors, ephedrine, norepinephrine, methylphenidate, tricyclic antidepressants, phenothiazines, or amphetamines may antagonize antihypertensive effects of guanadrel; concomitant use of alcohol may increase risk of guanadrel-induced orthostatic hypotension. Concomitant use of diuretics or other antihypertensive agents increases the antihypertensive effects of guanadrel.

Effects on diagnostic tests
None reported.

Adverse reactions
• CNS: fatigue, dizziness, drowsiness, syncope.
• CV: orthostatic hypotension, edema.
• EENT: blurred vision.
• GI: diarrhea.
• GU: impotence, ejaculation disturbances.

Overdose and treatment
Signs of overdose include hypotension, dizziness, blurred vision, and syncope.

After acute ingestion, empty stomach by induced emesis or gastric lavage. The effect of activated charcoal in absorbing guanadrel has not been determined. Further treatment is usually symptomatic and supportive.

▶ Special considerations
• Monitor supine and standing blood pressure, especially during periods of dosage adjustment.
• Assess for signs and symptoms of edema.
• Discontinue guanadrel 48 to 72 hours before surgery, to minimize risk of vascular collapse during anesthesia.
• Separate use of guanadrel and MAO inhibitors by at least 1 week.

Information for the patient
• Teach patient signs and symptoms of adverse effects and importance of reporting them; patient should also report excessive weight gain (more than 5 lb [2.25 kg] per week).
• Explain that orthostatic hypotension can be minimized by rising slowly from a supine position and avoiding sudden position changes; it may be aggravated by fever, hot weather, hot showers, prolonged standing, exercise, and alcohol.
• Warn patient to avoid hazardous activities that require mental alertness and to take drug at bedtime until tolerance develops to sedation, drowsiness, and other CNS effects.

- Advise patient to use ice chips, hard candy, or gum to relieve dry mouth.
- Warn patient to seek medical approval before taking nonprescription cold preparations.

Geriatric use
Elderly patients may be more sensitive to orthostatic hypotension.

Pediatric use
Safety and efficacy of guanadrel in children have not been established; use drug only if potential benefit outweighs risk.

Breast-feeding
It is not known whether guanadrel is distributed into breast milk. An alternative feeding method is recommended during therapy.

guanethidine sulfate
Ismelin

- Pharmacologic classification: adrenergic neuron blocking agent
- Therapeutic classification: antihypertensive
- Pregnancy risk category C

How supplied
Available by prescription only
Tablets: 10 mg, 25 mg

Indications, route, and dosage
Moderate to severe hypertension
Adults: Initially, 10 mg P.O. once daily; increase by 10 mg at weekly to monthly intervals, as necessary. Usual dosage is 25 to 50 mg once daily; some patients may require up to 300 mg.
Children: Initially, 200 mcg/kg or 6 mg/m² P.O. daily; increase gradually every 1 to 3 weeks to maximum of five to eight times initial dose.

Pharmacodynamics
Antihypertensive action: Guanethidine acts peripherally; it decreases arteriolar vasoconstriction and reduces blood pressure by inhibiting norepinephrine release and depleting norepinephrine stores in adrenergic nerve endings.

Pharmacokinetics
- *Absorption:* Guanethidine is absorbed incompletely from the GI tract. Maximal antihypertensive effects usually are not evident for 1 to 3 weeks.
- *Distribution:* Guanethidine is distributed throughout the body; it is not protein-bound but demonstrates extensive tissue binding.
- *Metabolism:* Guanethidine undergoes partial hepatic metabolism to pharmacologically less-active metabolites.
- *Excretion:* Guanethidine and metabolites are excreted primarily in urine; small amounts are excreted in feces. Elimination half-life after chronic administration is biphasic: initial half-life is 1½ days; a second half-life is 4 to 8 days.

Contraindications and precautions
Guanethidine is contraindicated in patients with known hypersensitivity to the drug; in patients with overt congestive heart failure (CHF) not caused by hypertension, because the drug may interfere with normal sympathetic compensation; and in patients with known or suspected pheochromocytoma, because the drug may increase sensitivity to circulating catecholamines.
Guanethidine should be used cautiously in patients with recent myocardial infarction, severe cardiac disease, cerebrovascular disease, peptic ulcer disease, impaired renal function, or bronchial asthma, because the drug may precipitate or worsen these conditions.

Interactions
Concomitant use of guanethidine with diuretics, other antihypertensive agents, levodopa, or alcohol may potentiate guanethidine's antihypertensive effect; guanethidine potentiates pressor effects of such agents as norepinephrine, metaraminol, and oral sympathomimetic nasal decongestants.
Concomitant use with digitalis glycosides may result in additive bradycardia; use with rauwolfia alkaloids may cause excessive postural hypotension, bradycardia, and mental depression.
Concomitant administration with monoamine oxidase (MAO) inhibitors, tricyclic antidepressants, or oral contraceptives may antagonize the antihypertensive effect of guanethidine.

Effects on diagnostic tests
None reported.

Adverse reactions
- CNS: dizziness, weakness, syncope.
- CV: orthostatic hypotension, bradycardia, CHF, arrhythmias, edema.
- EENT: nasal stuffiness, dry mouth.
- GI: diarrhea, weight gain.
- GU: interference with ejaculation.
- HEMA: anemia, thrombocytopenia, leukopenia.
Note: Drug should be discontinued if severe diarrhea develops.

Overdose and treatment
Signs of overdose include hypotension, blurred vision, syncope, bradycardia, and severe diarrhea.
After acute ingestion, empty stomach by induced emesis or gastric lavage and give activated charcoal to reduce absorption. Further treatment is usually symptomatic and supportive.

▶ Special considerations
- Dosage requirements may be reduced in the presence of fever.
- If diarrhea develops, atropine or paregoric may be prescribed.
- Discontinue drug 2 to 3 weeks before elective surgery, to reduce risk of cardiovascular collapse during anesthesia.
- When drug is replacing MAO inhibitors, wait at least 1 week before initiating guanethidine; if replacing ganglionic blocking agents, withdraw them slowly to prevent a spiking blood pressure response during the transfer period.
- Guanethidine has been used topically as a 5% ophthalmic solution to treat chronic open-angle glaucoma or endocrine ophthalmopathy.

Information for the patient
● Teach patient signs and symptoms of adverse reactions and importance of reporting them; patient should also report persistent diarrhea and excessive weight gain (5 lb/week). Advise patient not to discontinue the drug but to call for further instructions if adverse reactions occur.
● Warn patient to avoid hazardous activities that require mental alertness and to take drug at bedtime until tolerance develops to sedation, drowsiness, and other CNS effects.
● Advise patient to avoid sudden position changes, strenuous exercise, heat, and hot showers, to minimize orthostatic hypotension; and to relieve dry mouth with ice chips, hard candy, or gum.
● Advise patient not to double next scheduled dose if he misses one; he should take only the next scheduled dose.
● Advise patient to seek medical approval before taking nonprescription cold preparations.

Geriatric use
Elderly patients may be more sensitive to drug's antihypertensive effects.

Pediatric use
Safety and efficacy have not been established.

Breast-feeding
Small amounts of guanethidine are distributed into breast milk; an alternative feeding method is recommended during therapy.

guanfacine hydrochloride
Tenex

● Pharmacologic classification: centrally acting antiadrenergic
● Therapeutic classification: antihypertensive
● Pregnancy risk category B

How supplied
Available by prescription only
Tablets: 1 mg

Indications, route, and dosage
Mild to moderate hypertension
Adults: Initially, 0.5 to 1 mg P.O. daily, at bedtime. Average dose is 1 to 3 mg daily.

Pharmacodynamics
Antihypertensive action: Guanfacine is a centrally acting alpha$_2$-adrenoreceptor agonist whose mechanism of action is not clearly understood. It appears to stimulate central alpha$_2$-adrenergic receptors that decrease peripheral release of norepinephrine, thus decreasing peripheral vascular resistance and lowering blood pressure. Drug reduces heart rate by reducing sympathetic nerve impulses from the vasomotor center to the heart. Systolic and diastolic blood pressure are both decreased; cardiac output is not altered.
Elevated plasma renin activity and plasma catecholamine levels are lowered; however, there is no correlation with individual blood pressure. Single doses of guanfacine stimulate growth hormone secretion, but long-term use has no effect on growth hormone levels.

Pharmacokinetics
● *Absorption:* Guanfacine is absorbed well and completely after oral administration and is approximately 80% bioavailable. Peak plasma concentrations occur in 1 to 4 hours; average is about 2½ hours.
● *Distribution:* The drug is approximately 70% protein-bound; high distribution to tissues is suggested.
● *Metabolism:* The drug is metabolized in the liver.
● *Excretion:* About 50% is eliminated in urine as unchanged drug, the remainder as conjugates of metabolites.

Contraindications and precautions
Guanfacine is contraindicated in patients with known hypersensitivity to the drug.
The drug should be used cautiously in patients with cerebrovascular disease, coronary insufficiency, recent myocardial infarction (these conditions may be aggravated by reduced blood pressure); chronic hepatic function impairment, or a history of mental depression.

Interactions
Guanfacine may enhance the depressant effects of alcohol and other CNS depressants, such as phenothiazines, barbiturates, and benzodiazepines.
Concurrent use with other antihypertensive agents and/or diuretic combinations may potentiate the antihypertensive effects; this often is used to therapeutic advantage.
Nonsteroidal anti-inflammatory agents (especially indomethacin), estrogens, and sympathomimetics may reduce the antihypertensive effects of guanfacine. Indomethacin and other nonsteroidals may inhibit renal prostaglandin synthesis and/or cause sodium and fluid retention, thus antagonizing the antihypertensive activity of guanfacine. Blood pressure may be increased by estrogen-induced fluid retention; monitor patient carefully.

Effects on diagnostic tests
Guanfacine therapy alters urinary catecholamine concentrations and urinary vanillylmandelic acid (VMA) excretion (may be decreased during therapy but may increase on abrupt withdrawal). Plasma growth hormone levels may be increased after a single dose; chronic elevation does not follow long-term use.

Adverse reactions
● CNS: fatigue, somnolence, dizziness, headache, insomnia, asthenia, confusion, depression, amnesia.
● CV: bradycardia, palpitations, substernal pain, orthostatic hypotension, *rebound hypertension if abruptly discontinued.*
● DERM: dermatitis, pruritus, sweating.
● EENT: dry, itching, or burning eyes.
● GI: constipation, abdominal pain, nausea, vomiting, increased salivation, taste perversion.
● GU: testicular disorder, urinary incontinence, decreased libido.
● Other: dyspnea, leg cramps, dry mouth.

Overdose and treatment
Clinical manifestations of overdose include difficult breathing, extreme dizziness, faintness, slow heartbeat, severe or unusual tiredness or weakness.
Treat symptomatically, with careful cardiac monitor-

ing. Perform gastric lavage and infuse isoproterenol as appropriate. Guanfacine is dialyzed poorly.

▶ **Special considerations**
● Give at bedtime to reduce daytime drowsiness.
● Withdrawal syndrome may occur if guanfacine is stopped abruptly or discontinued before surgery; therefore, anesthesiologist must be informed if drug was withdrawn more than 2 days before surgery, or if drug has not been withdrawn.
● Dry mouth may contribute to development of dental caries, periodontal disease, oral candidiasis, and discomfort. Recommend use of sugarless gum or candy, ice, or saliva substitute.
● Monitor blood pressure at regular intervals.

Information for the patient
● Stress importance of diet and the possible need for sodium restriction and/or weight reduction.
● Tell patient to take medication as directed even if feeling well and to take daily dose at bedtime to minimize daytime drowsiness.
● Advise patient that medication may cause drowsiness or dizziness. Urge patient to avoid use of alcohol and other CNS depressants, which may add to this effect. Tell patient to avoid driving or performing other tasks that require alertness until effects of drug are known.
● Tell patient to take a missed dose as soon as possible; if taking more than one dose per day and it is almost time for next dose, skip the missed dose and return to regular schedule.
● Store drug away from heat and light, and out of children's reach.
● Tell patient to advise new physician that he is taking this medication before having surgery, including dental surgery, or emergency treatment.
● Advise chewing sugarless gum, candy, ice, or saliva substitute for treatment of dry mouth. If condition continues longer than 2 weeks, patient should call for further recommendations.
● Tell patient not to take other medications unless they have been prescribed. This is particularly important with medications for cough, cold, asthma, hay fever, or sinus.
● Tell patient not to stop taking medication abruptly; rebound hypertension may occur.

Geriatric use
Dizziness, drowsiness, hypotension, or faintness occurs more frequently in elderly patients, who may be more sensitive to effects of guanfacine.

Haemophilus b vaccines
(Haemophilus b vaccines)

Haemophilus b conjugate vaccine, diphtheria CRM₁₉₇ protein conjugate (HbOC)
HibTITER

Haemophilus b conjugate vaccine, diphtheria toxoid conjugate (PRP-D)
ProHIBIT

Haemophilus b conjugate vaccine, meningococcal protein conjugate (PRP-OMP)
PedvaxHIB

- Pharmacologic classification: vaccine
- Therapeutic classification: bacterial vaccine
- Pregnancy risk category C

How supplied
Available by prescription only
Conjugate vaccine, diphtheria CRM₁₉₇ protein conjugate
Injection: 10 mcg of purified *Haemophilus* b saccharide and approximately 25 mcg CRM₁₉₇ protein per 0.5 ml
Conjugate vaccine, diphtheria toxoid conjugate
Injection: 25 mcg of *Haemophilus influenzae* type B (Hib) capsular polysaccharide and 18 mcg of diphtheria toxoid protein per 0.5 ml
Conjugate vaccine, meningococcal protein conjugate
Powder for injection: 15 mcg *Haemophilus* b PRP, 250 mcg *Neisseria meningitidis* OMPC per dose

Indications, route, and dosage
Routine immunization
Haemophilus b conjugate vaccine, diphtheria CRM₁₉₇ protein conjugate
Infants age 6 weeks to 2 months: 0.5 ml I.M.; repeat at age 4 months and again at age 6 months. A booster dose is required at age 15 months.
Previously unvaccinated children age 2 to 6 months: Give 0.5 ml I.M.; repeat in 2 months and again in 4 months (for a total of three doses). A booster dose is required at age 15 months.
Previously unvaccinated children age 7 to 11 months: Give 0.5 ml I.M.; repeat in 2 months (for a total of two doses before age 15 months). A booster dose is required at age 15 months (but no sooner than 2 months after the last vaccination).
Previously unvaccinated children age 12 to 14 months: Give 0.5 ml I.M. A booster dose is required at age 15 months (but no sooner than 2 months after the last vaccination).

Haemophilus b conjugate vaccine, diphtheria toxoid conjugate
Children age 15 to 59 months: 0.5 ml I.M.
Haemophilus b conjugate vaccine, meningococcal protein conjugate
Infants age 6 weeks to 2 months: 0.5 ml I.M.; repeat at age 4 months. A booster dose is required at age 12 months.
Previously unvaccinated children age 2 to 6 months: 0.5 ml I.M.; repeat in 2 months. A booster dose is required at age 12 months. *Previously unvaccinated children age 7 to 11 months:* 0.5 ml I.M.; repeat in 2 months. A booster dose is required at age 15 months (but no sooner than 2 months after the last vaccination).
Previously unvaccinated children age 12 to 14 months: Give 0.5 ml I.M. A booster dose is required at age 15 months (but no sooner than 2 months after the last vaccination).

Pharmacodynamics
H. influenzae type b prophylaxis: This vaccine promotes active immunity to *H. influenzae* type b.

Pharmacokinetics
- *Absorption:* After I.M. or S.C. administration, increases in *H. influenzae* type b capsular antibody levels in serum are detectable in about 2 weeks and peak within 3 weeks.
- *Distribution:* Limited data indicate that antibodies to *H. influenzae* type b can be detected in fetal blood and in breast milk after administration of the vaccine to pregnant and breast-feeding women.
- *Metabolism:* No information available.
- *Excretion:* The vaccine polysaccharide has been detected in urine for up to 11 days after administration to children.

Contraindications and precautions
Haemophilus b vaccine is contraindicated in children with any febrile illness or active infection and in those with known hypersensitivity to thimerosal, a component of some of the commercially available preparations (check package insert). It also is contraindicated in children who are immunosuppressed or receiving immunosuppressive therapy.

Interactions
Concomitant use of *Haemophilus* b vaccine with corticosteroids or immunosuppressants may impair the immune response to the vaccine. Avoid vaccination under these circumstances.

Effects on diagnostic tests
None reported.

Adverse reactions
- Local: erythema and pain at injection site.
- Systemic: fever, *anaphylaxis*.

Overdose and treatment
No information available.

---

*Canada only   †Unlabeled clinical use   Italicized adverse reactions are life-threatening.

▶ **Special considerations**
• Obtain a thorough history of allergies and reactions to immunizations.
• Epinephrine solution 1:1,000 should be available to treat allergic reactions.
• Do not administer intradermally or I.V.
• This vaccine may be given simultaneously with diphtheria, tetanus, and pertussis (DTP) vaccine; measles, mumps, and rubella (MMR) vaccine; poliovirus vaccine, inactivated (IPV); meningococcal vaccine; or pneumococcal vaccine but should be administered at different sites. It may also be given concomitantly with oral poliovirus vaccine (OPV). It is generally not recommended in pregnancy.
• Store the vaccine in the refrigerator and protect it from light. Hib conjugate vaccine is produced by covalent bonding of the capsular polysaccharide of *Haemophilus influenzae* type b to a protein antigen, to produce an antigen resulting in both an enhanced antibody response and an immunologic memory.
• The ACIP currently recommends that beginning at age 2 months children receive one of the conjugate vaccines licensed for this age-group (*Haemophilus* b conjugate vaccine, diphtheria CRM$_{197}$ protein conjugate (HibTITER) or *Haemophilus* b conjugate vaccine, meningococcal protein conjugate (PedvaxHIB). Check the package insert to see if the vaccine is licensed for use in specific age-groups.
• Administer the same vaccine throughout the vaccination series; no data are available to support the interchangeability of the vaccines.
• Children under age 24 months who develop invasive HIB disease should be vaccinated because natural immunity may not develop.
• Vaccination should not be used to prevent secondary HIB disease because of the time required to develop immunity. Instead, chemoprophylaxis (with drugs such as rifampin) should be used in both vaccinated and unvaccinated individuals because children with immunity may carry and transmit the organism. However, if every child in a household or day-care group has been fully vaccinated, chemoprophylaxis is not necessary.
• Note that a conjugate vaccine containing meningococcal proteins will not prevent meningococcal disease; diphtheria proteins will not produce immunity against diphtheria. DTP vaccine should be administered according to the recommended schedule.

Information for the patient
• *H. influenzae* type b is a cause of meningitis in infants and preschool children. Explain to parents that this vaccine will protect children only against meningitis caused by this organism.
• Tell parents that children may experience swelling and inflammation at the injection site and fever. Recommend acetaminophen liquid for fever.
• Tell parents to report any worrisome or persistent adverse reactions promptly.

Pediatric use
• These vaccines are indicated only in children between age 2 months and 5 years.
• Check package insert for age limitations.

halazepam
Paxipam

• Pharmacologic classification: benzodiazepine
• Therapeutic classification: antianxiety agent
• Controlled substance schedule IV
• Pregnancy risk category D

How supplied
Available by prescription only
Tablets: 20 mg, 40 mg

Indications, route, and dosage
Relief of anxiety and tension
Adults: Usually, 20 to 40 mg P.O. t.i.d. or q.i.d.; optimal daily dosage is 80 to 160 mg. Daily doses up to 600 mg have been given. In elderly or debilitated patients, initial dosage is 20 mg once daily or b.i.d.

Pharmacodynamics
Anxiolytic action: Halazepam depresses the CNS at the limbic and subcortical levels of the brain. It produces an antianxiety effect by enhancing the effect of the neurotransmitter gamma-aminobutyric acid (GABA) on its receptor in the ascending reticular activating system, which increases inhibition and blocks both cortical and limbic arousal.

Pharmacokinetics
• *Absorption:* When administered orally, halazepam is absorbed through the GI tract. Peak levels occur in 1 to 3 hours.
• *Distribution:* Halazepam is distributed widely throughout the body. Drug is approximately 85% to 95% protein-bound.
• *Metabolism:* Halazepam is metabolized in the liver to the active metabolite desmethyldiazepam.
• *Excretion:* The metabolites of halazepam are excreted in urine as glucuronide conjugates. Although the half-life of halazepam is about 14 hours, the half-life of its metabolite, desmethyldiazepam, ranges from 30 to 200 hours.

Contraindications and precautions
Halazepam is contraindicated in patients with known hypersensitivity to the drug; in patients with acute narrow-angle glaucoma or untreated open-angle glaucoma, because of the drug's possible anticholinergic effect; in patients in shock or coma, because the drug's hypnotic or hypotensive effect may be prolonged or intensified; and in patients with acute alcohol intoxication who have depressed vital signs, because the drug will worsen CNS depression.
   Halazepam should be used cautiously in patients with psychoses, because the drug is rarely beneficial in such patients and may induce paradoxical reactions; in patients with myasthenia gravis or Parkinson's disease, because it may exacerbate the disorder; in patients with impaired renal or hepatic function, which prolongs elimination of the drug; in elderly or debilitated patients, who are usually more sensitive to the drug's CNS effects; and in individuals prone to addiction or drug abuse.

Interactions
Halazepam potentiates the CNS depressant effects of phenothiazines, narcotics, barbiturates, alcohol, antihistamines, monoamine oxidase inhibitors, general anesthetics, and antidepressants.

Concomitant use with cimetidine and possibly disulfiram causes diminished hepatic metabolism of halazepam, which increases its plasma concentration.

Heavy smoking accelerates halazepam's metabolism, thus lowering clinical effectiveness.

Effects on diagnostic tests
Halazepam therapy may elevate liver function test results. Minor changes in EEG patterns, usually low-voltage, fast activity, may occur during and after halazepam therapy.

Adverse reactions
● CNS: confusion, depression, drowsiness, lethargy, hangover effect, ataxia, dizziness, syncope, nightmares, fatigue, slurred speech, tremors, vertigo, headache, euphoria, irritability.
● CV: bradycardia, *cardiovascular collapse,* transient hypotension.
● DERM: rash, urticaria.
● EENT: diplopia, blurred vision, nystagmus.
● GI: constipation, dry mouth, anorexia, nausea, vomiting, abdominal discomfort.
● GU: urinary incontinence or retention.
● Other: *respiratory depression,* dysarthria, hepatic dysfunction, changes in libido.
   Note: Drug should be discontinued if hypersensitivity or the following paradoxical reactions occur: acute hyperexcited state, anxiety, hallucinations, increased muscle spasticity, insomnia, or rage.

Overdose and treatment
Clinical manifestations of overdose include somnolence, confusion, coma, hypoactive reflexes, dyspnea, labored breathing, hypotension, bradycardia, slurred speech, and unsteady gait or impaired coordination.

Support blood pressure and respiration until drug effects subside; monitor vital signs. Mechanical ventilatory assistance via endotracheal tube may be required to maintain a patent airway and support adequate oxygenation. Flumazenil, a specific benzodiazepine antagonist, may be useful. Use I.V. fluids and vasopressors such as dopamine and phenylephrine to treat hypotension as needed. If patient is conscious, induce emesis. Use gastric lavage if ingestion was recent, but only if an endotracheal tube is present to prevent aspiration. After emesis or lavage, administer activated charcoal with a cathartic as a single dose. Dialysis is of limited value.

▶ Special considerations
Besides those relevant to all *benzodiazepines,* consider the following recommendations.
● Assess hepatic function periodically to ensure adequate drug metabolism.
● Lower doses are effective in patients with renal or hepatic dysfunction.
● Store in a cool, dry place away from light.
● Discontinue the drug slowly (over 8 to 12 weeks) after long-term therapy.

Information for the patient
● Instruct patient in safety measures, such as to avoid sudden position changes and to dangle legs before getting out of bed to prevent injury.
● Advise patient of potential for physical and psychological dependence with chronic use.
● Advise patient to call before taking any nonprescription medications or making any changes in drug regimen.

Geriatric use
● Elderly patients are more sensitive to the CNS depressant effect of halazepam. Use with caution.
● Lower doses are usually effective in elderly patients because of decreased elimination.
● Elderly patients who receive this drug require supervision with ambulation and activities of daily living during initiation of therapy or after an increase in dose.

Pediatric use
Safe use has not been established in children under age 18.

Breast-feeding
Because a breast-fed infant may become sedated, have feeding difficulties, or lose weight, avoid use in breast-feeding women.

---

halcinonide
Halciderm*, Halog, Halog-E

● Pharmacologic classification: topical adrenocorticoid
● Therapeutic classification: anti-inflammatory
● Pregnancy risk category C

How supplied
Available by prescription only
Cream: 0.025%, 0.1%
Ointment: 0.1%
Topical solution: 0.1%

Indications, route, and dosage
Inflammation of acute and chronic corticosteroid-responsive dermatoses
Adults and children: Apply cream, ointment, or solution sparingly once daily to t.i.d. Occlusive dressing may be used for severe or resistant dermatoses.

Pharmacodynamics
Anti-inflammatory action: Halcinonide stimulates the synthesis of enzymes needed to decrease the inflammatory response. Depending on its strength, halcinonide is a group II (0.1%) or group III (0.025%) fluorinated corticosteroid.

Pharmacokinetics
● *Absorption:* The amount absorbed depends on the strength of the preparation, the amount applied, and the nature of the skin at the application site. It ranges from about 1% in skin with a thick stratum corneum (such as the palms, soles, elbows, and knees) to as high as 36% in areas of the thinnest stratum corneum (face, eyelids, and genitals). Absorption increases in areas of skin damage, inflammation, or occlusion. Some

systemic absorption of topical steroids may occur, especially through the oral mucosa.

● *Distribution:* After topical application, halcinonide is distributed throughout the local skin. Any drug absorbed into the circulation is distributed into muscle, liver, skin, intestines, and kidneys.

● *Metabolism:* After topical administration, halcinonide is metabolized primarily in the skin. The small amount absorbed into systemic circulation is metabolized primarily in the liver to inactive compounds.

● *Excretion:* Inactive metabolites are excreted by the kidneys, primarily as glucuronides and sulfates, but also as unconjugated products. Small amounts of the metabolites are also excreted in feces.

Contraindications and precautions
Halcinonide is contraindicated in patients who are hypersensitive to any component of the preparation and in patients with viral, fungal, or tubercular skin lesions.

Halcinonide should be used with extreme caution in patients with impaired circulation because the drug may increase the risk of skin ulceration.

Avoid using on the face or genital areas because increased absorption may result in striae.

Interactions
None significant.

Effects on diagnostic tests
None reported.

Adverse reactions
● Local: burning, itching, irritation, dryness, folliculitis, hypertrichosis, acneiform eruptions, hypopigmentation, perioral dermatitis, allergic contact dermatitis, maceration, secondary infection, atrophy, striae, miliaria.

Significant systemic absorption may produce the following reactions:

● CNS: euphoria, insomnia, headache, psychotic behavior, pseudotumor cerebri, mental changes, nervousness, restlessness.

● CV: congestive heart failure, hypertension, edema.

● EENT: cataracts, glaucoma, thrush.

● GI: peptic ulcer, irritation, increased appetite.

● Immune: immunosuppression, increased susceptibility to infection.

● Metabolic: hypokalemia, sodium retention, fluid retention, weight gain, hyperglycemia, osteoporosis, growth suppression in children.

● Musculoskeletal: muscle atrophy.

● Other: withdrawal syndrome (nausea, fatigue, anorexia, dyspnea, hypotension, hypoglycemia, myalgia, arthralgia, fever, dizziness, and fainting).

Note: Drug should be discontinued if local irritation, infection, systemic absorption, or hypersensitivity reaction occurs.

Overdose and treatment
No information available.

▶ Special considerations
Recommendations for use of halcinonide, for care and teaching of patient during therapy, and for use in elderly patients, children, and breast-feeding women are the same as those for all *topical adrenocorticoids.*

halobetasol propionate
Ultravate

● Pharmacologic classification: corticosteroid
● Therapeutic classification: topical anti-inflammatory
● Pregnancy risk category C

How supplied
Available by prescription only
Cream: 0.05%
Ointment: 0.05%

Indications, route, and dosage
Relief of inflammation and pruritus of corticosteroid-responsive dermatoses
Adults: Apply sparingly to affected areas b.i.d. and rub in gently and completely. Treatment beyond 2 consecutive weeks is not recommended; total dosage should not exceed 50 g weekly.

Pharmacodynamics
Anti-inflammatory action: Halobetasol is classified as a "super high potency" (group I) corticosteroid. Its anti-inflammatory response results from stimulation of the synthesis of enzymes needed to decrease inflammation.

Pharmacokinetics
● *Absorption:* The amount absorbed depends on the amount applied, the application site, vehicle, use of occlusive dressing, and integrity of skin. Some systemic absorption occurs.

● *Distribution:* Throughout the local skin.

● *Metabolism:* Metabolized primarily by the skin.

● *Excretion:* Information not available.

Contraindications and precautions
Halobetasol is contraindicated in patients with a history of hypersensitivity to the drug or any of its components and in patients with viral, fungal, herpetic, or tubercular skin lesions. Use with caution in children because of the increased susceptibility for systemic absorption and toxicity.

Interactions
None significant.

Effects on diagnostic tests
None significant.

Adverse reactions
● DERM: stinging, burning, itching, irritation, dryness, folliculitis, erythema, skin atrophy, leukoderma, vesicles, rash, hypertrichosis, acneiform eruptions, hypopigmentation, perioral dermatitis, allergic contact dermatitis, secondary infection, striae, miliaria.

Significant systemic absorption can produce the following reactions:

● CNS: euphoria, insomnia, headache, mental changes, nervousness, psychotic behavior, restlessness, pseudotumor cerebri, fatigue, dizziness, syncope.

● CV: *CHF,* hypertension, hypotension.

● EENT: cataracts, glaucoma, thrush.

- GI: peptic ulcer, GI irritation, increased appetite, nausea, anorexia.
- Other: edema, hypokalemia, weight gain, hyperglycemia, fluid retention, osteoporosis, muscle atrophy, myalgia, arthralgia, fever, growth suppression of children.

Overdose and treatment
Sufficient amounts can be absorbed to produce systemic effects – specifically, suppression of the hypothalamic-pituitary-adrenal (HPA) axis, Cushing's syndrome, hyperglycemia, and glucosuria – which are reversible after discontinuation of therapy.

▶ **Special considerations**
- Adrenocorticotropic hormone-stimulation, morning plasma cortisol, and urinary cortisol tests are useful in determining the extent of HPA axis suppression.
- Treatment should be limited to 2 weeks in dosage below 50 g weekly.
- Do not use occlusive dressings.
- Do not use to treat rosacea or perioral dermatitis. Discontinue drug if infection occurs.
- If HPA axis suppression occurs, discontinue drug·or reduce frequency of application or substitute a less potent corticosteroid.
- Do not use on face, groin, or axilla.

Information for the patient
- Warn patient to use externally and only as directed by physician and to avoid contact with eyes.
- Tell patient not to cover, bandage, or wrap treated area unless directed by physician.
- Tell patient to report any signs of stinging, burning, or irritation to physician.
- Caution patient to use halobetasol exactly as prescribed.

Pediatric use
Safety and effectiveness have not been established. Use with caution, as children are more susceptible to systemic absorption and effects because of higher ratio of skin surface area to body mass.

Breast-feeding
It is unknown if topically applied corticosteroids appear in breast milk; however, caution is advised because systemically administered corticosteroids appear in breast milk and could suppress the infant's growth.

haloperidol
Apo-Haloperidol*, Haldol, Novoperidol*, Peridol*

haloperidol decanoate
Haldol Decanoate, Haldol LA*

haloperidol lactate
Haldol, Haldol Concentrate

- Pharmacologic classification: butyrophenone
- Therapeutic classification: antipsychotic
- Pregnancy risk category C

How supplied
Available by prescription only
Haloperidol
Tablets: 0.5 mg, 1 mg, 2 mg, 5 mg, 10 mg, 20 mg
Injection: 5 mg/ml
Haloperidol lactate
Oral concentrate: 2 mg/ml
Haloperidol decanoate
Injection: 50 mg/ml, 100 mg/ml

Indications, route, and dosage
Psychotic disorders
Adults: Dosage varies for each patient. Initial dosage range is 0.5 to 5 mg P.O. b.i.d. or t.i.d.; or 2 to 5 mg I.M. q 4 to 8 hours, increased rapidly if necessary for prompt control. Maximum dosage is 100 mg P.O. daily. Doses over 100 mg have been used for patients with severely resistant conditions.
Chronic psychotic patients who require prolonged therapy
Adults: 50 to 100 mg I.M. of haloperidol decanoate q 4 weeks.
Control of tics, vocal utterances in Gilles de la Tourette's syndrome
Adults: 0.5 to 5 mg P.O. b.i.d. or t.i.d., increased p.r.n.
Children age 3 to 12: 0.05 to 0.075 mg/kg/day given b.i.d. or t.i.d.

Pharmacodynamics
Antipsychotic action: Haloperidol is thought to exert its antipsychotic effects by strong postsynaptic blockade of CNS dopamine receptors, thereby inhibiting dopamine-mediated effects; its pharmacologic effects are most similar to those of piperazine antipsychotics. Its mechanism of action in Gilles de la Tourette's syndrome is unknown.

Haloperidol has many other central and peripheral effects; it has weak peripheral anticholinergic effects and antiemetic effects, and produces both alpha and ganglionic blockade, and counteracts histamine- and serotonin-mediated activity. Its most prominent adverse reactions are extrapyramidal.

Pharmacokinetics
- *Absorption:* Rate and extent of absorption vary with route of administration: oral tablet absorption yields 60% to 70% bioavailability. I.M. dose is 70% absorbed within 30 minutes. Peak plasma levels after oral administration occur at 2 to 6 hours; after I.M. administration, 30 to 45 minutes; and after long-acting I.M. (decanoate) administration, 4 to 11 days.

● *Distribution:* Haloperidol is distributed widely into the body, with high concentrations in adipose tissue. Drug is 91% to 99% protein-bound.

● *Metabolism:* Haloperidol is metabolized extensively by the liver; there may be only one active metabolite that is less active than the parent drug.

● *Excretion:* About 40% of a given dose is excreted in urine within 5 days; about 15% is excreted in feces via the biliary tract.

Contraindications and precautions

Haloperidol is contraindicated in patients with known hypersensitivity to haloperidol, phenothiazines, and related compounds, including that expressed by jaundice because haloperidol may impair liver function; in patients with blood dyscrasias and bone marrow depression because *agranulocytosis* can occur; in patients with disorders accompanied by coma, brain damage, or CNS depression because of additive CNS depression; and in circulatory collapse or cerebrovascular disease because of the drug's hypotensive and arrhythmogenic effects.

Use haloperidol cautiously in patients with cardiac disease (arrhythmias, congestive heart failure, angina pectoris, valvular disease, or heart block), encephalitis, Reye's syndrome, head injury, respiratory disease, epilepsy and other seizure disorders, glaucoma, prostatic hypertrophy, urinary retention, hepatic or renal dysfunction, Parkinson's disease, pheochromocytoma, or hypocalcemia.

Some tablet formulations contain tartrazine, a yellow dye that may precipitate allergic reactions in certain hypersensitive individuals.

Interactions

Concomitant use of haloperidol with sympathomimetics, including epinephrine, phenylephrine, phenylpropanolamine, and ephedrine (often found in nasal sprays), and appetite suppressants may decrease their stimulatory and pressor effects.

Haloperidol may inhibit blood pressure response to centrally acting antihypertensive drugs, such as guanethidine, guanabenz, guanadrel, clonidine, methyldopa, and reserpine. Additive effects are likely after concomitant use of haloperidol with CNS depressants, including alcohol, analgesics, barbiturates, narcotics, tranquilizers, and general, spinal, or epidural anesthetics, or with parenteral magnesium sulfate (oversedation, respiratory depression, and hypotension); antiarrhythmic agents, quinidine, disopyramide, or procainamide (increased incidence of cardiac arrhythmias and conduction defects); atropine or other anticholinergic drugs, including antidepressants, monoamine oxidase inhibitors, phenothiazines, antihistamines, meperidine, and antiparkinsonian agents (oversedation, paralytic ileus, visual changes, and severe constipation); nitrates (hypotension); and metrizamide (increased risk of convulsions).

Beta-blocking agents may inhibit haloperidol metabolism, increasing plasma levels and toxicity.

Concomitant use with propylthiouracil increases risk of agranulocytosis; concomitant use with lithium may result in severe neurologic toxicity with an encephalitis-like syndrome, and a decreased therapeutic response to haloperidol.

Pharmacokinetic alterations and subsequent decreased therapeutic response to haloperidol may follow concomitant use with phenobarbital (enhanced renal excretion); aluminum- and magnesium-containing antacids and antidiarrheals (decreased absorption); and heavy smoking (increased metabolism).

Haloperidol may antagonize therapeutic effect of bromocriptine on prolactin secretion; it also may decrease the vasoconstricting effects of high-dose dopamine, and may decrease effectiveness and increase toxicity of levodopa (by dopamine blockade). Haloperidol may inhibit metabolism and increase toxicity of phenytoin.

Effects on diagnostic tests

None reported.

Adverse reactions

● CNS: extrapyramidal symptoms – dystonia, akathisia, torticollis, tardive dyskinesia (usually dose-related with long-term therapy, but it can develop rapidly), sedation, pseudoparkinsonism, drowsiness, *neuroleptic malignant syndrome* (dose-related; *fatal respiratory failure* in over 10% of patients if untreated), dizziness, headache, insomnia, exacerbation of psychotic symptoms.

● CV: *asystole*, orthostatic hypotension, tachycardia, dizziness and fainting, arrhythmias, ECG changes, increased anginal pain (after I.M. injection).

● EENT: blurred vision, tinnitus, mydriasis, increased intraocular pressure, ocular changes (retinal pigmentary change with long-term use).

● GI: dry mouth, constipation, nausea, vomiting, anorexia, diarrhea.

● GU: urinary retention, gynecomastia, hypermenorrhea, inhibited ejaculation.

● HEMA: transient leukopenia, *agranulocytosis*, thrombocytopenia, anemia (within 30 to 90 days).

● Local: contact dermatitis from concentrate or injectable form, muscle necrosis from I.M. injection more common with this drug.

● Other: hyperprolactinemia, photosensitivity, increased appetite or weight gain, hypersensitivity (rash, urticaria, drug fever, edema, cholestatic jaundice), decreased libido.

Note: Drug should be discontinued immediately if any of the following occurs: hypersensitivity, jaundice, agranulocytosis; neuroleptic malignant syndrome (marked hyperthermia, extrapyramidal effects, autonomic dysfunction); or if severe extrapyramidal symptoms occur even after dosage is lowered; and 48 hours before and 24 hours after myelography using metrizamide because of the risk of convulsions. When feasible, withdraw drug slowly and gradually; many drug effects persist after withdrawal.

Overdose and treatment

CNS depression is characterized by deep, unarousable sleep and possible coma, hypotension or hypertension, extrapyramidal symptoms, dystonia, abnormal involuntary muscle movements, agitation, seizures, arrhythmias, ECG changes (may show Q-T prolongation and torsades de pointes), hypothermia or hyperthermia, and autonomic nervous system dysfunction. Overdose with long-acting decanoate requires prolonged recovery time.

Treatment is symptomatic and supportive, including maintaining vital signs, airway, stable body temperature, and fluid and electrolyte balance. Ipecac may be used to induce vomiting, with due regard for haloperidol's antiemetic properties and hazard of aspiration. Gastric lavage also may be used, followed by activated charcoal and saline cathartics; dialysis does not help.

Regulate body temperature as needed. Treat hypotension with I.V. fluids: *do not give epinephrine.* Treat seizures with parenteral diazepam or barbiturates; arrhythmias, with parenteral phenytoin (1 mg/kg with rate titrated to blood pressure); extrapyramidal reactions with benztropine or parenteral diphenhydramine (2 mg/kg/minute).

▶ **Special considerations**
● Haloperidol has few cardiovascular adverse effects and may be preferred in patients with cardiac disease.
● Assess patient periodically for abnormal body movement.
● Tardive dyskinesia may occur after prolonged use. It may not appear until months or years later and may disappear spontaneously or persist for life.
● Protect medication from light. Slight yellowing of injection or concentrate is common; does not affect potency. Discard markedly discolored solutions.
● Do not withdraw drug abruptly unless required by severe adverse reactions.
● Dose of 2 mg is therapeutic equivalent of 100 mg chlorpromazine.
● When changing from tablets to decanoate injection, patient should receive 10 to 15 times the oral dose once a month (maximum 100 mg).
● Don't administer the decanoate form I.V.

Information for the patient
● Warn patient against activities that require alertness and good psychomotor coordination until CNS response to drug is determined. Drowsiness and dizziness usually subside after a few weeks.
● Patient should report adverse effects, such as extrapyramidal reactions.
● Avoid combining with alcohol or other depressants.

Geriatric use
● Especially useful for agitation associated with senile dementia.
● Elderly patients usually require lower initial doses and a more gradual dosage titration.

Pediatric use
Haloperidol is not recommended for children under age 3. Children are especially prone to extrapyramidal adverse reactions.

haloprogin
Halotex

● Pharmacologic classification: synthetic antifungal
● Therapeutic classification: topical antifungal
● Pregnancy risk category C

How supplied
Available by prescription only
Cream: 1%
Solution: 1%

Indications, route, and dosage
Tinea pedis, tinea cruris, tinea corporis, tinea manuum, and tinea versicolor
Adults: Apply liberally to affected area b.i.d. for 2 to 3 weeks.

Pharmacodynamics
Antifungal action: Haloprogin's mechanisms of action in yeast cells is thought to be inhibition of respiration and distruption of yeast cell membranes. Its mechanism of action in dermatophytes is unknown.

Pharmacokinetics
● *Absorption:* Insignificant.
● *Distribution:* None.
● *Metabolism:* Unknown.
● *Excretion:* Unknown.

Contraindications and precautions
Haloprogin is contraindicated in patients with known hypersensitivity to the drug.

Effects on diagnostic tests
None reported.

Interactions
None reported.

Adverse reactions
● Local: irritation, burning, vesicle formation, scaling, increased maceration, pruritus or exacerbation of existing lesions.
Note: Drug should be discontinued if hypersensitivity develops or if persistent irritation occurs.

Overdose and treatment
Not applicable.

▶ **Special considerations**
● Avoid contact with eyes.
● Intertriginous infections may require 4 weeks of therapy.

Information for the patient
● Advise patient to apply drug liberally to affected areas and to avoid contact with eyes. Tell patient to wash hands well after application, and advise him to discontinue use if condition worsens or irritation and burning persists.
● Tell patient to complete prescribed regimen, even if condition improves.

heparin calcium
Calciparine

heparin sodium
Heparin Lock Flush, Hep-Lock, Hep-Lock U/P, Liquaemin Sodium

● Pharmacologic classification: anticoagulant
● Therapeutic classification: anticoagulant
● Pregnancy risk category C

How supplied
Available products are derived from beef lung or porcine intestinal mucosa. All are injectable and available by prescription only.
Heparin calcium
Syringe: 5,000 units/0.2 ml
Ampule: 12,500 units/0.5 ml; 20,000 units/0.8 ml

Heparin sodium

Vials: 1,000 units/ml, 5,000 units/ml, 10,000 units/ml, 20,000 units/ml, 40,000 units/ml

Unit-dose ampules: 1,000 units/ml, 5,000 units/ml, 10,000 units/ml

Disposable syringes: 1,000 units/ml, 2,500 units/ml, 5,000 units/ml, 7,500 units/ml, 10,000 units/ml, 20,000 units/ml, 40,000 units/ml

Carpuject: 5,000 units/ml

Premixed I.V. solutions: 1,000 units in 500 ml normal saline solution; 2,000 units in 1,000 ml normal saline solution; 12,500 units in 250 ml 0.45% saline solution; 25,000 units in 250 ml 0.45% saline solution; 25,000 units in 500 ml 0.45% saline solution; 10,000 units in 100 ml 5% dextrose in water (D_5W); 12,500 units in 250 ml D_5W; 25,000 units in 250 ml D_5W; 25,000 units in 500 ml D_5W

Heparin sodium flush

Vials: 10 units/ml, 100 units/ml

Disposable syringes: 10 units/ml, 25 units/2.5 ml, 2,500 units/2.5 ml

Indications, route, and dosage
Deep vein thrombosis

Adults: Initially, 5,000 to 7,500 units I.V. push, then adjust dose according to partial thromboplastin time (PTT) results and give dose I.V. q 4 hours (usually 4,000 to 5,000 units); or 5,000 to 7,500 units I.V. bolus, then 1,000 units hourly by I.V. infusion pump. Wait 8 hours after bolus dose, and adjust hourly rate according to PTT.

Children: Initially, 50 units/kg I.V. drip. Maintenance dose is 50 to 100 units/kg I.V. drip q 4 hours. Constant infusion: 20,000 units/m² daily. Dosages adjusted according to PTT.

Pulmonary embolism

Adults: Initially, 7,500 to 10,000 units I.V. push, then adjust dose according to PTT results and give dose I.V. q 4 hours (usually 4,000 to 5,000 units); or 7,500 to 10,000 units I.V. bolus, then 1,000 units hourly by I.V. infusion pump. Wait 8 hours after bolus dose, and adjust hourly rate according to PTT.

Children: Initially, 50 units/kg I.V. drip. Maintenance dose 50 to 100 units/kg I.V. drip q 4 hours. Constant infusion: 20,000 units/m² daily. Dosages adjusted according to PTT.

Embolism prophylaxis

Adults: 5,000 units S.C. q 12 hours.

Open-heart surgery

Adults: (total body perfusion) 150 to 300 units/kg continuous I.V. infusion.

Disseminated intravascular coagulation

Adults: 50 to 100 units/kg I.V. q 4 hours as a single injection or constant infusion. Discontinue if no improvement in 4 to 8 hours.

Children: 25 to 50 units/kg I.V. q 4 hours, as a single injection or constant infusion. Discontinue if no improvement in 4 to 8 hours.

To maintain patency of I.V. indwelling catheters

10 to 100 units as an I.V. flush (not intended for therapeutic use).

Heparin dosing is highly individualized, depending upon disease state, age, and renal and hepatic status.

Pharmacodynamics

Anticoagulant action: Heparin accelerates formation of antithrombin III-thrombin complex; it inactivates thrombin and prevents conversion of fibrinogen to fibrin.

Pharmacokinetics

● *Absorption:* Heparin is not absorbed from the GI tract and must be given parenterally. After I.V. use, onset of action is almost immediate; after S.C. injection, onset of action occurs in 20 to 60 minutes.

● *Distribution:* Heparin is extensively bound to lipoprotein, globulins, and fibrinogen; it does not cross the placenta.

● *Metabolism:* Though metabolism is not completely described, heparin is thought to be removed by the reticuloendothelial system, with some metabolism occurring in the liver.

● *Excretion:* Little is known; a small fraction is excreted in urine as unchanged drug. Drug is not excreted into breast milk. Plasma half-life is between 1 and 2 hours.

Contraindications and precautions

Although clearly hazardous in the following conditions, use of heparin depends on the comparative risk of failure to treat the coexisting thromboembolic disorder. Heparin is thus conditionally contraindicated in active bleeding and in patients with blood dyscrasias or bleeding tendencies such as hemophilia, thrombocytopenia, or hepatic disease with hypoprothrombinemia; suspected intracranial hemorrhage; suppurative thrombophlebitis; inaccessible ulcerative lesions (especially GI); open ulcerative wounds; extensive denudation of skin; ascorbic acid deficiency and other conditions causing capillary permeability; during or after brain, eye, or spinal cord surgery; during continuous GI tube drainage; and in patients with subacute bacterial endocarditis, shock, advanced renal disease, threatened abortion, or severe hypertension.

Administer heparin cautiously during menstruation and immediately postpartum; to patients with mild hepatic or renal disease, GI ulcers, alcoholism, or occupations that risk physical injury; to patients with a history of allergy or asthma, because the drug is derived from potentially allergenic porcine or bovine sources; and to lactating women, because osteoporosis can occur in these patients after 2 to 4 weeks of therapy.

Interactions

Concomitant use with salicylates and oral anticoagulants increases anticoagulant effect; if it is not possible to avoid using these together, monitor prothrombin time (PT) and PTT.

Heparin may increase diazepam plasma levels and may antagonize the effects of adrenocorticotropic hormone (ACTH), insulin, or corticosteroids.

Large doses of vitamin C can antagonize the action of heparin.

Effects on diagnostic tests

Heparin therapy prolongs PT, may falsely elevate AST (SGOT) and serum ALT (SGPT) levels, and may cause false elevations in some tests for serum thyroxine levels.

Adverse reactions

● HEMA: *hemorrhage with excessive dosage, overly prolonged clotting time, thrombocytopenia.*

● Local: tissue irritation, mild pain, pruritus, ecchymosis.

● Other: *"white clot" syndrome (a type of arterial thrombosis);* hypersensitivity reactions including chills, fever, pruritus, rhinitis, burning of feet, conjunctivitis, lacrimation, arthralgia, urticaria. After long-term use with large doses: suppressed renal function, hyperkalemia,

---

*Canada only   †Unlabeled clinical use   Italicized adverse reactions are life-threatening.

rebound hyperlipidemia upon discontinuation of drug, osteoporosis (decrease in height, rib or back pain, spontaneous fractures).

Note: Drug should be discontinued if signs of hemorrhage or new thrombosis occur.

Overdose and treatment

The major sign of overdose is hemorrhage. Immediate withdrawal of the drug usually allows the hemorrhage to resolve; however, severe hemorrhage may require treatment with protamine sulfate. Usually, 1 mg protamine sulfate will neutralize 90 units of bovine heparin or 115 units of porcine heparin.

Heparin administered by the I.V. route disappears rapidly from the blood, so the protamine dose is dependent upon when heparin was administered. Protamine should be given slowly by I.V. injection (over 3 minutes), and not more than 50 mg should be given in any 10-minute period.

Heparin administered by the S.C. route will be slowly absorbed. Protamine should be given as a 25- to 50-mg loading dose, followed by constant infusion of the remainder of the calculated dose over 8 to 16 hours.

For severe bleeding, transfusions may be required.

▶ Special considerations

● Obtain pretherapy baseline thrombin time and PTT; measure PTT regularly. Anticoagulation is present when PTT values are 1.5 to 2 times control values; draw blood for PTT 4 to 6 hours after an I.V. bolus dose and 12 to 24 hours after an S.C. dose. Blood may be drawn at any time after 8 hours of constant I.V. infusion; if I.V. therapy is intermittent, draw blood ½ hour before next scheduled dose to avoid falsely prolonged PTT. Never draw blood for PTT from the I.V. tubing of the heparin infusion, or from vein of infusion; falsely prolonged PTT will result. Always draw blood from opposite arm.
● I.V. administration is preferred because of long-term effect and because S.C. and I.M. injections are irregularly absorbed. When possible, administer I.V. heparin by infusion pump for maximum safety.
● When using heparin flush solution, keep intermittent I.V. line patent by flushing it with saline solution before and after the heparin; many medications are incompatible with heparin, and may form precipitates if they come in contact with heparin.
● For S.C. injection, use one needle to withdraw solution from vial and another to inject drug. Give low-dose S.C. injections sequentially between iliac crests in lower abdomen; give slowly and deep into subcutaneous fat. After inserting needle into skin, do not withdraw plunger to check for blood, to reduce risk of tissue injury and hematoma; leave needle in place for 10 seconds after S.C. injection. Alternate site every 12 hours: right for morning, left for evening. Do not massage after S.C. injection; watch for local bleeding, hematoma, or inflammation. Rotate site.
● Check patient regularly for bleeding gums, bruises on arms or legs, petechiae, nosebleeds, melena, tarry stools, hematuria, or hematemesis. Monitor platelet counts regularly.
● Check I.V. infusions regularly, even when pumps are in good working order, to prevent overdose or underdose; do not piggyback other drugs into line while heparin infusion is running, because many antibiotics and other drugs inactivate heparin. Never mix any drug with heparin in syringe when bolus therapy is used.
● Avoid excessive I.M. injection of other drugs to prevent or minimize hematomas. If possible, do not give any I.M. injections.
● Abrupt withdrawal may increase coagulability; heparin is usually followed by prophylactic oral anticoagulant therapy.

Information for the patient

● Teach injection technique and methods of record-keeping if patient or family will be administering the drug.
● Encourage compliance with medication schedule, follow-up appointments, and need for routine monitoring of blood studies; teach patient and family signs of bleeding, and emphasize importance of calling immediately at first sign of excess bleeding.
● Caution patient not to take double dose if he misses one; tell patient to call for further instructions instead.
● Warn against use of aspirin and other nonprescription medications; stress need to seek medical approval before taking any new medication, and to tell all physicians and dentists about use of heparin.

Geriatric use

At least one manufacturer indicates that women over age 60 are at greatest risk of hemorrhage.

---

hepatitis B immune globulin, human (HBIG)
H-BIG, Hep-B-Gammagee, HyperHep

● Pharmacologic classification: immune serum
● Therapeutic classification: hepatitis B prophylaxis product
● Pregnancy risk category B

How supplied

Available by prescription only
Injection: 1-ml, 4-ml, and 5-ml vials

Indications, route, and dosage
Hepatitis B exposure

Adults and children: 0.06 ml/kg I.M. within 7 days after exposure. Repeat 28 days after exposure.
Neonates born to HB_sAg-positive women: 0.5 ml within 12 hours of birth. Initiation of HB vaccination is indicated as well.

The American College of Obstetricians and Gynecologists recommends use of HBIG in pregnancy for postexposure prophylaxis.

Pharmacodynamics

Postexposure prophylaxis of hepatitis B: HBIG provides passive immunity to hepatitis B.

Pharmacokinetics

● *Absorption:* HBIG is absorbed slowly after I.M. injection. Antibodies to hepatitis B surface antigen (HB_sAg) appear in serum within 1 to 6 days, peak within 3 to 11 days, and persist for about 2 to 6 months.
● *Distribution:* Evidence suggests that HBIG probably does not cross the placenta or distribute into breast milk.
● *Metabolism:* No information available.
● *Excretion:* The serum half-life for antibodies to HB_sAg is reportedly 21 days.

POSTEXPOSURE PROPHYLAXIS AGAINST HEPATITIS B

Because hepatitis B is so virulent, the Centers for Disease Control recommends that persons exposed to the virus receive prophylactic immunization. Typically, exposure to this virus is accidental and frequently involves health care workers. Accidental exposure may occur by direct mucous membrane contact (for example, from a splash or through sexual contact), by percutaneous exposure (needlestick), or by oral ingestion (pipette contact) of HB_sAg-positive blood, serum, or plasma.

Perinatal exposure occurs in infants born to mothers who are HB_sAg-positive. Such infants may become carriers for life. However, prophylactic immunization can help them quickly develop protective levels of hepatitis B antibodies. Follow the recommendations in the chart below for postexposure prophylaxis against hepatitis B.

TREATMENT	EXPOSURE	DOSAGE SCHEDULE
hepatitis B immune globulin (HBIG)	Percutaneous	Administer immediately.
	Perinatal	Administer within 12 hours of birth.
	Sexual	Administer within 14 days of sexual contact. (Administer second dose if patient is HB_sAg-positive for 3 months after initial detection.)
hepatitis B vaccine	Percutaneous	Administer within 7 days. (Administer second dose 1 month later and third dose 6 months after initial dose.)
	Perinatal	Administer within 12 hours of birth. (Administer second dose 1 month later and third dose 6 months after initial dose.) Initial dose can be administered at same time as HBIG, but at another site.
	Sexual	Administer within 14 days of sexual contact. (Administer second dose 1 month later and third dose 6 months after initial dose.)

Contraindications and precautions
HBIG is contraindicated in patients with known hypersensitivity to the drug or to thimerosal, a component of this immune serum.

Interactions
Concomitant use of HBIG may interfere with immune response to vaccination with live virus vaccines, such as measles, mumps, and rubella. Live virus vaccines should be administered 2 weeks before or 3 months after HBIG whenever possible.

Effects on diagnostic tests
None reported.

Adverse reactions
● Local: pain and tenderness at injection site.
● Systemic: urticaria, angioedema, *anaphylactic reactions* (rare; severe, potentially fatal reactions possible with I.V. administration).

Overdose and treatment
No information available.

▶ Special considerations
● Obtain a thorough history of allergies and reactions to immunizations.
● Epinephrine solution 1:1,000 should be available to treat allergic reactions.
● Administer this preparation I.M. only. Severe, even fatal, reactions may occur if it is administered I.V.
● Gluteal or deltoid areas are the preferred injection sites.

● HBIG may be given simultaneously, but at different sites, with hepatitis B vaccine.
● Store between 2° and 8° C (36° to 46° F). Do not freeze.
● Hospital staff should receive immunization if exposed to hepatitis B (for example, from a needlestick or direct contact).
● HBIG has not been associated with a higher incidence of acquired immunodeficiency syndrome (AIDS). The immune globulin is devoid of human immunodeficiency virus (HIV). Immune globulin recipients do not develop antibodies to HIV.

Information for the patient
● Explain to patient that his chances of getting AIDS after receiving HBIG are very small.
● Inform patient that HBIG provides temporary protection against hepatitis B only.
● Tell patient what to expect after vaccination: local pain, swelling, and tenderness at the injection site. Recommend acetaminophen to relieve minor discomfort.
● Encourage patient to promptly report headache, skin changes, or difficulty breathing.

Breast-feeding
It is unknown if HBIG distributes into breast milk. Administer with caution to breast-feeding women.

---

hepatitis B vaccine, recombinant (inactivated)
Engerix-B, Recombivax HB,
Recombivax HB Dialysis Formulation

- Pharmacologic classification: vaccine
- Therapeutic classification: viral vaccine
- Pregnancy risk category C

How supplied
Available by prescription only
Injection: 10 mcg $HB_sAg/0.5$ ml (Engerix-B, pediatric injection); 10 mcg HB_sAg/ml (Recombivax HB); 20 mcg HB_sAg/ml (Engerix-B); 40 mcg HB_sAg/ml (Recombivax HB Dialysis Formulation)

Indications, route, and dosage
Immunization against infection from all known subtypes of hepatitis B; primary preexposure prophylaxis against hepatitis B; or postexposure prophylaxis (when given with hepatitis B immune globulin)
Engerix-B
Adults and children over age 10: Initially, give 20 mcg (1-ml adult formulation) I.M., followed by a second dose of 20 mcg I.M. 30 days later. Give a third dose of 20 mcg I.M. 6 months after the initial dose.
Neonates and children up to age 10: Initially, give 10 mcg (0.5-ml pediatric formulation) I.M., followed by a second dose of 10 mcg I.M. 30 days later. Give a third dose of 10 mcg I.M. 6 months after the initial dose.
Adults undergoing dialysis or receiving immunosuppressant therapy: Initially, give 40 mcg I.M. (divided intotwo 20-mcg doses and administered at different sites). Follow with a second dose of 40 mcg I.M. in 30 days, a third dose after 2 months, and a final dose of 40 mcg I.M. 6 months after the initial dose.
   Note: Certain populations (neonates born to infected mothers, persons recently exposed to the virus, and travelers to high-risk areas) may receive the vaccine on an abbreviated schedule, with the initial dose followed by a second dose in 1 month and the third dose after 2 months. For prolonged maintenance of protective antibody titers, a booster dose is recommended 12 months after the initial dose.
Recombivax HB
Adults: Initially, give 10 mcg (1-ml adult formulation) I.M., followed by a second dose of 10 mcg I.M. 30 days later. Give a third dose of 10 mcg I.M. 6 months after the initial dose.
Children age 11 to 19: Initially, give 5 mcg (0.5-ml) I.M., followed by a second dose of 5 mcg I.M. 30 days later. Give a third dose of 5 mcg I.M. 6 months after the initial dose.
Neonates (born to HB_sAg-negative mothers) and children to age 10: Initially, give 2.5 mcg (0.25-ml) I.M., followed by a second dose of 2.5 mcg I.M. 30 days later. Give a third dose of 2.5 mcg I.M. 6 months after the initial dose.
Neonates born to HB_sAg-positive mothers: Initially, give 5 mcg (0.5-ml) I.M. with 0.5 ml hepatitis B immune globulin. Follow with a second dose of 5 mcg I.M. 30 days later. Give a third dose of 5 mcg I.M. 6 months after the initial dose. *Adults undergoing dialysis or receiving immunosuppressant therapy:* Initially, give 40 mcg I.M. (use dialysis formulation, which contains 40

mcg/ml). Follow with a second dose of 40 mcg I.M. in 30 days, and give a final dose of 40 mcg I.M. 6 months after the initial dose.

Pharmacodynamics
Hepatitis B prophylaxis: Hepatitis B vaccine promotes active immunity to hepatitis B.

Pharmacokinetics
Absorption, distribution, metabolism, and excretion have not been described. After I.M. administration, antibody to HB_sAg appears in serum within about 2 weeks, peaks after 6 months, and persists for at least 3 years.

Contraindications and precautions
Hepatitis B vaccine is contraindicated in patients with hypersensitivity to yeast or thimerosal, a component of the vaccine. (Some clinicians will use the vaccine cautiously in these patients.) It should be used cautiously in patients with any serious, active infection; in patients with compromised cardiac or pulmonary status; and in those for whom a febrile or systemic reaction could pose a serious risk.

Interactions
When used concomitantly, corticosteroids or immunosuppressants may impair the immune response to hepatitis B vaccine. Larger-than-usual doses of the vaccine may be necessary to develop adequate circulating antibody levels.

Effects on diagnostic tests
None reported.

Adverse reactions
- Local: soreness, swelling, warmth, and induration at injection site.
- Systemic: low-grade fever, rash, transient malaise, dizziness, nausea, vomiting, diarrhea, abdominal pain, myalgia, arthralgia, hypersensitivity reactions.

Overdose and treatment
No information available.

▶ Special considerations
- Obtain a thorough history of allergies and reactions to immunizations.
- Epinephrine solution 1:1,000 should be available to treat allergic reactions.
- The Centers for Disease Control report that response to hepatitis B vaccine is significantly better after injection into the deltoid rather than the gluteal muscle.
- Hepatitis B vaccine may be administered S.C., but only to persons, such as hemophiliacs and patients with thrombocytopenia, who are at risk of hemorrhage from I.M. injection. Do not administer I.V.
- Hepatitis B vaccine may be given simultaneously, but at different sites, with hepatitis B immune globulin, influenza virus vaccine, *Haemophilus influenzae* type B conjugate vaccine, polyvalent pneumococcal vaccine, or DTP.
- Although not necessary for most individuals, serologic testing (to confirm immunity to hepatitis B after the three-dose regimen) is recommended for persons over age 50, persons at high risk of needlestick injury (who might require postexposure prophylaxis), hemodialysis patients, immunocompromised patients, and those who inadvertently received one or more injections into the gluteal muscle.

- Thoroughly agitate vial just before administration to restore a uniform suspension (slightly opaque and white in color).
- Store opened and unopened vials in the refrigerator. Do not freeze.

Information for the patient
- Tell patient that there is no risk of contracting HIV or AIDS from hepatitis B vaccine because it is synthetically derived.
- Explain that hepatitis B vaccine provides protection against hepatitis B only, not against hepatitis A or hepatitis non-A, non-B.
- Tell patient to expect some discomfort at the injection site and possible fever, headache, or upset stomach. Recommend acetaminophen to relieve such effects. Encourage patient to report distressing adverse reactions.

Pediatric use
- Routine immunization is now recommended for all neonates, regardless of maternal HB$_s$Ag status. It is usually well tolerated and highly immunogenic in children and infants of all ages.

---

hetastarch (HES, hydroxyethyl starch)
Hespan

- Pharmacologic classification: amylopectin derivative
- Therapeutic classification: plasma volume expander
- Pregnancy risk category C

How supplied
Available by prescription only
Injection: 500 ml (6 g/100 ml in 0.9% sodium chloride solution)

Indications, route, and dosage
Plasma expander in shock and cardiopulmonary bypass surgery
Adults: 500 to 1,000 ml I.V. dependent on amount of blood lost and resultant hemoconcentration. Total dosage usually should not exceed 1,500 ml/day. Up to 20 ml/kg (1.2 g/kg)/hour may be used in hemorrhagic shock; in burns or septic shock, the rate should be reduced.
Leukapheresis adjunct
Hetastarch is an adjunct in leukapheresis to improve harvesting and increase the yield of granulocytes.

Hetastarch 250 to 700 ml is infused at a constant fixed ratio, usually 1:8 to venous whole blood during continous flow centrifugation (CFC) procedures. Up to 2 CFC procedures/week, with a total number of 7 to 10 procedures using hetastarch, have been found safe and effective. The safety of larger numbers of procedures is unknown.

Pharmacodynamics
- Plasma volume expander: Hetastarch has an average molecular weight of 450,000 and exhibits colloidal properties similar to human albumin. After an I.V. infusion of hetastarch 6%, the plasma volume expands slightly in excess of the volume infused because of the colloidal osmotic effect. Maximum plasma volume ex-

pansion occurs in a few minutes and decreases over 24 to 36 hours. Hemodynamic status may improve for 24 hours or longer.
- Leukapheresis adjunct: Hetastarch enhances the yield of granulocytes by centrifugal means.

Pharmacokinetics
- Absorption: After I.V. administration, the plasma volume expands within a few minutes.
- Distribution: Hetastarch is distributed in the blood plasma.
- Metabolism: Hetastarch molecules larger than 50,000 molecular weight are slowly enzymatically degraded to molecules that can be excreted.
- Excretion: 40% of hetastarch molecules smaller than 50,000 molecular weight are excreted in urine within 24 hours. Hetastarch molecules that are not hydroxyethylated are slowly degraded to glucose. Approximately 90% of the dose is eliminated from the body with an average half-life of 17 days; the remainder has a half-life of 48 days.

Contraindications and precautions
Hetastarch is contraindicated in patients with severe bleeding disorders, because it contains no clotting factors; in patients with severe congestive heart failure (CHF) or renal failure with oliguria or anuria, because it may worsen these conditions; or for treating shock in the absence of hypovolemia, because of the potential for volume overload.

Hetastarch should be used cautiously in patients with impaired renal or hepatic function, pulmonary edema, or CHF, to prevent circulatory overload; and in patients with thrombocytopenia, because the compound may interfere with platelet function. Large volumes of hetastarch may prolong prothrombin time (PT), partial thromboplastin time (PTT), bleeding time, and clotting time and may decrease hematocrit and protein concentrations.

Interactions
None reported.

Effects on diagnostic tests
When added to whole blood, hetastarch increases the erythrocyte sedimentation rate.

Adverse reactions
- CNS: headache.
- CV: peripheral edema of lower extremities; circulatory overload; heart failure; elevated PT, PTT, and clotting and bleeding times.
- DERM: urticaria, pruritus.
- EENT: periorbital edema, parotid gland enlargement.
- GI: nausea, vomiting.
- Other: muscle pain; anaphylactoid reaction, including wheezing, mild fever.
  Note: Drug should be discontinued if allergic or sensitivity reaction occurs.

Overdose and treatment
Clinical manifestations of overdose include the adverse reactions. Stop the infusion if an overdose occurs and treat supportively.

▶ Special considerations
- To avoid circulatory overload, carefully monitor patients with impaired renal function and those at high risk of pulmonary edema or CHF. Hetastarch 6% in

0.9% sodium chloride contains 77 mEq sodium and chloride per 500 ml.
● Do not administer as a substitute for blood or plasma.
● Discard partially used bottle because it does not contain a preservative.
● Monitor CBC, total leukocyte and platelet counts, leukocyte differential count, hemoglobin, hematocrit, PT and PTT, and electrolyte, BUN, and creatinine levels.
● Assess vital signs and cardiopulmonary status to obtain baseline at start of infusion to prevent fluid overload.
● Monitor I.V. site for signs of infiltration and phlebitis.
● Observe patient for edema.

Geriatric use
Use hetastarch with caution in elderly patients, who are more prone to fluid overload; a lower dosage may be sufficient to produce desired plasma volume expansion.

Pediatric use
Safety and efficacy in children have not been established.

Breast-feeding
Women receiving hetastarch should temporarily discontinue breast-feeding.

hexocyclium methylsulfate
Tral Filmtabs

● Pharmacologic classification: anticholinergic
● Therapeutic classification: antimuscarinic, gastrointestinal antispasmodic
● Pregnancy risk category C

How supplied
Available by prescription only
Tablets: 25 mg

Indications, route, and dosage
Adjunctive therapy in peptic ulcer
Adults: 25 mg q.i.d. before meals and h.s.

Pharmacodynamics
Anticholinergic action: Hexocyclium competitively blocks acetylcholine at cholinergic neuroeffector sites, decreasing GI motility and inhibiting gastric acid secretion.

Pharmacokinetics
● *Absorption:* Hexocyclium is poorly absorbed from the GI tract (10% to 25%).
● *Distribution:* Little is known of hexocyclium's distribution; however, drug does not cross the blood-brain barrier.
● *Metabolism:* Exact metabolic fate is unknown; duration of effect is about 3 to 4 hours.
● *Excretion:* Hexocyclium is excreted in urine and feces as unabsorbed drug.

Contraindications and precautions
Hexocyclium is contraindicated in patients with narrow-angle glaucoma, because drug-induced cycloplegia and mydriasis may increase intraocular pressure; in patients with obstructive uropathy, obstructive GI tract

disease, severe ulcerative colitis, myasthenia gravis, paralytic ileus, intestinal atony, or toxic megacolon, because the drug may exacerbate these conditions; in patients with known hypersensitivity to anticholinergics; and in patients who are allergic to tartrazine or aspirin.

Administer hexocyclium cautiously to patients with autonomic neuropathy, hyperthyroidism, coronary artery disease, cardiac arrhythmias, congestive heart failure, or ulcerative colitis, because drug may exacerbate symptoms of these disorders; to patients with hepatic or renal disease, because toxic accumulation can occur; to patients over age 40, because the drug may increase the glaucoma risk; to patients with hiatal hernia associated with reflux esophagitis, because the drug may decrease lower esophageal sphincter tone; and in hot or humid environments, because the drug may predispose the patient to heatstroke.

Interactions
Concurrent administration of antacids decreases oral absorption of anticholinergics. Administer hexocyclium at least 1 hour before antacids.

Concomitant administration of drugs with anticholinergic effects may cause additive toxicity.

Decreased GI absorption of many drugs has been reported after the use of anticholinergics (for example, levodopa and ketoconazole). Conversely, slowly dissolving digoxin tablets may yield higher serum digoxin levels when administered with anticholinergics.

Use cautiously with oral potassium supplements (especially wax-matrix formulations) because the incidence of potassium-induced GI ulcerations may be increased.

Effects on diagnostic tests
None reported.

Adverse reactions
● CNS: headache, insomnia, drowsiness, dizziness, confusion or excitement (in elderly patients), nervousness, weakness.
● CV: palpitations, tachycardia, orthostatic hypotension.
● DERM: urticaria, decreased sweating or anhidrosis, other dermal manifestations.
● EENT: blurred vision, mydriasis, increased ocular tension, cycloplegia, photophobia.
● GI: dry mouth, dysphagia, heartburn, taste loss, nausea, constipation, vomiting, abdominal distention, paralytic ileus.
● GU: urinary hesitancy and retention, impotence.
● Other: fever, allergic reactions.
Note: Drug should be discontinued if hypersensitivity, urinary retention, confusion or excitement, or curare-like symptoms develop.

Overdose and treatment
Clinical signs of overdose include curare-like symptoms and such peripheral effects as dilated, nonreactive pupils; blurred vision; flushed, hot, dry skin; dryness of mucous membranes; dysphagia; decreased or absent bowel sounds; urinary tension; hyperthermia; tachycardia; hypertension; and increased respiration.

Treatment is mainly symptomatic and supportive, as needed. If the patient is alert, induce emesis (or use gastric lavage) and follow with a saline cathartic and activated charcoal to prevent further drug absorption. In severe cases, physostigmine may be administered to block hexocyclium's antimuscarinic effects. Give fluids, as needed, to treat shock. If urinary retention occurs, catheterization may be necessary.

▶ **Special considerations**
Besides those relevant to all *anticholinergics,* consider the following recommendation.
● Some hexocyclium preparations contain tartrazine dye and may cause allergic reactions, especially in patients who are sensitive to aspirin.

Geriatric use
Hexocyclium should be administered cautiously to elderly patients. Lower doses are indicated.

Pediatric use
Hexocyclium is not intended for use in children.

Breast-feeding
Hexocyclium may be excreted in breast milk, possibly resulting in infant toxicity. Breast-feeding women should avoid this drug. Hexocyclium may also decrease milk production.

PHARMACOLOGIC CLASS

histamine₂-receptor antagonists

**cimetidine
famotidine
nizatidine
ranitidine**

The introduction of histamine₂ (H₂)-receptor antagonists has revolutionized the treatment of peptic ulcer disease. These drugs structurally resemble histamine and competitively inhibit histamine's action on gastric H₂-receptors. Cimetidine, approved for clinical use in 1977, is the prototype of this class.

Pharmacology
All H₂-receptor antagonists inhibit histamine's action at H₂-receptors in gastric parietal cells, reducing gastric acid output and concentration regardless of the stimulatory agent (histamine, food, insulin, caffeine) or basal conditions.

Clinical indications and actions
Duodenal ulcer
All four H₂-receptor antagonists are used to treat acute duodenal ulcer and to prevent ulcer recurrence.
Gastric ulcer
Cimetidine, famotidine, nizatidine, and ranitidine are indicated for acute gastric ulcer. However, the benefits of long-term therapy (greater than 8 weeks) with these drugs remain unproven.
Hypersecretory states
All four H₂-receptor antagonists are used to treat hypersecretory states such as Zollinger-Ellison syndrome. Because patients with these conditions require much higher doses than patients with peptic ulcer disease, they may experience more pronounced adverse effects.
Reflux esophagitis
H₂-receptor antagonists are used to provide short-term relief from gastroesophageal reflux in patients who don't respond to conventional therapy (life-style changes, antacids, diet modification). They act by raising the stomach pH. Some clinicians prefer to combine the H₂-receptor antagonist with metoclopramide, but further

study is necessary to confirm effectiveness of the combination.
Stress ulcer prophylaxis
H₂-receptor antagonists are used to prevent stress ulcers in critically ill patients, particularly those in intensive care units. However, this remains an unlabeled (FDA unapproved) indication; some physicians prefer intensive antacid therapy for such patients.
Other uses
H₂-receptor antagonists have been used for a number of other unlabeled indications, including short-bowel syndrome and prophylaxis for allergic reactions to I.V. contrast medium.

Overview of adverse reactions
H₂-receptor antagonists rarely cause adverse reactions. However, mild transient diarrhea, neutropenia, dizziness, fatigue, *cardiac arrhythmias,* and gynecomastia have been reported.

Cimetidine may inhibit hepatic enzymes, thereby impairing the metabolism of certain drugs. Ranitidine may also produce this effect, but to a lesser extent. Famotidine has not been shown to inhibit hepatic enzymes or drug clearance.

▶ **Special considerations**
● Give single daily dose at bedtime, b.i.d. doses morning and evening, and multiple doses with meals and at bedtime. Most clinicians prefer the once daily dosage at H.S. regimen for improved compliance.
● When administering drugs I.V., do not exceed recommended infusion rates because this may increase the risk of adverse cardiovascular effects. Continuous I.V. infusion may yield better suppression of acid secretion.
● Antacids may decrease drug absorption; give antacids at least 1 hour apart from H₂-receptor antagonists.
● Patients with renal disease may require a modified schedule.
● Avoid discontinuing these drugs abruptly.
● Smoking should be avoided while taking these drugs because smoking stimulates gastric acid secretion and worsens the disease.
● Many investigational uses for these drugs (particularly cimetidine) are being evaluated.
● Symptomatic response to therapy does not rule out gastric malignancy.

Geriatric use
Use caution when administering these drugs to elderly patients because of the increased risk of adverse reactions, particularly those affecting the CNS.

Pediatric use
Safety and efficacy have not been established.

Breast-feeding
H₂-receptor antagonists may be secreted in breast milk. Ratio of risk to benefit must be considered.

Representative combinations
None.

histoplasmin
Histolyn-CYL, Histoplasmin Diluted

- Pharmacologic classification: *Histoplasma capsulatum* antigen
- Therapeutic classification: skin test antigen
- Pregnancy risk category C

How supplied
Available by prescription only
Histolyn-CYL
Injection: vials containing 10 doses of 0.1 mg
Histoplasmin Diluted
Injection: vials containing 10 doses of 0.1 mg

Indications, route, and dosage
Suspected histoplasmosis; to assess cell-mediated immunity
Adults: 0.1 ml of 1:100 dilution intradermally 5 to 10 cm apart into the volar surface of the forearm. Use tuberculin syringe with 26G or 27G ⅝" to ½" needle.

Pharmacodynamics
Histoplasmin skin test is seldom used because it may increase the complement fixation titer, which is the preferred method to diagnose an active infection. A demonstration of the organism by histologic culture is required for diagnosis.

Histoplasmin is of little value in a fulminating infection because a negative reaction usually occurs. In mild infections, repeated negative reactions may suggest exclusion of *Histoplasma* as the causative agent. Histoplasmin testing should include laboratory and clinical examinations to exclude tuberculosis, Boeck's sarcoidosis, and Hodgkin's disease. The skin test may be negative in anergic patients or when prolonged periods of time have passed since infection.

The status of cell-mediated immunity can be determined from use of histoplasmin with other antigens. It can be given in a battery of at least four different antigens to which the patient has probably been exposed in the past. In vitro tests (such as lymphocyte stimulation or assays for T and B cells) are necessary to diagnose a specific disorder.

Pharmacokinetics
- *Absorption:* After histoplasmin is injected intradermally, the test site should be examined in 48 to 72 hours.
- *Distribution:* Injection must be given intradermally; subcutaneous injection invalidates the test.
- *Metabolism:* Not applicable.
- *Excretion:* Not applicable.

Contraindications and precautions
Histoplasmin is contraindicated in patients with a hypersensitivity to phenol or polysorbate 80. Excessive dosage may cause severe erythema and induration, followed by necrosis and ulceration that may last for weeks.

Interactions
None significant.

Effects of diagnostic tests
If serologic tests for histoplasmosis are indicated, take the blood sample before the application of the skin test. Intradermal injection of histoplasmin may result in elevation of serum antibody titer to histoplasmin.

Adverse reactions
- Local: immediate wheal reaction; occasionally, large reaction will result in vesiculation, local tissue necrosis, and scar formation.
- Systemic: urticaria, angioedema, shortness of breath, excessive perspiration.

Overdose and treatment
No information available.

▶ Special considerations
- Obtain history of allergies to eggs, feathers, and chicken, and reactions to skin tests. Also take history of travel to endemic areas (for example, central United States [Ohio Valley] and eastern United States).
- After injection of histoplasmin, observe patient for 15 minutes in case systemic allergic reaction occurs. Keep epinephrine 1:1,000 available to treat anaphylaxis.
- Accurate dosage (0.1 ml) and administration are essential with the use of histoplasmin.
- Read test in adequate light at 48 to 72 hours.
Positive reaction: Induration of 5 mm or more indicates a positive reaction (cell-mediated immunity response). Erythema without induration is considered negative. Read test at 48 and 72 hours. The usual delayed skin test reaction appears in 24 hours and peaks in 48 to 72 hours. A positive reaction indicates present or past infection with *H. capsulatum* or immunologically related organisms, such as *Blastomyces* or *Coccidioides* species.
Negative reaction: A negative test (induration of less than 5 mm) means the individual has not been sensitized to histoplasmin or has lost sensitivity.
Interpretation: To distinguish lesions associated with histoplasmin sensitivity from other causes, the skin should react to histoplasmin but not tuberculin, and lesions should last for at least 2 months.
- Reactivity to this test may be depressed or suppressed for as long as 6 weeks in individuals who have received concurrent virus vaccines, in those who are receiving a corticosteroid or immunosuppressive agents, and in those who have had viral infections. The histoplasmin skin test should not be performed within 3 weeks after the administration of a live virus.
- If local reaction occurs, cold packs or topical steroids may relieve the symptoms of pain, pruritus, and discomfort.
- Draw serologic test sample before administration of skin test.

Information for the patient
- Advise patient to report any unusual side effects.
- Explain that the induration will disappear in a few days.

Geriatric use
Elderly patients not experiencing a cell-mediated immune reaction to the test are considered anergic.

Pediatric use
Use in children is not indicated.

Breast-feeding
Benefit of the histoplasmin test to the breast-feeding woman should be weighed against possible risk to the infant.

histrelin acetate
Supprelin

- Pharmacologic classification: gonadotropin releasing hormone
- Therapeutic classification: posterior pituitary hormone
- Pregnancy risk category X

How supplied
Available by prescription only
Injection: 120 mcg/0.6 ml, 300 mcg/0.6 ml, 600 mcg/ 0.6 ml

Indications, route, and dosage
Centrally mediated (idiopathic or neurogenic) precocious puberty
Children (girls age 2 to 8; boys age 2 to 9½):10 mg/kg S.C. daily as a single injection.

Pharmacodynamics
Hormonal action: Histrelin mimics the effects of gonadotropin releasing hormone (GnRH; also called luteinizing hormone-releasing hormone, or LH-RH); however, it is more potent than the naturally occurring hormone. Chronic administration desensitizes the responsiveness of the pituitary gonadotropin, resulting in decreased sex hormone production by the testes or ovaries.

Pharmacokinetics
- *Absorption:* Because histrelin is a peptide, it is broken down in the GI tract when administered orally. Drug is usually administered S.C.
- *Distribution:* No information available. Drug acts within the CNS.
- *Metabolism:* No information available.
- *Excretion:* No information available. Decreases in follicle-stimulating hormone, LH, and sex steroid levels occur within 3 months.

Contraindications and precautions
Histrelin is contraindicated in patients with hypersensitivity to any component of the drug and during pregnancy or breast-feeding.
Drug is indicated only for patients who will comply with the daily administration schedule. Noncompliance or inadequate dosing may result in inadequate control of the pubertal process, which can cause recurrence of symptoms, including onset of menses, breast development, or testicular growth. Long-term consequences may involve decreased adult height.

Interactions
None reported.

Effects on diagnostic tests
None reported.

Adverse reactions
- CNS: migraine headache, headache, visual disturbances, mood changes, nervousness, dizziness, depression, libido changes, insomnia, anxiety, paresthesia, cognitive changes, syncope, somnolence, lethargy, impaired consciousness, tremor, hyperkinesia, increased frequency of seizures, hot flashes, conduct disorder.
- CV: vasodilation, edema, palpitations, tachycardia, hypertension, pallor.
- EENT: epistaxis, ear congestion, abnormal pupillary function, otalgia, hearing loss, polyopia, photophobia, pharyngitis, rhinorrhea, sinusitis.
- Endocrine: goiter.
- GI: abdominal pain, nausea, vomiting, diarrhea, flatulence, decreased appetite, dyspepsia, cramps, constipation, thirst, gastritis.
- GU: menstrual changes, vaginal dryness, leukorrhea, menorrhagia, breast pain or edema, breast discharge, decreased breast size, tenderness of female genitalia, glycosuria.
- HEMA: hyperlipidemia, anemia.
- Respiratory: upper respiratory infection, respiratory congestion, cough, asthma, breathing disorder, bronchitis, hyperventilation.
- Other: urticaria, pyrexia, arthralgia, muscle stiffness, muscle cramps, muscle pain, hypotonia, *acute hypersensitivity reactions (anaphylaxis, angioedema).*

Overdose and treatment
There is no experience with human overdosage. Doses up to 200 times the recommended daily dose in humans have been administered to mice with no adverse effects.

▶ Special considerations
- Reevaluate patient if prepubertal levels of sex steroids or GnRH test response are not achieved within 3 months of therapy.
- A complete physical and endocrinologic evaluation is necessary before drug therapy is initiated; several indices should be reexamined at 3 months, then every 6 to 12 months thereafter. Such evaluations should include determinations of height and weight, hand and wrist X-ray for bone age determination, sex steroid (estradiol or testosterone) levels, and GnRH stimulation test. These tests will be repeated periodically to determine effectiveness of therapy.
- Additional tests should be performed to rule out other causes of precocious puberty, including beta human chorionic gonadotropin levels (to rule out a chorionic gonadotropin-secreting tumor), pelvic/adrenal/testicular ultrasound (to rule out steroid-secreting tumor), and computed tomography of the head (to rule out intracranial tumor). Baseline evaluation should document the size of gonads for serial monitoring.

Information for the patient
- Drug is dispensed as a 7-day kit, which contains a patient information leaflet. Caregivers should read and understand the leaflet.
- Before initiating therapy, both patient and parents should understand the importance of strictly adhering to the daily administration schedules. To facilitate compliance and ensure adequate dosing, the drug should be given at about the same time each day.
- Explain the importance of rotating injection sites daily. Sites should include upper arms, thighs, and abdomen.
- Drug should be stored in its original container, in the

---

*Canada only   †Unlabeled clinical use   Italicized adverse reactions are life-threatening.

refrigerator (36° to 46° F [2° to 8° C]) and protected from light. Vials are to be used only once because the drug contains no preservatives. Allow drug to reach room temperature before injection.

• Be sure patient and parents understand that they should seek prompt medical attention for any signs of immediate hypersensitivity reactions, such as sudden development of skin rash, difficulty in breathing or swallowing, or rapid heartbeat. They should also report severe or persistent swelling, redness, or irritation at the injection site.

• Be sure patient and parents know the potential risks of therapy and adverse effects. During the first month of treatment, girls commonly experience a slight menstrual flow, which is probably related to decreasing estrogen levels brought on by treatment. As estrogen levels drop, menses begins because estrogens support the endometrium.

Pediatric use
Safety and efficacy in children under age 2 have not been established.

Breast-feeding
It is unknown if drug is excreted in breast milk. Do not use in breast-feeding women because of the risk to the infant.

---

homatropine hydrobromide
AK-Homatropine, I-Homatrine, Isopto Homatropine, Minims-Homatropine*

• Pharmacologic classification: anticholinergic agent
• Therapeutic classification: cycloplegic, mydriatic
• Pregnancy risk category C

How supplied
Available by prescription only
Ophthalmic solution: 2%, 5%

Indications, route, and dosage
Cycloplegic refraction
Adults: Instill 1 to 2 drops of 2% or 1 drop of 5% solution in eye; repeat in 5 to 10 minutes.
Children: Instill 1 drop of a 2% solution in the eye; repeat at 10-minute intervals.
Uveitis
Adults: Instill 1 to 2 drops of 2% or 5% solution in eye up to q 3 or 4 hours.
Children: Instill 1 drop of a 2% solution b.i.d. or t.i.d.

Pharmacodynamics
Cycloplegic and mydriatic action: Anticholinergic action prevents the sphincter muscle of the iris and the muscle of the ciliary body from responding to cholinergic stimulation, resulting in unopposed adrenergic influence and producing pupillary dilation (mydriasis) and paralysis of accommodation (cycloplegia).

Pharmacokinetics
• *Absorption:* Peak effect is reached in 40 to 60 minutes.
• *Distribution:* Unknown.
• *Metabolism:* Unknown.

• *Excretion:* Recovery from cycloplegic and mydriatic effects usually occurs within 1 to 3 days.

Contraindications and precautions
Homatropine is contraindicated in patients with narrow-angle glaucoma or hypersensitivity to belladonna alkaloids (such as atropine) or any other component. It should be used cautiously in patients with hypertension, cardiac disease, or increased intraocular pressure.

Interactions
Homatropine may interfere with the antiglaucoma effects of pilocarpine, carbachol, or cholinesterase inhibitors.

Effects on diagnostic tests
None significant.

Adverse reactions
• CNS: dysarthria, hallucinations, amnesia, ataxia, headache, somnolence.
• CV: tachycardia, hypotension, *arrhythmias,* vasodilation.
• DERM: allergic reaction, flushing, dryness, rash (children).
• Eye: irritation, blurred vision, stinging, allergic lid reactions, hyperemia, edema, exudate.
• GI: decreased GI motility, abdominal distention (infants). • GU: bladder distention, urine retention.
• Other: fever, *respiratory depression, coma, death.*
  Note: Drug should be discontinued if signs of systemic toxicity occur.

Overdose and treatment
Clinical manifestations of overdose include flushed dry skin, dry mouth, blurred vision, ataxia, dysarthria, hallucinations, tachycardia, and decreased bowel sounds.
  Treat accidental ingestion by emesis or activated charcoal. Use physostigmine to antagonize homatropine's anticholinergic activity in severe toxicity; propranolol may be used to treat symptomatic tachyarrhythmias unresponsive to physostigmine.

▶ Special considerations
• Homatropine may produce symptoms of atropine sulfate poisoning, such as severe mouth dryness and tachycardia.
• Drug should not be used internally.
• Patient may be photophobic and may benefit by wearing dark glasses to minimize discomfort.

Information for the patient
• Teach patient the correct way to instill drops and warn him not to touch eye with dropper.
• Tell patient that vision will be temporarily blurred after instillation, and advise him to use caution when driving or operating machinery.
• Inform patient that drug may produce drowsiness.

Geriatric use
Drug should be used with caution because of the possibility of undiagnosed glaucoma and increased sensitivity to the effects of homatropine.

Pediatric use
Drug should be used with caution in small children and infants. Increased chance of sensitivity in children with

---

Down's syndrome, spastic paralysis, or brain damage exists.

hyaluronidase
Wydase

- Pharmacologic classification: protein enzyme
- Therapeutic classification: adjunctive agent to increase absorption and dispersion of injected drugs
- Pregnancy risk category C

How supplied
Available by prescription only
Injection (lyophilized powder): 150 USP units/vial, 1,500 USP units/vial
Injection (solution): 150 USP units/ml in 1-ml and 10-ml vials

Indications, route, and dosage
Adjunct to increase absorption and dispersion of other injected drugs
Adults and children: Add 150 USP units to solution containing other medication.
Adjunct to increase the absorption rate of fluids given by hypodermoclysis
Adults and children: Add 150 USP units to each liter of clysis solution administered.
Adjunct in excretion urography
Adults and children: Administer 75 USP units S.C. over each scapula, before administration of the contrast medium.

Pharmacodynamics
Diffusing action: Hyaluronidase is a spreading or diffusing substance that modifies the permeability of connective tissue through the hydrolysis of hyaluronic acid. The drug enhances the diffusion of substances injected subcutaneously provided local interstitial pressure is adequate.

Pharmacokinetics
Absorption, distribution, metabolism, and *excretion* have not been described.

Contraindications and precautions
Hyaluronidase is contraindicated in patients with known hypersensitivity to the drug and for injection into infected, acutely inflamed, or cancerous areas.

Interactions
Concomitant use with local anesthetics may increase analgesia, hasten onset, and reduce local swelling; but may also increase systemic absorption, increase toxicity, and shorten duration of action.

Effects on diagnostic tests
None reported.

Adverse reactions
- Local: irritation, hypersensitivity reactions (erythema, wheal with pseudopods and urticaria).
Note: Drug should be discontinued if hypersensitivity occurs.

Overdose and treatment
Up to 75,000 units have been administered without ill effect; local adverse effects would be anticipated. Treat symptomatically.

▶ Special considerations
- Give skin test for sensitivity before use; a wheal with pseudopods appearing within 5 minutes after injection and lasting for 20 to 30 minutes along with urticaria indicates a positive reaction.
- Avoid contact with eyes; if it occurs, flood with water immediately.
- Hyaluronidase also may be used to diffuse local anesthetics at the site of injection, especially in nerve block anesthesia. It also has been used to enhance the diffusion of drugs in the management of I.V. extravasation.
- When considering administration of any other drug with hyaluronidase, consult appropriate references for compatibility.

Information for the patient
Instruct patient to report any unusual and significant side effects after injection.

Pediatric use
If administering hyaluronidase for hypodermoclysis, take care to avoid overhydration. In children younger than age 3, clysis should not exceed 200 ml; in premature neonates, clysis should not exceed 25 ml/kg and the rate should not exceed 2 ml/minute.

PHARMACOLOGIC CLASS

hydantoin derivatives

ethotoin
mephenytoin
phenacemide
phenytoin, phenytoin sodium

Hydantoins, of which phenytoin is the prototype, are used primarily to control tonic-clonic and partial seizures. Ethotoin and mephenytoin are used to treat partial seizures refractory to less toxic agents; because of its extreme toxicity, phenacemide usually is reserved for refractory seizures. Ethotoin is less toxic than phenytoin but also less effective. Mephenytoin is more likely to produce fatal blood dyscrasias than either ethotoin or phenytoin but is less likely to cause ataxia, gingival hyperplasia, hypertrichosis, or GI distress.

Pharmacology
The hydantoins exert their anticonvulsant effects by inhibiting the spread of seizure activity in the motor cortex; they stabilize seizure threshold against hyperexcitability produced by excessive stimulation and decrease post-tetanic potentiation (PTP) that accompanies abnormal focal discharge.

Phenytoin's antiarrhythmic effects are similar to those produced by quinidine or procainamide; it improves atrioventricular conduction, especially that depressed by digitalis, and prolongs the effective refractory period.

Clinical indications and actions
Seizure disorders
Hydantoins are used to control grand mal (tonic-clonic) and psychomotor seizures; phenytoin, the only par-

SELECTING ANTICONVULSANTS

The chart below lists some common anticonvulsant drugs and their various indications.

DRUGS	INDICATIONS	THERAPEUTIC SERUM LEVELS	TIME TO REACH STEADY STATE
carbamazepine	• tonic-clonic seizures • partial seizures • mixed seizures	6 to 14 mcg/ml	2 to 4 days
clonazepam	• absence seizures • myoclonic seizures • akinetic seizures	20 to 80 ng/ml	5 to 10 days
clorazepate	• partial seizures	Not established	5 to 10 days
diazepam	• status epilepticus	Not established	Not applicable
ethosuximide	• absence seizures	40 to 100 mcg/ml	4 to 7 days
ethotoin	• tonic-clonic seizures • complex partial seizures	15 to 50 mcg/ml	15 to 45 hours
mephenytoin	• tonic-clonic seizures • complex partial seizures • simple partial seizures	25 to 40 mcg/ml	Not established
methsuximide	• absence seizures	10 to 40 mcg/ml	8 to 16 hours
phenacemide	• severe mixed seizures • partial seizures	Not established	Not established
phenobarbital	• status epilepticus • tonic-clonic seizures	15 to 40 mcg/ml	14 to 21 days
phensuximide	• absence seizures	Not established	20 hours
phenytoin	• status epilepticus • tonic-clonic seizures • complex partial seizures	10 to 20 mcg/ml	5 to 10 days
primidone	• tonic-clonic seizures • partial seizures	5 to 12 mcg/ml (primidone) 10 to 40 mcg/ml (phenobarbital)	4 to 7 days
trimethadione	• absence seizures	700 to 800 mcg/ml	2 to 5 days
valproic acid	• absence seizures	50 to 100 mcg/ml	5 to 7 days

enteral hydantoin, is used to control status epilepticus and seizures occurring during neurosurgery and in patients who cannot receive oral therapy. Mephenytoin is used only for focal, jacksonian, and psychomotor seizures and in patients with refractory seizures.

Arrhythmias

Phenytoin is also used to counteract arrhythmias, especially those produced by digitalis. However, this is an unlabeled (FDA unapproved) use.

Overview of adverse reactions

The most common adverse reactions to hydantoins involve the CNS and are dose-related, especially drowsiness, headache, ataxia, and dizziness. Other adverse reactions include GI irritation, severe dermatologic and hematopoietic reactions, lymphadenopathy, gingival hyperplasia, and hepatotoxicity.

▶ **Special considerations**

• Monitor baseline liver function and hematologic laboratory studies and repeat at monthly intervals.

• Observe patient closely during therapy for possible adverse effects, especially at start of therapy. Hydantoins may cause gingival hyperplasia; good oral hygiene and gum care are essential to minimize effects.

• The hydantoin anticonvulsants should not be discontinued abruptly, but slowly over 6 weeks; abrupt discontinuation may cause status epilepticus.

• Drug interactions are frequently a problem, primarily with hepatically cleared drugs, such as chloramphenicol, digitoxin, isoniazid, and griseofulvin; be especially alert for toxic symptoms or breakthrough seizures in patients taking any of these drugs.

• Carefully follow manufacturer's directions for reconstitution, storage, and administration of all preparations.

Information for the patient

• Tell patient not to use alcohol while taking drug, as it may decrease drug's effectiveness and may increase CNS adverse reactions.

• Advise patient to avoid hazardous tasks that require mental alertness until degree of CNS sedative effect is determined.

• Tell patient to take oral drug with food if GI distress occurs.

• Teach patient signs and symptoms of hypersensitivity, liver dysfunction, and blood dyscrasias and to call at once if any of the following occurs: sore throat, fever, bleeding, easy bruising, lymphadenopathy, or rash.

• Tell patient to call immediately if pregnancy occurs.

• Warn patient never to discontinue drug suddenly or without medical supervision.

• Encourage patient to wear a Medic Alert bracelet or necklace, listing drug and seizure disorders, while taking anticonvulsants.

• Caution patient to consult pharmacist before changing brand or using generic drug; therapeutic effect may change.

• Explain that drug may increase gum growth and sensitivity (gingival hyperplasia); teach proper oral hygiene and urge patient or parent to establish good mouth care.

• Assure patient that pink or reddish brown discoloration of urine is normal and harmless.

Geriatric use

Use anticonvulsant drugs with caution. Elderly patients metabolize and excrete all drugs more slowly and may obtain therapeutic effect from lower dosages.

Pediatric use

Be sure to administer only dosage forms prepared for pediatric use.

Breast-feeding

Hydantoin anticonvulsants are excreted in breast milk; women should discontinue breast-feeding while taking these drugs.

Representative combinations

Phenytoin with phenobarbital: Dilantin sodium with phenobarbital.

---

hydralazine hydrochloride
Alazine Tabs, Apresoline

• Pharmacologic classification: peripheral vasodilator
• Therapeutic classification: antihypertensive
• Pregnancy risk category C

How supplied

Available by prescription only
Tablets: 10 mg, 25 mg, 50 mg, 100 mg
Injection: 20 mg/ml

Indications, route, and dosage
Moderate to severe hypertension

Adults: Initially, 10 mg P.O. q.i.d. for 2 to 4 days, then increased to 25 mg q.i.d. for the remainder of the week. If necessary, dosage is increased to 50 mg q.i.d. Max-

imum recommended dosage is 200 mg daily, but some patients may require 300 to 400 mg daily.

For severe hypertension, 10 to 50 mg I.M. or 10 to 20 mg I.V. repeated as necessary. Switch to oral antihypertensives as soon as possible.

For hypertensive crisis associated with pregnancy, initially 5 mg I.V., followed by 5 to 10 mg I.V. every 20 to 30 minutes until adequate reduction in blood pressure is achieved (usual range is 5 to 20 mg).

Children: Initially, 0.75 mg/kg P.O. daily in four divided doses (25 mg/m² daily); may increase gradually to 7.5 mg/kg daily.

I.M. or I.V. drug dosage is 1.7 to 3.5 mg/kg daily or 50 to 100 mg/m² daily in four to six divided doses.

†Short-term management of severe congestive heart failure

Adults: Initially 50 to 75 mg P.O.; then adjusted according to patient response. Most patients respond to 200 to 600 mg daily, divided every 6 to 12 hours, but dosages as high as 3 g daily have been used.

Pharmacodynamics

Antihypertensive action: Hydralazine has a direct vasodilating effect on vascular smooth muscle, thus lowering blood pressure. Hydralazine's effect on resistance vessels (arterioles and arteries) is greater than that on capacitance vessels (venules and veins).

Pharmacokinetics

• Absorption: Hydralazine is absorbed rapidly from the GI tract after oral administration; peak plasma levels occur in 1 hour. Antihypertensive effect occurs 20 to 30 minutes after oral dose, 5 to 20 minutes after I.V. administration, and 10 to 30 minutes after I.M. administration. Food enhances absorption.

• Distribution: Hydralazine is distributed widely throughout the body; drug is approximately 88% to 90% protein-bound.

• Metabolism: Hydralazine is metabolized extensively in the GI mucosa and the liver.

• Excretion: Most of a given dose of hydralazine is excreted in urine, primarily as metabolites; about 10% of an oral dose is excreted in feces. Antihypertensive effect persists 2 to 4 hours after an oral dose and 2 to 6 hours after I.V. or I.M. administration.

Contraindications and precautions

Hydralazine is contraindicated in patients with known hypersensitivity to the drug and in patients with mitral valve rheumatic heart disease or coronary artery disease. Drug should be used cautiously in patients with a history of stroke or severe renal damage because these conditions may be exacerbated by hypotension.

Interactions

Hydralazine may potentiate the effects of diuretics and other antihypertensive medications; profound hypotension may occur if drug is given with diazoxide.

Concomitant administration with monoamine oxidase inhibitors may synergistically decrease blood pressure; hydralazine may decrease the pressor response to epinephrine.

Effects on diagnostic tests

Hydralazine may cause positive antinuclear antibody (ANA) titer; positive lupus erythematosus (LE) cell preparation; blood dyscrasias, including leukopenia, agranulocytosis, and purpura; and hematologic abnor-

---

malities, including decreased hemoglobin and red blood cell count.

Adverse reactions
● CNS: peripheral neuritis, headache, dizziness.
● CV: orthostatic hypotension, tachycardia, arrhythmias, angina, palpitations, edema.
● DERM: rash.
● GI: nausea, vomiting, diarrhea, anorexia, weight gain.
● HEMA: neutropenia, leukopenia.
● Other: systemic lupus erythematosus (SLE) syndrome.
Note: Drug should be discontinued if patient develops signs or symptoms of SLE or blood dyscrasias, a positive ANA titer, or positive LE cell preparation.

Overdose and treatment
Clinical signs of overdose include hypotension, tachycardia, headache, and skin flushing; cardiac arrhythmias and shock may occur.

After acute ingestion, empty stomach by emesis or gastric lavage and give activated charcoal to reduce absorption. Follow with symptomatic and supportive care.

▶ Special considerations
● CBC, LE cell preparation, and ANA titer determinations should be performed before therapy and at regular intervals during long-term therapy.
● The incidence of hydralazine-induced SLE syndrome is greatest in patients receiving more than 200 mg/day for prolonged periods.
● Headache and palpitations may occur 2 to 4 hours after first oral dose but should subside spontaneously.
● Advise precautions for postural hypotension.
● Food enhances oral absorption and helps minimize gastric irritation; adhere to consistent schedule.
● Some preparations contain tartrazine, which may precipitate allergic reactions, especially in aspirin-sensitive patients.
● For I.V. administration: Monitor blood pressure every 5 minutes until stable, then every 15 minutes; put patient in Trendelenburg's position if he is faint or dizzy. Too-rapid reduction in blood pressure can cause mental changes from cerebral ischemia.
● Inject drug as soon as possible after draining through needle into syringe; drug changes color after contact with metal.
● Remember that patients with renal impairment may respond to lower maintenance doses of hydralazine.
● Sodium retention can occur with long-term use; observe for signs of weight gain and edema.

Information for the patient
● Teach patient about his disease and therapy, and explain why he must take drug exactly as prescribed, even when feeling well; advise him never to discontinue drug suddenly because severe rebound hypertension may occur.
● Explain adverse effects and advise patient to report any unusual effects, especially symptoms of SLE (sore throat, fever, muscle and joint pain, and skin rash).
● Explain how to minimize impact of adverse effects: to avoid operation of hazardous equipment until tolerance develops to sedation, drowsiness, and other CNS effects; to avoid sudden position changes, to minimize orthostatic hypotension; to avoid alcohol; and to take drug with meals to enhance absorption and minimize gastric irritation.

● Reassure patient that headaches and palpitations occurring 2 to 4 hours after initial dose usually subside spontaneously; if not, he should report such effects.
● Instruct patient to weigh himself at least weekly. Advise him to report weight gain that exceeds 5 lb (2.25 kg) per week.
● Warn patient to seek medical approval before taking nonprescription cold preparations.

Geriatric use
Elderly patients may be more sensitive to antihypertensive effects. Use with special caution in patients with history of stroke or impaired renal function; patients with renal impairment may respond to lower maintenance dosages.

Pediatric use
Hydralazine has had limited use in children, and its safety and efficacy in children have not been established; use only if potential benefit outweighs risk.

Breast-feeding
It is not known whether hydralazine is excreted into breast milk. An alternative feeding method is recommended during therapy.

---

hydrochlorothiazide
Apo-Hydro*, Aprozide, Chlorzide, Diaqua, Diuchlor-H*, Esidrix, HydroDIURIL, Hydromal, Hydro-Z-50, Hyperetic, Natrimax*, NeoCodema*, Novohydrazide*, Oretic, Ro-Hydrazide, SK-Hydrochlorothiazide, Urozide*

● Pharmacologic classification: thiazide diuretic
● Therapeutic classification: diuretic, antihypertensive
● Pregnancy risk category B

How supplied
Available by prescription only
Tablets: 25 mg, 50 mg, 100 mg
Solution: 50 mg/5 ml

Indications, route, and dosage
Edema
Adults: Initially, 25 to 100 mg P.O. daily or intermittently for maintenance.
Children over age 6 months: 2 to 2.2 mg/kg P.O. daily divided b.i.d.
Children under age 6 months: Up to 3.3 mg/kg P.O. daily divided b.i.d.
Hypertension
Adults: 12.5 to 50 mg P.O. once daily or in divided doses. Daily dosage increased or decreased according to blood pressure.

Pharmacodynamics
● *Diuretic action:* Hydrochlorothiazide increases urinary excretion of sodium and water by inhibiting sodium reabsorption in the cortical diluting tubule of the nephron, thus relieving edema.
● *Antihypertensive action:* The exact mechanism of hydrochlorothiazide's antihypertensive effect is unknown.

It may result partially from direct arteriolar vasodilation and a decrease in total peripheral resistance.

Pharmacokinetics
- *Absorption:* Hydrochlorothiazide is absorbed from the GI tract. The rate and extent of absorption vary with different formulations of this drug.
- *Distribution:* Unknown.
- *Metabolism:* None.
- *Excretion:* Hydrochlorothiazide is excreted unchanged in urine, usually within 24 hours.

Contraindications and precautions
Hydrochlorothiazide is contraindicated in patients with known hypersensitivity to the drug or to sulfonamide derivatives. Hydrochlorothiazide should be used cautiously in patients with severe renal disease because reduced glomerular filtration rate may cause azotemia and in patients with impaired hepatic function or liver disease because electrolyte alterations may precipitate hepatic coma. Hydrochlorothiazide-induced hypokalemia may predispose patients taking digoxin to digitalis toxicity.

Interactions
Hydrochlorothiazide potentiates the hypotensive effects of most other antihypertensive drugs; this may be used to therapeutic advantage.

Hydrochlorothiazide may potentiate hyperglycemic, hypotensive, and hyperuricemic effects of diazoxide, and its hyperglycemic effect may increase insulin or sulfonylurea requirements in diabetic patients.

Hydrochlorothiazide may reduce renal clearance of lithium, elevating serum lithium levels, and may necessitate reduction in lithium dosage by 50%.

Hydrochlorothiazide turns urine slightly more alkaline and may decrease urinary excretion of some amines, such as amphetamine and quinidine; alkaline urine also may decrease therapeutic efficacy of methenamine compounds such as methenamine mandelate.

Cholestyramine and colestipol may bind hydrochlorothiazide, preventing its absorption; give drugs 1 hour apart.

Effects on diagnostic tests
Hydrochlorothiazide therapy may alter serum electrolyte levels and may increase serum urate, glucose, cholesterol, and triglyceride levels. It also may interfere with tests for parathyroid function and should be discontinued before such tests.

Adverse reactions
- CV: volume depletion and dehydration, orthostatic hypotension, hypercholesterolemia, hypertriglyceridemia.
- DERM: dermatitis, photosensitivity, rash.
- GI: anorexia, nausea, pancreatitis.
- HEMA: *aplastic anemia, agranulocytosis,* leukopenia, thrombocytopenia.
- Hepatic: hepatic encephalopathy.
- Metabolic: asymptomatic hyperuricemia; gout; hyperglycemia and impairment of glucose tolerance; fluid and electrolyte imbalances, including hyponatremia, hypochloremia, hypercalcemia, and hypokalemia; metabolic alkalosis.
- Other: hypersensitivity reactions, such as pneumonitis and vasculitis.

Note: Drug should be discontinued if rising BUN and serum creatinine levels indicate renal impairment or if patient shows signs of impending coma.

Overdose and treatment
Clinical signs of overdose include GI irritation and hypermotility, diuresis, and lethargy, which may progress to coma.

Treatment is mainly supportive; monitor and assist respiratory, cardiovascular, and renal function as indicated. Monitor fluid and electrolyte balance. Induce vomiting with ipecac in conscious patient; otherwise, use gastric lavage to avoid aspiration. Do not give cathartics; these promote additional loss of fluids and electrolytes.

▶ Special considerations
Recommendations for preparation and use of hydrochlorothiazide and for care and teaching of the patient during therapy are the same as those for all *thiazide diuretics.*

Geriatric use
Elderly and debilitated patients require close observation and may require reduced dosages. They are more sensitive to excess diuresis because of age-related changes in cardiovascular and renal function. Excess diuresis promotes orthostatic hypotension, dehydration, hypovolemia, hyponatremia, hypomagnesemia, and hypokalemia.

Breast-feeding
Hydrochlorothiazide is distributed in breast milk; safety and effectiveness in breast-feeding women have not been established.

---

hydrocortisone (systemic)
Cortef, Cortenema, Hycort*, Hydrocortone

hydrocortisone acetate
Biosone, Colifoam*, Cortifoam, Hydrocortistab*

hydrocortisone cypionate
Cortef

hydrocortisone sodium phosphate
Efcortesol*, Hydrocortone Phosphate

hydrocortisone sodium succinate
A-hydroCort, Efcortelan Soluble*, Lifocort, Solu-Cortef

- Pharmacologic classification: glucocorticoid, mineralocorticoid
- Therapeutic classification: adrenocorticoid replacement
- Pregnancy risk category C

How supplied
Available by prescription only
Hydrocortisone
Tablets: 5 mg, 10 mg, 20 mg
Injection: 25 mg/ml, 50 mg/ml suspension

Enema: 100 mg/60 ml
Hydrocortisone acetate
Injection: 25 mg/ml, 50 mg/ml suspension
Enema: 10% aerosol foam (provides 90 mg/application)
Hydrocortisone cypionate
Oral suspension: 10 mg/5 ml
Hydrocortisone sodium phosphate
Injection: 50 mg/ml solution
Hydrocortisone sodium succinate
Injection: 100 mg, 250 mg, 500 mg, 1,000 mg/vial

Indications, route, and dosage
Severe inflammation, adrenal insufficiency
Adults: 5 to 30 mg P.O. b.i.d., t.i.d., or q.i.d. (as much as 80 mg P.O. q.i.d. may be given in acute situations). *Children:* 2 to 8 mg/kg or 60 to 240 mg/m² P.O. daily.
Hydrocortisone sodium succinate
Adults: Initially, 100 to 500 mg I.M. or I.V., then 50 to 100 mg I.M. as indicated.
Hydrocortisone sodium phosphate
Adults: 15 to 240 mg S.C., I.M., or I.V. q 12 hours.
Hydrocortisone acetate
Adults: 5 to 75 mg into joints or soft tissue at 2- or 3-week intervals. Dose varies with size of joint. In many cases, local anesthetics are injected with dose.
Shock (other than adrenal crisis)
Hydrocortisone sodium succinate
Adults: 500 mg to 2 g I.M. or I.V. q 2 to 6 hours.
Children: 0.16 to 1 mg/kg or 6 to 30 mg/m² I.M. or I.V. daily.
Hydrocortisone sodium phosphate
Children: 0.16 to 1 mg/kg I.M. daily or b.i.d.
Adjunctive treatment of ulcerative colitis and proctitis
Adults: One enema (100 mg) nightly for 21 days.

Pharmacodynamics
Adrenocorticoid replacement action: Hydrocortisone is an adrenocorticoid with both glucocorticoid and mineralocorticoid properties. It is a weak anti-inflammatory agent but a potent mineralocorticoid, having potency similar to that of cortisone and twice that of prednisone. Hydrocortisone (or cortisone) is usually the drug of choice for replacement therapy in patients with adrenal insufficiency. It is usually not used for immunosuppressant activity because of the extremely large doses necessary and the unwanted mineralocorticoid effects.

Hydrocortisone and hydrocortisone cypionate may be administered orally. Hydrocortisone sodium phosphate may be administered by I.M., subcutaneous, or I.V. injection or by I.V. infusion, usually at 12-hour intervals. Hydrocortisone sodium succinate may be administered by I.M. or I.V. injection or I.V. infusion every 2 to 10 hours, depending on the clinical situation. Hydrocortisone acetate is a suspension that may be administered by intra-articular, intrasynovial, intrabursal, intralesional, or soft tissue injection. It has a slow onset but a long duration of action. The injectable forms are usually used only when the oral dosage forms cannot be used.

Pharmacokinetics
● *Absorption:* Hydrocortisone is absorbed readily after oral administration. After oral and I.V. administration, peak effects occur in about 1 to 2 hours. The acetate suspension for injection has a variable absorption over 24 to 48 hours, depending on whether it is injected into an intra-articular space or a muscle, and the blood supply to that muscle.

● *Distribution:* Hydrocortisone is removed rapidly from the blood and distributed to muscle, liver, skin, intestines, and kidneys. Hydrocortisone is bound extensively to plasma proteins (transcortin and albumin). Only the unbound portion is active. Adrenocorticoids are distributed into breast milk and through the placenta.
● *Metabolism:* Hydrocortisone is metabolized in the liver to inactive glucuronide and sulfate metabolites.
● *Excretion:* The inactive metabolites and small amounts of unmetabolized drug are excreted by the kidneys. Insignificant quantities of drug are excreted in feces. The biological half-life of hydrocortisone is 8 to 12 hours.

Contraindications and precautions
Hydrocortisone is contraindicated in patients with systemic fungal infections (except in adrenal insufficiency) and in those with a hypersensitivity to ingredients of adrenocorticoid preparations. Patients who are receiving hydrocortisone should not be given live virus vaccines because hydrocortisone suppresses the immune response.

Hydrocortisone should be used with extreme caution in patients with GI ulceration, renal disease, hypertension, osteoporosis, diabetes mellitus, thromboembolic disorders, seizures, myasthenia gravis, congestive heart failure (CHF), tuberculosis, hypoalbuminemia, hypothyroidism, cirrhosis of the liver, emotional instability, psychotic tendencies, hyperlipidemias, glaucoma, or cataracts, because the drug may exacerbate these conditions.

Because adrenocorticoids increase the susceptibility to and mask symptoms of infection, hydrocortisone should not be used (except in life-threatening situations) in patients with viral or bacterial infections not controlled by anti-infective agents.

Interactions
When used concomitantly, hydrocortisone may in rare cases decrease the effects of oral anticoagulants by unknown mechanisms. Concomitant use of barbiturates, phenytoin, or rifampin may decrease corticosteroid effects because of increased hepatic metabolism. Cholestyramine, colestipol, and antacids decrease corticosteroid effect by adsorbing the corticosteroid, thereby decreasing the amount absorbed.

Hydrocortisone increases the metabolism of isoniazid and salicylates; this causes hyperglycemia, requiring dosage adjustment of insulin or oral hypoglycemic agents in diabetic patients. It may enhance hypokalemia associated with diuretic or amphotericin B therapy. The hypokalemia may increase the risk of toxicity in patients receiving digitalis.

Concomitant use of estrogens may reduce the metabolism of corticosteroids by increasing the concentration of transcortin. The half-life of the corticosteroid is then prolonged from increased protein binding. Concomitant administration of ulcerogenic drugs, such as nonsteroidal anti-inflammatory agents, may increase the risk of GI ulceration.

Effects on diagnostic tests
Hydrocortisone suppresses reactions to skin tests; causes false-negative results in the nitroblue tetrazolium tests for systemic bacterial infections; and decreases ^{131}I uptake and protein-bound iodine concentrations in thyroid function tests.

Hydrocortisone may increase glucose and cholesterol levels; may decrease serum potassium, calcium,

---

thyroxine, and triiodothyronine levels; and may increase urine glucose and calcium levels.

Adverse reactions

When administered in high doses or for prolonged therapy, hydrocortisone suppresses release of adrenocorticotropic hormone (ACTH) from the pituitary gland, and the adrenal cortex stops secreting endogenous corticosteroids. The degree and duration of hypothalamic-pituitary-adrenal (HPA) axis suppression produced by the drug is highly variable among patients and depends on the dose, frequency and time of administration, and duration of glucocorticoid therapy.

● CNS: euphoria, insomnia, headache, psychotic behavior, pseudotumor cerebri, mental changes, nervousness, restlessness.
● CV: CHF, hypertension, edema.
● DERM: delayed healing, acne, skin eruptions, striae.
● EENT: cataracts, glaucoma, thrush.
● GI: peptic ulcer, irritation, increased appetite.
● Immune: immunosuppression, increased susceptibility to infection.
● Metabolic: hypokalemia, sodium retention, fluid retention, weight gain, hyperglycemia, osteoporosis, growth suppression in children.
● Musculoskeletal: muscle atrophy.
● Other: muscle weakness, pancreatitis, hirsutism, cushingoid symptoms, withdrawal syndrome (nausea, fatigue, anorexia, dyspnea, hypotension, hypoglycemia, myalgia, arthralgia, fever, dizziness, and fainting). *Sudden discontinuation may be fatal or may exacerbate the underlying disease.* Acute adrenal insufficiency may occur with increased stress (infection, surgery, trauma) or abrupt withdrawal after long-term therapy.

Overdose and treatment

Acute ingestion, even in massive doses, is rarely a clinical problem. Toxic signs and symptoms rarely occur if drug is used for less than 3 weeks, even at large doses. However, chronic use causes adverse physiologic effects, including suppression of the HPA axis, cushingoid appearance, muscle weakness, and osteoporosis.

▶ Special considerations

Recommendations for use of hydrocortisone and for care and teaching of patients during therapy are the same as those for all *systemic adrenocorticoids.*

Pediatric use

Chronic use of hydrocortisone in children and adolescents may delay growth and maturation.

---

hydrocortisone (topical)
Acticort, Barriere-HC*, Calde CORT, Cetacort, Cortate*, Cort-Dome, Cortizone, Dermacort, Dermi Cort, Dermolate, Dermtex HC, Dioderm*, Efcortelan*, Emo-Cort*, HC-Jel, Hi-Cor, H₂ Cort, Hydro-Tex, Hytone, Nutracort, Penecort, Racet-SE, Rectocort*, Synacort, Unicort*

hydrocortisone acetate
Cortaid, Cort-Dome, Corticaine, Corticreme*, Cortiment*, Cortoderm*, Hyderm*, Lanacort, Novohydrocort*, Orabase-HCA, Pharma-Cort, Rhulicort

hydrocortisone butyrate
Locoid

hydrocortisone valerate
Westcort

● Pharmacologic classification: glucocorticoid
● Therapeutic classification: anti-inflammatory
● Pregnancy risk category C

How supplied
Available by prescription only
Hydrocortisone
Cream: 0.25%, 0.5%, 1%, 2.5%
Ointment: 0.5%, 1%, 2.5%
Lotion: 0.125%, 0.25%, 0.5%, 1%, 2%, 2.5%
Gel: 1%
Solution: 1%
Aerosol: 0.5%
Retention enema: 100 mg/60 ml unit
Hydrocortisone acetate
Cream: 0.5%
Ointment: 0.5%, 1%
Lotion: 0.5%
Suppositories: 10 mg, 15 mg, 25 mg
Rectal foam: 90 mg/application
Hydrocortisone butyrate
Cream, ointment: 0.1%
Hydrocortisone valerate
Cream, ointment: 0.2%

Available without prescription
Hydrocortisone
Cream, ointment, lotion: 0.5%
Hydrocortisone acetate
Cream, ointment, lotion, dental paste: 0.5%

Indications, route, and dosage
Inflammation of corticosteroid-responsive dermatoses, including those on face, groin, armpits, and under breasts; seborrheic dermatitis of scalp
Adults and children: Apply cream, lotion, ointment, foam, or aerosol sparingly once daily to q.i.d.
For aerosol
Shake can well. Direct spray onto affected area from a distance of 6″ (15 cm). Apply for only 3 seconds (to avoid freezing tissues). Apply to dry scalp after sham-

---

pooing; no need to massage or rub medication into scalp after spraying. Apply daily until acute phase is controlled, then reduce dosage to one to three times a week as needed to maintain control.

For rectal administration
Shake can well. Apply one application once daily or b.i.d. for 2 to 3 weeks, then every other day as necessary.

Dental lesions
Adults and children: Apply paste b.i.d. or t.i.d. and h.s.

Pharmacodynamics

Anti-inflammatory action: Hydrocortisone stimulates the synthesis of enzymes needed to decrease the inflammatory response. Hydrocortisone, a corticosteroid secreted by the adrenal cortex, is about 1.25 times more potent an anti-inflammatory agent than equivalent doses of cortisone, but both have twice the mineralocorticoid activity of the other glucocorticoids. As topical agents, hydrocortisone and hydrocortisone acetate are low-potency group VI glucocorticoids. Hydrocortisone valerate has group IV potency.

Hydrocortisone 0.5% and hydrocortisone acetate 0.5% are available without a prescription for the temporary relief of minor skin irritation, itching, and rashes caused by eczema, insect bites, soaps, and detergents.

Hydrocortisone is also administered rectally as a retention enema for the temporary treatment of acute ulcerative colitis. Hydrocortisone acetate suspension is also available as a rectal suppository or aerosol foam suspension for the temporary treatment of inflammatory conditions of the rectum such as hemorrhoids, cryptitis, proctitis, and pruritus ani.

Pharmacokinetics

● *Absorption:* Hydrocortisone absorption depends on the potency of the preparation, the amount applied, and the nature of the skin at the application site. It ranges from about 1% in areas with a thick stratum corneum, (such as the palms, soles, elbows, and knees) to as high as 36% in areas where the stratum corneum is thinnest (face, eyelids, and genitals). Absorption increases in areas of skin damage, inflammation, or occlusion. Some systemic absorption occurs, especially through the oral mucosa.
● *Distribution:* After topical application, hydrocortisone is distributed throughout the local skin layers. Any drug absorbed into circulation is removed rapidly from the blood and distributed into muscle, liver, skin, intestines, and kidneys.
● *Metabolism:* After topical administration, hydrocortisone is metabolized primarily in the skin. The small amount that is absorbed into systemic circulation is metabolized primarily in the liver to inactive compounds.
● *Excretion:* Inactive metabolites are excreted by the kidneys, primarily as glucuronides and sulfates, but also as unconjugated products. Small amounts of the metabolites are also excreted in feces.

Contraindications and precautions

Hydrocortisone is contraindicated in patients who are hypersensitive to any component of the preparation and in patients with viral, fungal, or tubercular skin lesions.

Drug should be used with extreme caution in patients with impaired circulation because it may increase the risk of skin ulceration.

Interactions
None significant.

Effects on diagnostic tests
None reported.

Adverse reactions
● Local: burning, itching, irritation, dryness, folliculitis, hypertrichosis, acneiform eruptions, hypopigmentation, perioral dermatitis, allergic contact dermatitis, maceration, secondary infection, atrophy, striae, miliaria.

Systemic absorption may produce the following reactions.
● CNS: euphoria, insomnia, headache, psychotic behavior, pseudotumor cerebri, mental changes, nervousness, restlessness.
● CV: congestive heart failure, hypertension, edema.
● DERM: delayed healing, acne, skin eruptions, striae.
● EENT: cataracts, glaucoma, thrush.
● GI: peptic ulcer, irritation, increased appetite.
● Immune: immunosuppression, increased susceptibility to infection.
● Metabolic: hypokalemia, sodium retention, fluid retention, weight gain, hyperglycemia, osteoporosis, growth suppression in children.
● Musculoskeletal: muscle atrophy.
● Other: withdrawal syndrome (nausea, fatigue, anorexia, dyspnea, hypotension, hypoglycemia, myalgia, arthralgia, fever, dizziness, and fainting).

Note: Drug should be discontinued if local irritation, infection, systemic absorption, or hypersensitivity reaction occurs.

Overdose and treatment
No information available.

▶ Special considerations
Recommendations for use of hydrocortisone, for care and teaching of patients during therapy, and for use in elderly patients, children, and breast-feeding women are the same as those for all *topical adrenocorticoids*.

---

hydroflumethiazide
Diucardin, Saluron

- Pharmacologic classification: thiazide diuretic
- Therapeutic classification: diuretic, antihypertensive
- Pregnancy risk category B

How supplied
Available by prescription only
Tablets: 50 mg

Indications, route, and dosage
Edema
Adults: 25 to 200 mg P.O. daily in divided doses; maintenance doses may be on intermittent or alternate-day schedule.
Children: 1 mg/kg P.O. daily.
Hypertension
Adults: 12.5 to 50 mg P.O. daily or b.i.d.

Pharmacodynamics
● *Diuretic action:* Hydroflumethiazide increases urinary excretion of sodium and water by inhibiting sodium reabsorption in the cortical diluting tubule of the nephron, thus relieving edema.
● *Antihypertensive action:* The exact mechanism of hydroflumethiazide's antihypertensive effect is unknown. It may be partially from direct arteriolar vasodilation and a decrease in total peripheral resistance.

Pharmacokinetics
Hydroflumethiazide is absorbed from the GI tract after oral administration. Limited data are available on other pharmacokinetic parameters.

Contraindications and precautions
Hydroflumethiazide is contraindicated in patients with anuria and in those with known sensitivity to the drug or to other sulfonamide derivatives.

Hydroflumethiazide should be used cautiously in patients with severe renal disease because it may decrease glomerular filtration rate and precipitate azotemia; in patients with impaired hepatic function or liver disease because electrolyte changes may precipitate coma; and in patients taking digoxin, because hypokalemia may predispose them to digitalis toxicity.

Interactions
Hydroflumethiazide potentiates the hypotensive effects of most other antihypertensive drugs; this may be used to therapeutic advantage.

Hydroflumethiazide may potentiate hyperglycemic, hypotensive, and hyperuricemic effects of diazoxide, and its hyperglycemic effect may increase insulin or sulfonylurea requirements in diabetic patients.

Hydroflumethiazide may reduce renal clearance of lithium, elevating serum lithium levels, and may necessitate reduction in lithium dosage by 50%.

Hydroflumethiazide turns urine slightly more alkaline and may decrease urinary excretion of some amines, such as amphetamine and quinidine; alkaline urine may also decrease therapeutic efficacy of methenamine compounds such as methenamine mandelate.

Cholestyramine and colestipol may bind hydroflumethiazide, preventing its absorption; give drugs 1 hour apart.

Effects on diagnostic tests
Hydroflumethiazide therapy may alter serum electrolyte levels and may increase serum urate, glucose, cholesterol, and triglyceride levels. It also may interfere with tests for parathyroid function and should be discontinued before such tests.

Adverse reactions
● CV: volume depletion and dehydration, orthostatic hypotension.
● DERM: dermatitis, photosensitivity, rash.
● GI: anorexia, nausea, pancreatitis.
● HEMA: *aplastic anemia, agranulocytosis,* leukopenia, thrombocytopenia.
● Hepatic: hepatic encephalopathy.
● Metabolic: asymptomatic hyperuricemia; hyperglycemia and impairment of glucose tolerance; fluid and electrolyte imbalances including hypokalemia, hyponatremia and hypochloremia; metabolic alkalosis; hypercalcemia.
● Other: hypersensitivity reactions, such as pneumonitis and vasculitis.

Note: Drug should be discontinued if rising BUN and serum creatinine levels indicate renal impairment or if patient shows signs of impending coma.

Overdose and treatment
Clinical signs of overdose include GI irritation and hypermotility, diuresis, and lethargy, which may progress to coma.

Treatment is mainly supportive; monitor and assist respiratory, cardiovascular, and renal function as indicated. Monitor fluid and electrolyte balance. Induce vomiting with ipecac in conscious patient; otherwise, use gastric lavage to avoid aspiration. Do not give cathartics; these promote additional loss of fluids and electrolytes.

▶ Special considerations
Recommendations for use of hydroflumethiazide and for care and teaching of the patient during therapy are the same as those for all *thiazide diuretics.*

Geriatric use
Elderly and debilitated patients require close observation and may require reduced dosages. They are more sensitive to excess diuresis because of age-related changes in cardiovascular and renal function. Excess diuresis promotes orthostatic hypotension, dehydration, hypovolemia, hyponatremia, hypomagnesemia, and hypokalemia.

Breast-feeding
Hydroflumethiazide is distributed in breast milk; its safety and effectiveness in breast-feeding women have not been established.

---

hydromorphone hydrochloride
Dilaudid, Dilaudid-HP

● Pharmacologic classification: opioid
● Therapeutic classification: analgesic, antitussive
● Controlled substance schedule II
● Pregnancy risk category C

How supplied
Available by prescription only
Tablets: 1 mg, 2 mg, 3 mg, 4 mg, 10 mg (contains tartrazine)
Injection: 1 mg/ml, 2 mg/ml, 3 mg/ml, 4 mg/ml
Suppository: 3 mg

Indications, route, and dosage
Moderate to severe pain
Adults: 1 to 6 mg P.O. q 4 to 6 hours, p.r.n. or around the clock; or 2 to 4 mg I.M., S.C., or I.V. q 4 to 6 hours, p.r.n. or around the clock (I.V. dose should be given over 3 to 5 minutes); or 3 mg rectal suppository h.s., p.r.n., or around the clock.
Cough
Adults: 1 mg P.O. q 3 to 4 hours, p.r.n.
Children age 6 to 12: 0.5 mg P.O. q 3 to 4 hours, p.r.n.

Pharmacodynamics
● *Antitussive action:* Hydromorphone acts directly on the cough center in the medulla, producing an antitussive effect.

• *Analgesic action:* Hydromorphone has analgesic properties related to opiate receptor affinity, and is recommended for moderate to severe pain. There is no intrinsic limit to the analgesic effect of hydromorphone, unlike the other opioids.

Pharmacokinetics
• *Absorption:* Hydromorphone is well absorbed after oral, rectal, or parenteral administration. Onset of action occurs in 15 to 30 minutes, with peak effect at ½ to 1 hour after dosing.
• *Distribution:* Unknown.
• *Metabolism:* Hydromorphone is metabolized primarily in the liver, where it undergoes conjugation with glucuronic acid.
• *Excretion:* Drug is excreted primarily in the urine as the glucuronide conjugate. Duration of action is 4 to 5 hours.

Contraindications and precautions
Hydromorphone is contraindicated in patients with known hypersensitivity to the drug or other phenanthrene opioids (codeine, hydrocodone, morphine, oxymorphone, or oxycodone).

Administer hydromorphone with extreme caution to patients with supraventricular arrhythmias; avoid, or administer drug with extreme caution to patients with head injury or increased intracranial pressure, because drug obscures neurologic parameters; and during pregnancy and labor, because drug readily crosses placenta (premature infants are especially sensitive to respiratory and CNS depressant effects).

Administer hydromorphone cautiously to patients with renal or hepatic dysfunction, because drug accumulation or prolonged duration of action may occur; to patients with pulmonary disease (asthma, chronic obstructive pulmonary disease), because drug depresses respiration and suppresses cough reflex; to patients undergoing biliary tract surgery, because drug may cause biliary spasm; to patients with convulsive disorders, because drug may precipitate seizures; to elderly or debilitated patients, who are more sensitive to both therapeutic and adverse drug effects; and to patients prone to physical or psychic addiction, because of the high risk of addiction to this drug.

Interactions
Concomitant use with other CNS depressants (narcotic analgesics, general anesthetics, antihistamines, phenothiazines, barbiturates, benzodiazepines, sedative-hypnotics, tricyclic antidepressants, alcohol, and muscle relaxants) potentiates drug's respiratory and CNS depression, sedation, and hypotensive effects. Concomitant use with cimetidine may also increase respiratory and CNS depression, causing confusion, disorientation, apnea, or seizures; such use usually requires reduced dosage of hydromorphone.

Drug accumulation and enhanced effects may result from concomitant use with other drugs that are extensively metabolized in the liver (rifampin, phenytoin, and digitoxin); combined use with anticholinergics may cause paralytic ileus.

Patients who become physically dependent on this drug may experience acute withdrawal syndrome if given a narcotic-antagonist.

Severe cardiovascular depression may result from concomitant use with general anesthetics.

Effects on diagnostic tests
Hydromorphone increases plasma amylase and lipase levels. Hydromorphone may delay gastric emptying; increased biliary tract pressure resulting from contraction of the sphincter of Oddi may interfere with hepatobiliary imaging studies.

Adverse reactions
• CNS: sedation, somnolence, clouded sensorium, dizziness, dysphoria, insomnia, agitation, confusion, headache, tremor, miosis, *seizures*, psychic dependence, lethargy, anxiety, fear, mood changes.
• CV: tachycardia, bradycardia, palpitations, chest wall rigidity, hypertension, hypotension, syncope, edema, *shock, cardiopulmonary arrest.*
• DERM: flushing, rashes, pruritus, pain and induration at injection site.
• GI: dry mouth, anorexia, biliary spasms (colic), ileus, nausea, vomiting, constipation.
• GU: urinary retention or hesitancy.
• Other: *respiratory depression.*
    Note: Drug should be discontinued if hypersensitivity, seizures, or cardiac arrhythmias occur.

Overdose and treatment
The most common signs and symptoms of hydromorphone overdose are CNS depression, respiratory depression, and miosis (pinpoint pupils). Other acute toxic effects include hypotension, bradycardia, hypothermia, shock, apnea, cardiopulmonary arrest, circulatory collapse, pulmonary edema, and seizures.

To treat an acute overdose, first establish adequate respiratory exchange via a patent airway and ventilation as needed; administer a narcotic antagonist (naloxone) to reverse respiratory depression. (Because the duration of action of hydromorphone is longer than that of naloxone, repeated dosing is necessary.) Naloxone should not be given unless the patient has clinically significant respiratory or cardiovascular depression. Monitor vital signs closely.

If the patient presents within 2 hours of ingestion of an oral overdose, empty the stomach immediately by inducing emesis (ipecac syrup) or using gastric lavage. Use caution to avoid any risk of aspiration. Administer activated charcoal via nasogastric tube for further removal of an oral overdose.

Provide symptomatic and supportive treatment (continued respiratory support, correction of fluid or electrolyte imbalance). Monitor laboratory parameters, vital signs, and neurologic status closely.

Contact the local or regional poison control center for further information.

▶ Special considerations
Besides those relevant to all *opioids,* consider the following recommendations.
• Before administration, visually inspect all parenteral products for particulate matter and extreme yellow discoloration.
• Oral dosage form is particularly convenient for patients with chronic pain, because tablets are available in several strengths, which enables patients to titrate their own dosage precisely.
• Dilaudid-HP, a highly concentrated form (10 mg/ml), may be administered in smaller volumes, preventing discomfort associated with large-volume injections.
• Store hydromorphone suppositories in refrigerator.

Geriatric use
Lower doses are usually indicated for elderly patients, because they may be more sensitive to the therapeutic and adverse effects of the drug.

Breast-feeding
It is unknown whether hydromorphone is excreted in breast milk; it should be used with caution in breast-feeding women.

hydroxychloroquine sulfate
Plaquenil Sulfate

- Pharmacologic classification: 4-amino-quinoline
- Therapeutic classification: antimalarial, anti-inflammatory agent
- Pregnancy risk category C

How supplied
Available by prescription only
Tablets: 200 mg (155 mg base)

Indications, route, and dosage
Suppressive prophylaxis of malarial attacks
Adults: 400 mg of sulfate (310 mg base) P.O. weekly on exactly the same day each week. (Begin 1 week before entering and continue for 4 weeks after leaving the endemic area.) If therapy begins after exposure, *double* the initial dose to 800 mg of sulfate (620 mg base) in two divided doses, 6 hours apart.
Infants and children: 5 mg (calculated as the base)/kg of body weight, not to exceed the adult dose (400 mg/week of the sulfate; 310 mg base). The schedule of prophylaxis is the same as for adults.
Acute malarial attacks
Adults and children over age 15: Initially, 800 mg (sulfate) P.O., then 400 mg after 6 to 8 hours, then 400 mg daily for 2 days (total of 2 g sulfate salt). Alternatively, a single 800-mg dose may prove effective.
Children age 11 to 15: 600 mg (sulfate) P.O. stat, then 200 mg 8 hours later, then 200 mg 24 hours later (total of 1 g sulfate salt).
Children age 6 to 10: 400 mg (sulfate) P.O. stat, then two doses of 200 mg at 8-hour intervals (total of 800 mg sulfate salt).
Children age 2 to 5: 400 mg (sulfate) P.O. stat, then 200 mg 8 hours later (total of 600 mg sulfate salt).
Children under age 1: 100 mg (sulfate) P.O. stat, then three doses of 100 mg 6 to 9 hours apart (total of 400 mg sulfate salt).
Lupus erythematosus (chronic discoid and systemic)
Adults: 400 mg P.O. daily or b.i.d., continued for several weeks or months, depending on response. Prolonged maintenance is 200 to 400 mg P.O. daily.
†Rheumatoid arthritis
Adults: Initially, 400 to 600 mg P.O. daily. When good response occurs (usually in 4 to 12 weeks), cut dosage in half.

Pharmacodynamics
- *Antimalarial action:* Hydroxychloroquine binds to DNA, interfering with protein synthesis. It also inhibits DNA and RNA polymerases. It is active against asexual erythrocytic forms of *Plasmodium malariae, P. ovale, P. vivax,* and many strains of *P. falciparum.*
- *Amebicidal action:* Mechanism of action is unknown.
- *Anti-inflammatory action:* Mechanism of action is unknown. Hydroxychloroquine may antagonize histamine and serotonin and inhibit prostaglandin effects by inhibiting conversion of arachidonic acid to prostaglandin F_2; it may also inhibit chemotaxis of polymorphonuclear leukocytes, macrophages, and eosinophils.

Pharmacokinetics
- *Absorption:* Hydroxychloroquine is absorbed readily and almost completely, with peak plasma concentrations occurring at 1 to 2 hours.
- *Distribution:* Hydroxychloroquine is bound to plasma proteins. It concentrates in the liver, spleen, kidneys, heart, and brain and is strongly bound in melanin-containing cells.
- *Metabolism:* Hydroxychloroquine is metabolized by the liver to desethylchloroquine and desethyl hydroxychloroquine.
- *Excretion:* Most of an administered dose is excreted unchanged in urine. The drug and its metabolites are excreted slowly in urine; unabsorbed drug is excreted in feces. Small amounts of the drug may be present in urine for months after the drug is discontinued. The drug is excreted in breast milk.

Contraindications and precautions
Hydroxychloroquine is contraindicated in patients who have experienced retinal or visual field changes or hypersensitivity reactions to 4-aminoquinoline compounds, unless these compounds are the only agents to which the malarial strain is sensitive.

Hydroxychloroquine should be used with caution in patients with psoriasis, porphyria, or G6PD deficiency because the drug may exacerbate these conditions. Because hydroxychloroquine concentrates in the liver and may cause adverse hepatic effects, it should be used with caution in patients with hepatic disease or alcoholism and in patients receiving other hepatotoxic drugs.

Interactions
Concomitant administration of kaolin or magnesium trisilicate may decrease absorption of hydroxychloroquine. Use with digoxin may increase serum digoxin levels.

Effects on diagnostic tests
Hydroxychloroquine may cause inversion or depression of the T wave or widening of the QRS complex on ECG. Rarely, it may cause decreased white blood cell, red blood cell, or platelet counts.

Adverse reactions
- CNS: irritability, nightmares, ataxia, *seizures,* psychic stimulation, *toxic psychosis,* vertigo, tinnitus, nystagmus, lassitude, fatigue, dizziness, hypoactive deep-tendon reflexes, skeletal muscle weakness, emotional changes, headache.
- DERM: pruritus, lichen planus-like eruptions, skin and mucosal pigmentary changes, pleomorphic skin eruptions, non-light-sensitive psoriasis.
- EENT: visual disturbances (blurred vision; difficulty in focusing; reversible corneal changes; generally irreversible, sometimes progressive or delayed, retinal changes, such as narrowing of arterioles; macular lesions; pallor of optic disk; optic atrophy; visual field

defects; patchy retinal pigmentation, often leading to blindness), ototoxicity (irreversible nerve deafness, tinnitus, labyrinthitis).

● GI: anorexia, abdominal cramps, diarrhea, nausea, vomiting.
● HEMA: *agranulocytosis, leukopenia,* thrombocytopenia, *aplastic anemia,* hemolysis in G6PD deficiency.
● Other: weight loss, bleaching of hair, alopecia, exacerbations of porphyria, immunoblastic lymphadenopathy.

Overdose and treatment

Symptoms of hydroxychloroquine overdose may appear within 30 minutes after ingestion and may include headache, drowsiness, visual changes, cardiovascular collapse, and seizures followed by respiratory and cardiac arrest.

Treatment is symptomatic. The stomach should be emptied by emesis or lavage. After lavage, activated charcoal in an amount at least five times the estimated amount of drug ingested may be helpful if given within 30 minutes of ingestion.

Ultra-short-acting barbiturates may help control seizures. Intubation may become necessary. Peritoneal dialysis and exchange transfusions may also be useful. Forced fluids and acidification of the urine are helpful after the acute phase.

▶ Special considerations

Besides those relevant to all *aminoquinolines,* consider the following recommendations.
● Baseline and periodic ophthalmologic examinations are necessary in prolonged or high-dosage therapy.
● Monitor for blurred vision, increased sensitivity to light, hearing loss, pronounced GI disturbances, or muscle weakness.
● Give immediately before or after meals on the same day each week to minimize gastric distress.

Information for the patient

To prevent drug-induced dermatoses, warn patient to avoid excessive exposure to the sun.

Pediatric use

Children are extremely susceptible to toxicity; monitor closely for adverse effects.

Breast-feeding

Safety has not been established. Use with caution in breast-feeding women.

hydroxyprogesterone caproate

Delalutin*, Duralutin, Gesterol L.A., Hy-Gestrone, Hylutin, Hyprogest 250, Hyproval P.A., Hyroxon, Pro-Depo

● Pharmacologic classification: progestin
● Therapeutic classification: progestin, antineoplastic
● Pregnancy risk category X

How supplied

Available by prescription only
Injection: 125 mg/ml, 250 mg/ml

Indications, route, and dosage

Amenorrhea and uterine bleeding

Adults: 375 mg I.M. May be repeated at 4-week intervals if needed. After 4 days of desquamation or if there is no bleeding within 21 days after administration, begin cyclic therapy with an estrogen.

Endometrial cancer

Adults: 1 g I.M. up to seven times per week for 12 weeks or as indicated. Therapy is discontinued if relapse occurs or if no objective response is seen after 12 weeks of therapy.

Test for endogenous estrogen production

250 mg at once; repeat for confirmation at 4 weeks. Bleeding should occur 7 to 14 days after the injection.

Pharmacodynamics

Progestational action: Hydroxyprogesterone suppresses ovulation, causes thickening of cervical mucus, and induces sloughing of the endometrium. It inhibits growth progression of progestin-sensitive uterine cancer tissue by an unknown mechanism.

Pharmacokinetics

This compound has a duration of action of 7 to 14 days when used as directed.
● *Absorption:* Hydroxyprogesterone is absorbed slowly after I.M. injection.
● *Distribution:* Unknown.
● *Metabolism:* Primarily hepatic; not well characterized.
● *Excretion:* Primarily renal; not well characterized.

Contraindications and precautions

Hydroxyprogesterone is contraindicated in patients with known hypersensitivity to progestins; in patients with a history of thromboembolic disorders because of its potential for causing thromboembolic disorders; in patients with severe hepatic disease because impaired hepatic metabolism may cause the drug to accumulate; in patient with breast or genital cancer because it may induce tumor growth; in patients with undiagnosed abnormal vaginal bleeding because the origin should be determined; and in pregnant or breast-feeding women.

Hydroxyprogesterone should be used cautiously in patients with existing conditions that might be aggravated by fluid and electrolyte retention, such as cardiac or renal disease, epilepsy, or migraine. Caution is also advised in administering this agent to diabetic patients (because decreased glucose tolerance may occur) or to patients with a history of mental depression.

Interactions

Concomitant use with bromocriptine may cause amenorrhea or galactorrhea, thus interfering with the action of bromocriptine. Concurrent use of these drugs is not recommended.

Effects on diagnostic tests

Glucose tolerance has been shown to decrease in a small percentage of patients receiving this drug. Abnormal thyroid or liver function tests may occur; the metyrapone test may be altered and the pregnanediol excretion may decrease.

Adverse reactions

● CNS: dizziness, headache, lethargy, depression, *cerebral thrombosis, embolism.*
● CV: hypertension, thrombophlebitis, *pulmonary embolism,* edema.

- DERM: melasma, chloasma rash.
- GI: nausea, vomiting.
- GU: breakthrough bleeding, dysmenorrhea, amenorrhea, cervical erosion or abnormal secretions.
- Hepatic: cholestatic jaundice.
- Local: irritation and pain at injection site.
- Other: decreased libido, cough, dyspnea, weight loss or gain, allergic reactions (with high doses).

Note: Drug should be discontinued if signs and symptoms of thromboembolic or thrombotic disorders, unexplained vision changes, migraine, or depression occur.

Overdose and treatment
No information available.

▶ Special considerations
Besides those relevant to all *progestins,* consider the following recommendations.
- Hydroxyprogesterone caproate is for I.M. administration only. Inject deep into large muscle mass, preferably the gluteal muscle.
- Women receiving hydroxyprogesterone should receive a copy of the manufacturer's package insert for the drug.
- Monitor diabetic patients during therapy for signs of decreased glucose tolerance.
- Patients receiving this drug should have a full physical examination, including a gynecologic exam and a Papanicolaou test, every 6 to 12 months.

Information for the patient
- Warn patient that edema and weight gain are likely.
- Remind patient that normal menstrual cycles may not resume for 2 to 3 months after discontinuing drug therapy.
- Advise patient of potential risks to the fetus if she becomes pregnant during therapy or is inadvertently exposed to the drug during the first 4 months of pregnancy.

Breast-feeding
Hydroxyprogesterone is contraindicated in breast-feeding women.

---

hydroxyurea
Hydrea

- Pharmacologic classification: antimetabolite (cell cycle-phase specific, S phase)
- Therapeutic classification: antineoplastic
- Pregnancy risk category C

How supplied
Available by prescription only
Capsules: 500 mg

Indications, route, and dosage
Dosage and indications may vary. Check current literature for recommended protocol.

Melanoma; chronic myelocytic leukemia; recurrent, metastatic, or inoperable ovarian cancer; squamous cell carcinoma of the head and neck; †*polycythemia vera;* †*essential thrombocytosis*
Adults: 60 to 80 mg/kg P.O. or 2,000 to 3,000 mg/m² P.O. as single dose q 3 days; or 20 to 30 mg/kg P.O. daily for a minimum of 6 weeks. Dosage is based on ideal body weight if patient is obese or has fluid retention.

†*To increase hemoglobin F production in patients with sickle cell trait*
Adults: 7.5 to 40 mg P.O. daily; the median dose reported in some studies is 20 mg/kg.

Pharmacodynamics
Antineoplastic action: The exact mechanism of hydroxyurea's cytotoxic action is unclear. Hydroxyurea inhibits DNA synthesis without interfering with RNA or protein synthesis. The drug may act as an antimetabolite, inhibiting the incorporation of thymidine into DNA, and may also damage DNA directly.

Pharmacokinetics
- *Absorption:* Hydroxyurea is well absorbed after oral administration, with peak serum levels occurring 2 hours after a dose. Higher serum levels are achieved if the drug is given as a large, single dose rather than in divided doses.
- *Distribution:* Hydroxyurea crosses the blood-brain barrier.
- *Metabolism:* Approximately 50% of an oral dose is degraded in the liver.
- *Excretion:* The remaining 50% is excreted in urine as unchanged drug. The metabolites are excreted through the lungs as carbon dioxide and in urine as urea.

Contraindications and precautions
Hydroxyurea is contraindicated in patients with a leukocyte count below 2,500/mm³; in those with a platelet count below 100,000/mm³; and in severely anemic patients because of the drug's hematologic toxicity. It is also contraindicated in pregnant patients because it may be fetotoxic.
Hydroxyurea should be used with extreme caution in patients with impaired renal function; they are susceptible to the development of visual and auditory hallucinations and pronounced hematologic toxicity. Hydroxyurea can impair fertility. Reversible germ cell toxicity has followed treatment with hydroxyurea.

Interactions
Concomitant use of hydroxyurea may decrease the activity of fluorouracil. Hydroxyurea appears to inhibit the conversion of fluorouracil to its active metabolite. A high incidence of neurotoxicity may occur when these two agents are administered together.

Effects on diagnostic tests
Hydroxyurea therapy elevates BUN, serum creatinine, and serum uric acid levels.

Adverse reactions
- CNS: drowsiness, hallucinations, *convulsions,* headache.
- DERM: rash, pruritus, facial erythema.
- GI: anorexia, nausea, vomiting, diarrhea, stomatitis, constipation.

● GU: increased BUN and serum creatinine levels.
● HEMA: *bone marrow depression* (dose-limiting), *leukopenia, thrombocytopenia,* anemia, megaloblastosis.
● Metabolic: hyperuricemia.
● Other: alopecia.
  Note: Drug should be discontinued if inflammation of the mucous membranes is severe; if leukocyte counts are less than 2,500/mm³; or if platelet counts are less than 100,000/mm³.

Overdose and treatment
Clinical manifestations of overdose include myelosuppression, ulceration of buccal and GI mucosa, facial erythema, maculopapular rash, disorientation, hallucinations, and impairment of renal tubular function.
  Treatment is usually supportive and includes transfusion of blood components.

▶ Special considerations
● If patient can't swallow capsule, he may empty contents into water and take immediately.
● Dose modification may be required following other chemotherapy or radiation therapy.
● Monitor intake and output levels; keep patient hydrated.
● Routinely measure BUN, uric acid, and serum creatinine levels.
● Drug may exacerbate postirradiation erythema.
● Auditory and visual hallucinations and blood toxicity increase when decreased renal function exists.
● Avoid all I.M. injections when platelet counts are below 100,000/mm³.
● Store capsules in tight container at room temperature. Avoid exposure to excessive heat.
● Drug is currently under investigation for the treatment of sickle cell anemia. Widespread use of the drug for this disease is not recommended because of the potential for toxicity.

Information for the patient
● Emphasize importance of continuing medication despite nausea and vomiting.
● Tell patient to call immediately if vomiting occurs shortly after taking a dose.
● Encourage daily fluid intake of 10 to 12 (8 oz) glasses, to increase urine output and facilitate excretion of uric acid.
● Tell patient to report unusual bruising or bleeding.
● Tell patient to avoid exposure to people with infections.

Geriatric use
Elderly patients may be more sensitive to the effects of the drug, requiring a lower dosage.

Pediatric use
Children may be more sensitive to the effects of the drug, requiring a lower dosage.

Breast-feeding
It is not known whether hydroxyurea distributes into breast milk. However, because of the potential for serious adverse reactions, mutagenicity, and carcinogenicity in the infant, breast-feeding is not recommended.

hydroxyzine hydrochloride
Anxanil, Atarax, Atozine, Durrax, E-Vista, Hydroxacen, Hyzine, Multipax★, Orgatrax, Quiess, Vistacon, Vistaject, Vistaquel, Vistazine

hydroxyzine pamoate
Hy-Pam, Vamate, Vistaril

● Pharmacologic classification: antihistamine (piperazine derivative)
● Therapeutic classification: antianxiety agent; sedative; antipruritic; antiemetic; antispasmodic
● Pregnancy risk category C

How supplied
Available by prescription only
Hydroxyzine hydrochloride
Capsules: 10 mg, 25 mg, 50 mg
Syrup: 10 mg/5 ml
Tablets: 10 mg, 25 mg, 50 mg, 100 mg
Injection: 25 mg/ml, 50 mg/ml
Hydroxyzine pamoate
Capsules: 25 mg, 50 mg, 100 mg
Oral suspension: 25 mg/5 ml

Indications, route, and dosage
Anxiety and tension
Adults: 25 to 100 mg P.O. t.i.d. or q.i.d.
Anxiety, tension, hyperkinesia
Children over age 6: 50 to 100 mg P.O. daily in divided doses.
Children under age 6: 50 mg P.O. daily in divided doses.
Preoperative and postoperative adjunctive sedation
Adults: 25 to 100 mg I.M. q 4 to 6 hours.
Children: 1.1 mg/kg I.M. q 4 to 6 hours.

Pharmacodynamics
● *Anxiolytic and sedative actions:* Hydroxyzine produces its sedative and antianxiety effects through suppression of activity at subcortical levels; analgesia occurs at high doses.
● *Antipruritic action:* Hydroxyzine is a direct competitor of histamine for binding at cellular receptor sites.
● *Other actions:* Hydroxyzine is used as a preoperative and postoperative adjunct for its sedative, antihistaminic, and anticholinergic activity.

Pharmacokinetics
● *Absorption:* Hydroxyzine is absorbed rapidly and completely after oral administration. Peak serum levels occur within 2 to 4 hours. Sedation and other clinical effects are usually noticed in 15 to 30 minutes.
● *Distribution:* The distribution of hydroxyzine in humans is not well understood.
● *Metabolism:* Hydroxyzine is metabolized almost completely in the liver.
● *Excretion:* Metabolites of hydroxyzine are excreted primarily in urine; small amounts of drug and metabolites are found in feces. Half-life of the drug is 3 hours. Sedative effects can last for 4 to 6 hours, and antihistaminic effects can persist for up to 4 days.

HYOSCYAMINE 549

Contraindications and precautions
Hydroxyzine is contraindicated in patients with known hypersensitivity to the drug. Hyroxyzine should be used cautiously in patients with open-angle glaucoma, urinary retention, or any other condition where anticholinergic effects would be detrimental.

Interactions
Hydroxyzine may add to or potentiate the effects of opioids, barbiturates, alcohol, tranquilizers, and other CNS depressants; the dose of CNS depressants should be reduced by 50%.

Concomitant use with other anticholinergic drugs causes additive anticholinergic effects.

Hydroxyzine may block the vasopressor action of epinephrine. If a vasoconstrictor is needed, use norepinephrine or phenylephrine.

Effects on diagnostic tests
Hydroxyzine therapy causes falsely elevated urinary 17-hydroxycorticosteroid levels. It also may cause false-negative skin allergen tests by attenuating or inhibiting the cutaneous response to histamine.

Adverse reactions
● CNS: sedation, dizziness, drowsiness, ataxia, weakness, slurred speech, headache, anxiety, tremor and *seizures* at high doses (rare).
● DERM: rash, urticaria.
● EENT: dry mouth, blurred vision, dental problems (with prolonged use).
● GI: constipation, nausea, bitter taste.
● GU: urinary retention.
● Local: marked irritation, sterile abscess, and tissue induration (after S.C. administration).
● Other: hypersensitivity (tightness of chest, wheezing).
Note: Drug should be discontinued if hypersensitivity with tightness of chest, wheezing, tremor, or seizures occurs.

Overdose and treatment
Clinical manifestations of overdose include excessive sedation and hypotension; seizures may occur.

Treatment is supportive only. For recent oral ingestion, empty gastric contents through emesis or lavage. Correct hypotension with fluids and vasopressors (phenylephrine or metaraminol). Do not give epinephrine, because hydroxyzine may counteract its effect.

▶ **Special considerations**
● Observe patients for excessive sedation, especially those receiving other CNS depressants.
● Inject deep I.M. only; not for I.V., intra-arterial, or S.C. use. Aspirate injection carefully to prevent inadvertent intravascular administration.

Information for the patient
● Tell patient to avoid tasks that require mental alertness or physical coordination until the CNS effects of the drug are known; advise against use of other CNS depressants with hydroxyzine unless prescribed. Patient should avoid alcohol ingestion.
● Instruct patient to seek medical approval before taking any nonprescription cold or allergy preparations that contain antihistamine, which may potentiate the effects of hydroxyzine.
● Recommend use of sugarless gum or candy to help relieve dry mouth; advise drinking plenty of water to help with dry mouth or constipation.

Geriatric use
Elderly patients may experience greater CNS depression and anticholinergic effects. Lower doses are indicated.

Breast-feeding
It is unknown whether hydroxyzine passes into breast milk. Safe use has not been established in breast-feeding women.

hyoscyamine
Cystospaz

hyoscyamine sulfate
Anaspaz, Bellaspaz, Cystospaz-M, Levsin, Levsin Drops, Levsinex Timecaps, Neoquess

● Pharmacologic classification: belladonna alkaloid
● Therapeutic classification: anticholinergic
● Pregnancy risk category C

How supplied
Available by prescription only
Hyoscyamine
Tablets: 0.150 mg
Hyoscyamine sulfate
Tablets: 0.125 mg, 0.130 mg
Capsules (timed-release): 0.375 mg
Oral solution: 0.125 mg/5 ml
Injection: 0.5 mg/ml

Indications, route, and dosage
GI tract disorders caused by spasm; adjunctive therapy for peptic ulcers
Adults: 0.125 to 0.25 mg P.O. or S.L. t.i.d. or q.i.d. before meals and h.s.; 0.375 mg P.O. (extended-release form) q 12 hours; or 0.25 to 0.5 mg (1 or 2 ml) I.M., I.V., or S.C. q 6 hours. (Substitute oral medication when symptoms are controlled.)
Children age 2 to 10: Half adult dose P.O.
Children under age 2: One-quarter adult dose P.O.

Pharmacodynamics
Antispasmodic and antiulcer action: Hyoscyamine competitively blocks acetylcholine at cholinergic neuroeffector sites, decreasing GI motility and inhibiting gastric acid secretion.

Pharmacokinetics
● *Absorption:* Hyoscyamine is well absorbed when taken orally; onset of action usually occurs in 20 to 30 minutes with tablets and 5 to 20 minutes with the elixir. Onset of action with parenteral administration usually occurs in 2 to 3 minutes.
● *Distribution:* Hyoscyamine is well distributed throughout the body and crosses the blood-brain barrier. About 50% of dose binds to plasma proteins.
● *Metabolism:* Hyoscyamine is metabolized in the liver. Usual duration of effect is up to 4 hours with standard oral and parenteral administration and up to 12 hours for the extended-release preparation.
● *Excretion:* Metabolites and unchanged drug are excreted in the urine.

Contraindications and precautions

Hyoscyamine is contraindicated in patients with narrow-angle glaucoma, because drug-induced cycloplegia and mydriasis may increase intraocular pressure; in patients with obstructive uropathy, obstructive GI tract disease, severe ulcerative colitis, myasthenia gravis, paralytic ileus, intestinal atony, or toxic megacolon, because the drug may exacerbate these conditions; and in patients with known hypersensitivity to anticholinergics.

Administer hyoscyamine cautiously to patients with autonomic neuropathy, hyperthyroidism, coronary artery disease, cardiac arrhythmias, congestive heart failure, or ulcerative colitis, because the drug may exacerbate the symptoms of these disorders; to patients with hepatic or renal disease, because toxic accumulation can occur; to patients over age 40, because the drug may increase the glaucoma risk; to patients with hiatal hernia associated with reflux esophagitis, because the drug may decrease lower esophageal sphincter tone; and in hot or humid environments, because the drug may predispose the patient to heatstroke.

Interactions

Concomitant use with amantadine may increase such adverse anticholinergic effects as confusion and hallucinations. Concomitant use with phenothiazines or haloperidol may reduce the antipsychotic effectiveness of these drugs, possibly by direct CNS antagonism; phenothiazines may also increase hyoscyamine's adverse anticholinergic effects. Antacids and antidiarrheals may decrease hyoscyamine's absorption. Administer hyoscyamine 1 hour prior to these agents.

Effects on diagnostic tests

None reported.

Adverse reactions

● CNS: headache, insomnia, drowsiness, dizziness, confusion or excitement (in elderly patients), nervousness, weakness.
● CV: palpitations, tachycardia, orthostatic hypotension.
● DERM: urticaria, decreased sweating or anhidrosis, other dermal manifestations.
● EENT: blurred vision, mydriasis, increased ocular tension, cycloplegia, photophobia.
● GI: dry mouth, dysphagia, constipation, heartburn, loss of taste, nausea, vomiting, paralytic ileus, abdominal distention.
● GU: urinary hesitancy and retention, impotence.
● Other: fever, allergic reactions.
  Note: Drug should be discontinued if hypersensitivity, confusion or excitement, urinary retention, or curare-like symptoms develop.

Overdose and treatment

Clinical signs of overdose include curare-like symptoms, central stimulation followed by depression, and such psychotic symptoms as disorientation, confusion, hallucinations, delusions, anxiety, agitation, and restlessness. Peripheral effects may include dilated, nonreactive pupils; blurred vision; flushed, hot, dry skin; dryness of mucous membranes; dysphagia; decreased or absent bowel sounds; urinary retention, hyperthermia; headache; tachycardia; hypertension; and increased respiration.

Treatment is primarily symptomatic and supportive, as needed. Maintain patent airway. If patient is alert, induce emesis (or use gastric lavage) and follow with a saline cathartic and activated charcoal to prevent further drug absorption. In severe cases, physostigmine may be administered to block antimuscarinic effects. Give fluids as needed, to treat shock; diazepam to control psychotic symptoms; and pilocarpine (instilled into the eyes) to relieve mydriasis. If urinary retention occurs, catheterization may be necessary.

▶ Special considerations

Besides those relevant to all *anticholinergics*, consider the following recommendations.
● Hyoscyamine is usually administered P.O. but may be given I.V., I.M., S.C., or sublingually when therapeutic effect is needed or if oral administration is not possible.
● Drug should be titrated according to patient's response and tolerance.

Geriatric use

Hyoscyamine should be administered cautiously to elderly patients. Lower doses are indicated.

Breast-feeding

Hyoscyamine may be excreted in breast milk, possibly resulting in infant toxicity. Breast-feeding women should avoid this drug. Hyoscyamine may also decrease milk production.

ibuprofen
Advil, Amersol*, Children's Advil,
Medipren, Motrin, Motrin IB, Nuprin,
PediaProfen, Rufen, Trendar

- Pharmacologic classification: nonsteroidal anti-inflammatory
- Therapeutic classification: nonnarcotic analgesic, antipyretic, anti-inflammatory
- Pregnancy risk category B (D in third trimester)

How supplied
Available without a prescription
Tablets: 200 mg

Available by prescription only
Tablets: 300 mg, 400 mg, 600 mg, 800 mg
Oral suspension: 100 mg/5 ml

Indications, route, and dosage
Arthritis, primary dysmenorrhea, gout, postextraction dental pain, mild to moderate pain
Adults: 200 to 800 mg P.O. t.i.d. or q.i.d. Do not exceed 3,200 mg as total daily dose.
Juvenile arthritis
Children: 30 to 40 mg/kg/day P.O., divided into three or four doses. Patients with milder disease may respond to 20 mg/kg daily in divided doses.
Fever reduction
Adults: 400 mg P.O. q 4 to 6 hours p.r.n.
Children: 5 mg/kg P.O. if the baseline temperature is 102.5° F (39.2° C) or below; 10 mg/kg P.O. if the baseline temperature is over 102.5° F The recommended daily maximum dose is 40 mg/kg. Alternatively, use the accompanying dosage table (see next page).

Pharmacodynamics
Analgesic, antipyretic, and anti-inflammatory actions: Mechanisms of action are unknown; ibuprofen is thought to inhibit prostaglandin synthesis.

Pharmacokinetics
- *Absorption:* Ibuprofen is absorbed rapidly and completely from the GI tract.
- *Distribution:* Ibuprofen is highly protein-bound.
- *Metabolism:* Ibuprofen undergoes biotransformation in the liver.
- *Excretion:* Ibuprofen is excreted mainly in urine, with some biliary excretion. Plasma half-life ranges from 2 to 4 hours.

Contraindications and precautions
Ibuprofen is contraindicated in patients with known hypersensitivity to the drug and in patients in whom aspirin or other nonsteroidal anti-inflammatory drugs (NSAIDs) induce symptoms of asthma, urticaria, or rhinitis.

Serious GI toxicity, especially ulceration or hemor-

rhage, can occur at any time in patients on chronic NSAID therapy. Ibuprofen should be administered cautiously to patients with a history of GI disease, hepatic or renal disease, cardiac decompensation, systemic lupus erythematosus, or bleeding abnormalities, because the drug may worsen these conditions.

Patients with known "triad" symptoms (aspirin hypersensitivity, rhinitis/nasal polyps, and asthma) are at high risk of bronchospasm. NSAIDs may mask the signs and symptoms of acute infection (fever, myalgia, erythema); carefully evaluate patients with high risk (for example, those with diabetes).

Interactions
Concomitant use of ibuprofen with anticoagulants and thrombolytic drugs (coumarin derivatives, heparin, streptokinase, or urokinase) may potentiate anticoagulant effects. Bleeding problems may occur if ibuprofen is used with other drugs that inhibit platelet aggregation, such as azlocillin, parenteral carbenicillin, dextran, dipyridamole, mezlocillin, piperacillin, sulfinpyrazone, ticarcillin, valproic acid, cefamandole, cefoperazone, moxalactam, plicamycin, aspirin, salicylates, or other anti-inflammatory agents. Concomitant use with salicylates, anti-inflammatory agents, alcohol, corticotropin, or steroids may cause increased GI adverse effects, including ulceration and hemorrhage. Aspirin may decrease the bioavailability of ibuprofen. Because of the influence of prostaglandins on glucose metabolism, concomitant use with insulin or oral hypoglycemic agents may potentiate hypoglycemic effects. Ibuprofen may displace highly protein-bound drugs from binding sites. Toxicity may occur with coumarin derivatives, phenytoin, verapamil, or nifedipine. Increased nephrotoxicity may occur with gold compounds, other anti-inflammatory agents, or acetaminophen. Ibuprofen may decrease the renal clearance of methotrexate and lithium. Antacids may decrease the absorption of ibuprofen. Ibuprofen may decrease effectiveness of diuretics and antihypertensives. Concomitant use with diuretics may increase nephrotoxicity.

Effects on diagnostic tests
The physiologic effects of ibuprofen may prolong bleeding time; decrease blood glucose concentrations; increase blood urea nitrogen, serum creatinine, and serum potassium levels; decrease serum uric acid, hemoglobin, and hematocrit levels; increase prothrombin time; and increase serum alkaline phosphatase, serum lactic dehydrogenase, and serum transaminase levels.

Adverse reactions
- CNS: headache, drowsiness, dizziness, aseptic meningitis, vertigo, weakness.
- CV: peripheral edema, congestive heart failure (CHF), hypotension, palpitations, tachycardia.
- DERM: pruritus, rash, urticaria.
- EENT: visual disturbances, tinnitus.
- GI: epigastric distress, nausea, vomiting, GI bleeding, constipation, anorexia, diarrhea, occult blood loss.
- GU: reversible renal failure (rare), hematuria, urinary

---

*Canada only   †Unlabeled clinical use   Italicized adverse reactions are life-threatening.

CHILDREN'S DOSAGE OF IBUPROFEN

AGE	WEIGHT (lb)	MG	TEASPOONS
5 mg/kg for fever <102.5° F. (39.2° C.)			
12 to 23 months	18 to 23	50	½
2 to 3 years	24 to 35	75	¾
4 to 5 years	36 to 47	100	1
6 to 8 years	48 to 59	125	1¼
9 to 10 years	60 to 71	150	1½
11 to 12 years	72 to 95	200	2
10 mg/kg for fever >102.5° F. (39.2° C.)			
12 to 23 months	18 to 23	100	1
2 to 3 years	24 to 35	150	1½
4 to 5 years	36 to 47	200	2
6 to 8 years	48 to 59	250	2½
9 to 10 years	60 to 71	300	3
11 to 12 years	72 to 95	350	4

tract infection, nocturia, elevated BUN, reduced creatinine clearance.
● HEMA: prolonged bleeding time.
● Hepatic: elevated liver enzymes.
● Other: *bronchospasm*, edema, thirst.
   Note: Drug should be discontinued if hypersensitivity or renal or hepatic toxicity occurs.

Overdose and treatment
Clinical manifestations of overdose include dizziness, drowsiness, paresthesia, vomiting, nausea, abdominal pain, headache, sweating, nystagmus, apnea, and cyanosis.
   To treat overdose of ibuprofen, empty stomach immediately by enducing emesis with ipecac syrup or by gastric lavage. Administer activated charcoal via nasogastric tube. Provide symptomatic and supportive measures (respiratory support and correction of fluid and electrolyte imbalances). Monitor laboratory parameters and vital signs closely. Alkaline diuresis may enhance renal excretion. Dialysis is of minimal value because ibuprofen is strongly protein-bound.

▶ Special considerations
Besides those relevant to all *NSAIDs,* consider the following recommendations.
● Maximum results in arthritis may require 1 to 2 weeks of continuous therapy with ibuprofen. Improvement may be seen, however, within 7 days.
● Administer on an empty stomach, 1 hour before or 2 hours after meals for maximum absorption. However, it may be administered with meals to lessen GI upset.
● Monitor cardiopulmonary status closely; monitor vital signs, especially heart rate and blood pressure. Observe for possible fluid retention.
● Establish safety measures, including raised side rails

and supervised walking, to prevent possible injury from CNS effects.
● Monitor auditory and ophthalmic functions periodically during ibuprofen therapy.

Information for the patient
● Instruct patient to seek medical approval before taking any nonprescription medications.
● Advise patient not to self-medicate with ibuprofen for longer than 10 days for analgesic use and not to exceed maximum dosage of six tablets (1.2 g) daily for self-medication. Caution patient not to take ibuprofen if fever lasts longer than 3 days unless prescribed.
● Tell patient to report any adverse reactions. They are usually dose-related.
● Instruct patient in safety measures to prevent injury. Caution him to avoid hazardous activities that require mental alertness until CNS effects are known.
● Encourage patient to adhere to prescribed drug regimen. Instruct him in need for medical follow-up.

Geriatric use
● Patients over age 60 may be more susceptible to the toxic effects of ibuprofen, especially adverse GI reactions. Use lowest possible effective dose.
● The effects of this drug on renal prostaglandins may cause fluid retention and edema, a significant drawback for elderly patients, especially those with CHF.

Pediatric use
Drug is not indicated for pain relief in children under age 12.

Breast-feeding
Ibuprofen does not enter breast milk in significant quantities. However, the manufacturer recommends alternate feeding methods during ibuprofen therapy.

---

idarubicin
Idamycin

- Pharmacologic classification: antibiotic antineoplastic
- Therapeutic classification: antineoplastic
- Pregnancy risk category D

How supplied
Available by prescription only
Injection: 5 mg, 10 mg (lyophilized powder) in single-dose vials with 50 or 100 mg lactose

Indications, route, and dosage
Treatment of acute myelocytic leukemia in adults, including fragment, antigen-binding, classifications M^1 through M^7, in combination with other approved antileukemic agents
Adults: 12 mg/m² daily by slow I.V. injection (over 10 to 15 minutes) for 3 days in combination with 100 mg/m² of cytarabine given daily by continuous infusion for 7 days or as a 25-mg/m² bolus followed by 200 mg/m² by continuous I.V. infusion daily for 5 days.

A second course may be administered if needed. If patient experiences severe mucositis, delay administration until recovery is complete and reduce dosage by 25%. Also reduce dosage in patients with hepatic or renal impairment. Idarubicin should not be given if bilirubin level is above 5 mg/dl.

Dosage and indications may vary. Check current literature for recommended protocol.

Pharmacodynamics
Antineoplastic action: Idarubicin inhibits nucleic acid synthesis by intercalation and interacts with the enzyme topoisomerase II. It is highly lipophilic, which results in an increased rate of cellular uptake.

Pharmacokinetics
- *Absorption:* Peak cellular concentrations are achieved within minutes of I.V. injection.
- *Distribution:* Idarubicin is highly lipophilic and excessively tissue-bound (97%), with highest concentrations in nucleated blood and bone marrow cells. Its metabolite, idarubicinol, is detected in CSF; clinical significance of this is under evaluation.
- *Metabolism:* Extensive extrahepatic metabolism is indicated. Metabolite has cytotoxic activity.
- *Excretion:* Predominantly by biliary excretion as its metabolite and, to a lesser extent, by renal elimination. The mean terminal half-life is 22 hours (range, 4 to 46 hours) when used as a single agent and 20 hours (range, 7 to 38 hours) when combined with cytarabine. Plasma levels of metabolite are sustained for longer than 8 days.

Contraindications and precautions
Idarubicin is contraindicated in patients with severe myelosuppression, preexisting cardiac disease, severe hemorrhagic conditions, or overwhelming infection. Use with extreme caution and reduced dosage in hepatic or renal function impairment.

Interactions
Idarubicin should not be mixed with other drugs unless specific compatibility data is available. Heparin causes precipitation. Degradation occurs with prolonged contact with alkaline solutions.

Adverse reactions
- CNS: headache, changed mental status, seizures.
- CV: *CHF,* atrial fibrillation, chest pain, *MI,* asymptomatic decline in left ventricular ejection fraction, myocardial insufficiency, *arrhythmias,* hemorrhage, myocardial toxicity.
- DERM: alopecia, rash, urticaria, bullous erythrodermatous rash of palms and soles, hives at injection site.
- GI: nausea, vomiting, cramps, diarrhea, mucositis, severe enterocolitis with perforation (rare).
- HEMA: *severe bone marrow depression.*
- Respiratory: pulmonary allergy.
- Other: infection, fever, changes in hepatic and renal functions, aplasia, local tissue necrosis (if extravasation occurs).

Overdose and treatment
Severe and prolonged myelosuppression and possibly increased severity of GI toxicity is anticipated. Supportive treatment, including platelet transfusions, antibiotics, and treatment of mucositis, is required. Acute cardiac toxicity with severe arrhythmias and delayed cardiac failure may also occur. Peritoneal or hemodialysis are not effective.

▶ Special considerations
- Frequently monitor hepatic and renal function and CBC.
- Hyperuricemia may result from rapid lysis of leukemic cells; take appropriate preventive measures (including adequate hydration) before starting treatment.
- Control systemic infections before therapy.
- Administer over 10 to 15 minutes into a free-flowing I.V. infusion of normal saline solution or dextrose 5% in water, which is running into a large vein.
- If extravasation or signs of extravasation occur, discontinue infusion immediately and restart in another vein. Treat with intermittent ice packs – one-half hour immediately, then one-half hour q.i.d. for 4 days – and evaluate affected extremity.
- Antiemetics may be used to prevent or treat nausea and vomiting.
- Reconstitute using 5 or 10 ml normal saline solution, for the 5- or 10-mg vial, respectively, to give a final concentration of 1 mg/ml. *Do not use bacteriostatic saline.*
- Follow usual chemotherapy mixing precautions. Vial is under negative pressure.
- Reconstituted solutions are stable for 3 days (72 hours) at room temperature (59 to 86 F. [15 to 30 C.]); 7 days, if refrigerated. Discard unused solutions appropriately.

Information for the patient
- Instruct patient to recognize signs and symptoms of extravasation and to notify physician or nurse promptly if these occur.
- Tell patient to report signs and symptoms of infection, including persistent fever or sore throat.
- Tell patient to minimize dangerous behavior that can cause bleeding and to report any bleeding or abnormal bruising.

Pediatric use
Safety and efficacy have not been established.

Breast-feeding
It is unknown if idarubicin is excreted in breast milk. The potential for serious adverse reactions in the infant must be considered. Breast-feeding should be discontinued before starting therapy with idarubicin.

idoxuridine (IDU)
Herplex Liquifilm, Stoxil Ophthalmic

- Pharmacologic classification: halogenated pyrimidine
- Therapeutic classification: antiviral agent
- Pregnancy risk category C

How supplied
Available by prescription only
Ophthalmic ointment: 0.5%
Ophthalmic solution: 0.1%

Indications, route, and dosage
Herpes simplex keratitis
Adults and children: Instill 1 drop of solution into conjunctival sac q 1 hour during day and q 2 hours at night until improvement; then decrease to 1 drop q 2 hours during day and q 4 hours at night. Or apply ointment to conjunctival sac q 4 hours or 5 times daily, with last dose at bedtime. Response should be seen within 7 days; if not, discontinue and begin alternate therapy. Continue therapy 5 to 7 days after healing appears to be complete. Therapy should not be continued longer than 21 days.

Pharmacodynamics
Antiviral action: Idoxuridine interferes with DNA synthesis, blocking viral reproduction.

Pharmacokinetics
- *Absorption:* Idoxuridine is poorly absorbed after instillation into the eye.
- *Distribution:* Unknown.
- *Metabolism:* Idoxuridine is metabolized to iodouracil and iodide in the liver.
- *Excretion:* Drug is excreted by the kidney.

Contraindications and precautions
Idoxuridine is contraindicated in patients with hypersensitivity to idoxuridine or to any component of the preparation.

Interactions
When used concomitantly with boric acid preparations, local irritation may occur. Avoid concomitant use.

Effects on diagnostic tests
None reported.

Adverse reactions
- *Eye:* temporary visual haze, irritation, pain, burning, or inflammation of eye; mild edema of eyelid or cornea; photophobia; small punctate defects in corneal epithelium; slowed corneal wound healing (with ointment).
- *Other:* hypersensitivity.
  Note: Drug should be discontinued if hypersensitivity reactions occur.

Overdose and treatment
The toxicity of ingested idoxuridine is unknown. If accidentally ingested, general measures, such as emesis, catharsis, or lavage may be used to remove drug from GI tract. Dermal exposure may be treated by washing the area with soap and water. Observe patient closely for possible signs and symptoms.

▶ Special considerations
- Drug is not intended for long-term use since it may damage corneal epithelium or inhibit ulcer healing. Do not use for more than 7 days after healing is complete, or 21 days total.
- Do not mix idoxuridine with other medications; do not use old solution, which may cause ocular burning and has no antiviral activity.
- Cleanse eye area of excessive exudate before application.

Information for the patient
- Tell patient to watch for signs of sensitivity, such as itching lids or constant burning and to stop drug and report such signs immediately.
- Inform patient to avoid sharing washcloths and towels with family members.
- Advise patient to wash hands before and after applying ointment or solution.
- Tell patient to apply finger pressure to inside corner of the eyes for 1 minute after solution instillation, to minimize systemic absorption; patient should not close eyes tightly or blink more than usual.

Breast-feeding
No data available; however, breast-feeding probably should be avoided during idoxuridine therapy.

ifosfamide
Ifex

- Pharmacologic classification: alkylating agent (cell cycle-phase nonspecific)
- Therapeutic classification: antineoplastic
- Pregnancy risk category C

How supplied
Injection: 1-g, 2-g, 3-g vials

Indications, route, and dosage
Dosage and indications may vary. Check current literature for recommended protocol.
Testicular cancer, †lung cancer, †Hodgkin's and †non-Hodgkin's lymphoma, †breast cancer, †acute and †chronic lymphocytic leukemia, †ovarian cancer, and †sarcomas
Adults and children: 700 to 1,000 mg/m²/day for 5 days; 2,400 mg/m²/day for 3 days; or up to 5,000 mg/m² as a single dose. Regimen is usually repeated q 3 weeks.
  The drug may be given by slow I.V. push, by intermittent infusion over at least 30 minutes, or by continuous infusion.

Pharmacodynamics
Antineoplastic action: Ifosfamide requires activation by hepatic microsomal enzymes to exert its cytotoxic activity. The active compound cross-links strands of DNA and also breaks the DNA chain.

---

*Canada only   †Unlabeled clinical use   Italicized adverse reactions are life-threatening.

Pharmacokinetics
• *Absorption:* Ifosfamide is not administered orally.
• *Distribution:* Ifosfamide cross the blood-brain barrier but its metabolites do not; therefore, alkylating activity does not occur in the cerebrospinal fluid.
• *Metabolism:* Approximately 50% of a dose is metabolized in the liver.
• *Excretion:* Ifosfamide and its metabolites are excreted primarily in the urine. The plasma elimination half-life is reported to be about 14 hours.

Contraindications and precautions
No contraindications are reported for ifosfamide. Dosage adjustments are necessary in renal impairment.

Interactions
Concomitant use with phenobarbital, phenytoin, and chloral hydrate may increase the activity of ifosfamide by induction of hepatic microsomal enzymes, increasing the conversion of ifosfamide to its active form. Concomitant corticosteroid therapy may decrease the effectiveness of ifosfamide by inhibiting the enzymes that convert the drug to its active form. Coadministration of allopurinol may increase the activity and bone marrow toxicity of ifosfamide, prolonging its half-life by an unknown mechanism.

Effects on diagnostic tests
Ifosfamide therapy may increase serum concentrations of AST (SGOT), ALT (SGPT), bilirubin, LDH, creatinine, BUN, and alkaline phosphatase.

Adverse reactions
• CNS: lethargy and confusion with high doses.
• GI: nausea, vomiting.
• GU: hemorrhagic cystitis (dose-limiting), nephrotoxicity, dysuria, frequency.
• HEMA: *leukopenia*, occasional thrombocytopenia.
• Hepatic: elevated liver enzymes.
• Other: alopecia, chemical phlebitis.

Overdose and treatment
Clinical manifestations of overdose include myelosuppression, nausea, vomiting, alopecia, and hemorrhagic cystitis.
Treatment is usually supportive and includes transfusion of blood components, antiemetics, and bladder irrigation.

▶ Special considerations
• Follow all established procedures for the safe handling, administration, and disposal of chemotherapeutic agents.
• To reconstitute 1-g vial, use 20 ml sterile water for injection to give a concentration of 50 mg/ml or 30 ml sterile water for injection to give a concentration of 100 mg/ml. Normal saline solution may also be used for reconstitution.
• Push fluids (3 liters daily) and administer with mesna (Mesnex) to prevent hemorrhagic cystitis. Avoid giving the drug at bedtime, because infrequent voiding during the night may increase the possibility of cystitis. Bladder irrigation with normal saline solution may decrease the possibility of cystitis.
• Use reconstituted solution within 8 hours, because it contains no preservatives.
• Drug can be further diluted with dextrose 5% in water or normal saline solution for I.V. infusion. This solution is stable for 7 days at room temperature.

• Drug may be given by I.V. push injection in a minimum of 75 ml normal saline solution over 30 minutes.
• I.V. infusions for periods up to 5 days can be used to administer ifosfamide.
• Infusing each dose over 2 hours or longer will decrease possibility of cystitis.
• Sterile phlebitis may occur at the injection site; apply warm compresses.
• Encourage patients to void every 2 hours during the day and twice during the night. Catheterization should be required for patients unable to void.
• Use cautiously in patients with renal impairment.
• Assess patient for changes in mental status and cerebellar dysfunction. Dose may have to be decreased.
• Monitor CBC and renal and liver function tests.

Information for the patient
• Tell patient to ensure adequate fluid intake to prevent bladder toxicity and to facilitate excretion of uric acid.
• Patient should avoid exposure to people with infections.
• Reassure patient that hair should grow back after treatment has ended.
• Tell patient to call immediately if blood appears in the urine.

Pediatric use
Children may be more sensitive to the effects of the drug, requiring a lower dosage.

Breast-feeding
It is not known whether ifosfamide distributes into breast milk. However, because of the potential for serious adverse reactions, mutagenicity, and carcinogenicity in the infant, breast-feeding is not recommended.

imipenem-cilastatin sodium
Primaxin I.M., Primaxin I.V.

• Pharmacologic classification: carbapenem (thienamycin class); beta-lactam antibiotic
• Therapeutic classification: antibiotic
• Pregnancy risk category C

How supplied
Available by prescription only
Powder for I.M. injection: 500-mg vial, 750-mg vial
Injection: 500-mg, 750-mg vials and infusion bottles.

Indications, route, and dosage
Mild to moderate lower respiratory tract, skin and skin-structure, or gynecologic infections
Adults: 500 to 750 mg I.M. q 12 hours.
Mild to moderate intra-abdominal infections
Adults: 750 mg I.M. q 12 hours.
Serious respiratory and urinary tract infections; intra-abdominal, gynecologic, bone, joint, or skin infections; bacterial septicemia; endocarditis
Adults: 250 mg to 1 g by I.V. infusion q 6 to 8 hours. Maximum daily dosage is 50 mg/kg/day or 4 g/day, whichever is less.
†Children: 60 to 100 mg/kg I.V. daily in divided doses q 6 hours.

Dosage in renal failure

● If creatinine clearance is 30 to 70 ml/minute, dosage in life-threatening infections is 500 mg q 6 hours; in moderate infections, 500 mg q 8 hours.
● If creatinine clearance is 20 to 30 ml/minute, dosage in life-threatening infections is 500 mg q 8 hours; in moderate infections, 500 mg q 12 hours.
● If creatinine clearance is 5 to 20 ml/minute, dosage in life-threatening infections is 500 mg q 12 hours; in moderate infections, 250 mg q 12 hours.
● If creatinine clearance is less than 5 ml/minute, dosage in life-threatening infections is 500 mg q 12 hours; in moderate infections, 250 mg q 12 hours.

Pharmacodynamics

Antibacterial action: A bactericidal drug, imipenem inhibits bacterial cell wall synthesis. Its spectrum of antimicrobial activity includes many gram-positive, gram-negative, and anaerobic bacteria, including *Staphylococcus* and *Streptococcus* species, *Escherichia coli*, *Klebsiella*, *Proteus*, *Enterobacter* species, *Pseudomonas aeruginosa*, and *Bacteroides* species including *B. fragilis*. Resistant bacteria include methicillin-resistant staphylococci, *Clostridium difficile*, and other *Pseudomonas* species.

Cilastatin inhibits imipenem's enzymatic breakdown in the kidneys, making it effective in treating urinary tract infections.

Pharmacokinetics

● *Absorption:* Following I.M. administration, imipenem blood levels peak within 2 hours; cilastatin levels reach their peak within 1 hour. After I.V. administration, peak levels of both agents appear in about 20 minutes. Imipenem is about 75% bioavailable and cilastatin is about 95% bioavailable after I.M. administration as compared to intravenous administration.
● *Distribution:* Imipenem-cilastatin is distributed rapidly and widely. Approximately 20% of imipenem is protein-bound; 40% of cilastatin is protein-bound.
● *Metabolism:* Imipenem is metabolized by kidney dehydropeptidase I, resulting in low urine concentrations. Cilastatin inhibits this enzyme, thereby reducing imipenem's metabolism.
● *Excretion:* About 70% of imipenem-cilastatin dose is excreted unchanged by the kidneys (when imipenem is combined with cilastatin) by tubular secretion and glomerular filtration. Imipenem is cleared by hemodialysis; therefore, a supplemental dose is required after this procedure. The half-life of the drug is about 1 hour after I.V. administration. The prolonged absorption that occurs after I.M. administration results in a longer half-life (2 to 3 hours).

Contraindications and precautions

Imipenem is contraindicated in patients with known hypersensitivity to the drug.

Imipenem should be administered cautiously to patients with a history of seizures, especially if they also have compromised renal function, because drug may induce seizures; and to patients who are allergic to penicillin or cephalosporins, because this drug is chemically similar to them. Chloramphenicol may impede the bactericidal effects of imipenem; give chloramphenicol a few hours after imipenem-cilastatin.

Interactions

Imipenem may be physically incompatible with aminoglycosides; avoid mixing together. Probenecid may prevent tubular secretion of cilastatin (but not imipenem) and thereby prolong plasma cilastatin half-life.

Effects on diagnostic tests

Serum levels of AST (SGOT), ALT (SGPT), alkaline phosphatase, lactic dehydrogenase, and bilirubin may be elevated, and erythrocyte, platelet, and leukocyte counts reduced during imipenem therapy.

Adverse reactions

● CNS: *seizures,* dizziness, encephalopathy, confusion.
● CV: hypotension.
● DERM: rash, urticaria, pruritus.
● GI: nausea, vomiting, diarrhea, *pseudomembranous colitis.*
● Local: thrombophlebitis, pain at injection site.
● Other: hypersensitivity, superinfection.
   Note: Drug should be discontinued if patient develops hypersensitivity reaction or if seizures or pseudomembranous colitis occurs.

Overdose and treatment

No information available.

▶ Special considerations

● Culture and sensitivity tests should be done before starting therapy.
● When reconstituting powder, shake until solution is clear. Solution may range from colorless to yellow; color variations within this range do not affect drug potency. After reconstitution, solution remains stable for 10 hours at room temperature and for 48 hours when refrigerated.
● Do not administer by direct I.V. bolus injection. Infuse 250- or 500-mg dose over 20 to 30 minutes; infuse 1-g dose over 40 to 60 minutes. If nausea occurs, slow infusion.
● Anticonvulsants should be continued in patients with known seizure disorders. Patients who exhibit CNS toxicity should receive phenytoin or benzodiazepines. Reduce dosage or discontinue drug if CNS toxicity continues.
● Drug has broadest antibacterial spectrum of any available antibiotic. It is most valuable for empiric treatment of unidentified infections and for mixed infections that would otherwise require combination of antibiotics, possibly including an aminoglycoside.
● Prolonged use may result in overgrowth of nonsusceptible organisms. In addition, use of imipenum-cilastatin as a sole course of therapy has resulted in resistance during therapy.

Geriatric use

Administer cautiously to elderly patients because they may also have renal dysfunction.

Pediatric use

Safety and effectiveness in children under age 12 have not been established; however, drug has been used in children age 3 months to 13 years. Dosage range is 15 to 25 mg/kg q 6 hours.

Breast-feeding

Imipenem is distributed into breast milk. Administer cautiously to breast-feeding women.

---

imipramine hydrochloride
Apo-Imipramine*, Impril*, Janimine,
Novopramine*, SK-Pramine, Tofranil,
Typramine

imipramine pamoate
Tofranil-PM

- Pharmacologic classification: dibenzazepine tricyclic antidepressant
- Therapeutic classification: antidepressant
- Pregnancy risk category D

How supplied
Available by prescription only
Tablets: 10 mg, 25 mg, 50 mg
Capsules: 75 mg, 100 mg, 125 mg, 150 mg
Injection: 12.5 mg/ml

Indications, route, and dosage
Depression, †neurogenic pain, †panic disorder, †generalized anxiety disorder
Adults: Initially, 75 to 100 mg P.O. or I.M. daily in divided doses, with 25- to 50-mg increments, up to 200 mg. Alternatively, some patients can start with lower doses (25 mg P.O.) and titrate slowly in 25-mg increments every other day. Maximum dosage is 300 mg daily. Alternatively, the entire dosage may be given at bedtime. (I.M. route rarely used.) Maximum dosage: 200 mg/day for outpatients, 300 mg/day for inpatients, 100 mg/day for elderly patients.
Childhood enuresis
Children age 6 or over: 25 to 75 mg P.O. daily, 1 hour before bedtime.

†Adjunctive treatment of detrusor instability in incontinent patients
Adults: 25 to 50 mg P.O. b.i.d. or 75 to 100 mg P.O. h.s.

Pharmacodynamics
Antidepressant action: Imipramine is thought to exert its antidepressant effects by inhibiting reuptake of norepinephrine and serotonin in CNS nerve terminals (presynaptic neurons), which results in increased concentrations and enhanced activity of these neurotransmitters in the synaptic cleft. Imipramine also has anticholinergic activity and is used to treat nocturnal enuresis in children over age 6.

Pharmacokinetics
- *Absorption:* Imipramine is absorbed rapidly from the GI tract and muscle tissue after oral and I.M. administration.
- *Distribution:* Imipramine is distributed widely into the body, including the CNS and breast milk. Drug is 90% protein-bound. Peak effect occurs in ½ to 2 hours; steady state is achieved within 2 to 5 days. Therapeutic plasma levels (parent drug and metabolite) are thought to range from 150 to 300 ng/ml.
- *Metabolism:* Imipramine is metabolized by the liver to the active metabolite desipramine. A significant first-pass effect may explain variability of serum concentrations in different patients taking the same dosage.
- *Excretion:* Most of drug is excreted in urine.

Contraindications and precautions
Imipramine is contraindicated in patients with known hypersensitivity to tricyclic antidepressants, trazodone, and related compounds; in the acute recovery phase of myocardial infarction (MI) because of its arrhythmogenic potential; in patients in coma or severe respiratory depression because of additive CNS depression; and during or within 14 days of therapy with monoamine oxidase inhibitors.

Imipramine should be used cautiously in patients with other cardiac disease (arrhythmias, congestive heart failure [CHF], angina pectoris, valvular disease, increased QRS intervals, or heart block); respiratory disorders; epilepsy and other seizure disorders; scheduled electroconvulsive therapy; bipolar disease; glaucoma; hyperthyroidism, or in those taking thyroid replacement; Type I and Type II diabetes; prostatic hypertrophy, paralytic ileus, or urinary retention; hepatic or renal dysfunction; Parkinson's disease; and in those undergoing surgery with general anesthesia.

Some formulations contain tartrazine and may provoke asthma in patients with aspirin allergy.

Interactions
Concomitant use of imipramine with sympathomimetics, including epinephrine, phenylephrine, phenylpropanolamine, and ephedrine (often found in nasal sprays) may increase blood pressure; use with warfarin may increase prothrombin time and cause bleeding. Concomitant use with thyroid medication, pimozide, and antiarrhythmic agents (quinidine, disopyramide, procainamide) may increase incidence of cardiac arrhythmias and conduction defects.

Imipramine may decrease hypotensive effects of centrally acting antihypertensive drugs, such as guanethidine, guanabenz, guanadrel, clonidine, methyldopa, and reserpine. Concomitant use with disulfiram or ethchlorvynol may cause delirium and tachycardia.

Additive effects are likely after concomitant use of imipramine with CNS depressants, including alcohol, analgesics, barbiturates, narcotics, tranquilizers, and anesthetics (oversedation); atropine or other anticholinergic drugs, including phenothiazines, antihistamines, meperidine, and antiparkinsonian agents (oversedation, paralytic ileus, visual changes, and severe constipation); or metrizamide (increased risk of convulsions).

Barbiturates and heavy smoking induce imipramine metabolism and decrease therapeutic efficacy; phenothiazines and haloperidol decrease its metabolism, decreasing therapeutic efficacy. Methylphenidate, cimetidine, oral contraceptives, propoxyphene, and beta blockers may inhibit imipramine metabolism, increasing plasma levels and toxicity.

Effects on diagnostic tests
Imipramine may prolong conduction time (elongation of Q-T and PR intervals, flattened T waves on ECG); it also may elevate liver function test results, decrease white blood cell counts, and decrease or increase serum glucose levels.

Adverse reactions
- CNS: drowsiness, dizziness, sedation, excitation, tremor, weakness, headache, nervousness, *seizures,* peripheral neuropathy, extrapyramidal symptoms, anxiety, vivid dreams, confusion (more marked in elderly patients), decreased libido, sexual dysfunction.
- CV: orthostatic hypotension, tachycardia, arrhyth-

mias, *MI, stroke, heart block, CHF,* palpitations, hypertension, ECG changes.
● EENT: blurred vision, tinnitus, mydriasis, increased intraocular pressure.
● GI: dry mouth, constipation, nausea, vomiting, anorexia, diarrhea, paralytic ileus, jaundice.
● GU: urine retention.
● Other: sweating, photosensitivity, hypersensitivity (rash, urticaria, drug fever, edema).

After abrupt withdrawal of long-term therapy, nausea, headache, or malaise (does not indicate addiction) may occur.

Note: Drug should be discontinued (not abruptly) if signs of hypersensitivity occur, such as urine retention, extreme dry mouth, rash, excessive sedation, seizures, tachycardia, sore throat, fever, or jaundice.

Overdose and treatment

Imipramine overdose is frequently life-threatening, particularly when combined with alcohol. The first 12 hours after acute ingestion are a stimulatory phase characterized by excessive anticholinergic activity (agitation, irritation, confusion, hallucinations, hyperthermia, parkinsonian symptoms, seizure, urine retention, dry mucous membranes, pupillary dilatation, constipation, and ileus). This is followed by CNS depressant effects, including hypothermia, decreased or absent reflexes, sedation, hypotension, cyanosis, and cardiac irregularities, including tachycardia, conduction disturbances, and quinidine-like effects on the ECG.

Severity of overdose is best indicated by widening of the QRS complex, which usually represents a serum level in excess of 1,000 ng/ml; serum concentrations are usually not helpful. Metabolic acidosis may follow hypotension, hypoventilation, and convulsions.

Treatment is symptomatic and supportive, including maintaining airway, stable body temperature, and fluid or electrolyte balance. Induce emesis if patient is conscious; follow with gastric lavage and activated charcoal to prevent further absorption. Dialysis is of little use. Treat seizures with parenteral diazepam or phenytoin; arrhythmias, with parenteral phenytoin or lidocaine; and acidosis, with sodium bicarbonate. Do not give barbiturates; these may enhance CNS and respiratory depressant effects.

▶ Special considerations

Besides those relevant to all *tricyclic antidepressants,* consider the following recommendations.
● Imipramine may be used to treat nocturnal enuresis in children.
● Imipramine is associated with a high incidence of orthostatic hypotension. Check sitting and standing blood pressures after initial dose.
● Do not give the full daily dosage at one time. Titrate patient to effect.
● I.M. administration may result in a more rapid onset of action than that with oral administration. However, oral therapy should be substituted for parenteral therapy as soon as possible.
● Drug should not be withdrawn abruptly, but tapered gradually over time.
● Do not give drug I.V.
● Tolerance to the sedative effects of this drug usually develops over several weeks.
● Drug should be discontinued at least 48 hours before surgical procedures.

Information for the patient
● Tell patient to take the medication exactly as prescribed, not to take the full daily dosage at one time, and not to double dose for missed doses.
● Explain that the full effects of the drug may not become apparent for up to 4 to 6 weeks after initiation of therapy.
● Warn patient not to discontinue drug abruptly, not to share drug with others, and not to drink alcoholic beverages while taking this drug.
● Suggest taking drug with food or milk if it causes stomach upset.
● Suggest relieving dry mouth with chewing gum or sugarless hard candy. Encourage good dental prophylaxis since persistent dry mouth may lead to increased incidence of dental caries.
● Encourage patient to report any unusual or troublesome effects immediately, including confusion, movement disorders, rapid heartbeat, dizziness, fainting, or difficulty urinating.

Geriatric use
Recommended dosage, 30 to 40 mg P.O. daily, not to exceed 100 mg daily. Initiate therapy at low doses (10 mg) and titrate slowly. Elderly patients may be at greater risk for adverse cardiac reactions.

Pediatric use
Not recommended for treating depression in patients younger than age 12. Do not use pamoate salt for enuresis in children.

Breast-feeding
Imipramine is excreted in breast milk in low concentrations. The potential benefit to the mother should outweigh possible risks to the infant.

immune globulin (gamma globulin; IG; immune serum globulin; ISG)

immune globulin for I.M. use (IGIM)
Gamastan, Gammar

immune globulin for I.V. use (IGIV)
Gamimune N, Gammagard, Gammar-IV, Iveegam, Sandoglobulin, Venoglobulin-I

- Pharmacologic classification: immune serum
- Therapeutic classification: immune serum
- Pregnancy risk category B

How supplied
Available by prescription only
IGIM
Injection: 2-ml and 10-ml vials
IGIV
I.V.: Gamimune N – 5% solution in 10-ml, 50-ml, and 100-ml single-use vials; Gammagard – 0.5-g, 2.5-g, 5-g, and 10-g single-use vials for reconstitution; Gammar-IV – 2.5-g vial with diluent; Iveegam – 0.5-g and 1-g vials

---

with diluent; 2.5-g and 5-g infusion bottles; Sandoglobulin – 1-g, 3-g, and 6-g single-use vials for reconstitution; Venoglobulin-I – 2.5-g and 5-g vials with diluent

Indications, route, and dosage
Agammaglobulinemia or hypogammaglobulinemia
IGIV

Adults and children: For Gamimune N only, 100 to 200 mg/kg or 2 to 4 ml/kg I.V. infusion monthly. Infusion rate is 0.01 to 0.02 ml/kg/minute for 30 minutes. Rate can then be increased to a maximum of 0.08 ml/kg/minute for remainder of infusion.

For Gammagard only, initially 200 to 400 mg/kg I.V., followed by 100 mg/kg at monthly intervals. Initiate infusion at 0.5 ml/kg/hour, gradually increasing to a maximum of 4 ml/kg/hour.

For Gammar-IV only, 100 to 200 mg/kg q 3 to 4 weeks. Infusion rate is 0.01 ml/kg/minute, increasing to 0.02 mg/kg/minute after 15 to 30 minutes, with gradual increase to 0.03 to 0.06 mg/kg/minute.

For Iveegam only, 200 mg/kg I.V. monthly. If response is inadequate, doses may be increased up to 800 mg/kg or the drug may be administered more frequently. Infuse at 1 to 2 ml/minute.

For Sandoglobulin only, 200 mg/kg I.V. monthly. Start with 0.5 to 1 ml/minute of a 30-mg/ml solution; increase up to 2.5 ml/minute gradually after 15 to 30 minutes.

For Venoglobulin-I only, 200 mg/kg I.V. monthly; may be increased to 300 to 400 mg/kg and may be repeated more frequently than once monthly. Infuse at 0.01 to 0.02 ml/kg/minute for 30 minutes, then increase to 0.04 ml/kg/minute or higher if tolerated.

IGIM
Adults: Initial dose 1.2 ml/kg, maximum one-time dose 30 to 50 ml.
Children: Initial dose 1.2 ml/kg, maximum one-time dose 20 to 30 ml.

Maintenance dose (adults and children) is 0.6 ml/kg q 2 weeks.

Hepatitis A exposure
Adults and children: 0.02 to 0.04 ml/kg I.M. as soon as possible after exposure. Up to 0.1 ml/kg may be given after prolonged or intense exposure.

Serum hepatitis posttransfusion
Adults and children: 10 ml I.M. within 1 week after transfusion and 10 ml I.M. 1 month later.

Measles exposure
Adults and children: 0.02 ml/kg within 6 days after exposure.

Modification of measles
Adults and children: 0.04 ml/kg I.M. within 6 days after exposure.

Measles vaccine complications
Adults and children: 0.02 to 0.04 ml/kg I.M.

Poliomyelitis exposure
Adults and children: 0.3 to 0.4 ml/kg I.M. within 7 days after exposure.

Chicken pox exposure
Adults and children: 0.2 to 1.3 ml/kg I.M. as soon as exposed.

Rubella exposure in first trimester of pregnancy
Women: 0.2 to 0.4 ml/kg I.M. as soon as exposed.

Idiopathic thrombocytopenic purpura
Adults: 0.4 g/kg Sandoglobulin I.V. for 5 consecutive days.

Pharmacodynamics
Immune action: Immune globulin provides passive immunity by increasing antibody titer.

Pharmacokinetics
● *Absorption:* After slow I.M. absorption, serum concentrations of gamma globulin peak within 2 days.
● *Distribution:* Gamma globulin distributes evenly between intravascular and extravascular spaces.
● *Metabolism:* Unknown.
● *Excretion:* The serum half-life of gamma globulin is reportedly 21 to 24 days in immunocompetent patients.

Contraindications and precautions
Immune globulin is contraindicated in patients known to have had an anaphylactic or severe systemic response to immune globulin and in patients with known hypersensitivity to thimerosal, maltose, or any component of the formulation.

Interactions
Concomitant use of immune globulin may interfere with the immune response to live virus vaccines (for example, measles, mumps, and rubella). Do not administer live virus vaccines within 3 months after administration of immune globulin.

Effects on diagnostic tests
None reported.

Adverse reactions
● Local: pain, erythema, and phlebitis at injection site.
● Systemic: headache, malaise, fever, chills, faintness, urticaria, *hypotension,* dyspnea, angioedema, *nephrotic syndrome, anaphylaxis.*
Note: Drug should be discontinued or the infusion rate of gamma globulin reduced if adverse reactions occur during infusion. When symptoms subside, resume at a rate the patient can tolerate.

Overdose and treatment
Excessively rapid I.V. infusion rate can precipitate an anaphylactoid reaction.

▶ Special considerations
● Obtain a thorough history of allergies and reactions to immunizations.
● Epinephrine solution 1:1,000 should be available to treat allergic reactions.
● Inject I.M. formulation into different sites, preferably into buttocks. Do not inject more than 3 ml per injection site.
● Do not give for hepatitis A exposure if 2 weeks or more have elapsed since exposure or after onset of clinical illness.
● Closely monitor blood pressure in patient receiving IGIV, especially if this is the patient's first infusion of immune globulin.
● Immune globulin has not been associated with an increased frequency of acquired immunodeficiency syndrome (AIDS). It is devoid of human immunodeficiency virus (HIV). Immune globulin recipients do not develop antibodies to HIV.
● Although pregnancy is not a contraindication to use, it is not known whether immune globulin can cause fetal harm.
● Store Sandoglobulin and Gammagard at room temperature not exceeding 77° F (25° C); Gamimune-N and Iveegam, at 36° to 46° F (2° to 8° C) but do not

---

freeze; Gammar-IV, at room temperature below 86° F (30° C) but do not freeze; Venoglobulin-I at room temperature below 86° F.

● Immune globulin has been studied in the treatment of various conditions, including Kawasaki disease, asthma, allergic disorders, autoimmune neutropenia, myasthenia gravis, and platelet transfusion rejection. It also has been used in the prophylaxis of infections in immunocompromised patients.

● Gamimune N can be diluted with dextrose 5% in water.

● Gammagard should be reconstituted with the diluent (sterile water for injection) and transfer device provided by the manufacturer. The administration set (provided) contains a 15-micron inline filter that must be used during administration.

● Sandoglobulin should be reconstituted with the diluent supplied (0.9% sodium chloride).

Information for the patient
● Explain to patient that his chances of getting AIDS or hepatitis after receiving immune globulin are minute.
● Tell patient what to expect after vaccination: some local pain, swelling, and tenderness at the injection site. Recommend acetaminophen to ease minor discomfort.
● Tell patient to promptly report headache, skin changes, or difficulty breathing.

Breast-feeding
It is unknown whether immune globulin distributes into breast milk. Use with caution in breast-feeding women.

---

indapamide
Lozol

● Pharmacologic classification: thiazide-like diuretic
● Therapeutic classification: diuretic, anti-hypertensive
● Pregnancy risk category B

How supplied
Available by prescription only
Tablets: 2.5 mg

Indications, route, and dosage
Edema, hypertension
Adults: 2.5 mg P.O. as a single daily dose taken in the morning; dosage may be increased to 5 mg daily.

Pharmacodynamics
● *Diuretic action:* Indapamide increases urinary excretion of sodium and water by inhibiting sodium reabsorption in the cortical diluting tubule of the nephron, thus relieving edema.
● *Antihypertensive action:* The exact mechanism of indapamide's antihypertensive effect is unknown. This effect may result from direct arteriolar vasodilatation, via calcium channel blockade. Indapamide also reduces total body sodium.

Pharmacokinetics
● *Absorption:* After oral administration, indapamide is absorbed completely from the GI tract; peak serum levels occur at 2 to 2½ hours.
● *Distribution:* Indapamide distributes widely into body

tissues as a result of its lipophilicity; drug is 71% to 79% plasma protein-bound.
● *Metabolism:* Indapamide undergoes significant hepatic metabolism.
● *Excretion:* About 60% of a dose of indapamide is excreted in urine within 48 hours; approximately 16% to 23% is excreted in feces.

Contraindications and precautions
Indapamide is contraindicated in patients with anuria or in those with a known sensitivity to the drug or to sulfonamide derivatives.

Indapamide should be used cautiously in patients with severe renal disease because it may decrease glomerular filtration rate and precipitate azotemia; in patients with impaired hepatic function or liver disease because electrolyte changes may precipitate coma; and in patients taking digoxin, because hypokalemia may predispose them to digitalis toxicity.

Interactions
Indapamide potentiates the hypotensive effects of most other antihypertensive drugs; this may be used to therapeutic advantage.

Indapamide may potentiate hyperglycemic, hypotensive, and hyperuricemic effects of diazoxide, and its hyperglycemic effect may increase insulin or sulfonylurea requirements in diabetic patients.

Indapamide may reduce renal clearance of lithium, elevating serum lithium levels, and may necessitate reduction in lithium dosage by 50%.

Indapamide turns urine slightly more alkaline and may decrease urinary excretion of some amines, such as amphetamine and quinidine; alkaline urine may also decrease therapeutic efficacy of methenamine compounds such as methenamine mandelate.

Cholestyramine and colestipol may bind indapamide, preventing its absorption; give drugs 1 hour apart.

Effects on diagnostic tests
Indapamide therapy may alter serum electrolyte levels and may increase serum urate, glucose, cholesterol, and triglyceride levels. It also may interfere with tests for parathyroid function and should be discontinued before such tests.

Adverse reactions
● CNS: headache, irritability, nervousness.
● CV: volume depletion and dehydration, orthostatic hypotension.
● DERM: dermatitis, photosensitivity, rash.
● GI: anorexia, nausea, pancreatitis.
● Metabolic: *asymptomatic hyperuricemia; gout;* fluid and electrolyte imbalances, including hypokalemia, hyponatremia and hypochloremia; metabolic alkalosis.
● Other: muscle cramps and spasms.
   Note: Drug should be discontinued if rising BUN and serum creatinine levels indicate renal impairment or if patient shows signs of impending coma.

Overdose and treatment
Clinical signs of overdose include GI irritation and hypermotility, diuresis, and lethargy, which may progress to coma.

Treatment is mainly supportive; monitor and assist respiratory, cardiovascular, and renal function as indicated. Monitor fluid and electrolyte balance. Induce vomiting with ipecac in conscious patient; otherwise, use gastric lavage to avoid aspiration. Do not give ca-

---

thartics; these promote additional loss of fluids and electrolytes.

▶ **Special considerations**
Recommendations for use of indapamide and for care and teaching of the patient during therapy are the same as those for all thiazide and thiazide-like diuretics.

Geriatric use
Elderly and debilitated patients require close observation and may require reduced dosages. They are more sensitive to excess diuresis because of age-related changes in cardiovascular and renal function. Excess diuresis promotes orthostatic hypotension, dehydration, hypovolemia, hyponatremia, hypomagnesemia, and hypokalemia.

Pediatric use
Safety and effectiveness have not been established.

Breast-feeding
Indapamide is distributed in breast milk; its safety and effectiveness in breast-feeding women have not been established.

indomethacin, indomethacin sodium trihydrate
Indocid, Indocin, Indocin SR, Indo-Lemmon, Indomed, Indameth

- Pharmacologic classification: nonsteroidal anti-inflammatory
- Therapeutic classification: nonnarcotic analgesic, antipyretic, anti-inflammatory
- Pregnancy risk category B (D in third trimester)

How supplied
Available by prescription only
Capsules: 25 mg, 50 mg
Capsules (sustained-release): 75 mg
Suspension: 25 mg/5 ml
Injection: 1-mg vials
Suppositories: 50 mg

Indications, route, and dosage
Moderate to severe arthritis, ankylosing spondylitis
Adults: 25 mg P.O. b.i.d. or t.i.d. with food or antacids; may increase dose by 25 mg daily q 7 days up to 200 mg daily; or 50 mg rectally q.i.d. Alternatively, sustained-release capsules (75 mg) may be given: 75 mg to start, in the morning or h.s., followed, if necessary, by 75 mg b.i.d.

Acute gouty arthritis
50 mg t.i.d. Reduce dose as soon as possible, then stop. Sustained-release capsules should not be used for this condition.

To close a hemodynamically significant patent ductus arteriosus in premature infants (I.V. form only)
Age less than 48 hours: 0.2 mg/kg I.V. followed by 2 doses of 0.1 mg/kg at 12- to 24-hour intervals.
Age 2 to 7 days: 0.2 mg/kg I.V. followed by 2 doses of 0.2 mg/kg at 12- to 24-hour intervals.

Over age 7 days: 0.2 mg/kg I.V. followed by 2 doses of 0.25 mg/kg at 12- to 24-hour intervals.

Pharmacodynamics
- *Analgesic, antipyretic, and anti-inflammatory actions:* Exact mechanisms of action are unknown; indomethacin is thought to produce its analgesic, antipyretic, and anti-inflammatory effects by inhibiting prostaglandin synthesis and possibly by inhibiting phosphodiesterase.
- *Closure of patent ductus arteriosus:* The exact mechanism of action is unknown, but is believed to be through inhibition of prostaglandin synthesis.

Pharmacokinetics
- *Absorption:* Indomethacin is absorbed rapidly and completely from the GI tract.
- *Distribution:* Indomethacin is highly protein-bound.
- *Metabolism:* Indomethacin is metabolized in the liver.
- *Excretion:* Indomethacin is excreted mainly in urine, with some biliary excretion.

Contraindications and precautions
Indomethacin is contraindicated in patients with known hypersensitivity to the drug; in patients in whom aspirin or other nonsteroidal anti-inflammatory drugs (NSAIDs) induce symptoms of asthma, urticaria, or rhinitis; in patients with active GI disorders because it may cause GI upset; in infants with untreated infection; in patients with active bleeding; in patients with coagulation defects or thrombocytopenia; in patients with necrotizing enterocolitis; and in patients with impaired renal function. Rectal form of indomethacin is contraindicated in patients with a history of recent rectal bleeding, proctitis, or ulcerative colitis.

Administer cautiously to patients with epilepsy, parkinsonism, hepatic or renal disease, cardiovascular disease, known intrinsic coagulation defects, infection, or a history of mental illness, because it may exacerbate the symptoms of these disorders.

Patients with known "triad" symptoms (aspirin hypersensitivity, rhinitis/nasal polyps, and asthma) are at high risk of bronchospasm. NSAIDs may mask the signs and symptoms of acute infection (fever, myalgia, erythema); carefully evaluate patients with high risk (such as those with diabetes).

Interactions
Concomitant use of indomethacin with anticoagulants and thrombolytic drugs (coumarin derivatives, heparin, streptokinase, or urokinase) may potentiate anticoagulant effects. Bleeding problems may occur if indomethacin is used with other drugs that inhibit platelet aggregation, such as azlocillin, parenteral carbenicillin, dextran, dipyridamole, mezlocillin, piperacillin, sulfinpyrazone, ticarcillin, valproic acid, cefamandole, cefoperazone, moxalactam, plicamycin, aspirin, salicylates, or other anti-inflammatory agents. Concomitant use with salicylates, anti-inflammatory agents, alcohol, corticotropin, or steroids may cause increased GI adverse effects, including ulceration and hemorrhage. Aspirin may decrease the bioavailability of indomethacin.

Because of the influence of prostaglandins on glucose metabolism, concomitant use with insulin or oral hypoglycemic agents may potentiate hypoglycemic effects. Indomethacin may displace highly protein-bound drugs from binding sites. Toxicity may occur with coumarin derivatives, phenytoin, verapamil, or nifedipine. Increased nephrotoxicity may occur with gold compounds, other anti-inflammatory agents, or acetaminophen. Indomethacin may decrease the renal clearance of methotrexate and lithium.

Concurrent use with antihypertensives and diuretics may decrease their effectiveness. Concurrent use with triamterene not recommended due to potential nephrotoxicity. Other diuretics may also predispose patients to nephrotoxicity.

Effects on diagnostic tests

Indomethacin may interfere with results of the dexamethasone suppression test. It may also interfere with urinary 5-hydroxyindoleacetic acid determinations.

Adverse reactions

● CNS: headache, drowsiness, dizziness, depression, confusion, peripheral neuropathy, convulsions, psychic disturbances, syncope, vertigo.
● CV: hypertension, edema.
● DERM: pruritus, rash, urticaria, *Stevens-Johnson syndrome*.
● EENT: blurred vision, corneal and retinal damage, hearing loss, tinnitus.
● GI: nausea, vomiting, anorexia, diarrhea, constipation, severe GI bleeding (with I.V. dose).
● GU: hematuria, hyperkalemia, *acute renal failure*, renal dysfunction (with I.V. dose).
● HEMA: *hemolytic anemia, aplastic anemia, agranulocytosis,* leukopenia, thrombocytopenic purpura, iron deficiency anemia, decreased platelet aggregation (with I.V. dose).
● Other: elevated liver enzymes, hypersensitivity (shocklike symptoms, rash, *respiratory distress, angioedema*); hyponatremia, hyperkalemia, hypoglycemia (with I.V. dose).
Note: Drug should be discontinued if hypersensitivity, significant GI symptoms, or signs of hepatotoxicity occur.

Overdose and treatment

Clinical manifestations of overdose include dizziness, nausea, vomiting, intense headache, mental confusion, drowsiness, tinnitus, sweating, blurred vision, paresthesias, and convulsions.

To treat indomethacin overdose, empty stomach immediately by inducing emesis with ipecac syrup or by gastric lavage. Administer activated charcoal via nasogastric tube. Provide symptomatic and supportive measures (respiratory support and correction of fluid and electrolyte imbalances). Monitor laboratory parameters and vital signs closely. Dialysis may be of little value because indomethacin is strongly protein-bound.

▶ Special considerations

Besides those relevant to all *NSAIDs*, consider the following recommendations.
● Do not mix oral suspension with liquids or antacids before administering.
● Patient should retain suppository in the rectum for at least 1 hour after insertion to ensure maximum absorption.
● Reconstitute 1 mg vial of I.V. dose with 1 to 2 ml of sterile water for injection or 0.9% sodium chloride injection. Prepare solution immediately before use to prevent deterioration. Do not use solution if it is discolored or contains a precipitate.
● Administer by direct I.V. injection over 5 to 10 seconds. Use a large vein to prevent extravasation.
● Monitor I.V. site for complications.
● Monitor cardiopulmonary status for significant

changes. Watch for signs and symptoms of fluid overload. Check weight and intake and output daily.
● Monitor renal function studies before start of therapy and frequently during therapy to prevent adverse effects.
● Severe headache may occur. If headache persists, dose should be decreased.
● I.V. administration should be used only for premature neonates with patent ductus arteriosus. Do not administer a 2nd or 3rd I.V. dose if anuria or marked oliguria is present.
● If ductus arteriosus reopens, a second course of one to three doses may be given. If ineffective, surgery may be necessary.
● Monitor carefully for bleeding and for reduced urine output.

Information for the patient

● Instruct patient in proper administration of dosage form prescribed, such as suppository, sustained-release capsule, or suspension.
● Advise patient to seek medical approval before taking any nonprescription medications.
● Caution patient to avoid hazardous activities that require alertness or concentration. Instruct him in safety measures to prevent injury.
● Tell patient to report any signs and symptoms of adverse reactions. Encourage patient to adhere to prescribed drug regimen and recommended follow-up.

Geriatric use

● Patients over age 60 may be more susceptible to the toxic effects of indomethacin.
● The effects of indomethacin on renal prostaglandins may cause fluid retention and edema, a significant drawback for elderly patients and those with congestive heart failure.

Pediatric use

● The safety of long-term indomethacin use in children under age 14 has not been established.
● Use of I.V. indomethacin in premature infants for patent ductus arteriosus is considered an alternative to surgery.

Breast-feeding

Indomethacin is secreted into breast milk in concentrations similar to those in maternal plasma; avoid use in breast-feeding women.

---

influenza virus vaccine, 1992-1993 trivalent types A & B (purified surface antigen)
Flu-Imune

influenza virus vaccine, 1992-1993 trivalent types A & B (subvirion or split virion)
Fluogen Split, Fluzone Split, Influenza Virus Vaccine (Split)

---

influenza virus vaccine, 1992-1993 trivalent types A & B (whole virion)
Fluzone (Whole)

- Pharmacologic classification: vaccine
- Therapeutic classification: viral vaccine
- Pregnancy risk category C

How supplied
Available by prescription only
Injection: 15 mcg A/Texas/36/91-like (H1N1), 15 mcg A/Beijing/353/89-like (H3N2), and 15 mcg B/Panama/45/90-like hemagglutinin antigens per 0.5 ml

Indications, route, and dosage
Annual influenza prophylaxis in high-risk patients

Adults and children over age 12: 0.5 ml whole or split virus I.M. (only one dose required).
Children age 9 to 12: 0.5 ml split virus or purified surface antigen I.M. (only one dose required).
Children age 3 to 8: 0.5 ml split virus or purified surface antigen I.M. Repeat dose in 4 weeks unless the child received the vaccine the previous year.
Children age 6 to 35 months: 0.25 ml split virus or purified surface antigen I.M. Repeat dose in 4 weeks unless the child received the vaccine the previous year.
  Check package insert for annual changes and additional dosing recommendations.

Pharmacodynamics
Influenza prophylaxis: This vaccine promotes active immunity to influenza by inducing production of antibodies. Protection is provided only against those strains of virus from which the vaccine is prepared (or closely related strains).

Pharmacokinetics
A protective effect is achieved in most patients 10 to 14 days after administration. The duration of immunity varies widely but usually lasts about 1 year.

Contraindications and precautions
Influenza vaccine is contraindicated in patients with a sensitivity to egg or chick embryo protein and in patients with an acute respiratory infection or any other active infection. This vaccine also is contraindicated in patients with a history of Guillain-Barré syndrome or a known hypersensitivity to thimerosal, a component of the vaccine.

Interactions
Concomitant use of influenza vaccine with corticosteroids or immunosuppressants may impair the immune response to the vaccine. Do not administer influenza vaccine to infants and children at the same time as DTP, or within 14 days after administering live attenuated measles virus vaccine. Influenza vaccine may decrease the elimination of some drugs, such as theophylline and warfarin, that are metabolized by the cytochrome P-450 system. This effect may occur for up to 3 weeks after influenza vaccination.

Effects on diagnostic tests
No information available.

Adverse reactions
- Local: erythema, induration (occurring most often in children and those not exposed to influenza viruses).
- Systemic: fever, malaise, myalgia, *Guillain-Barré syndrome, anaphylaxis.*

Overdose and treatment
No information available.

▶ Special considerations
- Annual influenza prophylaxis is recommended for elderly persons and for adults and children with chronic cardiovascular, pulmonary, or renal disorders; metabolic disease; severe anemia; or compromised immune function. This vaccine also is recommended for medical personnel who have extensive contact with high-risk patients, residents of nursing homes or other chronic care facilities, and teenagers or children (age 6 months through 18 years) who are receiving long-term aspirin therapy and may be at risk of Reye's syndrome following influenza. The vaccine should also be given to any person who wishes to reduce the chance of acquiring an influenza infection.
- Obtain a thorough history of allergies, especially to eggs or chicken feathers, and of reactions to immunizations.
- Patients with a known or suspected hypersensitivity to egg protein should have a skin test to assess sensitivity to the vaccine. Administer a scratch test with 0.05 to 0.1 ml of a 1:100 dilution in normal saline solution for injection. Patients with positive skin test reactions should not receive the influenza virus vaccine.
- Epinephrine solution 1:1,000 should be available to treat allergic reactions.
- Influenza vaccine should not be administered to a patient with active influenza infection. Such infection should be treated with amantadine.
- Preferred I.M. injection site is the deltoid muscle in adults and older children and the anterolateral thigh in infants and young children.
- To reduce the frequency of adverse reactions, use only the split virus vaccine in children.
- Pneumococcal vaccine may be given simultaneously but at a different injection site.
- Store vaccine between 2 and 8 C. (36 to 46 F.). Do not freeze.

Information for the patient
- Tell patient that he may experience discomfort at the injection site after immunization. He also may develop fever, malaise, and muscle aches 6 to 12 hours after vaccination that may persist for several days. Recommend acetaminophen to alleviate these effects.
- Encourage patient to report any distressing adverse reactions promptly.
- Warn patient that many cases of Guillain-Barré syndrome were reported after vaccination for the swine flu of 1976. This condition usually causes reversible paralysis and muscle weakness, but it can be fatal in some individuals. Influenza vaccines made after this date have not been associated with as high an incidence of Guillain-Barré syndrome; however, there is still a possibility, albeit small, that this condition may follow influenza vaccination.
- Tell patient that this vaccine will protect him only against the influenza A virus strains that will cause the majority of influenza cases in the given year and that he will need to be vaccinated annually.

Geriatric use
Annual vaccination is highly recommended for anyone over age 65.

Pediatric use
Influenza vaccine is contraindicated in children under age 6 months.

Breast-feeding
It is unknown whether this vaccine is distributed into breast milk. Use with caution in breast-feeding women.

insulin (regular)
Beef Regular Iletin II (acid neutral CZI), Humulin R, Iletin Regular*, Novolin R, Pork Regular Iletin II, Regular Iletin I, Regular (concentrated) Iletin II, Regular Pork Insulin, Velosulin, Velosulin Human

prompt insulin zinc suspension (semilente)
Iletin Semilente*, Semilente Iletin I, Semilente Purified Pork

isophane insulin suspension (NPH)
Beef NPH Iletin II, Humulin N, Iletin NPH*, Insulatard NPH, NPH*, NPH Iletin I, Novolin N, Pork NPH Iletin II, Protaphane NPH

insulin zinc suspension (lente)
Beef Lente Iletin II, Humulin L, Lentard, Lente Iletin I, Monotard, Novolin L, Pork Lente Iletin II

protamine zinc insulin suspension (PZI)
Beef Protamine Zinc Iletin II, Iletin PZI*, Pork Protamine Zinc Iletin II, Protamine Zinc Iletin I

extended insulin zinc suspension (ultralente)
Iletin Ultralente*, Ultralente*, Ultralente Iletin I, Ultralente Insulin, Ultralente Purified Beef

- Pharmacologic classification: pancreatic hormone
- Therapeutic classification: antidiabetic agent
- Pregnancy risk category B

How supplied
Available without prescription
Insulin (regular)
Injection (beef): 100 units/ml
Injection (pork): 100 units/ml, 500 units/ml
Injection (beef and pork): 40 units/ml, 100 units/ml
Injection (human): 100 units/ml
Prompt insulin zinc suspension (semilente)
Injection (beef): 100 units/ml
Injection (pork): 100 units/ml
Injection (beef and pork): 40 units/ml, 100 units/ml

Isophane insulin suspension (NPH)
Injection (beef): 100 units/ml
Injection (pork): 100 units/ml
Injection (beef and pork): 40 units/ml, 100 units/ml
Injection (human): 100 units/ml
Insulin zinc suspension (lente)
Injection (beef): 100 units/ml
Injection (pork): 100 units/ml
Injection (beef and pork): 40 units/ml, 100 units/ml
Injection (human): 100 units/ml
Protamine zinc insulin (PZI)
Injection (beef): 100 units/ml
Injection (pork): 100 units/ml
Injection (beef and pork): 40 units/ml, 100 units/ml
Extended zinc insulin suspension (ultralente)
Injection (beef): 100 units/ml
Injection (pork): 100 units/ml
Injection (beef and pork): 40 units/ml, 100 units/ml

Indications, route, and dosage
Diabetic ketoacidosis (regular insulin)
Adults: 25 to 150 units I.V. immediately, then additional doses may be given q 1 hour based on blood sugar levels until patient is out of acidosis; then give S.C. q 6 hours thereafter. Alternative dosage schedule is 50 to 100 units I.V. and 50 to 100 units S.C. immediately; additional doses may be given q 2 to 6 hours based on blood sugar levels; or 0.33 units/kg I.V. bolus, followed by 7 to 10 units/hour I.V. by continuous infusion. Continue infusion until blood sugar drops to 250 mg/dl then start S.C. insulin q 6 hours.
Children: 0.5 to 1 unit/kg in two divided doses, one given I.V. and the other S.C., followed by 0.5 to 1 unit/kg I.V. q 1 to 2 hours; or 0.1 unit/kg I.V. bolus, then 0.1 unit/kg/hour continuous I.V. infusion until blood sugar drops to 250 mg/dl, then start S.C. insulin.
Ketosis-prone and juvenile-onset diabetes mellitus, diabetes mellitus inadequately controlled by diet and oral hypoglycemics
Adults and children: Individualized dosage adjusted according to patient's blood and urine glucose concentrations.
Hyperkalemia
Adults: 5 to 10 units of regular insulin with 50 ml of $D_{50}W$ over 5 minutes. Alternatively, 25 units of regular insulin given S.C. and an infusion of 1000 ml $D_{10}W$ with 90 mEq sodium bicarbonate; infuse 330 ml over 30 minutes and the balance over 3 hours.

Pharmacodynamics
Insulin is used as a replacement for the physiologic production of endogenous insulin in patients with IDDM and diabetes mellitus inadequately controlled by diet and oral hypoglycemic agents. Insulin increases glucose transport across muscle and fat-cell membranes to reduce blood glucose levels. It also promotes conversion of glucose to its storage form, glycogen; triggers amino acid uptake and conversion to protein in muscle cells and inhibits protein degradation; stimulates triglyceride formation and inhibits release of free fatty acids from adipose tissue; and stimulates lipoprotein lipase activity, which converts circulating lipoproteins to fatty acids. Insulin is available in various forms and these differ mainly in onset, peak, and duration of action. Characteristics of the various insulin preparations are compared in the accompanying chart.

COMPARING INSULIN PREPARATIONS

The chart below lists the various forms of insulin and their times of onset, peak, and duration.

PREPARATION	PURIFIED*	ONSET	PEAK	DURATION
Rapid-acting Insulins				
Insulin injection (regular, crystalline zinc)				
Regular Iletin I	No	½ to 1 hr	2 to 4 hr	6 to 8 hr
Regular Insulin	No	½ hr	2½ to 5 hr	8 hr
Pork Regular Iletin II	Yes	½ to 1 hr	2 to 4 hr	6 to 8 hr
Beef Regular Iletin II	Yes	½ to 1 hr	2 to 4 hr	6 to 8 hr
Regular (concentrated) Iletin II	Yes	½ hr	varies	24 hr
Velosulin	Yes	½ hr	1 to 3 hr	8 hr
Purified Pork Insulin	Yes	½ hr	2½ to 5 hr	8 hr
Humulin R	N.A.	½ to 1 hr	2 to 4 hr	6 to 8 hr
Humulin B.R.	N.A.	½ hr	2 to 4 hr	6 to 8 hr
Novolin R	N.A.	½ hr	2½ to 5 hr	6 to 8 hr
Prompt insulin zinc suspension (semilente)				
Semilente Iletin I	No	1 to 2 hr	3 to 8 hr	10 to 16 hr
Semilente Insulin	No	1½ hr	5 to 10 hr	16 hr
Semilente Purified Pork Prompt Insulin	Yes	1½ hr	5 to 10 hr	16 hr
Intermediate-acting Insulins				
Isophane insulin suspension (NPH)				
NPH Iletin I	No	2 hr	6 to 12 hr	18 to 26 hr
NPH Insulin	No	1½ hr	4 to 12 hr	24 hr
Beef NPH Iletin II	Yes	2 hr	6 to 12 hr	18 to 26 hr
Pork NPH Iletin II	Yes	2 hr	6 to 12 hr	18 to 26 hr
NPH Purified Pork Isophane Insulin	Yes	1½ hr	4 to 12 hr	24 hr
Insulatard NPH	Yes	1½ hr	4 to 12 hr	24 hr
Humulin N	N.A.	1 to 2 hr	6 to 12 hr	18 to 24 hr
Novolin N	N.A.	1½ hr	4 to 12 hr	24 hr
Insulin zinc suspension (lente)				
Lente Iletin I	No	2 to 4 hr	6 to 12 hr	18 to 26 hr
Lente Insulin	No	2½ hr	7 to 15 hr	24 hr
Beef Lente Iletin II	Yes	2 to 4 hr	6 to 12 hr	18 to 36 hr
Pork Lente Iletin II	Yes	2 to 4 hr	6 to 12 hr	18 to 36 hr
Lente Purified Pork Insulin	Yes	2½ hr	7 to 15 hr	22 hr
Humulin L	N.A.	1 to 3 hr	6 to 12 hr	18 to 21 hr
Novolin L	N.A.	2½ hr	7 to 15 hr	22 hr
Isophane (NPH) 70%, regular insulin 30%				
Humulin 70/30	N.A.	½ hr	4 to 8 hr	24 hr
Mixtard	Yes	½ hr	4 to 8 hr	24 hr
Mixtard Human	N.A.	½ hr	4 to 8 hr	24 hr
Novolin 70/30	N.A.	½ hr	2 to 12 hr	24 hr
Long-acting Insulins				
Protamine zinc insulin suspension				
Protamine Zinc & Iletin I	No	4 to 8 hr	14 to 24 hr	28 to 36 hr
Beef Protamine Zinc & Iletin II	Yes	4 to 8 hr	14 to 24 hr	28 to 36 hr
Pork Protamine Zinc & Iletin II	Yes	4 to 8 hr	14 to 24 hr	28 to 36 hr
Extended insulin zinc suspension (ultralente)				
Ultralente Iletin I	No	4 to 8 hr	14 to 24 hr	28 to 36 hr
Ultralente Insulin	No	4 hr	10 to 30 hr	36 hr
Ultralente Purified Beef Insulin	Yes	4 hr	10 to 30 hr	36 hr

N.A. indicates not applicable
*Purified insulins contain < 10 ppm proinsulin.

Pharmacokinetics

● *Absorption:* Insulin must be given parenterally because it is destroyed in the GI tract. Commercially available preparations are formulated to differ in onset, peak, and duration after subcutaneous administration. They are classified as rapid-acting (½ to 1 hour onset), intermediate-acting (1 to 2 hour onset), and long-acting (4 to 8 hour onset). The accompanying table summarizes major pharmacokinetic differences.

● *Distribution:* Insulin is distributed widely throughout the body.

● *Metabolism:* Some insulin is bound and inactivated by peripheral tissues, but the majority appears to be degraded in the liver and kidneys.

● *Excretion:* Insulin is filtered by the renal glomeruli and undergoes some tubular reabsorption. The plasma half-life is about 9 minutes after I.V. administration.

Contraindications and precautions

Use only regular insulin in patients with circulatory collapse, diabetic ketoacidosis, or hyperkalemia. Do not administer regular insulin concentrated by I.V. Do not use intermediate- or long-acting insulins for coma or other emergency requiring rapid drug action.

Interactions

Alcohol, anabolic steroids, beta blockers, clofibrate, fenfluramine, MAO inhibitors, salicylates, and tetracycline can cause a prolonged hypoglycemic effect. Monitor blood glucose carefully.

Corticosteroids, dextrothyroxine sodium, epinephrine, and thiazide diuretics can diminish insulin response. Monitor for hyperglycemia.

Effects on diagnostic tests

The physiologic effects of insulin may decrease serum magnesium, potassium, or inorganic phosphate concentrations.

Adverse reactions

● DERM: urticaria.
● Metabolic: *hypoglycemia, hyperglycemia (rebound, or Somogyi, effect).*
● Local: lipoatrophy, lipohypertrophy, itching, swelling, redness, stinging, warmth at injection site.
● Other: *anaphylaxis.*

Overdose and treatment

Insulin overdose may produce signs and symptoms of hypoglycemia (tachycardia, palpitations, anxiety, hunger, nausea, diaphoresis, tremors, pallor, restlessness, headache, and speech and motor dysfunction). Treatment is directed towards treating hypoglycemia. Treatment depends on the patient's symptoms. If the patient is responsive, give 10 to 15 g of a fast-acting oral carbohydrate. If the patient's signs and symptoms persist after 15 minutes, give an additional 10 g carbohydrate. If the patient is unresponsive, an I.V. bolus of dextrose 50% solution should immediately increase blood glucose. Some clinicians prefer to use $D_{25}W$ because it is less irritating should extravasation occur. A common infusion rate is based on glucose content: 10 to 20 mg/kg/minute. You also may give glucagon parenterally or epinephrine subcutaneously; both drugs raise blood glucose levels in a few minutes by stimulating glycogenolysis. Fluid and electrolyte imbalance may require I.V. fluids and electrolyte (such as potassium) replacement.

▶ Special considerations

● Accuracy of measurement is very important, especially with regular insulin concentrated. Aids, such as magnifying sleeve, dose magnifier, or cornwall syringe, may help improve accuracy.
● With regular insulin concentrated, a secondary hypoglycemic reaction may occur 18 to 24 hours after injection. This may be caused by a repository effect of the drug and the high concentration of insulin in the preparation (500 units/ml).
● Dosage is always expressed in USP units.
● Do not interchange single-source beef or pork insulins without considering the need for dosage adjustment.
● Lente, semilente, and ultralente insulins may be mixed in any proportion.
● Regular insulin may be mixed with NPH or lente insulins in any proportion. However, in vitro binding will occur over time until an equilibrium is reached. These mixtures should be administered either immediately after preparation or after stability occurs (15 minutes for NPH regular, 24 hours for lente regular) in order to minimize variability in patient response. Note that switching from separate injections to a prepared mixture also may alter the patient's response.
● Advise patient not to alter the order of mixing insulins or change the model or brand of syringe or needle.
● Store insulin in cool area. Refrigeration desirable but not essential, except with regular insulin concentrated.
● Do not use insulin that has changed color or becomes clumped or granular in appearance.
● Check expiration date on vial before using contents.
● Administration route is S.C. because it allows slower absorption and causes less pain than I.M. injections. Ketosis-prone, juvenile-onset, severely ill, and newly diagnosed diabetics with very high blood sugar levels may require hospitalization and I.V. treatment with regular fast-acting insulin. Ketosis-resistant diabetics may be treated as outpatients with intermediate-acting insulin after they have received instructions on how to alter dosage according to self-performed urine or blood glucose determinations. Some patients, primarily pregnant or brittle diabetics, may use a dextrometer to perform fingerstick blood glucose tests at home.
● Press but do not rub site after injection. Rotate injection sites. Record sites to avoid overuse of one area. However, unstable diabetics may achieve better control if injection site is rotated within same anatomic region.
● To mix insulin suspension, swirl vial gently or rotate between palms or between palm and thigh. Do not shake vigorously; this causes bubbling and air in syringe.
● In pregnant diabetic patients, insulin requirements increase, sometimes drastically, then decline immediately postpartum.
● Some patients may develop insulin resistance and require large insulin doses to control symptoms of diabetes. U-500 insulin is available for such patients as Purified Pork Iletin Regular Insulin, U500. Although every pharmacy may not normally stock it, it is readily available. Patient should notify pharmacist several days before prescription refill is needed. Give hospital pharmacy sufficient notice before refill of inhouse prescription. Never store U-500 insulin in same area with other insulin preparations because of danger of severe overdose if given accidentally to other patients. U-500 insulin must be administered with a U-100 syringe because no syringes are made for this drug.
● Human insulin may be advantageous in patients who

are allergic to pork or beef forms. Humulin is synthesized by a genetically altered strain of *Escherichia coli.* Novolin brands are derived by enzymatic alteration of pork insulin.

Information for the patient
● Human insulin may be advantageous for patients who are allergic to pork or beef forms, for noninsulin-dependent patients requiring intermittent or short-term therapy (such as pregnancy, surgery, infection, or TPN therapy), for patients with insulin resistance, or for those who develop lipoatrophy.
● Be sure patient knows that insulin therapy relieves symptoms but does not cure the disease.
● Tell patient about the nature of disease, the importance of following the therapeutic regimen, specific diet, weight reduction, exercise, personal hygiene, avoiding infection, and timing of injection and eating.
● Tell patient to strictly adhere to manufacturer's instructions regarding assembly, administration, and care of specialized delivery systems, such as insulin pumps.
● Emphasize the importance of regular meal times and that meals must not be omitted.
● Teach patient that blood glucose monitoring is an essential guide to correct dosage and to therapeutic success.
● Emphasize the importance of recognizing hypoglycemic symptoms because insulin-induced hypoglycemia is hazardous and may cause brain damage if prolonged.
● Advise patient to always wear a medical identification bracelet or pendant, to carry ample insulin supply and syringes on trips, to have carbohydrates (sugar or candy) on hand for emergency, and to note any time-zone changes for dose schedule when traveling.
● Advise patient not to change the order of mixing insulins or change the model or brand of syringe or needle.
● Tell patient that use of marijuana may increase insulin requirements.
● Cigarette smoking decreases the absorption of insulin administered subcutaneously. Advise patient not to smoke within 30 minutes after insulin injection.

---

interferon alfa-n3
Alferon N

● Pharmacologic classification: biological response modifier
● Therapeutic classification: antineoplastic
● Pregnancy risk category C

How supplied
Available by prescription only
Injection: 5 million IU/ml, in 1-ml vials

Indications, route, and dosage
Note: Be sure to check literature for current protocol.
Treatment of condylomata acuminata
Adults: 0.5 ml (250,000 IU) per wart injected into the base of each wart twice weekly for up to 8 weeks. For large warts, inject at several points around the periphery of the wart using a total dose of 0.5 ml per wart. Maximum dose for each treatment is 0.5 ml per wart. Use a 30G needle.

Pharmacodynamics
Antineoplastic action: The interferons are naturally occurring small-protein molecules produced and secreted by cells in response to viral infections and biological inducers. They bind to specific membrane receptors on cell surfaces to initiate a series of events that include induction of protein synthesis, which is then followed by various cellular responses (inhibition of virus replication, suppression of cell proliferation, immunomodulation, enhanced phagocytosis, augmentation of lymphocytic cytotoxicity, and enhancement of human leukocyte antigen expression). The exact mechanism of action is undetermined.

Pharmacokinetics
● *Absorption:* After intralesional injection, plasma concentrations are below detectable levels, but systemic effects indicate that some systemic absorption does occur.
● *Distribution:* Unknown.
● *Metabolism:* Unknown.
● *Excretion:* Unknown.

Contraindications and precautions
Contraindicated in patients with hypersensitivity to human interferon alfa or any component of the injection and in patients who have anaphylactic sensitivity to mouse immunoglobulin G, egg protein, or neomycin. Use with caution in patients with debilitating medical conditions, such as cardiac disease, severe pulmonary disease, diabetes mellitus with ketoacidosis, coagulation disorders, seizure disorders, or severe myelosuppression because drug may worsen these conditions.

Interactions
None reported.

Effects on diagnostic tests
Decreases in WBC counts have been reported. The following laboratory values were abnormal in cancer patients: hemoglobin, WBC count, platelet counts, gamma-glutamyltransferase, AST (SGOT), alkaline phosphatase, and total bilirubin.

Adverse reactions
● CNS: dizziness, light-headedness, insomnia, sleepiness, fatigue, malaise, headache, depression.
● CV: hypotension, chest pain.
● DERM: generalized pruritus, photosensitivity.
● EENT: nose and sinus drainage, epistaxis, pharyngitis, blurred vision, ocular rotation pain.
● GI: nausea, vomiting, diarrhea, constipation, dyspepsia, heartburn, anorexia, stomatitis, mucositis.
● Other: flulike syndrome, fever, chills, sweating, vasovagal reaction, myalgia, arthralgia, sore injection site, back pain, left groin lymph node swelling.

Overdose and treatment
No information available.

▶ Special considerations
● Interferon alfa-n3 has been used for many unlabeled indications: hairy cell leukemia, bladder tumors, carcinoid tumors, chronic myelogenous leukemia, cutaneous T-cell lymphoma, essential thrombocythemia, non-Hodgkin's lymphoma (low grade), cervical carcinoma, chronic lymphocytic leukemia, acute leukemias, osteosarcoma, Kaposi's sarcoma related to acquired

---

immunodeficiency syndrome, malignant gliomas, melanoma, multiple myeloma, nasopharyngeal sarcoma, ovarian carcinoma, renal carcinoma, cutaneous warts, cytomegaloviruses, herpes keratoconjunctivitis, herpes simplex, papillomaviruses, rhinoviruses, vaccinia virus, varicella zoster, viral hepatitis B, and chronic non-A, non-B hepatitis.

• Different brands of interferons may not be therapeutically interchangeable.

• Almost all patients experience flulike symptoms, which diminish with continued therapy.

• Genital warts usually begin to disappear after several weeks of therapy, but treatment should continue for the full 8 weeks. In patients who experience partial resolution during treatment, further resolution occurs after treatment ends. Of those patients who experienced complete resolution, half had complete resolution by the end of treatment; the rest within 3 months post-treatment.

• Do not administer further treatment for 3 months after first course of therapy unless warts enlarge or new warts appear.

• Flulike symptoms are relieved by acetaminophen.

• Interferon alfa-n3 is manufactured from pooled units of human leukocytes induced by incomplete infection with an avian virus. Donors are screened to minimize risk of human immunodeficiency virus (HIV) and hepatitis B. There are no reported incidents of HIV or hepatitis B transmission.

• Advise patient of risks and benefits of therapy.

• Store in refrigerator; do not freeze. *Do not shake.*

• Use 30G needle to administer.

Information for the patient
Tell patient to watch for signs of anaphylaxis – local or generalized hives, tightness of the chest, wheezing, and dizziness or weakness – and to call physician if they develop.

Pediatric use
Safety and efficacy have not been established.

Breast-feeding
It is unknown if drug is excreted in breast milk; the potential for serious adverse reactions in the infant must be considered.

---

interferon alfa-2a, recombinant
Roferon-A

interferon alfa-2b, recombinant
Intron A

• Pharmacologic classification: biological response modifier
• Therapeutic classification: antineoplastic
• Pregnancy risk category C

How supplied
Roferon-A
3 million IU/vial; 18 million IU/multiple-dose vial for injection; 36 million IU/vial for injection
Intron A
3 million IU/vial with diluent for injection; 5 million IU/vial with diluent for injection; 10 million IU/vial with diluent for injection; 25 million IU/vial with diluent for injection; 50 million IU/vial with diluent for injection

Indications, route, and dosage
Hairy cell leukemia
alfa-2a
Adults: For induction, give 3 million units S.C. or I.M. daily for 16 to 24 weeks. For maintenance, 3 million units S.C. or I.M. three times weekly.
alfa-2b
Adults: 2 million units/m² I.M. or S.C. three times weekly (for both induction and maintenance).
Condylomata acuminata
alfa-2b
Adults: 1 million units per lesion, intralesionally, three times a week for 3 weeks.
Kaposi's sarcoma
Adults: For alfa-2a – induction: 36 million IU S.C. or I.M. daily for 10 to 12 weeks; maintenance: 36 million IU three times weekly. For alfa-2b, 30 million IU/m² S.C. or I.M. three times weekly. Maintain this dose unless the disease progresses rapidly or intolerance occurs.
Chronic hepatitis C (non-A, non-B)
Adults: 3 million (alfa-2b) IU S.C. or I.M. three times weekly. If response occurs, continue therapy for 6 months. If no response by 16 weeks, discontinue therapy.

Pharmacodynamics
Antineoplastic action: Interferon alfa is a sterile protein product produced by recombinant DNA techniques applied to genetically engineered *Escherichia coli* bacteria. The interferons are naturally occurring small protein molecules produced and secreted by cells in response to viral infections or synthetic and biological inducers. Their exact mechanism of action is unknown but appears to involve direct antiproliferative action against tumor cells or viral cells to inhibit replication and modulation of host immune response by enhancing the phagocytic activity of macrophages and augmenting specific cytotoxicity of lymphocytes for target cells. To date, three major classes of interferons have been identified: alfa, beta, and gamma.

Pharmacokinetics
• *Absorption:* More than 80% of the dose is absorbed after I.M. or S.C. injection.
• *Distribution:* Not applicable.
• *Metabolism:* The drug appears to be metabolized in the liver and kidney.
• *Excretion:* The drug is reabsorbed from glomerular filtrate with minor biliary elimination.

Contraindications and precautions
Interferons are contraindicated in patients with hypersensitivity to them or to any components of the product.

Drugs should be used cautiously in patients with severe hepatic or renal function impairment, seizure disorders, compromised CNS function, cardiac disease, or myelosuppression because the drugs may worsen these conditions.

Interactions
When used concomitantly, interferons may enhance the CNS effects of CNS depressants.

Concurrent use with a live virus vaccine may potentiate replication of vaccine virus, increase adverse effects, and decrease patient's antibody response.

Bone marrow depressant effects may be increased

---

when used with blood dyscrasia-causing medications, bone marrow depressant therapy, or radiation therapy. Dosage reduction may be required. Interferon may substantially increase the half-life of methylxanthines (including theophylline and aminophylline), perhaps by interfering with the cytochrome P-450 drug metabolizing enzymes.

Effects on diagnostic tests

Interferon therapy may cause mild and transient alterations of blood pressure (hypotension is likely). Interferons may decrease hemoglobin, hematocrit, leukocyte counts, platelets, and neutrophils (dose-related; recovery occurs within several days or weeks after withdrawal of interferon). Interferons may increase prothrombin time and partial thromboplastin time (dose-related); ALT (SGPT), AST (SGOT), LDH, and alkaline phosphatase levels (dose-related; reversible on withdrawal of interferon); and serum calcium, serum phosphorus, and fasting blood glucose levels.

Adverse reactions

- CNS: dizziness, confusion, paresthesia, numbness, lethargy, depression, nervousness, difficulty in thinking or concentrating, trouble sleeping, sedation, apathy, anxiety, irritability, fatigue.
- CV: hypotension, chest pain, arrhythmias, palpitations, syncope, congestive heart failure, hypertension, edema.
- DERM: rash, dryness, pruritus, partial alopecia, urticaria.
- GI: anorexia, nausea, diarrhea, vomiting, abdominal fullness, taste alteration.
- GU: transient impotence.
- HEMA: leukemia, mild thrombocytopenia.
- Other: pharyngitis, sneezing, dry or inflamed oropharynx, flulike symptoms (fever, headache, chills, muscle aches).

Overdose and treatment

No information available.

▶ Special considerations

- When preparing antineoplastic agents for injection, take special precautions because of their potential for carcinogenicity and mutagenicity. Use of a biological containment cabinet is recommended. Do not shake vials.
- Subcutaneous administration route should be used in patients whose platelet count is below 50,000/mm³.
- Different brands of interferons may not be therapeutically interchangeable.
- Almost all patients experience flulike symptoms at the beginning of therapy. These effects tend to diminish with continued therapy.
- Patient should be well hydrated, especially during initial stages of treatment. Premedicate with acetaminophen to minimize flulike symptoms.
- Dosage reduction may be needed if headache persists. Hypotension may result from fluid depletion; may require supportive treatment.
- Administration at bedtime minimizes inconvenience of fatigue.
- Monitor blood pressure, BUN, hematocrit, platelet count, ALT (SGPT), AST (SGOT), LDH, alkaline phosphatase, serum bilirubin, creatinine, uric acid, total and differential leukocyte count, and ECG.
- Monitor for CNS adverse reactions, such as de-

creased mental status and dizziness. Periodic neuropsychiatric monitoring is recommended.
- Special precautions required for patients who develop thrombocytopenia: exercise extreme care in performing invasive procedures; inspect injection site and skin frequently for signs of bruising; limit frequency of I.M. injections; test urine, emesis fluid, stool, and secretions for occult blood.
- Patient should avoid use of aspirin and excessive use of alcohol because they may increase the risk of GI bleeding.
- When using interferon alfa-2b for condylomata acuminata by intralesional injection, use only the 10 million-unit vial reconstituted with 1 ml of diluent. Using other strengths or more diluent would produce a hypertonic solution. For administration, use a 25G to 30G needle and a tuberculin syringe. Up to five lesions may be treated simultaneously.
- The following indications are not included in U.S. labeling, but the drug may be used for these applications: chronic myelocytic leukemia; treatment of renal carcinoma; superficial bladder carcinoma; treatment of non-Hodgkin's lymphomas, especially nodular, poorly differentiated types; malignant melanoma; multiple myeloma; mycosis fungoides; papillomas; laryngeal papillomatosis (interferon alfa-2b).

Information for the patient

- Review patient instruction sheet if patient is to self-administer, to ensure patient understanding of when and how to take medication. Stress importance of drinking extra fluids to prevent hypotension from fluid loss.
- Instruct patient in proper oral hygiene during treatment, because the bone marrow depressant effects of interferon may result in increased incidence of microbial infection, delayed healing, and gingival bleeding. A decrease in salivary flow may also occur.
- Advise patient not to take a missed dose or to double the next dose, but to call for further instructions.
- If patient is to self-administer drug, teach patient to prepare injection, how to use disposable syringe, proper administration technique, and stability of drug.
- Store drug in refrigerator; keep from freezing.
- Caution patient against driving or performing tasks requiring alertness until response to medication is known.
- Advise patient to seek medical approval before taking nonprescription medications for colds, coughs, allergies, and similar disorders; explain that interferons commonly cause flulike symptoms and patient may need to take acetaminophen before each dose.
- Emphasize need to follow instructions about taking and recording temperature, and how and when to take acetaminophen; not to have any immunization; and to avoid contact with persons who have taken oral polio vaccine. Because the body's resistance may be compromised, infection may occur.
- Tell patient drug may cause temporary loss of some hair. Normal hair growth should return when drug is withdrawn.

Geriatric use

Neurotoxicity and cardiotoxicity are more common in elderly patients, especially those with underlying CNS or cardiac impairment.

Breast-feeding

Risk-to-benefit ratio must be considered. Drug is usually not recommended in breast-feeding women because of the potential for serious adverse effects on breast-fed infants.

interferon gamma 1-B
Actimmune

- Pharmacologic classification: biological response modifier
- Therapeutic classification: antineoplastic
- Pregnancy risk category C

How supplied
Available by prescription only
Injection: 100 mcg (3 million units)/0.5 ml in single-dose vials

Indications, route, and dosage
Treatment of chronic granulomatous disease
Adults with body surface area > 0.5 m²: 50 mcg/m² (1.5 milliunits/m²) S.C. three times weekly (usually Monday, Wednesday, and Friday).
Adults with body surface area ≤ 0.5 m²: 1.5 mcg/kg S.C. three times weekly (usually Monday, Wednesday, and Friday).

Pharmacodynamics
Antineoplastic action: Interferon gamma 1-B is a single-chain polypeptide containing 140 amino acids, produced by fermentation of genetically engineered *Escherichia coli*. It has potent phagocyte activity not seen with other interferons. The exact mechanism of action is unknown, but growing evidence suggests it interacts functionally with other interleukin molecules and all form part of a complex lymphokine network. A broad range of biological activities have been noted, including enhancement of oxidative metabolism of tissue macrophages, antibody-dependent cellular cytotoxicity, natural killer cell activity, and effects on Fc receptor expression on monocytes and major histocompatibility antigen expression. In chronic granulomatous disease, interferon gamma 1-B provides enhancement of phagocyte function, including elevation of superoxide levels and improved killing of *Staphylococcus aureus*.

Pharmacokinetics
- *Absorption:* About 90% is absorbed after S.C. injection. Peak plasma concentrations are reached after 7 hours; no accumulation is noted after 12 consecutive daily doses.
- *Distribution:* Unknown.
- *Metabolism:* Unknown.
- *Excretion:* Unknown. Elimination half-life is 5.9 hours.

Contraindications and precautions
Contraindicated in patients with known hypersensitivity to interferon gamma, *E. coli*-derived products, or any component of the formulation. Use with caution in patients with preexisting cardiac disease, including ischemia, CHF, or arrhythmia; with known seizure disorders or compromised CNS function; and with myelosuppression.

Adverse reactions
- CNS: headache, fatigue; rarely: confusion, disorientation, gait disturbances, transient ischemic attacks, parkinsonian symptoms, seizures, hallucinations.
- CV: rarely: hypotension, syncope, tachyarrhythmias, *heart block, heart failure, MI.*
- DERM: rash, injection site erythema and tenderness, pain; rarely: exacerbation of dermatomyositis.
- GI: nausea, vomiting, diarrhea, constipation, anorexia, weight loss; rarely: bleeding, pancreatitis, hepatic insufficiency.
- Respiratory: flulike symptoms; rarely: interstitial pneumonitis, *pulmonary embolism,* tachypnea, bronchospasm.
- Other: fever, chills, myalgia, arthralgia; rarely: hyponatremia, hyperglycemia, reversible renal insufficiency, deep venous thrombosis.

Overdose and treatment
No information available.

Interactions
Interferon gamma 1-B can decrease hepatic microsomal cytochrome P-450 concentrations, which could lead to decreased metabolism of drugs that use this metabolic degradation pathway.
   Use with caution in patients receiving myelosuppressive agents.

▶ Special considerations
- Optimum injection sites are the right and left deltoids and anterior thigh.
- Flulike symptoms may be minimized by administering at bedtime and may be treated with acetaminophen.
- If acute hypersensitivity reaction occurs, discontinue drug immediately and institute symptomatic and supportive treatment.
- Transient cutaneous rashes have not required discontinuation of therapy.
- If home use is appropriate, instruct patient, family, and caregiver on safe and effective use of drug. Help them review contents of patient information package insert.
- Store drug in refrigerator immediately; do not freeze. Avoid excessive or vigorous agitation. *Do not shake.* Unopened or unentered vials should not be left at room temperature longer than 12 hours before use. Do not return vials that exceed these limits to refrigerator; they should be discarded.
- Each vial is designed for single use only. Discard unused portions of vials.
- Do not use after the stated expiration date on vial.
- If severe adverse reactions occur, dose should be reduced by 50% or therapy discontinued until reaction subsides.

Information for the patient
- Thoroughly review the patient information package insert with patient.
- For home use, teach correct procedures for collection and disposal of medical waste.

Pediatric use
Safety and efficacy have not been established in children under age 18.

Breast-feeding
It is unknown if interferon gamma 1-B is excreted in breast milk. Because of the potential for serious ad-

verse reactions in infants, a decision must be made whether to continue breast-feeding.

invert sugar
Travert

- Pharmacologic classification: carbohydrate
- Therapeutic classification: nonelectrolyte fluid replacement, fluid volume expander, caloric agent
- Pregnancy risk category C

How supplied
Available by prescription only
Injection: 1,000 ml (5%, 10%); 500 ml (10%); also available with electrolytes

Indications, route, and dosage
Nonelectrolyte fluid replacement and caloric supplementation solution
Adults and children: Dosage depends on patient's age, weight, and clinical need. I.V. infusion rate should not exceed 1 g/kg/hour. Single liter of 5% invert sugar yields 375 calories.

Pharmacodynamics
Metabolic action: Invert sugar is an equimolar mixture of dextrose (glucose) and fructose (levulose); therefore, this caloric source shares the actions of dextrose and fructose. Each gram provides about 4 calories. Fructose augments dextrose utilization. Invert sugar is used as a nonelectrolyte fluid and caloric replacement.

Pharmacokinetics
- *Absorption:* Invert sugar is administered intravenously.
- *Distribution:* As a source of water for hydration, invert sugar expands plasma volume.
- *Metabolism:* Dextrose is metabolized to carbon dioxide and water; fructose is converted to glycogen more rapidly than is dextrose.
- *Excretion:* Depending on the patient's hydration status, invert sugar can produce diuresis.

Contraindications and precautions
Rapid infusion of invert sugar can cause lactic acidosis; glycosuria and hypoglycemia can result. Electrolyte and fluid imbalances can occur.

Interactions
Invert sugar is contraindicated in patients with hereditary invert sugar intolerance. Many drugs may be incompatible when mixed in I.V. solutions; consult appropriate tables or pharmacist before preparing admixtures.

Effects on diagnostic tests
Several laboratory values may change as a result of patient's hydration status.

Adverse reactions
- CNS: confusion.
- CV: increased pulse rate, precipitation or exacerbation of congestive heart failure (CHF) in susceptible patients, *pulmonary edema*, hypertension.

- GU: glycosuria, osmotic diuresis.
- Metabolic: hyperglycemia, hypoglycemia, metabolic acidosis, dehydration, hypervolemia, hyperosmolar coma.
- Local: pain and inflammation at injection site.

Overdose and treatment
Discontinue infusion. Insulin may treat hyperglycemia caused by glucose component; fructose metabolism is not insulin-dependent. Diuresis or other therapeutic measures may be appropriate.

▶ Special considerations
- Infusion rate must be carefully controlled.
- Infusion sites should be changed regularly to avoid irritation with prolonged therapy and should be checked frequently to avoid extravasation.
- Watch closely for signs of fluid overload, pulmonary edema, or CHF. Monitor blood pressure frequently.
- Monitor serum glucose levels closely. Prolonged therapy can deplete pancreatic insulin production and secretion. In patients with diabetes mellitus, invert sugar must be used cautiously.
- Never discontinue treatment abruptly. If necessary, have dextrose 10% available to prevent rebound hyperinsulinemia and subsequent hypoglycemia.
- Monitor intake, output, and weight closely, especially if renal function is impaired.
- Monitor vital signs to detect adverse effects.

Pediatric use
- Safety and efficacy of this solution have not been established in children under age 12.
- Use cautiously in infants of diabetic mothers, except as may be indicated in newborn infants who are hypoglycemic.
- Make sure rate does not exceed 1 g/kg/hour in infants.

iodinated glycerol
Iophen, Organidin

- Pharmacologic classification: organic iodine complex
- Therapeutic classification: expectorant
- Pregnancy risk category X

How supplied
Available by prescription only
Tablets: 30 mg
Elixir: 60 mg/5 ml
Solution: 50 mg/ml

Indications, route, and dosage
Sputum liquification in bronchial asthma, bronchitis, emphysema (adjunct)
Adults: 60 mg P.O. q.i.d. (tablets); or 20 drops (solution) P.O. q.i.d. with fluids; or 5 ml (elixir) P.O. q.i.d.
Children: Up to half the adult dose based on child's weight.

Pharmacodynamics
Expectorant action: The exact mechanism of action is unknown; it is believed that iodinated glycerol reduces the viscosity of mucous secretions by increasing respiratory tract secretions.

Pharmacokinetics
● *Absorption:* Iodinated glycerol is absorbed from the GI tract.
● *Distribution:* Iodinated glycerol concentrates primarily in the respiratory tract and accumulates in the thyroid gland.
● *Metabolism:* Unknown.
● *Excretion:* Iodinated glycerol is excreted primarily in urine.

Contraindications and precautions
Iodinated glycerol is contraindicated in patients hypersensitive to iodides or iodine, in pregnant or nursing women, and in neonates because of potential for goitrogenic effects. Drug should be used with caution in children with cystic fibrosis because they are especially susceptible to the goitrogenic effects of iodides; in patients with thyroid disease, because of the hazard of hypothyroidism occurring with long-term use; drug also may induce goiter in iodide-sensitive hyperthyroid patients.

Interactions
Lithium potentiates hypothyroid and goitrogenic effects of iodinated glycerol. Concurrent administration with potassium-sparing diuretics and other potassium-containing drugs may cause hyperkalemia, arrhythmias, or cardiac arrest.

Effects on diagnostic tests
Long-term use of iodinated glycerol may alter the results of thyroid function tests; such alterations have not been reported with usual recommended dosage.

Adverse reactions
After long-term use:
● DERM: cutaneous and mucosal eruptions and hemorrhages.
● EENT: coryza, eye irritation, swollen eyelids, burning in nose and throat.
● Endocrine: thyroid enlargement, hypothyroidism.
● GI: nausea, gastrointestinal distress.
● Other: acute parotitis, upper respiratory inflammation, headache.
  Note: Drug should be discontinued if skin hypersensitivity or other evidence of hypersensitivity occurs.

Overdose and treatment
There have been no reports of acute overdose with iodinated glycerol. Iodism (chronic iodine poisoning) may occur after prolonged use. Symptoms include metallic taste, sore mouth, swollen eyelids, sneezing, skin eruptions, nausea, vomiting, epigastric pain, and diarrhea. Discontinue drug and treat supportively.

▶ Special considerations
● Give drug with a glass of water to help thin and loosen mucus in lungs.
● Monitor cough type and frequency, and encourage deep-breathing exercises.

Information for the patient
● Tell patient to mix oral solution in water or other liquid and drink all of liquid to get full dose.
● Tell patient to take tablets with full glass of water.
● Advise patient to use sugarless throat lozenges to decrease throat irritation and associated cough and to call if cough persists longer than 7 days.

● Recommend humidifier to filter out dust, smoke, and air pollutants.

Pediatric use
Drug is not recommended for neonates. Enlarged thyroid gland or goiter is more common in children with cystic fibrosis.

Breast-feeding
Safety in breast-feeding has not been established. An alternative feeding method is recommended during therapy.

---

iodoquinol (diiodohydroxyquin)
Amebaquin, Moebiquin, Yodoxin

● Pharmacologic classification: iodinated 8-hydroxyquinoline
● Therapeutic classification: amebicide
● Pregnancy risk category C

How supplied
Available by prescription only
Tablets: 210 mg, 650 mg
Powder: 25 g

Indications, route, and dosage
Intestinal amebiasis
Adults: 630 to 650 mg P.O. t.i.d. for 20 days. Total daily dosage should not exceed 2 g.
Children: Usual dosage is 30 to 40 mg/kg of body weight daily in two or three divided doses for 20 days.
  Frequently, iodoquinol is combined with metronidazole (750 mg P.O. q.i.d. for 5 to 10 days) for mild to moderate intestinal disease; and several other agents for invasive disease. It is useful only against the encysted form of the parasite, hence its use as a sole agent is limited to mild cases or asymptomatic carriers.
  Additional courses of iodoquinol therapy should not be repeated before a resting interval of 2 to 3 weeks.

Pharmacodynamics
Amebicidal action: Iodoquinol is amebicidal against protozoa, especially *Entamoeba histolytica.* It acts primarily in the intestinal lumen by an unknown mechanism.

Pharmacokinetics
● *Absorption:* About 8% of an oral dose is absorbed.
● *Distribution:* Unknown.
● *Metabolism:* Most of the absorbed dose appears to be glucuronidated or sulfated in the liver.
● *Excretion:* Glucuronide and sulfate conjugates of the drug are excreted in urine; parent drug is primarily excreted unchanged in feces. It is unknown if iodoquinol is excreted in breast milk.

Contraindications and precautions
Iodoquinol is contraindicated in patients with known hypersensitivity to 8-hydroxyquinolines or iodine-containing preparations because it contains iodine. It also is contraindicated in patients with hepatic or renal disease or optic neuropathy because it may exacerbate these conditions.
  Because of its iodine content, iodoquinol should be used with caution in patients with thyroid disease.

Long-term therapy is not recommended because of the potential hazard of visual and nerve damage.

Interactions
None reported.

Effects on diagnostic tests
Iodoquinol may increase protein-bound iodine levels and therefore interfere with thyroid function tests for up to 6 months after discontinuation of therapy.

Adverse reactions
● CNS: neurotoxicity, dysesthesia, weakness, vertigo, malaise, headache, agitation, retrograde amnesia, ataxia, *peripheral neuropathy.*
● DERM: pruritus, hives, papular and pustular eruptions, urticaria, discoloration of hair and nails.
● EENT: *optic neuritis,* optic atrophy, loss of vision.
● GI: anorexia, nausea, vomiting, abdominal cramps, diarrhea, increased motility, constipation, epigastric burning and pain, gastritis, anal irritation and itching.
● HEMA: *agranulocytosis.*
● Other: thyroid enlargement, fever, chills, generalized furunculosis, hair loss, muscle pain.
  Note: Drug should be discontinued if signs of hypersensitivity or toxicity occur.

Overdose and treatment
Overdose with iodoquinol may affect cardiovascular and respiratory function. Treatment is largely supportive. After recent ingestion (within 4 hours), empty stomach by induced emesis or gastric lavage. Follow with activated charcoal to decrease absorption. Saline or osmotic cathartics may also be helpful.

▶ Special considerations
● Patients should have periodic ophthalmologic examinations during therapy to detect optic neuropathy.
● Schedule dose after meals; tablets should be crushed and mixed with applesauce or chocolate syrup to facilitate swallowing.
● Monitor intake and output and renal function.
● Send fecal specimens to laboratory promptly; infection is detectable only in warm specimens.
● Monitor for diarrhea during first 3 days of therapy; if diarrhea continues beyond 3 days, consider alternate therapy.
● Monitor serum electrolyte levels and blood counts; replace fluids and electrolytes as necessary.
● Patient may be discharged when three consecutive daily stool specimens are normal.

Information for the patient
● Advise patient not to discontinue drug prematurely.
● Tell patient to report skin rash.
● Instruct patient about importance of follow-up appointments.
● Tell patient that stool specimens will be checked at 1, 3, and 6 months to ensure elimination of amebae.
● To help prevent reinfection, instruct patient and family members in proper hygiene, including disposal of feces and hand washing after defecation and before eating, and about the risks of eating raw foods and the control of contamination by flies.
● Advise use of liquid soap or reserved bar of soap to prevent cross contamination.
● Advise patient not to prepare, process, or handle food during treatment. Isolation of patient is unnecessary.

● Encourage other household members and suspected contacts to be tested and, if necessary, treated.

Breast-feeding
Safety has not been established.

---

ipecac syrup

● Pharmacologic classification: alkaloid emetic
● Therapeutic classification: emetic
● Pregnancy risk category C

How supplied
Available by prescription and without prescription
Syrup: 70 mg powdered ipecac/ml

Indications, route, and dosage
To induce vomiting in poisoning
Adults: 15 to 30 ml P.O., followed by 200 to 300 ml of water.
Children age 1 or older: 15 ml P.O., followed by about 200 ml of water or milk.
Children under age 1: 5 to 10 ml P.O., followed by 100 to 200 ml of water or milk.
  May repeat dose once after 20 minutes, if necessary.

Pharmacodynamics
Emetic action: Ipecac syrup directly irritates the GI mucosa and directly stimulates the chemoreceptor trigger zone through the effects of emetine and cephalin, its two alkaloids.

Pharmacokinetics
● *Absorption:* Ipecac syrup is absorbed in significant amounts mainly when it does not produce emesis. Onset of action usually occurs in 20 minutes.
● *Distribution:* Unknown.
● *Metabolism:* Unknown.
● *Excretion:* Emetine is excreted in urine slowly, over a period lasting up to 60 days. Duration of effect is 20 to 25 minutes.

Contraindications and precautions
Ipecac syrup is contraindicated in patients with poisoning caused by alkalis or corrosive agents because of hazard of further esophageal or mediastinal injury; in patients with poisoning from petroleum distillates; in patients who are semiconscious, unconscious, comatose, or in shock; and in patients with seizures, severe inebriation, depressed gag reflexes, or strychnine poisoning, because of hazards of aspiration: pneumonitis, bronchospasm, or pulmonary edema. Do not use in patients with heart disease because ipecac is potentially cardiotoxic.

Interactions
Activated charcoal may inactivate ipecac syrup; concomitant use with antiemetics or milk (or milk products) may decrease ipecac syrup's therapeutic effectiveness. Concomitant use with carbonated beverages may cause abdominal distention.

Effects on diagnostic tests
None reported.

Adverse reactions
● CNS: depression.
● CV: *cardiac arrhythmias, bradycardia, hypotension, atrial fibrillation,* or *fatal myocarditis* if drug is absorbed (for example, if patient doesn't vomit within 30 minutes) or after ingestion of excessive doses.
● GI: diarrhea.
   Note: Drug should be discontinued if emesis does not occur after second dose.

Overdose and treatment
Clinical effects of overdose include diarrhea, persistent nausea or vomiting (longer than 30 minutes), stomach cramps or pain, cardiac arrhythmias, hypotension, myocarditis, difficulty breathing, and unusual fatigue or weakness.
   Toxicity from chronic ipecac overdosage usually involves use of the concentrated fluid extract in dosage appropriate for the syrup. Clinical effects of cardiotoxicity include tachycardia, T-wave depression, atrial fibrillation, depressed myocardial contractility, congestive heart failure, and myocarditis. Other toxic effects include bloody stools and vomitus, hypotension, shock, seizures, and coma. Heart failure is the usual cause of death.
   Treatment requires discontinuation of the drug followed by symptomatic and supportive care, which may include digitalis and pacemaker therapy to treat cardiotoxic effects. However, no antidote exists for the cardiotoxic effects of ipecac, which may be fatal despite intensive treatment.

▶ Special considerations
● Administer ipecac syrup *before* giving activated charcoal, not after. Follow dose with 1 or 2 glasses of water. If vomiting does not occur after second dose, give activated charcoal to adsorb both ipecac syrup and ingested poison. Follow with gastric lavage.
● Inspect emesis for ingested substances, such as tablets or capsules.
● Ipecac syrup usually empties the stomach completely within 30 minutes (in over 90% of patients); average emptying time is 20 minutes.
● Be careful not to confuse ipecac syrup with ipecac fluid extract, which is rarely used but 14 times more potent. Never store these two drugs together – the wrong drug could cause death.
● In antiemetic toxicity, ipecac syrup is usually effective if less than 1 hour has passed since ingestion of antiemetic.
● Little if any systemic toxicity occurs with doses of 30 ml or less.
● Drug may be abused by patients with eating disorders (such as bulimia or anorexia nervosa).
● Ipecac syrup also may be used in small amounts as an expectorant in cough preparations; however, this use has doubtful therapeutic benefit.

Information for the patient
● Advise patient to get medical attention immediately when poisoning is suspected.
● Caution patient to call poison information center before taking ipecac syrup.
● Warn patient to avoid drinking milk or carbonated beverages with ipecac syrup because they may decrease drug's effectiveness; instead, instruct patient to take syrup with 1 or 2 glasses of water.
● Advise patient to take activated charcoal only after vomiting has stopped.

Pediatric use
Advise parents to keep ipecac syrup at home at all times but to keep it out of children's reach.

Breast-feeding
Hazard to breast-feeding infants has not been established; possible risks must be weighed against drug's benefits.

---

ipratropium bromide
Atrovent

● Pharmacologic classification: anticholinergic
● Therapeutic classification: bronchodilator
● Pregnancy risk category B

How supplied
Available by prescription only
Inhaler: Each metered dose supplies 18 mcg

Indications, route, and dosage
Bronchospasm in chronic bronchitis and emphysema
Adults: The usual dose is 1 or 2 inhalations (36 mcg) t.i.d. or q.i.d. Patients may take additional inhalations as needed, but should not exceed 12 inhalations in 24 hours.

Pharmacodynamics
Anticholinergic action: Ipratropium appears to inhibit vagally mediated reflexes by antagonizing the action of acetylcholine. Anticholinergics prevent the increases in intracellular concentration of cyclic guanosine monophosphate (cyclic GMP) that result from interaction of acetylcholine with the muscarinic receptor on bronchial smooth muscle.
   The bronchodilation following inhalation is primarily a local, site-specific effect, not a systemic one.

Pharmacokinetics
● *Absorption:* Ipratropium is not readily absorbed into the systemic circulation either from the surface of the lung or from the GI tract as confirmed by blood levels and renal excretion studies. Much of an inhaled dose is swallowed as shown by fecal excretion studies.
● *Distribution:* Not applicable.
● *Metabolism:* Hepatic; elimination half-life is about 2 hours.
● *Excretion:* Most of an administered dose is excreted unchanged in feces. Absorbed drug is excreted in urine and bile.

Contraindications and precautions
Ipratropium is contraindicated in patients allergic to atropine or its derivatives.
   Use cautiously in patients with narrow-angle glaucoma, prostatic hypertrophy, or bladder neck obstruction, because anticholinergics can worsen the symptoms associated with these disorders.
   Warning: Ipratropium is not indicated for the initial treatment of acute episodes of bronchospasm where rapid response is required.

Interactions
Concurrent use of ipratropium with antimuscarinic agents, including ophthalmic preparations, may produce additive effects. Increased risk of fluorocarbon toxicity may result from too-closely timed administration of ipratropium and other fluorocarbon propellant-containing oral inhalants such as glucocorticoids, adrenocorticoids, sympathomimetics, or cromolyn. A 5-minute interval between such agents is recommended.

Effects on diagnostic tests
None reported.

Adverse reactions
- CNS: nervousness, dizziness, headache, insomnia, fatigue.
- CV: palpitations.
- DERM: rash.
- EENT: blurred vision, dry mouth, mouth sores, irritation from aerosol, cough, hoarseness.
- GI: nausea, GI distress.
- GU: urinary difficulty.
- Other: cough, exacerbation of symptoms.

Overdose and treatment
Acute overdosage by inhalation is unlikely because ipratropium is not well-absorbed systemically after aerosol or oral administration.

▶ Special considerations
- Because of delayed onset of bronchodilation, ipratropium is not recommended to treat acute respiratory distress.
- Prolonged use of ipratropium inhalation may inhibit salivation and thereby promote dental caries, periodontal disease, and mouth pain. Patient should consult with dentist for special monitoring and preventive measures.

Information for the patient
- Tell patient to shake the drug well before using.
- Instruct patient to store drug away from heat and direct sunlight, and to protect it from freezing.
- Tell patient that temporary blurred vision may result if aerosol is sprayed into eyes.
- Advise patient to allow 1 minute between inhalations.
- Instruct patient to take a missed dose as soon as possible – unless it is almost time for the next scheduled dose, in which case he should skip the missed dose. Warn him to never double-dose.
- Suggest sugarless hard candy, gum, ice, or saliva substitute to relieve dry mouth. Tell patient to report dry mouth if it persists longer than 2 weeks.
- Instruct patient to call if he experiences no benefits within 30 minutes after administration, or if condition worsens.

Pediatric use
Safety and efficacy of use in children younger than age 12 have not been established.

Breast-feeding
It is not known whether this drug is excreted in breast milk. Although lipid-insoluble quaternary bases pass into breast milk, ipratropium is unlikely to reach the infant, especially when taken by aerosol. However, use caution when administering to breast-feeding women.

iron, oral supplements

ferrous fumarate
ferrous gluconate
ferrous sulfate

Iron has been used for medicinal purposes for centuries; an essential mineral, iron is a component of hemoglobin, myoglobin, and a number of enzymes needed for energy transfer. Most individuals ingest and absorb an adequate amount of iron per day from dietary sources.

Pharmacology
Iron is an essential component of hemoglobin. It is needed in adequate amounts for erythropoiesis and for efficient oxygen transport in the blood. Symptoms of iron deficiency that can be reversed with iron therapy include dysphagia, lip lesions, sore tongue, and skin lesions.

Clinical indications and actions
Iron-deficiency anemia
Oral iron supplements are indicated for the prevention and treatment of iron-deficiency anemias. Oral iron is available in various salts, providing different amounts of elemental iron: Ferrous fumarate provides 33% of elemental iron; ferrous gluconate provides 11.6% of elemental iron; ferrous sulfate provides 20%; the sulfate, exsiccated, provides 30% (approximate).

Overview of adverse reactions
Iron is corrosive, and GI intolerance is a common problem (5% to 20%) with ingestion of oral iron salts. Symptoms include nausea, vomiting, anorexia, constipation, and dark stools; liquid preparations may stain teeth.

▶ Special considerations
- Dilute liquid preparations in juice (preferably orange juice, which promotes absorption of iron) or water, but not in milk or antacids. Administer antacids 1 hour before or 2 hours after iron product, if possible, to prevent interference with absorption. To avoid staining teeth, give liquid preparations through a straw.
- Tablets or capsules should not be crushed; if patient has trouble swallowing, liquid form can be used.
- GI upset is dose-related, based on amount of elemental iron; between-meal dosage is preferred, but may increase GI intolerance.
- Food decreases absorption by 33% to 50%. Enteric-coated formulas and some sustained-release formulas may also decrease absorption significantly, because they transport iron past primary site of absorption.
- Monitor effect on bowel function.
- Oral iron may turn stools black. This is unabsorbed iron and is harmless unless there are signs of GI bleeding.
- Monitor hemoglobin and reticulocyte counts during therapy.

Information for the patient
- Explain rationale for therapy; teach possible adverse effects, and emphasize importance of reporting diarrhea or constipation for adjustment in dose, diet, or further work-up. Patient may need iron for 2 to 4 months after anemia resolves; encourage compliance.

- Advise patient to continue regular dosage schedule if he misses a dose and not to take double doses.
- Advise dilution of liquid dosage form in juice (preferably orange) or water, not milk or antacids, and drinking through a straw to avoid staining teeth.
- Explain toxicity of iron, and emphasize importance of keeping iron preparations away from children, because of hazard of iron poisoning.
- Teach patient dietary measures to help prevent constipation.
- Tell patient that oral iron may turn stools black; this is unabsorbed iron and is harmless.

Geriatric use
Iron-induced constipation is common in elderly patients; stress proper diet to minimize this adverse effect. Elderly patients may need higher doses, because reduced gastric secretions and achlorhydria may lower capacity for iron absorption.

Pediatric use
Caution parents about the potential lethal effects of iron overdose. Liquid preparations may stain the teeth.

Breast-feeding
Iron supplements are often recommended for breast-feeding women; no adverse effects have been documented.

Representative combinations
None.

---

iron dextran
Imferon, InFeD

- Pharmacologic classification: parenteral iron supplement
- Therapeutic classification: hematinic
- Pregnancy risk category C

How supplied
Available by prescription only
Injection: 50 mg elemental iron/ml

Indications, route, and dosage
Iron-deficiency anemia
Adults and children: Dosage is highly individualized and is based on the patient's weight and hemoglobin level. Drug is usually given I.M.; preservative-free solution can be given I.V.

Pharmacodynamics
Hematinic action: Iron dextran is a complex of ferric hydroxide and dextran in a colloidal solution. After I.M. injection, 10% to 50% remains in the muscle for several months; remainder enters bloodstream, increasing plasma iron concentration for up to 2 weeks. Iron is an essential component of hemoglobin.

Pharmacokinetics
- *Absorption:* I.M. doses are absorbed in two stages: 60% after 3 days, and up to 90% by 3 weeks. Remainder is absorbed over several months or longer.
- *Distribution:* During first 3 days, local inflammation facilitates passage of drug into the lymphatic system;

drug is then ingested by macrophages, which enter lymph and blood.
- *Metabolism:* After I.M. or I.V. administration, iron dextran is cleared from plasma by reticuloendothelial cells of the liver, spleen, and bone marrow.
- *Excretion:* In doses of 500 mg or less, half-life is 6 hours. Traces are excreted in breast milk, urine, bile, and feces. Drug cannot be removed by hemodialysis.

Contraindications and precautions
Iron dextran is contraindicated in patients with known hypersensitivity to any of the components and in patients with any anemia other than iron-deficiency anemia.

Administer iron dextran cautiously to patients with rheumatoid arthritis, because I.V. injections may exacerbate joint pain and swelling; and to patients with a significant history of allergies or asthma. Administer with extreme caution to patients with serious hepatic impairment because of potential for additional liver damage. *Do not administer simultaneously with oral iron.*

Interactions
None significant.

Effects on diagnostic tests
Large doses (over 100 mg iron) may color the serum brown.

Iron dextran may cause false elevations of serum bilirubin level and false reductions in serum calcium level.

Iron dextran prevents meaningful measurement of serum iron concentration and total iron binding capacity for up to 3 weeks; I.M. injection may cause dense areas of activity on bone scans using technetium 99m diphosphonate, for 1 to 6 days.

Adverse reactions
- CNS: headache, shivering, transitory paresthesia, arthralgia, myalgia, dizziness, malaise, syncope.
- CV: hypotensive reaction, peripheral vascular flushing (with overly rapid I.V. administration), tachycardia, precordial pain, *fatal arrhythmia.*
- DERM: rash, urticaria.
- GI: nausea, vomiting, metallic taste, transient loss of taste.
- GU: hematuria.
- Local: skin discoloration, soreness, inflammation, and sterile abscess at I.M. injection site; phlebitis at I.V. injection site.
- Other: *bronchospasm; anaphylaxis;* hemosiderosis; regional lymphadenopathy; I.V. administration may reactivate or exacerbate rheumatoid arthritis or ankylosing spondylitis.

Overdose and treatment
Injected iron has much greater bioavailability than oral iron, but data on acute overdose is limited.

▶ Special considerations
- Discontinue oral iron before giving iron dextran.
- Use 10-ml multi-dose vial only for I.M. injections, because it contains phenol as a preservative; use only 2- or 5-ml ampule without preservative for I.V. administration.
- Administer test dose of 0.5 ml iron dextrose I.M. or I.V. Be alert for anaphylaxis on test dose; monitor vital signs for drug reaction. Keep epinephrine (0.5 ml of a

---

1:1,000 solution) readily available for such an emergency.

● Inject I.M. preparation deeply into upper outer quadrant of buttocks (never an arm or other exposed area) using a 2- to 3-inch (5- to 8-cm), 19-gauge or 20-gauge needle. Use Z-track technique to avoid leakage into subcutaneous tissue and skin stains, and minimize staining by using a separate needle to withdraw drug from its container.

● I.V. use is controversial, and some hospitals do not allow it.

● Give drug I.V. if patient has insufficient muscle mass for deep injection, impaired absorption from muscle because of stasis or edema, a risk of uncontrolled I.M. bleeding from trauma (as in hemophilia), or need for massive and prolonged parenteral therapy (as in chronic substantial blood loss). Do not administer more than 50 mg of iron/minute (1 ml/minute) if using drug undiluted.

● After I.V. iron dextran administration, flush vein with 10 ml normal saline injection to minimize local irritation. Have patient rest for 15 to 30 minutes, since orthostatic hypotension may occur.

● Monitor hemoglobin, hematocrit, and reticulocyte count during therapy. An increase of about 1 g/dl/week in hemoglobin is usual.

Information for the patient
Warn patient of possibility of skin staining with I.M. injections.

Breast-feeding Traces of unmetabolized iron dextran are excreted in breast milk; impact on neonate is unknown.

---

isocarboxazid
Marplan

● Pharmacologic classification: monoamine oxidase inhibitor
● Therapeutic classification: antidepressant
● Pregnancy risk category C

How supplied
Available by prescription only
Tablets: 10 mg

Indications, route, and dosage
Severe depression unresponsive to other antidepressants or electroconvulsive therapy
Adults: 10 mg P.O. t.i.d.; reduce to 10 to 20 mg daily in divided doses when condition improves.

Pharmacodynamics
Antidepressant action: Depression is thought to result from low CNS concentrations of neurotransmitters, including norepinephrine and serotonin. Isocarboxazid inhibits monoamine oxidase (MAO), an enzyme that normally inactivates amine-containing substances, thus increasing the concentration and activity of these agents.

Pharmacokinetics
● *Absorption:* Isocarboxazid is absorbed rapidly and completely from the GI tract.
● *Distribution:* Not yet determined; dosage adjustments

are determined by therapeutic response and adverse reaction profile.
● *Metabolism:* Hepatic.
● *Excretion:* Isocarboxazid is excreted primarily in urine within 24 hours; some is excreted in feces via the biliary tract. Half-life is 2½ hours (relatively short), but enzyme inhibition is prolonged and unrelated to half-life.

Contraindications and precautions
Isocarboxazid is contraindicated in patients with uncontrolled hypertension and seizure disorders because the drug may precipitate hypertensive reactions and lower the seizure threshold.

Isocarboxazid should be used cautiously in patients with angina pectoris or other cardiovascular diseases, Type I and Type II diabetes, Parkinson's disease and other motor disorders, hyperthyroidism, pheochromocytoma, renal or hepatic insufficiency, and bipolar disease (reduce dosage during manic phase).

Interactions
Isocarboxazid enhances pressor effects of amphetamines, ephedrine, phenylephrine, phenylpropanolamine, and related drugs and may result in serious cardiovascular toxicity; most nonprescription cold, hay fever, and weight-reduction products contain these drugs.

Concomitant use of isocarboxazid with disulfiram may cause tachycardia, flushing, or palpitations. Concomitant use with general or spinal anesthetics, which are normally metabolized by MAO, may cause severe hypotension and excessive CNS depression; isocarboxazid should be discontinued for at least 1 week before using these agents. Isocarboxazid decreases effectiveness of local anesthetics (procaine, lidocaine, and so on), resulting in poor nerve block. Use cautiously and in reduced dosage with alcohol, barbiturates and other sedatives, narcotics, dextromethorphan, and tricyclic antidepressants. Cocaine and vasoconstrictors in local anesthetics may precipitate a hypertensive response.

Effects on diagnostic tests
Isocarboxazid therapy elevates liver function test results and urinary catecholamine levels.

Adverse reactions
● CNS: dizziness, vertigo, weakness, headache, overactivity, hyperreflexia, tremor, muscle twitching, mania, insomnia, confusion, memory impairment, fatigue, agitation, nervousness, altered libido.
● CV: orthostatic hypotension, arrhythmias, *paradoxical hypertension*, palpitations, tachycardia, *fatal intracranial hemorrhage during hypertensive crisis.*
● EENT: blurred vision.
● GI: dry mouth, anorexia, nausea, diarrhea, constipation, abdominal pain.
● GU: urine retention, dysuria, discolored urine.
● Hepatic: jaundice.
● Other: peripheral edema, sweating, weight changes, hypersensitivity (rash).
Note: Drug should be discontinued if signs of hypersensitivity occur; if rash or jaundice occurs; or if severe headache, palpitations, or fainting spells occur, indicating impending hypertensive crisis.

Overdose and treatment
Signs of overdose include exacerbations of adverse reactions or exaggerated responses to normal phar-

---

macologic activity; such symptoms become apparent slowly (in 24 to 48 hours) and may persist up to 2 weeks. Agitation, flushing, tachycardia, hypotension, hypertension, palpitations, motor activity, twitching, increased deep tendon reflexes, seizures, hyperpyrexia, cardiorespiratory arrest, and coma may occur.

Treat symptomatically and supportively: give 5 to 10 mg phentolamine I.V. push for hypertensive crisis; treat seizures, agitation, or tremors with I.V. diazepam; tachycardia with beta blockers; and fever with cooling blankets. Monitor vital signs and fluid and electrolyte balance. Use of sympathomimetics (such as norepinephrine and phenylephrine) is contraindicated in hypotension caused by MAO inhibitors.

▶ **Special considerations**
Besides those relevant to all *MAO inhibitors,* consider the following recommendations.
● Recommended only when tricyclic antidepressant or electroconvulsive therapy is ineffective or contraindicated.
● Watch for suicidal tendencies.
● Do not withdraw drug abruptly.
● Weigh patient biweekly; check for edema and urine retention.
● Have phentolamine (Regitine) available to counteract severe hypertension.
● Continue precautions 10 days after stopping drug, because of long-lasting effects.
● Expect time lag of 1 to 4 weeks before noticeable effect.
● Obtain baseline blood pressure readings, complete blood count, and liver function test results before beginning therapy, and continue to monitor throughout treatment.

Information for the patient
● Warn patient to avoid foods high in tyramine or tryptophan (aged hard cheese, Chianti wine, beer, hard liquor aged in wooden casks [such as whiskey], avocados, chicken livers, chocolate, bananas, soy sauce, meat tenderizers, salami, bologna, preserved meats), large amounts of caffeine, and self-medication with nonprescription drugs, especially cold, hay fever, or diet preparations.
● Warn patient about dizziness. Tell patient to get out of bed slowly, sitting up first for 1 minute.

Geriatric use
Isocarboxazid is contraindicated in elderly or debilitated patients.

Pediatric use
Isocarboxazid is not recommended for children under age 16.

Breast-feeding
Isocarboxazid may be excreted in breast milk. Use with caution in breast-feeding women.

isoetharine hydrochloride
Arm-a-Med, Beta-2, Bisorine, Bronkosol, Dey-Dose, Dey-Lute, Dispos-a-Med

isoetharine mesylate
Bronkometer

● Pharmacologic classification: adrenergic
● Therapeutic classification: bronchodilator
● Pregnancy risk category C

How supplied
Available by prescription only
Nebulizer inhaler: 0.062%, 0.08%, 0.1%, 0.125%, 0.14%, 0.167%, 0.17%, 0.2%, 0.25%, 0.5%, 1% solution
Aerosol inhaler: 340 mcg/metered spray

Indications, route, and dosage
Bronchial asthma and reversible bronchospasm that may occur with bronchitis and emphysema
Isoetharine hydrochloride
Adults: Administered by oxygen aerosolization, 0.5 to 1 ml of a 0.5% or 0.5 ml (range 0.25 to 0.5 ml) of a 1% solution diluted 1:3; or undiluted, 4 ml (range 2 to 4 ml) of a 0.125% solution, 2.5 ml of a 0.2% solution, or 2 ml of a 0.25% solution. Administered by IPPB solution, 0.5 to 1 ml of a 0.5% solution, or 0.5 ml (range 0.25 to 1 ml) of a 1% solution diluted 1:3; or undiluted 4 ml (range 2 to 4 ml) of a 0.125% solution, 2.5 ml of a 0.2% solution, or 2 ml of a 0.25% solution. Administered by hand-nebulizer, four inhalations (range 3 to 7 inhalations) of undiluted 0.5% or 1% solution.
Isoetharine mesylate
Adults: Administered by metered aerosol, one to two inhalations. Occasionally, more may be required.

Pharmacodynamics
Bronchodilating action: Isoetharine relaxes bronchial smooth muscle by direct action on beta$_2$-adrenergic receptors, resulting in relief of bronchospasm, increased vital capacity, and decreased airway resistance. It may also inhibit release of histamine. Isoetharine also relaxes the smooth muscles of the peripheral vasculature.

Pharmacokinetics
● *Absorption:* Isoetharine is absorbed rapidly from the respiratory tract after oral inhalation. Bronchodilation occurs immediately, peaks in 5 to 15 minutes, and persists 1 to 4 hours.
● *Distribution:* Isoetharine is distributed widely throughout the body.
● *Metabolism:* Isoetharine is metabolized in lungs, liver, GI tract, and other tissues.
● *Excretion:* Isoetharine is excreted in urine as unchanged drug and metabolites.

Contraindications and precautions
Isoetharine is contraindicated in patients with known hypersensitivity to the drug or to any ingredients in the formulation.

Administer cautiously to patients with hyperthyroidism, hypertension, acute coronary disease, angina, cardiac asthma, limited cardiac reserve, and cerebral arteriosclerosis, because the drug may worsen these conditions; and to patients with sulfite sensitivity, because some formulations contain sulfite preservatives.

Interactions
Concomitant use with epinephrine or other sympathomimetics may produce additive adverse cardiovascular effects. Beta-adrenergic blocking agents (such as propranolol) antagonize isoetharine's bronchodilating, cardiac, and vasodilating effects.

Effects on diagnostic tests
None reported.

Adverse reactions
● CNS: tremor, weakness, headache, anxiety, tension, restlessness, insomnia, dizziness, excitement.
● CV: increased heart rate, palpitations, *hypotension* or *hypertension*, angina.
● GI: nausea, vomiting.
● Other: cough, bronchial irritation, edema, paradoxical *bronchoconstriction*.
   Note: Drug should be discontinued if patient develops hypersensitivity to drug or sulfite preservatives, bronchoconstriction, or tachyphylaxis.

Overdose and treatment
Clinical manifestations of overdose include exaggeration of common adverse reactions, particularly nausea and vomiting, cardiac arrhythmias, hypertension, and extreme tremors.
   Treatment includes symptomatic and supportive measures. Monitor vital signs closely. Sedatives may be used to treat restlessness. Cardioselective beta blockers (like metoprolol) may be used to treat arrhythmias, but with caution (may induce asthmatic attack).

▶ **Special considerations**
Besides those relevant to all *adrenergic bronchodilators*, consider the following recommendations.
● Tolerance may develop after prolonged or excessive use.
● Therapy should be administered on arising in morning and before meals to reduce fatigue from activity by improving lung ventilation.
● Paradoxical airway resistance (sudden worsening of dyspnea) may follow repeated excessive use. If this occurs, patient or family should discontinue isoetharine and call for alternative therapy (such as epinephrine).
● Alternating therapy with isoetharine inhalation and epinephrine may be helpful. However, these drugs should not be administered simultaneously because of danger of excessive cardiac stimulation.
● Protect solutions from light, freezing, and heat. Store at controlled room temperature.

Information for the patient
● Instruct patient in correct use of inhaler.
● Tell patient to use only as directed, to take no more than two inhalations at one time with 1- to 2-minute intervals between, and to save applicator; refills may be available.
● Instruct patient to wait 1 full minute after initial one to two inhalations (Bronkometer) before inhaling another dose. Action should begin immediately and peak within 5 to 15 minutes.
● Warn patient to keep spray away from eyes.
● Urge patient to use inhalation therapy as prescribed.

If symptoms persist or worsen, patient should call for further instructions. Excessive use may decrease desired effect and cause distressing tachycardia, palpitations, headache, nausea, and dizziness.
● Tell patient to store drug away from heat and light (not in bathroom medicine cabinet where heat and humidity can cause drug to deteriorate) and out of children's reach.
● Ask patient about sensitivity to sulfites.

Geriatric use
Elderly patients may be more sensitive to isoetharine's effects; lower dose may be needed.

Pediatric use
Pediatric dosage recommendations not established by the manufacturer; however, some clinicians believe pediatric dosage is the same as the adult dosage.

Breast-feeding
It is unknown if drug is excreted in breast milk; therefore, use with caution in breast-feeding women.

isoniazid (INH)
Hyzyd, Isotamine*, Laniazid, Nydrazid, PMS-Isoniazid*, Rimifon*, Rolazid, Teebaconin

● Pharmacologic classification: isonicotinic acid hydrazine
● Therapeutic classification: antitubercular agent
● Pregnancy risk category C

How supplied
Available by prescription only
Oral solution: 50 mg/5 ml
Tablets: 50 mg, 100 mg, 300 mg
Injection: 100 mg/ml

Indications, route, and dosage
Primary treatment against actively growing tubercle bacilli
Adults: 5 to 10 mg/kg P.O. or I.M. daily single dose, up to 300 mg/day, continued for 9 months to 2 years.
Infants and children: 10 to 20 mg/kg P.O. or I.M. daily single dose, up to 300 to 500 mg/day, continued for 18 months to 2 years. Concomitant administration of at least one other effective antitubercular drug is recommended.
Prophylaxis against tubercle bacilli of those closely exposed or with positive skin test
Adults: 300 mg P.O. daily single dose, continued for 6 months to 1 year.
Infants and children: 10 mg/kg P.O. daily single dose, up to 300 mg/day, continued for 6 months to 1 year.

Pharmacodynamics
Antitubercular action: Isoniazid (INH) interferes with lipid and DNA synthesis, thus inhibiting bacterial cell wall synthesis. Its action is bacteriostatic or bactericidal, depending on organism susceptibility and drug concentration at infection site. INH is active against *Mycobacterium tuberculosis, M. bovis,* and some strains of *M. kansasii.*
   Resistance by *Mycobacterium tuberculosis* develops

---

*Canada only   †Unlabeled clinical use   Italicized adverse reactions are life-threatening.

rapidly when INH is used to *treat* tuberculosis, and it is usually combined with another antituberculosis agent to prevent or delay resistance. During prophylaxis, however, resistance is not a problem and isoniazid can be used alone.

Pharmacokinetics
● *Absorption:* INH is absorbed completely and rapidly from the GI tract after oral administration; peak serum concentrations occur 1 to 2 hours after ingestion. INH also is absorbed readily after I.M. injection.
● *Distribution:* INH is distributed widely into body tissues and fluids, including ascitic, synovial, pleural, and cerebrospinal fluids; lungs and other organs; and sputum and saliva. INH crosses the placenta as well as into breast milk in concentrations comparable to plasma.
● *Metabolism:* INH is inactivated primarily in the liver by genetically controlled acetylation. Rate of metabolism varies individually; fast acetylators metabolize drug five times as rapidly as others. About 50% of blacks and whites are slow acetylators of INH, whereas over 80% of Chinese, Japanese, and Eskimos are fast acetylators.
● *Excretion:* About 75% of a dose of INH is excreted in urine as unchanged drug and metabolites in 24 hours; some drug is excreted in saliva, sputum, feces, and breast milk. Plasma half-life in adults is 1 to 4 hours, depending on metabolic rate. INH is removed by peritoneal dialysis or hemodialysis.

Contraindications and precautions
INH is contraindicated in patients with known hypersensitivity to INH; in patients with history of INH-induced hepatic disease or other severe reactions, including arthralgias, fever, chills, or acute hepatic disease.

INH should be used cautiously in patients who ingest alcohol daily and in patients with chronic hepatic or renal disease, or a history of seizures.

Interactions
Concomitant daily use of alcohol may increase incidence of INH-induced hepatitis and seizures.

Concomitant use with cycloserine increases hazard of CNS toxicity, drowsiness, and dizziness from cycloserine.

INH-induced inhibition of metabolism and elevation of serum concentrations increases toxicity of benzodiazepines (such as diazepam), phenytoin, and carbamazepine.

Concomitant use of INH and disulfiram may cause coordination difficulties and psychotic episodes.

Concomitant use with antacids decreases oral absorption of INH; use with corticosteroids may decrease INH efficacy; use with rifampin may accelerate INH metabolism to hepatotoxic metabolites; because of rifampin-induced enzyme production; use with anticoagulants may increase anticoagulant activity.

Effects on diagnostic tests
INH alters results of urine glucose tests that use cupric sulfate method (Benedict's reagent or Clinitest).

Elevated liver function study results occur in about 15%; most abnormalities are mild and transient, but some persist throughout treatment.

Adverse reactions
● CNS: *peripheral neuropathy* (especially in malnourished, alcoholic, and diabetic patients, and in slow acety-

lators), usually preceded by paresthesias of hands and feet; psychosis; *seizures.*
● CV: postural hypotension.
● EENT: optic neuritis with atrophy.
● GI: nausea, vomiting, epigastric distress, constipation, dryness of the mouth.
● HEMA: *agranulocytosis,* hemolytic anemia, *aplastic anemia,* eosinophilia, leukopenia, neutropenia, thrombocytopenia, methemoglobinemia, pyridoxine-responsive hypochromic anemia.
● Hepatic: *hepatitis* (occasionally severe and sometimes fatal, especially in elderly), jaundice.
● Metabolic: hyperglycemia, metabolic acidosis, pyridoxine deficiency, gynecomastia.
● Local: irritation at injection site.
● Other: rheumatic syndrome and systemic lupus erythematosus-like syndrome, *hypersensitivity reactions* (fever, rash, lymphadenopathy, vasculitis).
Note: Drug should be discontinued if patient shows signs of hypersensitivity reaction or hepatic damage.

Overdose and treatment
Early signs of overdose include nausea, vomiting, slurred speech, dizziness, blurred vision, and visual hallucinations, occurring 30 minutes to 3 hours after ingestion; gross overdose causes CNS depression progressing from stupor to coma, with respiratory distress, intractable seizures, and death.

To treat, establish ventilation; control seizures with diazepam. Pyridoxine is administered to equal dose of INH. Initial dose is 1 to 4 g pyridoxine I.V., followed by 1 g every 30 minutes thereafter, until the entire dose is given. Clear drug with gastric lavage *after* seizure control, and correct acidosis with parenteral sodium bicarbonate; force diuresis with I.V. fluids and osmotic diuretics, and, if necessary, enhance clearance of the drug with hemodialysis or peritoneal dialysis.

▶ Special considerations
● At least 12 months of preventive therapy is recommended for persons with past tuberculosis and human immunodeficiency virus- (HIV-) infected individuals.
● If compliance is a problem, twice-weekly supervised drug administration may be effective. For adults, the recommended dose twice weekly is 15 mg/kg P.O., not to exceed 900 mg.
● Prescribe oral doses to be taken on empty stomach for maximum absorption, or with food if gastric irritation occurs.
● Aluminum-containing antacids or laxatives should be taken 1 hour after oral dose of INH.
● Obtain specimens for culture and sensitivity testing before first dose, but therapy may begin before test results are complete; repeat periodically to detect drug resistance.
● Monitor blood, renal, and hepatic function studies before and periodically during therapy to minimize toxicity; assess visual function periodically.
● Observe patient for adverse effects, especially hepatic dysfunction, CNS toxicity, and optic neuritis. Establish safety measures, in case postural hypotension occurs.
● INH may hinder stabilization of serum glucose level in patients with diabetes mellitus.
● Improvement usually evident after 2 to 3 weeks of therapy.
● Some clinicians recommend pyridoxine 50 mg P.O. daily to prevent peripheral neuropathy from large doses of INH. It may also be useful in patients at risk of de-

---

veloping peripheral neuropathy (malnutrition patients, diabetics, and alcohol abusers). Pyridoxine (50 to 200 mg daily) has been used to treat INH-induced neuropathy.
• Because INH is dialyzable, patients undergoing hemodialysis or peritoneal dialysis may need dosage adjustments.
• Hepatotoxicity appears to be age-related, and may limit use for prophylaxis. Ethanol consumption and history of alcohol-related liver disease also increases risk of hepatotoxicity.

Information for the patient
• Explain disease process and rationale for long-term therapy.
• Teach signs and symptoms of hypersensitivity and other adverse reactions, particularly visual disturbances, and emphasize need to report these; urge patient to report *any* unusual effects.
• Warn patient not to use alcohol; explain hazard of serious CNS toxicity and increased hazard of hepatitis.
• Teach patient how and when to take drug; instruct patient to take INH on an empty stomach, at least 1 hour before or 2 hours after meals. If GI irritation occurs, drug may be taken with food.
• Urge patient to comply with and complete prescribed regimen. Advise patient not to discontinue drug without medical approval; explain importance of follow-up appointments.
• INH therapy is usually continued for 18 months to 2 years for treatment of active tuberculosis; 12 months for prophylaxis; 9 months if INH and rifampin therapy are combined.
• Emphasize the importance of uninterrupted therapy to prevent relapse and spread of infection.

Geriatric use
Use with caution in elderly patients; incidence of hepatic effects is increased after age 35. INH prophylaxis in patients with a positive purified protein derivative (PPD) test may not be indicated in older patients because of risk of hepatotoxicity.

Pediatric use
Infants and children tolerate larger doses of the drug.

Breast-feeding
INH is excreted in breast milk; use with caution in breast-feeding women and monitor infants for possible INH-induced toxicity.

---

isopropamide iodide
Darbid

• Pharmacologic classification: anticholinergic
• Therapeutic classification: muscarinic, gastrointestinal antispasmodic
• Pregnancy risk category C

How supplied
Available by prescription only
Tablets: 5 mg

Indications, route, and dosage
Adjunctive therapy for peptic ulcer
Adults and children over age 12: 5 mg P.O. q 12 hours. Some patients may require 10 mg or more b.i.d. Dosage should be individualized to patient's need.

Pharmacodynamics
Anticholinergic action: Isopropamide competitively blocks acetylcholine at cholinergic neuroeffector sites, decreasing GI motility and inhibiting gastric acid secretion.

Pharmacokinetics
• *Absorption:* Isopropamide is poorly absorbed from the GI tract.
• *Distribution:* Isopropamide does not cross the blood-brain barrier; little else is known of its distribution.
• *Metabolism:* Exact metabolic fate is unknown.
• *Excretion:* Isopropamide is excreted in the urine as metabolites and in the feces as unchanged drug. Duration of effect is 10 to 12 hours.

Contraindications and precautions
Isopropamide is contraindicated in patients with narrow-angle glaucoma, because drug-induced cycloplegia and mydriasis may increase intraocular pressure; in patients with obstructive uropathy, obstructive GI tract disease, severe ulcerative colitis, myasthenia gravis, paralytic ileus, intestinal atony, or toxic megacolon, because the drug may exacerbate these conditions; and in patients with known hypersensitivity to anticholinergics.
Administer isopropamide cautiously to patients with autonomic neuropathy, hyperthyroidism, coronary artery disease, cardiac arrhythmias, congestive heart failure, or ulcerative colitis, because the drug may exacerbate the symptoms of these disorders; to patients with hepatic or renal disease, because toxic accumulation may occur; to patients over age 40, because the drug increases the glaucoma risk; to patients with hiatal hernia associated with reflux esophagitis, because the drug may decrease lower esophageal sphincter tone; and in hot or humid environments, because the drug may predispose the patient to heatstroke.

Interactions
Concurrent administration of antacids decreases oral absorption of anticholinergics. Administer isopropamide at least 1 hour before antacids.
Concomitant administration of drugs with anticholinergic effects may cause additive toxicity.
Decreased GI absorption of many drugs has been reported after the use of anticholinergics (for example, levodopa and ketoconazole). Conversely, slowly dissolving digoxin tablets may yield higher serum digoxin levels when administered with anticholinergics.
Use cautiously with slow-release solid oral potassium supplements (especially wax-matrix formulations) because the incidence of potassium-induced GI ulcerations may be increased.

Effects on diagnostic tests
Isopropamide may alter thyroid function test results and will suppress ^{131}I uptake; drug should be discontinued at least 1 week before such tests.

Adverse reactions

- CNS: headache, insomnia, drowsiness, dizziness, nervousness, weakness, confusion or excitement (in elderly).
- CV: palpitations, tachycardia, orthostatic hypotension.
- DERM: urticaria, decreased sweating or anhidrosis, iodine skin rash, other dermal manifestations.
- EENT: blurred vision, mydriasis, cycloplegia, increased ocular tension, photophobia.
- GI: dry mouth, dysphagia, heartburn, loss of taste, nausea, constipation, vomiting, paralytic ileus, abdominal distention.
- GU: urinary hesitancy and retention, impotence.
- Other: fever, allergic reaction.

Note: Drug should be discontinued if hypersensitivity, urinary retention, confusion or excitement, curare-like symptoms, or skin rash occurs.

Overdose and treatment

Clinical effects of overdose include curare-like symptoms and such peripheral effects as headache; dilated, nonreactive pupils; blurred vision; flushed, hot, dry skin; dryness of mucous membranes; dysphagia; decreased or absent bowel sounds; urinary retention; hyperthermia; tachycardia; hypertension; and increased respiration.

Treatment is primarily symptomatic and supportive, as needed. If patient is alert, induce emesis (or use gastric lavage) and follow with a saline cathartic and activated charcoal to prevent further drug absorption. In severe cases, physostigmine may be administered to block isopropamide's antimuscarinic effects. Give fluids, as needed, to treat shock. If urinary retention develops, catheterization may be necessary.

▶ Special considerations

Besides those relevant to all *anticholinergics,* consider the following recommendations.

- Discontinue isopropamide at least 1 week before thyroid function tests.
- Administer cautiously to patients with iodine hypersensitivity.

Geriatric use

- Administer isopropamide cautiously to elderly patients. Lower doses are indicated.

Breast-feeding

- Isopropamide may be excreted in breast milk, possibly resulting in infant toxicity. Breast-feeding women should avoid this drug.

isoproterenol
Aerolone, Isuprel, Vapo-Iso

isoproterenol hydrochloride
Isuprel, Isuprel Mistometer, Norisodrine

isoproterenol sulfate
Medihaler-Iso

- Pharmacologic classification: adrenergic
- Therapeutic classification: bronchodilator, cardiac stimulant
- Pregnancy risk category C

How supplied

Available by prescription only
Isoproterenol
Nebulizer inhaler: 0.25%, 0.5%, and 1%
Isoproterenol hydrochloride
Aerosol inhaler: 120 mcg or 131 mcg/metered spray
Tablets (sublingual): 10 mg, 15 mg
Injection: 20 mcg/ml, 200 mcg/ml
Isoproterenol sulfate
Aerosol inhaler: 80 mcg/metered spray

Indications, route, and dosage

Complete heart block after closure of ventricular septal defect
Adults: I.V. bolus, 0.04 to 0.06 mg (2 to 3 ml of a 1:50,000 dilution).
Children: I.V. bolus, 0.01 to 0.03 mg (0.5 to 1.5 ml of a 1:50,000 dilution).

To prevent heart block
Adults: 10 to 30 mg sublingually 4 to 6 times daily.

Maintenance therapy of AV block
Adults: Initially, 10 mg sublingually, followed by 5 to 50 mg p.r.n. Alternatively, 5 mg (half of a 10-mg tablet) administered rectally, followed by 5 to 15 mg p.r.n.

Bronchospasm during mild acute asthma attacks

Isoproterenol hydrochloride
Adults and children: Via aerosol inhalation, 1 inhalation initially, repeated as needed after 1 to 5 minutes, to a maximum 6 inhalations daily. Maintenance dose is 1 to 2 inhalations 4 to 6 times daily at 3- to 4-hour intervals. Via hand-bulb nebulizer, 5 to 15 deep inhalations of a 0.5% solution; if needed, may be repeated in 5 to 10 minutes. May be repeated up to 5 times daily. Alternatively, 3 to 7 deep inhalations of a 1% solution, repeated once in 5 to 10 minutes if needed. May be repeated up to 5 times daily.

Isoproterenol sulfate
Adults and children: For acute dyspneic episodes, inhalation initially; repeated if needed after 2 to 5 minutes. Maximum 6 inhalations daily. Maintenance dosage: 1 to 2 inhalations up to six times daily.

Bronchospasm in chronic obstructive pulmonary disease

Isoproterenol hydrochloride
Adults and children: Via hand-bulb nebulizer: 5 to 15 deep inhalations of a 0.5% solution, or 3 to 7 deep inhalations of a 1% solution give no more frequently than every 3 to 4 hours.

Bronchospasm during mild acute asthma attacks or in chronic obstructive pulmonary disease
Isoproterenol hydrochloride
Adults and children: 6 to 12 inhalations of a 0.025% nebulized solution, repeated at 15-minute intervals to a maximum of three treatments, not to exceed eight treatments in 24 hours.

Acute asthma attacks unresponsive to inhalation therapy or control of bronchospasm during anesthesia
Isoproterenol hydrochloride
Adults: 0.01 to 0.02 mg (0.5 to 1 ml of a 1:50,000 dilution) I.V. Repeat if needed.

For bronchodilation
Isoproterenol hydrochloride
Adults: 10 to 20 mg sublingually, not to exceed 60 mg daily.
Children: 5 to 10 mg sublingually, not to exceed 30 mg daily.

Emergency treatment of cardiac arrhythmias
Isoproterenol hydrochloride
Adults: Initially, 0.02 to 0.06 mg I.V. bolus. Subsequent doses 0.01 to 0.2 mg I.V. Alternatively, 5 mcg/minute titrated to patient's response. Range 2 to 20 mcg/minute. Alternatively, 0.2 mg I.M. or S.C.; subsequent doses 0.02 to 1 mg I.M. or 0.15 to 0.2 mg S.C. In *extreme* cases, 0.02 mg (0.1 of 1:5,000) intracardiac injection.
Children: May give half of initial adult dose.

Immediate temporary control of atropine-resistant hemodynamically significant bradycardia
Isoproterenol hydrochloride
Adults: 2 to 10 mcg/minute I.V. infusion, titrated to patient's response.
Children: 0.1 mcg/kg/minute, titrated to patient's response. Maximum rate is 1 mcg/kg/minute.

Adjunct in treatment of shock
Isoproterenol hydrochloride
Adults and children: 0.5 to 5 mcg/minute by continuous I.V. infusion titrated to patient's response.

Pharmacodynamics
● *Bronchodilator action:* Isoproterenol relaxes bronchial smooth muscle by direct action on beta$_2$-adrenergic receptors, relieving bronchospasm, increasing vital capacity, decreasing residual volume in lungs, and facilitating passage of pulmonary secretions. It also produces relaxation of GI and uterine smooth muscle via stimulation of beta$_2$ receptors. Peripheral vasodilation, cardiac stimulation, and relaxation of bronchial smooth muscle are the main therapeutic effects.
● *Cardiac stimulant action:* Isoproterenol acts on beta$_1$-adrenergic receptors in the heart, producing a positive chronotropic and inotropic effect; it usually increases cardiac output. In patients with AV block, isoproterenol AV node refractory and shortens conduction time and increases the rate and strength of ventricular contraction.

Pharmacokinetics
● *Absorption:* After injection or oral inhalation, isoproterenol is absorbed rapidly; after sublingual or rectal administration, absorption is variable and often unreliable. Onset of action is prompt after oral inhalation and persists up to 1 hour. Effects persist for a few minutes after I.V. injection, up to 2 hours after S.C. or sublingual administration, and up to 4 hours after rectal administration of sublingual tablet.

● *Distribution:* Isoproterenol is distributed widely throughout the body.
● *Metabolism:* Isoproterenol is metabolized by conjugation in the GI tract and by enzymatic reduction in liver, lungs, and other tissues.
● *Excretion:* Isoproterenol is excreted primarily in urine as unchanged drug and its metabolites.

Contraindications and precautions
Isoproterenol is contraindicated in patients with pre-existing cardiac arrhythmias, especially tachycardia (including tachycardia caused by digitalis toxicity), because of the drug's cardiac stimulant effects; and in those with known hypersensitivity to this drug or other sympathomimetics.

Administer cautiously to elderly patients, diabetic patients, those with renal or cardiovascular disease (hypertension, coronary insufficiency, angina, degenerative heart disease), or hyperthyroidism, because drug may worsen these conditions; and to sulfite-sensitive patients, because some formulations contain sulfite preservatives.

Interactions
Concomitant use of isoproterenol with epinephrine and other sympathomimetics may cause additive cardiovascular reactions. However, these drugs may be used together if at least 4 hours elapse between administration of the two drugs. Use with beta-adrenergic blockers antagonizes isoproterenol's cardiac-stimulating, bronchodilating, and vasodilating effects. Use with ergot alkaloids may increase blood pressure.

Arrhythmias may occur more readily when drug is administered to patients receiving digitalis, potassium-depleting drugs, or other drugs that affect cardiac rhythm. Isoproterenol should be used with caution in patients receiving cyclopropane or halogenated hydrocarbon general anesthetics.

Effects on diagnostic tests
Isoproterenol may reduce the sensitivity of spirometry in the diagnosis of asthma.

Adverse reactions
● CNS: nervousness, restlessness, insomnia, anxiety, tension, fear, excitement, weakness, dizziness, mild tremor, light-headedness, headache.
● CV: palpitation, tachycardia, angina, alterations in blood pressure, *arrhythmias.*
● GI: nausea, vomiting.
● Metabolic: hyperglycemia.
● Other: bronchial irritation and edema, sweating, flushing of face or skin, tinnitus.
Note: Drug should be discontinued if precordial distress, angina, ventricular arrhythmias, or swelling of parotids occurs or airway resistance develops.

Overdose and treatment
Clinical manifestations of overdose include exaggeration of common adverse reactions, particularly cardiac arrhythmias, extreme tremors, nausea and vomiting, and profound hypotension.

Treatment includes symptomatic and supportive measures. Monitor vital signs closely. Sedatives (barbiturates) may be used to treat CNS stimulation. Use cardioselective beta blocker to treat tachycardia and arrhythmias. These agents should be used with caution; they may induce asthmatic attack.

▶ **Special considerations**

Besides those relevant to all *adrenergics*, consider the following recommendations.

● Isoproterenol does not replace administration of blood, plasma, fluids, or electrolytes in patients with blood volume depletion.

● Severe paradoxical airway resistance may follow oral inhalations.

● Hypotension must be corrected before isoproterenol is administered.

● If three to five treatments within 6 to 12 hours provide minimal or no relief, re-evaluate therapy.

● Continuously monitor ECG during I.V. administration.

● Carefully monitor response to therapy by frequent determinations of heart rate, ECG pattern, blood pressure, and central venous pressure, as well as (for patients in shock) urine volume, blood pH, and Pco_2 levels.

● Prescribed I.V. infusion rate should include specific guidelines for regulating flow or terminating infusion in relation to heart rate, premature beats, ECG changes, precordial distress, blood pressure, and urine flow. Because of the danger of precipitating arrhythmias, rate of infusion is usually decreased or infusion may be temporarily discontinued if heart rate exceeds 110 beats/minute.

● Constant-infusion pump prevents sudden infusion of excessive amounts of drug.

● Sublingual doses should not be given more frequently than every 3 to 4 hours nor more than t.i.d.

● Sublingual tablet may be administered rectally, if indicated.

● Monitor for rebound bronchospasm when isoproterenol effects end.

● Isoproterenol has also been used to aid diagnosis of coronary artery disease and of mitral regurgitation.

● Do not inject solutions intended for oral inhalation.

Information for the patient

● Remind patient to save applicator; refills may be available.

● Urge patient to call if no relief is gained or condition worsens.

● Advise patient to store oral forms away from heat and light (not in bathroom medicine cabinet where heat and moisture will cause deterioration of the drug). Keep drug out of the reach of children.

Inhalation

● Give patient instructions on proper use of inhaler.

● Tell patient that saliva and sputum may appear red or pink after oral inhalation, because isoproterenol turns red on exposure to air.

● Advise patient to rinse mouth with water after drug is absorbed completely and between doses.

Sublingual

● Tell patient to allow sublingual tablet to dissolve under tongue, without sucking, and not to swallow saliva (may cause epigastric pain) until drug has been absorbed completely.

● Warn patient that frequent use of acidic sublingual tablets may damage teeth.

Geriatric use

Elderly patients may be more sensitive to the therapeutic and adverse effects of the drug.

Pediatric use

Use with caution.

Breast-feeding

It is unknown whether isoproterenol is excreted in breast milk; therefore, drug should be used with caution in breast-feeding women.

isosorbide
Ismotic

● Pharmacologic classification: osmotic diuretic
● Therapeutic classification: antiglaucoma agent
● Pregnancy risk category C

How supplied

Available by prescription only
Oral solution: 45% in 220-ml containers

Indications, route, and dosage
Short-term reduction of intraocular pressure from glaucoma

Adults: Initially, 1.5 g/kg P.O. Usual dosage range is 1 to 3 g/kg.

Pharmacodynamics

Diuretic action: Increases osmolarity of fluid presented to the kidney, decreasing reabsorption of water and resulting in diuresis. In the eye, isosorbide creates an osmotic gradient between plasma and ocular fluids.

Pharmacokinetics

● *Absorption:* Drug is absorbed rapidly after oral administration. Action begins within 10 to 30 minutes and peaks at 60 to 90 minutes.

● *Distribution:* Drug achieves good ocular penetration and is distributed to total body water.

● *Metabolism:* None.

● *Excretion:* Drug is eliminated unchanged by the kidney. Duration of action is 5 to 6 hours, and half-life is 7 to 8 hours.

Contraindications and precautions

Isosorbide is contraindicated in patients with anuria from severe renal disease, severe dehydration, acute pulmonary edema, or severe cardiac decompensation, because the osmotic effects of the drug may worsen the symptoms or disorders; and hypersensitivity to any components of the preparation.

Repeated doses should be used with caution in patients with diseases associated with sodium retention.

Interactions

None significant.

Effects on diagnostic tests

None reported.

Adverse reactions

● CNS: headache, confusion, disorientation, irritability, syncope, lethargy, light-headedness, vertigo.

● GI: nausea, vomiting, gastric discomfort, thirst, hiccups, diarrhea, anorexia.

● Other: hypernatremia, hyperosmolarity, rash.

Note: Drug should be discontinued if fluid or electrolyte imbalances occur or if urine output decreases drastically.

Overdose and treatment
Clinical effects of overdose include hypoglycemia, hyperuricemia, fluid and electrolyte imbalances, weakness, hyporeflexia, and arrhythmias.

Emesis may be indicated after substantial ingestion unless the patient is obtunded or comatose. Monitor the patient's fluid and electrolyte status closely.

▶ Special considerations
● Isosorbide carries less risk of nausea and vomiting than other oral hyperosmotics. Serving over cracked ice seems to improve palatability.
● Patient should be monitored for 5 to 10 minutes after administration.
● Drug may be used to interrupt acute attack of glaucoma before laser/surgical treatment.
● Additional antiemetics (I.M.) may be needed when isosorbide is used to lower intraocular pressure.

Information for the patient
● Tell patient to sip medication. This improves palatability.
● Tell patient that drug may cause him to feel thirsty.

Geriatric use
Drug should be used with caution in elderly patients because of increased risk of fluid and electrolyte imbalances.

Pediatric use
Drug should be used with caution in children because of increased risk of fluid and electrolyte imbalances.

isosorbide dinitrate
Apo-ISDN*, Coronex*, Dilatrate-SR, Iso-Bid, Isochron, Isonate, Isonate TR, Isordil, Isotrate, Novosorbide*, Onset-5; Sorate, Sorbide TD, Sorbitrate, Sorbitrate SA

● Pharmacologic classification: nitrate
● Therapeutic classification: antianginal agent, vasodilator
● Pregnancy risk category C

How supplied
Available by prescription only
Tablets: 5 mg, 10 mg, 20 mg, 30 mg, and 40 mg (oral); 2.5 mg, 5 mg, and 10 mg (sublingual); 40 mg (extended-release); 5 mg and 10 mg (chewable)
Capsules: (extended-release): 40 mg

Indications, route, and dosage
Treatment or prophylaxis of acute anginal attacks; treatment of chronic ischemic heart disease (by preload reduction)
Adults: Sublingual form – 2.5 to 10 mg under tongue for prompt relief of angina pain, repeated q 2 to 3 hours during acute phase, or q 4 to 6 hours for prophylaxis. Chewable form – 5 to 10 mg. p.r.n., for acute attack or q 2 to 3 hours for prophylaxis, but only after initial test dose of 5 mg to determine risk of severe hypotension.

Oral form – 5 to 30 mg P.O. q.i.d. for prophylaxis only (use smallest effective dose); sustained-release forms – 40 mg P.O. q 6 to 12 hours.

†Adjunctive treatment of congestive heart failure
Adults: 5 to 10 mg S.L. every 3 to 4 hours. Alternatively, give 20 to 40 mg P.O. (or chewable tablets) every 4 hours. Usually administered with vasodilators.

†Diffuse esophageal spasm without gastroesophageal reflux
Adults: 10 to 30 mg P.O. q 4 hours.

Pharmacodynamics
● *Antianginal action:* Isosorbide dinitrate reduces myocardial oxygen demand through peripheral vasodilation, resulting in decreased venous filling pressure (preload) and, to a lesser extent, decreased arterial impedance (afterload). These combined effects result in decreased cardiac work and, consequently, reduced myocardial oxygen demands. The drug also redistributes coronary blood flow from epicardial to subendocardial regions.
● *Vasodilating action:* The drug dilates peripheral vessels (primarily venous), helping to manage pulmonary edema and congestive heart failure (CHF) caused by decreased venous return to the heart (preload). Arterial vasodilatory effects also decrease arterial impedance (afterload) and thus left ventricular work, benefiting the failing heart. These combined effects may help some patients with acute myocardial infarction (MI). (Use of isosorbide dinitrate in patients with congestive heart failure and acute myocardial infarction is currently unapproved.)

Pharmacokinetics
● *Absorption:* Oral isosorbide dinitrate is well absorbed from the GI tract but undergoes first-pass metabolism, resulting in bioavailability of about 50% (depending on dosage form used). With sublingual and chewable forms, onset of action is 3 minutes; with other oral forms, 30 minutes; with extended-release form, 1 hour.
● *Distribution:* Limited information is available on drug's plasma protein binding and distribution. Like nitroglycerin, it is distributed widely throughout the body.
● *Metabolism:* Drug is metabolized in the liver to active metabolites.
● *Excretion:* Metabolites are excreted in the urine; elimination half-life is about 5 to 6 hours with oral administration; 2 hours with sublingual administration. About 80% to 100% of absorbed dose is excreted in the urine within 24 hours. Duration of effect is longer than that of sublingual preparations. With sublingual and chewable forms, duration of effect is 30 minutes to 2 hours; with other oral forms, 5 to 6 hours.

Contraindications and precautions
Isosorbide dinitrate is contraindicated in patients with a history of hypersensitivity or idiosyncratic reaction to nitrates; and in patients with severe anemia, because nitrate ions readily oxidize hemoglobin to methemoglobin.

Use caution when administering isosorbide dinitrate to patients with increased intracranial pressure or recent head trauma because the drug dilates meningeal vessels; in patients with open- or closed-angle glaucoma, although intraocular pressure is increased only briefly and aqueous humor drainage from the eye is impeded; in patients with diuretic-induced fluid depletion or low systolic blood pressure (below 90 mm Hg), because of the drug's hypotensive effect; and during

---

the initial days after acute myocardial infarction, because the drug may cause excessive hypotension and tachycardia.

Use of extended-release preparations in patients with malabsorption syndromes or gastrointestinal hypermotility is not recommended. Lack of response to three or more sublingual tablets may indicate acute myocardial infarction; this situation mandates immediate medical attention.

Interactions

Concomitant use of isosorbide with alcohol, antihypertensive drugs, beta blockers, or phenothiazines may cause additive hypotensive effects.

Effects on diagnostic tests

Isosorbide dinitrate may interfere with serum cholesterol determination tests using the Zlatkis-Zak color reaction, causing a falsely decreased value.

Adverse reactions

- CNS: headache (sometimes with throbbing), dizziness, blurred vision.
- CV: orthostatic hypotension, tachycardia, palpitations, ankle edema, syncope/fainting.
- DERM: cutaneous vasodilation with flushing, rash, dermatitis.
- GI: nausea, vomiting, dry mouth.
- Local: sublingual burning.
- Other: hypersensitivity.

Note: Drug should be discontinued if rash, dermatitis, blurred vision, or dry mouth occur.

Overdose and treatment

Clinical effects of overdose result primarily from vasodilation and methemoglobinemia and include hypotension; persistent throbbing headache; palpitations; visual disturbance; flushing of the skin and sweating (with skin later becoming cold and cyanotic); nausea and vomiting; colic and bloody diarrhea; orthostatis; initial hyperpnea; dyspnea; slow respiratory rate; bradycardia; heart block; increased intracranial pressure with confusion; fever; paralysis; and tissue hypoxia from methemoglobinemia, which can lead to cyanosis, metabolic acidosis, coma, clonic convulsions, and circulatory collapse. Death may result from circulatory collapse or asphyxia.

Treatment includes gastric lavage followed by administration of activated charcoal to remove remaining gastric contents. Blood gas measurements and methemoglobin levels should be monitored, as indicated. Supportive care includes respiratory support and oxygen administration, passive movement of extremities to aid venous return, recumbent positioning (Trendelenburg position, if necessary), maintenance of adequate body temperature, and administration of I.V. fluids.

An I.V. adrenergic agonist (such as phenylephrine) may be considered if further treatment is required. For methemoglobinemia, methylene blue (1 to 2 mg/kg I.V.) may be given. (Epinephrine and related compounds are contraindicated in isosorbide dinitrate overdose.)

▶ Special considerations

- Drug may cause headache, especially at first. Dose may need to be reduced temporarily, but tolerance usually develops to this effect. In the interim, patient may relive headache with aspirin or acetaminophen.
- Additional dose may be given before anticipated stress or at bedtime if angina is nocturnal.

- Monitor blood pressure and intensity and duration of patient's response to drug.
- Drug may cause orthostatic hypotension. To minimize this, have patient change to upright position slowly, walk up and down stairs carefully, and lie down at first sign of dizziness.
- Do not discontinue drug abruptly because this may cause coronary vasospasm.
- Store drug in cool place, in tightly closed container away from light.

Information for the patient

- Instruct patient to take medication regularly, as prescribed, and to keep it easily accessible at all times. Drug is physiologically necessary but not addictive.
- Warn patient that headache may occur initially, but may respond to usual headache remedies or dosage reduction. Assure patient that headache usually subsides gradually with continued treatment.
- If patient is taking oral tablet, tell him to take it on empty stomach, either 30 minutes before or 1 to 2 hours after meals; to swallow oral tablets whole; and to chew chewable tablets thoroughly before swallowing.
- Advise patient to sit when self-administering sublingual tablets. He should lubricate tablet with saliva or place a few milliliters of fluid under tongue with tablet. If patient experiences tingling sensation with drug placed sublingually, he may try to hold tablet in buccal pouch. Dose may be repeated every 10 to 15 minutes for maximum of three doses. If no relief occurs, patient should call or go to hospital emergency room.
- Warn patient to make positional changes gradually to avoid excessive dizziness.
- Instruct patient to avoid alcohol while taking this drug because severe hypotension and cardiovascular collapse may occur.
- Advise patient to report blurred vision, dry mouth, or persistent headache.
- Caution patient not to stop long-term therapy abruptly.

Pediatric use

Methemoglobinemia may occur in infants receiving large doses of isosorbate dinitrate.

---

isotretinoin
Accutane

- Pharmacologic classification: retinoic acid derivative
- Therapeutic classification: antiacne agent, keratinization stabilizer
- Pregnancy risk category X

How supplied

Available by prescription only
Capsules: 10 mg, 20 mg, 40 mg

Indications, route, and dosage
Severe cystic acne unresponsive to conventional therapy

Adults and adolescents: 0.5 to 2 mg/kg P.O. daily given in two divided doses and continued for 15 to 20 weeks.
†Keratinization disorders resistant to conventional therapy

Adults: Dosage varies with specific disease and severity of the disorder; dosages up to 4 mg/kg P.O. daily

---

have been used. Consult current literature for specific recommendations.

Pharmacodynamics

● *Antiacne action:* The exact mechanism of action is unknown; isotretinoin decreases the size and activity of sebaceous glands, which decreases secretion and probably explains the rapid clinical improvement. A reduction in *Propionibacterium acnes* in the hair follicles occurs as a secondary result of decreased nutrients.

● *Keratinizing action:* Isotretinoin has anti-inflammatory and keratinizing effects. The mechanism is unknown.

Pharmacokinetics

● *Absorption:* When administered orally, isotretinoin is absorbed rapidly from the GI tract. Peak concentrations occur in 3 hours, with peak concentrations of the metabolite 4-oxo-isotretinoin occurring in 6 to 20 hours. The therapeutic range for isotretinoin has not been established.

● *Distribution:* Isotretinoin, which has not been fully studied, is distributed widely. In animals, it is found in most organs and is known to cross the placenta. In humans, the degree of placental transfer and the degree of secretion in breast milk are unknown. Isotretinoin is 99.9% protein-bound, primarily to albumin.

● *Metabolism:* Isotretinoin is metabolized in the liver and possibly in the gut wall. The major metabolite is 4-oxo-isotretinoin, with tretinoin and 4-oxo-tretinoin also found in the blood and urine.

● *Excretion:* The elimination process is not fully known, although renal and biliary pathways are known to be used.

Contraindications and precautions

Drug is contraindicated in patients with sensitivity to isotretinoin, vitamin A, or other retinoids. Do not use in pregnant women, because of possible teratogenic effects, including hydrocephalus and microcephaly. Start therapy only after confirmation that patient is not pregnant and appropriate birth-control measures have been instituted. Any person taking isotretinoin should refrain from donating blood for at least 30 days after therapy has been discontinued. Frequent check of blood chemistry during therapy is also recommended.

Interactions

Isotretinoin will have a cumulative drying effect when used with medicated soaps and cleansers, medicated "cover-ups," topical peeling agents (benzoyl peroxide, resorcinol), and alcohol-containing preparations. Concurrent use of vitamin A products may have an additive toxic effect. Tetracyclines may increase the potential for the development of pseudotumor cerebri. Oral alcohol intake may increase plasma triglyceride levels.

Effects on diagnostic tests

The physiologic effects of the drug may alter liver function tests, blood counts, and blood glucose, uric acid, cholesterol, and triglyceride levels. May cause elevation of erythrocyte sedimentation rate.

Adverse reactions

● CNS: headache, fatigue, mood changes.
● DERM: dry skin, peeling of palms and toes, skin infection, photosensitivity, skin rash, burning, redness, irritation, pruritus.

● EENT: conjunctivitis, corneal deposits, dry eyes, decreased night vision, dry nose, epistaxis.
● Endocrine: hyperglycemia.
● GI: nausea, vomiting, diarrhea, rectal bleeding, abdominal or stomach pain, cheilitis (most frequent), dry mouth, nonspecific GI symptoms, gum bleeding and inflammation.
● HEMA: anemia, elevated platelet count.
● Hepatic: elevated AST (SGOT), ALT (SPGT), and alkaline phosphatase.
● Other: hypertriglyceridemia, musculoskeletal pain (skeletal hyperostosis), thinning of hair.

Note: Drug should be discontinued if symptoms of inflammatory bowel disease, visual disturbances, or pseudotumor cerebri are present, and if serum lipids are significantly elevated.

Overdose and treatment

Clinical manifestations of overdose are rare and would be extensions of adverse reactions.

▶ Special considerations

● Therapy usually lasts 15 to 20 weeks, followed by at least 8 weeks off drug before beginning a second course.
● Contact lenses may be uncomfortable during treatment; recommend use of artificial tears.
● Patient should take dose with or shortly after meals.
● Carefully monitor for visual problems.

Information for the patient

● Recommend taking drug with or shortly after meals to ease GI discomfort; chewing gum may relieve dryness of mouth.
● Warn patient that acne may worsen during the initial course of therapy and to call if the irritation becomes severe.
● Warn patient not to donate blood or become pregnant while taking this medication and for 30 days after discontinuing the drug.
● Caution against alcohol ingestion, to reduce the risk of hypertriglyceridemia.
● Warn patient to be cautious when driving, particularly at night because the drug causes decreased night vision.

Special instructions for female patients

● Isotretinoin is a potent teratogen and should not be given to female patients who are pregnant or may become pregnant during therapy. Patient selection is important—informed consent must be obtained from the patient or her legal guardian before initiating therapy. The patient or responsible adult must fully understand the consequences of fetal exposure to isotretinoin.
● Reliable methods of contraception are essential for sexually active females who are taking isotretinoin.
● Negative blood tests for pregnancy must be obtained before therapy.
● Schedule follow-up visits monthly during therapy. Do not prescribe more than a 6-week supply at a time. Pregnancy tests must be repeated monthly.
● Isotretinoin has been used in a limited number of patients to treat psoriasis (combined with psoralen and UV light); it has also been used to treat cutaneous neoplasms.

Breast-feeding

It is unknown whether isotretinoin passes into breast milk; breast-feeding is not recommended during drug therapy.

isoxsuprine hydrochloride
Rolisox, Vasodilan, Vasoprine

- Pharmacologic classification: beta-adrenergic agonist
- Therapeutic classification: peripheral vasodilator
- Pregnancy risk category C

How supplied
Available by prescription only
Tablets: 10 mg, 20 mg
Injection*: 5 mg/ml

Indications, route, and dosage
Cerebrovascular insufficiency, peripheral vascular diseases (such as arteriosclerosis obliterans, thromboangiitis obliterans, Raynaud's disease)
Adults: 10 to 20 mg P.O. t.i.d. or q.i.d.

Pharmacodynamics
Vasodilating action: Isoxsuprine produces peripheral vasodilation by a direct effect on vascular smooth muscle; drug produces cardiac stimulation and uterine relaxation. Isoxsuprine has beta-adrenergic agonist activity.

Pharmacokinetics
- *Absorption:* Isoxsuprine is absorbed well from the GI tract. After oral administration, action begins in 60 minutes; effects persist for about 3 hours.
- *Distribution:* Isoxsuprine crosses the placenta.
- *Metabolism:* Drug is conjugated partially in the blood.
- *Excretion:* Isoxsuprine is excreted primarily in urine; fecal excretion is insignificant. Half-life is about 1¼ hours.

Contraindications and precautions
Isoxsuprine is contraindicated in patients immediately postpartum and in the presence of arterial bleeding because of its uterine vasodilating relaxant effects.

Intravenous administration is contraindicated because it increases the incidence of adverse reactions; parenteral administration is not recommended for patients with hypotension or tachycardia because the drug may exacerbate these symptoms.

The efficacy of isoxsuprine in the treatment of peripheral vascular disease has not been established, and the drug should not be used as a substitute for appropriate medical or surgical therapy for the treatment of peripheral or cerebral vascular disease.

Interactions
None significant.

Effects on diagnostic tests
Isoxsuprine alters serum concentrations of blood glucose and free fatty acids.

Adverse reactions
- CNS: dizziness, nervousness.
- CV: hypotension, tachycardia, chest pain, irregular heartbeat.
- DERM: severe rash, flushing.
- GI: vomiting, abdominal distress, intestinal distention.

Note: Drug should be discontinued if rash appears.

Overdose and treatment
No specific recommendations are available. Treatment is supportive.

▶ Special considerations
The incidence of adverse reactions with isoxsuprine increases at higher doses and after parenteral administration.

Information for the patient
Advise patient to avoid rapid postural changes to minimize postural hypotension.

Geriatric use
Isoxsuprine-induced hypothermia may occur more commonly in elderly patients.

Pediatric use
Isoxsuprine crosses the placenta and may cause hypotension and tachycardia in neonates.

Breast-feeding
Safety in breast-feeding women has not been established.

---

isradipine
DynaCirc

- Pharmacologic classification: calcium channel blocker
- Therapeutic classification: antihypertensive
- Pregnancy risk category C

How supplied
Available by prescription only
Tablets: 2.5 mg, 5 mg

Indications, route, and dosage
Management of hypertension
Adults: Individualize dosage. Initially, 2.5 mg P.O. b.i.d. alone or with thiazide diuretic. Maximal response may require 2 to 4 weeks; therefore, dosage adjustments of 5 mg daily should be made at 2- to 4-week intervals up to a maximum of 20 mg daily. Dosages of 10 mg or more per day have not been shown to be more effective but rather to lead to increased incidence of adverse reactions. Same starting dosage is used in elderly, hepatic-impaired, and renal-impaired patients.

Pharmacodynamics
Antihypertensive action: A dihydropyridine calcium channel blocker, isradipine binds to calcium channels and inhibits calcium flux into cardiac and smooth muscle, which results in dilation of arterioles. This dilation reduces systemic resistance and lowers blood pressure while producing small increases in resting heart rate.

Pharmacokinetics
- *Absorption:* 90% to 95% absorbed after oral administration; peak concentrations are reached in 1.5 hours.
- *Distribution:* 95% is bound to plasma protein.
- *Metabolism:* Isradipine is completely metabolized before elimination with extensive first-pass metabolism.

● *Excretion:* 60% to 65% of the drug is excreted in urine; 25% to 30%, in feces.

Interactions
No clinically significant interactions have been reported. Severe hypotension has been reported with concomitant use of a beta blocker and a calcium channel blocker during fentanyl anesthesia but has not been seen with isradipine.

Adverse reactions
● CNS: headache, dizziness, fatigue, weakness, drowsiness, insomnia, lethargy, nervousness, depression, syncope, paresthesia, stroke.
● CV: palpitations, chest pain, tachycardia, hypotension, atrial fibrillation, *MI, heart failure,* transient ischemic attacks.
● DERM: flushing, rash.
● GI: nausea, vomiting, diarrhea, abdominal discomfort, constipation, dry mouth.
● GU: pollakiuria, nocturia, impotence, decreased libido.
● Respiratory: dyspnea, shortness of breath, cough.
● Other: visual disturbances, numbness, hyperhydrosis, throat discomfort.

Overdose and treatment
No well-documented cases of overdose have been reported; however, presumably excessive peripheral vasodilation with marked and prolonged systemic hypotension may occur. Symptomatic and supportive treatment should be provided, including active CV support, monitoring of input and output and cardiac and respiratory function, elevation of lower extremities, and fluid replacement as needed. Vasoconstrictors should be used *only when not specifically contraindicated.*

▶ Special considerations
● Isradipine has no significant effect on heart rate and no adverse effects on cardiac contractility, conduction or digitalis clearance, or lipid or renal function.
● Administration with food significantly increases the time to reach peak concentrations by about 1 hour. However, food has no effect on total bioavailability of drug.
● Elevated liver function test results have been reported in some patients.
● Individualize dosage. Allow 2 to 4 weeks between dosage adjustments.

Information for the patient
Instruct patient to notify physician of irregular heartbeat, shortness of breath, swelling of hands or feet, pronounced dizziness, constipation, nausea, or hypotension.

Geriatric use
No age-related problems have been reported.

Pediatric use
Safety and efficacy have not been established in children under age 18.

Breast-feeding
It is unknown if isradipine is excreted in breast milk. Consider the potential risk of serious adverse reactions in the infant.

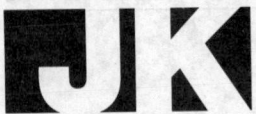

kanamycin sulfate
Anamid*, Kantrex, Klebcil

- Pharmacologic classification: aminoglycoside
- Therapeutic classification: antibiotic
- Pregnancy risk category D

How supplied
Available by prescription only
Capsules: 500 mg
Injection: 37.5 mg/ml (pediatric), 250 mg/ml, 333 mg/ml

Indications, route, and dosage
Serious infections caused by sensitive Escherichia coli, Proteus, Enterobacter aerogenes, Klebsiella pneumoniae, Serratia marcescens, mycobacterium and Acinetobacter
Adults and children with normal renal function: 15 mg/kg deep I.M. injection into upper outer quadrant of buttocks or I.V. infusion (diluted 500 mg/200 ml of normal saline solution or dextrose 5% in water infused over 30 to 60 minutes) daily divided q 8 to 12 hours. Maximum daily dose is 1.5 g.
Patients with impaired renal function: Doses and/or frequency of administration should be altered. In all patients, keep peak serum concentrations between 15 and 30 mcg/ml, and trough serum concentrations between 5 and 10 mcg/ml.
Neonates: 15 mg/kg I.M. or I.V. daily divided q 12 hours.
Adjunctive treatment in hepatic coma
Adults: 8 to 12 g P.O. daily in divided doses.
Preoperative bowel sterilization
Adults: 1 g P.O. q 1 hour for 4 doses, then q 4 hours for 4 doses; or 1 g P.O. q 1 hour for 4 doses, then q 6 hours for 36 to 72 hours.
Intraperitoneal irrigation
Instill 500 mg in 20 ml sterile distilled water via catheter into wound after patient fully recovers from anesthesia and neuromuscular blocking agent effects.
Wound irrigation
Up to 2.5 mg/ml in normal saline irrigation solution.
Dosage in renal failure
Adults: Initially, 7.5 mg/kg I.M. Subsequent doses and frequency determined by blood kanamycin concentrations and renal function studies. One method is to administer additional 7.5 mg/kg doses and adjust the dosing interval based upon steady-state serum creatinine:

$$\frac{\text{creatinine}}{(\text{mg/100 ml})} \times 9 = \frac{\text{dosing interval}}{(\text{in hours})}$$

Keep peak serum concentrations between 15 and 30 mcg/ml and trough serum concentration should not exceed 5 to 10 mcg/ml.

Pharmacodynamics
Antibiotic action: Kanamycin is bactericidal; it binds directly to the 30S ribosomal subunit, thus inhibiting bacterial protein synthesis. Its spectrum of activity includes many aerobic gram-negative organisms and some aerobic gram-positive organisms. Generally, kanamycin is far less active against many gram-negative organisms than are tobramycin, gentamicin, amikacin, and netilmicin. After oral administration, kanamycin inhibits ammonia-forming bacteria in the GI tract, decreasing ammonia and thus improving neurologic status of patients with hepatic encephalopathy.

Pharmacokinetics
- *Absorption:* Kanamycin is absorbed poorly after oral administration, although oral administration is enhanced in patients with impaired GI motility or mucosal ulcerations. Drug is usually given parenterally; peak serum concentrations occur 60 minutes after I.M. administration.
- *Distribution:* Kanamycin is distributed widely after parenteral administration; intraocular penetration is poor. CSF penetration is low, even in patients with inflamed meninges. Intraventricular administration produces high concentrations throughout the CNS. Protein binding is minimal. Kanamycin crosses the placenta.
- *Metabolism:* Not metabolized.
- *Excretion:* Kanamycin is excreted primarily in urine by glomerular filtration. Small amounts may be excreted in bile and breast milk. Elimination half-life in adults is 2 to 4 hours. In severe renal damage, half-life may extend to 80 hours.

Contraindications and precautions
Kanamycin is contraindicated in patients with known hypersensitivity to kanamycin or any other aminoglycoside, and when given orally, in patients with intestinal obstruction.

Kanamycin should be used cautiously in patients with intestinal mucosal ulcerations because of increased potential for pseudomembranous colitis; in patients with decreased renal function, tinnitus, vertigo, and high-frequency hearing loss who are susceptible to ototoxicity; in patients with dehydration, myasthenia gravis, parkinsonism, and hypocalcemia because the drug can exacerbate these symptoms or illnesses; in neonates and other infants; and in elderly patients.

Interactions
Concomitant use with the following drugs may increase the hazard of nephrotoxicity, ototoxicity, and/or neurotoxicity: methoxyflurane, polymyxin B, vancomycin, amphotericin B, cisplatin, cephalosporins, and other aminoglycosides; hazard of ototoxicity is also increased during use with ethacrynic acid, furosemide, bumetanide, urea, or mannitol. Dimenhydrinate and other antiemetics and antivertigo drugs may mask kanamycin-induced ototoxicity.

Concomitant use with penicillins results in a synergistic bactericidal effect against *Pseudomonas aeruginosa*, *E. coli*, *Klebsiella*, *Citrobacter*, *Enterobacter*, *Serratia*, and *Proteus mirabilis*. However, the drugs are physically and chemically incompatible and are inactivated when mixed or given together. In vivo inactivation has been reported when aminoglycosides and penicillins are used concomitantly.

Kanamycin may potentiate neuromuscular blockade of general anesthetics or neuromuscular blocking agents such as succinylcholine and tubocurarine. Oral kanamycin inhibits vitamin K-producing bacteria in GI tract and may potentiate action of oral anticoagulants; dosage adjustment of anticoagulants may be necessary.

Effects on diagnostic tests
Kanamycin-induced nephrotoxicity may elevate levels of blood urea nitrogen (BUN), nonprotein nitrogen, or serum creatinine and increase urinary excretion of casts.

Adverse reactions
● CNS: headache, lethargy, *neuromuscular blockade with respiratory depression.*
● EENT: ototoxicity (tinnitus, vertigo, hearing loss).
● GI: nausea, vomiting, diarrhea.
● GU: *nephrotoxicity* (cells or casts in the urine, oliguria, proteinuria, decreased creatinine clearance, increased BUN, serum creatinine and nonprotein nitrogen levels).
● Other: hypersensitivity reactions (eosinophilia, fever, rash, urticaria, pruritus), bacterial and fungal superinfections.
   Note: Drug should be discontinued if signs of ototoxicity, nephrotoxicity, or hypersensitivity occur; if severe diarrhea indicates pseudomembranous colitis; or if intestinal obstruction develops. Drug should be discontinued or serum levels monitored if intestinal ulcerations develop, especially in renal impairment.

Overdose and treatment
Clinical signs of overdose include ototoxicity, nephrotoxicity, and neuromuscular toxicity. Remove drug by hemodialysis or peritoneal dialysis. Treatment with calcium salts or anticholinesterases may reverse neuromuscular blockade. After recent ingestion (4 hours or less), empty the stomach by induced emesis or gastric lavage; follow with activated charcoal to reduce absorption.

▶ Special considerations
Besides those relevant to all *aminoglycosides,* consider the following recommendations.
● Oral kanamycin may potentiate effects of oral anticoagulants; monitor prothrombin times and adjust dosage if necessary.
● Darkening of vials does not indicate loss of potency.
● Because kanamycin is dialyzable, patients undergoing hemodialysis may need dosage adjustments.

---

kaolin and pectin mixtures
Donnagel MB*, Kao-Con*, Kaopectate, Kaopectate Concentrate, Kapectolin, K-P, K-Pek, Pectokay

● Pharmacologic classification: adsorbent
● Therapeutic classification: antidiarrheal
● Pregnancy risk category C

How supplied
Liquid: 190 mg kaolin/ml, 4.34 mg pectin/ml
Concentrated liquid: 290 mg kaolin/ml, 6.47 mg pectin/ml

Indications, route, and dosage
Mild, nonspecific diarrhea
Adults: 45 to 90 ml of the concentrate; or 60 to 120 ml of the regular strength suspension after each bowel movement.
Children over age 12: 45 ml concentrate; or 60 ml regular strength suspension after each bowel movement.
Children age 7 to 12: 30 ml concentrate; or 30 to 60 ml regular strength suspension after each bowel movement.
Children age 3 to 6: 15 ml concentrate; or 15 to 30 ml regular strength suspension after each bowel movement.

Pharmacodynamics
Antidiarrheal action: Kaolin/pectin is a clay-based adsorbent with antidiarrheal properties. It presumably adsorbs excess water that accumulates in the bowel during bowel dysfunction.

Pharmacokinetics
● *Absorption:* None.
● *Distribution:* None.
● *Metabolism:* None.
● *Excretion:* Kaolin/pectin is excreted in feces.

Contraindications and precautions
Kaolin/pectin is contraindicated in patients with bowel obstruction because it may exacerbate this condition. It should not be administered continuously for more than 48 hours.

Interactions
When used concomitantly, kaolin/pectin may impair absorption of the following drugs: antidyskinetics, antimuscarinics (especially atropine), chloroquine, dicyclomine, digoxin or digitalis glycosides, lincomycin, phenothiazines, tetracycline antibiotics, and xanthines (especially caffeine, theophylline, aminophylline, dyphylline, and oxtriphylline). Give kaolin/pectin at least 2 hours apart from tetracycline antibiotics or chloroquine; give it 2 hours before or 3 to 4 hours after administering other drugs listed above.

Effects on diagnostic tests
None reported.

Adverse reactions
● GI: constipation, intestinal obstruction; fecal impaction or ulceration in infants, elderly or debilitated patients; after chronic use, drug adsorbs nutrients.
   Note: Kaolin/pectin should be discontinued and therapy re-evaluated if diarrhea persists for more than 48 hours or if fever develops.

Overdose and treatment
No information available.

▶ Special considerations
After administration of the drug via nasogastric tube, tube should be flushed to clear it and ensure drug's passage to stomach.

Information for the patient
● Instruct patient regarding frequency of administration and tell him to shake liquid forms well before using.
● Warn patient to call if diarrhea persists for more than 48 hours or if fever develops.

Breast-feeding
Because kaolin/pectin is not absorbed, it presumably poses no risk to breast-feeding infants.

ketamine hydrochloride
Ketalar

- Pharmacologic classification: dissociative anesthetic
- Therapeutic classification: intravenous anesthetic
- Pregnancy risk category D

How supplied
Available by prescription only
Injection: 10 mg/ml, 50 mg/ml, 100 mg/ml

Indications, route, and dosage
Induction of general anesthesia, especially for short diagnostic or surgical procedures not requiring skeletal muscle relaxation; adjunct to other general anesthetics or low-potency agents, such as nitrous oxide
Adults and children: 1 to 4.5 mg/kg I.V. administered over 60 seconds; or 6.5 to 13 mg/kg I.M. To maintain anesthesia, repeat in increments of half to full initial dose.
To reduce the incidence of psychological manifestations during emergencies
Adults: 1 to 2 mg/kg may be administered at a rate of 0.5 mg/kg/minute with two to five I.V. doses (maximum 15 mg) of diazepam administered in a separate syringe.
†*To obtund consciousness in uncooperative patients ("stunning" effect)*
Adults: 2 to 5 mg/kg I.M.

Pharmacodynamics
Anesthetic action: Ketamine induces a profound sense of dissociation from the environment by direct action on the cortex and limbic system.

Pharmacokinetics
- *Absorption:* Ketamine is absorbed rapidly and well after I.M. injection. Drug induces surgical anesthesia in 30 seconds after I.V. administration, which lasts 5 to 10 minutes. After I.M. injection, anesthesia begins in 3 to 4 minutes and lasts 12 to 25 minutes.
- *Distribution:* Ketamine rapidly enters the CNS.
- *Metabolism:* Ketamine is metabolized by the liver to an active metabolite with one-third the potency of the parent drug.
- *Excretion:* Drug is excreted in the urine.

Contraindications and precautions
Ketamine is contraindicated in patients with schizophrenia or other acute psychosis, because it may exacerbate the condition; in patients with cardiovascular disease in which a sudden rise in blood pressure would be harmful; and in patients allergic to ketamine.

Interactions
Ketamine's cardiovascular effects may be blocked by concomitant use of halothane and, to a lesser extent, by enflurane, leading to significant myocardial depression and hypotension. Prolonged recovery time may occur if ketamine is used with barbiturates or narcotics.

Ketamine may increase the neuromuscular effects of tubocurarine and other nondepolarizing muscle relaxants if used concomitantly. This may result in prolonged respiratory depression. Concomitant use with thyroid hormones may cause hypertension and tachycardia.

Effects on diagnostic tests
None significant.

Adverse reactions
- CNS: tonic-clonic movements, respiratory depression, apnea (if administered too rapidly), hallucinations, confusion, excitement, dreamlike states, irrational behavior, psychic abnormalities.
- CV: hypertension; tachycardia; hypotension and bradycardia if used with halothane; *arrhythmias.*
- DERM: transient erythema, measles-like rash.
- EENT: diplopia, nystagmus, laryngospasm.
- GI: mild anorexia, nausea, vomiting, excessive salivation.
  Note: Drug should be discontinued if hypersensitivity, laryngospasm, or severe hypotension or hypertension occurs.

Overdose and treatment
Clinical signs include respiratory depression. Support respiration, using mechanical ventilation if necessary.

▶ Special considerations
- Patients require physical support because of rapid induction; monitor vital signs perioperatively. Blood pressure begins to rise shortly after injection, peaks at 10% to 50% above preanesthetic levels, and returns to baseline within 15 minutes. Ketamine's effects on blood pressure make it particularly useful in hypovolemic patients as an induction agent that supports blood pressure.
- Keep verbal, tactile, and visual stimulation to a minimum during induction and recovery. Emergence reactions occur in 12% of patients, including dreams, visual imagery, hallucinations, and delirium and may occur for up to 24 hours postoperatively. They may be reduced by using lower dosage of ketamine with I.V. diazepam and can be treated with short- or ultrashort-acting barbiturates. Incidence is lower in patients under age 15 or over age 65 and when drug is given I.M.
- Dissociative and hallucinatory side effects have led to drug abuse.
- Barbiturates are incompatible in the same syringe.
- For direct injection, dilute 100 mg/ml concentration with an equal volume of sterile water for injection, 0.9% sodium chloride, or dextrose 5% in water (D$_5$W). For continuous infusion, prepare a 1 mg/ml solution by adding 5 ml from the 100 mg/ml vial to 500 ml of D$_5$W or 0.9% sodium chloride.

Information for the patient
Warn patient to avoid tasks requiring motor coordination and/or mental alertness for 24 hours after anesthesia.

Geriatric use
Drug should be used with caution, especially in patients with suspected stroke, hypertension, or cardiac disease.

Pediatric use
Drug is safe and especially useful in managing minor surgical or diagnostic procedures or in repeated pro-

---

*Canada only   †Unlabeled clinical use   Italicized adverse reactions are life-threatening.

cedures that require large amounts of analgesia, such as the changing of burn dressings.

ketoconazole
Nizoral

- Pharmacologic classification: imidazole derivative
- Therapeutic classification: antifungal
- Pregnancy risk category C

How supplied
Available by prescription only
Tablets: 200 mg
Oral suspension: 100 mg/5 ml
Cream: 2%

Indications, route, and dosage
Severe fungal infections caused by susceptible organisms
Adults and children weighing more than 40 kg: Initially, 200 mg P.O. daily as a single dose. Dosage may be increased to 400 mg once daily in patients who do not respond to lower dosage.
Children: 5 to 10 mg/kg P.O. daily as a single dose or divided q 12 hours.
Topical treatment of tinea corporis, tinea cruris, and tinea versicolor
Adults and children: Apply once or twice daily for about 2 weeks.

Pharmacodynamics
Antifungal action: Ketoconazole is fungicidal and fungistatic, depending on drug concentrations. It inhibits demethylation of lanosterol, thereby altering membrane permeability and inhibiting purine transport. The in vitro spectrum of activity includes most pathogenic fungi. However, CSF concentrations following oral administration are not predictable. It should not be used to treat fungal meningitis, and specimens should be obtained for susceptibility testing before therapy. Currently available tests may not accurately reflect in vivo activity, so interpret results with caution.

It is used orally to treat disseminated or pulmonary coccidiomycosis, paracoccidiomycosis, or histoplasmosis; oral candidiasis; and candiduria (but low renal clearance may limit its usefulness).

It is also useful in some dermatophytoses, including tinea capitis, tinea cruris, tinea pedis, tinea manus, and tinea unguium (onychomycosis) caused by *Epidermophyton*, *Microsporum*, or *Trichophyton*.

Pharmacokinetics
- *Absorption:* Ketoconazole is converted to the hydrochloride salt before absorption. Absorption is erratic; it is decreased by raised gastric pH and may be increased in extent and consistency by food. Peak plasma concentrations occur at 1 to 4 hours.
- *Distribution:* Ketoconazole is distributed into bile, saliva, cerumen, synovial fluid, and sebum; CSF penetration is erratic and considered minimal. It is 84% to 99% bound to plasma proteins.
- *Metabolism:* Ketoconazole is converted into several inactive metabolites in the liver.
- *Excretion:* Over 50% of a ketoconazole dose is excreted in feces within 4 days; drug and metabolites are

secreted in bile. About 13% is excreted unchanged in urine. It is probably excreted in breast milk. The half-life is biphasic, initially 2 hours, with a terminal half-life of 8 hours.

Contraindications and precautions
Ketoconazole is contraindicated in patients with known hypersensitivity to the drug. It should be used with caution in patients with hepatic disease and in those taking other hepatotoxic drugs, because of possible added toxicity.

Because of the potential for serious hepatic toxicity, ketoconazole should be reserved for severe systemic fungal infections and should not be used for less serious fungal infections of the skin and nails.

Interactions
Concomitant use of ketoconazole with drugs that raise gastric pH (antacids, cimetidine, ranitidine, famotidine, and antimuscarinic agents) decreases absorption of ketoconazole; rifampin may decrease ketoconazole's serum concentration to ineffective levels.

Ketoconazole may enhance the toxicity of other hepatotoxic drugs and the anticoagulant effects of warfarin.

Ketoconazole may interfere with the metabolism of cyclosporine and thus raise serum levels of cyclosporine; concomitant use with phenytoin may alter serum levels of both drugs.

Ketoconazole may intensify the effects of oral sulfonylureas; may interact with ethanol to cause a disulfiram-like reaction.

Effects on diagnostic tests
Ketoconazole has been reported to cause transient elevations of AST (SGOT), ALT (SGPT), and alkaline phosphatase levels; it has also been reported to cause transient alterations of serum cholesterol and triglyceride levels.

Adverse reactions
- CNS: headache, nervousness, dizziness.
- DERM: pruritus.
- Endocrine: decreased serum estradiol, testosterone, or cortisol levels.
- GI: *nausea, vomiting,* abdominal pain, diarrhea, constipation, flatulence.
- Hepatic: elevated liver enzymes, *fatal hepatotoxicity,* hepatitis (in children).
- Other: gynecomastia with breast tenderness in males.
  Note: Drug should be discontinued if liver function tests show marked elevation or if clinical signs of hepatocellular dysfunction occur.

Overdose and treatment
Overdose may cause dizziness, tinnitus, headache, nausea, vomiting, or diarrhea; patients with adrenal hypofunction or patients on long-term corticosteroid therapy may show signs of adrenal crisis.

Treatment includes induced emesis and sodium bicarbonate lavage, followed by activated charcoal and a cathartic, and supportive measures as needed.

▶ Special considerations
- Identify organism, but do not delay therapy for results of laboratory tests.
- Give drug with citrus juice.
- Monitor for signs of hepatotoxicity: persistent nausea, unusual fatigue, jaundice, dark urine, and pale stools.

---

*Canada only †Unlabeled clinical use Italicized adverse reactions are life-threatening.

Information for the patient

● Ketoconazole requires acidity for absorption and is ineffective in patients with achlorhydria.

● Teach achlorhydric patients how to take ketoconazole: dissolve each tablet in 4 ml of aqueous solution of 0.2N hydrochloric acid, and administer through a glass or plastic straw to avoid damaging enamel on patient's teeth. Patient should drink a glass of water after each dose.

● Tell patient to avoid driving or performing other hazardous activities if dizziness or drowsiness occur; these often occur early in treatment but abate as treatment continues.

● Caution patient not to alter dose or dosage interval or to discontinue drug without medical approval. Explain that therapy must continue until active fungal infection is completely eradicated, to prevent recurrence.

● Reassure patient that nausea will subside; to minimize reaction, patient may take drug with food or may divide dosage into two doses.

● Advise patient to avoid self-prescribed preparations for GI distress; some may alter gastric pH levels and interfere with drug action.

● Encourage patient to get specific medical approval before taking any other drugs with ketoconazole.

Pediatric use

Safe use in children under age 2 has not been established.

Breast-feeding

Ketoconazole may be distributed in breast milk. Alternative feeding methods are recommended.

---

ketoprofen
Orudis

● Pharmacologic classification: nonsteroidal anti-inflammatory
● Therapeutic classification: nonnarcotic analgesic, antipyretic, anti-inflammatory
● Pregnancy risk category B (D in third trimester)

How supplied

Available by prescription only
Capsules: 25 mg, 50 mg, 75 mg
Suppositories: 100 mg

Indications, route, and dosage
Rheumatoid arthritis and osteoarthritis
Adults: 50 to 75 mg P.O. t.i.d. or q.i.d. Usual dose is 75 mg t.i.d. Maximum dosage is 300 mg/day.

Pharmacodynamics
Analgesic, antipyretic, and anti-inflammatory actions: Mechanisms of action are unknown; ketoprofen is thought to inhibit prostaglandin synthesis.

Pharmacokinetics
● *Absorption:* Ketoprofen is absorbed rapidly and completely from the GI tract.
● *Distribution:* The drug is highly protein-bound. The extent of body tissue fluid distribution is not known, but therapeutic levels appear to range from 0.4 to 6 mcg/ml.

● *Metabolism:* Ketoprofen is metabolized extensively in the liver.
● *Excretion:* Ketoprofen is excreted in urine as the parent drug and its metabolites.

Contraindications and precautions

Ketoprofen is contraindicated in patients with known hypersensitivity to the drug or in patients in whom aspirin or other nonsteroidal anti-inflammatory drugs (NSAIDs) induce symptoms of asthma, urticaria, or rhinitis.

Serious GI toxicity, such as ulceration or hemorrhage, can occur at any time in patients on chronic NSAID therapy. Ketoprofen should be administered cautiously to patients with a history of peptic ulcer disease, renal dysfunction, or hepatic dysfunction, because the drug may worsen these conditions; and to patients predisposed to fluid retention, such as those with congestive heart failure (CHF) and hypertension, because ketoprofen may increase the risk of fluid retention and edema.

Patients with known "triad" symptoms (aspirin hypersensitivity, rhinitis/nasal polyps, and asthma) are at high risk of bronchospasm. Patients with rectal or anal conditions may experience an exacerbation of these conditions when rectal suppository is used; administer cautiously. NSAIDs may mask the signs and symptoms of acute infection (fever, myalgia, erythema); carefully evaluate patients with high risk (such as those with diabetes).

Interactions

Concomitant use of ketoprofen with anticoagulants and thrombolytic drugs (coumarin derivatives, heparin, streptokinase, or urokinase) may potentiate anticoagulant effects. Bleeding problems may occur if ketoprofen is used with other drugs that inhibit platelet aggregation, such as azlocillin, parenteral carbenicillin, dextran, dipyridamole, mezlocillin, piperacillin, sulfinpyrazone, ticarcillin, valproic acid, cefamandole, cefoperazone, moxalactam, plicamycin, aspirin, salicylates, or other anti-inflammatory agents. Concomitant use with salicylates, anti-inflammatory agents, alcohol, corticotropin, or steroids may cause increased GI adverse effects, including ulceration and hemorrhage. Aspirin may decrease the bioavailability of ketoprofen.

Because of the influence of prostaglandins on glucose metabolism, concomitant use with insulin or oral hypoglycemic agents may potentiate hypoglycemic effects. Ketoprofen may displace highly protein-bound drugs from binding sites. Toxicity may occur with coumarin derivatives, phenytoin, verapamil, or nifedipine. Increased nephrotoxicity may occur with gold compounds, other anti-inflammatory agents, or acetaminophen. Ketoprofen may decrease the renal clearance of methotrexate and lithium. Ketoprofen may decrease the effectiveness of antihypertensive agents and diuretics. Concomitant use with diuretics may increase nephrotoxic potential.

Effects on diagnostic tests

In vitro interactions with glucose determinations have been reported with glucose oxidase and peroxidase methods.

The drug may interfere with serum iron determinations (false increases or decreases depending on method used) and produce false increases in serum bilirubin levels. These interactions were reported with

---

drug concentrations above those seen clinically (60 mg/ml).

Adverse reactions
- CNS: headache, dizziness, CNS inhibition or excitation.
- CV: peripheral edema, palpitations, CHF.
- DERM: rash, urticaria, pruritus.
- EENT: tinnitus, visual disturbances.
- GI: nausea, dyspepsia, abdominal pain, diarrhea, constipation, flatulence, anorexia, vomiting, stomatitis.
- GU: nephrotoxicity, increased BUN level, hematuria.
- HEMA: prolonged bleeding time, anemia.
- Other: elevated liver enzymes, muscle cramps, chills, fever.

Note: Drug should be discontinued if hypersensitivity or signs and symptoms of hepatotoxicity occur.

Overdose and treatment
Clinical manifestations of overdose include nausea and drowsiness.

To treat ketoprofen overdose, empty stomach immediately by inducing emesis with ipecac syrup or by gastric lavage. Administer activated charcoal via nasogastric tube. Provide symptomatic and supportive measures (respiratory support and correction of fluid and electrolyte imbalances). Monitor laboratory parameters and vital signs closely. Hemodialysis may be useful in removing ketoprofen and assisting in care of renal failure.

▶ Special considerations
Besides these relevant to all *NSAIDs*, consider the following recommendations.
- Administer ketoprofen tablets on an empty stomach either 30 minutes before or 2 hours after meals to ensure adequate absorption.
- Ketoprofen capsules may be taken with foods or antacids to minimize GI distress.
- Store ketoprofen suppositories in refrigerator.
- Monitor CNS effects of ketoprofen. Institute safety measures such as assisted walking, raised side rails, and gradual position changes, to prevent injury.
- Watch for possible photosensitivity reactions.
- Monitor laboratory test results for abnormalities.

Information for the patient
- Instruct patient in prescribed drug regimen and proper medication administration.
- Tell patient to seek medical approval before taking any nonprescription medications.
- Caution patient to avoid activities that require alertness or concentration. Instruct him in safety measures to prevent injury.
- Advise patient of potential photosensitivity reactions. Recommend use of sunscreen.
- Instruct patient to report any adverse reactions.

Geriatric use
- Patients over age 60 may be more susceptible to the toxic effects of ketoprofen. Use with caution.
- The effects of this drug on renal prostaglandins may cause fluid retention and edema, a significant drawback for elderly patients and those with congestive heart failure. The manufacturer recommends that the initial dose be reduced by 33% to 50% in geriatric patients.

Pediatric use
Safe use of ketoprofen in children under age 12 has not been established.

Breast-feeding
Most NSAIDs are distributed into breast milk; however, distribution of ketoprofen is unknown. Avoid use of ketoprofen in breast-feeding women.

ketorolac tromethamine
Toradol

- Pharmacologic classification: nonsteroidal anti-inflammatory drug (NSAID)
- Therapeutic classification: analgesic
- Pregnancy risk category B

How supplied
Available by prescription only
Tablets: 10 mg
Injection: 15 mg/ml, 30 mg/ml

Indications, route, and dosage
Short-term management of pain
Adults: Dosage should be based on patient response. Initially, give 30 or 60 mg I.M. as a loading dose, followed by half of the loading dose (15 or 30 mg) q 6 hours on a regular schedule or p.r.n. If pain recurs before 6 hours, dosage may be increased by as much as 50% (up to 60 mg); if drug relieves pain for 8 to 12 hours, increase dosage interval to q 8 to 12 hours, or reduce dose and maintain frequency. The recommended maximum dosage is 150 mg on the first day and 120 mg daily thereafter.

For oral therapy, give 10 mg P.O. q 4 to 6 hours. Maximum oral dose is 40 mg daily.

Pharmacodynamics
Analgesic action: Ketorolac is an NSAID that acts by inhibiting the synthesis of prostaglandins.

Pharmacokinetics
- Absorption: Ketorolac is completely absorbed after I.M. administration. After oral administration, food delays absorption but does not decrease total amount of drug absorbed.
- Distribution: Mean peak plasma levels occur about 30 minutes after a 50-mg dose and range from 2.2 to 3 mcg/ml. The drug is greater than 99% protein-bound.
- Metabolism: Primarily hepatic; a para-hydroxy metabolite and conjugates have been identified; less than 50% of a dose is metabolized. Liver impairment does not substantially alter drug clearance.
- Excretion: Primary excretion is in the urine (greater than 90%); the remainder, in feces. Terminal plasma half-life is 3.8 to 6.3 hours (average 4.5 hours) in young adults; it is substantially prolonged in patients with renal failure.

Contraindications and precautions
Ketorolac is contraindicated in patients hypersensitive to the drug and in those with the complete or partial triad syndrome (nasal polyps, angioedema, and bronchospasm after use of aspirin or other NSAIDs). Because NSAIDs can cause fluid retention and edema,

use cautiously in patients with cardiac disease or hypertension.

NSAIDs can cause serious GI toxicity, especially ulceration or hemorrhage, in patients on chronic therapy.

Use cautiously in patients with a history of GI disease, especially peptic ulcer disease. Long-term use of oral ketorolac is associated with a higher incidence of adverse GI effects than aspirin.

Carefully observe patients with coagulopathies and those receiving anticoagulants. Ketorolac inhibits platelet aggregation and can prolong bleeding time. This effect will disappear within 48 hours of discontinuing the drug. It will not alter platelet count, partial thromboplastin time, or prothrombin time.

Use with caution in patients with impaired hepatic or renal function. Safety in patients with serum creatinine above 5 g/dl or those undergoing dialysis has not been determined.

Interactions
Ketorolac may increase the levels of free (unbound) salicylates or warfarin in the blood. Clinical significance is unknown. NSAIDs increase lithium levels; they decrease methotrexate clearance and increase its toxicity.

Effects on diagnostic tests
Like other NSAIDs, ketorolac has been associated with borderline elevations of one or more liver function test results. Meaningful elevations of AST (SGOT) or ALT (SGPT) – three times the upper normal limit – occur in less than 1% of the patients. Because this drug inhibits platelet aggregation, it can prolong bleeding time.

Adverse reactions
● CNS: drowsiness, dizziness, headache, sweating.
● CV: edema.
● GI: nausea, dyspepsia, GI pain, diarrhea.
● Local: pain at the injection site.

Overdose and treatment
There is no experience with ketorolac overdose in humans. Animal studies revealed that high doses (greater than 100 mg/kg) decreased motor activity and caused diarrhea, pallor, crackles, labored breathing, and vomiting.

Withhold drug and provide supportive treatment.

▶ **Special considerations**
● The drug is intended for short-term management of pain. The rate and severity of adverse reactions should be less than that observed in patients taking NSAIDs on a chronic basis.
● I.M. injections in patients with coagulopathies or those receiving anticoagulants may cause bleeding and hematoma at the site of injection.
● When substituting oral for parenteral ketorolac, do not exceed a total dose of 120 mg (parenteral plus oral drug) on the day of transition and do not give more than 40 mg P.O., the maximum daily dosage for oral ketorolac.

Information for the patient
Warn patient that GI ulceration, bleeding, and perforation can occur at any time, with or without warning, in anyone taking NSAIDs on a chronic basis. Teach patient how to recognize the signs and symptoms of GI bleeding.

Pediatric use
Not recommended for use in children because safety and efficacy have not been established.

Geriatric use
Use lower initial doses (30 mg I.M.) in patients who are over age 65 or less than 110 lb (50 kg). In clinical trials, elderly subjects have exhibited a longer terminal half-life of the drug (average 7 hours in elderly patients as compared with 4.5 hours in healthy young adults).

Breast-feeding
Trace amounts of the drug have been detected in breast milk. Use with caution in breast-feeding women.

labetalol
Normodyne, Trandate

● Pharmacologic classification: alpha- and beta-adrenergic blocking agent
● Therapeutic classification: antihypertensive
● Pregnancy risk category C

How supplied
Available by prescription only
Tablets: 100 mg, 200 mg, 300 mg
Injection: 5 mg/ml in 20- and 40-ml vials

Indications, route, and dosage
Hypertension
Adults: 100 mg P.O. b.i.d. with or without a diuretic. Dosage may be increased by 100 mg b.i.d. daily every 2 or 4 days until optimum response is reached. Usual maintenance dosage is 200 to 400 mg b.i.d.
Severe hypertension and hypertensive emergencies; †pheochromocytoma; and †clonidine withdrawal hypertension
Adults: Initially, 20-mg I.V. bolus slowly over 2 minutes; may repeat injections of 40 to 80 mg every 10 minutes to a maximum dose of 300 mg.

Alternatively, may be given continuous I.V. infusion, at an initial rate of 2 mg/minute until satisfactory response is obtained. Usual cumulative dose is 50 to 200 mg.

Pharmacodynamics
Antihypertensive action: Labetalol inhibits catecholamine access to both beta- and postsynaptic alpha-adrenergic receptor sites. Drug may also have a vasodilating effect.

Pharmacokinetics
● *Absorption:* Oral absorption of labetalol is high (90% to 100%); however, drug undergoes extensive first-pass metabolism in the liver and only about 25% of an oral dose reaches systemic circulation unchanged. Antihypertensive effect is apparent in 20 minutes to 2 hours, peaking in 1 to 4 hours. After direct I.V. administration, antihypertensive effect occurs in 2 to 5 minutes; maximal effect occurs in 5 to 15 minutes.
● *Distribution:* Labetalol is distributed widely throughout the body; drug is approximately 50% protein-bound.
● *Metabolism:* Orally administered labetalol is metabolized extensively in the liver and possibly in GI mucosa.
● *Excretion:* Approximately 5% of a given dose is excreted unchanged in urine; remainder is excreted as

metabolites in urine and feces (biliary elimination). Antihypertensive effect of an oral dose persists for about 8 to 24 hours; after I.V. administration, it lasts about 2 to 4 hours. Plasma half-life is about 5½ hours after I.V. administration or 6 to 8 hours after oral administration.

Contraindications and precautions
Labetalol is contraindicated in patients with known hypersensitivity to the drug; and in patients with overt cardiac failure, severe bradycardia, second- or third-degree atrioventricular block, bronchial asthma, or cardiogenic shock, because the drug may worsen these conditions.

Labetalol should be used cautiously in patients with cardiomyopathy because beta blockade may precipitate congestive heart failure; in patients with pheochromocytoma because paradoxical hypertensive responses have been reported; in patients with diabetes mellitus or hyperthyroidism because labetalol may mask tachycardia (but not sweating or dizziness) caused by hypoglycemia or hyperthyroidism; and in patients with impaired hepatic function caused by increased metabolism (lower dosage may be necessary).

Interactions
Labetalol may potentiate antihypertensive effects of diuretics and other antihypertensive agents; concomitant use of I.V. labetalol and halothane may result in synergistic antihypertensive effect.

Oral cimetidine may increase bioavailability of oral labetalol; therefore, if used concomitantly, labetalol dosage should be adjusted. Glutethimide may decrease bioavailability of oral labetalol, requiring adjustment in labetalol dosage.

Labetalol may antagonize bronchodilation produced by beta-adrenergic agonists.

Concomitant use with tricyclic antidepressants may increase incidence of labetalol-induced tremor.

Effects on diagnostic tests
Labetalol therapy may cause a false-positive increase of urine free and total catecholamine levels when measured by a nonspecific trihydroxindole fluorometric method.

Adverse reactions
• CNS: vivid dreams, fatigue, headache.
• CV: orthostatic hypotension and dizziness, peripheral vascular disease, bradycardia.
• DERM: rash, tingling scalp.
• EENT: nasal stuffiness.
• Endocrine: hypoglycemia without tachycardia.
• GI: nausea, vomiting, dyspepsia.
• GU: sexual dysfunction, urinary retention.
• Hepatic: elevated liver function test results, hepatitis, jaundice.
• Other: increased airway resistance.
Note: Drug should be discontinued if patient develops signs of cardiac failure.

Overdose and treatment
Clinical signs of overdose include severe hypotension, bradycardia, heart failure, and bronchospasm.

After acute ingestion, empty stomach by induced emesis or gastric lavage, and give activated charcoal to reduce absorption. Subsequent treatment is usually symptomatic and supportive.

▶ Special considerations
Besides those relevant to all *beta-adrenergic blocking agents,* consider the following recommendations.
• Unlike other beta blockers, labetalol does not decrease resting heart rate or cardiac output.
• Dosage may need to be reduced in patients with hepatic insufficiency.
• Dizziness is the most troublesome adverse effect; it tends to occur in early stages of treatment, in patients taking diuretics, or in those receiving higher dosages.
• Transient scalp tingling occurs occasionally at the beginning of labetalol therapy. This usually subsides quickly.
• Investigational uses include managing chronic stable angina pectoris, excessive sympathetic activity associated with tetanus, and uncontrolled hypertension before and during anesthesia. Labetalol also may be used (with halothane anesthesia) to produce controlled hypotension.
• Do not mix labetalol with 5% sodium bicarbonate injection because they are not compatible.
• When titrating hospitalized patients from parenteral to oral labetalol, begin with 200 mg, then give 200 to 400 mg P.O. 6 to 12 hours later. Thereafter, give the same total daily dose orally that the patient received I.V., except divided t.i.d.

Information for the patient
Advise patient that transient scalp tingling may occur during initiation of therapy.

Geriatric use
Elderly patients may require lower maintenance dosages of labetalol because of increased bioavailability or delayed metabolism; they also may experience enhanced adverse effects. Use with caution in elderly patients.

Pediatric use
Safety and efficacy of labetalol in children have not been established; use only if potential benefit outweighs risk.

Breast-feeding
Small amounts of labetalol are distributed into breast milk; use drug with caution in breast-feeding women.

lactulose
Cephulac, Chronulac, Duphalac

• Pharmacologic classification: disaccharide
• Therapeutic classification: laxative
• Pregnancy risk category B

How supplied
Available by prescription only
Syrup: 10 g/15 ml

Indications, route, and dosage
Constipation
Adults: 15 to 30 ml P.O. daily.
To prevent and treat portal-systemic encephalopathy, including hepatic precoma and coma in patients with severe hepatic disease
Adults: Initially, 20 to 30 g P.O. (30 to 45 ml) t.i.d. or q.i.d., until two or three soft stools are produced daily.

Usual dosage is 60 to 100 g/day in divided doses; can also be given t.i.d. by retention enema in at least 100 ml of fluid.

Pharmacodynamics

Laxative action: Because lactulose is indigestible, it passes through the GI tract to the colon unchanged; there, it is digested by normally occurring bacteria. The weak acids produced in this manner increase the stool's fluid content and cause distention, thus promoting peristalsis and bowel evacuation.

Lactulose also is used to reduce serum ammonia levels in patients with hepatic disease. Lactulose breakdown acidifies the colon; this, in turn, converts ammonia (NH_3) to ammonium ($NH_4{}^+$), which is not absorbed and is excreted in the stool. Furthermore, this "ion trapping" effect causes ammonia to diffuse from the blood into the colon where it is excreted as well.

Pharmacokinetics

- *Absorption:* Lactulose is absorbed minimally.
- *Distribution:* Lactulose is distributed locally, primarily in the colon.
- *Metabolism:* Lactulose is metabolized by colonic bacteria (absorbed portion is not metabolized).
- *Excretion:* Most lactulose is excreted in feces; absorbed portion is excreted in urine.

Contraindications and precautions

Lactulose is contraindicated in patients who must restrict galactose intake and in patients with appendicitis, acute surgical abdomen, fecal impaction, or intestinal obstruction, because drug may aggravate symptoms of these disorders.

Lactulose should be used with caution in diabetic patients because of sugar content (lactose and galactose). Because of a theoretical potential for accumulation of hydrogen gas in the GI tract, patients receiving lactulose who undergo electrocautery procedures during proctoscopy and colonoscopy should receive a thorough bowel cleansing before the procedure to minimize the risk of explosion.

Interactions

When used concomitantly, neomycin and other antibiotics may theoretically decrease lactulose effectiveness by eliminating bacteria needed to digest it into the active form. Non-absorbable antacids may decrease lactulose effectiveness by preventing a decrease in the pH of the colon.

Effects on diagnostic tests

None reported.

Adverse reactions

- GI: abdominal cramps, belching, flatulence, gaseous distention, diarrhea.
  Note: Drug should be discontinued if severe abdominal pain occurs.

Overdose and treatment

No cases of overdose have been reported. Clinical effects include diarrhea and abdominal cramps.

▶ Special considerations

- After administration of the drug via nasogastric tube, the tube should be flushed with water to clear it and ensure drug's passage to stomach.

- Dilute drug with water or fruit juice to minimize its sweet taste.
- For administration by retention enema, 300 ml of drug should be diluted with 700 ml of water or normal saline solution and administered via rectal balloon catheter (may repeat every 4 to 6 hours). Patient should retain drug for 30 to 60 minutes. If retained less than 30 minutes, dose should be repeated immediately. Begin oral therapy before discontinuing retention enemas.
- Monitor frequency and consistency of stools.

Information for the patient

Advise patient to take drug with juice to improve taste.

Geriatric use

Monitor patient's serum electrolyte levels; elderly patients are more sensitive to possible hypernatremia.

---

leucovorin calcium (citrovorum factor or folinic acid)
Wellcovorin

- Pharmacologic classification: formyl derivative (active reduced form of folic acid)
- Therapeutic classification: vitamin; antidote
- Pregnancy risk category C

How supplied

Available by prescription only
Tablets: 5 mg, 10 mg, 15 mg, 25 mg
Injection: 1-ml ampule (3 mg/ml with 0.9% benzyl alcohol or 5 mg/ml, with methyl and propyl parabens); 50-mg vial (10 mg/ml after reconstitution, contains no preservatives); 5-ml ampule (5 mg/ml, with methyl and propyl parabens)

Indications, route, and dosage
Overdose of folic acid antagonist

Adults and children: P.O., I.M., or I.V. dose equivalent to the weight of the antagonist given as soon as possible after the overdose.
Leucovorin rescue after large methotrexate dose in treatment of cancer

Adults and children: Administer within 6 to 36 hours of last dose of methotrexate according to protocol. Some protocols use 10 mg/m² P.O., I.M., or I.V. q 6 hours for 72 hours. If at 24 hours serum creatinine increases by 50% over premethotrexate levels, leucovorin dose should be increased to 100 mg/m² q 3 hours until methotrexate level is less than 5×10^{-8} M.
Toxic effects of methotrexate used to treat severe psoriasis

Adults and children: 4 to 8 mg I.M. 2 hours after methotrexate dose.
Hematologic toxicity from pyrimethamine therapy

Adults and children: 5 to 15 mg P.O. or I.M. daily.
Hematologic toxicity from trimethoprim therapy

Adults and children: 400 mcg to 15 mg P.O. or I.M. daily.
Megaloblastic anemia from congenital enzyme deficiency

Adults and children: 3 to 6 mg I.M. daily, then 1 mg P.O. daily for life.

Folate-deficient megaloblastic anemias
Adults and children: Up to 1 mg of leucovorin P.O. or I.M. daily. Duration of treatment depends on hematologic response.

Pharmacodynamics
Reversal of folic acid antagonism: Leucovorin is a derivative of tetrahydrofolic acid, the reduced form of folic acid. Leucovorin performs as a cofactor in 1-carbon transfer reactions in the biosynthesis of purines and pyrimidines of nucleic acids. Impairment of thymidylate synthesis in patients with folic acid deficiency may account for defective DNA synthesis, megaloblast formation, and megaloblastic and macrocytic anemias. Leucovorin is a potent antidote for the hematopoietic and reticuloendothelial toxic effects of folic acid antagonists (trimethoprim, pyrimethamine, and methotrexate). "Leucovorin rescue" is used to prevent or decrease toxicity of massive methotrexate doses. Folinic acid "rescues" normal cells without reversing the oncolytic effect of methotrexate.

Pharmacokinetics
● *Absorption:* After oral administration, leucovorin is absorbed rapidly; peak serum folate concentrations occur less than 2 hours following a 15-mg dose. The increase in plasma and serum folate activity after oral administration is mainly from 5-methyltetrahydrofolate (the major transport and storage form of folate in the body).
● *Distribution:* Tetrahydrofolic acid and its derivatives are distributed throughout the body; the liver contains approximately half of the total body folate stores.
● *Metabolism:* Leucovorin is metabolized in the liver.
● *Excretion:* Leucovorin is excreted by the kidneys as 10-formyl tetrahydrofolate and 5,10-methenyl tetrahydrofolate. Duration of action is 3 to 6 hours.

Contraindications and precautions
Leucovorin calcium is contraindicated in patients with allergic reactions after oral and parenteral administration of folic acid. In patients with undiagnosed anemia, leucovorin may mask pernicious anemia by alleviating its hematologic effects while allowing neurologic complications to progress. When leucovorin rescue is used with high-dose methotrexate therapy, leucovorin must be administered until the blood concentration of methotrexate declines to nontoxic levels.

Interactions
Concomitant use of leucovorin with phenytoin will decrease serum phenytoin concentrations and increase frequency of seizures. Although this interaction has occurred solely in patients receiving folic acid, it should be considered when leucovorin is administered. The mechanism by which this occurs appears to be an increased metabolic clearance of phenytoin or a redistribution of phenytoin in the CSF and brain. Phenytoin and primidone may decrease serum folate levels, producing symptoms of folate deficiency. After chemotherapy with folic acid antagonists, parenteral administration is preferable to oral dosing because vomiting may cause loss of the leucovorin. To treat an overdose of folic acid antagonists, leucovorin should be administered within 1 hour if possible; it is usually ineffective after a 4-hour delay. Leucovorin has no effect on other methotrexate toxicities. When given concomitantly, leucovorin will increase toxicity of fluorouracil; lower doses of fluorouracil should be used.

Effects on diagnostic tests
Leucovorin may mask the diagnosis of pernicious anemia.

Adverse reactions
● DERM: rash, pruritus, erythema.
● Other: wheezing.

Overdose and treatment
Leucovorin is relatively nontoxic; no specific recommendations for overdose are reported. However, an excessive amount of leucovorin may nullify the chemotherapeutic effect of folic acid antagonists such as methotrexate.

▶ **Special considerations**
● Realize that leucovorin administration continues until plasma methotrexate levels are below 5 x 10^{-8} M.
● To prepare leucovorin for parenteral use, add 5 ml of bacteriostatic water for injection to vial containing 50 mg of base drug.
● Do not use as sole treatment of pernicious anemia or vitamin B_{12} deficiency.
● To treat overdose of folic acid antagonists, use the drug within 1 hour; it is not effective after a 4-hour delay.
● Monitor patient for rash, wheezing, pruritus, and urticaria, which can be signs of drug allergy.
● Monitor serum creatinine levels daily to detect possible renal function impairment.
● When giving more than 25 mg, drug should be administered parenterally.
● Store at room temperature in a light-resistant container, not in high-moisture areas.

Information for the patient
Emphasize importance of taking leucovorin only under medical supervision.

Pediatric use
● Drug may increase frequency of seizures in susceptible children.
● Do not use diluents containing benzyl alcohol when reconstituting drug for neonates.

Breast-feeding
It is unknown whether leucovorin is distributed into breast milk; use with caution in breast-feeding women.

---

leuprolide acetate
Lupron, Lupron Depot

● Pharmacologic classification: gonadotropic releasing hormone
● Therapeutic classification: antineoplastic, luteinizing hormone-releasing hormone (LHRH) analog
● Pregnancy risk category X

How supplied
Available by prescription only
Injection: 5 mg/ml in 2.8-ml multiple-dose vials
Suspension for depot injection: 3.75 mg, 7.5 mg

Indications, route, and dosage
Dosage and indications may vary. Check current literature for recommended protocol.
Management of advanced prostate cancer
Adults: 7.5 mg I.M. (depot injection) once monthly or 1 mg S.C. daily.
Treatment of endometriosis
Adults: 3.75 mg I.M. (depot injection) once monthly for a maximum of 6 months.

Pharmacodynamics
Antineoplastic action: Leuprolide is a synthetic analogue of luteinizing hormone-releasing hormone (LH-RH). It inhibits gonadotropin secretion and androgen or estrogen synthesis. Because of this effect, leuprolide may inhibit the growth of hormone-dependent tumors.
Hormonal action: Because leuprolide lowers levels of sex hormones, it causes a decrease in the size of endometrial implants, resulting in decreased dysmenorrhea and pelvic pain in women with endometriosis.

Pharmacokinetics
● *Absorption:* Leuprolide is a polypeptide molecule that is destroyed in the GI tract. After subcutaneous administration, the drug is rapidly, and essentially completely, absorbed.
● *Distribution:* Distribution in humans has not been determined; however, it is suggested that high concentrations distribute into kidney, liver, pineal, and pituitary tissue. Approximately 7% to 15% of a dose is bound to plasma proteins.
● *Metabolism:* The metabolic fate of leuprolide is unclear, but it may be metabolized in the anterior pituitary and hypothalamus, similar to endogenous gonadotropin-releasing hormone.
● *Excretion:* The plasma elimination half-life has been reported to be 3 hours.

Contraindications and precautions
Leuprolide is contraindicated in patients with hypersensitivity to gonadotropin hormone releasing hormone (GNRH) and GNRH analogs; in women with undiagnosed vaginal bleeding; and in pregnancy.

Use with caution in patients who are sensitive to benzyl alcohol, a preservative used in some formulations.

Interactions
None reported.

Effects on diagnostic tests
Serum acid phosphatase and testosterone levels initially increase then decrease with continued therapy.

Adverse reactions
● CNS: dizziness, numbness, headache, blurred vision, muscle pain.
● CV: angina, *MI, arrhythmias, CHF.*
● DERM: pruritus, rash.
● Endocrine: hot flashes, breast tenderness, gynecomastia.
● GI: nausea, vomiting, constipation, anorexia.
● GU: infertility, impaired spermatogenesis.
● Local: redness and induration at injection site.
● Other: alopecia, *pulmonary embolus,* peripheral edema, decreased libido, transient bone pain during first week of treatment.

Overdose and treatment
No information available.

▶ Special considerations
● Use a 22 gauge needle for injection.
● When treating endometriosis, administer for a maximum of 6 months. Safety and efficacy of retreatment is unknown.
● Discard solution if particulate matter is visible or if the solution is discolored.
● Erythema or induration may develop at injection site.
● When used for the treatment of prostate cancer, leuprolide may produce worsening of signs and symptoms of disease during the first 1 to 2 weeks of therapy. Temporary paresthesia and weakness may occur during the first week of therapy.
● Measure serum testosterone and acid phosphatase levels before and during therapy.
● No unusual adverse effects were observed in patients who had received 20 mg daily for 2 years.

Information for the patient
● Reassure patient that bone pain is transient and will disappear after about 1 week.
● Patient may experience a temporary reaction of burning, itching, and swelling at the injection site. Tell patient to report persistent reactions.
● Advise patient to continue taking medication even if he experiences a sense of well-being.

levamisole hydrochloride
Ergamisol

● Pharmacologic classification: immunomodulator
● Therapeutic classification: antineoplastic
● Pregnancy risk category C

How supplied
Available by prescription only
Tablets: 50 mg

Indications, route, and dosage
Adjuvant treatment in combination with fluorouracil after surgical resection in patients with Dukes' stage C colon cancer
Adults: Initially, 50 mg P.O. q 8 hours for 3 days starting 7 to 30 days after surgery. Repeat q 14 days for 1 year. Administer with fluorouracil 450 mg/m² daily by rapid I.V. push for 5 days concomitant with a 3-day course of levamisole, starting 21 to 34 days after surgery.

If levamisole therapy begins 7 to 20 days after surgery, start fluorouracil with the second course of levamisole at 21 to 24 days. If levamisole is initiated 21 to 30 days after surgery, start fluorouracil simultaneously with the first course of therapy.

Maintenance: 50 mg P.O. q 8 hours for 3 days q 2 weeks. Give with fluorouracil 450 mg/m² daily by rapid I.V. push weekly beginning 28 days after initiation of the 5-day course.

Pharmacodynamics
Antineoplastic action: Levamisole is an immunomodulator and its mechanism of action in combination with fluorouracil is unknown. Its effects on the immune sys-

tem are complete, but it appears to restore depressed immune function rather than stimulate response to above-normal levels. It can also stimulate antibody formation, enhance T-cell responses by stimulating T-cell activation and proliferation; potentiate monocyte and macrophage formation, including phagocytosis and chemotaxis; increase neutrophil mobility adherence and chemotaxis; and inhibit alkaline phosphatase. Levamisole also has cholinergic activity.

Pharmacokinetics
• *Absorption:* Levamisole is rapidly absorbed from the GI tract with peak plasma levels obtained within 1.5 to 2 hours.
• *Distribution:* Unknown.
• *Metabolism:* Extensively metabolized by the liver.
• *Excretion:* 70% of metabolites are excreted in urine over 3 days; 5%, in feces; less than 5% of unchanged drug is excreted in urine; less than 2%, in feces.

Contraindications and precautions
Contraindicated in patients with known hypersensitivity to levamisole or its components. Use with caution in patients with impaired renal or hepatic function.

Interactions
Disulfiram-like reaction occurs if used concurrently with alcohol. Concomitant administration with phenytoin has increased phenytoin levels. Monitor plasma phenytoin levels and decrease dosage as needed.

Adverse reactions
• CNS: fatigue, dizziness, headache, paresthesia, ataxia, somnolence, depression, nervousness, insomnia, anxiety, forgetfulness, blurred vision, confusion, paranoia, *seizures,* tremor.
• CV: chest pain.
• DERM: dermatitis, alopecia, pruritus, skin discoloration, urticaria.
• EENT: abnormal tearing, blurred vision, conjunctivitis, epistaxis, altered sense of smell.
• GI: nausea, vomiting, diarrhea, constipation, flatulence, stomatitis, anorexia, abdominal pain, dyspepsia.
• HEMA: *leukopenia, thrombocytopenia,* anemia, *granulocytopenia, agranulocytosis, neutropenia.*
• Other: fever, rigors, edema, taste perversion or metallic taste, infection, hyperbilirubinemia, flulike syndrome, arthralgia, myalgia.

Overdose and treatment
Fatalities have been reported after ingestion of 15 mg/kg by a 3-year-old child and of 32 mg/kg by an adult. No further clinical information is available. Gastric lavage is recommended along with symptomatic and supportive measures.

▶ Special considerations
• Levamisole should not be used in higher than recommended dosage or administered more frequently than indicated.
• Patient should be out of hospital, be ambulatory, maintaining normal oral nutrition, have well-healed wounds, and be fully recovered from any postsurgical complications before therapy with levamisole is initiated.
• If WBC count is 2,500 to 3,500/mm³, defer fluorouracil dose until the count is above 3,500/mm³. If WBC count is less than 2,500/mm³, defer fluorouracil until WBC count is above 3,500/mm³ and then reduce the dose

by 20%. If WBC count remains below 2,500/mm³ for more than 10 days even after deferring fluorouracil, discontinue levamisole. Defer both if platelet counts are below 100,000/mm³.
• If stomatitis or diarrhea develops during initial fluorouracil administration schedule, discontinue the course before the full 5 doses are administered. If stomatitis or diarrhea occurs during weekly maintenance therapy, defer the next dose of fluorouracil until it subsides. If adverse reactions are moderate to severe, reduce fluorouracil by 20% when treatment is resumed.
• Flulike syndrome frequently accompanies the onset of agranulocytosis but may also occur in the absence of agranulocytosis. Instruct patient to report any flulike symptoms immediately.
• Obtain CBC with differential, platelet counts, electrolytes, and liver function tests before initiation of therapy. CBC with differential and platelet counts should be performed weekly before each fluorouracil treatment; electrolyte and liver function tests, every 3 months for 1 year. Modify doses as needed.

Information for the patient
• Advise patient to use a soft toothbrush and electric razor to avoid trauma and excessive bleeding.
• Tell patient to report any unusual bruising or bleeding, persistent fever or flulike symptoms, sore throat, or weakness.

Pediatric use
Safety and efficacy have not been established.

Breast-feeding
It is unknown if levamisole is excreted in breast milk. The potential for serious adverse reactions in infants must be considered.

---

levobunolol hydrochloride
Betagan

• Pharmacologic classification: beta-adrenergic blocking agent
• Therapeutic classification: antiglaucoma agent
• Pregnancy risk category C

How supplied
Available by prescription only
Ophthalmic solution: 0.25%, 0.5%

Indications, route, and dosage
Chronic open-angle glaucoma and ocular hypertension
Adults: Instill 1 to 2 drops (0.5% solution) daily or 1 to 2 drops (0.25% solution) b.i.d. in eye(s).

Pharmacodynamics
Antiglaucoma action: Levobunolol is a nonselective beta-adrenergic blocking agent that reduces intraocular pressure. Exact mechanisms are unknown, but the drug appears to reduce formation of aqueous humor.

Pharmacokinetics
• *Absorption:* Onset of activity usually occurs within 60 minutes, with peak effect in 2 to 6 hours.
• *Distribution:* Unknown.

- *Metabolism:* Unknown.
- *Excretion:* Duration of effect is 24 hours.

Contraindications and precautions
Levobunolol is contraindicated in patients with hypersensitivity to any component of the preparation, or in patient with bronchial asthma, severe chronic obstructive pulmonary disease, sinus bradycardia, second- or third-degree AV block, cardiac failure, or cardiogenic shock, because it may worsen these symptoms or disorders.

It should be used with caution in patients with angle-closure glaucoma (use with a miotic), in patients with muscle weakness (myasthenic-like symptoms), and in patients with a history of heart failure, restricted pulmonary function, or diabetes mellitus.

Interactions
Levobunolol may increase the systemic effect of oral beta blockers, enhance the hypotensive and bradycardiac effect of reserpine and catecholamine-depleting agents, and increase reductions in intraocular pressure induced by pilocarpine, epinephrine, or carbonic anhydrase inhibitors.

Effects on diagnostic tests
Although oral beta blockers have been reported to decrease serum glucose levels from blockage of normal glycogen release after hypoglycemia, such instances have not been reported with the use of ophthalmic beta blockers.

Adverse reactions
- CNS: headache, dizziness, depression, syncope, lethargy, transient ataxia, *cerebral ischemia, cerebrovascular accident.*
- CV: bradycardia, *arrhythmias,* heart block, hypotension.
- DERM: urticaria, pruritus.
- Eye: transient burning and stinging, blepharoconjunctivitis, occasional tearing, itching, erythema, decreased visual acuity. Long-term use may decrease corneal sensitivity.
- GI: nausea, heartburn, diarrhea.
- Respiratory: *bronchospasm.*
  Note: Drug should be discontinued if symptoms of systemic toxicity occur.

Overdose and treatment
Overdose is extremely rare with ophthalmic use. However, usual manifestations include bradycardia, hypotension, bronchospasm, heart block, and cardiac failure.

After accidental ingestion, emesis is most effective if initiated within 30 minutes, providing the patient is not obtunded, comatose, or having seizures. Follow with activated charcoal. Treat bradycardia, conduction defects, and hypotension with I.V. fluids, glucagon, atropine, or isoproterenol. Treat bronchoconstriction with I.V. aminophylline, and seizures with I.V. diazepam.

▶ Special considerations
- Cardiac output is reduced in both healthy patients and those with heart disease. May decrease heart rate and blood pressure. Produces beta blockade in bronchi and bronchioles. No effect on pupil size or accommodation.
- In some patients, a few weeks' treatment may be required to stabilize pressure-lowering response; determine intraocular pressure after 4 weeks of treatment.
- Levobunolol is faster-acting than timolol.

Information for the patient
- Warn patient not to touch dropper to eye or surrounding tissue.
- Show patient how to instill drug. Teach patient to press lacrimal sac lightly for 1 minute after drug administration, to decrease chance of systemic absorption.
- Remind patient not to blink more than usual or to close eyes tightly during treatment.

Geriatric use
Drug should be used with caution in elderly patients with cardiac or pulmonary disease, who may experience exacerbation of symptoms, depending on the extent of systemic absorption.

---

levodopa (L-dopa)
Dopar, Larodopa

- Pharmacologic classification: precursor of dopamine
- Therapeutic classification: antiparkinsonism agent
- Pregnancy risk category C

How supplied
Available by prescription only
Tablets: 100 mg, 250 mg, 500 mg
Capsules: 100 mg, 250 mg, 500 mg

Indications, route, and dosage
Parkinsonism
Levodopa is indicated in treating idiopathic, postencephalitic, arteriosclerotic parkinsonism and symptomatic parkinsonism that may follow injury to the nervous system by carbon monoxide intoxication and manganese intoxication.
Adults: Initially, 0.5 to 1 g P.O. daily, given b.i.d., t.i.d., or q.i.d. with food; increase by no more than 0.75 g daily q 3 to 7 days, as tolerated. The usual optimal dose is 3 to 6 g daily divided into three doses. Do *not* exceed 8 g daily, except for exceptional patients. A significant therapeutic response may not be obtained for 6 months. Larger dose requires close supervision.

Pharmacodynamics
Antiparkinsonism action: Precise mechanism has not been established. A small percentage of each dose crossing the blood-brain barrier is decarboxylated. The dopamine then stimulates dopaminergic receptors in the basal ganglia to enhance the balance between cholinergic and dopaminergic activity, resulting in improved modulation of voluntary nerve impulses transmitted to the motor cortex.

Pharmacokinetics
- *Absorption:* Levodopa is absorbed rapidly from small intestine by an active amino acid transport system, with 30% to 50% reaching general circulation.
- *Distribution:* Levodopa is distributed widely to most body tissues, but not to the CNS, which receives less than 1% of dose because of extensive metabolism in the periphery.

- *Metabolism:* 95% of levodopa is converted to dopamine by L-aromatic amino acid decarboxylase enzyme in the lumen of the stomach and intestines and on the first pass through the liver.
- *Excretion:* Levodopa is excreted primarily in urine; 80% of dose is excreted within 24 hours as dopamine metabolites. The half-life is 1 to 3 hours.

Contraindications and precautions

Levodopa is contraindicated in patients with known hypersensitivity and in patients receiving monamine oxidase (MAO) inhibitors. Because levodopa may activate a malignant melanoma, do not use in patients with suspicious undiagnosed skin lesions or history of melanoma.

Drug should be used cautiously in patients with cardiovascular, renal, hepatic, or endocrine disease; in patients with history of myocardial infarction with residual arrhythmias, peptic ulcer, convulsions, psychiatric disorders, chronic wide-angle glaucoma, diabetes, pulmonary diseases, or bronchial asthma; and in patients receiving antihypertensives.

Interactions

Anesthetics or hydrocarbon inhalation may cause cardiac arrhythmias because of increased endogenous dopamine concentration. (Levodopa should be discontinued 6 to 8 hours before administration of anesthetics such as halothane.)

Antacids containing calcium, magnesium, or sodium bicarbonate may increase absorption of levodopa.

Concurrent use of anticonvulsants (such as hydantoin), benzodiazepines, phenothiazines, haloperidol, papaverine, rauwolfia alkaloids, or thioxanthenes may decrease therapeutic effects of levodopa.

Antihypertensives used concurrently with levodopa may produce increased hypotensive effect.

Methyldopa may alter the antiparkinsonian effects of levodopa and may produce additive toxic CNS effects.

Combined use with MAO inhibitors may cause a hypertensive crisis. MAO inhibitors should be discontinued for 2 to 4 weeks before starting levodopa.

Pyridoxine in a small dose (10 mg) reverses the antiparkinsonian effects of levodopa.

Sympathomimetics may increase the risk of cardiac arrhythmias (dosage reduction of the sympathomimetic is recommended; the administration of carbidopa with levodopa reduces the tendency of sympathomimetics to cause dopamine-induced cardiac dysrhythmias).

Anticholinergics used with levodopa may produce a mild synergy and increased efficacy (gradual reduction in anticholinergic dosage is necessary).

Tricyclic antidepressants may increase sympathetic activity, with sinus tachycardia and hypertension.

Effects on diagnostic tests

Coombs' test occasionally becomes positive during extended therapy. Colorimetric test for uric acid has shown false elevations. Copper-reduction method has shown false-positive results for urine glucose; glucose oxidase method has shown false-negative results. Levodopa also may interfere with tests for urine ketones.

Adverse reactions

- CNS: choreiform, dystonic, dyskinetic movements; involuntary grimacing, head movements, myoclonic body jerks, ataxia, tremors, muscle twitching; bradykinetic episodes; psychiatric disturbances, memory loss, nervousness, anxiety, disturbing dreams, euphoria, malaise, fatigue; severe depression, suicidal tendencies, dementia, delirium, hallucinations (may necessitate reduction or withdrawal of drug).
- CV: orthostatic hypotension, irregular heartbeat, tachycardia, palpitations, hypertension, phlebitis.
- DERM: diaphoresis, rash, alopecia, scleroderma-like skin changes.
- EENT: blepharospasm, diplopia, blurred vision, dilated pupils, rhinorrhea, dry mouth, bitter taste.
- GI: nausea, vomiting, anorexia, weight loss (at start of therapy), constipation, flatulence, diarrhea, epigastric pain, hiccups, sialorrhea, dry mouth, burning tongue, bitter taste, abdominal distress, dysphagia.
- GU: urinary frequency, retention, incontinence; darkened urine; priapism; increased libido.
- HEMA: hemolytic anemia, leukopenia, anemia, blood dyscrasias.
- Hepatic: hepatotoxicity.
- Other: transiently increased levels of BUN, AST (SGOT), ALT (SGPT), LDH, bilirubin, alkaline phosphatase; protein-bound iodine; decreased glucose tolerance; dark perspiration; and hyperventilation; leukopenia requiring temporary cessation of levodopa therapy.

Overdose and treatment

Clinical manifestations of overdose include spasm or closing of eyelids, irregular heartbeat or palpitations. Treatment includes immediate gastric lavage, maintenance of an adequate airway, and judicious administration of I.V. fluids and may include antiarrhythmic drugs if necessary. Pyridoxine P.O. 10 to 25 mg has been reported to reverse toxic and therapeutic effects of levodopa. (Its usefulness has not been established in acute overdose.)

▶ Special considerations

- Drug should be taken between meals and with low-protein snack to maximize drug absorption. Foods high in protein appear to interfere with transport of the drug.
- Maximum effectiveness of medication may not occur for several weeks or months after therapy begins.
- Carefully monitor patients also receiving antihypertensive medication or hypoglycemic agents for possible drug interactions. Stop MAO inhibitors at least 2 weeks before levodopa therapy begins.
- Adjust dosage according to patient's response and tolerance. Observe and monitor vital signs, especially while adjusting dose.
- Monitor patient for muscle twitching and blepharospasm (twitching of eyelids), which may be an early sign of drug overdose.
- Patients on long-term therapy should be tested regularly for diabetes and acromegaly; check blood tests and liver and kidney function studies periodically for adverse effects. Leukopenia may require cessation of therapy.
- Because of the risk of precipitating neuroleptic malignant levodopa dosage is reduced abruptly or discontinued.
- If restarting therapy after a long period of interruption, adjust drug dosage gradually to previous level.
- Patients who must undergo surgery should continue levodopa as long as oral intake is permitted, usually 6 to 24 hours before surgery. Drug should be resumed as soon as patient is able to take oral medication.

● Protect from heat, light, and moisture. If preparation darkens, it has lost potency and should be discarded.
● Monitor serum laboratory tests periodically for changes. Coombs' test occasionally becomes positive during extended use. Expect uric acid elevation with colorimetric method but not with uricase method.
● Alkaline phosphatase, AST (SGOT), ALT (SGPT), LDH, bilirubin, BUN, and protein-bound iodine levels show transient elevations in patients receiving levodopa; white blood cell, hemoglobin, and hematocrit levels show occasional reduction.
● Although controversial, a medically supervised period of drug discontinuance (drug holiday) may reestablish the effectiveness of a lower dose regimen.
● Combination of levodopa-carbidopa usually reduces amount of levodopa needed, thus reducing incidence of adverse reactions.
● Levodopa has also been used to relieve pain of herpes zoster.
● Pills may be crushed and mixed with applesauce or baby-food fruits for patients who have difficulty swallowing pills.

Information for the patient
● Warn patient and family not to increase drug dose without specific instruction. (They may be tempted to do this as disease symptoms of parkinsonism progress.)
● Explain that therapeutic response may not occur for up to 6 months.
● Advise patient and family that multivitamin preparations, fortified cereals, and certain nonprescription medications may contain pyridoxine (vitamin B_6), which can reverse the effects of levodopa.
● Warn patient of possible dizziness and orthostatic hypotension, especially at start of therapy. Tell patient to change position slowly and dangle legs before getting out of bed. Instruct patient in use of elastic stockings to control the adverse reaction if appropriate.
● Instruct patient in signs and symptoms of adverse reactions and therapeutic effects and the need to report any changes.
● Tell patient to take a missed dose as soon as possible; skip dose if next scheduled dose is within 2 hours, but do not double up doses.
● Advise the patient not to take levodopa with food, but that eating something about 15 minutes after administration may help reduce GI upset.

Geriatric use
● Smaller doses may be required because of reduced tolerance to the effects of levodopa.
● Elderly patients, especially those with osteoporosis, should resume normal activity gradually, because increased mobility may increase the risk of fractures.
● Elderly patients are more likely to develop psychic side effects such as anxiety, confusion, or nervousness; those with pre-existing coronary disease are more susceptible to levodopa's cardiac effects.

Pediatric use
Safe use of levodopa in children under age 12 has not been established.

Breast-feeding
Levodopa may inhibit lactation and should not be used by breast-feeding women.

levodopa-carbidopa
Sinemet

● Pharmacologic classification: decarboxylase inhibitor-dopamine precursor combination
● Therapeutic classification: antiparkinsonian agent
● Pregnancy risk category C

How supplied
Available by prescription only
Tablets: 10 mg carbidopa with 100 mg levodopa (Sinemet 10-100), 25 mg carbidopa with 100 mg levodopa (Sinemet 25-100), 25 mg carbidopa with 250 mg levodopa (Sinemet 25-250)

Indications, route, and dosage
Parkinsonism
Adults: 3 to 6 tablets of 25 mg carbidopa/250 mg levodopa daily in divided doses. Do not exceed 8 tablets of 25 mg carbidopa/250 mg levodopa daily. Optimum daily dosage must be determined by careful titration for each patient.

Most patients respond to a 100 mg/25 mg combination (one tablet t.i.d.). Dose may be increased q 1 or 2 days. Maintenance therapy must be carefully adjusted according to individual tolerance and desired therapeutic response.

The daily dose of carbidopa should be 70 mg or above to suppress the peripheral metabolism of levodopa but should not exceed 200 mg.

Pharmacodynamics
Decarboxylase inhibiting action: Carbidopa inhibits the peripheral decarboxylation of levodopa, thus slowing its conversion to dopamine in extracerebral tissues. This results in an increased availability of levodopa for transport to the brain, where it undergoes decarboxylation to dopamine.

Pharmacokinetics
● *Absorption:* 40% to 70% of the dose is absorbed after oral administration. Plasma levodopa concentrations are increased when carbidopa and levodopa are administered concomitantly because carbidopa inhibits the peripheral metabolism of levodopa.
● *Distribution:* Carbidopa is distributed widely in body tissues except the CNS. Levodopa is also distributed into breast milk.
● *Metabolism:* Carbidopa is not metabolized extensively. It inhibits metabolism of levodopa in the GI tract, thus increasing its absorption from the GI tract and its concentration in plasma.
● *Excretion:* 30% of dose is excreted unchanged in urine within 24 hours. When given with carbidopa, the amount of levodopa excreted unchanged in urine is increased by about 6%. The half-life is 1 to 2 hours.

Contraindications and precautions
Levodopa-carbidopa is contraindicated in patients known to be hypersensitive to either drug and in patients with bronchial asthma, emphysema, or other severe pulmonary disorders; severe cardiovascular disease; narrow-angle glaucoma; history of or suspected

---

melanoma; or history of myocardial infarction, because the drug may exacerbate symptoms of these disorders.

Interactions

Concomitant use with amantadine, benztropine, procyclidine, or trihexyphenidyl may increase the efficacy of levodopa. Bromocriptine may produce additive effects, allowing reduced levodopa dosage.

Anesthetics or hydrocarbon inhalation may cause cardiac arrhythmias because of increased endogenous dopamine concentration. (Levodopa-carbidopa should be discontinued 6 to 8 hours before administration of anesthetics such as halothane.)

Antacids containing calcium, magnesium, or sodium bicarbonate may increase absorption of levodopa.

Concurrent use of anticonvulsants (hydantoin), benzodiazepines, droperidol, haloperidol, loxapine, metyrosine, papaverine, phenothiazines, rauwolfia alkaloids, and thioxanthenes may decrease therapeutic effects of levodopa.

Concomitant use with antihypertensives may increase the hypotensive effect.

Methyldopa may alter the antiparkinsonian effects of levodopa and may produce additive toxic CNS effects. Molindone may inhibit antiparkinsonian effects of levodopa by blocking dopamine receptors in the brain.

Concurrent use of monoamine oxidase (MAO) inhibitors may cause a hypertensive crisis. MAO inhibitors should be discontinued for 2 to 4 weeks before starting levodopa-carbidopa.

Sympathomimetics may increase the risk of cardiac arrhythmias (reduced dosage of the sympathomimetic is recommended; however, the administration of carbidopa with levodopa reduces the tendency of sympathomimetics to cause dopamine-induced cardiac arrhythmias).

Effects on diagnostic tests

● Antiglobulin determinations (Coombs' test) are occasionally positive after long-term use.
● Levodopa-carbidopa therapy may elevate serum gonadotropin levels.
● Serum and urine uric acid determinations may show false elevations.
● Thyroid function determinations may inhibit thyroid stimulating hormone response to protirelin.
● Urine glucose determinations using copper reduction method may show false-positive results; with the glucose oxidase method, false-negative results.
● Urine ketone determination using dip-stick method, urine norepinephrine determinations, and urine protein determinations using Lowery test may show false-positive results.
● Systemic effects of this drug may elevate levels of BUN, ALT (SGPT), alkaline phosphatase, AST (SGOT), serum bilirubin, lactic dehydrogenase, and serum protein-bound iodine.

Adverse reactions

● CNS: choreiform, dystonic, dyskinetic movements; involuntary grimacing, head movements, myoclonic body jerks, ataxia, tremors, muscle twitching; bradykinetic episodes; psychiatric disturbances, confusion, memory loss, nervousness, anxiety, disturbing dreams, euphoria, malaise, weakness, fatigue; severe depression, *suicidal tendencies,* dementia, delirium, hallucinations (may necessitate reduction or withdrawal of drug).
● CV: orthostatic hypotension, cardiac irregularities, flushing, hypertension, phlebitis.
● EENT: blepharospasm, blurred vision, diplopia, mydriasis or miosis, widening of palpebral fissures, activation of latent Horner's syndrome, oculogyric crises, nasal discharge.
● GI: nausea, vomiting, anorexia, weight loss may occur at start of therapy; constipation; flatulence; diarrhea; epigastric pain; hiccups; sialorrhea; dry mouth; bitter taste.
● GU: urinary frequency, retention, incontinence; darkened urine; excessive and inappropriate sexual behavior; priapism.
● HEMA: *hemolytic anemia.*
● Hepatic: hepatotoxicity.
● Other: dark perspiration, hyperventilation.
Note: Drug should be discontinued if unusual and uncontrollable body movements, irregular heartbeat or palpitations, spasms or closing of eyelids, or severe and continuous nausea and vomiting occur.

Overdose and treatment

There have been no reports of overdosage with carbidopa. Clinical manifestations of levodopa overdose are irregular heartbeat and palpitations, severe continuous nausea and vomiting, spasm or closing of eyelids.

Treatment of overdose includes immediate gastric lavage and antiarrhythmic medication if necessary. Pyridoxine is not effective in reversing the actions of carbidopa and levodopa combinations.

▶ Special considerations

● Carefully monitor patients also receiving antihypertensive or hypoglycemic agents. Discontinue MAO inhibitors at least 2 weeks before therapy begins.
● Dosage is adjusted according to patient's response and tolerance to the drug. Therapeutic and adverse reactions occur more rapidly with levodopa-carbidopa combination than with levodopa alone. Observe and monitor vital signs, especially while dosage is being adjusted; report significant changes.
● Muscle twitching and blepharospasm (twitching of eyelids) may be an early sign of overdose.
● Patients on long-term therapy should be tested regularly for diabetes and acromegaly; periodically repeat blood test, liver and kidney function studies.
● If patient is being treated with levodopa, discontinue at least 8 hours before starting levodopa-carbidopa.
● The combination drug usually reduces the amount of levodopa needed by 75%, thereby reducing the incidence of adverse reactions.
● Pyridoxine (vitamin B6) does not reverse the beneficial effects of levodopa-carbidopa. Multivitamins can be taken without fear of losing control of symptoms.
● If therapy is interrupted temporarily, the usual daily dosage may be given as soon as patient resumes oral medications.
● Maximum effectiveness of medication may not occur for several weeks or months after therapy begins.

Information for the patient

● Instruct patient to report adverse reactions and therapeutic effects.
● Warn patient of possible dizziness or orthostatic hypotension, especially at the start of therapy. Patient should change position slowly and dangle legs before getting out of bed. Elastic stockings may control this adverse reaction in some patients.

- Tell patient to take food shortly after taking medication to relieve gastric irritation.
- Tell patient medication may cause darkening of the urine or sweat.
- Tell patient to take a missed dose as soon as possible, to skip a missed dose if next scheduled dose is within 2 hours, and never to double-dose.

Geriatric use
- In elderly patients, smaller doses may be required because of reduced tolerance to the effects of levodopa-carbidopa. Elderly patients, especially those with osteoporosis, should resume normal activity gradually because increased mobility may increase the risk of fractures.
- Elderly patients are especially vulnerable to psychic side effects, such as anxiety, confusion, or nervousness; those with preexisting coronary disease are more susceptible to cardiac effects.

Pediatric use
Safe use of levodopa-carbidopa in children under age 18 has not been established.

Breast-feeding
Because levodopa may inhibit lactation, the drug should not be used by breast-feeding women.

---

levonorgestrel
Norplant System

- Pharmacologic classification: progestin
- Therapeutic classification: contraceptive
- Pregnancy risk category X

How supplied
Available by prescription only
Implants: 36 mg in each of 6 silastic capsules; kits also include trocar, scalpel, forceps, syringe, two needles, package of skin closures, three packages of gauze sponges, stretch bandages, and surgical drape

Indications, route, and dosage
Long-term (up to 5 years), reversible prevention of pregnancy
Adults: Six silastic capsules are surgically implanted in the superficial plane beneath the skin of a woman's upper arm. Initially, 85 mcg/day of levonorgestrel is provided, declining to 50 mcg/day by 9 months, 35 mcg/day by 18 months, and 30 mcg/day thereafter.

Pharmacodynamics
Contraceptive action: Levonorgestrel is a synthetic, biologically active progestin, exhibiting no significant estrogenic activity. A continuous low dose of levonorgestrel is diffused through the wall of each capsule. Pregnancy is prevented by at least two mechanisms: inhibition of ovulation and thickening of the cervical mucus.

Pharmacokinetics
- *Absorption:* Maximum or near maximum concentrations are reached within 24 hours of implantation. Levonorgestrel is 100% bioavailable. Plasma concentrations average 0.3 ng/ml over 5 years but are highly variable as a function of individual metabolism and body weight.

- *Distribution:* Levonorgestrel is bound by the circulating protein sex hormone-binding globulin (SHBG).
- *Metabolism:* Metabolized by the liver.
- *Excretion:* Metabolites are excreted in the urine.

Contraindications and precautions
Levonorgestrel is contraindicated in women with active thrombophlebitis, thromboembolic disorders, undiagnosed abnormal genital bleeding, known or suspected pregnancy, acute liver disease, benign or malignant liver tumors, and known or suspected breast carcinoma. Use with caution in women with cardiac or renal disease, seizure disorders, migraines, or other conditions that might be aggravated by fluid and electrolyte retention. Also, use with caution in women who become significantly depressed or have a history of depression or emotional disorders because these conditions may worsen as a result of levonorgestrel; monitor such patients closely.

Interactions
Use in women taking carbamazepine or phenytoin results in reduced efficacy of levonorgestrel, which increases risk of pregnancy.

Effects on diagnostic tests
Decreased SHBG and thyroxine concentrations and increased triiodothyronine uptake have been reported.

Adverse reactions
- CNS: headache, nervousness, dizziness.
- DERM: infection at implant site, dermatitis, scalp hair loss, acne, hirsutism, hypertrichosis.
- GI: nausea, abdominal discomfort, change of appetite.
- GU: menstrual cycle irregularities – prolonged bleeding, spotting, amenorrhea, irregular onset of bleeding, frequent bleeding, scanty bleeding, cervicitis, vaginitis, leukorrhea.
- Other: pain or itching near implant site, implant removal difficulties, adnexal enlargement, mastalgia, weight gain, breast discharge, musculoskeletal pain.

Overdose and treatment
Overdose can occur if more than six silastic capsules are in situ, resulting in fluid retention with its associated effects and uterine bleeding irregularities. All previously implanted capsules should be removed before insertion of a new set.

▶ Special considerations
- The total implanted dose is 216 mg. Implantation of all six capsules should be performed during the first 7 days of the menstrual cycle. Insertion is subdermal in the midportion of the inside of the upper arm, 8 to 10 cm above the elbow crease.
- Each capsule is 2.4 mm in diameter and 34 mm in length.
- Determine if patient has any allergies to the antiseptic or anesthetic to be used or any contraindications to progestin-only contraception.
- During insertion, pay special attention to asepsis and correct placement of capsules; use careful technique, to minimize tissue trauma.
- Provide copy of patient information booklet; carefully review potential adverse reactions, risk and benefit of use of system, and other forms of contraception.

Information for the patient
- Tell patient that altered bleeding patterns tend to become more regular after 9 to 12 months.
- Warn patient to notify physician if heavy bleeding occurs.
- Advise patient to avoid bumping or wetting the insertion site for at least 3 days after insertion.
- Explain that some tenderness in the implant area may be experienced for 1 to 2 days.
- Tell patient that insertion usually takes 10 to 15 minutes and causes little or no discomfort because of the local anesthetic.
- Advise patient that, when laboratory studies are ordered, she should tell all health care providers that levonorgestrel implants are being used.
- Tell patient who takes phenytoin or carbamazepine that she may need to use additional contraceptive measures.
- Advise patient to thoroughly review patient information booklet.

---

levorphanol tartrate
Levo-Dromoran

- Pharmacologic classification: opioid
- Therapeutic classification: analgesic, adjunct to anesthesia
- Controlled substance schedule II
- Pregnancy risk category B (D if used at high doses or near term)

How supplied
Available by prescription only
Tablets: 2 mg
Injection: 2 mg/ml, in 1-ml ampules or 10-ml vials

Indications, route, and dosage
Moderate to severe pain
Adults: 2 to 3 mg P.O. or S.C. q 6 to 8 hours, p.r.n. or around the clock.

Pharmacodynamics
Analgesic action: Levorphanol is a synthetic morphinan derivative that produces analgesia by opiate receptor agonist activity and is recommended for moderate to severe pain.

Pharmacokinetics
- *Absorption:* Levorphanol is well absorbed after oral, S.C., or I.V. administration. Onset of action occurs in 20 to 90 minutes after parenteral administration. Duration of action is 4 to 8 hours.
- *Distribution:* Levorphanol is distributed widely throughout the body. It crosses the placenta and enters breast milk.
- *Metabolism:* Levorphanol is metabolized primarily in the liver, where it undergoes conjugation with glucuronic acid.
- *Excretion:* It is excreted principally in the urine as the glucuronide conjugate.

Contraindications and precautions
Levorphanol is contraindicated in patients with known hypersensitivity to the drug or other phenanthrene opioids (codeine, hydrocodone, morphine, oxymorphone, or oxycodone).

Administer levorphanol with extreme caution to patients with supraventricular arrhythmias; avoid or administer drug with extreme caution to patients with head injury or increased intracranial pressure, because drug obscures neurologic parameters; and during pregnancy and labor, because drug readily crosses placenta (premature infants are especially sensitive to respiratory and CNS depressant effects).

Administer levorphanol cautiously to patients with renal or hepatic dysfunction, because drug accumulation or prolonged duration of action may occur; to patients with pulmonary disease (asthma, chronic obstructive pulmonary disease), because drug depresses respiration and suppresses cough reflex; to patients undergoing biliary tract surgery, because drug may cause biliary spasm; to patients with convulsive disorders, because drug may precipitate seizures; to elderly or debilitated patients, who are more sensitive to both therapeutic and adverse drug effects; and to patients prone to physical or psychic addiction, because of the high risk of addiction to this drug.

Interactions
Concomitant use with other CNS depressants (narcotic analgesics, general anesthetics, antihistamines, phenothiazines, barbiturates, benzodiazepines, sedative-hypnotics, tricyclic antidepressants, alcohol, and muscle relaxants) potentiates drug's respiratory and CNS depression, sedation, and hypotensive effects. Concomitant use with cimetidine may also increase respiratory and CNS depression, causing confusion, disorientation, apnea, or seizures; such use requires reduced dosage of levorphanol.

Drug accumulation and enhanced effects may result from concomitant use with other drugs that are extensively metabolized in the liver (rifampin, phenytoin, and digitoxin); combined use with anticholinergics may cause paralytic ileus.

Patients who become physically dependent on this drug may experience acute withdrawal syndrome if given a narcotic antagonist.

Severe cardiovascular depression may result from the concomitant use with general anesthetics.

Effects on diagnostic tests
Levorphanol increases plasma amylase levels.

Adverse reactions
- CNS: sedation (most common), somnolence clouded sensorium, dysphoria, euphoria, insomnia, agitation, confusion, headache, tremor, miosis, *seizures,* psychic dependence.
- CV: tachycardia, *asystole,* bradycardia, palpitations, chest wall rigidity, hypertension, hypotension, syncope, edema, *shock.*
- DERM: flushing, rash, pruritus, pain at injection site.
- GI: dry mouth, anorexia, biliary spasms (colic), ileus, nausea, vomiting, constipation.
- GU: urinary retention or hesitancy, decreased libido.
- Other: *respiratory depression.*
  Note: Drug should be discontinued if hypersensitivity, seizures, or cardiac arrhythmias occur.

Overdose and treatment
The most common signs and symptoms of levorphanol overdose are CNS depression, respiratory depression, and miosis (pinpoint pupils). Other acute toxic effects include hypotension, bradycardia, hypothermia, shock,

---

apnea, cardiopulmonary arrest, circulatory collapse, pulmonary edema, and convulsions.

To treat acute overdose, first establish adequate respiratory exchange via a patent airway and ventilation as needed; administer narcotic antagonist (naloxone) to reverse respiratory depression. (Because the duration of action of levorphanol is longer than that of naloxone, repeated antagonist dosing is necessary.) Naloxone should not be given unless the patient has clinically significant respiratory or cardiovascular depression. Monitor vital signs closely.

If the patient presents within 2 hours of ingestion of an oral overdose, empty the stomach immediately by inducing emesis (ipecac syrup) or using gastric lavage. Use caution to avoid any risk of aspiration. Administer activated charcoal via nasogastric tube for further removal of the drug in an oral overdose.

Provide symptomatic and supportive treatment (continued respiratory support, correction of fluid or electrolyte imbalance). Monitor laboratory parameters, vital signs, and neurologic status closely.

Contact the local or regional poison information center for further information.

▶ **Special considerations**
Besides those relevant to all *opioids*, consider the following recommendations.
● Reduce levorphanol dosage when using with other drugs that depress CNS function. Use together with extreme caution. Monitor patient's response.

Information for the patient
Tell patient that the drug has a bitter taste.

Geriatric use
Lower doses usually are indicated for elderly patients, because they may be more sensitive to the therapeutic and adverse effects of the drug.

Breast-feeding
It is unknown whether levorphanol is excreted in breast milk; it should be used with caution in breast-feeding women.

---

levothyroxine sodium (T₄ or L-thyroxine sodium)
Eltroxin*, Levothroid, Levoxine, Synthroid, Synthrox, Syroxine

● Pharmacologic classification: thyroid hormone
● Therapeutic classification: thyroid hormone replacement agent
● Pregnancy risk category A

How supplied
Available by prescription only
Tablets: 25 mcg, 50 mcg, 75 mcg, 87 mcg, 100 mcg, 112 mcg, 125 mcg, 150 mcg, 175 mcg, 200 mcg, 300 mcg
Injection: 200 mcg/vial, 500 mcg/vial

Indications, route, and dosage
Cretinism
Children under age 1: Initially, 25 to 50 mcg P.O. daily, increased to 50 mcg.

Myxedema coma
Adults: 200 to 500 mcg I.V. If no response occurs in 24 hours, give an additional 100 to 300 mcg I.V. in 48 hours. A maintenance dose of 50 to 200 mcg may be given until the condition stabilizes and the drug can be given orally.

Thyroid hormone replacement for atrophy of gland, surgical removal, excessive radiation or anti-thyroid drugs, or congenital defect
Adults: For mild hypothyroidism – initially, 50 mcg P.O. daily, increased by 25 to 50 mcg P.O. daily q 2 to 4 weeks until desired response is achieved; may be administered I.V. or I.M. when P.O. ingestion is precluded for long periods. For severe hypothyroidism – 12.5 to 25 mcg daily, increased by 25 to 50 mcg daily q 2 to 4 weeks until desired response is achieved.
Adults over age 65: 25 mcg P.O. daily; may be increased by 25 mcg at 3- to 4-week intervals, depending on response.
Children: Therapy may be initiated at the full therapeutic dose. Incremental doses are not usually needed.
Children over age 12: Over 150 mcg or 2 to 3 mcg/kg/day.
Children age 6 to 12: 100 to 150 mcg or 4 to 5 mcg/kg/day.
Children age 1 to 5: 75 to 100 mcg or 5 to 6 mcg/kg/day.
Children age 6 to 12 months: 50 to 75 mcg or 6 to 8 mcg/kg/day.
Children up to 6 months: 25 to 50 mcg or 8 to 10 mcg/kg/day.

Pharmacodynamics
Thyroid hormone replacement: Levothyroxine affects protein and carbohydrate metabolism, promotes gluconeogenesis, increases the utilization and mobilization of glycogen stores, stimulates protein synthesis, and regulates cell growth and differentiation. The major effect of levothyroxine is to increase the metabolic rate of tissue.

Pharmacokinetics
● *Absorption:* Well absorbed from the GI tract. Full effects do not occur for 1 to 3 weeks after oral therapy begins. After I.M. administration, absorption is variable and poor. After an I.V. dose in patients with myxedema coma, increased responsiveness may occur within 6 to 8 hours, but maximum therapeutic effect may not occur for up to 24 hours.
● *Distribution:* Levothyroxine distribution has not been fully described; however, the drug is distributed into most body tissues and fluids. The highest levels are found in the liver and kidneys. Levothyroxine is 99% protein-bound.
● *Metabolism:* Levothyroxine is metabolized in peripheral tissues, primarily in the liver, kidneys, and intestines. About 85% of levothyroxine metabolized is deiodinated.
● *Excretion:* Fecal excretion eliminates 20% to 40% of levothyroxine. Half-life is 6 to 7 days.

Contraindications and precautions
Levothyroxine is contraindicated in patients with thyrotoxicosis, acute myocardial infarction, and uncorrected adrenal insufficiency because drug increases tissue metabolic demands. Levothyroxine also is contraindicated for treating obesity because it is ineffective and can cause life-threatening adverse reactions.

Levothyroxine should be used cautiously in patients with angina or other cardiovascular disease because of the risk of increased metabolic demands; in patients

---

with diabetes mellitus because of reduced glucose tolerance; in patients with malabsorption states because of decreased absorption; and in patients with long-standing hypothyroidism or myxedema because these patients may be more sensitive to the drug's effects.

Interactions

Concomitant use of levothyroxine with corticotropin causes changes in thyroid status. Changes in levothyroxine dosages may require dosage changes in corticotropin as well. Concomitant use with an anticoagulant may alter anticoagulant effect; an increase in levothyroxine dosage may necessitate a decrease in anticoagulant dosage. Concomitant use of levothyroxine with tricyclic antidepressants or sympathomimetics may increase the effects of any or all of these drugs and may lead to coronary insufficiency or cardiac arrhythmias.

Concomitant use of levothyroxine with oral antidiabetic agents or insulin may affect the dosage requirements of these agents. Beta blockers may decrease the conversion of levothyroxine to liothyronine. Cholestyramine may delay absorption of levothyroxine. Estrogens, which increase serum thyroxine-binding globulin levels, increase levothyroxine requirements. Hepatic enzyme inducers (such as phenytoin) may increase hepatic degradation of levothyroxine and raise dosage requirements of levothyroxine. Concomitant use with somatrem may accelerate epiphyseal maturation.

Effects on diagnostic tests

Levothyroxine therapy alters radioactive iodine (^{131}I) thyroid uptake, protein-bound iodine levels, and liothyronine uptake.

Adverse reactions

- CNS: nervousness, insomnia, tremor.
- CV: tachycardia, palpitations, *arrhythmias*, angina pectoris, *hypertension*, widened pulse pressure, *cardiac arrest*.
- GI: change in appetite, nausea, diarrhea.
- Other: headache, leg cramps, weight loss, sweating, heat intolerance, allergic skin reactions, fever, menstrual irregularities.

Note: Drug should be discontinued if allergic reactions or signs of hyperthyroidism occur.

Overdose and treatment

Clinical manifestations of overdose include signs and symptoms of hyperthyroidism, including weight loss, increased appetite, palpitations, nervousness, diarrhea, abdominal cramps, sweating, tachycardia, increased blood pressure, widened pulse pressure, angina, cardiac arrhythmias, tremor, headache, insomnia, heat intolerance, fever, and menstrual irregularities.

Treatment of overdose requires reduction of GI absorption and efforts to counteract central and peripheral effects, primarily sympathetic activity. Use gastric lavage or induce emesis (followed by activated charcoal up to 4 hours after ingestion). If the patient is comatose or is having seizures, inflate cuff on endotracheal tube to prevent aspiration. Treatment may include oxygen and artificial ventilation as needed to support respiration. It also should include appropriate measures to treat congestive heart failure and to control fever, hypoglycemia, and fluid loss. Propranolol (or another beta blocker) may be used to combat many of the effects of increased sympathetic activity. Levothyroxine should be gradually withdrawn over 2 to 6 days, then resumed at a lower dose.

▶ Special considerations

Besides those relevant to all *thyroid hormones,* consider the following recommendations.
- Administer as a single dose before breakfast.
- Carefully observe patient for adverse effects during initial titration phase.
- Monitor for aggravation of concurrent diseases, such as Addison's disease or diabetes mellitus.
- Patient with a history of lactose intolerance may be sensitive to Levothroid, which contains lactose.
- Synthroid 100- and 300-mcg tablets contain tartrazine, a dye that causes allergic reactions in susceptible individuals.
- When switching from levothyroxine to liothyronine, levothyroxine dosage should stop when liothyronine treatment begins. After residual effects of levothyroxine have disappeared, liothyronine dosage can be increased in small increments. When switching from liothyronine to levothyroxine, levothyroxine therapy should begin several days before withdrawing liothyronine to avoid relapse.
- Patient taking levothyroxine who requires ^{131}I uptake studies must discontinue drug 4 weeks before test.
- Protect drug from moisture and light. Prepare I.V. dose immediately before injection. Do not mix with other I.V. solutions.
- Levothyroxine has predictable effects because of standard hormonal content; therefore, it is the usual drug of choice for thyroid hormone replacement.

Information for the patient
- Instruct patient to take the medication at the same time each day; encourage morning dosing to avoid insomnia.
- Tell patient to report headache, diarrhea, nervousness, excessive sweating, heat intolerance, chest pain, increased pulse rate, or palpitations.
- Encourage patient to use the same product consistently because all brands do not have equal bioavailability.
- Advise patient not to store the drug in warm, humid areas, such as the bathroom, to prevent deterioration of the drug.

Geriatric use
Elderly patients are more sensitive to levothyroxine effects. In patients over age 60, initial dosage should be 25% lower than usual recommended dosage.

Pediatric use
Partial hair loss may occur during the first few months of therapy. Reassure child and parents that this is temporary.

Breast-feeding
Minimal amounts of levothyroxine are excreted in breast milk. Use with caution in breast-feeding women.

lidocaine (lignocaine)
Xylocaine

lidocaine hydrochloride
Alphacaine, Anestacon, Dalcaine, Dilocaine, L-caine, Lidoject, LidoPen Auto-Injector, Nervocaine, Nulicaine, Xylocaine, Xylocaine Viscous

- Pharmacologic classification: amide derivative
- Therapeutic classification: ventricular antiarrhythmic, local anesthetic
- Pregnancy risk category B

How supplied
Available without prescription
Ointment: 2.5%

Available by prescription only
Injection: 5 mg/ml, 10 mg/ml, 15 mg/ml, 20 mg/ml, 40 mg/ml, 100 mg/ml, and 200 mg/ml
Premixed solutions: dextrose 5% in water as 2 mg/ml, 4 mg/ml, and 8 mg/ml
Ointment: 5%
Topical solution: 2%, 4%, 10%
Jelly: 2%

Indications, route, and dosage
Ventricular arrhythmias from myocardial infarction, cardiac manipulation, or cardiac glycosides; ventricular tachycardia
Adults: 50 to 100 mg (1 to 1.5 mg/kg) I.V. bolus at 25 to 50 mg/minute. Give half this amount to elderly or lightweight patients and to those with congestive heart failure or hepatic disease. Repeat bolus q 3 to 5 minutes until arrhythmias subside or side effects develop. Do not exceed 300-mg total bolus during a 1-hour period. Simultaneously, begin constant infusion: 1 to 4 mg/minute. Use lower dosage in elderly patients, those with congestive heart failure or hepatic disease, or patients who weigh less than 50 kg. If single bolus has been given, repeat smaller bolus (usually one-half of the initial bolus) 15 to 20 minutes after start of infusion to maintain therapeutic serum level. After 24 hours of continuous infusion, decrease rate by half.
For I.M. administration: 200 to 300 mg in deltoid muscle has been used in early stages of acute myocardial infarction.
†*Children:* 1 mg/kg by I.V. bolus, followed by infusion of 30 mcg/kg/minute.
Local anesthesia of skin or mucous membranes, pain from dental extractions, stomatitis
Adults and children: Apply 2% to 5% solution or ointment or 15 ml of Xylocaine Viscous q 3 to 4 hours to oral or nasal mucosa.
Local anesthesia in procedures involving the male or female urethra
Adults: Instill about 15 ml (male) or 3 to 5 ml (female) into urethra.
Pain, burning, or itching caused by burns, sunburn, or skin irritation
Adults and children: Apply liberally.

Pharmacodynamics
- *Ventricular antiarrhythmic action:* One of the oldest antiarrhythmics, lidocaine remains among the most widely used drugs for treating acute ventricular dysrhythmias. According to the recently revised Advanced Cardiac Life Support guidelines (American Heart Association, 1986), lidocaine is the drug of choice to treat ventricular tachycardia and fibrillation. As a Class IB antiarrhythmic, it suppresses automaticity and shortens the effective refractory period and action potential duration of His-Purkinje fibers and suppresses spontaneous ventricular depolarization during diastole. Therapeutic concentrations do not significantly affect conductive atrial tissue and AV conduction. Unlike quinidine and procainamide, lidocaine does not significantly alter hemodynamics when given in usual doses. The drug seems to act preferentially on diseased or ischemic myocardial tissue; exerting its effects on the conduction system, it inhibits reentry mechanisms and halts ventricular arrhythmias.
- *Local anesthetic action:* As a local anesthetic, lidocaine acts to block initiation and conduction of nerve impulses by decreasing the permeability of the nerve cell membrane to sodium ions.

Pharmacokinetics
- *Absorption:* Lidocaine is absorbed after oral administration; however, a significant first-pass effect occurs in the liver and only about 35% of the drug reaches the systemic circulation. Oral doses high enough to achieve therapeutic blood levels result in an unacceptable toxicity, probably from high concentrations of lidocaine.
- *Distribution:* Lidocaine is distributed widely throughout the body; it has a high affinity for adipose tissue. After I.V. bolus administration, an early, rapid decline in plasma levels occurs; this is associated mainly with distribution into highly perfused tissues, such as the kidneys, lungs, liver, and heart, followed by a slower elimination phase in which metabolism and redistribution into skeletal muscle and adipose tissue occur. The first (early) distribution phase occurs rapidly, calling for initiation of a constant infusion after an initial bolus dose. Distribution volume declines in patients with liver and/or hepatic disease, resulting in toxic concentrations with usual doses. About 60% to 80% of circulating drug is bound to plasma proteins. Usual therapeutic drug level is 1.5 to 5 mcg/ml. Although toxicity may occur within this range, levels greater than 5 mcg/ml are considered toxic and warrant dosage reduction.
- *Metabolism:* Lidocaine is metabolized in the liver to two active metabolites. Less than 10% of a parenteral dose escapes metabolism and reaches the kidneys unchanged. Metabolism is affected by hepatic blood flow, which may decrease after myocardial infarction and with congestive heart failure. Liver disease also may limit metabolism.
- *Excretion:* Drug's half-life undergoes a biphasic process, with an initial phase of 7 to 30 minutes followed by a terminal half-life of 1.5 to 2 hours. Elimination half-life may be prolonged in patients with congestive heart failure or liver disease. Continuous infusions longer than 24 hours also may cause an apparent half-life increase.

Contraindications and precautions
Lidocaine is contraindicated in patients with Stokes-Adams syndrome or severe degrees of sinoatrial, atrioventricular, or intraventricular heart block who do not have an artificial pacemaker, because the drug may worsen these conditions; and in patients with known

---

hypersensitivity to this drug or other amide-type anesthetic agents.

Lidocaine is contraindicated in patients with inflammation or infection in puncture region, septicemia, severe hypertension, spinal deformities, and neurologic disorders. Use cautiously in debilitated, elderly, acutely ill, or obstetric patients; and in those with severe shock, heart block, general drug allergies, and paracervical block.

Lidocaine should be used with caution in patients with Wolff-Parkinson-White syndrome, bradycardia, or incomplete heart block, because the drug may exacerbate these conditions and precipitate other serious arrhythmias; and in patients with atrial fibrillation, because the drug may increase the ventricular rate.

Interactions
Concomitant use of lidocaine with cimetidine or beta blockers may cause lidocaine toxicity from reduced hepatic clearance. Concomitant use of high-dose lidocaine with succinylcholine may increase succinylcholine's neuromuscular effects. Concomitant use with other antiarrhythmic agents, including phenytoin, procainamide, propranolol, and quinidine, may cause additive or antagonist effects as well as additive toxicity.

Effects on diagnostic tests
Because I.M. lidocaine therapy may increase creatine phosphokinase levels, isoenzyme tests should be performed for differential diagnosis of acute myocardial infarction.

Adverse reactions
- CNS: anxiety, apprehension, nervousness, convulsions followed by drowsiness, unconsciousness, and *respiratory arrest*, confusion, tremors, lethargy, somnolence, stupor, restlessness, slurred speech, euphoria, depression, light-headedness, paresthesias, muscle twitching, *convulsions*.
- CV: myocardial depression, arrhythmias, *cardiac arrest*, hypotension, bradycardia.
- DERM: dermatologic reactions.
- EENT: tinnitus, blurred or double vision.
- GI: nausea, vomiting.
- Local: sensitization, rash.
- Other: edema, *status asthmaticus*, anaphylactoid reactions, *anaphylaxis*, soreness at injection site, cold sensation, diaphoresis.

Overdose and treatment
Clinical effects of overdose include signs and symptoms of CNS toxicity, such as convulsions and/or respiratory depression and cardiovascular toxicity (as indicated by hypotension).

Treatment includes general supportive measures and drug discontinuation. A patent airway should be maintained and other respiratory support measures carried out immediately. Diazepam or thiopental may be given to treat any convulsions. To treat significant hypotension, vasopressors (including dopamine and norepinephrine) may be administered.

▶ Special considerations
- Patient who is receiving I.V. lidocaine infusion should be attended and on cardiac monitor at all times. Use infusion pump or microdrip system and timer to monitor infusion precisely. Never exceed infusion rate of 4 mg/minute, if possible. A faster rate greatly increases risk of toxicity.

- Use drug with caution in elderly patients, those weighing less than 50 kg, and those with congestive heart failure or renal or hepatic disease. Such patients will need dosage reduction.
- Administration of lidocaine with epinephrine (for local anesthesia) to treat arrhythmias is contraindicated. Use solutions with epinephrine cautiously in cardiovascular disorders and in body areas with limited blood supply (ears, nose, fingers, toes).
- Monitor vital signs and serum electrolyte, BUN, and creatinine levels for abnormalities.
- Monitor ECG constantly if administering drug I.V., especially in patients with liver disease, congestive heart failure, hypoxia, respiratory depression, hypovolemia, or shock, because these conditions may affect drug metabolism, excretion, or distribution volume, predisposing patient to drug toxicity.
- Monitor for signs of excessive depression of cardiac conductivity (such as sinus node dysfunction, PR-interval prolongation, QRS-interval widening, and appearance or exacerbation of arrhythmias). If they occur, reduce dosage or discontinue drug.
- In many severely ill patients, convulsions may be the first sign of toxicity. However, severe reactions are usually preceded by somnolence, confusion, and paresthesias. Regard all signs and symptoms of toxicity as serious, and promptly reduce dosage and/or discontinue therapy. Continued infusion could lead to convulsions and coma. Give oxygen via nasal cannula, if not contraindicated. Keep oxygen and CPR equipment handy.
- Doses of up to 400 mg I.M. have been advocated in prehospital phase of acute myocardial infarction.
- Patient receiving lidocaine I.M. will show a sevenfold increase in serum CPK level. Such CPK originates in skeletal muscle, not the heart. Test isoenzyme levels to confirm myocardial infarction, if using I.M. route.
- Solutions containing preservatives should not be used for spinal, epidural, or caudal block.
- With epidural use, a 2- to 5-ml test dose should be injected at least 5 minutes before giving total dose, to check for intravascular or subarachnoid injection. Motor paralysis and extensive sensory anesthesia indicate subarachnoid injection.
- Therapeutic serum levels range from 2 to 5 mcg/ml.
- Discard partially used vials containing no preservatives.
- Drug has been used investigationally to treat refractory status epilepticus.

Geriatric use
Because of prevalence of concurrent disease states and declining organ system function in elderly patients, conservative lidocaine doses should be used.

Pediatric use
Safety and effectiveness in children have not been established. Use of an I.M. autoinjector device is not recommended.

---

lincomycin hydrochloride
Lincocin

- Pharmacologic classification: lincosamide
- Therapeutic classification: antibiotic
- Pregnancy risk category C

How supplied
Available by prescription only
Capsules: 500 mg
Pediatric capsules: 250 mg
Syrup: 250 mg/5 ml
Injection: 300 mg/ml in 2-ml and 10-ml vials and 2-ml U-Ject

Indications, route, and dosage
Respiratory, skin, soft-tissue, and urinary tract infections; osteomyelitis; septicemia caused by sensitive organisms
Adults: 500 mg P.O. q 6 to 8 hours (not to exceed 8 g/day); 600 mg I.M. daily or q 12 hours; or 600 mg to 1 g I.V. q 8 to 12 hours (not to exceed 8 g/day).
Children over age 1 month: 30 to 60 mg/kg P.O. daily, divided q 6 to 8 hours; 10 mg/kg I.M. daily or divided q 12 hours; or 10 to 20 mg/kg I.V. daily, divided q 6 to 8 hours. For I.V. infusion, dilute to 100 ml; infuse over 1 hour to avoid hypotension.

Pharmacodynamics
Antibacterial action: Lincomycin inhibits bacterial protein synthesis by binding to ribosome's 50S subunit. Spectrum of activity includes most *Streptococcus pneumoniae* and staphylococci, and several anaerobic gram-negative and gram-positive organisms.
Note: This spectrum of activity is similar to but less active than that of clindamycin. It should be reserved for infections with proven susceptibility, and it should not be used for CNS infections, or minor skin, dental, or respiratory infections. Although it demonstrates in vitro effectiveness, it is not considered the drug of choice in infections caused by gram-positive cocci.

Pharmacokinetics
- *Absorption:* With oral administration, only about 20% to 30% of lincomycin dose is absorbed; peak plasma levels occur in 2 hours. With I.M. administration, drug is absorbed rapidly; peak plasma levels occur in 30 minutes.
- *Distribution:* Lincomycin is well distributed in pleural fluid, synovial fluid, peritoneal fluid, bone, bile, and aqueous humor. It penetrates CSF poorly. Plasma protein-binding is concentration-dependent and ranges from about 57% to 72%.
- *Metabolism:* Lincomycin is metabolized partially in the liver.
- *Excretion:* Lincomycin is excreted by renal and biliary pathways; some is also excreted in breast milk. In patients with normal renal function, plasma half-life is 4 to 6 hours; in patients with impaired renal or hepatic function, plasma half-life may be prolonged.

Contraindications and precautions
Lincomycin is contraindicated in patients with known hypersensitivity to lincomycin or clindamycin.
Lincomycin should be administered cautiously to atopic patients because of potential for allergic reactions; to patients with preexisting hepatic disease because the drug may cause cholestatic jaundice; and to patients with a history of colitis because the drug may cause pseudomembranous colitis.

Interactions
When used concomitantly, lincomycin may potentiate the activity of neuromuscular blocking agents, warranting caution during anesthesia. Concomitant use with kaolin preparations reduces lincomycin absorption by 90%. Food decreases the rate and extent of lincomycin absorption.

Effects on diagnostic tests
Liver function test results may become abnormal and blood counts may decrease during lincomycin therapy.

Adverse reactions
- CNS: dizziness, headache.
- CV: hypotension or *cardiac arrest* (with rapid I.V. infusion).
- DERM: rashes, urticaria.
- EENT: glossitis, tinnitus.
- GI: nausea, vomiting, pseudomembranous colitis, persistent diarrhea, abdominal cramps, stomatitis, pruritus ani.
- GU: *nephrotoxicity* (albuminuria, azotemia, cylindruria, hematuria, proteinuria, decreased urine output, increased blood urea nitrogen level).
- HEMA: neutropenia, leukopenia, thrombocytopenia, purpura, *agranulocytosis.*
- Hepatic: cholestatic jaundice.
- Local: pain and phlebitis at injection site.
- Other: hypersensitivity, angioedema.
  Note: Drug should be discontinued if hypersensitivity reaction, severe diarrhea, or blood disorders occur.

Overdose and treatment
After rapid I.V. infusion, hypotension, syncope, and cardiac arrest have been reported. Specific recommendations for treatment of oral overdose are not available. Stop I.V. infusion and treat symptoms supportively.

▶ Special considerations
- Culture and sensitivity tests should be done before starting treatment.
- Give oral forms of drug 1 hour before or 2 hours after meals or a kaolin-containing medication.
- For I.M. route, give deep I.M. and rotate sites. Warn patient that I.M. injection may be painful.
- Dilute I.V. dose to at least 1 g/100 ml. Infuse over at least 1 hour to avoid adverse cardiovascular effects. Monitor blood pressure during I.V. infusion.
- Monitor liver function tests and complete blood counts (including platelet count).
- Do not treat drug-induced diarrhea with medications that reduce bowel motility (for example, anticholinergics and narcotics) because that will delay excretion of bacterial toxins.

Information for the patient
- Instruct patient to continue taking drug as directed, even after he feels better.
- For best absorption, advise patient taking oral form of drug to take drug with full glass of water 1 hour before or 2 hours after meals.
- Instruct patient to call if rash or diarrhea occurs; caution him not to treat diarrhea himself.

Pediatric use
Do not administer drug to neonates.

Breast-feeding
Drug is excreted in breast milk; alternative feeding method is recommended during therapy with lincomycin.

lindane (gamma benzene hexachloride)
G-Well, Kwell, Kwildane, Scabene

- Pharmacologic classification: chlorinated hydrocarbon insecticide
- Therapeutic classification: scabicide, pediculicide
- Pregnancy risk category B

How supplied
Available by prescription only
Cream: 1%
Lotion: 1%
Shampoo: 1%

Indications, route, and dosage
Scabies
Adults and children: After bathing with soap and water, apply a thin layer of cream or lotion and gently massage it on all skin surfaces, moving from the neck to the toes. After 8 to 12 hours, remove drug by bathing and scrubbing well. Treatment may be repeated after 1 week.
Pediculosis
Adults and children: After bathing with soap and water, apply lotion or cream to affected hairy areas and adjacent areas. After 8 to 12 hours, wash drug off with soap and water. Alternatively, apply shampoo to affected area, lather for 4 to 5 minutes, then rinse thoroughly. Comb hair to remove nits. Treatment may be repeated after 1 week.

Pharmacodynamics
Scabicide and pediculicide action: Lindane is toxic to the parasitic arthropod *Sarcoptes scabiei* and its eggs, and to *Pediculus capitis*, *Pediculus corporis*, and *Phthirus pubis*. The drug is absorbed through the organism's exoskeleton and causes its death.

Pharmacokinetics
- *Absorption:* 10% of topical dose may be absorbed in 24 hours.
- *Distribution:* Lindane is stored in body fat.
- *Metabolism:* Metabolism occurs in the liver.
- *Excretion:* Lindane is excreted in urine and feces.

Contraindications and precautions
Lindane is contraindicated in patients with sensitivity to the drug. It should be used with caution in pregnant women, as it can be absorbed systemically. Avoid contact with face, eyes and mucous membranes, and urethral meatus. Because lindane can be absorbed through the skin, the potential for CNS toxicity should be considered when the drug is used—particularly in children.

Interactions
None reported.

Effects on diagnostic tests
None reported.

Adverse reactions
- Local: irritation, contact dermatitis.
  Note: Drug should be discontinued if sensitization develops.

Overdose and treatment
Accidental ingestion may cause extreme CNS toxicity; reported symptoms include CNS stimulation, dizziness, and convulsions. To treat lindane ingestion, empty stomach by appropriate measures (emesis or lavage); follow with saline catharsis (do not use oil laxative). Treat seizures with pentobarbital, phenobarbital, or diazepam, as needed.

▶ **Special considerations**
- Warn patient that itching may continue for several weeks, even if treatment is effective, especially in scabies infestation.
- Patient's body should be clean (scrubbed well) and dry before application.
- If drug accidentally contacts eyes, patient should flush with water and call for further instructions. Patient should avoid inhaling vapor.
- Avoid applying drug to acutely inflamed skin, or raw, weeping surfaces.
- Place hospitalized patient in isolation with linen-handling precautions.

Information for the patient
- Explain correct use of medications.
- Explain that reapplication usually is not necessary unless live mites are found; advise reapplication if drug is accidentally washed off, but caution against overuse.
- Tell patient he may use lindane to clean combs and brushes, and to wash them thoroughly afterward; advise patient that all clothing and bed linen that may have been contaminated by the patient within the past 2 days should be machine washed in hot water and dried in hot dryer or dry-cleaned to avoid reinfestation or transmission of the organism.
- Discourage repeated use, which may irritate skin and cause systemic toxicity.
- Caution patient to avoid concomitant use of other oils or ointments.
- Advise patient that family and close contacts, including sexual contacts, should be treated concurrently.

Pediatric use
Drug should be used with caution, especially in infants and small children, who are much more susceptible to CNS toxicity. Discourage thumb-sucking in children using lindane, to prevent ingestion of the drug. The Centers for Disease Control recommends other scabicide therapies for children under age 10.

Breast-feeding
Because lindane can be absorbed systemically, it is not recommended for use in breast-feeding women.

liothyronine sodium (T₃)
Cytomel

- Pharmacologic classification: thyroid hormone
- Therapeutic classification: thyroid hormone replacement agent
- Pregnancy risk category A

How supplied
Available by prescription only
Tablets: 5 mcg, 25 mcg, 50 mcg

Indications, route, and dosage
Cretinism
Children age 3 and older: 50 to 100 mcg P.O. daily.
Children under age 3: 5 mcg P.O. daily, increased by 5 mcg q 3 to 4 days until desired response occurs.
Myxedema
Adults: Initially, 5 mcg daily, increased by 5 to 10 mcg q 1 to 2 weeks. Maintenance dosage is 50 to 100 mcg daily.
Nontoxic goiter
Adults: Initially, 5 mcg P.O. daily; may be increased by 12.5 to 25 mcg daily q 1 to 2 weeks. Usual maintenance dosage is 75 mcg daily.
Adults over age 65: Initially, 5 mcg P.O. daily, increased by 5-mcg increments q 1 to 2 weeks until dosage of 25 mcg is reached. Thereafter, dosages may be increased by 12.5 to 25 mcg daily q 1 to 2 weeks.
Children: Initially, 5 mcg P.O. daily, increased by 5-mcg increments at weekly intervals until desired response is achieved.
Thyroid hormone replacement
Adults: Initially, 25 mcg P.O. daily, increased by 12.5 to 25 mcg q 1 to 2 weeks until satisfactory response is achieved. Usual maintenance dosage is 25 to 75 mcg daily.
Liothyronine suppression test to differentiate hyperthyroidism from euthyroidism
Adults: 75 to 100 mcg daily for 7 days.

Pharmacodynamics
Thyroid hormone replacement: Liothyronine is usually a second-line drug in the treatment of hypothyroidism, myxedema, and cretinism. This component of thyroid hormone affects protein and carbohydrate metabolism, promotes gluconeogenesis, increases the utilization and mobilization of glycogen stores, stimulates protein synthesis, and regulates cell growth and differentiation. The major effect of liothyronine is to increase the metabolic rate of tissue. It may be most useful in syndromes of thyroid hormone resistance.

Pharmacokinetics
- *Absorption:* Liothyronine is 95% absorbed from the GI tract. Peak effect occurs within 24 to 72 hours.
- *Distribution:* Liothyronine is highly protein-bound. Its distribution has not been fully described.
- *Metabolism:* The metabolism of liothyronine is not fully understood.
- *Excretion:* Half-life is 1 to 2 days.

Contraindications and precautions
Liothyronine is contraindicated in patients with thyrotoxicosis, acute myocardial infarction, and uncorrected adrenal insufficiency because the drug increases tissue metabolic demands. Liothyronine also is contraindicated to treat obesity because it is ineffective and can cause life-threatening adverse reactions.

Liothyronine should be used cautiously in patients with angina or other cardiovascular disease because of the risk of increased metabolic demands; in patients with diabetes mellitus because of reduced glucose tolerance; in patients with malabsorption states caused by decreased absorption; and in patients with long-standing hypothyroidism or myxedema because these patients may be more sensitive to the drug's effects.

Interactions
Concomitant use of liothyronine with adrenocorticoids or corticotropin alters thyroid status. Changes in liothyronine dosages may require dosage changes in the adrenocorticoid or corticotropin as well.

Concomitant use of liothyronine with anticoagulants may impair the latter's effects; an increase in liothyronine dosage may require a lower dosage of the anticoagulant. Concomitant use of liothyronine with tricyclic antidepressants or sympathomimetics may increase the effects of any or all of these medications, causing coronary insufficiency or cardiac arrhythmias. Concomitant use of liothyronine with oral antidiabetic agents or insulin may affect dosage requirements of these agents. Estrogens, which increase serum thyroxine-binding globulin levels, increase liothyronine requirements.

Effects on diagnostic tests
Liothyronine therapy alters radioactive iodine (^{131}I) uptake, protein-bound iodine levels, and liothyronine uptake.

Adverse reactions
- CNS: nervousness, insomnia, tremor.
- CV: *tachycardia,* palpitations, *arrhythmias, angina pectoris, hypertension,* widened pulse pressure, *cardiac arrest.*
- GI: change in appetite, nausea, diarrhea.
- Other: headache, leg cramps, weight loss, sweating, heat intolerance, allergic skin reactions, fever, menstrual irregularities, hyperhidrosis.
  Note: Drug should be discontinued if allergic reactions or signs of hyperthyroidism occur.

Overdose and treatment
Clinical manifestations of overdose include signs and symptoms of hyperthyroidism, including weight loss, increased appetite, palpitations, diarrhea, nervousness, abdominal cramps, sweating, headache, tachycardia, increased blood pressure, widened pulse pressure, angina, cardiac arrhythmias, tremor, insomnia, heat intolerance, fever, and menstrual irregularities.

Treatment of overdose reduces GI absorption and counteracts central and peripheral effects, primarily sympathetic activity. Use gastric lavage or induce emesis (followed by activated charcoal up to 4 hours after ingestion). If the patient is comatose or having seizures, inflate the cuff on an endotracheal tube to prevent aspiration. Treatment may include oxygen and ventilation to maintain respiration. It also should include appropriate measures to treat congestive heart failure and to control fever, hypoglycemia, and fluid loss. Propranolol (or another beta blocker) may be used to counteract many of the effects of increased sympathetic activity.

Liothyronine should be withdrawn gradually over 2 to 6 days, then resumed at a lower dose.

▶ **Special considerations**
Besides those relevant to all *thyroid hormones,* consider the following recommendations.
● Liothyronine may be preferred when rapid effect is desired or when GI absorption or peripheral conversion of levothyroxine to liothyronine is impaired.
● Oral absorption may be reduced in patients with congestive heart failure.
● When switching from levothyroxine to liothyronine, levothyroxine should be discontinued and liothyronine started at low dosage, increasing in small increments after residual effects of levothyroxine have disappeared. When switching from liothyronine to levothyroxine, levothyroxine should be started several days before withdrawing liothyronine to avoid relapse.
● Patients taking liothyronine who require radioactive iodine uptake studies must discontinue drug 7 to 10 days before test.
● A parenteral formulation is available by special request for investigational use to treat myxedema coma. The usual initial dose is 200 mcg I.V., followed by 10 to 25 mcg I.V. q 8 to 12 hours until the P.O. form of the drug can be used.
● Use with caution in patients with heart disease.

Information for the patient
● Tell patient to report headache, diarrhea, nervousness, excessive sweating, heat intolerance, chest pain, increased pulse rate, or palpitations.
● Advise patient not to store liothyronine in warm, humid areas, such as the bathroom, to prevent deterioration of the drug.
● Encourage patient to take the drug at the same time each day, preferably in the morning, to avoid insomnia.

Geriatric use
Elderly patients are more sensitive to liothyronine's effects. In patients over age 60, initial dosage should be 25% lower than usual recommended dosage.

Pediatric use
● Partial hair loss may occur during the first few months of therapy. Reassure child and parents that this is temporary.
● Infants and children may experience an accelerated rate of bone maturation.

Breast-feeding
Minimal amounts of liothyronine are excreted in breast milk. Use with caution in breast-feeding women.

liotrix
Euthroid, Thyrolar

● Pharmacologic classification: thyroid hormone
● Therapeutic classification: thyroid hormone replacement agent
● Pregnancy risk category A

How supplied
Available by prescription only
Tablets: Euthroid-½ — levothyroxine sodium 30 mcg and liothyronine sodium 7.5 mcg
Euthroid-1 — levothyroxine sodium 60 mcg and liothyronine sodium 15 mcg
Euthroid-2 — levothyroxine sodium 120 mcg and liothyronine sodium 30 mcg
Euthroid-3 — levothyroxine sodium 180 mcg and liothyronine sodium 45 mcg
Thyrolar-¼ — levothyroxine sodium 12.5 mcg and liothyronine sodium 3.1 mcg
Thyrolar-½ — levothyroxine sodium 25 mcg and liothyronine sodium 6.25 mcg
Thyrolar-1 — levothyroxine sodium 50 mcg and liothyronine sodium 12.5 mcg
Thyrolar-2 — levothyroxine sodium 100 mcg and liothyronine sodium 25 mcg
Thyrolar-3 — levothyroxine sodium 150 mcg and liothyronine sodium 37.5 mcg

Indications, route, and dosage
Hypothyroidism
Dosages must be individualized to approximate the deficit in the patient's thyroid secretion.
Adults and children: Initially, 15 to 30 mg thyroid equivalent P.O. daily, increased by 15 to 30 mg thyroid equivalent q 1 to 2 weeks until desired response is achieved; increments in children's dosage q 2 weeks.
Adults over age 65: Initially, 15 to 30 mg thyroid equivalent. Usual adult dosage is doubled q 6 to 8 weeks until desired response is achieved.

Pharmacodynamics
Thyroid stimulant and replacement: Liotrix affects protein and carbohydrate metabolism, promotes gluconeogenesis, increases the utilization and mobilization of glycogen stores, stimulates protein synthesis, and regulates cell growth and differentiation. The major effect of liotrix is to increase the metabolic rate of tissue. It is used to treat hypothyroidism (myxedema, cretinism, and thyroid hormone deficiency).
   Liotrix is a synthetic preparation combining levothyroxine sodium and liothyronine sodium. Such combination products were developed because circulating liothyronine was assumed to result from direct release from the thyroid gland. About 80% of liothyronine is now known to be derived from deiodination of levothyroxine in peripheral tissues, and patients receiving only levothyroxine have normal serum liothyronine and levothyroxine levels. Therefore, there is no clinical advantage to combining thyroid agents; actually, it could result in excessive liothyronine concentration.

Pharmacokinetics
● *Absorption:* About 50% to 95% of liotrix is absorbed from the GI tract.

- *Distribution:* Distribution is not fully understood.
- *Metabolism:* Liotrix is metabolized partially in peripheral tissues (liver, kidneys, and intestines).
- *Excretion:* Liotrix is excreted partially in feces.

Contraindications and precautions

Liotrix is contraindicated in patients with thyrotoxicosis, acute myocardial infarction, and uncorrected adrenal insufficiency because liotrix increases tissue demands for adrenal hormones and may precipitate an acute adrenal crisis. Liotrix also is contraindicated to treat obesity because it is ineffective and can cause life-threatening adverse effects.

Liotrix should be used cautiously in patients with angina or other cardiovascular disease because of the risk of increased metabolic demands; in patients with diabetes mellitus because of reduced glucose tolerance; in patients with malabsorption states because of decreased absorption; and in patients with long-standing hypothyroidism or myxedema because these patients may be more sensitive to the drug's effects.

Interactions

Concomitant use of liotrix with corticotropin or an adrenocorticoid alters thyroid status; changes in liotrix dosage may require adrenocorticoid or corticotropin dosage changes as well. Concomitant use with an anticoagulant may alter anticoagulant effect; an increase in liotrix dosage may require a lower anticoagulant dose. Concomitant use of liotrix with tricyclic antidepressants or sympathomimetics may increase the effects of any or all of these drugs and may lead to coronary insufficiency or cardiac arrhythmias. Concomitant use with oral antidiabetic agents or insulin may affect dosage requirements of these agents. Beta blockers may decrease the conversion of T_4 to T_3. Cholestyramine may delay absorption of T_4. Estrogens, which increase serum thyroxine-binding globulin levels, increase liotrix dosage requirements. Hepatic enzyme inducers (such as phenytoin) may increase hepatic degradation of T_4, resulting in increased requirements of T_4. Concomitant use with somatrem may accelerate epiphyseal maturation.

Effects on diagnostic tests

Liotrix therapy alters radioactive iodine (^{131}I) thyroid uptake, protein-bound iodine levels, and T_3 uptake.

Adverse reactions

- CNS: nervousness, insomnia, tremor.
- CV: tachycardia, palpitations, *arrhythmias,* angina pectoris, *hypertension,* widened pulse pressure, *cardiovascular collapse, cardiac arrest.*
- GI: change in appetite, nausea, diarrhea.
- Other: headache, leg cramps, weight loss, sweating, heat intolerance, allergic skin reactions, fever, and menstrual irregularities. Hypersensitivity to the drug or tartrazine (a dye contained in Euthroid-½, -1 and -3) has also been reported.

Note: Drug should be discontinued if allergic reaction or signs of hyperthyroidism occur.

Overdose and treatment

Clinical manifestations of overdose include signs and symptoms of hyperthyroidism, including weight loss, increased appetite, palpitations, nervousness, diarrhea, abdominal cramps, sweating, tachycardia, increased pulse rate and blood pressure, angina, cardiac arrhythmias, tremor, headache, insomnia, heat intolerance, fever, and menstrual irregularities.

Treatment of overdose requires reduction of GI absorption and efforts to counteract central and peripheral effects, primarily sympathetic activity. Use gastric lavage or induce emesis, then follow with activated charcoal, if less than 4 hours since ingestion. If the patient is comatose or having seizures, inflate the cuff on an endotracheal tube to prevent aspiration. Treatment may include oxygen and artificial ventilation as needed to maintain respiration. It should also include appropriate measures to treat congestive heart failure and to control fever, hypoglycemia, and fluid loss. Propranolol (or atenolol, metoprolol, acebutolol, nadolol, or timolol) may be used to combat many of the effects of increased sympathetic activity. Thyroid therapy should be withdrawn gradually over 2 to 6 days, then resumed at a lower dosage.

▶ Special considerations

Besides those relevant to all *thyroid hormones,* consider the following recommendations.
- Note that levothyroxine (T_4) is the drug of choice for hypothyroidism. Hepatic conversion of T_4 to liothyronine (T_3) is usually adequate. Excessive exogenous supplementation of T_3 is usually associated with toxicity.
- The two commercially prepared liotrix brands contain different amounts of each ingredient; do not change from one brand to the other without considering the differences in potency.
- Monitor the patient's pulse rate and blood pressure.
- Protect liotrix from heat and moisture.

Information for the patient

- Tell patient to report headache, diarrhea, nervousness, excessive sweating, heat intolerance, chest pain, increased pulse rate, or palpitations.
- Advise patient not to store liotrix in warm and humid areas, such as the bathroom.
- Encourage patient to take a single daily dose in the morning to avoid insomnia.

Geriatric use

Elderly patients are more sensitive to the drug's effects. In patients over age 60, initial dosage should be 25% lower than usual recommended dosage.

Pediatric use

- Partial hair loss may occur during the first few months of therapy. Reassure child and parents that this is temporary.
- Infants and children may experience accelerated rate of bone maturation.

Breast-feeding

Minimal amounts of liotrix are excreted in breast milk. Use with caution in breast-feeding women.

---

lisinopril
Prinivil, Zestril

- Pharmacologic classification: angiotensin-converting enzyme (ACE) inhibitor
- Therapeutic classification: antihypertensive
- Pregnancy risk category C

How supplied
Available by prescription only
Tablets: 5 mg, 10 mg, 20 mg

Indications, route, and dosage
Mild to severe hypertension
Adults: Initially, 10 mg P.O. daily. Most patients are well-controlled on 20 to 40 mg daily as a single dose.

Pharmacodynamics
Antihypertensive action: Lisinopril inhibits angiotensin-converting enzyme (ACE), preventing pulmonary conversion of angiotensin I to angiotensin II, a potent vasoconstrictor. Reduced formation of angiotensin II decreases peripheral arterial resistance and aldosterone secretion, thereby reducing sodium and water retention and blood pressure.

Pharmacokinetics
- *Absorption:* Variable absorption occurs after oral administration; an average of about 25% of an oral dose has been absorbed by test subjects. Peak serum levels occur in about 7 hours. Onset of antihypertensive activity occurs in about 1 hour and peaks in about 6 hours.
- *Distribution:* Lisinopril is distributed widely in tissues. Plasma protein binding appears insignificant. Minimal amounts enter the brain. Preclinical studies indicate that it crosses the placenta.
- *Metabolism:* Lisinopril is not metabolized.
- *Excretion:* Lisinopril is excreted unchanged in the urine.

Contraindications and precautions
Lisinopril is contraindicated in patients hypersensitive to the drug. Use with caution in patients with impaired renal function because accumulation of the drug may occur. Use with caution in patients with severe congestive heart failure; because renal function may depend on the renin-angiotensin system, lisinopril may worsen oliguria or progressive azotemia.

Interactions
Concurrent use with diuretics may cause excessive hypotension. Indomethacin may attenuate the hypotensive effect of lisinopril. Concomitant use with potassium-sparing diuretics, potassium supplements, or potassium-containing salt substitutes may lead to hyperkalemia.

Effects on diagnostic tests
The drug's physiologic effects may lead to elevations of serum potassium, serum creatinine, blood urea nitrogen (BUN), and serum bilirubin levels; minor reductions of hemoglobin and hematocrit; and changes in liver enzymes.

Adverse reactions
- CNS: dizziness, headache, fatigue, depression, somnolence, paresthesia.
- CV: hypotension, orthostasis, chest pain.
- DERM: rash.
- EENT: nasal congestion.
- GI: diarrhea, nausea, dyspepsia.
- GU: impotence, decreased libido.
- HEMA: neutropenia.
- Metabolic: hyperkalemia.
- Other: upper respiratory symptoms, cough, muscle cramps.

Note: The drug should be discontinued if angioedema or a hypersensitivity response occurs.

Overdose and treatment
The most likely manifestation of overdose would be hypotension. Recommended treatment is intravenous infusion of normal saline solution.

▶ Special considerations
Besides those relevant to all *ACE inhibitors,* consider the following recommendations.
- Lisinopril is unaffected by food.
- Lisinopril attenuates potassium loss of thiazide diuretics. If patient is taking a diuretic, the diuretic should be discontinued 2 to 3 days before lisinopril therapy, or lisinopril dosage should be reduced to 5 mg once a day.
- If drug does not adequately control blood pressure, diuretics may be added.
- Review WBC and differential counts before treatment, every 2 weeks for 3 months, and periodically thereafter.
- Lower dosage is necessary in patients with impaired renal function.
- Beneficial effects of lisinopril may require several weeks of therapy.

Information for the patient
- Tell patient to report light-headedness, especially in first few days of treatment, so dose can be adjusted; signs of infection such as sore throat or fever, because drug may decrease WBC count; facial swelling or difficulty breathing, because drug may cause angioedema; and loss of taste, which may necessitate discontinuation of drug.
- Advise patient to avoid sudden postural changes to minimize orthostatic hypotension.
- Warn patient to seek medical approval before taking nonprescription cold preparations.

Geriatric use
Elderly patients may require lower doses due to impaired drug clearance. They may also be more sensitive to the hypotensive effects of lisinopril.

Pediatric use
Safety and efficacy of lisinopril in children have not been established; use only if potential benefits outweigh risks.

Breast-feeding
Lisinopril may be distributed into breast milk, but effect on breast-feeding infant is unknown; use drug with caution in breast-feeding women.

---

lithium carbonate
Carbolith*, Duralith*, Eskalith, Eskalith CR, Lithane, Lithizine*, Lithobid, Lithonate, Lithotabs

lithium citrate
Cibalith-S

- Pharmacologic classification: alkali metal
- Therapeutic classification: antimanic, antipsychotic
- Pregnancy risk category D

How supplied
Available by prescription only
Lithium carbonate
Capsules: 150 mg, 300 mg, 600 mg
Tablets: 300 mg
Tablets (sustained-release): 300 mg, 450 mg
Lithium citrate
Syrup (sugarless): 300 mg/5 ml (with 0.3% alcohol)

Indications, route, and dosage
Prevention or control of mania; prevention of depression in patients with bipolar illness
Adults: 300 to 600 mg or 5 to 10 ml lithium citrate (each 5 ml contains 8 mEq lithium, equivalent to 300 mg lithium carbonate) P.O. up to four times daily, increasing on the basis of blood levels and clinical response to achieve optimal dosage. Dosages to a maximum of 2.7 g daily divided t.i.d. or q.i.d. may be required in the acute manic phase of bipolar illness; for maintenance therapy the usual dosage is 900 mg to 1.2 g of lithium carbonate or 15 to 20 ml of lithium citrate (about 24 to 32 mEq) in two to four divided doses daily. Recommended therapeutic lithium blood levels: 1 to 1.5 mEq/liter for acute mania; 0.6 to 1.0 mEq/liter for maintenance therapy; and 2 mEq/liter as maximum. Dosage should be decreased rapidly when the acute attack has subsided.
†*Major depression,* †*schizoaffective disorder,* †*schizophrenic disorder,* †*alcohol dependence*
Adults: 300 mg lithium carbonate P.O. t.i.d. to q.i.d
Apparent mixed bipolar disorder in children
Children: Initially, 15 to 60 mg/kg or 0.5 to 1.5 g/m² lithium carbonate P.O. daily in three divided doses. Do not exceed usual adult dosage. Adjust dosage based on patient response and serum lithium levels; usual dosage range is 150 to 300 mg daily in divided doses.

Pharmacodynamics
Antimanic action: Lithium is thought to exert its antipsychotic and antimanic effects by competing with other cations for exchange at the sodium-potassium ionic pump, thus altering cationic exchange at the tissue level. It also inhibits adenyl cyclase, reducing intracellular levels of secondary messengers cyclic adenosine monophosphate (cAMP) and to a lesser extent, cyclic guanosine monophosphate (c6MP).

Pharmacokinetics
- *Absorption:* Rate and extent of absorption vary with dosage form: absorption is complete within 6 hours of oral administration.

- *Distribution:* Lithium is distributed widely into the body, including breast milk; concentrations in thyroid gland, bone, and brain tissue exceed serum levels. Peak effects occur at 30 minutes to 3 hours; liquid peaks at 15 minutes to 1 hour. Steady-state serum level is achieved in 12 hours, at which time trough levels should be drawn: therapeutic effect begins in 5 to 10 days and is maximal within 3 weeks. Therapeutic and toxic serum levels and therapeutic effects show good correlation. Therapeutic range is 0.6 to 1.2 mEq/liter; adverse reactions increase as level reaches 1.5 to 2 mEq/liter – such concentrations may be necessary in acute mania. Toxicity usually occurs at levels above 2 mEq/liter.
- *Metabolism:* Lithium is not metabolized.
- *Excretion:* Lithium is excreted 95% unchanged in urine; about 50% to 80% of a given dose is excreted within 24 hours. Level of renal function determines elimination rate.

Contraindications and precautions
Lithium is contraindicated in patients with known hypersensitivity to lithium.

Lithium should be used cautiously in patients with cardiovascular disease because drug causes ECG changes (including T wave depression in 20% to 30% of patients), heart block, and premature ventricular contractions; in patients with renal dysfunction, because delayed elimination may induce lithium toxicity and diabetes insipidus (characterized by extreme thirst and excessive urination in 30% to 50% of patients); in patients with hypovolemia, sodium depletion, or dehydration, which increase drug's effects; in patients with hypothyroidism because of risk of disease exacerbation or goiter formation; in patients with psoriasis, because lithium may exacerbate condition; and in patients with epilepsy and other seizure disorders, because drug may induce seizures. Many oral lithium products contain tartrazine, which may exacerbate asthma or respiratory disorders in aspirin-allergic patients.

Lithium has caused pseudotumor cerebri with papilledema and increased ICP in some patients. If this occurs, the drug should be discontinued, if possible. Some clinicians may elect to treat the patient with acetazolamide.

Interactions
Concomitant use of lithium with thiazide diuretics may decrease renal excretion and enhance lithium toxicity; diuretic dosage may need to be reduced by 30%. Indomethacin, phenylbutazone, piroxicam, and other nonsteroidal anti-inflammatory agents also decrease renal excretion of lithium and may require a 30% reduction in lithium dosage.

Mazindol, tetracyclines, phenytoin, carbamazepine, and methyldopa may increase lithium toxicity. Antacids and other drugs containing sodium, calcium, theophylline, aminophylline, or caffeine may increase lithium excretion by renal competition for elimination, thus decreasing lithium's therapeutic effect.

Lithium may interfere with pressor effects of sympathomimetic agents, especially norepinephrine; may potentiate the effects of neuromuscular blocking agents (such as succinylcholine, pancuronium, and atracurium); and may decrease the effects of chlorpromazine.

Concomitant use with haloperidol may result in severe encephalopathy characterized by confusion, tremors, extrapyramidal effects, and weakness. Use this combination with caution.

Dietary sodium may alter the renal elimination of lithium. Increased sodium intake may increase elimination of drug; decreased intake may decrease elimination.

Acute neurotoxicity with delirium has occurred in patients receiving lithium and electroconvulsive therapy (ECT). Lithium dosage should be reduced or withdrawn before ECT.

Effects on diagnostic tests

Lithium causes false-positive test results on thyroid function tests; drug also elevates neutrophil count.

Adverse reactions

● CNS: tremor, drowsiness, headache, confusion, restlessness, dizziness, psychomotor retardation, stupor, lethargy, coma, blackouts, *epileptiform seizures*, EEG changes, worsened organic brain syndrome, impaired speech, ataxia, muscle weakness, incoordination, hyperexcitability, exacerbation of psychotic symptoms, pseudotumor cerebri.
● CV: reversible ECG changes, *arrhythmias*, hypotension, *peripheral circulatory collapse*, allergic vasculitis, ankle and wrist edema, bradycardia.
● DERM: pruritus, rash, diminished or lost sensation, drying and thinning of hair.
● EENT: tinnitus, impaired vision.
● GI: nausea, vomiting, anorexia, diarrhea, dry mouth, thirst, metallic taste.
● GU: polyuria, glycosuria, incontinence, *nephrotoxicity with long-term use,* decreased renal concentrating capacity.
● Metabolic: transient hyperglycemia, goiter, hypothyroidism (lowered triiodothyronine, thyroxine, and protein-bound iodine levels; elevated iodine 131 uptake), hyponatremia.
● Other: weight gain (25%).
   The severity of lithium toxicity parallels serum concentration:
Less than 1.5 mEq/liter: thirst, nausea, vomiting, diarrhea, polyuria, slurred speech, hand tremors, weakness.
1.5 to 2 mEq/liter: GI distress, hand tremors, confusion, muscle twitching, ECG changes, incoordination.
2 to 2.5 mEq/liter: ataxia, polyuria, large volume of dilute urine, ECG changes, seizures, abnormal motor activity, tinnitus, hypotension, coma.
   Note: Drug should be discontinued if any of the following occurs: hypersensitivity, severe hypothyroidism or goiter, slurred speech, ataxia, incoordination, dysrhythmias, seizures, decreased renal function, or rash.

Overdose and treatment

Vomiting and diarrhea occur within 1 hour of acute ingestion (induce vomiting in noncomatose patients if it is not spontaneous). Death has occurred in patients ingesting 10 to 60 g of lithium; patients have ingested 6 g with minimal toxic effects. Serum lithium levels above 3.4 mEq/liter are potentially fatal.

Overdose with chronic lithium ingestion may follow altered pharmacokinetics, drug interactions, or volume or sodium depletion; sedation, confusion, hand tremors, joint pain, ataxia, muscle stiffness, increased deep tendon reflexes, visual changes, and nystagmus may occur. Symptoms may progress to coma, movement abnormalities, tremors, seizures, and cardiovascular collapse.

Treatment is symptomatic and supportive; closely monitor vital signs. If emesis is not feasible, treat with gastric lavage. Monitor fluid and electrolyte balance; correct sodium depletion with normal saline solution.

Institute hemodialysis if serum level is above 3 mEq/liter, and in severely symptomatic patients unresponsive to fluid and electrolyte correction, or if urine output decreases significantly. Serum rebound of tissue lithium stores (from high volume distribution) commonly occurs after dialysis and may necessitate prolonged or repeated hemodialysis. Peritoneal dialysis may help but is less effective.

▶ Special considerations

● Shake syrup formulation before administration.
● Lithium should be discontinued before electroconvulsive therapy.
● Patient should take drug with food or milk to reduce GI upset.
● Use cautiously with haloperidol, other antipsychotics, neuromuscular blocking agents, and diuretics; in elderly or debilitated persons; and in thyroid disease, brain damage, severe debilitation or dehydration, and sodium depletion.
● Monitor baseline ECG, thyroid, and renal studies, and electrolyte levels. Monitor lithium blood levels 8 to 12 hours after first dose, usually before morning dose, two or three times weekly first month, then weekly to monthly on maintenance therapy.
● Determination of lithium blood concentration is crucial to the safe use of the drug. Lithium shouldn't be used in patients who can't have regular lithium blood level checks. Be sure patient or responsible family member can comply with instructions.
● When lithium blood levels are below 1.5 mEq/liter, adverse reactions usually remain mild.
● Monitor fluid intake and output, especially when surgery is scheduled.
● Expect lag of 1 to 3 weeks before drug's beneficial effects are noticed. Other psychotropic medications (for example, Chlorpromazine) may be necessary during this interim period.
● Monitor for signs of edema or sudden weight gain.
● Adjust fluid and salt ingestion to compensate if excessive loss occurs through protracted sweating or diarrhea. Under normal conditions, patients should have fluid intake of 2,500 to 3,000 ml daily and a balanced diet with adequate salt intake.
● Arrange for outpatient follow-up of thyroid and renal functions every 6 to 12 months. Thyroid should be palpated to check for enlargement.
● Patient should carry identification/instruction card (available from pharmacy) with toxicity and emergency information.
● Check urine for specific gravity level below 1.015, which may indicate diabetes insipidus.
● Lithium may alter glucose tolerance in diabetic patients. Monitor blood glucose levels closely.
● Lithium is used investigationally to increase white blood cell count in patients undergoing cancer chemotherapy.
● Lithium is also used investigationally to treat cluster headaches, aggression, organic brain syndrome, and tardive dyskinesia. It has been used to treat syndrome of inappropriate secretion of antidiuretic hormone.
● Monitor serum levels and signs of impending toxicity.
● Lithane tablets contain tartrazine, a dye that may precipitate an allergic reaction in certain individuals, particularly asthmatics sensitive to aspirin.
● Lithium dosing should be carefully monitored when the patient's initial manic symptoms begin to subside because the ability to tolerate high serum lithium levels decreases as symptoms resolve.

---

*Canada only   †Unlabeled clinical use   Italicized adverse reactions are life-threatening.

Information for the patient
● Explain to patient that lithium has a narrow therapeutic margin of safety. A blood level that is even slightly too high can be dangerous.
● Warn patient and family to watch for signs of toxicity (diarrhea, vomiting, dehydration, drowsiness, muscle weakness, tremor, fever, and ataxia) and to expect transient nausea, polyuria, thirst, and discomfort during first few days. If toxic symptoms occur, patient should withhold one dose and call promptly.
● Warn ambulatory patient to avoid activities that require alertness and good psychomotor coordination until CNS response to drug is determined.
● Advise patient to maintain adequate water intake and adequate – but not excessive – salt in diet.
● Explain importance of regular follow-up visits to measure lithium serum levels.
● Tell patient to avoid large amounts of caffeine, which will interfere with drug's effectiveness.
● Advise patient to seek medical approval before initiating weight-loss program.
● Tell patient not to switch brands of lithium or take other drugs (prescription or nonprescription) without medical approval. Different brands may not provide equivalent effect.
● Warn patient against stopping drug abruptly.
● Tell patient to explain to close friend or family members the signs of lithium overdose, in case emergency aid is needed.

Geriatric use
Elderly patients are more susceptible to chronic overdose and toxic effects, especially dyskinesias. These patients usually respond to a lower dosages.

Pediatric use
Lithium is not recommended for use in children under age 12.

Breast-feeding
Lithium level in breast milk is 33% to 50% that of maternal serum level. Breast-feeding should be avoided during treatment with lithium.

---

lomefloxacin hydrochloride
Maxaquin

● Pharmacologic classification: fluoroquinolone
● Therapeutic classification: broad-spectrum antibiotic
● Pregnancy risk category C

How supplied
Available by prescription only
Tablets: 400 mg

Indications, route, and dosage
Acute bacterial exacerbations of chronic bronchitis caused by Haemophilus influenzae *or* Moraxella (Branhamella) catarrhalis
Adults: 400 mg P.O. daily for 10 days.

Uncomplicated urinary tract infections (cystitis) caused by Escherichia coli, Klebsiella pneumoniae, Proteus mirabilis, *or* Staphylococcus saprophyticus
Adults: 400 mg P.O. daily for 10 days.
Complicated urinary tract infections caused by E. coli, K. pneumoniae, P. mirabilis, *and* Pseudomonas aeruginosa; *possibly effective against infections caused by* Citrobacter diversus *or* Enterobacter cloacae
Adults: 400 mg P.O. daily for 14 days.
Prophylaxis of infections after transurethral surgical procedures
Adults: 400 mg P.O. 2 to 6 hours before surgery as a single dose.
Dosage adjustment for patients with renal failure
Adults: Patients with creatinine clearance of 10 to 40 ml/minute/1.73 m² should receive a loading dose of 400 mg P.O. on the first day, followed by 200 mg P.O. daily for duration of therapy. Periodic determination of blood levels of lomefloxacin is recommended. Hemodialysis removes negligible amounts of drug.

Pharmacodynamics
Antibiotic action: Lomefloxacin inhibits bacterial DNA gyrase, an enzyme necessary for bacterial replication. Lomefloxacin is bactericidal.

Pharmacokinetics
● *Absorption:* Lomefloxacin is absorbed rapidly from the GI tract; absolute bioavailability is 95% to 98%. Food impairs absorption by reducing total amount absorbed and slowing absorption rate.
● *Distribution:* Only 10% of drug is bound to plasma proteins.
● *Metabolism:* Drug is metabolized in the liver.
● *Excretion:* Most of drug is excreted unchanged in urine; about 10% is excreted as metabolites. Solubility in urine is pH dependent. About 10% of a dose appears unchanged in the feces. Half-life is 8 hours. Steady state is reached after 2 days of once-daily therapy.

Contraindications and precautions
Lomefloxacin is contraindicated in patients with hypersensitivity to the drug or other quinolones. Drug is also contraindicated in children and adolescents under age 18 and in pregnant and breast-feeding women. Lomefloxacin has caused arthropathy and lameness secondary to permanent cartilage damage when administered to juvenile animals.
   Use cautiously in patients with known or suspected CNS disorders, such as seizure disorder or cerebral arteriosclerosis, that may predispose to development of seizures.
   Several bacterial strains have demonstrated resistance to lomefloxacin, including *Streptococcus pneumoniae,* most group A, B, D, and G streptococci, *Pseudomonas cepacia, Ureaplasma urealyticum, Mycoplasma hominis,* and anaerobes.

Interactions
Antacids and sucralfate bind with lomefloxacin in the GI tract and impair its absorption. Administer no less than 4 hours before or 2 hours after a dose. Probenecid decreases excretion of lomefloxacin.
   When administered with cimetidine, other quinolones show substantially increased plasma half-lives. Other quinolones also increase the effects or serum levels of

---

warfarin and cyclosporine. Lomefloxacin has not been tested for these effects, however. Monitor for toxicity.

Effects on diagnostic tests
None reported.

Adverse reactions
● CNS: dizziness, fatigue, asthenia, headache, abnormal dreams, fatigue, malaise, asthenia, agitation, anorexia, anxiety, confusion, depersonalization, depression, increased appetite, insomnia, nervousness, somnolence, *seizures, coma,* hyperkinesia, tremor, vertigo, paresthesia.
● CV: flushing, hypotension, hypertension, edema, syncope, arrhythmias, tachycardia, bradycardia, extrasystole, cyanosis, *cardiac failure,* angina pectoris, *MI, pulmonary embolism, cerebrovascular disorder, cardiomyopathy,* phlebitis.
● DERM: pruritus, exfoliation, eczema, rash, urticaria, photosensitivity.
● EENT: epistaxis, abnormal vision, conjunctivitis, eye pain, earache, tinnitus, tongue discoloration.
● GI: diarrhea, nausea, dry mouth, abdominal pain, dyspepsia, vomiting, flatulence, constipation, inflammation, dysphagia, bleeding.
● GU: dysuria, hematuria, anuria, epididymitis, orchitis, vaginal moniliasis, perineal pain, intermenstrual bleeding, leukorrhea, vaginitis.
● HEMA: thrombocythemia, thrombocytopenia, lymphadenopathy, increased fibrinolysis.
● Metabolic: hypoglycemia, gout.
● Respiratory: cough, dyspnea, *bronchospasm,* respiratory disorder, respiratory infection, increased sputum, stridor.
● Other: *anaphylaxis,* increased sweating, taste perversion, leg cramps, arthralgia, myalgia, thirst, back pain, malaise, chills, allergic reaction, facial edema, influenza-like symptoms, decreased heat tolerance.

Overdose and treatment
Treatment of overdose includes emptying the stomach by induced vomiting or gastric lavage and observing the patient closely and providing supportive care. Drug is not significantly removed by hemodialysis or peritoneal dialysis.

▶ Special considerations
Lomefloxacin should not be used for empiric treatment of acute exacerbations of chronic bronchitis when the suspected pathogen is *Streptococcus pneumoniae* because this organism demonstrates resistance to the drug. Because blood levels of lomefloxacin do not readily exceed the minimum inhibitory concentration against *Pseudomonas aeruginosa,* drug should not be used to treat bacteremia caused by this organism; but it has been used successfully to treat complicated urinary tract *Pseudomonas* infections.

Information for the patient
● Remind patient to take all of the drug prescribed, even after he feels better.
● Advise patient to take drug on an empty stomach.
● Tell patient to avoid hazardous tasks that require alertness, such as driving, until adverse CNS effects of drug are known because it may cause dizziness or light-headedness.

Pediatric use
Because studies have shown that quinolones can cause arthropathy in immature animals, these drugs should be avoided in children.

Breast-feeding
It is unknown if drug is excreted in breast milk. Because of the risk of serious adverse effects on the infant, a decision should be made whether to discontinue the drug or discontinue breast-feeding.

---

lomustine (CCNU)
CeeNU

● Pharmacologic classification: alkylating agent, nitrosourea (cell cycle-phase nonspecific)
● Therapeutic classification: antineoplastic
● Pregnancy risk category C

How supplied
Available by prescription only
Capsules: 10 mg, 40 mg, 100 mg

Indications, route, and dosage
Dosage and indications may vary. Check current literature for recommended protocol.
Brain, colon, lung, and renal cell cancer; Hodgkin's disease; lymphomas; melanomas; multiple myeloma
Adults and children: 100 to 130 mg/m² P.O. as single dose q 6 weeks. Reduce dose according to bone marrow depression. Repeat doses should not be given until WBC count is more than 4,000/mm³ and platelet count is more than 100,000/mm³.

If leukocyte count is over 3,000/mm³ and platelet count is over 75,000/mm³, reduce subsequent doses by 25%; if leukocyte count is over 2,000/mm³ and platelet count is over 50,000/mm³, reduce subsequent doses by 50%; if leukocyte count is under 2,000/mm³ and platelet count is under 25,000/mm³, do not repeat dosage.

Pharmacodynamics
Antineoplastic action: Lomustine exerts its cytotoxic activity through alkylation, resulting in the inhibition of DNA and RNA synthesis. As with other nitrosourea compounds, lomustine is known to modify cellular proteins and alkylate proteins, resulting in an inhibition of protein synthesis. Cross-resistance exists between lomustine and carmustine.

Pharmacokinetics
● *Absorption:* Lomustine is rapidly and well absorbed across the GI tract after oral administration.
● *Distribution:* Lomustine is distributed widely into body tissues. Because of its high lipid solubility, the drug and its metabolites cross the blood-brain barrier to a significant extent.
● *Metabolism:* Lomustine is metabolized rapidly and extensively in the liver. Some of the metabolites have cytotoxic activity.
● *Excretion:* Metabolites of lomustine are excreted primarily in urine, with smaller amounts excreted in feces and through the lungs. The plasma elimination of lomustine is described as biphasic, with an initial phase half-life of 6 hours and a terminal phase of 1 to 2 days.

The extended half-life of the terminal phase is thought to be caused by enterohepatic circulation and protein-binding.

Contraindications and precautions
Lomustine is contraindicated in patients with a history of hypersensitivity to the drug.

Drug should be used cautiously in patients with renal and hepatic dysfunction because drug accumulation may occur; and in patients with hematologic compromise and those who have recently received cytotoxic or radiation therapy because the drug's adverse hematologic effects may be exacerbated. Administer with caution in patients with infection because the drug is myelosuppressive and may exacerbate infections.

Interactions
None reported.

Effects on diagnostic tests
Lomustine therapy may cause transient increases in liver function tests.

Adverse reactions
● CNS: lethargy, ataxia, dysarthria.
● GI: nausea and vomiting, beginning within 4 to 5 hours and lasting 24 hours; stomatitis.
● GU: nephrotoxicity, *progressive azotemia.*
● HEMA: anemia, *bone marrow depression* (dose-limiting); *leukopenia,* delayed up to 6 weeks, lasting 1 to 2 weeks; *thrombocytopenia,* delayed up to 4 weeks, lasting 1 to 2 weeks.
● Other: hepatotoxicity, alopecia.

Overdose and treatment
Clinical manifestations of overdose include myelosuppression, nausea, and vomiting.

Treatment is usually supportive and includes antiemetics and transfusion of blood components.

▶ Special considerations
Besides those relevant to all *alkylating agents,* consider the following recommendations.
● Give 2 to 4 hours after meals. Lomustine will be more completely absorbed if taken when the stomach is empty. To avoid nausea, give antiemetic before administering.
● Anorexia may persist for 2 to 3 days after a given dose.
● Alcoholic beverages should be avoided for a short period after a dose of lomustine.
● Dose modification may be required in patients with decreased platelets, leukocytes, or erythrocytes.
● Monitor CBC weekly. Drug is usually not administered more often than every 6 weeks; bone marrow toxicity is cumulative and delayed.
● Frequently assess renal and hepatic status.
● Avoid all I.M. injections when platelet count is below 100,000/mm³.
● Use anticoagulants cautiously. Watch closely for signs of bleeding.
● Because lomustine crosses the blood-brain barrier, it may be used to treat primary brain tumors.

Information for the patient
● Emphasize importance of continuing medication despite nausea and vomiting.
● Emphasize importance of taking the exact dose prescribed.
● Tell patient to call immediately if vomiting occurs shortly after a dose is taken.
● Advise patient to avoid exposure to people with infections.
● Warn patient to avoid aspirin-containing products.
● Tell patient to promptly report a sore throat, fever, or any unusual bruising or bleeding.

Breast-feeding
Metabolites of lomustine have been found in breast milk. Breast-feeding should be discontinued because of increased risk of serious adverse reactions, mutagenicity, and carcinogenicity in the infant.

loperamide hydrochloride
Imodium A-D, Imodium

● Pharmacologic classification: piperadine derivative
● Therapeutic classification: antidiarrheal
● Pregnancy risk category B

How supplied
Available by prescription only
Capsules: 2 mg
Available without prescription
Tablets: 2 mg
Solution: 1 mg/5 ml

Indications, route, and dosage
Acute, nonspecific diarrhea
Adults and children over age 12: Initially, 4 mg P.O., then 2 mg after each unformed stool. Maximum dosage is 16 mg daily.
Children age 9 to 11: 2 mg t.i.d. on first day.
Children age 6 to 8: 2 mg b.i.d. on first day.
Children age 2 to 5: 1 mg t.i.d. on first day.
Maintenance dose is ⅓ to ½ the initial dose.
Chronic diarrhea
Adults: Initially, 4 mg P.O., then 2 mg after each unformed stool until diarrhea subsides. Adjust dose to individual response.
Directions for patient self-medication
Adults: 4 mg after the first loose bowel movement, followed by 2 mg after each subsequent loose bowel movement, but no more than 8 mg daily for no more than 2 days.
Children age 9 to 11 (60-95 lbs): 2 mg after first loose bowel movement, followed by 1 mg after each subsequent loose bowel movement. Do not exceed 6 mg daily.
Children age 6 to 8 (48-59 lbs): 2 mg after first loose bowel movement, followed by 1 mg after each subsequent loose bowel movement. Do not exceed 4 mg daily.
Children age 2 to 5 (24-47 lbs): 1 mg after first loose bowel movement, followed by 1 mg after each subsequent loose bowel movement. Do not exceed 3 mg daily.

Pharmacodynamics
Antidiarrheal action: Loperamide reduces intestinal motility by acting directly on intestinal mucosal nerve endings; tolerance to antiperistaltic effect does not develop. The drug also may inhibit fluid and electrolyte secretion by an unknown mechanism. Although it is chemically related to opiates, it has not shown any physical dependance characteristics in humans, and it possesses no analgesic activity.

Pharmacokinetics
• *Absorption:* Loperamide is absorbed poorly from the GI tract.
• *Distribution:* Not well characterized.
• *Metabolism:* Absorbed loperamide is metabolized in the liver.
• *Excretion:* Loperamide is excreted primarily in feces; less than 2% is excreted in urine.

Contraindications and precautions
Loperamide is contraindicated in patients with diarrhea from pseudomembranous colitis or ulcerative colitis because it may precipitate toxic megacolon; in patients with diarrhea resulting from poisoning or infection by microbes that can penetrate the intestinal mucosa, because expulsion of intestinal contents may be a protective mechanism; and in patients with known hypersensitivity to the drug.

Loperamide should be used cautiously in patients with severe prostatic hypertrophy or hepatic disease because the drug may worsen the symptoms of this disorder.

Interactions
Concomitant use with an opioid analgesic may cause severe constipation.

Effects on diagnostic tests
None reported.

Adverse reactions
• CNS: drowsiness, fatigue, dizziness.
• GI: dry mouth, nausea, vomiting, abdominal cramps, abdominal distention, constipation.
• Other: rash.
Note: Drug should be discontinued if bowel sounds are absent, if abdominal distention occurs, or if patient does not improve within 48 hours (acute diarrhea) or 10 days (chronic diarrhea).

Overdose and treatment
Clinical effects of overdose include constipation, GI irritation, and CNS depression.

Treat with activated charcoal if ingestion was recent. If patient is vomiting, activated charcoal may be given in a slurry when patient can retain fluids. Alternately, gastric lavage may be performed, followed by administration of activated charcoal slurry. Monitor for CNS depression; treat respiratory depression with naloxone.

▶ Special considerations
After administration via nasogastric tube, tube should be flushed to clear it and ensure drug's passage to stomach.

Information for the patient
• Warn patient to take drug only as directed and not to exceed recommended dose.
• Caution patient to avoid driving and other tasks requiring alertness because drug may cause drowsiness and dizziness.
• Instruct patient to call if no improvement occurs in 48 hours or if fever develops.

Pediatric use
Drug is approved for use in children age 2 and older; however, children may be more susceptible to untoward CNS effects.

Breast-feeding
It is unknown if drug is excreted in breast milk. Use with caution.

---

lorazepam
Alzapam, Apo-Lorazepam*, Ativan, Loraz, Novolorazem*

• Pharmacologic classification: benzodiazepine
• Therapeutic classification: antianxiety agent; sedative-hypnotic
• Controlled substance schedule IV
• Pregnancy risk category D

How supplied
Available by prescription only
Tablets: 0.5 mg, 1 mg, 2 mg
Sublingual tablets:* 1 mg, 2 mg
Injection: 2 mg/ml, 4 mg/ml

Indications, route, and dosage
Anxiety, tension, agitation, irritability, especially in anxiety neuroses or organic (especially GI or CV) disorders
Adults: 2 to 6 mg P.O. daily in divided doses. Maximum dosage is 10 mg/day.
Insomnia
Adults: 2 to 4 mg P.O. h.s.
†*Preoperatively; treatment of status epilepticus*
Adults: 2 to 4 mg I.M. or I.V.

Pharmacodynamics
Anxiolytic and sedative actions: Lorazepam depresses the CNS at the limbic and subcortical levels of the brain. It produces an antianxiety effect by influencing the effect of the neurotransmitter gamma-aminobutyric acid (GABA) on its receptor in the ascending reticular activating system, which increases inhibition and blocks both cortical and limbic arousal after stimulation of the reticular formation.

Pharmacokinetics
• *Absorption:* When administered orally, lorazepam is well absorbed through the GI tract. Peak levels occur in 2 hours.
• *Distribution:* Lorazepam is distributed widely throughout the body. Drug is about 85% protein-bound.
• *Metabolism:* Lorazepam is metabolized in the liver to inactive metabolites.
• *Excretion:* The metabolites of lorazepam are excreted in urine as glucuronide conjugates.

Contraindications and precautions
Lorazepam is contraindicated in patients with known hypersensitivity to the drug or any ingredients in its formulation; in patients with acute narrow-angle glaucoma or untreated open-angle glaucoma, because of the drug's possible anticholinergic effect; in patients in coma, because the drug's hypnotic or hypotensive effect may be prolonged or intensified; and in patients with acute alcohol intoxication who have depressed vital signs, because the drug will worsen CNS depression.

Lorazepam should be used cautiously in patients

---

with psychoses because drug may induce paradoxical reactions; in patients with myasthenia gravis or Parkinson's disease because it may exacerbate the disorder; in patients with impaired hepatic function, which prolongs elimination of the drug; in elderly or debilitated patients, who are usually more sensitive to the drug's CNS effects; in individuals prone to addiction or drug abuse; and in patients with impaired respiratory function, such as chronic obstructive pulmonary disease.

Interactions
Lorazepam potentiates the CNS depressant effects of phenothiazines, narcotics, barbiturates, alcohol, antihistamines, monoamine oxidase inhibitors, general anesthetics, and antidepressants.

Concomitant use with cimetidine and possibly disulfiram causes diminished hepatic metabolism of lorazepam, which increases its plasma concentration.

Heavy smoking accelerates lorazepam's metabolism, thus lowering clinical effectiveness.

Combined use of parenteral lorazepam and scopolamine may be associated with an increased incidence of hallucinations, irrational behavior, and increased sedation.

Effects on diagnostic tests
Lorazepam therapy may increase the results of liver function tests.

Adverse reactions
● CNS: confusion, depression, drowsiness, lethargy, hangover effect, ataxia, dizziness, syncope, nightmares, fatigue, slurred speech, tremors, vertigo, behavior problems, paradoxical excitement, weakness, headache.
● CV: bradycardia, *circulatory collapse*, transient hypotension.
● DERM: rash, urticaria.
● EENT: diplopia, blurred vision, nystagmus.
● GI: constipation, dry mouth, anorexia, difficulty swallowing, nausea, vomiting, abdominal discomfort.
● GU: urinary incontinence or retention.
● Other: *respiratory depression*, dysarthria, hepatic dysfunction, changes in libido.
   Note: Drug should be discontinued if hypersensitivity or the following paradoxical reactions occur: acute hyperexcited state, anxiety, hallucinations, increased muscle spasticity, insomnia, or rage.

Overdose and treatment
Clinical manifestations of overdose include somnolence, confusion, coma, hypoactive reflexes, dyspnea, labored breathing, hypotension, bradycardia, slurred speech, and unsteady gait or impaired coordination.

Treatment requires support of blood pressure and respiration until drug effects subside; monitor vital signs. Mechanical ventilatory assistance via endotracheal tube may be required to maintain a patent airway and support adequate oxygenation. Flumazenil, a specific benzodiazepine antagonist, may be useful. Use I.V. fluids and vasopressors such as dopamine and phenylephrine to treat hypotension, if necessary. If patient is conscious, induce emesis. Use gastric lavage if ingestion was recent, but only if an endotracheal tube is present to prevent aspiration. After emesis or lavage, administer activated charcoal with a cathartic as a single dose. Dialysis is of limited value.

▶ Special considerations
Besides those relevant to all *benzodiazepines*, consider the following recommendations.
● Lorazepam is one of the preferred benzodiazepines for patients with hepatic disease.
● Use lowest possible effective dose to avoid oversedation.
● Parenteral lorazepam appears to possess potent amnestic effects.
● Administer oral lorazepam in divided doses, with the largest dose given before bedtime.
● Arteriospasm may result from intraarterial injection of lorazepam. Do not administer by this route.
● For I.V. administration, dilute lorazepam with an equal volume of a compatible diluent, such as dextrose 5% in water, sterile water for injection, or normal saline solution.
● Lorazepam may be injected directly into a vein or into the tubing of a compatible I.V. infusion, such as 0.9% saline solution or 5% dextrose solution. The rate of lorazepam I.V. injection should not exceed 2 mg/minute. Emergency resuscitative equipment should be available when administering I.V.
● Administer diluted lorazepam solutions immediately.
● Do not use lorazepam solutions if they are discolored or contain a precipitate.
● Administer I.M. dose of lorazepam undiluted, deep into a large muscle mass.
● Periodically assess hepatic function studies to prevent cumulative effects and to ensure adequate drug metabolism.
● No longer widely used as a preoperative medication because its effects are prolonged. May be useful for length procedures.

Information for the patient
● Caution patient not to make any changes in medication regimen without specific instructions.
● As appropriate, teach safety measures to protect from injury, such as gradual position changes and supervised walking.
● Advise patient of possible retrograde amnesia after I.V. or I.M. use.
● Advise patient to avoid large amounts of caffeine-containing products, which may interfere with lorazepam's effectiveness.
● Advise patient of potential for physical and psychological dependence with chronic use.
● Discontinue the drug slowly (over 8 to 12 weeks) after long-term therapy.

Geriatric use
● Elderly patients are more sensitive to lorazepam's CNS depressant effects. They may require supervision with ambulation and activities of daily living during initiation of therapy or after an increase in dose.
● Lower doses usually are effective in elderly patients because of decreased elimination.
● Parenteral administration of lorazepam is more likely to cause apnea, hypotension, bradycardia, and cardiac arrest in elderly patients.

Pediatric use
● Safe use of oral lorazepam in children under age 12 has not been established.
● Safe use of sublingual or parenteral lorazepam in children under age 18 has not been established.
● Closely observe neonate for withdrawal symptoms if

---

the mother took lorazepam for a prolonged period during pregnancy.

Breast-feeding
Lorazepam may be excreted in breast milk. Do not administer to breast-feeding women.

lovastatin
Mevacor

- Pharmacologic classification: lactone
- Therapeutic classification: cholesterol-lowering agent
- Pregnancy risk category X

How supplied
Available by prescription only
Tablets: 20 mg, 40 mg

Indications, route, and dosage
Reduction of low-density lipoprotein and total cholesterol levels in patients with primary hypercholesterolemia (types IIa and IIb)
Adults: Initially, 20 mg once daily with the evening meal. For patients with severely elevated cholesterol levels (for example, over 300 mg/dl), the initial dose should be 40 mg. The recommended range is 20 to 80 mg in single or divided doses.

Pharmacodynamics
Antilipemic action: Lovastatin, an inactive lactone, is hydrolyzed to the beta-hydroxy acid, which specifically inhibits 3-hydroxy-3-methylglutaryl-coenzyme A reductase (HMG-CoA reductase). This enzyme is an early (and rate-limiting) step in the synthetic pathway of cholesterol. At therapeutic doses, the enzyme is not blocked, and biologically necessary amounts of cholesterol can still be synthesized.

Pharmacokinetics
- *Absorption:* Animal studies indicate that about 30% of an oral dose is absorbed. Administration of drug with food improves plasma concentrations of total inhibitors by about 30%. Onset of action is about 3 days, with maximal therapeutic effects seen in 4 to 6 weeks.
- *Distribution:* Less than 5% of an oral dose reaches the systemic circulation because of extensive first-pass hepatic extraction; the liver is the drug's principal site of action. Both the parent compound and its principal metabolite are highly bound (more than 95%) to plasma proteins. Animal studies indicate that lovastatin can cross the placenta and the blood-brain barrier.
- *Metabolism:* Lovastatin is converted to the active B hydroxy acid form in the liver. Other metabolites include the 6' hydroxy derivative and two unidentified compounds.
- *Excretion:* About 80% of lovastatin is excreted primarily in feces, about 10% in urine.

Contraindications and precautions
Lovastatin is contraindicated in patients hypersensitive to the drug; in patients with active liver disease or unexplained persistent elevations of liver transaminase levels because the drug may be hepatotoxic; and in pregnant or breast-feeding women because the drug is teratogenic in animals.

Marked persistent elevations in serum transaminase levels have been noted. It is recommended that liver function tests be performed every 4 to 6 weeks during the first 15 months of therapy and periodically thereafter.

Drug should be used cautiously in patients with a history of liver disease and those who consume substantial quantities of alcohol; in patients at risk of developing renal failure secondary to rhabdomyolysis; in trauma patients; in patients undergoing major surgery; and in patients with severe acute infection, hypotension, severe metabolic, endocrine, or electrolyte disorders, or uncontrolled seizures.

Interactions
Concomitant administration with cholestyramine or colestipol may enhance lipid-reducing effects but may decrease bioavailability of lovastatin. Concomitant administration of cyclosporine, erythromycin, gemfibrozil, or niacin may increase risk of severe myopathy or rhabdomyolysis. Lovastatin may increase the anticoagulant effects of warfarin.

Effects on diagnostic tests
Lovastatin may elevate serum creatinine phosphokinase or serum transaminase levels.

Adverse reactions
- CNS: headache, dizziness.
- DERM: rash, pruritus.
- EENT: blurred vision, dysgeusia.
- GI: constipation, diarrhea, dyspepsia, flatus, abdominal pain or cramps, heartburn, nausea.
- Metabolic: elevated serum transaminase levels, abnormal liver tests.
- Musculoskeletal: muscle cramps, myalgia, myositis.
- Other: peripheral neuropathy.
  Note: Drug should be discontinued if liver function studies show signs of hepatotoxicity, or if patient develops myositis or renal failure secondary to rhabdomyolysis.

Overdose and treatment
None reported.

▶ Special considerations
- Initiate lovastatin only after diet and other nonpharmacologic therapies have proven ineffective. Patient should be on a standard cholesterol-lowering diet and continue on this diet during therapy.
- Lovastatin should be administered with the evening meal; absorption is enhanced and cholesterol biosynthesis is greater in the evening.
- Therapeutic response occurs in about 2 weeks, with maximum effects in 4 to 6 weeks.
- Monitor for signs of myositis; have patient report any muscle aches and pains.
- Liver function tests should be performed frequently during initiation of therapy and periodically thereafter.
- Store tablets at room temperature in a light-resistant container.

Information for the patient
- Stress importance of adhering to a cholesterol-lowering diet.
- Advise patient to restrict alcohol intake.
- Instruct patient to take drug with evening meal.
- Tell patient to report any adverse reactions, particularly muscle aches and pains.

---

*Canada only   †Unlabeled clinical use   Italicized adverse reactions are life-threatening.

Pediatric use
Safety and efficacy in children have not been established.

Breast-feeding
An alternative feeding method is recommended during therapy with lovastatin.

---

loxapine hydrochloride
Loxitane C, Loxitane I.M.

loxapine succinate
Loxapac*, Loxitane

- Pharmacologic classification: dibenzoxazepine
- Therapeutic classification: antipsychotic
- Pregnancy risk category C

How supplied
Available by prescription only
Capsules: 5 mg, 10 mg, 25 mg, 50 mg
Oral concentrate: 25 mg/ml
Injection: 50 mg/ml

Indications, route, and dosage
Psychotic disorders
Adults: 10 mg P.O. or I.M. b.i.d. to q.i.d., rapidly increasing to 60 to 100 mg P.O. daily for most patients; dose varies from patient to patient. Maximum daily dosage is 250 mg. Do not administer drug I.V.

Pharmacodynamics
Antipsychotic action: Loxapine is the only tricyclic antipsychotic; it is structurally similar to amoxapine. Loxapine is thought to exert its antipsychotic effects by postsynaptic blockade of CNS dopamine receptors, thus inhibiting dopamine-mediated effects. Loxapine has many other central and peripheral effects; its most prominent adverse reactions are extrapyramidal.

Pharmacokinetics
- *Absorption:* Loxapine is absorbed rapidly and completely from the GI tract. Sedation occurs in 30 minutes.
- *Distribution:* Loxapine is distributed widely into the body, including breast milk. Peak effect occurs at 1½ to 3 hours; steady-state serum level is achieved within 3 to 4 days. Drug is 91% to 99% protein-bound.
- *Metabolism:* Drug is metabolized extensively by the liver, forming a few active metabolites; duration of action is 12 hours.
- *Excretion:* Most of drug is excreted as metabolites in urine; some is excreted in feces via the biliary tract. About 50% of drug is excreted in urine and feces within 24 hours.

Contraindications and precautions
Loxapine is contraindicated in patients with known hypersensitivity to loxapine, and in patients with disorders accompanied by coma, CNS depression, brain damage, circulatory collapse, or cerebrovascular disease because of the potential hypotensive effects.

Loxapine should be used cautiously in patients with cardiac disease (arrhythmias, congestive heart failure, angina pectoris, valvular disease, or heart block), encephalitis, Reye's syndrome, head injury, respiratory disease, epilepsy and other seizure disorders, glaucoma, prostatic hypertrophy, urinary retention, hepatic or renal dysfunction, Parkinson's disease, pheochromocytoma, or hypocalcemia.

Interactions
Concomitant use of loxapine with sympathomimetics, including epinephrine, phenylephrine, phenylpropanolamine, and ephedrine (often found in nasal sprays), and with appetite suppressants may decrease their stimulatory and pressor effects. Loxapine may cause epinephrine reversal, an inhibition of epinephrine's vasopressor effect.

Loxapine may inhibit blood pressure response to centrally acting antihypertensive drugs, such as guanethidine, guanabenz, guanadrel, clonidine, methyldopa, and reserpine. Loxapine may antagonize therapeutic effect of bromocriptine on prolactin secretion; it may also decrease the vasoconstricting effects of high-dose dopamine, and may decrease effectiveness and increase toxicity of levodopa (by dopamine blockade).

Additive effects are likely after concomitant use of loxapine and CNS depressants, including alcohol, analgesics, barbiturates, narcotics, tranquilizers, anesthetics (general, spinal, epidural), and parenteral magnesium sulfate (oversedation, respiratory depression, and hypotension); antiarrhythmic agents, quinidine, disopyramide, and procainamide (increased incidence of cardiac arrhythmias and conduction defects); atropine and other anticholinergic drugs, including antidepressants, monoamine oxidase inhibitors, phenothiazines, antihistamines, meperidine, and antiparkinsonian agents (oversedation, paralytic ileus, visual changes, and severe constipation); and nitrates (hypotension).

Beta-blocking agents may inhibit loxapine metabolism, increasing plasma levels and toxicity.

Concomitant use with lithium may result in severe neurologic toxicity with an encephalitis-like syndrome and in decreased therapeutic response to loxapine. Aluminum- and magnesium-containing antacids and antidiarrheals decrease loxapine absorption and, thus, its therapeutic effects.

Effects on diagnostic tests
Loxapine causes false-positive test results for urinary porphyrins, urobilinogen, amylase, and 5-hydroxyindoleacetic acid (5-HIAA) because of darkening of urine by metabolites; it also causes false-positive urine pregnancy test results using human chorionic gonadotropin.

Loxapine elevates test results for liver enzymes and protein-bound iodine, and causes quinidine-like effects on the ECG.

Adverse reactions
- CNS: *extrapyramidal symptoms* dystonia, akathisia, torticollis (more common with I.M. administration), tardive dyskinesia (usually dose-related with long-term therapy, but it can develop rapidly), sedation, pseudoparkinsonism, drowsiness (frequent), *neuroleptic malignant syndrome* (dose-related; if untreated, fatal *respiratory failure* in over 10% of patients), dizziness, headache, insomnia, exacerbation of psychotic symptoms.
- CV: *asystole*, orthostatic hypotension, tachycardia, dizziness and fainting, *arrhythmias*, ECG changes, increased anginal pain after I.M. injection.
- EENT: blurred vision, tinnitus, mydriasis, increased

---

intraocular pressure, ocular changes (retinal pigmentary change on long-term use).
- GI: dry mouth, constipation, nausea, vomiting, anorexia, diarrhea.
- GU: urine retention, gynecomastia, hypermenorrhea, inhibited ejaculation.
- HEMA: transient leukopenia, *agranulocytosis,* thrombocytopenia, anemia (within 30 to 90 days).
- Local: contact dermatitis from concentrate or injectable, muscle necrosis from I.M. injection.
- Other: hyperprolactinemia, photosensitivity, increased appetite or weight gain, hypersensitivity (rash, urticaria, drug fever, edema), decreased libido.

Note: Drug should be discontinued immediately if any of the following occur: hypersensitivity, jaundice, agranulocytosis, neuroleptic malignant syndrome (marked hyperthermia, extrapyramidal effects, autonomic dysfunction), or severe extrapyramidal symptoms that occur even after dose is lowered. Drug should be discontinued 48 hours before and 24 hours after myelography using metrizamide, because of risk of convulsions. When feasible, drug should be withdrawn slowly and gradually; many drug effects persist after withdrawal.

Overdose and treatment
CNS depression is characterized by deep, unarousable sleep and possible coma, hypotension or hypertension, extrapyramidal symptoms, abnormal involuntary muscle movements, agitation, seizures, arrhythmias, ECG changes, hypothermia or hyperthermia, and autonomic nervous system dysfunction.

Treatment is symptomatic and supportive, including maintaining vital signs, airway, stable body temperature, and fluid and electrolyte balance.

Do not induce vomiting: drug inhibits cough reflex, and aspiration may occur. Use gastric lavage, then activated charcoal and saline cathartics; hemodialysis may be helpful. Regulate body temperature as needed. Treat hypotension with I.V. fluids: *do not give epinephrine.* Treat seizures with parenteral diazepam or barbiturates; arrhythmias with parenteral phenytoin (1 mg/kg with rate titrated to blood pressure); and extrapyramidal reactions with benztropine or parenteral diphenhydramine 2 mg/kg/minute.

▶ Special considerations
- Assess patient periodically for abnormal body movement.
- Tardive dyskinesia may occur, usually after prolonged use. It may not appear until months or years after treatment and may disappear spontaneously or persist for life.
- Avoid combining with alcohol or other depressants.
- Obtain baseline blood pressure measurements before starting therapy and monitor regularly.
- Dilute liquid concentrate with orange or grapefruit juice just before giving.
- Periodic ophthalmic tests are recommended.
- Dose of 10 mg is therapeutic equivalent of 100 mg chlorpromazine.
- Photosensitivity warnings may apply with loxapine.

Information for the patient
- Warn against activities that require alertness and good psychomotor coordination until CNS response to drug is determined. Drowsiness and dizziness usually subside after first few weeks.

- Sugarless gum or candy, mouthwash, ice chips, or artificial saliva may help alleviate dry mouth.
- Advise patient to get up slowly to avoid orthostatic hypotension.

Geriatric use
Elderly patients are highly sensitive to the antimuscarinic, hypotensive, and sedative effects of loxapine and have a higher risk of developing extrapyramidal adverse reactions, such as parkinsonism and tardive dyskinesia. These patients develop higher plasma concentrations and therefore require lower initial dosage and more gradual titration.

Pediatric use
Loxapine is not recommended for children under age 16.

---

lymphocyte immune globulin (antithymocyte globulin [equine])
Atgam

- Pharmacologic classification: immunoglobulin
- Therapeutic classification: immunosuppressive agent
- Pregnancy risk category C

How supplied
Available by prescription only
Injection: 50 mg of equine IgG per ml, in 5-ml ampules

Indications, route, and dosage
Prevention of acute renal allograft rejection
Adults and children: 15 mg/kg/day I.V. for 14 days, then same dosage every other day for the next 14 days (to a total of 21 doses in 28 days). The first dose of ATG should be administered within 24 hours before or after transplantation.
Treatment of acute renal allograft rejection
Adults and children: 10 to 15 mg/kg/day for 14 days; if necessary, the same dosage may be given every other day for another 14 days (to a total of 21 doses in 28 days). Therapy with ATG should begin at the first sign of acute rejection.
Aplastic anemia
Adults and children: 10 to 20 mg/kg I.V. daily for 8 to 14 days, followed by alternate day therapy for an additional 14 days (total of 21 doses in 28 days).
Skin allotransplantation
Adults: 10 mg/kg 24 hours before allograft; then 10 to 15 mg/kg every other day. Maintenance dosage is variable and can range from 5 to 40 mg/kg/day, depending upon clinical response and clinical indicators of immunosuppressive activity. Therapy usually continues until the allografts cover less than 20% of the total body surface area; in most cases, this requires 40 to 60 days of treatment.
Bone marrow allotransplantation
Adults: 7 to 10 mg/kg I.V. every other day for six doses.

Pharmacodynamics
Immunosuppressive action: The exact mechanism has not been fully defined but may involve elimination of antigen-reactive T cells (T-lymphocytes) in peripheral blood or alteration of T-cell function. The effects of antilymphocyte preparations, including ATG, on T cells are variable and complex. Whether the effects of ATG are mediated

through a specific subset of T cells has not been determined.

Pharmacokinetics

● *Absorption:* Peak plasma levels of equine IgG after I.V. administration of ATG vary, depending on the patient's ability to catabolize foreign IgG.
● *Distribution:* Distribution of ATG into body fluids and tissues has not been fully described. Since antilymphocyte serum reportedly is poorly distributed into lymphoid tissues (for example, spleen, lymph nodes), it is likely that ATG is also poorly distributed into these tissues.

No information is available on transplacental distribution of ATG. However, such distribution is likely because other immunoglobulins cross the placenta. Virtually all transplacental passage of immunoglobulins occurs during the last 4 weeks of pregnancy.
● *Metabolism:* Not known.
● *Excretion:* The plasma half-life of equine IgG reportedly averages about 6 days (range: 1.5 to 12 days). Approximately 1% of a dose of ATG is excreted in urine, principally as unchanged equine IgG. In one report, mean urinary concentration of equine IgG was approximately 4 mcg/ml after approximately 21 doses of ATG over 28 days.

Contraindications and precautions

ATG is contraindicated in patients who have had a severe systemic reaction during therapy with this drug or with another equine immunoglobulin G preparation. Anaphylaxis occurs in less than 1% of patients receiving ATG.

Note: Serum sickness reactions have occurred in patients receiving ATG. The incidence of serum sickness reactions to ATG in renal allograft recipients is unknown, in part because of the difficulty in diagnosing the reaction in these patients; but serum sickness reactions have occurred in a high percentage (85% to 100%) of patients receiving this drug for the treatment of aplastic anemia. Fever, nausea and vomiting, cutaneous lesions, and lymphadenopathy are common signs of serum sickness. Corticosteroids may be used to treat these reactions.

Interactions

Concomitant use of ATG with other immunosuppressive therapy (azathioprine, corticosteroids, graft irradiation), may intensify immunosuppression, an effect that can be used to therapeutic advantage; however, such therapy may increase vulnerability to infection and possibly the risk of lymphoma or lymphoproliferative disorders.

Effects on diagnostic tests

Elevations of hepatic serum enzymes have been reported.

Adverse reactions

● CNS: arthralgia, malaise, weakness, faintness, seizures, night sweats.
● CV: hypertension, hypotension, tachycardia, chest pain, edema, *pulmonary edema*, iliac vein obstruction, renal artery thrombosis.
● DERM: rash, pruritus, erythema.
● GI: nausea, vomiting, diarrhea, stomatitis, hiccups, epigastric pain, abdominal distention.
● Other: *anaphylaxis, serum sickness*, fever, chills, arthralgia, back pain, leukopenia, thrombocytopenia.

Note: Drug should be discontinued if signs and symptoms of anaphylaxis occur.

Overdose and treatment

No information available.

▶ Special considerations

● Dilute ATG concentrate for injection before I.V. infusion. Dilute the required dose of ATG in 0.45 or 0.9% sodium chloride injection (usually 250 to 1,000 ml); the final concentration preferably should not exceed 1 mg of equine IgG per ml. Infuse over at least 4 hours.
● Infusion in dextrose or highly acidic solutions is not recommended.
● Invert the I.V. infusion solution container into which ATG concentrate is added to prevent contact of undiluted ATG with air inside the container. Diluted solutions of ATG should be refrigerated at 2 to 8 C. if administration is delayed. Reconstituted solutions should not be used after 12 hours (including actual infusion time), even if stored at 2 to 8 C.
● Because of the risk of a severe systemic reaction (anaphylaxis), the manufacturer recommends an intradermal skin test before administration of the initial dose of ATG. The skin test procedure consists of intradermal injection of 0.1 ml of a 1:1,000 dilution of ATG concentrate for injection in 0.9% sodium chloride injection (5 mcg of equine IgG). A control test using 0.9% sodium chloride injection should be administered in the other arm to facilitate interpretation of the results. If a wheal or area of erythema greater than 10 mm in diameter (with or without pseudopod formation) and itching or marked local swelling develops, infusion of ATG requires extreme caution; severe and potentially fatal systemic reactions can occur in patients with a positive skin test. A systemic reaction to the skin test such as generalized rash, tachycardia, dyspnea, hypotension, or anaphylaxis rules out further administration of ATG. The predictive value of the ATG skin test has not been clearly established, and an allergic reaction may occur despite a negative skin test.
● Anaphylaxis may occur at any time during ATG therapy and may be indicated by hypotension, respiratory distress, or pain in the chest, flank, or back.
● The manufacturer has not yet determined the total number of ATG doses (10 to 20 mg/kg per dose) that can be administered safely to an individual patient. Some renal allograft recipients have received up to 50 doses in 4 months; others, up to four 28-day courses of 21 doses each without an increased incidence of adverse effects.
● ATG has been used to treat aplastic anemia, and as an adjunct in bone marrow and skin allotransplantation.
● Patients receiving ATG should be closely observed for signs of leukopenia, thrombocytopenia, and concurrent infection.
● To minimize the risks of leukopenia and infection, some clinicians recommend that azathioprine and corticosteroid dosages be reduced by 50% when ATG is used concomitantly with these drugs for the prevention or treatment of renal allograft rejection.
● Patients must be closely monitored for signs of infection during ATG therapy.
● Some clinicians elect to administer prophylactic platelet transfusion in patients receiving the drug for aplastic anemia because of the high risk of thrombocytopenia.

Information for the patient

Warn patient that a febrile reaction is likely.

Pediatric use

Safety and efficacy not established. Drug has had limited use in children age 3 months to 19 years.

Breast-feeding
Distribution into breast milk unknown but likely because other immunoglobulins are distributed into breast milk. Breast-feeding women should consider an alternative feeding method.

lypressin
Diapid

- Pharmacologic classification: posterior pituitary hormone
- Therapeutic classification: antidiuretic hormone
- Pregnancy risk category B

How supplied
Available by prescription only
Nasal spray: 0.185 mg/ml, in 8-ml bottle

Indications, route, and dosage
Nonnephrogenic diabetes insipidus
Adults and children: 1 or 2 sprays (approximately 2 USP posterior pituitary pressor units/spray) in either or both nostrils q.i.d. and an additional dose h.s., if needed, to prevent nocturia. If usual dosage is inadequate, increase frequency rather than number of sprays.

Pharmacodynamics
Antidiuretic action: Lypressin is used to control or prevent signs and complications of neurogenic diabetes insipidus. Acting primarily at the renal tubular level, lypressin increases cyclic 3',5'-adenosine monophosphate, which increases water permeability at the renal tubule and collecting duct, resulting in increased urine osmolality and decreased urinary flow rate.

Pharmacokinetics
- *Absorption:* Lypressin is destroyed by trypsin in the GI tract; therefore, it is given intranasally. Absorption is rapid from the nasal mucosa. Onset of effect is rapid after intranasal application and peaks within ½ to 2 hours.
- *Distribution:* Lypressin is distributed into the extracellular fluid.
- *Metabolism:* Lypressin is metabolized by the kidneys and liver.
- *Excretion:* A small amount of active drug and its inactive metabolites are excreted in urine. Duration of action is 3 to 8 hours. Half-life is about 15 minutes.

Contraindications and precautions
Lypressin is contraindicated in patients with known hypersensitivity to the drug. Large doses should be used with caution in patients with coronary artery disease because lypressin may cause coronary artery constriction. Although lypressin's pressor effects are minimal, the drug should be used with caution in patients in whom blood pressure elevation is hazardous.

Interactions
Concomitant use of lypressin with carbamazepine, chlorpropamide, or clofibrate may potentiate lypressin's antidiuretic effect; use with demeclocycline, lithium, norepinephrine, epinephrine, heparin, or alcohol may decrease the antidiuretic effect.

Effects on diagnostic tests
None reported.

Adverse reactions
- CNS: headache, dizziness, *seizures, coma.*
- DERM: hypersensitivity reaction.
- EENT: nasal congestion or ulceration, irritation, pruritus of nasal passages, rhinorrhea, conjunctivitis, periorbital edema.
- GI: heartburn from drip of excess spray into pharynx, abdominal cramps, frequent bowel movements.
- GU: possible transient fluid retention from overdose.
- Other: substernal tightness from inadvertent inhalation.
   Note: Drug should be discontinued if signs or symptoms of anaphylaxis, hypersensitivity, or water intoxication occur.

Overdose and treatment
Clinical manifestations of overdose include drowsiness, listlessness, headache, confusion, anuria, and weight gain (water intoxication). Treatment requires water restriction and temporary withdrawal of lypressin until polyuria occurs. Severe water intoxication may require osmotic diuresis with mannitol, hypertonic dextrose, or urea, either alone or with furosemide.

▶ Special considerations
Besides those relevant to all *posterior pituitary hormones,* consider the following recommendation.
- Observe for signs of early water intoxication – drowsiness, listlessness, headache, confusion, anuria, and weight gain – to prevent seizures, coma, and death.

Information for the patient
- Tell patient that drug should be applied topically to nasal mucosa as a spray; it should not be inhaled. Instruct patient about proper use: blow nose gently before using; hold bottle in an upright position; hold head upright and spray the medicine into each nostril by squeezing the bottle quickly and firmly; rinse the tip of the bottle with hot water and replace the cap after use; and do not allow water to enter bottle when rinsing.
- Instruct patient to carry medication at all times because of its fairly short duration of action.
- Tell patient to check the drug's expiration date.
- Tell patient to call if a cold or allergy develops because inflammation of the nasal mucosa will diminish the drug's absorption.

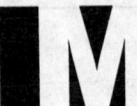

mafenide acetate
Sulfamylon Acetate

- Pharmacologic classification: synthetic anti-infective
- Therapeutic classification: topical antibacterial
- Pregnancy risk category C

How supplied
Available by prescription only
Cream: 8.5%

Indications, route, and dosage
Adjunctive treatment of second- and third-degree burns
Adults and children: Apply 1/16" (16 mm) daily or b.i.d. to cleansed, debrided wounds. Reapply as needed to keep burned area covered.

Pharmacodynamics
Antibacterial action: Mechanism of action of mafenide is undetermined; however, it appears that the drug interferes with bacterial cellular metabolism. Mafenide has a wide spectrum of activity and is bacteriostatic against many gram-negative and gram-positive organisms and several strains of anaerobes.

Pharmacokinetics
- *Absorption:* Drug diffuses through devascularized areas and is absorbed quickly.
- *Distribution:* Mafenide is distributed rapidly after topical application.
- *Metabolism:* Mafenide is metabolized rapidly to a weak carbonic anhydrase inhibitor metabolite.
- *Excretion:* Metabolite is excreted in the urine.

Contraindications and precautions
Mafenide acetate is contraindicated in patients with known hypersensitivity to mafenide acetate or to other sulfonamide derivatives (including furosemide, thiazide diuretics, carbonic anhydrase inhibitors, sulfites, parabens) and in women of childbearing age, unless benefit outweighs risk of hazard to fetus. Drug should be used with caution in patients with renal failure.

Drug is intended for topical use only; avoid contact with eyes and mucous membranes; use of mafenide may be followed by fungal colonization in and below eschar.

Interactions
None reported.

Effects on diagnostic tests
None reported.

Adverse reactions
- HEMA: bone marrow suppression, *fatal hemolytic anemia.*
- Metabolic: hyperchloremia, metabolic acidosis, porphyria.
- Pulmonary: hyperventilation, tachypnea.
- Local: pain, burning sensation, erythema, blisters, bleeding of new skin, excoriation.
- Other: hypersensitivity (rash, pruritus, itching, facial edema, urticaria, inflammation, eosinophilia).
   Note: Drug should be discontinued if sensitization develops.

Overdose and treatment
Accidental ingestion may cause diarrhea. To treat local overapplication, discontinue drug and clean skin thoroughly.

▶ Special considerations
- Apply to clean, debrided wound with sterile gloved hand, covering wound to approximately 1/16" (16 mm); reapply to areas if removed. Keep burned areas covered with cream at all times. Dressings usually are not required; if necessary, apply only a thin layer of dressing.
- Patient should be bathed daily to aid debridement; prior layer of cream should be removed before reapplication; whirlpool baths are extremely effective.
- Continue treatment until site is healed or ready for grafting.
- Monitor patient for overgrowth of nonsusceptible organisms; severe prolonged pain may indicate allergy.
- Monitor acid-base balance closely, especially in patients with pulmonary or renal dysfunction; if metabolic acidosis develops, discontinue drug for 24 to 48 hours.

Information for the patient
Instruct patient in proper care of burn sites; stress importance of calling promptly if condition worsens or adverse reactions occur.

Breast-feeding
Women should avoid breast-feeding while using mafenide.

magaldrate (aluminum-magnesium complex)
Antiflux*, Lowsium, Riopan, Riopan Plus

- Pharmacologic classification: aluminum-magnesium salt
- Therapeutic classification: antacid
- Pregnancy risk category C

How supplied
Available without prescription
Tablets (swallow): 480 mg
Tablets (chewable): 480 mg
Suspension: 540 mg/5 ml, 1,080 mg/5 ml

Indications, route, and dosage

Antacid

Suspension
Adults: 540 to 1,080 mg between meals and h.s. with water.

Tablets
Adults: 480 to 960 mg P.O. with water between meals and h.s.; or 1 to 2 chewable tablets (chewed before swallowing) between meals and h.s.

Pharmacodynamics

Antacid action: Magaldrate neutralizes gastric acid, reducing the direct acid irritant effect. This increases gastric pH, which inactivates pepsin. Magaldrate also enhances mucosal barrier integrity and improves gastroesophageal sphincter tone.

Pharmacokinetics

● *Absorption:* Aluminum may be absorbed systemically. Magnesium also may be absorbed, posing a risk to patients with renal failure. Absorption is unrelated to mechanism of action.
● *Distribution:* Primarily local.
● *Metabolism:* None.
● *Excretion:* Magaldrate is excreted in feces; some aluminum and magnesium may be excreted in breast milk. Duration of action is prolonged.

Contraindications and precautions

Magaldrate is contraindicated in patients with a colostomy or an ileostomy, renal failure or any degree of renal impairment, hypophosphatemia, appendicitis, undiagnosed rectal or GI bleeding, ulcerative colitis, diverticulitis, chronic diarrhea, or intestinal or gastric outlet obstruction, because this drug may exacerbate the symptoms of these conditions.

Magaldrate should be used cautiously in patients with decreased GI motility, such as elderly patients and those taking anticholinergics or antidiarrheals.

Interactions

When used concomitantly, magaldrate may increase levodopa absorption, increasing risk of toxicity.

The drug may inhibit absorption of phenothiazines (especially chlorpromazine) and may decrease absorption of quinolones, tetracycline, coumarin anticoagulants, chenodiol, antimuscarinics, diazepam, chlordiazepoxide, isoniazid, vitamin A, digoxin, and phosphates, thus lessening their effectiveness.

Magaldrate also may cause premature release of enterically coated drugs. Separate use of magaldrate and all oral drugs by 1 to 2 hours.

Effects on diagnostic tests

Magaldrate may antagonize pentagastrin's effect during gastric acid secretion tests; drug may decrease serum potassium levels, and increase serum gastrin and urine pH levels.

Adverse reactions

● GI: mild diarrhea, constipation.
● Other: unusual fatigue or weakness, unusual weight loss.

Overdose and treatment

No information available.

▶ Special considerations

● Shake suspension well; give with small amounts of water or fruit juice.
● After administration through nasogastric tube, tube should be flushed with water to clear it and ensure drug's passage to stomach.
● Give drug at least 1 hour apart from enterically coated medications.
● Chewable tablets contain sugar.
● Monitor renal function and serum phosphate, potassium, and magnesium levels in patients with renal disease.
● Most formulations contain less than 0.5 mg of sodium per tablet (or 5 ml of liquid).

Information for the patient

● Caution patient to take drug only as directed and 1 or 2 hours apart from other oral medications.
● Remind patient to shake suspension well or to chew tablets thoroughly.
● Warn patient not to take more than 18 teaspoonfuls or 20 tablets in a 24-hour period.

Pediatric use

Use of magaldrate as an antacid in children under age 6 requires a well-established diagnosis because children typically give vague descriptions of symptoms.

Breast-feeding

Some aluminum and magnesium may be excreted in breast milk. However, no problems have been associated with use in breast-feeding women.

---

magnesium hydroxide (milk of magnesia, magnesia magma)
Milk of Magnesia

● Pharmacologic classification: magnesium salt
● Therapeutic classification: antacid, antiulcer agent, laxative
● Pregnancy risk category B

How supplied

Available without prescription
Tablets: 300 mg, 600 mg
Suspension: 7.75%

Indications, route, and dosage

Constipation, bowel evacuation before surgery

Adults and children over age 6: 10 to 20 ml concentrated milk of magnesia P.O.; 15 to 60 ml milk of magnesia P.O.

Laxative

Adults: 30 to 60 ml P.O., usually h.s.
Children age 6 to 12: 15 to 30 ml P.O.
Children age 2 to 6: 5 to 15 ml P.O.

Antacid

Adults: 5 to 15 ml P.O. as needed.
Children: 2.5 to 5 ml P.O. as needed.

Pharmacodynamics

● *Antiulcer action:* Magnesium hydroxide neutralizes gastric acid, decreasing the direct acid irritant effect. This increases pH, which, in turn, leads to pepsin in-

activation. Magnesium hydroxide also enhances mucosal barrier integrity and improves gastric and esophageal sphincter tone.
- *Antacid action:* Magnesium hydroxide reacts rapidly with hydrochloric acid in the stomach to form magnesium chloride and water.
- *Laxative action:* Magnesium hydroxide produces its laxative effect by increasing the osmotic gradient in the gut and drawing in water, causing distention that stimulates peristalsis and bowel evacuation.

Pharmacokinetics
- *Absorption:* About 15% to 30% of magnesium may be absorbed systemically (posing a potential risk to patients with renal failure).
- *Distribution:* None.
- *Metabolism:* None.
- *Excretion:* Unabsorbed drug is excreted in feces; absorbed drug is excreted rapidly in urine.

Contraindications and precautions
Magnesium hydroxide is contraindicated in patients with renal failure because of decreased excretion of absorbed magnesium, which may lead to hypermagnesemia, and in patients with an ileostomy, a colostomy, abdominal pain, nausea, vomiting, fecal impaction, or intestinal obstruction or perforation, because the drug may worsen the symptoms associated with these disorders.

Interactions
When used concomitantly, magnesium hydroxide may decrease absorption of quinolones and tetracyclines and may cause premature release of enterically coated drugs.

Concomitant use of magnesium hydroxide with aluminum hydroxide may decrease the absorption rate and extent of chlordiazepoxide, chlorpromazine, dicumarol, digoxin, and isoniazid.

Effects on diagnostic tests
No information available.

Adverse reactions
- *GI:* diarrhea, abdominal cramps, nausea.
- *Metabolic:* hypermagnesemia, fluid and electrolyte disturbances (with prolonged use), dehydration.
- *Other:* laxative dependence in long-term or excessive use.
    Note: Drug should be discontinued if patient develops signs or symptoms of hypermagnesemia, such as hypotension, respiratory depression, narcosis, ECG changes, muscle weakness, sedation, or confusion.

Overdose and treatment
No information available.

▶ Special considerations
- Give drug at least 1 hour apart from enterically coated medications; shake suspension well.
- After administration of the drug through nasogastric tube, the tube should be flushed with water to clear it.
- Monitor for signs and symptoms of hypermagnesemia, especially if patient has impaired renal function.

Information for the patient
- Caution patient to avoid overuse to prevent laxative dependence.

- Instruct patient to shake suspension well or to chew tablets well.

Pediatric use
Use of magnesium hydroxide as an antacid in children younger than age 6 requires a well-established diagnosis because children tend to give vague descriptions of symptoms.

Breast-feeding
Some magnesium may be excreted in breast milk, but no problems have been reported with use by breast-feeding women.

---

magnesium salicylate
Analate, Arthrin, Doan's Pills, Efficin, Magan, Mobidin

- Pharmacologic classification: salicylate
- Therapeutic classification: nonnarcotic analgesic, antipyretic, anti-inflammatory
- Pregnancy risk category C

How supplied
Available by prescription only
Tablets: 480 mg, 545 mg, 600 mg, 650 mg

Available without prescription
Tablets: 325 mg, 500 mg

Indications, route, and dosage
Arthritis
Adults: 600 to 650 mg P.O. q 4 hours, or 1090 mg t.i.d.; 3.6 to 4.8 g/day may be given in three to four divided doses.
Mild pain or fever
Adults: 600 to 650 mg P.O. t.i.d. or q.i.d.

Pharmacodynamics
- *Analgesic action:* Drug produces analgesia by an ill-defined effect on the hypothalamus (central action) and by blocking generation of pain impulses (peripheral action). The peripheral action may involve inhibition of prostaglandin synthesis.
- *Anti-inflammatory action:* Drug is thought to exert its anti-inflammatory effect by inhibiting prostaglandin synthesis; it may also inhibit the synthesis or action of other mediators of inflammation.
- *Antipyretic action:* Drug relieves fever by acting on the hypothalamic heat-regulating center to produce peripheral vasodilation. This increases peripheral blood supply and promotes sweating, which leads to loss of heat and to cooling by evaporation.

Pharmacokinetics
- *Absorption:* Magnesium salicylate is absorbed rapidly and completely from the GI tract.
- *Distribution:* Drug is highly protein-bound.
- *Metabolism:* Drug is hydrolyzed in the liver.
- *Excretion:* Metabolites are excreted in urine.

Contraindications and precautions
Magnesium salicylate is contraindicated in patients with known hypersensitivity to salicylate or other nonsteroidal anti-inflammatory agents (NSAIDs), and in pa-

---

tients with GI ulcer, GI bleeding, or renal insufficiency, because of the risk of magnesium toxicity.

Magnesium salicylate should be used cautiously in patients with a history of GI disease, increased risk of GI bleeding, or decreased renal function.

Patients with known "triad" symptoms (aspirin hypersensitivity, rhinitis/nasal polyps, and asthma) are at high risk of bronchospasm. Salicylates may mask the signs and symptoms of acute infection (fever, myalgia, erythema); carefully evaluate patients with high risk (such as those with diabetes).

Interactions
Anticoagulants and thrombolytic drugs may to some degree potentiate the platelet-inhibiting effects of magnesium salicylate. Monitor therapy closely for both drugs. Concomitant use of magnesium salicylate with drugs that are highly protein-bound (such as phenytoin, sulfonylureas, warfarin) may cause displacement of either drug, and adverse effects. Monitor therapy closely for both drugs. Concomitant use with other GI-irritant drugs (steroids, antibiotics, other NSAIDs) may potentiate the adverse GI effects of magnesium salicylate. Use together with caution. Ammonium chloride and other urine acidifiers increase magnesium salicylate blood levels; monitor for magnesium salicylate toxicity. Antacids in high doses, and other urine alkalizers, decrease magnesium salicylate blood levels; monitor for decreased salicylate effect. Corticosteroids enhance magnesium salicylate elimination. Food and antacids delay and decrease absorption of magnesium salicylate.

Effects on diagnostic tests
Magnesium salicylate in high doses may cause false-positive urine glucose test results using copper sulfate method; it may cause false-negative urine glucose test results using glucose enzymatic method. False increases or decreases have been seen in urine VMA tests; false increases in serum uric acid have been seen. Magnesium salicylate may interfere with the Gerhardt test for urine aceto-acetic acid. Magnesium salicylate may increase serum levels of AST (SGOT), ALT (SGPT), alkaline phosphatase, and bilirubin.

Adverse reactions
● DERM: rash, bruising.
● EENT: tinnitus and hearing loss.
● GI: nausea, vomiting, GI distress, occult bleeding.
● Other: hypersensitivity manifested by *anaphylaxis* or asthma, abnormal liver function studies, hepatitis.
Note: Drug should be discontinued if hypersensitivity or signs and symptoms of hepatic dysfunction or salicylism occur.

Overdose and treatment
Clinical manifestations of overdose include metabolic acidosis with respiratory alkalosis, hyperpnea, and tachypnea from increased CO_2 production and direct stimulation of the respiratory center.

To treat overdose of magnesium salicylate, empty stomach immediately by inducing emesis with ipecac syrup if patient is conscious, or by gastric lavage. Administer activated charcoal via nasogastric tube. Provide symptomatic and supportive measures, such as respiratory support and correction of fluid and electrolyte imbalances. Monitor laboratory parameters and vital signs closely. Alkaline diuresis may enhance renal excretion.

▶ Special considerations
Besides those relevant to all *salicylates,* consider the following recommendations.
● Magnesium salicylate has been associated with a lower incidence of G.I. disturbances.
● Magnesium salicylate has a less profound effect on inhibiting platelet aggregation than other salicylates.
● Obtain hemoglobin and prothrombin tests periodically.
● Monitor serum magnesium levels to prevent magnesium toxicity, especially in patients with renal insufficiency.

Information for the patient
● Instruct patient to follow prescribed regimen and to report any problems.
● Advise patient not to take drug longer than 10 days without medical supervision.
● Caution patient to keep drug out of the reach of children.

Geriatric use
● Patients over age 60 may be more susceptible to the toxic effects of magnesium salicylate. Use with caution.
● The effects of salicylates on renal prostaglandins may cause fluid retention and edema, a significant drawback for elderly patients and those with congestive heart failure.

Pediatric use
● The safety of long-term magnesium salicylate use in children has not been established.
● Because of epidemiologic association with Reye's syndrome, the Centers for Disease Control recommend that children with chicken pox or flulike symptoms should not be given salicylates.
● Febrile, dehydrated children can develop toxicity rapidly.

Breast-feeding
Salicylates are distributed in breat milk; avoid use of magnesium salicylate in breast-feeding women.

magnesium sulfate

● Pharmacologic classification: mineral/electrolyte
● Therapeutic classification: anticonvulsant
● Pregnancy risk category B

How supplied
Injectable solutions: 10%, 12.5%, 25%, 50% in 2-ml, 5-ml, 10-ml, 20-ml, and 30-ml ampules, vials, and pre-filled syringes

Indications, route, and dosage
Hypomagnesemic seizures
Adults: 1 to 2 g (as 10% solution) I.V. over 15 minutes, then 1 g I.M. q 4 to 6 hours, based on patient's response and magnesium blood levels.
Seizures secondary to hypomagnesemia in acute nephritis
Children: 0.2 ml/kg of 50% solution I.M. q 4 to 6 hours, p.r.n., or 100 mg/kg of 10% solution I.V. given slowly. Titrate dosage according to magnesium blood levels and seizure response.

Prevention or control of seizures in preeclampsia or eclampsia

Adults: Initially, 4 g I.V. in 250 ml dextrose 5% in water and 4 g deep I.M. each buttock; then 4 g deep I.M. into alternate buttock q 4 hours, p.r.n. Alternatively, 4 g I.V. as a loading dose followed by 1 to 4 g hourly as an I.V. infusion.

Pharmacodynamics

Anticonvulsant action: Magnesium sulfate has CNS and respiratory depressant effects. It acts peripherally, causing vasodilation; moderate doses cause flushing and sweating, whereas high doses cause hypotension. It prevents or controls seizures by blocking neuromuscular transmission.

Magnesium sulfate is sometimes used in pregnant women to prevent or control preeclamptic or eclamptic seizures; it also is used to treat hypomagnesemic seizures in adults, and in children with acute nephritis.

Pharmacokinetics

• *Absorption:* I.V. magnesium sulfate acts immediately; effects last about 30 minutes. After I.M. injection, it acts within 60 minutes and lasts for 3 to 4 hours. Effective anticonvulsant serum levels are 2.5 to 7.5 mEq/liter.
• *Distribution:* Magnesium sulfate is distributed widely throughout the body.
• *Metabolism:* None.
• *Excretion:* Magnesium sulfate is excreted unchanged in urine; some is excreted in breast milk.

Contraindications and precautions

Magnesium sulfate is contraindicated in patients with known heart block, myocardial damage, respiratory depression, or renal failure; and in patients with eclampsia, for 2 hours preceding induced delivery, to prevent toxicity and respiratory and CNS depression in the newborn.

Patient's urine output should be maintained at 100 ml/4 hours; magnesium sulfate should be used with caution in patients with decreased renal function.

Interactions

Concomitant use with alcohol, narcotics, anxiolytics, barbiturates, antidepressants, hypnotics, antipsychotics, or general anesthetics may increase CNS depressant effects; reduced dosages may be required. Concomitant use of magnesium sulfate with succinylcholine or tubocurarine potentiates and prolongs neuromuscular blocking action of these drugs; use with caution.

Extreme caution should be used when magnesium sulfate is used concomitantly with cardiac glycosides; changes in cardiac conduction in digitalized patients may lead to heart block if I.V. calcium is administered.

Effects on diagnostic tests

None reported.

Adverse reactions

• CNS: sweating, drowsiness, depressed reflexes, flaccid paralysis, hypothermia.
• CV: hypotension, flushing, *circulatory collapse, depressed cardiac function, heart block.*
• Other: *respiratory paralysis,* hypocalcemia, pain at infusion site.
   Note: Drug should be discontinued if signs of hypersensitivity, anuria, toxic symptoms, or toxic serum levels occur.

Overdose and treatment

Clinical manifestations of overdose with magnesium sulfate include a sharp drop in blood pressure and respiratory paralysis, ECG changes (increased PR, QRS, and QT intervals), heart block, and asystole.

Treatment requires artificial ventilation and I.V. calcium salt to reverse respiratory depression and heart block. Usual dosage is 5 to 10 mEq of calcium (10 to 20 ml of a 10% calcium gluconate solution).

▶ Special considerations

• I.V. bolus *must* be injected slowly (to avoid respiratory or cardiac arrest).
• If available, administer by constant infusion pump; maximum infusion rate is 150 mg/minute. Rapid drip causes feeling of heat.
• Discontinue drug as soon as needed effect is achieved.
• When giving repeated doses, test knee jerk reflex before each dose; if absent, discontinue magnesium. Use of magnesium sulfate beyond this point risks respiratory center failure.
• Respiratory rate must be 16 breaths per minute or more before each dose. Keep I.V. calcium salts on hand.
• To calculate grams of magnesium in a percentage of solution: X% = X g/100 ml (for example, 25% = 25 g/100 ml = 250 mg/ml).
• Monitor serum magnesium load and clinical status to avoid overdose.
• After use in toxemic women within 24 hours before delivery, watch newborn for signs of magnesium toxicity, including neuromuscular and respiratory depression.

Pediatric use

Magnesium sulfate is not indicated for pediatric use.

Breast-feeding

Magnesium sulfate is excreted in breast milk; in patients with normal renal function, all magnesium sulfate is excreted within 24 hours of discontinuing drug. Alternative feeding method is recommended during therapy.

---

mannitol
Osmitrol

• Pharmacologic classification: osmotic diuretic
• Therapeutic classification: diuretic, prevention and management of acute renal failure or oliguria, reduction of intracranial or intraocular pressure, treatment of drug intoxication
• Pregnancy risk category C

How supplied

Available by prescription only
Injection: 5%, 10%, 15%, 20%, 25%

Indications, route, and dosage
Test dose for marked oliguria or suspected inadequate renal function

Adults and children over age 12: 200 mg/kg or 12.5 g as a 15% or 20% solution I.V. over 3 to 5 minutes. Response is adequate if 30 to 50 ml urine/hour is excreted over 2 to 3 hours.

Treatment of oliguria
Adults and children over age 12: 50 to 100 g as a 15% to 20% solution I.V. over 90 minutes to several hours.

Prevention of oliguria or acute renal failure
Adults and children over age 12: 50 to 100 g of a concentrated (5% to 25%) solution I.V. Exact concentration is determined by fluid requirements.

Edema
Adults and children over age 12: 100 g as a 10% to 20% solution I.V. over 2 to 6 hours.

To reduce intraocular pressure or intracranial pressure
Adults and children over age 12: 1.5 to 2 g/kg as a 15% to 25% solution I.V. over 30 to 60 minutes.

To promote diuresis in drug intoxication
Adults and children over age 12: up to 200 g as a 5% to 10% solution I.V. continuously, while maintaining 100 to 500 ml urine output/hour and positive fluid balance.

Pharmacodynamics
Diuretic action: Mannitol increases the osmotic pressure of glomerular filtrate, inhibiting tubular reabsorption of water and electrolytes, thus promoting diuresis. This action also promotes urinary elimination of certain drugs. This effect is useful for prevention and management of acute renal failure or oliguria. This action is also useful for reduction of intracranial or intraocular pressure because mannitol elevates plasma osmolality, enhancing flow of water into extracellular fluid.

Pharmacokinetics
● *Absorption:* Mannitol is not absorbed from the GI tract. I.V. mannitol lowers intracranial pressure in 15 minutes and intraocular pressure in 30 to 60 minutes; it produces diuresis in 1 to 3 hours.
● *Distribution:* Mannitol remains in the extracellular compartment. It does not cross the blood-brain barrier.
● *Metabolism:* Mannitol is metabolized minimally to glycogen in the liver.
● *Excretion:* Mannitol is filtered by the glomeruli; half-life in adults with normal renal function is about 100 minutes.

Contraindications and precautions
Mannitol is contraindicated in patients with established anuria who do not respond to a test dose and in patients with severe pulmonary congestion, pulmonary edema, severe congestive heart failure, or severe dehydration, because of the risk of circulatory overload.

Do not administer mannitol until adequate renal function and urine flow are determined by a test dose. Evaluate patient's cardiovascular status before and during drug administration; sudden expansion of extracellular fluid may precipitate congestive heart failure.

Interactions
Mannitol may enhance renal excretion of lithium and lower serum lithium levels.

Effects on diagnostic tests
Mannitol therapy alters electrolyte balance. It also may interfere with tests for inorganic phosphorus concentration or blood ethylene glycol.

Adverse reactions
● CNS: *rebound increase in intracranial pressure* 8 to 12 hours after diuresis, headache, confusion.
● CV: transient expansion of plasma volume during infusion, causing circulatory overload, CHF, or pul-

monary edema; tachycardia; angina-like chest pain; orthostatic hypotension.
● EENT: blurred vision, rhinitis.
● GI: thirst, nausea, vomiting.
● GU: urinary retention.
● Metabolic: fluid and electrolyte imbalance, water intoxication, cellular dehydration.

Note: Drug should be discontinued if patient's urine output continues to decline, if central venous pressure (CVP) rises, or if signs of tissue dehydration or circulatory overload occur.

Overdose and treatment
Clinical manifestations of overdose include polyuria, cellular dehydration, hypotension, and cardiovascular collapse.

Discontinue infusion and institute supportive measures. Hemodialysis removes mannitol and decreases serum osmolality.

▶ Special considerations
Besides those relevant to all *osmotic diuretics,* consider the following recommendations.
● Use with extreme caution in patients with compromised renal function; monitor vital signs (including CVP) hourly and input and output, weight, renal function, fluid balance, and serum and urinary sodium and potassium levels daily.
● For maximum pressure reduction during surgery, give drug 1 to 1½ hours preoperatively.
● Mannitol should be administered I.V. via an in-line filter, with great care to avoid extravasation.
● Do not administer with whole blood; agglutination will occur.
● Mannitol solutions commonly crystallize at low temperatures; place crystallized solutions in a hot water bath, shake vigorously to dissolve crystals, and cool to body temperature before use. Do not use solutions with undissolved crystals.

Information for the patient
● Tell patient he may feel thirsty or experience mouth dryness, and emphasize importance of drinking only the amount of fluids provided.
● With initial doses, warn patient to change position slowly, especially when rising from lying or sitting position, to prevent dizziness from orthostatic hypotension.
● Instruct patient to immediately report pain in the chest, back, or legs; shortness of breath; or apnea.

Geriatric use
Elderly or debilitated patients will require close observation and may require lower dosages. Excessive diuresis promotes rapid dehydration, leading to hypovolemia, hypokalemia, and hyponatremia.

Pediatric use
Dosage for children under age 12 has not been established.

Breast-feeding
Safety of mannitol in breast-feeding women has not been established.

---

maprotiline hydrochloride
Ludiomil

- Pharmacologic classification: tricyclic antidepressant
- Therapeutic classification: antidepressant
- Pregnancy risk category B

How supplied
Available by prescription only
Tablets: 25 mg, 50 mg, 75 mg

Indications, route, and dosage
Depression
Adults: Initial dosage is 75 mg daily for patients with mild to moderate depression. The dosage may be increased, as required, to 150 mg daily. Maximum dosage is 225 mg in patients who are hospitalized. Usually given t.i.d.; may be given in a single daily dose. Maintain initial dosage for 1 week before increasing; increase by 25-mg increments.

Pharmacodynamics
Antidepressant action: Maprotiline is thought to exert its antidepressant effects by inhibiting reuptake of norepinephrine and serotonin in CNS nerve terminals (presynaptic neurons), which results in increased concentration and enhanced activity of these neurotransmitters in the synaptic cleft. Maprotiline has minimal inhibitory effect on serotonin reuptake. Maprotiline is also anxiolytic.

Pharmacokinetics
- *Absorption:* Maprotiline is absorbed slowly but completely from the GI tract after oral administration.
- *Distribution:* Maprotiline is distributed widely into the body, including the CNS and breast milk. Drug is 88% protein-bound. Peak serum concentration levels occur 8 to 24 hours after oral dose; steady-state plasma levels and peak therapeutic effect usually occur within 2 weeks. Proposed therapeutic serum levels range between 200 and 300 ng/ml.
- *Metabolism:* Maprotiline is metabolized slowly by the liver to the active metabolite desmethylmaprotiline; a significant first-pass effect may account for variability of serum concentrations in different patients taking the same dosage.
- *Excretion:* Most of drug is excreted in urine as metabolites within 3 weeks. About 30% is excreted in feces via the biliary tract.

Contraindications and precautions
Maprotiline is contraindicated in patients with known hypersensitivity to tricyclic antidepressants, trazodone, and related compounds; in the acute recovery phase of myocardial infarction (MI) because of its arrhythmogenic potential; in coma or severe respiratory depression because of additive CNS depression; and during or within 14 days of therapy with monoamine oxidase inhibitors because the combination can precipitate hyperpyrexia, hypertension, and seizures.

Use maprotiline cautiously in patients with other cardiac disease (arrhythmias, congestive heart failure [CHF], angina pectoris, valvular disease, or heart block); respiratory disorders; alcoholism, epilepsy, and other seizure disorders; scheduled electroconvulsive therapy; bipolar disease; glaucoma; hyperthyroidism or in those taking thyroid replacement; Type I and Type II diabetes; prostatic hypertrophy, paralytic ileus, or urinary retention; hepatic or renal dysfunction; or Parkinson's disease; and in those undergoing surgery with general anesthesia.

Interactions
Concomitant use of maprotiline with sympathomimetics, including epinephrine, phenylephrine, phenylpropanolamine, and ephedrine (often found in nasal sprays), may increase blood pressure; use with warfarin may increase prothrombin time and cause bleeding. Concomitant use with thyroid hormones, pimozide, and antiarrhythmic agents (quinidine, disopyramide, procainamide) may increase incidence of cardiac dysrhythmias and conduction defects. Maprotiline may decrease hypotensive effects of centrally acting antihypertensive drugs, such as guanethidine, guanabenz, guanadrel, clonidine, methyldopa, and reserpine. Concomitant use with disulfiram or ethchlorvynol may cause delirium and tachycardia.

Additive effects are likely after concomitant use of maprotiline with CNS depressants, including alcohol, analgesics, barbiturates, narcotics, tranquilizers, and anesthetics (oversedation); atropine and other anticholinergic drugs, including phenothiazines, antihistamines, meperidine, and antiparkinsonian agents (oversedation, paralytic ileus, visual changes, and severe constipation); and metrizamide (increased risk of convulsions).

Barbiturates and heavy smoking induce maprotiline metabolism and decrease therapeutic efficacy; phenothiazines and haloperidol decrease its metabolism, decreasing therapeutic efficacy; methylphenidate, cimetidine, oral contraceptives, propoxyphene, and beta blockers may inhibit maprotiline metabolism, increasing plasma levels and toxicity.

Effects on diagnostic tests
Maprotiline may prolong conduction time (elongation of Q-T and PR intervals, flattened T waves on ECG); it also may elevate liver function test results, decrease white blood cell counts, and decrease or increase serum glucose levels.

Adverse reactions
- CNS: drowsiness, dizziness, sedation, excitation, tremors, weakness, headache, nervousness, *seizures* (high incidence), peripheral neuropathy, extrapyramidal symptoms, anxiety, vivid dreams, confusion (more marked in elderly patients), decreased libido.
- CV: orthostatic hypotension, tachycardia, arrhythmias, *stroke, heart block, CHF,* palpitations, hypertension, ECG changes.
- EENT: blurred vision, tinnitus, mydriasis, increased intraocular pressure.
- GI: dry mouth, constipation, nausea, vomiting, anorexia, diarrhea, paralytic ileus, jaundice.
- GU: urinary retention.
- Other: sweating, photosensitivity, hypersensitivity (rash, urticaria, drug fever, edema).

After abrupt withdrawal of long-term therapy, nausea, headache, malaise (does not indicate addiction) may occur.

Note: Drug should be discontinued (not abruptly) if signs of hypersensitivity occur. Monitor for urinary retention, extreme dry mouth, skin rash, excessive se-

---

*Canada only   †Unlabeled clinical use   Italicized adverse reactions are life-threatening.

dation, seizures, tachycardia, sore throat, fever, or jaundice.

Overdose and treatment
The first 12 hours after acute ingestion are a stimulatory phase characterized by excessive anticholinergic activity (agitation, irritation, confusion, hallucinations, hyperthermia, parkinsonian symptoms, seizure, urinary retention, dry mucous membranes, pupillary dilatation, constipation, and ileus). This is followed by CNS depressant effects, including hypothermia, decreased or absent reflexes, sedation, hypotension, cyanosis, and cardiac irregularities, including tachycardia, conduction disturbances, and quinidine-like effects on the ECG.

Severity of overdose is best indicated by prolongation of QRS complex beyond 100 ms; this usually indicates a serum level in excess of 1,000 ng/ml. Metabolic acidosis may follow hypotension, hypoventilation, and convulsions.

Treatment is symptomatic and supportive, including maintaining airway, stable body temperature, and fluid and electrolyte balance. Induce emesis with ipecac if patient is conscious; follow with gastric lavage and activated charcoal to prevent further absorption. Dialysis is of little use. Treat seizures with parenteral diazepam or phenytoin; arrhythmias, with parenteral phenytoin or lidocaine; and acidosis, with sodium bicarbonate. *Do not give barbiturates;* these may enhance CNS and respiratory depressant effects.

▶ Special considerations
Besides those relevant to all *tricyclic antidepressants,* consider the following recommendations.
● Maprotiline may possess a greater potential to induce seizures than other tricyclic antidepressants. Patients with abnormal EEGs should be watched closely.
● To minimize risk of seizures, total daily dosage should be less than 200 mg.

Information for the patient
● Tell patient not to take the full daily dosage at one time, and not to double doses for missed doses.
● Explain that the full effects of the drug may not become apparent for up to 4 weeks after initiation of therapy. Patient should take the medication exactly as prescribed.
● Warn patient not to discontinue drug abruptly; not to share drug with others; and not to drink alcoholic beverages while taking this drug.
● Encourage patient to report any unusual or troublesome effects immediately, including confusion, movement disorders, rapid heartbeat, dizziness, fainting, or difficulty urinating.
● Tell patient to store drug out of children's reach.

Geriatric use
Patients over age 60 should be given lower than average doses; 25 to 50 mg/day is usually satisfactory.

Pediatric use
Maprotiline is not recommended for children under age 18.

Breast-feeding
Maprotiline is excreted in breast milk in concentrations equal to or greater than those in woman's serum; potential benefit to woman must outweigh possible hazard to infant.

mazindol
Mazanor, Sanorex

● Pharmacologic classification: imidazoisoindol
● Therapeutic classification: anorexigenic agent
● Controlled substance schedule IV
● Pregnancy risk category C

How supplied
Available by prescription only
Tablets: 1 mg, 2 mg

Indications, route, and dosage
Short-term adjunct in exogenous obesity
Adults: 1 mg t.i.d. 1 hour before meals, or 2 mg daily 1 hour before lunch. Use lowest effective dosage.
†Adjunct treatment in cocaine abusers
Adults: 1 to 3 mg P.O. daily.
†Narcolepsy
Adults: 0.5 to 4 mg P.O. daily.

Pharmacodynamics
Anorexigenic action: Mazindol's chemical structure is different from that of amphetamines or other anorexigenics; it appears to act in the limbic system, inhibiting norepinephrine and dopamine uptake. Mazindol does not appear to produce euphoria and, therefore, has a low potential for abuse. Its appetite suppressant activity is comparable to that of amphetamines and diethylpropion.

Pharmacokinetics
● *Absorption:* Mazindol is absorbed readily after oral administration; onset of action is 30 to 60 minutes. Duration of action is 8 to 15 hours, permitting once-daily dosing.
● *Distribution:* Mazindol enters the CNS.
● *Metabolism:* Unknown.
● *Excretion:* Mazindol is excreted unchanged in urine.

Contraindications and precautions
Mazindol is contraindicated in patients with known hypersensitivity to the drug; in patients with glaucoma, because it can exacerbate the disease; in patients with a history of substance abuse; in agitated states; and for use with monoamine oxidase (MAO) inhibitors or within 14 days of such use.

Mazindol should be used with caution in patients with hypertension, severe cardiovascular disease, or diabetes mellitus, and in hyperexcitability states. Habituation or psychic dependence may follow prolonged use.

Interactions
Concomitant use with MAO inhibitors or within 14 days of such therapy may cause hypertensive crisis. Mazindol may decrease hypotensive effects of guanethidine and other antihypertensive agents; it also may alter insulin requirements in diabetic patients.

Concomitant use with pressor amines (norepinephrine or isoproterenol) during treatment for shock may cause hypertension; initiate therapy with lower doses, titrate slowly, and monitor blood pressure frequently.

Mazindol reportedly (one case) has increased lithium toxicity.

Concomitant use of mazindol and fenfluramine may increase risk of cardiac toxicity. Avoid concomitant use.

The use of this drug with caffeine or caffeinated beverages may enhance CNS effects. Avoid concomitant use.

Effects on diagnostic tests
None reported.

Adverse reactions
● CNS: nervousness, restlessness, dizziness, insomnia, dysphoria, headache, depression, drowsiness, weakness, tremors.
● CV: palpitations, tachycardia.
● DERM: rash, clamminess, pallor.
● GI: dry mouth, nausea, constipation, diarrhea, unpleasant taste.
● GU: difficulty initiating micturition, impotence.
● Other: shivering, excessive sweating, tolerance, physical and psychological dependence.

Note: Drug should be discontinued if signs of hypersensitivity occur.

Overdose and treatment
No data exist on acute overdose with mazindol in humans. However, anticipated symptoms include restlessness, tremor, hyperreflexia, fever, tachypnea, dizziness, nausea, vomiting, diarrhea, cramps, hypertension, tachycardia, and circulatory collapse.

Treat overdose supportively: monitor vital signs and fluid and electrolyte balance. Acidifying the urine may enhance mazindol excretion.

▶ Special considerations
● Administer mazindol with meals instead of 1 hour before meals if GI irritation occurs.
● Drug may alter insulin requirements. Monitor blood glucose levels.
● Tolerance or dependence may develop, but abuse potential is lower than that of other CNS stimulants.
● Concomitant use of mazindol and fenfluramine may increase risk of cardiac toxicity. Avoid concomitant use.
● Use with caffeine or caffeinated beverages may enhance CNS effects. Avoid concomitant use.

Information for the patient
● Instruct patient to take last daily dose at least 6 hours before bedtime to avoid insomnia.
● Tell patient to take drug with meals to prevent GI distress.

Geriatric use
Use with caution in elderly patients.

Pediatric use
Mazindol is not recommended for children under age 12.

Breast-feeding
Safety in breast-feeding has not been established. Alternative feeding method is recommended during therapy.

---

measles and rubella virus vaccine, live, attenuated
M-R-Vax II

● Pharmacologic classification: vaccine
● Therapeutic classification: viral vaccine
● Pregnancy risk category X

How supplied
Available by prescription only
Injection: Single-dose vial containing not less than 1,000 TCID^{50} (tissue culture infective doses) each of attenuated measles virus derived from Enders' attenuated Edmonston strain (grown in chick embryo culture) and the Wistar RA 27/3 strain of rubella virus (propagated in human diploid cell culture)

Note: 10-dose and 50-dose vials are available to government agencies and institutions only.

Indications, route, and dosage
Measles and rubella immunization
Adults and children age 15 months and over: 0.5 ml in outer aspect of the upper arm. For adequate protection against measles, a two-dose schedule is recommended (at least 1 month between doses).

Pharmacodynamics
Measles and rubella prophylaxis: This vaccine promotes active immunity to measles (rubeola) and German measles (rubella) virus by inducing production of antibodies.

Pharmacokinetics
Antibodies are usually detectable 2 to 3 weeks after injection. The duration of vaccine-induced immunity is expected to be lifelong.

Contraindications and precautions
Measles and rubella virus vaccine is contraindicated in patients with hypersensitivity (other than dermatitis) to neomycin, a component of the vaccine; in patients with infections, blood dyscrasias, or cancers of or affecting the bone marrow or lymphatic systems; in pregnant patients and those within 3 months of planned pregnancy; in patients in primary immunodeficiency states; and in patients receiving adrenocorticotropic hormone, corticosteroids (except in patients receiving corticosteroids as replacement therapy, for example, for Addison's disease), irradiation, or other immunosuppressant therapy. Use cautiously in children with a history of febrile seizures or cerebral injury, or in any febrile condition.

Interactions
Concomitant use of measles and rubella vaccine with immune serum globulin or transfusions of blood or blood products may interfere with the immune response to the vaccine. Defer vaccination for 3 months in these situations whenever possible.

The administration of immunosuppressive agents may interfere with the response to the vaccine.

Effects on diagnostic tests
Measles and rubella vaccine may temporarily decrease the response to tuberculin skin testing. If a tuberculin

---

skin test is necessary, administer it either before or simultaneously with measles and rubella vaccine.

Adverse reactions
- CNS: headache.
- GI: anorexia.
- Local: erythema, swelling, and tenderness at injection site.
- Systemic: fever and/or rash (occurring between the 5th and 12th day after vaccination), lymphadenopathy, *anaphylaxis,* febrile convulsions in susceptible children, anorexia.

Overdose and treatment
No information available.

▶ Special considerations
- Obtain a thorough history of allergies (especially to antibiotics, eggs, chicken, or chicken feathers) and of reactions to immunizations.
- Patients with a history of anaphylactoid reactions to eggs should have skin testing performed to assess vaccine sensitivity (against a control of normal saline solution in the opposing extremity). Administer a prick (intracutaneous) or scratch test with a 1:10 dilution. Read results after 5 to 30 minutes.
Positive reaction: wheal with or without pseudopodia and surrounding erythema.
- Epinephrine solution 1:1,000 should be available to treat allergic reactions.
- Do not administer I.V. Use a 25-gauge, ⅝" needle and inject S.C., preferably into the outer aspect of the upper arm.
- Use a sterile syringe free of preservatives, antiseptics, and detergents for each injection because these substances may inactivate the live virus vaccine.
- Use only diluent supplied. Discard reconstituted solution after 8 hours.
- Store at 2 to 8 C. (36 to 46 F.), and protect from light. Solution may be used if red, pink, or yellow, but it must be clear.
- Measles and rubella vaccine should not be given less than 1 month before or after immunization with other live virus vaccines, except for mumps virus vaccine and monovalent or trivalent live oral poliovirus vaccine, which may be administered simultaneously.
- The vaccine may not offer any protection when given within a few days' exposure to natural measles or rubella.
- According to Centers for Disease Control recommendations, measles, mumps and rubella (MMR) is the preferred vaccine.
- Give passive immunization with immune serum globulin when immediate protection against measles is required in patients who cannot receive the measles vaccine component. Do not administer either vaccine component simultaneously with immune serum globulin.
- Revaccination is not necessary if primary vaccine is given at or after age 15 months.

Information for the patient
- Tell patient what to expect: tingling sensations in the extremities or joint aches and pains that may resemble arthritis, beginning several days to several weeks after vaccination. These symptoms usually resolve within 1 week. Patients also may have pain and inflammation at the injection site and a low-grade fever, rash, or difficulty breathing. Recommend acetaminophen for relief of fever.

- Encourage patient to report distressing adverse reactions.

Pediatric use
Children under age 15 months may not respond to one or both of the vaccine components because retained maternal antibodies may interfere with the immune response.

Breast-feeding
- No data are available regarding distribution of measles and rubella virus components in breast milk. Some reports have demonstrated transfer of rubella virus or virus antigen into breast milk in appproximately 68% of patients.
- Few adverse effects have been associated with breast-feeding after immunization with rubella-containing vaccines. The risk-benefit ratio suggests that breast-feeding women may be immunized with the rubella component if necessary.

measles, mumps, and rubella virus vaccine, live
M-M-R II

- Pharmacologic classification: vaccine
- Therapeutic classification: viral vaccine
- Pregnancy risk category X

How supplied
Available by prescription only
Injection: Single-dose vial containing not less than 1,000 $TCID_{50}$ (tissue culture infective doses) of attenuated measles virus derived from Enders' attenuated Edmonston strain (grown in chick embryo culture); 5,000 $TCID_{50}$ of the Jeryl Lynn (B level) mumps strain (grown in chick embryo culture); and 1,000 $TCID_{50}$ of the Wistar RA 27/3 strain of rubella virus (propagated in human diploid cell culture)

Indications, route, and dosage
Measles, mumps, and rubella immunization
Adults (born after 1957) and children: 0.5 ml S.C. in outer aspect of the upper arm. Two doses are recommended for children. Give first dose, 0.5 ml S.C., when child is age 15 months or older and give the second dose when child enters school or first grade (age 4 to 6). Some local health officials may elect to give the second dose at an older age.

Pharmacodynamics
Measles, mumps, and rubella prophylaxis: This vaccine promotes active immunity to measles (rubeola), mumps, and German measles (rubella) by inducing production of antibodies.

Pharmacokinetics
Antibodies are usually evident 2 to 3 weeks after injection. The duration of vaccine-induced immunity is expected to be lifelong.

Contraindications and precautions
Measles, mumps, and rubella virus vaccine is contraindicated in patients with hypersensitivity (other than dermatitis) to neomycin, a component of the vaccine; in patients with infections, blood dyscrasias, cancers

of or affecting the bone marrow or lymphatic systems, or primary immunodeficiency states; in pregnant patients; and in patients receiving adrenocorticotropic hormone, corticosteroids (except in patients receiving corticosteroids as replacement therapy, for example, for Addison's disease), irradiation, or other immunosuppressant therapy.

Use cautiously in children with a history of febrile seizures or cerebral injury, or in any febrile situation.

Interactions

Concomitant use of measles, mumps, and rubella virus vaccine with immune serum globulin or transfusions of blood or blood products may interfere with the immune response to the vaccine. Whenever possible, vaccination should be deferred for 3 months in these situations.

The administration of immunosuppressive agents may interfere with the response to vaccine.

Effects on diagnostic tests

Measles, mumps, and rubella vaccine temporarily may decrease the response to tuberculin skin testing. If a tuberculin skin test is necessary, administer it either before or simultaneously with this vaccine.

Adverse reactions

● CNS: headache.
● GI: anorexia.
● Local: pain, burning, stinging, erythema, swelling, and tenderness at injection site.
● Systemic: fever and/or rash (occurring between the 5th and 12th day after vaccination), lymphadenopathy, malaise, urticaria, arthritis, arthralgia, paresthesia, *anaphylaxis, febrile convulsions in susceptible children.*

Overdose and treatment

No information available.

▶ Special considerations

● Obtain a thorough history of allergies, especially to antibiotics, eggs, chicken, or chicken feathers, and of reactions to immunizations.
● Patients with a history of anaphylactoid reactions to egg ingestion should first have a skin test to assess vaccine sensitivity (against a control of normal saline solution in the opposing extremity). Administer a prick (intracutaneous) or scratch test with a 1:10 dilution. Read results after 5 to 30 minutes.
Positive reaction: wheal with or without pseudopodia and surrounding erythema.
● Epinephrine solution 1:1,000 should be available to treat allergic reactions.
● Most adults born before 1957 are believed to have been infected with naturally occurring disease, and vaccination is not necessary; however, vaccination should be offered if they are considered susceptible.
● Do not administer I.V. Use a 25-gauge, ⅝" needle and inject S.C., preferably into the outer aspect of the upper arm. Use a sterile syringe free of preservatives, antiseptics, and detergents for each injection, because these substances may inactivate the live virus vaccine.
● Solution may be used if red, pink, or yellow, but it must be clear.
● Use only the diluent supplied. Discard reconstituted solution after 8 hours.
● Measles, mumps, and rubella vaccine should not be given less than 1 month before or after immunization with other live virus vaccines—except for monovalent

or trivalent live oral poliovirus vaccine, which may be administered simultaneously.
● The vaccine may not offer any protection when given within a few days after exposure to natural measles, mumps, or rubella.
● Give passive immunization with immune serum globulin, if ordered, when immediate protection against measles is required in patients who cannot receive the measles vaccine component. Do not administer any live virus vaccine component simultaneously with immune serum globulin.
● Revaccination is unnecessary if the child received two doses of vaccine at least 1 month apart, beginning after the first birthday.
● Store at 2 to 8 C. (36 to 46 F.), and protect from light.

Information for the patient

● Tell patient what to expect after vaccination: tingling sensations in the extremities or joint aches and pains that may resemble arthritis, beginning several days to several weeks after vaccination. These symptoms usually resolve within 1 week. The patient also may have pain and inflammation at the injection site and a low-grade fever, a rash, or difficulty breathing. Recommend acetaminophen to alleviate adverse reactions, such as fever.
● Tell patient to report distressing adverse reactions.

Pediatric use

Children under age 15 months may not respond to one, two, or all three of the vaccine components, because retained maternal antibodies may interfere with the immune response. However, vaccination at age 12 months is recommended if the child lives in a high-risk area, because the benefits outweigh the risk of a slightly lower efficacy of the vaccine.

Breast-feeding

● No data are available regarding distribution of measles or mumps virus components in breast milk. Some reports have demonstrated transfer of rubella virus or virus antigen into breast milk in approximately 68% of patients.
● Few adverse effects have been associated with breast-feeding after immunization with rubella-containing vaccines. The risk-benefit ratio suggests that breast-feeding women may be immunized with the rubella component if necessary.

---

measles virus vaccine, live, attenuated
Attenuvax

● Pharmacologic classification: vaccine
● Therapeutic classification: viral vaccine
● Pregnancy risk category X

How supplied

Available by prescription only
Injection: Single-dose vial containing not less than 1,000 $TCID_{50}$ (tissue culture infective doses) per 0.5 ml of attenuated measles virus derived from Enders' attenuated Edmonston strain grown in chick embryo culture (10- and 50-dose vials available to government agencies and institutions only)

Indications, route, and dosage
Immunization
Adults and children age 15 months and over: 0.5 ml (1,000 units) S.C. in outer aspect of the upper arm. Administer two doses at least 1 month apart. For children, the usual schedule is the first dose at age 15 months and a second dose at the entry of school (age 4 to 6 years).

Pharmacodynamics
Measles prophylaxis: Measles virus vaccine promotes active immunity to measles virus by inducing production of antibodies.

Pharmacokinetics
Antibodies are usually evident 2 to 3 weeks after injection. The duration of vaccine-induced immunity is at least 13 to 16 years and probably lifelong in most immunized persons.

Contraindications and precautions
Measles (rubeola) virus vaccine is contraindicated in patients with hypersensitivity (other than dermatitis) to neomycin, a component of the vaccine; in patients with infections, blood dyscrasias, or cancers of or affecting the bone marrow or lymphatic systems; in pregnant patients and those within 3 months of planned pregnancy; and in patients who are receiving adrenocorticotropic hormone, corticosteroids (except in patients receiving corticosteroids as replacement therapy, for example, for Addison's disease), irradiation, or other immunosuppressant therapy. Use cautiously in children with a history of febrile seizures or cerebral injury, or in any febrile condition.

Interactions
Concomitant use of measles vaccine with immune serum globulin or transfusions of blood or blood products may interfere with the immune response to the vaccine. Defer vaccination for 3 months in these situations.

The administration of immunosuppressive agents may interfere with the response to the vaccine.

Effects on diagnostic tests
Measles vaccine temporarily may decrease the response to tuberculin skin testing. Should a tuberculin skin test be necessary, administer it either before or simultaneously with the measles vaccine.

Adverse reactions
● CNS: headache.
● GI: anorexia.
● Local: erythema, swelling, and tenderness at injection site.
● Systemic: fever and/or rash (occurring between the 5th and 12th day after vaccination), lymphadenopathy, *anaphylaxis, febrile convulsions in susceptible children.*

Overdose and treatment
No information available.

▶ Special considerations
● Obtain a thorough history of allergies, especially to antibiotics, eggs, chicken, or chicken feathers, and of reactions to immunizations.
● Patients with a history of anaphylactoid reactions to eggs should first have skin testing performed to assess vaccine sensitivity (against a control of normal saline

solution in the other arm). Administer a prick (intracutaneous) or scratch test with a 1:10 dilution. Read results after 5 to 30 minutes.
Positive reaction: wheal with or without pseudopodia and surrounding erythema.
● Epinephrine solution 1:1,000 should be available to treat allergic reactions.
● Do not administer I.V. Use a 25-gauge, ⅝" needle and inject S.C., preferably into the outer aspect of the upper arm. Use a sterile syringe free of preservatives, antiseptics, and detergents for each injection, because these substances may inactivate the live virus vaccine.
● Use diluent supplied. Discard reconstituted solution after 8 hours.
● Measles vaccine should not be given less than 1 month before or after immunization with other live virus vaccines – except for mumps virus vaccine, rubella virus vaccine, or monovalent or trivalent live oral poliovirus vaccine, which may be administered simultaneously.
● The vaccine may offer some protection when given within a few days after exposure to natural measles.
● According to Centers for Disease Control recommendations, measles, mumps, and rubella (MMR) is the preferred vaccine.
● Give passive immunization with immune serum globulin if immediate protection against measles is required in patients who cannot receive the measles vaccine.
● Revaccination is unnecessary if primary vaccine is given at age 15 months or older.
● Store at 2 to 8 C. (35 to 46 F.), and protect from light. Solution may be used if red, pink, or yellow, but it must be clear.

Information for the patient
● Tell patient what to expect after vaccination: pain and inflammation at the injection site, fever, rash, general malaise, or difficulty breathing. Recommend acetaminophen for relief of fever.
● Encourage patient to report distressing adverse reactions.

Pediatric use
Children under age 15 months may not respond to the vaccine, because retained maternal antibodies may interfere with the immune response.

Breast-feeding
It is unknown whether measles virus vaccine is distributed into breast milk. Use with caution in breast-feeding women.

---

mebendazole
Vermox

● Pharmacologic classification: benzimidazole
● Therapeutic classification: anthelmintic
● Pregnancy risk category C

How supplied
Available by prescription only
Tablets (chewable): 100 mg

Indications, route, and dosage
Pinworm infections
Adults and children over age 2: 100 mg P.O. as a single dose. If infection persists 3 weeks later, repeat treatment.
Other roundworm, whipworm, and hookworm infections
Adults and children over age 2: 100 mg P.O. b.i.d. for 3 days. If infection persists 3 weeks later, repeat treatment.
†Trichinosis (second-line agent)
Adults: 200 to 400 mg t.i.d. for 3 days, then 400 to 500 mg t.i.d. for 10 days.
†Hydatid disease (second-line agent)
Adults: Limited use because of severe toxicity. 40 to 50 mg/kg/day for 3 to 8 months has been used to shrink cysts. Some clinicians maintain blood levels of 80 ng/ml with 100 mg/kg/day in four divided doses.

Pharmacodynamics
Anthelmintic action: Mebendazole inhibits uptake of glucose and other low-molecular weight nutrients in susceptible helminths, depleting the glycogen stores they need for survival and reproduction. It has a broad spectrum and may be useful in mixed infections. It is considered a drug of choice in the treatment of ascariasis, capillariasis, enterobiasis, trichuriasis, and uncinariasis; it has been used investigationally to treat echinococciasis, onchocerciasis, and trichinosis.

Pharmacokinetics
● *Absorption:* About 5% to 10% of an administered dose of mebendazole is absorbed; peak plasma concentrations occur at 2 to 4 hours. Absorption varies widely among patients.
● *Distribution:* Mebendazole is highly bound to plasma proteins; it crosses the placenta.
● *Metabolism:* Mebendazole is metabolized to inactive 2-amino-5(6)-benzimidazolyl phenylketone.
● *Excretion:* Most of a mebendazole dose is excreted in feces; 2% to 10% is excreted in urine in 48 hours as either unchanged drug or the 2-amine metabolite. Mebendazole's half-life is 3 to 9 hours. It is unknown if mebendazole is excreted in breast milk.

Contraindications and precautions
Mebendazole is contraindicated in patients with hypersensitivity to the drug.

Interactions
Concomitant use with anticonvulsants, including phenytoin and carbamazepine, may enhance the metabolism of mebendazole and decrease its efficacy.

Effects on diagnostic tests
None reported.

Adverse reactions
● GI: occasional, transient abdominal pain and diarrhea in massive infection.
● HEMA: reversible neutropenia.
● Other: fever, dizziness.
  Note: Drug should be discontinued if signs of hypersensitivity or toxicity occur.

Overdose and treatment
Signs and symptoms of overdose may include GI disturbances and altered mental status. No specific recommendations exist; treatment is supportive. After re-cent ingestion (within 4 hours), empty stomach by induced emesis or gastric lavage. Follow with activated charcoal to decrease absorption.

▶ Special considerations
● Tablets may be chewed, swallowed whole, or crushed and mixed with food.
● Laxatives, enemas, or dietary restrictions are unnecessary.
● Collect stool specimens in a clean, dry container and transfer to a properly labeled container to send to laboratory; ova may be destroyed by toilet bowl water, urine, and some drugs.
● Encourage patient's family and contacts to be checked for infestation and treated, if necessary.
● High dose treatment of hydatid disease and trichinosis is investigational. Frequently monitor white blood cell counts to detect drug toxicity, especially during initial therapy.

Information for the patient
● Teach patient and family members personal hygiene measures to prevent reinfection: washing perianal area and changing undergarments and bedclothes daily; washing hands and cleaning fingernails before meals and after defecation; and sanitary disposal of feces.
● Advise patient to bathe often, by showering, if possible.
● Advise patient to keep hands away from mouth, to keep fingernails short, and to wear shoes to avoid hookworm; explain that ova are easily transmitted directly and indirectly by hands, food, or contaminated articles. Washing clothes in household washing machine will destroy ova.
● Instruct patient to handle bedding carefully, because shaking will send ova into the air, and to disinfect toilet facilities and vacuum or damp-mop floors daily to reduce number of ova.

Pediatric use
Mebendazole should be given to children under age 2 only when potential benefits justify risks.

Breast-feeding
Safety in breast-feeding women has not been established.

mecamylamine hydrochloride
Inversine

● Pharmacologic classification: ganglionic blocking agent
● Therapeutic classification: antihypertensive
● Pregnancy risk category C

How supplied
Available by prescription only
Tablets: 2.5 mg

Indications, route, and dosage
Moderately severe to severe essential hypertension and uncomplicated malignant hypertension
Adults: Initially, 2.5 mg b.i.d. for 2 days, increasing (or decreasing) in increments of 2.5 mg/day at intervals of

---

not less than 2 days until desired response is achieved. Usual maintenance dosage is 25 mg/day in two to four divided doses.

Pharmacodynamics
Antihypertensive action: Mecamylamine competes with acetylcholine and causes vasodilation, thus reducing blood pressure, by blocking transmission of impulses at both sympathetic and parasympathetic ganglia.

Pharmacokinetics
● *Absorption:* Mecamylamine is absorbed almost completely from the GI tract. Antihypertensive effect begins gradually at ½ to 2 hours; maximal antihypertensive effect occurs at 3 to 5 hours.
● *Distribution:* Mecamylamine is distributed throughout the body; highest concentrations are in liver, kidneys, spleen, heart, and lungs.
● *Metabolism:* Unknown.
● *Excretion:* Approximately 50% of an oral dose of mecamylamine is excreted unchanged in urine; rate of renal elimination decreases when urine pH is 7.5 or higher. Negligible amounts of the drug are excreted in feces. Antihypertensive effect lasts for 6 to 12 hours; it may persist for 24 hours or more in patients with renal insufficiency.

Contraindications and precautions
Mecamylamine is contraindicated in patients with known hypersensitivity to the drug; in patients with coronary insufficiency, recent myocardial infarction, uremia, glaucoma, or pyloric stenosis, because the drug may exacerbate these conditions; in patients with chronic pyelonephritis or patients taking sulfonamides or antibiotics for pyelonephritis because of the manufacturer's recommendation; in patients on sodium restriction, because sodium depletion may enhance the drug's effects; and in breast-feeding women because of the high potential for adverse effects on the infant.

Mecamylamine should be used cautiously in patients with cerebral or coronary arteriosclerosis, renal insufficiency, or a history of recent cerebrovascular accident, because hypotensive effects may exacerbate these conditions. The drug's anticholinergic effects may exacerbate prostatic hypertrophy, bladder neck obstruction, and urethral stricture.

Interactions
Mecamylamine may potentiate the antihypertensive effects of diuretics and other antihypertensive agents; its antihypertensive effects may be potentiated by concomitant administration of alcohol or anesthesia.

Drugs that increase urine pH, such as sodium bicarbonate or acetazolamide, may inhibit mecamylamine excretion, predisposing patient to toxicity.

Effects on diagnostic tests
None reported.

Adverse reactions
● CNS: *convulsions,* choreiform movements, mental aberrations, tremors, paresthesias.
● CV: orthostatic dizziness and syncope, postural hypotension.
● EENT: glossitis, dry mouth, dilated pupils, blurred vision.
● GI: *ileus,* constipation, vomiting, nausea, anorexia.
● GU: urinary retention, sexual dysfunction, dysuria.
Note: Drug should be discontinued if hypotension is

excessive, if urinary retention occurs, and at the first sign of paralytic ileus.

Overdose and treatment
Clinical signs of overdose include hypotension, blurred vision, tachycardia, nausea, vomiting, urinary retention, and seizures.

After acute ingestion, empty stomach by induced emesis or gastric lavage and give activated charcoal to reduce absorption. Further treatment is usually symptomatic and supportive. Pressor amines may be needed to treat excessive hypotension; use small doses because mecamylamine-treated patients are extremely sensitive to vasopressors.

▶ Special considerations
● Do not withdraw drug suddenly; rebound hypertension may occur.
● Dosage adjustments may be necessary in patients with renal insufficiency.

Information for the patient
● Teach patient about his disease and explain why he must take drug exactly as prescribed, even when feeling well.
● Advise patient never to discontinue drug suddenly because severe rebound hypertension may occur.
● Explain adverse effects, and advise patient to report any unusual effects.
● Explain how to minimize adverse effects: to avoid hazardous activities that require mental alertness until tolerance develops to CNS adverse effects; to avoid sudden position changes to minimize orthostatic hypotension; to use ice chips, sugarless hard candy, or gum to relieve dry mouth; and to take drug after meals for more gradual absorption.
● When divided doses are taken, advise patient to take a relatively small dose in the morning (or omit it) and to take larger dose(s) at noon or in the evening because blood pressure response to mecamylamine may be greater in the morning.
● Warn patient to seek medical approval before taking nonprescription cold preparations.

Geriatric use
Administer drug with caution to elderly patients, because they are more likely to have a history of stroke or severe cerebral or coronary arteriosclerosis; evaluate renal and cardiovascular function carefully.

Pediatric use
Dosage in children has not been established.

Breast-feeding
Because of the potential for serious adverse reactions in breast-feeding infants, an alternative feeding method is recommended during mecamylamine therapy.

---

mechlorethamine hydrochloride (nitrogen mustard)
Mustargen

- Pharmacologic classification: alkylating agent (cell cycle-phase nonspecific)
- Therapeutic classification: antineoplastic
- Pregnancy risk category D

How supplied
Available by prescription only
Injection: 10-mg vials
Topical solution: 10 mg in 5 to 10 ml normal saline solution (must be prepared just before administration)
Ointment: 0.01% to 0.04%
Must be compounded: not commercially available in the United States or Canada

Indications, route, and dosage
Dosage and indications may vary. Check current literature for recommended protocols.
Hodgkin's disease; non-Hodgkin's lymphomas; breast, lung, and ovarian cancer; diffuse lymphocytic lymphoma; multiple myeloma; chronic lymphocytic leukemia; mycosis fungoides; and polycythemia vera
Adults: 0.4 mg/kg I.V. as a single dose or 0.1 mg/kg on 4 successive days q 3 to 6 weeks. Give through running I.V. infusion. Dose reduced in prior radiation or chemotherapy to 0.2 to 0.4 mg/kg. Dose based on ideal or actual body weight, whichever is less.
Mycosis fungoides
Adults: Apply sufficient lotion or ointment to cover lesion one to four times a day for 6 to 12 months after a complete response. Then, maintenance treatments continue for up to 3 years.
Intracavitary doses for neoplastic effusions
Adults: 0.2 to 0.4 mg/kg.

Pharmacodynamics
Antineoplastic action: Mechlorethamine exerts its cytotoxic activity through the basic processes of alkylation. The drug causes cross-linking of DNA strands, single-strand breakage of DNA, abnormal base pairing, and interruption of other intracellular processes, resulting in cell death.

Pharmacokinetics
- *Absorption:* Mechlorethamine is well absorbed after oral administration; however, because the drug is very irritating to tissue, it must be administered intravenously. After intracavitary administration, mechlorethamine is absorbed incompletely, probably from deactivation by body fluids in the cavity.
- *Distribution:* Mechlorethamine does not cross the blood-brain barrier.
- *Metabolism:* Mechlorethamine is converted rapidly to its active form, which reacts quickly with various cellular components before being deactivated.
- *Excretion:* Metabolites of mechlorethamine are excreted in urine. Less than 0.01% of an I.V. dose is excreted unchanged in urine.

Contraindications and precautions
Because of the potential of the drug to cause extensive and rapid development of amyloidosis, mechlorethamine is contraindicated in patients with foci of chronic or suppurative inflammation.

It may be necessary to adjust dosage or discontinue therapy in patients with infections, hematologic compromise, or bone marrow infiltration with malignant cells because of the drug's adverse hematologic effects.

Interactions
None reported.

Effects on diagnostic tests
Mechlorethamine therapy may increase blood and urine uric acid levels and may decrease serum pseudocholinesterase concentrations.

Adverse reactions
- CNS: drowsiness, vertigo, paresthesias (especially with high doses).
- EENT: tinnitus, metallic taste (immediately after dose), deafness.
- GI: nausea, vomiting, and anorexia begin within 1 hour and last 8 to 24 hours.
- GU: oligomenorrhea, amenorrhea, azoospermia, delayed spermatogenesis.
- HEMA: *bone marrow depression* (dose-limiting) occurs by days 4 to 10, lasting 10 to 21 days; mild anemia begins in 2 to 3 weeks, possibly lasting 7 weeks.
- Metabolic: hyperuricemia.
- Local: thrombophlebitis, sloughing, severe irritation if drug extravasates or touches skin, rash.
- Other: alopecia, herpes zoster.

Overdose and treatment
Clinical manifestations of overdose include lymphopenia and precipitation of uric acid crystals.

Treatment is usually supportive and includes transfusion of blood components, hydration, and allopurinol.

▶ Special considerations
Besides those relevant to all *alkylating agents*, consider the following recommendations.
- To reconstitute powder, use 10 ml of sterile water for injection or normal saline solution to give a concentration of 1 mg/ml.
- Solution is very unstable. It should be prepared immediately before infusion and used within 20 minutes. Discard unused solution.
- Drug may be administered I.V. push over a few minutes into the tubing of a freely flowing I.V. infusion.
- Dilution of mechlorethamine into a large volume of I.V. solution is not recommended, because the drug may react with the diluent and is not stable for a prolonged period.
- Treatment of extravasation includes local injections of a ⅙ M sodium thiosulfate solution. Prepare solution by mixing 4 ml of sodium thiosulfate 10% with 6 ml of sterile water for injection. Also, apply ice packs for 6 to 12 hours to minimize local reactions.
- During intracavitary administration, patient should be turned from side to side every 15 minutes for 1 hour to distribute drug.
- Avoid contact with skin or mucous membranes. Wear gloves when preparing solution and during administration to prevent accidental skin contact. If contact occurs, wash with copious amounts of water.
- Monitor uric acid levels and CBC.
- Use cautiously in the presence of severe anemia and depressed neutrophil or platelet count and in patients recently treated with radiation or chemotherapy.

• To prevent hyperuricemia with resulting uric acid nephropathy, allopurinol may be given; keep patient well hydrated.
• Anticoagulants should be used cautiously. Watch closely for signs of bleeding.
• Avoid all I.M. injections when platelet count is low.
• Mechlorethamine has been used topically to treat mycosis fungoides.

Information for the patient
• Tell patient to avoid exposure to people with infections.
• Adequate fluid intake is very important to facilitate excretion of uric acid.
• Reassure patient that hair should grow back after treatment has ended.
• Tell patient to promptly report any signs or symptoms of bleeding or infection.

Breast-feeding
It is not known whether mechlorethamine distributes into breast milk. However, because of the potential for serious adverse reactions, mutagenicity, and carcinogenicity in the infant, breast-feeding is not recommended.

---

meclizine hydrochloride
Antivert, Antrizine, Bonamine*, Bonine, Ru-Vert-M, Whevert

• Pharmacologic classification: piperazine-derivative antihistamine
• Therapeutic classification: antiemetic and antivertigo agent
• Pregnancy risk category B

How supplied
Available with or without prescription
Tablets: 12.5 mg, 25 mg, 50 mg
Tablets (chewable): 25 mg

Indications, route, and dosage
Dizziness
Adults: 25 to 100 mg P.O. daily in divided doses. Dosage varies with patient response.
Motion sickness
Adults: 25 to 50 mg P.O. 1 hour before travel; may repeat dose daily for duration of journey.

Pharmacodynamics
• *Antiemetic action:* Meclizine probably inhibits nausea and vomiting by centrally decreasing sensitivity of labyrinth apparatus that relays stimuli to the chemoreceptor trigger zone and stimulates the vomiting center in the brain.
• *Antivertigo action:* Drug decreases labyrinth excitability and conduction in vestibular-cerebellar pathways.

Pharmacokinetics
• *Absorption:* Onset of action is about 60 minutes.
• *Distribution:* Meclizine is well distributed throughout the body and crosses the placenta.
• *Metabolism:* Meclizine probably is metabolized in the liver.
• *Excretion:* Meclizine's half-life is about 6 hours; action

persists for 8 to 24 hours. Meclizine is excreted unchanged in feces; metabolites are found in urine.

Contraindications and precautions
Meclizine is contraindicated in patients with known hypersensitivity to this drug or other antiemetic antihistamines with a similar chemical structure, such as cyclizine, buclizine, or dimenhydrinate.
    Meclizine should be used with caution in patients with narrow-angle glaucoma, asthma, prostatic hypertrophy, or GU or GI obstruction because of anticholinergic effects. Drug may mask signs of intestinal obstruction or brain tumor.

Interactions
Additive sedative and CNS depressant effects may occur when meclizine is used concomitantly with other CNS depressants, such as alcohol, barbiturates, tranquilizers, sleeping agents, and antianxiety agents; drug should not be given to patients taking ototoxic medications, such as aminoglycosides, salicylates, vancomycin, loop diuretics, and cisplatin, because meclizine may mask signs of ototoxicity.

Effects on diagnostic tests
Meclizine should be discontinued 4 days before diagnostic skin tests, to avoid preventing, reducing, or masking test response.

Adverse reactions
• CNS: drowsiness, fatigue.
• EENT: blurred vision, dry nose and throat.
• GI: constipation, diarrhea, nausea, vomiting, anorexia.

Overdose and treatment
Clinical manifestations of moderate overdose may include hyperexcitability alternating with drowsiness. Seizures, hallucinations, and respiratory paralysis may occur in profound overdose. Anticholinergic symptoms, such as dry mouth, flushed skin, fixed and dilated pupils, and GI symptoms, are common, especially in children.
    Treat overdose by administering gastric lavage to empty stomach contents; emesis with ipecac syrup may be ineffective. Treat hypotension with vasopressors, and control seizures with diazepam or phenytoin. *Do not give stimulants.*

▶ Special considerations
Besides those relevant to all *antihistamines,* consider the following recommendations.
• Tablets may be placed in mouth and allowed to dissolve without water, or they may be chewed or swallowed whole.
• Abrupt withdrawal of drug after long-term use may cause paradoxical reactions or sudden reversal of improved state.

Geriatric use
Elderly patients are usually more sensitive to adverse effects of antihistamines and are especially likely to experience a greater degree of dizziness, sedation, hyperexcitability, dry mouth, and urinary retention than younger patients.

Pediatric use
Safety and efficacy for use in children have not been established. Do not use in children under age 12; infants

---

and children under age 6 may experience paradoxical hyperexcitability.

Breast-feeding
Safety in breast-feeding has not been established.

meclofenamate
Meclomen

- Pharmacologic classification: nonsteroidal anti-inflammatory
- Therapeutic classification: nonnarcotic analgesic, antipyretic, anti-inflammatory
- Pregnancy risk category B (D in third trimester)

How supplied
Available by prescription only
Capsules: 50 mg, 100 mg

Indications, route, and dosage
Rheumatoid arthritis and osteoarthritis
Adults: 200 to 400 mg P.O. daily in three or four equally divided doses.
Mild to moderate pain
Adults: 50 to 100 mg P.O. q 4 to 6 hours. Do not exceed 400 mg daily.

Pharmacodynamics
Analgesic, antipyretic, and anti-inflammatory actions: Mechanisms of action are unknown; meclofenamate is thought to inhibit prostaglandin synthesis.

Pharmacokinetics
- *Absorption:* Drug is absorbed rapidly and completely from the GI tract.
- *Distribution:* Drug is highly bound (more than 99%) to plasma proteins.
- *Metabolism:* Drug is oxidized in the liver to active and inactive metabolites.
- *Excretion:* Drug is excreted in urine, with some biliary excretion; plasma half-life after repeated doses is about 3 hours.

Contraindications and precautions
Meclofenamate is contraindicated in patients with known hypersensitivity to the drug, and in patients in whom aspirin or other nonsteroidal anti-inflammatory drugs (NSAIDs) induce symptoms of asthma, urticaria, or rhinitis.

Serious GI toxicity, including ulceration or hemorrhage, can occur at any time with NSAID use, especially in patients on chronic therapy. Meclofenamate should be used cautiously in patients with a history of GI bleeding, hepatic or renal disease, blood dyscrasias, or diabetes mellitus, because the drug may worsen these disorders; and in asthmatic patients with nasal polyps, because patients with known "triad" symptoms (aspirin hypersensitivity, rhinitis/nasal polyps, and asthma) are at high risk of cross-sensitivity to meclofenamate with precipitation of bronchospasm.

Interactions
Concomitant use of meclofenamate with anticoagulants and thrombolytic drugs (coumarin derivatives, heparin, streptokinase, or urokinase) may potentiate

anticoagulant effects. Bleeding problems may occur if used with other drugs that inhibit platelet aggregation, such as azlocillin, parenteral carbenicillin, dextran, dipyridamole, mezlocillin, piperacillin, sulfinpyrazone, ticarcillin, valproic acid, cefamandole, cefoperazone, moxalactam, plicamycin, aspirin, salicylates, or other anti-inflammatory agents. Concomitant use with salicylates, anti-inflammatory agents, alcohol, corticotropin, or steroids may cause increased GI adverse effects, including ulceration and hemorrhage. Aspirin may decrease the bioavailability of meclofenamate.

Because of the influence of prostaglandins on glucose metabolism, concomitant use with insulin or oral hypoglycemic agents may potentiate hypoglycemic effects. Meclofenamate may displace highly protein-bound drugs from binding sites. Toxicity may occur with coumarin derivatives, phenytoin, verapamil, or nifedipine. Meclofenamate may decrease the renal clearance of methotrexate and lithium. Meclofenamate may decrease the clinical effectiveness of diuretics and antihypertensives. Concomitant use with diuretics may increase nephrotoxicity.

Effects on diagnostic tests
False-positive test results for urine bilirubin by the Di-Azo tablet test have been reported.

Adverse reactions
- CNS: headache, dizziness, drowsiness, vertigo, nervousness, confusion.
- CV: edema.
- DERM: rash, urticaria.
- EENT: blurred vision, eye irritation, tinnitus.
- GI: nausea, diarrhea, vomiting, flatulence, anorexia, bleeding.
- GU: nephrotoxicity, dysuria, hematuria.
- HEMA: leukopenia, thrombocytopenia, *agranulocytosis, aplastic anemia.*
- Other: elevated liver function tests, hepatotoxicity.
  Note: Drug should be discontinued if hypersensitivity, rash or diarrhea, or signs and symptoms of hepatotoxicity appear.

Overdose and treatment
Clinical manifestations of meclofenamate overdose include CNS stimulation, irrational behavior, marked agitation, and generalized seizures. Renal toxicity may follow this phase of CNS stimulation.

To treat overdose of meclofenamate, empty stomach immediately by inducing emesis with ipecac syrup or by gastric lavage. Administer activated charcoal via nasogastric tube. Provide symptomatic and supportive measures (respiratory support and correction of fluid and electrolyte imbalances). Appropriate therapy for seizure control with I.V. diazepam may be indicated. Monitor laboratory parameters and vital signs closely. Dialysis may prove beneficial in correcting azotemia or electrolyte abnormalities but not in removing the drug because of its protein-binding ability.

▶ Special considerations
Besides those relevant to all *NSAIDs,* consider the following recommendations.
- Adjust dose according to patient response.
- Check GI elimination patterns. Monitor for complaints of diarrhea.
- Check hydration status. Monitor for signs and symptoms of dehydration and electrolyte imbalance resulting from possible diarrhea.

---

*Canada only   †Unlabeled clinical use   Italicized adverse reactions are life-threatening.

● Meclofenamate contains sodium. Monitor patient for signs of fluid retention. Check weight and intake and output daily for significant changes. Restrict sodium intake as necessary.
● Institute safety measures to prevent injury if CNS effects occur.

Information for the patient
● Instruct patient to avoid use of nonprescription medications, especially those containing aspirin and sodium. Tell patient to call before using any nonprescription medication.
● Reinforce signs and symptoms of possible adverse effects. Instruct patient to report them.
● Advise patient to record his weight two or three times weekly and to report any weight gain of 3 to 4 pounds in 1 week.
● Instruct patient in diet therapy to assist with control of possible diarrhea. Reinforce need for fluids and bland frequent meals if diarrhea occurs.
● Encourage patient to follow prescribed regimen and recommended schedule of follow-up. Warn female patient to call promptly if she becomes pregnant while taking meclofenamate.
● Caution patient that drowsiness may occur and to use care in activities requiring alertness, especially with initial exposure.
● Instruct patient in safety measures to prevent injury.

Geriatric use
● Patients over age 60 may be more susceptible to the toxic effects of meclofenamate.
● The effects of this drug on renal prostaglandins may cause fluid retention and edema, a significant drawback for elderly patients, especially those with congestive heart failure.

Pediatric use
The safe use of long-term meclofenamate therapy in children under age 14 has not been established.

Breast-feeding
Most NSAIDs are distributed into breast milk; however, it is not known if meclofenamate is. Avoid use of meclofenamate in breast-feeding women.

---

medium-chain triglycerides
M.C.T. Oil

● Pharmacologic classification: modular supplement
● Therapeutic classification: enteral nutrition therapy
● Pregnancy risk category C

How supplied
Available without prescription
Oil: 960 ml (115 calories/15 ml)

Indications, route, and dosage
Inadequate digestion or absorption of food fats, chylous ascites, or chylous thorax
Adults: 15 ml P.O. t.i.d. or q.i.d. Maximum of 100 ml/ day.

Pharmacodynamics
Metabolic action: Medium-chain triglycerides are indicated as a supplementary fat source when conventional fats are not tolerated. Medium-chain triglycerides are more rapidly hydrolyzed than conventional food fat, require less bile for digestion, are carried by the portal circulation, and are not dependent on chylomicron formation or lymphatic transport. Medium-chain triglycerides are a useful energy source in malabsorption patients but do not provide essential fatty acids.

Pharmacokinetics
● *Absorption:* Medium-chain triglycerides are absorbed by the portal circulation; they are not dependant upon chylomicron formation or lymphatic transport for absorption. As compared to dietary fat, they require less bile acid for digestion.
● *Distribution:* Triglycerides are transported by lipoproteins to storage sites in adipose tissue.
● *Metabolism:* Triglycerides are broken down by lipase to free fatty acids and glycerol. The free fatty acids are used to produce energy through the fatty acid cycle.
● *Excretion:* Excess fat is excreted in feces; ketone bodies may appear in urine.

Contraindications and precautions
Medium-chain triglycerides are contraindicated in patients with advanced hepatic cirrhosis. Large amounts may elevate blood and spinal fluid levels of medium-chain fatty acids because of impaired hepatic clearance. These elevated levels have caused reversible coma and precoma in patients with advanced cirrhosis. Use cautiously in patients with hepatic cirrhosis, encephalopathy, or other precipitating factors.

Interactions
No information available.

Effects on diagnostic tests
None reported.

Adverse reactions
● CNS: reversible coma in susceptible patients with advanced cirrhosis.
● GI: nausea, vomiting, diarrhea, abdominal distention, cramps.

Overdose and treatment
No information available.

▶ Special considerations
● Medium-chaim triglycerides provide 7.7 calories/ml.
● To minimize GI adverse effects, give smaller doses more frequently with meals, or mixed with salad dressing or chilled fruit juice.
● Use metal, glass, or ceramic containers and utensils.
● Medium-chain triglycerides do not provide essential fatty acids.

Information for the patient
Provide counseling with the dietitian so the patient can learn how to incorporate this substance into his diet.

---

medroxyprogesterone acetate
Amen, Curretab, Depo-Provera,
Provera

- Pharmacologic classification: progestin
- Therapeutic classification: progestin,
antineoplastic
- Pregnancy risk category X

How supplied
Available by prescription only
Tablets: 2.5 mg, 5 mg, 10 mg
Injection: 100 mg/ml and 400 mg/ml

Indications, route, and dosage
Abnormal uterine bleeding from hormonal imbalance
Adults: 5 to 10 mg P.O. daily for 5 to 10 days beginning on day 16 or 21 of menstrual cycle. If patient has received estrogen, then 10 mg P.O. daily for 10 days beginning on day 16 of cycle.
Secondary amenorrhea
Adults: 5 to 10 mg P.O. daily for 5 to 10 days.
Endometrial or renal carcinoma
Adults: 400 to 1,000 mg/week I.M.

Pharmacodynamics
- *Progestational action:* Medroxyprogesterone suppresses ovulation, causes thickening of cervical mucus, and induces sloughing of the endometrium.
- *Antineoplastic action:* Medroxyprogesterone may inhibit growth progression of progestin-sensitive endometrial or renal cancer tissue by an unknown mechanism.

Pharmacokinetics
- *Absorption:* Slow absorption after I.M. administration.
- *Distribution:* Not well characterized.
- *Metabolism:* Primarily hepatic; not well characterized.
- *Excretion:* Primarily renal; not well characterized.

Contraindications and precautions
Medroxyprogesterone is contraindicated in patients with known hypersensitivity to progestins, a history of thromboembolic disorders, severe hepatic disease, breast or genital cancer, or undiagnosed abnormal vaginal bleeding because it may worsen these disorders; and in pregnant or breast-feeding women.

Medroxyprogesterone should be used cautiously in patients with existing conditions that might be aggravated by fluid and electrolyte retention, such as cardiac or renal disease, epilepsy, or migraine, because drug may worsen these conditions. Caution is also advised in administering this agent to diabetic patients (because decreased glucose tolerance may occur) or to patients with a history of mental depression (because drug may induce depression).

Interactions
In patients receiving bromocriptine, progestins may cause amenorrhea or galactorrhea, thus interfering with the action of bromocriptine. Concurrent use of these drugs is not recommended.

Effects on diagnostic tests
Pregnanediol excretion may decrease; serum alkaline phosphatase and amino acid levels may increase. Glucose tolerance has been shown to decrease in a small percentage of patients receiving this drug.

Adverse reactions
- CNS: dizziness, headache, lethargy, depression.
- CV: thrombophlebitis, *pulmonary embolism,* edema.
- DERM: melasma, rash.
- GU: breakthrough bleeding, dysmenorrhea, amenorrhea, cervical erosion or abnormal secretions.
- Hepatic: cholestatic jaundice.
- Metabolic: hyperglycemia, decreased libido.
- Local: pain, induration, sterile abscesses.
- Other: breast tenderness, acne, galactorrhea.
Note: Drug should be discontinued if hypersensitivity, thromboembolic or thrombotic disorders, visual disturbances, migraine or severe depression develops.

Overdose and treatment
No information available.

▶ Special considerations
Besides those relevant to all *progestins,* consider the following recommendations.
- Parenteral form is for I.M. administration only. Inject deep into large muscle mass, preferably the gluteal muscle. Monitor for development of sterile abscesses. Medroxyprogesterone suspension must be shaken vigorously immediately before each use to ensure complete suspension of the drug.
- Medroxyprogesterone has been used to treat obstructive sleep apnea and to manage paraphilia.
- Parenteral form has been used as a long-acting contraceptive in females.

Breast-feeding
Medroxyprogesterone is contraindicated in breast-feeding women.

medrysone
HMS Liquifilm Ophthalmic

- Pharmacologic classification: corticosteroid
- Therapeutic classification: ophthalmic anti-inflammatory
- Pregnancy risk category C

How supplied
Available by prescription only
Suspension: 1%

Indications, route, and dosage
Allergic conjunctivitis, vernal conjunctivitis, episcleritis, ophthalmic epinephrine sensitivity reaction
Adults and children: Instill 1 drop in conjunctival sac b.i.d. to q.i.d. May use q hour during first 1 to 2 days if needed.

Pharmacodynamics
Anti-inflammatory action: Medrysone, a synthetic corticosteroid, stimulates the synthesis of enzymes needed to decrease the inflammatory response. Conjunctival

administration of medrysone effectively reduces local inflammation. Because medrysone has not been proven to be effective in iritis and uveitis, it is not recommended for treatment of these conditions.

Pharmacokinetics
• *Absorption:* After ophthalmic administration, medrysone is absorbed through the aqueous humor. Because of the low doses used, very little drug is absorbed systemically.
• *Distribution:* Medrysone is distributed through the local tissue layers. Any drug that is absorbed into circulation is distributed rapidly into muscle, liver, skin, intestines, and kidneys.
• *Metabolism:* Medrysone is primarily metabolized locally. The small amount that is absorbed into systemic circulation is metabolized primarily in the liver to inactive compounds.
• *Excretion:* Inactive metabolites are excreted by the kidneys, primarily as glucuronides and sulfates, but also as unconjugated products. Small amounts of the metabolites are also excreted in feces.

Contraindications and precautions
Medrysone is contraindicated in patients who are hypersensitive to any component of the preparation; in patients with fungal infections of the eye; and in patients with acute, untreated purulent bacterial, viral, or fungal ocular infections. It should be used cautiously in patients with corneal abrasions. If a bacterial infection does not respond promptly to appropriate anti-infective therapy, the corticosteroid should be discontinued and another therapy applied.

Intraocular pressure should be measured every 2 to 4 weeks for the first 2 months of ophthalmic corticosteroid therapy and then, if no increase in pressure has occurred, about every 1 to 2 months thereafter.

Interactions
None reported.

Effects on diagnostic tests
None reported.

Adverse reactions
• Eye: transient burning or stinging on administration; mydriasis, ptosis, epithelial punctate keratitis, and corneal or scleral malacia (rare); increased intraocular pressure, thinning of the cornea, interference with corneal wound healing, increased susceptibility to viral or fungal corneal infection, corneal ulceration; glaucoma, cataracts, defects in visual acuity and visual field with (long-term use).
• Systemic: rare, but may occur with excessive doses or long-term use.
Note: Drug should be discontinued if topical application results in local irritation, infection, significant systemic absorption, or hypersensitivity reaction; if visual acuity decreases or visual field is diminished; or if burning, stinging, or watering of eyes does not quickly resolve after administration.

Overdose and treatment
No information available.

▶ Special considerations
Recommendations for use of medrysone and for care and teaching of patient during therapy are the same as those for all *ophthalmic adrenocorticoids*.

mefenamic acid
Ponstan*, Ponstel

• Pharmacologic classification: nonsteroidal anti-inflammatory
• Therapeutic classification: nonnarcotic analgesic, antipyretic, anti-inflammatory
• Pregnancy risk category C (D in third trimester)

How supplied
Available by prescription only
Capsules: 250 mg

Indications, route, and dosage
Mild to moderate pain, dysmenorrhea
Adults and children over age 14: 500 mg P.O. initially, then 250 mg q 4 hours, p.r.n. Maximum therapy 1 week.

Pharmacodynamics
Analgesic, antipyretic, and anti-inflammatory actions: Mechanisms of action are unknown; mefenamic acid is thought to inhibit prostaglandin synthesis.

Pharmacokinetics
• *Absorption:* Mefenamic acid is absorbed rapidly and completely from the GI tract.
• *Distribution:* Drug is highly protein-bound.
• *Metabolism:* Drug is metabolized in the liver.
• *Excretion:* Mefenamic acid is excreted mainly in urine, with some biliary excretion. The plasma half-life is around 2 hours.

Contraindications and precautions
Mefenamic acid is contraindicated in patients with known hypersensitivity to this drug or in patients in whom aspirin or other nonsteroidal anti-inflammatory drugs (NSAIDs) induce symptoms of asthma, urticaria, or rhinitis.

Serious GI toxicity, especially ulceration or hemorrhage, can occur at any time with NSAID use, especially in patients on chronic therapy. This drug should be administered cautiously in patients with a history of GI disease, cardiac disease, hepatic or renal disease, blood dyscrasias, or diabetes mellitus, because it may worsen these conditions.

Patients with known "triad" symptoms (aspirin hypersensitivity, rhinitis/nasal polyps, and asthma) are at high risk of bronchospasm. NSAIDs may mask the signs and symptoms of acute infection (fever, myalgia, erythema); carefully evaluate patients with high risk (such as those with diabetes).

Interactions
Concomitant use of mefenamic acid with anticoagulants and thrombolytic drugs (coumarin derivatives, heparin, streptokinase, or urokinase) may potentiate anticoagulant effects. Bleeding problems may occur if used with other drugs that inhibit platelet aggregation, such as azlocillin, parenteral carbenicillin, dextran, dipyridamole, mezlocillin, piperacillin, sulfinpyrazone, ticarcillin, valproic acid, cefamandole, cefoperazone, moxalactam, plicamycin, aspirin, salicylates, or other anti-inflammatory agents. Concomitant use with salicylates, anti-inflammatory agents, alcohol, corticotropin, or steroids may cause increased GI adverse reactions,

including ulceration and hemorrhage. Aspirin may decrease the bioavailability of mefenamic acid.

Because of the influence of prostaglandins on glucose metabolism, concomitant use with insulin or oral hypoglycemic agents may potentiate hypoglycemic effects. Mefenamic acid may displace highly protein-bound drugs from binding sites. Toxicity may occur with coumarin derivatives, phenytoin, verapamil, or nifedipine. Increased nephrotoxicity may occur with gold compounds, other anti-inflammatory agents, or acetaminophen. Mefenamic acid may decrease the renal clearance of methotrexate and lithium. Mefenamic acid may decrease the clinical effectiveness of diuretics and antihypertensives. Concomitant use with diuretics may increase nephrotoxicity.

Effects on diagnostic tests
False-positive results for urine bilirubin by the Di-Azo tablet test have been reported. Serum BUN, transaminase, and potassium levels may be increased by the drug; hematocrit may be decreased. Mefenamic acid may also increase prothrombin time.

Adverse reactions
● CNS: headache, dizziness, drowsiness, vertigo, nervousness, insomnia.
● CV: edema.
● DERM: rash, urticaria.
● EENT: blurred vision, eye irritation.
● GI: nausea, diarrhea, vomiting, flatulence, anorexia, *bleeding*.
● GU: nephrotoxicity, dysuria, hematuria.
● HEMA: leukopenia, thrombocytopenia, *agranulocytosis, aplastic anemia, hemolytic anemia.*
● Hepatic: hepatotoxicity.
Note: Drug should be discontinued if hypersensitivity, rash, or diarrhea develops.

Overdose and treatment
Clinical manifestations of overdose include CNS stimulation, irrational behavior, marked agitation, and generalized seizures. Renal toxicity may follow this phase of CNS stimulation.

To treat overdose of mefenamic acid, empty stomach immediately by inducing emesis with ipecac syrup or by gastric lavage. Administer activated charcoal via nasogastric tube. Provide symptomatic and supportive measures (respiratory support and correction of fluid and electrolyte imbalances). Appropriate therapy for seizure control with I.V. diazepam may be indicated. Monitor laboratory parameters and vital signs closely. Mefenamic acid is not dialyzable.

▶ **Special considerations**
Besides those relevant to all *NSAIDs*, consider the following recommendations.
● Monitor GI elimination patterns for complaints of diarrhea.
● Monitor for signs and symptoms of fluid retention, dehydration, or electrolyte imbalance. Check weight frequently for significant changes.
● Insulin-dependent diabetic patients on mefenamic acid may have increased insulin requirements. Monitor serum glucose levels frequently.
● For acute pain therapy, mefenamic acid should not be used longer than 1 week to avoid adverse effects of prolonged use.
● Institute safety measures to prevent injury that may occur because of CNS effects.

Information for the patient
● Tell patient to call for instructions before using any nonprescription medication.
● Teach signs and symptoms of possible adverse effects. Instruct patient to call if any occur.
● Advise patient to record his weight two or three times weekly and to report any weight gain of 3 pounds or more within 1 week.
● Teach patient dietary measures to control possible diarrhea.
● Advise patient of need for medical follow-up while taking mefenamic acid.
● Warn patient that drowsiness may occur and to avoid hazardous activities that require alertness.

Geriatric use
● Patients over age 60 may be more susceptible to the toxic effects of mefenamic acid.
● The effects of this drug on renal prostaglandins may cause fluid retention and edema, a significant drawback for elderly patients and those with congestive heart failure. Elderly patients are more likely to develop severe diarrhea with mefenamic acid.

Pediatric use
Do not use long-term mefenamic acid therapy in children under age 14; safety of this use has not been established.

Breast-feeding
Because mefenamic acid is distributed into breast milk, avoid use in breast-feeding women.

---

mefloquine hydrochloride
Lariam

● Pharmacologic classification: quinine derivative
● Therapeutic classification: antimalarial
● Pregnancy risk category C

How supplied
Available by prescription only
Tablets: 250 mg

Indications, route, and dosage
Malaria treatment
Adults: 1,250 mg P.O. as a single dose. Patients with *Plasmodium vivax* infections should receive subsequent therapy with primaquine or other 8-aminoquinolones to avoid relapse.
Malaria prophylaxis
Adults: 250 mg P.O. once weekly for 4 weeks, then 250 mg every other week. Initiate prophylaxis 1 week before entering endemic area, and continue for 4 weeks after return. For prolonged visits to endemic areas, prophylaxis should continue for three doses after return.
Dosage in renal failure
No adjustment is necessary.

Pharmacodynamics
Antimalarial action: Mefloquine acts as a blood schizonticide. Its exact mechanism of action has not been identified. Mefloquine is effective against all human types of malaria, including chloroquine-resistant ma-

laria, and *Plasmodium falciparum* and *P. vivax* infections.

Pharmacokinetics
● *Absorption:* Mefloquine is well absorbed after oral administration.
● *Distribution:* Mefloquine concentrates in the red blood cells and is approximately 98% protein-bound.
● *Metabolism:* Mefloquine is metabolized by the liver.
● *Excretion:* Mefloquine is primarily excreted via the liver. Small amounts can be found in the urine and breast milk. The half-life in normal adults is approximately 21 days.

Contraindications and precautions
Mefloquine is contraindicated in patients with a known hypersensitivity to mefloquine or related compounds.

Interactions
Mefloquine may have cardiovascular effects when taken with beta blockers (propranolol). To prevent cardiac problems resulting from concomitant use with quinine or quinidine, mefloquine dose should follow the last quinine dose by at least 12 hours. Seizures may occur with concomitant use of mefloquine and chloroquine; loss of seizure control may occur with concomitant use of valproic acid.

Adverse reactions
● CNS: dizziness, syncope, asthenia, *seizures*, hallucinations, confusion, depression, disorientation.
● CV: bradycardia, *cardiac arrest, arrhythmias.*
● DERM: pruritus, rash.
● GI: nausea, vomiting.

Overdose and treatment
Treatment usually includes induced vomiting and management of symptoms. Major problems are related to cardiotoxic effects. Treat vomiting or diarrhea with standard fluid therapy.

▶ **Special considerations**
● Monitor liver function tests with prolonged therapy.
● Ophthalmologic examinations are recommended during prolonged therapy because ocular lesions have been noted in laboratory animals.

Information for the patient
● Advise patient to use caution when performing potentially hazardous tasks because drug may cause dizziness and altered sense of balance.
● To facilitate compliance, advise patient taking mefloquine for prophylaxis to take the drug on the same day of the week.
● Patients taking mefloquine prophylaxis should discontinue the drug if they notice signs or symptoms of unexplained anxiety, depression, confusion, or restlessness. These symptoms may indicate impending toxicity.
● Tell patient not to take the drug on an empty stomach and always to take it with a full (at least 8 oz, or 240 ml) glass of water.

Pediatric use
Safety and efficacy in children have not been demonstrated.

megestrol acetate
Megace, Pallace

● Pharmacologic classification: progestin
● Therapeutic classification: antineoplastic
● Pregnancy risk category X

How supplied
Available by prescription only
Tablets: 20 mg, 40 mg

Indications, route, and dosage
Dosage and indications may vary. Check current literature for recommended protocol.
Breast carcinoma
Adults: 40 mg P.O. q.i.d.
Endometrial carcinoma
Adults: 10 to 80 mg P.O. q.i.d.

Pharmacodynamics
Antineoplastic action: Megestrol inhibits growth and causes regression of progestin-sensitive breast and endometrial cancer tissue by an unknown mechanism.

Pharmacokinetics
● *Absorption:* Megestrol is well absorbed across the GI tract after oral administration.
● *Distribution:* Megestrol appears to be stored in fatty tissue and is highly bound to plasma proteins.
● *Metabolism:* Megestrol is completely metabolized in the liver.
● *Excretion:* The metabolites are eliminated primarily through the kidneys.

Contraindications and precautions
Megestrol is contraindicated in patients with known hypersensitivity to progestins; in patients with a history of thromboembolic disorder because the drug may be associated with thromboembolic disease; in patients with severe hepatic disease because drug accumulation may occur; in patients with undiagnosed abnormal vaginal bleeding because drug may stimulate growth of some tumors; and in pregnant or breast-feeding women because of the potential for adverse effects on the fetus or neonate.
    Drug should be used cautiously in patients with conditions that might be aggravated by fluid and electrolyte retention such as cardiac or renal disease, epilepsy, or migraine. Caution is also advised in administering this agent to diabetic patients because decreased glucose tolerance may occur or to patients with a history of mental depression because drug may exacerbate these effects.

Interactions
Concomitant use with bromocriptine may cause amenorrhea or galactorrhea, thus interfering with the action of bromocriptine. Concurrent use of these drugs is not recommended.

Effects on diagnostic tests
Pregnanediol excretion may decrease; serum alkaline phosphatase and amino acid concentrations may increase. Glucose tolerance has been shown to decrease in a small percentage of patients receiving megestrol.

---

*Canada only   †Unlabeled clinical use   Italicized adverse reactions are life-threatening.

Adverse reactions
● CV: thrombophlebitis.
● Other: carpal tunnel syndrome, alopecia.

Overdose and treatment
No information available.

▶ Special considerations
Recommendations for administration of megestrol and for care and teaching of the patient during therapy are the same as those for all *progestins*.

---

melphalan (phenylalanine mustard)
Alkeran

● Pharmacologic classification: alkylating agent (cell cycle-phase nonspecific)
● Therapeutic classification: antineoplastic
● Pregnancy risk category D

How supplied
Available by prescription only
Tablets (scored): 2 mg

Indications, route, and dosage
Dosage and indications may vary. Check current literature for recommended protocol.
Multiple myeloma, testicular seminoma, non-Hodgkin's lymphoma, osteogenic sarcoma, breast cancer
Adults: 150 mcg/kg/day P.O. for 7 days, followed by a 3-week rest period. When leukocyte counts begin to rise, give maintenance dose of 50 mcg/kg. Alternatively, 100 to 500 mcg/kg/day P.O. for 2 to 3 weeks or 250 mcg/kg/day for 4 days, followed by a 2- to 4-week rest period. When leukocyte counts begin to rise above 3,000/mm³ and platelet counts are greater than 100,000/mm³, give maintenance dose of 2 to 4 mg/day. Or 250 mcg/kg/day P.O. or 7 mg/m²/day P.O. for 5 days every 5 to 6 weeks. Adjust dose to maintain mild leukopenia and thrombocytopenia.
Nonresectable advanced ovarian cancer
Adults: 200 mcg/kg/day P.O. for 5 days, repeated q 4 to 6 weeks if blood counts return to normal.

Pharmacodynamics
Antineoplastic action: Melphalan exerts its cytotoxic activity by forming cross-links of strands of DNA and RNA and inhibiting protein synthesis.

Pharmacokinetics
● *Absorption:* The absorption of melphalan from the GI tract is incomplete and variable. One study found that absorption ranged from 25% to 89% after an oral dose of 0.6 mg/kg.
● *Distribution:* Melphalan distributes rapidly and widely into total body water. The drug initially is 50% to 60% bound to plasma proteins and eventually increases to 80% to 90% over time.
● *Metabolism:* Melphalan is extensively deactivated by the process of hydrolysis.
● *Excretion:* The elimination of melphalan has been described as biphasic, with an initial half-life of 8 minutes and a terminal half-life of 2 hours. Melphalan and

its metabolites are excreted primarily in urine, with 10% of an oral dose excreted as unchanged drug.

Contraindications and precautions
Melphalan is contraindicated in patients with a history of hypersensitivity to the drug or resistance to previous therapy with it. A cross-sensitivity, which manifests as a rash, may occur between melphalan and chlorambucil.
Drug should be used with caution in patients with hematologic compromise or recent exposure to cytotoxic or radiation therapy because of the drug's myelosuppressive effects; and in patients with renal dysfunction because accumulation and excessive toxicity may occur.

Interactions
No clinically significant drug interactions have been reported with melphalan.

Effects on diagnostic tests
Melphalan therapy may increase blood and urine levels of uric acid.

Adverse reactions
● DERM: dermatitis.
● GI: mild nausea and vomiting, diarrhea, stomatitis.
● HEMA: *bone marrow depression* (dose-limiting); *leukopenia, thrombocytopenia, agranulocytosis;* acute nonlymphocytic leukemia may develop with chronic use.
● Other: alopecia, pneumonitis, *pulmonary fibrosis*.
Note: Drug should be discontinued at the first signs of bone marrow depression.

Overdose and treatment
Clinical manifestations of overdose include myelosuppression and hypocalcemia.
Treatment is usually supportive and includes transfusion of blood components.

▶ Special considerations
Besides those relevant to all *alkylating agents*, consider the following recommendations.
● Oral dose may be taken all at one time.
● Administer melphalan on an empty stomach because absorption is decreased by food.
● Frequent hematologic monitoring, including a CBC, is necessary for accurate dosage adjustments and prevention of toxicity.
● Discontinue therapy temporarily or reduce dosage if leukocyte count falls below 3,000/mm³ or platelet count falls below 100,000/mm³.
● Avoid I.M. injections when platelet count is below 100,000/mm³.
● Anticoagulants, aspirin, and aspirin-containing products should be used cautiously.

Information for the patient
● Tell patient it is vital to continue medication despite nausea and vomiting.
● Tell patient to call immediately if vomiting occurs shortly after taking a dose.
● Explain that adequate fluid intake is important to facilitate excretion of uric acid.
● Patient should avoid exposure to people with infections.
● Reassure patient that hair should grow back after treatment has ended.

---

*Canada only   †Unlabeled clinical use   Italicized adverse reactions are life-threatening.

• Tell patient to promptly report any signs and symptoms of infection or bleeding.

Breast-feeding
It is not known whether melphalan distributes into breast milk. However, because of the potential for serious adverse reactions, mutagenicity, and carcinogenicity in the infant, breast-feeding is not recommended.

---

meningitis vaccine
Menomune-A/C/Y/W-135

• Pharmacologic classification: vaccine
• Therapeutic classification: bacterial vaccine
• Pregnancy risk category C

How supplied
Available by prescription only
Injection: a killed bacterial vaccine in 10-dose and 50-dose vials with vial of diluent

Indications, route, and dosage
Meningococcal meningitis prophylaxis
Adults and children over age 2: 0.5 ml S.C.

Pharmacodynamics
Meningitis prophylaxis: This vaccine promotes active immunity to meningitis caused by *Neisseria meningitidis.*

Pharmacokinetics
No information available.

Contraindications and precautions
Meningitis vaccine is contraindicated in patients with infections or immunodeficiency states and those receiving corticosteroids or other immunosuppressants. Meningitis vaccine also is contraindicated in pregnancy unless clearly required.

Interactions
None reported.

Effects on diagnostic tests
None reported.

Adverse reactions
• Local: pain, erythema, induration, axillary lymphadenopathy.
• Systemic: headache, malaise, chills, fever (usually resolves in 48 hours), cramps, *anaphylaxis.*

Overdose and treatment
No information available.

▶ **Special considerations**
• Obtain a thorough history of allergies and reactions to immunizations.
• Do not give meningitis vaccine intradermally, I.M., or I.V.
• Epinephrine solution 1:1,000 should be available to treat allergic reactions.
• Reconstitute with diluent provided. Shake until dissolved. Discard reconstituted solution after 5 days.
• Store between 2 to 8 C. (36 to 46 F.).

Information for the patient
• Tell patient what to expect after vaccination: pain and inflammation at the injection site. Recommend acetaminophen to alleviate adverse reactions, such as fever.
• Encourage patient to report distressing adverse reactions.
• Tell female patient of childbearing age to avoid pregnancy for 3 months after vaccination. Provide contraceptive information if necessary.
• Explain that this vaccine will provide immunity only to meningitis caused by one type of bacteria.

Pediatric use
Meningitis vaccine is not recommended for children under age 2.

Breast-feeding
It is unknown whether meningitis vaccine is distributed into breast milk. Use with caution in breast-feeding women.

---

menotropins
Pergonal

• Pharmacologic classification: gonadotropin
• Therapeutic classification: ovulation stimulant, spermatogenesis stimulant
• Pregnancy risk category X

How supplied
Available by prescription only
Injection: 75 IU of luteinizing hormone (LH) and 75 IU of follicle-stimulating hormone (FSH) activity per ampule; 150 IU of LH and 150 IU of FSH activity per ampule

Indications, route, and dosage
Production of follicular maturation
Adults: 75 IU each of FSH and LH I.M. daily for 9 to 12 days, followed by 10,000 USP units chorionic gonadotropin, human (HCG) I.M. 1 day after last dose of menotropins; repeat for two menstrual cycles. Then, if ovulation and/or follicular development does not occur, increase to 150 IU each of FSH and LH I.M. daily for 9 to 12 days, followed by 10,000 USP units HCG I.M. 1 day after last dose of menotropins; repeat for two menstrual cycles.
Stimulation of spermatogenesis
Adults: After 4 to 6 months of treatment with HCG, 1 ampule (75 IU) I.M. three times weekly (given concomitantly with 2,000 USP units HCG twice weekly) for at least 4 months.

Pharmacodynamics
• *Ovulation stimulant action:* Menotropins causes growth and maturation of the ovarian follicle in women who do not have primary ovarian failure by mimicking the action of endogenous LH and FSH. Additional treatment with human chorionic gonadotropin is usually required to achieve ovulation.
• *Spermatogenesis stimulant action:* Menotropins causes spermatogenesis when coadministered with HCG in men with primary or secondary pituitary hypofunction.

Pharmacokinetics
● *Absorption:* Drug must be administered parenterally for effectiveness.
● *Distribution:* Unknown.
● *Metabolism:* Not fully known.
● *Excretion:* Menotropins is excreted in the urine.

Contraindications and precautions
Menotropins is contraindicated in women with primary ovarian failure and infertility not resulting from anovulation because therapy will not correct infertility; in women with overt adrenal or thyroid disease, pituitary tumors, undiagnosed abnormal vaginal bleeding, or ovarian cysts; and in pregnant or breast-feeding women.

Menotropins is contraindicated in men with normal pituitary function, primary testicular failure, or infertility from any cause other than hypogonadotropic hypogonadism because therapy will not correct infertility.

Use caution in initiating therapy with menotropins. In women, primary ovarian failure or early pregnancy must be ruled out, and anovulation confirmed, before treatment may begin. In men, primary testicular failure must be ruled out, and abnormally low gonadotropin levels must be present. Menotropins should be prescribed only by physicians thoroughly familiar with infertility disorders. To avoid causing hyperstimulation syndrome, only the lowest possible effective dose of menotropins should be used.

Interactions
None reported.

Effects on diagnostic tests
None reported.

Adverse reactions
● GI: nausea, vomiting, diarrhea.
● GU: *in females:* ovarian enlargement with pain and abdominal distention, ovarian hyperstimulation syndrome (sudden ovarian enlargement, ascites with or without pain, or pleural effusion), follicular cysts; *in males:* gynecomastia.
● Other: fever, *arterial thromboembolism.*
   Note: Drug should be discontinued if hyperstimulation syndrome or abdominal pain occurs or if ovaries become abnormally enlarged.

Overdose and treatment
The most common dose-related adverse effect appears to be ovarian hyperstimulation syndrome. Drug should be discontinued. Symptomatic and supportive care should include bed rest, fluid and electrolyte replacement, and analgesics.

▶ Special considerations
● Menotropins is administered by I.M. route only.
● Reconstitute with 1 to 2 ml of sterile saline injection. Use immediately.
● Pregnancy usually occurs 4 to 6 weeks after therapy.
● Pregnancies that follow ovulation induced with menotropins show a relatively high frequency of multiple births.

Information for the patient
● Teach patient signs and tests that indicate time of ovulation, such as increase in basal body temperature and increase in the appearance and volume of cervical mucus.
● Warn patient to report immediately symptoms of hyperstimulation syndrome: abdominal distention and pain, dyspnea, and vaginal bleeding.
● Tell patient multiple births are possible.
● In infertility, encourage daily intercourse from day before chorionic gonadotropin is given until ovulation occurs.
● Advise patient that she should be examined at least every other day for signs of excessive ovarian stimulation during therapy and for 2 weeks after treatment is discontinued.

Breast-feeding
Not indicated for use by breast-feeding women.

mepenzolate bromide
Cantil

● Pharmacologic classification: anticholinergic
● Therapeutic classification: antimuscarinic, gastrointestinal antispasmodic
● Pregnancy risk category C

How supplied
Available by prescription only
Tablets: 25 mg

Indications, route, and dosage
Adjunctive therapy in peptic ulcer, irritable bowel syndrome, and neurologic bowel disturbances
Adults: 25 to 50 mg P.O. q.i.d. with meals and h.s. Adjust dosage to individual patient's needs.

Pharmacodynamics
Anticholinergic action: Mepenzolate competitively blocks acetylcholine at cholinergic neuroeffector sites, decreasing GI tract motility and inhibiting gastric acid secretion.

Pharmacokinetics
● *Absorption:* Mepenzolate is poorly absorbed from the GI tract.
● *Distribution:* Mepenzolate does not cross the blood-brain barrier; little else is known about its distribution.
● *Metabolism:* Exact metabolic fate is unknown.
● *Excretion:* From 3% to 22% of dose is excreted in urine over a 5-day period; the remainder is excreted in feces as unabsorbed drug.

Contraindications and precautions
Mepenzolate is contraindicated in patients with narrow-angle glaucoma, because drug-induced cycloplegia and mydriasis may increase intraocular pressure; in patients with obstructive uropathy, obstructive GI tract disease, severe ulcerative colitis, myasthenia gravis, paralytic ileus, intestinal atony, or toxic megacolon, because the drug may exacerbate these conditions; and in patients with known hypersensitivity to anticholinergics or bromides.

Administer mepenzolate cautiously to patients with autonomic neuropathy, hyperthyroidism, coronary artery disease, cardiac arrhythmias, congestive heart failure, or ulcerative colitis, because the drug may exacerbate the symptoms of these disorders; to patients with hepatic or renal disease, because toxic accumu-

---

lation may occur; to patients over age 40, because the drug increases the glaucoma risk; to patients with hiatal hernia associated with reflux esophagitis, because the drug may decrease lower esophageal sphincter tone; and in hot or humid environments, because the drug may predispose the patient to heatstroke.

Interactions
Concurrent administration of antacids decreases oral absorption of anticholinergics. Administer mepenzolate at least 1 hour before antacids.

Concomitant administration of drugs with anticholinergic effects may cause additive toxicity.

Decreased GI absorption of many drugs has been reported after the use of anticholinergics (for example, levodopa and ketoconazole). Conversely, slowly dissolving digoxin tablets may yield higher serum digoxin levels when administered with anticholinergics.

Use cautiously with oral potassium supplements (especially wax-matrix formulations) because the incidence of potassium-induced GI ulcerations may be increased.

Effects on diagnostic tests
None reported.

Adverse reactions
• CNS: headache, insomnia, drowsiness, dizziness, weakness, confusion and excitement (in elderly).
• CV: palpitations, tachycardia, orthostatic hypotension.
• DERM: urticaria, decreased sweating or anhidrosis, other dermal manifestations.
• EENT: blurred vision, mydriasis, cycloplegia, increased ocular tension, photophobia.
• GI: dry mouth, dysphagia, heartburn, loss of taste, nausea, constipation, vomiting, paralytic ileus, abdominal distention.
• GU: urinary hesitancy and retention, impotence.
• Other: fever, allergic reaction.
Note: Drug should be discontinued if hypersensitivity, urinary retention, confusion or excitement, curarelike symptoms, or skin rash occurs.

Overdose and treatment
Clinical signs of overdose include curare-like symptoms and such peripheral effects as headache; dilated, nonreactive pupils; blurred vision; flushed, hot, dry skin; dry mucous membranes; dysphagia; decreased or absent bowel sounds; urinary retention; hyperthermia; tachycardia; hypertension; and increased respiration.

Treatment is primarily symptomatic and supportive, as needed. If the patient is alert, induce emesis (or use gastric lavage) and follow with a saline cathartic and activated charcoal to prevent further drug absorption. In severe cases, physostigmine may be administered to block mepenzolate's antimuscarinic effects. Give fluids, as needed, to treat shock. If urinary retention occurs, catheterization may be necessary.

▶ Special considerations
Besides those relevant to all *anticholinergics*, consider the following recommendations.
• Store mepenzolate in a dark, tight container to protect it from excessive moisture, light, and heat.
• Drug contains tartrazine dye, which may cause allergic reactions, especially in patients sensitive to aspirin.

Geriatric use
Mepenzolate should be administered cautiously to elderly patients. Lower doses are indicated.

Breast-feeding
Mepenzolate may be excreted in breast milk, possibly resulting in infant toxicity. Breast-feeding women should avoid this drug. Mepenzolate may also decrease milk production.

meperidine hydrochloride (pethidine hydrochloride)
Demerol

• Pharmacologic classification: opioid
• Therapeutic classification: analgesic, adjunct to anesthesia
• Controlled substance schedule II
• Pregnancy risk category B

How supplied
Available by prescription only
Tablets: 50 mg, 100 mg
Liquid: 50 mg/ml
Injection: 10 mg/ml, 25 mg/ml, 50 mg/ml, 75 mg/ml, 100 mg/ml

Indications, route, and dosage
Moderate to severe pain
Adults: 50 to 150 mg P.O., I.M., I.V., or S.C. q 3 to 4 hours. Continuous I.V. infusion: 15 to 35 mg/hour p.r.n. or around the clock.
Children: 1.1. to 1.8 mg/kg P.O., I.M., I.V., or S.C. q 4 to 6 hours or 175 mg/m² daily in 6 divided doses. Maximum single dose for children should not exceed 100 mg.
Preoperatively
Adults: 50 to 100 mg I.M., I.V., or S.C. 30 to 90 minutes before surgery. Do not exceed adult dose.
Children: 1 to 2.2 mg/kg I.M., I.V., or S.C. 30 to 90 minutes before surgery. Do not exceed adult dose.

Pharmacodynamics
Analgesic action: Meperidine is a narcotic agonist with actions and potency similar to those of morphine, with principle actions at the opiate receptors. It is recommended for the relief of moderate to severe pain.

Pharmacokinetics
• *Absorption:* Meperidine given orally is only half as effective as it is parenterally. Onset of analgesia occurs within 10 to 45 minutes. Duration of action is 2 to 4 hours.
• *Distribution:* Meperidine is distributed widely throughout the body.
• *Metabolism:* Meperidine is metabolized primarily by hydrolysis in the liver.
• *Excretion:* About 30% of a dose of meperidine is excreted in the urine as the N-demethylated derivative; about 5% is excreted unchanged. Excretion is enhanced by acidifying the urine.

Contraindications and precautions
Meperidine is contraindicated in patients with known hypersensitivity to the drug or any phenylpiperidine opioid (meperidine or its analogs).

Administer meperidine with extreme caution to patients with supraventricular arrhythmias; avoid, or administer drug with extreme caution to patients with head injury or increased intracranial pressure, because drug obscures neurologic parameters; and during pregnancy and labor, because drug readily crosses placenta (premature infants are especially sensitive to respiratory and CNS depressant effects of narcotic agonists).

Administer meperidine cautiously to patients with renal or hepatic dysfunction, because drug accumulation or prolonged duration of action may occur; to patients with pulmonary disease (asthma, chronic obstructive pulmonary disease), because drug depresses respiration and suppresses cough reflex; to patients undergoing biliary tract surgery, because drug may cause biliary spasm; to patients with convulsive disorders, because drug may precipitate seizures; in elderly or debilitated patients, who are more sensitive to both therapeutic and adverse drug effects; and to patients prone to physical or psychic addiction, because of the high risk of addiction to this drug.

Meperidine has atropine-like effects. Administer cautiously to patients with glaucoma.

Interactions

Concomitant use with other CNS depressants (narcotic analgesics, general anesthetics, antihistamines, phenothiazines, barbiturates, benzodiazepines, sedative-hypnotics, tricyclic antidepressants, alcohol, and muscle relaxants) potentiates drug's respiratory and CNS depression, sedation, and hypotensive effects. Concomitant use with cimetidine may also increase respiratory and CNS depression, causing confusion, disorientation, apnea, or seizures; such use requires reduced dosage of meperidine.

Drug accumulation and enhanced effects may result from concomitant use with other drugs that are extensively metabolized in the liver (rifampin, phenytoin, and digitoxin); combined use with anticholinergics may cause paralytic ileus.

Patients who become physically dependent on this drug may experience acute withdrawal syndrome if given a narcotic antagonist.

Severe cardiovascular depression may result from concomitant use with general anesthetics; meperidine can potentiate the adverse effects of isoniazid.

Concomitant use with monoamine oxidase (MAO) inhibitors may precipitate unpredictable and occasionally fatal reactions, even in patients who may receive MAO inhibitors within 14 days of receiving meperidine. Some reactions have been characterized by coma, respiratory depression, cyanosis, and hypotension; in others, hyperexcitability, convulsions, tachycardia, hyperpyrexia, and hypertension have occurred.

Effects on diagnostic tests

Meperidine increases plasma amylase or lipase levels through increased biliary tract pressure; levels may be unreliable for 24 hours after meperidine administration.

Adverse reactions

● CNS: sedation, somnolence, clouded sensorium, light-headedness, dizziness, paradoxical excitement, euphoria, insomnia, agitation, confusion, headache, tremor, miosis, seizures, psychic dependence, *convulsions* (at high doses); inadvertent injection about a nerve trunk may result in sensory-motor paralysis which is usually but not always temporary.

● CV: tachycardia, *asystole*, bradycardia, palpitations, hypotension, syncope.
● DERM: sweating, flushing, rash, pruritus, pain at injection site, local irritation and induration after subcutaneous injection (especially when repeated).
● GI: dry mouth, anorexia, biliary spasms (colic), ileus, nausea, vomiting, constipation.
● GU: urinary retention or hesitancy.
● Other: *respiratory depression.*
Note: Drug should be discontinued if hypersensitivity, seizures, or cardiac arrhythmias occur.

Overdose and treatment

The most common signs and symptoms of meperidine overdose are CNS depression, respiratory depression, skeletal muscle flaccidity, cold and clammy skin, mydriasis, bradycardia, and hypotension. Other acute toxic effects include hypothermia, shock, apnea, cardiopulmonary arrest, circulatory collapse, pulmonary edema, and convulsions.

To treat acute overdose, first establish adequate respiratory exchange via a patent airway and ventilation as needed; administer a narcotic antagonist (naloxone) to reverse respiratory depression. (Because the duration of action of meperidine is longer than that of naloxone, repeated dosing is necessary.) Naloxone should not be given unless the patient has clinically significant respiratory or cardiovascular depression. Monitor vital signs closely.

If the patient presents within 2 hours of ingestion of an oral overdose, empty the stomach immediately by inducing emesis (ipecac syrup) or using gastric lavage. Use caution to avoid any risk of aspiration. Administer activated charcoal via nasogastric tube for further removal of meperidine, and acidify urine to help remove meperidine.

Provide symptomatic and supportive treatment (continued respiratory support, correction of fluid or electrolyte imbalance). Monitor laboratory parameters, vital signs, and neurologic status closely.

▶ Special considerations

Besides those relevant to all *opioids,* consider the following recommendations.
● Meperidine may be administered to some patients who are allergic to morphine.
● Meperidine and its active metabolite normeperidine accumulate. Monitor for toxic effects, especially in patients with poor renal function.
● Because meperidine toxicity commonly appears after several days of treatment, this drug is not recommended for treatment of chronic pain.
● Meperidine may be given slow I.V., preferably as a diluted solution. S.C. injection is very painful. During I.V. administration, tachycardia may occur, possibly as a result of the drug's atropine-like effects.
● Oral dose is less than half as effective as parenteral dose. Give I.M. if possible. When changing from parenteral to oral route, dosage should be increased.
● Syrup has local anesthetic effect. Give with water.
● Alternating meperidine with a peripherally active non-narcotic analgesic (aspirin, acetaminophen, NSAIDs) may improve pain control while allowing lower narcotic dosages.
● Injectable meperidine is compatible with saline and dextrose 5% solutions and their combinations, and with lactated Ringer's and sodium lactate solution.
● Question patients carefully regarding possible use of MAO inhibitors within the past 14 days.

Geriatric use
Lower doses are usually indicated for elderly patients, because they may be more sensitive to the therapeutic and adverse effects of the drug.

Pediatric use
Meperidine should not be administered to infants under age 6 months.

Breast-feeding
Meperidine is excreted in breast milk. It should be used with caution in breast-feeding women.

---

mephentermine sulfate
Wyamine

- Pharmacologic classification: adrenergic
- Therapeutic classification: vasopressor
- Pregnancy risk category C

How supplied
Available by prescription only
Injection: 15 mg/ml, 30 mg/ml parenteral

Indications, route, and dosage
Hypotension
Adults and children: Average dosage 0.5 mg/kg for adults; 0.4 mg/kg for children; range 10 to 80 mg I.M., or 20 to 60 mg I.V. bolus followed by slow infusion of a solution containing 1.2 mg/ml.
Hypotension caused by spinal anesthesia
Adults: 30 to 45 mg I.V.; additional doses of 30 mg may be given to maintain blood pressure.
Prevention of hypotension during spinal anesthesia
Adults: 30 to 40 mg I.M. administered 10 to 20 minutes before administration of spinal anesthesic.

Pharmacodynamics
Vasopressor action: The mechanism of action has not been determined. Reportedly, mephentermine indirectly stimulates beta- and alpha-adrenergic receptors by releasing norepinephrine from its storage site. It produces a positive inotropic effect, increasing cardiac output, coronary blood flow, force of contraction, and stroke volume. It also shortens atrioventricular (AV) nodal conduction time and increases ventricular conduction velocity.

By directly dilating arteries and arterioles in skeletal muscle and mesenteric vascular beds, mephentermine increases venous return to the heart and systolic and diastolic blood pressure.

Pharmacokinetics
- Absorption: Pressor response occurs almost immediately and persists 15 to 30 minutes after I.V. injection; after I.M. injection, onset is within 5 to 15 minutes, persisting 1 to 4 hours.
- Distribution: Unknown.
- Metabolism: Mephentermine is metabolized in liver by N-demethylation and p-hydroxylation.
- Excretion: Mephentermine is excreted in urine within 24 hours as unchanged drug and metabolites. Acidic urine may increase excretion.

Contraindications and precautions
Mephentermine is contraindicated in patients with hypersensitivity to drug. Administer cautiously to patients with cardiovascular disease, hypertension, hyperthyroidism, hypovolemic states, or chronic illness (because of increased potential for adverse reactions).

Interactions
Concomitant use of mephentermine with general anesthetics, especially cyclopropane or inhalation hydrocarbon anesthetics, may result in arrhythmias. Digitalis may sensitize myocardium to effects of mephentermine. Phenothiazines may antagonize pressor effects of mephentermine; monoamine oxidase inhibitors may potentiate these effects and should not be used with mephentermine. Reserpine and guanethidine may reduce pressor response to mephentermine.

Effects on diagnostic tests
None significant.

Adverse reactions
- CNS: nervousness, anxiety, seizures.
- CV: tachycardia, *arrhythmias*, AV block, hypertension.
  Note: Drug should be discontinued if patient develops hypersensitivity or cardiac arrhythmias.

Overdose and treatment
Clinical manifestations of overdose include visual hallucinations of colored geometric forms, paranoid psychosis, euphoria, drowsiness, weeping, incoherence, weakness, and numbness and tingling of extremities.

These adverse CNS effects rapidly disappear when drug is withdrawn.

▶ Special considerations
Besides those relevant to all *adrenergics*, consider the following recommendations.
- Hypovolemia should be treated and corrected before administration of mephentermine. Drug is not a replacement for blood, fluid, plasma, or electrolytes.
- Mephentermine may increase uterine contractions during third trimester of pregnancy.
- Hypercapnea, hypoxia, and acidosis may reduce effectiveness or increase adverse effects of mephentermine. Identify and correct such conditions before administration.
- Closely observe patient and monitor blood pressure, heart rate, ECG, and central venous pressure.
- During I.V. administration, check blood pressure and pulse every 2 minutes until patient is stabilized, and every 5 minutes thereafter. Continue monitoring vital signs for the duration of drug action or longer if indicated.
- Mephentermine is incompatible with epinephrine and hydralazine. Do not mix together or administer through same I.V. line.

Information for the patient
Advise patient to report any adverse reactions.

Geriatric use
Administer at lower doses and with caution to elderly patients.

Pediatric use
Use with caution in children.

---

mephenytoin
Mesantoin

- Pharmacologic classification: hydantoin derivative
- Therapeutic classification: anticonvulsant
- Pregnancy risk category C

How supplied
Available by prescription only
Tablets: 100 mg

Indications, route, and dosage
Generalized tonic-clonic or complex-partial seizures
Adults: 50 to 100 mg P.O. daily; may increase by 50 to 100 mg at weekly intervals, up to 200 mg P.O. q 8 hours. Dosages up to 800 mg/day may be required.
Children: Initial dosage is 50 to 100 mg P.O. daily (3 to 15 mg/kg/day or 100 to 450 mg/m²) in three divided doses. May increase slowly by 50 to 100 mg at weekly intervals up to 200 mg P.O. t.i.d., divided q 8 hours. Dosage must be adjusted individually. Usual maintenance dosage in children is 100 to 400 mg/day divided q 8 hours.

Pharmacodynamics
Anticonvulsant action: Like other hydantoin derivatives, mephenytoin stabilizes the neuronal membranes and limits seizure activity either by increasing efflux or by decreasing influx of sodium ions across cell membranes in the motor cortex during generation of nerve impulses. Like phenytoin, mephenytoin appears to have antiarrhythmic effects.

Mephenytoin is used for prophylaxis of tonic-clonic (grand mal), psychomotor, focal, and jacksonian-type partial seizures in patients refractory to less toxic agents. It usually is combined with phenytoin, phenobarbital, or primidone; phenytoin is preferred because it causes less sedation than barbiturates. Mephenytoin also is used with succinimides to control combined absence and tonic-clonic disorders; combined use with oxazolidines is not recommended because of the increased hazard of blood dyscrasias.

Pharmacokinetics
- *Absorption:* Mephenytoin is absorbed from the GI tract. Onset of action occurs in 30 minutes and persists for 24 to 48 hours.
- *Distribution:* Mephenytoin is distributed widely throughout the body; good seizure control without toxicity occurs when serum concentrations of drug and major metabolite reach 25 to 40 mcg/ml.
- *Metabolism:* Mephenytoin is metabolized by the liver.
- *Excretion:* Mephenytoin is excreted in urine.

Contraindications and precautions
Mephenytoin is contraindicated in patients with hypersensitivity to hydantoins. Generally it is used when other anticonvulsants have failed. It should be used with caution, and patients should be monitored carefully for toxic reactions, including potentially fatal blood dyscrasias and mucocutaneous syndromes. Such have occurred within 2 weeks to 2 years after initiation of therapy.

Interactions
Mephenytoin's therapeutic effects and toxicity may be increased by concomitant use with oral anticoagulants, antihistamines, chloramphenicol, cimetidine, diazepam, diazoxide, disulfiram, isoniazid, phenylbutazone, salicylates, sulfamethizole, or valproate. Mephenytoin's therapeutic effects may be decreased by concomitant use of alcohol or folic acid. Mephenytoin may decrease the effects of oral contraceptives.

Effects on diagnostic tests
Mephenytoin may elevate liver function test results.

Adverse reactions
- CNS: ataxia, drowsiness, fatigue, irritability, choreiform movements, depression, tremor, sleeplessness, dizziness, (usually transient).
- DERM: rashes, *exfoliative dermatitis.*
- EENT: photophobia, conjunctivitis, diplopia, nystagmus.
- GI: gingival hyperplasia, nausea and vomiting (with prolonged use).
- HEMA: *leukopenia,* neutropenia, *agranulocytosis,* thrombocytopenia, pancytopenia, eosinophilia.
- Other: alopecia, weight gain.
Note: Drug should be discontinued if signs of hypersensitivity or hepatotoxicity occur; if neutrophil count decreases by 1,600 to 2,500/mm³ or other signs of hematologic abnormalities occur; or if lymphadenopathy or rash occurs.

Overdose and treatment
Signs of acute mephenytoin toxicity may include restlessness, dizziness, drowsiness, nausea, vomiting, nystagmus, ataxia, dysarthria, tremor, and slurred speech; hypotension, respiratory depression, and coma may follow. Death may result from respiratory and circulatory depression.

Treat overdose with gastric lavage or emesis and follow with supportive treatment. Carefully monitor vital signs and fluid and electrolyte balance. Forced diuresis is of little or no value. Hemodialysis or peritoneal dialysis may be helpful.

▶ Special considerations
Besides those relevant to all *hydantoin derivatives,* consider the following recommendations.
- Decreased alertness and coordination are most pronounced at start of treatment. Patient may need help with walking and other activities for first few days.
- Drug should not be discontinued abruptly. Transition from mephenytoin to other anticonvulsant drug should progress over 6 weeks.

Information for the patient
- Tell patient never to discontinue drug or change dosage except as prescribed and to avoid alcohol, which decreases effectiveness of drug and increases sedative effects.
- Explain to patient that follow-up laboratory tests are essential for safe use.
- Instruct patient to report any unusual changes immediately (cutaneous reaction, sore throat, glandular swelling, fever, mucous membrane swelling).

Pediatric use
Children usually require from 100 to 400 mg/day.

Breast-feeding
Safe use in breast-feeding has not been established. Alternative feeding method is recommended during therapy with mephenytoin.

---

mephobarbital
Mebaral, Mentaban, Mephoral

- Pharmacologic classification: barbiturate
- Therapeutic classification: anticonvulsant, nonspecific CNS depressant
- Controlled substance schedule IV
- Pregnancy risk category D

How supplied
Available by prescription only
Tablets: 32 mg, 50 mg, 100 mg

Indications, route, and dosage
Generalized tonic-clonic or absence seizures
Adults: 400 to 600 mg P.O. daily or in divided doses.
Children: 6 to 12 mg/kg P.O. daily, divided q 6 to 8 hours (smaller doses are given initially and increased over 4 to 5 days as needed).

Pharmacodynamics
Anticonvulsant action: Mephobarbital increases seizure threshold in the motor cortex. It is indicated to treat generalized tonic-clonic (grand mal), absence (petit mal), myoclonic, and mixed-type seizures and, as a sedative, to relieve anxiety and tension. It is used chiefly to replace phenobarbital when less sedation is needed (no data support this rationale) and in children with hyperexcitability states or other mood disturbances.

Pharmacokinetics
- *Absorption:* About 50% of an oral dose of mephobarbital is absorbed from the GI tract; action begins within 30 to 60 minutes and lasts 10 to 16 hours.
- *Distribution:* Mephobarbital is distributed widely throughout the body.
- *Metabolism:* Mephobarbital is metabolized by the liver to phenobarbital; about 75% of a given dose is converted in 24 hours. Therapeutic blood levels of phenobarbital are 15 to 40 mcg/ml.
- *Excretion:* Mephobarbital is excreted primarily in urine; small amounts are excreted in breast milk.

Contraindications and precautions
Mephobarbital is contraindicated in patients with known hypersensitivity to barbiturates; in suspected pregnancy and pregnancy near term because of the hazard of respiratory depression and neonatal coagulation defects; in patients with severe respiratory disease or status asthmaticus because it may cause respiratory depression; or in patients with a history of porphyria or marked hepatic impairment because it may exacerbate porphyria. Drug should be used with caution in patients taking alcohol, CNS depressants, monoamine oxidase (MAO) inhibitors, narcotic analgesics, or anticoagulants.

Interactions
Alcohol and other CNS depressants, including narcotic analgesics, cause excessive depression in patients taking mephobarbital. Although concrete data are lacking, mephobarbital is assumed to be an enzyme inducer (like phenobarbital); therefore all cautions for phenobarbital drug interactions apply. Barbiturates can induce hepatic metabolism of oral anticoagulants, combination oral contraceptives, and doxycycline. Concomitant use with MAO inhibitors potentiates CNS depressant effects of barbiturates; rifampin may decrease barbiturate levels and thereby decrease efficacy.

Effects on diagnostic tests
Mephobarbital may elevate liver function test results.

Adverse reactions
- CNS: dizziness, headache, hangover, confusion, paradoxical excitation, exacerbation of existing pain, drowsiness, nightmares, hallucinations.
- CV: hypotension.
- DERM: urticaria, morbilliform rash, blisters, purpura, *erythema multiforme, Stevens-Johnson syndrome.*
- GI: nausea, vomiting, epigastric pain, constipation.
- HEMA: megaloblastic anemia, *agranulocytosis,* thrombocytopenia.
- Other: allergic reactions (facial edema).
  Note: Drug should be discontinued if signs of hypersensitivity or hepatic dysfunction occur.

Overdose and treatment
Symptoms of acute overdose include CNS and respiratory depression, areflexia, oliguria, tachycardia, hypotension, hypothermia, and coma. Shock may occur. In massive overdose, ECG may be flat, even if patient is not clinically dead.

Treat overdose symptomatically and supportively: in conscious patient with intact gag reflex, induce emesis with ipecac; follow in 30 minutes with repeated doses of activated charcoal. Forced diuresis and alkalinization of urine may hasten excretion. Hemodialysis may be necessary. Monitor vital signs and fluid and electrolyte balance.

▶ Special considerations
Besides those relevant to all *barbiturates,* consider the following recommendations.
- Monitor for signs of bleeding if patient is on stable anticoagulant regimen.
- Do not withdraw drug abruptly; after long-term use, lower dosage gradually.
- Mephobarbital impairs ability to perform tasks requiring mental alertness, such as driving a car.

Information for the patient
- Explain rationale for therapy and the potential risks and benefits.
- Teach patient how to recognize signs and symptoms of adverse reactions and what to do if they occur.
- Tell patient to avoid alcohol and other sedatives to prevent added CNS depression.
- Barbiturates carry a risk of physical and psychic dependence; warn patient not to discontinue drug abruptly or to alter dosage.
- Explain that barbiturates may render oral contraceptives ineffective; advise consideration of different birth control method.
- Advise patient to avoid hazardous tasks that require mental alertness until degree of sedative effect is determined.

Geriatric use
Reduce dosage in elderly patients; they are usually more sensitive to CNS depressants. Some clinicians avoid using mephobarbital in elderly patients because it can cause excessive CNS depression or paradoxical excitement.

Pediatric use
Mephobarbital is not recommended for children under age 6.

Breast-feeding
Some mephobarbital is excreted in breast milk. Alternative feeding method is recommended during therapy with mephobarbital.

---

meprobamate
Apo-Meprobamate*, Equanil, Meditran*, Meprospan, Miltown, Neo-Tran*, Neuramate, Neurate, Novomepro*, Sedabamate, SK-Bamate, Tranmep

- Pharmacologic classification: carbamate
- Therapeutic classification: antianxiety agent
- Controlled substance schedule IV
- Pregnancy risk category D

How supplied
Available by prescription only
Tablets: 200 mg, 400 mg, 600 mg
Capsules: 200 mg, 400 mg
Capsules (sustained-release): 200 mg, 400 mg

Indications, route, and dosage
Anxiety and tension
Adults: 1.2 to 1.6 g P.O. in three or four equally divided doses. Maximum dosage is 2.4 g daily.
Children age 6 to 12: 100 to 200 mg P.O. b.i.d. or t.i.d. Not recommended for children under age 6.

Pharmacodynamics
Anxiolytic action: While the cellular mechanism of meprobamate is unknown, the drug causes nonselective CNS depression similar to that seen with use of barbiturates. Meprobamate acts at multiple sites in the CNS, including the thalamus, hypothalamus, limbic system, and spinal cord, but not the medulla or reticular activating system.

Pharmacokinetics
- *Absorption:* After oral administration, meprobamate is well absorbed; peak serum levels occur in 1 to 3 hours. Sedation usually occurs within 1 hour.
- *Distribution:* Meprobamate is distributed throughout the body; 20% is protein-bound. The drug occurs in breast milk at two to four times the serum concentration; meprobamate crosses the placenta.
- *Metabolism:* Meprobamate is metabolized rapidly in the liver to inactive glucuronide conjugates.
- *Excretion:* The metabolites of meprobamate and 10% to 20% of a single dose as unchanged drug are excreted in urine.

Contraindications and precautions
Meprobamate is contraindicated in patients with known hypersensitivity to the drug or other carbamates and in patients with intermittent porphyria. Some formulations contain tartrazine, which is contraindicated in patients allergic to aspirin (because significant cross-reactivity has been demonstrated).

Meprobamate should be used cautiously in patients with impaired renal or hepatic function; and in patients with depression, suicidal tendencies, or a history of drug abuse or addiction.

Meprobamate may precipitate seizures or lower seizure threshold. Use cautiously, if at all, in patients with a history of seizures or an active seizure disorder.

Interactions
Meprobamate may add to or potentiate the effects of alcohol, barbiturates, antihistamines, tranquilizers, narcotics, or other CNS depressants.

Effects on diagnostic tests
Meprobamate therapy may falsely elevate urinary 17-ketosteroids, 17-ketogenic steroids (as determined by the Zimmerman reaction), and 17-hydroxycorticosteroid levels (as determined by the Glenn-Nelson technique).

Adverse reactions
- CNS: dizziness, drowsiness, ataxia, slurred speech, headache, vertigo, weakness, euphoria, paradoxical excitation.
- CV: palpitations, arrhythmias, syncope, hypotension, tachycardia.
- DERM: pruritus, urticaria, dermatitis, erythematous maculopapular rash, *exfoliative dermatitis, erythema multiforme.*
- EENT: blurred vision.
- GI: anorexia, nausea, vomiting, diarrhea, stomatitis.
- HEMA: *agranulocytosis,* thrombocytopenic purpura, *aplastic anemia,* pancytopenia (rare).
- Other: hypersensitivity (eosinophilia, hyperpyrexia, chills, *bronchospasm,* angioedema, *Stevens-Johnson syndrome, anaphylaxis).*

   Note: Drug should be discontinued if hypersensitivity, paradoxical excitation with EEG changes, severe prolonged hypotension, skin rash, sore throat, or unusual bleeding or bruising occurs.

Overdose and treatment
Clinical manifestations of overdose include drowsiness, lethargy, ataxia, coma, hypotension, shock, and respiratory depression.

   Treatment of overdose is supportive and symptomatic including maintaining adequate ventilation and a patent airway, with mechanical ventilation if needed.

   Treat hypotension with fluids and vasopressors as needed. Empty gastric contents by emesis or lavage if ingestion is recent, followed by activated charcoal and a cathartic. Treat seizures with parenteral diazepam. Peritoneal and hemodialysis may effectively remove the drug. Serum levels greater than 100 mcg/ml may be fatal.

▶ Special considerations
- Assess level of consciousness and vital signs frequently.
- Impose safety precautions, such as raised bed rails, especially for elderly patients, when initiating treatment or increasing the dose. Patient may need assistance when walking.

• Periodic evaluation of complete blood count is recommended during long-term therapy.
• The possibility of abuse and addiction exists.
• Withdraw drug gradually; otherwise, withdrawal symptoms may occur if patient has been taking the drug for a long time.

Information for the patient
• Tell patient to avoid other CNS depressants, such as antihistamines, narcotics, and tranquilizers, while taking this drug, unless prescribed. Tell patient to avoid alcoholic beverages while on drug.
• Advise patient not to increase the dose or frequency and not to abruptly discontinue or decrease the dose unless prescribed.
• Tell patient to avoid tasks that require mental alertness or physical coordination until the drug's CNS effects are known.
• Advise patient that sugarless candy or gum, or ice chips can help relieve dry mouth.
• Advise patient to report any sore throat, fever, or unusual bleeding or bruising.
• Advise patient of the potential for physical or psychological dependence with chronic use.

Geriatric use
Elderly patients may have more pronounced CNS effects. Use lowest dose possible.

Pediatric use
Safety has not been established in children under age 6.

Breast-feeding
The drug is found in breast milk at two to four times the serum concentration. Do not use in breast-feeding women.

---

mercaptopurine (6-MP)
Purinethol

• Pharmacologic classification: antimetabolite (cell cycle-phase specific, S phase)
• Therapeutic classification: antineoplastic
• Pregnancy risk category D

How supplied
Available by prescription only
Tablets (scored): 50 mg

Indications, route, and dosage
Dosage and indications may vary. Check current literature for recommended protocols.
Acute lymphoblastic leukemia (in children), acute myeloblastic leukemia, chronic myelocytic leukemia
Adults: 2.5 mg/kg or 80 to 100 mg/m² P.O. daily as a single dose, up to 5 mg/kg daily. Maintenance dosage is 1.5 to 2.5 mg/kg daily.
Children age 5 and over: 1.5 mg/kg or 75 mg/m² P.O. daily. Maintenance dosage is 1.5 to 2.5 mg/kg daily.

Pharmacodynamics
Antineoplastic action: Mercaptopurine is converted intracellularly to its active form, which exerts its cytotoxic antimetabolic effects by competing for an enzyme required for purine synthesis. This results in inhibition of DNA and RNA synthesis. Cross-resistance exists between mercaptopurine and thioguanine.

Pharmacokinetics
• *Absorption:* The absorption of mercaptopurine after an oral dose is incomplete and variable; approximately 50% of a dose is absorbed. Peak serum levels occur 2 hours after a dose.
• *Distribution:* Mercaptopurine distributes widely into total body water. The drug crosses the blood-brain barrier, but the cerebrospinal fluid concentration is too low for treatment of meningeal leukemias.
• *Metabolism:* Mercaptopurine is extensively metabolized in the liver. The drug appears to undergo extensive first-pass metabolism, contributing to its low bioavailability.
• *Excretion:* Mercaptopurine and its metabolites are excreted in urine.

Contraindications and precautions
Mercaptopurine should not be used in patients whose disease has shown resistance to therapy with this drug. There is usually complete cross-resistance between mercaptopurine and thioguanine.
  Bone marrow suppression, resulting in anemia, leukopenia, or thrombocytopenia, is usually the most consistent dose-related toxicity. Patients should understand the symptoms associated with these adverse effects and report them immediately. Weekly evaluations of hematocrit or hemoglobin, WBC count, differential count, and platelet count should be performed during therapy.
  The incidence of hepatotoxicity increases when doses exceed 2.5 mg/kg/day. Clinical jaundice usually occurs early in treatment, but there have been reports of patients taking the drug for 8 years before jaundice develops. Close monitoring of liver function tests may allow early detection of hepatotoxicity.

Interactions
When used concomitantly, allopurinol, at doses of 300 to 600 mg/day, increases the toxic effects of mercaptopurine, especially myelosuppression. This interaction is due to the inhibition of mercaptopurine metabolism by allopurinol. Reduce dosage of mercaptopurine to 25% to 30% when administering concomitantly with allopurinol.
  Concomitant use with mercaptopurine decreases the anticoagulant activity of warfarin. The mechanism of this interaction is unknown.
  Mercaptopurine should be used cautiously with other hepatotoxic drugs because of the increased potential for hepatotoxicity.

Effects on diagnostic tests
Mercaptopurine therapy may also cause falsely elevated serum glucose and uric acid values when sequential multiple analyzer is used.

Adverse reactions
• DERM: hyperpigmentation, rash.
• GI: nausea, vomiting, and anorexia in 25% of patients; painful oral ulcers.
• HEMA: *bone marrow depression* (dose-limiting), decreased RBC count, *leukopenia, thrombocytopenia,* anemia (all may persist several days after drug is stopped).
• Hepatic: jaundice, *hepatic necrosis.*

● Metabolic: hyperuricemia.
● Other: fever, headache.
   Note: Drug should be discontinued if signs of bone marrow toxicity or toxic hepatitis are evident.

Overdose and treatment
Clinical manifestations of overdose include myelosuppression, nausea, vomiting, and hepatic necrosis.

   Treatment is usually supportive and includes transfusion of blood components and antiemetics. Mercaptopurine is dialyzable.

▶ Special considerations
● Warn patient that improvement may take 2 to 4 weeks or longer.
● Monitor weekly blood counts; watch for precipitous fall.
● Store tablets at room temperature and protect from light.
● Dose modifications may be required following chemotherapy or radiation therapy, in depressed neutrophil or platelet count, and in impaired hepatic or renal function.
● Monitor intake and output. Push fluids (3 liters daily).
● Drug is sometimes called 6-mercaptopurine or 6-MP.
● Monitor hepatic function and hematologic values weekly during therapy.
● Monitor serum uric acid levels. If allopurinol is necessary, use very cautiously.
● Observe for signs of bleeding and infection.
● Hepatic dysfunction is reversible when drug is stopped. Watch for jaundice, clay-colored stools, and frothy dark urine. Drug should be stopped if hepatic tenderness occurs.
● Avoid all I.M. injections when platelet count is below 100,000/mm³.
● Mercaptopurine has been used to treat regional enteritis (Crohn's disease) and ulcerative colitis. Usual dosage is 1.5 mg/kg/day, gradually increased to 2.5 mg/kg/day if tolerated.

Information for the patient
● Tell patient to continue medication despite nausea and vomiting.
● Tell patient to call immediately if vomiting occurs shortly after taking a dose.
● Warn patient to avoid alcoholic beverages while taking this medication.
● Urge patient to ensure adequate fluid intake, to increase urine output and facilitate the excretion of uric acid.
● Patient should avoid exposure to people with infections.

Pediatric use
Adverse GI reactions are less common in children than in adults.

Breast-feeding
It is not known whether mercaptopurine distributes into breast milk. However, because of the potential for serious adverse reactions, mutagenicity, and carcinogenicity in the infant, breast-feeding is not recommended.

mesalamine
Asacol, Rowasa

● Pharmacologic classification: salicylate
● Therapeutic classification: anti-inflammatory
● Pregnancy risk category B

How supplied
Available by prescription only
Tablets, delayed release: 400 mg
Suppositories: 500 mg
Rectal suspension: 4 g/60 ml, in units of 7 disposable bottles

Indications, route, and dosage
Treatment of active mild to moderate distal ulcerative colitis, proctosigmoiditis, or proctitis
Adults: 800 mg P.O. t.i.d. for 6 weeks. Alternatively, use 1 rectal suppository b.i.d. for 3 to 6 weeks. For maximum benefit, the suppository should be retained for 1 to 3 hours or longer. The usual dosage of mesalamine suspension enema in 60-ml units is one rectal instillation (4 g) once a day, preferably at bedtime, and retained for approximately 8 hours.

Pharmacodynamics
Anti-inflammatory action: The mechanism of action of mesalamine (and sulfasalazine) is unknown, but appears to be topical rather than systemic. Mucosal production of arachidonic acid (AA) metabolites, both through cyclooxygenase pathways (for example, prostanoids) and through lipoxygenase pathways (for example, leukotrienes [LTs] and hydroxyeicosatetraenoic acids [HETEs] is increased in patients with chronic inflammatory bowel disease; possibly, mesalamine may diminish inflammation by blocking cyclooxygenase and inhibiting prostaglandin (PG) production in the colon.
   Sulfasalazine is split by bacterial action in the colon into sulfapyridine (SP) and mesalamine (5-ASA). The mesalamine component is considered therapeutically active in ulcerative colitis. The usual oral dose of sulfasalazine for active ulcerative colitis in adults is 2 to 4 g per day in divided doses; 4 g of sulfasalazine provide 1.6 g of free mesalamine to the colon.

Pharmacokinetics
● *Absorption:* Mesalamine administered rectally as a suppository or suspension enema is poorly absorbed from the colon. The extent of absorption depends on the retention time with considerable individual variation. Oral tablets are coated with an acrylic resin that delays the release of the drug until the tablet is beyond the terminal ileum. About 72% of a dose reaches the colon; 28% of a dpse is absorbed. Absorption is not affected by food.
● *Distribution:* Maximum plasma levels of mesalamine and N-acetyl 5-aminosalicylic acid are about twice as high as those seen with sulfisalazine therapy. At steady state, approximately 10% to 30% of the daily 4-g rectal dose can be recovered in cumulative 24 hour urine collections.
● *Metabolism:* Mesalamine undergoes acetylation, but whether this takes place at colonic or systemic sites is unknown. Whatever the metabolic site, most absorbed mesalamine is excreted in urine as the N-acetyl-5-ASA metabolite. Patients demonstrated plasma levels of 2 mcg/ml 10 to 12 hours after rectal administration. About two-

thirds of this was the N-acetyl metabolite. The elimination half-life of mesalamine is 0.5 to 1.5 hour; half-life of the acetylated metabolite is 5 to 10 hours. Steady-state plasma levels showed no accumulation of either free or metabolized drug during repeated daily administrations.

• *Excretion:* After rectal administration, most of the drug is excreted in the feces as parent drug and metabolite. After oral administration, most of the drug is excreted in the urine as metabolite.

Contraindications and precautions

Mesalamine is contraindicated in patients with hypersensitivity to the drug or any component of the formulation including sulfites.

Mesalamine has been associated with an acute intolerance syndrome, marked by cramping, acute abdominal pain and bloody diarrhea; sometimes fever, headache, and a rash. This reaction requires prompt withdrawal of the drug. The patient's history of sulfasalazine intolerance, if any, should be re-evaluated. Rechallenge to validate the hypersensitivity should be attempted only if clearly necessary, under close medical supervision, and with due consideration of reduced dosage. One patient previously sensitive to sulfasalazine was rechallenged with 400 mg oral mesalamine; within 8 hours she experienced headache, fever, intensive abdominal colic, and profuse diarrhea and was readmitted as an emergency. She responded poorly to steroid therapy; 2 weeks later, a pancolectomy was required.

Because preclinical studies showed the kidneys to be the major target organ for mesalamine toxicity, consider the possibility of increased absorption and renal tubular damage. Monitor urinalysis, BUN, and creatinine levels, especially in patients receiving concurrent drugs that liberate mesalamine, and in those with preexisting renal disease. When mesalamine is given rectally, absorption is poor and limited to the distal colon; overt renal toxicity has not been observed with such use.

Most patients hypersensitive to sulfasalazine are able to take mesalamine enemas without any allergic reaction. Nevertheless, exercise caution when mesalamine is initially used in patients known to be allergic to sulfasalazine. Instruct these patients to discontinue therapy if signs of rash or fever become apparent.

While using mesalamine some patients have developed pancolitis. However, extension of upper disease boundary or flare-ups occurred less often in mesalamine patients than in placebo patients.

In patients with sulfite sensitivity, mesalamine may cause allergic-type reactions (hives, itching, wheezing, and anaphylaxis). Sulfite sensitivity is seen more frequently in asthmatics or in atopic nonasthmatic persons.

Epinephrine is the preferred treatment for serious allergic or emergency situations even though epinephrine injection contains sodium or potassium metabisulfite. The alternatives to using epinephrine in a life-threatening situation may not be satisfactory. The presence of a sulfite in epinephrine injection should not deter the administration of the drug for treatment of serious allergic or other emergency situation.

Interactions
None reported.

Effects on diagnostic test
None reported.

Adverse reactions
• GI: flatulence, rectal pain, itching, hemorrhoids.
• Other: hair loss, flulike syndrome.

Overdose and treatment
No information available.

▶ Special considerations

While the effect of the drug may be evident in 3 to 21 days, the usual course of therapy is 3 to 6 weeks depending on symptoms and sigmoidoscopic findings. Clinical studies have not determined if suspension enema will modify relapse rates after the 6-week short-term treatment.

Information for the patient
• Tell the patient to swallow the tablets whole, and not to crush or chew them.
• For maximum effectiveness, the suppository should be retained as long as possible (at least 1 to 3 hours).
• Instruct patient in correct use of rectal suspension:
—Shake the bottle well to make sure the suspension is homogeneous.
—Remove the protective sheath from the applicator tip. Holding the bottle at the neck will not cause any of the medication to be discharged.
—To administer, lie on the left side (to facilitate migration into the sigmoid colon) with the lower leg extended and the upper right leg flexed forward for balance; or may use the knee-chest position.
—Gently insert the applicator tip in the rectum pointing toward the umbilicus.
—Steadily squeeze the bottle to discharge the preparation into the colon.
• Patient instructions are included with every 7 units.

Pediatric use
Safety and efficacy for use in children have not been established.

Breast-feeding
It is not known whether mesalamine or its metabolites are excreted in human milk. As a general rule, breast-feeding should be avoided during drug therapy because many drugs are excreted in human milk.

---

mesna
Mesnex

• Pharmacologic classification: thiol derivative
• Therapeutic classification: uroprotectant
• Pregnancy risk category B

How supplied
Available by prescription only
Injection: 100 mg/ml in 2-, 4-, and 10-ml ampules

Indications, route, and dosage
Prevention of ifosfamide-induced hemorrhagic cystitis
Calculate the daily dose as 60% of the ifosfamide dose. It is then administered in three equally divided bolus doses: The first dose is given at the time of ifosfamide injection. Subsequent doses are given at 4 and 8 hours following ifosfamide.

Protocols that use 1.2 g/m² ifosfamide would employ 240 mg/m² mesna at 0, 4, and 8 hours after ifosfamide.

Pharmacodynamics
Uroprotectant action: Mesna disulfide is reduced to mesna in the kidney and reacts with the urotoxic metabolites of ifosfamide to detoxify the drug and protect the urinary system.

Pharmacokinetics
● *Absorption:* Mesna is administered I.V.
● *Distribution:* Remains in the vascular compartment. Mesna doesn't distribute through tissues.
● *Metabolism:* Rapidly metabolized to mesna disulfide, its only metabolite.
● *Excretion:* In the kidneys, 33% of the dose is eliminated in the urine in 24 hours; the half-life of mesna and mesna disulfide are 0.36 and 1.17 hours respectively.

Contraindications and precautions
Mesna is contraindicated in patients with known hypersensitivity to mesna or other thiol compounds.

Note that the drug does not reduce the other toxicities associated with ifosfamide therapy, nor is it effective in all patients.

Interactions
Mesna is physically incompatible with cisplatin. Do not add mesna to cisplatin infusions.

Effects on diagnostic tests
Mesna may produce a false-positive test for urinary ketones. A red-violet color will return to violet with the addition of acetic acid.

Adverse reactions
● CNS: headache, fatigue.
● CV: hypotension.
● GI: bad taste, soft stools, diarrhea, nausea, vomiting.
● Other: allergy.
Note: Because mesna is usually administered with antineoplastic agents, it is difficult to identify adverse reactions attributable to mesna alone.

Overdose and treatment
None reported. There is no known antidote for mesna.

▶ Special considerations
● Discard any unused mesna from open ampules. It will form an inactive oxidation product (dimesna) upon exposure to oxygen.
● Dilute the appropriate dose in 5% dextrose injection, 0.9% sodium chloride injection, or lactated Ringer's injection to a concentration of 20 mg/ml. Once diluted, the solution is stable for 24 hours at room temperature.

Information for the patient
Instruct the patient to report hematuria immediately.

Pediatric use
Safety in children has not been established.

Breast-feeding
It is not known whether mesna is excreted in breast milk.

mesoridazine besylate
Serentil

● Pharmacologic classification: phenothiazine (piperidine derivative)
● Therapeutic classification: antipsychotic
● Pregnancy risk category C

How supplied
Available by prescription only
Tablets: 10 mg, 25 mg, 50 mg, 100 mg
Oral concentrate: 25 mg/ml (0.6% alcohol)
Injection: 25 mg/ml

Indications, route, and dosage
Psychoneurotic manifestations (anxiety)
Adults and children over age 12: 10 mg P.O. t.i.d. up to a maximum of 150 mg/day.
Schizophrenia
Adults and children over age 12: Initially, 50 mg P.O. t.i.d. to a maximum of 400 mg/day; or 25 mg I.M. repeated in 30 to 60 minutes, p.r.n., not to exceed 200 mg I.M. daily.
Alcoholism
Adults and children over age 12: 25 mg P.O. b.i.d., up to a maximum of 200 mg/day.
Behavioral problems associated with chronic brain syndrome
Adults and children over age 12: 25 mg P.O. t.i.d., up to a maximum of 300 mg/day. I.M. dosage form is irritating.

Pharmacodynamics
Antipsychotic action: Mesoridazine, a metabolite of thioridazine, is thought to exert its antipsychotic effects by postsynaptic blockade of CNS dopamine receptors, thereby inhibiting dopamine-mediated effects.

Mesoridazine has many other central and peripheral effects; it produces both alpha and ganglionic blockade and counteracts histamine- and serotonin-mediated activity. Its most prominent adverse reactions are antimuscarinic and sedative; it causes fewer extrapyramidal effects than other antipsychotics.

Pharmacokinetics
● *Absorption:* Rate and extent of absorption vary with route of administration. Oral tablet absorption is erratic and variable, with onset ranging from ½ to 1 hour. Oral liquids are much more predictable; I.M. dosage form is absorbed rapidly.
● *Distribution:* Mesoridazine is distributed widely into the body, including breast milk. Peak effects occur at 2 to 4 hours; steady-state serum level is achieved within 4 to 7 days. Drug is 91% to 99% protein-bound.
● *Metabolism:* Mesoridazine is metabolized extensively by the liver; no active metabolites are formed. Duration of action is 4 to 6 hours.
● *Excretion:* Most of drug is excreted as metabolites in urine; some drug is excreted in feces via the biliary tract.

Contraindications and precautions
Mesoridazine is contraindicated in patients with known hypersensitivity to phenothiazines and related compounds, including allergic reactions involving hepatic function, because it is potentially hepatotoxic; in patients with blood dyscrasias and bone marrow depression because it may induce agranulocytosis; in patients with disorders accompanied by coma, brain damage, or CNS

depression because of additive CNS depression; in patients with circulatory collapse or cerebrovascular disease because of its hypotensive effects; and for use with adrenergic-blocking agents or spinal or epidural anesthetics because of its alpha-blocking activity.

Mesoridazine should be used cautiously in patients with cardiac disease (arrhythmias, congestive heart failure, angina pectoris, valvular disease, or heart block), encephalitis, Reye's syndrome, head injury, respiratory disease, epilepsy and other seizure disorders, glaucoma, prostatic hypertrophy, urinary retention, hepatic or renal dysfunction, Parkinson's disease, pheochromocytoma, and hypocalcemia.

Oral dosage forms may contain tartrazine; dye may cause allergic reaction in aspirin-allergic patients.

Interactions

Concomitant use of mesoridazine with sympathomimetics, including epinephrine, phenylephrine, phenylpropanolamine, and ephedrine (often found in nasal sprays), or appetite suppressants may decrease their stimulatory and pressor effects. Phenothiazines can cause epinephrine reversal and produce hypotension when epinephrine is used as a pressor agent.

Mesoridazine may inhibit blood pressure response to centrally acting antihypertensive drugs, such as guanethidine, guanabenz, guanadrel, clonidine, methyldopa, and reserpine. Additive effects are likely after concomitant use of mesoridazine with CNS depressants, including alcohol, analgesics, barbiturates, narcotics, tranquilizers, and general, spinal, or epidural anesthetics, or parenteral magnesium sulfate (oversedation, respiratory depression, and hypotension); antiarrhythmic agents, quinidine, disopyramide, or procainamide (increased incidence of cardiac arrhythmias and conduction defects); atropine and other anticholinergic drugs, including antidepressants, monoamine oxidase inhibitors, phenothiazines, antihistamines, meperidine, and antiparkinsonian agents (oversedation, paralytic ileus, visual changes, and severe constipation); nitrates (hypotension); and metrizamide (increased risk of convulsions).

Beta-blocking agents may inhibit mesoridazine metabolism, increasing plasma levels and toxicity. Concomitant use with propylthiouracil increases risk of agranulocytosis; concomitant use with lithium may result in severe neurologic toxicity with an encephalitis-like syndrome, and a decreased therapeutic response to mesoridazine.

Pharmacokinetic alterations and subsequent decreased therapeutic response to mesoridazine may follow concomitant use with phenobarbital (enhanced renal excretion); aluminum- and magnesium-containing antacids and antidiarrheals (decreased absorption); caffeine; or heavy smoking (increased metabolism).

Mesoridazine may antagonize therapeutic effect of bromocriptine on prolactin secretion; it also may decrease the vasoconstricting effects of high-dose dopamine, and may decrease effectiveness and increase toxicity of levodopa (by dopamine blockade). Mesoridazine may inhibit metabolism and increase toxicity of phenytoin.

Effects on diagnostic tests

Mesoridazine causes false-positive test results for urinary porphyrins, urobilinogen, amylase, and 5-hydroxyindoleacetic acid, because of darkening of urine by metabolites; it also causes false-positive urine pregnancy test results using human chorionic gonadotropin.

Mesoridazine elevates tests for liver function and protein-bound iodine and causes quinidine-like effects on the ECG.

Adverse reactions

● CNS: extrapyramidal symptoms – dystonia, akathisia, torticollis, tardive dyskinesia (usually dose-related with long-term therapy, but it can develop rapidly), sedation (high incidence), pseudoparkinsonism, drowsiness (frequent), *neuroleptic malignant syndrome* (if untreated, *fatal respiratory failure* in over 10% of patients), dizziness, headache, insomnia, exacerbation of psychotic symptoms.

● CV: *asystole*, orthostatic hypotension (high incidence), tachycardia, dizziness/fainting, *arrhythmias,* ECG changes, increased anginal pain after I.M. injection.

● EENT: blurred vision, tinnitus, mydriasis, increased intraocular pressure, ocular changes (retinal pigmentary change with long-term use).

● GI: dry mouth, constipation, nausea, vomiting, anorexia, diarrhea.

● GU: urinary retention, gynecomastia, hypermenorrhea, inhibited ejaculation.

● HEMA: transient leukopenia, *agranulocytosis*, thrombocytopenia, anemia (within 30 to 90 days).

● Local: contact dermatitis from concentrate or injectable form, muscle necrosis from I.M. injection.

● Other: hyperprolactinemia, photosensitivity, increased appetite/weight gain, hypersensitivity (rash, urticaria, drug fever, edema, cholestatic jaundice [in 2% to 4% of patients within first 30 days]), decreased libido.

After abrupt withdrawal of long-term therapy, gastritis, nausea, vomiting, dizziness, tremors, feeling of heat or cold, sweating, tachycardia, headache, or insomnia may occur.

Note: Drug should be discontinued if hypersensitivity, jaundice, agranulocytosis, neuroleptic malignant syndrome (marked hyperthermia, extrapyramidal effects, autonomic dysfunction), or severe extrapyramidal symptoms occur even after dosage is lowered. Drug should be discontinued 48 hours before and 24 hours after myelography using metrizamide because of risk of convulsions. When feasible, drug should be withdrawn slowly and gradually; many drug effects persist after withdrawal.

Overdose and treatment

CNS depression is characterized by deep, unarousable sleep and possible coma, hypotension or hypertension, extrapyramidal symptoms, abnormal involuntary muscle movements, agitation, seizures, arrhythmias, ECG changes, hypothermia or hyperthermia, and autonomic nervous system dysfunction.

Treatment is symptomatic and supportive, including maintaining vital signs, airway, stable body temperature, and fluid/electrolyte balance.

Do not induce vomiting: drug inhibits cough reflex, and aspiration may occur. Use gastric lavage, then activated charcoal and saline cathartics; dialysis does not help. Regulate body temperature as needed. Treat hypotension with I.V. fluids: *do not give epinephrine*. Treat seizures with parenteral diazepam or barbiturates; arrhythmias, with parenteral phenytoin (1 mg/kg with rate titrated to blood pressure); extrapyramidal reactions, with benztropine or parenteral diphenhydramine at 2 mg/kg/minute.

▶ Special considerations

Recommendations for administration of mesoridazine, for care and teaching of the patient during therapy, and for use in elderly and breast-feeding patients are the same as those for all *phenothiazines*.

Pediatric use

Drug is not recommended in children under age 12.

---

*Canada only　　　†Unlabeled clinical use　　　Italicized adverse reactions are life-threatening.

metaprotereol sulfate
Alupent, Metaprel

- Pharmacologic classification: adrenergic
- Therapeutic classification: bronchodilator
- Pregnancy risk category C

How supplied
Available by prescription only
Tablets: 10 mg, 20 mg
Solution: 10 mg/5 ml
Aerosol inhaler: 0.65 mg/metered spray
Nebulizer inhaler: 0.4%, 0.6%, 5% solution

Indications, route, and dosage
Bronchial asthma and reversible broncho-spasm

Adults and children over age 9 or weighing more than 60 lb (27.3 kg): 20 mg P.O. t.i.d. or q.i.d.
Children age 6 to 9 or weighing less than 60 lb: 10 mg P.O. t.i.d. or q.i.d.
Adults and children age 12 and older: Administered by metered aerosol, 2 or 3 inhalations, with at least 2 minutes between inhalations; no more than 12 inhalations in 24 hours. Administered by hand-bulb nebulizer, 10 inhalations of an undiluted 5% solution or alternatively, administered by IPPB, 0.3 ml (range 0.2 to 0.3 ml) of a 5% diluted solution or 2.5 ml of a 0.6% solution. These doses need not be repeated more often than every 4 hours for an acute attack. For chronic therapy, these doses may be administered t.i.d. or q.i.d.

Pharmacodynamics
Bronchodilator action: Metaproterenol relaxes bronchial smooth muscle and peripheral vasculature by stimulating beta$_2$-adrenergic receptors, thus decreasing airway resistance via bronchodilation. It has lesser effect on beta$_1$ receptors and has little or no effect on alpha-adrenergic receptors. In high doses, it may cause CNS and cardiac stimulation, resulting in tachycardia, hypertension, or tremors.

Pharmacokinetics
- *Absorption:* Metaproterenol is well-absorbed from the GI tract. Onset of action occurs within 1 minute after oral inhalation, 5 to 30 minutes after nebulization, and 15 to 30 minutes after oral administration, with peak effects seen in about 1 hour. Duration of action after oral inhalation is 1 to 4 hours after single dose; 1 to 2½ hours after multiple doses; after nebulization, 2 to 6 hours after single dose, 4 to 6 hours after repeated doses; after oral administration, 1 to 4 hours.
- *Distribution:* Metaproterenol is widely distributed throughout the body.
- *Metabolism:* Metaproterenol is extensively metabolized on first pass through the liver.
- *Excretion:* Metaproterenol is excreted in urine, mainly as glucuronic acid conjugates.

Contraindications and precautions
Metaproterenol is contraindicated in patients with pre-existing cardiac arrhythmias associated with tachycardia, because of the drug's cardiac stimulant effects, and in those with hypersensitivity to the drug or ingredients in formulation.

Administer with extreme caution to patients with hypertension, coronary artery disease, congestive heart failure, hyperthyroidism, or diabetes, because the drug may worsen these conditions, or to patients who are sensitive to the effects of other sympathomimetics.

Administer cautiously to patients with sulfite sensitivity, because some preparations contain sulfite preservatives.

Interactions
Concomitant use with other sympathomimetics may produce additive effects and toxicity. Use of metaproterenol with general anesthetics (especially chloroform, cyclopropane, halothane, and trichlorethylene), theophylline derivatives, digitalis glycosides, levodopa, other sympathomimetics, or thyroid hormones may increase the potential for cardiac effects, including severe ventricular tachycardia, cardiac arrhythmias, and coronary insufficiency.

Beta-adrenergic blockers, especially propranolol, antagonize metaproterenol's bronchodilating effects.

Increased CNS stimulation may result from concomitant use with xanthines, other sympathomimetics, and other CNS stimulating drugs.

Effects on diagnostic tests
Metaproterenol may reduce the sensitivity of spirometry in the diagnosis of asthma.

Adverse reactions
- CNS: weakness, drowsiness, tremor, nervousness, headache, dizziness.
- CV: tachycardia, palpitations, hypertension; *with excessive use, cardiac arrest.*
- GI: nausea, vomiting, bad taste in mouth.
- Other: *paradoxical bronchoconstriction with excessive use,* muscle cramps in legs, hypersensitivity reactions.

Note: Drug should be discontinued if bronchoconstriction or hypersensitivity to drug or sulfite preservatives occurs.

Overdose and treatment
Clinical manifestations of overdose include exaggeration of common adverse reactions, particularly nausea and vomiting, cardiac arrhythmias, angina, hypertension, and seizures.

Treatment includes supportive and symptomatic measures. Monitor vital signs closely. Support cardiovascular status. Use cardioselective beta$_1$-adrenergic blockers (acebutolol, atenolol, metoprolol) to treat symptoms with extreme caution; they may induce severe bronchospasm or asthmatic attack.

▶ Special considerations
Besides those relevant to all *adrenergics,* consider the following recommendations.
- Adverse reactions are dose-related, characteristic of sympathomimetics, and may persist a long time because of the long duration of action of metaproterenol.
- Excessive or prolonged use may lead to decreased effectiveness.
- Avoid simultaneous administration of adrenocorticoid inhalation aerosol. Allow at least 5 minutes to lapse between using the two aerosols.
- Monitor patient for signs and symptoms of toxic effects (nausea and vomiting, tremors, and cardiac dysrhythmias).
- Aerosol treatments may be used with oral tablet dosing.

Information for the patient

• Instruct patient to use only as directed and to take no more than two inhalations at one time with 1- to 2-minute intervals between. Remind patient to save applicator; refills may be available.

• Tell patient to take missed dose if remembered within 1 hour. If beyond 1 hour, patient should skip dose and resume regular schedule. The patient should *not* double dose.

• Tell patient to store drug away from heat and light, and safely out of children's reach.

• If no relief is obtained or condition worsens, patient should call immediately.

• Warn patient to avoid simultaneous use of adrenocorticoid aerosol, and to allow at least 5 minutes to lapse between using the two aerosols.

• Tell the patient that he may experience bad taste in mouth after using oral inhaler.

• Instruct patient to shake container, exhale through nose as completely as possible, then administer aerosol while inhaling deeply through mouth, and hold breath for 10 seconds before exhaling slowly. Patient should wait 1 to 2 minutes before repeating inhalations.

• Tell patient that drug may have shorter duration of action after prolonged use. Advise patient to report failure to respond to usual dose.

• Warn patient not to increase dose or frequency unless prescribed; serious adverse reactions are possible.

Geriatric use

Elderly patients may be more sensitive to the therapeutic and adverse effects of the drug.

Pediatric use

Safety and efficacy of oral inhalation in children under age 12 not established. Safety and efficacy of oral preparations in children under age 6 not established.

---

metaraminol bitartrate
Aramine

• Pharmacologic classification: adrenergic
• Therapeutic classification: vasopressor
• Pregnancy risk category C

How supplied

Available by prescription only
Injection: 10 mg/ml parenteral

Indications, route, and dosage
Hypotension

Adults: 2 to 10 mg I.M. or S.C.
Children: 0.1 mg/kg or 3 mg/m² S.C. or I.M.

Hypotension in severe shock

Adults: 0.5 to 5 mg direct I.V. followed by I.V. infusion. If necessary, mix 15 to 100 mg in 500 ml normal saline solution or dextrose 5% in water; titrate infusion based on blood pressure response.
Children: 0.01 mg/kg or 0.03 mg/m² direct I.V. followed by I.V. infusion, if necessary, of 0.4 mg/kg or 12 mg/m² diluted and titrated to maintain desired blood pressure.

Pharmacodynamics

Vasopressor action: Metaraminol acts predominantly by direct stimulation of alpha-adrenergic receptors, which constrict both capacitance and resistance blood vessels, resulting in increased total peripheral resistance; increased systolic and diastolic blood pressure; decreased blood flow to vital organs, skin, and skeletal muscle; and constriction of renal blood vessels, which reduces renal blood flow. It also has a direct stimulating effect on beta₁ receptors of the heart, producing a positive inotropic response, and an indirect effect, releasing norepinephrine from its storage sites, which, with repeated use, may result in tachyphylaxis. Metaraminol also acts as a weak or false neurotransmitter by replacing norepinephrine in sympathetic nerve endings. Its main effects are vasoconstriction and cardiac stimulation. It does not usually cause CNS stimulation but may cause contraction of pregnant uterus and uterine blood vessels because of its alpha-adrenergic effects.

Pharmacokinetics

• *Absorption:* Onset of action after I.M. injection occurs within 10 minutes; after I.V. injection, within 1 to 2 minutes; after S.C. injection, 5 to 20 minutes. Pressor effects may persist 20 to 90 minutes, depending on route of administration and patient variability.

• *Distribution:* Not completely known.

• *Metabolism:* In vitro tests suggest that metaraminol is not metabolized. Effects appear to be terminated by uptake of drug into tissues and by urinary excretion.

• *Excretion:* Metaraminol is excreted in urine; may be accelerated by acidifying urine.

Contraindications and precautions

Metaraminol is contraindicated in patients with peripheral or mesenteric vascular thrombosis (may increase ischemia and extend area of infarction), in patients with profound hypoxia or hypercapnea, and in those undergoing general anesthesia with cyclopropane and other inhalation hydrocarbon anesthetics (risk of inducing cardiac arrhythmias).

Administer cautiously to hypertensive or hyperthyroid patients (increased adverse reaction) and to those with diabetes, heart disease, cirrhosis, Buerger's disease, peripheral vascular disease, acidosis, or history of malaria (relapse may occur). Also administer cautiously in patients with known sensitivity to sulfites because commercially available formulations contain sulfites.

Interactions

Concomitant use may prolong and intensify cardiac stimulant and vasopressor effects of monoamine oxidase (MAO) inhibitors. Do not administer metaraminol until 14 days after MAO inhibitors have been discontinued.

Increased cardiac effects may result when metaraminol is used with general anesthetics, maprotiline, digitalis glycosides, levodopa, other sympathomimetics, or thyroid hormones.

When metaraminol is used with the alpha-adrenergic blocking agents, pressor effects may be decreased (but not completely blocked). When metaraminol is used with doxapram, trimethaphan, mazindol, methylphenidate, or ergot alkaloids, pressor effects may be increased.

Concomitant use of beta blockers with metaraminol may result in mutual inhibition of therapeutic effects, with increased potential for hypertension, and excessive bradycardia with possible heart block.

Metaraminol may also decrease the hypotensive effects of guanadrel, guanethidine, rauwolfia alkaloids, and diuretics used as antihypertensives. Concomitant

---

use with atropine blocks the reflex bradycardia caused by metaraminol and enhances its pressor response.

Effects on diagnostic tests
None reported.

Adverse reactions
● CNS: apprehension, anxiety, tremor, restlessness, weakness, faintness, dizziness, headache, *convulsions* (excessive use).
● CV: precordial pain, peripheral and visceral vasoconstriction, palpitations, arrhythmias, sinus or *ventricular tachycardia,* bradycardia, hypotension, hypertension.
● GI: nausea, vomiting.
● GU: decreased urine output.
● Other: hyperglycemia, pallor, sweating, *respiratory distress,* fever.
   Note: Drug should be discontinued if patient is hypersensitive to drugs or sulfites, or if infiltration or thrombosis occurs during I.V. administration.

Overdose and treatment
Clinical manifestations of overdose include severe hypertension, arrhythmias, seizures, cerebral hemorrhage, acute pulmonary edema, and cardiac arrest.
   Treatment requires discontinuation of drug followed by supportive and symptomatic measures. Monitor vital signs closely. Use atropine for reflex bradycardia and propranolol for arrhythmias.

▶ Special considerations
Besides those relevant to all *adrenergics,* consider the following recommendations.
● Monitor blood pressure and heart rate and rhythm during and after metaraminol administration until patient is stable.
● Correct blood volume depletion before administration. Metaraminol is not a substitute for blood, plasma, fluids, or electrolyte replacement.
● Drug must be diluted before use. Preferred solutions for dilution are normal saline solution or dextrose 5% injection. Select injection site carefully. I.V. route is preferred, using large veins. Avoid extravasation. Monitor infusion rate; use of infusion controlling device preferred. Withdraw drug gradually; recurrent hypotension may follow abrupt withdrawal.
● Allow at least 10 minutes to elapse before administering additional doses because maximum effect is not immediately apparent.
● To treat extravasation, infiltrate site promptly with 10 to 15 ml normal saline solution containing 5 to 10 mg phentolamine, using fine needle.
● Cumulative effect possible after prolonged use. Excessive vasopressor response may persist after drug is withdrawn.
● Keep emergency drugs on hand to reverse effect of metaraminol: atropine for reflex bradycardia, phentolamine for extravasation, and propranolol for dysrhythmias.
● Monitor diabetic patients closely. Insulin adjustments may be needed.
● Closely monitor fluid and electrolyte status.
● Do not mix in bag or syringe with other medications.

Information for the patient
● Ask patient about allergy to sulfites before administering.

● Inform patient that he'll need frequent assessment of vital signs.
● Tell patient to report any adverse reactions.

Geriatric use
Elderly patients may be more sensitive to the effects of the drug.

Pediatric use
Use with caution. Solutions for I.V. infusion can be prepared to contain 1 mg of metaraminol per 25 ml of diluent.

---

metaxalone
Skelaxin

● Pharmacologic classification: oxazolidinone derivative
● Therapeutic classification: skeletal muscle relaxant
● Pregnancy risk category C

How supplied
Available by prescription only
Tablets (scored): 400 mg

Indications, route, and dosage
Skeletal muscle relaxant; adjunct for relief of acute musculoskeletal conditions
Adults and children over age 12: 800 mg P.O. t.i.d. or q.i.d.

Pharmacodynamics
Skeletal muscle relaxant action: Metaxalone is a CNS depressant, which produces skeletal muscle relaxant effects through an unknown mechanism. Its effects may be related to its sedative actions.

Pharmacokinetics
● *Absorption:* Onset of action occurs within 1 hour and persists for 4 to 6 hours.
● *Distribution:* Peak serum concentrations occur in 2 hours.
● *Metabolism:* Metaxalone is metabolized in the liver.
● *Excretion:* Metaxalone is excreted in urine as metabolites; plasma half-life is 2 to 3 hours.

Contraindications and precautions
Metaxalone is contraindicated in patients with impaired hepatic or renal function because of the potential for accumulation of drug after repeated doses, in patients with known hypersensitivity to the drug or history of drug-induced hemolytic anemias, or in patients with other anemias, because the drug may induce hemolytic anemia.
   Administer cautiously to patients with history of hepatic disease.

Interactions
Concomitant use of metaxalone with other CNS depressants, including alcohol, narcotics, anxiolytics, antipsychotics, or tricyclic antidepressants, may produce additive CNS depression.

Effects on diagnostic tests

Metaxalone therapy alters cupric sulfate urine glucose test results (false-positive results with Benedict's solution, Clinitest, and Fehling's solution), but does not interfere with glucose tests using glucose oxidase (Clinistix, Diastix, Tes-Tape). Patients receiving metaxalone may develop abnormalities in liver function tests.

Adverse reactions

● CNS: drowsiness, dizziness, headache, nervousness, confusion, irritability.
● GI: nausea, anorexia, dry mouth, vomiting, GI upset.
● Other: urinary retention, exacerbation of tonic-clonic seizures, hypersensitivity reactions, rash, pruritus, leukopenia, hemolytic anemias, jaundice.
   Note: Drug should be discontinued if patient develops hypersensitivity, rash, elevated liver enzyme levels, or signs of hepatotoxicity.

Overdose and treatment

Clinical manifestations of overdose include exaggerated adverse reactions, particularly nausea and vomiting, seizures, and extreme drowsiness. Treat with gastric lavage and other supportive measures as needed. Monitor vital signs closely.

▶ Special considerations

Liver function tests should be performed periodically throughout therapy.

Information for the patient

● Tell patient drug may cause drowsiness. Patient should avoid hazardous activities that require alertness until degree of CNS depression can be determined.
● Advise patient to avoid alcoholic beverages and to use care with cough and cold preparations because some may contain alcohol.
● Patient may take missed dose if remembered within 1 hour. If beyond 1 hour, patient should skip dose and return to regular schedule. Warn patient not to double dose.

Geriatric use

Lower doses are indicated, because elderly patients are more sensitive to drug's effects.

Pediatric use

Safety has not been established in children under age 12.

Breast-feeding

It is unknown whether drug is excreted in breast milk. Breast-feeding should be avoided during treatment with metaxalone.

methadone hydrochloride

Dolophine, Methadose, Physeptone*

● Pharmacologic classification: opioid
● Therapeutic classification: analgesic, narcotic detoxification adjunct
● Controlled substance schedule II
● Pregnancy risk category C

How supplied

Available by prescription only
Tablets: 5 mg, 10 mg, 40 mg for oral solution (for narcotic abstinence syndrome)
Oral solution: 5 mg/5 ml, 10 mg/5 ml, 10 mg/ml
Injection: 10 mg/ml

Indications, route, and dosage

Severe pain
Adults: 2.5 to 10 mg P.O., I.M., or S.C. q 4 to 12 hours, p.r.n. or around the clock.
Narcotic abstinence syndrome
Adults: 15 to 40 mg P.O. daily (highly individualized). Maintenance dosage: 20 to 120 mg P.O. daily. Adjust dose as needed. Daily doses greater than 120 mg require special state and federal approval.

Pharmacodynamics

Analgesic action: Methadone is an opiate agonist that has analgesic activity via an affinity for the opiate receptors similar to that of morphine. It is recommended for severe, chronic pain and is also used in detoxification and maintenance of patients with opiate abstinence syndrome.

Pharmacokinetics

● *Absorption:* Methadone is well absorbed from the GI tract. Oral administration delays onset and prolongs duration of action as compared to parenteral administration. Onset of action occurs within 30 to 60 minutes; peak effect is seen at ½ to 1 hour.
● *Distribution:* Methadone is highly bound to tissue protein, which may explain its cumulative effects and slow elimination.
● *Metabolism:* Methadone is metabolized primarily in the liver by N-demethylation.
● *Excretion:* Duration of action is 4 to 6 hours. Urinary excretion, the major route, is dose-dependent. Methadone metabolities are also excreted in the feces via the bile.

Contraindications and precautions

Methadone is contraindicated in patients with known hypersensitivity to the drug.
   Administer methadone with extreme caution to patients with supraventricular arrhythmias; avoid, or administer drug with extreme caution to patients with head injury or increased intracranial pressure, because drug obscures neurologic parameters; and during pregnancy and labor, because drug readily crosses placenta (premature infants are especially sensitive to respiratory and CNS depressant effects).
   Administer methadone cautiously to patients with renal or hepatic dysfunction, because drug accumulation or prolonged duration of action may occur; to patients with pulmonary disease (asthma, chronic obstructive pulmonary disease), because drug depresses

respiration and suppresses cough reflex; to patients undergoing biliary tract surgery, because drug may cause biliary spasm; to patients with convulsive disorders, because drug may precipitate seizures; to elderly or debilitated patients, who are more sensitive to both therapeutic and adverse drug effects; and to patients prone to physical or psychic addiction, because of the high risk of addiction to this drug.

Interactions
Concomitant use with other CNS depressants (narcotic analgesics, general anesthetics, antihistamines, phenothiazines, barbiturates, benzodiazepines, sedative-hypnotics, antidepressants, alcohol, and muscle relaxants) potentiates drug's respiratory and CNS depression, sedation, and hypotensive effects. Concomitant use with cimetidine may also increase respiratory and CNS depression, causing confusion, disorientation, apnea, or seizures. Such use usually requires reduced dosage of methadone.

Drug accumulation and enhanced effects may result from concomitant use with other drugs that are extensively metabolized in the liver (rifampin, phenytoin, and digitoxin); combined use with anticholinergics may cause paralytic ileus.

Patients who become physically dependent on this drug may experience acute withdrawal syndrome if given a narcotic antagonist. Use with caution, and monitor closely.

Effects on diagnostic tests
Methadone increases plasma amylase levels.

Adverse reactions
● CNS: sedation, light-headedness, dizziness, clouded sensorium, euphoria, insomnia, agitation, confusion, dysphoria, psychic dependence, choreic movements.
● CV: bradycardia, palpitations, faintness, syncope, edema.
● DERM: sweating, flushing, rash, pruritus, pain at injection site.
● GI: dry mouth, anorexia, biliary spasms (colic), nausea, vomiting, constipation
● GU: urinary retention or hesitancy, decreased libido.
● Other: *respiratory depression*, physical dependence.

Overdose and treatment
The most common signs and symptoms of methadone overdose are CNS depression, respiratory depression, and miosis (pinpoint pupils). Others include hypotension, bradycardia, hypothermia, shock, apnea, cardiopulmonary arrest, circulatory collapse, pulmonary edema, and convulsions. Toxicity may result from accumulation of the drug over several weeks.

To treat acute overdose, first establish adequate respiratory exchange via a patent airway and ventilation as needed; administer a narcotic antagonist (naloxone) to reverse respiratory depression. (Because the duration of action of methadone is longer than that of naloxone, repeated naloxone dosing is necessary.) The antagonist naloxone should not be given unless the patient has clinically significant respiratory or cardiovascular depression. Monitor vital signs closely.

If the patient presents within 2 hours of ingestion of an oral overdose, empty the stomach immediately by inducing emesis (ipecac syrup) or using gastric lavage. Use caution to avoid any risk of aspiration. Administer activated charcoal via nasogastric tube for further removal of the drug in an oral overdose.

Provide symptomatic and supportive treatment (continued respiratory support, correction of fluid or electrolyte imbalance). Monitor laboratory parameters, vital signs, and neurologic status closely.

▶ Special considerations
Besides those relevant to all *opioids*, consider the following recommendations.
● Ascertain if the patient is in a methadone maintenance program for management of narcotic addiction and, if so, at what dosage, and continue that program appropriately.
● Dispersable tablets may be dissolved in 120 ml (4 oz) of water or fruit juice; oral concentrate must be diluted to at least 90 ml with water before administration.
● Oral liquid form (not tablets) is legally required and is the only form available in drug maintenance programs.
● Regimented scheduling (around the clock) is beneficial in severe, chronic pain. When used for severe, chronic pain, tolerance may develop with long-term use, requiring a higher dose to achieve the same degree of analgesia.
● Patient treated for narcotic abstinence syndrome will usually require an additional analgesic if pain control is necessary.
● If used with general anesthetics, tranquilizers, sedatives, hypnotics, alcohol, tricyclic antidepressants, or monoamine oxidase inhibitors, respiratory depression, hypotension, profound sedation, or coma may occur. Use together with extreme caution. Monitor patient's response.

Information for the patient
If appropriate, tell patient that constipation is often severe during maintenance with methadone. Instruct him to take a stool softener or other laxative.

Geriatric use
Lower doses are usually indicated for elderly patients, because they may be more sensitive to the therapeutic and adverse effects of the drug.

Pediatric use
Methadone is not recommended for use in children. Safe use as maintenance drug in adolescent addicts not established.

Breast-feeding
Methadone is excreted in breast milk; it may cause physical dependence in breast-feeding infants of women on methadone maintenance therapy.

methamphetamine hydrochloride
Desoxyn, Methampex

- Pharmacologic classification: amphetamine
- Therapeutic classification: CNS stimulant, short-term adjunctive anorexigenic agent, sympathomimetic amine
- Controlled substance schedule II
- Pregnancy risk category C

How supplied
Available by prescription only
Tablets: 5 mg
Tablets (long-acting): 5 mg, 10 mg, 15 mg

Indications, route, and dosage
Attention deficit disorder with hyperactivity
Children age 6 and older: 2.5 to 5 mg P.O. once daily or b.i.d., with 5-mg increments weekly, p.r.n. Usual effective dosage is 20 to 25 mg daily.
Short-term adjunct in exogenous obesity
Adults: 2.5 to 5 mg P.O. once daily to t.i.d. 30 minutes before meals; or one long-acting 5- to 15-mg tablet daily before breakfast.

Pharmacodynamics
- *CNS stimulant action:* Amphetamines are sympathomimetic amines with CNS stimulant activity; in hyperactive children, they have a paradoxical calming effect.
- *Anorexigenic action:* Anorexigenic effects are thought to occur in the hypothalamus, where decreased smell and taste acuity decreases appetite; they may involve other systemic and metabolic effects. They may be tried for short-term control of refractory obesity, with caloric restriction and behavior modification.

The cerebral cortex and reticular activating system appear to be the primary sites of activity; amphetamines release nerve terminal stores of norepinephrine, promoting nerve impulse transmission. At high dosages, effects are mediated by dopamine.

Amphetamines are used to treat narcolepsy and as adjuncts to psychosocial measures in attention deficit disorder in children. The precise mechanisms of action in these conditions are unknown.

Pharmacokinetics
- *Absorption:* Methamphetamine hydrochloride is rapidly absorbed from the GI tract after oral administration; effects last 6 to 12 hours.
- *Distribution:* Widely distributed throughout the body. Crosses the placenta and enters breast milk.
- *Metabolism:* Metabolized in the liver to at least seven metabolites.
- *Excretion:* Excreted in urine.

Contraindications and precautions
Methamphetamine is contraindicated in patients with hypersensitivity or idiosyncratic reaction to sympathomimetic amines; in patients with hyperthyroidism, glaucoma, angina pectoris, or any degree of hypertension or other severe cardiovascular disease because it may cause hazardous arrhythmias and changes in blood pressure; and in patients with a history of substance abuse. They also are contraindicated for concomitant

use with monoamine oxidase (MAO) inhibitors or within 14 days of discontinuing such therapy.

Methamphetamine should be used with caution in patients with diabetes mellitus; in patients who are elderly, debilitated, asthenic, or psychopathic; in patients who have a history of suicidal or homicidal tendencies, and in children with Gilles de la Tourette's syndrome. Amphetamine-induced CNS stimulation superimposed on CNS depression can cause seizures. Some formulations (Desoxyn Gradumet, 15 mg) may contain tartrazine, which may precipitate an allergic reaction in sensitive individuals.

Interactions
Concomitant use with MAO inhibitors (or drugs with MAO-inhibiting activity, such as furazolidone), or within 14 days of such therapy, may cause hypertensive crisis; use with antihypertensives may antagonize their effects.

Concomitant use with antacids, sodium bicarbonate, or acetazolamide enhances reabsorption of methamphetamine and prolongs duration of action, whereas use with ascorbic acid enhances methamphetamine excretion and shortens duration of action. Use with phenothiazines or haloperidol decreases methamphetamine effects; barbiturates antagonize methamphetamine by CNS depression, whereas caffeine or other CNS stimulants produce additive effects.

Patients using methamphetamine have an increased risk of arrhythmias during general anesthesia.

Methamphetamine may alter insulin requirements.

Effects on diagnostic tests
Methamphetamine may elevate plasma corticosteroid levels and may interfere with urinary steroid determinations.

Adverse reactions
- CNS: nervousness, insomnia (common), irritability, talkativeness, dizziness, headache, hyperexcitability, tremors, psychosis.
- CV: hypertension or hypotension, tachycardia, palpitations, cardiac arrhythmias.
- DERM: urticaria.
- EENT: blurred vision, mydriasis.
- GI: nausea, vomiting, abdominal cramps, diarrhea or constipation, dry mouth, anorexia, metallic aftertaste.
- GU: impotence, changes in libido.
- Other: exacerbation of tics, tolerance, physical and psychological dependence.

Note: Drug should be discontinued if signs of hypersensitivity or idiosyncrasy occur.

Overdose and treatment
Symptoms of overdose include increasing restlessness, tremor, hyperreflexia, tachypnea, confusion, aggressiveness, hallucinations, and panic; fatigue and depression usually follow the excitement stage. Other symptoms may include arrhythmias, shock, alterations in blood pressure, nausea, vomiting, diarrhea, and abdominal cramps; death is usually preceded by convulsions and coma.

Treat overdose symptomatically and supportively: if ingestion is recent (within 4 hours), use gastric lavage or emesis and sedate with barbiturate; monitor vital signs and fluid and electrolyte balance. Urinary acidification may enhance excretion. Saline catharsis (magnesium citrate) may hasten GI evacuation of unabsorbed long-acting forms. Hemodialysis or peritoneal dialysis may be effective in severe cases.

▶ **Special considerations**
Besides those relevant to all *amphetamines,* consider the following recommendations.
● Methamphetamine is not recommended for first-line treatment of obesity.
● Do not crush long-acting dosage forms.
● When treating behavioral disorders in children, consider a periodic discontinuation of the drug to evaluate effectiveness and the need for continued therapy.
● Rapid withdrawal after prolonged use may lead to depression, somnolence, and increased appetite.

Information for the patient
● Warn patient that potential for abuse is high. Discourage use to combat fatigue.
● Advise patient to avoid caffeine-containing drinks and alcohol, to take drug 1 hour before next meal, and to take last daily dose at least 6 hours before bedtime to prevent insomnia.
● Warn patient not to increase dosage unless prescribed.

Geriatric use
Elderly or debilitated patients may be especially sensitive to methamphetamine's effects. Drug should be used with caution.

Pediatric use
Methamphetamine is not recommended for weight reduction in children under age 12.

---

methantheline bromide
Banthine

● Pharmacologic classification: anticholinergic
● Therapeutic classification: antimuscarinic, gastrointestinal antispasmodic
● Pregnancy risk category C

How supplied
Available by prescription only
Tablets: 50 mg

Indications, route, and dosage
Adjunctive therapy in peptic ulcer; uninhibited, hypertonic, neurogenic bladder
Adults: 50 to 100 mg P.O. q 6 hours.
Children over age 1: 12.5 to 50 mg q.i.d.
Children under age 1: 12.5 to 25 mg q.i.d.
Neonates: 12.5 mg b.i.d., then t.i.d.

Pharmacodynamics
Antispasmodic action: Methantheline competitively blocks acetylcholine at cholinergic neuroeffector sites, inhibiting gastric acid secretion and pancreatic secretions.

Pharmacokinetics
● *Absorption:* Methantheline is poorly absorbed from the GI tract.
● *Distribution:* Methantheline does not cross the blood-brain barrier; little else is known about its distribution.

● *Metabolism:* Exact metabolic fate is unknown.
● *Excretion:* Methantheline is thought to be excreted in urine as metabolites and unchanged drug and in feces in large percentages as unabsorbed drug.

Contraindications and precautions
Methantheline is contraindicated in patients with narrow-angle glaucoma, because drug-induced cycloplegia and mydriasis may increase intraocular pressure; in patients with obstructive uropathy, obstructive GI tract disease, severe ulcerative colitis, myasthenia gravis, paralytic ileus, intestinal atony, or toxic megacolon, because the drug may exacerbate these conditions; and in patients with known hypersensitivity to anticholinergics or bromides.

Administer methantheline cautiously to patients with autonomic neuropathy, hyperthyroidism, coronary artery disease, cardiac arrhythmias, congestive heart failure, or ulcerative colitis, because the drug may exacerbate the symptoms of these disorders; to patients with hepatic or renal disease, because toxic accumulation may occur; to patients over age 40, because the drug increases the glaucoma risk; to patients with hiatal hernia associated with reflux esophagitis, because the drug may decrease lower esophageal sphincter tone; and in hot or humid environments, because the drug may predispose the patient to heatstroke.

Interactions
Concurrent administration of antacids decreases oral absorption of anticholinergics. Administer methantheline at least 1 hour before antacids.

Concomitant administration of drugs with anticholinergic effects may cause additive toxicity.

Decreased GI absorption of many drugs has been reported after the use of anticholinergics (for example, levodopa and ketoconazole). Conversely, slowly dissolving digoxin tablets may yield higher serum digoxin levels when administered with anticholinergics.

Use cautiously with oral potassium supplements (especially wax-matrix formulations) because the incidence of potassium-induced GI ulcerations may be increased.

Effects on diagnostic tests
None reported.

Adverse reactions
● CNS: headache, insomnia, drowsiness, dizziness, weakness, confusion and excitement (in elderly).
● CV: palpitations, tachycardia, orthostatic hypotension.
● DERM: urticaria, decreased sweating or anhidrosis, other dermal manifestations.
● EENT: blurred vision, mydriasis, cycloplegia, increased ocular tension, photophobia.
● GI: dry mouth, dysphagia, heartburn, loss of taste, nausea, constipation, vomiting, paralytic ileus, abdominal distention.
● GU: urinary hesitancy and retention, impotence.
● Other: fever, allergic reaction.
Note: Drug should be discontinued if hypersensitivity, urinary retention, confusion or excitement, curare-like symptoms, or skin rash occurs.

Overdose and treatment
Clinical signs of overdose include curare-like symptoms and such peripheral effects as headache; dilated, nonreactive pupils; blurred vision; flushed, hot, dry skin;

---

dryness of mucous membranes; dysphagia; decreased or absent bowel sounds; urinary retention; hyperthermia; tachycardia; hypertension; and increased respiration.

Treatment is primarily symptomatic and supportive, as needed. If the patient is alert, induce emesis (or use gastric lavage) and follow with a saline cathartic and activated charcoal to prevent further drug absorption. In severe cases, physostigmine may be administered to block methantheline's antimuscarinic effects. Give fluids, as needed, to treat shock. If urinary retention occurs, catheterization may be necessary.

▶ **Special considerations**
Besides those relevant to all *anticholinergics*, consider the following recommendations.
● Administer methantheline P.O. only.
● Drug should be titrated until therapeutic effect is obtained or adverse effects become intolerable.

Information for the patient
Advise patients to swallow tablets whole instead of chewing them.

Geriatric use
Methantheline should be administered cautiously to elderly patients. Lower doses are indicated.

Breast-feeding
Methantheline may be excreted in breast milk, possibly resulting in infant toxicity. Breast-feeding women should avoid this drug. Methantheline may also decrease milk production.

methazolamide
Neptazane

● Pharmacologic classification: carbonic anhydrase inhibitor
● Therapeutic classification: adjunctive treatment for open-angle glaucoma, perioperatively for acute angle-closure glaucoma
● Pregnancy risk category C

How supplied
Available by prescription only
Tablets: 25 mg, 50 mg

Indications, route, and dosage
Glaucoma (open-angle or preoperatively in obstructive or angle-closure)
Adults: 50 to 100 mg P.O. b.i.d. or t.i.d.

Pharmacodynamics
Anti-glaucoma action: In open-angle glaucoma and perioperatively for acute angle-closure glaucoma, methazolamide decreases the formation of aqueous humor, lowering intraocular pressure.

Pharmacokinetics
● *Absorption:* Methazolamide is absorbed more slowly than acetazolamide.
● *Distribution:* Methazolamide distributes into plasma, erythrocytes, extracellular fluid, bile, aqueous humor, and CSF.

● *Metabolism:* Methazolamide is metabolized partially by the liver.
● *Excretion:* About 20% to 30% of a methazolamide dose is excreted in urine.

Contraindications and precautions
Methazolamide is contraindicated in patients with hepatic insufficiency, low potassium or sodium levels, hyperchloremic acidosis, or severe renal impairment, because of the potential for enhanced electrolyte imbalances.

Methazolamide should be used cautiously in patients with respiratory acidosis or other severe respiratory problems because the drug may produce acidosis; in patients with diabetes because it may cause hyperglycemia and glycosuria; in patients taking cardiac glycosides because they are more susceptible to digitalis toxicity from methazolamide-induced hypokalemia; and in patients taking other diuretics.

Interactions
Methazolamide alkalizes urine, thus decreasing excretion of amphetamines, procainamide, quinidine, and flecainide. Methazolamide increases excretion of salicylates, phenobarbital, and lithium, lowering plasma levels of these drugs and necessitating dosage adjustments.

Effects on diagnostic tests
Because methazolamide alkalizes urine, it may cause false-positive proteinuria when Albustix or Albutest test are performed. Methazolamide also may decrease iodine uptake by the thyroid.

Adverse reactions
● CNS: drowsiness, paresthesias.
● DERM: rash.
● EENT: transient myopia.
● GI: nausea, vomiting, anorexia.
● GU: crystalluria, renal calculi.
● HEMA: *aplastic anemia,* hemolytic anemia, leukopenia.
● Metabolic: *hyperchloremic acidosis,* hypokalemia, asymptomatic hyperuricemia.
Note: Drug should be discontinued if blood pH level is below 7.2 or Pco$_2$ level is markedly elevated.

Overdose and treatment
Specific recommendations are unavailable. Treatment is supportive and symptomatic. Carbonic anhydrase inhibitors increase bicarbonate excretion and may cause hypokalemia and hyperchloremic acidosis. Induce emesis or perform gastric lavage. Do not induce catharsis because this may exacerbate electrolyte disturbances. Monitor fluid and electrolyte levels.

▶ **Special considerations**
Besides those relevant to all *carbonic anhydrase inhibitors*, consider the following recommendations.
● Diuretic effect is increased in acidosis.
● Monitor patients with glaucoma for eye pain to ensure drug efficacy.

Geriatric use
Elderly and debilitated patients require close observation because they are more susceptible to drug-induced diuresis. Excessive diuresis promotes rapid dehydration, hypovolemia, hypokalemia, and hyponatre-

mia, and may cause circulatory collapse. Reduced dosages may be indicated.

Breast-feeding
Safety of methazolamide in breast-feeding women has not been established.

---

methdilazine
Dilosyn*

methdilazine hydrochloride
Tacaryl

- Pharmacologic classification: phenothiazine derivative
- Therapeutic classification: antihistamine (H₁-receptor antagonist), antipruritic
- Pregnancy risk category C

How supplied
Available by prescription only
Tablets: 8 mg methdilazine hydrochloride
Tablets (chewable): 3.6 mg methdilazine (equal to 4 mg methdilazine hydrochloride)
Syrup: 4 mg/5 ml methdilazine hydrochloride

Indications, route, and dosage
Pruritus
Adults: 8 mg P.O. b.i.d. to q.i.d. or (chewable tablets) 7.2 mg P.O. b.i.d. to q.i.d.
Children over age 3: 4 mg P.O. b.i.d. to q.i.d. or (chewable tablets) 3.6 mg P.O. b.i.d. to q.i.d.

Pharmacodynamics
Antihistamine action: Antihistamines compete with histamine for histamine H₁-receptor sites on the smooth muscle of the bronchi, GI tract, uterus, and large blood vessels; by binding to cellular receptors, they prevent access of histamine and suppress histamine-induced allergic symptoms, even though they do not prevent its release.

Pharmacokinetics
Absorption, distribution, metabolism, and excretion have not been reported.

Contraindications and precautions
Methdilazine is contraindicated in patients with known hypersensitivity to this medication or other antihistamines or phenothiazines with a similar chemical structure, such as promethazine or trimeprazine; during acute asthmatic attack, because it thickens bronchial secretions; in acutely ill or dehydrated children, because they are at increased risk of developing dystonias; and in patients who have taken monoamine oxidase (MAO) inhibitors within the preceding 2 weeks.

Methdilazine should be used with caution in patients with narrow-angle glaucoma; in those with pyloroduodenal obstruction or urinary bladder obstruction from prostatic hypertrophy or narrowing of the bladder neck, because of its significant anticholinergic effects; in patients with cardiovascular disease or hypertension, because of risks of palpitations and tachycardia; and in patients with acute or chronic respiratory dysfunction (especially children) because methdilazine may suppress the cough reflex.

Methdilazine should be used with caution in children with a history of sleep apnea, a family history of sudden infant death syndrome, or Reye's syndrome.

Interactions
MAO inhibitors interfere with the detoxification of methdilazine and thus prolong and intensify its central depressant and anticholinergic effects; added sedation and CNS depression may occur when methdilazine is used concomitantly with other antihistamines, alcohol, barbiturates, tranquilizers, sleeping aids, or antianxiety agents.

Phenothiazines potentiate the CNS depressant and analgesic effect of narcotics; the phenothiazine activity of methdilazine is potentiated by oral contraceptives, progesterone, reserpine, and nylidrin hydrochloride.

Do not give epinephrine to reverse methdilazine-induced hypotension; partial adrenergic blockade may cause a further fall in blood pressure.

Effects on diagnostic tests
Methdilazine should be discontinued 4 days before diagnostic skin tests, to avoid preventing, reducing, or masking positive test response.

Adverse reactions
- CNS: extrapyramidal symptoms (especially at high doses), dizziness, drowsiness, headache, tinnitus, insomnia, euphoria, tremors, excitation, *tonic-clonic convulsions,* catatonia, increased appetite.
- CV: postural hypotension, reflex tachycardia, ECG changes.
- DERM: photosensitivity, rash, systemic lupus erythematosus-like symptoms.
- GI: anorexia, constipation, cholestatic jaundice.
- GU: urinary frequency and retention, dysuria.
- HEMA: leukopenia, *agranulocytosis.*
- Respiratory: thickened bronchial secretions.
- Chronic use: skin pigmentation, corneal opacities, impaired vision.

Overdose and treatment
Clinical manifestations of overdose may include either CNS depression (sedation, reduced mental alertness, apnea, and cardiovascular collapse) or CNS stimulation (insomnia, hallucinations, tremor, or convulsions). Atropine-like symptoms, such as dry mouth, flushed skin, fixed and dilated pupils, and GI symptoms, are common, especially in children.

Treat overdose by inducing emesis with ipecac syrup (in conscious patient), followed by activated charcoal to reduce further drug absorption. Use gastric lavage if patient is unconscious or ipecac fails. Treat hypotension with vasopressors, and control seizures with diazepam or phenytoin. *Do not give stimulants.*

▶ Special considerations
Besides those relevant to all *antihistamines,* consider the following recommendations.

Information for the patient
Advise patient to chew and swallow chewable tablets promptly, because local anesthetic effect may cause choking.

Geriatric use
Elderly patients are likely to be more sensitive to the phenothiazine-type adverse reactions — excessive sedation, hypotension, confusion, and extrapyramidal

signs, especially parkinsonism and dyskinesia. Elderly patients are usually more sensitive to adverse effects of antihistamines and are especially likely to experience a greater degree of dizziness, sedation, hyperexcitability, dry mouth, and urinary retention than younger patients; such symptoms usually respond to a decrease in medication dosage.

Pediatric use
Drug should be used with caution in children. Methdilazine is not indicated for use in premature infants or neonates. Infants and children under age 6 may experience paradoxical hyperexcitability.

Breast-feeding
Antihistamines such as methdilazine should not be used during breast-feeding. Many of these drugs are secreted in breast milk, exposing the infant to risks of unusual excitability; premature infants are at particular risk for convulsions.

---

methenamine hippurate
Hiprex, Urex

methenamine mandelate
Mandameth, Mandelamine, Mandelamine Forte (suspension)

- Pharmacologic classification: formaldehyde pro-drug
- Therapeutic classification: urinary tract antiseptic
- Pregnancy risk category C

How supplied
Available by prescription only
Methenamine hippurate
Tablets: 1 g
Methenamine mandelate
Tablets: 500 mg, 1 g
Tablets (enteric-coated): 500 mg, 1 g
Tablets (film-coated): 500 mg, 1 g
Suspension: 250 mg/5 ml, 500 mg/5 ml (Forte)
Granules: 500 mg, 1 g

Indications, route, and dosage
Long-term prophylaxis or suppression of chronic urinary tract infections
Methenamine hippurate
Adults and children over age 12: 1 g P.O. q 12 hours.
Children age 6 to 12: 500 mg to 1 g P.O. q 12 hours.
Urinary tract infections, infected residual urine in patients with neurogenic bladder
Methenamine mandelate
Adults: 1 g P.O. q.i.d.
Children age 6 to 12: 500 mg P.O. q.i.d.
Children under age 6: 50 mg/kg daily, in divided doses after meals and h.s.

Pharmacodynamics
Antibacterial action: Methenamine is hydrolyzed to formaldehyde and ammonia in the urine. Formaldehyde acts as a nonspecific antibacterial agent and is bactericidal.

Pharmacokinetics
- *Absorption:* About 10% to 30% of an oral dose is hydrolyzed by gastric acid to ammonia and formaldehyde;
enteric-coated tablets undergo less degradation, but extent and rate of absorption is reduced.
- *Distribution:* Methenamine crosses the placenta and enters breast milk.
- *Metabolism:* About 10% to 25% of methenamine is metabolized in the liver.
- *Excretion:* Most of dose is excreted by the kidneys via glomerular filtration and tubular secretion. In the urine, methenamine is converted to formaldehyde. Peak formaldehyde concentrations occur in approximately 2 hours (after dose of hippurate) and 3 to 8 hours (after dose of mandelate). Plasma half-life of parent drug is 3 to 6 hours.

Contraindications and precautions
Methenamine is contraindicated in patients with severe renal or hepatic dysfunction because the drug may worsen these conditions; in patients who are severely dehydrated because crystalluria may occur in patients with reduced urine flow rates; and in patients with known hypersensitivity to the drug.

Interactions
When used concomitantly, urine alkalinizing agents, such as sodium bicarbonate and acetazolamide, reduce methenamine's effectiveness by elevating urine pH and inhibiting methenamine's conversion to its active agent, formaldehyde. Concomitant use with sulfonamides causes formaldehyde to form an insoluble precipitate in acidic urine.

Effects on diagnostic tests
Formaldehyde formation from methenamine may cause false elevations in catecholamine and 17-hydroxycorticosteroid levels and false decreases in 5-hydroxyindoleacetic acid and estriol levels in urine.
Liver function test results may become abnormal during methenamine therapy.

Adverse reactions
- DERM: rashes.
- GI: nausea, vomiting, diarrhea.
- GU: urinary tract irritation, dysuria, urinary frequency, hematuria, albuminuria (all with high doses).
Note: Drug should be discontinued if patient develops hypersensitivity reaction.

Overdose and treatment
No information available.

▶ Special considerations
- Obtain a clean-catch urine specimen for culture and sensitivity tests before starting therapy and repeat as needed.
- Do not administer methenamine concomitantly with sulfonamides.
- Drug is ineffective against *Candida* infection.
- Oral suspension contains vegetable oil. Use cautiously in elderly or debilitated patients because aspiration may cause lipid pneumonia.
- Monitor fluid intake and output. Maintain fluid intake of 1,500 to 2,000 ml daily.
- For best results, maintain urine pH at 5.5 or less. Use Nitrazine paper to check pH. To effectively acidify

---

urine, large doses of ascorbic acid (6 to 12 g/day) may be necessary.
● Obtain liver function studies periodically during long-term therapy.
● *Proteus* and *Pseudomonas* infections tend to raise urine pH; urinary acidifiers are usually necessary when treating these infections.
● If rash appears, discontinue drug and re-evaluate therapy.
● Some products (such as Hiprex) may contain tartrazine dye, which may induce allergic reactions in certain individuals.

Information for the patient
● Instruct patient to limit intake of alkaline foods, such as vegetables, milk, and peanuts. Encourage him to drink cranberry, plum, and prune juices; these juices or ascorbic acid may be used to acidify urine.
● Warn patient not to take antacids, including Alka-Seltzer and sodium bicarbonate.
● Instruct patient to take drug after meals to minimize GI upset.
● Encourage patient to drink plenty of fluids to ensure adequate urine flow.

Breast-feeding
Methenamine is excreted in breast milk. Peak levels, which occur about 1 hour after dose, are approximately equivalent to maternal serum levels. No adverse reactions in infants have been reported.

---

methicillin sodium
Staphcillin

● Pharmacologic classification: penicillinase-resistant penicillin
● Therapeutic classification: antibiotic
● Pregnancy risk category B

How supplied
Available by prescription only
Injection: 1 g, 4 g, 6 g
Pharmacy bulk package: 10 g
I.V. infusions piggyback: 1 g, 4 g

Indications, route, and dosage
Systemic infections caused by susceptible organisms
Adults: 4 to 12 g I.M. or I.V. daily, divided into doses given q 4 to 6 hours.
Children: 150 to 200 mg/kg I.M. or I.V. daily, divided into doses given q 4 to 6 hours.

Pharmacodynamics
Antibiotic action: Methicillin is bactericidal; it adheres to bacterial penicillin-binding proteins, thus inhibiting bacterial cell wall synthesis. Methicillin resists the effects of penicillinases – enzymes that inactivate penicillin – and is thus active against many strains of penicillinase-producing bacteria. This activity is most important against penicillinase-producing staphylococci; some strains may remain resistant. Methicillin is also active against a few gram-positive aerobic and anaerobic bacilli but has no significant effect on gram-negative bacilli.

Pharmacokinetics
● *Absorption:* Methicillin is inactivated by gastric secretions and must be given parenterally. Peak plasma concentrations occur 30 to 60 minutes after I.M. injection.
● *Distribution:* Methicillin is distributed widely. CSF penetration is poor but enhanced by meningeal inflammation. Methicillin crosses the placenta; it is 30% to 50% protein-bound.
● *Metabolism:* Methicillin is metabolized only partially.
● *Excretion:* Methicillin and metabolites are excreted in urine by renal tubular secretion and glomerular filtration. They are also excreted in breast milk and in bile. Elimination half-life in adults is about ½ hour, prolonged to 2½ hours in severe renal impairment; it is prolonged to 4 to 6 hours in anuric patients.

Contraindications and precautions
Methicillin is contraindicated in patients with known hypersensitivity to any other penicillin or to cephalosporins.

Interactions
Concomitant use of methicillin with aminoglycosides produces synergistic bactericidal effects against *Staphylococcus aureus*. However, the drugs are physically and chemically incompatible and are inactivated when mixed or given together.

Probenecid blocks renal tubular secretion of penicillin, raising its serum concentrations.

Effects on diagnostic tests
Methicillin falsely shows increases in serum uric acid concentration levels (copper-chelate method); it interferes with measurement of 17-hydroxycorticosteroids (Porter-Silber test). Positive Coombs' tests have been reported. Methicillin may cause transient reductions in red blood cell, white blood cell, and platelet counts. Abnormal urinalysis result may indicate drug-induced interstitial nephritis. Methicillin may falsely decrease serum aminoglycoside concentrations.

Adverse reactions
● CNS: neuropathy, *seizures* (with high doses).
● GI: glossitis, stomatitis, *pseudomembranous colitis*, intrahepatic cholestasis, diarrhea.
● GU: *interstitial nephritis*.
● HEMA: *eosinophilia*, hemolytic anemia, transient neutropenia, thrombocytopenia, *agranulocytosis*.
● Local: vein irritation, thrombophlebitis.
● Other: *hypersensitivity reactions* (chills, fever, edema, rash, urticaria, *anaphylaxis*), bacterial or fungal superinfection.
   Note: Drug should be discontinued if immediate hypersensitivity reactions occur or if signs of acute interstitial nephritis or pseudomembranous colitis occur. Patient may require alternate therapy if any of the following occurs: drug fever, eosinophilia, hematuria, neutropenia, or unexplained elevations in serum creatinine or BUN levels.

Overdose and treatment
Clinical signs of overdose include neuromuscular irritability or seizures. Methicillin can be removed by gastric lavage, but is not appreciably removed by hemodialysis or peritoneal dialysis.

▶ **Special considerations**
Besides those relevant to all *penicillins*, consider the following recommendations.
• Schedule for administration around the clock to maintain adequate plasma levels.
• Frequently monitor results of urinalysis for signs of adverse renal effects.
• Monitor neurologic status. High blood concentrations may cause seizures.
• Periodically check renal, hepatic, and hematopoietic function during prolonged therapy.

Information for the patient
Encourage pateint to report all adverse reactions.

Pediatric use
Elimination of methicillin is reduced in neonates; safe use of drug in neonates has not been established.

Breast-feeding
Methicillin is excreted in breast milk; drug should be used with caution in breast-feeding women.

---

methimazole
Tapazole

• Pharmacologic classification: thyroid hormone antagonist
• Therapeutic classification: antihyperthyroid agent
• Pregnancy risk category D

How supplied
Available by prescription only
Tablets: 5 mg, 10 mg

Indications, route, and dosage
Hyperthyroidism
Adults: 15 mg P.O. daily if mild; 30 to 40 mg P.O. daily if moderately severe; 60 mg P.O. daily if severe. Continue until patient is euthyroid, then start maintenance dosage of 5 mg daily to b.i.d. Maximum dosage is 150 mg daily.
Children: 0.4 mg/kg/day divided q 8 hours. Continue until patient is euthyroid, then start maintenance dosage of 0.2 mg/kg/day divided q 8 hours.
Preparation for thyroidectomy
Adults and children: Same dosages as for hyperthyroidism until patient is euthyroid; then iodine may be added for 10 days before surgery.
Thyrotoxic crisis
Adults and children: Same dosages as for hyperthyroidism, with concomitant iodine therapy and propranolol. Propylthiouracil is preferred for thyroid "storm."

Pharmacodynamics
Antithyroid action: In treating hyperthyroidism, methimazole inhibits synthesis of thyroid hormone by interfering with the incorporation of iodide into tyrosine. Methimazole also inhibits the formation of iodothyronine. As preparation for thyroidectomy, methimazole inhibits synthesis of the thyroid hormone and causes a euthyroid state, reducing surgical problems during thyroidectomy; as a result, the mortality for a single-stage thyroidectomy is low. Iodide reduces the vascularity of the gland, making it less friable. For treating thyrotoxic

crisis (thyrotoxicosis), propylthiouracil (PTU) theoretically is preferred over methimazole because it inhibits peripheral deiodination of thyroxine to triiodothyronine.

Pharmacokinetics
• *Absorption:* Methimazole is absorbed rapidly from the GI tract (70% to 80% bioavailable). Peak plasma levels are reached within 1 hour.
• *Distribution:* Methimazole readily crosses the placenta and is distributed into breast milk. It is concentrated in the thyroid. Methimazole is not protein-bound.
• *Metabolism:* Methimazole undergoes hepatic metabolism.
• *Excretion:* About 80% of the drug and its metabolites are excreted renally; 7% is excreted unchanged. Half-life is between 5 and 13 hours.

Contraindications and precautions
Methimazole is contraindicated in patients with hypersensitivity to the drug and in breast-feeding women. It should be used with caution in patients over age 40 and at dosages greater than 40 mg/day because of increased risk of agranulocytosis; in patients receiving other agents known to cause agranulocytosis; and in patients with infection or hepatic dysfunction.

Interactions
Concomitant use of methimazole with PTU and adrenocorticoids or ACTH may require a dosage adjustment of the steroid when thyroid status changes. Concomitant use with other bone marrow depressant agents causes an increased risk of agranulocytosis. Concomitant use with other hepatotoxic agents increases the risk of hepatotoxicity. Concurrent use with iodinated glycerol, lithium, or potassium iodide may potentiate hypothyroid and goitrogenic effects.

Effects on diagnostic tests
Methimazole therapy alters selenomethionine (^{75}Se) uptake by the pancreas and ^{123}I or ^{131}I uptake by the thyroid. Hepatotoxicity may be evident by elevations of prothrombin time and of serum alanine aminotransferase, serum aspartate aminotransferase, bilirubin, alkaline phosphatase, and lactic dehydrogenase levels.

Adverse reactions
• CNS: headache, drowsiness, vertigo, depression, paresthesias.
• DERM: rash, urticaria, skin discoloration, pruritus, lupus-like syndrome, *exfoliative dermatitis.*
• GI: diarrhea, nausea, vomiting, epigastric distress, sialadenopathy (appear to be dose-related).
• HEMA: *agranulocytosis,* leukopenia, granulocytopenia, thrombocytopenia (appear to be dose-related).
• Hepatic: jaundice, *hepatitis.*
• Renal: nephritis.
• Other: arthralgia, myalgia, salivary gland enlargement, loss of taste, drug fever, lymphadenopathy, hair loss, edema.
Note: Drug should be discontinued at the first sign of hepatotoxicity or if the patient develops agranulocytosis, pancytopenia, hepatitis (fever, swelling of cervical lymph nodes), or exfoliative dermatitis.

Overdose and treatment
Clinical manifestations of overdose include nausea, vomiting, epigastric distress, fever, headache, arthralgia, pruritus, edema, and pancytopenia. Treatment is supportive; gastric lavage should be performed or eme-

sis should be induced if possible. If bone marrow depression develops, fresh whole blood, corticosteroids, and anti-infectives may be required.

▶ Special considerations
Besides those relevant to all *thyroid hormone antagonists*, consider the following recommendations.
● Best response occurs if dosage is administered around the clock and given at the same time each day in respect to meals.
● Dosages of over 40 mg/day increase the risk of agranulocytosis.
● A beta blocker, usually propranolol, usually is given to manage the peripheral signs of hyperthyroidism, primarily tachycardia.
● Euthyroid state may take several months to develop.

Information for the patient
● Tell patient to take drug at regular intervals around the clock and to take it at the same time each day in relation to meals.
● If GI upset occurs, tell patient to take drug with meals.
● Tell patient to call promptly if fever, sore throat, malaise, unusual bleeding, yellowing of eyes, nausea, or vomiting occurs.
● Advise patient not to store drug in bathroom; heat and humidity cause it to deteriorate.
● Tell patient to inform all other physicians and dentists of methimazole therapy.
● Teach patient how to recognize the signs of hyperthyroidism and hypothyroidism and what to do if they occur.

Breast-feeding
Patient should discontinue breast-feeding before beginning therapy because methimazole is excreted into breast milk. However, if breast-feeding is necessary, PTU is the preferred antithyroid agent.

---

methocarbamol
Delaxin, Robamol, Robaxin

● Pharmacologic classification: carbonate derivative of guaifenesin
● Therapeutic classification: skeletal muscle relaxant
● Pregnancy risk category C

How supplied
Available by prescription only
Tablets: 500 mg, 750 mg
Injection: 100 mg/ml parenteral

Indications, route, and dosage
Adjunct in acute, painful musculoskeletal conditions
Adults: 1.5 g P.O. q.i.d. for 2 to 3 days. Maintenance dosage, 4 to 4.5 g P.O. daily in three to six divided doses. Alternatively, 1 g I.M. or I.V. Maximum dosage, 3 g daily I.M. or I.V. for 3 consecutive days.
Supportive therapy in tetanus management
Adults: 1 to 2 g direct I.V. at a rate of 300 mg/minute. Additional 1 to 2 g dose may be administered. Total initial I.V. dosage, 3 g. Repeat I.V. infusion of 1 to 2 g q 6 hours until nasogastric tube can be inserted. Total P.O. dosage, 24 g daily.

Children: 15 mg/kg or 500 mg/m² I.V. Don't inject faster than 180 mg/m × 2/minute. May be repeated q 6 hours if necessary to a total dosage of 1.8 g daily for 3 consecutive days.

Pharmacodynamics
Skeletal muscle relaxant action: Methocarbamol does not relax skeletal muscle directly. Its effects appear to be related to its sedative action; however, the exact mechanism of action is unknown.

Pharmacokinetics
● *Absorption:* Methocarbamol is rapidly and completely absorbed from the GI tract. Onset of action after single oral dose is within ½ hour. Onset of action after single I.V. dose is achieved immediately.
● *Distribution:* Methocarbamol is widely distributed throughout the body.
● *Metabolism:* Methocarbamol is extensively metabolized in liver via dealkylation and hydroxylation.
● *Excretion:* Methocarbamol is rapidly and almost completely excreted in urine, mainly as its glucuronide and sulfate metabolites (40% to 50%), as unchanged drug (10% to 15%), and the rest as unidentified metabolites.

Contraindications and precautions
Methocarbamol is contraindicated in patients with known hypersensitivity to the drug.
Administer injectable methocarbamol with caution, if at all, to patients with known or suspected epilepsy, because of the potential for seizures; and to those with impaired renal function (propylene glycol vehicle may irritate the kidneys).

Interactions
Concomitant use of methocarbamol with other CNS depressant drugs, including alcohol, narcotics, anxiolytics, tricyclic antidepressants, and psychotics, may cause additive CNS depression. When used with other depressants, exercise care to avoid overdose. Patients with myasthenia gravis who receive anticholinesterase agents may experience severe weakness if given methocarbamol.

Effects on diagnostic tests
Methocarbamol therapy alters results of laboratory tests for urine 5-hydroxyindoleacetic acid (5-HIAA) using quantitative method of Udenfriend (false-positive) and for urine vanillylmandelic acid (false-positive when Gitlow screening test used; no problem when quantitative method of Sunderman used).

Adverse reactions
● CNS: drowsiness, dizziness, light-headedness, headache, vertigo, mild muscular incoordination, syncope, *seizures.*
● CV: hypotension, bradycardia.
● EENT: blurred vision, nystagmus, diplopia, conjunctivitis with nasal congestion.
● GI: nausea, adynamic ileus, metallic taste, GI upset, anorexia.
● Other: fever, allergic reactions, rash, pruritus, urticaria, flushing.
After I.M. or I.V. administration, *anaphylaxis,* thrombophlebitis, sloughing, pain at injection site, hemolysis, increased hemoglobin and red blood cells in urine, *seizures.*
Note: Drug should be discontinued if patient develops hypersensitivity, rash, or seizures.

Overdose and treatment

Clinical manifestations of overdose include extreme drowsiness, nausea and vomiting, and cardiac arrhythmias.

Treatment includes symptomatic and supportive measures. If ingestion is recent, empty stomach by emesis or gastric lavage (may reduce absorption). Maintain adequate airway; monitor urine output and vital signs; administer I.V. fluids if needed.

▶ Special considerations

• Do not administer subcutaneously. Give I.V. undiluted at a rate not exceeding 300 mg per minute. May also be given by I.V. infusion after diluting in D_5W or normal saline solution.

• Patient should be supine during and for at least 10 to 15 minutes after I.V. injection.

• To give via nasogastric tube, crush tablets and suspend in water or normal saline solution.

• When used in tetanus, follow manufacturer's instructions.

• Patient's urine may turn black, blue, brown, or green on standing.

• Patient needs assistance in walking after parenteral administration.

• Extravasation of I.V. solution may cause thrombophlebitis and sloughing from hypertonic solution.

• Oral administration should replace parenteral use as soon as feasible.

• Adverse reactions after oral administration are usually mild and transient and subside with dosage reduction.

Information for the patient

• Tell patient urine may turn black, blue, green, or brown.

• Warn patient drug may cause drowsiness. Patient should avoid hazardous activities that require alertness until degree of CNS depression can be determined.

• Advise patient to make position changes slowly, particularly from recumbent to upright position, and to dangle legs before standing.

• Advise patient to avoid alcoholic beverages and use cold or cough preparations carefully because some contain alcohol.

• Tell patient to store drug away from heat and light (not in bathroom medicine cabinet) and safely out of reach of children.

• Tell patient to take missed dose if remembered within 1 hour. Beyond 1 hour, patient should skip that dose and resume regular schedule. Do not double dose.

• Inform athletes that skeletal muscle relaxants are banned in competition and tested for by the U.S. Olympic Committee and the National Collegiate Athletic Association.

Geriatric use

Lower doses are indicated, because elderly patients are more sensitive to the drug's effects.

Pediatric use

For children under age 12, use only as recommended for tetanus.

Breast-feeding

Methocarbamol is excreted in breast milk in small amounts. Patient should not breast-feed during treatment with methocarbamol.

---

methohexital sodium
Brevital Sodium

• Pharmacologic classification: barbiturate
• Therapeutic classification: I.V. anesthetic
• Controlled substance schedule IV
• Pregnancy risk category C

How supplied

Available by prescription only
Injection: 500 mg, 2.5 g, 5 g powder for injection

Indications, route, and dosage
Induction of anesthesia; anesthesia for short procedures (such as electroconvulsive therapy [ECT])
Dosage is highly individualized.

Adults and children: For induction of anesthesia, a 1% solution is administered at a rate of about 1 ml/5 seconds, possibly with inhalant anesthetics and/or skeletal muscle relaxants. The induction dose may vary from 50 to 120 mg or more but averages about 70 mg; it usually provides anesthesia for 5 to 7 minutes. Maintenance of anesthesia may be achieved via intermittent injections of about 20 to 40 mg (2 to 4 ml of 1% solution), as needed, usually every 4 to 7 minutes; or by continuous I.V infusion of a 0.2% solution (average rate of about 3 ml of a 0.2% solution [1 drop/second]).

Pharmacodynamics

Anesthetic action: Methohexital produces anesthesia by direct depression of the polysynaptic midbrain reticular activating system; drug decreases presynaptic (via decreased neurotransmitter release) and postsynaptic excitation. These effects may be subsequent to increased gamma-aminobutyric acid (GABA), enhancement of GABA's effects, or a direct effect on GABA receptor sites.

Pharmacokinetics

• *Absorption:* Methohexital is only given I.V.; it is an ultrashort-acting barbiturate; peak concentrations in the brain occur between 30 seconds and 2 minutes after administration.

• *Distribution:* Methohexital distributes throughout the body; highest initial concentrations occur in vascular areas of the brain, primarily gray matter. Methohexital is 80% protein-bound.

• *Metabolism:* Methohexital is metabolized extensively in the liver.

• *Excretion:* Unchanged methohexital is not excreted in significant amounts. Duration of action depends on tissue redistribution.

Contraindications and precautions

Methohexital is contraindicated in patients with acute intermittent or variegate porphyria; in patients with known hypersensitivity to the drug; and whenever general anesthesia is contraindicated.

It should be used cautiously in patients with respiratory obstruction; circulatory, cardiac, renal, or hepatic dysfunction; severe anemia; marked obesity or status asthmaticus (use *extreme* caution), because the drug worsens these conditions. Use with caution in patients with a full stomach because it blocks airway reflexes and may predispose the patient to aspiration.

Interactions
Methohexital may potentiate or add to CNS depressant effects of sedatives, hypnotics, antihistamines, narcotics, phenothiazines, benzodiazepines, and alcohol.

Concomitant use with ketamine for anesthesia may cause profound respiratory depression, because ketamine potentiates methohexital.

Effects on diagnostic tests
Methohexital causes dose-dependent alteration of EEG patterns.

Adverse reactions
● CNS: skeletal muscle hyperactivity, anxiety, restlessness, headache, emergence delirium.
● CV: transient hypotension, tachycardia, *circulatory depression, peripheral vascular collapse.*
● DERM: pain, swelling, ulceration and necrosis on extravasation.
● GI: abdominal pain, nausea, vomiting, excessive salivation.
● Respiratory: *respiratory depression, apnea, laryngospasm, bronchospasm,* hiccups.
● Local: thrombophlebitis and pain at injection site, injury to adjacent nerves.
   Note: Drug should be discontinued if peripheral vascular collapse, respiratory arrest, or hypersensitivity reaction occurs.

Overdose and treatment
Clinical signs include respiratory depression, respiratory arrest, hypotension, and shock. Treat supportively, using, as needed, mechanical ventilation and I.V. fluids or vasopressors (dopamine, phenylephrine) for hypotension. Monitor vital signs closely.

▶ Special considerations
● Avoid extravasation or intra-arterial injection because of possible tissue necrosis and gangrene.
● Drug is physically incompatible with lactated Ringer's solution; with acidic solutions, such as atropine, metocurine, and succinylcholine; and with silicone. Avoid contact with rubber stoppers or parts of syringes that have been treated with silicone. The preferred diluent is sterile water, but dextrose 5% or 0.9% sodium chloride may be used.

Geriatric use
Lower doses may be indicated.

Pediatric use
Use with caution.

---

methotrexate, methotrexate sodium
Folex, Mexate

● Pharmacologic classification: antimetabolite (cell cycle-phase specific, S phase)
● Therapeutic classification: antineoplastic
● Pregnancy risk category D

How supplied
Available by prescription only
Tablets (scored): 2.5 mg

Injection: 20-mg, 25-mg, 50-mg, 100-mg, 250-mg, 1-g vials, lyophilized powder, preservative-free; 25-mg/ml vials, preservative-free solution; 2.5-mg/ml, 25-mg/ml vials, lyophilized powder, preserved

Indications, route, and dosage
Dosage and indications may vary. Check current literature for recommended protocols.
Trophoblastic tumors (choriocarcinoma, hydatidiform mole)
Adults: 15 to 30 mg P.O. or I.M. daily for 5 days. Repeat after 1 or more weeks, according to response or toxicity.
Tumors of head and neck, refractory lymphomas
Adults and children: High-dose methotrexate – up to 6 gm/m² as an infusion over 6 to 12 hours.
Acute lymphoblastic and lymphatic leukemia
Adults and children: 3.3 mg/m² P.O., I.M., or I.V. daily for 4 to 6 weeks or until remission occurs; then 20 to 30 mg/m² P.O. or I.M. twice weekly or 2.5 mg/kg I.V. q 14 days.
Meningeal leukemia
Adults and children: 12 mg/m²intrathecally to a maximum dose of 15 mg q 2 to 5 days until cerebrospinal fluid is normal. Use only vials of powder with no preservatives; dilute using normal saline solution injection *without* preservatives or Elliot's B solution. Use only new vials of drug and diluent. Use immediately after reconstitution.
Burkitt's lymphoma (Stage I or Stage II)
Adults: 10 to 25 mg P.O. daily for 4 to 8 days with 1-week rest intervals.
Lymphosarcoma (Stage III; non-Hodgkin's lymphoma)
Adults: 0.625 to 2.5 mg/kg daily P.O., I.M., or I.V.
Breast cancer
Adults: 40 to 60 mg/m² I.V. as a single dose. Usually used in combination with other agents.
Mycosis fungoides (advanced)
Adults: 2.5 to 10 mg P.O. daily or 50 mg I.M. weekly; or 25 mg I.M. twice weekly.
Psoriasis (severe)
Adults: 10 to 25 mg P.O., I.M., or I.V. as single weekly dose.
Rheumatoid arthritis (severe, refractory)
Adults: 7.5 to 15 mg/week in divided doses.

Pharmacodynamics
Antineoplastic action: Methotrexate exerts its cytotoxic activity by tightly binding with dihydrofolic acid reductase, an enzyme crucial to purine metabolism, resulting in an inhibition of DNA, RNA, and protein synthesis.

Pharmacokinetics
● *Absorption:* The absorption of methotrexate across the GI tract appears to be dose related. Lower doses are essentially completely absorbed, while absorption of larger doses is incomplete and variable. Intramuscular doses are absorbed completely. Peak serum levels are achieved 30 minutes to 2 hours after an intramuscular dose and 1 to 4 hours after an oral dose.
● *Distribution:* Methotrexate is distributed widely throughout the body, with the highest concentrations found in the kidneys, gallbladder, spleen, liver, and skin. The drug crosses the blood-brain barrier but does not achieve therapeutic levels in the CSF. Approximately 50% of the drug is bound to plasma protein.
● *Metabolism:* Methotrexate is metabolized only slightly in the liver.

---

*Canada only   †Unlabeled clinical use   Italicized adverse reactions are life-threatening.

- *Excretion:* Methotrexate is excreted primarily into urine as unchanged drug. The elimination has been described as biphasic, with a first-phase half-life of 45 minutes and a terminal phase half-life of 4 hours.

Contraindications and precautions

Methotrexate is contraindicated in pregnant patients because drug may be fetotoxic. It is also contraindicated in nursing women because of the risk of serious adverse effects to the infant.

Use cautiously in patients with impaired renal, hepatic, or hematologic status because of the drug's adverse hematologic effects. Close monitoring during therapy is required.

Administer by intrathecal injection with extreme caution. Large doses may cause seizures. Serum levels of the drug following intrathecal injection may be high enough to cause systemic toxicity.

Adverse GI effects may cause severe nausea and vomiting or stomatitis. Monitor patient for dehydration. Use with extreme caution in patients with peptic ulcer disease or ulcerative colitis.

Because the drug has the potential for both acute and chronic hepatotoxicity, use with extreme caution in patients with preexisting liver damage or impaired hepatic function. Chronic toxicity, characterized by hepatic fibrosis and cirrhosis, is potentially fatal. It is usually seen following long-term use (2 years or longer) and cumulative doses of 1.5 g.

Methotrexate therapy should be discontinued if the patient experiences pulmonary symptons, such as a dry, non-productive cough or evidence of a non-specific pneumonitis. Fever, cough, dyspnea, hypoxemia, and radiologic evidence of a pulmonary infiltrate are typical findings.

Methotrexate redistributes slowly from third space compartments, such as asciti fluid or pleural effusions. This slow redistribution can result in prolonged, high blood levels of methotrexate and toxicity. Before administering methotrexate to patietns with significant third space lesions, evacuate the fluid. Monitor plasma levels closely.

Interactions

Concomitant use with probenecid increases the therapeutic and toxic effects of methotrexate by inhibiting the renal tubular secretion of methotrexate; salicylates also increase the therapeutic and toxic effects of methotrexate by the same mechanism. Combined use of these agents requires a lower dosage of methotrexate.

NSAIDs, sulfonamides, salicylates, and sulfonylureas may increase the therapeutic and toxic effects of methotrexate by displacing methotrexate from plasma proteins, increasing the concentrations of free methotrexate. Concurrent use of these agents with methotrexate should be avoided if possible.

Immunizations may not be effective when given during methotrexate therapy. Because of the risk of disseminated infections, live virus vaccines are generally not recommended during therapy.

Phenytoin serum levels may be decreased by chemotherapeutic regimens that employ methotrexate, resulting in an increased risk of seizures.

Effects on diagnostic tests

Methotrexate therapy may increase blood and urine concentrations of uric acid. Methotrexate may alter results of the laboratory assay for folate by inhibiting the

organism used in the assay, thus interfering with the detection of folic acid deficiency.

Adverse reactions

- CNS: *arachnoiditis within hours of intrathecal use;* subacute neurotoxicity may begin a few weeks later; necrotizing demyelinating leukoencephalopathy a few years later.
- DERM: exposure to sun may aggravate psoriatic lesions, photosensitivity; urticaria, pruritus, hyperpigmentation, rash.
- GI: stomatitis; diarrhea leading to hemorrhagic enteritis and intestinal perforation; nausea; vomiting; gingivitis; pharyngitis.
- GU: *tubular necrosis.*
- HEMA: *bone marrow depression* (dose-limiting); *leukopenia* and *thrombocytopenia* (nadir occurring on day 7), anemia.
- Hepatic: hepatic dysfunction leading to cirrhosis or hepatic fibrosis.
- Metabolic: hyperuricemia.
- Other: alopecia, *pulmonary interstitial infiltrates;* long-term use in children may cause osteoporosis.

Note: Drug should be discontinued if diarrhea or ulcerative stomatitis occurs.

Overdose and treatment

Clinical manifestations of overdose include myelosuppression, anemia, nausea, vomiting, dermatitis, alopecia, and melena.

The antidote for the hematopoietic toxicity of methotrexate is calcium leucovorin, started within 1 hour after the administration of methotrexate. The dosage of leucovorin should be high enough to produce plasma concentrations higher than those of methotrexate.

▶ Special considerations

- Methotrexate may be given undiluted by I.V. push injection.
- Drug can be diluted to a higher volume with normal saline solution for I.V. infusion.
- Use reconstituted solutions of preservative-free drug within 24 hours after mixing.
- For intrathecal administration, use preservative-free formulations only. Dilute with unpreserved normal saline and further dilute with either lactated Ringer's or Elliott's B solution, to a final concentration of 1 mg/ml.
- Dose modification may be required in impaired hepatic or renal function, bone marrow depression, aplasia, leukopenia, thrombocytopenia, or anemia. Use cautiously in infection, peptic ulcer, ulcerative colitis, and in very young, old, or debilitated patients.
- GI adverse reactions may require stopping drug.
- Rash, redness, or ulcerations in mouth or pulmonary adverse reactions may signal serious complications.
- Monitor uric acid levels.
- Monitor intake and output daily. Force fluids (2 to 3 liters daily).
- Alkalinize urine by giving sodium bicarbonate tablets to prevent precipitation of drug, especially with high doses. Maintain urine pH at more than 6.5. Reduce dose if BUN level is 20 to 30 mg/dl or serum creatinine level is 1.2 to 2 mg/dl. Stop drug if BUN level is more than 30 mg/dl or serum creatinine level is more than 2 mg/dl.
- Watch for increases in AST (SGOT), ALT (SGPT), and alkaline phosphatase levels, which may signal hepatic dysfunction. Methotrexate should not be used when the potential for "third spacing" exists.

---

*Canada only   †Unlabeled clinical use   Italicized adverse reactions are life-threatening.

● Watch for bleeding (especially GI) and infection.
● Monitor temperature daily, and watch for cough, dyspnea, and cyanosis.
● Avoid all I.M. injections in patients with thrombocytopenia.
● Leucovorin rescue is necessary with high-dose protocols (doses greater than 100 mg).

Information for the patient

● Emphasize importance of continuing medication despite nausea and vomiting. Advise patient to call immediately if vomiting occurs shortly after taking a dose.
● Encourage adequate fluid intake to increase urine output, to prevent nephrotoxicity, and to facilitate excretion of uric acid.
● Warn patient to avoid alcoholic beverages during therapy with methotrexate.
● Warn patient to avoid conception during and immediately after therapy because of possible abortion or congenital anomalies.
● Tell patient to avoid prolonged exposure to sunlight and to use a highly protective sunscreen when exposed to sunlight.
● Teach patient good mouth care to prevent superinfection of oral cavity.
● Advise patient that hair should grow back after treatment has ended.
● Recommend salicylate-free analgesics for pain relief or fever reduction.
● Tell patient to avoid exposure to people with infections.
● Advise patient report any unusual bruising or bleeding promptly.

Breast-feeding

Methotrexate is distributed into breast milk. Therefore, because of the potential for serious adverse reactions, mutagenicity, and carcinogenicity in the infant, breast-feeding should be discontinued.

---

methotrimeprazine hydrochloride
Levoprome, Nozinan∗

● Pharmacologic classification: propylamino phenothiazine
● Therapeutic classification: sedative, analgesic agent, antipruritic
● Pregnancy risk category C

How supplied
Available by prescription only
Injection: 20 mg/ml in 10-ml vial, 25 mg/ml∗
Tablets∗: 2 mg, 5 mg, 25 mg, 50 mg
Drops∗: 40 mg/ml
Solution∗: 20 mg/ml

Indications, route, and dosage
Postoperative analgesia
Adults and children over age 12: Initially, 2.5 to 7.5 mg I.M. q 4 to 6 hours, then adjust dose.
Preanesthetic medication
Adults and children over age 12: 2 to 20 mg I.M. 45 minutes to 3 hours before surgery.

Sedation, analgesia
Adults and children over age 12: 10 to 20 mg deep I.M. q 4 to 6 hours as required.
Adults over age 65: 5 to 10 mg I.M. q 4 to 6 hours.

Pharmacodynamics
Sedative and analgesic actions: Methotrimeprazine depresses the subcortical area of the brain at the levels of the thalamus, hypothalamus, and reticular and limbic systems. The resulting suppression of sensory impulses causes the marked sedation seen with the drug. Studies have not shown methotrimeprazine's analgesic effects to be independent of the sedative effects.

Pharmacokinetics
● *Absorption:* After I.M. injection, peak serum levels are attained in 30 to 90 minutes; maximum analgesic effects occur in 20 to 40 minutes.
● *Distribution:* Methotrimeprazine is distributed throughout the body, including the CNS. The drug also crosses the placenta into umbilical cord blood.
● *Metabolism:* Methotrimeprazine is metabolized in the liver to less active metabolites.
● *Excretion:* The metabolites of methotrimeprazine are excreted unchanged. Duration of sedation or analgesia is only 4 hours.

Contraindications and precautions
Methotrimeprazine is contraindicated in patients with known phenothiazine hypersensitivity; in patients hypersensitive to sulfites because the parenteral form of the drug contains sodium metabisulfite; in patients with severe renal or hepatic disease, because drug accumulation may occur; in patients with cardiac disease, because the drug may exacerbate the disease; and in patients with seizure disorders, because it may lower the seizure threshold.

Methotrimeprazine should be used cautiously in elderly or debilitated patients with cardiovascular disease or in any patient in whom a sudden decrease in blood pressure might lead to serious complications. Use drug with great caution in patients with clinically significant hypotension or those who are receiving antihypertensives, because excessive hypotension may occur; or in those receiving monoamine oxidase inhibitors, because it may prolong sedative effects.

Interactions
Methotrimeprazine may add to or potentiate the effects of other CNS depressants such as opiates, benzodiazepines, antihistamines, tranquilizers, barbiturates, alcohol, and general anesthetics.

The drug may potentiate the anticholinergic effects of a number of drugs, including succinylcholine, atropine, and scopolamine. Increased CNS stimulation, including delirium and hallucinations, may occur.

Use of methotrimeprazine in patients receiving antihypertensives may cause a profound decrease in blood pressure.

Do not treat methotrimeprazine-induced hypotension with mixed alpha- and beta-adrenergic agonists such as epinephrine; that would cause an even greater decrease in blood pressure.

Effects on diagnostic tests
Methotrimeprazine therapy alters provocative and blocking tests for pheochromocytoma by producing sedation and orthostatic hypotension.

Adverse reactions
- **CNS:** disorientation, drowsiness, dizziness, euphoria, excessive sedation, headache, fainting, weakness, slurred speech, amnesia.
- **CV:** orthostatic hypotension, tachycardia, palpitations.
- **DERM:** local inflammation, swelling at injection site.
- **EENT:** blurred vision, dry mouth, nasal congestion.
- **GI:** nausea, vomiting, abdominal discomfort, constipation.
- **GU:** urinary retention.
- **HEMA:** *agranulocytosis* and other blood dyscrasias (with prolonged use).
- **Hepatic:** cholestatic jaundice with prolonged use.
- **Other:** phenothiazine adverse effects (*neuroleptic malignant syndrome* characterized by fever, leukocytosis, catatonia, and rigidity), dystonic reactions, akathisia, altered temperature regulation, pain and swelling at injection site.

Note: Drug should be discontinued if hypersensitivity, paradoxical euphoria, dystonic reactions, or severe prolonged hypotension occur.

Overdose and treatment
Clinical manifestations of overdose include excessive sedation, stupor, coma, hypotension, extrapyramidal reactions, and seizures.

Treat supportively. Maintain patent airway and adequate ventilation; maintain cardiovascular function with fluids and alpha-adrenergic agonists such as phenylephrine or norepinephrine. Do not use epinephrine for blood pressure control, because it may exacerbate hypotension. Treat seizures with parenteral diazepam, and extrapyramidal reactions with parenteral benztropine or diphenhydramine.

▶ Special considerations
Besides those relevant to all *phenothiazines*, consider the following recommendations.
- Administer the drug deep I.M. into a large muscle mass and rotate sites. Do not give I.V.
- Methotrimeprazine may be mixed in the same syringe with scopolamine or atropine; do not mix with other drugs.
- Monitor level of consciousness and vital signs frequently.
- Check blood pressure frequently when first starting the drug or increasing the dose; blood pressure will fall within 10 to 20 minutes after injection; fainting, weakness, or dizziness may occur.
- Patient should be in bed and observed closely for 6 to 12 hours after administration.
- As necessary, institute safety measures – for example, raised side rails – to prevent injury.
- Monitor complete blood count and liver function tests during long-term use.
- Do not administer methotrimeprazine for longer than 30 days.
- Store drug in a cool, dry place away from direct light.

Information for the patient
Tell patient drug may cause dizziness. Advise patient to stay in bed after drug administration, or to arise slowly, first to the sitting position, then pause before standing to prevent falls and injury.

Geriatric use
Elderly patients with cardiovascular disease are at greater risk of hypotension. Lower doses are indicated.

Pediatric use
Safe use in children under age 12 has not been established.

Breast-feeding
Safe use of methotrimeprazine in breast-feeding women has not been established.

---

methoxsalen
8-MOP, Oxsoralen, Oxsoralen-Ultra

- Pharmacologic classification: psoralen derivative
- Therapeutic classifications: pigmenting, antipsoriatic
- Pregnancy risk category C

How supplied
Available by prescription only
Capsules: 10 mg
Lotion: 1%

Indications, route, and dosage
Induce repigmentation in vitiligo
Adults and children over age 12: 20 mg P.O. 2 to 4 hours before measured periods of exposure to sunlight or ultraviolet light on alternate days. Alternatively, for small well-defined lesions, apply lotion 1 to 2 hours before exposure to ultraviolet light, no more than once weekly.
Psoriasis
Adults: 10 to 70 mg P.O. 1.5 to 2 hours before exposure to high intensity ultraviolet A light, 2 to 3 times weekly, at least 48 hours apart. Dosage is based upon patient's weight.

Pharmacodynamics
- *Pigmenting action:* The exact mechanism of action of methoxsalen is not known; it is dependent on the presence of functioning melanocytes and UV light. Methoxsalen may stimulate the enzymes that catalyze melanin precursors. Also, the inflammatory response generated may stimulate melanin production.
- *Antipsoriatic action:* Methoxsalen probably exerts its antipsoriatic effects by inhibiting DNA synthesis and decreasing cell proliferation. Cell-regulating, leukocyte, and vascular effects may also be involved in this action.

The oral dosage form produces greater erythemic and melanogenic effects, while the topical preparation causes a more intense photosensitizing response.

Pharmacokinetics
- *Absorption:* Following oral administration, methoxsalen is absorbed well but variably, with peak serum concentrations in 1½ to 3 hours. Food increases both absorption and peak concentration. The extent of topical absorption has not been determined. Skin sensitivity to UV light occurs in about 1 to 2 hours, reaches a maximum effect in 1 to 4 hours, and persists for 3 to 8 hours. Topical administration yields a UV sensitivity in 1 to 2 hours, which may persist for several days.
- *Distribution:* Methoxsalen is distributed throughout the body, with epidermal cells preferentially taking up the drug. It is 75% to 91% bound to serum proteins, most commonly albumin. Distribution across the placenta or in breast milk is unknown.

---

*Canada only   †Unlabeled clinical use   Italicized adverse reactions are life-threatening.

- *Metabolism:* Methoxsalen is activated by long-wavelength UV light and is metabolized in the liver.
- *Excretion:* Methoxsalen is excreted almost entirely as metabolites in the urine, with 80% to 90% eliminated within the first 8 hours.

Contraindications and precautions
Methoxsalen is contraindicated in patients hypersensitive to psoralens and in those with diseases associated with photosensitivity because of the drug's photosensitization. Do not use in patients with melanoma, history of melanoma, or invasive squamous cell carcinoma, because the drug may be a photocarcinogen. Oral methoxsalen is contraindicated in patients with aphakia, because increased retinal damage may occur.

Oxsoralen capsules contain tartarazine; therefore, use cautiously in patients with tartrazine or asprin sensitivity.

Interactions
Methoxsalen reacts with other photosensitizing drugs and foods including sulfonamides, tetracyclines, phenothiazines, thiazides, griseofulvin, nalidixic acid, trioxsalen, and coal tar products to yield an additive photosensitizing effect. The ingestion of foods such as carrots, limes, figs, celery, mustard, parsley, and parsnips should be avoided. These foods contain furocoumarin, which may cause an additive effect. No serious reactions have been reported with these foods, but caution should be exercised.

Effects on diagnostic tests
Abnormal liver function test results have been reported, but the exact relationship is unknown.

Adverse reactions
- CNS: dizziness, headache, depression, nervousness, trouble sleeping.
- DERM: burns, blistering, peeling, swelling of extremities, itching, erythema, photosensitivity.
- GI: nausea, abdominal discomfort, diarrhea.
- Other: *cataracts, toxic hepatitis,* leg cramps.
  Note: Drug should be discontinued if signs of overexposure to sunlight occur.

Overdose and treatment
Clinical manifestations of overdose include serious burning and blistering of skin, which may occur from overdose of drug or overexposure to UV light. Treat acute oral overdose with gastric lavage, which, however, is effective only in the first 2 to 3 hours. Place patient in a darkened room for 8 to 24 hours or until cutaneous reactions subside. Treat burns as necessary.

▶ **Special considerations**
- Wear gloves when applying lotion to patient.
- Temporary withdrawal of therapy is the recommended procedure in case of burning or blistering of the skin.
- Oxsoralen-Ultra should not be used interchangeably with regular Oxsoralen because it exhibits significantly greater bioavailability.
- The treatment regimen of psoralen and ultraviolet radiation in the range of 320 to 400 nm wavelength (UVA) is known as PUVA. Preleukemia and acute myeloid leukemia have been associated with PUVA therapy.
- Complete blood count with differential, antinuclear antibody, liver function, BUN, and creatinine tests should be performed at baseline and repeated every 6 months.
- Patient should wear UVA protective glasses for several hours after treatment.
- Periodic ophthalmologic exams are recommended during therapy.

Information for the patient
- Teach patient how and when to use product; tell patient to wear gloves to avoid photosensitization and possible burns. Stress adherence to correct dosage schedule. If a dose is missed, patient should not increase the next dose. If more than one dose is missed, a proportionately lower dose should be given when therapy is resumed.
- Advise taking with food and milk to reduce GI irritation and, possibly, increase absorption.
- Tell patient to use proper protective precautions, including sunglasses and sunscreens. However, sunscreens may be only partially effective. Tell patient to protect skin for 8 hours after oral administration.
- Explain that drug may take several months to work. Tell patient *not* to increase the dose or UV light exposure during this time.

Pediatric use
Use in children under age 12 is not recommended.

Breast-feeding
It is unknown whether methoxsalen is distributed in breast milk; therefore, the drug should be used cautiously in breast-feeding women.

---

methscopolamine bromide
Pamine

- Pharmacologic classification: anticholinergic
- Therapeutic classification: antimuscarinic, gastrointestinal antispasmodic
- Pregnancy risk category C

How supplied
Available by prescription only
Tablets: 2.5 mg

Indications, route, and dosage
Adjunctive therapy in peptic ulcer and irritable bowel syndrome
Adults: 2.5 to 5 mg P.O. ½ hour before meals and h.s.

Pharmacodynamics
Antiulcer action: Methscopolamine competitively blocks acetylcholine at cholinergic neuroeffector sites, inhibiting gastric acid secretion and decreasing GI motility.

Pharmacokinetics
- *Absorption:* Methscopolamine is poorly absorbed from the GI tract.
- *Distribution:* Largely unknown.
- *Metabolism:* Unknown.
- *Excretion:* Methscopolamine is believed to be excreted in the urine as metabolites and unchanged drug, and in the feces in large amounts as unabsorbed drug.

Contraindications and precautions

Methscopolamine is contraindicated in patients with narrow-angle glaucoma, because drug-induced cycloplegia and mydriasis may increase intraocular pressure; in patients with obstructive uropathy, obstructive GI tract disease, severe ulcerative colitis, myasthenia gravis, paralytic ileus, intestinal atony, or toxic megacolon, because the drug may exacerbate these conditions; and in patients with known hypersensitivity to anticholinergics or bromides.

Administer methscopolamine cautiously to patients with autonomic neuropathy, hyperthyroidism, coronary artery disease, cardiac arrhythmias, congestive heart failure, or ulcerative colitis, because the drug may exacerbate the symptoms of these disorders; to patients with hepatic or renal disease, because toxic accumulation may occur; to patients over age 40, because the drug increases the glaucoma risk; to patients with hiatal hernia associated with reflux esophagitis, because the drug may reduce lower esophageal sphincter tone; and in hot or humid environments, because the drug may predispose the patient to heatstroke.

Interactions

Concurrent administration of antacids decreases oral absorption of anticholinergics. Administer methscopolamine at least 1 hour before antacids.

Concomitant administration of drugs with anticholinergic effects may cause additive toxicity.

Decreased GI absorption of many drugs has been reported after the use of anticholinergics (for example, levodopa and ketoconazole). Conversely, slowly dissolving digoxin tablets may yield higher serum digoxin levels when administered with anticholinergics.

Use cautiously with oral potassium supplements (especially wax-matrix formulations) because the incidence of potassium-induced GI ulcerations may be increased.

Effects on diagnostic tests

None reported.

Adverse reactions

● CNS: headache, insomnia, drowsiness, dizziness, weakness, confusion or excitement (in elderly).
● CV: palpitations, tachycardia, orthostatic hypotension.
● DERM: urticaria, decreased sweating or anhidrosis, other dermal manifestations, iodine skin rash.
● EENT: blurred vision, mydriasis, cycloplegia, increased ocular tension, photophobia.
● GI: dry mouth, dysphagia, heartburn, loss of taste, nausea, constipation, vomiting, paralytic ileus, abdominal distention.
● GU: urinary hesitancy and retention, impotence.
● Other: fever, allergic reaction.
Note: Drug should be discontinued if hypersensitivity, urinary retention, confusion or excitement, curarelike symptoms, or skin rash occurs.

Overdose and treatment

Clinical signs of overdose include curare-like symptoms and such peripheral effects as headache; dilated, nonreactive pupils; blurred vision; flushed, hot, dry skin; dry mucous membranes; dysphagia; decreased or absent bowel sounds; urinary retention; hypothermia; tachycardia; hypertension; and increased respiration.

Treatment is primarily symptomatic and supportive, as needed. If patient is alert, induce emesis (or use

gastric lavage) and follow with a saline cathartic and activated charcoal to prevent further drug absorption. In severe cases, physostigmine may be administered to block methscopolamine's antimuscarinic effects. Give fluids, as needed, to treat shock. If urinary retention develops, catheterization may be necessary.

▶ Special considerations

Besides those relevant to all *anticholinergics*, consider the following recommendations.
● Methscopolamine should be titrated until the therapeutic effect is obtained or adverse effects become intolerable.
● Administer drug before meals and at bedtime.

Geriatric use

Administer methscopolamine cautiously to elderly patients. Lower doses are indicated.

Breast-feeding

Methscopolamine may be excreted in breast milk, possibly resulting in infant toxicity. Breast-feeding women should avoid this drug.

---

methsuximide
Celontin Half-Strength Kapseals, Celontin Kapseals

● Pharmacologic classification: succinimide derivative
● Therapeutic classification: anticonvulsant
● Pregnancy risk category C

How supplied

Available by prescription only
Capsules: 150 mg, 300 mg

Indications, route, and dosage
Refractory absence seizures
Adults and children: 10 mg/kg or 600 mg/m² P.O. daily. Maximum daily dosage is 1.2 g.

Pharmacodynamics
Anticonvulsant action: Methsuximide raises the seizure threshold; it suppresses characteristic spike-and-wave pattern by depressing neuronal transmission in the motor cortex and basal ganglia. It is indicated for absence (petit mal) seizures refractory to other drugs.

Pharmacokinetics
● *Absorption:* Methsuximide is absorbed from the GI tract; peak plasma concentrations occur in 1 to 4 hours.
● *Distribution:* Methsuximide is distributed widely throughout the body. Therapeutic plasma concentration levels appear to be 10 to 40 mcg/ml.
● *Metabolism:* Methsuximide is metabolized in the liver to several metabolites; N-demethyl methsuximide is a potent CNS depressant and may be the active metabolite.
● *Excretion:* Methsuximide is excreted in urine.

Contraindications and precautions
Methsuximide is contraindicated in patients with known hypersensitivity to succinimides; and in patients with mixed forms of epilepsy, because it may precipitate grand mal seizures.

Methsuximide should be used with caution in patients with hepatic or renal disease and in patients taking other CNS depressants or anticonvulsants. Abrupt withdrawal may precipitate petit mal seizures. Use of anticonvulsants during pregnancy has been associated with increased incidence of birth defects.

Interactions
Concomitant use of methsuximide with other CNS depressants (alcohol, narcotics, anxiolytics, antidepressants, antipsychotics, and other anticonvulsants) causes additive sedative and CNS depressant effects.

Effects on diagnostic tests
Methsuximide may elevate liver enzymes and cause abnormal renal function test results.

Adverse reactions
● CNS: drowsiness, ataxia, dizziness, irritability, nervousness, headache, insomnia, confusion, depression, aggressiveness, psychosis.
● DERM: urticaria, pruritic and erythematous rashes, *Stevens-Johnson syndrome*, systemic lupus erythematosus.
● EENT: blurred vision, photophobia, periorbital edema.
● GI: nausea, vomiting, anorexia, diarrhea, weight loss, abdominal or epigastric pain, constipation.
● HEMA: eosinophilia, leukopenia, monocytosis, pancytopenia.
Note: Drug should be discontinued if signs of hypersensitivity, rash or unusual skin lesions, or any of the following signs of blood dyscrasia occur: joint pain, fever, sore throat, or unusual bleeding or bruising.

Overdose and treatment
Symptoms of overdose may include dizziness and ataxia (beginning within 1 hour after overdose); condition may progress to stupor and coma.

Treat overdose supportively. Monitor vital signs and fluid and electrolyte balance carefully. Charcoal hemoperfusion or hemodialysis may be used for severe cases.

▶ Special considerations
Besides those relevant to all *succinimide derivatives*, consider the following recommendations.
● Methsuximide may be hemodialyzable. Dosage adjustments may be necessary in patients undergoing hemodialysis.
● Never change or withdraw drug suddenly. Abrupt withdrawal may precipitate petit mal seizures.
● Obtain CBC every 3 months; urinalysis and liver function tests every 6 months.
● Protect capsules from excessive heat (104° F. [40° C.]).

Information for the patient
● Tell patient to store capsules away from excessive heat and humidity to maintain effectiveness of drug. For example, tell patient not to store drug in the bathroom or in the glove compartment of a car.
● Warn patient not to use capsules that are not full or seem to have melted.
● Tell patient to take drug with milk or food if GI upset occurs.
● Tell patient to avoid alcoholic beverages.
● Warn patient not to discontinue medication abruptly or to change dosage unless prescribed.
● Advise patient to wear a Medic Alert necklace or bracelet indicating medication use and epilepsy.

● Tell patient to promptly report skin rash, pregnancy, sore throat, joint pains, unexplained fever, or unusual bleeding or bruising.
● Warn patient to avoid activities that require alertness and good psychomotor coordination until CNS response to drug has been determined.

methyclothiazide
Aquatensen, Enduron, Ethon

● Pharmacologic classification: thiazide diuretic
● Therapeutic classification: diuretic, antihypertensive
● Pregnancy risk category B

How supplied
Available by prescription only
Tablets: 2.5 mg, 5 mg

Indications, route, and dosage
Edema, hypertension
Adults: 2.5 to 10 mg P.O. daily.
Children: 0.05 to 0.2 mg/kg P.O. daily.

Pharmacodynamics
● *Diuretic action:* Methyclothiazide increases urinary excretion of sodium and water by inhibiting sodium reabsorption in the cortical diluting tubule of the nephron, thus relieving edema.
● *Antihypertensive action:* The exact mechanism of methyclothiazide's antihypertensive effect is unknown. It may partially result from direct arteriolar vasodilatation and a decrease in total peripheral resistance.

Pharmacokinetics
● *Absorption:* Methyclothiazide is absorbed rapidly from the GI tract.
● *Distribution:* Methyclothiazide is thought to be distributed into extracellular space.
● *Metabolism:* Insignificant.
● *Excretion:* Methyclothiazide is excreted unchanged in urine.

Contraindications and precautions
Methyclothiazide is contraindicated in patients with anuria and in those with known sensitivity to the drug or to other sulfonamide derivatives. Methyclothiazide should be used with caution in patients with severe renal disease because it may decrease glomerular filtration rate and precipitate azotemia; in patients with impaired hepatic function or liver disease because electrolyte changes may precipitate coma; and in patients taking digoxin, because hypokalemia may predispose them to digitalis toxicity.

Interactions
Methyclothiazide potentiates the hypotensive effects of most other antihypertensive drugs; this may be used to therapeutic advantage.

Methyclothiazide may potentiate hyperglycemic, hypotensive, and hyperuricemic effects of diazoxide, and its hyperglycemic effect may increase insulin or sulfonylurea requirements in diabetic patients.

Methyclothiazide may reduce renal clearance of lith-

---

ium, elevating serum lithium levels, and may necessitate a 50% reduction in lithium dosage.

Methyclothiazide turns urine slightly more alkaline and may decrease urinary excretion of some amines, such as amphetamine and quinidine; alkaline urine may also decrease therapeutic efficacy of methenamine compounds such as methenamine mandelate.

Cholestyramine and colestipol may bind methyclothiazide, preventing its absorption; give drugs 1 hour apart.

Effects on diagnostic tests
Methyclothiazide therapy may alter serum electrolyte levels and may increase serum urate, glucose, cholesterol, and triglyceride levels. It also may interfere with tests for parathyroid function and should be discontinued before such tests.

Adverse reactions
● CV: volume depletion and dehydration, orthostatic hypotension, hypercholesterolemia, hypertriglyceridemia.
● DERM: dermatitis, photosensitivity.
● GI: anorexia, nausea, pancreatitis.
● HEMA: aplastic anemia, agranulocytosis, leukopenia, thrombocytopenia.
● Hepatic: hepatic encephalopathy.
● Metabolic: asymptomatic hyperuricemia; gout; hyperglycemia and impairment of glucose tolerance; fluid and electrolyte imbalances, including hyponatremia, hypochloremia, hypokalemia, and hypercalcemia; metabolic alkalosis.
● Other: hypersensitivity reactions, such as pneumonitis and vasculitis.
Note: Drug should be discontinued if rising BUN and serum creatinine levels indicate renal impairment or if patient shows signs of impending coma.

Overdose and treatment
Clinical signs of overdose include GI irritation and hypermotility, diuresis, and lethargy, which may progress to coma.

Treatment is mainly supportive; monitor and assist respiratory, cardiovascular, and renal function as indicated. Monitor fluid and electrolyte balance. Induce vomiting with ipecac in conscious patient; otherwise, use gastric lavage to avoid aspiration. Do not give cathartics; these promote additional loss of fluids and electrolytes.

▶ Special considerations
Recommendations for use of methyclothiazide and for care and teaching of the patient during therapy are the same as those for all thiazide diuretics.

Geriatric use
Elderly and debilitated patients require close observation and may require reduced dosages. They are more sensitive to excess diuresis because of age-related changes in cardiovascular and renal function. Excess diuresis promotes orthostatic hypotension, dehydration, hypovolemia, hyponatremia, hypomagnesemia, and hypokalemia.

Breast-feeding
Methyclothiazide may be distributed in breast milk; its safety and effectiveness in breast-feeding women have not been established.

methylcellulose
Cellothyl, Citrucel, Cologel

● Pharmacologic classification: adsorbent
● Therapeutic classification: bulk-forming laxative
● Pregnancy risk category C

How supplied
Available without prescription
Powder: 105 mg/g

Indications, route, and dosage
Chronic constipation
Adults: 1 heaping tablespoon powder in 240 ml (8 oz) water daily to t.i.d.
Children age 6 to 12: 1 level tablespoon powder in 120 ml (4 oz) water daily to t.i.d.
Chronic diarrhea
Adults and children: 1 tablespoon powder in 80 ml (approximately 3 oz) water daily to t.i.d.

Pharmacodynamics
Laxative action: Methylcellulose adsorbs intestinal fluid and serves as a source of indigestible fiber, stimulating peristaltic activity.

Pharmacokinetics
● Absorption: Methylcellulose is not absorbed. Action begins in 12 to 24 hours, but full effect may not occur for 2 to 3 days.
● Distribution: Methylcellulose is distributed locally, in the intestine.
● Metabolism: None.
● Excretion: Methylcellulose is excreted in feces.

Contraindications and precautions
Methylcellulose is contraindicated in patients with abdominal pain, acute surgical abdomen, or intestinal obstruction or perforation, because the drug may exacerbate the symptoms of these conditions.

Interactions
When used concomitantly, methylcellulose may absorb oral medications; separate administration by at least 1 hour.

Effects on diagnostic tests
None reported.

Adverse reactions
● GI: abdominal cramps, diarrhea, nausea, vomiting, intestinal obstruction (if chewed or taken dry).
Note: Drug should be discontinued if abdominal pain occurs.

Overdose and treatment
No information available.

▶ Special considerations
● Administer drug with water or juice (at least 8 oz).
● Drug may absorb oral medications; schedule at least 1 hour apart from all other drugs.
● Bulk laxatives most closely mimic natural bowel function and do not promote laxative dependence.
● Methylcellulose is especially useful in patients with

postpartum constipation, chronic laxative abuse, irritable bowel syndrome, diverticular disease, or colostomies; in debilitated patients; and to empty colon before barium enema examinations.

Information for the patient
● Instruct patient to take other oral medications 1 hour before or after methylcellulose.
● Explain that the drug's full effect may not occur for 2 to 3 days.

Breast-feeding
Because methylcellulose is not absorbed, use probably poses no risk to breast-feeding infants.

---

methyldopa
Aldomet, Amodopa Tabs, Apo-Methyldopa*, Dopamet*, Novomedopa*

● Pharmacologic classification: centrally acting antiadrenergic agent
● Therapeutic classification: antihypertensive
● Pregnancy risk category C

How supplied
Available by prescription only
Tablets: 125 mg, 250 mg, 500 mg
Oral suspension: 250 mg/5 ml
Injection (as methyldopate hydrochloride): 250 mg/5 ml in 5-ml vials

Indications, route, and dosage
Moderate to severe hypertension (generally considered a Step 2 agent)
Adults: Initially, 250 mg P.O. b.i.d. to t.i.d. in first 48 hours, then increased or decreased as needed every 2 days. Entire daily dose may be given in the evening or at bedtime. Dosages may need adjustment if other antihypertensive drugs are added to or deleted from therapy.
Maintenance dose: 500 mg to 2 g daily in two to four divided doses. Maximum recommended daily dosage is 3 g. I.V. infusion dosage is 250 to 500 mg given over 30 to 60 minutes q 6 hours. Maximum I.V. dosage is 1 g q 6 hours.
Children: Initially, 10 mg/kg P.O. daily or 300 mg/m² P.O. daily in two to four divided doses; or 20 to 40 mg/kg I.V. daily or 0.6 to 1.2 g/m² I.V. daily in four divided doses. Increase dose at least every 2 days until desired response occurs. Maximum daily dosage is 65 mg/kg, 2 g/m², or 3 g, whichever is least.

Pharmacodynamics
Antihypertensive action: The exact mechanism of methyldopa's antihypertensive effect is unknown; it is thought to be caused by methyldopa's metabolite, alpha-methylnorepinephrine, which stimulates central inhibitory alpha-adrenergic receptors, decreasing total peripheral resistance; drug may also act as a false neurotransmitter.

Pharmacokinetics
● *Absorption:* Methyldopa is absorbed partially from the GI tract. Absorption varies, but usually about 50%

of an oral dose is absorbed. After oral administration, maximal decline in blood pressure occurs in 3 to 6 hours; however, full effect is not evident for 2 to 3 days. No correlation exists between plasma concentration and antihypertensive effect. After I.V. administration, blood pressure usually begins to fall in 4 to 6 hours.
● *Distribution:* Methyldopa is distributed throughout the body and is bound weakly to plasma proteins.
● *Metabolism:* Methyldopa is metabolized extensively in the liver and intestinal cells.
● *Excretion:* Methyldopa and its metabolites are excreted in urine; unabsorbed drug is excreted unchanged in feces. Elimination half-life is approximately 2 hours. Antihypertensive activity usually persists up to 24 hours after oral administration and 10 to 16 hours after I.V. administration.

Contraindications and precautions
Methyldopa is contraindicated in patients with known hypersensitivity to the drug and in patients with active hepatic disease, such as hepatitis or cirrhosis. Drug is also contraindicated in patients who developed hepatic dysfunction during previous methyldopa therapy; such patients may have impaired drug metabolism and may be predisposed to methyldopa-induced hepatic dysfunction.

Methyldopa should be used cautiously in patients taking diuretics and other antihypertensive drugs; in patients with renal failure, because accumulation of active metabolites may lead to prolonged hypotension; in patients with previous hepatic dysfunction, who may be predisposed to methyldopa-induced hepatic dysfunction; and in patients taking levodopa, because an additive antihypertensive effect may occur.

Interactions
Methyldopa may potentiate the antihypertensive effects of other antihypertensive agents and the pressor effects of sympathomimetic amines such as phenylpropanolamine.

Concomitant use with phenothiazines or tricyclic antidepressants may cause a reduction in antihypertensive effects; use with haloperidol may produce dementia and sedation; use with phenoxybenzamine may cause reversible urinary incontinence.

Fenfluramine and verapamil may potentiate the effects of methyldopa.

Methyldopa may impair tolbutamide metabolism, enhancing tolbutamide's hypoglycemic effect.

Patients undergoing surgery may require reduced dosages of anesthetics.

Effects on diagnostic tests
Methyldopa alters urine uric acid, serum creatinine, and AST (SGOT) levels; it may also cause falsely high levels of urine catecholamines, interfering with the diagnosis of pheochromocytoma. A positive direct antiglobulin (Coombs') test may also occur.

Adverse reactions
● CNS: sedation, headache, weakness, dizziness, decreased mental acuity, involuntary choreoathetoid movements, psychic disturbances, depression, nightmares.
● CV: bradycardia, orthostatic hypotension, aggravated angina, *myocarditis*, edema, weight gain.
● EENT: dry mouth, nasal stuffiness.
● GI: diarrhea, pancreatitis.

---

*Canada only   †Unlabeled clinical use   Italicized adverse reactions are life-threatening.

- HEMA: *hemolytic anemia*, reversible granulocytopenia, *thrombocytopenia*.
- Hepatic: *hepatic necrosis* (rare), abnormal liver function test results.
- Other: gynecomastia, lactation, rash, drug-induced fever, impotence.

Note: Drug should be discontinued if any of the following occur: abnormalities in liver function tests results, jaundice, positive Coombs' test, or choreoathetoid movements.

Overdose and treatment

Clinical signs of overdose include sedation, hypotension, impaired atrioventricular conduction, and coma. After recent (within 4 hours) ingestion, empty stomach by induced emesis or gastric lavage. Give activated charcoal to reduce absorption; then treat symptomatically and supportively. In severe cases, hemodialysis may be considered.

▶ Special considerations

- Patients with impaired renal function may require smaller maintenance dosages of the drug.
- Methyldopa hydrochloride is administered I.V.; I.M. or subcutaneous administration is not recommended because of unpredictable absorption.
- Patients receiving methyldopa may become hypertensive after dialysis because drug is dialyzable.
- At the initiation of, and periodically throughout therapy, monitor hemoglobin, hematocrit, and red blood cell count for hemolytic anemia; also monitor liver function tests.
- Take blood pressure in supine, sitting, and standing positions during dosage adjustment; take blood pressure at least every 30 minutes during I.V. infusion until patient is stable.
- Sedation and drowsiness usually disappear with continued therapy; bedtime dosage will minimize this effect. Orthostatic hypotension may indicate a need for dosage reduction.
- Monitor intake and output and daily weights to detect sodium and water retention; voided urine exposed to air may darken because of the breakdown of methyldopa or its metabolites.
- Tolerance may develop after 2 to 3 weeks.
- Signs of hepatotoxicity may occur 2 to 4 weeks after therapy begins.
- Monitor for signs and symptoms of drug-induced depression.

Information for the patient

- Teach patient signs and symptoms of adverse effects, such as "jerky" movements, and about the need to report them; patient should also report excessive weight gain (5 lb [2.25 kg] per week), signs of infection, or fever.
- Teach patient to minimize adverse effects by taking drug at bedtime until tolerance develops to sedation, drowsiness, and other CNS effects; by avoiding sudden position changes to minimize orthostatic hypotension; and by using ice chips, hard candy, or gum to relieve dry mouth.
- Warn patient to avoid hazardous activities that require mental alertness until sedative effects subside.
- Warn patient to call for instructions before taking nonprescription cold preparations.

Geriatric use

Dosage reductions may be necessary in elderly patients because they are more sensitive to sedation and hypotension.

Pediatric use

Safety and efficacy of methyldopa in children have not been established; use only if potential benefits outweigh risks.

Breast-feeding

Methyldopa is distributed into breast milk; an alternative feeding method is recommended during therapy.

---

methylene blue
Urolene Blue

- Pharmacologic classification: thiazine dye
- Therapeutic classification: urinary tract antiseptic, cyanide poisoning antidote, treatment of methemoglobinemia
- Pregnancy risk category C

How supplied

Available by prescription only
Tablets: 55 mg, 65 mg
Injection: 10 mg/ml

Indications, route, and dosage
Cystitis, urethritis, chronic urolithiasis
Adults: 55 mg to 130 mg P.O. t.i.d. after meals with glass of water.
Methemoglobinemia and cyanide poisoning
Adults and children: 1 to 2 mg/kg by slow I.V. infusion over several minutes. Dose may be repeated in 1 hour if necessary.
Chronic methemoglobinemia
Adults: 100 to 300 mg P.O. daily.

Pharmacodynamics

- *Urinary tract antiseptic action:* Methylene blue is a mildly antiseptic dye.
- *Cyanide poisoning antidote:* High concentrations convert the ferrous iron of reduced hemoglobin to ferric iron, forming methemoglobin. Methemoglobin forms a complex with cyanide, preventing cyanide's interference in cellular respiration; this permits drug's use as an antidote in cyanide poisoning. Low methylene blue concentrations can hasten methemoglobin's conversion to hemoglobin.

Pharmacokinetics

- *Absorption:* When administered orally, methylene blue is well absorbed from the GI tract.
- *Distribution:* Methylene blue distribution is unknown.
- *Metabolism:* Methylene blue is reduced to leukomethylene blue by the tissues.
- *Excretion:* Methylene blue is excreted in urine and bile; approximately 70% of oral dose is excreted in urine as leukomethylene blue.

Contraindications and precautions

Methylene blue is contraindicated in patients with renal insufficiency because drug accumulation may occur; in patients with glucose-6-phosphate dehydrogenase

(G6PD) deficiency because the drug may cause hemolysis; and in patients with known hypersensitivity to the drug.

Interactions
None reported.

Effects on diagnostic tests
Methemoglobinemia may occur during therapy with large I.V. doses of methylene blue.

Adverse reactions
● GI: nausea, vomiting, diarrhea.
● GU: dysuria, bladder irritation, urine discoloration (blue-green).
● HEMA: anemia (with long-term use).
● Other: fever (with high oral doses).
   Note: Drug should be discontinued if patient develops hypersensitivity reaction.

Overdose and treatment
Clinical effects of large I.V. doses include nausea, vomiting, abdominal pain, precordial pain, headache, dizziness, hypertension, profuse sweating, confusion, methemoglobinemia, and cyanosis. Large oral doses may cause fever.
   Treatment is supportive.

▶ Special considerations
● Monitor hemoglobin concentration for evidence of anemia, which may result from accelerated erythrocyte destruction.
● Monitor fluid intake and output. Maintain intake of at least 2,000 ml daily.
● Necrotic abscess may develop if drug is injected subcutaneously or if extravasation occurs.
● Drug is rarely used as urinary tract antiseptic because more effective agents are available.
● Drug, a dye, is occasionally used to diagnose gastroesophageal reflux.
● Skin stains may be removed with hypochlorite solutions.

Information for the patient
● Warn patient that drug turns urine and stool blue-green.
● Instruct patient to take drug after meals with glass of water.

methylergonovine maleate
Methergine

● Pharmacologic classification: ergot alkaloid
● Therapeutic classification: oxytocic

How supplied
Available by prescription only
Tablets: 0.2 mg
Injection: 0.2 mg/ml ampule

Indications, route, and dosage
Prevent and treat postpartum hemorrhage due to uterine atony or subinvolution
Adults: 0.2 mg I.M. or I.V. q 2 to 4 hours for maximum of 5 doses. Following initial I.M. or I.V. dose, may give

0.2 to 0.4 mg P.O. q 6 to 12 hours for 2 to 7 days. Decrease dose if severe cramping occurs.

Pharmacodynamics
Oxytocic action: Methylergonovine maleate stimulates contractions of uterine and vascular smooth muscle. The intense uterine contractions are followed by periods of relaxation. The drug produces vasoconstriction primarily of capacitance blood vessels, causing increased central venous pressure and elevated blood pressure. The drug increases the amplitude and frequency of uterine contractions and tone, which therefore impedes uterine blood flow.

Pharmacokinetics
● *Absorption:* Absorption is rapid, with 60% of an oral dose appearing in the bloodstream. Peak plasma concentrations occur in approximately 3 hours. Onset of action is immediate for I.V., 2 to 5 minutes for I.M., and 5 to 15 minutes for oral doses.
● *Distribution:* The distribution of this drug is not fully known.
● *Metabolism:* Extensive first-pass metabolism precedes hepatic metabolism.
● *Excretion:* The drug is excreted primarily in the feces, with a small amount in urine.

Contraindications and precautions
Drug is contraindicated in patients sensitive to ergot preparations and in threatened spontaneous abortion, induction of labor, and before delivery of placenta. Use cautiously in patients with hypertension, sepsis, obliterative vascular disease, and hepatic, renal, and cardiac disease, because of the potential for adverse cardiovascular effects.

Interactions
Methylergonovine maleate enhances the vasoconstrictor potential of other ergot alkaloids and sympathomimetic amines. Combined use of local anesthetics with vasoconstrictors (lidocaine with epinephrine) or smoking (nicotine) will enhance vasoconstriction.

Effects on diagnostic tests
Methylergonovine maleate therapy may decrease serum prolactin concentrations.

Adverse reactions
● CNS: headache, confusion, dizziness, ringing in ears.
● CV: chest pain, weakness in legs (peripheral vasospasm), hypertension, palpitations.
● GI: nausea, vomiting, diarrhea, cramping.
● Respiratory: shortness of breath.
● Other: itching; sweating; pain in arms, legs, or lower back; hypersensitivity.
   Note: Drug should be discontinued if hypertension or allergic reactions occur.

Overdose and treatment
Clinical manifestations of overdose include seizures and gangrene, with nausea, vomiting, diarrhea, dizziness, fluctuations in blood pressure, weak pulse, chest pain, tingling, and numbness and coldness in extremities. Treatment of oral overdose requires that the patient drink tap water, milk, or vegetable oil to delay absorption, then follow with gastric lavage or emesis, then activated charcoal and cathartics. Treat seizures with anticonvulsants and hypercoagulability with heparin;

use vasodilators to improve blood flow as required. Gangrene may require surgical amputation.

▶ **Special considerations**
● Contractions begin 5 to 15 minutes after P.O. administration, 2 to 5 minutes after I.M. injection, and immediately following I.V. injection; continue 3 hours or more after P.O. or I.M. administration, 45 minutes after I.V.
● Monitor blood pressure, pulse rate, and uterine response; watch for sudden change in vital signs or frequent periods of uterine relaxation, and character and amount of vaginal bleeding.
● High doses during delivery may also cause uterine tetany and possible infant hypoxia or intracranial hemorrhage.
● Store tablets in tightly closed, light-resistant containers. Discard if discolored.
● Store I.V. solutions below 46.4° F. (8° C.). Daily stock may be kept at room temperature for 60 to 90 days.

Information for the patient
● Advise patient not to smoke while taking this medication.
● Advise patient of adverse reactions.

Breast-feeding
Ergot alkaloids inhibit lactation. Drug is excreted in breast milk, and ergotism has been reported in breast-fed infants.

methylphenidate hydrochloride
Methidate, Ritalin, Ritalin SR

● Pharmacologic classification: piperidine CNS stimulant
● Therapeutic classification: CNS stimulant (analeptic)
● Controlled substance schedule II
● Pregnancy risk category C

How supplied
Available by prescription only
Tablets: 5 mg, 10 mg, 20 mg
Tablets (sustained-release): 20 mg

Indications, route, and dosage
Attention deficit disorder with hyperactivity (ADDH)
Children age 6 and older: Initially, 5 to 10 mg P.O. daily before breakfast and lunch, with 5- to 10-mg increments weekly as needed until an optimum daily dosage of 2 mg/kg is reached, not to exceed 60 mg/day. The usual effective dosage is 10 to 20 mg/day.
Narcolepsy
Adults: 10 mg P.O. b.i.d. or t.i.d. ½ hour before meals. Dosage varies with patient needs, average dose is 20 to 30 mg/day (dosage range 5 to 60 mg/day).

Pharmacodynamics
Analeptic action: The cerebral cortex and reticular activating system appear to be the primary sites of activity; methylphenidate releases nerve terminal stores of norepinephrine, promoting nerve impulse transmission. At high doses, effects are mediated by dopamine.
Methylphenidate is used to treat narcolepsy and as

an adjunctive to psychosocial measures in ADDH. Like amphetamine, it has a paradoxical calming effect in hyperactive children.

Pharmacokinetics
● *Absorption:* Methylphenidate is absorbed rapidly and completely after oral administration; peak plasma concentrations occur at 1 to 2 hours. Duration of action is usually 4 to 6 hours (with considerable individual variation); sustained-release tablets may act for up to 8 hours.
● *Distribution:* Unknown.
● *Metabolism:* Methylphenidate is metabolized by the liver.
● *Excretion:* Methylphenidate is excreted in urine.

Contraindications and precautions
Methylphenidate is contraindicated in patients with known hypersensitivity to sympathomimetic amines; in patients with symptomatic cardiovascular disease, hyperthyroidism, angina pectoris, moderate to severe hypertension, or advanced arteriosclerosis because it may cause dangerous arrhythmias and blood pressure changes; in patients with severe exogenous or endogenous depression, glaucoma, parkinsonism, or agitated states; in patients with a history of marked anxiety, tension, or agitation because it can exacerbate such conditions; or in patients with a history of substance abuse.
Methylphenidate should be used with caution in patients with a history of diabetes mellitus, cardiovascular disease, motor tics, seizures, or Gilles de la Tourette's syndrome (drug may precipitate disorder); and in elderly, debilitated, or hyperexcitable patients.

Interactions
Concomitant use with caffeine may decrease efficacy of methylphenidate in ADDH; use with monoamine oxidase (MAO) inhibitors (or drugs with MAO-inhibiting activity) or within 14 days of such therapy may cause severe hypertension.
Methylphenidate may inhibit metabolism and increase the serum levels of anticonvulsants (phenytoin, phenobarbital, primidone), coumarin anticoagulants, phenylbutazone, and tricyclic antidepressants; it also may decrease the hypotensive effects of guanethidine and bretylium.
Caffeine may enhance methylphenidate's CNS stimulant effects. Avoid concomitant use.

Effects on diagnostic tests
None reported.

Adverse reactions
● CNS: nervousness, insomnia, dizziness, headache, akathisia, dyskinesia, Gilles de la Tourette's syndrome, psychotic episodes.
● CV: palpitations, angina, tachycardia, changes in blood pressure and pulse rate, arrhythmias.
● DERM: rash, urticaria, *exfoliative dermatitis*, erythema multiforme.
● EENT: difficulty with accommodation, blurring of vision.
● GI: nausea, dry throat, abdominal pain, anorexia, weight loss.
● Other: growth suppression, tolerance, physical and psychological dependence.
Note: Drug should be discontinued if signs of hy-

persensitivity or seizures occur or if no improvement is noticed within 1 month at maintenance dosage level.

Overdose and treatment

Symptoms of overdose may include euphoria, confusion, delirium, coma, toxic psychosis, agitation, headache, vomiting, dry mouth, mydriasis, self-injury, fever, diaphoresis, tremors, hyperreflexia, muscle twitching, seizures, flushing, hypertension, tachycardia, palpitations, and arrhythmias.

Treat overdose symptomatically and supportively: use gastric lavage or emesis in patients with intact gag reflex. Maintain airway and circulation. Closely monitor vital signs and fluid and electrolyte balance. Maintain patient in cool room, monitor temperature, minimize external stimulation, and protect him against self-injury. External cooling blankets may be needed.

▶ Special considerations

● Methylphenidate is the drug of choice for ADDH. Therapy is usually discontinued after puberty.
● Monitor initiation of therapy closely; drug may precipitate Gilles de la Tourette's syndrome.
● If paradoxical aggravation of symptoms occurs during therapy, reduce dosage or discontinue drug.
● Check vital signs regularly for increased blood pressure or other signs of excessive stimulation; avoid late-day or evening dosing, especially of long-acting dosage forms, to minimize insomnia.
● Monitor blood and urine glucose levels in diabetic patients; drug may alter insulin requirements.
● Drug may decrease seizure threshold in seizure disorders.
● Monitor complete blood count, differential, and platelet counts when patient is taking drug long-term.
● Intermittent drug-free periods when stress is least evident (weekends, school holidays) may help prevent development of tolerance and permit decreased dosage when drug is resumed. Sustained-release form allows convenience of single, at-home dosing for school children.
● Drug has abuse potential; discourage use to combat fatigue. Some abusers dissolve tablets and inject drug.
● After high-dose and long-term use, abrupt withdrawal may unmask severe depression. Lower dosage gradually to prevent acute rebound depression.
● Methylphenidate impairs ability to perform tasks requiring mental alertness.
● Be sure patient obtains adequate rest; fatigue may result as drug wears off.
● Monitor height and weight; drug has been associated with growth suppression.
● Discourage methylphenidate use for analeptic effect; CNS stimulation superimposed on CNS depression may cause neuronal instability and seizures.

Information for the patient

● Explain rationale for therapy and the risks and benefits that may be anticipated.
● Tell patient to avoid drinks containing caffeine to prevent added CNS stimulation and not to alter dosage unless prescribed.
● Advise narcoleptic patient to take first dose on awakening; advise ADDH patient to take last dose several hours before bedtime to avoid insomnia.
● Tell patient not to chew or crush sustained-release dosage forms.
● Warn patient not to use drug to mask fatigue, to be sure to obtain adequate rest, and to call if excessive CNS stimulation occurs.
● Advise diabetic patients to monitor blood glucose levels, as drug may alter insulin needs.
● Advise patient to avoid hazardous activities that require mental alertness until degree of sedative effect is determined.

Pediatric use
Methylphenidate is not recommended for ADDH in children under age 6. Drug has been associated with growth suppression; all patients should be monitored.

---

methylprednisolone (systemic)
Medrol, Medrone*

methylprednisolone acetate
dep-Medalone, Depoject, Depo-Medrone*, Depo-Medrol, Depopred, Depo-Predate, Duralone, Durameth, Medralone, Medrone, M-Prednisol, Rep-Pred

methylprednisolone sodium succinate
A-methaPred, Solu-Medrane*, Solu-Medrol

● Pharmacologic classification: glucocorticoid
● Therapeutic classification: anti-inflammatory, immunosuppressant
● Pregnancy risk category C

How supplied
Available by prescription only
Methylprednisolone
Tablets: 2 mg, 4 mg, 8 mg, 16 mg, 24 mg, 32 mg
Methylprednisolone acetate
Injection: 20 mg/ml, 40 mg/ml, 80 mg/ml suspension
Methylprednisolone sodium succinate
Injection: 40 mg, 125 mg, 500 mg, 1,000 mg, 2,000 mg/vial

Indications, route, and dosage
Severe inflammation or immunosuppression
Adults: 4 to 48 mg P.O. daily in a single dose or in divided doses.
Children: 117 mcg/kg/day to 1.66 mg/kg/day P.O. in three or four divided doses.
Methylprednisolone acetate
Adults: 10 to 80 mg I.M. daily; or 4 to 80 mg into joints and soft tissue p.r.n. q 1 to 5 weeks; or 20 to 60 mg intralesionally.
Children: 117 mcg/kg I.M. q 3 days; or 140 to 835 mcg/kg I.M. q 12 to 24 hours.
Methylprednisolone sodium succinate
Adults: 10 to 250 mg I.M. or I.V. q 4 hours.
Children: 0.03 to 0.2 mg/kg or 1 to 6.25 mg/m² I.M. or I.V. daily in divided doses.
Shock
Methylprednisolone sodium succinate
Adults: 100 to 250 mg I.V. at 2- to 6-hour intervals.
Children: 0.03 to 0.2 mg/kg or 1 to 6.25 mg/m² I.M. or I.V. daily in divided doses.

Pharmacodynamics

Anti-inflammatory action: Methylprednisolone stimulates the synthesis of enzymes needed to decrease the inflammatory response. It suppresses the immune system by reducing activity and volume of the lymphatic system, thus producing lymphocytopenia (primarily of T-lymphocytes), decreasing immunoglobulin and complement concentrations, decreasing passage of immune complexes through basement membranes, and possibly by depressing reactivity of tissue to antigen-antibody interactions.

Methylprednisolone is an intermediate-acting glucocorticoid. It has essentially no mineralocorticoid activity but is a potent glucocorticoid, with five times the potency of an equal weight of hydrocortisone. It is used primarily as an anti-inflammatory agent and immunosuppressant.

Methylprednisolone may be administered orally. Methylprednisolone sodium succinate may be administered by I.M. or I.V. injection or by I.V. infusion, usually at 4- to 6-hour intervals. Methylprednisolone acetate suspension may be administered by intra-articular, intrasynovial, intrabursal, intralesional, or soft tissue injection. It has a slow onset but a long duration of action. The injectable forms are usually used only when the oral dosage forms cannot be used.

Pharmacokinetics

● *Absorption:* Methylprednisolone is absorbed readily after oral administration. After oral and I.V. administration, peak effects occur in about 1 to 2 hours. The acetate suspension for injection has a variable absorption over 24 to 48 hours, depending on whether it is injected into an intra-articular space or a muscle, and on the blood supply to that muscle.
● *Distribution:* Methylprednisolone is distributed rapidly to muscle, liver, skin, intestines, and kidneys. Adrenocorticoids are distributed into breast milk and through the placenta.
● *Metabolism:* Methylprednisolone is metabolized in the liver to inactive glucuronide and sulfate metabolites.
● *Excretion:* The inactive metabolites and small amounts of unmetabolized drug are excreted by the kidneys. Insignificant quantities of drug are excreted in feces. The biological half-life of methylprednisolone is 18 to 36 hours.

Contraindications and precautions

Methylprednisolone is contraindicated in patients with hypersensitivity to ingredients of adrenocorticoid preparations, and in those with systemic fungal infections (except in adrenal insufficiency). Patients who are receiving methylprednisolone should not be given live virus vaccines because methylprednisolone suppresses the immune response.

Methylprednisolone should be used with extreme caution in patients with GI ulceration, renal disease, hypertension, osteoporosis, diabetes mellitus, thromboembolic disorders, seizures, myasthenia gravis, congestive heart failure (CHF), tuberculosis, hypoalbuminemia, hypothyroidism, cirrhosis of the liver, emotional instability, psychotic tendencies, hyperlipidemias, glaucoma, or cataracts, because the drug may exacerbate these conditions.

Because adrenocorticoids increase the susceptibility to and mask symptoms of infection, methylprednisolone should not be used (except in life-threatening situations) in patients with viral or bacterial infections not controlled by anti-infective agents.

Interactions

When used concomitantly, adrenocorticoids may decrease the effects of oral anticoagulants by unknown mechanisms.

Glucocorticoids increase the metabolism of isoniazid and salicylates; cause hyperglycemia, requiring dosage adjustment of insulin or oral hypoglycemic agents in diabetic patients; and may enhance hypokalemia associated with diuretic or amphotericin B therapy. The hypokalemia may increase the risk of toxicity in patients concurrently receiving digitalis glycosides.

Barbiturates, phenytoin, and rifampin may cause decreased corticosteroid effects because of increased hepatic metabolism. Cholestyramine, colestipol, and antacids decrease the corticosteroid effect by adsorbing the corticosteroid, decreasing the amount absorbed.

Concomitant use with estrogens may reduce the metabolism of corticosteroids by increasing the concentration of transcortin. The half-life of the corticosteroid is then prolonged because of increased protein binding. Concomitant administration of ulcerogenic drugs such as nonsteroidal anti-inflammatory agents may increase the risk of GI ulceration.

Effects on diagnostic tests

Methylprednisolone suppresses reactions to skin tests; causes false-negative results in the nitroblue tetrazolium test for systemic bacterial infections; decreases ^{131}I uptake and protein-bound iodine concentrations in thyroid function tests; may increase glucose and cholesterol levels; may decrease serum potassium, calcium, thyroxine, and triiodothyronine levels; and may increase urine glucose and calcium levels.

Adverse reactions

When administered in high doses or for prolonged therapy, methylprednisolone suppresses release of adrenocorticotropic hormone (ACTH) from the pituitary gland; in turn, the adrenal cortex stops secreting endogenous corticosteroids. The degree and duration of hypothalamic-pituitary-adrenal (HPA) axis suppression produced by the drug is highly variable among patients and depends on the dose, frequency and time of administration, and duration of glucocorticoid therapy.
● CNS: euphoria, insomnia, headache, psychotic behavior, pseudotumor cerebri, mental changes, nervousness, restlessness.
● CV: CHF, hypertension, edema.
● DERM: delayed healing, acne, skin eruptions, striae.
● EENT: cataracts, glaucoma, thrush.
● GI: peptic ulcer, irritation, increased appetite.
● Immune: immunosuppression, increased susceptibility to infection.
● Metabolic: hypokalemia, sodium retention, fluid retention, weight gain, hyperglycemia, osteoporosis, growth suppression in children.
● Musculoskeletal: muscle atrophy, weakness.
● Other: pancreatitis, hirsutism, cushingoid symptoms, withdrawal syndrome (nausea, fatigue, anorexia, dyspnea, hypotension, hypoglycemia, myalgia, arthralgia, fever, dizziness, and fainting). *Sudden withdrawal may be fatal or may exacerbate the underlying disease.* Acute adrenal insufficiency may occur with increased stress (infection, surgery, trauma) or abrupt withdrawal after long-term therapy.

Overdose and treatment

Acute ingestion, even in massive doses, is rarely a clinical problem. Toxic signs and symptoms rarely occur if drug is used for less than 3 weeks, even at large doses. However, chronic use causes adverse physiologic effects, including suppression of the HPA axis, cushingoid appearance, muscle weakness, and osteoporosis.

▶ Special considerations

Recommendations for use of methylprednisolone and for care and teaching of patients during therapy are the same as those for all *systemic adrenocorticoids.*

Pediatric use

Chronic use of adrenocorticoids in children and adolescents may delay growth and maturation.

---

methylprednisolone acetate (topical)
Medrol

- Pharmacologic classification: adrenocorticoid
- Therapeutic classification: anti-inflammatory
- Pregnancy risk category C

How supplied

Available by prescription only
Ointment: 0.25%, 1%
Powder (for enema): 40 mg

Indications, route, and dosage
Inflammation of corticosteroid-responsive dermatoses

Adults and children: Apply ointment sparingly in a thin film once daily to q.i.d. (Occlusive dressings may be used for severe or resistant dermatoses.) Rub gently into affected area.
Adjunctive treatment of mild to moderate acute ulcerative colitis

Adults: Rectally, as a retention enema or continuous drip three to seven times a week for 2 weeks or more.

Pharmacodynamics

Anti-inflammatory action: Methylprednisolone acetate stimulates the synthesis of enzymes needed to decrease the inflammatory response. Topical methylprednisolone ointment is classified as a group VI potency corticosteroid.

Pharmacokinetics

- *Absorption:* Methylprednisolone absorption depends on the potency of the preparation, the amount applied, and the nature of the skin at the application site. It ranges from about 1% in areas with a thick stratum corneum (such as the palms, soles, elbows, and knees) to as high as 36% in areas of the thinnest stratum corneum (face, eyelids, and genitals). Absorption increases in areas of skin damage, inflammation, or occlusion. Some systemic absorption of topical steroids occurs, especially through the oral mucosa.
- *Distribution:* After topical application, methylprednisolone is distributed throughout the local skin. Any drug absorbed into circulation is distributed rapidly into muscle, liver, skin, intestines, and kidneys.
- *Metabolism:* After topical administration, methylprednisolone is metabolized primarily in the skin. The small amount that is absorbed into systemic circulation is metabolized primarily in the liver to inactive compounds.
- *Excretion:* Inactive metabolites are excreted by the kidneys, primarily as glucuronides and sulfates, but also as unconjugated products. Small amounts of the metabolites are also excreted in feces.

Contraindications and precautions

Methylprednisolone is contraindicated in patients who are hypersensitive to any component of the preparation and in patients with viral, fungal, or tubercular skin lesions.

Drug should be used with extreme caution in patients with impaired circulation because it may increase the risk of skin ulceration.

Interactions

None significant.

Effects on diagnostic tests

None significant.

Adverse reactions

- Local: burning, itching, irritation, dryness, folliculitis, hypertrichosis, acneiform eruptions, hypopigmentation, perioral dermatitis, allergic contact dermatitis, maceration, secondary infection, atrophy, striae, miliaria.

Significant systemic absorption may produce the following effects.
- CNS: euphoria, insomnia, headache, psychotic behavior, pseudotumor cerebri, mental changes, nervousness, restlessness.
- CV: congestive heart failure, hypertension, edema.
- EENT: cataracts, glaucoma, thrush.
- GI: peptic ulcer, irritation, increased appetite.
- Immune: increased susceptibility to infection.
- Musculoskeletal: muscle atrophy.
- Other: hypokalemia, sodium retention, fluid retention, weight gain, hyperglycemia, osteoporosis, growth suppression in children, withdrawal syndrome (nausea, fatigue, anorexia, dyspnea, hypotension, hypoglycemia, myalgia, arthralgia, fever, dizziness, and fainting).

Note: Drug should be discontinued if local irritation, infection, systemic absorption, or hypersensitivity reaction occurs.

Overdose and treatment

No information available.

▶ Special considerations

Recommendations for use of methylprednisolone acetate, for care and teaching of patients during therapy, and for use in elderly patients, children, and breastfeeding women are the same as those for all *topical adrenocorticoids.*

---

methyltestosterone
Android 5, Android 10, Android 25, Metandren, Metandren Linguets, Oreton-Methyl, Testred, Virilon

- Pharmacologic classification: androgen
- Therapeutic classification: androgen replacement
- Controlled substance schedule III
- Pregnancy risk category X

How supplied
Available by prescription only
Tablets: 10 mg, 25 mg
Buccal tablets: 5 mg, 10 mg
Capsules: 10 mg

Indications, route, and dosage
Prevention of postpartum breast engorgement and pain
Adults: 80 mg P.O. daily, or 40 mg buccal daily for 3 to 5 days.
Breast cancer in women
Adults: 50 to 200 mg P.O. daily, or 25 to 100 mg buccal daily.
Male hypogonadism
Adults and adolescents: 10 to 50 mg P.O. daily, or 5 to 25 mg buccal daily.
Postpubertal cryptorchidism
Adults: 30 mg P.O. daily, or 15 mg buccal daily.

Pharmacodynamics
Androgenic action: Methyltestosterone mimics the action of the endogenous androgen testosterone by stimulating receptors in androgen-responsive organs and tissues. It exerts inhibitory, antiestrogenic effects on hormone-responsive breast tumors and metastases.

Pharmacokinetics
Methyltestosterone is eliminated primarily by hepatic metabolism. Its pharmacokinetics are otherwise poorly described.

Contraindications and precautions
Methyltestosterone is contraindicated in patients with known sensitivity to the drug; and in patients with severe renal or cardiac disease, which may be aggravated by fluid and electrolyte retention caused by this drug; in patients with hepatic disease because impaired elimination may cause toxic accumulation of drug; in male patients with prostatic or breast cancer or benign prostatic hypertrophy with obstruction because this drug can stimulate the growth of cancerous breast or prostate tissue in males; in pregnant and breast-feeding women because animal studies have shown that administration of androgens during pregnancy causes masculinization of the fetus; and in patients with undiagnosed abnormal genital bleeding, as this drug can stimulate the growth of malignant neoplasms. Metandren 10 mg linguets and 25 mg tablets contain tartrazine which may cause allergic reactions in sensitive patients. Use with caution.

Interactions
In patients with diabetes, decreased blood glucose levels may require adjustment of insulin or oral hypoglycemic drug dosage.

Methyltestosterone may potentiate the effects of warfarin-type anticoagulants, resulting in increased prothrombin time. Use with adrenocorticosteroids or ACTH increases potential for fluid and electrolyte accumulation. Concurrent administration with oxyphenbutazone may increase serum oxyphenbutazone concentrations.

Effects on diagnostic tests
Methyltestosterone may cause abnormal results of fasting plasma glucose (FBS), glucose tolerance (GTT), and metyrapone tests. Sulfobromophthalein (BSP) retention may be increased. Thyroid function test results (protein-bound iodine, radioactive iodine uptake, thyroid-binding capacity) and 17-ketosteroid levels may decrease. Liver function test results, prothrombin time (especially in patients on anticoagulant therapy), and serum creatinine may be elevated. Because of this agent's anabolic activity, serum sodium, potassium, calcium, phosphate, and cholesterol levels may all rise.

Adverse reactions
- Androgenic: *in females:* deepening of voice, clitoral enlargement, changes in libido; *in males:* prepubertal – premature epiphyseal closure, priapism, phallic enlargement; postpubertal – testicular atrophy, oligospermia, decreased ejaculatory volume, impotence, gynecomastia, epididymitis.
- CNS: headache, anxiety, mental depression, generalized paresthesia.
- CV: edema.
- DERM: acne, oily skin, hirsutism, flushing, sweating, male pattern baldness.
- GI: gastroenteritis, constipation, nausea, vomiting, diarrhea, change in appetite, weight gain.
- GU: bladder irritability, vaginitis, menstrual irregularities.
- HEMA: polycythemia, suppression of clotting factors II, V, VII, and X.
- Hepatic: cholestatic hepatitis or jaundice.
- Local: irritation of oral mucosa with buccal administration.
- Other: hypercalcemia, *hepatocellular cancer* (long-term use), anaphylactoid reactions (rare).
Note: Drug should be discontinued if hypercalcemia, edema, hypersensitivity reaction, priapism, or excessive sexual stimulation occurs, or if virilization occurs in females.

Overdose and treatment
No information available.

▶ Special considerations
Besides those relevant to all *androgens,* consider the following recommendations.
- Carefully observe female patients for signs of excessive virilization. If possible, discontinue therapy at the first sign of virilization because some adverse effects (deepening of the voice, clitoral enlargement) are irreversible.
- Observe for signs and symptoms of hypoglycemia in patients with diabetes, and for signs and symptoms of bleeding such as ecchymoses or petechiae in patients receiving oral anticoagulants.

Information for the patient
● Tell patient to place buccal tablets in upper or lower buccal pouch between cheek and gum and to allow 30 to 60 minutes to dissolve. The patient should never chew or swallow the tablets, and should change tablet absorption site with each buccal dose to minimize risk of buccal irritation.
● Advise patient not to eat, drink, chew, or smoke while buccal tablet is in place. Patient should rinse mouth with water after use of buccal tablets.
● Tell patient to report inflamed or painful oral membranes or any discomfort. Emphasize good oral hygiene.
● Advise patient to report signs and symptoms of virilization (in females), too frequent or persistent erections (in males), or GI distress immediately.

Geriatric use
Observe elderly male patients for the development of prostatic hypertrophy. Development of prostatic hypertrophy or prostatic carcinoma mandates discontinuing the drug.

Pediatric use
Use with extreme caution in children to avoid precocious puberty and premature closure of the epiphyses. X-ray examinations every 6 months are recommended to assess skeletal maturation.

Breast-feeding
Methyltestosterone is contraindicated in breast-feeding women.

---

methyprylon
Noludar

- Pharmacologic classification: piperidine-dione derivative
- Therapeutic classification: sedative-hypnotic
- Controlled substance schedule III
- Pregnancy risk category B

How supplied
Available by prescription only
Tablets: 50 mg, 200 mg
Capsules: 300 mg

Indications, route, and dosage
Insomnia
Adults: 200 to 400 mg P.O. 15 minutes before bedtime.
Children over age 12: 50 mg P.O. h.s., increased to 200 mg, if necessary. Maximum dosage is 400 mg/day.

Pharmacodynamics
Hypnotic action: The cellular mechanism(s) of action of methyprylon is not known. Methyprylon increases the threshold of the arousal centers in the brain in a manner similar to the barbiturates. The drug causes nonspecific CNS depression.

Pharmacokinetics
● *Absorption:* Methyprylon is absorbed rapidly and completely after oral administration. Peak concentrations after a single 650-mg dose are 5.7 to 10 mg/dl

and occur in 1 to 2 hours. A concentration of 10 mg/dl is considered therapeutic. Action begins in about 1 hour.
● *Distribution:* Very little is known about the distribution of methyprylon; it is approximately 60% protein-bound.
● *Metabolism:* Methyprylon is metabolized in the liver to inactive metabolites, which are excreted in the bile and reabsorbed.
● *Excretion:* Inactive metabolites of methyprylon are excreted in urine. Less than 3% is excreted unchanged. Methyprylon's half-life is 3 to 6 hours. The duration of sleep produced is 5 to 8 hours.

Contraindications and precautions
Methyprylon is contraindicated in patients with known hypersensitivity to the drug or those with intermittent porphyria. Drug should be used cautiously in patients with hepatic or renal failure, which may result in impaired elimination.

Use caution when long-term therapy is being considered in patients with low platelet or white blood cell counts, because drug may cause further depressions of blood count.

Use cautiously in patients with a history of mental depression, suicidal ideation or drug abuse.

Interactions
Methyprylon may add to or potentiate the effects of alcohol, barbiturates, antihistamines, tranquilizers, narcotics, benzodiazepines, and other CNS depressants.

Effects on diagnostic tests
Methyprylon may interfere with urinary steroid determination (17-ketosteroid determinations using Holtorff Koch modification of the Zimmerman reaction and 17-hydroxycorticosteroids using the modified Glenn-Nelson technique).

Adverse reactions
● CNS: morning drowsiness, dizziness, vertigo, ataxia, pyrexia, headache, paradoxical excitation, nightmares, depression, confusion.
● CV: hypotension, syncope.
● DERM: rash, pruritus.
● EENT: diplopia, blurred vision.
● GI: esophagitis, vomiting, nausea, diarrhea, constipation.
● HEMA: *aplastic anemia,* thrombocytopenic purpura, neutropenia.
● Other: cholestatic jaundice.
  Note: Drug should be discontinued if hypersensitivity, paradoxical excitation, or acute organic brain syndrome occur or if platelet or neutrophil counts decline.

Overdose and treatment
Clinical manifestations of overdose include somnolence, confusion, coma, hypotension, shock, tachycardia, constricted pupils, edema, and respiratory depression.

Support respiration and cardiovascular function; empty stomach by emesis or lavage if ingestion was recent. Hemodialysis removes methyprylon. Excitation, seizures, delirium, and hallucinations may be seen upon recovery. Use barbiturates cautiously for control.

▶ Special considerations
● Methyprylon is not a first-line drug because of its potential for adverse reactions and toxicity.
● Like many other hypnotic agents, this drug is asso-

---

ciated with diminished effectiveness during prolonged use. It is not recommended for use longer than 7 days.
- Periodic blood counts are advisable during long-term treatment to prevent possible adverse effects.
- Institute safety measures: supervised walking and raised bed rails, especially for elderly patients.
- Take precautions to prevent drug hoarding or self-dosing by patients who are depressed or suicidal or who have a history of drug abuse or addiction.
- Abrupt discontinuation may cause withdrawal symptoms; discontinue by reducing dose gradually. Continued use for long periods may cause addiction.
- Store in a cool, dry place.

Information for the patient
- Tell patient to avoid the use of other CNS depressants unless prescribed. Warn the patient about the dangers of combining this drug with alcohol. An excessive depressant effect is possible even if the drug is taken the evening before ingestion of alcohol.
- Warn patient not to increase dose or frequency unless prescribed, and not to abruptly stop taking the drug if he has been taking it for a prolonged period, because withdrawal symptoms may occur.
- Tell patient to call for instructions before taking any nonprescription cold or allergy preparations, which may potentiate the drug's CNS depressant effects.
- Advise patient not to attempt tasks that require mental alertness or physical coordination until the drug's CNS effects are known.
- Advise patient of potential for psychological or physical dependence with chronic use.

Geriatric use
Elderly patients, especially those with hepatic or renal disease, may experience greater CNS depression. Use lowest effective dose.

Pediatric use
Safe use in children under age 12 has not been established.

Breast-feeding
Safe use of methyprylon in breast-feeding women has not been established.

methysergide maleate
Sansert

- Pharmacologic classification: ergot alkaloid
- Therapeutic classification: vasoconstrictor
- Pregnancy risk category X

How supplied
Available by prescription only
Tablets: 2 mg

Indications, route, and dosage
Prevention and treatment of vascular headaches, including migraine and cluster headaches
Adults: 4 to 8 mg P.O. daily in divided doses with meals.

†**To control diarrhea in patients with carcinoid disease**
Adults: 2 mg P.O. t.i.d. Adjust dosage as needed and tolerated. Usual dosage range is 4 to 16 mg P.O. t.i.d.

Pharmacodynamics
Vasoconstrictor action: Methysergide competitively blocks serotonin peripherally and may act as a serotonin agonist in the CNS (brain stem). Its antiserotonin effects result in inhibition of peripheral vasoconstrictor and pressor effects of serotonin, inflammation induced by serotonin, and a reduction in the increased rate of platelet aggregation caused by serotonin.
    The mechanism involved in prophylaxis of vascular headaches by methysergide is unknown; however, its effectiveness may result from humoral factors affecting the pain threshold and from its central serotonin-agonist effect.

Pharmacokinetics
- Absorption: Methysergide is rapidly absorbed from the GI tract.
- Distribution: Methysergide is widely distributed in body tissues.
- Metabolism: Methysergide is metabolized in the liver to methylergonovine and glucuronide metabolites.
- Excretion: 56% of a dose is excreted in urine as unchanged drug and its metabolites. Plasma elimination half-life is 10 hours.

Contraindications and precautions
Methysergide is contraindicated in patients with peripheral vascular disease, severe arteriosclerosis, severe hypertension, coronary artery disease, phlebitis or cellulitis of lower limbs, pulmonary disease, collagen disease, and valvular heart disease, because of the potential for adverse cardiovascular effects; in patients with impaired renal or hepatic function, or fibrotic processes, because of the potential for accumulation after chronic administration; and in patients with peptic ulcer, serious infections, previous sensitivity to ergot drugs, and those in debilitated states. Methysergide is contraindicated during pregnancy.
    Long-term, uninterrupted therapy is associated with fibrosis in pulmonary, cardiac, and retroperitoneal tissues. Methysergide must not be administered continuously for longer than 6 months, and a drug-free interval of 3 to 4 weeks must follow each 6-month course of therapy.
    Administer cautiously to patients sensitive to tartrazine dye as tablets contain tartrazine. Tartrazine sensitivity often occurs in patients sensitive to aspirin.

Interactions
None significant.

Effects on diagnostic tests
None reported.

Adverse reactions
- CV: vascular insufficiencies; *coronary insufficiency;* precipitation or aggravation of angina; claudication in legs; abdominal angina; cold, numb, painful extremities; postural hypotension; tachycardia.
- CNS: insomnia, overstimulation, drowsiness, dizziness, light-headedness, vertigo, ataxia, restlessness, nervousness, rapid speech, visual disturbances, confusion, lethargy, mental depression, psychic disturbances similar to those experienced with LSD.

● GI: nausea, vomiting, diarrhea, heartburn, abdominal pain, constipation.
● Other: facial flushing; rash; dermatitis; hair loss; peripheral edema; weight gain; arthralgia; myalgia; weakness; thickened, reddened, orange-peel skin; neutropenia; eosinophilia; *fibrosis of retroperitoneal, pleuro-pulmonary, and cardiac tissue.*
   Note: Drug should be discontinued if signs or symptoms of impaired circulation or fibrosis occur or if hypersensitivity develops.

Overdose and treatment
Clinical manifestations of overdose include hyperactivity, euphoria, dizziness, peripheral vasospasm with diminished or absent pulses, and coldness, mottling, and cyanosis of extremities.
   Treatment requires supportive measures with prolonged and careful monitoring. If patient is conscious and ingestion recent, induce emesis; if unconscious, insert cuffed endotracheal tube and perform gastric lavage followed by saline (magnesium sulfate) cathartic. Administer I.V. fluids if needed. Monitor vital signs.
   Apply warmth (not direct heat) to ischemic extremities if vasospasm occurs. Administer vasodilators (nitroprusside, tolazoline, or prazosin) if needed.
   Contact local or regional poison control center for more information.

▶ Special considerations
Besides those relevant to all *ergot alkaloids,* consider the following recommendations.
● GI effects may be reduced by gradual introduction of medication and by giving with food or milk.
● Do not use drug to treat acute episodes of migraine, vascular headache, or muscle contraction headache.
● Dosage should be reduced gradually for 2 to 3 weeks before discontinuing drug.
● If drug is given for cluster headaches, it is usually administered only during the cluster.
● Methysergide has also been used to control diarrhea in patients with carcinoid disease.

Information for the patient
● Tell patient not to take drug for longer than 6 months at any one time and to wait 3 to 4 weeks before restarting.
● Tell patient to report immediately any signs of numbness or tingling in hands or feet; red or violet blisters on hands and feet; or any other signs or symptoms of impaired circulation.
● Warn patient to avoid alcoholic beverages, because alcohol may worsen headaches; to avoid smoking, because it may increase adverse effects of drug; and to avoid prolonged exposure to very cold temperatures, because cold may increase adverse effects of drug.
● Tell patient to report illness or infection, which may increase sensitivity to drug effects.
● Explain that after discontinuing this drug, body may need time to adjust depending on the amount used and the duration of time involved.

Geriatric use
Use with caution.

Pediatric use
Not recommended for use in children because of risk of fibrosis.

Breast-feeding
May be excreted in breast milk. Breast-feeding should be avoided during treatment with methysergide.

---

metipranolol hydrochloride
OptiPranolol

● Pharmacologic classification: beta-adrenergic blocker
● Therapeutic classification: antiglaucoma agent
● Pregnancy risk category C

How supplied
Available by prescription only
Ophthalmic solution: 0.3% in 5- or 10-ml dropper bottles with 0.004% benzalkonium chloride and ethylenediaminetetraacetic acid

Indications, route, and dosage
Treatment of ocular conditions in which lowering of intraocular pressure (IOP) would be beneficial (ocular hypertension, chronic open-angle glaucoma)
Adults: Instill 1 drop into affected eye(s) b.i.d. Larger dosage or more frequent administration is not known to be of benefit. If IOP is not satisfactory, concomitant therapy to lower IOP may be instituted.

Pharmacodynamics
Antiglaucoma action: The exact mechanism of ocular antihypertensive action is not known but appears to be a reduction of aqueous humor production. A slight increase in outflow facility has been demonstrated with metipranolol. Like other noncardioselective beta blockers, metipranolol does not have significant local anesthetic (membrane-stabilizing) actions or intrinsic sympathomimetic activity. It does reduce elevated and normal IOP with or without glaucoma with little or no effect on pupil size or accommodation. In patients with IOP above 24 mm Hg, pressure is reduced an average of 20% to 26%.

Pharmacokinetics
● *Absorption:* Drug is intended to act locally, but some systemic absorption may occur. Onset of action occurs in less than 30 minutes.
● *Distribution:* Local.
● *Metabolism:* Unknown.
● *Excretion:* Unknown; maximum effect occurs in about 2 hours; duration of effect is 12 to 24 hours.

Contraindications and precautions
Metipranolol is contraindicated in patients with known hypersensitivity to the drug or any of its components and in patients with bronchial asthma, history of bronchial asthma or severe chronic obstructive pulmonary disease, second- and third-degree AV block, cardiac failure, and cardiogenic shock. Use with caution in patients with nonallergic bronchospasm, chronic bronchitis, emphysema, diabetes mellitus (especially in those subject to spontaneous hypoglycemia), hyperthyroidism, or cerebrovascular insufficiency.

Interactions
Use with caution in patients taking systemic beta blockers because of potential for additive effects. The following agents may interact with ophthalmic beta blockers: antithyroid agents, calcium channel blockers, catecholamine-depleting drugs, cimetidine, clonidine, oral contraceptives, digoxin, haloperidol, hydralazine, insulin, lidocaine, morphine, nondepolarizing neuromuscular blocking agents, NSAIDs, phenobarbital, phenothiazines, prazosin, rifampin, salicylates, sympathomimetics, theophylline, and thyroid hormones. Smoking may also interfere with drug's effect.

Adverse reactions
● CNS: headache, anxiety, dizziness, depression, somnolence, nervousness, asthenia.
● CV: hypertension, *MI*, atrial fibrillation, angina, palpitations, bradycardia.
● DERM: rash.
● EENT: transient local discomfort, tearing, conjunctivitis, eyelid dermatitis, blurred vision, blepharitis, browache, abnormal vision, photophobia, edema, rhinitis, epistaxis.
● GI: nausea.
● Respiratory: dyspnea, bronchitis, cough.
● Other: allergic reaction, myalgia.

Overdose and treatment
If ocular overdose occurs, flush eye(s) with copious amounts of water or normal saline solution.

Systemic overdose, after accidental ingestion, may cause bradycardia, hypotension, bronchospasm, or acute cardiac failure. Discontinue therapy, institute supportive and symptomatic measures, and decrease further absorption, for example, by gastric lavage.

▶ Special considerations
● Concomitant pilocarpine and other miotics, dipivefrin, or systemic carbonic anhydrase inhibitors may be administered if IOP is not adequately controlled.
● Proper administration is essential for optimal therapeutic response; instruct patient in correct techniques. The normal eye can retain only about 10 microliters (µl) of fluid; the average dropper delivers 25 to 50 µl/drop. Thus, the value of more than 1 drop is questionable. If multiple-drop therapy is indicated, the best interval between drops is 5 minutes.

Information for the patient
● Tell patient to wash hands thoroughly before administration and then to follow these directions:
— Tilt head back or lie down and gaze upward.
— Gently grasp lower eyelid below eyelashes and pull eyelid away from eye to form a pouch.
— Place dropper directly over eye, avoiding contact of dropper with eye or any surface.
— Look up just before applying drop; look down for several seconds after applying drop. Slowly release eyelid.
— Close eyes gently for 1 to 2 minutes. Closing eyes tightly after instillation may expel medication from "pouch." Apply gentle pressure to inside corner of eye at bridge of nose to retard drainage of solution from intended area.
● Tell the patient to avoid rubbing the eye and to minimize blinking.
● Tell patient not to rinse dropper after use.
● Advise patient to check expiration date on bottle before use and not to use eye drops that have changed color.
● Tell patient who must use more than one medication to wait at least 5 minutes between instillations.

Pediatric use
Safety and efficacy have not been established.

Breast-feeding
It is unknown if metipranolol is excreted in breast milk. Use with caution in breast-feeding women because systemic beta blockers are excreted in breast milk.

---

metoclopramide hydrochloride
Clopra, Emex*, Maxeran*, Maxolon, Reclomide, Reglan

● Pharmacologic classification: para-aminobenzoic acid (PABA) derivative
● Therapeutic classification: antiemetic, gastrointestinal stimulant
● Pregnancy risk category B

How supplied
Available by prescription only
Tablets: 5 mg, 10 mg
Syrup: 5 mg/5 ml
Injection: 5 mg/5 ml

Indications, route, and dosage
To prevent or reduce nausea and vomiting induced by cisplatin and other chemotherapy
Adults: 2 mg/kg I.V. q 2 hours for 5 doses, beginning 30 minutes before cisplatin administration.
To facilitate small-bowel intubation and to aid in radiologic examinations
Adults: 10 mg I.V. as a single dose over 1 to 2 minutes.
Children age 6 to 14: 2.5 to 5 mg I.V.
Children under age 6: 0.1 mg/kg I.V.
Delayed gastric emptying secondary to diabetic gastroparesis
Adults: 10 mg P.O. 30 minutes before meals and h.s. for 2 to 8 weeks, depending on response.
Gastroesophageal reflux
Adults: 10 to 15 mg P.O. q.i.d., p.r.n., taken 30 minutes before meals.

Pharmacodynamics
● *Antiemetic action:* Metoclopramide inhibits dopamine receptors in the brain's chemoreceptor trigger zone to inhibit or reduce nausea and vomiting.
● *Gastrointestinal stimulant action:* Metoclopramide relieves esophageal reflux by increasing lower esophageal sphincter tone and reduces gastric stasis by stimulating motility of the upper GI tract, thus reducing gastric emptying time.

Pharmacokinetics
● *Absorption:* After oral administration, metoclopramide is absorbed rapidly and thoroughly from the G.I. tract; action begins in 30 to 60 minutes. After I.M. administration, about 74% to 96% of the drug is bioavailable; action begins in 10 to 15 minutes. After I.V. administration, onset of action occurs in 1 to 3 minutes.
● *Distribution:* Metoclopramide is distributed to most

---

body tissues and fluids, including the brain. It crosses the placenta and is distributed in breast milk.
● *Metabolism:* Metoclopramide is not metabolized extensively; a small amount is metabolized in the liver.
● *Excretion:* Most metoclopramide is excreted in urine and feces. Hemodialysis and renal dialysis remove minimal amounts. Duration of effect is 1 to 2 hours.

Contraindications and precautions
Metoclopramide is contraindicated in patients with known hypersensitivity to the drug or to sulfonamides; in patients with pheochromocytoma because it may induce hypertensive crisis; and in patients with seizure disorders, renal failure, liver failure, Parkinson's disease, GI hemorrhage, or intestinal obstruction or perforation, because the drug may exacerbate symptoms of these disorders.

Metoclopramide should be used cautiously in children because they may have a higher incidence of CNS adverse effects and in patients with a history of breast cancer because the drug stimulates prolactin secretion.

Do not use the drug for more than 12 weeks.

Interactions
Metoclopramide may increase or decrease absorption of other drugs, depending on changes in transit time through intestinal tract; it may increase absorption of aspirin, acetaminophen, diazepam, ethanol, levodopa, lithium, and tetracycline and may decrease absorption of digoxin.

Anticholinergics and opiates may antagonize metoclopramide's effect on GI motility. Concomitant use with antihypertensives and CNS depressants (such as alcohol, sedatives, and tricyclic antidepressants) may lead to increased CNS depression.

Concomitant use with phenothiazine and butyrophenone antipsychotics may potentiate extrapyramidal reactions.

Effects on diagnostic tests
Metoclopramide may increase serum aldosterone and prolactin levels.

Adverse reactions
● CNS: restlessness, anxiety, drowsiness, fatigue, lassitude, insomnia, headache, dizziness, extrapyramidal symptoms, tardive dyskinesia, dystonic reactions, sedation.
● CV: transient hypertension.
● DERM: rash.
● Endocrine: prolactin secretion, loss of libido.
● GI: nausea, bowel disturbances.
● Other: fever.
    Note: Drug should be discontinued if extrapyramidal effects occur.

Overdose and treatment
Clinical effects of overdose (which is rare) include drowsiness, dystonia, seizures, and extrapyramidal effects.

Treatment includes administration of antimuscarinics, antiparkinsonian agents, or antihistamines with antimuscarinic activity (for example, 50 mg diphenhydramine, given I.M.).

▶ **Special considerations**
● For I.V. *push* administration, use undiluted and inject over a 1- to 2-minute period. For I.V. *infusion*, dilute with 50 ml of dextrose 5% in water, dextrose 5% in

0.45% sodium chloride, sodium chloride injection, Ringer's injection, or lactated Ringer's injection, and infuse over at least 15 minutes.
● Administer by I.V. infusion 30 minutes before chemotherapy.
● Drug may be used to facilitate nasoduodenal tube placement.
● Diphenhydramine may be used to counteract extrapyramidal effects of high-dose metoclopramide.
● Drug is not recommended for long-term use.
● Metoclopramide has been used investigationally to treat anorexia nervosa, dizziness, migraine, intractable hiccups, and to promote postpartum lactation; oral dose form is being used investigationally to treat nausea and vomiting.

Information for the patient
● Warn patient to avoid driving for 2 hours after each dose because drug may cause drowsiness. Until extent of CNS effect is known, advise patient not to consume alcohol.
● Tell patient to report any twitching or involuntary movement.

Geriatric use
Use drug with caution, especially if patient has impaired renal function; dosage may need to be decreased. Elderly patients are more likely to experience extrapyramidal symptoms and tardive dyskinesia.

Pediatric use
Children have an increased incidence of adverse CNS effects.

Breast-feeding
Because drug is distributed in breast milk, use caution when administering it to breast-feeding women.

metocurine iodide
Metubine

● Pharmacologic classification: nondepolarizing neuromuscular blocking agent
● Therapeutic classification: skeletal muscle relaxant
● Pregnancy risk category C

How supplied
Available by prescription only
Injection: 2 mg/ml

Indications, route, and dosage
Adjunct to anesthesia to induce skeletal muscle relaxation, to facilitate intubation and ventilation, and to reduce fractures and dislocations
Dose depends on anesthetic used, individual needs, and response. Doses are representative and must be adjusted. Administer as sustained injection over 30 to 60 seconds.
Adults: Initially, 0.2 to 0.4 mg/kg I.V. Additional doses of 0.5 to 1 mg I.V. may be administered as indicated.
To weaken muscle contractions in pharmacologically or electrically induced convulsions
Adults: 1.75 to 5.5 mg I.V. slowly as a sustained injection until a head-drop response occurs.

Pharmacodynamics

Skeletal muscle relaxant action: Prevents acetylcholine (ACh) from binding to the receptors on the motor endplate, thus blocking depolarization. Produces effects nearly identical to tubocurarine.

Pharmacokinetics

• *Absorption:* Skeletal muscle relaxation is apparent within 1 to 4 minutes after I.V. administration. Maximum effect persists 35 to 60 minutes. Duration of action ranges from 15 to 90 minutes, depending on dose and anesthetic used. Cumulative effect may occur with repeated doses.

• *Distribution:* Metocurine is 35% plasma protein-bound, mainly as globulins.

• *Metabolism:* Metocurine is metabolized in the plasma.

• *Excretion:* About 50% of a dose is excreted unchanged in urine within 48 hours, and 2% is excreted unchanged in feces via biliary elimination.

Contraindications and precautions

Metocurine is contraindicated in patients with known hypersensitivity to the drug or iodides and in whom histamine release may be hazardous.

Administer with extreme caution to patients with poor renal perfusion or severe renal disease because of the potential for impaired elimination and prolonged effects. Exercise caution in elderly or debilitated patients and in those with cardiovascular, hepatic or pulmonary impairment, hypotension, shock, or respiratory depression, because of the potential for compromised respiratory function and adverse hemodynamic effects; in those with myasthenia gravis or myasthenic syndrome of lung cancer, because of the potential for prolonged neuromuscular blockade; in those with dehydration, thyroid disorders, collagen diseases, porphyria, electrolyte disturbances, or hyperthermia, because the drug may worsen these disorders; and in those with hepatitis or renal failure, because the drug may accumulate and prolong neuromuscular blockade.

Interactions

Comcomitant use with aminoglycoside antibiotics, clindamycin, lincomycin, polymyxin antibiotics, local anesthetics (especially lidocaine and procaine), beta-adrenergic blockers, general anesthetics, furosemide, parenteral magnesium salts, depolarizing neuromuscular blocking agents, other nondepolarizing neuromuscular blocking agents, quinidine or quinine, thiazide diuretics, and other potassium-depleting medications may enhance the neuromuscular blocking ability of metocurine.

Effects on diagnostic tests

None reported.

Adverse reactions

• CV: hypotension.
• GI: decreased motility and tone.
• Other: histamine release (and subsequent sequelae: wheezing or troubled breathing, hypotension, increased salivation, *bronchospasm*, edema, circulatory collapse), *respiratory depression*.

Note: Drug should be discontinued if the patient develops hypersensitivity to drug or iodides.

Overdose and treatment

Clinical manifestations of overdose include prolonged respiratory depression, apnea, and cardiovascular collapse. A sudden release of histamine may also occur, causing hypotension and bronchospasm.

A peripheral nerve stimulator is recommended to monitor response and to evaluate neuromuscular blockade. Maintain adequate airway and manual or mechanical ventilation until patient maintains unassisted ventilation. Monitor vital signs and ECG closely.

Anticholinesterase agent (edrophonium, neostigmine, or pyridostigmine) may be used to reverse effects of metocurine.

▶ **Special considerations**
• Monitor vital signs, especially respiration, and fluid intake and output.
• Monitor baseline electrolytes levels (especially potassium, calcium, and magnesium).
• A 1-mg dose is therapeutic equivalent of 1.8 mg tubocurarine.
• Keep airway clear; have emergency respiratory support equipment available.
• Determine whether patient has iodide allergy.
• Store solution away from heat and light.
• Do not mix in same syringe or give through same needle with alkaline solutions. When combined with barbiturates, precipitation may occur.
• Use fresh solution only.
• I.V. infusion requires direct medical supervision.
• Drug does not relieve pain nor affect consciousness; therefore, assess need for pain medication or sedation.

Geriatric use
Administer cautiously to elderly patients.

Pediatric use
Use with caution because metocurine is twice as potent as tubocurarine in children, but the recovery rate is the same.

Breast-feeding
It is unknown if metocurine is excreted in breast milk. No problems have been reported in humans.

metolazone
Diulo, Zaroxolyn

• Pharmacologic classification: quinazoline derivative (thiazide-like) diuretic
• Therapeutic classification: diuretic, antihypertensive
• Pregnancy risk category D

How supplied

Available by prescription only
Tablets: 0.5 mg, 2.5 mg, 5 mg, 10 mg

Indications, route, and dosage

Edema (heart failure)
Adults: 5 to 10 mg P.O. daily.
Edema (renal disease)
Adults: 5 to 20 mg P.O. daily.
Hypertension
Adults: 2.5 to 5 mg P.O. daily; maintenance dosage determined by patient's blood pressure.

Pharmacodynamics
● *Diuretic action:* Metolazone increases urinary excretion of sodium and water by inhibiting sodium reabsorption in the cortical diluting tubule of the nephron, thus relieving edema. Metolazone may be more effective in edema associated with impaired renal function than thiazide or thiazide-like diuretics.
● *Antihypertensive action:* The exact mechanism of metolazone's antihypertensive effect is unknown; it may result from direct arteriolar vasodilatation. Metolazone also reduces total body sodium levels and total peripheral resistance.

Pharmacokinetics
● *Absorption:* About 65% of a given dose of metolazone is absorbed after oral administration to healthy subjects; in cardiac patients, absorption falls to 40%. However, rate and extent of absorption vary among preparations.
● *Distribution:* Metolazone is 50% to 70% erythrocyte-bound and about 33% protein-bound.
● *Metabolism:* Insignificant.
● *Excretion:* About 70% to 95% of metolazone is excreted unchanged in urine. Half-life is about 14 hours in healthy subjects; it may be prolonged in patients with decreased creatinine clearance.

Contraindications and precautions
Metolazone is contraindicated in patients with anuria and in those with known sensitivity to the drug.
　Metolazone should be used cautiously in patients with severe renal disease because it may decrease glomerular filtration rate and precipitate azotemia; in patients with impaired hepatic function or liver disease because electrolyte changes may precipitate coma; and in patients taking digoxin, because hypokalemia may predispose them to digitalis toxicity.

Interactions
Metolazone potentiates the hypotensive effects of most other antihypertensive drugs; this may be used to therapeutic advantage.
　Metolazone may potentiate hyperglycemic, hypotensive, and hyperuricemic effects of diazoxide, and its hyperglycemic effect may increase insulin or sulfonylurea requirements in diabetic patients.
　Metolazone may reduce renal clearance of lithium, elevating serum lithium levels, and may necessitate a 50% reduction in lithium dosage.
　Metolazone turns urine slightly more alkaline and may decrease urinary excretion of some amines, such as amphetamine and quinidine; alkaline urine may also decrease therapeutic efficacy of methenamine compounds such as methenamine mandelate.
　Cholestyramine and colestipol may bind metolazone, preventing its absorption; give drugs 1 hour apart.

Effects on diagnostic tests
Metolazone therapy may alter serum electrolyte levels and may increase serum urate, glucose, cholesterol, and triglyceride levels. It also may interfere with tests for parathyroid function and should be discontinued before such tests.

Adverse reactions
● CV: volume depletion and dehydration, orthostatic hypotension, hypercholesterolemia, hypertriglyceridemia.
● DERM: dermatitis, photosensitivity.
● GI: anorexia, nausea, pancreatitis.
● HEMA: *aplastic anemia, agranulocytosis,* leukopenia, thrombocytopenia.
● Hepatic: hepatic encephalopathy.
● Metabolic: asymptomatic hyperuricemia; gout; hyperglycemia and impairment of glucose tolerance; fluid and electrolyte imbalances, including hyponatremia, hypochloremia, hypercalcemia, and hypokalemia; metabolic alkalosis.
● Other: hypersensitivity reactions, such as pneumonitis and vasculitis.
　Note: Drug should be discontinued if rising BUN and serum creatinine levels indicate renal impairment or if patient shows signs of impending coma.

Overdose and treatment
Clinical signs of overdose include GI irritation and hypermotility, diuresis, and lethargy, which may progress to coma.
　Treatment is mainly supportive; monitor and assist respiratory, cardiovascular, and renal function as indicated. Monitor fluid and electrolyte balance. Induce vomiting with ipecac in conscious patient; otherwise, use gastric lavage to avoid aspiration. Do not give cathartics; these promote additional loss of fluids and electrolytes.

▶ Special considerations
Besides those relevant to all *thiazide and thiazide-like diuretics,* consider the following recommendations.
● Metolazone is effective in patients with decreased renal function.
● Metolazone is used as an adjunct in furosemide-resistant edema.

Geriatric use
Elderly and debilitated patients require close observation and may require reduced dosages. They are more sensitive to excess diuresis because of age-related changes in cardiovascular and renal function. Excess diuresis promotes orthostatic hypotension, dehydration, hypovolemia, hyponatremia, hypomagnesemia, and hypokalemia.

Pediatric use
Safety and effectiveness have not been established.

Breast-feeding
Metolazone may be distributed in breast milk; its safety and effectiveness in breast-feeding women have not been established.

metoprolol tartrate
Lopressor

● Pharmacologic classification: beta-adrenergic blocking agent
● Therapeutic classification: antihypertensive, adjunctive treatment of acute myocardial infarction (MI)
● Pregnancy risk category B

How supplied
Available by prescription only
Tablets: 50 mg, 100 mg
Injection: 1 mg/ml in 5-ml ampules or prefilled syringes

---

*Canada only　　　†Unlabeled clinical use　　　Italicized adverse reactions are life-threatening.

Indications, route, and dosage
Mild to severe hypertension
Adults: Initially, 100 mg P.O. daily in single or divided doses. Usual maintenance dosage is 100 to 450 mg daily.
Early intervention in acute MI
Adults: Three 5-mg I.V. boluses q 2 minutes. Then, beginning 15 minutes after last dose, 50 mg P.O. q 6 hours for 48 hours. *Maintenance dose:* 100 mg P.O. b.i.d.
Angina
Adults: 100 mg in two divided doses. *Maintenance dose:* 100 to 400 mg daily.

Pharmacodynamics
• *Antihypertensive action:* Metoprolol is classified as a cardioselective beta$_1$ antagonist; exact mechanism of metoprolol's antihypertensive effect is unknown. The drug may reduce blood pressure by blocking adrenergic receptors, thus decreasing cardiac output; by decreasing sympathetic outflow from the CNS; or by suppressing renin release.
• *Action after acute MI:* The exact mechanism by which metoprolol decreases mortality after MI is unknown. In patients with MI, metoprolol reduces heart rate, systolic blood pressure, and cardiac output. The drug also appears to decrease the occurrence of ventricular fibrillation in these patients.

Pharmacokinetics
• *Absorption:* Orally administered metoprolol is absorbed rapidly and almost completely from GI tract; food enhances absorption. Peak plasma concentrations occur in 90 minutes. After I.V. administration, maximum beta blockade occurs in 20 minutes. Maximum therapeutic effect occurs after 1 week of treatment.
• *Distribution:* Metoprolol is distributed widely throughout the body; drug is about 12% protein-bound.
• *Metabolism:* Metoprolol is metabolized in the liver.
• *Excretion:* About 95% of a given dose of metoprolol is excreted in urine. Beta blockade persists for about 24 hours after oral administration and 5 to 8 hours after I.V. administration.

Contraindications and precautions
Metoprolol is contraindicated in patients with known hypersensitivity to the drug; and in patients with overt cardiac failure, second- or third-degree atrioventricular block, and cardiogenic shock, because the drug may worsen these conditions.

Metoprolol should be used cautiously in patients with coronary insufficiency because beta-adrenergic blockade may precipitate congestive heart failure (CHF); in patients with impaired hepatic function (dosage reduction may be necessary); in patients with diabetes mellitus or hyperthyroidism, because metoprolol may mask the tachycardia associated with hypoglycemia and hyperthyroidism (drug will not mask dizziness and sweating from hypoglycemia); in patients with bronchospastic disease (dosages higher than 100 mg/day may inhibit bronchodilating effects of endogenous catecholamines [at lower doses, metoprolol selectively inhibits beta$_1$-receptors]); and in patients with sinus node dysfunction because depression of sinoatrial node automaticity may occur.

Interactions
Concomitant use with cardiac glycosides may cause excessive bradycardia. Metoprolol may potentiate antihypertensive effects of diuretics or other antihypertensive agents. Metoprolol may antagonize the beta-adrenergic effects of sympathomimetic agents.

Effects on diagnostic tests
Metoprolol may elevate serum transaminase, alkaline phosphatase, lactic dehydrogenase, and uric acid levels.

Adverse reactions
• CNS: fatigue, lethargy.
• CV: bradycardia, hypotension, *CHF*, peripheral vascular disease, shortness of breath.
• DERM: rash.
• GI: nausea, diarrhea.
• HEMA: eosinophilia, *agranulocytosis*, nonthrombocytopenic and thrombocytopenic purpura.
• Other: fever, arthralgias, dyspnea, wheezing.
Note: Drug should be discontinued if patient develops signs of heart failure or mental depression.

Overdose and treatment
Clinical signs of overdose include severe hypotension, bradycardia, heart failure, and bronchospasm.

After acute ingestion, empty stomach by induced emesis or gastric lavage, and give activated charcoal to reduce absorption. Subsequent treatment is usually symptomatic and supportive.

▶ **Special considerations**
Besides those relevant to all *beta-adrenergic blocking agents,* consider the following recommendations.
• Metoprolol may be administered daily as a single dose or in divided doses. If a dose is missed, patient should take only the next scheduled dose.
• Drug should be given with meals to enhance absorption.
• Dosage may need to be reduced in patients with impaired hepatic function.
• Most patients with asthma or bronchitis can safely use this drug in low doses (for example, daily doses of less than 100 mg) without fear of worsening their condition.
• Avoid late-evening doses to minimize insomnia.
• Observe patient for signs of mental depression.

Geriatric use
Elderly patients may require lower maintenance dosages of metoprolol because of delayed metabolism; they may also experience enhanced adverse effects. Use with caution.

Pediatric use
Safety and efficacy of metoprolol in children have not been established. No dosage recommendation exists for children.

Breast-feeding
Metoprolol is distributed into breast milk. An alternative feeding method is recommended during therapy.

metronidazole
Apometronidazole*, Femazole, Flagyl, Metric 21, Metronid, Metryl, Neo-metric*, Novonidazol*, PMS Metronidazole*, Protostat, Satric

metronidazole hydrochloride
Flagyl I.V., Flagyl I.V. RTU, Metro I.V., Metronidazole Redi-Infusion

- Pharmacologic classification: nitroimidazole
- Therapeutic classification: antibacterial, antiprotozoal, amebicide
- Pregnancy risk category B

How supplied
Available by prescription only
Tablets: 250 mg, 500 mg
Powder for injection: 500-mg single-dose vials
Injection: 500 mg/dl ready to use

Indications, route, and dosage
Amebic hepatic abscess
Adults: 500 to 750 mg P.O. t.i.d. for 5 to 10 days.
Children: 35 to 50 mg/kg daily (in three doses) for 10 days.
Intestinal amebiasis
Adults: 750 mg P.O. t.i.d. for 5 to 10 days. Centers for Disease Control recommends addition of iodoquinol 650 mg P.O. t.i.d. for 20 days.
Children: 35 to 50 mg/kg daily (in three doses) for 5 to 10 days. Follow this therapy with oral iodoquinol.
Trichomoniasis
Adults (both men and women concurrently): 250 mg P.O. t.i.d. for 7 days or 2 g P.O. as a single dose; 4 to 6 weeks should elapse between courses of therapy.
Refractory trichomoniasis
Adults (women): 500 mg P.O. b.i.d. for 7 days.
Bacterial infections caused by anaerobic microorganisms
Adults: Loading dose is 15 mg/kg I.V. infused over 1 hour (approximately 1 g for a 70-kg adult). Maintenance dose is 7.5 mg/kg I.V. or P.O. q 6 hours (approximately 500 mg for a 70-kg adult). The first maintenance dose should be administered 6 hours after the loading dose. Maximum dosage should not exceed 4 g daily.
Children: 7.5 mg/kg I.V. q 6 hours.
Giardiasis
Adults: 250 mg P.O. t.i.d. for 5 days.
Children: 5 mg/kg P.O. t.i.d. for 5 days.
Prevention of postoperative infection in contaminated or potentially contaminated colorectal surgery
Adults: 15 mg/kg infused over 30 to 60 minutes and completed approximately 1 hour before surgery. Then 7.5 mg/kg infused over 30 to 60 minutes at 6 and 12 hours after the initial dose.

Pharmacodynamics
Bactericidal, amebicidal, and trichomonicidal action: The nitro group of metronidazole is reduced inside the infecting organism; this reduction product disrupts DNA and inhibits nucleic acid synthesis. The drug is active in intestinal and extraintestinal sites. It is active against most anaerobic bacteria and protozoa, including *Bac-*

teroides fragilis, B. melaninogenicus, Fusobacterium, Veillonella, Clostridium, Peptococcus, Peptostreptococcus, Entamoeba histolytica, Trichomonas vaginalis, Giardia lamblia, and *Balantidium coli.*

Pharmacokinetics
- *Absorption:* About 80% of an oral dose is absorbed, with peak serum concentrations occurring at about 1 hour; food delays peak concentrations to about 2 hours.
- *Distribution:* Metronidazole is distributed into most body tissues and fluids, including cerebrospinal fluid (CSF), bone, bile, saliva, pleural and peritoneal fluids, vaginal secretions, seminal fluids, middle ear fluid, and hepatic and cerebral abscesses. CSF levels approach serum levels in patients with inflamed meninges; they reach about 50% of serum levels in patients with uninflamed meninges. Less than 20% of metronidazole is bound to plasma proteins. It readily crosses the placenta.
- *Metabolism:* Metronidazole is metabolized to an active 2-hydroxymethyl metabolite and also to other metabolites.
- *Excretion:* About 60% to 80% of the dose is excreted as the parent compound or its metabolites. About 20% of a metronidazole dose is excreted unchanged in urine; about 6% to 15% is excreted in feces. Metronidazole's half-life is 6 to 8 hours in adults with normal renal function; the half-life may be prolonged in patients with impaired hepatic function. It is secreted into breast milk.

Contraindications and precautions
Metronidazole is contraindicated in patients with hypersensitivity to nitroimidazole derivatives. It is also contraindicated during the first trimester of pregnancy because its safety for such use has not been studied.

Metronidazole should be used with caution in patients with a history of blood dyscrasias because drug can cause leukopenia; in patients receiving corticosteroids; and in those predisposed to edema from the sodium content of the administered solution.

It should be used with extreme caution (at lower than recommended doses) in patients with severe hepatic impairment because metronidazole and its metabolites accumulate in the plasma. Administer with caution to patients with CNS diseases because seizures and peripheral neuropathy have been reported. Metronidazole should not be used indiscriminately because animal studies suggest carcinogenicity.

Interactions
Concomitant use of metronidazole with oral anticoagulants prolongs prothrombin time. Concomitant use with alcohol inhibits alcohol dehydrogenase activity, causing a disulfiram-like reaction (nausea, vomiting, headache, cramps, and flushing) in some patients; it is not recommended. Concomitant use with disulfiram may precipitate psychosis and confusion and should be avoided.

Concomitant use with barbiturates and phenytoin may diminish the antimicrobial effectiveness of metronidazole by increasing its metabolism and may require higher doses of metronidazole.

Concomitant use with cimetidine may decrease the clearance of metronidazole, thereby increasing its potential for causing adverse effects.

Effects on diagnostic tests
Metronidazole may interfere with the chemical analyses of aminotransferases and triglyceride, leading to falsely

decreased values. Rarely, it has been reported to flatten the T waves on ECG.

Adverse reactions
• CNS: vertigo, headache, ataxia, incoordination, confusion, irritability, depression, restlessness, weakness, fatigue, drowsiness, insomnia, sensory neuropathy, paresthesias of extremities, psychic stimulation, neuromyopathy, and seizures.
• CV: ECG changes, (flattened T wave), edema (with I.V. RTU preparation).
• DERM: pruritus, flushing, urticaria.
• GI: abdominal cramping, stomatitis, *nausea, vomiting, anorexia,* diarrhea, constipation, proctitis, dry mouth, pseudomembranous colitis.
• GU: darkened urine, polyuria, dysuria, pyuria, incontinence, cystitis, decreased libido, dyspareunia, dryness of vagina and vulva, sense of pelvic pressure.
• HEMA: transient leukopenia, neutropenia.
• Local: *thrombophlebitis after I.V. infusion.*
• Other: bacterial and fungal superinfection, especially *Candida* (glossitis, furry tongue), metallic taste, fever, gynecomastia, nasal congestion.

Overdose and treatment
Clinical signs of overdose include nausea, vomiting, ataxia, seizures, and peripheral neuropathy.

There is no known antidote for metronidazole; treatment is supportive. If patient does not vomit spontaneously, induced emesis or gastric lavage is indicated for an oral overdose; activated charcoal and a cathartic may be used. Diazepam or phenytoin may be used to control seizures.

▶ Special considerations
• Trichomoniasis should be confirmed by wet smear and amebiasis by culture before giving metronidazole.
• If indicated during pregnancy for trichomoniasis, the 7-day regimen is preferred over the single-dose regimen. Treatment with metronidazole should be avoided during the first trimester.
• The I.V. form should be administered by slow infusion only; if used with a primary I.V. fluid system, discontinue the primary fluid during the infusion; *do not give by I.V. push.*
• Monitor patient on I.V. metronidazole for candidiasis.
• A 1% solution may be effective topically to treat decubitus ulcers.
• When treating amebiasis, monitor number and character of stools; send fecal specimens to laboratory promptly; infestation is detectable only in warm specimens. Repeat fecal examinations at 3-month intervals to ensure elimination of amebae.
• When preparing powder for injection, follow manufacturer's instructions carefully; use solution prepared from powder within 24 hours. I.V. solutions must be prepared in three steps: reconstitution with 4.4 ml of 0.9% sodium chloride injection (with or without bacteriostatic water); dilution with lactated Ringer's injection, 5% dextrose in water, or 0.9% sodium chloride; and neutralization with sodium bicarbonate, 5 mEq per 500 mg metronidazole.

Information for the patient
• Tell patient that drug may cause metallic taste and discolored (red-brown) urine.
• Tell patient to take tablets with meals to minimize GI distress and that tablets may be crushed to facilitate swallowing.

• Counsel patient on need for medical follow-up after discharge.
• Advise patient to report any adverse effects.
• Tell patient to avoid alcohol and alcohol-containing medications during therapy and for at least 48 hours after the last dose to prevent disulfiram-like reaction.
Amebiasis patients:
• Explain to patient that follow-up examinations of stool specimens are necessary for 3 months after treatment is discontinued, to ensure elimination of amebae.
• To help prevent reinfection, instruct patient and family members in proper hygiene, including disposal of feces and hand washing after defecation and before handling, preparing, or eating food, and about the risks of eating raw food and the control of contamination by flies.
• Encourage other household members and suspected contacts to be tested and, if necessary, treated.
Trichomoniasis patients:
• Teach correct personal hygiene, including perineal care.
• Explain that asymptomatic sexual partners of patients being treated for trichomoniasis should be treated simultaneously to prevent reinfection; patient should refrain from intercourse during therapy or have partner use condom.

Pediatric use
Neonates may eliminate the drug more slowly than older infants and children.

Breast-feeding
Patient should discontinue breast-feeding while taking this drug.

metronidazole (topical)
MetroGel

• Pharmacologic classification: nitroimidazole
• Therapeutic classification: antiprotozoal, antibacterial
• Pregnancy risk category B

How supplied
Available by prescription only
Topical gel: 0.75%

Indications, route, and dosage
Topical treatment of acne rosacea
Adults: Apply a thin film twice daily to affected area during the morning and evening. Significant results should be seen within 3 weeks and continue for the first 9 weeks of therapy.

Pharmacodynamics
Anti-inflammatory action: Although its exact mechanism of action is unknown, topical metronidazole probably exerts an anti-inflammatory effect through its antibacterial and antiprotozoal actions.

Pharmacokinetics
Under normal conditions, serum levels of metronidazole after topical administration are negligible.

Contraindications and precautions
Contraindicated in patients allergic to the drug or other ingredients of the formulation (such as parabens).

Use cautiously in patients with history or evidence of blood dyscrasias, because chemically related compounds are associated with blood dyscrasias.

Interactions
Concomitant use with oral anticoagulants may potentiate the anticoagulant effect. Monitor patient for potential adverse effects.

Effects on diagnostic tests
None reported.

Adverse reactions
● DERM: transient redness, burning, irritation.
● EENT: tearing (if applied around the eyes).

Overdose and treatment
None reported. Overdose after topical application is unlikely.

▶ **Special considerations**
Topical metronidazole therapy has not been associated with the adverse reactions observed with parenteral or oral metronidazole therapy (including disulfiram-like reaction following alcohol ingestion). However, some of the drug can be absorbed following topical use. Limited clinical experience has not shown any of these adverse effects.

Information for the patient
● Advise patient to cleanse area thoroughly before applying the drug. Patient may use cosmetics after applying the drug.
● Instruct patients to avoid use of the drug on the eyelids and to apply it cautiously if drug must be used around the eyes.
● If local reactions occur, advise patient to apply drug less frequently or to discontinue use and call for specific instructions.

Pediatric use
Safety has not been established.

Breast-feeding
Safety has not been established. Metronidazole is excreted in breast milk. A decision should be made whether to discontinue the drug or to recommend discontinuing breast-feeding, after assessing the importance of the drug to the mother.

metyrosine
Demser

● Pharmacologic classification: tyrosine hydroxylase inhibitor
● Therapeutic classification: antihypertensive in pheochromocytoma
● Pregnancy risk category C

How supplied
Available by prescription only
Capsules: 250 mg

Indications, route, and dosage
Short-term management of pheochromocytoma before surgery, or long-term management when surgery is contraindicated or tumor is malignant
Adults and children over age 12: 250 mg P.O. q.i.d.; may be increased by 250 to 500 mg every day to a maximum of 4 g/day in divided doses. For preoperative preparation, give optimally effective dosage for at least 5 to 7 days.

Pharmacodynamics
Antihypertensive action: Metyrosine competitively inhibits tyrosine hydroxylase, thereby decreasing endogenous catecholamine concentrations in patients with normal or increased catecholamine production. Metyrosine decreases the frequency and severity of hypertensive attacks and the resultant headache, nausea, sweating, and tachycardia in patients with pheochromocytoma.

Pharmacokinetics
● *Absorption:* Metyrosine is absorbed well from the GI tract. In patients with pheochromocytoma, gradual decrease in blood pressure occurs during first 2 days of therapy.
● *Distribution:* Complete distribution pattern is unknown; drug crosses the blood-brain barrier.
● *Metabolism:* Minimal.
● *Excretion:* From 53% to 88% of a given dose is excreted unchanged in urine within 24 hours. Blood pressure gradually returns to pretreatment levels within 2 to 3 days after metyrosine therapy is discontinued.

Contraindications and precautions
Metyrosine is contraindicated in patients with known hypersensitivity to the drug and in patients with hypertension of unknown etiology.

Metyrosine should be used cautiously in patients with impaired hepatic or renal function and in patients receiving phenothiazines or butyrophenones, because increased inhibition of catecholamine synthesis may increase incidence of extrapyramidal symptoms.

Interactions
Metyrosine may increase sedation caused by alcohol or other CNS depressants.

Effects on diagnostic tests
Metyrosine therapy may cause false elevations of urine catecholamine levels in patients without pheochromocytoma.

Adverse reactions
● CNS: sedation, extrapyramidal symptoms such as speech difficulty and tremors, disorientation, mental depression, psychological disturbances.
● GI: diarrhea, nausea, vomiting, abdominal pain.
● GU: crystalluria, hematuria.
● Other: impotence, hypersensitivity.
 Note: Drug should be discontinued if signs of hypersensitivity occur.

Overdose and treatment
Overdose is manifested primarily by hypotension. After acute ingestion, empty stomach by induced emesis or gastric lavage, and give activated charcoal to reduce absorption. Further treatment is usually symptomatic and supportive.

▶ **Special considerations**
• Although metyrosine decreases blood pressure in patients with pheochromocytoma, it does not decrease blood pressure in most patients with hypertension unrelated to pheochromocytoma. Do not use to treat hypertension of unknown etiology.
• Monitor blood pressure and ECG continuously during surgery.
• Metyrosine (1.5 to 3 g daily, in divided doses) has been used with phenothiazines to treat chronic schizophrenia.

Information for the patient
• Warn the patient that sedation almost always occurs but usually subsides after several days of treatment; insomnia may occur when drug is discontinued.
• Instruct patient to increase daily fluid intake to prevent crystalluria; daily urine volume should be 2,000 ml or more.
• Advise patient to avoid hazardous activities while CNS adverse effects persist, to report persistent diarrhea, and to avoid alcohol.
• Warn patient to call for instruction before taking nonprescription cold preparations.

Geriatric use
Administer with caution to elderly patients because of decreased drug elimination.

Pediatric use
Experience with metyrosine in children under age 12 is limited; dosage schedules have not been established.

Breast-feeding
It is not known whether metyrosine is distributed into breast milk; drug is not recommended for use by breast-feeding women.

mexiletine hydrochloride
Mexitil

• Pharmacologic classification: lidocaine analogue, sodium channel antagonist
• Therapeutic classification: ventricular antiarrhythmic
• Pregnancy risk category C

How supplied
Available by prescription only
Capsules: 150 mg, 200 mg, 250 mg

Indications, route, and dosage
Refractory ventricular arrhythmias, including ventricular tachycardia and premature ventricular contractions
Adults: 200 to 400 mg P.O. followed by 200 mg q 8 hours. May increase dose to 400 mg q 8 hours if satisfactory control is not obtained. Some patients may respond well to 450 mg q 12 hours.

Pharmacodynamics
Antiarrhythmic action: Mexiletine is structurally similar to lidocaine and exerts similar electrophysiologic and hemodynamic effects. A Class IB antiarrhythmic, it suppresses automaticity and shortens the effective refractory period and action potential duration of His-Purkinje

fibers and suppresses spontaneous ventricular depolarization during diastole. At therapeutic serum levels, the drug does not affect conductive atrial tissue or AV conduction.

Unlike quinidine and procainamide, mexiletine does not significantly alter hemodynamics when given in usual doses. Its effects on the conduction system inhibit reentry mechanisms and halt ventricular arrhythmias. The drug does not have a significant negative inotropic effect.

Pharmacokinetics
• *Absorption:* About 90% of drug is absorbed from the GI tract; peak serum levels occur in 2 to 3 hours. Absorption rate decreases with conditions that speed gastric emptying.
• *Distribution:* Mexiletine is distributed widely throughout the body. Distribution volume declines in patients with liver and/or hepatic disease, resulting in toxic serum drug levels with usual doses. About 50% to 60% of circulating drug is bound to plasma proteins. Usual therapeutic drug level is 0.5 to 2 mcg/ml. Although toxicity may occur within this range, levels above 2 mcg/ml are considered toxic and are associated with an increased frequency of adverse CNS effects, warranting dosage reduction.
• *Metabolism:* Mexiletine is metabolized in the liver to relatively inactive metabolites. Less than 10% of a parenteral dose escapes metabolism and reaches the kidneys unchanged. Metabolism is affected by hepatic blood flow, which may be reduced in patients who are recovering from myocardial infarction and in those with congestive heart failure. Liver disease also limits metabolism.
• *Excretion:* In healthy patients, drug's half-life is 10 to 12 hours. Elimination half-life may be prolonged in patients with congestive heart failure or liver disease. Urinary excretion increases with urine acidification and slows with urine alkalinization.

Contraindications and precautions
Mexiletine is contraindicated in patients with cardiogenic shock, because the drug has a mild negative inotropic effect and may increase systemic vascular resistance slightly, thereby exacerbating this condition; in patients with preexisting second- or third-degree heart block without an artificial pacemaker, because the drug may further depress cardiac conduction; and in patients with hypersensitivity to the drug.

Mexiletine should be used with caution in patients with severe degrees of sinoatrial, atrioventricular, or intraventricular heart block who do not have an artificial pacemaker, because the drug may worsen these conditions; in patients with hepatic or myocardial failure, because the drug may accumulate and cause toxicity; in patients with seizure disorders, because the drug may induce seizures; and in patients with bradycardia or hypotension, because the drug may worsen these conditions.

Interactions
Concomitant use of mexiletine with drugs that alter gastric emptying time (such as narcotics, antacids containing aluminum-magnesium hydroxide, and atropine) may delay mexiletine absorption; concomitant use with metoclopramide may increase absorption.

Concomitant use with drugs that alter hepatic enzyme function (such as rifampin, phenobarbital, and phenytoin) may induce hepatic metabolism of mexiletine and thus reduce serum drug levels. Concomitant use with cimetidine may decrease mexiletine metabolism, resulting in increased serum levels. Concomitant use with drugs that acidify the urine (such as ammonium chloride) enhances mexiletine excretion; concomitant use with drugs that alkalinize urine (such as high-dose antacids, carbonic anhydrase inhibitors, and sodium bicarbonate) decreases mexiletine excretion.

Effects on diagnostic tests
Liver function test results may be transiently altered during mexiletine therapy.

Adverse reactions
● CNS: tremor, dizziness, blurred vision, ataxia, diplopia, confusion, nystagmus, nervousness, headache.
● CV: hypotension, bradycardia, arrhythmias, angina.
● DERM: rash.
● GI: nausea, vomiting.
● Respiratory: dyspnea.
● Other: elevation of liver function test values.

Overdose and treatment
Clinical effects of overdose are primarily extensions of adverse CNS effects. Convulsions are the most serious effect.

  Treatment usually involves symptomatic and supportive measures. In acute overdose, emesis induction or gastric lavage should be performed. Urine acidification may accelerate drug elimination. If patient has bradycardia and hypotension, atropine may be given.

▶ Special considerations
● Dosage should be administered with meals, if possible.
● Avoid administering drug within 1 hour of antacids containing aluminum-magnesium hydroxide.
● When changing from lidocaine to mexiletine, stop infusion when first mexiletine dose is given. Keep infusion line open, however, until dysrhythmia appears to be satisfactorily controlled.
● Patients who are not controlled by dosing every 8 hours may respond to dosing every 6 hours.
● Many patients who respond well to mexiletine can be maintained on an every-12-hour schedule. Twice-daily doses improve patient compliance.
● Monitor blood pressure and heart rate and rhythm for significant change.
● Tremor (usually a fine hand tremor) is commonly evident in patients taking higher doses of mexiletine.
● Therapeutic serum drug levels range from 0.75 to 2 mcg/ml.

Information for the patient
● Instruct patient to take drug with food to reduce risk of nausea.
● Instruct patient to report any of the following: unusual bleeding or bruising, signs of infection (such as fever, sore throat, stomatitis, or chills), or fatigue.

Geriatric use
Most elderly patients require reduced dosages, because of reduced hepatic blood flow and therefore, decreased metabolism. Elderly patients also may be more susceptible to CNS side effects.

Breast-feeding
Mexiletine is excreted in breast milk. Alternative feeding form should be used during therapy with this drug.

mezlocillin sodium
Mezlin

● Pharmacologic classification: extended-spectrum penicillin, acyclaminopenicillin
● Therapeutic classification: antibiotic
● Pregnancy risk category B

How supplied
Available by prescription only
Injection: 1 g, 2 g, 3 g, 4 g
Infusion: 2 g, 3 g, 4 g
Pharmacy bulk package: 20 g

Indications, route, and dosage
Infections caused by susceptible organisms
Adults: 100 to 300 mg/kg I.V. or I.M. daily given in four to six divided doses. Usual dose is 3 g q 4 hours or 4 g q 6 hours. For serious infections, up to 24 g daily may be administered.
Children under age 12: 200 to 300 mg/kg per day I.M. or I.V. in divided doses q 4 to 6 hours.
Dosage in renal failure
Adults: If creatinine clearance is 10 to 30 ml/min, give 3 g q 8 hours. If creatinine clearance is < 10 ml/min, give 2 g q 8 hours. (If the infection is life-threatening, the above doses may be given every 6 hours.) Patients on hemodialysis should be given 3 to 4 g after each dialysis session, then q 12 hours. Patients on peritoneal dialysis may receive 3 g q 12 hours.

Pharmacodynamics
Antibiotic action: Mezlocillin is bactericidal; it adheres to bacterial penicillin-binding proteins, thereby inhibiting bacterial cell wall synthesis.

  Extended-spectrum penicillins are more resistant to inactivation by certain beta-lactamases, especially those produced by gram-negative organisms, but are still liable to inactivation by certain others.

  Mezlocillin's spectrum of activity includes many gram-negative aerobic and anaerobic bacilli, many gram-positive and gram-negative aerobic cocci, and some gram-positive aerobic and anaerobic bacilli, but a large number of these organisms are resistant to mezlocillin. Mezlocillin may be effective against some strains of carbenicillin-resistant and ticarcillin-resistant gram-negative bacilli. Mezlocillin should not be used as sole therapy because of the rapid development of resistance. Some clinicians feel that there is no evidence that it has any advantages over ticarcillin or carbenicillin, at least with respect to cure rates. Mezlocillin is less active against *Pseudomonas aeruginosa* than other members of this class, such as azlocillin and piperacillin; however, both mezlocillin and piperacillin are more effective against *Enterobacteriaceae* than is azlocillin.

Pharmacokinetics
● *Absorption:* After an I.M. dose, peak plasma concentrations occur at ¾ to 1½ hours.
● *Distribution:* Mezlocillin is distributed widely. It penetrates minimally into CSF with uninflamed meninges. Mezlocillin crosses the placenta and is 16% to 42% protein-bound.
● *Metabolism:* Mezlocillin is metabolized partially; about 15% of a dose is metabolized to inactive metabolites.
● *Excretion:* Mezlocillin is excreted primarily (39% to

72%) in urine by glomerular filtration and renal tubular secretion; up to 30% of a dose is excreted in bile, and some is excreted in breast milk. Elimination half-life in adults is about ¾ to 1½ hours; in extensive renal impairment, half-life is extended to 2 to 14 hours. Mezlocillin is removed by hemodialysis but not by peritoneal dialysis.

Contraindications and precautions
Mezlocillin is contraindicated in patients with known hypersensitivity to any other penicillin or to cephalosporins.

Mezlocillin should be used cautiously in patients with renal impairment because it is excreted in urine; decreased dosage is required in moderate to severe renal failure.

Interactions
Concomitant use with aminoglycoside antibiotics results in a synergistic bactericidal effect against *Pseudomonas aeruginosa, Escherichia coli, Klebsiella, Citrobacter, Enterobacter, Serratia,* and *Proteus mirabilis.* However, the drugs are physically and chemically incompatible and are inactivated when mixed or given together.

Concomitant use of mezlocillin (and other extended-spectrum penicillins) with clavulanic acid also produces a synergistic bactericidal effect against certain beta-lactamase producing bacteria.

Probenecid blocks tubular secretion of penicillins, raising their serum concentrations.

Large doses of penicillins may interfere with renal tubular secretion of methotrexate, thus delaying elimination and elevating serum concentrations of methotrexate.

Effects on diagnostic tests
Mezlocillin alters tests for urinary or serum proteins; it interferes with turbidimetric methods that use sulfosalicylic acid, trichloroacetic acid, acetic acid, or nitric acid.

Mezlocillin does not interfere with tests using bromophenol blue (Albustix, Albutest, MultiStix).

Positive Coombs' tests have been reported in patients taking carbenicillin disodium.

Mezlocillin may falsely decrease serum aminoglycoside concentrations. Mezlocillin may cause hypokalemia and hypernatremia and prolong prothrombin times; it may also cause transient elevations in liver function studies and transient reductions in red blood cell, white blood cell, and platelet counts.

Adverse reactions
● CNS: neuromuscular irritability, seizures.
● GI: nausea, diarrhea, vomiting, *pseudomembranous colitis.*
● GU: *acute interstitial nephritis.*
● HEMA: *bleeding with high doses,* neutropenia, eosinophilia, leukopenia, thrombocytopenia.
● Metabolic: hypokalemia.
● Local: pain at injection site, vein irritation, phlebitis.
● Other: *hypersensitivity reactions* (edema, fever, chills, rash, pruritus, urticaria, *anaphylaxis*), bacterial and fungal superinfection.
Note: Drug should be discontinued if immediate hypersensitivity reactions occur; if bleeding complications occur; or if severe diarrhea occurs, as this may indicate pseudomembranous colitis.

Overdose and treatment
Clinical signs of overdose include neuromuscular sensitivity or seizures; a 4- to 6-hour hemodialysis will remove 20% to 30% of mezlocillin.

▶ Special considerations
Beside those relevant to all *penicillins,* consider the following recommendations.
● Mezlocillin may be more suitable than carbenicillin or ticarcillin for patients on salt-free diets; mezlocillin contains only 1.85 mEq of sodium per gram.
● Monitor serum potassium level and liver function studies.
● Patient with high serum concentrations may have convulsions.
● This drug is almost always used with another antibiotic, such as an aminoglycoside, in life-threatening infections.
● Inject I.M. dose slowly over 12 to 15 seconds to minimize pain. Do not exceed 2 g per site.
● If precipitate forms during refrigerated storage, warm to 98.6° F. (37° C.) in warm water bath and shake well. Solution should be clear.
● Because mezlocillin is partially dialyzable, patients undergoing hemodialysis may need dosage adjustments.

Geriatric use
Half-life may be prolonged in elderly patients because of impaired renal function.

Breast-feeding
Mezlocillin is distributed readily into breast milk; safe use in breast-feeding women has not been established. Alternative feeding method is recommended during therapy.

---

miconazole
Monistat I.V.

miconazole nitrate
Micatin, Monistat 3, Monistat 7, Monistat-Derm

● Pharmacologic classification: imidazole derivative
● Therapeutic classification: antifungal
● Pregnancy risk category B

How supplied
Available by prescription only
Injection: 10 mg/ml
Vaginal suppositories: 200 mg
Vaginal cream: 2%

Available without prescription
Cream: 2%
Lotion: 2%
Powder: 2%
Spray: 2%
Vaginal suppositories: 100 mg

Indications, route, and dosage

Systemic fungal infections caused by susceptible organisms

Adults: 200 to 3,600 mg daily. I.V. dosages may vary with diagnosis and with infective agent. May divide daily dosage over three infusions, 200 to 1,200 mg per infusion. Dilute in at least 200 ml of 0.9% NaCl. Repeated courses may be needed because of relapse or reinfection.

Children: 20 to 40 mg/kg daily. Do not exceed 15 mg/kg per infusion.

Bladder instillation: 200 mg diluted and instilled into the bladder b.i.d. to q.i.d. or by continuous irrigation.

Fungal meningitis

Adults: 20 mg intrathecally as an adjunct to intravenous administration.

Cutaneous or mucocutaneous fungal infections caused by susceptible organisms

Topical use

Adults: Cover affected areas twice daily for 2 to 4 weeks.

Vaginal use

Adults: Insert 200-mg suppository at bedtime for 3 days, or 100-mg suppository or cream at bedtime for 7 days.

Pharmacodynamics

Antifungal action: Miconazole is both fungistatic and fungicidal, depending on drug concentration, in *Coccidioides immitis, Candida albicans, Cryptococcus neoformans, Histoplasma capsulatum, Candida tropicalis, Candida parapsilosis, Paracoccidioides brasiliensis, Sporothrix schenckii, Aspergillus flavus, A. ustus, Microsporum canis, Curvularia, Pseudallescheria boydii,* dermatophytes, and some gram-positive bacteria. Miconazole causes thickening of the fungal cell wall, altering membrane permeability; it also may kill the cell by interference with peroxisomal enzymes, causing accumulation of peroxide within the cell wall. It attacks virtually all pathogenic fungi.

In clinical use, miconazole is considered an alternative to amphotericin B to treat coccidiomycosis, but ketoconazole is preferred. Its clinical effectiveness in blastomycosis and histoplasmosis is highly variable. Its broad spectrum of activity makes it useful in treating superficial cutaneous infections and vaginal candidal infections.

Pharmacokinetics

- *Absorption:* About 50% of an oral miconazole dose is absorbed; however, no oral dosage form is currently available. A small amount of drug is systemically absorbed after vaginal administration.
- *Distribution:* Miconazole penetrates well into inflamed joints, vitreous humor, and the peritoneal cavity. Distribution into sputum and saliva is poor, and CSF penetration is unpredictable. Miconazole is over 90% bound to plasma proteins.
- *Metabolism:* Miconazole is metabolized in the liver, predominantly to inactive metabolites.
- *Excretion:* Miconazole elimination is triphasic; terminal half-life is about 24 hours. Between 10% and 14% of an oral dose is excreted in urine; 50%, in feces. Up to 1% of a vaginal dose is excreted in urine; 14% to 22% of an I.V. dose is excreted in urine. It is unknown whether it is excreted in breast milk.

Contraindications and precautions

Miconazole is contraindicated in patients with known hypersensitivity to the drug. It should be used with caution in patients with hepatic disease.

Interactions

Miconazole enhances the anticoagulant effect of warfarin. It may antagonize the effects of amphotericin B.

Effects on diagnostic tests

Miconazole may cause a transient decrease in hematocrit levels and an increase or decrease in platelet counts; it frequently causes erythrocyte aggregation. Miconazole also may cause hyponatremia, hyperlipidemia, and hypertriglyceridemia; abnormalities in lipoprotein and immunoelectrophoretic patterns are from the polyoxyl 35 castor oil vehicle.

Adverse reactions

- CNS: dizziness, drowsiness.
- DERM: pruritic rash, irritation, contact dermatitis.
- GI: nausea, vomiting, diarrhea, anorexia.
- HEMA: transient decreases in hematocrit levels, thrombocytopenia, erythrocyte aggregation.
- Metabolic: transient decrease in serum sodium levels, hyperlipidemia.
- Local: phlebitis at injection site.
- Other: fever, flushing, *anaphylaxis*.

   Note: Drug should be discontinued if condition worsens or irritation or signs of toxicity occur.

Overdose and treatment

Symptoms of overdose include GI complaints and altered mental status. Treatment after recent oral ingestion (within 4 hours) includes emesis or lavage followed by activated charcoal and an osmotic cathartic; subsequent care is supportive, as needed.

▶ Special considerations

- Identify causative organism by culture and sensitivity studies before I.V. or topical therapy is started.
- Initial I.V. therapy requires direct medical supervision; cardiorespiratory arrest has been reported with first dose.
- Check for possible hypersensitivity to drug before I.V. infusion; be prepared for anaphylaxis.
- Infuse over 30 to 60 minutes; rapid injection of undiluted miconazole may cause arrhythmias.
- Premedication with an antiemetic may lessen nausea and vomiting.
- Monitor CBC and electrolyte, triglyceride, and cholesterol levels before and frequently throughout therapy to detect adverse effects.
- Pruritic rash may persist for weeks after drug is discontinued; it may be controlled with oral or I.V. diphenhydramine.
- Cleanse affected area before applying cream or lotion. After application, massage area gently until cream disappears. Use lotion rather than cream in intertriginous areas to prevent maceration.
- Continue topical therapy for at least 1 month; improvement should begin in 1 to 2 weeks. If no improvement occurs by 4 weeks, reevaluate diagnosis.
- Insert vaginal applicator high into vagina.
- Patients with fungal meningitis require I.V. and intrathecal therapy.
- Miconazole has the advantage of causing fewer and less severe adverse reactions than other antifungals.

Information for the patient

- Teach patient the symptoms of fungal infection, and explain treatment rationale.
- Encourage patient to adhere to prescribed regimen and follow-up visits and to report any adverse effects.

● Teach patient correct procedure for intravaginal or topical applications.

● To prevent vaginal reinfection, teach correct perineal hygiene and recommend that patient abstain from sexual intercourse during therapy.

Pediatric use
Safe use in children under age 1 has not been established.

Breast-feeding
Safety has not been established.

midazolam hydrochloride
Versed

● Pharmacologic classification: benzodiazepine
● Therapeutic classification: preoperative sedative, agent for conscious sedation, adjunct for induction of general anesthesia, amnesic agent
● Controlled substance schedule IV
● Pregnancy risk category D

How supplied
Available by prescription only
Injection: 1 mg/ml in 2-ml, 5-ml, and 10-ml vials; 5 mg/ml in 1-ml, 2-ml, 5-ml, and 10-ml vials; 5 mg/ml in 2-ml disposable syringe

Indications, route, and dosage
Preoperative sedation (to induce sleepiness or drowsiness and relieve apprehension)
Adults: 0.035 mg to 0.04 mg/kg I.M. approximately 1 hour before surgery. May be administered with atropine or scopolamine and reduced doses of narcotics.
Conscious sedation before short diagnostic or endoscopic procedures
Adults: 1 to 2 mg by slow I.V. injection immediately before the procedure. May give up to 4 mg when concomitant narcotics are omitted.
Induction of general anesthesia
Adults: 0.3 to 0.35 mg/kg I.V. over 20 to 30 seconds. Additional increments of 25% of the initial dose may be needed to complete induction. Up to 0.6 mg/kg total dose may be given.

Pharmacodynamics
● *Sedative and anesthetic action:* Although the exact mechanism is unknown, midazolam, like other benzodiazepines, is thought to facilitate the action of gamma-aminobutyric acid (GABA) to provide a short-acting CNS depressant action.
● *Amnesic action:* The mechanism of action by which midazolam causes amnesia is not known.

Pharmacokinetics
● *Absorption:* Absorption after I.M. administration appears to be 80% to 100%; peak serum concentrations occur in 45 minutes and are about one-half of those after I.V. administration. Sedation begins within 15 minutes after an I.M. dose and within 2 to 5 minutes after I.V. injection. After I.V. administration, induction of anesthesia occurs in 1½ to 2½ minutes.
● *Distribution:* Midazolam has a large volume of dis-

tribution and is approximately 97% protein-bound. The drug crosses the placenta and enters fetal circulation.
● *Metabolism:* Midazolam is metabolized in the liver.
● *Excretion:* The metabolites of midazolam are excreted in urine. The half-life of midazolam is 2 to 6 hours. Duration of sedation is usually 1 to 4 hours.

Contraindications and precautions
Midazolam is contraindicated in patients with known hypersensitivity to benzodiazepines. Do not administer to patients with severe hypotension or shock, or to patients with alcohol intoxication and depressed vital signs.

Midazolam should be used cautiously in patients with severe hepatic dysfunction, renal failure, or congestive heart failure, because these patients eliminate the drug more slowly, and increased effects may be seen; and in patients with glaucoma, because midazolam may elevate intraocular pressure. Debilitated patients and elderly patients, especially those with chronic obstructive pulmonary disease (COPD), are at greatly increased risk for hypotension or respiratory depression with the use of midazolam.

Interactions
Midazolam may add to or potentiate the effects of alcohol, barbiturates, narcotics, antihistamines, tranquilizers, antidepressants, and other CNS and respiratory depressants.

Fentanyl, droperidol, and narcotics, used as preoperative medications, potentiate the hypnotic effect of midazolam. Midazolam may decrease the needed dose of inhaled anesthetics by depressing respiratory drive. Isoniazid may decrease the metabolism of midazolam.

Effects on diagnostic tests
None reported.

Adverse reactions
● CNS: retrograde amnesia, euphoria, confusion, emergence delirium or agitation, tonic-clonic movements, ataxia, slurred speech, paresthesia, headache, oversedation, yawning.
● CV: hypotension, tachycardia.
● DERM: hives, rash, pruritus.
● EENT: blurred vision, diplopia, nystagmus, pinpoint pupils, "blocked ears."
● GI: acid taste, excessive salivation, vomiting, nausea, hiccups.
● Local: warmth or cold at injection site, swelling, burning, redness, induration, phlebitis.
● Other: fluctuations in vital signs, chills, *laryngospasm, bronchospasm, respiratory depression, apnea.*
Note: Drug should be discontinued if hypersensitivity reactions occur.

Overdose and treatment
Clinical manifestations of overdose include confusion, stupor, coma, respiratory depression, and hypotension. Treatment is supportive. Maintain patent airway, and ensure adequate ventilation with mechanical support if necessary. Monitor vital signs. Use I.V. fluids or ephedrine to treat hypotension.

▶ Special considerations
Besides those relevant to all *benzodiazepines,* consider the following recommendations.
● Individualize dosage; use smallest effective dose possible. Use with extreme caution and reduced dosage in elderly and debilitated patients.

● Medical personnel who administer midazolam should be familiar with airway management. Close monitoring of cardiopulmonary function is required. Continuously monitor patients who have received midazolam to detect potentially life-threatening respiratory depression.
● Solutions of dextrose 5% in water (D_5W), 0.9% sodium chloride, and lactated Ringer's solution are compatible with midazolam.
● Before I.V. administration, ensure the immediate availability of oxygen and resuscitative equipment. Apnea and death have been reported with rapid I.V. administration. Avoid intraarterial injection because the hazards of this route are unknown. Avoid extravasation. Administer I.V. dose slowly to prevent respiratory depression.
● Administer I.M. dose deep into a large muscle mass to prevent tissue injury.
● Do not use any solution that is discolored or contains a precipitate.
● Hypotension occurs more frequently in patients premedicated with narcotics. Monitor vital signs closely.
● Laryngospasm and bronchospasm may occur rarely; countermeasures should be available.
● Midazolam can be mixed in the same syringe with morphine, meperidine, atropine, and scopolamine.

Information for the patient
● Advise patient to postpone tasks that require mental alertness or physical coordination until the drug's effects have worn off.
● As necessary, instruct patient in safety measures, such as supervised walking and gradual position changes, to prevent injury.
● Advise patient to call for instructions before taking any nonprescription drugs.

Geriatric use
Elderly or debilitated patients, especially those with COPD, are at significantly increased risk for respiratory depression and hypotension. Lower doses are indicated. Use with caution.

Pediatric use
Safety and efficacy of midazolam have not been established in children.

Breast-feeding
It is unknown whether midazolam passes into breast milk; it should be used with caution in breast-feeding women.

---

mineral oil
Agoral, Kondremul∗, Kondremul Plain, Lansoyl∗, Milkinol, Neo-Cultol, Nujol, Petrogalar Plain, Zymenol

● Pharmacologic classification: lubricant oil
● Therapeutic classification: laxative
● Pregnancy risk category C

How supplied
Available without prescription
Jelly: 55% w/w
Emulsion: 2.5 ml/5 ml
Suspension: 1.4 ml/5 ml, 2.75 ml/5 ml

Indications, route, and dosage
Constipation, preparation for bowel studies or surgery
Adults: 5 to 45 ml P.O. h.s., or 4-oz enema.
Children: 5 to 20 ml P.O. h.s., or 1- to 2-oz enema.

Pharmacodynamics
Laxative action: Mineral oil acts mainly in the colon, lubricating the intestine and retarding colonic fluid absorption.

Pharmacokinetics
● *Absorption:* Mineral oil normally is absorbed minimally; with emulsified drug form, significant absorption occurs. Action begins in 6 to 8 hours.
● *Distribution:* Mineral oil is distributed locally, primarily in the colon.
● *Metabolism:* None.
● *Excretion:* Mineral oil is excreted in feces.

Contraindications and precautions
Mineral oil is contraindicated in patients with fluid and electrolyte disturbances, appendicitis, acute surgical abdomen, fecal impaction, or intestinal obstruction or perforation, because the drug may exacerbate these symptoms or these conditions.
   The enema form is contraindicated in children under age 2 because of potential for adverse effects.
   Oral forms should be avoided in elderly bedridden patients and in children under age 6 because of the risk of oil droplet aspiration. Repeated use is not recommended in pregnant patients because the drug may cause hypoprothrombinemia and hemorrhagic disease of the neonate.

Interactions
Stool softeners such as docusate increase mineral oil absorption to potentially toxic levels; avoid concomitant use, which may cause lipoid pneumonia. Mineral oil may impair absorption of fat-soluble vitamins (A, D, E, and K), anticoagulants, oral contraceptives, digitalis glycosides, and sulfonamides, thus lessening their therapeutic effects.

Effects on diagnostic tests
None reported.

Adverse reactions
● GI: nausea; vomiting; diarrhea in excessive use; abdominal cramps, especially in severe constipation; decreased absorption of nutrients and fat-soluble vitamins, resulting in deficiency; slowed healing after hemorrhoidectomy; anal itching.
● Other: pruritus, laxative dependence in long-term or excessive use.
   Note: Drug should be discontinued if abdominal pain occurs.

Overdose and treatment
No information available.

▶ Special considerations
● Avoid administering drug to patients lying flat because if drug is aspirated into the lungs, pneumonitis may result.
● Do not give drug with food because this may delay gastric emptying, resulting in delayed drug action and increased aspiration risk. Separate by at least 2 hours.

- To improve taste, give emulsion and suspension with fruit juice or carbonated beverages.
- Prescribe cleansing enema 30 minutes to 1 hour after retention enema.
- Reduce or divide dose or use emulsified drug form to avoid leakage through anal sphincter.
- Mineral oil may impair absorption of fat-soluble vitamins (A, D, E, and K).

Information for the patient
- Instruct patient not to take mineral oil with stool softeners.
- Warn patient that mineral oil may leak through anal sphincter, especially with repeated use or with enema form. Undergarment protection may be desired.

Geriatric use
Because of the increased aspiration risk, use caution when administering drug to elderly patients.

Pediatric use
Mineral oil is not recommended for children under age 6 because of the risk of aspiration. The enema form is contraindicated in children under age 2.

---

minocycline hydrochloride
Minocin

- Pharmacologic classification: tetracycline
- Therapeutic classification: antibiotic
- Pregnancy risk category D

How supplied
Available by prescription only
Capsules: 50 mg, 100 mg
Tablets: 50 mg, 100 mg
Suspension: 50 mg/5 ml
Injection: 100 mg/vial

Indications, route, and dosage
Infections caused by sensitive organisms
Adults: Initially, 200 mg P.O., I.V.; then 100 mg q 12 hours or 50 mg P.O. q 6 hours.
Children over age 8: Initially, 4 mg/kg P.O., I.V.; then 4 mg/kg P.O. daily, divided q 12 hours. Give I.V. in 500 to 1,000 ml solution without calcium, over 6 hours.
Gonorrhea in patients sensitive to penicillin
Adults: Initially, 200 mg; then 100 mg q 12 hours for 4 days.
Syphilis in patients sensitive to penicillin
Adults: Initially, 200 mg; then 100 mg q 12 hours for 10 to 15 days.
Meningococcal carrier state
Adults: 100 mg P.O. q 12 hours for 5 days.
Uncomplicated urethral, endocervical, or rectal infection
Adults: 100 mg b.i.d. for at least 7 days.
Uncomplicated gonoccocal urethritis in men
Adults: 100 mg b.i.d. for 5 days.

Pharmacodynamics
Antibacterial action: Minocycline is bacteriostatic; it binds reversibly to ribosomal units, thus inhibiting bacterial protein synthesis.

Minocycline is active against many gram-negative and gram-positive organisms, *Mycoplasma, Rickettsia, Chlamydia,* and spirochetes; it may be more active against staphylococci than other tetracyclines.

The potential vestibular toxicity and cost of minocycline limits its usefulness. It may be more active than other tetracyclines against *Nocardia asteroides;* it is also effective against *Mycobacterium marinum* infections. It has been used for meningococcal meningitis prophylaxis because of its activity against *Neisseria meningitidis.*

Pharmacokinetics
- *Absorption:* Minocycline is 90% to 100% absorbed after oral administration; peak serum levels occur at 2 to 3 hours.
- *Distribution:* Minocycline is distributed widely into body tissues and fluids, including synovial, pleural, prostatic, and seminal fluids, bronchial secretions, saliva, and aqueous humor; CSF penetration is poor. Minocycline crosses the placenta; it is 55% to 88% protein-bound.
- *Metabolism:* Minocycline is metabolized partially.
- *Excretion:* Minocycline is excreted primarily unchanged in urine by glomerular filtration. Plasma half-life is 11 to 26 hours in adults with normal renal function. Some drug is excreted in breast milk.

Contraindications and precautions
Minocycline is contraindicated in patients with known hypersensitivity to any tetracycline; during the second half of pregnancy; and in children under age 8 because of the risk of permanent discoloration of teeth, enamel defects, and retardation of bone growth.

Use drug with caution in patients likely to be exposed to direct sunlight or ultraviolet light because of the risk of photosensitivity reactions.

Interactions
Concomitant use of minocycline with antacids containing aluminum, calcium, or magnesium or with laxatives containing magnesium decreases oral absorption of minocycline (because of chelation); concomitant use with oral iron products or sodium bicarbonate also decreases absorption. Foods and milk and other dairy products may also decrease absorption of minocycline, but less so than with other tetracyclines.

Tetracyclines may antagonize bactericidal effects of penicillin, inhibiting cell growth through bacteriostatic action; administer penicillin 2 to 3 hours before tetracycline.

Concomitant use of tetracycline necessitates lowered dosage of oral anticoagulants due to enhanced effects, and lowered dose of digoxin due to increased bioavailability.

Effects on diagnostic tests
Minocycline causes false-negative results in urine glucose tests using glucose oxidase reagent (Clinistix or Tes-Tape).

Minocycline causes false elevations in fluorometric test results for urinary catecholamines.

Adverse reactions
- CNS: light-headedness, dizziness from vestibular toxicity.
- CV: pericarditis.
- DERM: maculopapular and erythematous rashes, photosensitivity, increased pigmentation, urticaria, discolored nails and teeth.

- EENT: dysphagia, glossitis.
- GI: anorexia, epigastric distress, nausea, vomiting, diarrhea, enterocolitis, inflammatory lesions in ano-genital region.
- GU: reversible nephrotoxicity (Fanconi's syndrome) from *outdated* tetracyclines.
- HEMA: neutropenia, eosinophilia.
- Metabolic: increased BUN level.
- Local: *thrombophlebitis.*
- Other: hypersensitivity, bacterial and fungal super-infection.

Note: Drug should be discontinued if signs of toxicity, hypersensitivity, or superinfection occur; if erythema follows exposure to sunlight or ultraviolet light; or if severe diarrhea indicates pseudomembranous colitis.

Overdose and treatment
Clinical signs of overdose are usually limited to GI tract; give antacids or empty stomach by gastric lavage if ingestion occurred within the preceding 4 hours.

▶ **Special considerations**
Besides those relevant to all *tetracyclines,* consider the following recommendations.
- Reconstitute 100 mg powder with 5 ml sterile water for injection, with further dilution of 500 to 1,000 ml for I.V. infusion.
- Reconstituted solution is stable for 24 hours at room temperature. However, final diluted solution should be used immediately.

Pediatric use
Drug is not recommended for use in children younger than age 9.

Breast-feeding
Avoid use in breast-feeding women.

minoxidil (systemic)
Loniten

- Pharmacologic classification: peripheral vasodilator
- Therapeutic classification: antihypertensive
- Pregnancy risk category C

How supplied
Available by prescription only
Tablets: 2.5 mg, 10 mg

Indications, route, and dosage
Severe hypertension
Adults and children older than age 12: Initially, 5 mg P.O. as a single daily dose. Effective dosage range is usually 10 to 40 mg daily. Maximum dosage is 100 mg/day.
Children under age 12: 0.2 mg/kg (maximum 5 mg) as a single daily dose. Effective dosage range is usually 0.25 to 1 mg/kg daily in one or two doses. Maximum dosage is 50 mg/day.

Pharmacodynamics
Antihypertensive action: Minoxidil produces its antihypertensive effect by a direct vasodilating effect on vascular smooth muscle; the effect on resistance vessels (arterioles and arteries) is greater than that on capacitance vessels (venules and veins).

Pharmacokinetics
- *Absorption:* Minoxidil is absorbed rapidly from the GI tract; antihypertensive effect occurs in 30 minutes, peaking at 2 to 8 hours.
- *Distribution:* Minoxidil is distributed widely into body tissues; it is not bound to plasma proteins.
- *Metabolism:* Approximately 90% of a given dose is metabolized.
- *Excretion:* Drug and metabolites are excreted primarily in urine. Antihypertensive action persists for 2 to 5 days.

Contraindications and precautions
Minoxidil is contraindicated in patients with known hypersensitivity to the drug, and in patients with pheochromocytoma because it may stimulate catecholamine secretion from the tumor.

Minoxidil should be used cautiously in patients with recent myocardial infarction because vasodilation may increase myocardial oxygen demand via reflex tachycardia; and in patients with pulmonary hypertension, congestive heart failure (CHF), or significant renal impairment, because pulmonary artery pressure may increase.

Interactions
Minoxidil may potentiate the effects of diuretics or other antihypertensive drugs; concomitant use with guanethidine may cause profound orthostatic hypotension.

Effects on diagnostic tests
Minoxidil may elevate serum alkaline phosphatase, serum creatinine, and BUN levels, as well as antinuclear antibody titers; drug may transiently decrease hemoglobin and hematocrit levels. Minoxidil may also alter direction and magnitude of T waves on ECG.

Adverse reactions
- CV: edema, tachycardia, *pericardial effusion and cardiac tamponade,* CHF, ECG changes.
- DERM: rash, *Stevens-Johnson syndrome.*
- HEMA: *thrombocytopenia and leukopenia* (rare).
- Other: reversible hypertrichosis (elongation, thickening, and enhanced pigmentation of fine body hair), breast tenderness.

Note: Drug should be discontinued if pericardial effusion develops.

Overdose and treatment
Clinical signs of overdose include hypotension, tachycardia, headache, and skin flushing.

After acute ingestion, empty stomach by induced emesis or gastric lavage, and give activated charcoal to reduce absorption. Further treatment is usually symptomatic and supportive.

▶ **Special considerations**
- Minoxidil therapy is usually given concomitantly with two or more other antihypertensive drugs, such as diuretics, beta blockers, or sympathetic nervous system suppressants.
- Monitor blood pressure and pulse after administration, and report significant changes; assess intake, output, and body weight for sodium and water retention.
- Monitor for CHF, pericardial effusion, and cardiac

tamponade; have phenylephrine, dopamine, and vasopressin on hand to treat hypotension.

• Patients with renal failure or on dialysis may require smaller maintenance doses of minoxidil. Because minoxidil is removed by dialysis, it is recommended that on the day of dialysis, the drug be administered immediately after dialysis if dialysis is at 9 a.m.; if dialysis is after 3 p.m., the daily dose is given at 7 a.m. (8 hours before dialysis).

• Minoxidil has been used in 1% and 5% topical solutions to promote hair growth.

Information for the patient
• Explain that minoxidil is usually taken with other antihypertensive medications; emphasize importance of taking medication as prescribed.
• Caution patient to report the following cardiac symptoms promptly: increased heart rate (> 20 beats/minute over normal), rapid weight gain, shortness of breath, chest pain, severe indigestion, dizziness, light-headedness, or fainting.
• Tell patient to call for instructions before taking nonprescription cold preparations.
• Advise patient that hypertrichosis will disappear 1 to 6 months after stopping drug.

Geriatric use
Elderly patients may be sensitive to drug's antihypertensive effects. Dosage adjustment may be necessary because of altered drug clearance.

Pediatric use
Because of limited experience in children, use with caution. Cautious drug titration is necessary.

Breast-feeding
Minoxidil is distributed into breast milk. An alternative feeding method is recommended during therapy.

---

minoxidil (topical)
Rogaine

• Pharmacologic classification: direct acting vasodilator
• Therapeutic classification: hair-growth stimulant
• Pregnancy risk category C

How supplied
Available by prescription only
Topical solution: 2%

Indications, route, and dosage
Treatment of male pattern baldness (alopecia androgenetica)
Adults: Apply 1 ml to affected area b.i.d.

Pharmacodynamics
Hair-growth stimulation: The exact mechanism by which minoxidil promotes hair growth is unknown. It may alter androgen metabolism in the scalp, or it may exert a local vasodilatation and enhance the microcirculation around the hair follicle. It may also directly stimulate the hair follicle.

Pharmacokinetics
• *Absorption:* Minoxidil is poorly absorbed through intact skin. Approximately 0.3% to 4.5% of a topically applied dose reaches the systemic circulation.
• *Distribution:* Serum levels are generally negligible. Steady state levels are reached after 3 days of administering the drug b.i.d.
• *Metabolism:* Has not been fully described.
• *Excretion:* Minoxidil is eliminated primarily by the kidneys. About 95% of a topically applied dose is eliminated after 4 days.

Contraindications and precautions
Minoxidil is contraindicated in patients with a history of hypersensitivity to minoxidil, propylene glycol, or ethanol.

Decreased integrity of the epidermal barrier caused by inflammation or disease of the skin, such as excoriations, psoriasis, or severe sunburn, may increase minoxidil absorption.

Although extensive use of topical minoxidil has not revealed evidence that enough minoxidil is absorbed to have systemic effects, greater absorption due to misuse, individual variability, or unusual sensitivity could, at least theoretically, produce a systemic effect.

Experience with oral minoxidil has shown the following major cardiovascular effects: salt and water retention; generalized and local edema; pericardial effusion, pericarditis, and tamponade; tachycardia; and increased incidence of angina or new onset of angina. Patients with underlying heart disease are at special risk of these effects. Additive effects are possible in patients being treated for hypertension.

Interactions
None reported. Theoretically, absorbed minoxidil may potentiate orthostatic hypotension in patients taking guanethidine.

Effect on diagnostic tests
None reported.

Adverse reactions
• CNS: headache, dizziness, faintness, light-headedness, anxiety, depression, fatigue.
• CV: edema, chest pain, blood pressure increases/decreases, palpitations, pulse rate increases/decreases.
• DERM: irritant dermatitis, allergic contact dermatitis, eczema, hypertrichosis, local erythema, pruritus, dry skin, scalp flaking, exacerbation of hair loss, alopecia.
• GI: diarrhea, nausea, vomiting.
• GU: urinary tract infections, renal calculi, urethritis, prostatitis, epididymitis.
• HEMA: lymphadenopathy, thrombocytopenia.
• Metabolic: edema, weight gain.
• Musculoskeletal: fractures, back pain, tendinitis.
• Respiratory: bronchitis, upper respiratory infection, sinusitis.
• Special senses: conjunctivitis, ear infections, vertigo, visual disturbances and diminished visual acuity.
• Other: hypersensitivity (nonspecific allergic reactions, hives, allergic rhinitis, facial swelling), sexual dysfunction.

Overdose and treatment
None reported. However, if topical use produces systemic adverse effects, wash application site thoroughly with soap and water and treat symptoms, as appro-

---

priate. Treatment is symptomatic. Clinical signs of oral overdose include hypotension, tachycardia, headache, and skin flushing.

After acute ingestion, empty stomach by induced emesis or gastric lavage, and give activated charcoal to reduce absorption. Further treatment is usually symptomatic and supportive.

▶ **Special considerations**
● Do not use with other topical agents such as corticosteroids, retinoids, and petrolatum or agents that enhance percutaneous absorption. Rogaine is for topical use only; each ml contains 20 mg minoxidil and accidental ingestion could cause adverse systemic effects.
● Monitor patients 1 month after starting topical minoxidil therapy and at least every 6 months afterward. Discontinue topical minoxidil if systemic effects occur.
● The alcohol base will burn and irritate the eye and other sensitive surfaces (eye, abraded skin, and mucous membranes). If topical minoxidil contacts sensitive areas, flush with copious cool water.
● Before starting treatment, check that patient has a normal, healthy scalp. Local abrasion or dermatitis may increase absorption and the risk of adverse effects.
● Before treatment with topical minoxidil patient should have a history and physical and should be advised of potential risks; a risk-benefit decision should be made. Patients with cardiac disease should realize that adverse effects may be especially serious. Alert patients to the possibility of tachycardia and fluid retention, and monitor for increased heart rate, weight gain, or other systemic effects.

Information for the patient
● Tell patient to avoid inhaling the spray.
● Teach patient to apply topical minoxidil as follows: Hair and scalp should be dry before application. 1 ml should be applied to the total affected areas twice daily. Total daily dose should not exceed 2 ml. If the fingertips are used to apply the drug, wash the hands afterwards.
● Encourage patient to carefully review patient information leaflet, which is included with each package and in the full product information.

Pediatric use
Safety and effectiveness have not been established for patients under age 18.

Breast-feeding
Topical minoxidil should not be administered to breast-feeding women.

---

misoprostol
Cytotec

● Pharmacologic classification: prostaglandin E₁ analog
● Therapeutic classification: antiulcer agent, gastric mucosal protectant
● Pregnancy risk category X

How supplied
Available by prescription only
Tablets: 100 mcg, 200 mcg

Indications, route, and dosage
Prevention of gastric ulcer induced by NSAIDs
Adults: 200 mcg P.O. q.i.d. with meals and h.s. Dosage may be reduced to 100 mg P.O. q.i.d. in patients who cannot tolerate this dosage.
†*Treatment of duodenal or gastric ulcer*
Adults: 200 mg P.O. q.i.d. with meals and h.s.

Pharmacodynamics
Antiulcer action: Misoprostol enhances the production of gastric mucus and bicarbonate, and decreases basal, nocturnal, and stimulated gastric acid secretion.

Pharmacokinetics
● *Absorption:* Rapid after oral administration.
● *Distribution:* Highly bound (about 90%) to plasma proteins. Peak levels are reached in about 12 minutes.
● *Metabolism:* Rapidly de-esterified to misoprostol acid, the biologically active metabolite. The de-esterified metabolite undergoes further oxidation in several body tissues.
● *Excretion:* About 15% of an oral dose appears in the feces; the balance is excreted in the urine. Terminal half-life is 20 to 40 minutes.

Contraindications and precautions
Misoprostol is contraindicated in pregnant women because of its abortifacient property. Patients must be warned about this potential and be advised not to give the drug to anyone else. It should not be used in women of childbearing age unless they require NSAID therapy, are at high risk of developing gastric ulcers, and are aware of risks of using the drug during pregnancy.

Misoprostol is also contraindicated in patients allergic to prostaglandin derivatives.

Interactions
Misoprostol levels are diminished by concomitant administration with food or antacid, and misoprostol diminishes the availability of aspirin. None of these effects is believed to be significant.

Effects on diagnostic tests
Misoprostol produces a modest decrease in basal pepsin secretion.

Adverse reactions
● CNS: headache.
● GI: abdominal pain, diarrhea, nausea, flatulence, dyspepsia, vomiting, constipation.
● GU: spotting, cramps, hypermenorrhea, menstrual disorder, dysmenorrhea, postmenopausal vaginal bleeding.

Overdose and treatment
There has been little clinical experience with overdose. Cumulative daily doses of 1,600 mcg have been administered, with only minor GI discomfort noted. Treatment should be supportive.

▶ **Special considerations**
● Misoprostol is sold only as a unit of use package with patient information enclosed.
● Misoprostol should not be prescribed for a female patient of childbearing age unless she:
– needs NSAID therapy, and is at high risk of developing gastric ulcers.
– is capable of complying with effective contraception.

– has received both oral and written warnings regarding the hazards of misoprostol therapy, the risk of possible contraception failure, and the hazards this drug would pose to other women of childbearing age who might take this drug by mistake.

– has had a negative serum pregnancy test within 2 weeks before beginning therapy, and she will begin therapy on the second or third day of her next normal menstrual period.

● Diarrhea is usually dose-related and develops within the first 2 weeks of therapy. It can be minimized by administering the drug after meals and at bedtime, and by avoiding magnesium-containing antacids.

● Misoprostol has been used for treatment and prophylaxis of reflux esophagitis, alcohol-induced gastritis, hemorrhagic gastritis, and fat malabsorption in cystic fibrosis.

Information for the patient
Explain to the patient the importance of not giving this drug to anyone else. Make sure the patient understands that a pregnant woman who takes the drug may experience a miscarriage. The miscarriage could be incomplete and the patient may experience life-threatening bleeding.

Pediatric use
Safety has not been established in children under age 18.

Breast-feeding
Breast-feeding is not recommended because of the potential for misoprostol-induced diarrhea in the infant.

---

mitomycin
Mutamycin

● Pharmacologic classification: antineoplastic antibiotic (cell cycle-phase nonspecific)
● Therapeutic classification: antineoplastic
● Pregnancy risk category C

How supplied
Available by prescription only
Injection: 5-mg, 20-mg, 40-mg vials

Indications, route, and dosage
Dosage and indications may vary. Check current literature for recommended protocol.
Stomach, pancreatic, breast, colon, head, neck, lung, and hepatic cancer
Adults: 2 mg/m² I.V. daily for 5 days. Stop drug for 2 days, then repeat dose for 5 more days; or 10 to 20 mg/m² as a single dose. Repeat cycle q 6 to 8 weeks. Stop drug if WBC count is below 3,000/mm³ or platelet count is below 75,000/mm³.

Pharmacodynamics
Antineoplastic action: Mitomycin exerts its cytotoxic activity by a mechanism similar to that of the alkylating agents. The drug is converted to an active compound which forms cross-links between strands of DNA, inhibiting DNA synthesis. Mitomycin also inhibits RNA and protein synthesis to a lesser extent.

Pharmacokinetics
● *Absorption:* Because of its vesicant nature, mitomycin must be administered intravenously.
● *Distribution:* Mitomycin distributes widely into body tissues; animal studies show that the highest concentrations are found in the muscle, eyes, lungs, intestines, and stomach. The drug does not cross the blood-brain barrier.
● *Metabolism:* Mitomycin is metabolized by hepatic microsomal enzymes and is also deactivated in the kidneys, spleen, brain, and heart.
● *Excretion:* Mitomycin and its metabolites are excreted in urine. A small portion is eliminated in bile and feces.

Contraindications and precautions
Mitomycin is contraindicated in patients with a history of hypersensitivity to the drug; in patients with a WBC count below 3,000/mm³, platelet count below 75,000/mm³, or serum creatinine level above 1.7 mg/100 ml; and in those with coagulation disorders, prolonged prothrombin time, or serious infections, because of the potential for adverse effects.

Interactions
Concomitant use with dextran and urokinase enhances the cytotoxic activity of mitomycin. Through a series of enzymatic processes, these agents increase autolysis of cells, adding to the cell death caused by mitomycin.

Effects on diagnostic tests
Mitomycin therapy, through drug-induced renal toxicity, may increase serum creatinine and BUN concentrations.

Adverse reactions
● CNS: paresthesias.
● GI: nausea, vomiting, anorexia, stomatitis.
● HEMA: *bone marrow depression* (dose-limiting), *thrombocytopenia, leukopenia* (may be delayed up to 8 weeks and may be cumulative with successive doses).
● Local: desquamation, induration, pruritus, pain at site of injection; with extravasation, cellulitis, ulceration, sloughing.
● Other: reversible alopecia; purple coloration of nail beds; fever; syndrome characterized by microangiopathic hemolytic anemia, *thrombocytopenia,* renal toxicity, and hypertension.
Note: Drug should be discontinued if WBC count is below 3,000/mm³ or platelet count is below 75,000/mm³.

Overdose and treatment
Clinical manifestations of overdose include myelosuppression, nausea, vomiting, and alopecia.
Treatment is usually supportive and includes transfusion of blood components, antiemetics, and antibiotics for infections that may develop.

▶ Special considerations
● To reconstitute 5-mg vial, use 10 ml of sterile water for injection; to reconstitute 20-mg vial, use 40 ml of sterile water for injection, to give a concentration of 0.5 mg/ml.
● Drug may be administered by I.V. push injection slowly over 5 to 10 minutes into the tubing of a freely flowing I.V. infusion.
● Drug can be further diluted to 100 to 150 ml with

---

normal saline solution or dextrose 5% in water for I.V. infusion (over 30 to 60 minutes or longer).
● Reconstituted solution remains stable for 1 week at room temperature and for 2 weeks if refrigerated.
● Mitomycin has been used intraarterially to treat certain tumors, for example, into hepatic artery for colon cancer. It has also been given as a continuous daily infusion.
● An unlabeled use of this drug is to treat small bladder papillomas. It is instilled directly into the bladder in a concentration of 20 mg/20 ml sterile water.
● Ulcers caused by extravasation develop late and dorsal to the extravasation site. Apply cold compresses for at least 12 hours.
● Continue CBC and blood studies at least 7 weeks after therapy is stopped. Monitor for signs of bleeding.

Information for the patient
● Tell patient to avoid exposure to people with infections.
● Warn patient not to receive immunizations during therapy and for several weeks afterward. Members of the same household should not receive immunizations during the same period.
● Reassure patient that hair should grow back after treatment has been discontinued.
● Tell patient to call promptly if he develops a sore throat or fever or notices any unusual bruising or bleeding.

Breast-feeding
It is not known whether mitomycin distributes into breast milk. However, because of the potential for serious adverse reactions, mutagenicity, and carcinogenicity in the infant, breast-feeding is not recommended.

---

mitotane
Lysodren

● Pharmacologic classification: chlorophenothane (DDT) analogue
● Therapeutic classification: antineoplastic, antiadrenal agent
● Pregnancy risk category C

How supplied
Available by prescription only
Tablets (scored): 500 mg

Indications, route, and dosage
Dosage and indications may vary. Check current literature for recommended protocol.
Inoperable adrenocortical cancer
Adults: Initially, 1 to 6 g P.O. daily in divided doses t.i.d. or q.i.d. Increase to 9 to 10 g daily as tolerated. If severe adverse reactions appear, reduce dosage until maximum tolerated dosage is achieved (varies from 2 to 16 g daily but is usually 8 to 10 g daily).
Cushing's syndrome
Adults: 1 to 12 g P.O. daily in divided doses; maintenance dosage ranges from 500 mg twice weekly to 2 g daily.

Pharmacodynamics
● *Antineoplastic action:* The exact mechanism of mitotane's activity is unclear. Possibly, a metabolite binds to mitochondrial proteins in the adrenal cortex, resulting in cell death.
● *Adrenocortical action:* Mitotane also inhibits the production of corticosteroids and alters extraadrenal metabolism of endogenous and exogenous steroids.

Pharmacokinetics
● *Absorption:* After oral administration, 35% to 40% of a dose is absorbed across the GI tract.
● *Distribution:* Mitotane is widely distributed in body tissue; fatty tissue is the primary storage site. Slow release of mitotane from fatty tissue into the plasma occurs after the drug is discontinued. A metabolite of mitotane has been detected in the cerebrospinal fluid.
● *Metabolism:* Mitotane is metabolized in the liver and other tissue.
● *Excretion:* Mitotane and its metabolites are excreted in urine and bile. The plasma elimination half-life is reported to be 18 to 159 days.

Contraindications and precautions
Mitotane is contraindicated in patients with a history of hypersensitivity to the drug. It should be used cautiously in patients with impaired liver function; the drug may accumulate in the body because of impaired metabolism.

Interactions
When used concomitantly, mitotane may decrease the effect of barbiturates, coumarin anticoagulants, and phenytoin through the induction of hepatic microsomal enzymes, increasing the metabolism of these agents to inactive compounds. Concomitant use with CNS depressants can cause an additive CNS depression. Spironolactone may block the actions of mitotane.

Effects on diagnostic tests
Mitotane therapy may decrease concentrations of urinary 17-hydroxycorticosteroid, plasma cortisol, protein-bound iodine, and serum uric acid.

Adverse reactions
● CNS: depression; somnolence; vertigo; brain damage and dysfunction in long-term, high-dose therapy; fatigue.
● CV: flushing.
● DERM: maculopapular rash, pruritus, pigmentation, dermatitis.
● GI: severe nausea, vomiting, diarrhea, anorexia.
● GU: *hemorrhagic cystitis,* hematuria.
● Metabolic: adrenal insufficiency.
● Other: adrenal insufficiency, blurred vision, diplopia, fever.
 Note: Drug should be discontinued if patient suffers from shock, severe trauma, infection, or another condition that would be adversely affected by adrenocortical insufficiency.

Overdose and treatment
Clinical manifestations of overdose include vomiting, weakness, numbness of extremities, diarrhea, apprehension, and excitement.
 Treatment is usually supportive and includes activated charcoal, saline cathartic, induction of emesis with ipecac, intestinal lavage with mannitol 20%, and appropriate symptomatic therapy.

▶ Special considerations
• Mitotane can be administered with or without food in the stomach. Avoid administering the drug with a fatty meal because the drug distributes mostly to body fat.
• Give an antiemetic before administering mitotane, to reduce nausea.
• Dosage may be reduced if GI or skin reactions are severe.
• Dose modification may be required in hepatic disease.
• Obese patients may need higher dosage and may have longer-lasting adverse reactions, because drug distributes mostly to body fat.
• Evaluate efficacy by reduction in pain, weakness, anorexia, and tumor mass.
• Monitor for symptoms of hepatotoxicity.
• Drug should not be used in a patient with shock or trauma. Use of corticosteroids may avoid acute adrenocorticoid insufficiency.
• Glucocorticoid therapy is usually required. During periods of physiologic stress (such as infection or surgery), glucocorticoid dosage should be increased.
• Monitor behavioral and neurologic signs daily throughout therapy.
• Adequate trial is at least 3 months, but therapy can continue if clinical benefits are observed.

Information for the patient
• Tell patient it is important to continue medication despite nausea and vomiting.
• Warn patient to avoid alcoholic beverages after taking a dose of medication because excessive drowsiness may occur.
• Tell patient drug may cause drowsiness. Patient should use caution when performing activities that require mental alertness.
• Patient should call immediately if vomiting occurs shortly after taking a dose.

Breast-feeding
It is not known whether mitotane distributes into breast milk. However, because of the potential for serious adverse reactions in the infant, breast-feeding is not recommended.

mitoxantrone hydrochloride
Novantrone

• Pharmacologic classification: antibiotic antineoplastic
• Therapeutic classification: antineoplastic
• Pregnancy risk category D

How supplied
Available by prescription only
Injection: 2 mg mitoxantrone base/ml in 10-ml, 12.5-ml, 15-ml vials

Indications, route, and dosage
Initial treatment in combination with other approved drugs for acute nonlymphocytic leukemia
Adults: For induction (in combination chemotherapy), 12 mg/m² daily by I.V. infusion on days 1 to 3, and 100 mg/m² of cytosine arabinoside by continuous I.V. infusion (over 24 hours) on days 1 to 7 for 7 days.
Most complete remissions follow initial course of induction therapy. A second course may be given if antileukemic response is incomplete: give mitoxantrone for 2 days and cytosine for 5 days using the same daily dosage levels. Second course of therapy should be withheld until toxicity clears if severe or life-threatening nonhematologic toxicity occurs.

Pharmacodynamics
Antineoplastic action: Mitoxantrone's mechanism of action is not completely established. It is a DNA-reactive agent that has cytocidal effects on proliferating and nonproliferating cells, suggestive of lack of cell-phase specificity.

Pharmacokinetics
• *Absorption:* Not applicable. Administered only by I.V. infusion.
• *Distribution:* Mitoxantrone is 78% plasma protein-bound.
• *Metabolism:* Metabolized by the liver.
• *Excretion:* Excretion is via renal and hepatobiliary systems; 6% to 11% of dose is excreted in urine within 5 days: 65% is unchanged drug; 35% is two inactive metabolites. Within 5 days, 25% of dose is excreted in feces.

Contraindications and precautions
Mitoxantrone is contraindicated in patients with known hypersensitivity to the drug. It should not be used in patients with preexisting myelosuppression resulting from prior drug therapy unless possible benefit warrants risk of further myelosuppression. Use with caution in patients with hepatic or renal impairment or preexisting cardiac disease.

Adverse reactions
• CNS: seizures, headache.
• CV: *CHF, arrhythmia,* ECG changes, chest pain, tachycardia, hypotension, asymptomatic decreases in left ventricular ejection fraction.
• DERM: alopecia, petechiae, ecchymosis, urticaria, rashes.
• EENT: conjunctivitis.
• GI: nausea, vomiting, diarrhea, abdominal pain, mucositis, stomatitis, bleeding.
• GU: urinary tract infection, renal failure.
• HEMA: thrombocytopenia, leukopenia.
• Respiratory: cough, dyspnea, pneumonia.
• Other: jaundice, sepsis, fungal infections, fever, phlebitis at injection site (rare), tissue necrosis after extravasation (rare).

Overdose and treatment
Accidental overdoses have occurred and have caused severe leukopenia with infection. Monitor hematologic parameters and treat symptomatically. Antimicrobial therapy may be necessary.

▶ Special considerations
• Close and frequent monitoring of hematologic and chemical laboratory parameters, including serial CBC and liver function tests, with frequent patient observation is recommended.
• Safety of administration by routes other than I.V. has not been established. Do not use intrathecally.
• Hyperuricemia may result from rapid lysis of tumor

cells. Monitor serum uric acid levels. Institute hypouricemic therapy before antileukemic therapy.
● Transient elevations of AST (SGOT) and ALT (SGPT) have occurred 4 to 24 days after mitoxantrone therapy.
● To prepare, dilute solutions to at least 50 ml with either 0.9% sodium chloride solution or dextrose 5% in water (D₅W). Inject slowly into tubing of a freely running I.V. solution of 0.9% sodium chloride solution or D₅W over not less than 3 minutes. Discard unused infusion solutions appropriately. Do not mix for infusion with heparin; a precipitate may form. Specific compatibility data are not available.
● If extravasation occurs, discontinue I.V. and restart in another vein. Mitoxantrone is a nonvesicant and the possibility of severe local reactions is minimal.
● Urine may appear blue-green for 24 hours after administration.
● Bluish discoloration of sclera may occur. Advise patient of this as well as how to recognize signs of myelosuppression.

Information for the patient
● Tell patient urine may appear blue-green for 24 hours after administration and sclera may appear bluish.
● Advise patient to notify physician promptly if signs and symptoms of myelosuppression develop (fever, sore throat, easy bruising, or excessive bleeding).

Pediatric use
Safety and efficacy have not been established.

Breast-feeding
It is unknown if mitoxantrone is excreted in breast milk. Because of potential for serious adverse reactions in infants, breast-feeding should be discontinued before therapy.

---

mivacurium chloride
Mivacron

● Pharmacologic classification: nondepolarizing neuromuscular blocker
● Therapeutic classification: skeletal muscle relaxant
● Pregnancy risk category C

How supplied
Available by prescription only
Injection: 2 mg/ml in 5-ml and 10-ml vials
Infusion: 0.5 mg/ml, in 50 ml dextrose 5% in water (D₅W)

Indications, route, and dosage
Adjunct to general anesthesia, to facilitate endotracheal intubation and to provide skeletal muscle relaxation during surgery or mechanical ventilation
Dosage is highly individualized. Note that all times of onset and duration of neuromuscular blockade are averages and considerable individual variation is normal.
Adults: Usually, 0.15 mg/kg I.V. push over 5 to 15 seconds provides adequate muscle relaxation within 2½ minutes for endotracheal intubation. Supplemental doses of 0.1 mg/kg I.V. q 15 minutes usually maintains muscle relaxation. Alternatively, maintain neuromuscular blockade with a continuous infusion of 4 mcg/kg/

minute started simultaneously with initial dose, or 9 to 10 mcg/kg/minute started after evidence of spontaneous recovery of initial dose. When used with isoflurane or enflurane anesthesia, dosage is usually reduced about 25%.
Children age 2 to 12: 0.20 mg/kg I.V. push administered over 5 to 15 seconds. Neuromuscular blockade is usually evident in less than 2 minutes. Although supplemental doses of 0.1 mg/kg I.V. q 15 minutes usually maintains muscle relaxation in adults, maintenance doses are usually required more frequently in children. Alternatively, maintain neuromuscular blockade with a continuous infusion titrated to effect. Most children respond to 5 to 31 mcg/kg/minute (average 14 mcg/kg/minute).

Pharmacodynamics
Neuromuscular blocking action: Mivacurium competes with acetylcholine for receptor sites at the motor endplate. Because this action may be antagonized by cholinesterase inhibitors, mivacurium is considered a competitive antagonist. Drug is a mixture of three stereoisomers, each possessing neuromuscular blocking activity: the cis-trans isomer (36% of the total) and the trans-trans isomer (57% of the total) are about 10 times as potent as the cis-cis isomer (only 6% of the total). The isomers do not interconvert in vivo.

Pharmacokinetics
● *Absorption:* No information available.
● *Distribution:* Mivacurium's volume of distribution is small, indicating that it does not extensively distribute to tissues.
● *Metabolism:* Mivacurium is rapidly hydrolyzed by plasma pseudocholinesterase to inactive components.
● *Excretion:* Drug is excreted in bile and urine. Of the highly active isomers, the cis-trans and trans-trans isomers each have an elimination half-life of under 2.3 minutes. The less active cis-cis isomer, which is only a small portion of the total drug, has an elimination half-life of 55 minutes.

Contraindications and precautions
Mivacurium is contraindicated in patients with hypersensitivity to the drug. Drug should be administered only by personnel familiar with use of neuromuscular blockers and techniques involved in maintaining a patent airway. It should not be used unless facilities and equipment for artificial respiration, mechanical ventilation, oxygen therapy, and intubation and an antagonist are within reach.
Use very cautiously, if at all, in patients who are homozygous for the atypical plasma pseudocholinesterase gene because drug is metabolized to inactive compounds by plasma pseudocholinesterase.
Use cautiously in patients with significant cardiovascular disease and in those who may be adversely affected by release of histamine (such as asthmatic patients). In such patients, initial dose should be lower or given over longer periods (60 seconds) to avoid hypotension.
Also use cautiously, possibly at reduced dosage, in debilitated patients; in patients with metastatic cancer, severe electrolyte disturbances, or neuromuscular diseases; and in those in whom potentiation or difficulty in reversal of neuromuscular blockade is anticipated. Patients with myasthenia gravis or myasthenic syndrome (Eaton-Lambert syndrome) are particularly sensitive to the effects of nondepolarizing relaxants. Test

doses of 0.015 to 0.020 mg/kg may be used to assess such patients' sensitivity to the drug.

Patients with severe burns often develop resistance to nondepolarizing neuromuscular blockers; however, they may also have reduced plasma pseudocholinesterase activity. Administer a test dose to assess patients' sensitivity to the drug.

Interactions
Administration to patients receiving aminoglycosides (kanamycin, neomycin, streptomycin, and gentamicin), bacitracin, colistin, polymyxin B, colistimethate, magnesium salts, or tetracyclines may result in increased muscle weakness. Phenytoin and carbamazepine may prolong the time to maximal block or shorten the duration of blockade with neuromuscular blockers.

Quinidine or inhalational anesthetics (especially isoflurane or enflurane) may enhance the activity (or prolong action) of nondepolarizing neuromuscular blockers.

Mivacurium is physically incompatible with alkaline solutions (such as barbiturate solutions) and may form a precipitate. Do not administer through the same I.V. line with any of these drugs.

Effects on diagnostic tests
None reported.

Adverse reactions
● CNS: dizziness.
● CV: flushing, hypotension, tachycardia, bradycardia, arrhythmias.
● DERM: rash, urticaria, erythema.
● Respiratory: *bronchospasm*, wheezing, *respiratory insufficiency or apnea*.
● Other: prolonged muscle weakness, phlebitis, muscle spasms.

Overdose and treatment
Overdosage may result in prolonged neuromuscular blockade. Maintain a patent airway and control respirations until patient recovers neuromuscular function. Antagonists should not be administered until there is some evidence of spontaneous recovery. In clinical trials, administration of 0.3 to 0.64 mg/kg neostigmine methylsulfate or 0.5 mg/kg edrophonium chloride to patients with spontaneous recovery of muscle function resulted in increased muscle strength of about 10% recovery to about 95% recovery within 10 minutes.

▶ Special considerations
● When mivacurium is administered I.V. push to adults receiving anesthetic combinations of nitrous oxide and opiates, neuromuscular blockade usually lasts 15 to 20 minutes; most patients recover 95% of muscle strength in 25 to 30 minutes.
● Duration of drug effect is increased about 150% in patients with end-stage renal disease and 300% in patients with hepatic dysfunction.
● Dosage should be adjusted to ideal body weight in obese patients (patients 30% or more above their ideal weight) because of reported prolonged neuromuscular blockade.
● A nerve stimulator and train-of-four monitoring are recommended to document antagonism of neuromuscular blockade and recovery of muscle strength. Before attempting pharmacologic reversal with neostigmine methylsulfate or edrophonium chloride, some evidence of spontaneous recovery should be evident.

● Experimental evidence suggests that acid-base and electrolyte balance may influence actions of and response to nondepolarizing neuromuscular blockers. Alkalosis may counteract paralysis; acidosis may enhance it.
● Note that mivacurium, like other neuromuscular blockers, does not have an effect on consciousness or pain threshold. To avoid patient distress, this drug should not be administered until the patient's consciousness is obtunded by the general anesthetic.
● Drug is compatible with D_5W, 0.9% sodium chloride injection, dextrose 5% in 0.9% sodium chloride injection, lactated Ringer's injection, and dextrose 5% in lactated Ringer's injection. Diluted solutions are stable for 24 hours at room temperature.
● When diluted as directed, mivacurium is compatible with alfentanil, fentanyl, sufentanil, droperidol, and midazolam.
● Drug is available as premixed infusion in D_5W. After removing the protective outer wrap, check container for minor leaks by squeezing the bag before administering. Do not add any other drugs to the container, and do not use the container in series connections.

Pediatric use
Like other neuromuscular blockers, dosage requirements for children are higher on a mg/kg basis as compared with adults. Onset and recovery of neuromuscular blockade occur more rapidly in children.

Breast-feeding
It is unknown if drug is excreted in breast milk. Use with caution in breast-feeding women.

---

molindone hydrochloride
Moban

● Pharmacologic classification: dihydroindolone
● Therapeutic classification: antipsychotic
● Pregnancy risk category C

How supplied
Available by prescription only
Tablets: 5 mg, 10 mg, 25 mg, 50 mg, 100 mg
Oral solution: 20 mg/ml

Indications, route, and dosage
Psychotic disorders
Adults: 50 to 75 mg P.O. daily, increased to a maximum of 225 mg daily. Doses up to 400 mg may be required.

Pharmacodynamics
Antipsychotic action: Molindone is unrelated to all other antipsychotic drugs; it is thought to exert its antipsychotic effects by postsynaptic blockade of CNS dopamine receptors, thereby inhibiting dopamine-mediated effects.

Molindone has many other central and peripheral effects; it also produces alpha and ganglionic blockade. Its most prominent adverse reactions are extrapyramidal.

Pharmacokinetics
● *Absorption:* Data are limited, but absorption appears rapid; peak effects occur within 1½ hours.

- *Distribution:* Molindone is distributed widely into the body.
- *Metabolism:* Molindone is metabolized extensively; drug effects persist for 24 to 36 hours.
- *Excretion:* Most of drug is excreted as metabolites in urine; some is excreted in feces via the biliary tract. Overall, 90% of a given dose is excreted within 24 hours.

Contraindications and precautions

Molindone is contraindicated in patients with known hypersensitivity to molindone; and in patients with disorders accompanied by coma, CNS depression, brain damage, circulatory collapse, or cerebrovascular disease because of additive CNS depression and adverse effects on blood pressure. Use molindone cautiously in patients with cardiac disease (dysrhythmias, congestive heart failure, angina pectoris, valvular disease, or heart block); Reye's syndrome; encephalitis, head injury, or related conditions because drug may mask signs and symptoms; in patients with respiratory disease because molindone may worsen glaucoma; in patients with prostatic hypertrophy; in patients with urinary retention; in patients with hepatic or renal dysfunction; in patients with Parkinson's disease; and in patients with pheochromocytoma, because drug may cause excessive buildup of transmitters, resulting in adverse cardiovascular effects.

Molindone lowers seizure threshold and may cause seizures in patients with epilepsy and other seizure disorders.

Patients with hypocalcemia are more likely to develop extrapyramidal reactions. Administration of molindone may influence the CNS thermoregulatory center and predispose the patient to hyperthermia or hypothermia.

In patients with hepatic or renal dysfunction, decreased metabolism and excretion may cause the drug to accumulate in plasma.

Sulfite preservatives in oral solution could induce acute asthmatic attack in asthma patients.

Interactions

Concomitant use with sympathomimetics, including epinephrine, phenylephrine, phenylpropanolamine, and ephedrine (often found in nasal sprays), or appetite suppressants may decrease their stimulatory and pressor effects. Because of its alpha-blocking potential, molindone may cause epinephrine reversal – a hypotensive response to epinephrine.

Molindone may inhibit blood pressure response to centrally acting antihypertensive drugs, such as guanethidine, guanabenz, guanadrel, clonidine, methyldopa, and reserpine. Additive effects are likely after concomitant use of molindone with CNS depressants, including alcohol, analgesics, barbiturates, narcotics, tranquilizers, and general, spinal, or epidural anesthetics, or parenteral magnesium sulfate (oversedation, respiratory depression, and hypotension); antiarrhythmic agents, quinidine, disopyramide, or procainamide (increased incidence of cardiac arrhythmias and conduction defects); atropine or other anticholinergic drugs, including antidepressants, monoamine oxidase inhibitors, phenothiazines, antihistamines, meperidine, and antiparkinsonian agents (oversedation, paralytic ileus, visual changes, and severe constipation); nitrates (hypotension); and metrizamide (increased risk of convulsions).

Beta-blocking agents may inhibit molindone metabolism, increasing plasma levels and toxicity.

Concomitant use with propylthiouracil increases risk of agranulocytosis; concomitant use with lithium may result in severe neurologic toxicity with an encephalitis-like syndrome, and a decreased therapeutic response to molindone.

Decreased therapeutic response to molindone may follow concomitant use with calcium-containing drugs, such as phenytoin and tetracyclines, aluminum- and magnesium-containing antacids, or antidiarrheals (decreased absorption); or caffeine (increased metabolism).

Molindone may antagonize therapeutic effect of bromocriptine on prolactin secretion; it may also decrease the vasoconstricting effects of high-dose dopamine and may decrease effectiveness and increase toxicity of levodopa (by dopamine blockade). Calcium sulfate in molindone tablets may inhibit the absorption of phenytoin or tetracyclines.

Effects on diagnostic tests

Molindone causes false-positive results in urine pregnancy tests using human chorionic gonadotropin and additive potential for causing convulsions with metrizamide myelography.

Molindone elevates levels of liver enzymes (AST [SGOT] and ALT [SGPT]), free fatty acids, and BUN; drug may alter white blood cell (WBC) counts and may increase or decrease serum glucose levels.

Adverse reactions

- CNS: extrapyramidal symptoms – dystonia, akathisia, torticollis, tardive dyskinesia (usually dose-related with long-term therapy, but it can develop rapidly), sedation (high incidence), pseudoparkinsonism, drowsiness (frequent), *neuroleptic malignant syndrome* (dose-related; if untreated, *fatal respiratory failure* in over 10% of patients), dizziness, headache, insomnia (early awakening), exacerbation of psychotic symptoms.
- CV: *asystole,* orthostatic hypotension, tachycardia, dizziness/fainting, arrhythmias, ECG changes, increased anginal pain after I.M. injection.
- EENT: blurred vision, tinnitus, mydriasis, increased intraocular pressure, ocular changes (retinal pigmentary change with long-term use).
- GI: dry mouth, constipation, nausea, vomiting, anorexia, diarrhea.
- GU: urine retention, gynecomastia, hypermenorrhea, inhibited ejaculation.
- HEMA: transient leukopenia, *agranulocytosis,* thrombocytopenia, anemia (within 30 to 90 days).
- Hepatic: cholestatic jaundice.
- Local: contact dermatitis from concentrate or injectable form, muscle necrosis from I.M. injection.
- Other: hyperprolactinemia, photosensitivity, increased appetite or weight gain, neuroleptic malignant syndrome, hypersensitivity (rash, urticaria, drug fever, edema, decreased libido.

  Note: Drug should be discontinued if hypersensitivity, jaundice, agranulocytosis, or neuroleptic malignant syndrome (marked hyperthermia, extrapyramidal effects, autonomic dysfunction) occurs; if WBC count falls below 4,000; or if severe extrapyramidal symptoms occur even after dosage is lowered. Drug should be discontinued 48 hours before and 24 hours after myelography using metrizamide because of the additive risk of convulsions. When feasible, withdraw drug slowly and gradually; many drug effects persist after withdrawal.

Overdose and treatment
CNS depression is characterized by deep, unarousable sleep and possible coma, hypotension or hypertension, extrapyramidal symptoms, abnormal involuntary muscle movements, agitation, seizures, arrhythmias, ECG changes, hypothermia or hyperthermia, and autonomic nervous system dysfunction.

Treatment is symptomatic and supportive, including maintaining vital signs, airway, stable body temperature, and fluid/electrolyte balance.

Do not induce vomiting: drug inhibits cough reflex, and aspiration may occur. Use gastric lavage, then activated charcoal and saline cathartics; dialysis does not help. Regulate body temperature as needed. Treat hypotension with I.V. fluids: *do not give epinephrine.* Treat seizures with parenteral diazepam or barbiturates; arrhythmias, with parenteral phenytoin (1 mg/kg with rate titrated to blood pressure); extrapyramidal reactions, with benztropine or parenteral diphenhydramine at 2 mg/kg/minute.

▶ Special considerations
● Oral formulations may cause GI distress and should be administered with food or fluids.
● Dilute concentrate in 2 to 4 oz of liquid, preferably soup, water, juice, carbonated drinks, milk, or puddings.
● Drug may cause pink to brown discoloration of urine.
● Protect liquid forms from light.

Information for the patient
● Explain the risks of dystonic reaction and tardive dyskinesia, and advise patient to report abnormal body movements.
● Warn patient to avoid spilling liquid preparations on the skin; rash and irritation may result.
● Advise the patient to avoid temperature extremes (hot or cold baths, sunlamps, or tanning beds) because drug may cause thermoregulatory changes.
● Suggest sugarless gum or candy, ice chips, or artificial saliva to relieve dry mouth.
● Warn patient not to take drug with antacids or antidiarrheals; not to drink alcoholic beverages or take other drugs that cause sedation; not to stop taking the drug or take *any* other drug except as instructed; and to take drug exactly as prescribed, without doubling after missing a dose.
● Warn patient about sedative effect. Tell patient to report difficult urination, sore throat, dizziness, or fainting.

Geriatric use
Lower doses are recommended; 30% to 50% of usual dose may be effective. Elderly patients are at greater risk for tardive dyskinesia and other extrapyramidal effects.

Pediatric use
Drug is not recommended for children under age 12.

monoamine oxidase inhibitors

**isocarboxazid
pargyline hydrochloride
phenelzine sulfate
selegiline hydrochloride
tranylcypromine sulfate**

Antidepressant effects of monoamine oxidase (MAO) inhibitors were first noted in 1952 during studies with iproniazid, a hydrazine derivative of the antitubercular agent isoniazid. Because of excessive hepatotoxicity, iproniazid was never used clinically. Currently available MAO inhibitors include two hydrazine derivatives, isocarboxazid and phenelzine sulfate, and two nonhydrazine derivatives, tranylcypromine sulfate and pargyline hydrochloride, all of which are less hepatotoxic than iproniazid. All four have antihypertensive activity and antidepressant effects; only pargyline is used (rarely) to treat severe hypertension.

MAO inhibitors can cause serious adverse reactions and interact adversely with many foods and drugs. They are useful drugs for treating affective illness, especially "atypical" major depression disorders (particularly depression with hypersomnia, hyperphagia, or severe anxiety) or depression unresponsive to tricyclic antidepressants. They are also useful for panic disorder.

Pharmacology
Some forms of depression are thought to result from low CNS levels of neurotransmitters, including norepinephrine and serotonin. MAO inhibitors, as their name implies, depress the effects of MAO, an enzyme that is present principally in the CNS and inactivates amine-containing substances, including the neurotransmitters. Many adverse effects from MAO inhibitors are attributed to gradual buildup and increased activity of neurotransmitters after enzyme inhibition.

Selegiline specifically inhibits MAO type B, which is found only in the CNS.

Clinical indications and actions
Depression
MAO inhibitors are used to treat severe, atypical depression refractory to tricyclic antidepressants. Data suggest that depressed patients with coexisting obsessive-compulsive behavior, histrionic personality, or phobia respond more favorably to MAO inhibitors than to tricyclic antidepressants.
Hypertension
Pargyline is used to treat moderate to severe hypertension. Although rarely used, it may be effective in some patients refractory to other agents.
Parkinson's disease
Selegiline is used as an adjunct to carbidopa-levodopa in the treatment of Parkinson's disease.

Overview of adverse reactions
MAO inhibitors' most serious adverse reactions involve blood pressure. Hypotensive reactions appear to follow gradual accumulation of false neurotransmitters (phenylethylamines) in adrenergic nerve terminals; normal breakdown of these agents is also inhibited by MAO. Severe hypertension also may result from interaction with drugs with sympathomimetic activity, such as pseudoephedrine, phenylephrine, and phenylpropa-

nolamine, other false neurotransmitters, and other drugs with vasoconstrictive effects.

Ingestion of food or beverages containing tyramine may provoke hypertensive crisis – a rapid and severe increase in blood pressure. Hypertensive crisis is attributed to displacement of norepinephrine by false neurotransmitters; prodromal symptoms include severe occipital headache, tachycardia, sweating, and visual disturbances.

All MAO inhibitors cause CNS adverse reactions, including restlessness, hyperexcitability, insomnia, and headache. Over time, tolerance develops to most adverse reactions.

▶ **Special considerations**
● Implement all precautions for use of MAO inhibitors, given alone or with other drugs, for 14 days after discontinuation of drug. Check for potential interactions with other drugs patient may be taking, and especially avoid concomitant use of MAO inhibitors with alcohol or alcohol-containing drugs, phenothiazines, other CNS stimulants, and food and beverages containing tyramine.
● MAO inhibitors impair ability to perform tasks requiring mental alertness, such as driving a car.
● Check vital signs regularly for increased blood pressure or other signs of excessive CNS stimulation.
● Patient should be observed to be sure each dose of drug is swallowed; as depressed patients begin to improve, they may hoard pills for suicide attempt.
● MAO inhibitors may be used with electroconvulsive therapy.

Information for the patient
● Explain rationale for therapy and the risks and benefits that may be anticipated; also explain that full therapeutic effect of drug may not occur for several weeks.
● Advise patient to promptly report any unusual reactions, especially severe headache, rash, dark urine, pale stools, or jaundice.
● Tell patient to avoid beverages and drugs containing alcohol and not to take any other drug (including nonprescription products) unless prescribed.
● Give patient a list of tyramine-containing foods and beverages, and explain why patient should avoid these.
● Tell patient during initial therapy to rise slowly from recumbent position (take at least 2 minutes when getting out of bed) to avoid dizziness from orthostatic hypotension.
● Teach patient how and when to take drug, not to increase dosage unless prescribed, and never to discontinue drug abruptly.
● Advise diabetic patient to monitor serum glucose levels, as drug may alter insulin needs.
● Advise patient to avoid hazardous tasks that require mental alertness until full effect of drug is determined.
● Urge patient to obtain Medic Alert or similar bracelet or necklace identification listing therapy with MAO inhibitors.

Geriatric use
MAO inhibitors are not recommended for use in patients over age 60.

Pediatric use
MAO inhibitors are not recommended for children under age 16.

Breast-feeding
Safety has not been established.

Representative combinations
Pargyline hydrochloride with methylclothiazide: Eutron.

---

monoctanoin
Moctanin

● Pharmacologic classification: esterified glycerol
● Therapeutic classification: cholelitholytic
● Pregnancy risk category C

How supplied
Available by prescription only
Solution: 120-ml bottles

Indications, route, and dosage
To solubilize cholesterol gallstones that are retained in the biliary tract after cholecystectomy
Adults: Administered as a continuous perfusion through a catheter inserted directly into the common bile duct via a T tube. Perfusion rate should not exceed 3 to 5 ml/hour at a pressure of 10 cm water. Duration of perfusion is 2 to 10 days.
Do *not* administer I.V. or I.M.

Pharmacodynamics
Cholelitholytic action: This agent is hydrolyzed rapidly into fatty acids, which increases the solubility of gallstones. Monoctanoin acts only on cholesterol stones.

Pharmacokinetics
● *Absorption:* Monoctanoin is perfused directly into the common bile duct.
● *Distribution:* None.
● *Metabolism:* Monoctanoin is hydrolyzed by pancreatic and other digestive lipases to produce fatty acids.
● *Excretion:* None.

Contraindications and precautions
Monoctanoin is contraindicated in patients with jaundice, significant biliary tract infection, recent jejunitis, pancreatitis, or duodenal ulcer because these disorders are irritating to the GI and biliary tracts. Monitor patients with impaired liver function for metabolic acidosis.

Interactions
None reported.

Effects on diagnostic tests
None reported.

Adverse reactions
● GI: nausea, vomiting, diarrhea, pain, indigestion, anorexia.
● HEMA: leukopenia.
● Other: fever, chills, diaphoresis, headache, pruritus, lethargy, metabolic acidosis.
Note: Drug should be discontinued if anorexia, chills, fever, leukocytosis, jaundice, or severe right upper quadrant pain appears or if there is no improvement in 10 days.

Overdose and treatment
No information available.

▶ **Special considerations**
● Baseline liver function tests should be performed prior to perfusion.
● The drug is irritating. To minimize this effect on the biliary and GI tracts, the rate should not exceed 3 to 5 ml/hour and the pressure should be 10 cm H_2O (never exceeding 15 cm H_2O).
● Average duration of therapy is 5 days. If there is no change in 10 days, therapy is discontinued.
● Slowing rate of perfusion or discontinuing perfusion during meals will reduce GI discomfort.
● Warm medication before use (65 to 80 F.]18.3 to 26.7 C.[); keep temperature of medication above 65 F. during perfusion.
● Monoctanoin therapy usually follows cholecystectomy. Gallstones should be analyzed for solubility in monoctanoin.

Breast-feeding
It is unknown whether monoctanoin is excreted in breast milk; it should be used with caution in breast-feeding women.

---

moricizine hydrochloride
Ethmozine

● Pharmacologic classification: sodium channel blocker
● Therapeutic classification: antiarrhythmic
● Pregnancy risk category: B

How supplied
Available by prescription only
Tablets: 200 mg, 250 mg, 300 mg

Indications, route, and dosage
Treatment of documented, life-threatening ventricular arrhythmias when benefit of treatment outweighs risks
Adults: Dosage must be individualized. Usual range is 600 to 900 mg daily given q 8 hours in equally divided doses. Dosage may be adjusted within this range in increments of 150 mg daily at 3-day intervals until desired effect is obtained. Hospitalization is recommended for initiation of therapy because patient will be at high risk.

Pharmacodynamics
Antiarrhythmic action: Although moricizine is chemically related to the neuroleptic phenothiazines, it has no demonstrated dopaminergic activities. It does have potent local anesthetic activity and myocardial membrane stabilizing effects. A class I antiarrhythmic agent, it reduces the fast inward current carried by sodium ions. In patients with ventricular tachycardia, moricizine prolongs AV conduction but has no significant effect on ventricular repolarization. Intra-atrial conduction or atrial effective refractory periods are not consistently affected and moricizine has minimal effect on sinus cycle length and sinus node recovery time. This may be significant in patients with sinus node dysfunction.

In patients with impaired left ventricular function,

moricizine has minimal effects on measurements of cardiac performance: cardiac index, stroke volume, pulmonary capillary wedge pressure, systemic or pulmonary vascular resistance, and ejection fraction either at rest or during exercise. A small but consistent increase in resting blood pressure and heart rate are seen. Moricizine has no effect on exercise tolerance in patients with ventricular arrhythmias, CHF, or angina pectoris.

Moricizine has antiarrhythmic activity similar to that of disopyramide, propranolol, and quinidine. Arrhythmia "rebound" is not noted after discontinuation of therapy.

Pharmacokinetics
● *Absorption:* Peak plasma concentrations are usually reached within 0.5 to 2 hours. Administration within 30 minutes of mealtime delays absorption and lowers peak plasma levels but has no effect on extent of absorption.
● *Distribution:* Moricizine is 95% plasma protein-bound.
● *Metabolism:* Moricizine undergoes significant first-pass metabolism and at least 26 metabolites have been identified with no single one representing at least 1% of the administered dose. Moricizine has been shown to induce its own metabolism.
● *Excretion:* 56% is excreted in feces; 39%, in urine; some is also recycled through enterohepatic circulation.

Contraindications and precautions
Moricizine is contraindicated in patients with known hypersensitivity to the drug and in those with preexisting second- or third-degree AV block, with right bundle branch block when associated with left hemiblock (unless a pacemaker is present), and in cardiogenic shock. Use with extreme caution in patients with sick sinus syndrome as it may cause sinus bradycardia, sinus pause, or sinus arrest. Use with caution in patients with hepatic or renal impairment, CHF, and preexisting conduction abnormalities and when concomitant medications that affect cardiac conduction are initiated; monitor such patients carefully.

Interactions
Concomitant use with cimetidine decreases moricizine clearance by 49%; no significant changes in efficacy or tolerance were observed. Use with propranolol may produce a small additive increase in the PR interval. Theophylline clearance increases and plasma half-life decreases with concomitant therapy; monitor when moricizine is added or discontinued. Concomitant digoxin therapy prolongs the PR interval.

Adverse reactions
● CNS: dizziness, headache, nervousness, somnolence, fatigue.
● CV: *proarrhythmia*, palpitations, hypotension, hypertension, supraventricular tachycardia, chest pain, *CHF, ventricular tachyarrhythmias.*
● EENT: sinusitis.
● GI: nausea, vomiting, dry mouth, diarrhea, constipation.
● Respiratory: dyspnea, apnea, hyperventilation, cough.
● Other: pain, hypesthesia, blurred vision, urine retention, drug fever, hypothermia, allergic reactions (rash, pruritus, urticaria, swelling of lips and tongue, periorbital edema).

---

*Canada only   †Unlabeled clinical use   Italicized adverse reactions are life-threatening.

Overdose and treatment
Symptoms of overdose include emesis, lethargy, coma, syncope, hypotension, conduction disturbances, exacerbation of CHF, MI, sinus arrest, arrhythmias, and respiratory failure. No specific antidote has been identified. Treatment should be supportive and include careful monitoring of cardiac, respiratory, and CNS changes. Gastric evacuation with care to avoid aspiration may be used as well.

▶ **Special considerations**
● When transferring from another antiarrhythmic to moricizine, previous therapy should be withdrawn 1 to 2 half-lives before initiating moricizine.
● Patients with renal or hepatic impairment should be started at 600 mg daily or lower and closely monitored (with ECG) before making dosage adjustments.
● Hypokalemia, hyperkalemia, or hypomagnesemia may alter moricizine's effects; correct electrolyte imbalances before start of therapy.

Pediatric use
Safety and efficacy have not been established

Breast-feeding
Moricizine is excreted in breast milk. Because of the potential for adverse reactions in the breast-fed infant, a decision whether or not to continue therapy must be made.

---

morphine hydrochloride*
M.O.S.*, Morphitec*

morphine sulfate
Astramorph, Duramorph, Epimorph*, MS Contin, RMS Uniserts, Roxanol, Statex*

● Pharmacologic classification: opioid
● Therapeutic classification: narcotic analgesic
● Controlled substance schedule II
● Pregnancy risk category C

How supplied
Available by prescription only
Morphine hydrochloride*
Tablets: 10 mg, 20 mg, 40 mg, 60 mg
Oral solution: 1 mg/ml, 5 mg/ml, 10 mg/ml, 20 mg/ml, 50 mg/ml
Syrup: 1 mg/ml, 5 mg/ml
Suppositories: 20 mg, 30 mg
Morphine sulfate
Tablets: 10 mg, 15 mg, 30 mg
Tablets (extended release): 30 mg
Oral solution: 10 mg/5 ml, 20 mg/5 ml, 20 mg/ml
Syrup: 1 mg/ml, 5 mg/ml
Injection (with preservative): 2 mg/ml, 4 mg/ml, 8 mg/ml, 10 mg/ml, 15 mg/ml
Injection (without preservative): 500 mcg/ml, 1 mg/ml
Soluble tablets: 10 mg, 15 mg, 30 mg
Suppositories: 5 mg, 10 mg, 20 mg

Indications, route, and dosage
Severe pain
Adults: 4 to 15 mg S.C. or I.M., or 30 to 60 mg P.O. or by rectum q 4 hours, p.r.n. or around the clock. May be injected slow I.V. (over 4 to 5 minutes) diluted in 4 to 5 ml water for injection. May also administer controlled-release tablets q 8 to 12 hours. As an epidural injection, 5 mg via an epidural catheter every 24 hours.
Children: 0.1 to 0.2 mg/kg S.C. Maximum dose: 15 mg. In some situations, morphine may be administered by continuous I.V. infusion or by intraspinal and intrathecal injection.
Preoperative sedation and adjunct to anesthesia
Adults: 8 to 10 mg I.M., S.C., or I.V.
To control pain associated with acute myocardial infarction
Adults: 8 to 15 mg I.M., S.C., or I.V. Additional, smaller doses may be given in 3- to 4-hour intervals as needed.
†*Adjunctive treatment of acute pulmonary edema*
Adults: 10 to 15 mg I.V. at a rate not exceeding 2 mg/minute.

Pharmacodynamics
Analgesic action: Morphine is the principal opium alkaloid, the standard for opiate agonist analgesic activity. The mechanism of action is thought to be via the opiate receptors, altering the patient's perception of pain. Morphine is particularly useful in severe, acute pain or severe, chronic pain. Morphine also has a central depressant effect on respiration and on the cough reflex center.

Pharmacokinetics
● *Absorption:* Morphine is absorbed variably from the GI tract. Onset of analgesia occurs within 15 to 60 minutes. Peak analgesia occurs ½ to 1 hour after dosing.
● *Distribution:* Morphine is distributed widely through the body.
● *Metabolism:* Morphine is metabolized primarily in the liver.
● *Excretion:* Duration of action is 3 to 7 hours. Morphine is excreted in the urine and bile.

Contraindications and precautions
Morphine is contraindicated in patients with known hypersensitivity to the drug or other phenanthrene opioids (codeine, hydrocodone, hydromorphone, oxycodone, oxymorphone).

Administer morphine with extreme caution to patients with supraventricular arrhythmias; avoid, or administer drug with extreme caution to patients with head injury or increased intracranial pressure, because it obscures neurologic parameters; and during pregnancy and labor, because drug readily crosses placenta (premature infants are especially sensitive to respiratory and CNS depressant effects).

Administer morphine cautiously to patients with renal or hepatic dysfunction, because drug accumulation or prolonged duration of action may occur; to patients with pulmonary disease (asthma, chronic obstructive pulmonary disease), because drug depresses respiration and suppresses cough reflex; to patients undergoing biliary tract surgery, because drug may cause biliary spasm; to patients with convulsive disorders, because drug may precipitate seizures; to elderly or debilitated patients, who are more sensitive to both therapeutic

---

*Canada only   †Unlabeled clinical use   Italicized adverse reactions are life-threatening.

and adverse drug effects; and to patients prone to physical or psychic addiction, because of the high risk of addiction to this drug.

Interactions

Concomitant use with other CNS depressants (narcotic analgesics, general anesthetics, antihistamines, monoamine oxidase inhibitors, phenothiazines, barbiturates, benzodiazepines, sedative-hypnotics, tricyclic antidepressants, alcohol, and muscle relaxants) potentiates drug's respiratory and CNS depression, sedation, and hypotensive effects. Concomitant use with cimetidine also may increase respiratory and CNS depression, causing confusion, disorientation, apnea, or seizures. Reduced dosage of morphine is usually necessary.

Drug accumulation and enhanced effects may result from concomitant use with other drugs that are extensively metabolized in the liver (rifampin, phenytoin, and digitoxin); combined use with anticholinergics may cause paralytic ileus.

Patients who become physically dependent on this drug may experience acute withdrawal syndrome if given a narcotic antagonist.

Severe cardiovascular depression may result from concomitant use with general anesthetics.

Effects on diagnostic tests

Morphine increases plasma amylase levels.

Adverse reactions

● CNS: sedation, somnolence, clouded sensorium, euphoria, insomnia, agitation, confusion, headache, tremor, miosis, seizures, psychic dependence, nightmares (with long-acting dosage form).
● CV: tachycardia, *asystole*, bradycardia, palpitations, chest wall rigidity, hypertension, hypotension, syncope, edema.
● DERM: flushing (with epidural use), rashes, pruritus, pain at injection site.
● GI: dry mouth, anorexia, biliary spasms (colic), ileus, nausea, vomiting, constipation.
● GU: urinary retention or hesitancy, decreased libido.
● Other: *respiratory depression.*
   Note: Drug should be discontinued if hypersensitivity, seizures, or cardiac arrhythmias occur.

Overdose and treatment

Rapid I.V. administration may result in overdose because of the delay in maximum CNS effect (30 minutes). The most common signs and symptoms of morphine overdose is respiratory depression with or without CNS depression, respiratory depression, and miosis (pinpoint pupils). Other acute toxic effects include hypotension, bradycardia, hypothermia, shock, apnea, cardiopulmonary arrest, circulatory collapse, pulmonary edema, and convulsions.

To treat acute overdose, first establish adequate respiratory exchange via a patent airway and ventilation as needed; administer a narcotic antagonist (naloxone) to reverse respiratory depression. (Because the duration of action of morphine is longer than that of naloxone, repeated naloxone dosing is necessary.) Naloxone should not be given in the absence of clinically significant respiratory or cardiovascular depression. Monitor vital signs closely.

If the patient presents within 2 hours of ingestion of an oral overdose, empty the stomach immediately by inducing emesis (ipecac syrup) or using gastric lavage. Use caution to avoid any risk of aspiration. Administer activated charcoal via nasogastric tube for further removal of the drug in an oral overdose.

Provide symptomatic and supportive treatment (continued respiratory support, correction of fluid or electrolyte imbalance). Monitor laboratory parameters, vital signs, and neurologic status closely.

▶ Special considerations

Besides those relevant to all *opioids*, consider the following recommendations.
● Morphine is the drug of choice in relieving pain of myocardial infarction; may cause transient decrease in blood pressure.
● Regimented scheduling (around the clock) is beneficial in severe, chronic pain.
● Oral solutions of various concentrations are available, as well as a new intensified oral solution.
● Note the disparity between oral and parenteral doses.
● For sublingual administration, measure out oral solution with tuberculin syringe, and administer dose a few drops at a time to allow maximal sublingual absorption and to minimize swallowing.
● Refrigeration of rectal suppositories is not necessary. Note that in some patients, rectal and oral absorption may not be equivalent.
● Preservative-free preparations are now available for epidural and intrathecal administration. The use of the epidural route is increasing.
● Epidural morphine has proven to be an excellent analgesic for patients with postoperative pain. After epidural administration, monitor closely for respiratory depression up to 24 hours after the injection. Check respiratory rate and depth according to protocol (for example, every 15 minutes for 2 hours, followed by every hour for 18 hours). Some clinicians advocate a dilute naloxone infusion (5 to 10 mcg/kg/hr) during the first 12 hours to minimize respiratory depression without altering pain relief.
● Morphine may worsen or mask gallbladder pain.

Information for the patient

● Tell patient that oral liquid form of morphine may be mixed with a glass of fruit juice immediately before it is taken, if desired, to improve the taste.
● Tell patients taking long-acting morphine tablets to swallow them whole. They should not break, crush, or chew the tablets before swallowing them.

Geriatric use

Lower doses are usually indicated for elderly patients, who may be more sensitive to the therapeutic and adverse effects of the drug.

Breast-feeding

Morphine is excreted in breast milk. A woman should wait 2 to 3 hours after last dose before breast-feeding to avoid sedation in the infant.

moxalactam
Moxam

- Pharmacologic classification: third-generation cephalosporin
- Therapeutic classification: antibiotic
- Pregnancy risk category B

How supplied
Available by prescription only
Injection: 1 g, 2 g
Pharmacy bulk package: 20 g

Indications, route, and dosage
Serious respiratory, urinary, CNS, intra-abdominal, gynecologic, and skin infections; bacteremia; and septicemia
Adults: Usual daily dose is 2 to 6 g I.M. or I.V. administered in divided doses q 8 hours for 5 to 10 days, or up to 14 days. Up to 12 g/day may be needed in life-threatening infections or in infections caused by less susceptible organisms.
Children: 50 mg/kg I.M. or I.V. q 6 to 8 hours.
Total daily dosage is same for I.M. or I.V. administration and depends on susceptibility of organism and severity of infection. In patients with impaired renal function, doses or frequency of administration must be modified according to degree of impairment, severity of infection, and susceptibility of organism. Moxalactam should be injected deep I.M. into the gluteus or lateral aspect of the thigh.

Pharmacodynamics
Antibacterial action: Moxalactam is 1-oxa-beta-lactam and has a mechanism of action similar to other cephalosporins. Moxalactam is primarily bactericidal; however, it may be bacteriostatic. Activity depends on the organism, tissue penetration, drug dosage, and rate of organism multiplication. It acts by adhering to bacterial penicillin-binding proteins, thereby inhibiting cell wall synthesis. Third-generation cephalosporins appear more active against some beta-lactamase-producing gram-negative organisms.
Moxalactam is active against some gram-positive organisms and many enteric gram-negative bacilli and some strains of *Pseudomonas aeruginosa, Bacteroides,* and other anaerobes. *Acinetobacter* and *Listeria* are usually resistant to moxalactam.

Pharmacokinetics
- *Absorption:* Moxalactam is not absorbed from the GI tract and must be given parenterally; peak serum levels occur ½ to 1 hour after an I.M. dose.
- *Distribution:* Moxalactam is distributed widely into most body tissues and fluids, including the gallbladder, liver, kidneys, bone, sputum, bile, and pleural and synovial fluids; unlike most other cephalosporins, it has good CSF penetration. Moxalactam crosses the placenta; it is 45% to 60% protein-bound.
- *Metabolism:* Moxalactam is not metabolized.
- *Excretion:* Moxalactam is excreted primarily in urine by glomerular filtration; small amounts of drug are excreted in breast milk. Elimination half-life is 2 to 3½ hours in normal adults; severe renal disease prolongs half-life to about 5 to 10 hours. Hemodialysis removes moxalactam, but peritoneal dialysis does not.

Contraindications and precautions
Moxalactam is contraindicated in patients with known hypersensitivity to any cephalosporin.
Use moxalactam with caution in patients with penicillin allergy, who are usually more susceptible to such reactions; and in patients with coagulopathy and elderly, debilitated, or malnourished patients, who are usually at greater risk of bleeding complications.

Interactions
Concomitant use with aminoglycosides results in synergistic activity against *Pseudomonas aeruginosa* and *Serratia marcescens;* such combined use slightly increases risk of nephrotoxicity.
Concomitant use with alcohol may cause disulfiram-type reactions (flushing, sweating, tachycardia, headache, abdominal cramping).

Effects on diagnostic tests
Moxalactam causes positive Coombs' tests and may elevate liver function test results and prothrombin times.

Adverse reactions
- CNS: headache, malaise, paresthesias, dizziness, seizures.
- DERM: maculopapular and erythematous rashes, *urticaria.*
- GI: *pseudomembranous colitis,* nausea, anorexia, vomiting, diarrhea, glossitis, dyspepsia, abdominal cramps, tenesmus, pruritus ani.
- GU: genital pruritus.
- HEMA: transient neutropenia, eosinophilia, hemolytic anemia, *hypoprothrombinemia, bleeding.*
- Local: pain at injection site, induration, sterile abscesses, tissue sloughing; phlebitis and thrombophlebitis with I.V. injection.
- Other: hypersensitivity, dyspnea, fever, bacterial and fungal superinfection.
  Note: Drug should be discontinued if signs of toxicity, immediate hypersensitivity reaction, or hypoprothrombinemia occur or if severe diarrhea indicates pseudomembranous colitis; alternative therapy should be considered if the patient develops fever, eosinophilia, hematuria, or neutropenia.

Overdose and treatment
Clinical signs of overdose include neuromuscular hypersensitivity. Seizure may follow high CNS concentrations. Hypoprothrombinemia and bleeding may occur and may require treatment with vitamin K or blood products. Moxalactam may be removed by hemodialysis.

▶ Special considerations
Besides those relevant to all *cephalosporins,* consider the following recommendations.
- For patients on sodium restriction, note that moxalactam injection contains 3.8 mEq of sodium chloride per gram of drug.
- Moxalactam does not interfere with urine glucose determinations.
- Dilute I.M. dose with sterile or bacteriostatic water, 0.9% NaCl, or 0.5% or 1% lidocaine HCl injection.
- Administer deep I.M. into large muscle mass to prevent tissue damage. Aspirate before injection to avoid inadvertent entry into blood vessel. Rotate injection sites to prevent tissue damage. Apply ice to site to minimize pain.
- For direct intermittent I.V. administration, add 10 ml

of sterile water for injection, dextrose 5% injection, or 0.9% NaCl injection per gram of moxalactam. Administer slowly over 3 to 5 minutes or through tubing of free-flowing compatible I.V. solution.

• Monitor for signs and symptoms of overt or occult bleeding. Monitor complete blood count, platelet count, and prothrombin time for abnormalities.

• Bleeding associated with hypoprothrombinemia can be prevented with vitamin K, 10 mg per week to be given prophylactically. Bleeding can be promptly reversed with the administration of vitamin K.

• Because moxalactam is hemodialyzable, patients undergoing treatment with hemodialysis may require dosage adjustments.

• Concomitant use with alcohol can lead to disulfiram-like reaction. Use this drug cautiously in patients on home I.V. antibiotic therapy who drink alcohol, or consider alternative drug therapy.

Geriatric use
Reduced dosage may be necessary in elderly patients with diminished renal function. Hypoprothrombinemia and bleeding have been reported most frequently in elderly patients, particularly those who are debilitated or malnourished.

Pediatric use
Moxalactam may be used in infants and children, but it is not often used because of the availability of better alternatives.

Breast-feeding
Moxalactam is distributed into breast milk and should be used with caution in breast-feeding women. Safe use has not been established.

---

mumps skin test antigen
MSTA

• Pharmacologic classification: viral antigen
• Therapeutic classification: skin test antigen
• Pregnancy risk category C

How supplied
Available by prescription only
Injection: 20 complement-fixing units/ml suspension; 10 tests/1-ml vial

Indications, route, and dosage
To assess cell-mediated immunity
Adults and children: 0.1 ml intradermally into the volar surface of the forearm.

Pharmacodynamics
Antigenic action: Mumps skin test is not indicated for the immunization, diagnosis, or treatment of mumps virus infection.

The status of cell-mediated immunity can be determined from use of mumps with other antigens. In vitro tests (such as lymphocyte stimulation and assays for T and B cells) are necessary to diagnose a specific disorder.

Pharmacokinetics
• *Absorption:* After intradermal injection of mumps skin test antigen, the test site should be examined in 48 to 72 hours.
• *Distribution:* Injection must be given intradermally; subcutaneous injection invalidates the test.
• *Metabolism:* Not applicable.
• *Excretion:* Not applicable.

Contraindications and precautions
Mumps skin test antigen is contraindicated in persons sensitive to avian protein (chicken, eggs, or feathers) and in those hypersensitive to thimerosal.

Interactions
None reported.

Effects on diagnostic tests
None reported.

Adverse reactions
• Systemic: nausea, headache, anorexia, drowsiness.
• Local: tenderness, pruritus, and rash occur at injection site. Occasionally, a severe delayed-hypersensitivity reaction will produce vesiculation, local tissue necrosis, abscess, and scar formation.
• Other: *anaphylaxis,* Arthus reaction, urticaria, angioedema, shortness of breath, excessive perspiration.

Overdose and treatment
Administer epinephrine 1:1,000 if anaphylaxis occurs.

▶ **Special considerations**
• Obtain history of allergies and reactions to skin tests. In patients hypersensitive to feathers, eggs, or chicken, a severe reaction may follow administration of mumps skin test antigen.
• After injection of mumps skin test antigen, observe the patient for 15 minutes for possible immediate-type systemic allergic reaction. Keep epinephrine 1:1,000 available.
• Accurate dosage (0.1 ml) and administration are essential with the use of mumps skin test antigen.
• Examine injection site within 48 to 72 hours, interpreting as follows:
Positive reaction: An area of erythema 1.5 cm or more in diameter, with or without induration, indicates sensitivity.
Negative reaction: Erythema of less than 1.5 cm or induration less than 5 mm means the individual has not been sensitized to mumps or is anergic.
• Reactivity to this test may be depressed or suppressed for as long as 6 weeks in individuals who have received concurrent virus vaccines, in those who are receiving a corticosteroid or other immunosuppressive agents, in those who have had viral infections, and in malnourished patients.
• Mumps skin test antigen is not used to assess exposure to mumps. It is used in assessing T cell function for immunocompetence since most normal individuals will exhibit a positive reaction.
• Cold packs or topical steroids may give relief from the symptoms of pain, pruritus, and discomfort if a local reaction occurs.
• Store vial in refrigerator.

Information for the patient
● Have patient report any unusual side effects.
● Explain that the induration will disappear in a few days.

Geriatric use
Elderly patients who do not react to this test are considered anergic.

Breast-feeding
Benefit of the mumps skin test to the breast-feeding woman should be weighed against possible risk to the infant.

---

mumps virus vaccine, live
Mumpsvax

● Pharmacologic classification: vaccine
● Therapeutic classification: viral vaccine
● Pregnancy risk category X

How supplied
Available by prescription only
Injection: single-dose vial containing not less than 5,000 TCID$_{50}$s0 (tissue culture infective doses) of attenuated mumps virus derived from Jeryl Lynn mumps strain (grown in chick embryo culture), and vial of diluent

Indications, route, and dosage
Immunization
Adults and children over age 1: 1 vial (5,000 units) S.C. in outer aspect of the upper arm.

Pharmacodynamics
Mumps prophylaxis: This vaccine promotes active immunity to mumps.

Pharmacokinetics
Antibodies usually are evident 2 to 3 weeks after injection. The duration of vaccine-induced immunity is at least 20 years and probably lifelong.

Contraindications and precautions
Live mumps virus vaccine is contraindicated in patients with hypersensitivity (other than dermatitis) to neomycin, a component of the vaccine; in patients with infections, blood dyscrasias, or cancers of or affecting the bone marrow or lymphatic systems; in patients in primary immunodeficiency states; in pregnant patients; and in those receiving adrenocorticotropic hormone, corticosteroids (except in patients receiving corticosteroids as replacement therapy, for example, for Addison's disease), irradiation, or other immunosuppressant therapy.

Interactions
Concomitant use of mumps vaccine with immune serum globulin or transfusions of blood or blood products may interfere with the immune response to the vaccine. If possible, vaccination should be deferred for 3 months in these situations.

The administration of immunosuppressive agents may interfere with the response to the vaccine.

Effects on diagnostic tests
Mumps vaccine temporarily may decrease the response to tuberculin skin testing. Should a tuberculin skin test be necessary, administer it either before or simultaneously with mumps vaccine.

Adverse reactions
● CNS: *seizures, optic neuritis* (rare).
● Local: burning, stinging, and inflammation at injection site.
● Systemic: low-grade fever, rash, malaise, parotitis, orchitis.

Overdose and treatment
No information available.

▶ Special considerations
● Mumps vaccine should not be used in delayed hypersensitivity (anergy) skin testing.
● Obtain a thorough history of allergies, especially to antibiotics, eggs, chicken, or chicken feathers, and of reactions to immunizations.
● Patients with a history of anaphylactoid reactions to egg ingestion should first have skin testing performed to assess vaccine sensitivity (against a control of normal saline solution in the opposite arm). Administer an intradermal or scratch test with a 1:10 dilution. Read results after 5 to 30 minutes.
Positive reaction: wheal with or without pseudopodia and surrounding erythema. If sensitivity test is positive, consider desensitization.
● Epinephrine solution 1:1,000 should be available to treat allergic reactions.
● Do not administer vaccine I.V. Use a 25-gauge, ⅝″ needle and inject S.C., preferably into the outer aspect of the upper arm.
● Use only diluent supplied. Discard reconstituted solution after 8 hours.
● Store in refrigerator and protect from light. Solution may be used if red, pink, or yellow, but it must be clear.
● Mumps vaccine should not be given less than 1 month before or after immunization with other live virus vaccines — except for live, attenuated measles virus vaccine, live rubella virus vaccine, or monovalent or trivalent live oral poliovirus vaccine, which may be administered simultaneously.
● The vaccine will not offer protection when given after exposure to natural mumps.
● Revaccination is not required if primary vaccine was given at age 1 or older.

Information for the patient
● Tell patient that he may experience pain and inflammation at the injection site and a low-grade fever, rash, or general malaise.
● Encourage patient to report distressing adverse reactions.
● Recommend acetaminophen to alleviate adverse reactions, such as fever.
● Tell female patients of childbearing age to avoid pregnancy for 3 months after vaccination. Provide contraceptive information if necessary.

Pediatric use
Mumps vaccine is not recommended for children under age 1 because retained maternal mumps antibodies may interfere with the immune response.

Breast-feeding

It is unknown whether mumps vaccine is distributed into breast milk. No problems have been documented. Use mumps vaccine with caution in breast-feeding women.

---

mupirocin (pseudomonic acid A)
Bactroban

- Pharmacologic classification: antibiotic
- Therapeutic classification: topical antibacterial
- Pregnancy risk category B

How supplied
Available by prescription only
Ointment: 2%

Indications, route, and dosage
Topical treatment of impetigo due to Staphylococcus aureus, *beta-hemolytic* Streptococcus, *and* Streptococcus pyogenes
Adults and children: Apply a small amount to the affected area, t.i.d. The area treated may be covered with a gauze dressing if desired.

Pharmacodynamics
Antibacterial action: Mupirocin is structurally unrelated to other agents and is produced by fermentation of the organism *Pseudomonas fluorescens.* Mupirocin inhibits bacterial protein synthesis by reversibly and specifically binding to bacterial isoleucyl transfer-RNA synthetase. Mupirocin shows no cross-resistance with chloramphenicol, erythromycin, gentamicin, lincomycin, methicillin, neomycin, novobiocin, penicillin, streptomycin, or tetracycline.

Pharmacokinetics
- *Absorption:* Normal subjects showed no absorption after 24-hour application under occlusive dressings.
- *Distribution:* Mupirocin is highly protein-bound (about 95%). A substantial decrease in activity can be expected in the presence of serum (as in exudative wounds).
- *Metabolism:* Mupirocin is metabolized locally in the skin to monic acid.
- *Excretion:* Mupirocin is eliminated locally by desquamation of the skin.

Contraindications and precautions
Mupirocin is contraindicated in any patient who is sensitive to the drug or ingredients in the formulation. This drug should not be used in the eyes.

Interactions
None reported.

Effects on diagnostic tests
None reported.

Adverse reactions
- DERM: rash, erythema, dry skin, contact dermatitis.
- Local: itching, pain, burning, tenderness, swelling.

Overdose and treatment
No information available.

▶ Special considerations
- Reevaluate patients not showing a clinical response within 3 to 5 days.
- If sensitivity or chemical irritation occurs, discontinue treatment and institute appropriate alternative therapy.
- When used on burns or to treat extensive open wounds, absorption of polyethylene glycol vehicle is possible and may result in serious renal toxicity.
- Monitor for superinfection. Use of antibiotics (prolonged or repeated) may result in bacterial or fungal overgrowth of nonsusceptible organisms. Such overgrowth may lead to a secondary infection.

Information for the patient
Advise patient to wash and dry affected areas thoroughly. Then apply thin film, rubbing in gently.

Breast-feeding
It is not known whether mupirocin is present in breast milk. Use with caution.

---

muromonab-CD3
Orthoclone OKT3

- Pharmacologic classification: monoclonal antibody
- Therapeutic classification: immunosuppressive agent
- Pregnancy risk category C

How supplied
Injection: 5 mg/5 ml in 5-ml ampules

Indications, route, and dosage
Treatment of acute allograft rejection in renal transplant patients
Adults: 5 mg/day, for 10 to 14 days. Begin treatment once acute renal rejection is diagnosed.
Children younger than age 12: 2.5 mg/day rapid I.V. for 10 to 14 days or 100 mcg (0.1 mg) per kg of body weight for 10 to 14 days.

Pharmacodynamics
Immunosuppressive action: Muromonab-CD3 reverses graft rejection, probably by interfering with T cell function that promotes acute renal rejection. It interacts with, and prevents the function of, the T cell antigen receptor complex in the cellular membrane, which influences antigen recognition and is essential for signal transduction. Muromonab-CD3 reacts with most peripheral T cells in blood and in body tissues, and blocks all known T cell functions.

Pharmacokinetics
- *Absorption:* Immediate after I.V. administration.
- *Distribution:* Unknown.
- *Metabolism:* Unknown.
- *Excretion:* Unknown.

Contraindications and precautions
Contraindicated in patients allergic to muromonab-CD3 and in patients with fluid overload. Use with extreme caution in patients allergic to products of murine origin.
  This drug contains polysorbate 80 and should not be used for the in vitro treatment of bone marrow. Because this drug is a heterologous protein, it induces antibod-

---

ies, which could limit its efficacy and may cause serious reactions upon readmission. A second course should be administered with caution.

Monitor patient closely for 48 hours after the first dose. Administration of methylprednisolone sodium succinate 1 mg/kg I.V. before muromonab-CD3 and I.V. hydrocortisone sodium succinate 100 mg given 30 minutes after is strongly recommended to minimize the first-dose reaction. Acetaminophen and antihistamines, given concomitantly, may reduce early reactions.

The most serious first-dose reaction, potentially fatal severe pulmonary edema, has occurred infrequently (in fewer than 5% of the first 107 patients and in none of the subsequent 311 patients treated with first-dose restrictions). In every patient who developed pulmonary edema, fluid overload was present before treatment. Therefore, carefully evaluate patients for fluid overload by chest X-ray or weight gain of > 3%. The patient's weight should be less than 3% above minimum weight the week before treatment begins.

Interactions
Muromonab-CD3 may potentiate immunosuppressive effects of other immunosuppressant drugs (azathioprine, cyclosporine).

Effects on diagnostic tests
None reported.

Adverse reactions
● CNS: pyrexia, chills, tremor, severe headaches, aseptic meningitis.
● CV: chest pain, *severe pulmonary edema.*
● EENT: wheezing.
● GI: nausea, vomiting, diarrhea.
● Other: dyspnea, infections, *anaphylaxis*, serum sickness.

Overdose and treatment
No information available.

▶ Special considerations
● Preparation of solution: Draw solution into a syringe through a low protein-binding 0.2 or 0.22 micrometer (mcm) filter. Discard filter and attach needle for I.V. bolus injection.
● Because this drug is a protein solution, it may develop a few fine translucent particles, which do not affect its potency.
● Administer as an I.V. bolus in less than 1 minute. Do not give by I.V. infusion or combined with other drug solutions.
● The manufacturer recommends if the patient's temperature exceeds 37.8° C. (100° F.), lower with antipyretics before muromonab-CD3 administration.
● Chest X-ray taken within 24 hours before treatment must be clear of fluid; monitor WBCs and differentials at intervals during treatment. Monitor the drug's effect on circulating T cells using flow cytometry or by expressing the CD3 antigen by in vitro assay.
● Immunosuppressive therapy increases susceptibility to infection and to lymphoproliferative disorders. Lymphomas may follow immunosuppressive therapy; their occurrence seems related to the intensity and duration of immunosuppression rather than the use of specific agents since most patients receive a combination of treatments.
● A "first-dose" reaction is common within ½ to 6 hours after the first dose, consisting of significant fever, chills,

dyspnea, and malaise. Pulmonary edema may occur if patient is not pretreated with a corticosteroid.
● Concomitant immunosuppressive therapy should be reduced to a daily dose of prednisone 0.5 mg/kg and azathioprine 25 mg. Cyclosporine should be reduced or discontinued. Maintenance immnuosuppression can resume 3 days before discontinuation of muromonab-CD3.
● Storage and stability: Refrigerate at 2° to 8° C. (36° to 46° F.). Do not freeze or shake.

Information for the patient
Inform patients of expected first-dose effects (fever, chills, dyspnea, chest pain, nausea and vomiting).

Pediatric use
Safety and efficacy for use in children have not been established. Patients as young as age 2 have had no unexpected adverse effects.

Breast-feeding
Safety in breast-feeding women has not been established.

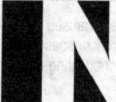

nabumetone
Relafen

- Pharmacologic classification: nonsteroidal anti-inflammatory
- Therapeutic classification: antiarthritic agent
- Pregnancy risk category C

How supplied
Available by prescription only
Tablets: 500 mg, 750 mg

Indications, route, and dosage
Acute and chronic treatment of rheumatoid arthritis or osteoarthritis
Adults: Initially, 1,000 mg P.O. daily as a single dose or in divided doses b.i.d. Adjust dosage according to patient response. Maximum recommended daily dose is 2,000 mg.

Pharmacodynamics
Anti-inflammatory action: Nabumetone probably acts by inhibiting the synthesis of prostaglandins.

Pharmacokinetics
- *Absorption:* Nabumetone is well absorbed from the GI tract. After absorption, about 35% of drug is rapidly transformed to 6-methoxy-2-naphthylacetic acid (6MNA), the principal active metabolite; the balance is transformed to unidentified metabolites. Administration with food increases the absorption rate and peak levels of 6MNA but doesn't change total drug absorbed.
- *Distribution:* 6MNA is more than 99% bound to plasma proteins.
- *Metabolism:* 6MNA is metabolized to inactive metabolites in the liver.
- *Excretion:* Metabolites are excreted primarily in the urine. About 9% appears in the feces. Elimination half-life is about 24 hours. Half-life is increased in patients with renal failure.

Contraindications and precautions
Nabumetone is contraindicated in patients with hypersensitivity to the drug and in patients with asthma, urticaria, or other allergic reactions to nabumetone, other NSAIDs, or aspirin.

Use cautiously in patients with renal or hepatic impairment; CHF, hypertension, or other conditions that may predispose the patient to fluid retention; and a history of peptic ulcer disease.

Serious GI toxicity, such as bleeding and ulceration, can occur during chronic use of NSAIDs; it can occur at any time, sometimes without warning.

Interactions
Concomitant use with drugs that are highly bound to plasma proteins (such as warfarin) increase the risk of adverse reactions because nabumetone may displace drug. Use together with caution.

Effects on diagnostic tests
None reported.

Adverse reactions
- CNS: dizziness, headache, fatigue, increased sweating, insomnia, nervousness, somnolence.
- DERM: pruritus, rash.
- GI: diarrhea, dyspepsia, abdominal pain, constipation, flatulence, nausea, dry mouth, gastritis, stomatitis, vomiting.
- Other: tinnitus, edema.

Overdose and treatment
After an accidental overdose, empty the stomach by induced emesis or lavage. Activated charcoal may limit the amount of drug absorbed.

▶ Special considerations
Besides those relevant to all *NSAIDs,* consider the following recommendations.
- Because NSAIDs impair the synthesis of renal prostaglandins, they can decrease renal blood flow and lead to reversible renal function impairment, especially in patients with preexisting renal failure, liver dysfunction, and heart failure; in elderly patients; and in those taking diuretics. These patients should be monitored closely during therapy.
- During long-term therapy, periodically monitor renal and liver function, CBC, and hematocrit. Monitor carefully for signs and symptoms of GI bleeding.

Information for the patient
- Tell patient to take drug with food, milk, or antacids. Studies have shown that drug is absorbed more rapidly when administered with food or milk.
- Stress the importance of follow-up examinations to detect adverse GI effects.
- Teach patient the signs and symptoms of GI bleeding, and tell him to report them immediately.
- Advise patient to limit alcohol intake because of the risk of additive GI toxicity.

Geriatric use
No differences in safety or efficacy have been noted in elderly patients.

Pediatric use
Safety and efficacy have not been established.

Breast-feeding
The active metabolite of nabumetone, 6MNA, has been found in the milk of laboratory rats. Because of the risk of serious toxicity to the infant, use in breast-feeding women is not recommended.

nadolol
Corgard

- Pharmacologic classification: beta-adrenergic blocking agent
- Therapeutic classification: antihypertensive, antianginal
- Pregnancy risk category C

How supplied
Available by prescription only
Tablets: 20 mg, 40 mg, 80 mg, 120 mg, 160 mg

Indications, route, and dosage
Hypertension
Adults: Initially, 40 mg P.O. once daily. Dosage may be increased in 40- to 80-mg increments until optimum response occurs. Usual maintenance dosage is 40 or 80 mg once daily. Doses of up to 240 or 320 mg daily and, rarely, 640 mg daily may be necessary.
Long-term prophylactic management of chronic stable angina pectoris
Adults: Initially, 40 mg P.O. once daily. Dosage may be increased in 40- to 80-mg increments until optimum response occurs. Usual maintenance dosage is 40 or 80 mg once daily. Doses of up to 160 or 240 mg daily may be needed.

Pharmacodynamics
- *Antihypertensive action:* The mechanisms of nadolol's antihypertensive effect are unknown. The drug may reduce blood pressure by blocking adrenergic receptors, thus decreasing cardiac output; or by decreasing sympathetic outflow from the CNS; or by suppressing renin release.
- *Antianginal action:* Nadolol decreases myocardial oxygen consumption, thus relieving angina, by blocking catecholamine-induced increases in heart rate, myocardial contraction, and blood pressure.

Pharmacokinetics
- *Absorption:* From 30% to 40% of a dose of nadolol is absorbed from the GI tract; peak plasma concentrations occur in 2 to 4 hours. Absorption is not affected by food.
- *Distribution:* Nadolol is distributed throughout the body; drug is about 30% protein-bound.
- *Metabolism:* None.
- *Excretion:* Most of a given dose is excreted unchanged in urine; the remainder is excreted in feces. Plasma half-life is about 20 hours. Antihypertensive and antianginal effects persist for about 24 hours.

Contraindications and precautions
Nadolol is contraindicated in patients with known hypersensitivity to the drug; and in patients with sinus bradycardia, overt cardiac failure, second- or third-degree atrioventricular block, or bronchial asthma, because the drug may worsen these conditions.

Nadolol should be used cautiously in patients with impaired hepatic or renal function (decrease dose if creatinine clearance falls below 50 ml/minute); in patients with coronary insufficiency, because beta-adrenergic blockade may precipitate congestive heart failure (CHF); in patients with diabetes mellitus and hyperthyroidism, because drug may mask tachycardia (it does not mask sweating and dizziness caused by hypoglycemia); and in patients with bronchospastic diseases. High doses may inhibit bronchodilating effects of endogenous catecholamines.

Interactions
Concomitant use with other antiarrhythmic agents may have additive or antagonistic cardiac effects and additive toxic effects.

Nadolol may potentiate antihypertensive effects of diuretics and other antihypertensive agents and, at high doses, the neuromuscular blocking effect of tubocurarine and related agents.

Nadolol may antagonize beta-adrenergic stimulating effects of sympathomimetic agents such as isoproterenol; concomitant use with epinephrine may cause a decrease in pulse rate with first- and second-degree heart block and hypertension.

Antimuscarinic agents such as atropine may antagonize nadolol-induced bradycardia.

Effects on diagnostic tests
None reported.

Adverse reactions
- CNS: dizziness, fatigue, sedation, behavioral changes, paresthesias, headache, reversible mental depression with catatonia, visual disturbances, depression, nightmares.
- CV: hypotension, *bradycardia, CHF,* peripheral vascular disease.
- DERM: rash, pruritus, reversible alopecia.
- EENT: dry mouth, cough, nasal stuffiness, tinnitus.
- GI: nausea, vomiting, diarrhea, constipation, indigestion, anorexia, bloating, flatulence, abdominal discomfort.
- Metabolic: hypoglycemia without tachycardia.
- Other: *bronchospasm,* decreased libido, Peyronie's disease.
  Note: Drug should be discontinued if patient develops signs of heart failure.

Overdose and treatment
Clinical signs of overdose include severe hypotension, bradycardia, heart failure, and bronchospasm.

After acute ingestion, empty stomach by induced emesis or gastric lavage, and give activated charcoal to reduce absorption. Magnesium sulfate may be given orally as a cathartic. Subsequent treatment is usually symptomatic and supportive.

▶ Special considerations
Besides those relevant to all *beta-adrenergic blocking agents,* consider the following recommendations.
- Dosage adjustments may be necessary in patients with renal impairment.
- Nadolol has been used as an antiarrhythmic agent and as a prophylactic agent for migraine headaches.

Geriatric use
Elderly patients may require lower maintenance dosages of nadolol because of increased bioavailability or delayed metabolism; they also may experience enhanced adverse effects.

Pediatric use
Safety and efficacy in children have not been established; use only if potential benefit outweighs risk.

Breast-feeding

Nadolol is distributed into breast milk; an alternative feeding method is recommended during therapy.

---

nafarelin acetate
Synarel

- Pharmacologic classification: synthetic decapeptide
- Therapeutic classification: gonadotropin-releasing hormone (GnRH) analog
- Pregnancy risk category X

How supplied

Available by prescription only
Nasal solution: 2 mg/ml (200 mcg/metered spray)

Indications, route, and dosage
Management of endometriosis, pain relief, reduction of endometriotic lesions

Adults: Usual daily dose is 400 mcg administered as one 200-mcg spray into one nostril in a.m. and one 200-mcg spray into the other nostril in p.m. If menstruation persists after 2 months, may increase dose to 800 mcg daily as one spray in each nostril in a.m. and one spray in each nostril in p.m.

Note: Recommended duration of therapy is 6 months. Retreatment is not recommended; safety data for retreatment not available. Clinical experience is limited to women age 18 years and older.

Pharmacodynamics
Hormonal action: Nafarelin stimulates release of luteinizing hormone and follicle-stimulating hormone, which temporarily increases ovarian steroid production. Repeated dosing abolishes the stimulatory effect on the pituitary gland; after about 4 weeks, decreased secretion of gonadal steroids results in quiescence of the tissues and functions that depend on gonadal steroids.

Pharmacokinetics
- *Absorption:* After intranasal administration, nafarelin is rapidly absorbed through the nasal mucosa into systemic circulation. Maximum serum concentrations are achieved in 10 to 40 minutes. Average serum half-life is about 3 hours.
- *Distribution:* 80% is bound to plasma proteins.
- *Metabolism:* Degraded by peptidase.
- *Excretion:* Unknown.

Contraindications and precautions

Nafarelin is contraindicated in patients with known hypersensitivity to GnRH and GnRH agonist analogs; with undiagnosed abnormal vaginal bleeding; and in patients who are or may become pregnant or who are breast-feeding.

Because of the risk of pregnancy, patients should use nonhormonal methods of contraception. Pregnancy must be excluded before starting treatment. If patient becomes pregnant during therapy, discontinue drug and inform patient of potential risk to fetus.

Interactions
None reported.

Effects on diagnostic tests
Tests of pituitary gonadotropin and gonadal functions may be misleading during treatment and as long as 4 to 8 weeks after treatment.

Adverse reactions
- CNS: headaches, depression, paresthesia, emotional lability, insomnia.
- CV: palpitations.
- DERM: seborrhea, acne, maculopapular rash, urticaria.
- EENT: nasal irritation, eye pain.
- GI: weight gain.
- GU: decreased libido, vaginal dryness.
- HEMA: elevated plasma phosphorus and eosinophil counts; decreased serum calcium and WBC counts.
- Other: hot flashes, myalgia, lactation, breast size reduction, breast engorgement, hirsutism, decreased bone density.

Note: Nafarelin may cause increases in plasma enzymes (AST [SGOT], ALT [SGPT]). Serum cholesterol and triglyceride levels were also elevated after treatment.

Overdose and treatment
No information available.

▶ Special considerations
- Pregnancy must be excluded before treatment.
- No evidence of favorable or adverse effects on pregnancy rates.
- Loss of bone density may not be reversible after treatment; chronic use of alcohol and/or tobacco, strong family history of osteoporosis, chronic use of corticosteroid or anticonvulsant drugs represent major risk factor for loss of bone density.

Information for the patient
- Instruct patient to carefully read information packet included in drug package.
- Tell patient that regular menstruation should stop with continued use of drug.
- Instruct patient to notify physician if menstruation continues after 2 months of treatment.
- Inform patient that breakthrough bleeding may occur, especially if successive doses are missed.
- Tell patient to discontinue use if she suspects that she has become pregnant and to notify physician promptly. Inform patient of potential risk to fetus and instruct her to use nonhormonal contraception during therapy.
- Explain adverse effects of hypoestrogenism.
- Instruct patient to consult physician if she experiences intercurrent rhinitis. If rhinitis requires a topical nasal decongestant, it must be used at least 30 minutes after nafarelin dose.

Breast-feeding
It is not known whether nafarelin is excreted in breast milk; however, use in breast-feeding women is not recommended.

---

nafcillin sodium
Nafcil, Nallpen, Unipen

- Pharmacologic classification: penicillin-ase-resistant penicillin
- Therapeutic classification: antibiotic
- Pregnancy risk category B

How supplied
Available by prescription only
Capsules: 250 mg
Solution: 250 mg/5 ml (after reconstitution)
Tablets: 500 mg
Injection: 500 mg, 1 g, 2 g
Pharmacy bulk package: 10 g
I.V. infusion piggyback: 1 g, 1.5 g, 2 g, 4 g

Indications, route, and dosage
Systemic infections caused by susceptible organisms (methicillin-sensitive S. aureus*)*
Adults: 2 to 4 g P.O. daily, divided into doses given q 6 hours; 2 to 12 g I.M. or I.V. daily, divided into doses given q 4 to 6 hours.
Children: 50 to 100 mg/kg P.O. daily, divided into doses given q 4 to 6 hours; 100 to 200 mg/kg I.M. or I.V. daily, divided into doses given q 4 to 6 hours.

Pharmacodynamics
Antibiotic action: Nafcillin is bactericidal; it adheres to bacterial penicillin-binding proteins, thus inhibiting bacterial cell wall synthesis.

Nafcillin resists the effects of penicillinases — enzymes that inactivate penicillin — and is thus active against many strains of penicillinase-producing bacteria; this activity is most important against penicillinase-producing staphylococci; some strains may remain resistant. Nafcillin is also active against a few gram-positive aerobic and anerobic bacilli but has no significant effect on gram-negative bacilli.

Pharmacokinetics
- *Absorption:* Nafcillin is absorbed erratically and poorly from the GI tract; peak serum levels occur at ½ to 2 hours after an oral dose and 30 to 60 minutes after an I.M. dose. Food decreases absorption.
- *Distribution:* Nafcillin is distributed widely; CSF penetration is poor but enhanced by meningeal inflammation. Nafcillin crosses the placenta and is 70% to 90% protein-bound.
- *Metabolism:* Nafcillin is metabolized primarily in the liver; it undergoes enterohepatic circulation. No dosage adjustment is necessary for patients in renal failure.
- *Excretion:* Nafcillin and metabolites are excreted primarily in bile; about 25% to 30% is excreted in urine unchanged. It may also be excreted in breast milk. Elimination half-life in adults is ½ to 1½ hours.

Contraindications and precautions
Nafcillin is contraindicated in patients with known hypersensitivity to any other penicillin or to cephalosporins.

Interactions
Concomitant use of nafcillin with aminoglycosides produces synergistic bactericidal effects against *Staphylococcus aureus.* However, the drugs are physically and chemically incompatible and are inactivated when mixed or given together.

Probenecid blocks renal tubular secretion of penicillins; however, this interaction has only a small effect on the excretion of nafcillin.

Effects on diagnostic tests
Nafcillin alters tests for urinary and serum proteins; turbidimetric urine and serum proteins are often falsely positive or elevated in tests using sulfosalicylic acid or trichloroacetic acid.

Nafcillin may cause transient reductions in red blood cell, white blood cell, and platelet counts. Abnormal urinalysis results may indicate drug-induced interstitial nephritis.

Adverse reactions
- GI: nausea, vomiting, diarrhea, *pseudomembranous colitis.*
- GU: *hematuria, acute interstitial nephritis.*
- HEMA: transient leukopenia, *neutropenia,* granulocytopenia, thrombocytopenia with high doses.
- Local: vein irritation, thrombophlebitis.
- Other: *hypersensitivity reactions* (chills, fever, rash, pruritus, urticaria, *anaphylaxis*), bacterial or fungal superinfection.
  Note: Drug should be discontinued if immediate hypersensitivity reactions occur or if signs of interstitial nephritis or pseudomembranous colitis occur. Patient may require alternate therapy if any of the following occurs: drug fever, eosinophilia, hematuria, neutropenia, or unexplained elevations in serum creatinine concentrations, BUN levels, or liver function studies.

Overdose and treatment
Clinical signs of overdose include neuromuscular irritability or seizures. No specific recommendations. Treatment is supportive. After recent ingestion (4 hours or less), empty stomach by induced emesis or gastric lavage; follow with activated charcoal to reduce absorption. Nafcillin is not appreciably removed by hemodialysis.

▶ Special considerations
Besides those relevant to all *penicillins,* consider the following recommendations.
- Drug should be given with water only; acid in fruit juice or carbonated beverage may inactivate drug.
- Give dose on empty stomach; food decreases absorption.

Information for the patient
Tell patient to report severe diarrhea or allergic reactions promptly.

Geriatric use
Half-life may be prolonged in elderly patients because of impaired hepatic and renal function.

Pediatric use
Nafcillin that has been reconstituted with bacteriostatic water for injection with benzyl alcohol should not be used in neonates because of toxicity.

Breast-feeding
Nafcillin is excreted into breast milk; drug should be used with caution in breast-feeding women.

---

nalbuphine hydrochloride
Nubain

- Pharmacologic classification: narcotic agonist-antagonist; opioid partial agonist
- Therapeutic classification: analgesic; adjunct to anesthesia
- Pregnancy risk category C

How supplied
Available by prescription only
Injection: 10 mg/ml, 20 mg/ml

Indications, route, and dosage
Moderate to severe pain
Adults: 10 to 20 mg S.C., I.M., or I.V. q 3 to 6 hours, p.r.n. or around the clock. Maximum dosage: 160 mg/day.

Pharmacodynamics
Analgesic action: The analgesic effect of nalbuphine is believed to result from the drug's action at opiate receptor sites in the CNS, relieving moderate to severe pain. The narcotic antagonist effect may result from competitive inhibition at opiate receptors. Like other opioids, nalbuphine causes respiratory depression, sedation, and miosis. In patients with coronary artery disease or myocardial infarction (MI), it appears to produce no substantial changes in heart rate, pulmonary artery or wedge pressure, left ventricular end-diastolic pressure, pulmonary vascular resistance, or cardiac index.

Pharmacokinetics
- *Absorption:* When administered orally, nalbuphine is about one-fifth as effective as an analgesic as it is when given I.M., apparently because of "first-pass" metabolism in the GI tract and liver. Onset of action is within 15 minutes, with peak effect seen at ½ to 1 hour.
- *Distribution:* Nalbuphine is not appreciably bound to plasma proteins.
- *Metabolism:* Nalbuphine is metabolized in the liver; duration of action is 3 to 6 hours.
- *Excretion:* Nalbuphine is excreted in urine and to some degree in bile.

Contraindications and precautions
Nalbuphine is contraindicated in patients with known hypersensitivity to the drug or other phenanthrene opioids (codeine, hydrocodone, hydromorphone, morphine, oxycodone, oxymorphone).

Administer nalbuphine with extreme caution to patients with supraventricular arrhythmias; avoid, or administer drug with extreme caution to patients with head injury or increased intracranial pressure, because drug obscures neurologic parameters; and during pregnancy and labor, because drug readily crosses placenta (premature infants are especially sensitive to respiratory and CNS depressant effects of opioids).

Administer nalbuphine cautiously to patients with MI who are nauseated or vomiting because it may induce nausea and vomiting; to patients with renal or hepatic dysfunction, because drug accumulation or prolonged duration of action may occur; to patients with pulmonary disease (asthma, chronic obstructive pulmonary disease), because drug depresses respiration and suppresses cough reflex; to patients undergoing biliary tract surgery, because drug may cause biliary spasm; to patients with convulsive disorders, because drug may precipitate seizures; to elderly or debilitated patients, who are more sensitive to both therapeutic and adverse drug effects; and to patients prone to physical or psychic addiction, because of the high risk of addiction to this drug.

Nalbuphine has a lower potential for abuse than do narcotic agonists, but the risk still exists.

Nalbuphine contains sulfites as preservatives and should not be used in patients who are allergic to sulfites.

Interactions
If administered within a few hours of barbiturate anesthetics such as thiopental, nalbuphine may produce additive CNS and respiratory depressant effects and, possibly, apnea.

According to some reports, cimetidine may increase narcotic nalbuphine toxicity, causing disorientation, respiratory depression, apnea, and seizures. Because data are limited, this combination is not contraindicated; however, be prepared to administer a narcotic antagonist if toxicity occurs.

Reduced doses of nalbuphine are usually necessary when drug is used concomitantly with other CNS depressants (narcotic analgesics, antihistamines, phenothiazines, barbiturates, benzodiazepines, sedative-hypnotics, alcohol, tricyclic antidepressants, and muscle relaxants), which may potentiate the drug's respiratory and CNS depression, sedation, and hypotensive effects; use with general anesthetics may also cause severe cardiovascular depression.

Drug accumulation and enhanced effects may result if drug is given concomitantly with other drugs that are extensively metabolized in the liver (rifampin, phenytoin, and digitoxin).

Patients who become physically dependent on this drug may experience acute withdrawal syndrome if given high doses of a narcotic antagonist. Use with caution, and monitor closely.

Effects on diagnostic tests
None reported.

Adverse reactions
- CNS: sedation, dizziness, vertigo, nervousness, depression, restlessness, hostility, unusual dreams, hallucinations (less than with pentazocine), euphoria, dysphoria, feeling of heaviness, numbness, tingling, disorientation, confusion, headache, faintness, psychic dependence.
- CV: tachycardia, bradycardia, hypertension, hypotension.
- DERM: flushing, rashes, pruritus, sweaty or clammy feeling, urticaria.
- GI: dry mouth, biliary spasms (colic), cramps, dyspepsia, bitter taste, nausea, vomiting.
- GU: urinary urgency.
- Other: *respiratory depression,* dyspnea, asthma, speech difficulty, blurred vision.
Note: Drug should be discontinued if hypersensitivity, seizures, or cardiac arrhythmias occur.

Overdose and treatment
The most common signs and symptoms of nalbuphine overdose are CNS depression, respiratory depression, and miosis (pinpoint pupils). Other acute toxic effects

include hypotension, bradycardia, hypothermia, shock, apnea, cardiopulmonary arrest, circulatory collapse, pulmonary edema, and convulsions.

To treat acute overdose, first establish adequate respiratory exchange via a patent airway and ventilation as needed; administer a narcotic antagonist (naloxone) to reverse respiratory depression. (Because the duration of action of nalbuphine is longer than that of naloxone, repeated naloxone dosing is necessary. Naloxone should not be given in the absence of clinically significant respiratory or cardiovascular depression. Monitor vital signs closely.

Provide symptomatic and supportive treatment (continued respiratory support, correction of fluid or electrolyte imbalance). Monitor laboratory parameters, vital signs, and neurologic status closely.

▶ Special considerations
Besides those relevant to all *narcotic agonist-antagonists*, consider the following recommendations.
● Nalbuphine may obscure the signs and symptoms of an acute abdominal condition or worsen gallbladder pain.
● Nalbuphine may cause orthostatic hypotension in ambulatory patients.
● Before administration, visually inspect all parenteral products for particulate matter and discoloration.
● Parenteral administration of nalbuphine provides better analgesia than oral administration. Intravenous doses should be given by slow I.V. injection, preferably in diluted solution. Rapid I.V. injection increases the incidence of adverse effects.
● Nalbuphine causes respiratory depression, which at 10 mg is equal to the respiratory depression produced by 10 mg of morphine.
● Nalbuphine also acts as a narcotic antagonist; it may precipitate abstinence syndrome in narcotic-dependent patients.

Geriatric use
Lower doses are usually indicated for elderly patients, who may be more sensitive to the therapeutic and adverse effects of the drug.

Pediatric use
Safety in children under age 18 is not established.

Breast-feeding
It is not known whether nalbuphine is excreted in breast milk; it should be used with caution in breast-feeding women.

---

nalidixic acid
NegGram

● Pharmacologic classification: quinolone antibiotic
● Therapeutic classification: urinary tract antiseptic
● Pregnancy risk category B

How supplied
Available by prescription only
Tablets: 250 mg, 500 mg, 1 g
Suspension: 250 mg/5 ml

Indications, route, and dosage
Acute and chronic urinary tract infections caused by susceptible gram-negative organisms
Adults: 1 g P.O. q.i.d. for 7 to 14 days; 2 g P.O. daily for long-term use.
Children over age 3 months: 55 mg/kg P.O. daily divided q.i.d. for 7 to 14 days; 33 mg/kg P.O. daily divided q.i.d. for long-term use.

Pharmacodynamics
Antimicrobial action: Drug is bactericidal and inhibits microbial synthesis of deoxyribonucleic acid (DNA). Spectrum of action includes most gram-negative organisms except *Pseudomonas*. (Approximately 10% of patients develop nalidixic acid-resistant organisms during therapy.)

Pharmacokinetics
● *Absorption:* Nalidixic acid is well absorbed from the GI tract; peak concentrations occur in 1 to 2 hours.
● *Distribution:* Nalidixic acid concentrates in renal tissue and seminal fluid; it does not penetrate prostatic tissue and only minimal amounts appear in CSF and the placenta. The drug is highly protein-bound.
● *Metabolism:* Nalidixic acid is metabolized to the more active hydroxynalidixic acid and inactive conjugates in the liver.
● *Excretion:* 13% of metabolites and 2% to 3% of unchanged drug are excreted via the kidneys. In patients with normal renal function, plasma half-life of nalidixic acid is 1 to 2½ hours. In an anuric patient, the half-life is prolonged up to 21 hours.

Contraindications and precautions
Nalidixic acid is contraindicated in patients with a history of seizure disorders because the drug may induce seizures; in patients with glucose-6-phosphate dehydrogenase deficiency because drug may induce hemolytic anemia; and in patients with known hypersensitivity to the drug.

Nalidixic acid should be administered cautiously to patients with renal or hepatic dysfunction because of potential for drug accumulation, and to patients with severe cerebral arteriosclerosis because of potential for CNS toxicity. Cross-resistance with cinoxacin has been reported.

Interactions
When used concomitantly with warfarin or dicumarol, nalidixic acid may displace clinically significant amounts of these anticoagulants from serum albumin binding sites, possibly causing excessive anticoagulation. When taken with other photosensitizing drugs, additive effects may occur.

Effects on diagnostic tests
False-positive reactions may occur in urine glucose tests using cupric sulfate reagents (such as Benedict's test, Fehling's test, and Clinitest), from reaction between glucuronic acid (liberated by urinary metabolites of nalidixic acid) and cupric sulfate. Urine 17-ketosteroid and urine 17-ketogenic steroid levels may be falsely elevated because nalidixic acid interacts with *m*-dinitro benzene, used to measure these urine metabolites. Urinary vanillylmandelic acid levels may also be falsely elevated.

Circulating erythrocyte, platelet, and leukocyte counts may decrease transiently during nalidixic acid therapy.

Adverse reactions
- CNS: drowsiness, weakness, headache, dizziness, vertigo, convulsions in epileptic patients, confusion, hallucinations.
- DERM: pruritus, photosensitivity, urticaria, rash.
- EENT: sensitivity to light, change in color perception, diplopia, blurred vision.
- GI: abdominal pain, nausea, vomiting, diarrhea.
- HEMA: eosinophilia, thrombocytopenia, leukopenia, hemolytic anemia.
- Other: angioedema, arthralgia, fever, chills, increased intracranial pressure (ICP), and bulging fontanelles in infants and children.

Note: Drug should be discontinued if patient develops hypersensitivity reaction, seizures, toxic psychosis, evidence of increased ICP, or photosensitivity reaction.

Overdose and treatment
Clinical effects of overdose include toxic psychosis, seizures, increased ICP, metabolic acidosis, lethargy, nausea, and vomiting. However, because nalidixic acid is rapidly excreted, such reactions usually resolve in 2 to 3 hours.

Gastric lavage may be performed after recent ingestion. However, if drug absorption has occurred, supportive measures, including increased fluid administration, should be initiated. Anticonvulsants may be used to treat nalidixic acid–induced seizures; however, this measure is rarely required.

▶ **Special considerations**
- Obtain culture and sensitivity tests before starting therapy, and repeat as needed.
- Obtain complete blood count and renal and liver function studies periodically during long-term therapy.
- Drug is ineffective against *Pseudomonas* infection or infection found outside urinary tract.
- Resistant bacteria may emerge after first 48 hours of therapy (especially if inadequate doses are prescribed).
- Although CNS toxicity is rare, brief convulsions, increased ICP, and toxic psychosis may occur in infants, children, and elderly patients.

Information for the patient
- Instruct patient to report visual disturbances; these usually disappear with dosage reduction.
- Warn patient that exposure to sunlight may cause photosensitivity. Inform him that photosensitivity reactions usually resolve within 2 to 8 weeks after drug therapy ends. Also warn that bullae may continue to follow subsequent exposure to sunlight or mild skin trauma for up to 3 months after drug therapy ends.
- Advise patient that he may take drug with food or milk to avoid GI upset.
- Warn patient to observe caution while driving because drug may produce drowsiness or blurred vision.

Pediatric use
Do not administer drug to infants under age 3 months because safety has not been established; do not administer to prepubertal children because drug may be toxic to cartilage in weight-bearing joints.

Breast-feeding
Drug is excreted in breast milk in low concentrations. In one case, hemolytic anemia occurred in infant of uremic mother taking 1 g q.i.d. Lower drug excretion and elevated serum level resulted in higher excretion in milk.

---

naloxone hydrochloride
Narcan

- Pharmacologic classification: narcotic (opioid) antagonist
- Therapeutic classification: narcotic antagonist
- Pregnancy risk category B

How supplied
Available by prescription only
Injection: 0.4 mg/ml, 1 mg/ml, 0.02 mg/ml, 0.4 mg/ml (paraben free)

Indications, route, and dosage
Known or suspected narcotic-induced respiratory depression, including that caused by pentazocine and propoxyphene
Adults: 0.4 to 2 mg I.V., S.C., or I.M., repeated q 2 to 3 minutes, p.r.n. If no response is observed after 10 mg has been administered, the diagnosis of narcotic-induced toxicity should be questioned.
Postoperative narcotic depression
Adults: 0.1 to 0.2 mg I.V. q 2 to 3 minutes, p.r.n. Adult concentration is 0.4 mg/ml. Some clinicians advocate much smaller doses: dilute to 40 mcg/ml and administer in 40 mcg doses. These small doses are used to reverse respiratory depression while maintaing analgesia.
Children: 0.01 mg/kg dose I.M., I.V., or S.C., repeated q 2 to 3 minutes p.r.n. Note: If initial dose does not result in clinical improvement, up to 10 times this dose (0.1 mg/kg) may be needed to be effective.
Neonates (asphyxia neonatorum): 0.01 mg/kg I.V. into umbilical vein repeated q 2 to 3 minutes for three doses. Concentration for use in neonates and children is 0.02 mg/ml.

Pharmacodynamics
Narcotic (opioid) antagonism: Naloxone is essentially a pure antagonist. In patients who have received an opioid agonist or other analgesic with narcotic-like effects, naloxone antagonizes most of the opioid effects, especially respiratory depression, sedation, and hypotension. Because the duration of action of naloxone in most cases is shorter than that of the opioid, opiate effects may return as those of naloxone dissipate. Naloxone does not produce tolerance or physical or psychological dependence. The precise mechanism of action is unknown, but is thought to involve competitive antagonism of more than one opiate receptor in the CNS.

Pharmacokinetics
- *Absorption:* Naloxone is rapidly inactivated after oral administration; therefore, it is given parenterally. Its onset of action is 1 to 2 minutes after I.V. administration, and 2 to 5 minutes after I.M. or S.C. administration. The duration of action is longer after I.M. use and higher doses, when compared to I.V. use and lower doses.
- *Distribution:* Naloxone is rapidly distributed into body tissues and fluids.
- *Metabolism:* Naloxone is rapidly metabolized in the liver, primarily by conjugation.

• *Excretion:* Duration of action is approximately 45 minutes, depending on route and dose. Drug is excreted in urine. The plasma half-life has been reported to be from 30 to 90 minutes in adults, and 3 hours in neonates.

Contraindications and precautions

Naloxone is contraindicated in patients with known hypersensitivity to the drug.

Administer naloxone with extreme caution to patients with supraventricular arrhythmias; avoid or administer drug with extreme caution to patients with a head injury or increased intracranial pressure, because drug obscures neurologic parameters; and during pregnancy and labor, because drug readily crosses the placenta (premature infants appear especially sensitive to its respiratory and CNS depressant effects when the drug is used during delivery).

Administer cautiously to patients with convulsive disorders, because naloxone can precipitate seizures; and to elderly or debilitated patients, who are more sensitive to the drug's therapeutic and adverse effects.

Naloxone should be administered cautiously to narcotic addicts, including newborns of women with narcotic dependence, in whom it may produce an acute abstinence syndrome.

Because the duration of action of naloxone is shorter than that of most opiates, continued surveillance of the patient is mandatory, and repeated naloxone doses are often necessary. Other supportive therapy, with attention to maintenance of adequate respiratory and cardiovascular function, is imperative.

Interactions

When given to a narcotic addict, naloxone may produce an acute abstinence syndrome. Use with caution, and monitor closely.

Effects on diagnostic tests

None reported.

Adverse reactions

• CV: tachycardia, increased blood pressure.
• GI: nausea and vomiting (with high doses).
• Other: tremors, sweating, pulmonary edema (postoperatively).

Note: Drug should be discontinued if signs of a severe acute abstinence syndrome appear.

Overdose and treatment

No serious adverse reactions to naloxone overdose are known, except those of acute abstinence syndrome in narcotic dependent persons.

▶ Special considerations

Besides those relevant to all *narcotic antagonists,* consider the following recommendations.
• Before administering, visually inspect all parenteral products for particulate matter and discoloration.
• Take a careful drug history to rule out possible narcotic addiction, to avoid inducing withdrawal symptoms (apply cautions also to the baby of an addicted woman).
• Because naloxone's duration of activity is shorter than that of most narcotics, vigilance and repeated doses are usually necessary in the management of an acute narcotic overdose in a nonaddicted patient.
• Avoid relying on the drug too much, that is, do not neglect attention to the ABCs (airway, breathing, and circulation). Maintain adequate respiratory and cardiovascular status at all times. Respiratory "overshoot"

may occur; monitor for respiratory rate higher than before respiratory depression. Respiratory rate increases in 1 to 2 minutes, and effect lasts 1 to 4 hours.
• Naloxone is not effective in treating respiratory depression caused by nonopioid drugs.
• Naloxone can be diluted in dextrose 5% or normal saline solution. Use within 24 hours after mixing.
• Naloxone is the safest drug to use when cause of respiratory depression is uncertain.
• Naloxone may be administered by continuous I.V. infusion, which is necessary in many cases to control the adverse effects of epidurally administered morphine.
• Naloxone has been used investigationally to treat Alzheimer's disease. It has also been shown to improve circulation in refractory shock, and has been used by some researchers to relieve certain cases of chronic constipation.

Geriatric use

Lower doses are usually indicated for elderly patients, because they may be more sensitive to the therapeutic and adverse effects of the drug.

Pediatric use

Administer with extreme caution to children. Adult concentration (0.4 mg/ml) may be diluted by mixing 0.5 ml with 9.5 ml sterile water or saline solution for injection to make neonatal concentration (0.02 mg/ml).

Breast-feeding

It is not known whether naloxone is excreted in breast milk.

---

naltrexone hydrochloride
Trexan

• Pharmacologic classification: narcotic (opioid) antagonist
• Therapeutic classification: narcotic detoxification adjunct
• Pregnancy risk category C

How supplied

Available by prescription only
Tablets: 50 mg

Indications, route, and dosage
Adjunct for maintenance of opioid-free state in detoxified individuals

Adults: Initially, 25 mg P.O. If no withdrawal signs occur within 1 hour, administer an additional 25 mg. Once patient has been started on 50 mg q 24 hours, flexible maintenance schedule may be used. From 50 to 150 mg may be given daily, depending on the schedule prescribed.

Pharmacodynamics

Opioid antagonism: Naltrexone is essentially a pure opiate (narcotic) antagonist. Like naloxone, it has little or no agonist activity. Its precise mechanism of action is unknown, but it is thought to involve competitive antagonism of more than one opiate receptor in the CNS. When administered to patients who have not recently received opiates, it exhibits little or no pharmacologic effect. At oral doses of 30 to 50 mg daily, it produces minimal analgesia, only slight drowsiness, and no respiratory depression. However, pharmacologic effects, including psychotomimetic effects, increased systolic or diastolic blood pressure, respiratory depression, and decreased oral temperature, which are suggestive of opiate agonist activity, have reportedly occurred in a few patients. In patients who have received single or repeated large doses of opiates, naltrexone attenuates or produces a complete but reversible block of the pharmacologic effects of the narcotic. Naltrexone does not produce physical or psychological dependence, and tolerance to its antagonist activity reportedly does not develop.

Pharmacokinetics

- *Absorption:* Naltrexone is well absorbed after oral administration, reaching peak plasma levels after 1 hour, although it does undergo extensive first-pass hepatic metabolism (only 5% to 20% of an oral dose reaches the systemic circulation unchanged). Peak effect occurs within 1 hour.
- *Distribution:* The extent and duration of the antagonist activity of naltrexone appear directly related to plasma and tissue concentrations of the drug. It is widely distributed throughout the body, but considerable interindividual variation exists.
- *Metabolism:* Oral naltrexone undergoes extensive first-pass hepatic metabolism. Its major metabolite is believed to be a pure antagonist also, and may contribute to its efficacy. Drug and hepatic metabolites may undergo enterohepatic recirculation.
- *Excretion:* Naltrexone is excreted primarily by the kidneys. Elimination half-life is about 10 hours, that of its major active metabolite is about 14 hours.

Contraindications and precautions

Naltrexone is contraindicated in patients with known hypersensitivity to the drug.

Administer naltrexone with extreme caution to patients with allergy to another drug in the same chemical class; to patients receiving narcotic analgesics or to those who are narcotic-dependent or are undergoing narcotic withdrawal; to any individual who fails a naloxone challenge or who has a positive urinary screen for opioids; and to patients with acute hepatitis or liver failure (naltrexone can cause dose-related hepatocellular injury.)

Naltrexone is a potent antagonist with a prolonged pharmacologic effect (48 to 72 hours), but the blockade produced is surmountable; any attempt by a patient to overcome the antagonism by taking narcotics is very dangerous and could lead to fatal overdose.

Interactions

When naltrexone is taken with opioid-containing medications (cough and cold preparations, antidiarrheals, and opioid analgesics), opioid activity will be attenuated.

Effects on diagnostic tests

Because of its hepatotoxicity, naltrexone may alter the results of liver function tests.

Adverse reactions

No serious adverse reactions have been identified with the use of naltrexone at any dose for a patient who is opioid free, but this drug does have the capacity to cause hepatocellular injury if given at higher than recommended doses. Naltrexone can precipitate or exacerbate signs and symptoms of abstinence in anyone not completely opioid free.

Note: Drug should be discontinued if adverse changes in liver function tests, hypersensitivity, or seizures occur.

Overdose and treatment

Naltrexone overdose has not been documented. In one study, subjects who received 800 mg/day (16 tablets) for up to 1 week showed no evidence of toxicity. In case of overdose, provide symptomatic and supportive treatment in a closely supervised environment. Contact the local or regional poison control center for further information.

▶ Special considerations

Besides those relevant to all *narcotic (opioid) antagonists,* consider the following recommendations.
- Administer a naloxone (Narcan) challenge test to the patient before naltrexone use. Naloxone (0.8 to 2 mg, S.C. or I.V., incremental doses) is administered and the patient closely monitored for signs and symptoms of opiate withdrawal. If acute abstinence signs and symptoms are present, do not administer naltrexone.
- Before administering, take a careful drug history to rule out possible narcotic use. Do not attempt treatment until the patient has been opiate-free for 7 to 10 days. Verify self-reporting of abstinence from narcotics by urinalysis. No withdrawal signs or symptoms should be reported by the patient or be evident.
- Perform liver function tests before naltrexone use to establish a baseline and to evaluate possible drug-induced hepatotoxicity. In an emergency situation requiring analgesia that can only be achieved with opiates, patient who has been receiving naltrexone may need a higher dose than usual of narcotic, and the resulting respiratory depression may be deeper and more prolonged.

Information for the patient

- Patients taking naltrexone may not benefit from opioid medications, such as cough and cold preparations, antidiarrheal products, and, of course, narcotic analgesics; recommend nonnarcotic alternative if available.
- Warn patient not to self-administer narcotics while taking naltrexone, because serious injury, coma, or death may result.
- Explain that naltrexone has no tolerance or dependence liability.
- Tell patient to report any withdrawal signs and symptoms (tremors, vomiting, bone or muscle pains, sweating, abdominal cramps).
- Tell patient to carry an identification card that alerts medical personnel that naltrexone is taken, and to inform any new physician that he is receiving naltrexone therapy.

Geriatric use

Use in elderly patients is not documented, but they would probably require reduced dosage.

Pediatric use

Safe use of naltrexone in patients under age 18 has not been established.

Breast-feeding

It is unknown whether naltrexone is excreted in breast milk. It should be used with caution in breast-feeding women, especially in view of its known hepatotoxicity.

---

*Canada only   †Unlabeled clinical use   Italicized adverse reactions are life-threatening.

nandrolone decanoate
Anabolin LA-100, Androlone-D 100, Deca-Durabolin, Hybolin Decanoate, Kabolin, Nandrobolic L.A., Neo-Durabolic

nandrolone phenpropionate
Anabolin-I.M., Androlone, Androlone 50, Durabolin, Hybolin Improved, Nandrobolic

- Pharmacologic classification: anabolic steroid
- Therapeutic classification: erythropoietic (nandrolone decanoate), anabolic (nandrolone decanoate), antineoplastic (nandrolone phenpropionate)
- Controlled substance schedule III
- Pregnancy risk category X

How supplied
Available by prescription only
Decanoate
Injection: 50 mg/ml, 100 mg/ml, 200 mg/ml (in oil)
Phenpropionate
Injection: 25 mg/ml, 50 mg/ml (in oil)

Indications, route, and dosage
Anemia associated with renal insufficiency
Decanoate
Adults: 100 mg to 200 mg I.M. weekly in males; 50 to 100 mg/week in females.
Children age 2 to 13: 25 to 50 mg I.M. every 3 to 4 weeks.
Metastatic breast cancer
Phenpropionate
Adults: 50 to 100 mg I.M. weekly.

Pharmacodynamics
- *Androgenic action:* Nandrolone exerts inhibitory effects on hormone-responsive breast tumors and metastases.
- *Erythropoietic action:* Nandrolone stimulates the kidneys' production of erythropoietin, leading to increases in red blood cell mass and volume.
- *Anabolic action:* Nandrolone may reverse corticosteroid-induced catabolism and promote tissue development in severely debilitated patients.

Pharmacokinetics
Nandrolone is metabolized by the liver. Its pharmacokinetics are otherwise poorly described.

Contraindications and precautions
Nandrolone is contraindicated in patients with severe renal or cardiac disease because fluid and electrolyte retention caused by this agent may aggravate these disorders; in patients with hepatic disease because impaired elimination of the drug may cause toxic accumulation; in male patients with prostatic or breast cancer or benign prostatic hypertrophy with obstruction and in patients with undiagnosed abnormal genital bleeding because this drug can stimulate the growth of cancerous breast or prostate tissue in males; and in pregnant or breast-feeding women because animal studies have shown that administration of anabolic steroids during pregnancy causes masculinization of the female fetus. Administer nandrolone decanoate cautiously in patients with a history of coronary artery disease because the drug has hypercholesterolemic effects.

Interactions
In patients with diabetes, decreased blood glucose levels may require adjustment of insulin or oral hypoglycemic drug dosage.

Nandrolone decanoate may potentiate the effects of warfarin-type anticoagulants, causing increases in prothrombin time. Use with adrenocorticosteroids or adrenocorticotropic hormone increases the potential for fluid and electrolyte retention.

Effects on diagnostic tests
Nandrolone may cause abnormal results of fasting plasma glucose, glucose tolerance, and metyrapone tests. It may increase sulfobromophthalein retention. Thyroid function test results (protein-bound iodine, radioactive iodine uptake, thyroid-binding capacity) and 17-ketosteroid levels may decrease. Liver function test results, prothrombin time (especially in patients receiving anticoagulant therapy), and serum creatinine levels may be elevated. Because of this agent's anabolic activity, serum sodium, potassium, calcium, phosphate, and cholesterol levels may all rise.

Adverse reactions
- Androgenic: *in females:* deepening of voice, clitoral enlargement, decreased or increased libido; *in males:* prepubertal—premature epiphyseal closure, priapism, phallic enlargement; postpubertal—testicular atrophy, oligospermia, decreased ejaculatory volume, impotence, gynecomastia, epididymitis.
- CNS: headache, mental depression.
- CV: edema.
- DERM: acne, oily skin, hirsutism, flushing, sweating.
- GI: gastroenteritis, nausea, vomiting, diarrhea, change in appetite, weight gain.
- GU: bladder irritability, vaginitis, menstrual irregularities.
- Hepatic: reversible jaundice, hepatotoxicity.
- Local: pain at injection site, induration.
- Other: hypercalcemia, hypercalciuria.

  Note: Drug should be discontinued if hypercalcemia, edema, hypersensitivity reaction, priapism, or excessive sexual stimulation occurs or if virilization occurs in females.

Overdose and treatment
No information available.

▶ Special considerations
Besides those relevant to all *anabolic steroids*, consider the following recommendations.
- Nandrolone injections should be administered deeply into the gluteal muscle.
- An adequate iron intake is necessary for maximum response when patient is receiving nandrolone decanoate injections.

Geriatric use
Observe elderly male patients for the development of prostatic hypertrophy.

Pediatric use
Do not use in prepubertal children because of risk of premature epiphyseal closure, masculinization of females, or precocious development in males.

Breast-feeding
To avoid potential toxicity in the infant, drug should not be used by breast-feeding women.

---

naphazoline hydrochloride
Ak-Con, Albalon Liquifilm, Allerest, Allergy Drops, Clear Eyes, Comfort Eye Drops, Degest 2, I-Naphline, Muro's Opcon, Naphcon A, Naphcon Forte, Privine Hydrochloride, VasoClear, Vasocon

- Pharmacologic classification: sympatho-mimetic agent
- Therapeutic classification: decongestant, vasoconstrictor
- Pregnancy risk category C

How supplied
Available by prescription only
Ophthalmic solution: 0.1%

Available without prescription
Ophthalmic solution: 0.012%, 0.02%, 0.03%
Nasal drops or sprays: 0.05% (solution)

Indications, route, and dosage
Ocular congestion, irritation, itching
Adults: Instill 1 to 3 drops (0.1% solution) or 1 to 2 drops (0.012% to 0.03% solution) in eye daily to q.i.d.
Nasal congestion
Adults and children over age 12: 1 or 2 drops or sprays (0.05% solution) as needed. Do not use drops more than q 3 hours or spray more often than q 4 to 6 hours.

Pharmacodynamics
Decongestant action: Naphazoline produces vasoconstriction by local and alpha-adrenergic action on blood vessels of the conjunctiva or nasal mucosa; therefore, it reduces blood flow and nasal congestion.

Pharmacokinetics
Unknown.

Contraindications and precautions
Naphazoline is contraindicated in patients with hypersensitivity to any component of the preparation and in patients with narrow-angle glaucoma. It should be used with caution in patients with hyperthyroidism, cardiac disease, hypertension, or diabetes mellitus and in elderly patients.

Interactions
Concomitant use with MAO inhibitors may result in an increased adrenergic response and hypertensive crisis.

Effects on diagnostic tests
None reported.

Adverse reactions
- CNS: headache, dizziness, nervousness, *coma.*
- CV: hypertension, *cardiovascular collapse.*
- ENT: transient burning, stinging, dryness or ulceration of mucosa, anosmia, sneezing, rebound nasal congestion (with excessive or long-term use).
- Eye: transient stinging, pupillary dilation, irritation, hyperemia, increased or decreased intraocular pressure.
- Other: nausea, weakness, nasal congestion, sweating.
  Note: Drug should be discontinued if systemic symptoms occur.

Overdose and treatment
Clinical manifestations of overdose include CNS depression, sweating, decreased body temperature, bradycardia, shocklike hypotension, decreased respirations, cardiovascular collapse, and coma.

Activated charcoal or gastric lavage may be used initially to treat accidental ingestion (administer early before sedation occurs). Monitor vital signs and ECG, as ordered. Treat seizures with I.V. diazepam.

▶ Special considerations
- Naphazoline is the most widely used ocular decongestant.
- Monitor for blurred vision, pain, or lid edema.
- Do not shake container.

Information for the patient
- Teach patient how to instill ophthalmic or nasal medication; tell patient not to share medication with others.
- Advise patient to report blurred vision, eye pain, or lid swelling that occurs when using ophthalmic product.
- Advise patient using ophthalmic solution that photophobia may follow pupil dilation; tell patient to report this effect promptly.
- Warn patient not to exceed recommended dosage; rebound nasal congestion and conjunctivitis also may occur with frequent or prolonged use.
- Tell patient to call if nasal congestion persists after 5 days of using nasal solution.

Geriatric use
Drug should be used with caution in elderly patients with severe cardiac disease or poorly controlled hypertension and in diabetics prone to diabetic ketoacidosis.

Pediatric use
Use in infants and children may result in CNS depression, leading to coma and marked reduction in body temperature. Although available without prescription, parents should not use 0.05% nasal solution or spray in children under age 6 or 0.025% solution in children under age 2 unless directed by physician.

---

naproxen
Naprosyn

naproxen sodium
Anaprox

- Pharmacologic classification: nonsteroidal anti-inflammatory
- Therapeutic classification: nonnarcotic analgesic, antipyretic, anti-inflammatory
- Pregnancy risk category B

How supplied
Available by prescription only
Naproxen
Tablets: 250 mg, 375 mg, 500 mg
Oral suspension: 125 mg/5 ml
Naproxen sodium
Tablets (film-coated): 275 mg, 550 mg
Note: 275 mg naproxen sodium 250 mg naproxen

Indications, route, and dosage
Mild to moderately severe musculoskeletal or soft tissue irritation
Naproxen
Adults: 250 to 375 mg b.i.d.
Naproxen sodium
Adults: 275 mg in the morning and 375 mg in the evening.
Mild to moderate pain; primary dysmenorrhea
Naproxen sodium
Adults: 500 to 550 mg P.O. to start, followed by 250 to 275 mg q 6 to 8 hours p.r.n. Maximum daily dose should not exceed 1.25 g of naproxen or 1.375 g of naproxen sodium.
Acute gout
Naproxen
Adults: 750 mg initially, then 250 mg q 8 hours until episode subsides.
Naproxen sodium
Adults: 825 mg initially, then 275 mg q 8 hours until attack has subsided.
Juvenile rheumatoid arthritis
Naproxen
Children: 10 mg/kg/day in two divided doses.

Pharmacodynamics
Analgesic, antipyretic, and anti-inflammatory actions: Mechanisms of action are unknown; naproxen is thought to inhibit prostaglandin synthesis.

Pharmacokinetics
- *Absorption:* Naproxen is absorbed rapidly and completely from the GI tract. Effect peaks at 2 to 4 hours.
- *Distribution:* Naproxen is highly protein-bound.
- *Metabolism:* Naproxen is metabolized in the liver.
- *Excretion:* Naproxen is excreted in urine.

Contraindications and precautions
Naproxen and naproxen sodium are contraindicated in patients with known hypersensitivity and in patients in whom aspirin or other nonsteroidal anti-inflammatory drugs (NSAIDs) induce symptoms of asthma, urticaria, or rhinitis.

Serious GI toxicity, especially ulceration or hemorrhage, can occur at any time in patients on chronic NSAID therapy. Naproxen should be used cautiously in patients with a history of angioedema or of GI disease, peptic ulcer, or renal or cardiovascular disease, because the drug may worsen these conditions. Avoid use during pregnancy (especially the third trimester) because these drugs may prolong labor.

Patients with known "triad" symptoms (aspirin hypersensitivity, rhinitis/nasal polyps, and asthma) are at high risk of cross-sensitivity to naproxen with precipitation of bronchospasm.

The signs and symptoms of acute infection (fever, myalgias, erythema) may be masked by the use of naproxen. Carefully evaluate patients with high infection risk (such as diabetic patients).

Interactions
Concomitant use of naproxen with anticoagulants and thrombolytic drugs (coumarin derivatives, heparin, streptokinase, or urokinase) may potentiate anticoagulant effects. Bleeding problems may occur if used with other drugs that inhibit platelet aggregation, such as azlocillin, parenteral carbenicillin, dextran, dipyridamole, mezlocillin, piperacillin, sulfinpyrazone, ticarcillin, valproic acid, cefamandole, cefoperazone, moxalactam, plicamycin, aspirin, salicylates, or other anti-inflammatory agents. Concomitant use with salicylates, anti-inflammatory agents, alcohol, corticotropin, or steroids may cause increased GI adverse reactions, including ulceration and hemorrhage. Aspirin may decrease the bioavailability of naproxen.

Because of the influence of prostaglandins on glucose metabolism, concomitant use with insulin or oral hypoglycemic agents may potentiate hypoglycemic effects. Naproxen may displace highly protein-bound drugs from binding sites. Toxicity may occur with coumarin derivatives, phenytoin, verapamil, or nifedipine. Increased nephrotoxicity may occur with gold compounds, other anti-inflammatory agents, or acetaminophen. Naproxen may decrease the renal clearance of methotrexate and lithium. Naproxen may decrease the clinical effectiveness of antihypertensive agents and diuretics. Concomitant use may increase risk of nephrotoxicity.

Effects on diagnostic tests
Naproxen and its metabolites may interfere with urinary 5-hydroxyindoleacetic acid (5-HIAA) and 17-hydroxycorticosteroid determinations. The physiologic effects of naproxen may lead to an increase in bleeding time (may persist for 4 days after withdrawal of drug); serum creatinine and potassium, BUN, and serum transaminase levels may also increase.

Adverse reactions
- **CNS:** headache, drowsiness, pulmonary infiltrates, light-headedness, vertigo, excitation, dizziness.
- **CV:** peripheral edema, congestive heart failure (CHF), hypotension, palpitations.
- **DERM:** pruritus, rash, urticaria.
- **EENT:** visual disturbances.
- **GI:** nausea, epigastric pain, dyspepsia, vomiting, constipation, GI bleeding or perforation, occult blood loss.
- **GU:** hematuria, cystitis, nocturia, nephrotoxicity.
- **HEMA:** prolonged bleeding time, *aplastic anemia*, neutropenia.
- **Hepatic:** elevated liver enzymes.
  Note: Drug should be discontinued if hypersensitivity or signs and symptoms of hepatotoxicity occur.

Overdose and treatment
Clinical manifestations of overdose include drowsiness, heartburn, indigestion, nausea, and vomiting.

To treat overdose of naproxen, empty stomach immediately by inducing emesis with ipecac syrup or by gastric lavage. Administer activated charcoal via nasogastric tube. Provide symptomatic and supportive measures (respiratory support and correction of fluid and electrolyte imbalances). Monitor laboratory parameters and vital signs closely. Hemodialysis is ineffective in naproxen removal.

▶ Special considerations
Besides those relevant to all *NSAIDs*, consider the following recommendations.
● Use lowest possible effective dose; 250 mg of naproxen is equivalent to 275 mg of naproxen sodium.
● Relief usually begins within 2 weeks after beginning therapy with naproxen.
● Institute safety measures to prevent injury resulting from possible CNS effects.
● Monitor fluid balance. Monitor for signs and symptoms of fluid retention, especially significant weight gain.

Information for the patient
● Caution patient to avoid concomitant use of nonprescription drugs.
● Reinforce signs and symptoms of possible adverse reactions. Instruct patient to report them promptly.
● Instruct patient to check weight every 2 to 3 days and to report any weight gain of 3 pounds or more within 1 week.
● Instruct patient in safety measures; advise him to avoid activities that require alertness until CNS effects are known.
● Warn patient against combining naproxen (Naprosyn) with naproxen sodium (Anaprox) because both circulate in the blood as naproxen anion.

Geriatric use
● Patients over age 60 are more sensitive to the adverse effects (especially GI toxicity) of naproxen.
● Naproxen's effect on renal prostaglandins may cause fluid retention and edema. This may be significant in elderly patients, especially those with CHF.

Pediatric use
Safe use of naproxen in children under age 2 has not been established. Safe use of naproxen sodium in children has not been established. No age-related problems reported.

Breast-feeding
Because they are distributed into breast milk, naproxen and naproxen sodium should be avoided during breast-feeding.

natamycin
Natacyn

● Pharmacologic classification: polyene macrolide antibiotic
● Therapeutic classification: antifungal agent
● Pregnancy risk category C

How supplied
Available by prescription only
Ophthalmic suspension: 5%

Indications, route, and dosage
Conjuctivitis and keratitis caused by susceptible fungi
Adults: Initially, 1 drop instilled in conjunctival sac q 1 to 2 hours. After 3 to 4 days, reduce dosage to 1 drop 6 to 8 times daily.
Blepharitis caused by susceptible fungi
Adults: 1 drop instilled in conjunctival sac q 4 to 6 hours.

Pharmacodynamics
Antifungal action: Natamycin increases fungal cell membrane permeability, causing leakage of essential cellular contents.

Pharmacokinetics
● *Absorption:* Systemic absorption is unlikely after topical administration; drug is not absorbed from the GI tract.
● *Distribution:* Topical administration produces effective concentrations within the corneal stroma but not in intraocular fluid.
● *Metabolism:* Unknown.
● *Excretion:* Unknown.

Contraindications and precautions
Natamycin is contraindicated in patients with hypersensitivity to any component of the formulation. Concomitant treatment with topical corticosteroids is contraindicated in fungal eye infections because of the potential for acceleration of the infection.

Caution: If keratitis fails to improve after a 7- to 10-day course, the infection may be caused by an organism unsusceptible to natamycin. Monitor tolerance to natamycin twice weekly. Determine initial and sustained therapy by laboratory diagnosis and response to the drug.

Interactions
None reported.

Effects on diagnostic tests
None reported.

Adverse reactions
● Eye: ocular edema and hyperemia.
Note: Drug should be discontinued if eye pain occurs.

Overdose and treatment
The toxicity of ingested natamycin is unknown; if accidentally ingested, use general measures such as emesis, cathartic, or lavage to remove drug from the GI tract. Treat dermal exposure by washing the area

---

with soap and water. Observe the patient closely for possible signs and symptoms.

▶ **Special considerations**
● Natamycin is the only antifungal available in an ophthalmic preparation; it is the treatment of choice for fungal keratitis.
● Continue therapy for 14 to 21 days or until active disease subsides; then, reduce dosage gradually at 4- to 7-day intervals to assure that organism has been eliminated; if infection does not improve within 7 to 10 days, reevaluate diagnosis.
● Remove excessive exudate before application.

Information for the patient
● Show patient how to apply drug. He should apply light finger pressure on lacrimal sac for 1 minute after drops are instilled. Stress importance of compliance with recommended therapy.
● Advise patient not to share eye medications with family members.
● Instruct patient to shake suspension well before using and to store it in refrigerator or at room temperature.
● Warn patient that drug may cause blurred vision and photosensitivity.

neomycin sulfate
Mycifradin Sulfate, Myciguent

● Pharmacologic classification: aminoglycoside
● Therapeutic classification: antibiotic
● Pregnancy risk category C

How supplied
Available by prescription only
Tablets: 500 mg
Oral solution: 125 mg/5 ml
Otic: 5 mg/ml (with polymyxin B sulfate 10,000 units/ml and hydrocortisone 1%)

Available without prescription
Cream: 0.5%
Ointment: 0.5%

Indications, route, and dosage
Infectious diarrhea caused by enteropathogenic Escherichia coli
Adults: 50 mg/kg P.O. daily in 4 divided doses for 2 to 3 days.
Children: 50 to 100 mg/kg P.O. daily divided q 4 to 6 hours for 2 to 3 days.
Suppression of intestinal bacteria preoperatively
Adults: 1 g P.O. q 1 hour for 4 doses, then 1 g q 4 hours for the balance of the 24 hours. A saline cathartic should precede therapy.
Children: 40 to 100 mg/kg P.O. daily divided q 4 to 6 hours. First dose should be preceded by saline cathartic.
Adjunctive treatment in hepatic coma
Adults: 1 to 3 g P.O. q.i.d. for 5 to 6 days; 200 ml of 1% or 100 ml of 2% solution as enema retained for 20 to 60 minutes q 6 hours.

External ear canal infection
Adults and children: Two to five drops into ear canal t.i.d. or q.i.d.
Topical bacterial infections, burns, wounds, skin grafts, following surgical procedure, lesions, pruritus, trophic ulcerations, and edema
Adults and children: Rub in small amount gently b.i.d., t.i.d., or as directed.
Dosage in renal failure
Adults and children: Reduce dosage. Specific recommendations are not available.

Pharmacodynamics
Antibiotic action: Neomycin is bactericidal; it binds directly to the 30S ribosomal subunit, thus inhibiting bacterial protein synthesis. Its spectrum of action includes many aerobic gram-negative organisms and some aerobic gram-positive organisms. Generally, neomycin is far less active against many gram-negative organisms than are tobramycin, gentamicin, amikacin, and netilmicin. Given orally or as retention enema, neomycin inhibits ammonia-forming bacteria in the GI tract, reducing ammonia and improving neurologic status of patients with hepatic encephalopathy. It is rarely given systemically because of its high potential for ototoxicity and nephrotoxicity. The FDA recently revoked licensing of the parenteral preparation for this reason.

Pharmacokinetics
● *Absorption:* Neomycin is absorbed poorly (about 3%) after oral administration, although oral administration is enhanced in patients with impaired GI motility or mucosal intestinal ulcerations. After oral administration, peak serum levels occur at 1 to 4 hours. Neomycin is not absorbed through intact skin; it may be absorbed from wounds, burns, or skin ulcers.
● *Distribution:* Neomycin is distributed widely after parenteral administration into synovial, pleural, peritoneal, pericardial, ascitic, and abscess fluids, and bile. Intraocular penetration is poor; CSF penetration is low even in patients with inflamed meninges. Protein binding is minimal. Neomycin crosses the placenta. Oral administration restricts distribution to the GI tract.
● *Metabolism:* Not metabolized.
● *Excretion:* Neomycin is excreted primarily in urine by glomerular filtration. Elimination half-life in adults is 2 to 3 hours; in severe renal damage, half-life may extend to 24 hours. After oral administration, neomycin is excreted primarily unchanged in feces.

Contraindications and precautions
Neomycin is contraindicated in patients with known hypersensitivity to neomycin or any other aminoglycoside and, when given orally, in patients with intestinal obstruction. Otic preparation is contraindicated in perforated eardrum.
   Neomycin should be used cautiously in patients with intestinal mucosal ulcerations; in patients with large skin wounds; in patients with decreased renal function; in patients with tinnitus, vertigo, and high-frequency hearing loss, who are susceptible to ototoxicity; in patients with dehydration, myasthenia gravis, parkinsonism, and hypocalcemia; in neonates and other infants; and in elderly patients.
   Chronic application to inflamed skin increases hazard of sensitization to neomycin.

Interactions
Concomitant use with the following drugs may increase the hazard of nephrotoxicity, ototoxicity, and neurotoxicity: methoxyflurane, polymyxin B, vancomycin, amphotericin B, cisplatin, cephalosporins, and other aminoglycosides; hazard of ototoxicity is also increased during use with ethacrynic acid, furosemide, bumetanide, urea, or mannitol. Dimenhydrinate and other antiemetics and antivertigo drugs may mask neomycin-induced ototoxicity.

Concomitant use with penicillins results in a synergistic bactericidal effect against *Pseudomonas aeruginosa, Escherichia coli, Klebsiella, Citrobacter, Enterobacter, Serratia,* and *Proteus mirabilis.* However, the drugs are physically and chemically incompatible and are inactivated when mixed or given together.

Neomycin may potentiate neuromuscular blockade from general anesthetics or neuromuscular blocking agents such as succinylcholine and tubocurarine.

Oral neomycin inhibits vitamin K-producing bacteria in GI tract and may potentiate action of oral anticoagulants; dosage adjustment of anticoagulants may be necessary.

Effects on diagnostic tests
Neomycin-induced nephrotoxicity may elevate levels of blood urea nitrogen (BUN), nonprotein nitrogen, or serum creatinine; it may increase urinary excretion of casts, if systemic absorption occurs.

Adverse reactions
● CNS: headache, lethargy, neuromuscular blockage with respiratory depression.
● DERM: rash, urticaria, contact dermatitis. Systemic absorption possible when used on extensive areas.
● EENT: ototoxicity (tinnitus, vertigo, hearing loss); if used in ear, burning, erythema, vesicular dermatitis.
● GI: nausea, vomiting, *diarrhea, pseudomembranous colitis.*
● GU: *nephrotoxicity* (cells or casts in the urine, oliguria, proteinuria, decreased creatinine clearance, increased BUN, serum creatinine, and nonprotein nitrogen levels).
● Other: hypersensitivity reactions (eosinophilia, fever, rash, urticaria, pruritus), bacterial or fungal superinfection.
Note: Drug should be discontinued if signs of ototoxicity, nephrotoxicity, or hypersensitivity occur; if severe diarrhea indicates pseudomembranous colitis; or if intestinal obstruction develops. Drug should be discontinued or serum concentrations monitored if intestinal ulcerations develop, especially in renal impairment.

Overdose and treatment
Clinical signs of overdose include ototoxicity, nephrotoxicity, and neuromuscular toxicity. Remove drug by hemodialysis or peritoneal dialysis; treatment with calcium salts or anticholinesterases reverses neuromuscular blockade. After recent ingestion (4 hours or less), empty the stomach by induced emesis or gastric lavage; follow with activated charcoal to reduce absorption.

▶ Special considerations
Beside those relevant to all *aminoglycosides,* consider the following recommendations.
Preoperative bowel contamination
● Provide low-residue diet and cathartic immediately

before administration of oral neomycin; follow-up enemas may be necessary to completely empty bowel.
Topical therapy
● Do not apply to more than 20% of body surface.
● Do not apply to any body surface of patient with decreased renal function without considering risk/benefit ratio.
● Monitor patient for hypersensitivity or contact dermatitis.
Otic therapy
● Reculture persistent drainage.
● Drug best used in combination with other antibiotics.
● Avoid touching ear with dropper.

---

neostigmine bromide
neostigmine methylsulfate
Prostigmin

● Pharmacologic classification: cholinesterase inhibitor
● Therapeutic classification: muscle stimulant
● Pregnancy risk category C

How supplied
Available by prescription only
Tablets: 15 mg
Injection: 0.25 mg/ml, 0.5 mg/ml, 1 mg/ml

Indications, route, and dosage
Antidote for tubocurarine
Adults: 0.5 to 2.5 mg slow I.V. Repeat p.r.n. Give 0.6 to 1.2 mg atropine sulfate I.V. before antidote dose.
Postoperative abdominal distention and bladder atony
Adults: 0.5 to 1 mg I.M. or S.C. q 4 to 6 hours.
Postoperative ileus
Adults: 0.25 to 1 mg I.M. or S.C. q 4 to 6 hours.
Neonates and infants: 0.04 mg/kg I.M. q 6 hours.
Myasthenia gravis
Adults: 15 to 30 mg t.i.d. (range 15 to 375 mg daily); or 0.5 to 2 mg I.M. or I.V. q 1 to 3 hours. Dosage must be individualized, depending on response and tolerance of adverse effects. Therapy may be required day and night.
Children: 7.5 to 15 mg P.O. t.i.d. to q.i.d.

Pharmacodynamics
Muscle stimulant action: Neostigmine blocks acetylcholine's hydrolysis by cholinesterase, resulting in acetylcholine accumulation at cholinergic synapses. That leads to increased cholinergic receptor stimulation at the myoneural junction.

Pharmacokinetics
● *Absorption:* Neostigmine is poorly absorbed (1% to 2%) from GI tract after oral administration. Action usually begins 2 to 4 hours after oral administration and 10 to 30 minutes after injection.
● *Distribution:* About 15% to 25% of dose binds to plasma proteins.
● *Metabolism:* Drug is hydrolyzed by cholinesterases and metabolized by microsomal liver enzymes. Duration of effect varies considerably, depending on patient's physical and emotional status and on disease severity.
● *Excretion:* About 80% of dose is excreted in urine as

---

unchanged drug and metabolites in the first 24 hours after administration.

Contraindications and precautions

Neostigmine is contraindicated in patients with mechanical obstruction of the urinary or intestinal tract, because of its stimulatory effect on smooth muscle; in patients with bradycardia or hypotension, because the drug may exacerbate these conditions; and in patients with known hypersensitivity to cholinergics or bromides.

Administer neostigmine with extreme caution to patients with bronchial asthma, because the drug may precipitate bronchospasm. Administer cautiously to patients with epilepsy, because it may stimulate the CNS; to patients with peritonitis, vagotonia, hyperthyroidism, or cardiac arrhythmias, because it may exacerbate these conditions; to patients with peptic ulcer disease, because it may increase gastric acid secretion; and to patients with recent coronary occlusion, because drug stimulates the cardiovascular system.

Interactions

Concomitant use with procainamide or quinidine may reverse neostigmine's cholinergic effect on muscle. Corticosteroids may also decrease cholinergic effects; when corticosteroids are stopped, however, neostigmine's cholinergic effects may increase, possibly affecting muscle strength.

Concomitant use with succinylcholine may result in prolonged respiratory depression from plasma esterase inhibition, causing delayed succinylcholine hydrolysis; use with other cholinergic drugs may cause additive toxicity. Use with ganglionic blockers, such as mecamylamine, may critically decrease blood pressure; effect is usually preceded by abdominal symptoms.

Magnesium has a direct depressant effect on skeletal muscle and may antagonize neostigmine's beneficial effects.

Effects on diagnostic tests

None reported.

Adverse reactions

● CNS: headache, dizziness, muscle weakness, confusion, nervousness, sweating.
● CV: arrhythmias, bradycardia, hypotension.
● DERM: rash (bromide).
● EENT: miosis, lacrimation, spasm of accommodation, diplopia, conjunctival hyperemia.
● GI: nausea, vomiting, diarrhea, abdominal cramps, excessive salivation.
● Other: *bronchospasm*, bronchoconstriction, *respiratory depression*, muscle cramps.
  Note: Drug should be discontinued if hypersensitivity, skin rash, or difficulty breathing occurs.

Overdose and treatment

Clinical signs of overdose include headache, nausea, vomiting, diarrhea, blurred vision, miosis, excessive tearing, bronchospasm, increased bronchial secretions, hypotension, incoordination, excessive sweating, muscle weakness, cramps, fasciculations, paralysis, bradycardia or tachycardia, excessive salivation, and restlessness or agitation.

Support respiration; bronchial suctioning may be performed. The drug should be discontinued immediately. Atropine may be given to block neostigmine's muscarinic effects but will not counter the drug's paralytic effects on skeletal muscle. Avoid atropine overdose, because it may lead to bronchial plug formation.

▶ Special considerations

Besides those relevant to all *cholinesterase inhibitors*, consider the following recommendations.
● Monitor patient's vital signs, particularly pulse.
● If muscle weakness is severe, determine if this stems from drug toxicity or from exacerbation of myasthenia gravis. A test dose of edrophonium I.V. will aggravate drug-induced weakness but will temporarily relieve weakness resulting from the disease.
● Hospitalized patients may be able to manage a bedside supply of tablets to take themselves.
● Give neostigmine with food or milk to reduce the chance for GI adverse effects.
● When administering drug to patient with myasthenia gravis, schedule largest dose before anticipated periods of fatigue. For example, if patient has dysphagia, schedule this dose 30 minutes before each meal.
● Stop all other cholinergic drugs during neostigmine therapy because of the risk of additive toxicity.
● When administering neostigmine to prevent abdominal distention and GI distress, insertion of a rectal tube may be indicated to help passage of gas.
● Administering atropine concomitantly with neostigmine can relieve or eliminate adverse reactions; these symptoms may indicate neostigmine overdose and will be masked by atropine.
● Patients may develop resistance to this drug.

Information for the patient

Instruct patient to observe and record changes in muscle strength.

Geriatric use

Elderly patients may be more sensitive to neostigmine's effects. Use with caution.

Pediatric use

Recommendations for use in children are the same as those for all *cholinergics*.

Breast-feeding

Neostigmine may be excreted in breast milk, possibly resulting in infant toxicity. The woman's clinical status should determine whether she should discontinue breast-feeding or the use of this drug.

netilmicin sulfate

Netromycin

● Pharmacologic classification: aminoglycoside
● Therapeutic classification: antibiotic
● Pregnancy risk category D

How supplied

Available by prescription only
Injection: 10 mg/ml, 25 mg/ml, 100 mg/ml

Indications, route, and dosage
Serious infections caused by aerobic gram-negative bacilli (P. aeruginosa and some Enterobacteriaceae) resistant to gentamicin or tobramycin

Adults and children over age 12: 3 to 6.5 mg/kg/day by I.M. injection or I.V. infusion. May be given q 12 hours to treat serious urinary tract infections and q 8 to 12 hours to treat serious systemic infections.

Children age 6 weeks to 12 years: 5.5 to 8 mg/kg/day by I.M. injection or I.V. infusion given either as 1.8 to 2.7 mg/kg q 8 hours or as 2.7 to 4 mg/kg q 12 hours.

Neonates under age 6 weeks: 4 to 6.5 mg/kg/day by I.M. injection or I.V. infusion given as 2 to 3.25 mg/kg q 12 hours.

Dosage in renal failure
In all patients, monitor serum blood levels to keep peak serum concentrations between 6 and 12 mcg/ml and trough serum concentrations not to exceed 0.5 mcg/ml. Several methods are available for calculating dosage in renal failure. One source recommends decreasing both dose and interval:

DOSAGE IN ADULTS

Creatinine clearance (ml/min/ 1.73 m²)	Percentage of usual dose	Interval
>50	50 to 90	q 8 to 12 hours
10 to 50	20 to 60	q 12 hours
<10	10 to 20	q 24 to 48 hours

Pharmacodynamics
Antibiotic action: Netilmicin is bactericidal; it binds directly to the 30S ribosomal subunit, thus inhibiting bacterial protein synthesis. Its spectrum of activity includes many aerobic gram-negative organisms (including most strains of *P. aeruginosa*) and some aerobic gram-positive organisms and generally is similar to gentamicin and tobramycin in spectrum. Netilmicin may act against some bacterial strains resistant to other aminoglycosides but generally amikacin is preferred.

Pharmacokinetics
● *Absorption:* Netilmicin is absorbed poorly after oral administration and is given parenterally; peak serum concentrations occur 30 to 60 minutes after I.M. administration.
● *Distribution:* Netilmicin is distributed widely after parenteral administration; intraocular penetration is poor. CSF penetration is low, even in patients with inflamed meninges. Protein binding is minimal. Netilmicin crosses the placenta.
● *Metabolism:* Not metabolized.
● *Excretion:* Netilmicin is excreted primarily in urine by glomerular filtration; small amounts may be excreted in bile and breast milk. Elimination half-life in adults is 2 to 2½ hours. In severe renal damage, half-life may extend beyond 30 hours.

Contraindications and precautions
Netilmicin is contraindicated in patients with known hypersensitivity to netilmicin or any other aminoglycoside, or bisulfites.

Netilmicin should be used cautiously in patients with decreased renal function; in patients with tinnitus, vertigo, and high-frequency hearing loss who are susceptible to ototoxicity; in patients with dehydration, myasthenia gravis, parkinsonism, and hypocalcemia; in neonates and other infants; and in elderly patients.

Interactions
Concomitant use of netilmicin with the following drugs may increase the hazard of nephrotoxicity, ototoxicity, and neurotoxicity: methoxyflurane, polymyxin B, vancomycin, capreomycin, cisplatin, cephalosporins, amphotericin B, and other aminoglycosides; hazard of ototoxicity is also increased during use with ethacrynic acid, furosemide, bumetanide, urea, or mannitol. Dimenhydrinate or other antiemetic and antivertigo drugs may mask netilmicin-induced ototoxicity.

Concomitant use with penicillins results in a synergistic bactericidal effect against *P. aeruginosa, E. coli, Klebsiella, Citrobacter, Enterobacter, Serratia,* and *Proteus mirabilis.* However, the drugs are physically and chemically incompatible and are inactivated when mixed or given together. In vivo inactivation has been reported when aminoglycosides and penicillins are used concomitantly.

Netilmicin may potentiate neuromuscular blockade due to general anesthetics or neuromuscular blocking agents such as succinylcholine and tubocurarine.

Effects on diagnostic tests
Netilmicin-induced nephrotoxicity may elevate levels of blood urea nitrogen (BUN), nonprotein nitrogen, or serum creatinine and increase urinary excretion of casts.

Adverse reactions
● CNS: headache, lethargy, *neuromuscular blockade with respiratory depression.*
● EENT: ototoxicity (tinnitus, vertigo, hearing loss).
● GI: diarrhea, *pseudomembranous colitis.*
● GU: *nephrotoxicity* (cells or casts in the urine; oliguria; proteinuria; decreased creatinine clearance; increased BUN, nonprotein nitrogen, and serum creatinine levels).
● Other: hypersensitivity reactions (eosinophilia, fever, rash, urticaria, pruritus), bacterial or fungal superinfection.

Note: Drug should be discontinued if signs of ototoxicity or nephrotoxicity occur or if severe diarrhea indicates pseudomembranous colitis.

Overdose and treatment
Clinical signs of overdose include ototoxicity, nephrotoxicity, and neuromuscular blockade. Remove drug by hemodialysis or peritoneal dialysis. Treatment with calcium salts or anticholinesterases reverses neuromuscular blockade.

▶ Special considerations
Besides those relevant to all *aminoglycosides,* consider the following recommendations.
● Animal data suggest that netilmicin may be less ototoxic than other aminoglycosides.
● Because netilmicin is dializable, patients undergoing hemodialysis or peritoneal dialysis may need dosage adjustment.

niacin (vitamin B₃, nicotinic acid)
Niac, Nico-400, Nicobid, Nicolar,
Nicotinex, Span-Niacin, Vitamin B-3

- Pharmacologic classification: B-complex vitamin
- Therapeutic classification: vitamin B₃, antilipemic, peripheral vasodilator
- Pregnancy risk category A (C if greater than recommended daily allowance [RDA])

How supplied
Available by prescription only
Injection: 30-ml vials, 100 mg/ml
Capsules: 500 mg
Available without prescription
Tablets: 25 mg, 50 mg, 100 mg, 250 mg, 500 mg
Tablets (timed-release): 250 mg, 500 mg, 750 mg
Capsules (timed-release): 125 mg, 250 mg, 300 mg, 400 mg, 500 mg, 750 mg
Elixir: 50 mg/5 ml

Indications, route, and dosage
Pellagra
Adults: 10 to 20 mg P.O., S.C., I.M., or I.V. infusion daily, depending on severity of niacin deficiency. Maximum recommended daily dosage is 500 mg; should be divided into 10 doses, 50 mg each.
Children: Up to 300 mg P.O. or 100 mg I.V. infusion daily, depending on severity of niacin deficiency.

To prevent recurrence after symptoms subside, advise adequate nutrition and adequate supplements to meet RDA.
Peripheral vascular disease and circulatory disorders
Adults: 250 to 800 mg P.O. daily in divided doses.
Adjunctive treatment of hyperlipidemias, especially those associated with hypercholesterolemia
Adults: 1.5 to 3 g daily in three divided doses with or after meals, increased at intervals to 6 g daily to a maximum of 9 g daily.
Dietary supplement
Adults: 10 to 20 mg P.O. daily.

Pharmacodynamics
- *Vitamin replacement:* As a vitamin, niacin functions as a coenzyme essential to tissue respiration, lipid metabolism, and glycogenolysis. Niacin deficiency causes pellagra, which manifests as dermatitis, diarrhea, and dementia; administration of niacin cures pellagra. Niacin lowers cholesterol and triglyceride levels by an unknown mechanism.
- *Vasodilating action:* Niacin acts directly on peripheral vessels, dilating cutaneous vessels and increasing blood flow, predominantly in the face, neck, and chest.
- *Antilipemic effect:* Mechanism of action is unknown. Nicotinic acid inhibits lipolysis in adipose tissues, decreases hepatic esterification of triglyceride, and increases lipoprotein lipase activity. It reduces serum cholesterol and triglyceride levels.

Pharmacokinetics
- *Absorption:* Niacin is absorbed rapidly from the GI tract. Peak plasma levels occur in 45 minutes. Cholesterol and triglyceride levels decrease after several days.
- *Distribution:* Niacin coenzymes are distributed widely in body tissues; niacin is distributed in breast milk.
- *Metabolism:* Niacin is metabolized by the liver to active metabolites.
- *Excretion:* Niacin is excreted in urine.

Contraindications and precautions
Niacin is contraindicated in patients with known hypersensitivity to the drug and with liver disease because large doses may cause liver damage; in patients with peptic ulcer, which niacin may activate; and in patients with arterial hemorrhage, severe hypotension, or niacin hypersensitivity.

Use niacin cautiously in patients with gout, diabetes mellitus, or gallbladder disease because it may exacerbate the symptoms associated with these disorders.

Interactions
Concomitant use with sympathetic blocking agents may cause added vasodilation and hypotension.

Effects on diagnostic tests
Niacin therapy alters fluorometric test results for urine catecholamines and results for urine glucose tests using cupric sulfate (Benedict's reagent).

Adverse reactions
Most adverse reactions are dose-dependent.
- CNS: dizziness, syncope, transient headache.
- CV: tachycardia, hypotension, excessive peripheral vasodilation.
- DERM: flushing, warmth, burning, tingling, rash, dryness, pruritus.
- GI: nausea, stomach pain, vomiting, diarrhea, bloating, flatulence, activation of peptic ulcer, hepatotoxicity.
- Metabolic: hyperglycemia, hyperuricemia.
- Other: blurred vision.
Note: Drug should be discontinued if abnormal liver function tests signal hepatotoxicity.

Overdose and treatment
Niacin is a water-soluble vitamin; these seldom cause toxicity in patients with normal renal function.

▶ Special considerations
- Recommended daily allowance of niacin in adult males is 19 mg; in adult females, 15 mg; and in children, 5 to 20 mg.
- For I.V. infusion, use concentration of 10 mg/ml or dilute in 500 ml normal saline solution; give slowly, no faster than 2 mg/minute.
- I.V. administration of niacin may cause fibrinolysis, metallic taste in mouth, and anaphylactic shock.
- Megadoses of niacin are not usually recommended.
- Monitor hepatic function and blood glucose levels during initial therapy.
- Aspirin may reduce flushing response.

Information for the patient
- Explain disease process and rationale for therapy; stress fact that use of niacin to treat hyperlipidemia or to dilate peripheral vessels is not "just taking a vitamin," but serious medicine. Emphasize importance of complying with therapy.
- Explain that cutaneous flushing and warmth com-

monly occur in the first 2 hours; they will cease on continued therapy.
● Advise patient not to make sudden postural changes to minimize effects of postural hypotension.
● Instruct patient to avoid hot liquids when initially taking drug to reduce flushing response.
● Recommend taking niacin with meals to minimize GI irritation.

Breast-feeding
No problems have been reported in humans taking normal daily doses as dietary requirement.

---

niacinamide (nicotinamide)

● Pharmacologic classification: B-complex vitamin
● Therapeutic classification: vitamin B$_3$
● Pregnancy risk category C

How supplied
Available by prescription only
Injection: 30-ml vials, 100 mg/ml

Available without prescription
Tablets: 50 mg, 100 mg, 500 mg
Tablets (timed-release): 1,000 mg

Indications, route, and dosage
Pellagra
Adults: 10 to 20 mg P.O., S.C., I.M., or I.V. infusion daily, depending on severity of niacin deficiency. Maximum daily dose recommended, 500 mg; should be divided into 10 doses, 50 mg each.
Children: Up to 300 mg P.O. or 100 mg I.V. infusion daily, depending on severity of niacin deficiency.
　To prevent recurrence after symptoms subside, advise adequate nutrition and supplements to meet RDA.

Pharmacodynamics
Vitamin replacement: Niacinamide is used by the body as a source of niacin; it is essential for tissue respiration, lipid metabolism, and glycogenolysis, but lacks the vasodilating and antilipemic effects of niacin.

Pharmacokinetics
● *Absorption:* Niacinamide is absorbed readily from the GI tract.
● *Distribution:* Niacinamide is distributed widely in body tissues.
● *Metabolism:* Niacinamide is metabolized in the liver.
● *Excretion:* Niacinamide is excreted in the urine.

Contraindications and precautions
Niacinamide is contraindicated in patients with known hypersensitivity to the drug or liver disease because the drug may be hepatotoxic; or in patients with active peptic ulcer because niacinamide may exacerbate peptic ulcer disease.

Interactions
None reported.

Effects on diagnostic tests
Niacinamide alters liver function and serum bilirubin test results.

Adverse reactions
● CNS: mild headache, dizziness.
● GI: activation of peptic ulcer, vomiting, stomach pain, bloating, fatulence, diarrhea, *hepatotoxicity.*
　Note: Drug should be discontinued if liver function tests indicate abnormalities.

Overdose and treatment
Niacinamide is a water-soluble vitamin; these seldom cause toxicity in patients with normal renal function.

▶ Special considerations
● When giving I.V. infusion, use a concentration of 10 mg/ml or, as an infusion, in 500 ml normal saline solution. Inject slowly, no faster than 2 mg/minute.
● Megadoses of niacinamide are not usually recommended.
● Monitor hepatic function and blood glucose levels during initial therapy.
● Niacinamide has no vasodilating or antilipemic effects.

Information for the patient
Recommend taking niacinamide with meals to minimize GI irritation.

Breast-feeding
No problems have been reported in humans taking normal daily requirements.

---

nicardipine hydrochloride
Cardene

● Pharmacologic classification: calcium channel blocking agent
● Therapeutic classification: antianginal, antihypertensive
● Pregnancy risk category C

How supplied
Available by prescription only
Capsules: 20 mg, 30 mg

Indications, route, and dosage
Hypertension; management of chronic stable angina
Adults: Initially, 20 mg P.O. t.i.d. Titrate dosage according to patient response. Usual dosage range is 20 to 40 mg t.i.d.

Pharmacodynamics
Antihypertensive and antianginal action: Nicardipine inhibits the transmembrane flux of calcium ions into cardiac and smooth muscle cells. The drug appears to act specifically on vascular muscle, and may cause a smaller decrease in cardiac output than other calcium channel blockers because of its vasodilatory effect.

Pharmacokinetics
● *Absorption:* Completely absorbed after oral administration. Plasma levels are detectable within 20 minutes, and peak in about 1 hour. Absorption may be decreased if drug is taken with food. Therapeutic serum levels are 28 to 50 ng/ml.
● *Distribution:* Extensively (> 95%) bound to plasma proteins.

● *Metabolism:* A substantial first-pass effect reduces absolute bioavailability to about 35%. The drug is extensively metabolized in the liver, and the process is saturable. Increasing dosage yields non-linear increases in plasma levels.

● *Excretion:* Elimination half-life is about 8.6 hours after steady state levels are reached.

Contraindications and precautions

Nicardipine is contraindicated in patients hypersensitive to the drug. It is also contraindicated in patients with advanced aortic stenosis because the decrease in afterload produced by the drug may worsen myocardial oxygen balance in these patients. Some patients experience worsened severity, frequency, or duration of angina upon initiation of therapy.

Use cautiously in patients with congestive heart failure because the drug has a negative inotropic effect. Careful monitoring of blood pressure during initiation of therapy is recommended.

Interactions

Concomitant administration of cimetidine results in higher plasma levels of nicardipine. Serum levels of digoxin should be carefully monitored because some calcium channel antagonists may increase plasma levels of digitalis preparations.

Concomitant administration of cyclosporine results in increased plasma levels of cyclosporine. Careful monitoring is recommended.

Severe hypotension has been reported in patients taking calcium channel blocking agents who undergo fentanyl anesthesia.

Effects on diagnostic tests

None reported.

Adverse reactions

● CNS: dizziness, headache, asthenia, somnolence, paresthesia, malaise, nervousness, tremor.
● CV: pedal edema, flushing, increased angina, palpitations, tachycardia, edema, *sustained tachycardia,* syncope, dyspnea, abnormal ECG.
● DERM: rash.
● GI: nausea, dyspepsia, dry mouth, constipation.

Overdose and treatment

Overdosage may produce hypotension, bradycardia, drowsiness, confusion, and slurred speech. Treatment is supportive, with vasopressors administered as needed. Intravenous calcium gluconate may be useful to counteract the effects of the drug.

▶ Special considerations

Besides those relevant to all *calcium channel blockers,* consider the following recommendations.
● At least 3 days should be allowed between dosage changes to ensure achievement of steady state plasma levels.
● When treating patients with chronic stable angina, sublingual nitroglycerin, prophylactic nitrate therapy, and beta-adrenergic blocking agents may be continued, as indicated.
● When treating hypertension, blood pressure measurements should be made during times of plasma level trough (approximately 8 hours after a dose, or immediately before subsequent doses). Because of the prominent effects that may occur during plasma level peaks, additional blood pressure measurements should be made 1 to 2 hours after a dose.
● In patients with hepatic dysfunction, therapy should begin at 20 mg b.i.d.; subsequent dosage should be carefully titrated according to patient response.

Pediatric use
Safe use in children under age 18 has not been established.

Breast-feeding
Substantial levels of nicardipine have been found in the milk of animals given nicardipine. Breast-feeding is not recommended.

niclosamide
Niclocide

● Pharmacologic classification: salicylanilide
● Therapeutic classification: anthelmintic
● Pregnancy risk category B

How supplied
Available by prescription only
Tablets (chewable): 500 mg

Indications, route, and dosage
Tapeworms (fish and beef)
Adults: 4 tablets (2 g) chewed thoroughly as a single dose.
Children weighing more than 34 kg: 3 tablets (1.5 g) chewed thoroughly as a single dose.
Children weighing 11 to 34 kg: 2 tablets (1 g) chewed thoroughly as a single dose.
Dwarf tapeworm
Adults: 4 tablets chewed thoroughly as a single daily dose for 7 days.
Children weighing more than 34 kg: 3 tablets chewed thoroughly on the 1st day, then 2 tablets for the next 6 days.
Children weighing 11 to 34 kg: 2 tablets chewed thoroughly on the 1st day, then 1 tablet daily for the next 6 days.

Pharmacodynamics
Anthelmintic action: Niclosamide inhibits mitochondrial oxidative phosphorylation in tapeworms; it also decreases uptake of glucose, decreasing anaerobic generation of adenosine triphosphate needed for cell function. Niclosamide is active against *Diphyllobothrium latum, Dipylidium caninum, Hymenolepis diminuta, H. nana, Taenia saginata, T. solium,* and *Enterobius vermicularis.*

Pharmacokinetics
● *Absorption:* An oral dose of niclosamide is absorbed poorly.
● *Distribution:* Distribution of the small amount of drug absorbed has not been studied.
● *Metabolism:* Niclosamide is not appreciably metabolized by the mammalian host but may be metabolized in the GI tract by the worm.
● *Excretion:* Niclosamide is excreted in feces. It is unknown if it is excreted in breast milk.

Contraindications and precautions
Niclosamide is contraindicated in patients who are hypersensitive to the drug.

Interactions
None reported.

Effects on diagnostic tests
Transient elevation of AST (SGOT) levels was reported in an I.V. narcotics addict taking niclosamide. No other effects have been reported.

Adverse reactions
- CNS: drowsiness, dizziness, headache.
- DERM: rash, pruritus ani, alopecia.
- EENT: oral irritation, bad taste in mouth.
- GI: *nausea, vomiting, anorexia,* diarrhea, constipation, rectal bleeding.
- Other: fever, sweating, palpitations, backache.
  Note: Drug should be discontinued if signs of hypersensitivity or toxicity occur.

Overdose and treatment
Treat overdose by giving a fast-acting laxative and an enema. Do not induce vomiting.

▶ Special considerations
- Tablets should be taken as a single dose after breakfast; they can be crushed and mixed with water or applesauce for small children.
- A mild laxative is indicated in constipated patients to cleanse bowel before starting drug.
- Persistent tapeworm segments or ova excreted on or after the 7th day of therapy indicate failure; repeat course of treatment.
- Protect drug from light.

Information for the patient
- Inform patient about sources of tapeworm and means to avoid them.
- Teach patient and family members proper hygiene measures to prevent reinfection, including daily bathing of perianal area, washing hands after defecation and before eating, and sanitary disposal of feces.
- Explain importance of keeping follow-up appointments for repeat stool examinations 1 and 3 months after drug is discontinued, to ensure that worms and ova are completely eliminated.
- Urge patient with dwarf tapeworms to drink fruit juices; this helps eliminate accumulated intestinal mucus that harbors them.

Pediatric use
Safety and efficacy in children under age 2 have not been established.

Breast-feeding
Safety has not been established.

nicotine polacrilex (nicotine resin complex)
Nicorette

- Pharmacologic classification: nicotinic agonist
- Therapeutic classification: smoking cessation aid
- Pregnancy risk category X

How supplied
Available by prescription only
Chewing gum: 2 mg nicotine resin complex per square

Indications, route, and dosage
Aid in managing nicotine dependence
Temporary aid to the cigarette smoker seeking to give up smoking while participating in a behavior modification program under medical supervision. In general, the smoker with the "physical" type of nicotine dependence is the most likely to benefit from the use of nicotine chewing gum.
Adults: Chew one piece of gum slowly and intermittently for 30 minutes whenever the urge to smoke occurs. Most patients require approximately 10 pieces of gum per day during the first month. Do not exceed 30 pieces of gum per day.

Pharmacodynamics
Nicotine replacement action: Nicotine polacrilex is an agonist at the nicotinic receptors in the peripheral and central nervous systems and produces both behavioral stimulation and depression. It acts on the adrenal medulla to aid in overcoming physical dependence on nicotine during withdrawal from habitual smoking.
  Nicotine's cardiovascular effects are usually dose dependent. Nonsmokers have experienced CNS-mediated symptoms of hiccuping, nausea, and vomiting, even with a small dose. A smoker chewing a 2-mg piece of gum every hour usually does not experience cardiovascular side effects.

Pharmacokinetics
- *Absorption:* The nicotine is bound to ion-exchange resin and is released only during chewing. The blood level depends upon the vigor with which the gum is chewed.
- *Distribution:* Nicotine's distribution into tissues has not been fully characterized. Nicotine crosses the placenta and is distributed into the breast milk.
- *Metabolism:* Nicotine is metabolized mainly by the liver and somewhat by the kidney and lung. The main metabolites are cotinine and nicotine-1′-N-oxide.
- *Excretion:* Both nicotine and its metabolites are excreted in urine, with approximately 10% to 20% excreted unchanged. Excretion of nicotine is increased in acid urine and by high urine output.

Contraindications and precautions
Nicotine polacrilex is contraindicated in nonsmokers; in patients recovering from a myocardial infarction, in those with life-threatening arrhythmias, and in those with severe or worsening angina pectoris (Buerger's disease, Prinzmetal variant angina), because it may exacerbate the symptoms of these disorders; and in

patients with active temporomandibular joint disease, because the drug is released by vigorous chewing.

Nicotine is contraindicated in pregnant women. Nicotine resin complex may cause fetal harm when administered to a pregnant woman. Use Nicorette gum with caution in patients having pharyngeal inflammation and in those with a history of peptic ulcer or esophagitis.

Use cautiously in patients with dental problems that may be exacerbated by vigorous chewing.

To minimize the risk of dependence to Nicorette gum, encourage patient to stop its use after 3 months; additional time is not associated with further success in smoking cessation.

Interactions
Smoking may increase the metabolism of the following drugs: caffeine, theophylline, imipramine, and pentazocine. Smoking cessation either with or without nicotine substitutes may reverse this effect. Smoking cessation may reduce the first-pass metabolism of propoxyphene.

Nicorette gum and smoking can increase the circulating levels of cortisol and catecholamines. Therapy with adrenergic agonists or adrenergic blockers may require adjustments.

Effects on diagnostic tests
None significant.

Adverse reactions
● CNS: dizziness, light-headedness, headache, irritability, euphoria, tinnitus.
● DERM: flushing.
● EENT: throat soreness, jaw muscle ache (from chewing).
● GI: nausea, vomiting, indigestion, heartburn.
● Other: hiccups, palpitations.

Overdose and treatment
The risk of overdose is minimized by early nausea and vomiting that result from excessive nicotine intake. Poisoning manifests as nausea, vomiting, salivation, abdominal pain, diarrhea, cold sweats, headache, dizziness, disturbed hearing and vision, mental confusion, and weakness.

Treatment includes emesis – give ipecac syrup if it has not occurred. A saline cathartic will speed the gum's passage through the GI tract. Give gastric lavage followed by activated charcoal in unconscious patients. Provide supportive treatment of respiratory paralysis and cardiovascular collapse as needed.

▶ Special considerations
● Nicorette resin complex is the only smoking cessation aid that has been proven safe and effective.
● Smokers most likely to benefit from Nicorette gum are those with a high physical dependence. Typically, such smokers smoke more than 15 cigarettes daily; prefer brands of cigarettes with high nicotine levels; usually inhale the smoke; smoke the first cigarette within 30 minutes of arising; and find the first morning cigarette the hardest to give up.
● Instruct patient to chew the gum slowly and intermittently for about 30 minutes to promote slow and even buccal absorption of nicotine. Fast chewing allows faster absorption and produces more adverse reactions.
● At the initial visit, instruct patient to chew one piece of gum whenever the urge to smoke occurs instead of having a cigarette. Most patients will require approximately 10 pieces of gum per day during the first month of treatment.
● Successful abstainers will begin gradually withdrawing gum usage after 3 months. Use of the gum for longer than 6 months is not recommended.
● The gum is sugar-free and usually does not stick to dentures.

Information for the patient
● Instruct patient to not exceed 30 pieces of gum per day.
● Advise patient not to drink liquids while chewing the gum because the drug's absorption will be altered.
● Patients should also participate in a formal stop smoking program.
● A patient instruction sheet is included in the package dispensed to the patient. Allow the patient adequate time to read it and ask questions.

Geriatric use
Reduced doses of Nicorette gum may be necessary in older patients.

Breast-feeding
Because nicotine freely passes to breast milk and has the potential for serious adverse effects, this drug should not be used by breast-feeding women.

---

nicotine transdermal system
Habitrol, Nicoderm, Nicotrol, Prostep

● Pharmacologic classification: nicotinic cholinergic agonist
● Therapeutic classification: smoking cessation aid
● Pregnancy risk category D

How supplied
Available by prescription only
Transdermal system: designed to release nicotine at a fixed rate
　Habitrol: 21 mg/day, 14 mg/day, 11 mg/day
　Nicoderm: 21 mg/day, 14 mg/day, 11 mg/day
　Nicotrol: 15 mg/day, 10 mg/day, 5 mg/day
　Prostep: 22 mg/day, 11 mg/day

Indications, route, and dosage
Relief of nicotine withdrawal symptoms in patients attempting smoking cessation
Adults: 1 transdermal system applied to a nonhairy part of the upper trunk or upper outer arm. Dosage varies slightly with product selected.
Nicoderm, Habitrol: Initially, apply 1 21-mg/day system daily for 6 weeks. After 24 hours, the system should be removed and a new system applied to a different site. Then, taper dosage to 14 mg/day for 2 to 4 weeks. Finally, taper dosage to 7 mg/day if necessary. Nicotine substitution and gradual withdrawal should take 8 to 12 weeks.

Patients who weigh under 100 lb, patients who have cardiovascular disease, and those who smoke less than half a pack of cigarettes per day should start therapy with the 14-mg/day system.
Nicotrol: Initially, apply 1 15-mg/day system daily for 12 weeks. The system should be applied upon waking and removed at bedtime. Then, taper dosage to 10 mg/

---

day for 2 weeks. Finally, taper dosage to 5 mg/day for 2 weeks if necessary. As an alternative to this schedule, patients who have successfully abstained from smoking should have their dosage reduced q 2 to 4 weeks until the 5-mg/day dosage has been used for 2 weeks. Nicotine substitution and gradual withdrawal should take 14 to 20 weeks.

Prostep: Initially, apply 1 22-mg/day system daily for 4 to 8 weeks. After 24 hours, the system should be removed and a new system applied to a different site. Patients who weigh under 100 lb should start therapy with the 11-mg/day system. Those who have successfully stopped smoking during this period may discontinue drug. If therapy was initiated with the 22-mg/day system, patient may be treated for an additional 2 to 4 weeks at the lower dosage (11 mg/day). Nicotine substitution and gradual withdrawal should take 6 to 12 weeks.

Pharmacodynamics
Nicotinic cholinergic action: The nicotine transdermal system provides nicotine, the chief stimulant alkaloid found in tobacco products, which stimulates nicotinic acetylcholine receptors in the CNS, neuromuscular junction, autonomic ganglia, and adrenal medulla.

Pharmacokinetics
● *Absorption:* Drug is rapidly absorbed after application of the transdermal system.
● *Distribution:* Plasma protein-binding of drug is below 5%.
● *Metabolism:* Drug is metabolized by the liver, kidney, and lung. Over 20 metabolites have been identified. Primary metabolites are cotinine (15%) and trans-3-hydroxycotinine (45%).
● *Excretion:* Drug is excreted primarily in the urine as metabolites; about 10% is excreted unchanged. With high urine flow rates or acidified urine, up to 30% can be excreted unchanged.

Contraindications and precautions
Drug is contraindicated in patients with hypersensitivity to nicotine or any component of the transdermal system. Use with extreme caution and only after educational and behavioral interventions have failed in patients with recent MI, serious arrhythmias, or worsening angina pectoris or during pregnancy. Use cautiously in elderly patients and in those with renal or hepatic insufficiency, endocrine disease, peptic ulcer disease, or hypertension.

Because nicotine can be addictive and toxic, use cautiously in all patients. The risks of nicotine administration must be weighed against the potential hazards if patient continues to smoke while using the transdermal system. Patients should be warned that if they continue to smoke while using the system, they may experience adverse effects because peak serum nicotine levels will be substantially higher than those achieved by smoking alone.

Interactions
Cessation of smoking may decrease induction of hepatic enzymes responsible for metabolizing certain drugs, such as acetaminophen, caffeine, imipramine, oxazepam, pentazocine, propranolol, and theophylline; dosage reduction of such drugs may be necessary. Cessation of smoking may increase the amount of subcutaneous insulin absorbed and may require reduction of insulin dosage.

Cessation of smoking may decrease levels of circulating catecholamines and may require lower doses of adrenergic antagonists (such as prazosin or labetalol) or higher doses of adrenergic agonists (such as isoproterenol or phenylephrine).

Effects on diagnostic tests
None reported.

Adverse reactions
● CNS: somnolence, dizziness, headache, insomnia.
● DERM: erythema, pruritus, burning at application site, local erythema, cutaneous hypersensitivity, rash, sweating.
● EENT: pharyngitis, sinusitis.
● GI: abdominal pain, constipation, dyspepsia, nausea.
● GU: dysmenorrhea.
● Other: back pain, myalgia.

Overdose and treatment
Overdosage could produce symptoms associated with acute nicotine poisoning, including nausea, vomiting, diarrhea, weakness, respiratory failure, hypotension, and seizures. Treat symptomatically. Barbiturates or benzodiazepines may be used to treat seizures, and atropine may attenuate excessive salivation or diarrhea. Administer fluids to treat hypotension; increase urine flow to enhance elimination of the drug.

▶ Special considerations
● Use of the transdermal system for more than 3 months should be discouraged. Chronic nicotine consumption by any route can be dangerous and habit-forming.
● Patients who cannot stop cigarette smoking during the initial 4 weeks of therapy will probably not benefit from continued use of drug. Patients who were unsuccessful may benefit from counseling to identify factors that led to the unsuccessful attempt. Encourage patient to minimize or eliminate the factors that contributed to treatment failure and to try again, possibly after some interval, before the next attempt.
● Health care workers' exposure to the nicotine within the transdermal systems should be minimal; however, avoid unnecessary contact with the system. After contact, wash hands with water alone because soap can enhance absorption.

Information for the patient
● Tell patient to discontinue use of the patch and to call immediately if he experiences a generalized rash or persistent or severe local skin reactions (pruritus, edema, or erythema).
● Make sure patient understands that nicotine can evaporate from the transdermal system once it is removed from its protective packaging. The patch should not be altered in any way (folded or cut) before it is applied. It should be applied promptly after removal of the system's protective packaging. Do not store at temperatures above 86° F (30° C).
● Teach patient how to dispose of the transdermal system. After removal, fold the patch in half, bringing the adhesive sides together. If the system comes in a protective pouch, dispose of the used patch in the pouch that contained the new system. Careful disposal is necessary to prevent accidental poisoning of children or pets.
● Patient information is dispensed with drug at the time the prescription is filled. Be sure that patient reads and understands this material.

---

*Canada only   †Unlabeled clinical use   Italicized adverse reactions are life-threatening.

Pediatric use
Safety and efficacy in children have not been established. Note that the amount of nicotine contained in a patch could prove fatal to a child if ingested; even used patches contain a substantial amount of residual nicotine. Patients should take care to ensure that both used and unused transdermal systems are out of the reach of children.

Breast-feeding
Nicotine passes freely into breast milk and is readily absorbed after oral administration. Weigh the infant's risk of exposure to nicotine from a transdermal patch against his risk of exposure from continued smoking by the mother.

nicotinyl alcohol
Roniacol*, Roniacol Timespan*

- Pharmacologic classification: vitamin B₃ (nicotinic acid) precursor
- Therapeutic classification: peripheral vasodilator, vasospastic therapy adjunct
- Pregnancy risk category C

How supplied
Available by prescription only
Tablets: 50 mg
Tablets (timed-release): 150 mg

Indications, route, and dosage
Conditions of deficient circulation, such as peripheral vascular disease, vascular spasm, varicose ulcers, decubital ulcers, Meniere's syndrome, vertigo
Adults: 50- to 100-mg regular tablets P.O. b.i.d. or t.i.d. (may increase to 150 to 200 mg P.O. t.i.d. or q.i.d.); 150- to 300-mg timed-release tablets P.O. b.i.d.; 5 to 10 ml of elixir P.O. t.i.d.

Pharmacodynamics
Peripheral vasodilating action: Nicotinyl alcohol is converted to nicotinic acid (niacin), which produces peripheral vasodilation by a direct effect on vascular smooth muscle.

Pharmacokinetics
- *Absorption:* Vasodilation occurs 5 to 30 minutes after oral administration of standard tablets; timed-release tablets act in 30 minutes. Clinical improvement may occur gradually over several weeks.
- *Distribution:* After conversion to niacin, drug is distributed widely in body tissues.
- *Metabolism:* After conversion to niacin, drug is metabolized by the liver.
- *Excretion:* Niacin is excreted in urine.

Contraindications and precautions
Nicotinyl alcohol is contraindicated in patients with active peptic ulcer, severe cerebrovascular disease, or recent myocardial infarction.

Use cautiously in patients with severe obliterative coronary artery disease; a "steal effect" may further decrease blood flow to ischemic areas, since nicotinyl alcohol has a greater effect on peripheral vessels than on cerebral and coronary vessels.

Interactions
None reported.

Effects on diagnostic tests
Nicotinyl alcohol therapy alters serum concentrations of ALT (SGPT), alkaline phosphatase, AST (SGOT), and bilirubin. Drug may elevate blood and urinary glucose levels in diabetic patients with hypercholesterolemia.

Long-term use at high doses may elevate serum lactate dehydrogenase levels, indicating hepatotoxicity.

Adverse reactions
- CV: transient flushing, hypotension.
- GI: diarrhea, nausea, vomiting.
- Other: allergic reactions, jaundice, dependent edema, increased hair loss.

Note: Drug should be discontinued if patient shows signs of hepatic hypersensitivity (jaundice, eosinophilia, and altered liver function tests).

Overdose and treatment
No specific recommendations are available. After recent ingestion (4 hours or less), empty stomach by induced emesis or gastric lavage. Follow with activated charcoal to decrease absorption. Subsequent treatment is supportive.

▶ Special considerations
- Monitor vital signs during therapy.
- Antihyperlipidemic effects may occur gradually, over a period of several weeks.

Information for the patient
- Warn patient of possible adverse reactions; advise patient to report pronounced adverse reactions.
- Encourage patient to stop smoking. Nicotine reverses the effects of nicotinyl alcohol on blood vessels.

Geriatric use
The risk of hypothermia is increased in elderly patients.

Pediatric use
Safe use in children has not been established.

Breast-feeding
Safety in breast-feeding women has not been established. Encourage use of alternative feeding method.

nifedipine
Adalat, Procardia, Procardia XL

- Pharmacologic classification: calcium channel blocker
- Therapeutic classification: antianginal
- Pregnancy risk category C

How supplied
Available by prescription only
Capsules: 10 mg, 20 mg
Tablets (extended-release): 30 mg, 60 mg, 90 mg

Indications, route, and dosage
Management of Prinzmetal's or variant angina or chronic stable angina pectoris
Adults: Starting dose is 10 mg P.O. t.i.d. Usual effective dosage range is 10 to 20 mg t.i.d. Some patients may require up to 30 mg q.i.d. Maximum daily dose is 180 mg.
Hypertension
Adults: Initially, 30 to 60 mg P.O. once daily (extended-release tablets). Adjust dosage at 7- to 14-day intervals according to patient tolerance and response. Maximum dosage is 120 mg daily.

Pharmacodynamics
Antianginal action: Nifedipine dilates systemic arteries, resulting in decreased total peripheral resistance, and modestly decreased systemic blood pressure with a slightly increased heart rate, decreased afterload, and increased cardiac index. Reduced afterload and the subsequent decrease in myocardial oxygen consumption probably account for nifedipine's value in treating chronic stable angina. In Prinzmetal's angina, nifedipine inhibits coronary artery spasm, increasing myocardial oxygen delivery.

Pharmacokinetics
● *Absorption:* Approximately 90% of a dose of nifedipine is absorbed rapidly from the gastrointestinal tract after oral administration; however, only about 65% to 70% of drug reaches the systemic circulation because of a significant first-pass effect in the liver. Peak serum levels occur in about 30 minutes to 2 hours. Hypotensive effects may occur 5 minutes after sublingual administration. Therapeutic serum levels are 25 to 100 ng/ml.
● *Distribution:* About 92% to 98% of circulating nifedipine is bound to plasma proteins.
● *Metabolism:* Nifedipine is metabolized in the liver.
● *Excretion:* Nifedipine is excreted in the urine and feces as inactive metabolites. Elimination half-life is 2 to 5 hours. Duration of effect ranges from 4 to 12 hours.

Contraindications and precautions
Nifedipine is contraindicated in patients with known hypersensitivity to the drug. It should be used with caution when administered to patients with congestive heart failure or aortic stenosis (especially if they are receiving concomitant beta blockers), because the drug may precipitate or worsen heart failure and cause excessive hypotension (from its peripheral vasodilatory effects), possibly exacerbating angina symptoms when therapy begins or dosage is increased.

Interactions
Concomitant use of nifedipine with beta blockers may exacerbate angina, congestive heart failure, hypotension, and arrhythmias. Concomitant use with fentanyl may cause excessive hypotension. Concomitant use with digoxin may cause increased serum digoxin levels. Use with hypotensive agents may precipitate excessive hypotension.

Effects on diagnostic tests
Mild to moderate increase in serum concentrations of alkaline phosphate, LDH, AST (SGOT), and ALT (SGPT) have been noted.

Adverse reactions
● CNS: dizziness, light-headedness, flushing, headache, weakness, syncope.
● CV: peripheral edema, hypotension, palpitations, worsening of angina, *myocardial infarction, congestive heart failure.*
● EENT: nasal congestion.
● GI: nausea, heartburn, diarrhea.
● Other: muscle cramps, dyspnea.

Overdose and treatment
Clinical effects of overdose are extensions of the drug's pharmacologic effects, primarily peripheral vasodilation and hypotension.
    Treatment includes such basic support measures as hemodynamic and respiratory support. If patient requires blood pressure support by a vasoconstrictor, norepinephrine may be administered. Extremities should be elevated and any fluid deficit corrected.

▶ Special considerations
● Initial doses or dosage increase may exacerbate angina briefly. Reassure patient that this symptom is temporary.
● Nifedipine is not available in sublingual form. However, liquid in oral capsule may be withdrawn by puncturing capsule with needle, and the drug may be instilled into the buccal pouch. Or, a punctured capsule may be chewed.
● Monitor blood pressure regularly, especially if patient is also taking beta blockers or antihypertensives.
● Although rebound effect has not been observed when drug is stopped, dosage should be reduced slowly under medical supervision.
● Use with caution in patients with unstable angina who are not currently taking a beta blocker. Some clinicians report a higher incidence of myocardial infarction in such patients.

Information for the patient
● Instruct patient to swallow capsules whole without breaking, crushing, or chewing them.
● Patients may experience annoying hypotensive effects during titration of dose. Urge compliance.

Geriatric use
Drug should be used with caution in elderly patients because they may be more sensitive to drug's effects and duration of effect may be prolonged.

nimodipine
Nimotop

● Pharmacologic classification: calcium channel blocking agent
● Therapeutic classification: cerebral vasodilator
● Pregnancy risk category C

How supplied
Available by prescription only
Capsules: 30 mg

Indications, route, and dosage
Improvement of neurological deficits after subarachnoid hemorrhage from ruptured congenital aneurysms
Adults: 60 mg P.O. q 4 hours for 21 days. Therapy should begin within 96 hours of the subarachnoid hemorrhage.

Dosage in patients with hepatic impairment
Adults: 30 mg P.O. q 4 hours.

Pharmacodynamics
Neuronal sparing action: Nimodipine inhibits calcium ion influx across cardiac and smooth muscle cells, thus decreasing myocardial contractility and oxygen demand, and dilates coronary arteries and arterioles. Initially thought to relieve vasospasm in patients after subarachnoid hemorrhage, its mechanism of action is not fully known.

Pharmacokinetics
- *Absorption:* Well absorbed after oral administration. However, because of extensive first-pass metabolism, bioavailability is only about 3% to 30%.
- *Distribution:* Greater than 95% protein-bound.
- *Metabolism:* Extensively metabolized in the liver. The drug and metabolites undergo enterohepatic recycling.
- *Excretion:* Less than 1% as the parent drug. Elimination half-life is 1 to 9 hours.

Contraindications and precautions
There are no known contraindications to nimodipine therapy, and the drug was relatively well tolerated in clinical trials. Nimodipine should be reserved for patients who are in good neurological condition post-ictus (for example, Hunt and Hess grades I to III).

Interactions
Concomitant use with antihypertensives may enhance the hypotensive effect; use with calcium channel blocking agents may enhance these drugs' cardiovascular effects.

Effects on diagnostic tests
None reported.

Adverse reactions
- CNS: headaches.
- CV: decreased blood pressure, flushing, edema.
- DERM: rash.
- GI: abdominal discomfort, constipation.
- HEMA: thrombocytopenia and anemia (< 1%).
- Hepatic: increased serum transaminase levels.

Overdose and treatment
Nausea, weakness, drowsiness, confusion, bradycardia, and decreased cardiac output can be expected. Treatment should be supportive. Administer pressor amines to counter hypotension; cardiac pacing, atropine or sympathomimetics to treat bradycardia. Calcium gluconate I.V. has been used to treat calcium channel blocker overdose.

▶ Special considerations
Besides those relevant to all *calcium channel blockers,* consider the following recommendations.
- Unlike other calcium channel blockers, nimodipine is not used for angina pectoris or hypertension.
- Patients with hepatic failure should receive lower doses. Initiate therapy at 30 mg P.O. every 4 hours, with close monitoring of blood pressure and heart rate.
- Monitor blood pressure and heart rate in all patients, especially at the initiation of therapy.
- If the patient cannot swallow capsules, the ends of the liquid-filled capsule should be punctured with an 18G needle and the contents drawn up into a syringe.

The dose can then be instilled into the patient's nasogastric tube and the tube rinsed with 30 ml of normal saline.

Information for the patient
Advise the patient to rise from the supine position slowly to avoid dizziness and hypotension, especially at the beginning of therapy.

Pediatric use
Safety and efficacy have not been established.

Breast-feeding
Substantial amounts of the drug are found in the milk of lactating animals. Breast-feeding is not recommended during therapy.

PHARMACOLOGIC CLASS

nitrates

amyl nitrate
erythrityl tetranitrate
isosorbide dinitrate
nitroglycerin
pentaerythritol tetranitrate

Nitrates have been recognized as effective vasodilators for over 100 years. The best known drug of this group, nitroglycerin, remains the therapeutic mainstay for classic and variant angina. With the availability of a commercial I.V. nitroglycerin form, the drug's use in reducing afterload and preload in various cardiac disorders has generated renewed enthusiasm. Various other dosage forms of nitroglycerin and of the other nitrates also are available, thereby improving and extending their clinical usefulness.

Pharmacology
Nitrates' major pharmacologic property is vascular smooth muscle relaxation, resulting in generalized vasodilation. Venous effects predominate; however, nitroglycerin produces dose-dependent dilatation of both arterial and venous beds. Decreased peripheral venous resistance results in venous pooling of blood and decreased venous return to the heart (preload); decreased arteriolar resistance reduces systemic vascular resistance and arterial pressure (afterload). These vascular effects lead to reduction of myocardial oxygen consumption, promoting a more favorable oxygen supply-demand ratio. (Although nitrates reflexively increase heart rate and myocardial contractility, reduced ventricular wall tension results in a net decrease in myocardial oxygen consumption). In the coronary circulation, nitrates redistribute circulating blood flow along collateral channels and preferentially increase subendocardial blood flow, improving perfusion to the ischemic myocardium.

Nitrates relax all smooth muscle — not just vascular smooth muscle — regardless of autonomic innervation, including bronchial, biliary, gastrointestinal, ureteral, and uterine smooth muscle.

Clinical indications and actions
Angina pectoris
By relaxing vascular smooth muscle in both the venous and arterial beds, nitrates cause a net decrease in myocardial oxygen consumption; by dilating coronary

---

Canada only   †Unlabeled clinical use   Italicized adverse reactions are life-threatening.

vessels, they lead to redistribution of blood flow to ischemic tissue. Although systemic and coronary vascular effects may vary slightly, depending on which nitrate is used, both smooth muscle relaxation and vasodilation probably account for nitrates' value in treating angina. Because individual nitrates have similar pharmacologic and therapeutic properties, the best nitrate to use in a specific situation depends mainly on the onset of action and duration of effect required.

Sublingual nitroglycerin is considered the drug of choice to treat acute angina pectoris because of its rapid onset of action, relatively low cost, and well-established effectiveness. Lingual or buccal nitroglycerin and other rapidly acting nitrates (amyl nitrate and sublingual or chewable isosorbide dinitrate) also may prove useful for this indication. Amyl nitrate is rarely used because it is expensive, inconvenient, and carries a high risk of adverse effects. Sublingual, lingual, or buccal nitroglycerin or sublingual or chewable isosorbide dinitrate or erythritol tetranitrate typically prove effective in circumstances likely to provoke an angina attack.

Long-acting nitrates and/or beta-adrenergic blockers usually are considered the drugs of choice in the prophylactic management of angina pectoris. Nitrates with a relatively long duration of effect include oral preparations of erythrityl tetranitrate, isosorbide dinitrate, pentaerythritol tetranitrate, and oral or topical nitroglycerin.

The effectiveness of oral nitrates is debatable, although isosorbide dinitrate and nitroglycerin generally are now considered effective. However, the effectiveness of erythrityl tetranitrate, pentaerythritol tetranitrate, and topical nitroglycerin preparations has not been fully determined. Some experts believe oral nitrates are ineffective or less effective than rapidly acting I.V. nitrates in reducing frequency of angina and increasing exercise tolerance. Also, prolonged use of oral nitrates may cause cross-tolerance to sublingual nitrates.

I.V. nitroglycerin may be used to treat unstable angina pectoris, Prinzmetal's angina, and angina pectoris in patients who have not responded to recommended doses of nitrates and/or a beta-adrenergic blocker.

Sedatives may be useful in the adjunctive management of angina pectoris associated with psychogenic factors. However, if combination therapy is required, each drug should be adjusted individually; fixed combinations of oral nitrates and sedatives should be avoided.

Acute myocardial infarction
The hemodynamic effects of I.V., sublingual, or topical nitroglycerin may prove beneficial in treating left ventricular failure and pulmonary congestion associated with acute myocardial infarction. However, the drugs' effects on morbidity and mortality in patients with these conditions is controversial.

I.V., sublingual, and topical nitroglycerin and isosorbide dinitrate are effective adjunctive agents in managing acute and chronic heart failure. Sublingual administration can quickly reverse the signs and symptoms of pulmonary congestion in acute pulmonary edema; however, the I.V. form may control hemodynamic status more accurately.

Overview of adverse reactions
Headache, the most common adverse effect, is most common early in therapy. Possibly severe, it usually diminishes rapidly. Postural hypotension may occur and may result in dizziness and/or weakness. Patients who are especially sensitive to hypotensive effects may ex-

perience nausea, vomiting, weakness, restlessness, pallor, cold sweats, tachycardia, syncope, or cardiovascular collapse. Alcohol may intensify these effects. Transient flushing may occur; GI upset may be controlled by a temporary dosage reduction. If blurred vision, dry mouth, or rash develops, therapy should be discontinued (rash occurs more commonly with pentaerythritol). Both tolerance and dependence to these agents can occur with repeated, prolonged use.

Tolerance to both the vascular and antianginal effects of the drugs can develop, and cross-tolerance between the nitrates and nitrites has been demonstrated. Tolerance is associated with a high or sustained plasma drug concentration and occurs most frequently with oral, I.V., and topical therapy. It rarely occurs with intermittent sublingual use. However, patients taking oral isosorbide dinitrate or topical nitroglycerin have not exhibited cross-tolerance to sublingual nitroglycerin.

Development of tolerance can be prevented by using the lowest effective dose and maintaining an intermittent dosing schedule. A nitrate-free interval of 10 to 12 hours daily (for example, by removing the transdermal nitroglycerin patch in the early evening and not reapplying until the next morning) may also help prevent tolerance.

▶ Special considerations
Oral dosage forms
● Best absorption will occur if taken on an empty stomach (1 hour before or 2 hours after meals) and with a full glass of water.
● Dosage should be titrated to patient response. Patients should avoid switching brands after they are stabilized on a particular formulation.

Buccal dosage form
● The tablet should be placed between the upper lip or cheek and gum.
● Dissolution rate varies, but will usually range from 3 to 5 hours. Hot liquids will increase dissolution rate and should be avoided.
● Patient should not use buccal form at bedtime because of risk of aspiration.

Sublingual dosage form
● Only the sublingual and translingual forms should be used to relieve acute angina attack. Although a burning sensation was formerly an indication of drug's potency, many current preparations do not produce this sensation.

Topical dosage form
● To apply ointment, spread in uniform thin layer to any hairless part of the skin except distal parts of arms and legs, because absorption will not be maximal at these sites. Do not rub in. Cover with plastic film to aid absorption and to protect clothing. If using Tape-Surrounded Appli-Ruler (TSAR) system, keep TSAR on skin to protect patient's clothing and ensure that ointment remains in place. If serious adverse reactions develop in patients using ointment or transdermal system, remove product at once or wipe ointment from skin. Be sure to avoid contact with ointment.
● Be sure to remove transdermal patch before defibrillation. Because of the patch's aluminum backing, electric current may cause patch to explode.

Information for the patient
● Instruct patient to avoid alcohol while taking nitrates, because severe hypotension and cardiovascular collapse may occur.
● Instruct patient to sit when taking nitrates, to prevent injury from transient episodes of dizziness, syncope, or other signs of cerebral ischemia that the drug may cause.
● Advise patient to treat headache with aspirin or acetaminophen.
● Tell patient to report blurred vision, dry mouth, or persistent headache.
● Warn patient not to stop taking drug abruptly, because this may cause withdrawal symptoms.

Pediatric use
The safety and effectiveness of nitrates in children have not been established.

Breast-feeding
Excretion into breast milk is unknown. Use with caution.

Representative combinations
None.

---

nitrofurantoin macrocrystals
Macrodantin

nitrofurantoin microcrystals
Furadantin, Furalan, Furan, Furanite, Nitrofan

● Pharmacologic classification: nitrofuran
● Therapeutic classification: urinary tract antiseptic
● Pregnancy risk category B

How supplied
Available by prescription only
Macrocrystals
Capsules: 25 mg, 50 mg, 100 mg
Microcrystals
Tablets: 50 mg, 100 mg
Capsules: 50 mg, 100 mg
Suspension: 25 mg/5 ml

Indications, route, and dosage
Initial or recurrent urinary tract infections caused by susceptible organisms
Adults and children over age 12: 50 to 100 mg P.O. q.i.d., with meals and h.s.
Children age 1 month to 12 years: 5 to 7 mg/kg P.O. daily, divided q.i.d.
Long-term suppression therapy
Adults: 50 to 100 mg P.O. daily h.s. as a single dose.
Children: As low as 1 mg/kg/day in a single dose or two divided doses.

Pharmacodynamics
Antibacterial action: Nitrofurantoin has bacteriostatic action in low concentrations and possible bactericidal action in high concentrations. Although its exact mechanism of action is unknown, it may inhibit bacterial enzyme systems. Drug is most active at an acidic pH.
Drug's spectrum of activity includes many common gram-positive and gram-negative urinary pathogens,

including *Escherichia coli*, *Staphylococcus aureus*, enterococci, and certain strains of *Klebsiella*, and *Enterobacter*. Organisms that usually resist nitrofurantoin include *Pseudomonas*, *Acinetobacter*, *Serratia*, *Providencia*, and *Proteus*.

Pharmacokinetics
● *Absorption:* When administered orally, nitrofurantoin is well absorbed (mainly by the small intestine) from the GI tract. Presence of food aids drug's dissolution and speeds absorption. The macrocrystal form exhibits slower dissolution and absorption; it causes less GI distress.
● *Distribution:* Nitrofurantoin crosses into bile and placenta. From 20% to 60% binds to plasma proteins. Plasma half-life is approximately 20 minutes. Peak urine concentrations occur in about 30 minutes when drug is given as microcrystals, somewhat later when given as macrocrystals.
● *Metabolism:* Nitrofurantoin is metabolized partially in the liver.
● *Excretion:* About 30% to 50% of dose is eliminated by glomerular filtration and tubular secretion into urine as unchanged drug within 24 hours. Some drug may be excreted in breast milk.

Contraindications and precautions
Nitrofurantoin is contraindicated in patients with severe renal dysfunction (creatinine clearance below 40 ml/minute) because urine concentrations of the drug will be ineffective and toxicity may occur; in infants under age 1 month, in pregnant patients, and in patients with glucose-6-phosphate dehydrogenase (G6PD) deficiency because of the potential for hemolytic anemias; and in patients with known hypersensitivity to the drug.
Nitrofurantoin should be administered cautiously to patients with diabetes mellitus, anemia, vitamin B deficiency, or electrolyte imbalance, because it increases the risk of peripheral neuropathy.

Interactions
When used concomitantly, probenecid and sulfinpyrazone reduce renal excretion of nitrofurantoin, leading to increased serum and decreased urine nitrofurantoin concentrations. Increased serum concentration may lead to increased toxicity; decreased urine concentration may reduce drug's antibacterial effectiveness.
Concomitant use with magnesium-containing antacids may decrease nitrofurantoin absorption. Concomitant use with nalidixic acid antagonizes nalidixic acid's antibacterial activity.
Anticholinergic drugs and foods enhance nitrofurantoin's bioavailability by slowing GI motility, thereby increasing the drug's dissolution and absorption.
Concomitant use with quinolone derivatives (cinoxacin, norfloxacin, ciprofloxacin, nalidixic acid) may antagonize the anti-infective effects.

Effects on diagnostic tests
Nitrofurantoin may cause false-positive results in urine glucose tests using cupric sulfate reagents (such as Benedict's test, Fehling's test, or Clinitest) because it reacts with these reagents.
Anemia and abnormal results of liver function tests may occur during nitrofurantoin therapy.

Adverse reactions
● CNS: peripheral neuropathy, headache, dizziness, drowsiness, ascending polyneuropathy.

• DERM: maculopapular, erythematous, or eczematous eruption; pruritus; urticaria; *exfoliative dermatitis;* *Stevens-Johnson syndrome.*
• GI: anorexia, nausea, vomiting, abdominal pain, diarrhea, hepatitis.
• HEMA: hemolysis in patients with G6PD deficiency, *agranulocytosis,* thrombocytopenia.
• Other: asthma attacks in patients with history of asthma, *anaphylaxis,* hypersensitivity, transient alopecia, drug fever, overgrowth of nonsusceptible organisms in urinary tract, pulmonary sensitivity reactions (cough, chest pains, fever, chills, dyspnea).
Note: Drug should be discontinued if patient develops hypersensitivity, hemolysis, peripheral neuropathy, or pulmonary reaction.

Overdose and treatment
Acute overdosage may result in nausea and vomiting. Treat symptomatically. No specific antidote is known. Increase fluid intake to promote urinary excretion of drug.

▶ Special considerations
• Obtain culture and sensitivity tests before starting therapy, and repeat as needed.
• Give oral preparations 1 hour apart from magnesium-containing antacids. Oral suspension may be mixed with water, milk, fruit juice, and formulas.
• Monitor complete blood count regularly.
• Monitor fluid intake and output and pulmonary status.
• Drug may turn urine brown or rust-yellow.
• Avoid administering drug with nalidixic acid.
• Continue treatment for at least 3 days after sterile urine specimens have been obtained.
• Long-term therapy may cause overgrowth of nonsusceptible organisms, especially *Pseudomonas.*

Information for the patient
• Instruct patient to take drug with food or milk to minimize GI distress.
• Caution patient that drug may cause false-positive results in urine glucose tests using cupric sulfate reduction method (Clinitest) but not in glucose oxidase test (Tes-Tape, Diastix, Clinistix).
• Emphasize that bedtime dose is important because drug will remain in bladder longer.
• Warn patient that drug may turn urine brown or rust-yellow.

Pediatric use
Drug is contraindicated in infants under age 1 month because their immature enzyme systems increase the risk of hemolytic anemia.

Breast-feeding
Safety has not been established. Although drug is excreted in low concentrations in breast milk, no adverse reactions have been reported, except in infants with G6PD deficiency, who may develop hemolytic anemia.

nitrofurazone
Furacin

• Pharmacologic classification: synthetic antibacterial nitrofuran derivative
• Therapeutic classification: topical antibacterial
• Pregnancy risk category C

How supplied
Available by prescription only
Topical solution: 0.2%
Ointment: 0.2% soluble dressing
Cream: 0.2%

Indications, route, and dosage
Adjunct for major burns (especially when resistance to other anti-infectives occurs); prevention of skin graft infection before or after surgery
Adults and children: Apply directly to lesion or to dressings used to cover the affected area daily or as indicated, depending on severity of burn.

Pharmacodynamics
Antibacterial action: The exact mechanism of action is unknown. However, it appears that the drug inhibits bacterial enzymes involved in carbohydrate metabolism. Nitrofurazone has a broad spectrum of activity.

Pharmacokinetics
• *Absorption:* Limited with topical use.
• *Distribution:* None.
• *Metabolism:* None.
• *Excretion:* None.

Contraindications and precautions
Use may result in bacterial or fungal overgrowth of nonsusceptible organisms, which may lead to secondary infections.
Drug should be used with caution in patients with renal impairment. Nitrofurazone is contraindicated in patients with hypersensitivity to the drug.

Interactions
None reported.

Effects on diagnostic tests
None reported.

Adverse reactions
• Local: allergic contact dermatitis.
Note: Drug should be discontinued if sensitization, superinfection, or irritation develops.

Overdose and treatment
Discontinue use and cleanse area with mild soap and water.

▶ Special considerations
• Avoid contact with eyes and mucous membranes.
• Monitor patient for overgrowth of nonsusceptible organisms, including fungi.
• Use diluted solutions within 24 hours after preparation; discard diluted solution that becomes cloudy.

Information for the patient
● Teach patient proper application of drug. Apply directly on lesion or place on gauze.
● Tell patient to avoid exposure of drug to direct sunlight, excessive heat, strong fluorescent lighting, and alkaline materials.

Breast-feeding
Safety has not been established. Potential benefits to mother must be weighed against risks to infant.

---

nitroglycerin (glyceryl trinitrate)
Oral, extended release
Ang-O-Span, Klavikordal, N-G-C,
Niong, Nitro-Bid, Nitrocap, Nitrocap
T.D., Nitroglyn, Nitrolin, Nitronet,
Nitrong, Nitrong SR*, Nitrospan,
Nitrostat SR

Sublingual
Nitrostabilin*, Nitrostat

Translingual
Nitrolingual

I.V.
Nitrobid IV, Nitrol IV, Nitrostat IV, Tridil

Topical
Nitrobid, Nitrol, Nitrong, Nitrostat

Transdermal
Nitrodisc, Nitro-Dur, Nitro-Dur II, NTS,
Transderm-Nitro

Transmucosal
Nitrogard

● Pharmacologic classification: nitrate
● Therapeutic classification: antianginal, vasodilator
● Pregnancy risk category C

How supplied
Available by prescription only
Tablets: 2.6 mg, 6.5 mg, 9 mg (sustained-release); 0.15 mg, 0.3 mg, 0.4 mg, 0.6 mg (sublingual); 1 mg, 2 mg, 3 mg (buccal, controlled-release)
Aerosol (lingual): 0.4 mg/metered spray
Capsules (sustained-release): 2.5 mg, 6.5 mg, 9 mg
I.V.: 0.5 mg/ml, 0.8 mg/ml, 5 mg/ml
Topical: 2% ointment
Transdermal: 2.5 mg, 5 mg, 7.5 mg, 10 mg, 15 mg/24 hour systems

Indications, route, and dosage
Prophylaxis against chronic anginal attacks
Adults: 1 sustained-release capsule q 8 to 12 hours; or 2% ointment. Start with ½" ointment, increasing with ½" increments until headache occurs, then decreasing to previous dose. Range of dosage with ointment is 2" to 5". Usual dose is 1" to 2". Alternatively, transdermal disc or pad may be applied to hairless site once daily. However, to prevent tolerance, topical forms should not be worn overnight.

Relief of acute angina pectoris; prophylaxis to prevent or minimize anginal attacks when taken immediately before stressful events
Adults: 1 sublingual tablet (gr ¼₀₀, ½₀₀, ⅟₁₅₀, ⅟₁₀₀) dissolved under the tongue or in the buccal pouch immediately upon indication of anginal attack. May repeat q 5 minutes for 15 to 30 minutes. Or, using Nitrolingual spray, spray one or two doses into mouth, preferably onto or under the tongue. May repeat every 3 to 5 minutes to a maximum of 3 doses within a 15-minute period. Or, transmucosally, 1 to 3 mg every 3 to 5 hours during waking hours.
Hypertension, congestive heart failure, angina
Nitroglycerin is indicated to control hypertension associated with surgery, to treat congestive heart failure associated with myocardial infarction, to relieve angina pectoris in acute situations, and to produce controlled hypotension during surgery (by I.V. infusion).
Adults: Initial infusion rate is 5 mcg/minute. May be increased by 5 mcg/minute q 3 to 5 minutes until a response is noted. If a 20 mcg/minute rate doesn't produce desired response, dosage may be increased by as much as 20 mcg/minute q 3 to 5 minutes.

Pharmacodynamics
● *Antianginal action:* Nitroglycerin relaxes vascular smooth muscle of both the venous and arterial beds, resulting in a net decrease in myocardial oxygen consumption. It also dilates coronary vessels, leading to redistribution of blood flow to ischemic tissue. The drug's systemic and coronary vascular effects (which may vary slightly with the various nitroglycerin forms) probably account for its value in treating angina.
● *Vasodilating action:* Nitroglycerin dilates peripheral vessels, making it useful (in I.V. form) in producing controlled hypotension during surgical procedures and in controlling blood pressure in perioperative hypertension. Because peripheral vasodilation decreases venous return to the heart (preload), nitroglycerin also helps to treat pulmonary edema and congestive heart failure. Arterial vasodilation decreases arterial impedance (afterload), thereby decreasing left ventricular work and aiding the failing heart. These combined effects may prove valuable in treating some patients with acute myocardial infarction. (Use of nitroglycerin in congestive heart failure and myocardial infarction currently are unapproved indications.)

Pharmacokinetics
● *Absorption:* Nitroglycerin is well absorbed from the GI tract. However, because it undergoes first-pass metabolism in the liver, the drug is incompletely absorbed into the systemic circulation. Onset of action for oral preparations is slow (except for sublingual tablets). After sublingual administration, absorption from the oral mucosa is relatively complete. Nitroglycerin is also well absorbed after topical administration as an ointment or transdermal system. Onset of action for various preparations is as follows: I.V., 1 to 2 minutes; sublingual, 1 to 3 minutes; translingual spray, 2 minutes; transmucosal tablet, 3 minutes; ointment, 20 to 60 minutes; oral (sustained-release), 40 minutes; transdermal, 40 to 60 minutes.
● *Distribution:* Nitroglycerin is distributed widely throughout the body. About 60% of circulating drug is bound to plasma proteins.
● *Metabolism:* Nitroglycerin is metabolized in the liver and serum to 1,3 glyceryl dinitrate, 1,2 glyceryl dini-

---

trate, and glyceryl mononitrate. Dinitrate metabolites have a slight vasodilatory effect.

• *Excretion:* Nitroglycerin metabolites are excreted in the urine; elimination half-life is about 1 to 4 minutes. Duration of effect for various preparations is as follows: I.V., 30 minutes; sublingual, up to 30 minutes; translingual spray, 30 to 60 minutes; transmucosal tablet, 5 hours; ointment, 3 to 6 hours; oral (sustained-release), 4 to 8 hours; transdermal, 18 to 24 hours.

Contraindications and precautions

Nitroglycerin is contraindicated in patients with head trauma or cerebral hemorrhage, because of potential for increased intracranial pressure; in patients with severe anemia, because nitrate ions can readily oxidize hemoglobin to methemoglobin; and in patients with a history of hypersensitivity or idiosyncratic reaction to nitrates.

I.V. nitroglycerin is contraindicated in patients with hypotension or uncorrected hypovolemia, because the drug may cause severe hypotension and shock; and in patients with constrictive pericarditis and pericardial tamponade, because the drug may cause hypotension, reduce preload, and decrease cardiac output.

Nitroglycerin should be used with caution in patients with increased intracranial pressure, because the drug dilates meningeal vessels; in patients with open- or closed-angle glaucoma, although intraocular pressure is increased only briefly and drainage of aqueous humor from the eye is unimpeded; in patients with diuretic-induced fluid depletion or low systolic blood pressure (less than 90 mm Hg), because of the drug's hypotensive effect; and during the initial days after acute myocardial infarction because the drug may cause excessive hypotension and tachycardia. (However, nitroglycerin has been used with some success to decrease myocardial ischemia and possibly reduce the extent of infarction.)

Tolerance to both the vascular and antianginal effects of the drugs can develop, and cross-tolerance between the nitrates and nitrites has been demonstrated. Tolerance is associated with a high or sustained plasma drug concentration and occurs most frequently with oral, I.V., and topical therapy. It rarely occurs with intermittent sublingual use. However, patients taking oral isosorbide dinitrate or topical nitroglycerin have not exhibited cross-tolerance to sublingual nitroglycerin.

Development of tolerance can be prevented by using the lowest effective dose and maintaining an intermittent dosing schedule. A nitrate-free interval of 10 to 12 hours daily (for example, by removing the transdermal nitroglycerin patch in the early evening and not reapplying until the next morning) may also help prevent tolerance.

Interactions

Concomitant use of nitroglycerin with alcohol, antihypertensive drugs, or phenothiazines may cause additive hypotensive effects. Concomitant use with ergot alkaloids may precipitate angina. Oral nitroglycerin may increase the bioavailability of ergot alkaloids.

Effects on diagnostic tests

Nitroglycerin may interfere with serum cholesterol determination tests using the Zlatkis-Zak color reaction, resulting in falsely decreased values.

Adverse reactions

• CNS: headache (sometimes throbbing), dizziness, weakness, blurred vision.
• CV: orthostatic hypotension, tachycardia, flushing, palpitations, fainting.
• DERM: cutaneous vasodilation, skin irritation (topical form).
• GI: nausea, vomiting.
• Local: sublingual burning, dry mouth.
• Other: hypersensitivity reactions (rash, dermatitis).
  Note: Drug should be discontinued if rash, dermatitis, blurred vision, or dry mouth occurs.

Overdose and treatment

Clinical effects of overdose result primarily from vasodilation and methemoglobinemia and include hypotension, persistent throbbing headache, palpitations, visual disturbances, flushing of the skin, sweating (with skin later becoming cold and cyanotic), nausea and vomiting, colic, bloody diarrhea, orthostasis, initial hyperpnea, dyspnea, slow respiratory rate, bradycardia, heart block, increased intracranial pressure with confusion, fever, paralysis, tissue hypoxia (from methemoglobinemia) leading to cyanosis, and metabolic acidosis, coma, clonic convulsions, and circulatory collapse or asphyxia. Death may result from circulatory collapse or asphyxia.

Treatment includes gastric lavage followed by administration of activated charcoal to remove remaining gastric contents. Blood gas measurements and methemoglobin levels should be monitored, as indicated. Supportive care includes respiratory support and oxygen administration, passive movement of the extremities to aid venous return, and recumbent positioning.

▶ Special considerations

• Only the sublingual and translingual forms should be used to relieve acute angina attack.
• To apply ointment, spread in uniform thin layer to any hairless part of the skin except distal parts of arms or legs, because absorption will not be maximal at these sites. Do not rub in. Cover with plastic film to aid absorption and to protect clothing. If using Tape-Surrounded Appli-Ruler (TSAR) system, keep TSAR on skin to protect patient's clothing and ensure that ointment remains in place. If serious adverse effects develop in patients using ointment or transdermal system, remove product at once or wipe ointment from skin. Be sure to avoid contact with ointment.
• Administration as I.V. infusion requires special nonabsorbent tubing supplied by manufacturer, because regular plastic tubing may absorb up to 80% of drug. Infusion should be prepared in glass bottle or container.
• If drug causes headache (especially likely with initial doses), aspirin or acetaminophen may be indicated. Dosage may need to be reduced temporarily.
• Sublingual dose may be administered before anticipated stress or at bedtime if angina is nocturnal.
• Drug may cause orthostatic hypotension. To minimize this, patient should change to upright position slowly, go up and down stairs carefully, and lie down at the first sign of dizziness.
• When administering drug to patients during initial days after acute myocardial infarction, monitor hemodynamic and clinical status carefully.
• Monitor blood pressure and intensity and duration of patient's response to drug.
• Be sure to remove transdermal patch before defi-

brillation. Because of the patch's aluminum backing, electric current may cause patch to explode.

● When terminating transdermal nitroglycerin treatment for angina, gradually reduce dosage and frequency of application over 4 to 6 weeks.

● To prevent withdrawal symptoms, reduce dosage gradually after long-term use of oral or topical preparations.

● Store drug in cool, dark place in tightly closed container. To ensure freshness, replace supply of sublingual tablets every 3 months. Remove cotton from container because it absorbs drug.

Information for the patient

● Instruct patient to take medication regularly, as prescribed and to keep sublingual form accessible at all times. The drug is physiologically necessary but not addictive.

● Teach patient to take oral tablet on empty stomach, either 30 minutes before or 1 to 2 hours after meals, to swallow oral tablets whole, and to chew chewable tablets thoroughly before swallowing.

● Instruct patient to take sublingual tablet at first sign of angina attack. Tell him to wet tablet with saliva, place it under the tongue until completely absorbed, and sit down and rest. If no relief occurs, he should call or go to hospital emergency room. If he complains of tingling sensation with drug placed sublingually, he may try holding tablet in buccal pouch.

● Advise patient to store nitroglycerin sublingual tablets in original container or other container specifically approved for this use.

● Instruct patient to place transmucosal tablet under upper lip or in buccal pouch, to let it dissolve slowly over a 3- to 5-hour period, and not to chew or swallow tablet. Advise him that dissolution rate may increase if he touches tablet with tongue or drinks hot liquids.

● If patient is receiving nitroglycerin lingual aerosol (Nitrolingual), instruct him how to use this device correctly. Remind him not to inhale spray but to release it onto or under the tongue. Also tell him not to swallow immediately after administering the spray but to wait about 10 seconds before swallowing.

● Instruct patient to use caution when wearing transdermal patch near microwave oven. Leaking radiation may heat patch's metallic backing and cause burns.

● Warn patient that headache may follow initial doses but that this symptom may respond to usual headache remedies or dosage reduction (however, dose should be reduced only with medical approval). Assure patient that headache usually subsides gradually with continued treatment.

● Instruct patient to avoid alcohol while taking this drug because severe hypotension and cardiovascular collapse may occur.

● Warn patient that drug may cause dizziness or flushing and to move to an upright position slowly.

● Tell patient to report blurred vision, dry mouth, or persistent headache.

Pediatric use

Methemoglobinemia may occur in infants receiving large doses of nitroglycerin.

nitroprusside sodium
Nipride, Nitropress

● Pharmacologic classification: vasodilator
● Therapeutic classification: antihypertensive
● Pregnancy risk category C

How supplied
Available by prescription only
Injection: 50 mg/5-ml vial

Indications, route, and dosage
Hypertensive emergencies
Adults and children: I.V. infusion titrated to blood pressure; average dose is 3 mcg/kg/minute, with a range of 0.5 to 10 mcg/kg/minute. Maximum infusion rate is 10 mcg/kg/minute.

Pharmacodynamics
Antihypertensive action: Nitroprusside acts directly on vascular smooth muscle, causing peripheral vasodilation.

Pharmacokinetics
● *Absorption:* Drug is administered by I.V. route and, therefore, is not absorbed. I.V. infusion of nitroprusside reduces blood pressure almost immediately.
● *Distribution:* Unknown.
● *Metabolism:* Nitroprusside is metabolized rapidly in erythrocytes and tissues and is converted to thiocyanate in the liver.
● *Excretion:* Nitroprusside is excreted primarily in urine, entirely as metabolites. Blood pressure returns to pretreatment level 1 to 10 minutes after completion of infusion.

Contraindications and precautions
Nitroprusside is contraindicated in patients with known hypersensitivity to the drug and in patients with compensatory hypertension secondary to arteriovenous shunt or coarctation of the aorta, because a decrease in blood pressure may be harmful to these patients.

Nitroprusside should be used cautiously in patients with renal insufficiency because thiocyanate, one of the metabolic products of nitroprusside, is excreted by the kidney, and may accumulate; in patients with hepatic insufficiency because drug metabolism may be impaired; in patients with hypothyroidism because thiocyanate inhibits iodine uptake and binding; and in patients with low vitamin B_{12} concentrations because the drug may interfere with vitamin B_{12} distribution and metabolism.

Interactions
Nitroprusside may potentiate antihypertensive effects of other antihypertensive medications; its antihypertensive effects may be potentiated by general anesthetics, particularly halothane and enflurane, and by ganglionic blocking agents. Pressor agents such as epinephrine may cause an increase in blood pressure during nitroprusside therapy.

Effects on diagnostic tests
An increase in serum creatinine concentration may occur during therapy.

Adverse reactions
The following adverse reactions usually indicate overdose:
- CNS: headache, dizziness, ataxia, loss of consciousness, *coma*, weak pulse, absent reflexes, widely dilated pupils, restlessness, muscle twitching, diaphoresis.
- CV: distant heart sounds, palpitations, *dyspnea*, shallow breathing, *hypotension*.
- DERM: pink color.
- GI: vomiting, nausea, abdominal pain.
- GU: may aggravate renal insufficiency.
- Metabolic: *acidosis*.
- Respiratory: pulmonary shunting.

Note: Drug should be discontinued if metabolic acidosis occurs; it may indicate cyanogen toxicity.

Overdose and treatment
Clinical manifestations of overdose include the adverse reactions listed above and increased tolerance to the drug's antihypertensive effects.

Treat overdose by giving nitrites to induce methemoglobin formation. Discontinue the nitroprusside and administer amyl nitrite inhalations for 15 to 30 seconds each minute until a 3% sodium nitrite solution can be prepared. Administer amyl nitrite cautiously to minimize risk of additional hypotension secondary to vasodilation. Then administer the sodium nitrite solution by I.V. infusion at a rate not exceeding 2.5 to 5 ml/minute up to a total dose of 10 to 15 ml. Follow with I.V. sodium thiosulfate infusion (12.5 g in 50 ml of dextrose 5% in water [D_5W] solution) over 10 minutes. If necessary, repeat infusions of sodium nitrite and sodium thiosulfate at half the initial doses. Further treatment involves symptomatic and supportive care.

▶ Special considerations
- Blood pressure should be checked at least every 5 minutes at the start of the infusion and at least every 15 minutes thereafter during infusion.
- Prepare solution using D_5W solution; do not use bacteriostatic water for injection or sterile saline solution for reconstitution; because of light sensitivity, foil-wrap I.V. solution (but not tubing). Fresh solutions have faint brownish tint; discard after 24 hours.
- Infuse drug with infusion pump.
- This drug is best run piggyback through a peripheral line with no other medications; do not adjust rate of main I.V. line while drug is running because even small boluses can cause severe hypotension.
- Nitroprusside can cause cyanide toxicity; therefore, check serum thiocyanate levels every 72 hours; levels above 100 mcg/ml are associated with cyanide toxicity, which can produce profound hypotension, metabolic acidosis, dyspnea, ataxia, and vomiting. If such symptoms occur, discontinue infusion and re-evaluate therapy.
- Nitroprusside also may be used to produce controlled hypotension during anesthesia, to reduce bleeding from the surgical procedure.
- Hypertensive patients are more sensitive to nitroprusside than normotensive patients. Also, patients taking other antihypertensive drugs are extremely sensitive to nitroprusside. Nitroprusside has been used in patients with acute myocardial infarction, refractory heart failure, and severe mitral regurgitation. It has also been used orally as an antihypertensive.

Information for the patient
Ask patient to report any CNS symptoms (such as headache or dizziness) promptly.

Geriatric use
Elderly patients may be more sensitive to the drug's antihypertensive effects.

Breast-feeding
It is not known if nitroprusside is distributed into breast milk; administer drug with caution to breast-feeding women.

nizatidine
Axid

- Pharmacologic classification: histamine H_2-receptor antagonist
- Therapeutic classification: antiulcer agent
- Pregnancy risk category C

How supplied
Available by prescription only
Capsules: 150 mg, 300 mg

Indications, route, and dosage
Treatment of active duodenal ulcer
Adults: 300 mg P.O. once daily h.s. Alternatively, may give 150 mg P.O. b.i.d.
Maintenance therapy for duodenal ulcer patients
Adults: 150 mg P.O. once daily h.s.
Dosage in renal failure

DOSAGE IN ADULTS		
Creatinine clearance (ml/min/ 1.73 m²)	Active duodenal ulcer	Maintenance
20 to 50	150 mg/day	150 mg every other day
< 20	150 mg every other day	150 mg every 3 days

Pharmacodynamics
Antiulcer action: Nizatidine is a competitive, reversible inhibitor of histamine H_2 receptors, particularly those in the gastric parietal cells.

Pharmacokinetics
- *Absorption:* Nizatidine is well absorbed (> 90%) after oral administration. Absorption may be slightly enhanced by food, and slightly impaired by antacids.
- *Distribution:* Approximately 35% of nizatidine is bound to plasma protein. Peak plasma concentrations (700 to 1,800 mcg/liter for a 150-mg dose and 1,400 to 3,600 mcg/liter for a 300-mg dose) occur from 0.5 to 3 hours after the dose. A concentration of 1,000 mcg/liter is equivalent to 3 mol/liter, a dose of 300 mg is equivalent to 905 moles.
- *Metabolism:* Nizatidine probably undergoes hepatic

metabolism. About 40% of excreted drug is metabolized; the remainder is excreted unchanged.

● *Excretion:* More than 90% of an oral dose of nizatidine is excreted in the urine within 12 hours. Renal clearance is about 500 ml/min, which indicates excretion by active tubular secretion. Less than 6% of an administered dose is eliminated in the feces.

Elimination half-life is 1 to 2 hours. Moderate to severe renal impairment significantly prolongs the half-life and decreases the clearance of nizatidine. In anephric persons, the half-life is 3.5 to 11 hours; the plasma clearance is 7 to 14 liters per hour.

Contraindications and precautions
Nizatidine is contraindicated in patients with hypersensitivity to the drug. Use with caution in patients with hypersensitivity to other H_2-receptor antagonists.

Interactions
Because nizatidine does not inhibit the cytochrome P-450-linked drug metabolizing enzyme system, drug interactions mediated by inhibition of hepatic metabolism are not expected. Concomitant use of high doses of aspirin (3,900 mg/day) with nizatidine (150 mg b.i.d.) increases serum salicylate levels.

Effects on diagnostic tests
False-positive tests for urobilinogen may occur during nizatidine therapy.

Adverse reactions
● CNS: somnolence.
● CV: short episodes of asymptomatic ventricular tachycardia.
● DERM: rash, urticaria, sweating, *exfoliative dermatitis.*
● Endocrine: gynecomastia.
● HEMA: thrombocytopenia.
● Hepatic: hepatocellular injury, reversible liver-enzyme abnormalities.
● Other: hyperuricemia.

Overdose and treatment
Expected clinical effects of overdose are cholinergic, including lacrimation, salivation, emesis, miosis and diarrhea. Treatment may include use of activated charcoal, emesis, or lavage, with clinical monitoring and supportive therapy.

▶ Special considerations
● Because nizatidine is excreted primarily by the kidneys, reduce dosage in patients with moderate to severe renal insufficiency.
● Nizatidine is partially metabolized in the liver. In patients with normal renal function and uncomplicated hepatic dysfunction, the disposition of nizatidine is similar to that in patients with normal hepatic function.
● For patients on maintenance therapy, consider that the effects of continuous therapy with nizatidine for longer than 1 year are not known.

Information for the patient
Advise patient not to smoke as this may increase gastric acid secretion and worsen the disease.

Geriatric use
Safety and efficacy appear similar to those in younger patients. However, consider that elderly patients have reduced renal functions.

Pediatric use
Safety and efficacy in children have not been established.

Breast-feeding
Use with caution in women who are breast-feeding. Consider that nizatidine is secreted and concentrated in the milk of lactating rats.

PHARMACOLOGIC CLASS

nonsteroidal anti-inflammatory drugs (NSAIDs)

**diflunisal
etodolac
fenoprofen calcium
flurbiprofen
ibuprofen
indomethacin
indomethacin sodium trihydrate
ketoprofen
ketorolac tromethamine
meclofenamate
mefenamic acid
nabumetone
naproxen
naproxen sodium
oxyphenbutazone
phenylbutazone
piroxicam
sulindac
tolmetin sodium**

Nonsteroidal anti-inflammatory drugs (NSAIDs) are a growing class of drugs that are prescribed widely for their analgesic and anti-inflammatory effects; some members of this class have an antipyretic effect.

Pharmacology
The analgesic effect of NSAIDs may result from interference with the prostaglandins involved in pain. Prostaglandins appear to sensitize pain receptors to mechanical stimulation or to other chemical mediators. NSAIDs inhibit synthesis of prostaglandins peripherally and possibly centrally. Their anti-inflammatory action may also contribute indirectly to their analgesic effect.

Like the salicylates, the anti-inflammatory effects of NSAIDs may result in part from inhibition of prostaglandin synthesis and release during inflammation. The exact mechanism has not been clearly established, but the anti-inflammatory effect of NSAIDs correlates with their ability to inhibit prostaglandin synthesis.

Clinical indications and actions
Pain, inflammation, and fever
NSAIDs are used principally for symptomatic relief of mild to moderate pain and inflammation. These agents usually provide temporary relief of mild to moderate pain, especially that associated with inflammation. NSAIDs are used to treat low-intensity pain of headache, arthralgia, myalgia, neuralgia, and mild to moderate pain from dental or surgical procedures or dysmenorrhea.

Oral NSAIDs are also used for long-term treatment of rheumatoid arthritis, juvenile arthritis, and osteoarthritis. In osteoarthritis, NSAIDs are used primarily for analgesia. NSAIDs offer only symptomatic treatment

---

for rheumatoid conditions, and do not reverse or arrest the disease process. NSAIDs reduce pain, stiffness, swelling, and tenderness.

Overview of adverse reactions

Adverse reactions to oral NSAIDs chiefly involve the GI tract, particularly erosion of the gastric mucosa. Most common symptoms are dyspepsia, heartburn, epigastric distress, nausea, and abdominal pain. GI symptoms usually occur in the first few days of therapy, and often subside with continuous treatment. They can be minimized by administering NSAIDs with meals or food, antacids, or large quantities of water or milk.

CNS side effects (headache, dizziness, drowsiness) may also occur. Flank pain with other signs and symptoms of nephrotoxicity has occasionally been reported. Fluid retention may aggravate preexisting hypertension or CHF. NSAIDs should not be used in patients with renal insufficiency.

▶ Special considerations

● Use NSAIDs cautiously in patients with a history of GI disease, increased risk of GI bleeding, or decreased renal function.
● Patients with known "triad" symptoms (aspirin hypersensitivity, rhinitis/nasal polyps, and asthma) are at high risk of bronchospasm.
● NSAIDs may mask the signs and symptoms of acute infection (fever, myalgia, erythema); carefully evaluate patients at high risk for infection (for example, those with diabetes).
● Administer oral NSAIDs with a full 8-oz glass of water to assure adequate passage into stomach. Have patient sit up for 15 to 30 minutes after taking the drug to prevent lodging of the drug in the esophagus.
● Tablets may be crushed and mixed with food or fluids to aid swallowing, and with antacids to minimize gastric upset.
● Assess level of pain and inflammation before start of therapy. Evaluate patient for relief or reduction of these symptoms.
● Monitor for signs and symptoms of bleeding. Assess bleeding time if surgery is required.
● Monitor ophthalmic and auditory function before and periodically during therapy to prevent toxicity.
● Monitor CBC, platelets, prothrombin times, and hepatic and renal function studies periodically to detect abnormalities.
● Patients who do not respond to one NSAID may respond to another NSAID.
● Use of an NSAID with an opioid analgesic has an additive effect. Use of lower doses of the opioid analgesic may be possible.

Information for the patient

● Tell patient to take medication with 8 oz of water 30 minutes before or 2 hours after meals, or with food or milk if gastric irritation occurs.
● Explain that taking the drug as directed is necessary to achieve the desired effect; 2 to 4 weeks of treatment may be needed before benefit is seen.
● Advise patients on chronic NSAID therapy to arrange for monitoring of laboratory parameters, especially BUN, serum creatinine, liver function tests, and CBC.
● Warn patients with current or history of rectal bleeding to avoid using rectal NSAID suppositories. Because they must be retained in the rectum for at least 1 hour, they may cause irritation and bleeding.
● Warn pregnant patients to avoid the use of all NSAIDs,

especially during the third trimester, when prostaglandin inhibition may cause prolonged gestation, dystocia, and delayed parturition.
● Warn patient that use of alcoholic beverages while on NSAID therapy may cause increased GI irritation and, possibly, GI bleeding.

Geriatric use

● Patients over age 60 may be more susceptible to the toxic effects of NSAIDs because of decreased renal function, resulting in NSAID accumulation.
● The effects of NSAIDs on renal prostaglandins may cause fluid retention and edema, a significant drawback for elderly patients, especially those with congestive heart failure.

Pediatric use

Do not use long-term NSAID therapy in children under age 14; safety of such use has not been established.

Breast-feeding

Most NSAIDs are distributed into breast milk; NSAID therapy is not recommended during breast-feeding.

Representative combinations

None.

---

norepinephrine bitartrate
(formerly levarterenol bitartrate)
Levophed

● Pharmacologic classification: adrenergic (direct acting)
● Therapeutic classification: vasopressor
● Pregnancy risk category D

How supplied

Available by prescription only
Injection: 1 mg/ml parenteral

Indications, route, and dosage
To maintain blood pressure in acute hypotensive states
Adults: Initially, 8 to 12 mcg/minute I.V. infusion, then titrated to maintain desired blood pressure; maintenance dosage, 2 to 4 mcg/minute.
Children: Initially, 2 mcg/minute or 2 mcg/m²/minute I.V. infusion, then titrated to maintain desired blood pressure. For advanced cardiac life support, initial infusion rate is 0.1 mcg/kg/minute.

Pharmacodynamics

Vasopressor action: Norepinephrine acts predominantly by direct stimulation of alpha-adrenergic receptors, constricting both capacitance and resistance blood vessels. That results in increased total peripheral resistance; increased systolic and diastolic blood pressure; decreased blood flow to vital organs, skin, and skeletal muscle; and constriction of renal blood vessels, which reduces renal blood flow. It also has a direct stimulating effect on beta, receptors of the heart, producing a positive inotropic response. Its main therapeutic effects are vasoconstriction and cardiac stimulation.

Pharmacokinetics
● *Absorption:* Pressor effect occurs rapidly after infusion, is of short duration, and stops within 1 to 2 minutes after infusion is stopped.
● *Distribution:* Norepinephrine localizes in sympathetic nerve tissues.
● *Metabolism:* Norepinephrine is metabolized in the liver and other tissues to inactive compounds.
● *Excretion:* Norepinephrine is excreted in urine primarily as sulfate and glucuronide conjugates. Small amounts are excreted unchanged in urine.

Contraindications and precautions
Norepinephrine is contraindicated in patients with peripheral or mesenteric vascular thrombosis (may increase ischemia and extend area of infarction), profound hypoxia or hypercapnea, hypovolemia, and in those undergoing general anesthesia with cyclopropane and other inhalation hydrocarbon anesthetics (risk of inducing cardiac arrhythmias). Norepinephrine is also contraindicated for use with local anesthetics in fingers, toes, ears, nose, or genitalia.

Administer cautiously to hypertensive or hyperthyroid patients (increased risk of adverse reactions). Also administer cautiously to patients with known hypersensitivity to sulfites; commercially available formulation contains sodium metabisulfite.

Interactions
When used concomitantly with general anesthetics, norepinephrine may cause increased cardiac arrhythmias; when used with tricyclic antidepressants, monoamine oxidase inhibitors, some antihistamines, parenteral ergot alkaloids, guanethidine, and methyldopa, norepinephrine may cause severe, prolonged hypertension.

Use with beta blockers may result in an increased potential for hypertension. (Propranolol may be used to treat cardiac arrhythmias occurring during norepinephrine administration.) Use with furosemide or other diuretics may decrease arterial responsiveness.

Concomitant use with atropine blocks the reflex bradycardia caused by norepinephrine and enhances its pressor effects.

Effects on diagnostic tests
None reported.

Adverse reactions
● CNS: headache, weakness, dizziness, restlessness, anxiety, insomnia, tremor.
● CV: precordial pain, *severe hypertension,* severe peripheral and visceral vasoconstriction, arrhythmias, bradycardia.
● GI: nausea, vomiting.
● GU: decreased urine output.
● Local: severe irritation and necrosis with extravasation.
● Other: *respiratory difficulty, apnea,* pallor, swelling and engorgement of thyroid, photophobia, sweating, *cerebral hemorrhage, convulsions, metabolic acidosis,* hyperglycemia, hyperthermia.
Note: Drug should be discontinued if hypersensitivity, infiltration, or thrombosis occurs.

Overdose and treatment
Clinical manifestations of overdose include severe hypertension, photophobia, retrosternal or pharyngeal pain, intense sweating, vomiting, cerebral hemorrhage, convulsions, and cardiac arrhythmias. Monitor vital signs closely.

Treatment includes supportive and symptomatic measures. Use atropine for reflex bradycardia, phentolamine for extravasation, and propranolol for arrhythmias.

▶ Special considerations
Besides those relevant to all *adrenergics,* consider the following recommendations.
● Correct blood volume depletion before administration. Norepinephrine is not a substitute for blood, plasma, fluid, or electrolyte replacement.
● Select injection site carefully. Administration by I.V. infusion requires an infusion pump or other device to control flow rate. If possible, infuse into antecubital vein of the arm or the femoral vein. Change injection sites for prolonged therapy. Must be diluted before use with 5% dextrose with or without sodium chloride. (Dilution with sodium chloride alone not recommended.) Monitor infusion rate. Withdraw drug gradually; recurrent hypotension may follow abrupt withdrawal.
● Prepare infusion solution by adding 4 mg norepinephrine to 1 liter of 5% dextrose. The resultant solution contains 4 mcg/ml.
● Extravasation: To treat, infiltrate site promptly with 10 to 15 ml saline solution containing 5 to 10 mg phentolamine, using a fine needle.
● Some physicians add phentolamine (5 to 10 mg) to each liter of infusion solution as a preventive against sloughing, should extravasation occur.
● Monitor intake and output. Norepinephrine reduces renal blood flow, which may cause decreased urine output initially.
● Patient should be attended constantly during administration of norepinephrine. Baseline blood pressure and pulse should be taken before therapy, then repeated every 2 minutes until stabilization; then repeated every 5 minutes during drug administration.
● In addition to vital signs, monitor patient's mental state, skin temperature of extremities, and skin color (especially earlobes, lips, and nail beds).
● In patients with previously normal blood pressure, adjust flow rate to maintain blood pressure at low normal (usually 80 to 100 mm Hg systolic); in hypertensive patients, maintain systolic no higher than 40 mm Hg below preexisting pressure level.
● Protect solution from light. Discard solution that is discolored or contains a precipitate.
● Norepinephrine has been used to control upper GI hemorrhage with 8 mg of norepinephrine in 100 ml of normal saline solution instilled through a nasogastric tube q hour for 6 to 8 hours, then q 2 hours for 4 to 6 hours, then gradually reduced until drug is discontinued. Alternatively, 8 mg of norepinephrine in 250 ml of normal saline solution administered intraperitoneally.

Information for the patient
● Inform patient that he'll need frequent monitoring of vital signs.
● Tell patient to report any adverse reactions.

Geriatric use
Elderly patients are more sensitive to the effects of the drug. Decreased cardiac output may be harmful to elderly patients with poor cerebral or coronary circulation.

Pediatric use
Use with caution in children.

norethindrone
Micronor, Norlutin, Nor-Q.D.

norethindrone acetate
Aygestin, Norlutate

- Pharmacologic classification: progestin
- Therapeutic classification: contraceptive
- Pregnancy risk category X

How supplied
Available by prescription only
Norethindrone
Tablets: 0.35 mg, 5 mg
Norethindrone acetate
Tablets: 5 mg

Indications, route, and dosage
Amenorrhea, abnormal uterine bleeding, endometriosis
Norethindrone
Adults: 5 to 20 mg P.O. daily on days 5 to 25 of menstrual cycle.
Norethindrone acetate
Adults: 2.5 to 10 mg P.O. daily on days 5 to 25 of menstrual cycle.
Endometriosis
Norethindrone
Adults: 10 mg P.O. daily for 14 days, then increase by 5 mg P.O. daily q 2 weeks up to 30 mg/day.
Norethindrone acetate
Adults: 5 mg P.O. daily for 14 days, then increase by 2.5 mg/day q 2 weeks up to 15 mg/day.
Contraception
Adults: 0.35 mg norethindrone P.O. daily, beginning day 1 of menstrual cycle and continuing uninterrupted thereafter.

Pharmacodynamics
Contraceptive action: Norethindrone suppresses ovulation, causes thickening of cervical mucus, and induces sloughing of the endometrium.

Pharmacokinetics
- *Absorption:* Norethindrone is well absorbed after oral administration.
- *Distribution:* Drug is distributed widely. It is about 80% protein-bound and distributes into bile and breast milk.
- *Metabolism:* Norethindrone is primarily hepatic; it undergoes extensive first-pass metabolism.
- *Excretion:* Drug is excreted primarily in feces. Elimination half-life is 5 to 14 hours.

Contraindications and precautions
Norethindrone is contraindicated in patients with known hypersensitivity to progestins, a history of thromboembolic disorders, severe hepatic disease, breast cancer, or undiagnosed abnormal vaginal bleeding; and in pregnant and breast-feeding women.
Norethindrone should be used cautiously in patients with existing conditions that might be aggravated by fluid and electrolyte retention, such as cardiac or renal disease, epilepsy, or migraine; in patients because decreased glucose tolerance may occur; and in patients with a history of mental depression because norethindrone may worsen this condition.

Interactions
Concomitant use with bromocriptine may cause amenorrhea or galactorrhea, thus interfering with the action of bromocriptine. Concurrent use of these drugs is not recommended.

Effects on diagnostic tests
Pregnanediol excretion may decrease; serum alkaline phosphatase and amino acid levels may increase. Glucose tolerance has been shown to decrease in a small percentage of patients receiving this drug.

Adverse reactions
- CNS: dizziness, headache, lethargy, depression.
- CV: thrombophlebitis, *pulmonary embolism,* edema.
- DERM: melasma, rash.
- GU: breakthrough bleeding, dysmenorrhea, amenorrhea, cervical erosion or abnormal secretions.
- Hepatic: cholestatic jaundice.
- Metabolic: hyperglycemia, decreased libido.
  Note: Drug should be discontinued if hypersensitivity, thromboembolic or thrombotic disorders, visual disturbances, migraine headache, or severe depression occurs.

Overdose and treatment
No information available.

▶ Special considerations
Recommendations for administration of norethindrone, and for care and teaching of the patient during therapy, are the same as those for all *progestins*.

norfloxacin (ophthalmic)
Chibroxin

- Pharmacologic classification: fluoroquinolone
- Therapeutic classification: broad-spectrum antibiotic
- Pregnancy risk category C

How supplied
Available by prescription only
Ophthalmic solution: 0.3% in 5-ml containers

Indications, route, and dosage
Conjunctivitis caused by susceptible strains of bacteria
Adults and children age 1 and over: 1 or 2 drops in the affected eye q.i.d. for up to 7 days. If condition warrants, 2 drops may be applied q 2 hours during the waking hours of the first day of treatment.

Pharmacodynamics
Antibiotic action: Ophthalmic norfloxacin inhibits bacterial DNA gyrase, an enzyme necessary for bacterial replication. Drug is bacteriostatic or bactericidal, depending on concentration.

Pharmacokinetics
- *Absorption:* Systemic absorption of ophthalmic norfloxacin is limited.
- *Distribution:* No information available.
- *Metabolism:* No information available.
- *Excretion:* No information available.

Contraindications and precautions

Ophthalmic norfloxacin is contraindicated in patients with a history of hypersensitivity to norfloxacin or other quinolone antibiotics. This drug should not be injected into the eye.

Serious hypersensitivity reactions, including anaphylaxis, have occurred in patients receiving systemic quinolone therapy. Discontinue drug at the first sign of hypersensitivity, such as irritation.

Prolonged use may result in overgrowth of nonsusceptible organisms, including fungi. Institute appropriate therapy if superinfection occurs.

Interactions

Drug interactions with the ophthalmic form have not been studied. Systemically administered drug interferes with metabolism of theophylline, caffeine, and cyclosporine; it may also enhance the effects of oral anticoagulants. Use cautiously in patients receiving these drugs.

Effects on diagnostic tests

None reported.

Adverse reactions

● EENT: local burning or discomfort, itching, chemosis, photophobia, conjunctival hyperemia.
● Other: bad taste in mouth.

Overdose and treatment

A topical overdose of the drug may be flushed from the eye with warm tap water.

▶ Special considerations

Drug is indicated for treatment of conjunctivitis when caused by susceptible bacteria. Known susceptible strains include *Acinetobacter calcoaceticus, Aeromonas hydrophila, Haemophilus influenzae, Proteus mirabilis, Serratia marcescens, Staphylococcus aureus, Staphylococcus epidermidis, Staphylococcus warnerii,* and *Streptococcus pneumoniae.*

Information for the patient

● Teach patient how to instill drug correctly. Remind him not to touch the tip of the bottle with his hands and to avoid contact of the tip with the eye or surrounding tissue.
● Remind patient not to share washcloths or towels with other family members to avoid spreading infection. Tell him not to share the drug with others.
● Advise patient to wash hands before and after instilling solution.
● Tell patient to store drug at room temperature and to protect the drug from light.

Pediatric use

Systemically administered quinolones have caused arthropathy in young animals; however, ophthalmic norfloxacin has not produced this adverse effect.

Breast-feeding

It is unknown if drug is excreted in breast milk. Use with caution in breast-feeding women.

norfloxacin (systemic)
Noroxin

● Pharmacologic classification: fluoroquinolone
● Therapeutic classification: broad-spectrum antibiotic
● Pregnancy risk category C

How supplied

Available by prescription only
Tablets: 400 mg

Indications, route, and dosage
Complicated and uncomplicated urinary tract infections caused by various gram-negative and gram-positive bacteria, bacterial prostatitis
Adults: Complicated infection—400 mg P.O. b.i.d. for 10 to 21 days; uncomplicated infection—400 mg P.O. b.i.d. for 7 to 10 days. Do not exceed 800 mg/day. Patients with creatinine clearance below 30 ml/minute should receive 400 mg/day for appropriate duration of therapy.

Pharmacodynamics
Antibacterial action: Norfloxacin is generally bactericidal. It inhibits DNA gyrase, blocking DNA synthesis. Drug's spectrum of activity includes most aerobic gram-positive and gram-negative urinary pathogens, including *Pseudomonas aeruginosa.*

Pharmacokinetics
● *Absorption:* About 30% to 40% of norfloxacin dose is absorbed from the GI tract (as dose increases, percentage of absorbed drug decreases). Food may reduce absorption.
● *Distribution:* Norfloxacin is distributed into renal tissue, liver, galladder, prostatic fluid, testicles, seminal fluid, bile, and sputum. From 10% to 15% binds to plasma proteins.
● *Metabolism:* Norfloxacin's metabolism is unknown.
● *Excretion:* Most systemically absorbed drug is excreted by the kidneys, with about 30% appearing in bile. In patients with normal renal function, plasma half-life is 3 to 4 hours; up to 8 hours in severe renal impairment.

Contraindications and precautions
Norfloxacin is contraindicated in pregnant women because it has demonstrated embryotoxic effects in animals; in children because it has exhibited neurotoxic effects in young animals; and in patients with known hypersensitivity to other quinolones (nalidixic acid or cinoxacin).

Norfloxacin should be administered cautiously to patients with a history of seizures because drug's effects on the brain are unknown.

Interactions
When used concomitantly, probenecid may increase serum norfloxacin levels. Concomitant use with nitrofurantoin antagonizes norfloxacin's antibacterial activity. Concomitant use with antacids is not recommended by manufacturer. Food interferes with norfloxacin's absorption.

Concomitant use with xanthine derivatives (theophylline, aminophylline) may increase theophylline concentration and the risk of xanthine-related toxicities.

NORGESTREL 771

Effects on diagnostic tests
Blood urea nitrogen (BUN), serum creatinine, and ALT (SGPT), AST (SGOT), and alkaline phosphatase may increase; hematocrit may decrease; and eosinophilia and neutropenia may occur during norfloxacin therapy.

Adverse reactions
● CNS: headache, dizziness, somnolence, depression, insomnia, tinnitus.
● DERM: rash, erythema.
● GI: dry mouth, nausea, abdominal pain, dyspepsia, constipation, flatulence, heartburn, diarrhea.
● GU: crystalluria with higher dosages.
● HEMA: leukopenia.
● Hepatic: transient elevations of AST (SGOT) and ALT (SGPT) levels.
● Other: fatigue, fever, arthralgia.

Overdose and treatment
No information available.

▶ Special considerations
● Obtain culture and sensitivity tests before starting therapy, and repeat as needed throughout therapy.
● Make sure patient is well hydrated before and during therapy to avoid crystalluria.
● Arrange for baseline and follow-up BUN, creatinine clearance, complete blood count, and liver function tests.
● Evaluate patient for signs and symptoms of resistant infection or reinfection.

Information for the patient
● Instruct patient to continue taking drug as directed, even if he feels better.
● Advise patient to take drug 1 hour before or 2 hours after meals and antacids.
● Warn patient that drug may cause dizziness that impairs his ability to perform tasks that require alertness and coordination.

Pediatric use
Drug is contraindicated in children because animal studies suggest a potential risk of arthropathy.

Breast-feeding
Safety has not been established; alternative feeding method is recommended during treatment with norfloxacin.

norgestrel
Ovrette

● Pharmacologic classification: progestin
● Therapeutic classification: contraceptive
● Pregnancy risk category X

How supplied
Available by prescription only
Tablets: 0.075 mg

Indications, route, and dosage
Contraception
Adults: 1 tablet P.O. daily.

Pharmacodynamics
Contraceptive action: Norgestrel suppresses ovulation and causes thickening of cervical mucus.

Pharmacokinetics
Norgestrel is well-absorbed after oral administration. Distribution, metabolism, and excretion have not been described.

Contraindications and precautions
Norgestrel is contraindicated in patients with known hypersensitivity to progestins; in patients with a history of thromboembolic disorders because the drug may induce thromboembolic disorders; in patients with severe hepatic disease because it may worsen liver damage; in patients with breast or genital cancer or undiagnosed abnormal vaginal bleeding because the drug may stimulate growth of hormone-sensitive tumors; and in pregnant and breast-feeding women.

Norgestrel should be used cautiously in patients with existing conditions that might be aggravated by fluid and electrolyte retention, such as cardiac or renal disease, epilepsy, or migraine. Caution also is advised in administering this agent to diabetic patients (because decreased glucose tolerance may occur) or to patients with a history of mental depression (because norgestrel may worsen this condition).

Interactions
Concomitant use with bromocriptine may cause amenorrhea or galactorrhea, thus interfering with the action of bromocriptine. Concurrent use of these drugs is not recommended.

Effects on diagnostic tests
Pregnanediol excretion may decrease; serum alkaline phosphatase and amino acid levels may increase. Glucose tolerance has been shown to decrease in a small percentage of patients receiving this drug.

Adverse reactions
● CNS: cerebral thrombosis or hemorrhage, migraine headache, lethargy, depression.
● CV: hypertension, thrombophlebitis, pulmonary embolism, edema.
● DERM: melasma, rash.
● GU: breakthrough bleeding, change in menstrual flow, dysmenorrhea, spotting, amenorrhea, cervical erosion.
● Hepatic: cholestatic jaundice.
● Other: breast tenderness, enlargement, or secretions.

Overdose and treatment
No information available.

▶ Special considerations
Besides those relevant to all progestins, consider the following recommendations.
● Failure rate of the progestin-only contraceptive is about three times higher than that of the combination contraceptives.
● Ovrette tablets contain tartrazine. Use cautiously in patients with tartrazine or aspirin sensitivity.

Information for the patient
● Tell patient to take drug at the same time every day, even if menstruating. Norgestrel is also known as the "minipill."
● Advise patient of increased risk of serious cardio-

vascular adverse reactions associated with heavy smoking, especially while taking oral contraceptives.

● Risk of pregnancy increases with each tablet missed. A patient who misses 1 tablet should take it as soon as she remembers; she should then take the next tablet at the regular time. A patient who misses 2 tablets should take one as soon as she remembers and then take the next regular dose at the usual time; she should use a nonhormonal method of contraception in addition to norgestrel until 14 tablets have been taken. A patient who misses 3 or more tablets should discontinue the drug and use a nonhormonal method of contraception until after her menses. If her menstrual period does not occur within 45 days, pregnancy testing is necessary.

● Advise patient to report immediately excessive bleeding or bleeding between menstrual cycles.

● Advise patient to use a second method of birth control for the first cycle on norgestrel, or for 3 weeks after starting the hormonal contraceptive, to ensure full protection.

● Advise patient who wishes to become pregnant to wait at least 3 months after discontinuing norgestrel, to prevent birth defects.

Breast-feeding
Norgestrel is contraindicated in breast-feeding women.

nortriptyline hydrochloride
Aventyl, Pamelor

● Pharmacologic classification: tricyclic antidepressant
● Therapeutic classification: antidepressant
● Pregnancy risk category D

How supplied
Available by prescription only
Capsules: 10 mg, 25 mg, 50 mg, 75 mg
Solution: 10 mg/5 ml (4% alcohol)

Indications, route, and dosage
Depression, †panic disorder
Adults: 25 mg P.O. t.i.d. or q.i.d., gradually increasing to a maximum of 150 mg/day. Alternatively, entire dosage may be given h.s.

Pharmacodynamics
Antidepressant action: Nortriptyline is thought to exert its antidepressant effects by inhibiting reuptake of norepinephrine and serotonin in CNS nerve terminals (presynaptic neurons), which results in increased concentrations and enhanced activity of these neurotransmitters in the synaptic cleft. Nortriptyline inhibits reuptake of serotonin more actively than norepinephrine; it is less likely than other tricyclic antidepressants to cause orthostatic hypotension.

Pharmacokinetics
● *Absorption:* Nortriptyline is absorbed rapidly from the GI tract after oral administration.
● *Distribution:* Nortriptyline is distributed widely into the body, including the CNS and breast milk. Drug is 95% protein-bound. Peak plasma levels occur within 8 hours after a given dose; steady-state serum levels are achieved within 2 to 4 weeks. Therapeutic serum level ranges from 50 to 150 ng/ml.

● *Metabolism:* Nortriptyline is metabolized by the liver; a significant first-pass effect may account for variability of serum concentrations in different patients taking the same dosage.
● *Excretion:* Most of drug is excreted in urine; some is excreted in feces, via the biliary tract.

Contraindications and precautions
Nortriptyline is contraindicated in patients with known hypersensitivity to tricyclic antidepressants, trazodone, and related compounds; in the acute recovery phase of myocardial infarction (MI) because it can cause arrhythmias and depress cardiac function; in patients in coma or severe respiratory depression because of additive CNS depression; and during or within 14 days of therapy with monoamine oxidase inhibitors because this combination may cause excessive sympathetic stimulation with hypertensive crisis, high fevers, and seizures.

Nortriptyline should be used cautiously in patients with other cardiac disease (arrhythmias, congestive heart failure [CHF], angina pectoris, valvular disease, or heart block); in patients with respiratory disorders; in patients with alcoholism, epilepsy, and other seizure disorders because this drug may lower the seizure threshold; in patients receiving electroconvulsive therapy because of added risk of hypomania and delirium; in bipolar disease; in patients with glaucoma because drug may increase intraocular pressure, even in normal doses; in patients with hyperthyroidism or in those taking thyroid replacement; in patients with Type I and Type II diabetes; in patients with prostatic hypertrophy, paralytic ileus, or urinary retention because drug may worsen these conditions; in patients with hepatic or renal dysfunction because impaired metabolism and excretion may result in drug accumulation; in patients with Parkinson's disease; and in those undergoing surgery with general anesthesia.

Interactions
Concomitant use of nortriptyline with sympathomimetics, including epinephrine, phenylephrine, phenylpropanolamine, and ephedrine (often found in nasal sprays), may increase blood pressure; use with warfarin may increase prothrombin time and cause bleeding. Concomitant use with thyroid medication, pimozide, or antiarrhythmic agents (quinidine, disopyramide, procainamide) may increase incidence of cardiac arrhythmias and conduction defects.

Nortriptyline may decrease hypotensive effects of centrally acting antihypertensive drugs, such as guanethidine, guanabenz, guanadrel, clonidine, methyldopa, and reserpine.

Concomitant use with disulfiram or ethchlorvynol may cause delirium and tachycardia.

Additive effects are likely after concomitant use of nortriptyline with CNS depressants, including alcohol, analgesics, barbiturates, narcotics, tranquilizers, and anesthetics (oversedation); atropine and other anticholinergic drugs, including phenothiazines, antihistamines, meperidine, and antiparkinsonian agents (oversedation, paralytic ileus, visual changes, and severe constipation); and metrizamide (increased risk of convulsions).

Barbiturates and heavy smoking induce nortriptyline metabolism and decrease therapeutic efficacy; phenothiazines and haloperidol decrease its metabolism, decreasing therapeutic efficacy; methylphenidate, cimetidine, oral contraceptives, propoxyphene, and beta blockers may inhibit nortriptyline metabolism, increasing plasma levels and toxicity.

Effects on diagnostic tests
Nortriptyline may prolong conduction time (elongation of Q-T and PR intervals, flattened T waves on ECG); it also may elevate liver function test results, decrease white blood cell count, and decrease or increase serum glucose levels.

Adverse reactions
● CNS: drowsiness, dizziness, sedation, excitation, tremors, weakness, headache, nervousness, seizures, peripheral neuropathy, extrapyramidal symptoms, anxiety, vivid dreams, confusion (more marked in the elderly), decreased libido.
● CV: orthostatic hypotension, tachycardia, *arrhythmias, MI, stroke, heart block, CHF,* palpitations, hypertension, ECG changes.
● DERM: rash, urticaria, drug fever, edema.
● EENT: blurred vision, tinnitus, mydriasis, increased intraocular pressure.
● GI: dry mouth, constipation, nausea, vomiting, anorexia, diarrhea, paralytic ileus, jaundice.
● GU: urine retention.
● Other: sweating, photosensitivity, hypersensitivity (rash, urticaria, drug fever, edema).
    After abrupt withdrawal of long-term therapy, nausea, headache, and malaise may occur (does not indicate addiction).
    Note: Drug should be discontinued (not abruptly) if signs of hypersensitivity occur. Monitor for urine retention, extreme dry mouth, rash, excessive sedation, seizures, tachycardia, sore throat, fever, or jaundice.

Overdose and treatment
The first 12 hours after acute ingestion are a stimulatory phase characterized by excessive anticholinergic activity (agitation, irritation, confusion, hallucinations, hyperthermia, parkinsonian symptoms, seizures, urine retention, dry mucous membranes, pupillary dilation, constipation, and ileus). This is followed by CNS depressant effects, including hypothermia, decreased or absent reflexes, sedation, hypotension, cyanosis, and cardiac irregularities, including tachycardia, conduction disturbances, and quinidine-like effects on the ECG.
    Severity of overdose is best indicated by prolonging QRS complex beyond 100 ms, which usually indicates a serum level above 1,000 ng/ml. Metabolic acidosis may follow hypotension, hypoventilation, and convulsions.
    Treatment is symptomatic and supportive, including maintaining a patent airway, stable body temperature, and fluid and electrolyte balance. Induce emesis with ipecac syrup if patient is conscious; follow with gastric lavage and activated charcoal to prevent further absorption. Dialysis is usually ineffective. Treat seizures with parenteral diazepam or phenytoin; arrhythmias with parenteral phenytoin or lidocaine; and acidosis with sodium bicarbonate. *Do not give barbiturates;* these may enhance CNS and respiratory depressant effects.

▶ Special considerations
Besides those relevant to all *tricyclic antidepressants,* consider the following recommendations.
● Nortriptyline may be administered at bedtime to reduce daytime sedation. Tolerance to sedative effects usually develops over the initial weeks of therapy.
● Drug should be withdrawn gradually over a few weeks;

however, it should be discontinued at least 48 hours before surgical procedures.
● Drug is available in liquid forms.

Information for the patient
● Explain that patient may not see full effects of drug therapy for up to 4 weeks after start of therapy.
● Warn patient about sedative effects.
● Suggest taking full daily dose at bedtime to prevent daytime sedation.
● Tell patient not to drink alcoholic beverages, not to double doses after missing one, and not to discontinue the drug abruptly, except as instructed.
● Warn patient about possible dizziness. Tell patient to lie down for about 30 minutes after each dose at start of therapy and to avoid sudden postural changes, to avoid dizziness. Postural hypotension is usually less severe than with amitriptyline.
● Urge patient to report unusual reactions promptly: confusion, movement disorders, fainting, rapid heartbeat, or difficulty urinating.
● Tell patient to store drug away from children.

Geriatric use
Lower dosages may be indicated. Elderly patients are at greater risk for adverse cardiac effects.

Pediatric use
Not recommended for children. Lower dosages may be indicated for adolescents.

Breast-feeding
Nortriptyline is excreted in breast milk in low concentrations; potential benefit to woman should outweigh potential harm to infant.

---

novobiocin sodium
Albamycin

● Pharmacologic classification: polycyclic antibiotic
● Therapeutic classification: antibiotic
● Pregnancy risk category C

How supplied
Available by prescription only
Capsules: 250 mg

Indications, route, and dosage
Infections caused by sensitive Staphylococcus aureus *and* Proteus *when other antibiotics are contraindicated*
Adults: 250 mg P.O. q 6 hours or 500 mg P.O. q 12 hours. In severe infections, adults may receive 500 mg q 6 hours or 1 g q 12 hours. Maximum recommended dosage is 2 g/day.
Children: 15 to 45 mg/kg/day in divided doses q 6 to 12 hours.
    Therapy should be continued to 48 hours after resolution of symptoms.

Pharmacodynamics
Antibacterial action: Drug interferes with synthesis of the bacterial cell wall, protein, and nucleic acid, producing bacteriostatic effects on susceptible gram-positive bacteria and certain gram-negative bacteria. It is

---

currently used rarely because of the availability of less toxic alternatives.

Pharmacokinetics
• *Absorption:* Novobiocin is well absorbed, reaching peak levels in about 2 hours.
• *Distribution:* Novobiocin is distributed poorly into pleural, ascitic, and joint fluid but tends to concentrate in biliary fluid. It does not distribute into CSF well, even in patients with inflamed meninges. More than 90% is bound to plasma proteins.
• *Metabolism:* Novobiocin's metabolism is unknown.
• *Excretion:* Novobiocin is excreted mainly in bile and feces.

Contraindications and precautions
Novobiocin is contraindicated in infants and in patients with known hypersensitivity to drug.

Novobiocin should be administered cautiously to patients with a history of drug allergies, to patients with hepatic disease, and to patients with blood disorders, because drug may exacerbate these symptoms or disorders.

Interactions
None reported.

Effects on diagnostic tests
A yellow-colored metabolite of novobiocin interferes with Evelyn-Malloy method of serum bilirubin determination. Serum enzyme levels in liver function tests increase and blood elements decrease during novobiocin therapy (however, eosinophil levels increase).

Adverse reactions
• DERM: rash.
• GI: jaundice, nausea, vomiting, diarrhea.
• HEMA: leukopenia, eosinophilia, anemia, thrombocytopenia.
• Other: alopecia, hypersensitivity (common), fever.
  Note: Drug should be discontinued if patient develops signs or symptoms of blood dyscrasias, such as rash, fever, jaundice, or GI distress.

Overdose and treatment
No information available.

▶ Special considerations
• Obtain culture and sensitivity tests before starting therapy.
• Monitor liver function tests (serum glutamic-oxaloacetic transaminase [SGOT], serum glutamic-pyruvic transaminase [SGPT], bilirubin, and serum alkaline phosphatase levels) and hematologic tests (complete blood count, platelet count, and reticulocyte count) before and during therapy.

Information for the patient
• Instruct patient to take drug on an empty stomach, 1 hour before or 2 hours after meals, with a full glass of water.
• Caution patient to continue taking drug as directed, even if he feels better.
• Tell patient to report symptoms of blood dyscrasias, such as rash, fever, jaundice, or GI distress.

Pediatric use
Novobiocin should not be used in term or premature neonates because it may adversely affect bilirubin levels.

Breast-feeding
Because drug is excreted into breast milk, alternative feeding method is recommended during novobiocin therapy.

---

nylidrin hydrochloride
Arlidin

• Pharmacologic classification: beta-adrenergic agonist
• Therapeutic classification: peripheral vasodilator
• Pregnancy risk category C

How supplied
Available by prescription only
Tablets: 6 mg, 12 mg

Indications, route, and dosage
Peripheral vascular disorders
Indications include arteriosclerosis obliterans, thromboangiitis obliterans, diabetic vascular disease, night leg cramps, Raynaud's phenomenon and disease, ischemic ulcer, frostbite, acrocyanosis, acroparesthesia, and sequelae of thrombophlebitis.
Circulatory disturbances of the middle ear
Indications include primary cochlear ischemia, cochlear striae, vascular ischemia, and macular or ampullar ischemia; and in other circulatory disturbances from labyrinth artery spasm or obstruction.
Adults: 3 to 12 mg P.O. t.i.d. or q.i.d.

Pharmacodynamics
Vasodilating action: Nylidrin dilates arterioles in skeletal muscle by beta-adrenergic stimulation; drug may also act directly to relax vascular smooth muscle. Nylidrin also increases cerebral blood flow.

Pharmacokinetics
• *Absorption:* Nylidrin is absorbed readily from the GI tract. Action begins in about 10 minutes, peaks in 30 minutes, and lasts for 2 hours.
• *Distribution:* Unknown.
• *Metabolism:* Unknown.
• *Excretion:* Nylidrin is excreted in urine.

Contraindications and precautions
Nylidrin is contraindicated in patients with acute myocardial infarction (AMI), paroxysmal tachycardia, progressive angina pectoris, or thyrotoxicosis because the drug may exacerbate these disorders. In AMI, drug may have a "steal effect"; that is, a further decrease in blood flow to ischemic areas may occur because the drug has a greater dilating effect on peripheral blood vessels than on coronary vessels.

Use nylidrin cautiously in patients with decompensated heart disease; in patients with peptic ulcer because the drug increases gastric acid secretion; and in pregnant women because increased blood glucose levels have been reported in pregnant women (espe-

---

cially diabetic women) receiving nylidrin during the last trimester.

The efficacy of nylidrin and other vasodilators in the treatment of peripheral vascular disease, circulatory disturbances of the inner ear, and cerebrovascular disorders has not been established.

Interactions
None significant.

Effects on diagnostic tests
None reported.

Adverse reactions
● CNS: trembling, nervousness, weakness, dizziness unrelated to labyrinth artery insufficiency.
● CV: palpitations, hypotension, flushing, tachycardia, postural hypotension.
● GI: nausea, vomiting.
● Other: chilliness, anemia.

Overdose and treatment
Clinical signs of overdose include transient headache, flushing, dyspnea, palpitations, tachycardia, transient absence of diastolic blood pressure, and transient non-radiating chest pain. The lethal dose of nylidrin is estimated to be 2 g in adults and 200 mg in children under age 2. Blood pressure may increase noticeably, followed by hypotension accompanied by inability to urinate. Nausea, vomiting, fever, chills, cyanosis, restlessness, tremors, confusion, metallic taste, blurred vision, convulsions, coma, respiratory failure, and circulatory collapse may also occur.

Treatment is supportive and symptomatic; emesis, gastric lavage, and activated charcoal may help in recent ingestion.

▶ Special considerations
Nylidrin increases heart rate and cardiac output; it also increases gastric juice volume and gastric acid secretion.

Information for the patient
● Tell patient to avoid sudden postural changes to minimize effects of orthostatic hypotension.
● Warn patient to avoid tasks requiring alertness.

Breast-feeding
Safety has not been established.

---

nystatin
Korostatin, Mycostatin, Mykinac, Nilstat, Nystex, O-V Statin

● Pharmacologic classification: polyene macrolide
● Therapeutic classification: antifungal
● Pregnancy risk category B

How supplied
Available by prescription only
Tablets: 500,000 units
Suspension: 100,000 units/ml
Vaginal suppositories: 100,000 units
Cream: 100,000 units/g
Ointment: 100,000 units/g

Powder: 100,000 units/g

Indications, route, and dosage
Gastrointestinal infections
Adults: 500,000 to 1 million units as oral tablets, t.i.d.
Oral, vaginal, and intestinal infections caused by susceptible organisms
Adults: 400,000 to 600,000 units of oral suspension q.i.d. for oral candidiasis.
Children and infants over age 3 months: 250,000 to 500,000 units of oral suspension q.i.d.
Newborn and premature infants: 100,000 units of oral suspension q.i.d.
Cutaneous or mucocutaneous candidal infections
Topical use: Apply to affected areas two or three times daily until healing is complete.
Vaginal use: 100,000 units, as vaginal tablets, inserted high into vagina daily or b.i.d. for 14 days.

Pharmacodynamics
Antifungal action: Nystatin is both fungistatic and fungicidal. It binds to sterols in the fungal cell membrane, altering its permeability and allowing leakage of intracellular components. It acts against various yeasts and fungi, including Candida albicans.

Pharmacokinetics
● Absorption: Nystatin is not absorbed from the GI tract, nor through the intact skin or mucous membranes.
● Distribution: No detectable amount of the drug is available for tissue distribution.
● Metabolism: No detectable amount of drug is systemically available for metabolism.
● Excretion: Oral nystatin is excreted almost entirely unchanged in feces.

Contraindications and precautions
Nystatin is contraindicated in patients with known hypersensitivity to the drug.

Interactions
None reported.

Effects on diagnostic tests
None reported.

Adverse reactions
● GI: transient nausea, vomiting, diarrhea (usually with large oral dosage).
Note: Drug should be discontinued if skin irritation or signs of toxicity occur.

Overdose and treatment
Nystatin overdose may result in nausea, vomiting, and diarrhea. Treatment is unnecessary because toxicity is negligible.

▶ Special considerations
● Vaginal tablets may be used by pregnant women up to 6 weeks before term.
● Avoid hand contact with drug; hypersensitivity is rare but can occur.
● For treatment of oral candidiasis, patient should have clean mouth, and should hold suspension in mouth for several minutes before swallowing; for infant thrush, medication should be swabbed on oral mucosa.
● Immunosuppressed patient may be given vaginal tablets (100,000 units) by mouth to provide prolonged drug

contact with oral mucosa; alternatively, use clotrimazole troche.
● For candidiasis of the feet, patient should dust powder on shoes and stockings as well as feet for maximal contact and effectiveness.
● Avoid occlusive dressings or ointment on moist covered body areas that favor yeast growth.
● To prevent maceration, use cream on intertriginous areas, and powder on moist lesions.
● Cleanse affected skin gently before topical application; cool, moist compresses applied for 15 minutes between applications help soothe and dry skin.
● Cleansing douches may be used by nonpregnant women for aesthetic reasons; they should use preparations that do not contain antibacterials, which may alter flora and promote reinfection.
● Protect drug from light, air, and heat.
● Nystatin is ineffective in systemic fungal infection.

Information for the patient
● Teach patient signs and symptoms of candidal infection. Inform patient about predisposing agents: use of antibiotics, oral contraceptives, and corticosteroids; diabetes; infected sexual partners; and tight-fitting pantyhose and undergarments.
● Teach good oral hygiene. Explain that overuse of mouthwash and poorly fitting dentures, especially in elderly patients, may alter flora and promote infection.
● Tell patient to continue using vaginal cream through menstruation; emphasize importance of washing applicator thoroughly after each use.
● Advise patient to change stockings and undergarments daily; teach good skin care.
● Teach patient how to administer each dosage form prescribed.
● Tell patient to continue drug for 1 to 2 weeks after symptoms clear, to prevent reinfection.

Breast-feeding
Safety has not been established.

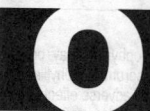

octreotide acetate
Sandostatin

- Pharmacologic classification: synthetic octapeptide
- Therapeutic classification: somatotropic hormone
- Pregnancy risk category B

How supplied
Available by prescription only
Injection: 0.05 mg, 0.1 mg, 0.5 mg

Indications, route, and dosage
Symptomatic treatment of flushing and diarrhea associated with carcinoid tumors
Adults: Initially, 100 to 600 mcg daily S.C. in two to four divided doses for the first 2 weeks of therapy (usual daily dosage is 300 mcg). Subsequent dosage is based on individual response.
Symptomatic treatment of watery diarrhea associated with Vasoactive Intestinal Peptide-secreting tumors (VIPomas)
Adults: Initially, 200 to 300 mcg daily S.C. in two to four divided doses for the first 2 weeks of therapy. Subsequent dosage is based on individual response, but usually will not exceed 450 mcg daily.

Pharmacodynamics
Antidiarrheal action: Octreotide mimics the action of naturally occurring somatostatin and decreases the secretion of gastroenterohepatic peptides that may contribute to the adverse signs and symptoms seen in patients with metastatic carcinoid tumors and VIPomas. It is not known if the drug affects the tumor directly.

Pharmacokinetics
- *Absorption:* Octreotide is absorbed rapidly and completely after injection. Peak plasma levels occur in less than 30 minutes.
- *Distribution:* Drug is distributed to the plasma, where it binds to serum lipoprotein and albumin.
- *Metabolism:* Eliminated from the plasma at a slower rate than the naturally occuring hormone. Apparent half-life is about 1.5 hours, with a duration of effect of up to 12 hours.
- *Excretion:* About 35% of the drug appears unchanged in the urine.

Contraindications and precautions
Octreotide is contraindicated in patients allergic to the drug or any of its components.

Octreotide therapy may be associated with the development of cholelithiasis by altering gallbladder motility or fat absorption. Monitor patient regularly for gallbladder disease.

Interactions
Octreotide may decrease plasma levels of cyclosporine. Concomitant use with insulin, oral hypoglycemics (sulfonylureas), or oral diazoxide may require dosage adjustments during therapy. Use with octreotide may require dosage adjustment of other drugs used to control symptoms of the disease (such as beta blockers).

Effects on diagnostic tests
Octreotide suppresses secretion of growth hormone and of the gastroenterohepatic peptides gastrin, vasoactive intestinal peptide (VIP), insulin, glucagon, secretin, motilin, and pancreatic polypeptide.

Adverse reactions
- CNS: dizziness, light-headedness, fatigue, headache.
- DERM: flushing; edema; wheal, erythema, or pain at injection site.
- GI: nausea, diarrhea, abdominal pain or discomfort, loose stools, vomiting, fat malabsorption.
- Metabolic: hyperglycemia, hypoglycemia, hypothyroidism.

Overdose and treatment
Doses of 1,000 mcg have been administered as an I.V. bolus in volunteers without adverse effects. The drug may produce metabolic changes in certain patients.

▶ Special considerations
- Fluid and electrolyte balance may be altered after initiation of octreotide therapy.
- Half-life may be altered in patients with end-stage renal failure who are undergoing dialysis. Dosage adjustment may be necessary.
- Baseline and periodic tests of thyroid function are advised because the drug's long-term effects on hypothalamic-pituitary function are not known.
- Laboratory values that are frequently monitored during therapy include urinary 5-hydroxyindoleacetic acid (5-HIAA), plasma serotonin, plasma substance P for carcinoid tumors, and plasma VIP for VIPomas.
- Mild, transient hypoglycemia or hyperglycemia may be seen during octreotide therapy. Observe patient for signs of glucose imbalance and monitor closely during therapy.
- Octreotide may alter fat absorption and aggravate fat malabsorption. Periodic assessment of 72-hour fecal fat and serum carotene is recommended.

Information for the patient
Because the drug may cause gallstones, tell patient to report any abdominal discomfort promptly.

Pediatric use
Doses of 1 to 10 mcg/kg appear to be well-tolerated in children.

Breast-feeding
Safety has not been established. It is not known if the drug is excreted in breast milk.

---

ofloxacin
Floxin

- Pharmacologic classification: fluoroquin-
olone
- Therapeutic classification: antibiotic
- Pregnancy risk category C

How supplied
Available by prescription only
Tablets: 200 mg, 300 mg, 400 mg
Injection: 200 mg in 50 ml dextrose 5% in water; 400
mg in water for injection in 10 and 20 ml single use
vials; 400 mg in 100 ml dextrose 5% in water.

Indications, route, and dosage
*Acute bacterial exacerbations of chronic
bronchitis and pneumonia caused by susceptible organisms*
Adults: 400 mg P.O. or I.V. q 12 hours for 10 days.
*Sexually transmitted diseases, such as acute
uncomplicated urethral and cervical gonorrhea, nongonococcal urethritis and cervicitis,
and mixed infections of urethra and cervix*
Adults: Acute uncomplicated gonorrhea – 400 mg P.O.
or I.V. once as a single dose; cervicitis and urethritis –
300 mg P.O. or I.V. q 12 hours for 7 days.
*Mild to moderate skin and skin-structure in-
fections*
Adults: 400 mg P.O. or I.V. q 12 hours for 10 days.
Urinary tract infections
Adults: Cystitis caused by *Escherichia coli* or *Klebsiella
pneumoniae* – 200 mg P.O. or I.V. q 12 hours for 3 days;
cystitis caused by other organisms – 200 mg P.O. or
I.V. q 12 hours for 7 days.
Complicated urinary tract infections
Adults: 20 mg P.O. or I.V. q 12 hours for 10 days.
Prostatitis
Adults: 300 mg P.O. or I.V. q 12 hours for 6 weeks.

Pharmacodynamics
Antibacterial action: Ofloxacin interferes with DNA gyrase, which is needed for synthesis of bacterial DNA.

Pharmacokinetics
- *Absorption:* Ofloxacin is well absorbed after oral administration, with maximum serum concentrations
achieved within 1 to 2 hours. Because the oral bioavailability is about 98%, the oral and I.V. dosage is the
same.
- *Distribution:* Widely distributed to body tissues and
fluids.
- *Metabolism:* Pyridobenzoxazine ring decreases extent of metabolism in liver.
- *Excretion:* 70% to 80% is excreted unchanged in
urine; less than 5%, in feces.

Contraindications and precautions
Contraindicated in patients with a history of or known
sensitivity to quinolone antibiotics (including ciprofloxacin, cinoxacin, nalidixic acid, and norfloxacin). Use
with caution in patients with known or suspected CNS
disorders, such as cerebral arteriosclerosis, seizure
disorders, or other factors that predispose to seizures
because seizures have been linked with the use of other
quinolone derivatives.

Interactions
Concomitant therapy with theophylline may prolong
theophylline half-life, increase serum theophylline levels, and risk theophylline-related adverse effects. Monitor closely and adjust theophylline dosage as needed.
Concomitant administration with antacids interferes with
GI absorption of ofloxacin, resulting in decreased serum
levels; separate administration by 2 to 4 hours.

Adverse reactions
- CNS: insomnia, headache, dizziness, asthenia, mal-
aise, anxiety, fatigue, sleep disorders, nervousness,
syncope, vertigo.
- CV: edema, hypertension, palpitations, vasodilation.
- GI: nausea, diarrhea, weight loss, dyspepsia, con-
stipation, dry mouth.
- GU: urinary frequency, external genital pruritus in
femals, vaginitis, vaginal discharge.
- Respiratory: cough, rhinorrhea.
- Other: arthralgia, myalgia, pruritus, rash.

Overdose and treatment
In case of overdose, empty the stomach and maintain
hydration. Observe patient and treat symptomatically.

▶ Special considerations
- Adjust dosage in patients with creatinine clearance
of 50 ml/minute or less. Give initial dose as recommended, additional doses as follows: if creatinine clearance is above 50 ml/minute, no dosage adjustment at
12-hour intervals; if 10 to 50 ml/minute, no dosage adjustment at 24-hour intervals; if below 10 ml/minute,
50% of recommended dose q 24 hours.
- Periodic assessment of organ system functions is
recommended during prolonged therapy.
- Give I.V. ofloxacin by slow infusion only; do not give
I.M., S.C., intrathecally, or by intraperitoneal injection.
Administer over at least 60 minutes and avoid rapid or
bolus injection. Compatible with most common I.V. solutions, including dextrose 5% in water injection, 0.9%
sodium chloride injection, dextrose 5% in 0.9% sodium
chloride injection, dextrose 5% in 0.45% sodium chloride injection, 5% dextrose in lactated Ringer's solution,
and 5% sodium bicarbonate injection.
- Ofloxacin is not recommended for syphilis.

Information for the patient
- Advise patient to drink fluids liberally.
- Advise patient to separate doses of antacids, vitamins, and ofloxacin by 2 hours.
- Advise patient to take on an empty stomach one-half
hour before or 2 hours after meals.
- Tell patient dizziness and light-headedness may occur. Advise caution when driving or operating hazardous machinery until effects of drug are known.
- Warn patient that hypersensitivity reactions may follow first dose; patient should discontinue at first sign
of skin rash or other allergic reaction and notify physician immediately.
- Because photosensitivity reactions have occurred,
advise patient to avoid prolonged exposure to direct
sunlight and to use a sunscreen when outdoors.

Pediatric use
Safety and efficacy in children and adolescents under
age 18 have not been established. Similar drugs have
caused arthropathy in juvenile animals.

Breast-feeding
Safety has not been established. Ofloxacin is excreted in breast milk in levels similar to those found in plasma.

---

olsalazine sodium
Dipentum

- Pharmacologic classification: salicylate
- Therapeutic classification: anti-inflammatory
- Pregnancy risk category C

How supplied
Available by prescription only
Capsules: 250 mg

Indications, route, and dosage
Maintenance of remission of ulcerative colitis in patients intolerant of sulfasalazine
Adults: 1 g P.O. daily in two divided doses.

Pharmacodynamics
Anti-inflammatory action: The mechanism of action is unknown but appears to be topical rather than systemic. Olsalazine is converted to mesalamine (5-aminosalicylic acid; 5-ASA) in the colon. Presumably, mesalamine diminishes inflammation by blocking cyclooxygenase and inhibiting prostaglandin production in the colon.

Pharmacokinetics
- *Absorption:* After oral administration, approximately 2.4% of a single dose is absorbed; maximum concentrations appear in about 2 hours.
- *Distribution:* Liberated mesalamine is absorbed slowly from the colon, resulting in very high local concentrations.
- *Metabolism:* 0.1% is metabolized in the liver; remainder will reach the colon, where it is rapidly converted to mesalamine by colonic bacteria.
- *Excretion:* Less than 1% is recovered in urine.

Contraindications and precautions
Olsalazine is contraindicated in patients with known hypersensitivity to salicylates.

Interactions
None reported.

Adverse reactions
- CNS: headache, fatigue, drowsiness, lethargy, depression, vertigo, dizziness, insomnia, paresthesia.
- DERM: rash, itching.
- EENT: dry eyes, blurred vision.
- GI: diarrhea, abdominal pain, cramps, nausea, dyspepsia, bloating, anorexia, vomiting, stomatitis, blood in stool, dry mouth.
- Other: elevated AST (SGOT) and ALT (SGPT), muscle cramps, peripheral edema, photosensitivity.

Overdose and treatment
Decreased motor activity and diarrhea can occur. Treat overdosage symptomatically and supportively.

▶ Special considerations
- Diarrhea was noted in 17% of patients, but it is difficult to distinguish from underlying condition.
- Monitor CBC with differential and liver function tests periodically.

Information for the patient
- Advise patient to take drug with food and in evenly divided doses.
- Advise patient to contact physician if diarrhea develops.

Pediatric use
Safety and efficacy have not been established.

Breast-feeding
It is unknown if olsalazine is excreted in breast milk. Use with caution.

---

omeprazole
Prilosec

- Pharmacologic classification: substituted benzimidazole
- Therapeutic classification: gastric acid suppressant
- Pregnancy risk category C

How supplied
Available by prescription only
Capsules (delayed-release): 20 mg

Indications, route, and dosage
Severe erosive esophagitis; symptomatic, poorly responsive gastroesophageal reflux disease (GERD)
Adults: 20 mg P.O. daily for 4 to 8 weeks. Patients with GERD should have failed initial therapy with a histamine$_2$ antagonist.
Pathological hypersecretory conditions (such as Zollinger-Ellison syndrome)
Adults: Initial dosage is 60 mg P.O. daily, with dosage titrated according to patient response. Daily dosages exceeding 80 mg should be administered in divided doses. Doses up to 120 mg t.i.d. have been administered. Therapy should continue as long as clinically indicated.

Pharmacodynamics
Antisecretory action: Omeprazole inhibits the activity of the acid (proton) pump, H^+/K^+ adenosine triphosphatase (ATPase), located at the secretory surface of the gastric parietal cell. This blocks the formation of gastric acid.

Pharmacokinetics
- *Absorption:* Omeprazole is acid-labile, and the formulation contains enteric-coated granules that permit absorption after the drug leaves the stomach. Absorption is rapid, with peak levels occurring in less than 3.5 hours. Bioavailability is about 40% because of instability in gastric acid as well as a substantial first-pass effect. Bioavailability increases slightly with repeated dosing, possibly because of the drug's effect on gastric acidity.
- *Distribution:* Protein binding is about 95%.

● *Metabolism:* Metabolism is primarily hepatic.
● *Excretion:* Primarily renal. Plasma half-life is 0.5 to 1 hour, but drug effects may persist for days.

Contraindications and precautions
Omeprazole is contraindicated in patients hypersensitive to the drug or any component of the enteric formulation. Prolonged (2-year) studies in rats revealed a dose-related increase in gastric carcinoid tumors; studies in humans have not detected a risk from short-term exposure to the drug. Further study is needed to assess the impact of sustained hypergastrinemia and hypochlorhydria. The manufacturer recommends that duration of omeprazole therapy not exceed the recommended period.

Interactions
Elimination of drugs metabolized by hepatic oxidation, including diazepam, warfarin, and phenytoin, may be impaired by omeprazole. Patients taking these drugs or others that are metabolized by the hepatic microsomal enzyme system (including propranolol and theophylline) should be monitored closely.
Drugs that depend on low gastric pH for absorption (including ketoconazole, iron derivatives, and ampicillin esters) may exhibit poor bioavailability in patients taking omeprazole.

Effects on diagnostic tests
Serum gastrin levels rise in most patients during the first 2 weeks of therapy.

Adverse reactions
● CNS: headache, dizziness.
● DERM: rash.
● GI: diarrhea, abdominal pain, nausea, vomiting, constipation, flatulence, increased liver enzyme levels.
● HEMA: *agranulocytosis, pancytopenia.*
● Respiratory: cough.
● Other: back pain, muscle cramps.

Overdose and treatment
There has been no experience with overdose. Dosages up to 360 mg daily have been well-tolerated. Dialysis is believed to be of little value because of the extent of binding to plasma proteins. Treatment should be symptomatic and supportive.

▶ Special considerations
● Omeprazole increases its own bioavailability with repeated administration. The drug is labile in gastric acid, and less of the drug is lost to hydrolysis as the drug raises gastric pH.
● Dosage adjustments are not required for patients with renal or hepatic impairment.
● Capsule should not be crushed.

Information for the patient
● Explain the importance of taking the drug exactly as prescribed.
● Take before meals and do not crush the capsule.

Pediatric use
Safe use in children has not been established.

Breast-feeding
It is not known if omeprazole is excreted in breast milk. Animal studies have shown decreased weight gain in pups receiving milk from females fed high doses of omeprazole.

---

ondansetron hydrochloride
Zofran

● Pharmacologic classification: serotonin (5-HT₃) receptor antagonist
● Therapeutic classification: antiemetic
● Pregnancy risk category B

How supplied
Available by prescription only
Injection: 2 mg/ml in 20-ml multidose vials

Indications, route, and dosage
Prevention of nausea and vomiting associated with initial and repeat courses of emetogenic cancer chemotherapy, including high-dose cisplatin
Adults and children ages 4 to 18: Three I.V. doses of 0.15 mg/kg with first dose infused over 15 minutes beginning 30 minutes before start of chemotherapy. Subsequent doses are administered 4 and 8 hours after the first dose.

Pharmacodynamics
Antiemetic action: The mechanism of action is not fully defined; however, ondansetron is *not* a dopamine-receptor antagonist. Because serotonin receptors of the 5-HT₃ type are present both peripherally on vagal nerve terminals and centrally in the chemoreceptor trigger zone, it is not certain if ondansetron's antiemetic action is mediated centrally, peripherally, or in both sites.

Pharmacokinetics
● *Absorption:* Ondansetron is administered I.V.
● *Distribution:* 70% to 76% is plasma protein-bound.
● *Metabolism:* Extensively metabolized by hydroxylation on the indole ring, followed by glucuronide or sulfate conjugation.
● *Excretion:* 5% of dose is recovered in urine as parent compound.

Contraindications and precautions
Ondansetron is contraindicated in patients with known hypersensitivity to the drug. Use with caution in patients with hepatic impairment.

Interactions
Ondansetron is metabolized by cytochrome P-450; thus, inducers or inhibitors of this enzyme may change clearance and half-life of ondansetron; however, no dosage adjustment is required. Cisplatin, carmustine, and etoposide do not affect ondansetron's pharmacokinetics.

Adverse reactions
● CNS: headache, akathisia, acute dystonic reactions, generalized seizures (rare).
● CV: tachycardia (rare), angina (rare), ECG alterations (rare).
● GI: diarrhea, constipation.
● Other: rash; bronchospasm, hypokalemia (rare).

Overdose and treatment
Doses more than 10 times the recommended dose have been given without incident. There is no recommended antidote. If overdose is suspected, manage with supportive therapy.

▶ Special considerations
Ondansetron is stable at room temperature for 48 hours after dilution with 0.9% sodium chloride, dextrose 5% in water, 5% dextrose and 0.9% sodium chloride, 5% dextrose and 0.45% sodium chloride, or 3% sodium chloride.

Geriatric use
No age-related problems have been reported.

Pediatric use
Little information is available for use in children age 3 and under.

Breast-feeding
It is unknown if drug is excreted in breast milk; caution is recommended.

PHARMACOLOGIC CLASS

opioids

alfentanil hydrochloride
codeine phosphate
codeine sulfate
difenoxin
diphenoxylate
fentanyl citrate
hydromorphone hydrochloride
levorphanol tartrate
meperidine hydrochloride
methadone hydrochloride
morphine sulfate
oxycodone hydrochloride
oxymorphone hydrochloride
propoxyphene hydrochloride
propoxyphene napsylate
sufentanil citrate

Opioids, previously called narcotic agonists, are usually understood to include natural and semisynthetic alkaloid derivatives from opium and their synthetic surrogates, whose actions mimic those of morphine. Except for propoxyphene, which is Schedule IV, these drugs are classified as Schedule II by the federal Drug Enforcement Agency, because they have a high potential for addiction and abuse. Until relatively recently, opioids were used indiscriminately for analgesia and sedation and to control diarrhea and cough.

Pharmacology
Opioids act as agonists at specific opiate receptor binding sites in the CNS and other tissues; these are the same receptors occupied by endogenous opioid peptides (enkephalins and endorphins) to alter CNS response to painful stimuli. Opiate agonists do not alter the cause of pain, but only the patient's perception of the pain; they relieve pain without affecting other sensory functions. Opiate receptors are present in highest concentrations in the limbic system, thalamus, striatum, hypothalamus, midbrain, and spinal cord.

Opioids produce respiratory depression by a direct effect on the respiratory centers in the brain stem, resulting in decreased sensitivity and responsiveness to increases in carbon dioxide tension. These drugs' antitussive effects are mediated by a direct suppression of the cough reflex center. They cause nausea, probably by stimulation of the chemoreceptor trigger zone in the medulla oblongata; through orthostatic hypotension, which causes dizziness; and possibly by increasing vestibular sensitivity.

Opioids also cause drowsiness, sedation, euphoria, dysphoria, mental clouding, and EEG changes; higher than usual analgesic doses cause anesthesia. Most opioids cause miosis, although meperidine and its derivatives may also cause mydriasis, or no pupillary change.

Because opioids decrease gastric, biliary, and pancreatic secretions and delay digestion, constipation is a common adverse reaction. At the same time, these drugs increase tone in the biliary tract and may cause biliary spasms. Some patients may have no biliary effects, while others may have biliary spasms that increase plasma amylase and lipase levels up to 15 times the normal values.

Opioids increase smooth muscle tone in the urinary tract and induce spasms, causing urinary urgency. These drugs have little cardiovascular effect in a supine patient, but may cause orthostatic hypotension when the patient assumes upright posture. These drugs are also associated with manifestations of histamine release or peripheral vasodilation, including pruritus, flushing, red eyes, and sweating. These effects are often mistakenly attributed to allergy and should be evaluated carefully.

The opiates can be divided chemically into four groups: phenanthrenes (codeine, hydrocodone, hydromorphone, morphine, oxycodone, and oxymorphone); phenylheptylamines (methadone and propoxyphene); phenylpiperidines (alfentanil, diphenoxylate, fentanyl, meperidine, and sufentanil); and morphinans (levorphanol). If a patient is hypersensitive to an opioid, agonist-antagonist, or antagonist of a given chemical group, use extreme caution in considering the use of another agent from the same chemical group; however, a drug from the other groups might be well tolerated.

Some of the opioids are well absorbed after oral or rectal administration; others must be administered parenterally. Intravenous dosing is the most rapidly effective and reliable; absorption after I.M. or S.C. dosing may be erratic. Opioids vary in onset and duration of action; they are removed rapidly from the bloodstream and distributed, in decreasing order of concentration, into skeletal muscle, kidneys, liver, intestinal tract, lungs, spleen, and brain; they readily cross the placenta.

Opioids are metabolized mainly in the microsomes in the endoplasmic reticulum of the liver (first-pass effect) and also in the CNS, kidneys, lungs, and placenta. They undergo conjugation with glucuronic acid, hydrolysis, oxidation, or N-dealkylation. They are excreted primarily in the urine; small amounts are excreted in the feces.

Clinical indications and actions
The opioids produce varying degrees of analgesia and have antitussive, antidiarrheal, and sedative effects. Clinical response is dose-related and varies with each patient.
Analgesia
Opioids may be used in the symptomatic management of moderate to severe pain associated with acute and

---

some chronic disorders, including renal or biliary colic, myocardial infarction, acute trauma, postoperative pain, or terminal cancer. They also may be used to provide analgesia during diagnostic and orthopedic procedures and during labor. Drug selection, route of administration, and dosage depend on a variety of factors. For example, in mild pain, oral therapy with codeine or oxycodone usually suffices. In acute pain of known short duration, such as that associated with diagnostic procedures or orthopedic manipulation, a short-acting drug such as meperidine, or fentanyl is effective. These drugs are often given to alleviate postoperative pain, but because they influence CNS function require special care to monitor the course of recovery and to detect early signs of complications. Opioids are commonly used to manage severe, chronic pain associated with terminal cancer; this requires careful evaluation and titration of drug used and dosage and route of administration.

Pulmonary edema
Morphine, meperidine, oxymorphone, hydromorphone, and other similar drugs have been used to relieve anxiety in patients with dyspnea associated with acute pulmonary edema and acute left ventricular failure. These drugs should not be used to treat pulmonary edema resulting from a chemical respiratory stimulant. Opioids decrease peripheral resistance, causing pooling of blood in the extremities and decreased venous return, cardiac work load, and pulmonary venous pressure; blood is thus shifted from the central to the peripheral circulation.

Preoperative sedation
Routine use of opioids for preoperative sedation in patients without pain is not recommended, because it may cause complications during and after surgery. To allay preoperative anxiety, a barbiturate or benzodiazepine is equally effective, with a lower incidence of postoperative vomiting.

Anesthesia
Certain opioids, including alfentanil, fentanyl, and sufentanil, may be used for induction of anesthesia, as an adjunct in the maintenance of general and regional anesthesia, or as a primary anesthetic agent in surgery.

Cough suppression
Some opioids, most commonly codeine and its derivative, hydrocodone, are used as antitussives to relieve dry, nonproductive cough.

Diarrhea
Diphenoxylate and other opioids are used as antidiarrheal agents. All opioids cause constipation to some degree; however, only a few are indicated for this use. Usually, opiate antidiarrheals are empirically combined with antacids, absorbing agents, and belladonna alkaloids in commercial preparations.

Overview of adverse reactions
Respiratory depression and, to a lesser extent, circulatory depression (including orthostatic hypotension) are the major hazards of treatment with opioids. Rapid I.V. administration increases the incidence and severity of these serious adverse effects. Respiratory arrest, shock, and cardiac arrest have occurred. It is likely that equianalgesic doses of individual opiates produce a comparable degree of respiratory depression, but its duration may vary. Other adverse CNS effects include dizziness, visual disturbances, mental clouding or depression, sedation, coma, euphoria, dysphoria, weakness, faintness, agitation, restlessness, nervousness, seizures, and, rarely, delirium and insomnia. Adverse effects seem to be more prevalent in ambulatory patients and those not experiencing severe pain. Adverse GI effects include nausea, vomiting, and constipation, as well as increased biliary tract pressure that may result in biliary spasm or colic. Tolerance, psychological dependence, and physical dependence (addiction) may follow prolonged, high-dose therapy (more than 100 mg of morphine daily for more than 1 month).

Use opiate agonists with extreme caution during pregnancy and labor, because they readily cross the placenta. Premature infants appear especially sensitive to their respiratory and CNS depressant effects when used during delivery.

Opiate agonists have a high potential for addiction and should always be administered with caution in patients prone to physical or psychic dependence. The agonist-antagonists have a lower potential for addiction and abuse, but the liability still exists.

▶ Special considerations
● Administer with extreme caution to patients with head injury, increased intracranial pressure, seizures, asthma, chronic obstructive pulmonary disease, alcoholism, prostatic hypertrophy, severe hepatic or renal disease, acute abdominal conditions, cardiac arrhythmias, hypovolemia, or psychiatric disorders, and to elderly or debilitated patients. Reduced doses may be necessary.
● Consider possible interactions with other drugs the patient is taking.
● Keep resuscitative equipment and a narcotic antagonist (naloxone) available. Be prepared to provide support of ventilation and gastric lavage.
● Parenteral administration of opiates provides better analgesia than oral administration. Intravenous administration should be given by slow injection, preferably in diluted solution. Rapid I.V. injection increases the incidence of adverse effects.
● Parenteral injections by I.M. or S.C. route should be given cautiously to patients who are chilled, hypovolemic, or in shock, because decreased perfusion may lead to accumulation of the drug and toxic effects. Rotate I.M. or S.C. injection sites to avoid induration.
● Before administration, visually inspect all parenteral products for particulate matter and discoloration.
● Oral solutions of varying concentrations are available. Carefully note the strength of the solution.
● A regular dosage schedule (rather than "p.r.n. pain") is preferred to alleviate the symptoms and anxiety that accompany pain.
● The duration of respiratory depression may be longer than the analgesic effect. Monitor the patient closely with repeated dosing.
● With chronic administration, evaluate the patient's respiratory status before each dose. Because severe respiratory depression may occur (especially with accumulation from chronic dosing), watch for respiratory rate below the patient's baseline level. Evaluate the patient for restlessness, which may be a sign of compensatory response for hypoxia.
● Opiates or agonist-antagonists may cause orthostatic hypotension in ambulatory patients. Have the patient sit or lie down to relieve dizziness or fainting.
● Since opiates depress respiration when they are used postoperatively, encourage patient turning, coughing, and deep breathing to avoid atelectases.
● If gastric irritation occurs, give oral products with food; food delays absorption and onset of analgesia.
● Opiates may obscure the signs and symptoms of an acute abdominal condition or worsen gallbladder pain.

---

*Canada only   †Unlabeled clinical use   Italicized adverse reactions are life-threatening.

COMPARING OPIOIDS

DRUG	ROUTE	ONSET	PEAK	DURATION
codeine	I.M., P.O., S.C.	15 to 30 min	30 to 60 min	4 to 6 hours
hydrocodone	P.O.	30 min	60 min	4 to 6 hours
hydromorphone	I.M., I.V., S.C.	15 min	30 min	4 to 5 hours
	P.O., rectal	30 min	60 min	4 to 5 hours
levorphanol	I.V.	15 min	20 min	4 to 8 hours
	P.O.	≤60 min	90 min	4 to 8 hours
	S.C.	≤60 min	60 to 90 min	4 to 8 hours
meperidine	I.M.	10 to 15 min	30 to 50 min	2 to 4 hours
	P.O.	15 to 30 min	60 min	2 to 4 hours
	S.C.	10 to 15 min	40 to 60 min	2 to 4 hours
methadone	I.M., P.O., S.C.	30 to 60 min	30 to 60 min	4 to 6 hours †
morphine	I.M.	≤20 min	30 to 60 min	3 to 7 hours
	P.O., rectal	≤20 min	≤60 min	3 to 7 hours
	S.C.	≤20 min	50 to 90 min	3 to 7 hours
oxycodone	P.O.	15 to 30 min	30 to 60 min	4 to 6 hours
oxymorphone	I.M., S.C.	10 to 15 min	30 to 60 min	3 to 6 hours
	I.V.	5 to 10 min	30 to 60 min	3 to 6 hours
	rectal	15 to 30 min	30 to 60 min	3 to 6 hours
propoxyphene	P.O.	20 to 60 min	2 to 2½ hours	4 to 6 hours

†Due to cumulative effects, duration of action increases with repeated doses.

• The antitussive activity of opiates is used to control persistent, exhausting cough or dry, nonproductive cough.
• The first sign of tolerance to the therapeutic effect of opioid agonists or agonist-antagonists is usually a shortened duration of effect.
• Administration of an opiate to a woman shortly before delivery may cause respiratory depression in the neonate. Monitor closely and be prepared to resuscitate.
• Preservative-free morphine (Astramorph, Duramorph) is now available for epidural or intrathecal use.

Information for the patient
• Opioids may produce drowsiness and sedation. Tell patient to use drug with caution and to avoid hazardous activities that require full alertness and coordination.
• Tell patient to avoid ingestion of alcohol when taking opioid agonists, because it will cause additive CNS depression.
• Explain that constipation may result from taking an opiate. Suggest measures to increase dietary fiber content, or recommend a stool softener.
• If patient's condition allows, instruct patient to breathe deeply, cough, and change position every 2 hours to avoid respiratory complications.
• Encourage patient to void at least every 4 hours to avoid urinary retention.
• Tell the patient to take the medication as prescribed and to call if significant adverse effects occur.
• Tell patient not to increase dosage if he is not experiencing the desired effect, but to call for prescribed dosage adjustment.

• Instruct the patient not to double dose. Tell him to take a missed dose as soon as he remembers unless it's almost time for the next dose. If this is so, the patient should skip the missed dose and go back to the regular dosage schedule.
• Tell the patient to call immediately for emergency help if he thinks he or someone else has taken an overdose.
• Explain the signs of overdose to the patient and his family.

Geriatric use
Lower doses are usually indicated for elderly patients, who may be more sensitive to the therapeutic and adverse effects of the drug.

Pediatric use
Safety and effectiveness in children have not been established.

Breast-feeding
Codeine, meperidine, methadone, morphine, and propoxyphene are excreted in breast milk and should be used with caution in breast-feeding women. Methadone has been shown to cause physical dependence in breast-feeding infants of women maintained on methadone.

Representative combinations
Codeine with acetaminophen: Phenaphen with codeine, Proval, Stopain, Baypap with codeine, Tylenol with codeine, Capital with codeine, Empracet with codeine, Emtec*, Phenaphen with codeine, Rovnox with

codeine*, Ty-tab with codeine, Acetaco, Aceta with codeine, Coastaldyne, Codap; with alcohol: Pavadon elixir; with caffeine: Tylenol No. 1 Forte*, Atasol with codeine, Exdol with codeine, Lenoltec; with salicylamide: Codalon; with butalbital: Bancap with codeine, G-2, G-3; with promethazine: Maxigesic; with calcium iodide and alcohol: Calcidrine.

Codeine phosphate with guaifenesin: Baytussin A.C., Cheracol, Gydeine Cough, Guiatuss A.C., Guiatussin with codeine Liquid, Mytussin AC, Nortussin with codeine, Robitussin AC, Tolu-Sed Cough; with iodinated glixerol: Iophen-C Liquid, Tussi-Organidin Liquid; with phenylephrine hydrochloride, chlorpheniramine maleate, and ammonium chloride: Ru-Tuss; with tripolidine hydrochloride and pseudoephedrine hydrochloride: Actifed-C; with ephedrine and theophylline: Co-Xan; with pheniramine maleate and alcohol: Partuss AC.

Codeine sulfate with terpin hydrate: Prunicodeine.

Codeine with aspirin: Anexia with codeine, Codasa, Empirin with codeine.

Codeine and aspirin with caffeine: Fiorinal with codeine; with phenacetin and caffeine: APC with codeine; with magnesium hydroxide and aluminum hydroxide: Ascriptin with codeine; with butalbital and caffeine: Buffa-comp No. 3; with acetophenetidin and caffeine: Aspodyne with codeine.

Dihydrocodeine with acetaminophen and caffeine: Compal, Synalgos-DC-A.

Fentanyl with droperidol: Innovar.

Hydrocodone bitartrate with acetaminophen: Bancap-HC, Dolacet, Hydrocet, Lorcet HD, Propain-HC, Zydone, Lortab, Amacodone, Anexia, Co-gesic, Damacet-P, Dolo-pap, Duradyne DHC, Hydrogesic, HY-PHEN, Norcet, Vicodin; with aspirin and caffeine: Damason-P; with aspirin, acetaminophen, and caffeine: Diagesic, Hyco-pap; with guaifenesin: Entuss tablets, Hycotuss liquid (with alcohol); with guaifenesin and pseudophedrine hydrochloride: Detussin expectorant, Entuss-D, Tussero expectorant (with alcohol); with guaifenesin and phenindamine tartrate: P-V Tussin tablets; with guaifenesin and phenylephrine: Donatussin DC; with potassium guaiacosulfonate: Codiclear DH, Entuss Liquid; with pseudophedrine hydrochloride: Detussin Liquid, Tussero; with homatropine methylbromide: Hycodan; with phenylephrine hydrochloride and pyrilamine maleate: Codimal DH syrup; with phenylpropanolamine hydrochloride: Hycomine; with phenylephrine hydrochloride, pyrilamine maleate, chlorpheniramine maleate salicylamide, citric acid, and caffeine: Citra forte capsules; with phenindamine tartrate, ammonium chloride, and alcohol: P-V Tussin syrup; with pheniramine maleate, pyrilamine maleate, potassium citrate, and ascorbic acid: Citra forte; with phenylephrine hydrochloride, phenylpropanolamine hydrochloride, pheniramine maleate, pyrilamine maleate, and alcohol: Ru-Tuss with hydrocodone; with guaifenesin and alcohol: S-T forte; with phenyl toloxamine: Tussionex.

Meperidine with acetaminophen: Demerol-APAP; with promethazine: Mepergan, Mepergan fortis.

Methadone with aspirin, phenacetin, and caffeine: Nodalin.

Oxycodone hydrochloride with acetaminophen: Tylox, Roxicet, Oxycocet*, Percocet, Percocet-Demi; with oxycodone terephthalate and aspirin: Percodan, Percodan-Demi.

Propoxyphene with acetaminophen: Dolene AP-65, Dolene-AP, Lorcet, Wygesic, Darvocet-N, Propacet SK; with aspirin and caffeine: Darvon Compound, Darvon

Compound-65, Dolene Compound 65, Propoxyphene Compound 65, Ropoxy Compound 65; with aspirin, phenacetin, and caffeine: Doraphen Compound 65, Procomp-65.

PHARMACOLOGIC CLASS

opioid (narcotic) agonist-antagonists

**buprenorphine
butorphanol
dezocine
nalbuphine
pentazocine**

The term "narcotic (or opiate) agonist-antagonist" is somewhat imprecise. This class of drugs has varying degrees of agonist and antagonist activity. These drugs are potent analgesics, with somewhat less addiction potential than the pure narcotic agonists.

Pharmacology

The detailed pharmacology of these drugs is poorly understood. Each agent is believed to act on different opiate receptors in the CNS to a greater or lesser degree, thus yielding slightly different effects. Like the opioid agonists, these drugs can be divided into related chemical groups. Buprenorphine, butorphanol, and nalbuphine are phenanthrenes, like morphine, whereas dezocine is an aminotetralin and pentazocine falls into a unique class, the benzmorphans.

Clinical indications and actions
Pain

Opioid agonist-antagonists are primarily used as analgesics, particularly in patients at high risk for drug dependence or abuse. Some are used as preoperative or preanesthetic medication, to supplement balanced anesthesia or to relieve prepartum pain.

Contraindications and precautions

Opioid agonist-antagonists are contraindicated in patients with known hypersensitivity to any drug of the same chemical group. Use these drugs with extreme caution in patients with supraventricular arrhythmias; avoid or administer drug with extreme caution in patients with head injury or increased intracranial pressure, because neurologic parameters are obscured; during pregnancy and labor, because drug crosses placenta readily (premature infants are especially sensitive to respiratory and CNS depressant effects of narcotic agonists-antagonists).

Use opioid agonist-antagonists cautiously in patients with renal or hepatic dysfunction, because drug accumulation and/or prolonged duration of action may occur; in patients with pulmonary disease (asthma, chronic obstructive pulmonary disease) because drug depresses respiration and suppresses cough reflex; in patients undergoing biliary tract surgery, because drug may cause biliary spasm; in patients with convulsive disorders, because drug may precipitate seizures; in elderly and debilitated patients who are more sensitive to both therapeutic and adverse drug effects; and in patients prone to physical or psychic addiction, because of the high risk of addiction to this drug.

Opioid agonist-antagonists have a lower potential for abuse than do narcotic agonists, but the risk still exists.

Overview of adverse reactions

Major hazards of agonist-antagonists are respiratory depression, apnea, shock, and cardiopulmonary arrest, possibly causing death. All opioid agonist-antagonists can cause respiratory depression, but the severity of such depression each drug can cause has a "ceiling"; for example, each drug depresses respiration to a certain point, but increased doses do not depress it further. All of the opioid agonist-antagonists have been reported to cause withdrawal symptoms after abrupt discontinuation of long-term use; they appear to have some addiction potential, but less than that of the pure opioid agonists.

CNS effects are the most common adverse reactions and may include drowsiness, sedation, light-headedness, dizziness, hallucinations, disorientation, agitation, euphoria, dysphoria, insomnia, confusion, headache, tremor, miosis, seizures, and psychic dependence. Cardiovascular reactions may include tachycardia, bradycardia, palpitations, chest wall rigidity, hypertension, hypotension, syncope, and edema. GI reactions may include nausea, vomiting, and constipation (most common), dry mouth, anorexia, and biliary spasms (colic). Other effects include urinary retention or hesitancy, decreased libido, flushing, rash, pruritus, and pain at the injection site.

Opioid agonist-antagonists can produce morphine-like dependence and thus have abuse potential. Psychic and physiological dependence with drug tolerance can develop upon chronic repeated administration. Patients with dependence or tolerance to narcotic agonist-antagonists usually present with an acute abstinence syndrome or withdrawal signs and symptoms, of which the severity is related to the degree of dependence, abruptness of withdrawal, and the drug used.

Commonly, signs and symptoms of withdrawal are yawning, lacrimation, and sweating (early); mydriasis, piloerection, flushing of face, tachycardia, tremor, irritability, and anorexia (intermediate); and muscle spasms, fever, nausea, vomiting, and diarrhea (late).

▶ Special considerations

● The opioid agonist-antagonists, as well as the opioid antagonists, can reverse the desired effects of opioids, thus, members of different pharmacologic groups (for example, meperidine and buprenorphine) should not be prescribed at the same time.
● Always keep resuscitative equipment and an opioid antagonist (naloxone) available. Be prepared to provide ventilation, and gastric lavage.
● Parenteral administration of opioid agonist-antagonists provides better analgesia than does oral dosing. Intravenous dosing should be given by very slow injections, preferably in diluted solution. Rapid intravenous injection increases the incidence of adverse effects.
● Give I.M. or S.C. injections cautiously to patients who are chilled, hypovolemic, or in shock, because decreased perfusion may lead to accumulation.
● Before administration, visually inspect all parenteral products for particles and discoloration and note the strength of the solution.
● Patient tolerance may develop to the opiate agonist activity but does not develop to opiate antagonist activity.
● A regular dosing schedule (rather than "p.r.n. pain") is preferable to alleviate the symptoms and anxiety that accompany pain.
● The duration of respiratory depression may be longer

than the analgesic effect. Monitor patient closely with repeated dosing.
● During chronic administration, regularly evaluate the patient's respiratory status. Because severe respiratory depression may occur (especially with accumulation on chronic dosing), watch for respiratory rate that is less than the patient's baseline respiratory rate. Also evaluate the patient for restlessness, which may be a compensatory response to hypoxia.
● Opioid agonist-antagonists may cause orthostatic hypotension in ambulatory patients. Have patient sit or lie down to relieve dizziness or fainting.
● Because opioid agonist-antagonists can depress respiration when used postoperatively, strongly encourage patient turning, coughing, and deep breathing to avoid atelectases. Monitor respiratory status.
● Oral opioid agonist-antagonists may be taken with food to prevent gastric irritation. Food will delay absorption and the onset of analgesia.
● Opioid agonist-antagonists may obscure the signs and symptoms of an acute abdominal condition or worsen gallbladder pain.
● The first sign of tolerance to the therapeutic effect of agonist-antagonists is usually a reduced duration of effect.
● Administering an opiate agonist-antagonist to the mother shortly before delivery may cause respiratory depression in the neonate. Monitor the infant closely and be prepared to resuscitate.

Information for the patient

● Warn ambulatory patients to be cautious when performing tasks that require alertness, such as driving, if they are taking an opioid agonist-antagonist.
● Warn patient not to stop taking an opioid agonist-antagonist abruptly if he has been taking it for a prolonged period and/or at a high dose.
● Tell patient not to increase dosage if it is not producing the desired effect, but to call for prescribed dosage adjustment.
● Tell patient to avoid ingesting alcohol when taking opioid agonist-antagonists, since additive CNS depression will occur.
● Tell patient that constipation may result. Suggest measures to increase dietary fiber content or recommend a stool softener.
● Instruct patient not to double dose. Tell him to take a missed dose as soon as he remembers unless it's almost time for next dose. If this is so, tell him to skip the missed dose and go back to regular dosage schedule.
● Tell patient to call for emergency help if he thinks he or someone else has taken an overdose.
● Explain the signs of overdose to patient and to his family.
● Instruct patient to breathe deeply, cough, and change position every 2 hours to avoid respiratory complications.
● Encourage patient to void at least every 4 hours to avoid urinary retention.
● Tell patient to take the medication as prescribed and to promptly report significant adverse effects.
● Inform woman taking an opioid agonist-antagonist to call promptly if she is planning or suspects pregnancy; warn her that her fetus also may become addicted to the drug.

Geriatric use
Lower doses are usually indicated for elderly patients, who may be more sensitive to the therapeutic and adverse effects of these drugs.

Pediatric use
Neonates may be more susceptible to the respiratory depressant effects of opiate agonist-antagonists.

Breast-feeding
Usually, these drugs are not recommended for use in breast-feeding women.

Representative combinations
Pentazocine with acetaminophen: Talacen; with aspirin: Talwin compound; with naloxone: Talwin NX.

PHARMACOLOGIC CLASS

opioid (narcotic) antagonists

naloxone
naltrexone

The narcotic antagonists naloxone and naltrexone do not produce analgesia; they produce few effects in the absence of an opioid agonist.

Pharmacology
Naloxone and naltrexone are phenanthrine derivatives, chemically related to the opioid agonist oxymorphone. Their pharmacologic actions depend on whether an opioid agonist has been administered previously, the actions of that opioid, and the extent of physical dependence to it.

Naloxone is a competitive antagonist at several opioid receptors. Low S.C. doses produce no discernible subjective effects; higher doses produce only slight drowsiness. Naltrexone is more effective in oral doses and has a longer duration of action.

At higher dosages, naloxone and naltrexone may have some agonist effects, but these are clinically insignificant.

Clinical indications and actions
Opioid-induced respiratory depression
Narcotic antagonists are used to reverse or block the effects of narcotic agonists (and, acutely, narcotic agonist-antagonists). Naloxone is used in acute, emergency situations, primarily to treat opioid-induced respiratory depression, though naloxone-treated patients may not show complete reversal of the opiate sedative effects.

Adjunct in treating opiate addiction
Naltrexone is used as part of long-term treatment for opioid addiction. By preventing the euphoria that normally results from the use of opioids, use of naltrexone helps discourage their illicit use.

Overview of adverse reactions
Nausea and vomiting may occur with high doses. Abrupt reversal of narcotic agonist effects may result in nausea, vomiting, sweating, tachycardia, increased blood pressure, and tremulousness. In postoperative patients, excessive dosage may reverse analgesia and cause excitement, with arrhythmias and fluctuations in blood pressure. When given to a narcotic addict, opioid antagonists may produce an acute abstinence syndrome.

Drug should be discontinued if signs of a severe acute abstinence syndrome appear.

▶ Special considerations
● Use with extreme caution in patients with head injury, increased intracranial pressure, seizures, asthma, alcoholism, prostatic hypertrophy, severe hepatic or renal disease, acute abdominal conditions, cardiac arrhythmias, hypovolemia, or psychiatric disorders; and in elderly or debilitated patients. Reduced doses may be necessary.
● Opioid antagonists should not be used in narcotic addicts, including newborns or mothers with narcotic dependence, in whom they may produce an acute abstinence syndrome.
● Keep resuscitative equipment available. Be prepared to provide supported ventilation and gastric lavage.
● Because naloxone's duration of activity is shorter than that of most narcotics, vigilance and repeated doses are usually necessary to manage an acute narcotic overdose in a nonaddicted patient.
● Maintain airway and monitor circulatory status.

Geriatric use
No specific recommendations available.

Pediatric use
No specific recommendations available.

Breast-feeding
No specific recommendations available.

Representative combinations
None.

opium tincture (laudanum)
opium tincture, camphorated (paregoric)

● Pharmacologic classification: opiate
● Therapeutic classification: antidiarrheal
● Controlled substance schedule II
● Pregnancy risk category B (D when used long-term or in high doses)

How supplied
Available by prescription only
Opium tincture
Alcoholic solution: equivalent to morphine 10 mg/ml
Opium tincture, camphorated
Alcoholic solution: Each 5 ml contains morphine, 2 mg; anise oil, 0.2 ml; benzoic acid, 20 mg; camphor, 20 mg; glycerin, 0.2 ml; and ethanol to make 5 ml

Indications, route, and dosage
Acute, nonspecific diarrhea
Adults: 0.6 ml opium tincture (range 0.3 to 1 ml) P.O. q.i.d. (maximum dosage 6 ml daily), or 5 to 10 ml camphorated opium tincture daily, b.i.d., t.i.d., or q.i.d. until diarrhea subsides.
Children: 0.25 to 0.5 ml/kg camphorated opium tincture daily, b.i.d., t.i.d., or q.i.d. until diarrhea subsides.

Opium tincture has been used to treat withdrawal symptoms in infants whose mothers are narcotic addicts.

---

*Canada only   †Unlabeled clinical use   Italicized adverse reactions are life-threatening.

Pharmacodynamics
Antidiarrheal action: Opium, derived from the opium poppy, contains several ingredients. The most active ingredient, morphine, increases GI smooth muscle tone, inhibits motility and propulsion, and diminishes secretions. By inhibiting peristalsis, the drug delays passage of intestinal contents, increasing water resorption and relieving diarrhea.

Pharmacokinetics
• *Absorption:* Morphine is absorbed variably from the gut.
• *Distribution:* Although opium alkaloids are distributed widely in the body, the low doses used to treat diarrhea act primarily in the GI tract. Camphor crosses the placenta.
• *Metabolism:* Opium is metabolized in the liver.
• *Excretion:* Opium is excreted in urine; opium alkaloids (especially morphine) enter breast milk. Drug effect persists 4 to 5 hours.

Contraindications and precautions
Opium tincture and camphorated opium tincture are contraindicated in patients with known hypersensitivity to morphine alkaloids; in patients with acute respiratory depression because they may worsen this condition; in patients with diarrhea resulting from pseudomembranous colitis or ulcerative colitis because of the potential for toxic megacolon; and in patients with diarrhea resulting from poisoning or from certain bacterial or parasitic infections because expulsion of intestinal contents may be beneficial (until toxic agent has been eliminated from the GI tract).

Opium tincture and camphorated opium tincture should be used cautiously in patients with asthma or severe prostatic hypertrophy because the drugs may exacerbate symptoms associated with these disorders; in patients with hepatic disease because of the potential for drug accumulation; and in patients with narcotic or alcohol dependence because the drugs contain alcohol and opiates.

Interactions
When used concomitantly with other CNS depressants, opium tincture and camphorated opium tincture result in an additive effect. Concomitant use with metoclopramide may antagonize the effects of metoclopramide.

Effects on diagnostic tests
Opium tincture and camphorated opium tincture may prevent delivery of technetium-99m disofenin to the small intestine during hepatobiliary imaging tests; delay test until 24 hours after last dose. The drugs also may increase serum amylase and lipase levels by inducing contractions of the sphincter of Oddi and increasing biliary tract pressure.

Adverse reactions
• CNS: sedation, dizziness, lethargy, euphoria.
• GI: nausea, vomiting, abdominal cramps, dry mouth, anorexia.
• Other: physical dependence in long-term use.
Note: Drugs should be discontinued if signs of CNS or respiratory depression occur.

Overdose and treatment
Clinical effects of overdose include drowsiness, hypotension, seizures, and apnea. Empty stomach by induced emesis or gastric lavage; maintain patent airway.

Use naloxone to treat respiratory depression. Monitor patient for signs and symptoms of CNS or respiratory depression.

▶ Special considerations
• Mix drug with sufficient water to ensure passage to stomach.
• Opium tincture is 25 times more potent than camphorated opium tincture (Paregoric); take care not to confuse these drugs.
• Monitor patient's vital signs.
• Monitor bowel function.
• Risk of physical dependence on drug increases with long-term use.
• Do not refrigerate drug.

Information for the patient
• Warn patient that physical dependence may result from long-term use.
• Warn patient to use caution when driving a car or performing other tasks requiring alertness because drug may cause drowsiness, dizziness, and blurred vision.
• Because drug is indicated only for short-term use, instruct patient to report diarrhea that persists longer than 48 hours.
• Advise patient to take drug with food if it causes nausea, vomiting, or constipation.
• Instruct patient to call immediately if he has difficulty breathing or shortness of breath.
• Instruct patient to drink adequate fluids while diarrhea persists.

Breast-feeding
Because opium alkaloids (especially morphine) are excreted in breast milk, drug's possible risks must be weighed against benefits.

---

orphenadrine citrate
Banflex, Flexoject, Flexon, Marflex, Myolin, Neocyten, Noradex, Norflex, Orflagen, Orphenate

orphenadrine hydrochloride
Disipal

• Pharmacologic classification: diphenhydramine analog
• Therapeutic classification: skeletal muscle relaxant
• Pregnancy risk category C

How supplied
Available by prescription only
Tablets: 50 mg, 100 mg
Tablets (extended-release): 100 mg
Injection: 30 mg/ml parenteral

Indications, route, and dosage
Adjunct in painful, acute musculoskeletal conditions
Adults: 100 mg P.O. b.i.d., or 60 mg I.V. or I.M. q 12 hours.
Symptomatic treatment of parkinsonian syndrome
Adults: 50 mg P.O. t.i.d.

Pharmacodynamics

Skeletal muscle relaxant action: Orphenadrine does not relax skeletal muscle directly. Atropine-like central action on cerebral motor centers or on the medulla may be the mechanism by which it reduces skeletal muscle spasm. Its reported analgesic effect may add to its skeletal muscle relaxant properties.

Orphenadrine also has mild antimuscarinic activity (of benefit in Parkinson's disease), postganglionic anticholinergic effects, antihistamine activity (less than diphenhydramine), and local anesthetic action.

Pharmacokinetics

● *Absorption:* Orphenadrine is rapidly absorbed from the GI tract; its onset of action occurs within 1 hour, peaks within 2 hours, and persists for 4 to 6 hours.
● *Distribution:* Orphenadrine is widely distributed throughout the body.
● *Metabolism:* Its metabolic fate is unknown, but orphenadrine is almost completely metabolized to at least eight metabolites.
● *Excretion:* Orphenadrine is excreted in urine, mainly as its metabolites. Small amounts are excreted unchanged. Its half-life is about 14 hours.

Contraindications and precautions

Orphenadrine is contraindicated in patients with known hypersensitivity to the drug, and in patients in whom anticholinergic and antimuscarinic effects are undesirable: those with achalasia, bladder neck obstruction, glaucoma, myasthenia gravis, peptic ulcer, prostate hypertrophy, or pyloric or duodenal obstruction.

Administer cautiously to patients with cardiac, hepatic, or renal function impairment.

Interactions

Concomitant use with propoxyphene or CNS depressants, including alcohol, anxiolytics, tricyclic antidepressants, narcotics, and antipsychotics, may produce additive CNS effects; concurrent use requires reduction of both agents. Use with other anticholinergic agents may increase anticholinergic effects; with monoamine oxidase inhibitors, may increase CNS adverse effects.

Effects on diagnostic tests

None reported.

Adverse reactions

● CNS: drowsiness, dizziness, weakness, headache, restlessness, irritability, confusion (especially in elderly patients), disorientation, hallucinations, insomnia.
● CV: tachycardia, palpitations, transient syncope.
● GI: nausea, dry mouth, constipation, paralytic ileus, epigastric distress, difficulty swallowing.
● GU: urinary retention or hesitancy.
● Other: blurred vision, allergic reactions, rash, pruritus, urticaria, *anaphylaxis, aplastic anemia,* increased intraocular pressure, mydriasis.
Note: Drug should be discontinued if hypersensitivity or cardiac arrhythmias occur.

Overdose and treatment

Clinical manifestations of overdose include dry mouth, blurred vision, urinary retention, tachycardia, confusion, paralytic ileus, deep coma, seizures, shock, respiratory arrest, cardiac arrhythmias, and death.

Treatment includes symptomatic and supportive measures. If ingestion is recent, induce emesis or gas-tric lavage followed by activated charcoal. Monitor vital signs and fluid and electrolyte balance.

▶ Special considerations

● Periodic blood, urine, and liver function tests are recommended in prolonged therapy.
● Monitor vital signs, especially intake and output, noting any urinary retention.
● When giving orphenadrine I.V., inject slowly over 5 minutes. Keep patient supine during and 5 to 10 minutes after injection. Paradoxical initial bradycardia may occur when giving I.V.; usually disappears in 2 minutes.

Information for the patient

● Advise patient to relieve dry mouth with ice chips, sugarless gum, hard candy, or saliva substitutes.
● Orphenadrine may cause drowsiness. Tell patient to avoid hazardous activities that require alertness or physical coordination until CNS depressant effects can be determined.
● Warn patient to avoid alcoholic beverages and to use cough and cold preparations cautiously, because some contain alcohol.
● Tell patient to store drug away from heat and light (not in bathroom medicine cabinet) and safely out of reach of children.
● Instruct patient to take missed dose if remembered within 1 hour. If beyond 1 hour, patient should skip that dose and return to regular schedule. Do not double dose.

Geriatric use

Elderly patients may be more sensitive to drug's effects.

Pediatric use

Safety and efficacy in children under age 12 have not been established.

oxacillin sodium
Bactocill, Prostaphlin

● Pharmacologic classification: penicillinase-resistant penicillin
● Therapeutic classification: antibiotic
● Pregnancy risk category B

How supplied

Available by prescription only
Capsules: 250 mg, 500 mg
Oral solution: 250 mg/5 ml (after reconstitution)
Injection: 250 mg, 500 mg, 1 g, 2 g, 4 g
Pharmacy bulk package: 10 g
I.V. infusion: 1 g, 2 g, 4 g

Indications, route, and dosage
Systemic infections caused by Staphylococcus aureus

Adults: 2 to 4 g P.O. daily, divided into doses given q 6 hours; 2 to 12 g I.M. or I.V. daily, divided into doses given q 4 to 6 hours.
Children: 50 to 100 mg/kg P.O. daily, divided into doses given q 6 hours; 150 to 200 mg/kg I.M. or I.V. daily, divided into doses given q 4 to 6 hours.

Pharmacodynamics

Antibiotic action: Oxacillin is bactericidal; it adheres to bacterial penicillin-binding proteins, thus inhibiting bacterial cell wall synthesis. Oxacillin resists the effects of penicillinases—enzymes that inactivate penicillin—and is thus active against many strains of penicillinase-producing bacteria; this activity is most important against penicillinase-producing staphylococci; some strains may remain resistant. Oxacillin is also active against a few gram-positive aerobic and anaerobic bacilli but has no significant effect on gram-negative bacilli.

Pharmacokinetics

● *Absorption:* Oxacillin is absorbed rapidly but incompletely from the GI tract; it is stable in an acid environment. Peak serum concentrations occur within ½ to 2 hours after an oral dose and 30 minutes after an I.M. dose. Food decreases absorption.
● *Distribution:* Oxacillin is distributed widely. CSF penetration is poor but enhanced by meningeal inflammation. Oxacillin crosses the placenta; it is 89% to 94% protein-bound.
● *Metabolism:* Oxacillin is metabolized partially.
● *Excretion:* Oxacillin and metabolites are excreted primarily in urine by renal tubular secretion and glomerular filtration; it is also excreted in breast milk and in small amounts in bile. Elimination half-life in adults is ½ to 1 hour, extended to 2 hours in severe renal impairment. Dosage adjustments are not required in patients with renal impairment.

Contraindications and precautions

Oxacillin is contraindicated in patients with known hypersensitivity to any other penicillin or to cephalosporins.

Interactions

Concomitant use of oxacillin with aminoglycosides produces synergistic bactericidal effects against *Staphylococcus aureus.* However, the drugs are physically and chemically incompatible and are inactivated when mixed or given together. In vivo inactivation has been reported when aminoglycosides and penicillins are used concomitantly.

Probenecid blocks renal tubular secretion of penicillins, raising their serum levels.

Effects on diagnostic tests

Oxacillin alters tests for urinary and serum proteins; turbidimetric urine and serum proteins are often falsely positive or elevated in tests using sulfosalicylic acid or trichloroacetic acid.

Oxacillin may cause transient reductions in red blood cell, white blood cell, and platelet counts. Elevations in liver function tests may indicate drug-induced hepatitis or cholestasis. Abnormal urinalysis results may indicate drug-induced interstitial nephritis.

Oxacillin may falsely decrease serum aminoglycoside concentrations.

Adverse reactions

● CNS: neuropathy, neuromuscular irritability, *seizures.*
● GI: oral lesions, diarrhea, *pseudomembranous colitis,* intrahepatic cholestasis.
● GU: interstitial nephritis, transient hematuria, proteinuria.
● HEMA: granulocytopenia, thrombocytopenia, eosinophilia, *hemolytic anemia,* transient neutropenia.
● Hepatic: hepatitis, elevated enzymes.
● Local: *thrombophlebitis.*
● Other: *hypersensitivity reactions (fever, chills, rash, urticaria, anaphylaxis),* bacterial or fungal superinfection.

Note: Drug should be discontinued if immediate hypersensitivity reactions occur or if signs of interstitial nephritis or pseudomembranous colitis occur. Patient may require alternate therapy if any of the following occurs: drug fever, eosinophilia, hematuria, neutropenia, or unexplained elevations in serum creatinine concentration, BUN levels, or liver function studies.

Overdose and treatment

Clinical signs of overdose include neuromuscular sensitivity or seizures. No specific recommendations. Treatment is supportive. After recent ingestion (within 4 hours), empty the stomach by induced emesis or gastric lavage; follow with activated charcoal to reduce absorption. Oxacillin is not appreciably removed by peritoneal or hemodialysis.

▶ Special considerations

Besides those relevant to all *penicillins,* consider the following recommendations.
● Give oral drug with water only; acid in fruit juice or carbonated beverage may inactivate drug.
● Give oral dose on empty stomach; food decreases absorption.
● Except in osteomyelitis, do not give I.M. or I.V. unless patient can't take oral dose.
● Assess renal and hepatic function; watch for elevated SGOT and SGPT and report significant changes.

Information for the patient
● Explain need to take oral preparations without food and to follow with water only because of acid content of fruit juice and carbonated beverages.
● Tell patient to report any allergic reactions or severe diarrhea promptly.

Geriatric use
Half-life may be prolonged in elderly patients because of impaired renal function.

Pediatric use
Elimination of oxacillin is reduced in neonates. Transient hematuria, azotemia, and albuminuria have occurred in some neonates receiving oxacillin; monitor renal function closely.

Breast-feeding
Oxacillin is excreted into breast milk; drug should be used with caution in breast-feeding women.

oxamniquine
Vansil

● Pharmacologic classification: tetrahydroquinoline
● Therapeutic classification: anthelmintic
● Pregnancy risk category C

How supplied
Available by prescription only
Capsules: 250 mg

Indications, route, and dosage
Schistosomiasis caused by Schistosoma mansoni
Adults and children: Individualize dosage based upon geographic location of source of infection: if African or Middle Eastern origin, 30 to 60 mg/kg daily, divided b.i.d. or q.i.d., for 1 to 2 days. West African strains can generally be treated with a single dose of 15 mg/kg.

Pharmacodynamics
Anthelmintic action: Oxamniquine paralyzes worm musculature; worms subsequently are dislodged from mesenteric veins and killed by host tissue reactions. Female worms cease to lay eggs after treatment. Oxamniquine is active against *Schistosoma mansoni.*

Pharmacokinetics
● *Absorption:* Oxamniquine is well absorbed, with peak plasma concentrations reached at 1 to 3 hours. Food decreases the rate and extent of absorption.
● *Distribution:* The distribution of oxamniquine is not clearly defined.
● *Metabolism:* Oxamniquine is metabolized extensively to inactive acid metabolites in the GI lumen and mucosa.
● *Excretion:* Oxamniquine and its metabolites are excreted primarily in urine; plasma half-life is 1 to 2½ hours. It is unknown if oxamniquine is excreted in breast milk.

Contraindications and precautions
Oxamniquine should be used with caution in patients with seizure disorders because it may cause seizures.

Interactions
Concomitant use of oxamniquine and praziquantel may result in synergistic antischistosomal activity; the clinical significance of such action is unknown.

Effects on diagnostic tests
Oxamniquine therapy may interfere with spectometric urinalysis; it also may cause transient elevation of liver enzyme levels. It may increase erythrocyte sedimentation rate and the reticulocyte count and may increase or decrease the leukocyte count. Rarely, electroencephalogram changes and minor ECG and pulmonary X-ray changes have been reported.

Adverse reactions
● CNS: seizures, *dizziness, drowsiness, headache,* excitation, hallucinations, insomnia.
● DERM: urticaria, rash, pruritus.
● GI: nausea, vomiting, abdominal pain, anorexia.
● Renal: proteinuria, hematuria, bilirubinuria.
● Other: joint pain, malaise, fever (usually occurs 5 to 7 days after treatment).
   Note: Drug should be discontinued if signs of hypersensitivity or toxicity occur.

Overdose and treatment
Treatment of overdose is largely supportive, particularly of cardiovascular and respiratory functions. After recent ingestion (within 4 hours), empty stomach by induced emesis or gastric lavage. Follow with activated charcoal to decrease absorption. Osmotic cathartics may be helpful.

▶ Special considerations
● Give drug after meals or with food to minimize GI distress.
● Monitor neurologic function; if patient has history of seizures, be alert to possible drug-induced recurrences.

Information for the patient
● Tell patient to take drug with food to decrease the incidence of adverse reactions, espcially dizziness, drowsiness, and nausea.
● Tell patient not to drive or perform other hazardous activities if drug causes dizziness or drowsiness.
● Tell patient that oxamniquine may cause orange-red discoloration of urine.

Breast-feeding
Safety has not been established.

---

oxazepam
Apo-Oxazepam*, Novoxapam*, Oxpam*, Serax, Zapex*

● Pharmacologic classification: benzodiazepine
● Therapeutic classification: antianxiety agent, sedative-hypnotic
● Controlled substance schedule IV
● Pregnancy risk category D

How supplied
Available by prescription only
Tablets: 15 mg
Capsules: 10 mg, 15 mg, 30 mg

Indications, route, and dosage
Alcohol withdrawal
Adults: 15 to 30 mg P.O. t.i.d. or q.i.d.
Severe anxiety
Adults: 10 to 30 mg P.O. t.i.d. or q.i.d.
Tension, mild to moderate anxiety
Adults: 10 to 15 mg P.O. t.i.d. or q.i.d.

Pharmacodynamics
Anxiolytic and sedative-hypnotic action: Oxazepam depresses the CNS at the limbic and subcortical levels of the brain. It produces an antianxiety effect by enhancing the effect of the neurotransmitter gamma-aminobutyric acid (GABA) on its receptor in the ascending reticular activating system, which increases inhibition and blocks both cortical and limbic arousal.

Pharmacokinetics
● *Absorption:* When administered orally, oxazepam is well absorbed through the GI tract. Peak levels occur in 1 to 4 hours. Onset of action occurs at 60 to 120 minutes.
● *Distribution:* Oxazepam is distributed widely throughout the body. Drug is 85% to 95% protein-bound.
● *Metabolism:* Oxazepam is metabolized in the liver to inactive metabolites.
● *Excretion:* The metabolites of oxazepam are excreted in urine as glucuronide conjugates. The half-life of oxazepam ranges from 5 to 13 hours.

Contraindications and precautions

Oxazepam is contraindicated in patients with known hypersensitivity to the drug; in patients with acute narrow-angle glaucoma or untreated open-angle glaucoma, because of the drug's possible anticholinergic effects; in patients in coma, because the drug's hypnotic effect may be prolonged or intensified; and in patients with acute alcohol intoxication who have depressed vital signs, because the drug will worsen CNS depression. Oxazepam tablets contain tartrazine, which may induce allergic reaction in hypersensitive individuals. Patients allergic to aspirin exhibit a high incidence of cross-sensitivity.

Oxazepam should be used cautiously in patients with psychoses, because the drug is rarely beneficial in such patients and may induce paradoxical reactions; in patients with myasthenia gravis or Parkinson's disease, because it may exacerbate the disorder; in patients with impaired renal or hepatic function, which prolongs elimination of the drug; in elderly or debilitated patients, who are usually more sensitive to the drug's CNS effects; and in individuals prone to addiction or drug abuse.

Interactions

Oxazepam potentiates the CNS depressant effects of phenothiazines, narcotics, antihistamines, monoamine oxidase inhibitors, barbiturates, alcohol, general anesthetics, and antidepressants.

Concomitant use with cimetidine and possibly disulfiram causes diminished hepatic metabolism of oxazepam, which increases its plasma concentration.

Heavy smoking accelerates oxazepam metabolism, thus lowering clinical effectiveness.

Antacids may decrease the rate of oxazepam absorption.

Oxazepam may inhibit the therapeutic effects of levodopa.

Effects on diagnostic tests

Oxazepam therapy may increase liver function test results. Changes in EEG patterns, usually low-voltage, fast activity, may occur during and after oxazepam therapy.

Adverse reactions

● CNS: confusion, depression, drowsiness, lethargy, hangover effect, ataxia, dizziness, syncope, nightmares, fatigue, slurred speech, tremors, vertigo, headache, behavior problems.
● CV: bradycardia, *circulatory collapse*, transient hypotension.
● DERM: rash, urticaria.
● EENT: diplopia, blurred vision, nystagmus.
● GI: constipation, dry mouth, anorexia, nausea, vomiting, abdominal discomfort.
● GU: urinary incontinence or retention.
● Other: *respiratory depression*, dysarthria, hepatic dysfunction, changes in libido.
Note: Drug should be discontinued if the following paradoxical reactions occur: acute hyperexcited state, anxiety, hallucinations, increased muscle spasticity, insomnia, or rage.

Overdose and treatment

Clinical manifestations of overdose include somnolence, confusion, coma, hypoactive reflexes, dyspnea, labored breathing, hypotension, bradycardia, slurred speech, and unsteady gait or impaired coordination.

Support blood pressure and respiration until the drug effects have subsided; monitor vital signs. Mechanical ventilatory assistance via endotracheal tube may be required to maintain a patent airway and support adequate oxygenation. Flumazenil, a specific benzodiazepine antagonist, may be useful. As needed, use I.V. fluids and vasopressors such as dopamine and phenylephrine to treat hypotension. If the patient is conscious, induce emesis. Use gastric lavage if ingestion was recent, but only if an endotracheal tube is present to prevent aspiration. After emesis or lavage, administer activated charcoal with a cathartic as a single dose. Dialysis is of limited value.

▶ Special considerations

Besides those relevant to all *benzodiazepines*, consider the following recommendations.
● Monitor hepatic and renal function studies to ensure normal function.
● Oxazepam tablets contain tartrazine dye; check patient's history for allergy to this substance.
● Store in a cool, dry place away from light.

Information for the patient
● Advise patient not to change any part of medication regimen without medical approval.
● Instruct patient in safety measures, such as gradual position changes and supervised ambulation, to prevent injury.
● Sleepiness may not occur for up to 2 hours after taking oxazepam; tell patient to wait before taking an additional dose.
● Advise patient of potential for physical and psychological dependence with chronic use of oxazepam.
● Reduce dosage gradually (over 8 to 12 weeks) after long-term use.

Geriatric use
● Elderly patients are more susceptible to the CNS depressant effects of oxazepam. Some may require supervision with ambulation and activities of daily living during initiation of therapy or after an increase in dose.
● Tell patient not to discontinue drug suddenly if he's been taking it for prolonged periods.
● Lower doses are usually effective in elderly patients because of decreased elimination.

Pediatric use
Safe use in children under age 12 has not been established. Closely observe neonate for withdrawal symptoms if mother took oxazepam for a prolonged period during pregnancy.

Breast-feeding
The breast-fed infant of a mother who uses oxazepam may become sedated, have feeding difficulties, or lose weight; avoid use in breast-feeding women.

PHARMACOLOGIC CLASS

oxazolidinedione derivatives

paramethadione
pemoline
trimethadione

Oxazolidinediones, which are similar in structure to hydantoins, are used primarily to control absence seizures; because of their greater toxicity, they usually are reserved for seizures refractory to other anticonvulsants. This class has been replaced largely by the less toxic succinimides.

Pharmacology
Oxazolidinediones elevate the seizure threshold in the cerebral cortex and basal ganglia; they are less effective than either hydantoins or barbiturates. They cause CNS sedation, which may lead to ataxia at high doses; paramethadione has the least sedative effect.

Clinical indications and actions
Seizure disorders
Oxazolidinediones are used to control absence (petit mal) seizures refractory to anticonvulsants, especially in patients with mixed epilepsy. They have no value in tonic-clonic seizures and may precipitate a first tonic-clonic seizure.

Overview of adverse reactions
The most common adverse effects from oxazolidinediones include blurred vision, drowsiness, and such GI disturbances as nausea and vomiting. Toxic effects include fatal hematologic and renal reactions, lupus-like syndromes, and lymphadenopathy resembling malignant lymphoma. Strict medical supervision is necessary during the first year of treatment. Because of their potential teratogenicity and toxic adverse effects, these drugs should be reserved for severely refractory seizure disorders.

▶ Special considerations
● Oxazolidinediones are contraindicated during pregnancy, because of their potential to cause fetal malformations, and in patients with known hypersensitivity to oxazolidinedione. These drugs should be used with caution in patients with renal or hepatic dysfunction, severe blood dyscrasias, and retinal or optic nerve disease because of their potential to cause severe toxicities in these organs and systems.
● Monitor baseline liver and renal function and complete blood count at beginning of therapy and monthly during therapy.
● Drug should be discontinued if neutrophil count falls below 2,500/mm³ or if any of the following occur: hypersensitivity, scotomata, hepatitis, systemic lupus erythematosus, lymphadenopathy, rash, nephrosis, alopecia, or grand mal seizures.
● Anticonvulsants should not be discontinued abruptly.

Information for the patient
● Explain rationale for treatment and the need for close medical supervision.
● Teach patient signs and symptoms of hypersensitivity, liver dysfunction, and blood dyscrasias and to report any of the following: sore throat, fever, malaise, bleeding, easy bruising, petechiae, lymphadenopathy, scotomata, or rash.
● Tell patient to call immediately if pregnancy occurs.
● Warn patient never to discontinue drug without medical supervision.
● Advise patient not to use alcohol while taking drug, as it may decrease drug's effectiveness and increase CNS adverse effects.
● Advise patient to avoid tasks that require mental alertness, such as driving a car, until degree of sedative effect is determined. Drug may cause dizziness, drowsiness, or blurred vision.
● Tell patient to take drug with food if GI distress occurs.

● Encourage patient to wear a Medic Alert bracelet or necklace, listing the drug and seizure disorder, while taking anticonvulsants.
● Advise patient to wear dark glasses if photophobia occurs and to apply sunscreen if photosensitivity develops.

Geriatric use
Use anticonvulsant drugs with caution. Elderly patients metabolize and excrete all drugs slowly and may obtain therapeutic effect from lower doses.

Pediatric use
Be sure to administer only dosage forms prepared for pediatric use; these drugs are not recommended for children under age 2.

Breast-feeding
It is unknown if oxazolidinediones are excreted in breast milk. Alternative feeding method is recommended during therapy.

Representative combinations
None.

oxiconazole nitrate
Oxistat

● Pharmacologic classification: ergosterol synthesis inhibitor
● Therapeutic classification: antifungal agent
● Pregnancy risk category B

How supplied
Available by prescription only
Topical cream: 1%

Indications, route, and dosage
Topical treatment of dermal infections caused by Trichophyton rubrum *and* T. mentagrophytes *(tinea pedis, tinea cruris, and tinea corporis)*
Adults and children: Apply to affected area once daily (in the evening) for 2 weeks (1 month for tinea pedis).

Pharmacodynamics
Antifungal action: Oxiconazole inhibits ergosterol synthesis in susceptible fungal organisms, thereby weakening cytoplasmic membrane integrity.

Pharmacokinetics
● *Absorption:* Systemic absorption is low. Less than 0.3% is recovered in the urine up to 5 days after application.
● *Distribution:* Most of the drug concentrates in the epidermis, with smaller amounts in the upper and deeper corneum.
● *Metabolism:* Unknown.
● *Excretion:* Urine recovery of the drug has been demonstrated. It is unknown if the drug is excreted in the feces.

Contraindications and precautions
Drug is contraindicated in patients hypersensitive to oxiconazole nitrate. This drug is not for ophthalmic use.

Interactions
None reported.

Effects on diagnostic tests
None reported.

Adverse reactions
● DERM: itching, burning, irritation, maceration, erythema, fissuring.

Overdose and treatment
Oral or parenteral administration to animals resulted in CNS stimulation and tissue irritation. Specific treatment recommendations are unavailable.

▶ **Special considerations**
If the patient shows no response after treatment for 2 weeks to 1 month, the diagnosis should be reviewed.

Information for the patient
● Be sure patient understands that the drug is for external use only.
● Instruct patient not to use drug near the eyes.

Breast-feeding
Animal studies have shown that oxiconazole is excreted in breast milk. Exercise caution when prescribing the drug to a breast-feeding woman.

***

oxtriphylline
Apo-Oxtriphylline*, Choledyl,
Novotriphyl*

● Pharmacologic classification: xanthine derivative
● Therapeutic classification: bronchodilator
● Pregnancy risk category C

How supplied
Available by prescription only
Tablets: 100 mg, 200 mg
Tablets (sustained release): 400 mg, 600 mg
Syrup: 50 mg/5 ml
Elixir: 100 mg/5 ml

Indications, route, and dosage
To relieve acute bronchial asthma and reversible bronchospasm associated with chronic bronchitis and emphysema
Adults and children over age 12: 200 mg P.O. q 6 hours, or 400 or 600 mg sustained-release tablet q 12 hours.
Children age 2 to 12: 4 mg/kg P.O. q 6 hours. Increase as needed to maintain therapeutic levels of theophylline (generally regarded as 10 to 20 mcg/ml but some patients may respond to lower plasma levels).

Pharmacodynamics
Bronchodilating action: Oxtriphylline exerts its bronchodilating action after it is converted to theophylline. (Oxtriphylline is 64% anhydrous theophylline.) Theophylline antagonizes adenosine receptors in the bronchi, and may inhibit phosphodiesterase and increase levels of cyclic adenosine monophosphate (CAMP), thus relaxing smooth muscle of the respiratory tract.

Pharmacokinetics
● *Absorption:* Drug is well absorbed; rate of absorption and onset of action depend on dosage form.
● *Distribution:* Drug is distributed rapidly throughout body fluids and tissues.
● *Metabolism:* Oxtriphylline, the choline salt of theophylline, is converted to theophylline, then metabolized to inactive compounds.
● *Excretion:* Drug is excreted in the urine as theophylline (10%) and theophyllic metabolites.

Contraindications and precautions
Oxtriphylline is contraindicated in patients with hypersensitivity to xanthines. Use cautiously in patients with compromised cardiac or circulatory function, diabetes, glaucoma, hypertension, hyperthyroidism, peptic ulcer, or gastroesophageal reflux, because drug may worsen these symptoms or conditions.

Interactions
When used concomitantly, oxtriphylline increases the excretion of lithium. Cimetidine, allopurinol (high dose), propranolol, erythromycin, and troleandomycin may increase serum concentration of oxtriphylline by decreasing hepatic clearance. Barbiturates, nicotine, marijuana, and aminoglutethimide decrease effects of oxtriphylline by enhancing its metabolism. Beta blockers exert antagonistic pharmacologic effect.

Effects on diagnostic tests
Oxtriphylline may falsely elevate serum uric acid levels measured by colorimetric methods. Theophylline levels may be falsely elevated in patients using furosemide, phenylbutazone, probenecid, some cephalosporins, sulfa medications, theobromine, caffeine, tea, chocolate, cola beverages, and acetaminophen, depending on assay method used.

Adverse reactions
● CNS: Irritability, restlessness, headache, insomnia, dizziness, *convulsions*, depression, light-headedness, muscle twitching.
● CV: palpitations, marked flushing, hypotension, sinus tachycardia, *ventricular tachycardia* and other life-threatening arrhythmias, extrasystoles, *circulatory failure*.
● GI: nausea, vomiting, epigastric pain, loss of appetite, diarrhea.
● Respiratory: tachypnea, *respiratory arrest*.
● Other: fever, urinary retention, hyperglycemia.
   Note: Drug should be discontinued if any adverse reaction intensifies; this signals impending overdose.

Overdose and treatment
Clinical manifestations of overdose include nausea, vomiting, insomnia, irritability, tachycardia, extrasystoles, tachypnea, or tonic-clonic seizures. The onset of toxicity may be sudden and severe, with arrhythmias and seizures as the first signs. Induce emesis except in convulsing patients; follow with activated charcoal and cathartics. Treat arrhythmias with lidocaine and seizures with I.V. benzodiazepine; support cardiovascular and respiratory systems.

▶ **Special considerations**
● Do not crush sustained-release tablets.
● Monitor vital signs and intake and output. Observe for CNS stimulation and CV adverse reactions.

***

*Canada only   †Unlabeled clinical use   Italicized adverse reactions are life-threatening.

● Store at 59° to 86° F. (15° to 30° C.) away from heat and light.

Information for the patient
● Instruct patient about the drug and dosage schedule; if a dose is missed, he should take it as soon as possible. However, he should never double-dose.
● Advise patient of the adverse effects and possible signs of toxicity, and to report sign of excessive CNS stimulation (nervousness, tremors, akathisia).
● Warn patient to avoid consuming large quantities of xanthine-containing foods and beverages.

Geriatric use
Decrease dose and monitor closely.

Pediatric use
Use with caution in neonates.

Breast-feeding
Drug is excreted in the milk and may cause irritability, insomnia, or fretfulness in the breast-fed infant.

oxybutynin chloride
Ditropan

● Pharmacologic classification: synthetic tertiary amine
● Therapeutic classification: antispasmodic
● Pregnancy risk category C

How supplied
Available by prescription only
Tablets: 5 mg
Syrup: 5 mg/5 ml

Indications, route, and dosage
Antispasmodic for neurogenic bladder
Adults: 5 mg P.O. b.i.d. to t.i.d. to maximum of 5 mg q.i.d.
Children over age 5: 5 mg P.O. b.i.d. to maximum of 5 mg t.i.d.

Pharmacodynamics
Antispasmodic action: Oxybutynin reduces the urge to void, increases bladder capacity, and reduces the frequency of contractions to the detrusor muscle. The drug exerts a direct spasmolytic action and an antimuscarinic action on smooth muscle.

Pharmacokinetics
● *Absorption:* Oxybutynin is absorbed rapidly, with peak levels occurring in 3 to 6 hours. Action begins in 30 to 60 minutes and persists for 6 to 10 hours.
● *Distribution:* No data available.
● *Metabolism:* Drug is metabolized by the liver.
● *Excretion:* Drug is excreted principally in urine.

Contraindications and precautions
Oxybutynin is contraindicated in patients with partial or complete GI tract obstruction, glaucoma, myasthenia gravis, adynamic ileus, megacolon, or severe or ulcerative colitis, because it may worsen these symptoms or disorders; in debilitated and elderly patients with intestinal atony; in hemorrhaging patients with unstable cardiovascular status; and in patients with obstructive uropathy.

Oxybutynin should be used with caution in elderly patients, in patients with autonomic neuropathy or hepatic or renal disease, and in patients with reflux esophagitis because drug may aggravate these conditions.

Interactions
Oxybutynin intensifies the antimuscarinic effects of atropine and related compounds. There is a possibility of an additive sedative effect with other CNS depressants.

Effects on diagnostic tests
None reported.

Adverse reactions
● CNS: drowsiness, dizziness, insomnia, flushing.
● CV: palpitations, tachycardia.
● DERM: urticaria, rash, severe allergic reactions in patients sensitive to anticholinergics.
● EENT: transient blurred vision; mydriasis; cycloplegia; dry mouth, nose, and throat; increased intraocular pressure.
● GI: nausea, vomiting, constipation, bloated feeling.
● GU: impotence, urinary hesitance or retention.
● Other: decreased sweating, fever, suppression of lactation.
    Note: Drug should be discontinued if a hypersensitivity reaction occurs or if signs and symptoms of circulatory or respiratory distress or CNS excitation occur.

Overdose and treatment
Clinical manifestations of overdose include restlessness, excitement, psychotic behavior, flushing, hypotension, circulatory failure, and fever. In severe cases, paralysis, respiratory failure, and coma may occur. Treatment requires gastric lavage followed by physostigmine 0.5 to 2 mg slow I.V. push repeated up to 5 mg if necessary. Use ice packs or alcohol sponges to control fever. Counteract CNS excitation, if necessary, with a slow I.V. drip of 2% thiopental or 2% chloral hydrate rectal suspension (100 to 200 ml). Maintain artificial respiration if paralysis of respiratory muscles occurs.

▶ Special considerations
● Oxybutynin may cause gastric irritation when taken on an empty stomach. Food or milk may relieve the symptoms.
● Cystometry and other appropriate urologic procedures are performed prior to starting therapy and periodically to evaluate patient response.
● Store in tightly closed containers between 59° and 86° F. (15° and 30° C.).

Information for the patient
● Instruct patient regarding medication and dosage schedule; tell patient to take a missed dose as soon as possible and not to double up on doses.
● Warn patient about the possibility of decreased mental alertness or visual changes.
● Remind patient to use caution while taking drug when in warm climates, to minimize chance of heatstroke.

Geriatric use
Elderly patients may be more sensitive to the antimuscarinic effects. The drug is contraindicated in elderly and debilitated patients with intestinal atony.

---

*Canada only   †Unlabeled clinical use   Italicized adverse reactions are life-threatening.

Pediatric use
Dosage guidelines have not been established for children under age 5.

Breast-feeding
No problems have been reported, but oxybutynin may inhibit lactation.

---

oxycodone hydrochloride
Roxicodone, Supeudol*

- Pharmacologic classification: opioid
- Therapeutic classification: analgesic
- Controlled substance schedule II
- Pregnancy risk category C

How supplied
Available by prescription only
Tablets: 5 mg/5 ml
Oral solution: 5 mg/ml
Suppositories: 10 mg, 20 mg

Indications, route, and dosage
Moderate to severe pain
Adults: 5 mg P.O. every 3 to 6 hours; alternatively 10 to 40 mg p.r.n. (by rectum) 3 or 4 times per day.
Children over age 12: 2.44 mg P.O. every 6 hours.
Children age 6 to 12: 1.22 mg P.O. every 6 hours.

Pharmacodynamics
Analgesic action: Oxycodone acts on opiate receptors providing analgesia for moderate to moderately severe pain. Episodes of acute pain, rather than chronic pain, appear to be more responsive to treatment with oxycodone.

Pharmacokinetics
- *Absorption:* After oral administration, the onset of analgesic effect occurs within 15 to 30 minutes and peak effect is reached within 1 hour.
- *Distribution:* Rapid.
- *Metabolism:* Drug is metabolized in the liver.
- *Excretion:* Oxycodone is excreted principally by the kidneys. Duration of analgesia is 4 to 6 hours.

Contraindications and precautions
Oxycodone is contraindicated in patients with known hypersensitivity to the drug or other phenanthrene opioids (codeine, hydrocodone, hydromorphone, or oxymorphone).

Administer oxycodone with extreme caution to patients with supraventricular arrhythmias; avoid, or administer drug with extreme caution to patients with head injury or increased intracranial pressure, because drug obscures neurologic parameters; and during pregnancy and labor, because drug readily crosses placenta (premature infants are especially sensitive to respiratory and CNS depressant effects of opioids).

Administer oxycodone cautiously to patients with renal or hepatic dysfunction, because drug accumulation or prolonged duration of action may occur; to patients with pulmonary disease (asthma, chronic obstructive pulmonary disease), because drug depresses respiration and suppresses cough reflex; to patients undergoing biliary tract surgery, because drug may cause biliary spasm; to patients with convulsive disorders, because drug may precipitate seizures; to elderly or debilitated patients, who are more sensitive to both therapeutic and adverse drug effects; and to patients prone to physical or psychic addiction, because of the high risk of addiction to this drug.

Interactions
Concomitant with other CNS depressants (narcotic analgesics, general anesthetics, antihistamines, phenothiazines, barbiturates, benzodiazepines, sedative-hypnotics, tricyclic antidepressants, alcohol, and muscle relaxants), potentiates the drug's respiratory and CNS depression, sedation, and hypotensive effects. Concomitant use with cimetidine may also increase respiratory and CNS depression, causing confusion, disorientation, apnea, or seizures.

Drug accumulation and enhanced effects may result from concomitant use with other drugs that are extensively metabolized in the liver (rifampin, phenytoin, and digitoxin); combined with anticholinergics may cause paralytic ileus.

Patients who become physically dependent on this drug may experience acute withdrawal syndrome if given high doses of an opioid agonist-antagonist or a single dose of an antagonist.

Severe cardiovascular depression may result from concomitant use with general anesthetics.

Oxycodone products containing aspirin may increase anticoagulant's effect. Monitor clotting times, and use together cautiously.

Effects on diagnostic tests
Oxycodone increases plasma amylase and lipase and liver enzyme levels.

Adverse reactions
- CNS: sedation, euphoria, dysphoria, light-headedness (common), dizziness.
- DERM: rashes, pruritus.
- GI: nausea, vomiting, constipation.
- Other: *respiratory depression.*

At high doses, oxycodone hydrochloride produces many morphine-like adverse reactions.

Note: Drug should be discontinued if the following occur: hypersensitivity, seizures, or life-threatening cardiac arrhythmias.

Overdose and treatment
The most common signs and symptoms of a severe overdose are CNS depression, respiratory depression, and miosis (pinpoint pupils). Other acute toxic effects include hypotension, bradycardia, hypothermia, shock, apnea, cardiopulmonary arrest, circulatory collapse, pulmonary edema, and convulsions.

To treat acute overdose, first establish adequate respiratory exchange via a patent airway and ventilation as needed; administer a narcotic antagonist (naloxone) to reverse respiratory depression. (Because the duration of action of oxycodone is longer than that of naloxone, repeated naloxone dosing is necessary.) Naloxone should not be given unless patient has clinically significant respiratory or cardiovascular depression. Monitor vital signs closely.

If patient presents within 2 hours of ingestion of an oral overdose, empty the stomach immediately by inducing emesis (ipecac syrup) or using gastric lavage. Use caution to avoid any risk of aspiration. Administer activated charcoal via nasogastric tube for further removal of the drug in an oral overdose.

---

*Canada only   †Unlabeled clinical use   Italicized adverse reactions are life-threatening.

Provide symptomatic and supportive treatment (continued respiratory support, correction of fluid or electrolyte imbalance). Monitor laboratory parameters, vital signs, and neurologic status closely.

Dialysis may be helpful if combination products with aspirin or acetaminophen are involved.

▶ **Special considerations**
Besides those relevant to all *opioids*, consider the following recommendations.
● For full analgesic effect, give before patient has intense pain.
● Single-agent oxycodone solution or tablets is especially good for patients who shouldn't take aspirin or acetaminophen.
● Oxycodone has high abuse potential.
● Oxycodone may obscure the signs and symptoms of an acute abdominal condition or worsen gallbladder pain.
● Consider prescribing a stool softener for patients on long-term therapy.

Geriatric use
Lower doses are usually indicated for elderly patients, who may be more sensitive to the therapeutic and adverse effects of the drug.

Pediatric use
Dosage may be individualized for children; however, safety and effectiveness in children have not been established.

Breast-feeding
It is unknown whether oxycodone is excreted in breast milk; it should be used with caution in breast-feeding women.

oxymetazoline hydrochloride
Afrin, Allerest 12-Hour Nasal, Coricidin Nasal Mist, Dristan Long Lasting Nasal Mist, Duramist Plus, Duration, 4-Way Long-Acting Nasal Spray, Nafrine*, Neo-Synephrine 12 Hour Nasal Spray, Nöstrilla Long Acting Nasal Decongestant, NTZ Long Acting Nasal, Sinarest 12-Hour, Sinex Long-Lasting

● Pharmacologic classification: sympathomimetic agent
● Therapeutic classification: decongestant, vasoconstrictor
● Pregnancy risk category C

How supplied
Available without prescription
Nasal solution: 0.025% (drops) for children
Nasal drops or spray: 0.05%

Indications, route, and dosage
Nasal congestion
Adults and children over age 6: Apply 2 to 4 drops or sprays of 0.05% solution to nasal mucosa b.i.d.
Children age 2 to 6: Apply 2 to 3 drops of 0.025% solution to nasal mucosa b.i.d. Use no longer than 3 to 5 days. Dosage for younger children has not been established.

Pharmacodynamics
Decongestant action: Produces local vasoconstriction of arterioles through alpha receptors to reduce blood flow and nasal congestion.

Pharmacokinetics
Unknown.

Contraindications and precautions
Oxymetazoline hydrochloride is contraindicated in patients with narrow-angle glaucoma or hypersensitivity to any components of the preparation.

It should be used with caution in patients with hyperthyroidism, cardiac disease, hypertension, diabetes mellitus, and advanced arteriosclerosis.

Interactions
Oxymetazoline hydrochloride may potentiate the pressor effects of tricyclic antidepressants from significant systemic absorption of the decongestant.

Effects on diagnostic tests
None reported.

Adverse reactions
● CNS: headache, drowsiness, dizziness, insomnia, tremor, psychological disturbances, seizures, CNS depression, weakness, hallucinations, prolonged psychosis.
● CV: palpitations, *hypotension with cardiovascular collapse,* tachycardia, precordial pain.
● EENT: rebound nasal congestion or irritation (with excessive or long-term use), dryness of nose and throat, increased nasal discharge, stinging, sneezing, blurred vision, ocular irritation, tearing, photophobia.
● Other: dysuria, orofacial dystonia, pallor, sweating.
Note: Drug should be discontinued if symptoms of systemic toxicity occur.

Overdose and treatment
Clinical manifestations of overdose include somnolence, sedation, sweating, CNS depression with hypertension, bradycardia, decreased cardiac output, rebound hypotension, cardiovascular collapse, depressed respirations, coma.

Because of rapid onset of sedation, emesis is not recommended unless given early. Activated charcoal or gastric lavage may be utilized initially. Monitor vital signs and ECG. Treat seizures with I.V. diazepam.

▶ **Special considerations**
Monitor carefully for adverse reactions in patients with cardiovascular disease, diabetes mellitus, or prostatic hypertrophy, because systemic absorption can occur.

Information for the patient
● Emphasize that only one person should use dropper bottle or nasal spray.
● Advise patient not to exceed recommended dosage and to use drug only when needed.
● Tell patient nasal mucosa may sting, burn, or become dry.
● Warn patient that excessive use may cause bradycardia, hypotension, dizziness, and weakness.
● Show patient how to apply: have patient bend head forward and sniff spray briskly.

---

*Canada only   †Unlabeled clinical use   Italicized adverse reactions are life-threatening.

Geriatric use
Drug should be used with caution in elderly patients with cardiac disease, poorly controlled hypertension, or diabetes mellitus.

Pediatric use
Children may exhibit increased side effects from systemic absorption.

oxymetholone
Anadrol, Anapolon

- Pharmacologic classification: anabolic steroid
- Therapeutic classification: antianemic
- Controlled substance schedule III
- Pregnancy risk category X

How supplied
Available by prescription only
Tablets: 50 mg

Indications, route, and dosage
Aplastic anemia
Adults and children: 1 to 5 mg/kg P.O. daily. Dose highly individualized; response not immediate. Trial of 3 to 6 months required. Although the maximum dosage is 5 mg/kg/day, most patients respond to 1 to 2 mg/kg/day.
Premature infants and neonates: 0.175 mg/kg of body weight, or 5 mg/m² of body surface area, daily, as a single dose.

Pharmacodynamics
Erythropoietic action: Oxymetholone stimulates the kidneys' production of erythropoietin, leading to increases in red blood cell number, mass, and volume.

Pharmacokinetics
Oxymetholone is metabolized by the liver. Its pharmacokinetics are otherwise poorly described.

Contraindications and precautions
Oxymetholone is contraindicated in patients with severe renal or cardiac disease which may be worsened by the fluid and electrolyte retention this drug may cause; in patients with hepatic disease, because impaired elimination may cause toxic accumulation of the drug; in male patients with prostatic or breast cancer, benign prostatic hypertrophy with obstruction, or undiagnosed abnormal genital bleeding because this drug can stimulate the growth of cancerous breast or prostate tissue in males; and in pregnant and breast-feeding women because animal studies have shown that administration of anabolic steroids during pregnancy causes masculinization of the female fetus.
Because of its hypercholesterolemic effects, this drug should be administered cautiously in patients with a history of coronary artery disease.

Interactions
In patients with diabetes, decreased blood glucose levels may require adjustment of insulin or oral hypoglycemic drug dosage.
Oxymetholone may potentiate the effects of warfarin-type anticoagulants, prolonging prothrombin time. Use with adrenocorticosteroids or adrenocorticotropic hormone results in increased potential for fluid and electrolyte retention.

Effects on diagnostic tests
Oxymetholone may cause abnormal results of fasting plasma glucose, glucose tolerance, and metyrapone tests. It may increase sulfobromophthalein retention. Thyroid function test results (protein-bound iodine, radioactive iodine uptake; thyroid-binding capacity) and 17-ketosteroid levels may decrease. Liver function test results, prothrombin time (especially in patients receiving anticoagulant therapy), and serum creatinine levels may be elevated. Because of this agent's anabolic activity, serum sodium, potassium, calcium, phosphate, and cholesterol levels may all rise.

Adverse reactions
- Androgenic: *in females:* deepening of voice, clitoral enlargement, changes in libido; *in males:* prepubertal – premature epiphyseal closure, priapism, phallic enlargement; postpubertal – testicular atrophy, oligospermia, decreased ejaculatory volume, impotence, gynecomastia, epididymitis.
- CNS: headache, mental depression.
- CV: edema.
- DERM: acne, oily skin, hirsutism, flushing, sweating.
- GI: gastroenteritis, nausea, vomiting, constipation, diarrhea, change in appetite, weight gain.
- GU: bladder irritability, vaginitis, menstrual irregularities.
- Hepatic: reversible jaundice, hepatotoxicity.
- Other: hypercalcemia.
  Note: Drug should be discontinued if hypercalcemia, edema, hypersensitivity reaction, priapism, or excessive sexual stimulation occurs or if virilization occurs in females.

Overdose and treatment
No information available.

▶ Special considerations
Besides those relevant to all *anabolic steroids*, consider the following recommendations.
- Effects in osteoporosis are usually seen in 4 to 6 weeks.

Geriatric use
Observe elderly male patients for the development of prostatic hypertrophy.

Pediatric use
Use with extreme caution to avoid premature epiphyseal closure, masculinization of females, or precocious development of males.

oxymorphone hydrochloride
Numorphan

- Pharmacologic classification: opioid
- Therapeutic classification: analgesic
- Controlled substance schedule II
- Pregnancy risk category C

How supplied
Available by prescription only
Injection: 1 mg/ml, 1.5 mg/ml

Suppository: 5 mg

Indications, route, and dosage
Moderate to severe pain
Adults: 1 to 1.5 mg I.M. or S.C. q 4 to 6 hours, p.r.n. or around the clock; 0.5 mg I.V. q 4 to 6 hours, p.r.n. or around the clock; or 2.5 to 5 mg rectally q 4 to 6 hours, p.r.n. or around the clock.

Note: Parenteral administration of this drug is also indicated for preoperative medication, for support of anesthesia, for obstetrical analgesia, and for relief of anxiety in dyspnea associated with acute left ventricular failure and pulmonary edema.

Pharmacodynamics
Analgesic action: Oxymorphone effectively relieves moderate to severe pain via agonist activity at the opiate receptors. It has little or no antitussive effect.

Pharmacokinetics
● *Absorption:* Oxymorphone is well absorbed after rectal, S.C., I.M., or I.V. administration. The onset of action usually occurs within 15 to 30 minutes. Peak analgesic effect is seen at ½ to 1 hour.
● *Distribution:* Oxymorphone is widely distributed.
● *Metabolism:* Oxymorphone is primarily metabolized in the liver.
● *Excretion:* Duration of action is 3 to 6 hours. Drug is excreted primarily in the urine as oxymorphone hydrochloride.

Contraindications and precautions
Oxymorphone is contraindicated in patients with known hypersensitivity to the drug or any phenanthrene opioid (codeine, hydrocodone, hydromorphone, morphine, oxycodone).

Administer oxymorphone with extreme caution to patients with supraventricular arrhythmias; avoid, or administer drug with extreme caution to patients with head injury or increased intracranial pressure, because drug obscures neurologic parameters; and during pregnancy and labor, because drug readily crosses placenta (premature infants are especially sensitive to respiratory and CNS depressant effects).

Administer oxymorphone cautiously to patients with renal or hepatic dysfunction, because drug accumulation or prolonged duration of action may occur; to patients with pulmonary disease (asthma, chronic obstructive pulmonary disease), because drug depresses respiration and suppresses cough reflex; to patients undergoing biliary tract surgery, because drug may cause biliary spasm; to patients with convulsive disorders, because drug may precipitate seizures; to elderly or debilitated patients, who are more sensitive to both therapeutic and adverse drug effects; and to patients prone to physical or psychic addiction, because of the high risk of addiction to this drug.

Interactions
Concomitant use with other CNS depressants (opiates, general anesthetics, antihistamines, phenothiazines, barbiturates, benzodiazepines, sedative-hypnotics, tricyclic antidepressants, alcohol, and muscle relaxants) potentiates the drug's respiratory and CNS depression, sedation, and hypotensive effects.

Concomitant use with cimetidine may also increase respiratory and CNS depression, causing confusion, disorientation, apnea, or seizures. Reduced dosage of oxymorphone is usually necessary.

Drug accumulation and enhanced effects may result from concomitant use with other drugs that are extensively metabolized in the liver (rifampin, phenytoin, and digitoxin); combined use with anticholinergics may cause paralytic ileus.

Patients who become physically dependent on this drug may experience acute withdrawal syndrome if given a narcotic antagonist.

Severe cardiovascular depression may result from concomitant use with general anesthetics.

Effects on diagnostic tests
Oxymorphone increases plasma amylase levels.

Adverse reactions
● CNS: sedation, drowsiness, headache, miosis, dysphoria, light-headedness.
● GI: nausea, vomiting.
● Other: *respiratory depression.*

Note: Drug should be discontinued if hypersensitivity, seizures, or cardiac arrhythmias occur.

Overdose and treatment
The most common signs and symptoms of oxymorphone overdose are CNS depression (extreme somnolence progressing to stupor and coma), respiratory depression, and miosis (pinpoint pupils). Other acute toxic effects include hypotension, bradycardia, hypothermia, shock, apnea, cardiopulmonary arrest, circulatory collapse, pulmonary edema, and seizures.

To treat acute overdose, first establish adequate respiratory exchange via a patent airway and ventilation as needed; administer a narcotic antagonist (naloxone) to reverse respiratory depression. (Because the duration of action of oxymorphone is longer than that of naloxone, repeated naloxone dosing is necessary.) Naloxone should not be given unless the patient has clinically significant respiratory or cardiovascular depression. Monitor vital signs closely.

Provide symptomatic and supportive treatment (continued respiratory support, correction of fluid or electrolyte imbalance). Monitor laboratory parameters, vital signs, and neurologic status closely.

▶ Special considerations
Besides those relevant to all *opioids,* consider the following recommendations.
● Refrigerate oxymorphone suppositories.
● Oxymorphone is well absorbed rectally and is an alternative to opioids with more limited dosage forms.
● Oxymorphone may worsen gallbladder pain.

Geriatric use
Lower doses are usually indicated for elderly patients, who may be more sensitive to the therapeutic and adverse effects of the drug.

Pediatric use
Oxymorphone should not be administered to children under age 12.

Breast-feeding
It is not known whether oxymorphone is excreted in breast milk; it should be used with caution in breast-feeding women.

oxyphenbutazone

- Pharmacologic classification: nonsteroidal anti-inflammatory
- Therapeutic classification: nonnarcotic analgesic, antipyretic, anti-inflammatory, uricosuric
- Pregnancy risk category C

How supplied
Available by prescription only
Tablets: 100 mg

Indications, route, and dosage
Pain, inflammation in arthritis, ankylosing spondylitis
Adults: Initially, 300 to 600 mg daily in three or four divided doses; then 100 mg q.i.d.
Acute gouty arthritis
Adults: Initially, 400 mg as a single dose, then 100 mg q 4 hours; not to exceed 4 to 5 days.

Pharmacodynamics
Analgesic, antipyretic, and anti-inflammatory actions: The mechanisms of action of oxyphenbutazone, a metabolite of phenylbutazone, are unknown; oxyphenbutazone is thought to inhibit prostaglandin synthesis.

Pharmacokinetics
- *Absorption:* Drug is absorbed rapidly and completely from the GI tract.
- *Distribution:* Oxyphenbutazone is 98% protein-bound.
- *Metabolism:* Drug is metabolized in the liver.
- *Excretion:* Oxyphenbutazone is excreted in urine. Plasma half-life ranges from 50 to 100 hours.

Contraindications and precautions
Oxyphenbutazone is contraindicated in patients with known hypersensitivity to oxyphenbutazone or phenylbutazone; in patients in whom aspirin or other nonsteroidal anti-inflammatory drugs (NSAIDs) induce symptoms of asthma, urticaria, or rhinitis; in patients under age 14, because safety has not been established; and in patients with senility, GI bleeding, blood dyscrasias, or renal, hepatic, cardiac, or thyroid disease, because drug may mask symptoms associated with these disorders or worsen these conditions. Drug should not be used in patients on long-term anticoagulant therapy because of its potential for adverse hematologic effects.

Serious GI toxicity, especially ulceration or hemorrhage, can occur at any time in patients on chronic NSAID therapy. Use with caution in patients with a history of GI disease (especially peptic ulcer disease).

Patients with known "triad" symptoms (aspirin hypersensitivity, rhinitis/nasal polyps, and asthma) are at high risk of cross-sensitivity to oxyphenbutazone with precipitation of bronchospasm.

Because of the potential for serious blood dyscrasias, oxyphenbutazone is not recommended for initial therapy.

Interactions
When used concomitantly, anticoagulants and thrombolytic drugs may be potentiated by the platelet-inhibiting effect of oxyphenbutazone. Concomitant use of oxyphenbutazone with highly protein-bound drugs (phenytoin, sulfonylureas, warfarin) may cause displacement of either drug, and adverse effects. Monitor therapy closely for both drugs. Concomitant use with other GI-irritating drugs (steroids, antibiotics, NSAIDs) may potentiate the adverse GI effects of oxyphenbutazone. Use together with caution.

Antacids and food delay and decrease the absorption of oxyphenbutazone. NSAIDs are known to decrease renal clearance of lithium carbonate, thus increasing lithium serum levels and risks of adverse effects. Oxyphenbutazone is known to induce liver microsomal enzyme activity. Use with caution with other highly metabolized drugs (digitoxin). Concomitant use with other NSAIDs increases the risk of nephrotoxicity and decreases uricosuric effects.

Effects on diagnostic tests
Oxyphenbutazone interferes with thyroid function test results. It may decrease ^{131}I uptake, decrease serum thyroxine concentrations, and increase resin or erythrocyte triiodothyronine uptake.

The physiologic effects of the drug may prolong bleeding time, increase blood glucose concentrations, decrease serum uric acid concentrations, and increase AST (SGOT) and ALT (SGPT) levels.

Adverse reactions
- CNS: confusion, restlessness, lethargy, headache, dizziness.
- CV: hypertension, pericarditis, myocarditis, cardiac decompensation, CHF.
- DERM: petechiae, pruritus, purpura, dermatoses ranging from rash to *toxic necrotizing epidermolysis.*
- EENT: optic neuritis, blurred vision, retinal hemorrhage or detachment, hearing loss, tinnitus.
- GI: nausea, vomiting, anorexia, diarrhea, ulceration, bleeding, constipation.
- GU: proteinuria, hematuria, glomerulonephritis, nephrotic syndrome, *renal failure.*
- HEMA: *aplastic anemia, agranulocytosis,* bone marrow depression, *thrombocytopenia,* leukopenia.
- Other: toxic and nontoxic goiter, respiratory alkalosis, metabolic acidosis, hepatitis, elevated liver enzymes, hepatotoxicity, jaundice.
Note: Drug should be discontinued if the following occur: fever, sore throat, mouth ulcers, GI discomfort, black or tarry stools, bleeding, bruising, rash, weight gain, signs and symptoms of hepatotoxicity, or abnormal CBC.

Overdose and treatment
Clinical manifestations of overdose include nausea, abdominal pain, and drowsiness; vomiting, hematemesis, diarrhea, restlessness, dizziness, agitation, hallucinations, psychosis, coma, convulsions, hyperpyrexia, electrolyte disturbances, hyperventilation, respiratory arrest, and cyanosis.

To treat overdose of oxyphenbutazone, empty stomach immediately by inducing emesis with ipecac syrup if patient is conscious, or by gastric lavage. Administer activated charcoal via nasogastric tube. Provide symptomatic and supportive measures (respiratory support and correction of fluid and electrolyte imbalances). Use I.V. fluids with caution to prevent fluid overload. Monitor laboratory parameters and vital signs closely. If seizures occur, benzodiazepines may help to control them. Hemodialysis may be helpful in removing drug.

---

*Canada only   †Unlabeled clinical use   Italicized adverse reactions are life-threatening.

▶ **Special considerations**

Besides those relevant to all *NSAIDs*, consider the following recommendations.

● Complete physical examination and laboratory evaluation are recommended before therapy.

● Administer oxyphenbutazone with meals or food to minimize GI upset.

● Assess cardiopulmonary status closely. Monitor vital signs for significant changes.

● Monitor for signs and symptoms of fluid retention.

● Check results of laboratory tests before start of therapy to establish a baseline. Monitor CBC and renal and hepatic studies every 2 weeks to detect any abnormalities.

● Impose safety measures, such as supervised ambulation and raised side rails, to prevent injury.

● Response should be seen in 2 to 3 days. Drug should be stopped if no response in 1 week. Use lowest possible effective dose.

● Administer cautiously to patients over age 40. Serious blood dyscrasias appear more frequently in women, the elderly, and with long-term use.

Information for the patient

● Warn patient to remain under close medical supervision.

● Warn patient against exceeding prescribed dosage.

● Caution patient to avoid concomitant use of alcohol with oxyphenbutazone. Tell patient to call for specific instructions before using any nonprescription medications.

● Warn patient of possible CNS effects and to avoid hazardous activities that require alertness. Instruct patient in safety measures to prevent injury.

● Instruct patient to record daily weight and to report any weight gain of 2 pounds or more within a few days.

● Advise patient to immediately report any adverse reactions.

Geriatric use

● Patients over age 60 are more sensitive to the drug's adverse effects.

● Through its effect on renal prostaglandins, oxyphenbutazone may cause fluid retention and edema. This may be significant in elderly patients, especially those with congestive heart failure.

● Monitor CBC weekly in elderly patients. Report any abnormality immediately.

● Patients over age 60 should not receive drug longer than 1 week.

Pediatric use

Oxyphenbutazone is contraindicated in children under age 14.

Breast-feeding

Oxyphenbutazone is distributed into breast milk; an alternative feeding method should be considered during therapy with this drug.

---

oxyphencyclimine hydrochloride
Daricon

● Pharmacologic classification: anticholinergic
● Therapeutic classification: gastrointestinal antispasmodic
● Pregnancy risk category C

How supplied

Available by prescription only
Tablets: 10 mg

Indications, route, and dosage
Adjunctive treatment of peptic ulcer and irritable bowel syndrome

Adults: 10 mg P.O. b.i.d. in the morning and h.s., or 5 mg P.O. b.i.d. or t.i.d.

Pharmacodynamics

Antispasmodic action: Oxyphencyclimine competitively blocks acetylcholine at cholinergic neuroeffector sites, decreasing gastric acid secretion and GI motility. Oxyphencyclimine also exerts a nonspecific, direct spasmolytic action on smooth muscle and has some local anesthetic properties that may contribute to spasmolysis of the GI and biliary tracts.

Pharmacokinetics

● *Absorption:* Oxyphencyclimine is incompletely absorbed from the GI tract.

● *Distribution:* Presumably, oxyphencyclimine is widely distributed throughout the body. Because it is a quaternary ammonium compound, significant amounts of drug probably don't enter the CNS.

● *Metabolism:* Oxyphencyclimine's exact metabolic fate is unknown. Usual duration of effect is up to 12 hours.

● *Excretion:* Oxyphencyclimine is probably primarily excreted in urine; exact excretion mode is unknown.

Contraindications and precautions

Oxyphencyclimine is contraindicated in patients with narrow-angle glaucoma, because drug-induced cycloplegia and mydriasis may increase intraocular pressure; in patients with obstructive uropathy, obstructive GI tract disease, severe ulcerative colitis, myasthenia gravis, paralytic ileus, intestinal atony, or toxic megacolon, because the drug may exacerbate these conditions; and in patients with known hypersensitivity to anticholinergics.

Administer oxyphencyclimine cautiously to patients with autonomic neuropathy, hyperthyroidism, coronary artery disease, cardiac arrhythmias, congestive heart failure, chronic pulmonary disease, or ulcerative colitis, because the drug may exacerbate the symptoms of these conditions; to patients with hepatic or renal disease, because toxic accumulation may occur; to patients over age 40, because the drug increases the glaucoma risk; to patients with hiatal hernia associated with reflux esophagitis, because the drug may decrease lower esophageal sphincter tone; and in hot or humid environments, because the drug may predispose the patient to heatstroke.

Interactions
Concurrent administration of antacids decreases oral absorption of anticholinergics. Administer oxyphencyclimine at least 1 hour before antacids.

Concomitant administration of drugs with anticholinergic effects may cause additive toxicity.

Decreased GI absorption of many drugs has been reported after the use of anticholinergics (for example, levodopa and ketoconazole). Conversely, slowly dissolving digoxin tablets may yield higher serum digoxin levels when administered with anticholinergics.

Use cautiously with oral potassium supplements (especially wax-matrix formulations) which may increase the incidence of potassium-induced GI ulcerations.

Effects on diagnostic tests
None reported.

Adverse reactions
● CNS: headache, insomnia, drowsiness, dizziness, nervousness, weakness, confusion or excitement (in elderly).
● CV: palpitations, tachycardia, orthostatic hypotension.
● DERM: urticaria, decreased sweating or anhidrosis, other dermal manifestations.
● EENT: blurred vision, mydriasis, increased intraocular pressure, cycloplegia, photophobia.
● GI: constipation, nausea, vomiting, paralytic ileus, dry mouth, dysphagia, loss of taste, abdominal distention, heartburn.
● GU: urinary hesitancy and retention, impotence.
● Other: fever, allergic reaction.
Note: Drug should be discontinued if hypersensitivity, urinary retention, or curare-like symptoms develop.

Overdose and treatment
Clinical signs of overdose include curare-like symptoms, central stimulation followed by depression, and such psychotic symptoms as disorientation, confusion, hallucinations, delusions, anxiety, agitation, and restlessness. Peripheral effects may include dilated, nonreactive pupils; blurred vision; flushed, hot, dry skin; dryness of mucous membranes; dysphagia; decreased or absent bowel sounds; urinary retention; hyperthermia; headache; tachycardia; hypertension; and increased respiration.

Treatment is primarily symptomatic and supportive, as needed. Maintain a patent airway. If the patient is alert, induce emesis (or use gastric lavage) and follow with saline cathartic and activated charcoal to prevent further drug absorption. In severe cases, physostigmine may be administered to block oxyphencyclimine's antimuscarinic effects. Give fluids, as needed, to treat shock; diazepam to control psychotic symptoms; and pilocarpine (instilled into the eyes) to relieve mydriasis. If urinary retention develops, catheterization may be necessary.

▶ **Special considerations**
Besides those relevant to all *anticholinergics,* consider the following recommendation.
● Drug should be titrated until therapeutic effect is obtained or adverse effects become intolerable.

Geriatric use
Oxyphencyclimine should be administered cautiously to elderly patients. Lower doses are indicated.

Breast-feeding
Oxyphencyclimine may be excreted in breast milk, possibly resulting in infant toxicity. Breast-feeding women should avoid this drug. Drug may also decrease milk production.

oxytetracycline hydrochloride
Dalimycin, E.P. Mycin, Oxlopar, Oxy-Kesso-Tetra, Oxymycin, Oxytetrachlor, Terramycin, Uri-Tet

- Pharmacologic classification: tetracycline
- Therapeutic classification: antibiotic
- Pregnancy risk category D

How supplied
Available by prescription only
Capsules: 250 mg
Tablets: 250 mg
Injection: 50 mg/ml with lidocaine 2%; 125 mg/ml with lidocaine 2%

Indications, route, and dosage
Infections caused by sensitive organisms
Adults: 250 mg P.O. q 6 hours; 100 mg I.M. q 8 to 12 hours; 250 mg I.M. as a single dose.
Children over age 8: 25 to 50 mg/kg P.O. daily, divided q 6 hours; or 15 to 25 mg/kg I.M. daily, divided q 8 to 12 hours.
Brucellosis
Adults: 500 mg P.O. q.i.d. for 3 weeks with streptomycin 1 g I.M. q 12 hours first week, once daily second week.
Syphilis in patients sensitive to penicillin
Adults: 30 to 40 g total dose P.O., divided equally over 15 days.
Gonorrhea in patients sensitive to penicillin
Adults: Initially, 1.5 g P.O. followed by 0.5 g q.i.d. for a total of 9 g.
Dosage in renal failure
Specific recommendations are unavailable. Decreased dosage and/or increased intervals between doses is recommended by the manufacturer for patients with significant renal impairment.

Pharmacodynamics
Antibacterial action: Oxytetracycline is bacteriostatic; it binds reversibly to ribosomal units, thereby inhibiting bacterial protein synthesis.

Oxytetracycline is active against many gram-negative and gram-positive organisms, *Mycoplasma, Rickettsia, Chlamydia,* and spirochetes. Its spectrum of antibiotic action is similar to other tetracyclines, and many clinicians feel it offers no advantages over less expensive tetracycline alternatives.

Tetracyclines are drugs of choice in brucellosis, glanders, cholera, relapsing fever, melioidosis, leptospirosis, and early stages of Lyme disease. They are preferred drugs for chlamydial infections, granuloma inguinale, and urethritis due to *Ureaplasma urealyticum* (but some clinicians prefer erythromycin).

Pharmacokinetics
● *Absorption:* Oxytetracycline is 60% absorbed from the GI tract after oral administration in fasting adults; peak serum levels occur at 2 to 4 hours. Absorption is

significantly reduced by food or milk and other dairy products. I.M. absorption is erratic and incomplete.
- *Distribution:* Oxytetracycline is distributed widely into body tissues and fluids, including synovial, pleural, prostatic, and seminal fluids, bronchial secretions, saliva, and aqueous humor; CSF penetration is poor. Oxytetracycline crosses the placenta; it is 10% to 40% protein-bound.
- *Metabolism:* Oxytetracycline is not metabolized.
- *Excretion:* Systemically absorbed oxytetracycline is excreted primarily unchanged in urine by glomerular filtration; some drug may be excreted in breast milk. Plasma half-life is 6 to 10 hours in adults with normal renal function. Only minimal amounts are removed by hemodialysis or peritoneal dialysis.

Contraindications and precautions
Oxytetracycline is contraindicated in patients with known hypersensitivity to any tetracycline; during the second half of pregnancy; and in children under age 8 because of the risk of permanent discoloration of teeth, enamel defects, and retardation of bone growth.

Use drug with caution in patients with decreased renal function because drug may elevate BUN levels and exacerbate dysfunction; and in patients apt to be exposed to sunlight or ultraviolet light because of the risk of photosensitivity reactions.

Interactions
Concomitant use of oxytetracycline with antacids containing aluminum, calcium, or magnesium or with laxatives containing magnesium decreases absorption of oxytetracycline (because of chelation); concomitant use with food, milk and other dairy products, oral iron products, or sodium bicarbonate also impairs oral absorption.

Tetracyclines may antagonize bactericidal effects of penicillin, inhibiting cell growth through bacteriostatic action; administer penicillin 2 to 3 hours before oxytetracycline.

Oxytetracycline enhances the risk of nephrotoxicity from methoxyflurane; it also necessitates lowered dosage of oral anticoagulants because of enhanced effects, and lowered dosage of digoxin because of increased bioavailability.

Effects on diagnostic tests
Oxytetracycline causes false-negative results in urine glucose tests utilizing glucose oxidase reagent (Clinistix or Tes-Tape); parenteral dosage form may cause false-negative results on Clinitest.

Oxytetracycline causes false elevations in fluorometric tests for urinary catecholamines.

Oxytetracycline may elevate BUN level in patients with decreased renal function.

Adverse reactions
- CNS: *intracranial hypertension.*
- CV: *pericarditis.*
- DERM: maculopapular and erythematous rashes, urticaria, photosensitivity, increased pigmentation, discolored nails and teeth.
- EENT: dysphagia, glossitis.
- GI: anorexia, nausea, vomiting, diarrhea, enterocolitis, anogenital inflammation.
- GU: reversible nephrotoxicity (Fanconi's syndrome) with *outdated* tetracyclines.
- HEMA: neutropenia, eosinophilia.
- Metabolic: *increased BUN levels.*

- Local: irritation after I.M. injection, thrombophlebitis.
- Other: hypersensitivity, bacterial and fungal superinfection.
Note: Drug should be discontinued if signs of toxicity, hypersensitivity, progressive renal dysfunction, or superinfection occur; if erythema follows exposure to sunlight or ultraviolet light; or if severe diarrhea indicates pseudomembranous colitis.

Overdose and treatment
Clinical signs of overdose are usually limited to GI tract; give antacids or empty stomach by gastric lavage if ingestion occurred within the preceding 4 hours.

▶ **Special considerations**
Besides those relevant to all *tetracyclines,* consider the following recommendations.
- Inject I.M. dose deeply into large muscle mass to reduce pain. Rotate injection sites. Because I.M. preparations contain a local anesthetic, rule out hypersensitivity to local anesthetics before injecting.
- Reconstituted solution is stable for 48 hours in refrigerator.
- Store dry powder at room temperature; store syrup in cool place, protected from light.

Pediatric use
Drug should not be used in children younger than age 8.

Breast-feeding
Avoid use in breast-feeding women.

oxytocin
Pitocin, Syntocinon

- Pharmacologic classification: exogenous hormone
- Therapeutic classification: oxytocic, lactation stimulant

How supplied
Available by prescription only
Injection: 10-units/ml ampules, vials, and Tubex
Nasal solution: 40 units/ml

Indications, route, and dosage
Induction of labor
Adults: Initially, 1 to 2 milliunit/minute I.V. infusion. Rate of infusion may be increased slowly to a maximum of 20 milliunits/minute. Decrease rate when labor is firmly established.
Augmentation of labor
Adults: Initially, 2 milliunits/minute I.V. infusion. Rate of infusion may be increased slowly to a maximum of 20 milliunits/minute.
Reduction of postpartum bleeding after expulsion of placenta
Adults: 20 to 40 milliunits/minute I.V. infusion after delivery of the placenta.
Induce abortion
Adults: 20 to 100 milliunits/minute I.V infusion.
To promote initial milk ejection
Adults: One spray or three drops nasal solution into one or both nostrils 2 or 3 minutes before breast-feeding or pumping breasts.

†*Oxytocin challenge test to assess fetal distress in high-risk pregnancies greater than 31 weeks' gestation*

Adults: Prepare solution by adding 5 to 10 units oxytocin to 1 liter of 5% dextrose injection (yielding a solution of 5 to 10 milliunits per ml). Infuse 0.5 milliunits per minute, gradually increasing at 15 minute intervals to a maximum infusion infusion of 20 milliunits/minute. Discontinue infusion when three moderate uterine contractions occur in a 10 minute interval.

Pharmacodynamics

● *Oxytocic action:* Oxytocin increases the sodium permeability of uterine myofibrils, indirectly stimulating the contraction of uterine smooth muscle. The threshold for response is lowered in the presence of high estrogen concentrations. Uterine response increases with the length of the pregnancy and increases further during active labor. Response mimics labor contractions.

● *Lactation stimulation:* By contracting the myoepithelial cells surrounding the alveoli of the breasts, oxytocin forces milk from the alveoli into the larger ducts and facilitates milk ejection.

Pharmacokinetics

● *Absorption:* Onset is immediate following I.V. injection and occurs within 3 to 5 minutes of an I.M. injection. Absorption through the nasal mucosa is rapid but may be erratic; it acts within a few minutes.

● *Distribution:* Drug is distributed throughout the extracellular fluid; small amounts may enter the fetal circulation.

● *Metabolism:* Oxytocin is metabolized rapidly in the kidneys and liver. In early pregnancy, a circulating enzyme, oxytocinase, can inactivate the drug.

● *Excretion:* Only small amounts are excreted in the urine as oxytocin. The half-life is 3 to 5 minutes and the duration of action is 1 hour following I.V. infusion; 2 to 3 hours I.M.; and 20 minutes intranasal.

Contraindications and precautions

Oxytocin is contraindicated in patients with hypersensitivity to the drug. The nasal preparation is contraindicated during pregnancy.

Oxytocin should not be used to induce labor when the benefit-to-risk ratio for the mother or child favors surgical intervention, when labor is progressing normally during the first and second stages of labor, when hypertonic patterns of labor occur, or when vaginal delivery is contraindicated.

Interactions

Cyclopropane anesthesia may modify oxytocin's cardiovascular effects. It may also delay the induction of thiopental anesthesia.

Effects on diagnostic tests

None reported.

Adverse reactions

Maternal

● CNS: *subarachnoid hemorrhage* resulting from hypertension; *convulsions or coma resulting from water intoxication.*

● CV: hypotension; increased heart rate, systemic venous return, and cardiac output; arrhythmia.

● GI: nausea, vomiting.

● HEMA: afibrinogenemia; may be related to increased postpartum bleeding, pelvic hematoma.

● Other: hypersensitivity, tetanic contractions, abruptio placentae, impaired uterine blood flow, increased uterine motility, uterine rupture.

Fetal

● CV: bradycardia, tachycardia, premature ventricular contractions, cardiac arrhythmias.

● HEMA: hyperbilirubinemia.

● Other: *anoxia, asphyxia.*

   Note: Drug should be discontinued if the uterine response is severe, because this may result in adverse effects on both the mother and the fetus.

Overdose and treatment

Clinical manifestations of overdose include hyperstimulation of the uterus, causing tetanic contractions and possible uterine rupture, cervical laceration, abruptio placentae, impaired uterine blood flow, amniotic fluid embolism, and fetal trauma. The drug has a very short half-life; therefore, therapy should be halted and supportive care initiated.

▶ Special considerations

● Administer by I.V. infusion, not I.V. bolus injection.

● Never give oxytocin by more than one route simultaneously.

● Monitor and record uterine contractions, heart rate, blood pressure, intrauterine pressure, fetal heart rate, and character of blood loss every 15 minutes.

● When administering oxytocin challenge test, monitor fetal heart rate and uterine contractions immediately before and during infusion. If fetal heart rate does not change during test, repeat in 1 week. If late deceleration in fetal heart rate is noted, consider terminating pregnancy.

● May produce an antidiuretic effect; monitor fluid intake and output.

● During long infusions, watch for signs of water intoxication.

● Have magnesium sulfate (20% solution) available for relaxation of the myometrium.

● Not recommended for routine I.M. use. However, 10 units may be administered I.M. after delivery of the placenta to control postpartum uterine bleeding.

● Solution containing 10 milliunits/ml may be prepared by adding 10 units of oxytocin to 1 liter of 0.9 sodium chloride or dextrose 5% in water solutions. Solution containing 20 milliunits/ml may be prepared by adding 10 units of oxytocin to 500 ml of 0.9 sodium chloride or dextrose 5% in water solutions.

Information for the patient

● Explain possible adverse effects of the drug.

● For nasal use: Instruct patient to clear nasal passages before using drug. With head in vertical position, patient should hold squeeze bottle upright and eject solution into nostril. If preferred, the solution can be instilled in drop form by inverting the squeeze bottle and exerting gentle pressure.

Breast-feeding

Minimal amounts of drug enter breast milk. Risks must be evaluated.

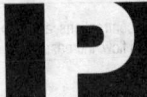

pamidronate disodium
Aredia

- Pharmacologic classification: biphosphonate; pyrophosphate analog
- Therapeutic classification: antihypercalcemic
- Pregnancy risk category C

How supplied
Available by prescription only
Injection: 30 mg/vial

Indications, route, and dosage
Moderate to severe hypercalcemia associated with malignancy (with or without metastases)
Adults: Dosage depends on severity of hypercalcemia. Serum calcium levels should be corrected for serum albumin. Corrected serum calcium (CCa) is calculated using the following formula:

$$\underset{\text{(in mg/dl)}}{CCa} = \underset{\text{(mg/dl)}}{serum\ Ca} + 0.8\ \underset{\text{(in g/dl)}}{(4 - serum\ albumin)}$$

Patients with moderate hypercalcemia (CCa levels of 12 to 13.5 mg/dl) may receive 60 to 90 mg by I.V. infusion over 24 hours. Patients with severe hypercalcemia (CCa levels over 13.5 mg/dl) may receive 90 mg as the initial dose.

Pharmacodynamics
Antihypercalcemic action: Pamidronate inhibits the resorption of bone. Drug adsorbs to hydroxyapatite crystals in bone and may directly block the dissolution of calcium phosphate. Drug apparently does not inhibit bone formation or mineralization.

Pharmacokinetics
- *Distribution:* After I.V. administration in animals, about 50% to 60% of a dose is rapidly absorbed by bone; drug is also taken up by the kidneys, liver, spleen, teeth, and tracheal cartilage.
- *Metabolism:* None.
- *Excretion:* Pamidronate is excreted by the kidneys; an average of 51% of a dose is excreted in urine within 72 hours of administration.

Contraindications and precautions
Pamidronate is contraindicated in patients with hypersensitivity to the drug or other biphosphonates, such as etidronate. Use with extreme caution and consider risk:benefit in patients with renal impairment.

Drug should be used only after patient has been vigorously hydrated with saline. In patients with mild to moderate hypercalcemia, hydration alone may be sufficient.

Interactions
Pamidronate may form a precipitate when mixed with solutions that contain calcium.

Effects on diagnostic tests
Pamidronate therapy may alter serum electrolyte levels, including serum calcium, potassium, magnesium, and phosphate.

Adverse reactions
- CNS: *seizures.*
- CV: fluid overload, hypertension.
- GI: abdominal pain, anorexia, constipation, nausea, vomiting.
- GU: urinary tract infection.
- HEMA: anemia.
- Local: redness, swelling, pain.
- Other: hypophosphatemia, hypokalemia, hypomagnesemia, hypocalcemia, bone pain, fever.

Overdose and treatment
Symptomatic hypocalcemia could result from overdosage; treat with I.V. calcium. In one reported case, a 209-lb (95-kg) woman who received 285 mg daily for 3 days experienced hyperpyrexia (103 °F [39.5° C]), hypotension, and transient taste perversion. Fever and hypotension were rapidly corrected with steroids.

▶ Special considerations
- Because drug can cause electrolyte disturbances, careful monitoring of serum electrolytes (especially calcium, phosphate, and magnesium) is essential. Short-term administration of calcium may be necessary in patients with severe hypocalcemia. Also monitor creatinine, CBC, differential, hematocrit, and hemoglobin levels.
- Carefully monitor patients with preexisting anemia, leukopenia, or thrombocytopenia during the first 2 weeks after therapy.
- Monitor patient's temperature. In clinical trials, 27% of patients experienced an elevation of 1° C for 24 to 48 hours after therapy.
- Reconstitute vial with 10 ml sterile water for injection. Once drug is completely dissolved, add to 1,000 ml 0.45% or 0.9% sodium chloride injection or dextrose 5% in water. Do not mix with infusion solutions that contain calcium, such as Ringer's injection or lactated Ringer's injection. Visually inspect for precipitate before administering.
- Injection solution is stable for 24 hours at room temperature. Give only by I.V. infusion. Animal studies have shown evidence of nephropathy when drug is given as a bolus.

Pediatric use
Safety and efficacy in children have not been established.

Breast-feeding
It is unknown if drug is excreted in breast milk. Use with caution in breast-feeding women.

---

*Canada only   †Unlabeled clinical use   Italicized adverse reactions are life-threatening.

pancreatic enzymes

pancreatin
pancrelipase

Pancreatic enzymes, principally amylase, protease, and lipase, are extracted from fresh hog pancreas. Preparations are processed in enteric formulations to prevent destruction by pepsin and gastric acid.

Pharmacology

The pancreatic enzymes, like the endogenous pancreatic enzymes, provide the enzymes necessary to digest protein, starches, and fats in enzyme-deficient patients.

Clinical indications and actions
Pancreatic insufficiency

All pancreatic enzymes provide supplemental or replacement enzymes to promote digestion in enzyme-deficient patients and help correct malabsorption in patients after pancreatectomy and bowel resection or other conditions that prohibit mixing of pancreatic enzymes high in the intestine.

Overview of adverse reactions

Since drugs are not absorbed, adverse reactions are all local to the GI tract and usually consist of nausea, vomiting, diarrhea, and stomach cramps.

▶ Special considerations

● Contraindicated in patients with severe pork hypersensitivity.
● Use only after confirmed diagnosis of exocrine pancreatic insufficiency. Not effective in GI disorders unrelated to enzyme deficiency.
● For maximal effect, administer dose just prior to or during a meal.
● Adequate replacement decreases number of bowel movements and improves stool consistency.
● The preparations are coated to protect the enzymes from gastric juices; do not crush or chew.
● Antacids or H$_2$ blockers, such as cimetidine or ranitidine, may be administered concurrently to prevent inactivation of non-enteric-coated drug products; enteric coating on some products may reduce availability of enzyme in upper portion of jejunum.
● For young children, mix powders (including contents of capsule) with applesauce and give at mealtime. Avoid inhalation of powder. Older children may swallow capsules with food.

Representative combinations

Pancreatin with ox bile extract, oxidized mixed ox bile acids, and desoxycholic acid: Bilogen; with dehydrocholic acid and pepsin: Canz, Digestozyme; with ox bile extract, papain, and duodenal substances (dessicated and defatted): Digenzyme; with bile salts (in core), hyoscyamine sulfate, atropine sulfate, hyoscine hydrobromide, phenobarbital, and pepsin (in outer layer): Donnazyme; with pepsin and bile salts: Entozyme; with pepsin and taurocholic acid: Enzymet; with pepsin, bile salts, dehydrocholic acid, and desoxycholic acid: Pepsatal; with ox bile salts and activated charcoal: Karbokoff.

pancreatin
Dizymes, Hi-Vegi-Lip, Pancreatin Enseals, Pancreatin Tablets

● Pharmacologic classification: pancreatic enzyme
● Therapeutic classification: digestant
● Pregnancy risk category C

How supplied

Available without prescription
Dizymes
Tablets (enteric-coated): 250 mg pancreatin, 6,750 units lipase, 41,250 units protease, 43,750 units amylase
Hi-Vegi-Lip
Tablets (enteric-coated): 2,400 mg pancreatin, 12,000 units lipase, 60,000 units protease, and 60,000 units amylase
Pancreatin Enseals
Tablets (enteric-coated): 1,000 mg pancreatin, 2,000 units lipase, 25,000 units protease, 25,000 units amylase
Pancreatin Tablets
Tablets (enteric-coated): 325 mg pancreatin, 650 units lipase, 8,125 units protease, 8,125 units amylase

Indications, route, and dosage
Exocrine pancreatic secretion insufficiency, digestive aid in cystic fibrosis, steatorrhea and other disorders of fat metabolism secondary to insufficient pancreatic enzymes
Adults and children: 1 to 3 tablets P.O. with meals.

Pharmacodynamics

Digestive action: The proteolytic, amylolytic, and lipolytic enzymes enhance the digestion of proteins, starches, and fats. This agent is sensitive to acids and is more active in neutral or slightly alkaline environments.

Pharmacokinetics

● *Absorption:* Drug is not absorbed; it acts locally in the GI tract.
● *Distribution:* None.
● *Metabolism:* None.
● *Excretion:* Drug is excreted in feces.

Contraindications and precautions

Pancreatin is contraindicated in patients with hypersensitivity to hog protein.

Interactions

Pancreatin activity may be reduced by calcium- or magnesium-containing antacids; however, antacids or H$_2$ blockers (such as cimetidine) may reduce the inactivation of the enzymes by gastric acid. Pancreatin decreases absorption of iron-containing products.

Effects on diagnostic tests

Pancreatin, particularly in large doses, increases serum uric acid concentrations.

Adverse reactions

There are usually no reactions to normal doses.
● GI: nausea, vomiting, diarrhea, stomach cramps.

Note: Drug should be discontinued if an allergic reaction occurs.

Overdose and treatment
Clinical manifestations of overdose include hyperuricosuria and hyperuricemia.

▶ Special considerations
● For maximal effect, administer dose just before or during a meal.
● Tablets may not be crushed or chewed.
● Diet should balance fat, protein, and starch intake properly to avoid indigestion. Dosage varies according to degree of maldigestion and malabsorption, amount of fat in diet, and enzyme activity of individual preparations.
● Adequate replacement decreases number of bowel movements and improves stool consistency.
● Use only after confirmed diagnosis of exocrine pancreatic insufficiency. Not effective in GI disorders unrelated to pancreatic enzyme deficiency.
● Enteric coating may reduce availability of enzyme in upper portion of jejunum.

Information for the patient
● Explain use of drug, and advise storage away from heat and light.
● Be sure patient or family understands special dietary instructions for the particular disease.

---

pancrelipase
Cotazym, Cotazym-S, Festal II, Ilozyme, Ku-Zyme HP, Pancrease, Pancrease MT4, Pancrease MT10, Pancrease MT16, Viokase

● Pharmacologic classification: pancreatic enzyme
● Therapeutic classification: digestant
● Pregnancy risk category C

How supplied
Available by prescription only
Cotazym
Capsules: 8,000 units lipase, 30,000 units protease, 30,000 units amylase
Cotazym-S
Capsules: 5,000 units lipase, 20,000 units protease, 20,000 units amylase
Ilozyme
Tablets: 11,000 units lipase, 30,000 units protease, 30,000 units amylase

Available without prescription
Festal II
Tablets: 6,000 units lipase, 20,000 units protease, 30,000 units amylase
Ku-Zyme HP
Capsules: 8,000 units lipase, 30,000 units protease, 30,000 units amylase
Pancrease
Capsules: 4,000 units lipase, 25,000 units protease, 20,000 units amylase
Pancrease MT4
Tablets (enteric-coated microtablets): 4,000 units lipase, 12,000 units protease, 12,000 units amylase

Pancrease MT10
Tablets (enteric-coated microtablets): 10,000 units lipase, 30,000 units protease, 30,000 units amylase
Pancrease MT16
Tablets (enteric-coated microtablets): 16,000 units lipase, 48,000 units protease, 48,000 units amylase
Viokase
Powder: 16,800 units lipase, 70,000 units protease, 70,000 units amylase

Indications, route, and dosage
Exocrine pancreatic secretion insufficiency, cystic fibrosis in adults and children, steatorrhea and other disorders of fat metabolism secondary to insufficient pancreatic enzymes
Adults and children: Dosage range is 1 to 3 capsules or tablets P.O. before or with meals and 1 capsule or tablet with snack; or 1 to 2 powder packets before meals or snacks. Dose must be titrated to patient's response.

Pharmacodynamics
Digestive action: The proteolytic, amylolytic, and lipolytic enzymes enhance the digestion of proteins, starches, and fats. This agent is sensitive to acids and is more active in neutral or slightly alkaline environments.

Pharmacokinetics
● *Absorption:* Drug is not absorbed and acts locally in the GI tract.
● *Distribution:* None.
● *Metabolism:* None.
● *Excretion:* Drug is excreted in feces.

Contraindications and precautions
Pancrelipase is contraindicated in patients with hypersensitivity to pork or pork derivatives. The powder is extremely irritating if inhaled.

Interactions
When used concomitantly, pancrelipase activity may be reduced by calcium- or magnesium-containing antacids; however, antacids or H₂ blockers (such as cimetidine) may reduce inactivation of the enzymes by gastric acid. Pancrelipase decreases absorption of iron-containing products.

Effects on diagnostic tests
Pancrelipase therapy increases serum uric acid concentrations, particularly with large doses.

Adverse reactions
There are usually no reactions to normal doses.
● GI: nausea, vomiting, diarrhea, stomach cramps.
   Note: Drug should be discontinued if an allergic reaction occurs.

Overdose and treatment
Clinical manifestations of overdose include hyperuricosuria and hyperuricemia.

▶ Special considerations
● For maximal effect, administer dose just before or during a meal.
● Preparations may not be crushed or chewed.
● Use only after confirmed diagnosis of exocrine pancreatic insufficiency. Not effective in GI disorders unrelated to enzyme deficiency.
● For young children, mix powders (including content

---

*Canada only   †Unlabeled clinical use   Italicized adverse reactions are life-threatening.

of capsules) with applesauce and give at mealtime. Avoid inhalation of powder. Older children may swallow capsules with food.
● Dosage varies with degree of maldigestion and malabsorption, amount of fat in diet, and enzyme activity of individual preparations.
● Adequate replacement decreases number of bowel movements and improves stool consistency.
● Enteric coating on some products may reduce availability of enzyme in upper portion of jejunum.

Information for the patient
● Teach patient or family proper use of drug, and advise storage away from heat and light.
● Be sure patient or family understands special dietary instructions for the particular disease.

Pediatric use
Capsules may be opened to facilitate swallowing. They may be sprinkled on food, but a pH of 5.5 or greater is necessary to ensure stability.

---

pancuronium bromide
Pavulon

● Pharmacologic classification: nondepolarizing neuromuscular blocking agent
● Therapeutic classification: skeletal muscle relaxant
● Pregnancy risk category C

How supplied
Available by prescription only
Injection: 1 mg/ml, 2 mg/ml parenteral

Indications, route, and dosage
Adjunct to anesthesia to induce skeletal muscle relaxation, facilitate intubation and ventilation, and to weaken muscle contractions in induced convulsions
Dose depends on anesthetic used, individual needs, and response. Doses are representative and must be adjusted.
Adults and children over age 1 month: Initially, 0.04 to 0.1 mg/kg I.V.; then 0.01 mg/kg q 30 to 60 minutes if needed.

Pharmacodynamics
Skeletal muscle relaxant action: Pancuronium prevents acetylcholine (ACh) from binding to the receptors on the motor end-plate, thus blocking depolarization. It may increase heart rate through direct blocking effect on the ACh receptors of the heart; increase is dose-related. Pancuronium causes little or no histamine release and no ganglionic blockade.

Pharmacokinetics
● *Absorption:* After I.V. administration, onset of action occurs within 30 to 45 seconds, with peak effects seen in 3 to 4½ minutes. Onset and duration are dose-related. After 0.06 mg/kg dose, effects begin to subside in 35 to 45 minutes. Repeated doses may increase the magnitude and duration of action.
● *Distribution:* Very low protein binding regardless of dose.

● *Metabolism:* Unknown metabolism; small amounts may be metabolized by the liver.
● *Excretion:* Mainly excreted unchanged in urine; some through biliary excretion.

Contraindications and precautions
Pancuronium is contraindicated in patients with known hypersensitivity to the drug or to bromides, and in patients with pre-existing tachycardia or in whom minor elevation in heart rate is undesirable. Administer with extreme caution to patients with poor renal perfusion or severe renal disease. Administer with caution to patients with bronchogenic carcinoma, dehydration or electrolyte imbalances, electrolyte disturbances, hepatic or pulmonary function impairment, hyperthermia, hypothermia, or myasthenia gravis. Administer cautiously at reduced dosage in pregnant women receiving magnesium sulfate.

Interactions
Concomitant use of pancuronium with succinylcholine may enhance and prolong neuromuscular blocking effects of pancuronium. The effects of pancuronium may also be potentiated by aminoglycoside antibiotics, clindamycin, lincomycin, polymyxin antibiotics, general anesthetics, beta-blocking agents, furosemide, lithium, parenteral magnesium salts, depolarizing neuromuscular blocking agents, other nondepolarizing neuromuscular blocking agents, quinidine or quinine, thiazide diuretics, and potassium-depleting agents. Concomitant use with opioid analgesics may increase respiratory depression.

Effects on diagnostic tests
None significant.

Adverse reactions
● CV: elevated pulse rate, especially after high doses or when administered in combination with ketamine; slight elevation in blood pressure (dose-related).
● Local: burning sensation along vein (rare).
● Other: excessive salivation and sweating (particularly in children), transient rash, wheezing, *prolonged dose-related apnea,* residual muscular weakness.
   Note: Drug should be discontinued if hypersensitivity or cardiovascular collapse occurs.

Overdose and treatment
Clinical manifestations of overdose include prolonged respiratory depression, apnea, and cardiovascular collapse.
   Use a peripheral nerve stimulator to monitor response and to evaluate neuromuscular blockade. Maintain an adequate airway and manual or mechanical ventilation until patient can maintain adequate ventilation unassisted.

▶ Special considerations
● Monitor baseline electrolyte levels, intake and output, and vital signs, especially heart rate and respiration.
● Administration requires direct medical supervision, with emergency respiratory support available.
● If using succinylcholine, allow its effects to subside before administering pancuronium.
● Store drug in refrigerator and not in plastic container or syringes. Plastic syringes may be used to administer dose.
● Do not mix in same syringe or give through same needle with barbiturates or other alkaline solutions.

● Use fresh solution only.
● Neostigmine, edrophonium, or pyridostigmine may be used to reverse effects.
● Dosage should be reduced when ether or other inhalation anesthetics that enhance neuromuscular blockade are used.
● Large doses may increase frequency and severity of tachycardia.
● Drug does not relieve pain or affect consciousness; be sure to assess need for analgesic or sedative.

Geriatric use
The usual adult dose must be individualized depending on response.

Pediatric use
Dosage for neonates under age 1 month must be carefully individualized. For infants over age 1 month and children, see adult dosage.

Breast-feeding
It is unknown if pancuronium is excreted in breast milk. Use with caution in breast-feeding women.

papaverine hydrochloride
Cerebid, Cerespan, Delapav, Myobid, Papacon, Pavabid, Pavacap, Pavacen, Pavadur, Pavadyl, Pavagen, Pava-Par, Pava-Rx, Pavased, Pavasule, Pavatine, Paverolan, P-200, Vasal

● Pharmacologic classification: benzylisoquinoline derivative, opiate alkaloid
● Therapeutic classification: peripheral vasodilator
● Pregnancy risk category C

How supplied
Available by prescription only
Tablets: 30 mg, 60 mg, 100 mg, 200 mg, 300 mg
Tablets (sustained-release): 200 mg
Capsules (sustained-release): 150 mg
Injection: 30 mg/ml in 2- and 10-ml ampules

Indications, route, and dosage
Relief of cerebral and peripheral ischemia associated with arterial spasm and myocardial ischemia; treatment of coronary occlusion and certain cerebral angiospastic states
Adults: 75 to 300 mg P.O. three to five times daily or 150 to 300 mg sustained-release preparations q 8 to 12 hours; 30 to 120 mg I.M. or I.V. q 3 hours, as indicated.
Children: 6 mg/kg I.M.or I.V. q.i.d.

Pharmacodynamics
Vasodilating action: Papaverine relaxes smooth muscle directly by inhibiting phosphodiesterase, thus increasing concentration of cyclic adenosine monophosphate. There is considerable controversy regarding the clinical effectiveness of papaverine. Some clinicians find little objective evidence of any clinical value.

Pharmacokinetics
● *Absorption:* 54% of orally administered papaverine is bioavailable. Peak plasma levels occur 1 to 2 hours after an oral dose; half-life varies from ½ to 24 hours, but levels can be maintained by giving drug at 6-hour intervals. Sustained-release forms are sometimes absorbed poorly and erratically.
● *Distribution:* Papaverine tends to localize in adipose tissue and in the liver; the remainder is distributed throughout the body. About 90% of the drug is protein-bound.
● *Metabolism:* Papaverine is metabolized by the liver.
● *Excretion:* Papaverine is excreted in urine as metabolites.

Contraindications and precautions
Papaverine is contraindicated in patients with complete atrioventricular (AV) heart block because large doses may depress AV and intraventricular conduction, causing serious arrhythmias.
Use drug cautiously in patients with glaucoma.
Papaverine is not recommended as a substitute for nitroglycerin during anginal attacks.

Interactions
Papaverine may decrease the antiparkinsonian effects of levodopa and exacerbate such symptoms as rigidity and tremors. Heavy tobacco smoking may interfere with the therapeutic effect of papaverine because nicotine constricts the blood vessels. Papaverine's effects may be potentiated by CNS depressants and may have a synergic response with morphine.

Effects on diagnostic tests
Papaverine therapy alters serum concentrations of eosinophils, ALT (SGPT), alkaline phosphatase, and bilirubin. Elevated serum bilirubin levels signal hepatic hypersensitivity to papaverine.

Adverse reactions
● CNS: headache, drowsiness, dizziness, depression, sedation, or lethargy.
● CV: increased heart rate, hypertension (with parenteral use), depressed AV and intraventricular conduction, *arrhythmias.*
● GI: nausea, constipation, diarrhea, abdominal distress, anorexia.
● Other: hepatic hypersensitivity, sweating, flushing, increased depth of respiration.
Note: Drug should be discontinued if signs of hepatic hypersensitivity occur (jaundice, eosinophilia, and altered liver function test results).

Overdose and treatment
Clinical signs of overdose include drowsiness, weakness, nystagmus, diplopia, incoordination, and lassitude, progressing to coma with cyanosis and respiratory depression.
To slow drug absorption, give activated charcoal, tap water, or milk, then evacuate stomach contents by gastric lavage or emesis, and follow with catharsis. If coma and respiratory depression occur, take appropriate measures; maintain blood pressure. Hemodialysis may be helpful.

▶ Special considerations
● Papaverine is an opiate; however, it has strikingly different pharmacologic properties than other drugs in this group.
● Papaverine may be given orally, I.M. or, when immediate effect is needed, by slow I.V. injection. Inject

---

I.V. slowly over 1 to 2 minutes; arrhythmias and fatal apnea may follow rapid injection.
- Papaverine injection is incompatible with lactated Ringer's injection; a precipitate will form.

Information for the patient
- Advise patient to avoid sudden postural changes to minimize possible orthostatic hypotension.
- Instruct patient to report nausea, abdominal distress, anorexia, constipation, diarrhea, jaundice, rash, sweating, tiredness, or headache.

Geriatric use
Elderly patients are at greater risk of papaverine-induced hypothermia.

Pediatric use
Children's doses are administered parenterally.

Breast-feeding
Safety in breast-feeding women has not been established.

---

para-aminosalicylate sodium (PAS)
Parasal Sodium, Pasdium, P.A.S. Sodium, Teebacin

- Pharmacologic classification: aminobenzoic acid analogue
- Therapeutic classification: antitubercular agent
- Pregnancy risk category C

How supplied
Available by prescription only
Tablets: 500 mg, 1 g
Powder: 4.18-g packets

Indications, route, and dosage
Adjunctive treatment of tuberculosis
Adults: 12 to 15 g P.O. daily, divided in three or four doses.
Children: 240 to 360 mg/kg P.O. daily, divided in three or four doses.

Pharmacodynamics
Antibiotic action: PAS is bacteriostatic; it interferes with folic acid synthesis by enzyme inhibition. PAS is active only against Mycobacterium tuberculosis.

PAS is considered adjunctive therapy in tuberculosis and is given with another antitubercular agent to prevent or delay development of drug resistance by M. tuberculosis.

Pharmacokinetics
- Absorption: PAS is absorbed readily from the GI tract after oral administration; peak serum concentrations occur 30 to 60 minutes after ingestion.
- Distribution: PAS is distributed widely into body tissues and fluids, including pleural, synovial, and peritoneal fluids. PAS does not penetrate CSF in uninflamed meninges but may do so in inflamed meninges. PAS is 50% to 75% protein-bound; it is not known if PAS crosses the placenta.
- Metabolism: PAS is acetylated by intestinal mucosa

and liver enzymes to N-acetyl-para-aminosalicylic acid and para-aminosalicyluric acid.
- Excretion: PAS is excreted primarily in urine by glomerular filtration and renal tubular secretion; small amounts of drug may be excreted in breast milk. Plasma half-life in adults is 1 hour.

Contraindications and precautions
PAS is contraindicated in patients with known hypersensitivity to aminosalicylic acid or its salts. It should be used cautiously in patients with congestive heart failure or glucose-6-phosphate dehydrogenase deficiency, in whom excess sodium could be harmful, and in patients with hepatic or renal disease or a history of gastric ulcer.

Interactions
Aminosalicylic acid and its salts may decrease oral absorption of rifampin and vitamin B_{12}; PAS may increase effects of oral anticoagulants.

Probenecid increases aminosalicylic acid serum concentrations by blocking renal tubular secretion. Diphenhydramine decreases oral absorption of PAS.

Ascorbic acid and ammonium chloride may acidify urine in PAS-treated patients, causing crystalluria.

Effects on diagnostic tests
PAS alters urine glucose testing by cupric sulfate method (Benedict's reagent or Clinitest) and may cause false-positive elevations of urine urobilinogen (Ehrlich's reagent method), urinary protein, and vanillylmandelic acid.

Adverse reactions
- CNS: encephalopathy.
- CV: vasculitis.
- DERM: rash, pruritus.
- GI: nausea, vomiting, diarrhea, abdominal pain, peptic ulcer, gastric ulcer, malabsorption (folic acid, vitamin B_{12}, iron, lipids).
- GU: albuminuria, hematuria, crystalluria.
- HEMA: leukopenia, agranulocytosis, eosinophilia, thrombocytopenia, hemolytic anemia.
- Hepatic: jaundice, hepatitis.
- Metabolic: acidosis, hypokalemia, goiter.
- Other: infectious mononucleosis-like syndrome, fever, lymphadenopathy.
Note: Drug should be discontinued if patient shows signs of hypersensitivity reaction, bone marrow toxicity, or hepatic failure.

Overdose and treatment
Signs of overdose include nausea, vomiting, hypokalemia, and acidosis. No specific recommendations for treatment are available. Treatment is supportive. After recent ingestion (within 4 hours), empty the stomach by induced emesis or gastric lavage. Follow with activated charcoal to decrease absorption.

It is not known if the drug is removed by hemodialysis or peritoneal dialysis.

▶ Special considerations
- Drug may be taken with or after meals, or with antacids to avoid gastric irritation.
- Obtain specimens for culture and sensitivity testing before first dose, but therapy may begin before test results are completed; repeat tests periodically to detect drug resistance.
- Observe patients for adverse reactions and monitor

---

serum electrolyte levels and hematologic, renal, and liver function studies to minimize toxicity.
● Avoid PAS in patients on sodium-restricted diets; a 15 g dose contains 1.6 g sodium.
● Observe patient for edema.
● Store drug in tight, light-resistant container in a dry place. Use solutions within 24 hours. Drug deteriorates rapidly with exposure to heat, air, or moisture. Discard if drug turns brown or purple.

Information for the patient
● Explain disease process and rationale for long-term therapy.
● Teach signs and symptoms of hypersensitivity and other adverse reactions, and emphasize need to report *any* unusual effects.
● Tell patient to call promptly if loss of appetite, fatigue, malaise, jaundice, dark urine, rash, or itching occurs.
● Teach patient how and when to take drug and to discard drug if it turns brown or purple.
● To prevent bitter aftertaste, tell patient to rinse mouth with clear water or to chew sugarless gum after taking drug.
● Urge patient to comply with prescribed regimen, and not to discontinue drug without medical approval; explain importance of follow-up appointments.

Breast-feeding
May be excreted in breast milk; use with caution in breast-feeding women.

---

paramethadione
Paradione

● Pharmacologic classification: oxazolidinedione derivative
● Therapeutic classification: anticonvulsant
● Pregnancy risk category D

How supplied
Available by prescription only
Capsules: 150 mg, 300 mg

Indications, route, and dosage
Refractory absence seizures
Adults: Initially, 300 mg P.O. t.i.d; may increase by 300 mg daily at weekly intervals, up to 600 mg q.i.d., if needed.
Children over age 6: 0.9 g P.O. daily in divided doses t.i.d. or q.i.d.
Children age 2 to 6: 0.6 g P.O. daily in divided doses t.i.d. or q.i.d.
Children under age 2: 0.3 g P.O. daily in divided doses b.i.d.

Pharmacodynamics
Anticonvulsant action: Paramethadione raises the threshold for cortical seizures but does not modify the seizure pattern. It decreases projection of focal activity and reduces both repetitive spinal cord transmission and spike-and-wave patterns of absence (petit mal) seizures.

Pharmacokinetics
● *Absorption:* Paramethadione is absorbed from the GI tract.

● *Distribution:* Paramethadione is distributed widely throughout the body.
● *Metabolism:* Paramethadione is demethylated in the liver to active metabolites.
● *Excretion:* Paramethadione is excreted in urine; it is unknown whether drug is excreted in breast milk.

Contraindications and precautions
Paramethadione is contraindicated during pregnancy and in patients with known hypersensitivity to oxazolidinedione derivatives; use paramethadione with extreme caution in patients with severe hepatic or renal disease, severe blood dyscrasias, or diseases of the retina or optic nerve because the drug may exacerbate diseases of the optic nerve. Preparation contains tartrazine; use with caution in patients with asthma or aspirin allergy because of possible allergic reactions.

Interactions
Concomitant use of paramethadione and mephenytoin or phenacemide may result in a high incidence of toxicity; such combinations should be avoided.

Effects on diagnostic tests
Paramethadione may cause abnormalities in liver function test results.

Adverse reactions
● CNS: drowsiness, sedation, fatigue, vertigo, headache, paresthesia, irritability.
● CV: hypertension, hypotension.
● DERM: acneiform or morbilliform rash, *exfoliative dermatitis, erythema multiforme,* petechiae, alopecia.
● EENT: hemeralopia, photophobia, diplopia, epistaxis, retinal hemorrhage.
● GI: nausea, vomiting, abdominal pain, weight loss, bleeding gums.
● GU: albuminuria, vaginal bleeding, nephrotic syndrome.
● HEMA: neutropenia, leukopenia, eosinophilia, thrombocytopenia, pancytopenia, *agranulocytosis, hypoplastic* and *aplastic anemia.*
● Hepatic: abnormal liver function test results.
● Other: lymphadenopathy, lupus erythematosus.
  Note: Drug should be discontinued if signs of hypersensitivity, any rash (even acneiform), or unusual skin lesions occur; if scotomata occur; if neutrophil count falls to or below 2,500/mm^3; if any of the following signs of blood dyscrasias occur: joint pain, fever, sore throat, or unusual bleeding or bruising; if patient has persistent or increasing albuminuria; if jaundice or other signs of hepatic dysfunction occur; or if syndromes resembling systemic lupus erythematosus, malignant lymphoma, or myasthenia gravis occur.

Overdose and treatment
Symptoms of overdose include nausea, drowsiness, ataxia, and visual disturbances; coma may follow massive overdose.
  Treat overdose with immediate gastric lavage or emesis, and with supportive measures. Monitor vital signs and fluid and electrolyte balance carefully. Alkalinization of urine may hasten renal excretion. Monitor blood counts and hepatic and renal function after recovery.

▶ Special considerations
● Paramethadione should be used only after less toxic alternatives have failed.

• Drug should not be withdrawn abruptly because this may precipitate seizures.
• Perform CBC, hepatic function tests, and urinalysis before therapy at monthly intervals for the first year and periodically thereafter.

Information for the patient
• Emphasize need for close medical supervision.
• Advise women of childbearing age to use an effective contraceptive method and to call promptly if they suspect pregnancy.
• Tell patient to take drug with food or milk to prevent GI distress.
• Urge patient to report the following reactions promptly: visual disturbance, excessive dizziness or drowsiness, sore throat, fever, bleeding or bruising, or skin rash.
• Inform patient that hemeralopia (day blindness) may be relieved with dark glasses.

paramethasone acetate
Haldrone

• Pharmacologic classification: glucocorticoid
• Therapeutic classification: anti-inflammatory, immunosuppressant
• Pregnancy risk category C

How supplied
Available by prescription only
Tablets: 1 mg, 2 mg

Indications, route, and dosage
Inflammatory conditions
Adults: 0.5 to 6 mg P.O. t.i.d. or q.i.d.
Children: 58 to 800 mcg/kg daily divided t.i.d. or q.i.d.

Pharmacodynamics
• *Immunosuppressant action:* Paramethasone stimulates the synthesis of enzymes needed to decrease the inflammatory response. It suppresses the immune system by reducing activity and volume of the lymphatic system, thus producing lymphocytopenia (primarily of T-lymphocytes), decreasing passage of immune complexes through basement membranes, and possibly by depressing reactivity of tissue to antigen-antibody interactions.
• *Anti-inflammatory action:* Paramethasone is a long-acting steroid with anti-inflammatory potency 10 times that of an equal weight of hydrocortisone. It has essentially no mineralocorticoid activity. Paramethasone tablets are used as oral anti-inflammatory agents.

Pharmacokinetics
• *Absorption:* Paramethasone is absorbed readily after oral administration. Peak effects occur within 1 to 2 hours.
• *Distribution:* Paramethasone is distributed rapidly to muscle, liver, skin, intestines, and kidneys. Paramethasone is bound weakly to plasma proteins (transcortin and albumin). Only the unbound portion is active. Adrenocorticoids are distributed into breast milk and through the placenta.
• *Metabolism:* Paramethasone is metabolized in the liver to inactive glucuronide and sulfate metabolites.
• *Excretion:* The inactive metabolites and small

amounts of unmetabolized drug are excreted by the kidneys. Insignificant quantities of drug are excreted in feces. The biological half-life of paramethasone is 36 to 54 hours.

Contraindications and precautions
Paramethasone is contraindicated in patients with systemic fungal infections (except in adrenal insufficiency) or a hypersensitivity to ingredients of adrenocorticoid preparations. Patients receiving paramethasone should not be given live-virus vaccines because paramethasone suppresses the immune response.

Paramethasone should be used with extreme caution in patients with GI ulceration, renal disease, hypertension, osteoporosis, diabetes mellitus, thromboembolic disorders, seizures, myasthenia gravis, congestive heart failure (CHF), tuberculosis, hypoalbuminemia, hypothyroidism, cirrhosis of the liver, emotional instability, psychotic tendencies, hyperlipidemias, glaucoma, or cataracts, because the drug may exacerbate these conditions.

Because adrenocorticoids increase the susceptibility to and mask symptoms of infection, paramethasone should not be used (except in life-threatening situations) in patients with viral or bacterial infections not controlled by anti-infective agents.

Interactions
When used concomitantly, paramethasone rarely may decrease the effects of oral anticoagulants by unknown mechanisms.

Glucocorticoids increase the metabolism of isoniazid and salicylates; they cause hyperglycemia, requiring dosage adjustment of insulin or oral hypoglycemic agents in diabetic patients; and may enhance hypokalemia associated with diuretic or amphotericin B therapy. The hypokalemia may increase the risk of toxicity in patients concurrently receiving digitalis glycosides.

Barbiturates, phenytoin, and rifampin may cause decreased paramethasone effects because of increased hepatic metabolism. Cholestyramine, colestipol, and antacids decrease the corticosteroid effect by adsorbing the corticosteroid, decreasing the amount absorbed.

Concomitant use with estrogens may reduce the metabolism of paramethasone by increasing the concentration of transcortin. The half-life of paramethasone is then prolonged because of increased protein binding. Concomitant administration of ulcerogenic drugs, such as nonsteroidal anti-inflammatory agents, may increase the risk of GI ulceration.

Effects on diagnostic tests
Paramethasone suppresses reactions to skin tests; causes false-negative results in the nitroblue tetrazolium test for systemic bacterial infections; decreases ^{131}I uptake and protein-bound iodine concentrations in thyroid function tests; may increase glucose and cholesterol levels; may decrease serum potassium, calcium, thyroxine, and triiodothyronine levels; and may increase urine glucose and calcium levels.

Adverse reactions
When administered in high doses or for prolonged therapy, the glucocorticoids suppress release of adrenocorticotropic hormone (ACTH) from the pituitary gland; in turn, the adrenal cortex stops secreting endogenous corticosteroids. The degree and duration of hypothalamic-pituitary-adrenal (HPA) axis suppression pro-

duced by the drugs is highly variable among patients and depends on the dose, frequency and time of administration, and duration of glucocorticoid therapy.

• CNS: euphoria, insomnia, headache, psychotic behavior, pseudotumor cerebri, mental changes, nervousness, restlessness.
• CV: CHF, hypertension, edema.
• DERM: delayed healing, acne, skin eruptions, striae.
• EENT: cataracts, glaucoma, thrush.
• GI: peptic ulcer, irritation, increased appetite.
• Immune: immunosuppression, increased susceptibility to infection.
• Metabolic: hypokalemia, sodium retention, fluid retention, weight gain, hyperglycemia, osteoporosis, growth suppression in children.
• Musculoskeletal: muscle atrophy, weakness.
• Other: pancreatitis, hirsutism, cushingoid symptoms, withdrawal syndrome (nausea, fatigue, anorexia, dyspnea, hypotension, hypoglycemia, myalgia, arthralgia, fever, dizziness, and fainting). Sudden withdrawal may be fatal or may exacerbate the underlying disease. Acute adrenal insufficiency may occur with increased stress (infection, surgery, trauma) or abrupt withdrawal after long-term therapy.

Overdose and treatment
Acute ingestion, even in massive doses, is rarely a clinical problem. Toxic signs and symptoms rarely occur if drug is used for less than 3 weeks, even at large dosage ranges. However, chronic use causes adverse physiologic effects, including suppression of the HPA axis, cushingoid appearance, muscle weakness, and osteoporosis.

▶ Special considerations
Recommendations for use of paramethasone and for care and teaching of patients during therapy are the same as those for all systemic adrenocorticoids.

Pediatric use
Long-acting glucocorticoids such as paramethasone are likely to inhibit maturation and growth in adolescents and children. Long-term use in children is not recommended.

Breast-feeding
Excretion in breast milk unknown. Consider risks versus benefits in breast-feeding women.

---

paromomycin sulfate
Humatin

• Pharmacologic classification: aminoglycoside
• Therapeutic classification: antibacterial, amebicide
• Pregnancy risk category C

How supplied
Available by prescription only
Capsules: 250 mg

Indications, route, and dosage
Intestinal amebiasis (acute and chronic) in patients who cannot take metronidazole
Adults and children: 25 to 35 mg/kg P.O. daily in three doses for 5 to 10 days after meals.
Tapeworm (fish, beef, pork, and dog) infections in patients who cannot take praziquantel or niclosamide
Adults: 1 g P.O. q 15 minutes for four doses.
Children: 11 mg/kg P.O. q 15 minutes for four doses.
Adjunctive management of hepatic coma
Adults: 4 g P.O. daily in two to four divided doses for 5 to 6 days. Higher daily doses (up to 8 g) have been used, but usually cause serious adverse effects.
†Dientamoeba fragilis infections
Adults and children: 25 to 30 mg/kg P.O. daily in three divided doses for 7 days.

Pharmacodynamics
• Amebicidal action: Paromomycin acts on contact in the intestinal lumen by an unknown mechanism. It is effective against the trophozoite and encysted forms of Entamoeba histolytica and against Diphyllobothrium latum (fish tapeworm), Dipylidium caninum (dog and cat tapeworm), Hymenolepis nana (dwarf tapeworm), Taenia saginata (beef tapeworm), and T. solium (pork tapeworm).
• Adjunct in hepatic coma: Paromomycin inhibits nitrogen-forming bacteria in the GI tract by inhibiting protein synthesis at the 30S subunit of the ribosome.

Pharmacokinetics
• Absorption: Very small amounts of an oral dose of paromomycin are absorbed by the intact GI tract; however, larger amounts may be absorbed in patients with ulcerative intestinal disorders or renal insufficiency.
• Distribution: Distribution of paromomycin has not been characterized adequately.
• Metabolism: No metabolites have been detected.
• Excretion: Almost 100% of paromomycin is excreted unchanged in the feces; systemically absorbed drug is excreted in urine and may accumulate in patients with renal dysfunction. It is unknown if paromomycin is excreted in breast milk.

Contraindications and precautions
Paromomycin is contraindicated in patients with impaired renal function because of its potential for nephrotoxicity; in patients with intestinal obstruction; and in patients with known hypersensitivity to the drug.
  Paromomycin should be administered cautiously to patients with ulcerative intestinal lesions because of potential absorption that could exaggerate the risk of ototoxicity and nephrotoxicity.

Interactions
None reported.

Effects on diagnostic tests
None reported.

Adverse reactions
• CNS: headache, vertigo.
• DERM: rash, exanthema, pruritus.
• EENT: ototoxicity.
• GI: anorexia, nausea, vomiting, epigastric pain and burning, abdominal cramps, diarrhea, constipation, increased motility, steatorrhea, pruritus ani, malabsorption syndrome.

- GU: hematuria, nephrotoxicity.
- HEMA: eosinophilia.
- Other: bacterial and fungal superinfection.
  Note: Drug should be discontinued if signs of hypersensitivity or toxicity occur.

Overdose and treatment
Paromomycin overdose may affect cardiovascular and respiratory function. Treatment is largely supportive. After recent ingestion (within 4 hours), empty stomach by induced emesis or gastric lavage. Follow with activated charcoal to decrease absorption. Osmotic cathartics also may help.

▶ Special considerations
- Administer paromomycin after meals to prevent GI upset.
- Watch for signs of bacterial or fungal superinfection.
- Monitor patients with GI ulceration or renal dysfunction; drug absorption may impair renal clearance.
- Criterion of cure is absence of fecal amebae in specimen examined weekly for 6 weeks after discontinuation of treatment and thereafter monthly for 2 years.
- Not effective in the treatment of extraintestinal amebiasis.
- Many clinicians prefer praziquantel or niclosamide for the treatment of tapeworm infection. Paromomycin may cause disintegration of worm segments, and possibly release of viable eggs.

Information for the patient
- Counsel patient on need for medical follow-up after discharge.
- Advise patient to report any adverse effects.
- Tell patient how disease is transmitted.
- To help prevent reinfection, instruct patient in proper hygiene, including disposal of feces and hand washing after defecation and before eating, and about the risks of eating raw food and the control of contamination by flies. Advise patient not to prepare, process, or serve food until treatment is completed.
- Advise use of liquid soap or reserved bar of soap to prevent cross-contamination.
- Tell patient to encourage other household members and suspected contacts to be tested and, if necessary, treated.
- Isolating patient is unnecessary.

Geriatric use
Drug should be used with caution because of the possibility of decreased renal function and baseline hearing impairment in this age-group.

Breast-feeding
Safety has not been established.

pemoline
Cylert

- Pharmacologic classification: oxazolidinedione derivative, CNS stimulant
- Therapeutic classification: analeptic
- Controlled substance schedule IV
- Pregnancy risk category B

How supplied
Available by prescription only
Tablets: 18.75 mg, 37.5 mg, 75 mg
Tablets (chewable and containing povidine): 37.5 mg

Indications, route, and dosage
Attention deficit disorder (ADD)
Children age 6 and older: Initially, 37.5 mg P.O. given in the morning. Daily dosage can be raised by 18.75 mg weekly. Effective dosage range is 56.25 to 75 mg daily; maximum is 112.5 mg daily.
Narcolepsy
Adults: 50 to 200 mg daily, in divided doses after breakfast and lunch.
†*Mild stimulant in elderly patients*
Adults: 20 to 50 mg P.O. daily in divided doses after breakfast and lunch.

Pharmacodynamics
Analeptic action: Pemoline differs structurally from methylphenidate and amphetamines; however, like those drugs, pemoline has a paradoxical calming effect in children with ADD.

Pemoline's mechanism of action is unknown; it may be mediated by enhanced cerebral neurotransmission.

Pemoline is used primarily to treat ADD in children over age 6; investigationally, its CNS stimulant effect has been studied in narcolepsy in adults, in fatigue, in depressed and schizophrenic states, and in elderly patients.

Pharmacokinetics
- *Absorption:* Pemoline is well absorbed after oral administration. Peak therapeutic effects occur at 4 hours and persist about 8 hours.
- *Distribution:* Distribution is unknown. Drug is 50% protein-bound.
- *Metabolism:* Pemoline is metabolized by the liver to active and inactive metabolites.
- *Excretion:* Pemoline and its metabolites are excreted in urine; 75% of an oral dose is excreted within 24 hours.

Contraindications and precautions
Pemoline is contraindicated in patients with hypersensitivity to pemoline; in those with impaired hepatic function because it may have an adverse effect on liver function; and in children under age 6. It should be used with caution in patients with decreased renal function and in patients with a history of Gilles de la Tourette's syndrome because it may precipitate this disorder.

Interactions
Concomitant use with caffeine may decrease efficacy of pemoline in ADD; concomitant use with anticonvulsants may decrease the seizure threshold.

Effects on diagnostic tests
Pemoline may cause abnormalities in liver function test results.

Adverse reactions
● CNS: insomnia, malaise, irritability, fatigue, mild depression, dizziness, headache, drowsiness, hallucinations, nervousness (large doses), *seizures*, nystagmus, oculogyric crisis, unusual facial movement, Gilles de la Tourette's syndrome, psychosis.
● CV: tachycardia (with large doses).
● DERM: rash.
● GI: anorexia, abdominal pain, nausea, diarrhea.
● GU: prostatic hyperplasia.
● Hepatic: liver enzyme elevations, jaundice.
● Other: weight loss on initial therapy; weight gain after 3 to 6 months, tolerance, physical and psychological dependence.
   Note: Drug should be discontinued if signs of hypersensitivity occur or if markedly elevated liver function test results and jaundice occur concurrently.

Overdose and treatment
Symptoms of overdose may include irregular respiration, hyperreflexia, restlessness, tachycardia, hallucinations, excitement, and agitation.
   Treat overdose symptomatically and supportively: use gastric lavage if symptoms are not severe (hyperexcitability or coma). Monitor vital signs and fluid and electrolyte balance. Maintain patient in a cool room, monitor temperature, and minimize external stimulation; protect patient from self-injury. Chlorpromazine or haloperidol usually can reverse CNS stimulation. Hemodialysis may help.

▶ Special considerations
● Monitor initiation of therapy closely; drug may precipitate Gilles de la Tourette's syndrome.
● Check vital signs regularly for increased blood pressure or other signs of excessive stimulation.
● Give drug in a single morning dose for maximum daytime benefit and to minimize insomnia.
● Monitor blood and urine glucose levels in diabetic patients; drug may alter insulin requirement.
● Monitor complete blood counts, differential, and platelet counts while patient is on long-term therapy.
● Determine baseline and periodically assess liver function tests. If abnormalities occur, discontinue therapy.
● Explain that therapeutic effects may not appear for 3 to 4 weeks and that intermittent drug-free periods when stress is least evident (weekends, school holidays) may help assess patient's condition and prevent development of tolerance and permit decreased dosage when drug is resumed.
● Monitor height and weight; drug has been associated with growth suppression.
● Abrupt withdrawal after high-dose long-term use may unmask severe depression. Lower dosage gradually to prevent acute rebound depression.
● Pemoline impairs ability to perform tasks requiring mental alertness.
● Be sure patient obtains adequate rest; fatigue may result as drug wears off.
● Discourage pemoline use for analeptic effect, as drug has abuse potential; CNS stimulation superimposed on CNS depression may cause neuronal instability and seizures.
● Carefully follow manufacturer's directions for reconstitution, storage, and administration of all preparations. Pemoline has been used to treat narcolepsy in adults (50 to 200 mg divided b.i.d.) as well as depression and schizophrenia, but these uses are controversial.

Information for the patient
● Explain rationale for therapy and the anticipated risks and benefits; teach signs and symptoms of adverse reactions and need to report these.
● Tell patient to avoid drinks containing caffeine, to prevent added CNS stimulation, and not to alter dosage without medical approval.
● Teach patient how and when to use drug; tell patient not to chew or crush sustained-release dosage form.
● Warn patient not to use drug to mask fatigue, to be sure to obtain adequate rest, and to report excessive CNS stimulation.
● Advise diabetic patients to monitor blood glucose levels, as drug may alter insulin needs.
● Advise patient to avoid tasks that require mental alertness until degree of sedative effect is determined.

Pediatric use
Pemoline is not recommended for ADD in children under age 6.

----

penbutolol sulfate
Levatol

● Pharmacologic classification: beta-adrenergic blocking agent
● Therapeutic classification: antihypertensive
● Pregnancy risk category C

How supplied
Available by prescription only
Tablets: 20 mg

Indications, route, and dosage
Treatment of mild to moderate hypertension
Adults: 20 mg P.O. once daily. Usually given with other antihypertensive agents, such as thiazide diuretics.

Pharmacodynamics
Antihypertensive action: Penbutolol blocks both $beta_1$- and $beta_2$-adrenergic receptors. Its antihypertensive effects may be related to its peripheral antiadrenergic effects that lead to decreased cardiac output, a central effect that leads to decreased sympathetic tone, or decreased renin secretion by the kidneys.

Pharmacokinetics
● *Absorption:* Penbutolol is almost completely absorbed after oral administration. Peak plasma levels occur 2 to 3 hours after administration.
● *Distribution:* 80% to 98% of the drug is bound to plasma proteins.
● *Metabolism:* Drug is metabolized by the liver. Several metabolites have been identified; some retain partial pharmacologic activity.
● *Excretion:* Average elimination half-life of the parent drug is 5 hours; some metabolites persist for 20 hours or more. Most metabolites are excreted in the urine.

Contraindications and precautions

Penbutolol is contraindicated in patients allergic to this drug or other beta blockers. It is also contraindicated in those with sinus bradycardia, cardiogenic shock, congestive heart failure(CHF), overt cardiac failure, and patients with greater than first-degree heart block. Beta-adrenergic blocking agents should be avoided in patients with pheochromocytoma unless alpha-adrenergic blocking agents are also used. They should also be avoided in patients with chronic airway disease, such as chronic bronchitis or emphysema. Administer cautiously to patients with a history of CHF controlled by digitalis glycosides and diuretics.

Advise patients not to discontinue the drug abruptly, because sudden withdrawal of other beta blockers has precipitated angina and myocardial infarction. However, clinical experience has shown that withdrawal of beta blockers in patients who have had a myocardial infarction does not present major problems.

Interactions

Oral calcium antagonists may enhance the hypotensive effects of beta-adrenergic blocking agents as well as predispose the patient to bradycardia and dysrhythmias. Clonidine may cause paradoxical hypertension when combined with beta-adrenergic blocking agents. Also, beta blockers may enhance rebound hypertension when clonidine is withdrawn.

Beta-adrenergic blocking agents may alter the hypoglycemic response to insulin or oral hypoglycemic agents. Monitor the patient closely.

Beta blockers may enhance the "first dose" orthostatic hypotension seen with prazocin and terazocin. Avoid the concomitant use of reserpine or other catecholamine-depleting drugs.

Concomitant use may decrease the hypotensive response to sympathomimetics (including isoproterenol, dopamine, dobutamine, and norepinephrine) and may decrease the bronchodilator effect of theophylline.

Penbutolol has been shown to increase the volume of distribution of lidocaine in normal patients, implying that it may increase the loading dose requirements in some patients.

Effects on diagnostic tests

None reported.

Adverse reactions

● CNS: syncope, dizziness, vertigo, headache, fatigue, mental depression, paresthesias, hypoesthesia or hyperesthesia, lethargy, anxiety, nervousness, diminished concentration, sleep disturbances, nightmares, bizarre or frequent dreams, sedation, changes in behavior, reversible mental depression, catatonia, hallucinations, alteration of time perception, memory loss, emotional lability, light-headedness.
● CV: bradycardia, chest pain, asymptomatic hypotension, peripheral ischemia, worsening of angina or arterial insufficiency, peripheral vascular insufficiency, claudication, CHF, *cerebrovascular accident*, edema, pulmonary edema, vasodilation, symptomatic postural hypotension, tachycardia, palpitations, conduction disturbances, first- and third-degree heart block, intensification of AV block.
● DERM: pallor, flushing, rash.
● GI: gastric pain, flatulence, nausea, constipation, dry mouth, heartburn, vomiting, dysgeusia.
● GU: impotence, nocturia, urinary retention.
● Metabolic: hyperglycemia, hypoglycemia.

● Respiratory: pharyngitis, *laryngospasm*, respiratory distress, shortness of breath.
● Other: allergic reactions, *anaphylaxis*, eye discomfort, decreased libido.

Overdose and treatment

Clinical signs of overdose may include bradycardia, bronchospasm, heart failure, and severe hypotension.

After emptying the stomach by lavage (for acute oral ingestion), administer symptomatic and supportive care. Bradycardia may be treated with atropine or cautious use of isoproterenol. Digitalis and diuretics may be useful in treating heart failure, and vasopressors (such as epinephrine or alpha-adrenergic agonists) may be used to counter severe hypotension. Treat bronchospasm with aminophylline or isoproterenol.

▶ Special considerations

Besides those relevant to all *beta-adrenergic blockers,* consider the following recommendations.
● Like other beta blockers, penbutolol may cause patients to exhibit hypersensitivity to catecholamines upon withdrawal.
● To discontinue this drug, dosage should be slowly tapered over a period of 1 to 2 weeks, especially in patients with ischemic heart disease. If symptoms of angina develop, immediately reinstitute therapy, at least temporarily, and take steps to control the patient's unstable angina.

Information for the patient

● Advise patient not to discontinue the drug abruptly, because sudden withdrawal of other beta blockers has precipitated angina and myocardial infarction.
● Patient should report adverse effects immediately, particularly slow heart rate, chest congestion, cough, wheezing, or shortness of breath from mild exertion.
● Teach patient about disease and therapy. Explain why it is important to continue taking this drug, even when feeling well.
● Advise patient to report unpleasant side effects promptly.
● Advise patient to check with physician or pharmacist before taking any OTC medications.

Geriatric use

Pharmacokinetic studies indicate no difference in plasma half-life in healthy elderly patients as compared to patients on renal dialysis.

Pediatric use

Safety and effectiveness in children have not been established.

Breast-feeding

It is not known if penbutolol is excreted in breast milk. Use with caution in breast-feeding women.

penicillamine
Cuprimine, Depen

- Pharmacologic classification: chelating agent
- Therapeutic classification: heavy metal antagonist, antirheumatic agent
- Pregnancy risk category C

How supplied
Available by prescription only
Capsules: 125 mg, 250 mg
Tablets: 250 mg

Indications, route, and dosage
Wilson's disease
Adults: 250 mg P.O. q.i.d. 30 to 60 minutes before meals and at least 2 hours after the evening meal. Adjust dosage to achieve urinary copper excretion of 0.5 to 1 mg daily. Dosage greater than 2 g is seldom necessary.
Children: 20 mg/kg P.O. daily divided q.i.d. 30 to 60 minutes before meals and at least 2 hours after the evening meal. Adjust dosage to achieve urinary copper excretion of 0.5 to 1 mg daily.
Cystinuria
Adults: 250 mg P.O. daily in 4 divided doses, then gradually increasing dosage. Usual dosage is 2 g daily (range is 1 to 4 g daily). Adjust dosage to achieve urinary cystine excretion of less than 100 mg daily when renal calculi are present, or 100 to 200 mg daily when no calculi are present.
Children: 30 mg/kg P.O. divided q.i.d. 30 to 60 minutes before meals and at least 2 hours after the evening meal. Adjust dosage to achieve urinary cystine excretion of less than 100 mg daily when renal calculi are present, or 100 to 200 mg daily when no calculi are present.
Rheumatoid arthritis, †Felty's syndrome
Adults: Initially, 125 to 250 mg P.O. daily, with increases of 125 to 250 mg daily at 1- to 3-month intervals if necessary. Maximum dosage is 1.5 g daily.
†Adjunctive treatment of heavy metal poisoning
Adults: 500 to 1,500 mg P.O. daily for 1 to 2 months.
Children: 30 to 40 mg/kg or 600 to 750 mg/m² P.O. daily for 1 to 6 months.

Pharmacodynamics
- *Antirheumatic action:* Mechanism of action in rheumatoid arthritis is unknown; penicillamine depresses circulating IgM rheumatoid factor (but not total circulating immunoglobulin levels) and depresses T-cell but not B-cell activity. It also depolymerizes some macroglobulins (for example, rheumatoid factors).
- *Chelating agent:* Penicillamine forms stable, soluble complexes with copper, iron, mercury, lead, and other heavy metals that are excreted in urine; it is particularly useful in chelating copper in patients with Wilson's disease. Penicillamine also combines with cystine to form a complex more soluble than cystine alone, thereby reducing free cystine below the level of urinary stone formation.

Pharmacokinetics
- *Absorption:* Drug is well absorbed after oral administration; peak serum levels occur at 1 hour. Food and mineral supplements, especially those containing iron, decrease absorption by complexing in the gut.
- *Distribution:* Only limited data available.
- *Metabolism:* Uncomplexed penicillamine is metabolized in the liver to inactive disulfides.
- *Excretion:* Only small amounts of penicillamine are excreted unchanged; after 24 hours, 50% of the drug is excreted in urine, 20% in feces, and 30% is unaccounted for.

Contraindications and precautions
Penicillamine is contraindicated in patients with known hypersensitivity to the drug; in patients with a history of penicillamine-related aplastic anemia or agranulocytosis; in patients with significant renal or hepatic insufficiency; in pregnant women; and in patients receiving gold salts, immunosuppressants, antimalarials, or phenylbutazone because of the increased risk of serious hematologic effects.

Penicillamine should be used with caution in patients allergic to penicillin (cross reaction is rare); in patients who receive a second course of therapy and who may have become sensitized and are more likely to have allergic reactions; and in patients who develop proteinuria not associated with Goodpasture's syndrome.

Interactions
Iron salts and antacids decrease absorption of penicillamine.

Effects on diagnostic tests
Penicillamine therapy may cause positive test results for antinuclear antibody (ANA) with or without clinical systemic lupus erythematosus-like syndrome.

Penicillamine may (rarely) elevate LDH, AST (SGOT), ALT (SGPT), and alkaline phosphatase levels. Such elevations do not necessarily indicate significant hepatotoxicity.

Adverse reactions
- DERM: pruritus; erythematous rash; intensely pruritic rash with scaly, macular lesions on trunk; pemphigoid reactions; urticaria; *exfoliative dermatitis;* increased skin friability; purpuric or vesicular ecchymoses; wrinkling.
- EENT: oral ulcerations, glossitis, cheilosis.
- GI: anorexia, nausea, vomiting, dyspepsia, diarrhea, dysgeusia or hypogeusia.
- HEMA: eosinophilia, leukopenia, granulocytopenia, *thrombocytopenia, aplastic anemia, agranulocytosis,* thrombotic thrombocytopenia, purpura, hemolytic anemia or iron deficiency anemia, lupus-like syndrome.
- Hepatic: cholestatic jaundice, *pancreatitis,* hepatic dysfunction.
- Other: proteinuria, arthralgia, lymphadenopathy, pneumonitis, alteration in sense of taste (salty and sweet), metallic taste, Goodpasture's syndrome, alopecia, drug fever, myasthenia gravis (with prolonged use).

Note: Drug should be discontinued if patient has signs of hypersensitivity or drug fever, usually in conjunction with other allergic manifestations (if Wilson's disease, may rechallenge); or if any of the following occur: rash developing 6 months or more after start of therapy; pemphigoid reaction; hematuria or proteinuria with hemoptysis or pulmonary infiltrates; gross or persistent microscopic hematuria or proteinuria greater than 2 g/day in patients with rheumatoid arthritis; platelet count below 100,000/mm³ or leukocyte count below

3,500 mm³, or if either shows three consecutive decreases (even within normal range).

Overdose and treatment
There are no reports of significant overdose with penicillamine. To treat penicillamine overdose, induce emesis unless unconscious or gag reflex is absent; otherwise empty stomach by gastric lavage and then administer activated charcoal and sorbitol. Thereafter, treat supportively. Treat seizures with diazepam (or pyridoxine if previously successful). Hemodialysis will remove penicillamine.

▶ Special considerations
● Perform urinalyses, CBC including differential blood count every 2 weeks for 4 to 6 months, then monthly; kidney and liver functions studies also should be performed, usually every 6 months. Report fever or allergic reactions (rash, joint pains, easy bruising) immediately. Check routinely for proteinuria, and handle patient carefully to avoid skin damage.
● About one third of patients receiving penicillamine experience an allergic reaction. Monitor patient for signs and symptoms of allergic reaction.
● Patients with Wilson's disease or cystinuria may require daily pyridoxine (vitamin B_6) supplementation.
● Prescribe drug to be taken 1 hour before or 2 hours after meals or other medications to facilitate absorption.
● For the initial treatment of Wilson's disease, 10 to 40 mg of sulfurated potash should be administered with each meal during penicillamine therapy for 6 months to 1 year, then discontinued.
● Penicillamine also has been used to treat lead poisoning and primary biliary cirrhosis.

Information for the patient
● Provide health education for patients with Wilson's disease, rheumatoid arthritis, or cystinuria; explain disease process and rationale for therapy and explain that clinical results may not be evident for 3 months.
● Encourage patient compliance with therapy and follow-up visits.
● Stress importance of immediate reporting of any fever, chills, sore throat, bruising, bleeding, or allergic reaction.
● Tell patient to take the medication on an empty stomach 30 minutes to 1 hour before meals or 2 hours after ingesting food, antacids, mineral supplements, vitamins, or other medications. Tell patient to drink large amounts of water, especially at night.
● Advise patient receiving penicillamine for rheumatoid arthritis that an exacerbation of the disease may occur during therapy. This usually can be controlled by the concomitant administration of nonsteroidal anti-inflammatory drugs.
● Advise patient taking penicillamine for Wilson's disease to maintain a low-copper (less than 2 mg daily) diet by excluding foods with high copper content, such as chocolate, nuts, liver, and broccoli. Also, sulfurated potash may be administered with meals to minimize copper absorption.

Geriatric use
Lower doses may be indicated. Monitor renal and hepatic function closely.

Pediatric use
Check for possible iron deficiency resulting from chronic use.

Breast-feeding
Safety has not been established in breast-feeding; alternative feeding method is recommended during therapy.

PHARMACOLOGIC CLASS

penicillins

Natural penicillin
penicillin G benzathine; potassium; procaine; sodium
penicillin V potassium

Aminopenicillin
amoxicillin trihydrate; clavulanate
ampicillin
ampicillin sodium; sulbactam
ampicillin sodium; trihydrate
bacampicillin hydrochloride

Penicillinase-resistant
cloxacillin sodium
dicloxacillin sodium
methicillin sodium
nafcillin sodium
oxacillin sodium

Extended-spectrum
azlocillin sodium
carbenicillin sodium; indanyl sodium
mezlocillin sodium
piperacillin sodium
ticarcillin clavulanate
ticarcillin disodium

Penicillins are very effective antibiotics with low toxicity. Their activity was first discovered by Sir Alexander Fleming in 1928, but they were not developed for use against systemic infections until 1940. Penicillin is naturally derived from *Penicillium chrysogenum*. New synthetic derivatives are created by chemical reactions that modify their structure, resulting in increased GI absorption, resistance to destruction by beta-lactamase (penicillinase), and a broader spectrum of susceptible organisms.

Pharmacology
The basic structure of penicillin is a thiazolidine ring connected to a beta-lactam ring that contains a side chain. This nucleus is the main structural requirement for antibacterial activity; modifications of the side chain alter penicillin's antibacterial and pharmacologic effects.

Penicillins are generally bactericidal. They inhibit synthesis of the bacterial cell wall, causing rapid cell lysis, and are most effective against fast-growing susceptible bacteria.

The sites of action for penicillins are enzymes known as penicillin-binding proteins (PBP). The affinity of certain penicillins for PBP in various microorganisms helps explain differing spectra of activity in this class of antibiotics.

Bacterial resistance to beta-lactam antibiotics is conferred most significantly by bacterial production of beta-lactamase enzymes, which destroy the beta-lactam ring and thus inactivate penicillin; decreased cell wall permeability and alteration in binding affinity to PBP also contribute to such resistance.

Oral absorption of penicillin varies widely; the most acid labile is penicillin G. Side-chain modifications in penicillin V, ampicillin, amoxicillin, and other orally administered penicillins are more stable in gastric acid and permit better absorption from the GI tract.

Penicillins are distributed widely throughout the body; CSF penetration is minimal but is enhanced in patients with inflamed meninges. Most penicillins are only partially metabolized. With the exception of nafcillin, penicillins are excreted primarily in urine, chiefly via renal tubular effects; nafcillin undergoes enterohepatic circulation and is excreted chiefly through the biliary tract.

Clinical indications and actions
Infection caused by susceptible organisms

● *Natural penicillins:* Penicillin G is the prototype of this group; derivatives such as penicillin V are more acid stable and thus better absorbed by the oral route. All natural penicillins are vulnerable to inactivation by beta-lactamase producing bacteria. Natural penicillins act primarily against gram-positive organisms.

Clinical indications for natural penicillins include streptococcal pneumonia, enterococcal and nonenterococcal Group D endocarditis, diphtheria, anthrax, meningitis, tetanus, botulism, actinomycosis, syphilis, relapsing fever, Lyme disease, and others. Natural penicillins are used prophylactically against pneumococcal infections, rheumatic fever, bacterial endocarditis, and neonatal Group B streptococcal disease.

Susceptible aerobic gram-positive cocci include *Staphylococcus aureus;* nonenterococcal Group D streptococci, Groups A, B, D, G, H, K, L, and M streptococci, *S. viridans;* and enterococcus (usually in combination with an aminoglycoside). Susceptible aerobic gram-negative cocci include *Neisseria meningitidis* and non-penicillinase-producing *N. gonorrhoeae.*

Susceptible aerobic gram-positive bacilli include *Corynebacterium* (both diphtheria and opportunistic species), *Listeria,* and *Bacillus anthracis.* Susceptible anaerobes include *Peptococcus, Peptostreptococcus, Actinomyces, Clostridium, Fusobacterium, Veillonella,* and non-beta-lactamase-producing strains of *S. pneumoniae.*

Susceptible spirochetes include *Treponema pallidum, T. pertenue, Leptospira,* and *Borrelia recurrentis.*

● *Aminopenicillins* (amoxicillin, ampicillin, and bacampicillin) offer a broader spectrum of activity including many gram-negative organisms. Like natural penicillins, aminopenicillins are vulnerable to inactivation by penicillinase. They are primarily used to treat septicemia, gynecologic infections, and infections of the urinary, respiratory, and GI tracts, and skin, soft tissue, bones, and joints. Their activity spectrum includes *Escherichia coli, Proteus mirabilis, Shigella, Salmonella, S. pneumoniae, N. gonorrhoeae, Haemophilus influenzae, Staphylococcus aureus, Staphylococcus epidermidis,* and *Listeria monocytogenes.*

● *Penicillinase-resistant penicillins* (cloxacillin, dicloxacillin, oxacillin, and nafcillin) are semisynthetic penicillins designed to remain stable against hydrolysis by most staphylococcal penicillinases and thus are the drugs of choice against susceptible penicillinase-producing staphylococci. They also retain activity against most organisms susceptible to natural penicillins. Clinical indications are much the same as for aminopenicillins.

● *Extended-spectrum penicillins* (azlocillin, carbenicillin, mezlocillin, piperacillin, and ticarcillin), as their name implies, offer a wider range of bactericidal action than the other three classes, are used in hard-to-treat gram-negative infections, and are usually given in combination with aminoglycosides. They are used most often against susceptible strains of *Enterobacter, Klebsiella, Citrobacter, Serratia, Bacteroides fragilis,* and *Pseudomonas aeruginosa;* their gram-negative spectrum also includes *Proteus vulgaris, Providencia rettgeri,* and *Morganella morganii.* These penicillins are also vulnerable to destruction by beta-lactamase or penicillinases.

Overview of adverse reactions

● *Systemic reactions:* Hypersensitivity reactions occur with all penicillins; they range from mild rashes, fever and eosinophilia to fatal anaphylaxis. Hematologic reactions include hemolytic anemia, transient neutropenia, leukopenia, and thrombocytopenia.

Certain adverse reactions are more common with specific classes of penicillin: bleeding episodes are usually seen at high-dose levels of extended-spectrum penicillins; acute interstitial nephritis is reported most often with methicillin; GI adverse effects are most common with but not limited to ampicillin. High doses, especially of penicillin G, irritate the CNS in patients with renal disease, causing confusion, twitching, lethargy, dysphagia, seizures, and coma. Hepatotoxicity is most common with penicillinase-resistant penicillins; hyperkalemia and hypernatremia with extended-spectrum penicillins.

Jarisch-Herxheimer reaction can occur when penicillin G is used in secondary syphilis; it presents as chills, fever, headache, myalgia, tachycardia, malaise, sweating, hypotension, and sore throat and is attributed to release of endotoxin following spirochete death.

● *Local reactions:* Local irritation from parenteral therapy may be severe enough to require discontinuation of the drug or administration by subclavian catheter if drug therapy is to continue.

▶ Special considerations

● Assess patient's history of allergies; do not give a penicillin to any patient with a history of hypersensitivity reactions to either penicillins or cephalosporins. Try to ascertain whether previous reactions were true hypersensitivity reactions or merely an adverse reaction, such as GI distress, which the patient has interpreted as allergy.

● Keep in mind that a negative history for penicillin hypersensitivity does not preclude future allergic reactions; monitor patient continuously for possible allergic reactions or other untoward effects.

● In patients with renal impairment, dosage should be reduced if creatinine clearance is below 10 ml/minute.

● Assess level of consciousness, neurologic status, and renal function when high doses are used, because excessive blood levels can cause CNS toxicity.

● Obtain results of cultures and sensitivity tests before first dose; however, therapy may begin before test results are complete. Repeat tests periodically to assess drug efficacy.

● Monitor vital signs, electrolytes, and renal function studies; monitor body weight for fluid retention with extended-spectrum penicillins for possible hypokalemia or hypernatremia.

● Coagulation abnormalities, even frank bleeding, can follow high doses, especially of extended-spectrum penicillins; monitor prothrombin times and platelet

COMPARING PENICILLINS

DRUG	ROUTE	ADULT DOSAGE	FREQUENCY	PENICILLINASE RESISTANT
amoxicillin	P.O.	250 to 500 mg	q 8 hours	No
		3 g with 1 g probenecid for gonorrhea	single dose	
amoxicillin/ clavulanate potassium	P.O.	250 to 500 mg	q 8 hours	Yes
ampicillin	I.M., I.V.	2 to 14 g daily	divided doses given q 4 to 6 hours	No
	P.O.	250 to 500 mg	q 6 hours	
		3.5 g with 1 g probenecid (for gonorrhea)	single dose	
ampicillin sodium/ sulbactum sodium	I.M., I.V.	1.5 to 3 g	q 6 to 8 hours	Yes
azlocillin	I.V.	200 to 350 mg/kg daily	divided doses given q 4 to 6 hours	No
bacampicillin	P.O.	400 to 800 mg	q 12 hours	No
carbenicillin	I.M., I.V.	200 mg/kg daily (for urinary infections)	divided doses given q 4 to 6 hours	No
		30 to 40 g daily (for systemic infections)	divided doses given q 4 to 6 hours	
	P.O.	382 to 764 mg	q 6 hours	No
cloxacillin	P.O.	250 mg to 1 g	q 6 hours	Yes
dicloxacillin	P.O.	125 to 500 mg	q 6 hours	Yes
methicillin	I.M., I.V.	1 to 2 g	q 4 to 6 hours	Yes
mezlocillin	I.M., I.V.	3 to 4 g	q 4 to 6 hours	No
nafcillin	I.M., I.V.	250 mg to 2 g	q 4 to 6 hours	Yes
	P.O.	500 mg to 1 g	q 6 hours	
oxacillin	I.M., I.V.	250 mg to 2 g	q 4 to 6 hours	Yes
	P.O.	500 mg to 1 g	q 6 hours	
penicillin G benzathine	I.M.	1.2 to 2.4 million units	single dose	No
penicillin G potassium	I.M., I.V.	200,000 to 4 million units	q 4 hours	No
	P.O.	400,000 to 800,000 units	q 6 hours	
penicillin G procaine	I.M.	600,000 to 1.2 million units	q 1 to 3 days	No
		4.8 million units with 1 g probenecid (for syphilis)	single dose for primary, secondary, and early latent syphilis; weekly for 3 weeks for late latent syphilis	
penicillin G sodium	I.M., I.V.	200,000 to 4 million units	q 4 hours	No

*Canada only   †Unlabeled clinical use   Italicized adverse reactions are life-threatening.

COMPARING PENICILLINS *(continued)*

DRUG	ROUTE	ADULT DOSAGE	FREQUENCY	PENICILLINASE RESISTANT
penicillin V potassium	P.O.	250 to 500 mg	q 6 to 8 hours	No
piperacillin	I.M., I.V.	100 to 300 mg/kg daily	divided doses given q 4 to 6 hours	No
ticarcillin	I.M., I.V.	150 to 300 mg/kg daily	divided doses given q 3 to 6 hours	No
ticarcillin/clavulanate potassium	I.V.	3 g	q 4 to 6 hours	Yes

counts, and assess patient for signs of occult or frank bleeding.

• Monitor patients on long-term therapy for possible superinfection, especially elderly and debilitated patients and others receiving immunosuppressants or radiation therapy; monitor closely, especially for fever.

Oral and parenteral administration

• Give penicillins at least 1 hour before giving bacteriostatic antibiotics (tetracyclines, erythromycins, and chloramphenicol); these drugs inhibit bacterial cell growth, decreasing rate of penicillin uptake by bacterial cell walls.

• Always consult manufacturer's directions for reconstitution, dilution, and storage of drugs; check expiration dates.

• Give oral penicillin at least 1 hour before or 2 hours after meals to enhance gastric absorption; food may or may not decrease absorption.

• Refrigerate oral suspensions (stable for 14 days); shake well before administering, to assure correct dosage.

• Administer I.M. dose deep into large muscle mass (gluteal or midlateral thigh); rotate injection sites to minimize tissue injury; do not inject more than 2 g of drug per injection site. Apply ice to injection site for pain.

• Do not add or mix other drugs with I.V. infusions—particularly aminoglycosides, which will be inactivated if mixed with penicillins; they are chemically and physically incompatible. If other drugs must be given I.V., temporarily stop infusion of primary drug.

• Infuse I.V. drug continuously or intermittently (over 30 minutes) and assess I.V. site frequently to prevent infiltration or phlebitis; rotate infusion site q 48 hours; intermittent I.V. infusion may be diluted in 50 to 100 ml sterile water, 0.9% sodium chloride, dextrose 5% in water, dextrose 5% in water and half normal saline, or lactated Ringer's solution.

• Solutions should always be clear, colorless to pale yellow, and free of particles; do not give solutions containing precipitates or other foreign matter.

Information for the patient

• Explain disease process and rationale for therapy.

• Teach signs and symptoms of hypersensitivity and other adverse reactions, and emphasize need to report *any* unusual reactions.

• Teach signs and symptoms of bacterial and fungal superinfection to patients, especially elderly and debilitated patients and others with low resistance from immunosuppressants or irradiation; emphasize need to report signs of infection.

• Be sure patient understands how and when to take drugs; urge patient to complete entire prescribed regimen, to comply with instructions for around-the-clock dosage, and to keep follow-up appointments.

• Counsel patient to check expiration date of drug and to discard unused drug and not give it to family member or friends.

Geriatric use

• Use with caution; elderly patients are susceptible to superinfection.

• Many elderly patients have renal impairment, which decreases excretion of penicillins; lower the dosage in elderly patients who have diminished creatinine clearance.

Pediatric use

Specific dosage recommendations have been established for most penicillins.

Breast-feeding

Consult individual drug recommendations.

Representative combinations

Amoxicillin with clavulanate potassium: Augmentin.

Ampicillin trihydrate with probenecid: Polycillin PRB, Principen with Probenecid, Probampacin, Trojacillin-Plus.

Penicillin G benzathine with penicillin G procaine: Bicillin, Curacillin F.A., Duracillin Fortified, Bicillin C-R, Bicillin 900/300.

Penicillin G procaine with dihydrostreptomycin sulfate: Intramammary infusion USP XXI; with novobiocin sodium: USP XXI; with aluminum stearate: USP XXI.

---

penicillin G benzathine
Bicillin L-A, Megacillin Suspension, Permapen

penicillin G potassium
Cryspen, Deltapen, Lanacillin, Parcillin, Pensorb, Pentids, Pfizerpin

penicillin G procaine
Crysticillin A.S., Duracillin A.S., Pfizerpen A.S., Wycillin

penicillin G sodium
Crystapen*

- Pharmacologic classification: natural penicillin
- Therapeutic classification: antibiotic
- Pregnancy risk category B

How supplied
Available by prescription only
Penicillin G benzathine
Tablets: 200,000 units
Injection: 300,000 units/ml, 600,000 units/ml
Penicillin G procaine
Injection: 300,000 units/ml, 500,000 units/ml, 600,000 units/ml
Penicillin G potassium
Tablets: 200,000 units, 250,000 units, 400,000 units, 500,000 units, 800,000 units
Oral suspension: 200,000 units/5 ml, 250,000 units/5 ml, 400,000 units/5 ml (after reconstitution) suspension
Injection: 200,000 units, 500,000 units, 1 million units, 5 million units, 10 million units, 20 million units
Penicillin G sodium
Injection: 5 million units

Indications, route, and dosage
Congenital syphilis
Penicillin G benzathine
Children under age 2: 50,000 units/kg I.M. as a single dose.
Group A streptococcal upper respiratory infections
Penicillin G benzathine
Adults: 1.2 million units I.M. in a single injection.
Children who weigh 27 kg or more: 900,000 units I.M. in a single injection.
Children under 27 kg: 300,000 to 600,000 units I.M. in a single injection.
Prophylaxis of poststreptococcal rheumatic fever
Penicillin G benzathine
Adults and children: 1.2 million units I.M. once a month or 600,000 units twice a month.
Syphilis of less than 1 year's duration
Penicillin G benzathine
Adults: 2.4 million units I.M. in a single dose.
Syphilis of more than 1 year's duration
Penicillin G benzathine
Adults: 2.4 million units I.M. weekly for 3 successive weeks.

Moderate to severe systemic infections
Penicillin G potassium
Adults: 1.6 to 3.2 million units P.O. daily, divided int doses given q 6 hours (1 mg = 1,600 units); or 1.2 t 24 million units I.M. or I.V. daily, divided into doses give q 4 hours.
Children: 25,000 to 100,000 units/kg P.O. daily, divide into doses given q 6 hours; or 25,000 to 300,000 units kg I.M. or I.V. daily, divided into doses given q 4 hours
Moderate to severe systemic infections
Penicillin G procaine
Adults: 600,000 to 1.2 million units I.M. daily as a single dose.
Children: 300,000 units I.M. daily as a single dose.
Uncomplicated gonorrhea
Penicillin G procaine
Adults and children over age 12: 1 g probenecid, ther 30 minutes later, 4.8 million units of penicillin G procaine I.M., divided into two injection sites.
Pneumococcal pneumonia
Penicillin G procaine
Adults and children over age 12: 300,000 to 600,000 units I.M. daily q 6 to 12 hours.
Moderate to severe systemic infections
Penicillin G sodium
Adults: 1.2 to 24 million units I.M. or I.V. daily, divided into doses given q 4 hours.
Children: 25,000 to 300,000 units/kg I.M. or I.V. daily, divided into doses given q 4 hours.
Endocarditis prophylaxis for dental surgery
Penicillin G sodium
Adults: 2 million units I.V. or I.M. 30 to 60 minutes before procedure, then 1 million units 6 hours later.
Dosage in renal failure

Creatinine clearance (ml/min/ 1.73 m²)	Dosage
10 to 50	50% of the usual dose every 4 to 5 hours; alternatively, give the usual dose every 8 to 12 hours.
< 10	50% of the usual dose every 8 to 12 hours; alternatively, give the usual dose every 12 to 18 hours.

Pharmacodynamics
Antibiotic action: Penicillin G is bactericidal; it adheres to penicillin-binding proteins, thus inhibiting bacterial cell wall synthesis. Penicillin G's spectrum of activity includes most non-penicillinase-producing strains of gram-positive and gram-negative aerobic cocci; spirochetes; and some gram-positive aerobic and anaerobic bacilli.

Pharmacokinetics
Penicillin G is available as four salts, each having the same bactericidal action, but designed to offer greater oral stability (potassium salt) or to prolong duration of action by slowing absorption after I.M. injection (benzathine and procaine salts).
- *Absorption:* Oral—penicillins are hydrolyzed by gastric acids; only 15% to 30% of an oral dose of penicillin G potassium is absorbed; the remainder is hydrolyzed

by gastric secretions. Peak serum concentrations of penicillin G potassium occur at 30 minutes. Food in stomach reduces rate and extent of absorption. Penicillin V is absorbed better after oral administration than penicillin G potassium.

Intramuscular—sodium and potassium salts of penicillin G are absorbed rapidly after I.M. injection; peak serum concentrations occur within 15 to 30 minutes. Absorption of other salts is slower. Peak serum concentrations of penicillin G procaine occur at 1 to 4 hours, with drug detectable in serum for 1 to 2 days; peak serum concentrations of penicillin G benzathine occur at 13 to 24 hours, with serum concentrations detectable for 1 to 4 weeks.

• *Distribution:* Penicillin G is distributed widely into synovial, pleural, pericardial, and ascitic fluids and bile, and into liver, skin, lungs, kidneys, muscle, intestines, tonsils, maxillary sinuses, saliva, and erythrocytes. CSF penetration is poor but is enhanced in patients with inflamed meninges. Pencillin G crosses the placenta; it is 45% to 68% protein-bound.

• *Metabolism:* Between 16% and 30% of an I.M. dose of penicillin G is metabolized to inactive compounds.

• *Excretion:* Penicillin G is excreted primarily in urine by tubular secretion; 20% to 60% of dose is recovered in 6 hours. Some drug is excreted in breast milk. Elimination half-life in adults is about ½ to 1 hour. Severe renal impairment prolongs half-life; penicillin G is removed by hemodialysis and only minimally removed by peritoneal dialysis.

Contraindications and precautions
Penicillin G is contraindicated in patients with known hypersensitivity to any other penicillin or to cephalosporins.

Penicillin G should be used cautiously in patients with renal impairment because it is excreted in urine; decreased dosage is required in patient with moderate to severe renal failure.

Interactions
Concomitant use with aminoglycosides produces synergistic therapeutic effects, chiefly against enterococci; this combination is most effective in enterococcal bacterial endocarditis. However, the drugs are physically and chemically incompatible and are inactivated when mixed or given together. In vivo inactivation has been reported when aminoglycosides and penicillins are used concomitantly.

Probenecid blocks tubular secretion of penicillin, raising its serum concentrations.

Concomitant use of penicillin G with clavulanate appears to enhance effect of penicillin G against certain beta-lactamase-producing bacteria.

Large doses of penicillin may interfere with renal tubular secretion of methotrexate, thus delaying elimination and elevating serum concentrations of methotrexate.

Concomitant use of penicillin G with some nonsteroidal anti-inflammatory drugs prolongs penicillin half-life by competition for urinary excretion or displacement of penicillin from protein-binding sites; similarly, concomitant use with sulfinpyrazone, which inhibits tubular secretion of penicillin G, also prolongs its half-life.

Concomitant use of parenteral penicillin G potassium with potassium-sparing diuretics may cause hyperkalemia; penicillin G potassium is contraindicated in patients with renal failure.

Effects on diagnostic tests
Penicillin G alters test results for urine and serum protein levels; it interferes with turbidimetric methods using sulfosalicylic acid, trichloracetic acid, acetic acid, and nitric acid. Penicillin G does not interfere with tests using bromophenol blue (Albustix, Albutest, Multistix).

Penicillin G alters urine glucose testing using cupric sulfate (Benedict's reagent); use Clinistix or Tes-Tape instead. Penicillin G may cause falsely elevated results of urine specific gravity tests in patients with low urine output and dehydration, and falsely elevated Norymberski and Zimmermann test results for 17-ketogenic steroids; it causes false-positive CSF protein test results (Folin-Ciocalteau method) and may cause positive Coombs' test results.

Penicillin G may falsely decrease serum aminoglycoside concentrations. Adding beta-lactamase to the sample inactivates the penicillin, rendering the assay more accurate. Alternatively, the sample can be spun down and frozen immediately after collection.

Adverse reactions
• CNS: neuropathy, seizures at high doses.
• CV: *congestive heart failure with high doses (penicillin G sodium).*
• GI: *diarrhea,* epigastric distress, vomiting, nausea.
• HEMA: hemolytic anemia, leukopenia, eosinophilia, thrombocytopenia.
• Metabolic: *possible potassium poisoning (hyperreflexia, convulsions, coma).*
• Local: vein pain and irritation, injection-site sterile abscess or thrombophlebitis.
• Other: *hypersensitivity* (rash, urticaria, maculopapular eruptions, exfoliative dermatitis, chills, fever, edema, *anaphylaxis*), arthralgia, bacterial or fungal superinfection.
Note: Drug should be discontinued if immediate hypersensitivity reactions occur or if severe diarrhea indicates pseudomembranous colitis.

Overdose and treatment
Clinical signs of overdose include neuromuscular irritability or seizures. No specific recommendations available. Treatment is supportive. After recent ingestion (within 4 hours), empty stomach by induced emesis or gastric lavage. Follow with activated charcoal to decrease absorption. Pencillin G can be removed by hemodialysis.

▶ Special considerations
Beside those relevant to all *penicillins,* consider the following recommendations.
• Give oral drug on empty stomach for maximum drug absorption because food may interfere with absorption; follow drug only with water because acid in citrus juices and carbonated beverages impairs absorption.
• Monitor closely for possible hypernatremia with sodium salt or hyperkalemia with potassium salt.
• Patients with poor renal function are predisposed to high blood concentrations, which may cause seizures. Monitor renal function.
• Have emergency equipment on hand to manage possible anaphylaxis.
• Because penicillins are dialyzable, patients undergoing hemodialysis may need dosage adjustments.
• Commercially available penicillin G benzathine tablets contain tartrazine, which may induce an allergic reaction in certain individuals.

Geriatric use
Half-life is prolonged in elderly patients because of impaired renal function.

Breast-feeding
Penicillin G is excreted in breast milk; use in breast-feeding women may sensitize infant to penicillin.

penicillin V

penicillin V potassium
Betapen-VK, Biotic-V Powder, Bopen V-K, Cocillin V-K, Lanacillin VK, Ledercillin VK, LV, Nadopen-V★, Novopen VK★, Penapar VK, Penbec-V★, Pen-Vee K, Pfizerpen VK, PVF K★, Robicillin VK, Uticillin VK, V-Cillin K, Veetids

- Pharmacologic classification: natural penicillin
- Therapeutic classification: antibiotic
- Pregnancy risk category B

How supplied
Available by prescription only
Penicillin V
Suspension: 125 mg/5 ml, 250 mg/5 ml (after reconstitution)
Tablets: 250 mg, 500 mg
Penicillin V potassium
Suspension: 125 mg/5 ml, 250 mg/5 ml (after reconstitution)
Tablets: 125 mg, 250 mg, 500 mg
Tablets (film-coated): 250 mg, 500 mg

Indications, route, and dosage
Mild to moderate susceptible infections
Adults: 250 to 500 mg (400,000 to 800,000 units) P.O. q 6 hours.
Children: 15 to 50 mg/kg (25,000 to 90,000 units/kg) P.O. daily, divided into doses given q 6 to 8 hours.
Endocarditis prophylaxis for dental surgery
Adults: 2 g P.O. 30 to 60 minutes before procedure, then 500 mg P.O. q 6 hours for eight doses.
Children under 30 kg: Half the adult dose.

Pharmacodynamics
Antibiotic action: Penicillin V is bactericidal; it adheres to penicillin-binding proteins, thus inhibiting bacterial cell wall synthesis.

Penicillin V's spectrum of activity includes most non-penicillinase-producing strains of gram-positive and gram-negative aerobic cocci; spirochetes; and some gram-positive aerobic and anaerobic bacilli.

Pharmacokinetics
- *Absorption:* Penicillin V has greater acid stability and is absorbed more completely than penicillin G after oral administration. About 60% to 75% of an oral dose of penicillin V is absorbed. Peak serum concentrations occur at 60 minutes in fasting subjects; food has no significant effect.
- *Distribution:* Penicillin V is distributed widely into synovial, pleural, pericardial, and ascitic fluids and bile, and into liver, skin, lungs, kidneys, muscle, intestines, tonsils, maxillary sinuses, saliva, and erythrocytes. CSF penetration is poor but is enhanced in patients with inflamed meninges. Pencillin V crosses the placenta; it is 75% to 89% protein-bound.
- *Metabolism:* Between 35% and 70% of a penicillin V dose is metabolized to inactive compounds.
- *Excretion:* Penicillin V is excreted primarily in urine by tubular secretion; 26% to 65% of dose is recovered in 6 hours. Some drug is excreted in breast milk. Elimination half-life in adults is ½ hour. Severe renal impairment prolongs half-life.

Contraindications and precautions
Penicillin V is contraindicated in patients with known hypersensitivity to any other penicillin or to cephalosporins.

Penicillin V should be used cautiously in patients with renal impairment because it is excreted in urine; decreased dosage is required in patients with moderate to severe renal failure.

Interactions
Penicillin V may decrease efficacy of estrogen-containing oral contraceptives; breakthrough bleeding may occur.

Concomitant use with aminoglycosides produces synergistic therapeutic effects, chiefly against enterococci; however, the drugs are physically and chemically incompatible and are inactivated when mixed or given together. In vivo inactivation has been reported when aminoglycosides and pencillins are used concomitantly.

Probenecid blocks tubular secretion of penicillin, resulting in higher serum concentrations of drug.

Concomitant use of penicillin V with sulfinpyrazone, which inhibits tubular secretion of penicillin V, prolongs its half-life.

Effects on diagnostic tests
Penicillin V alters test results for urine and serum protein levels; it interferes with turbidimetric methods using sulfosalicylic acid, trichloracetic acid, acetic acid, and nitric acid. Penicillin V does not interfere with tests using bromophenol blue (Albustix, Albutest, MultiStix). Penicillin V may falsely decrease serum aminoglycoside concentrations.

Adverse reactions
- CNS: neuropathy, *seizures at high doses.*
- GI: *diarrhea,* epigastric distress, vomiting, nausea.
- HEMA: *hemolytic anemia,* leukopenia, *eosinophilia,* thrombocytopenia.
- Other: *hypersensitivity* (rash, urticaria, maculopapular eruptions, *exfoliative dermatitis,* chills, fever, edema, *anaphylaxis),* arthralgia, bacterial or fungal superinfection.

Note: Drug should be discontinued if immediate hypersensitivity reactions occur or if severe diarrhea indicates pseudomembranous colitis.

Overdose and treatment
Clinical signs of overdose include neuromuscular sensitivity or seizures. No specific recommendations are available. Treatment is supportive. After recent ingestion (within 4 hours), empty stomach by induced emesis or gastric lavage; follow with activated charcoal to reduce absorption.

▶ **Special considerations**
Besides those relevant to all *penicillins*, consider the following recommendations.
● Give oral dose 1 hour before or 2 hours after meals for maximum absorption.
● After reconstitution, oral suspension is stable for 14 days if refrigerated.

Geriatric use
Half-life may be prolonged in elderly patients because of impaired renal function.

Breast-feeding
Penicillin V is excreted in breast milk; use in breast-feeding women may sensitize the infant to pencillins.

---

pentaerythritol tetranitrate
Duotrate, Naptrate, Pentol, Pentol SA, Pentritol, Pentylan, Peritrate, Peritrate SA, PETN

● Pharmacologic classification: nitrate
● Therapeutic classification: antianginal, vasodilator
● Pregnancy risk category C

How supplied
Available by prescription only
Tablets: 10 mg, 20 mg, 40 mg, 80 mg; 80 mg (extended-release)
Capsules (extended-release): 30 mg, 45 mg, 60 mg, 80 mg

Indications, route, and dosage
Prophylaxis of angina pectoris
Adults: 10 to 20 mg P.O. t.i.d. to q.i.d.; may be titrated upward to 40 mg P.O. q.i.d. 30 minutes before or 1 hour after meals and h.s.; 80 mg of sustained-release preparation P.O. b.i.d.

Pharmacodynamics
Antianginal action: Pentaerythritol tetranitrate shares the antianginal and vasodilator actions of other nitrates. However, it is ineffective in relieving acute angina.

Pharmacokinetics
● *Absorption:* Drug is absorbed from the gastrointestinal tract, with bioavailability of about 50%. Onset of action of hemodynamic effects is about 20 to 60 minutes.
● *Distribution:* Little is known about drug's distribution; however, it is probably similar to that of nitroglycerin and other nitrates.
● *Metabolism:* Drug is metabolized in the liver and serum to pentaerythritol mononitrate, pentaerythritol dinitrate, pentaerythritol trinitrate, and pentaerythritol. Pentaerythritol trinitrate, the only active metabolite, has a plasma half-life of about 10 minutes.
● *Excretion:* Drug is excreted in the urine primarily as inactive metabolites. Duration of effect is 4 to 5 hours.

Contraindications and precautions
Pentaerythritol tetranitrate is contraindicated in patients with severe anemia, because nitrate ions can readily oxidize hemoglobin to methemoglobin; in patients with head trauma or cerebral hemorrhage, be-

cause it may increase intracranial pressure; severe anemia, because the hypotensive effects of the drug may further worsen tissue perfusion; and in patients with a history of hypersensitivity or idiosyncratic reaction to nitrates.
Drug should be used with caution in patients with hypotension, because the drug may worsen this condition; in patients with increased intracranial pressure, because drug dilates meningeal vessels; in patients with open-angle or narrow-angle glaucoma, although introcular pressure is increased only briefly and drainage of aqueous humor from the eye is unimpeded; in patients with diuretic-induced fluid depletion or low systolic blood pressure (below 90 mm Hg), because of drug's hypotensive effect; and in patients who have had acute myocardial infarction in the past several days, because drug may cause excessive hypotension and tachycardia.

Interactions
Concomitant use of pentaerythritol tetranitrate with alcohol, antihypertensive drugs, beta blockers, phenothiazines, other nitrates, pentaerythritol tetranitrate may cause additive hypotensive effects. Concomitant use with ergot alkaloids increases ergot alkaloid bioavailability, possibly precipitating angina.

Effects on diagnostic tests
Pentaerythritol tetranitrate may interfere with serum cholesterol determination methods involving Zlatkis-Zak color reaction, causing falsely decreased values.

Adverse reactions
● CNS: headache (possibly throbbing), dizziness, weakness, blurred vision.
● CV: orthostatic hypotension, tachycardia, flushing, palpitations, fainting.
● DERM: cutaneous vasodilation.
● GI: nausea, vomiting, dry mouth.
● Other: hypersensitivity reactions (rash, dermatitis).
Note: Drug should be discontinued if rash, dermatitis, blurred vision, or dry mouth occurs.

Overdose and treatment
Clinical effects of overdose result mainly from vasodilation and methemoglobinemia and include hypotension; persistent throbbing headache; palpitations; visual disturbances; flushing of skin and sweating (with later skin coldness and cyanosis); nausea and vomiting; colic and bloody diarrhea; orthostasis; initial hyperpnea; dyspnea and slow respiratory rate; bradycardia; heart block; increased intracranial pressure with confusion; fever; paralysis; and tissue hypoxia caused by methemoglobinemia, possibly leading to cyanosis, metabolic acidosis, coma, clonic convulsions, and circulatory collapse. Death may follow circulatory collapse or asphyxia.
Treatment involves gastric lavage followed by administration of activated charcoal to remove remaining gastric contents. Blood gas measurements and methemoglobin levels should be monitored as indicated. Supportive measures may include respiratory support and oxygen administration, passive movement of extremities to aid venous return, recumbent positioning (Trendelenburg's position, if necessary), I.V. fluid administration, and maintenance of warm body temperature. An I.V. adrenergic agonist may be considered if patient requires further treatment. For methemoglobinemia, methylene blue (1 to 2 mg/kg I.V.) may be ad-

---

*Canada only   †Unlabeled clinical use   Italicized adverse reactions are life-threatening.

ministered. (Epinephrine and related compounds are contraindicated.)

▶ **Special considerations**

• Administer medication before meals, if possible.
• Medication may cause headache, especially at first. Administer aspirin or acetaminophen. Dosage may need to be reduced temporarily, but tolerance usually develops.
• If necessary, administer additional doses before anticipated stress or at bedtime for nocturnal angina.
• Do not administer drug for relief of acute angina attacks.
• Monitor blood pressure and intensity and duration of patient's response to drug.
• Medication may cause orthostatic hypotension. To minimize this effect, have patient change to upright position slowly, walk down stairs carefully, and lie down at first sign of dizziness.
• Do not discontinue drug abruptly after long-term therapy, because this may cause coronary vasospasm.
• Store medication in cool place in tightly covered, light-resistant container.

Information for the patient

• Instruct patient that drug should be taken before meals for optimal effect.
• Warn patient that, initially, drug may cause headache, which may respond to usual headache remedies. Assure patient that headache usually subsides with continued treatment.
• Inform patient that medication should be taken regularly, even long-term if ordered. Drug is physiologically necessary but not addictive.
• Instruct patient to avoid alcohol because severe hypotension and cardiovascular collapse may occur.
• Warn patient that drug may cause dizziness or flushing. Instruct patient to change positions gradually to avoid excessive dizziness.

---

pentamidine isethionate
NebuPent, Pentam 300

• Pharmacologic classification: diamidine derivative
• Therapeutic classification: antiprotozoal
• Pregnancy risk category C

How supplied
Available by prescription only
Injection: 300-mg vials
Solution for inhalation: 300 mg

Indications, route, and dosage
Pneumonia caused by Pneumocystis carinii
Adults and children: 4 mg/kg I.V. or I.M. once a day for 14 days. As alternate dose in children, 150 mg/m² daily for 5 days, then 100 mg/m² for duration of therapy.
Prophylaxis against Pneumocystis carinii *pneumonia (PCP) in persons at high risk for the disease*
Adults: 300 mg by inhalation once every 4 weeks. The aerosol form of the drug should be administered by the Respirgard II jet nebulizer.

Pharmacodynamics
Antiprotozoal action: Mechanism is unknown. However, pentamidine may work by inhibiting synthesis of ribonucleic acid (RNA), deoxyribonucleic acid (DNA), proteins, or phospholipids. It may also interfere with several metabolic processes, particularly certain energy-yielding reactions and reactions involving folic acid. Drug's spectrum of activity includes *P. carinii* and *Trypanosoma* organisms.

Pharmacokinetics
• *Absorption:* Daily I.M. doses (4 mg/kg) produce surprisingly few plasma level fluctuations. Plasma levels usually increase slightly 1 hour after I.M. injection. Little information exists regarding pharmacokinetics with I.V. administration. Absorption is limited after aerosol administration.
• *Distribution:* Pentamidine appears to be extensively tissue-bound. CNS penetration is poor. Extent of plasma protein-binding is unknown.
• *Metabolism:* Pentamidine's metabolism is unknown.
• *Excretion:* Most of drug is excreted unchanged in the urine. Drug's extensive tissue-binding may account for its appearance in urine 6 to 8 weeks after therapy ends.

Contraindications and precautions
Because of its potentially toxic effect, pentamidine is only used as a second-line agent for *P. carinii* pneumonia.

Pentamidine should be administered cautiously to patients with hypertension, hypotension, hyperglycemia, hypoglycemia, hypocalcemia, leukopenia, thrombocytopenia, anemia, or hepatic or renal dysfunction because of risk of serious adverse effects.

Patients who have developed serious or life-threatening reactions to systemic pentamidine may not be good candidates for treatment with the aerosol form.

The Centers for Disease Control recommends against administering pentamidine prophylaxis to HIV-infected pregnant women because of the risk to the fetus; however, such treatment may be considered postpartum.

Interactions
When used concomitantly, pentamidine may have additive nephrotoxic effects with aminoglycosides, amphotericin B, capreomycin, colistin, cisplatin, methoxyflurane, polymyxin B, and vancomycin.

Effects on diagnostic tests
Blood urea nitrogen (BUN), serum creatinine, AST (SGOT), and ALT (SGPT) levels may increase during pentamidine therapy.

Other abnormal findings may include hyperkalemia and hypocalcemia. Hypoglycemia may occur initially (possibly from stimulation of endogenous insulin release); later, hyperglycemia may result from direct pancreatic cell damage.

Adverse reactions
• CNS: confusion, hallucinations, dizziness.
• CV: *hypotension* (possibly severe and fatal), dysrhythmias (*ventricular tachycardia*).
• DERM: flushing, rash, pruritus, *toxic epidermal necrolysis, Stevens-Johnson syndrome*.
• Endocrine: hypoglycemia within first 5 to 7 days (possibly severe and prolonged, requiring I.V. dextrose infusion); latent hyperglycemia (may occur several months after therapy, possibly causing insulin-dependent diabetes mellitus); hypocalcemia; hyperkalemia.

- GI: nausea, vomiting, diarrhea, anorexia, metallic taste, acute pancreatitis, elevated liver enzyme levels.
- GU: elevated BUN and serum creatinine levels, renal toxicity (usually reversible).
- HEMA: leukopenia, thrombocytopenia, neutropenia, anemia, megaloblastic changes (secondary to folate decrease).
- Inhalation: metallic taste, pharyngitis, cough, nausea, bronchospasm, shortness of breath, rhinitis, laryngitis.
- Local: pain, sterile abscess, induration at injection site, phlebitis (with I.V. infusion).
- Other: fever, *anaphylaxis*.

Overdose and treatment
No information available.

▶ Special considerations
- Make sure patient has adequate fluid status before administering drug; dehydration may lead to hypotension and renal toxicity.
- I.V. infusion avoids risk of local reactions and proves as safe as I.M. injection when given slowly, over at least 60 minutes. To prepare drug for I.V. infusion, add 3 to 5 ml of sterile water for injection or dextrose 5% in water (D_5W) to 300-mg vial to yield 100 mg/ml or 60 mg/ml, respectively. Withdraw desired dose and dilute further into 50 to 250 ml of D_5W; infuse over at least 60 minutes. Diluted solution remains stable for 5 days.
- To prepare drug for I.M. injection, add 3 ml of sterile water for injection to 300-mg vial to yield 100 mg/ml. Withdraw desired dose and inject deep I.M.
- Patient should be supine during I.V. administration to minimize hypotension risk. Because patient may develop sudden, severe hypotension after I.M. injection or during I.V. infusion, closely monitor blood pressure during infusion and several times thereafter until patient is stable.
- Keep emergency drugs and equipment (including emergency airway, vasopressors, and I.V. fluids) on hand.
- Monitor daily blood glucose, BUN, and serum creatinine levels.
- Monitor periodic electrolyte levels, complete blood count, platelet count, and liver function tests.
- Observe patient for signs and symptoms of hypoglycemia.
- When inhalation solution is used for prophylaxis against PCP, high-risk individuals include HIV-infected persons with a history of PCP; patients who have never had an episode of PCP but whose CD4 cells are below 20% of total lymphocytes, or whose CD4 cell count is below 200/mm^2.
- To administer by inhalation, the dose should be diluted in 6 ml of sterile water and delivered at 6 liters/minute from a 50-p.s.i. compressed air source until the reservoir is dry. Alternate delivery systems (other than the Respirgard II) are under investigation but are currently not recommended.
- Patients who develop wheezing or cough during pentamidine aerosol therapy may benefit by pretreatment (at least 5 minutes before pentamidine administration) with a bronchodilator.

pentazocine hydrochloride
Fortral, Talwin*, Talwin-Nx (with naloxone hydrochloride)

pentazocine lactate
Fortral*

- Pharmacologic classification: narcotic agonist-antagonist, opioid partial agonist
- Therapeutic classification: analgesic, adjunct to anesthesia
- Controlled substance schedule IV
- Pregnancy risk category C

How supplied
Available by prescription only
Tablets: 50 mg
Injection: 30 mg/ml

Indications, route, and dosage
Moderate to severe pain
Adults: 50 to 100 mg P.O. q 3 to 4 hours, p.r.n. or around the clock. Maximum oral dosage: 600 mg daily. Or 30 mg I.M., I.V., or S.C. q 3 to 4 hours, p.r.n. or around the clock. Maximum parenteral dosage: 360 mg daily. Doses above 30 mg I.V. or 60 mg I.M. or S.C. not recommended.

Pharmacodynamics
Analgesic action: The exact mechanisms of action of pentazocine are unknown. It is believed to be a competitive antagonist at some, and an agonist at other receptors, resulting in relief of moderate pain. Pentazocine can produce respiratory depression, sedation, miosis, and antitussive effects. It also may cause psychotomimetic and dysphoric effects. In patients with coronary artery disease, it elevates mean aortic pressure, left ventricular end-diastolic pressure, and mean pulmonary artery pressure. In patients with acute MI, I.V. pentazocine increases systemic and pulmonary arterial pressures and systemic vascular resistance.

Pharmacokinetics
- *Absorption:* Pentazocine is well absorbed after oral or parenteral administration. However, orally administered drug undergoes first-pass metabolism in the liver and less than 20% of a dose reaches the systemic circulation unchanged. Bioavailability is increased in patients with hepatic dysfunction; patients with cirrhosis absorb 60% to 70% of the drug. Onset of analgesia is 15 to 30 minutes, with peak effect at 15 to 60 minutes.
- *Distribution:* Pentazocine appears to be widely distributed in the body.
- *Metabolism:* Pentazocine is metabolized in the liver, mainly by oxidation and secondarily by glucuronidation. Metabolism may be prolonged in patients with impaired hepatic function.
- *Excretion:* Duration of effect is 3 hours. There is considerable interpatient variability in its urinary excretion. Very small amounts of the drug are excreted in the feces after oral or parenteral administration.

Contraindications and precautions
Pentazocine is contraindicated in patients with known hypersensitivity to the drug or other opiate partial agonists.

Administer pentazocine with extreme caution after MI or to patients with supraventricular arrhythmias; avoid, or administer drug with extreme caution to patients with head injury or increased intracranial pressure, because drug obscures neurologic parameters; and during pregnancy and labor, because drug readily crosses placenta (premature infants are especially sensitive to respiratory and CNS depressant effects of narcotic agonist-antagonists).

Administer pentazocine cautiously to patients with renal or hepatic dysfunction, because drug accumulation or prolonged duration of action may occur; to patients with pulmonary disease (asthma, chronic obstructive pulmonary disease), because drug depresses respiration and suppresses cough reflex; to patients undergoing biliary tract surgery, because drug may cause biliary spasm; to patients with convulsive disorders, because drug may precipitate seizures; to elderly or debilitated patients, who are more sensitive to both thereutic and adverse drug effects; and to patients prone to physical or psychic addiction, because of the high abuse potential for this drug.

Narcotic agonist-antagonists have a lower potential for abuse than do narcotic agonists, but the risk still exists.

Interactions

If administered within a few hours of barbiturates, such as thiopental, pentazocine may produce additive CNS and respiratory depressant effects and, possibly, apnea.

Cimetidine may increase pentazocine toxicity, causing disorientation, respiratory depression, apnea, and seizures. Because data are limited, this combination is not contraindicated; however, be prepared to administer naloxone if toxicity occurs.

Reduced doses of pentazocine usually are necessary when drug is used concomitantly with other CNS depressants (narcotic analgesics, antihistamines, phenothiazines, barbiturates, benzodiazepines, sedative-hypnotics, tricyclic antidepressants, alcohol, and muscle relaxants), because such use potentiates drug's respiratory and CNS depression, sedation, and hypotensive effects; use with general anesthetics also may cause severe cardiovascular depression.

Drug accumulation and enhanced effects may result from concomitant use with other drugs that are extensively metabolized in the liver (rifampin, phenytoin, and digitoxin).

Patients who become physically dependent on this drug may experience acute withdrawal syndrome if given high doses of a narcotic agonist-antagonist or a single dose of an antagonist. Use with caution, and monitor closely.

Effects on diagnostic tests
None reported.

Adverse reactions
● CNS: sedation, dizziness (common), light-headedness (common), euphoria, hallucinations, headache, insomnia, irritability, tremor, tinnitus, disorientation, confusion, *seizures,* parasthesia, syncope.
● CV: hypertension, tachycardia, shock.
● DERM: dermatitis, pruritus, diaphoresis, soft-tissue induration, nodules, and cutaneous depression can occur at injection sites; severe sclerosis of skin, subcutaneous tissue, and underlying muscle at site of multiple injections.

● GI: constipation, dry mouth, nausea, vomiting.
● GU: urinary retention.
Note: Drug should be discontinued if hypersensitivity, seizures, or cardiac arrhythmias occur.

Overdose and treatment
The signs of pentazocine hydrochloride overdose have not been defined because of a lack of clinical experience with overdosage. If overdose should occur, all supportive measures (oxygen, I.V. fluids, vasopressors) should be used as necessary. Mechanical ventilation should be considered. Parenteral naloxone is an effective antagonist for respiratory depression because of pentazocine.

▶ Special considerations
Besides those relevant to all *narcotic agonist-antagonists,* consider the following recommendations.
● Tablets are not well absorbed.
● Do not mix in same syringe with soluble barbiturates.
● Pentazocine may obscure the signs and symptoms of an acute abdominal condition or worsen gallbladder pain.
● Pentazocine may cause orthostatic hypotension in ambulatory patients. Have patient sit down to relieve symptoms.
● Pentazocine possesses narcotic antagonist properties. May precipitate abstinence syndrome in narcotic-dependent patients.
● Talwin Nx, the available oral pentazocine, contains the narcotic antagonist naloxone, which prevents illicit I.V. use.

Information for the patient
● Tell patient to report skin rash, confusion, disorientation, or other serious adverse effects.
● Warn patient that Talwin Nx is for oral use only. Severe reactions may result if tablets are crushed, dissolved, and injected.

Geriatric use
Lower doses are usually indicated for elderly patients, who may be more sensitive to the therapeutic and adverse effects of the drug.

Pediatric use
Use of pentazocine is not recommended in children under age 12.

Breast-feeding
It is unknown whether pentazocine is excreted in breast milk; it should be used with caution in breast-feeding women.

---

pentobarbital sodium
Nembutal

- Pharmacologic classification: barbiturate
- Therapeutic classification: anticonvulsant, sedative-hypnotic
- Controlled substance schedule II (suppositories schedule III)
- Pregnancy risk category D

How supplied
Available by prescription only
Elixir: 18.2 mg/5 ml
Capsules: 50 mg, 100 mg
Injection: 50 mg/ml, 1-ml and 2-ml disposable syringes; 2-ml, 20-ml, and 50-ml vials
Suppositories: 30 mg, 60 mg, 120 mg, 200 mg

Indications, route, and dosage
Sedation
Adults: 20 to 40 mg P.O. b.i.d., t.i.d., or q.i.d.
Children: 2 to 6 mg/kg P.O. daily in divided doses, to a maximum of 100 mg/dose.
Insomnia
Adults: 100 to 200 mg P.O. h.s. or 150 to 200 mg deep I.M.; 120 to 200 mg rectally.
Children: 2 to 6 mg/kg I.M., up to a maximum of 100 mg/dose. Or 30 mg rectally (age 2 months to 1 year), 30 to 60 mg rectally (age 1 to 4), 60 mg rectally (age 5 to 12), 60 to 120 mg rectally (age 12 to 14).
Preanesthetic medication
Adults: 150 to 200 mg I.M. or P.O. in two divided doses.
Anticonvulsant
Adults: Initially, 100 mg I.V.; after 1 minute additional doses may be given. Maximum dosage is 500 mg.
Children: Initially, 50 mg I.M. or I.V.; after 1 minute additional doses may be given.
†Treatment of cerebral ischemia or cerebral edema following stroke, head trauma, or Reye's syndrome (barbiturate coma)
Adults: 1 to 3 mg/kg/hour by I.V. infusion after an initial loading dose sufficient to produce burst suppression of the electroencephalogram (5 to 34 mg/kg).

Pharmacodynamics
- *Sedative-hypnotic action:* The exact cellular site and mechanism(s) of action are unknown. Pentobarbital acts throughout the CNS as a nonselective depressant with a fast onset of action and short duration of action. Particularly sensitive to this drug is the reticular activating system, which controls CNS arousal. Pentobarbital decreases both presynaptic and postsynaptic membrane excitability by facilitating the action of gamma-aminobutyric acid (GABA).
- *Anticonvulsant action:* Pentobarbital suppresses the spread of seizure activity produced by epileptogenic foci in the cortex, thalamus, and limbic systems by enhancing the effect of GABA. Both presynaptic and postsynaptic excitability are decreased, and the seizure threshold is raised.

Pharmacokinetics
- *Absorption:* Pentobarbital is absorbed rapidly after oral and rectal administration, with an onset of action of 10 to 15 minutes. Peak serum concentrations occur between 30 and 60 minutes after oral administration.

After I.M. injection, the onset of action occurs within 10 to 25 minutes. After I.V. administration, the onset of action occurs immediately. Serum concentrations needed for sedation and hypnosis are 1 to 5 mcg/ml and 5 to 15 mcg/ml, respectively. After oral or rectal administration, duration of hypnosis is 1 to 4 hours.
- *Distribution:* Pentobarbital is distributed widely throughout the body. Approximately 35% to 45% is protein-bound. Drug accumulates in fat with long-term use.
- *Metabolism:* Pentobarbital is metabolized in the liver by penultimate oxidation.
- *Excretion:* 99% of pentobarbital is eliminated as glucuronide conjugates and other metabolites in the urine. Terminal half-life ranges from 35 to 50 hours. Duration of action is 3 to 4 hours.

Contraindications and precautions
Pentobarbital is contraindicated in patients with known hypersensitivity to barbiturates and in patients with bronchopneumonia, status asthmaticus, or severe respiratory distress, because of the potential for respiratory depression. Pentobarbital should not be used in patients who are depressed or have suicidal ideation because the drug can worsen depression; in patients with uncontrolled acute or chronic pain, because exacerbation of pain and paradoxical excitement can occur; or in patients with porphyria, because this drug can trigger symptoms of this disease.

Pentobarbital should be used cautiously in patients who must perform hazardous tasks requiring mental alertness, because the drug causes drowsiness. Administer parenteral pentobarbital slowly and with extreme caution to patients with hypotension or severe pulmonary or cardiovascular disease because of potential adverse hemodynamic effects. Because tolerance and physical or psychological dependence can occur, prolonged use of high doses should be avoided. Pentobarbital capsules may contain tartrazine, which may cause an allergic reaction in certain individuals, especially those who are sensitive to aspirin. Prenatal exposure to barbiturates is associated with an increased incidence of fetal abnormalities and, possibly, brain tumors. Use of barbiturates in the third trimester may be associated with physical dependence in neonates. Risk-benefit must be considered.

Interactions
Pentobarbital may potentiate or add to CNS and respiratory depressant effects of other sedative-hypnotics, antihistamines, narcotics, antidepressants, tranquilizers, and alcohol.

Pentobarbital enhances the enzymatic degradation of warfarin and other oral anticoagulants; patients may require increased doses of the anticoagulants. Drug also enhances hepatic metabolism of some drugs, including digitoxin (not digoxin), corticosteroids, oral contraceptives and other estrogens, theophylline and other xanthines, and doxycycline. Pentobarbital impairs the effectiveness of griseofulvin by decreasing absorption from the GI tract.

Valproic acid, phenytoin, disulfiram, and monoamine oxidase inhibitors decrease the metabolism of pentobarbital and can increase its toxicity. Rifampin may decrease pentobarbital levels by increasing hepatic metabolism.

Effects on diagnostic tests
Pentobarbital may cause a false-positive phentolamine test. The drug's physiologic effects may impair the ab-

---

sorption of cyanocobalamin ^{57}Co; it may decrease serum bilirubin concentrations in neonates, epileptic patients, and in patients with congenital nonhemolytic unconjugated hyperbilirubinemia. EEG patterns show a change in low-voltage, fast activity; changes persist for a time after discontinuation of therapy.

Adverse reactions
● CNS: drowsiness, lethargy, vertigo, headache, CNS depression, rebound insomnia, increased dreams or nightmares, possibly *seizures* (after acute withdrawal or reduction in dosage), mental confusion, paradoxical excitement, confusion and agitation (especially in elderly patients).
● CV: hypotension (after rapid I.V. administration), bradycardia, *circulatory collapse*.
● DERM: urticaria, rash, *exfoliative dermatitis, Stevens-Johnson syndrome*.
● EENT: miosis.
● GI: nausea, vomiting, diarrhea, constipation.
● Local: thrombophlebitis, pain and possible tissue damage at the site of extravascular injection.
● Other: laryngospasm, *bronchospasm, respiratory depression*, angioedema; vitamin K deficiency and bleeding have occurred in newborns of mothers treated during pregnancy. Hyperalgesia occurs in low doses or in patients with chronic pain.
Note: Drug should be discontinued if hypersensitivity reaction, profound CNS or respiratory depression, or skin eruptions occur.

Overdose and treatment
Clinical manifestations of overdose include unsteady gait, slurred speech, sustained nystagmus, somnolence, confusion, respiratory depression, pulmonary edema, areflexia, and coma. Typical shock syndrome with tachycardia and hypotension may occur. Jaundice, hypothermia followed by fever, and oliguria also may occur. Serum concentrations greater than 10 mcg/ml may produce profound coma; concentrations greater than 30 mcg/ml may be fatal.

To treat, maintain and support ventilation and pulmonary function as necessary; support cardiac function and circulation with vasopressors and I.V. fluids, as needed. If patient is conscious and gag reflex is intact, induce emesis (if ingestion was recent) by administering ipecac syrup. If emesis is contraindicated, perform gastric lavage while a cuffed endotracheal tube is in place to prevent aspiration. Follow with administration of activated charcoal or saline cathartic. Measure intake and output, vital signs, and laboratory parameters. Maintain body temperature.

Alkalinization of urine may be helpful in removing drug from the body. Hemodialysis may be useful in severe overdose.

▶ Special considerations
Besides those relevant to all *barbiturates*, consider the following recommendations.
● I.V. injection should be reserved for emergency treatment and should be given under close supervision. Be prepared for emergency resuscitative measures.
● Avoid I.V. administration at a rate greater than 50 mg/minute to prevent hypotension and respiratory depression.
● High dose therapy for elevated intracranial pressure may require mechanically assisted ventilation.
● Administer I.M. dose deep into large muscle mass. Do not administer more than 5 ml into any one site.

● Discard any solution that is discolored or contains precipitate.
● Administration of full loading doses over short periods of time to treat status epilepticus will require ventilatory support in adults.
● To assure accuracy of dosage, do not divide suppositories.
● Drug has no analgesic effect and may cause restlessness or delirium in patients with pain.
● Nembutal tablets contain tartrazine dye, which may cause allergic reactions in susceptible persons.
● To prevent rebound of rapid-eye-movement sleep after prolonged therapy, discontinue gradually over 5 to 6 days.

Information for the patient
● Advise pregnant patient of potential hazard to fetus or neonate when taking pentobarbital late in pregnancy. Withdrawal symptoms can occur.
● Tell patient not to take drug continuously for longer than 2 weeks.
● Emphasize the dangers of combining this drug with alcohol. An excessive depressant effect is possible even if the drug is taken the evening before ingestion of alcohol.

Geriatric use
Elderly patients usually require lower doses because of increased susceptibility to CNS depressant effects of pentobarbital. Confusion, disorientation, and excitability may occur in elderly patients. Use with caution.

Pediatric use
Barbiturates may cause paradoxical excitement in children. Use with caution.

Breast-feeding
Pentobarbital passes into breast milk. Do not administer to breast-feeding women.

pentostatin (2'-deoxycoformycin; DCF)
Nipent

● Pharmacologic classification: adenosine deaminase inhibitor
● Therapeutic classification: antileukemic agent
● Pregnancy risk category D

How supplied
Available by prescription only
Powder for injection: 10 mg/vial

Indications, route, and dosage
Alpha-interferon-refractory hairy-cell leukemia
Adults: 4 mg/m² I.V. every other week.

Pharmacodynamics
Antileukemic action: Pentostatin inhibits the enzyme adenosine deaminase (ADA), causing an increase in intracellular levels of deoxyadenosine triphosphate. This increase leads to cell damage and death. Because ADA is most active in cells of the lymphoid system (especially malignant T cells), drug is useful in treating leukemias.

Pharmacokinetics

● *Distribution:* Plasma protein-binding is low (about 4%); distribution half-life is about 11 minutes.
● *Metabolism:* Unknown.
● *Excretion:* Over 90% of drug is excreted in urine. Clearance depends on renal function; mean terminal half-life is about 6 hours in patients with normal renal function; increases to 18 hours or more in patients with renal impairment (creatinine clearance below 50 ml/minute).

Contraindications and precautions

Pentostatin is contraindicated in patients with hypersensitivity to the drug. It should be used cautiously and only under supervision of a physician qualified and experienced in the use of cancer chemotherapeutic agents. Adverse reactions to pentostatin therapy are common.

Withhold or discontinue drug in patients with evidence of CNS toxicity; also withhold drug if patient has a severe rash. Do not give to patients who have an active infection; drug may be resumed when infection clears. Avoid use in patients with renal damage (creatinine clearance of 60 ml/minute or less).

Temporarily withhold drug if absolute neutrophil count falls below 200 cells/mm³ if the pretreatment level was over 500 cells/mm³. There are no recommendations regarding dosage adjustments in patients with anemia, neutropenia, or thrombocytopenia.

Interactions

Concomitant use with fludarabine increases the risk of severe or fatal pulmonary toxicity. Don't use together. Concomitant use with vidarabine increases the incidence or severity of adverse effects associated with either drug.

Effects on diagnostic tests

None reported.

Adverse reactions

● CNS: headache, neurologic symptoms, anxiety, confusion, depression, dizziness, insomnia, nervousness, paresthesia, somnolence, abnormal thinking.
● CV: *arrhythmias,* abnormal ECG, thrombophlebitis, hemorrhage.
● DERM: ecchymosis, petechiae, rash, skin disorder, eczema, dry skin, herpes simplex, herpes zoster, maculopapular rash, vesiculobullous rash, pruritus, seborrhea, discoloration, sweating.
● EENT: abnormal vision, conjunctivitis, ear pain, eye pain, epistaxis, pharyngitis, rhinitis, sinusitis.
● GI: nausea, vomiting, anorexia, diarrhea, constipation, flatulence, stomatitis.
● GU: GU disorder, hematuria, dysuria, increased BUN level, increased creatinine level.
● HEMA: *myelosuppression,* leukopenia, anemia, thrombocytopenia, lymphadenopathy.
● Hepatic: elevated liver function tests.
● Metabolic: weight loss, peripheral edema, increased lactate dehydrogenase levels.
● Respiratory: cough, upper respiratory disorder, *lung disorder,* bronchitis, dyspnea, *lung edema, pneumonia.*
● Other: fever, infection, fatigue, pain, *allergic reactions,* chills, sepsis, chest pain, abdominal pain, back pain, flulike syndrome, asthenia, malaise, myalgia, arthralgia.

Overdose and treatment

High dosage of pentostatin (20 to 50 mg/m² in divided doses over 5 days) has been associated with deaths from severe CNS, hepatic, pulmonary, and renal toxicity. No specific antidote is known. If overdosage occurs, treat symptoms and provide supportive care.

▶ Special considerations

● Drug should be used only in patients who have hairy-cell leukemia refractory to alpha interferon: disease that progresses after a minimum of 3 months of treatment with alpha interferon or does not respond after 6 months of therapy.
● Optimal duration of therapy is unknown. Current recommendations call for two additional courses of therapy after a complete response. If patient hasn't had a partial response after 6 months of therapy, discontinue drug. If patient has had only a partial response, continue drug for another 6 months or for two courses of therapy after a complete response.
● Store powder for injection in the refrigerator (36° to 46° F [2° to 8° C]). Reconstituted and diluted solutions should be used within 8 hours because drug contains no preservative.
● Follow appropriate guidelines for proper handling, administration, and disposal of chemotherapeutic agents. Treat all spills and waste products with 5% sodium hypochlorite solution. Wear protective clothing and polyethylene gloves. To prepare and administer: Add 5 ml sterile water for injection to the vial containing pentostatin powder for injection. Mix thoroughly to make a solution of 5 mg/ml. Administer drug by I.V. bolus injection, or dilute further in 25 or 50 ml of dextrose 5% in water (D₅W) or 0.9% sodium chloride injection and infuse over 20 to 30 minutes.
● Be sure patient is adequately hydrated before therapy. Administer 500 to 1,000 ml of D₅W in 0.45% sodium chloride injection. Give 500 ml of D₅W after drug is given.
● Before therapy, assess renal function with a serum creatinine or creatinine clearance assay; repeat determinations periodically. Perform baseline and periodic determinations of CBC. Bone marrow aspirates and biopsies may be required at 2- to 3-month intervals to assess response to treatment.

Pediatric use

Safe use in children or adolescents has not been established.

Breast-feeding

It is unknown if drug is excreted in breast milk. Because of the risk of serious toxicity to the breast-feeding infant, a decision should be made whether to discontinue drug or discontinue breast-feeding.

pentoxifylline
Trental

- Pharmacologic classification: xanthine derivative
- Therapeutic classification: hemorrheologic agent
- Pregnancy risk category C

How supplied
Available by prescription only
Tablets (extended-release): 400 mg

Indications, route, and dosage
Intermittent claudication from chronic occlusive vascular disease
Adults: 400 mg P.O. t.i.d. with meals.

Pharmacodynamics
Hemorrheologic action: Pentoxifylline improves capillary blood flow by increasing erythrocyte flexibility and reducing blood viscosity.

Pharmacokinetics
- *Absorption:* Pentoxifylline is absorbed almost completely from the GI tract but undergoes first-pass hepatic metabolism. Absorption is slowed by food. Peak concentrations occur in 2 to 4 hours, but clinical effect requires 2 to 4 weeks of continuous therapy.
- *Distribution:* Distribution of pentoxifylline is unknown; drug is bound to erythrocyte membrane.
- *Metabolism:* Pentoxifylline is metabolized extensively by erythrocytes and the liver.
- *Excretion:* Metabolites are excreted principally in urine; less than 4% of drug is excreted in feces. Half-life of unchanged drug is about ½ to ¾ hour; half-life of metabolites is about 1 to 1½ hours.

Contraindications and precautions
Pentoxifylline is contraindicated in patients with known hypersensitivity to this or other xanthine derivatives, such as caffeine, theophylline, or theobromine.

Use drug cautiously in patients at high hemorrhagic risk, such as surgical patients or those with peptic ulcers.

Interactions
Concomitant use of pentoxifylline and antihypertensives may increase hypotensive response; some patients taking pentoxifylline have had small decreases in blood pressure.

Although a causal relationship has not been proved, bleeding and prolonged prothrombin time have been reported in patients treated with pentoxifylline; patients taking oral anticoagulants (such as warfarin) or drugs that inhibit platelet aggregation with pentoxifylline may have bleeding abnormalities.

Effects on diagnostic tests
None reported.

Adverse reactions
- CNS: headache, dizziness, tremor, agitation, nervousness, dowsiness, insomnia.
- CV: mild hypotension, arrhythmias, tachycardia, palpitations, flushing, edema, dyspnea, increased prothrombin time.
- GI: dyspepsia, nausea, vomiting.
Note: Drug should be discontinued if adverse reactions persist after dosage reduction.

Overdose and treatment
Clinical signs of overdose include flushing, hypotension, convulsions, somnolence, loss of consciousness, fever, and agitation. There is no known antidote. Empty stomach by gastric lavage; treat symptoms and support respiration and blood pressure.

▶ Special considerations
- Monitor blood pressure regularly, especially in patients taking antihypertensive agents; also monitor prothrombin time, especially in patients taking anticoagulants such as warfarin.
- If GI and CNS adverse effects occur, decrease the dosage to twice daily. If adverse effects persist, the drug should be discontinued.
- Drug is useful in patients who are not good candidates for surgery.
- Do not crush or break timed-release tablets; make certain patient swallows them whole.

Information for the patient
- Explain need for continuing therapy for at least 8 weeks; warn patient not to discontinue drug during this period without medical approval.
- Advise taking drug with meals to minimize GI distress.
- Tell patient to report any GI or CNS adverse reactions; they may require dosage reduction.

Geriatric use
Elderly patients may have increased bioavailability and decreased excretion of pentoxifylline and, thus, are at higher risk for drug toxicity; adverse reactions may be more common in the elderly.

Pediatric use
Safety and efficacy have not been established for patients under age 18.

Breast-feeding
Pentoxifylline enters breast milk. Alternative feeding method is recommended during therapy.

pergolide mesylate
Permax

- Pharmacologic classification: dopaminergic agonist
- Therapeutic classification: antiparkinson agent
- Pregnancy risk category B

How supplied
Available by prescription only
Tablets: 0.05 mg, 0.25 mg, 1 mg

Indications, route, and dosage
Adjunct to levodopa-carbidopa in the management of Parkinson's disease
Adults: Initially, 0.05 mg P.O. daily for the first 2 days. Gradually increase dosage by 0.1 to 0.15 mg every third day over the next 12 days of therapy. Subsequent dosage can be increased by 0.25 mg every third day until optimum response occurs. The mean therapeutic daily dose is 3 mg.

The drug is usually administered in divided doses t.i.d. Gradual reductions in levodopa-carbidopa dosage may be made during dosage titration.

Pharmacodynamics
Antiparkinson action: Pergolide stimulates dopamine receptors at both D_1 and D_2 sites. It acts by directly stimulating postsynaptic receptors in the nigrostriatal system.

Pharmacokinetics
● *Absorption:* Well absorbed after oral administration.
● *Distribution:* Pergolide is approximately 90% bound to plasma proteins.
● *Metabolism:* It is metabolized to at least 10 different compounds, some of which retain some pharmacologic activity.
● *Excretion:* Primarily by the kidneys.

Contraindications and precautions
Pergolide is contraindicated in patients allergic to the drug or ergot alkaloids.

Symptomatic orthostatic or sustained hypotension may occur in some patients, especially at initial therapy.

Hallucinosis may occur in some patients. Tolerance to this adverse effect was not seen in early clinical trials.

In premarketing trials, over 140 of approximately 2,300 patients died while taking pergolide. However, these deaths did not appear to be linked to use of the drug, since these patients were elderly and debilitated.

Interactions
Concomitant use of drugs that are dopamine antagonists, including phenothiazines, butyrophenones, thioxanthines and metoclopramide, may antagonize the effects of pergolide.

Effects on diagnostic tests
None reported.

Adverse reactions
● CNS: headache, asthenia, dyskinesia, dizziness, hallucinations, dystonia, confusion, somnolescence, insomnia, anxiety, depression, tremors, abnormal dreams, personality disorder, psychosis, abnormal gait, akathisia, extrapyramidal syndrome, incoordination, paresthesia, akinesia, hypertonia, neuralgia, speech disorder.
● CV: postural hypotension, vasodilation, palpitation, hypotension, syncope, hypertension, arrhythmias, *myocardial infarction.*
● DERM: rash, sweating.
● EENT: rhinitis, epistaxis, abnormal vision, diplopia, taste perversion, eye disorder.
● GI: abdominal pain, nausea, constipation, diarrhea, dyspepsia, anorexia, vomiting, dry mouth.
● GU: urinary frequency, urinary tract infection, hematuria.
● Other: taste alteration; accident or injury; flu syndrome; chills; infection; facial, peripheral, or generalized edema; weight gain; arthralgia; bursitis; myalgia; twitching; chest, neck, and back pain.

Note: The above adverse reactions, although not always attributable to the drug, occurred in less than 1% of the study population.

Overdose and treatment
One patient who intentionally ingested 60 mg of pergolide presented with hypotension and vomiting. Other cases of overdose revealed symptoms of hallucinations, involuntary movements, palpitations, and arrhythmias.

Treatment should be supportive. Monitor cardiac function and protect the patient's airway. Antiarrhythmics and sympathomimetics may be necessary to support cardiovascular function. Adverse CNS effects may be treated with dopaminergic antagonists (such as phenothiazines). If indicated, gastric lavage or induced emesis may be used to empty the stomach of its contents. Orally administered activated charcoal may be useful in attenuating absorption.

▶ Special considerations
In early clinical trials, 27% of the patients who attempted pergolide therapy did not finish the trial because of adverse effects (primarily hallucinations and confusion).

Information for the patient
● Inform patients of the potential for adverse effects. Warn them to avoid activities that could expose them to injury secondary to orthostatic hypotension and syncope.
● Caution the patient to rise slowly to avoid orthostatic hypotension, particularly at the beginning of therapy.

Pediatric use
Safety has not been established.

Breast-feeding
Safety has not been established.

---

permethrin
Elimite, Nix

● Pharmacologic classification: synthetic pyrethroid
● Therapeutic classification: pediculocide
● Pregnancy risk category B

How supplied
Available without a prescription
Liquid: 60 ml (1%)
Cream: 5%

Indications, route, and dosage
Pediculosis
Adults and children: Apply sufficient volume to saturate the hair and scalp. Allow to remain on the hair for 10 minutes before rinsing. A second application is sometimes necessary in 5 to 7 days.

Pharmacodynamics
Permethrin acts on the parasites' nerve cell membranes to disrupt the sodium channel current and thereby paralyze them.

Pharmacokinetics
- *Absorption:* Not entirely investigated but probably less than 2% of the amount applied.
- *Distribution:* Systemic distribution is unknown.
- *Metabolism:* Rapidly metabolized by ester hydrolysis to inactive metabolites.
- *Excretion:* Metabolites are excreted in the urine. Residual persistence on the hair is detectable for up to 10 days.

Contraindications and precautions
Permethrin is contraindicated in persons with hypersensitivity to any synthetic pyrethroid or pyrethrin, to chrysanthemums, or to any component of the product.

Interactions
None reported.

Effects on diagnostic tests
None reported.

Adverse reactions
- Local: pruritus, burning or stinging, tingling, numbness, scalp discomfort, erythema, edema, rash.

Overdose and treatment
With accidental ingestion, perform gastric lavage and employ general supportive measures.

▶ Special considerations
- Tell patient or caregiver to first wash hair with shampoo, rinse it thoroughly, and then towel dry.
- Tell patient or caregiver to apply sufficient volume to saturate the hair and scalp.
- A single treatment is usually all that is necessary. Combing of nits is not required for effectiveness, but drug package supplies a fine-tooth comb for cosmetic use as desired.
- A second application may be necessary if lice are observed 7 days after the initial application.
- Permethrin has been shown to be at least as effective as lindane (Kwell) in treating head lice.

Information for the patient
Itching, redness, or swelling of the scalp may occur; if irritation persists, notify the physician.

Pediatric use
Safety and efficacy for use in children under age 2 have not been established.

Breast-feeding
It is not known whether permethrin is excreted in breast milk. Consider discontinuing breast-feeding temporarily or not using the medication.

perphenazine
Apo-Perphernazine*, Trilafon

- Pharmacologic classification: phenothiazine (piperazine derivative)
- Therapeutic classification: antipsychotic; antiemetic
- Pregnancy risk category C

How supplied
Available by prescription only
Tablets: 2 mg, 4 mg, 8 mg, 16 mg
Repetabs (sustained-release): 8 mg
Oral concentrate: 16 mg/5 ml
Injection: 5 mg/ml

Indications, route, and dosage
Psychosis
Adults: Initially, 8 to 16 mg P.O. b.i.d., t.i.d., or q.i.d., increasing to 64 mg daily.
Children over age 12: 6 to 12 mg P.O. daily in divided doses.
Mental disturbances, acute alcoholism, nausea, vomiting, hiccups
Adults and children over age 12: 5 to 10 mg I.M., p.r.n. Maximum dosage is 15 mg I.M. in ambulatory patients, 30 mg daily in hospitalized patients.

Perphenazine may be given slowly by I.V. drip at a rate of 1 mg/2 minutes with continuous blood pressure monitoring (rarely used). A maximum of 5 mg I.V. diluted to 0.5 mg/ml with normal saline solution may be given for severe hiccups or vomiting. Extended-release preparation may be given 8 to 16 mg P.O. b.i.d. for outpatients; 8 to 32 mg P.O. b.i.d. for inpatients.

Pharmacodynamics
Antipsychotic action: Perphenazine is thought to exert its antipsychotic effects by postsynaptic blockade of CNS dopamine receptors, thus inhibiting dopamine-mediated effects; antiemetic effects are attributed to dopamine receptor blockade in the medullary chemoreceptor trigger zone. Perphenazine has many other central and peripheral effects: it produces both alpha and ganglionic blockade and counteracts histamine- and serotonin-mediated activity. Its most serious adverse reactions are extrapyramidal.

Pharmacokinetics
- *Absorption:* Rate and extent of absorption vary with administration route: oral tablet absorption is erratic and variable, with onset of action ranging from ½ to 1 hour; oral concentrate absorption is much more predictable. I.M. drug is absorbed rapidly.
- *Distribution:* Perphenazine is distributed widely into the body, including breast milk. Drug is 91% to 99% protein-bound. After oral tablet administration, peak effect occurs at 2 to 4 hours; steady-state serum levels are achieved within 4 to 7 days.
- *Metabolism:* Perphenazine is metabolized extensively by the liver, but no active metabolites are formed.
- *Excretion:* Most of drug is excreted in urine via the kidneys; some is excreted in feces via the biliary tract.

Contraindications and precautions
Perphenazine is contraindicated in patients with known hypersensitivity to phenothiazines and related com-

pounds, including allergic reactions involving hepatic function because perphenazine may be hepatotoxic; in patients with blood dyscrasias and bone marrow depression because drug may have adverse effects on bone marrow and blood cell lines; in disorders accompanied by coma, brain damage, or CNS depression because of additive CNS and respiratory depression; in patients with circulatory collapse or cerebrovascular disease because drug may adversely affect blood pressure through its alpha blocking effects; and with adrenergic blocking agents or spinal or epidural anesthetics because of the potential for alpha blockade.

Perphenazine should be used cautiously in patients with cardiac disease (arrhythmias, congestive heart failure, angina pectoris, valvular disease, or heart block); encephalitis; Reye's syndrome; head injury; respiratory disease; epilepsy and other seizure disorders (drug may lower seizure threshold); glaucoma (drug may raise intraocular pressure); prostatic hypertrophy, Parkinson's disease, urinary retention (drug may worsen these conditions); hepatic or renal dysfunction (impaired metabolism and excretion may cause drug accumulation); pheochromocytoma; or hypocalcemia (increased risk of extrapyramidal reactions). Exposure to temperature extremes may predispose the patient to hyperthermia or hypothermia.

Interactions

Concomitant use of perphenazine with sympathomimetics, including epinephrine, phenylephrine, phenylpropanolamine, and ephedrine (often found in nasal sprays), and with appetite suppressants may decrease their stimulatory and pressor effects. Phenothiazines can cause epinephrine reversal and a hypotensive response when epinephrine is used for its pressor effects.

Perphenazine may inhibit blood pressure response to centrally acting antihypertensive drugs, such as guanethidine, guanabenz, guanadrel, clonidine, methyldopa, and reserpine. Additive effects are likely after concomitant use of perphenazine with CNS depressants, including alcohol, analgesics, barbiturates, narcotics, tranquilizers, and general, spinal, or epidural anesthetics, or parenteral magnesium sulfate (oversedation, respiratory depression, and hypotension); antiarrhythmic agents, quinidine, disopyramide, and procainamide (increased incidence of cardiac dysrhythmias and conduction defects); atropine or other anticholinergic drugs, including antidepressants, monoamine oxidase inhibitors, phenothiazines, antihistamines, meperidine, and antiparkinsonian agents (oversedation, paralytic ileus, visual changes, and severe constipation); nitrates (hypotension); and metrizamide (increased risk of convulsions).

Beta-blocking agents may inhibit perphenazine metabolism, increasing plasma levels and toxicity.

Concomitant use with propylthiouracil increases risk of agranulocytosis; concomitant use with lithium may result in severe neurologic toxicity with an encephalitis-like syndrome, and a decreased therapeutic response to perphenazine.

Pharmacokinetic alterations and subsequent decreased therapeutic response to perphenazine may follow concomitant use with phenobarbital (enhanced renal excretion), aluminum and magnesium-containing antacids and antidiarrheals (decreased absorption), caffeine, or heavy smoking (increased metabolism).

Perphenazine may antagonize therapeutic effect of bromocriptine on prolactin secretion; it may also decrease vasoconstricting effects of high-dose dopamine

and may decrease effectiveness and increase toxicity of levodopa (by dopamine blockade). Perphenazine may inhibit metabolism and increase toxicity of phenytoin.

Effects on diagnostic tests

Perphenazine causes false-positive test results for urinary porphyrins, urobilinogen, amylase, and 5-hydroxyindoleacetic acid, because of darkening of urine by metabolites; it also causes false-positive urine pregnancy test results using human chorionic gonadotropin.

Perphenazine elevates test results for liver enzymes and protein-bound iodine and causes quinidine-like effects on the ECG.

Adverse reactions

● CNS: extrapyramidal symptoms – dystonia, akathisia, torticollis, tardive dyskinesia (usually dose-related with long-term therapy, but it can develop rapidly), sedation (low incidence), pseudoparkinsonism, drowsiness (frequent), *neuroleptic malignant syndrome* (dose-related; fatal *respiratory failure* in over 10% of patients, if untreated), dizziness, fainting, headache, insomnia, exacerbation of psychotic symptoms.
● CV: *asystole*, orthostatic hypotension, tachycardia, arrhythmias, ECG changes, increased anginal pain after I.M. injection.
● EENT: blurred vision, tinnitus, mydriasis, increased intraocular pressure, ocular changes (retinal pigmentary change on long-term use).
● GI: dry mouth, constipation, nausea, vomiting, anorexia, diarrhea.
● GU: urine retention, gynecomastia, hypermenorrhea, inhibited ejaculation.
● HEMA: transient leukopenia, *agranulocytosis*, thrombocytopenia, anemia (within 30 to 90 days).
● Local: contact dermatitis from concentrate or injectable form, muscle necrosis from I.M. injection.
● Other: hyperprolactinemia, photosensitivity, increased appetite or weight gain, hypersensitivity (rash, urticaria, drug fever, edema, cholestatic jaundice [in 0.1% to 4% of patients within first 30 days]), decreased libido.

After abrupt withdrawal of long-term therapy, gastritis, nausea, vomiting, dizziness, tremors, feeling of heat or cold, sweating, tachycardia, headache, or insomnia may occur.

Note: Drug should be discontinued if hypersensitivity, jaundice, agranulocytosis, or neuroleptic malignant syndrome (marked hyperthermia, extrapyramidal effects, autonomic dysfunction) occurs or if severe extrapyramidal symptoms occur even after dose is lowered. Drug should be discontinued 48 hours before and 24 hours after myelography using metrizamide because of the risk of convulsions. When feasible, drug should be withdrawn slowly and gradually; many drug effects persist after withdrawal.

Overdose and treatment

CNS depression is characterized by deep, unarousable sleep and possible coma, hypotension or hypertension, extrapyramidal symptoms, dystonia, abnormal involuntary muscle movements, agitation, seizures, arrhythmias, ECG changes, hypothermia or hyperthermia, and autonomic nervous system dysfunction.

Treatment is symptomatic and supportive, including maintaining vital signs, airway, stable body temperature, and fluid and electrolyte balance.

Do not induce vomiting: drug inhibits cough reflex, and aspiration may occur. Use gastric lavage, then activated charcoal and saline cathartics; dialysis is usually ineffective. Regulate body temperature as needed. Treat hypotension with I.V. fluids: *do not give epinephrine.* Treat seizures with parenteral diazepam or barbiturates; arrhythmias with parenteral phenytoin (1 mg/kg with rate titrated to blood pressure); and extrapyramidal reactions with benztropine or parenteral diphenhydramine 2 mg/kg/minute.

▶ Special considerations
Besides those relevant to all *phenothiazines,* consider the following recommendations.

- Oral formulations may cause stomach upset; administer with food or fluid.
- Dilute the concentrate in 2 to 4 oz of liquid (water, carbonated drinks, fruit juice, tomato juice, milk, or puddings). Dilute every 5 ml of concentrate with 60 ml of suitable fluid.
- Liquid formulation may cause rash upon contact with skin.
- I.M. injection may cause skin necrosis; avoid extravasation.
- Administer I.M. injection deep into upper outer quadrant of buttocks. Massaging the injection site may prevent formation of abscesses.
- Do not administer drug for injection if it is excessively discolored or contains precipitate.
- Monitor blood pressure before and after parenteral administration.
- Shake oral concentrate before administration.

Information for the patient
- Explain the risks of dystonic reactions and tardive dyskinesia, and tell patient to report abnormal body movements.
- Tell patient to avoid sun exposure and to wear sunscreen when going outdoors, to prevent photosensitivity reactions; and to avoid using heat lamps and tanning beds, which may cause burning of the skin or skin discoloration.
- Tell patient to avoid spilling the liquid; contact with skin may cause rash and irritation.
- Warn patient not to take extremely hot or cold baths and to avoid exposure to temperature extremes, sunlamp, or tanning beds; the drug may cause thermoregulatory changes.
- Advise patient to take drug exactly as prescribed and not to double doses for missed doses.
- Tell patient that interactions with many other drugs are possible. Advise patient to seek medical approval before taking any self-prescribed medication.
- Tell patient not to stop taking the drug suddenly; any adverse reactions may be alleviated by a dosage reduction. Patient should promptly report difficulty urinating, sore throat, dizziness, or fainting.
- Tell patient to avoid hazardous activities that require alertness until the drug's effect is established. Reassure patient that sedative effects of the drug should become tolerable in several weeks.
- Tell patient not to drink alcohol or take other medications that may cause excessive sedation.
- Explain which fluids are appropriate for diluting the concentrate (not apple juice or caffeine-containing drinks); explain dropper technique of measuring dose.
- Suggest sugarless hard candy or chewing gum, ice chips, or artificial saliva to relieve dry mouth.
- Tell patient not to crush or chew sustained-release form.

Geriatric use
Elderly patients tend to require lower doses. Dose must be titrated to effects; 30% to 50% of the usual dose may be effective. Elderly patients are at greater risk for adverse effects, especially tardive dyskinesia and other extrapyramidal effects.

Pediatric use
Drug is not recommended for children under age 12.

Breast-feeding
Perphenazine may enter breast milk. Use with caution. Potential benefits to the mother should outweigh the potential harm to the infant.

---

phenacemide
Phenurone

- Pharmacologic classification: substituted acetylurea derivative, open-chain hydantoin
- Therapeutic classification: anticonvulsant
- Pregnancy risk category D

How supplied
Available by prescription only
Tablets: 500 mg

Indications, route, and dosage
Refractory, complex-partial, generalized tonic-clonic, absence, and atypical absence seizures
Adults: 500 mg P.O. t.i.d; may increase by 500 mg weekly up to 5 g daily, p.r.n.
Children age 5 to 10: 250 mg P.O. t.i.d.; may increase by 250 mg weekly, up to 1.5 g daily, p.r.n.
    Satisfactory seizure control may occur with dosages as low as 250 mg t.i.d.

Pharmacodynamics
Anticonvulsant action: Phenacemide elevates the seizure threshold by an unknown mechanism. It elevates the threshold for maximal ECT seizures and maximizes their tonic phase.

Pharmacokinetics
- *Absorption:* Phenacemide is absorbed well from the GI tract; duration of action is about 5 hours.
- *Distribution:* Unknown.
- *Metabolism:* Phenacemide is metabolized by the liver.
- *Excretion:* Phenacemide is excreted in urine. It is unknown whether drug is excreted in breast milk.

Contraindications and precautions
Phenacemide is contraindicated in patients with known hypersensitivity to phenacemide and in patients with jaundice or other signs of liver dysfunction because it may be hepatotoxic.

    Use phenacemide with caution in patients with a history of drug allergy, especially to anticonvulsants; and in patients with personality disorders, as suicide attempts have occurred. Use phenacemide with extreme caution in patients taking other anticonvulsants. Paranoid symptoms have developed in patients receiving phenacemide and ethotoin concurrently.

Interactions

Concomitant use of phenacemide with ethotoin may cause paranoid symptoms; use with other anticonvulsants (mephenytoin, trimethadione, or paramethadione) may markedly increase toxicity.

Effects on diagnostic tests

Phenacemide may cause abnormalities in liver enzyme test results.

Adverse reactions

- CNS: drowsiness, dizziness, insomnia, headaches, paresthesias, *depression, suicidal tendencies,* aggressiveness, psychic changes.
- DERM: rashes.
- GI: anorexia, weight loss.
- GU: nephritis with marked albuminuria.
- HEMA: aplastic anemia, agranulocytosis, leukopenia.
- Hepatic: *hepatitis,* jaundice.

Note: Drug should be discontinued if signs of hypersensitivity, jaundice, or other hepatotoxicity occur; if marked depression of white blood cell (WBC) count (leukocyte level below 4,000/mm³) occurs; if albumin, blood, casts, or leukocytes occur in urine; if rash occurs; or if patient shows new or exacerbated personality disorder.

Overdose and treatment

Symptoms of overdose include initial excitement followed by drowsiness, nausea, ataxia, and coma.

Treat overdose with gastric lavage or emesis and follow with supportive treatment. Monitor vital signs and fluid and electrolyte balance carefully. Hemodialysis or total exchange transfusion has been used for severe cases and pediatric patients. Careful evaluation of renal, hepatic, and hematologic status is crucial after recovery.

▶ **Special considerations**

Besides those relevant to all *hydantoin derivatives,* consider the following recommendations.

- This drug is extremely toxic and is usually reserved for patients with severe epilepsy (especially mixed forms) resistant to other anticonvulsants.
- Obtain baseline liver function tests, complete blood counts, and urinalyses before and at monthly intervals during treatment; discontinue drug if a marked depression of blood count is observed.

Information for the patient

- Advise patient of potential serious toxicity with phenacemide. Urge patient to report any of the following immediately: pregnancy, jaundice, abdominal pain, pale stools, dark urine, fever, sore throat, mouth sores, rashes, unusual bleeding or bruising, or loss of appetite. All such reports mandate immediate review of laboratory studies.
- Inform patient about possible psychological reactions, and tell him to report immediately any changes in mood or affect, such as decreased interest in himself or his surroundings, depression, or aggression.

Pediatric use

Safety is not established for children under age 5.

Breast-feeding

Phenacemide is not known to be excreted in breast milk; however, because of potential for serious toxicity, alternative feeding method is recommended during phenacemide therapy.

---

phenazopyridine hydrochloride

Azo-Standard, Baridium, Di-Azo, Diridone, Phenazo*, Phenazodine, Pyridiate, Pyridium, Pyronium*, Urodine

- Pharmacologic classification: azo dye
- Therapeutic classification: urinary analgesic
- Pregnancy risk category B

How supplied

Available by prescription only
Tablets: 100 mg, 200 mg

Indications, route, and dosage
Pain with urinary tract irritation or infection
Adults: 100 to 200 mg P.O. t.i.d.
Children: 4 mg/kg t.i.d.; or 100 mg P.O. t.i.d.

Pharmacodynamics

Analgesic action: Phenazopyridine has a local anesthetic effect on urinary tract mucosa via an unknown mechanism.

Pharmacokinetics

- *Absorption* and *distribution* have not been described, although traces are thought to enter CSF and cross the placenta.
- *Metabolism:* Drug is metabolized in the liver.
- *Excretion:* Phenazopyridine is excreted in urine.

Contraindications and precautions

Drug is contraindicated in patients with known hypersensitivity to phenazopyridine and in patients with renal and hepatic insufficiency because of the potential for drug accumulation.

Interactions

None significant.

Effects on diagnostic tests

Drug may alter results of Clinistix, Tes-Tape, Acetest, and Ketostix. Clinitest should be used to obtain accurate urine glucose test results.

Phenazopyridine may also interfere with Ehrlich's test for urine urobilinogen; phenolsulfonphthalein (PSP) excretion tests of kidney function; sulfobromophthalein (BSP) excretion tests of liver function; and urine tests for protein, steroids, or bilirubin.

Adverse reactions

- CNS: headache, vertigo.
- DERM: rash.
- GI: nausea.
- GU: renal stones.
- Other: anemia.

Note: Drug should be discontinued if skin or sclera becomes yellow-tinged. This may indicate accumulation or hepatotoxicity from impaired renal excretion.

Overdose and treatment
Clinical manifestations of overdose include methemoglobinemia (most obvious as cyanosis), along with renal and hepatic impairment and failure.

To treat overdose of phenazopyridine, empty stomach immediately by inducing emesis with ipecac syrup or by gastric lavage. Administer methylene blue, 1 to 2 mg/kg I.V., or 100 to 200 mg ascorbic acid P.O. to reverse methemoglobinemia. Provide symptomatic and supportive measures (respiratory support and correction of fluid and electrolyte imbalances). Monitor laboratory parameters and vital signs closely. Contact local or regional poison information center for specific instructions.

▶ Special considerations
● Drug colors urine red or orange; it may stain fabrics.
● Use only as an analgesic.
● May be used with an antibiotic to treat urinary tract infections.
● Phenazopyridine should be discontinued in 2 days with concurrent antibiotic use.

Information for the patient
● Instruct patient in measures to prevent urinary tract infection.
● Advise patient of possible adverse reactions; caution that drug colors urine red or orange and may stain clothing.
● Tell patient that stains on clothing may be removed with a 0.25% solution of sodium dithionate or hydrosulfite.
● Advise patient to take a missed dose as soon as possible and not to double doses.
● Instruct patient to report symptoms that worsen or do not resolve.

Geriatric use
● Use with caution in elderly patients because of possible decreased renal function.
● Administer with food or fluids to reduce GI upset.
● Evaluate response to medication therapy; assess urinary function, such as output, complaints of burning, pain, and frequency.
● Monitor vital signs, especially temperature.
● Encourage patient to force fluids (if not contraindicated). Monitor intake and output.

Breast-feeding
Safe use in breast-feeding women has not been established.

phendimetrazine hydrochloride
Adipost, Anorex, Bacarate, Bontril, Delcozine, Di-ap-trol, Obalan, Obezine, PDM, Phenzine, Prelu-2, Sprx-1, Sprx-2, Sprx-3, Statobex, Trimtabs, Wehless-105

● Pharmacologic classification: amphetamine congener
● Therapeutic classification: short-term anorexigenic agent for exogenous obesity, indirect-acting sympathomimetic amine
● Controlled substance schedule III
● Pregnancy risk category C

How supplied
Available by prescription only
Tablets: 35 mg
Capsules: 35 mg
Capsules (sustained-release): 105 mg

Indications, route, and dosage
Short-term adjunct in exogenous obesity
Adults: 35 mg P.O. b.i.d. or t.i.d. 1 hour before meals. Maximum dosage is 70 mg t.i.d. Use lowest effective dosage adjusted to individual response. Dosage for 9sustained-release capsule is 105 mg once daily in the morning 1 hour before breakfast.

Pharmacodynamics
Anorexigenic action: Phendimetrazine is an indirect-acting sympathomimetic amine; it is considered a second-line drug for weight control because it causes euphoria, has a high abuse potential, and often causes unacceptable CNS stimulation. Anorexigenic effects are thought to follow direct stimulation of the hypothalamus and may involve other CNS and metabolic effects.

Pharmacokinetics
● *Absorption:* Phendimetrazine is absorbed readily after oral administration; therapeutic effects persist for 4 hours with regular tablets, longer with the sustained-release preparation.
● *Distribution:* Phendimetrazine is distributed widely throughout the body.
● *Metabolism:* Phendimetrazine is metabolized by the liver.
● *Excretion:* Phendimetrazine is excreted in urine. Half-life ranges from 2 hours for the regular dosage forms to 10 hours for the sustained-release capsules.

Contraindications and precautions
Phendimetrazine is contraindicated in patients with known hypersensitivity to phendimetrazine; in patients with hyperthyroidism, all degrees of hypertension, angina pectoris or other severe cardiovascular disease, glaucoma, and advanced arteriosclerosis; in agitated or highly nervous patients; and in patients with a history of drug abuse.

Phendimetrazine also is contraindicated for use with monoamine oxidase (MAO) inhibitors or within 14 days of such use because this combination may cause hypertensive crisis; or with other CNS stimulants. Some phendimetrazine formulations may contain tartrazine and are contraindicated in patients with asthma or aspirin allergy.

It should be used with caution in patients with known hypersensitivity to sympathomimetic amines and in hyperexcitability states. Habituation or psychic dependence may occur on prolonged use.

Interactions
Concomitant use with MAO inhibitors (or drugs with MAO-inhibiting potential) or within 14 days of such therapy may cause hypertensive crisis.

Phendimetrazine may decrease hypotensive effects of guanethidine and other antihypertensive agents; it also may alter insulin requirements in diabetic patients. Concomitant use with excessive caffeine may cause additive CNS stimulation; use with general anesthetics may result in cardiac arrhythmias.

Use with antacids, sodium bicarbonate, or acetazolamide increases renal reabsorption of phendimetrazine and prolongs its duration of action; use with phenothiazines or haloperidol decreases effects of phendimetrazine.

Effects on diagnostic tests
None reported.

Adverse reactions
● CNS: nervousness, dizziness, insomnia, tremor, headache, euphoria, overstimulation.
● CV: tachycardia, palpitations, arrhythmias, hypertension.
● EENT: blurred vision.
● GI: dry mouth, nausea, abdominal cramps, diarrhea or constipation, glossitis, stomatitis.
● GU: dysuria, changes in libido.
● Other: tolerance, physical and psychological dependence.

Note: Drug should be discontinued if signs of hypersensitivity occur.

Overdose and treatment
Symptoms of acute overdose include restlessness, tremor, hyperreflexia, fever, tachypnea, dizziness, confusion, aggressive behavior, hallucinations, panic, blood pressure changes, arrhythmias, nausea, vomiting, diarrhea, and cramps. Fatigue and depression usually follow CNS stimulation; convulsions, coma, and death may follow.

Treat overdose symptomatically and supportively: treatment may include sedation with barbiturates. Acidification of urine may hasten excretion. Monitor vital signs and fluid and electrolyte balance.

▶ Special considerations
Besides those relevant to all *amphetamines,* consider the following recommendations.
● Give morning dose 2 hours after breakfast.
● Give last daily dose at least 6 hours before bedtime to prevent insomnia.
● Abrupt discontinuation may lead to extreme fatigue and depression.

Information for the patient
● Tell patient to avoid caffeine-containing drinks, not to take drug more frequently than prescribed, and to take last dose at least 6 hours before bedtime to prevent insomnia.
● Advise patient to call if palpitations occur.

Geriatric use
Lower dosages may be indicated for elderly patients.

Pediatric use
Phendimetrazine is not recommended for children under age 12.

---

phenelzine sulfate
Nardil

● Pharmacologic classification: monoamine oxidase inhibitor
● Therapeutic classification: antidepressant
● Pregnancy risk category C

How supplied
Available by prescription only
Tablets: 15 mg

Indications, route, and dosage
Severe depression, †panic disorder
Adults: 15 mg P.O. t.i.d. Increase rapidly to 60 mg/day; maximum daily dose is 90 mg. Onset of maximum therapeutic effect is 2 to 6 weeks. Some clinicians reduce dosage after response occurs; maintenance dosage may be as low as 15 mg daily or every other day.

Not recommended for children under age 16.

Pharmacodynamics
Antidepressant action: Depression is thought to result from low CNS concentrations of neurotransmitters, including norepinephrine and serotonin. Phenelzine inhibits monoamine oxidase (MAO), an enzyme that normally inactivates amine-containing substances, thus increasing the concentration and activity of these agents.

Pharmacokinetics
● *Absorption:* Phenelzine is absorbed rapidly and completely from the GI tract.
● *Distribution:* Not yet determined; dose adjustments are determined by therapeutic response and adverse reaction profile.
● *Metabolism:* Hepatic.
● *Excretion:* Phenelzine is excreted primarily in urine within 24 hours; some drug is excreted in feces via the biliary tract. Half-life is relatively short, but enzyme inhibition is prolonged and unrelated to drug half-life.

Contraindications and precautions
Phenelzine is contraindicated in patients with uncontrolled hypertension and seizure disorders because it may provoke hypertensive crisis and lowers the seizure threshold, even in patients controlled with anticonvulsant therapy.

Phenelzine should be used cautiously in patients with angina pectoris and other cardiovascular disease; in patients with Type I and Type II diabetes; in patients with Parkinson's disease and other motor disorders or hyperthyroidism because it may worsen these conditions; in patients with pheochromocytoma because of risk of hypertensive crisis; in patients with renal or hepatic insufficiency because diminished metabolism and excretion can cause drug accumulation; and in patients with bipolar illness because drug may provoke sudden mood change from depression to mania (reduce dosage during manic phase).

Interactions
Phenelzine enhances pressor effects of amphetamines, ephedrine, phenylephrine, phenylpropanolamine, and related drugs and may result in serious cardiovascular toxicity; most nonprescription cold, hay fever, and weight-reduction products contain these drugs.

Concomitant use of phenelzine with disulfiram may cause tachycardia, flushing, or palpitations. Concomitant use with general or spinal anesthetics, which are normally metabolized by MAO, may cause severe hypotension and excessive CNS depression. Phenelzine decreases effectiveness of local anesthetics (procaine, lidocaine), resulting in poor nerve block, and should be discontinued for at least 1 week before use of these agents.

Use cautiously and in reduced dosage with alcohol, barbiturates and other sedatives, narcotics, dextromethorphan, and tricyclic antidepressants.

Effects on diagnostic tests
Phenelzine therapy elevates liver function test results and urinary catecholamine levels and may elevate white blood cell count.

Adverse reactions
● CNS: dizziness, vertigo, headache, overactivity, hyperreflexia, tremors, muscle twitching, mania, jitters, agitation, nervousness, insomnia, confusion, memory impairment, drowsiness, weakness, fatigue.
● CV: palpitations, tachycardia, *fatal intracranial hemorrhage during hypertensive crisis,* paradoxical hypertension, orthostatic hypotension, arrhythmias.
● GI: dry mouth, anorexia, nausea, constipation, abdominal pain.
● GU: urinary retention, dysuria, discolored urine.
● Hepatic: jaundice.
● Other: peripheral edema, sweating, weight changes.
Note: Drug should be discontinued if any of the following occurs: signs of hypersensitivity; rash; jaundice; or severe headache, palpitations, or fainting spells, indicating impending hypertensive crisis.

Overdose and treatment
Signs of overdose include exacerbations of adverse reactions or exaggerated responses to normal pharmacologic activity; such symptoms become apparent slowly (within 24 to 48 hours) and may persist for up to 2 weeks. Agitation, flushing, tachycardia, hypotension, hypertension, palpitations, increased motor activity, twitching, increased deep tendon reflexes, seizures, hyperpyrexia, cardiorespiratory arrest, and coma may occur. Doses of 375 mg to 1.5 g have been ingested with fatal and nonfatal results.

Treat symptomatically and supportively: give 5 to 10 mg phentolamine I.V. push for hypertensive crisis; treat seizures, agitation, or tremors with I.V. diazepam; tachycardia, with beta blockers; and fever, with cooling blankets. Monitor vital signs and fluid and electrolyte balance. Use of sympathomimetics (such as norepinephrine or phenylephrine) is contraindicated in hypotension caused by MAO inhibitors.

▶ Special considerations
Besides those relevant to all *MAO inhibitors,* consider the following recommendations.
● Consider the inherent risk of suicide until significant improvement of depressive state occurs. High-risk patients should have close supervision during initial drug therapy. To reduce risk of suicidal overdose, prescribe the smallest quantity of tablets consistent with good management.
● At start of therapy, patient should lie down for about 1 hour after taking phenelzine; to prevent dizziness from orthostatic blood pressure changes, patient should avoid sudden changes to standing position.
● Unlike that with other MAO inhibitors, combination therapy with phenelzine and tricyclic antidepressants is generally well tolerated.

Information for the patient
● Warn patient not to take alcohol, other CNS depressants, or any self-prescribed medications (such as cold, hay fever, or diet preparations) without medical approval.
● Explain that many foods and beverages – such as wine, beer, cheeses, preserved fruits, meats, and vegetables – may interact with this drug. A list of foods to avoid can usually be obtained from the dietary department or pharmacy at most hospitals.
● Tell patient to avoid hazardous activities that require alertness until the drug's full effect on the CNS is known. Suggest taking drug at bedtime to minimize daytime sedation.
● Tell patient to take the drug exactly as prescribed, and not to double doses if a dose is missed.
● Tell patient not to discontinue the drug abruptly and to report any problems; dosage reduction can relieve most adverse reactions.

Geriatric use
Phenelzine is not recommended for patients over age 60.

phenobarbital
Barbita, Gardenal*, Solfoton

phenobarbital sodium
Luminal

● Pharmacologic classification: barbiturate
● Therapeutic classification: anticonvulsant, sedative-hypnotic
● Controlled substance schedule IV
● Pregnancy risk category D

How supplied
Available by prescription only
Tablets: 8 mg, 15 mg, 16 mg, 30 mg, 32 mg, 60 mg, 65 mg, 100 mg
Capsules: 16 mg
Oral solution: 15 mg/5 ml; 20 mg/5 ml
Elixir: 20 mg/5 ml
Injection: 30 mg/ml, 60 mg/ml, 65 mg/ml, 130 mg/ml
Powder for injection: 120 mg/ampule

Indications, route, and dosage
All forms of epilepsy, febrile seizures in children
Adults: 100 to 200 mg P.O. daily, divided t.i.d. or given as single dose h.s.
Children: 4 to 6 mg/kg P.O. daily, usually divided q 12 hours. It can, however, be administered once daily.

Status epilepticus
Adults: 10 mg/kg as I.V. infusion no faster than 60 mg/minute. May give up to 20 mg/kg total. Administer in acute care or emergency area only.
Children: 5 to 10 mg/kg I.V. May repeat q 10 to 15 minutes up to total of 20 mg/kg. I.V. injection rate should not exceed 50 mg/minute.

Sedation
Adults: 30 to 120 mg P.O. daily in two or three divided doses.
Children: 6 mg/kg P.O. divided t.i.d.

Insomnia
Adults: 100 to 320 mg P.O. or I.M.
Children: 3 to 6 mg/kg.

Preoperative sedation
Adults: 100 to 200 mg I.M. 60 to 90 minutes before surgery.
Children: 16 to 100 mg I.M. 60 to 90 minutes before surgery.

†Hyperbilirubinemia
Neonates: 5 to 10 mg/kg P.O. daily or 5 to 10 mg/kg I.M. daily for the first few days after birth.

†Chronic cholestasis
Adults: 90 to 180 mg P.O. daily in two or three divided doses.
Children under age 12: 3 to 12 mg/kg P.O. daily in two or three divided doses.

Pharmacodynamics
• *Anticonvulsant action:* Phenobarbital suppresses the spread of seizure activity produced by epileptogenic foci in the cortex, thalamus, and limbic systems by enhancing the effect of gamma-aminobutyric acid (GABA). Both presynaptic and postsynaptic excitability are decreased; also, phenobarbital raises the seizure threshold.
• *Sedative-hypnotic action:* Phenobarbital acts throughout the CNS as a nonselective depressant with a slow onset of action and a long duration of action. Particularly sensitive to this drug is the reticular activating system, which controls CNS arousal. Phenobarbital decreases both presynaptic and postsynaptic membrane excitability by facilitating the action of GABA. The exact cellular site and mechanism(s) of action are unknown.

Pharmacokinetics
• *Absorption:* Phenobarbital is absorbed well after oral and rectal administration, with 70% to 90% reaching the bloodstream. Absorption after I.M. administration is 100%. After oral administration, peak serum levels are reached in 1 to 2 hours, and peak levels in the CNS are achieved at 1 to 3 hours. Onset of action occurs 1 hour or longer after oral dosing; onset after I.V. administration is about 5 minutes. A serum concentration of 10 mcg/ml is needed to produce sedation; 40 mcg/ml usually produces sleep. Concentrations of 20 to 40 mcg/ml are considered therapeutic for anticonvulsant therapy.
• *Distribution:* Phenobarbital is distributed widely throughout the body. Phenobarbital is approximately 25% to 30% protein-bound.
• *Metabolism:* Phenobarbital is metabolized by the hepatic microsomal enzyme system.
• *Excretion:* 25% to 50% of a phenobarbital dose is eliminated unchanged in urine. The remainder is excreted as metabolites of glucuronic acid. Phenobarbital's half-life is 5 to 7 days.

Contraindications and precautions
Phenobarbital is contraindicated in patients with known hypersensitivity to barbiturates and in patients with bronchopneumonia, status asthmaticus, or other severe respiratory distress because of the potential for respiratory depression. Phenobarbital should not be used in patients who are depressed or have suicidal ideation, because the drug can worsen depression; in patients with uncontrolled acute or chronic pain, because exacerbation of pain or paradoxical excitement can occur; or in patients with porphyria, because this drug can trigger symptoms of this disease.

Phenobarbital should be used cautiously in patients who must perform hazardous tasks requiring mental alertness, because the drug causes drowsiness; and in patients with impaired renal function, because up to 50% of phenobarbital is excreted in urine. Administer parenteral phenobarbital slowly and with extreme caution to patients with hypotension or severe pulmonary or cardiovascular disease because of potential adverse hemodynamic effects. Because tolerance and physical or psychological dependence may occur, prolonged use of high doses should be avoided.

Prenatal exposure to barbiturates is associated with an increased incidence of fetal abnormalities and, possibly, brain tumors. Use of barbiturates in the third trimester may be associated with physical dependence in neonates. Risk-benefit must be considered.

Interactions
Phenobarbital may add to or potentiate CNS and respiratory depressant effects of other sedative-hypnotics, antihistamines, narcotics, phenothiazines, antidepressants, tranquilizers, and alcohol.

Phenobarbital enhances the enzymatic degradation of warfarin and other oral anticoagulants; patients may require increased doses of the anticoagulant. Drug also enhances hepatic metabolism of some drugs, including digitoxin (not digoxin), corticosteroids, oral contraceptives and other estrogens, theophylline and other xanthines, and doxycycline.

Phenobarbital impairs the effectiveness of griseofulvin by decreasing absorption from the GI tract.

Valproic acid, phenytoin, disulfiram, and monoamine oxidase inhibitors decrease the metabolism of phenobarbital and can increase its toxicity.

Rifampin may decrease phenobarbital levels by increasing hepatic metabolism.

Effects on diagnostic tests
Phenobarbital may cause a false-positive phentolamine test. The physiologic effects of the drug may impair the absorption of cyanocobalamin ^{57}Co; it may decrease serum bilirubin concentrations in neonates, epileptics, and in patients with congenital nonhemolytic unconjugated hyperbilirubinemia. Barbiturates may increase sulfobromophthalein retention. EEG patterns show a change in low-voltage, fast activity; changes persist for a time after discontinuation of therapy.

Adverse reactions
• CNS: drowsiness, lethargy, vertigo, headache, CNS depression, paradoxical excitement, confusion and agitation (in elderly patients); hyperexcitability in children; rebound insomnia, increased dreams or nightmares, possibly seizures (after acute withdrawal or reduction in dosage).
• CV: hypotension (after rapid I.V. administration), bradycardia, *circulatory collapse.*

- DERM: urticaria, rash, *exfoliative dermatitis*, and *Stevens-Johnson syndrome*.
- EENT: miosis.
- GI: epigastric pain, nausea, vomiting, diarrhea, constipation.
- Local: thrombophlebitis, pain and possible tissue damage at site of extravascular injection.
- Other: *respiratory depression*, laryngospasm, *bronchospasm*, vitamin K deficiency and bleeding have occurred in newborns of mothers treated during pregnancy. Hyperalgesia may occur in low doses or in patients with chronic pain.

Note: Drug should be discontinued if hypersensitivity reaction, profound CNS or respiratory depression, or skin eruptions occur.

Overdose and treatment

Clinical manifestations of overdose include unsteady gait, slurred speech, sustained nystagmus, somnolence, confusion, respiratory depression, pulmonary edema, areflexia, and coma. Typical shock syndrome with tachycardia and hypotension along with jaundice, oliguria, and chills followed by fever may occur.

Treatment is aimed at the maintenance and support of ventilation and pulmonary function as necessary; support of cardiac function and circulation with vasopressors and I.V. fluids as needed. If patient is conscious and gag reflex is intact, induce emesis (if ingestion was recent) by administering ipecac syrup. If emesis is contraindicated, perform gastric lavage while a cuffed endotracheal tube is in place to prevent aspiration. Follow with administration of activated charcoal or saline cathartic. Measure intake and output, vital signs, and laboratory parameters. Maintain body temperature.

Alkalinization of urine may be helpful in removing drug from the body; hemodialysis may be useful in severe overdose. Oral activated charcoal may enhance phenobarbital elimination regardless of its route of administration.

▶ Special considerations

Besides those relevant to all *barbiturates,* consider the following recommendations.
- Oral solution may be mixed with water or juice to improve taste.
- Do not crush or break extended-release form; this will impair drug action.
- Reconstitute powder for injection with 2.5 to 5 ml sterile water for injection. Roll vial in hands; do not shake.
- Use a larger vein for I.V. administration to prevent extravasation.
- Avoid I.V. administration at a rate greater than 60 mg/minute to prevent hypotension and respiratory depression. It may take up to 30 minutes after I.V. administration to achieve maximum effect.
- Administer parenteral dose within 30 minutes of reconstitution because phenobarbital hydrolyzes in solution and on exposure to air.
- Keep emergency resuscitation equipment on hand when administering phenobarbital I.V.
- Administer I.M. dose deep into a large muscle mass to prevent tissue injury.
- Only parenteral solutions prepared from powder may be given S.C.; however, this route is not recommended.
- Do not use injectable solution if it contains a precipitate.
- Administration of full loading doses over short periods

of time to treat status epilepticus will require ventilatory support in adults.
- Full therapeutic effects are not seen for 2 to 3 weeks, except when loading dose is used.

Information for the patient

- Advise patient of potential for physical and psychological dependence with prolonged use.
- Warn the patient to avoid alcohol and other CNS depressants while taking this drug. An excessive depressant effect is possible even if the drug is taken the evening before ingestion of alcohol.
- Warn patient not to stop taking the drug suddenly because this could cause a withdrawal reaction.
- Advise the patient to avoid driving and other hazardous activities that require alertness until the adverse CNS effects of the drug are known.

Geriatric use

Elderly patients are more sensitive to the effects of phenobarbital and usually require lower doses. Confusion, disorientation, and excitability may occur in elderly patients.

Pediatric use

Paradoxical hyperexcitability may occur in children. Use with caution. Use of phenobarbital extended-release capsules is not recommended in children under age 12.

Breast-feeding

Phenobarbital passes into breast milk; avoid administering to breast-feeding women.

phenolphthalein

Alophen, Correctol, Espotabs, Evac-U-Gen, Evac-U-Lax, Ex-Lax, Feen-a-Mint, Modane, Phenolax, Prulet

- Pharmacologic classification: anthraquinone derivative
- Therapeutic classification: stimulant laxative
- Pregnancy risk category C

How supplied

Available without prescription
White phenolphthalein
Tablets: 60 mg
Tablets (chewable): 60 mg, 64.8 mg
Yellow phenolphthalein
Chewing gum: 97.2 mg
Tablets (chewable): 80 mg, 90 mg, 97.2 mg

Indications, route, and dosage
Constipation
Adults: 60 to 200 mg P.O., preferably h.s.

Pharmacodynamics

Laxative action: Phenolphthalein has a direct irritant effect on the colon, which stimulates peristalsis and bowel evacuation; it also promotes intestinal fluid accumulation. Although not confirmed in clinical studies, yellow phenolphthalein is said to be three times more potent than white phenolphthalein.

Pharmacokinetics
● *Absorption:* Approximately 15% of a dose is absorbed and enters the enterohepatic circulation. Action begins in 6 to 10 hours.
● *Distribution:* Primary site of action is the colon; drug enters breast milk.
● *Metabolism:* Absorbed portion is metabolized in the liver.
● *Excretion:* Phenolphthalein is excreted in feces, urine, and breast milk; effect may last several days.

Contraindications and precautions
Phenolphthalein is contraindicated in patients with appendicitis, abdominal pain or cramps, nausea, vomiting, acute surgical abdomen, intestinal obstruction or perforation, or fecal impaction, because the drug may exacerbate these symptoms or conditions; and in patients with known hypersensitivity to the drug.

Phenolphthalein should be used cautiously in patients with rectal bleeding because it may worsen this condition. Some formulations contain tartrazine, which may precipitate an allergic reaction, especially in persons allergic to aspirin.

Interactions
None reported.

Effects on diagnostic tests
Phenolphthalein may increase rate of phenolsulfonphthalein (PSP) excretion during PSP excretion tests and may cause false-positive results on urine urobilinogen and estrogen tests using Kolber procedure.

Adverse reactions
● DERM: dermatitis, pruritus, rash.
● GI: diarrhea, abdominal cramps, nausea, colic (with large doses), melanotic pigmentation of colonic mucosa, malabsorption of nutrients; "cathartic colon" (syndrome resembling ulcerative colitis radiologically and pathologically) in chronic misuse; reddish discoloration in alkaline feces.
● Other: laxative dependence in long-term or excessive use, *hypersensitivity;* reddish discoloration of urine.
Note: Drug should be discontinued if abdominal pain or hypersensitivity occurs.

Overdose and treatment
No cases of overdose have been reported; probable clinical effects include abdominal pain and diarrhea.

▶ Special considerations
● Before recommending laxative use, review the patient's medications and diet for possible causes of constipation.
● Yellow phenolphthalein is two to three times more potent than white phenolphthalein.

Information for the patient
● Inform patient that drug's laxative effect may persist for several days and that drug may discolor urine and feces.
● Warn patient to discontinue use if rash develops.
● Warn patients that chronic laxative use may cause laxative dependence and electrolyte depletion, which may result in weakness, incoordination, and orthostatic hypotension.

Pediatric use
Phenolphthalein and other stimulant laxatives usually are not recommended for children. Children may mistake the drug for candy; keep it out of their reach.

Breast-feeding
Although phenolphthalein is excreted in breast milk, no adverse effects have been reported in breast-feeding infants.

PHARMACOLOGIC CLASS

phenothiazines

Aliphatic derivatives
chlorpromazine
ethopropazine
promazine
promethazine
propiomazine
triflupromazine
trimeprazine

Piperazine derivatives
acetophenazine
fluphenazine
perphenazine
prochlorperazine
thiethylperazine
trifluoperazine

Piperadine derivatives
mesoridazine
thioridazine

Pyrollidine derivatives
methdilazine

Thioxanthenes
chlorprothixene
thiothixene

The phenothiazines were originally synthesized by European scientists seeking aniline-like dyes in the late 1800s. Several decades later, in the 1930s, promethazine was identified and found to have sedative, antihistaminic, and narcotic-potentiating effects. Chlorpromazine was synthesized in the 1950s; this drug proved to have many effects, among them strong antipsychotic activity.

Pharmacology
Phenothiazines are classified in terms of chemical structure: the aliphatic agents (chlorpromazine, promazine, and triflupromazine) have a greater sedative, hypotensive, allergic, and convulsant activity; the piperazines (acetophenazine, perphenazine, prochlorperazine, fluphenazine, and trifluoperazine) are more likely to produce extrapyramidal symptoms; the piperidines (thioridazine and mesoridazine) have intermediate effects. Thioxanthenes are chemically similar to phenothiazines, and pharmacologically similar to piperazine phenothiazines.

All antipsychotics have fundamentally similar mechanisms of action; they are believed to function as dopamine antagonists, blocking postsynaptic dopamine receptors in various parts of the CNS; their antiemetic effects result from blockage of the chemoreceptor trigger zone. They also produce varying degrees of anticholinergic and alpha-adrenergic receptor blocking actions. The drugs are structurally similar to tricyclic antidepressants (TCAs) and share many adverse reactions.

All antipsychotics have equal clinical efficacy when given in equivalent doses; choice of specific therapy is determined primarily by the individual patient's response and adverse reaction profile. A patient who does not respond to one drug may respond to another.

Onset of full therapeutic effects requires 6 weeks to 6 months of therapy; therefore, dosage adjustment is recommended at not less than weekly intervals.

Clinical indications and actions
Psychoses
The phenothiazines (except ethopropazine, methdilazine, promethazine, propiomazine, thiethylperazine, and trimeprazine) and thioxanthenes (chlorprothixene and thiothixene) are indicated to treat agitated psychotic states. They are especially effective in controlling hallucinations in schizophrenic patients, the manic phase of manic-depressive illness, and excessive motor and autonomic activity.
Nausea and vomiting
Chlorpromazine, perphenazine, prochlorperazine, thiethylperazine, and triflupromazine are effective in controlling severe nausea and vomiting induced by CNS disturbances. They do not prevent motion sickness or vertigo.
†Anxiety
Chlorpromazine, mesoridazine, promethazine, propiomazine, prochlorperazine, and trifluoperazine also may be used for short-term treatment of moderate anxiety in selected nonpsychotic patients, for example, to control anxiety before surgery.
Severe behavior problems
Chlorpromazine and thioridazine are indicated to control combativeness and hyperexcitability in children with severe behavior problems. They also are used in hyperactive children for short-term treatment of excessive motor activity with labile moods, impulsive behavior, aggressiveness, attention deficit, and poor tolerance of frustration. Mesoridazine is used to manage hypersensitivity and to promote cooperative behavior in patients with mental deficiency and chronic brain syndrome.
Tetanus
Chlorpromazine is an effective adjunct in treating tetanus.
Porphyria
Because of its effects on the autonomic nervous system, chlorpromazine is effective in controlling abdominal pain in patients with acute intermittent porphyria.
Intractable hiccups
Chlorpromazine has been used to treat patients with intractable hiccups. The mechanism is unknown.
Neurogenic pain
Fluphenazine is a useful adjunct managing selected chronic pain states (such as narcotic withdrawal).
Parkinson's disease
Ethopropazine, because of its potent anticholinergic effects, is useful in the adjunctive treatment of Parkinson's disease.
Allergies and pruritus
Because of their potent antihistaminic effects, many of these drugs (including methdilazine, promethazine, and trimeprazine) are used to relieve itching or symptomatic rhinitis.

Overview of adverse reactions
Phenothiazines may produce extrapyramidal symptoms (dystonic movements, torticollis, oculogyric crises, parkinsonian symptoms) from akathisia during early treatment, to tardive dyskinesia after long-term use. In some cases, such symptoms can be alleviated by dosage reduction or treatment with diphenhydramine, trihexyphenidyl, or benztropine mesylate. Dystonia usually occurs on initial therapy or at increased dosage in children and younger adults; parkinsonian symptoms and tardive dyskinesia more often affect older patients, especially women.

A neuroleptic malignant syndrome resembling severe parkinsonism may occur (most often in young men taking fluphenazine); it consists of rapid onset of hyperthermia, muscular hyperreflexia, marked extrapyramidal and autonomic dysfunction, arrhythmias, sweating, and several other unpleasant reactions. Although rare, this condition carries a 10% mortality and requires immediate treatment, including cooling blankets, neuromuscular blocking agents, dantrolene, and supportive measures.

Other adverse reactions are similar to those seen with TCAs, including varying degrees of sedative and anticholinergic effects, orthostatic hypotension with reflex tachycardia, fainting and dizziness, and dysrhythmias; GI reactions including anorexia, nausea, vomiting, abdominal pain and local gastric irritation; seizures; endocrine effects; hematologic disorders; ocular changes and other visual disturbances; skin eruptions; and photosensitivity. Allergic manifestations are usually marked by elevation of liver enzymes progressing to obstructive jaundice.

Generally, the piperidine derivatives mesoridazine and thioridazine have the most pronounced cardiovascular effects, and piperazine derivatives have the least. As might be anticipated, parenteral administration is more often associated with cardiovascular effects because of more rapid absorption. Seizures are most common with aliphatic derivatives.

▶ Special considerations
● Phenothiazines are contraindicated in patients with known hypersensitivity to phenothiazines and related compounds, including allergic reactions involving hepatic function; in patients with blood dyscrasias and bone marrow depression; in patients with coma, liver damage, CNS depression, circulatory collapse, or cerebrovascular disease, since additive CNS depression and accompanying blood pressure alteration may seriously worsen these states; and in conjunction with adrenergic blocking agents or spinal or epidural anesthesia because of the potential for excessive postural hypotension.
● Phenothiazines should be used cautiously in patients with cardiac disease (arrhythmias, congestive heart failure, angina pectoris, valvular disease, or heart block) to avoid further compromise of cardiac function from alpha blockade; such reactions are particularly likely in patients with preexisting cardiac compromise or a history of arrhythmias.
● Phenothiazines should be used cautiously in patients with encephalitis, Reye's syndrome, or head injury, because these drugs' antiemetic and CNS depressant effects may mask signs and symptoms and obscure diagnosis; in patients with respiratory disease, because of hazard of respiratory depression and suppression of cough reflex subsequent to additive CNS depression; and in patients with epilepsy and other seizure disor-

---

ders, because these drugs lower seizure threshold and may require additional dosage of anticonvulsants.

• Phenothiazines should be used cautiously in patients with glaucoma, prostatic hypertrophy, paralytic ileus, and urine retention, because drugs have significant antimuscarinic effect that may exacerbate these conditions; in patients with hepatic or renal dysfunction because of hazard of drug accumulation; in patients with Parkinson's disease, because drugs may aggravate tremors and other symptoms; in patients with pheochromocytoma, because of possible adverse cardiovascular effects; and in patients with hypocalcemia, because of increased risk of extrapyramidal symptoms.

• Check vital signs regularly for decreased blood pressure (especially before and after parenteral therapy) or tachycardia; observe patient carefully for other adverse reactions.

• Check intake and output for urine retention or constipation, which may require dosage reduction.

• Monitor bilirubin levels weekly for first 4 weeks; monitor complete blood count, ECG (for quinidine-like effects), liver and renal function studies, electrolyte levels (especially potassium), and eye examinations at baseline and periodically thereafter, especially in patients on long-term therapy.

• Observe patient for mood changes to monitor progress; benefits may not be apparent for several weeks.

• Monitor for involuntary movements. Check patient receiving prolonged treatment at least once every 6 months.

• Do not withdraw drug abruptly; although physical dependence does not occur with antipsychotic drugs, rebound exacerbation of psychotic symptoms may occur, and many drug effects persist.

• Carefully follow manufacturer's instructions for reconstitution, dilution, administration, and storage of drugs; slightly discolored liquids may or may not be all right to use. Check with pharmacist.

Information for the patient

• Explain rationale and anticipated risks and benefits of therapy, and that full therapeutic effect may not occur for several weeks.

• Teach signs and symptoms of adverse reactions and importance of reporting *any* unusual effects, especially involuntary movements.

• Tell patient to avoid beverages and drugs containing alcohol, and not to take any other drug (especially CNS depressants) including nonprescription products without medical approval.

• Instruct diabetic patients to monitor blood sugar, as drug may alter insulin needs.

• Teach patient how and when to take drug, not to increase dose without medical approval, and never to discontinue drug abruptly; suggest taking full dose at bedtime if daytime sedation is troublesome.

• Advise patient to lie down for 30 minutes after first dose (1 hour if I.M.) and to rise slowly from sitting or supine position to prevent orthostatic hypotension.

• Warn patient to avoid tasks requiring mental alertness and psychomotor coordination, such as driving, until full effects of drug are established; emphasize that sedative effects will lessen after several weeks.

• Drugs are locally irritating; advise taking with milk or food to minimize GI distress. Warn that oral concentrates and solutions will irritate skin, and tell patient not to crush or open sustained-release products, but to swallow them whole.

• Warn patient that excessive exposure to sunlight, heat lamps, or tanning beds may cause photosensitivity reactions (burn and abnormal hyperpigmentation).

• Tell patient to avoid exposure to extremes of heat or cold, because of risk of hypothermia or hyperthermia induced by alteration in thermoregulatory function.

• Recommend sugarless gum or hard candy, ice chips, or artificial saliva to relieve dry mouth.

• Explain that phenothiazines may cause pink to brown discoloration of urine.

Geriatric use

Lower doses are indicated in geriatric patients, who are more sensitive to therapeutic and adverse effects, especially cardiac toxicity, tardive dyskinesia, and other extrapyramidal effects. Titrate dosage to patient response.

Pediatric use

Unless otherwise specified, antipsychotics are not recommended for children under age 12; be very careful when using phenothiazines for nausea and vomiting, as acutely ill children (chicken pox, measles, CNS infections, dehydration) are at greatly increased risk of dystonic reactions.

Breast-feeding

If feasible, patient should not breast-feed while taking antipsychotics; most phenothiazines are excreted in breast milk and have a direct effect on prolactin levels. Benefit to mother must outweigh hazard to infant.

Representative combinations

None.

---

phenoxybenzamine hydrochloride
Dibenzyline

• Pharmacologic classification: alpha-adrenergic blocking agent
• Therapeutic classification: antihypertensive for pheochromocytoma; cutaneous vasodilator
• Pregnancy risk category C

How supplied

Available by prescription only
Capsules: 10 mg

Indications, route, and dosage

To control or prevent paroxysmal hypertension and sweating in patients with pheochromocytoma

Adults: Initially, 10 mg P.O. b.i.d., then increased every other day until desired response is achieved. Usual maintenance dosage is 20 to 40 mg b.i.d or t.i.d daily.
Children: Initially, 0.2 mg/kg or 6 mg/m² P.O. daily in a single dose. Maintenance dosage is 0.4 to 1.2 mg/kg or 12 to 36 mg/m² daily.

†*Adjunctive therapy in the treatment of Raynaud's syndrome, frostbite, and acrocyanosis*
Adults: Initially, 10 mg P.O., then increased by 10 mg q 4 days to a maximum of 60 mg/day.

Pharmacodynamics
• *Antihypertensive action:* Phenoxybenzamine non-competitively blocks stimulation of alpha-adrenergic receptors, causing long-acting sympathetic blockade. The drug acts on vascular smooth muscle to block epinephrine- and norepinephrine-induced vasoconstriction, causing peripheral vasodilation and reflex tachycardia. Phenoxybenzamine reverses the pressor effect of epinephrine (epinephrine reversal) and blocks, but does not reverse, the vasoconstrictor effects of norepinephrine.
• *Cutaneous vasodilator action:* Phenoxybenzamine blocks epinephrine- and norepinephrine-induced vasodilation.

Pharmacokinetics
• *Absorption:* After oral administration, phenoxybenzamine is absorbed variably from the GI tract; its effects begin gradually over several hours.
• *Distribution:* Phenoxybenzamine is highly lipid-soluble and may accumulate in fat after large doses.
• *Metabolism:* Dealkylation, probably in the liver. Half-life is 24 hours.
• *Excretion:* Phenoxybenzamine is excreted in urine and bile; alpha-adrenergic blocking effects may persist for up to 7 days after therapy is discontinued.

Contraindications and precautions
Phenoxybenzamine is contraindicated in patients with known hypersensitivity to the drug.
   The drug should be used cautiously in patients with cerebrovascular or coronary insufficiency, because decreased blood pressure may precipitate stroke or angina; in patients with congestive heart failure, coronary artery disease, or advanced renal disease, because hypotension may exacerbate these conditions; and in patients in shock, because additional fluid replacement will be needed.

Interactions
Phenoxybenzamine may antagonize the effects of alpha-adrenergic stimulating sympathomimetic agents. Concomitant use with drugs that stimulate both alpha- and beta-adrenergic receptors—for example, epinephrine—may cause vasodilation, an increased hypotensive response, and tachycardia.

Effects on diagnostic tests
None reported.

Adverse reactions
• CNS: lethargy, drowsiness.
• CV: orthostatic hypotension, *tachycardia, shock.*
• EENT: nasal stuffiness, dry mouth, miosis.
• GI: vomiting, abdominal distress.
• Other: impotence, inhibition of ejaculation.
   Note: Drug should be discontinued if patient shows signs of overdose.

Overdose and treatment
Clinical signs of overdose include postural hypotension, dizziness, tachycardia, vomiting, lethargy, and shock. After acute ingestion, empty stomach by induced emesis or gastric lavage, and give activated charcoal to reduce absorption. Further treatment is usually symptomatic and supportive. Most vasopressors are ineffective; however, adequate doses of norepinephrine may overcome phenoxybenzamine-induced alpha

blockade. Because drug effects are cumulative, extended monitoring of patients is necessary.

▶ Special considerations
Besides those relevant to all *alpha-adrenergic blocking agents,* consider the following recommendations.
• During dosage adjustment, monitor pulse rate and rhythm; check blood pressure in recumbent and standing positions.
• Monitor respiratory status carefully; symptoms of pneumonia and asthma may be aggravated.
• Place patient in Trendelenburg's position if faintness or dizziness occurs.
• Optimal effect may require several weeks; monitor patient closely for adverse effects.
• Nasal congestion and adverse effects on male sexual function usually subside during continued therapy.
• Administer drug with milk or in divided doses to reduce GI irritation.
• Phenoxybenzamine has been used to establish adequacy of fluid volume replacement in patients in shock; to treat micturition disorders; and intravenously to treat hypertensive crisis caused by sympathomimetic amines, foods, or drugs in patients taking monoamine oxidase inhibitors.

Information for the patient
• Teach patient about disease and rationale for therapy; explain that he must continue drug even if he feels well, never discontinue it suddenly, and report any unusual symptoms or malaise.
• Explain that postural hypotension may be minimized by rising slowly and avoiding sudden position changes; dry mouth may be relieved by ice chips, hard candy, or sugarless gum; and taking drug with milk in divided doses will minimize gastric irritation.
• Tell patient to avoid alcohol.
• Warn patient to seek medical approval before taking nonprescription cold preparations.

Geriatric use
Elderly patients are more apt to have marked cerebral or coronary atherosclerosis or renal insufficiency; give drug with caution.

Pediatric use
Administer cautiously to children.

Breast-feeding
It is not known whether phenoxybenzamine is distributed into breast milk; an alternative feeding method is recommended during therapy.

phensuximide
Milontin

• Pharmacologic classification: succinimide derivative
• Therapeutic classification: anticonvulsant
• Pregnancy risk category D

How supplied
Available by prescription only
Capsules: 500 mg

Indications, route, and dosage
Absence seizures
Adults and children: 500 mg to 1 g P.O. b.i.d. or t.i.d.

Pharmacodynamics
Anticonvulsant action: Phensuximide raises the seizure threshold; it suppresses characteristic spike-and-wave pattern by depressing neuronal transmission in the motor cortex and basal ganglia. It is indicated for absence (petit mal) seizures refractory to other drugs.

Pharmacokinetics
- *Absorption:* Phensuximide is absorbed from the GI tract; peak plasma concentrations occur at 1 to 4 hours.
- *Distribution:* Phensuximide is distributed widely throughout the body.
- *Metabolism:* Little is known about phensuximide's metabolism; hydroxy metabolite has been isolated.
- *Excretion:* Excretion of phensuximide has not been studied; it is at least partially excreted in urine.

Contraindications and precautions
Phensuximide is contraindicated in patients with known hypersensitivity to succinimide derivatives. It should be use with caution in patients with hepatic or renal disease and in patients taking other CNS depressants or anticonvulsants.

Phensuximide may increase the incidence of generalized tonic-clonic seizures if used alone to treat mixed seizures; abrupt withdrawal may precipitate petit mal seizures. Use of anticonvulsants during pregnancy has been associated with an increased incidence of birth defects.

Interactions
Concomitant use of phensuximide and other CNS depressants (alcohol, narcotics, anxiolytics, antidepressants, antipsychotics, and other anticonvulsants) may increase sedative effects.

Effects on diagnostic tests
None reported.

Adverse reactions
- CNS: muscular weakness, drowsiness, dizziness, ataxia, headache, insomnia, confusion, psychosis.
- DERM: pruritus, eruptions, erythema, *Stevens-Johnson syndrome.*
- GI: nausea, vomiting, anorexia, abdominal pain, diarrhea.
- GU: urinary frequency, renal damage, hematuria.
- HEMA: transient leukopenia, pancytopenia, *agranulocytosis,* eosinophilia.
- Other: periorbital edema.
  Note: Drug should be discontinued if signs of hypersensitivity, rash, or unusual skin lesions occur; or if any of the following signs of blood dyscrasia occur: joint pain, fever, sore throat, or unusual bleeding or bruising.

Overdose and treatment
Symptoms of overdose may include dizziness and ataxia, which may progress to stupor and coma. Treat overdose supportively. Carefully monitor vital signs and fluid and electrolyte balance. Charcoal hemoperfusion or hemodialysis may be used for severe cases.

▶ Special considerations
Besides those relevant to all *succinimide derivatives,* consider the following recommendations.

- Patient should have periodic tests for hematologic and liver function. Complete blood counts are recommended every 3 months; urinalysis and liver function tests, every 6 months.
- Observe patient for signs of hematologic or other severe adverse reactions. Drug can cause symptoms of SLE.
- Phensuximide may be removed by hemodialysis. Dosage adjustments may be necessary in patients undergoing dialysis.

Information for the patient
- Tell patient that drug may color urine pink, red, or brown. This is not harmful.
- Tell patient to take drug with food or milk to avoid GI upset, to avoid use of alcoholic beverages, and not to discontinue the drug abruptly or change dose except as directed.
- Encourage patient immediately to report skin rash, joint pain, fever, sore throat, bleeding, or bruising.

Breast-feeding
Excretion into breast milk unknown. Consider alternative feeding methods during therapy.

---

phentermine hydrochloride
Adipex-P, Anoxine, Dapex, Fastin, Ionamin, Obe-nix, Obermine, Obiphen, Parmine, Phentrol, Rolaphent, Unicelles, Wilpowr

- Pharmacologic classification: amphetamine congener
- Therapeutic classification: short-term adjunctive anorexigenic agent, indirect-acting sympathomimetic amine
- Controlled substance schedule IV
- Pregnancy risk category C

How supplied
Available by prescription only
Capsules and tablets: 8 mg, 15 mg, 18.75 mg, 30 mg, 37.5 mg
Capsules (resin complex, sustained-release): 15 mg, 30 mg

Indications, route, and dosage
Short-term adjunct in exogenous obesity
Adults: 8 mg P.O. t.i.d. ½ hour before meals; or 15 to 37.5 mg daily before breakfast (resin complex).

Pharmacodynamics
Anorexigenic action: Phentermine is an indirect-acting sympathomimetic amine; it causes fewer and less severe adverse reactions from CNS stimulation than do amphetamines, and its potential for addiction is lower.

Anorexigenic effects are thought to follow direct stimulation of the hypothalamus; they may involve other CNS and metabolic effects.

Pharmacokinetics
- *Absorption:* Phentermine is absorbed readily after oral administration; therapeutic effects persist for 4 to 6 hours.
- *Distribution:* Phentermine is distributed widely throughout the body.

- *Metabolism:* Unknown.
- *Excretion:* Phentermine is excreted in urine.

Contraindications and precautions
Phentermine is contraindicated in patients with known hypersensitivity to phentermine, and in patients with hyperthyroidism, all degrees of hypertension, angina pectoris or other severe cardiovascular disease, glaucoma, or advanced arteriosclerosis. Phentermine also is contraindicated for use with monoamine oxidase (MAO) inhibitors or within 14 days of such use.

It should be used with caution in patients with known hypersensitivity to sympathomimetic amines; in hyperexcitability and agitated states; and in patients with a history of substance abuse. Habituation or psychic dependence may follow prolonged use.

Interactions
Concomitant use with MAO inhibitors (or drugs with MAO-inhibiting effects) or within 14 days of such therapy may cause hypertensive crisis. Phentermine may decrease hypotensive effects of guanethidine and other antihypertensive agents; it also may alter insulin requirements in diabetic patients. Concomitant use with excessive amounts of caffeine may cause additive CNS stimulation.

Concomitant use with general anesthetics may result in cardiac arrhythmias. Antacids, sodium bicarbonate, and acetazolamide increase renal reabsorption of phentermine and prolong its duration of action. Phenothiazines and haloperidol decrease phentermine effects.

Effects on diagnostic tests
None reported.

Adverse reactions
- CNS: nervousness, dizziness, insomnia, fainting, euphoria, depression.
- CV: palpitations, tachycardia, increased blood pressure, arrhythmias.
- DERM: urticaria, rash, burning sensation, hair loss.
- GI: dry mouth, unpleasant taste, nausea, constipation, diarrhea.
- GU: libido changes, impotence, polyuria, menstrual changes.
- HEMA: bone marrow depression.
- Other: dyspnea, blurred vision, gynecomastia, sweating, chills, fever, tolerance, physical and psychological dependence.
Note: Drug should be discontinued if signs of hypersensitivity occur.

Overdose and treatment
Symptoms of acute overdose include restlessness, tremor, hyperreflexia, fever, tachypnea, dizziness, confusion, aggressive behavior, hallucinations, blood pressure changes, arrhythmias, nausea, vomiting, diarrhea, and cramps. Fatigue and depression usually follow CNS stimulation; convulsions, coma, and death may follow.

Treat overdose symptomatically and supportively: sedation may be necessary. Chlorpromazine may antagonize CNS stimulation. Acidification of urine may hasten excretion. Monitor vital signs and fluid and electrolyte balance.

▶ Special considerations
Besides those relevant to all *amphetamines*, consider the following recommendations.

- Intermittent courses of treatment (6 weeks on, followed by 4 weeks off) are equally effective as continuous use.
- Greatest weight loss occurs in the first weeks of therapy and diminishes in succeeding weeks. When such tolerance to drug effect develops, drug should be discontinued instead of increasing the dosage.
- Do not crush sustained-release dosage forms.
- Give morning dose 2 hours after breakfast.

Information for the patient
- Advise patient to take morning dose 2 hours after breakfast, not to crush or chew sustained-release products, and to avoid caffeine-containing drinks.
- Tell patient to take last daily dose at least 6 hours before bedtime to prevent insomnia.
- Warn patient not to take drug more frequently than prescribed.
- Advise patient that drug may produce dizziness, fatigue, or drowsiness.
- Tell patient to call if palpitations occur.
- Tell diabetic patients to closely monitor blood glucose. Results may require adjustment in eating habits, body weight and activity and change in dosage of antidiabetic drug.

Pediatric use
Phentermine is not recommended for children under age 12.

phentolamine mesylate
Regitine

- Pharmacologic classification: alpha-adrenergic blocking agent
- Therapeutic classification: antihypertensive agent for pheochromocytoma; cutaneous vasodilator
- Pregnancy risk category C

How supplied
Available by prescription only
Injection: 5 mg/ml in 1-ml vials

Indications, route, and dosage
Aid for diagnosis of pheochromocytoma
Adults: 5 mg I.V. or I.M.
Children: 1 mg I.V., 3 mg I.M., or 0.1 mg/kg or 3 mg/m² I.V.
Control or prevention of paroxysmal hypertension immediately before or during pheochromocytomectomy
Adults: 5 mg I.M. or I.V. 1 to 2 hours preoperatively, repeated as necessary; 5 mg I.V. during surgery if indicated.
Children: 1 mg, 0.1 mg/kg, or 3 mg/m² I.M. or I.V. 1 to 2 hours preoperatively, repeated as necessary; 1 mg, 0.1 mg/kg, or 3 mg/m² I.V. during surgery if indicated.
Prevention of dermal necrosis and sloughing or extravasation after I.V. administration of norepinephrine
Inject 5 to 10 mg in 10 ml of normal saline solution into the affected area, or add 10 mg to each liter of I.V. fluids containing norepinephrine.

---

†*Adjunctive treatment of CHF secondary to acute MI*
Adults: 170 to 400 mcg/minute by I.V. infusion.
†*Treatment adjunct for males with impotence (neurogenic or vascular)*
Adults: 0.5 to 1 mg by intracavernosal injection. Usually administered with 30 mg papaverine injection.

Pharmacodynamics
● *Antihypertensive action:* Phentolamine competitively antagonizes endogenous and exogenous amines at presynaptic and postsynaptic alpha-adrenergic receptors, decreasing both preload and afterload.
● *Cutaneous vasodilation:* Phentolamine blocks epinephrine- and norepinephrine-induced vasodilation.

Pharmacokinetics
● *Absorption:* Antihypertensive effect is immediate after I.V. administration.
● *Distribution:* Unknown.
● *Metabolism:* Unknown.
● *Excretion:* About 10% of a given dose of phentolamine is excreted unchanged in urine; excretion of remainder is unknown. Phentolamine has a short duration of action; plasma half-life is 19 minutes after I.V. administration.

Contraindications and precautions
Phentolamine is contraindicated in patients with known hypersensitivity to the drug and in patients with coronary artery disease or recent myocardial infarction (MI), because the drug may exacerbate these conditions.
  Drug should be given cautiously to patients with gastritis or peptic ulcer and to patients receiving other antihypertensives.

Interactions
Phentolamine antagonizes vasoconstrictor and hypertensive effects of epinephrine and ephedrine.

Effects on diagnostic tests
None reported.

Adverse reactions
● CNS: dizziness, lethargy, flushing.
● CV: hypotension, *shock*, arrhythmias, palpitations, tachycardia, angina pectoris.
● GI: diarrhea, abdominal pain, nausea, vomiting, hyperperistalsis.
● Other: nasal stuffiness, hypoglycemia.
  Note: Drug should be discontinued if severe hypotension develops.

Overdose and treatment
Signs of overdose include hypotension, dizziness, fainting, tachycardia, vomiting, lethargy, and shock.
  Treat supportively and symptomatically. Use norepinephrine if necessary to increase the blood pressure. *Do not* use epinephrine; it stimulates both alpha and beta receptors and will cause vasodilation and a further drop in blood pressure.

▶ Special considerations
Besides those relevant to all *alpha-adrenergic blocking agents*, consider the following recommendations.
● Usual doses of phentolamine have little effect on the blood pressure of normal individuals or patients with essential hypertension.
● Before test for pheochromocytoma, have the patient rest in supine position until blood pressure is stabilized. When phentolamine is administered I.V., inject dose rapidly after effects of the venipuncture on the blood pressure have passed. A marked decrease in blood pressure will be seen immediately, with the maximum effect seen within 2 minutes. Record blood pressure immediately after the injection, at 30-second intervals for the first 3 minutes, and at 1-minute intervals for the next 7 minutes. When phentolamine is administered I.M., maximum effect occurs within 20 minutes. Record blood pressure every 5 minutes for 30 to 45 minutes after injection.
● A positive test response occurs when the patient's blood pressure decreases at least 35 mm Hg systolic and 25 mm Hg diastolic; a negative test response occurs when the patient's blood pressure remains unchanged, is elevated, or decreases less than 35 mm Hg systolic and 25 mm Hg diastolic.
● When possible, sedatives, analgesics, and all other medication should be withdrawn at least 24 hours (preferably 48 to 72 hours) before the phentolamine test; antihypertensive drugs should be withdrawn and test should not be performed until blood pressure returns to pretreatment levels; rauwolfia drugs should be withdrawn at least 4 weeks before test.
● Phentolamine has been used to treat hypertension resulting from clonidine withdrawal and to treat the reaction to sympathetic amines or other drugs or foods in patients taking monoamine oxidase inhibitors.
● Phentolamine also has been used in patients with MI associated with left ventricular failure in an attempt to reduce infarct size and decrease left ventricular ejection impedance. It also has been used to treat supraventricular premature contractions.

Information for the patient
● Teach patient about phentolamine test, if indicated.
● Tell patient to report adverse effects at once.
● Tell patient not to take sedatives or narcotics for at least 24 hours before phentolamine test.

Geriatric use
Administer cautiously.

Pediatric use
Administer cautiously.

Breast-feeding
It is not known if phentolamine is distributed into breast milk; because of possible adverse reactions in the infant, a decision should be made whether to discontinue breast-feeding or the drug, depending on the importance of the drug for the lactating woman.

---

*Canada only   †Unlabeled clinical use   Italicized adverse reactions are life-threatening.

phenylbutazone
Algoverine*, Azolid, Butagen, Butazolidin, Butazone, Intrabutazone*, Malgesic*, Neo-Zoline*

- Pharmacologic classification: nonsteroidal anti-inflammatory
- Therapeutic classification: nonnarcotic analgesic, antipyretic, anti-inflammatory, uricosuric
- Pregnancy risk category C

How supplied
Available by prescription only
Tablets: 100 mg
Capsules: 100 mg

Indications, route, and dosage
Pain, inflammation in arthritis, ankylosing spondylitis
Adults: Initially, 100 to 200 mg P.O. t.i.d. or q.i.d. Maximum dosage is 600 mg/day. When improvement is obtained, decrease dose to 100 mg t.i.d. or q.i.d.
Acute, gouty arthritis
Adults: 400 mg initially as single dose, then 100 mg q 4 hours for 4 days or until relief is obtained.

Pharmacodynamics
Analgesic, antipyretic, and anti-inflammatory actions: Mechanisms of action are unknown, but phenylbutazone is thought to inhibit prostaglandin synthesis.

Pharmacokinetics
- *Absorption:* Phenylbutazone is absorbed rapidly and completely from the GI tract.
- *Distribution:* The drug is 98% protein-bound.
- *Metabolism:* Phenylbutazone is metabolized in the liver. Oxyphenbutazone is an active metabolite.
- *Excretion:* Phenylbutazone is excreted in urine. Plasma half-life ranges from 50 to 100 hours.

Contraindications and precautions
Phenylbutazone is contraindicated in patients with known hypersensitivity to phenylbutazone or oxyphenbutazone; in patients in whom aspirin or other nonsteroidal anti-inflammatory drugs (NSAIDs) induce symptoms of asthma, urticaria, or rhinitis; in patients under age 14 because safety has not been established; and in patients with senility, GI ulcer, blood dyscrasias, or renal, hepatic, cardiac, and thyroid disease, because the drug may mask symptoms of or worsen these conditions. Do not use in patients on long-term anticoagulant therapy because of the potential for adverse hematologic effects.

Patients with known "triad" symptoms (aspirin hypersensitivity, rhinitis/nasal polyps, and asthma) are at high risk of bronchospasm. NSAIDs may mask the signs and symptoms of acute infection (fever, myalgia, erythema); carefully evaluate patients with high risk (such as those with diabetes).

Serious GI toxicity, especially ulceration or hemorrhage, can occur at any time in patients on chronic NSAID therapy. Use with caution in patients with a history of GI disease, particularly peptic ulcer disease.

Because of the potential for serious blood dyscrasias, phenylbutazone is not recommended for initial therapy.

Interactions
When used concomitantly, anticoagulants and thrombolytic drugs may be potentiated by the platelet-inhibiting effect of phenylbutazone. Concomitant use of phenylbutazone with highly protein-bound drugs (phenytoin, sulfonylureas, warfarin) may cause displacement of either drug, and adverse effects. Monitor therapy closely for both drugs. Concomitant use with other GI-irritating drugs (steroids, antibiotics, NSAIDs) may potentiate the adverse GI effects of phenylbutazone. Use together with caution.

Antacids and food may decrease the absorption of phenylbutazone. NSAIDs are known to decrease renal clearance of lithium carbonate, thus increasing lithium serum levels and risks of adverse effects. Phenylbutazone is a known inducer of microsomal enzymes in the liver. Use with caution in combination with highly metabolized drugs (digitoxin). When phenylbutazone is used concomitantly with other NSAIDs, there is a potential for increased uricosuric effect.

Effects on diagnostic tests
Phenylbutazone interferes with the results of thyroid function tests. It may decrease ^{131}I uptake, decrease serum thyroxine concentrations, and increase resin or erythrocyte triiodothyronine uptake.

The physiologic effects of the drug may prolong bleeding time, increase blood glucose concentrations, decrease serum uric acid concentrations, and increase liver function test values of AST (SGOT) and ALT (SGPT).

Adverse reactions
- CNS: confusion, restlessness, lethargy, headache, dizziness, drowsiness, peripheral neuropathy.
- CV: hypertension, pericarditis, myocarditis, *cardiac decompensation,* congestive heart failure (CHF), pulmonary edema.
- DERM: petechiae, pruritus, purpura, dermatoses ranging from rash to *toxic necrotizing epidermolysis.*
- EENT: optic neuritis, blurred vision, retinal hemorrhage or detachment, hearing loss, tinnitus.
- GI: nausea, vomiting, anorexia, diarrhea, ulceration, GI bleeding, constipation.
- GU: proteinuria, hematuria, glomerulonephritis, nephrotic syndrome, *renal failure.*
- HEMA: *bone marrow depression (hemolytic or aplastic anemia, agranulocytosis, thrombocytopenia),* leukopenia.
- Other: toxic and nontoxic goiter, respiratory alkalosis, metabolic acidosis, elevated liver enzymes, jaundice, hepatitis.
   Note: Drug should be discontinued if the following occur: fever, sore throat, mouth ulcers, GI discomfort, black or tarry stools, bleeding, bruising, rash, or weight gain. If patient shows signs and symptoms of hepatotoxicity or abnormal CBC discontinue drug immediately.

Overdose and treatment
Clinical manifestations of overdose include drowsiness, abdominal pain, nausea, vomiting, hematemesis, diarrhea, restlessness, dizziness, agitation, hallucinations, psychosis, coma, convulsions, hyperpyrexia, electrolyte disturbances, hyperventilation, respiratory arrest, and cyanosis.

To treat phenylbutazone overdose, empty stomach immediately, if patient is conscious, by inducing emesis

---

with ipecac syrup or by gastric lavage. Administer activated charcoal via nasogastric tube. Provide symptomatic and supportive measures (respiratory support and correction of fluid and electrolyte imbalances). Use I.V. fluids with caution to prevent fluid overload. Monitor laboratory parameters and vital signs closely. If seizures occur, benzodiazepines may help to control them. Hemodialysis may help remove drug.

▶ **Special considerations**
Besides those relevant to all *NSAIDs*, consider the following recommendations.
● Complete physical examination and laboratory evaluation are recommended before therapy.
● Administer phenylbutazone with meals or food to minimize GI upset.
● Assess cardiopulmonary status closely. Monitor vital signs for any significant changes.
● Monitor for fluid retention.
● Record patient's weight and intake and output daily.
● Review laboratory parameters to establish baseline before initiation of therapy. Monitor serum lab values, especially CBC and renal and liver function studies, every 2 weeks.
● Institute safety measures, such as supervised ambulation and raised side rails, to prevent injury.
● Response should be seen in 2 to 3 days. Drug should be stopped if no response is seen within 1 week.
● Administer cautiously to patients over age 40.

Information for the patient
● Warn patient to remain under close medical supervision and to keep all follow-up and laboratory appointments.
● Warn patient against exceeding prescribed dosage.
● Caution patient to avoid concomitant use of alcohol with phenylbutazone. Tell him to seek medical approval before using any nonprescription medications.
● Warn patient of possible CNS effects and to avoid hazardous activities that require alertness. Instruct him in safety measures to prevent injury.
● Instruct patient to record daily weight and to notify you of any weight gain of 2 pounds or more within a few days.
● Advise patient to report any adverse reactions immediately.

Geriatric use
● Patients over age 60 are more sensitive to the adverse effects of salicylates and NSAIDs.
● Through the effect on renal prostaglandins, salicylates and NSAIDs may cause fluid retention and edema. This may be significant in elderly patients and those with CHF.
● Discontinue drug after 1 week in patients over age 60.

Pediatric use
Phenylbutazone is contraindicated in children under age 14.

Breast-feeding
Phenylbutazone is distributed into breast milk; an alternative feeding method should be considered during therapy with the drug.

phenylephrine hydrochloride
Nasal products
Allerest, Neo-Synephrine, Sinex

Parenteral
Neo-Synephrine

Ophthalmic
Ak-Dilate, Ak-Nefrin, Isopto Frin, Mydfrin, Neo-Synephrine, Prefin Liquifilm

● Pharmacologic classification: adrenergic
● Therapeutic classification: vasoconstrictor
● Pregnancy risk category C

How supplied
Available by prescription only
Injection: 10 mg/ml parenteral
Ophthalmic solution: 0.12%, 2.5%, 10%

Available without prescription
Nasal solution: 0.123%, 0.16%, 0.2%, 0.5%, 1%
Nasal spray: 0.2%, 0.25%, 0.5%

Indications, route, and dosage
Hypotensive emergencies during spinal anesthesia
Adults: Initially, 0.1 to 0.2 mg I.V.; subsequent doses should also be low (0.1 mg)
Children: 0.044 to 0.088 mg/kg I.M. or S.C.
Prevention of hypotension during spinal or inhalation anesthesia
Adults: 2 to 3 mg S.C. or I.M. 3 or 4 minutes before anesthesia.
Mild to moderate hypotension
Adults: 1 to 10 mg S.C. or I.M. (initial dose should not exceed 5 mg). Additional doses may be given in 1 to 2 hours if needed. Or, 0.1 to 0.5 mg slow I.V. injection (initial dose should not exceed 0.5 mg). Additional doses may be given q 10 to 15 minutes.
Children: 0.1 mg/kg or 3 mg/m² I.M. or S.C.
Paroxysmal supraventricular tachycardia
Adults: Initially, 0.5 mg rapid I.V.; subsequent doses may be increased in increments of 0.1 to 0.2 mg. Maximum dose should not exceed 1 mg.
Prolongation of spinal anesthesia
Adults: 2 to 5 mg added to anesthetic solution.
Adjunct in the treatment of severe hypotension or shock
Adults: 0.1 to 0.18 mg/minute I.V. infusion. After blood pressure stabilizes, maintain at 0.04 to 0.06 mg/minute, adjusted to patient response.
Vasoconstrictor for regional anesthesia
Adults: 1 mg phenylephrine added to 20 ml local anesthetic.
Mydriasis (without cycloplegia)
Adults: Instill 1 or 2 drops 2.5% or 10% solution in eye before procedure. May be repeated in 10 to 60 minutes if needed.
Posterior synechia (adhesion of iris)
Adults: Instill 1 drop 10% solution in eye 3 or more times daily with atropine sulfate.
Diagnosis of Horner's or Raeder's syndrome
Adults: Instill a 1% or 10% solution in both eyes.

Initial treatment of postoperative malignant glaucoma
Adults: Instill 1 drop of a 10% solution with 1 drop of a 1% to 4% atropine sulfate solution 3 or more times daily.

Nasal, †sinus, or eustachian tube congestion
Adults and children over age 12: Apply 2 to 3 drops or 1 to 2 sprays of 0.25% to 1% solution instilled in each nostril; or a small quantity of 0.5% nasal jelly applied into each nostril. Apply jelly or spray to nasal mucosa.
Children age 6 to 12: Apply 2 to 3 drops or 1 to 2 sprays in each nostril.
Children under age 6: Apply 2 to 3 drops or sprays of 0.125% or 0.16% solution in each nostril.

Drops, spray, or jelly can be given q 4 hours, p.r.n.

Conjunctival congestion
Adults: 1 to 2 drops of 0.12% to 0.25% solution applied to conjunctiva q 3 to 4 hours p.r.n.

Pharmacodynamics
Vasopressor action: Phenylephrine acts predominantly by direct stimulation of alpha-adrenergic receptors, which constrict resistance and capacitance blood vessels, resulting in increased total peripheral resistance; increased systolic and diastolic blood pressure; decreased blood flow to vital organs, skin, and skeletal muscle; and constriction of renal blood vessels, reducing renal blood flow. Its main therapeutic effect is vasoconstriction.

It may also act indirectly by releasing norepinephrine from its storage sites. Phenylephrine does not stimualte beta receptors except in large doses (activates beta$_1$ receptors). Tachyphylaxis (tolerance) may follow repeated injections.

Other alpha-adrenergic effects include action on the dilator muscle of the pupil (producing contraction) and local decongestant action in the arterioles of the conjunctiva (producing constriction).

Phenylephrine acts directly on alpha-adrenergic receptors in the arterioles of conjunctiva nasal mucosa, producing constriction. Its vasoconstricting action on skin, mucous membranes, and viscera slows the vascular absorption rate of local anesthetics, which prolongs their action, localizes anesthesia, and decreases the risk of toxicity.

Phenylephrine may cause contraction of pregnant uterus and constriction of uterine blood vessels.

Pharmacokinetics
● *Absorption:* Pressor effects occur almost immediately after I.V. injection and persist 15 to 20 minutes; after I.M. injection, onset is within 10 to 15 minutes, persisting ½ to 2 hours; after S.C. injection, onset is within 10 to 15 minutes, with effects persisting 50 to 60 minutes. Nasal or conjunctival decongestant effects persist 30 minutes to 4 hours. Peak effects for mydriasis are 15 to 60 minutes for the 2.5% solution; 10 to 90 minutes for the 10% solution. Mydriasis recovery time is 3 hours for the 2.5% solution; 3 to 7 hours for the 10% solution.
● *Distribution:* Unknown.
● *Metabolism:* Phenylephrine is metabolized in the liver and intestine by the enzyme monoamine oxidase.
● *Excretion:* Unknown.

Contraindications and precautions
Phenylephrine is contraindicated in patients with severe coronary disease, cardiovascular disease including myocardial infarction, or peripheral or mesenteric vascular thrombosis (may increase ischemia or extend area

of infarction); in patients with severe hypertension or ventricular tachycardia; or for use with local anesthetics on fingers, toes, ears, nose, and genitalia.

Administer with extreme caution to elderly or debilitated patients, and those with hyperthyroidism, bradycardia, partial heart block, myocardial disease, diabetes mellitus, narrow-angle glaucoma, severe arteriosclerosis, acute pancreatitis, or hepatitis (may increase ischemia in liver or pancreas).

Also administer cautiously to patients with known hypersensitivity to sulfites because phenylephrine contains sulfite preservatives.

Interactions
Phenylephrine may increase risk of cardiac arrhythmias, including tachycardia, when used concomitantly with epinephrine or other sympathomimetics, digitalis glycosides, levodopa, guanadrel or guanethidine, tricyclic antidepressants, monoamine oxidase (MAO) inhibitors, or general anesthetics (chloroform, cyclopropane, and halothane).

Pressor effects are potentiated when phenylephrine is used with oxytocics, doxapram, MAO inhibitors, methyldopa, trimethaphan, mecamylamine, mazindol, and ergot alkaloids.

Decreased pressor response (hypotension) may result when phenylephrine is used with alpha-adrenergic blockers, antihypertensives, diuretics used as antihypertensives, guanadrel or guanethidine, rauwolfia alkaloids, or nitrates.

Use of phenylephrine with thyroid hormones may increase effects of either drug; with nitrates, it may reduce antianginal effects.

The mydriatic response to phenylephrine is decreased in concomitant use of levodopa and increased in concomitant use with cycloplegic antimuscarinic drugs, such as atropine.

Effects on diagnostic tests
Phenylephrine may lower intraocular pressure in normal eyes or in open-angle glaucoma. The drug also may cause false-normal tonometry readings.

Adverse reactions
● CNS: restlessness, insomnia, anxiety, nervousness, light-headedness, weakness, dizziness, tremor, paresthesias in extremities and coolness in skin (after injection), headache, browache, *seizures.*
● CV: *precordial pain or discomfort,* peripheral and visceral vasoconstriction, bradycardia, tachycardia, decreased cardiac output, *hypertension,* palpitations, anginal pain.
● EENT: blurred vision; transient burning and stinging on instillation; increased sensitivity of eyes to light; iris floaters; glaucoma; rebound miosis; dermatitis; burning, stinging, and dryness of nasal mucosa; rebound nasal congestion.
● GI: vomiting.
● Local: tissue sloughing with extravasation.
● Other: *respiratory distress,* sweating, blanching of skin, tolerance with prolonged use.
   Note: Drug should be discontinued if hypersensitivity or cardiac arrhythmias occur.

Overdose and treatment
Clinical manifestations of overdose include exaggeration of common adverse reactions, palpitations, paresthesia, vomiting, cardiac arrhythmias, hypertension.

To treat, discontinue drug and provide symptomatic

---

and supportive measures. Monitor vital signs closely. Use atropine sulfate to block reflex bradycardia; phentolamine to treat excessive hypertension; and propranolol to treat cardiac arrhythmias, or levodopa to reduce an excessive mydriatic effect of an ophthalmic preparation as necessary.

▶ **Special considerations**

Besides those relevant to all *adrenergics*, consider the following recommendations.
● Give I.V. through large veins, and monitor flow rate. To treat extravasation ischemia, infiltrate site promptly and liberally with 10 to 15 ml of saline solution containing 5 to 10 mg of phentolamine through fine needle. Topical nitroglycerin has also been used.
● During I.V. administration, pulse, blood pressure, and central venous pressure should be monitored (every 2 to 5 minutes). Control flow rate and dosage to prevent excessive increases. I.V. overdoses can induce ventricular arrhythmias.
● Hypovolemic states should be corrected before administration of drug; phenylephrine should not be used in place of fluid, blood, plasma, and electrolyte replacement.
● Phenylephrine is chemically incompatible with butacaine, sulfate, alkalies, ferric salts, and oxidizing agents and metals.

Ophthalmic
● Apply digital pressure to lacrimal sac during and for 1 to 2 minutes after instillation to prevent systemic absorption.
● Prolonged exposure to air or strong light may cause oxidation and discoloration. Do not use if solution is brown or contains precipitate.
● To prevent contamination, do not touch applicator tip to any surface. Instruct patient in proper technique.

Nasal
● Prolonged or chronic use may result in rebound congestion and chronic swelling of nasal mucosa.
● To reduce risk of rebound congestion, use weakest effective dose.
● After use, rinse tip of spray bottle or dropper with hot water and dry with clean tissue. Wipe tip of nasal jelly container with clean, damp tissues.

Information for the patient
● Tell patient to store away from heat, light, and humidity (not in bathroom medicine cabinet) and out of children's reach.
● Warn patient to use only as directed. If using nonprescription product, the patient should follow directions on label and not use more often or in larger doses than prescribed or recommended.
● Caution patient not to exceed recommended dosage regardless of formulation; patient should not double, decrease, or omit doses nor change dosage intervals unless so instructed.
● Tell patient to call if drug provides no relief in 2 days after using phenylephrine ophthalmic solution or 3 days after using the nasal solution.
● Explain that systemic absorption from nasal and conjunctival membranes can occur. Patient should report systemic reactions such as dizziness and chest pain and discontinue drug.

Ophthalmic
● Tell patient not to use if solution is brown or contains a precipitate.
● Tell patient to wash hands before applying and to use finger to apply pressure to lacrimal sac during and for 1 to 2 minutes after instillation to decrease systemic absorption.
● Tell patient to avoid touching tip to any surface to prevent contamination.
● Tell patient that after applying drops, pupils will become unusually large. Patient should use sunglasses to protect eyes from sunlight and other bright lights, and call if effects persist 12 hours or more.

Nasal
● After use, patient should rinse tip of spray bottle or dropper with hot water and dry with clean tissue or wipe tip of nasal jelly container with clean, damp tissues.
● Instruct patient to blow nose gently (with both nostrils open) to clear nasal passages well, before using medication.
● Teach patient correct instillation
– drops: tilt head back while sitting or standing up, or lie on bed and hang head over side. Stay in position a few minutes to permit medication to spread through nose.
– spray: with head upright, squeeze bottle quickly and firmly to produce 1 or 2 sprays into each nostril; wait 3 to 5 minutes, blow nose and repeat dose.
– jelly: place in each nostril and sniff it well back into nose.
● Tell patient that increased fluid intake helps keep secretions liquid.
● Warn patient to avoid using nonprescription medications with phenylephrine to prevent possible hazardous interactions.

Geriatric use
Effects may be exaggerated in elderly patients. In patients over age 50, phenylephrine (ophthalmic solution) appears to alter the reponse of the dilator muscle of the pupil so that rebound miosis may occur the day after the drug is administered.

Pediatric use
Infants and children may be more susceptible than adults to drug effects. Because of the risk of precipitating severe hypertension, only ophthalmic solutions containing 0.5% or less should be used in infants under age 1. The 10% ophthalmic solution is contraindicated in infants. Most manufacturers recommend that the 0.5% nasal solution not be used in children under age 12 except under medical supervision, and the 0.25% nasal solution should not be used in children under age 6 except under medical supervision.

Breast-feeding
It is not known if phenylephrine is distributed into breast milk; drug should be used with caution in breast-feeding women.

phenytoin, phenytoin sodium, phenytoin sodium (extended)
Dilantin

phenytoin sodium (prompt)
Di-Phen, Diphenylan

- Pharmacologic classification: hydantoin derivative
- Therapeutic classification: anticonvulsant
- Pregnancy risk category D

How supplied
Available by prescription only
Phenytoin
Tablets (chewable): 50 mg
Oral suspension: 30 mg/5 ml, 125 mg/5 ml
Phenytoin sodium
Injection: 50 mg/ml
Phenytoin sodium, extended
Capsules: 30 mg, 100 mg
Phenytoin sodium, prompt
Capsules: 30 mg, 100 mg

Indications, route, and dosage
Generalized tonic-clonic seizures, status epilepticus, nonepileptic seizures (post-head trauma, Reye's syndrome)
Adults: Loading dosage is 10 to 15 mg/kg I.V. slowly, not to exceed 50 mg/minute; oral loading dosage consists of 1 g divided into three doses (400 mg, 300 mg, 300 mg) given at 2-hour intervals. Maintenance dosage is 300 mg P.O. daily (extended only) or divided t.i.d. (extended or prompt).
Children: Loading dosage is 15 mg/kg I.V. at 50 mg/minute, or P.O. divided q 8 to 12 hours; then start maintenance dosage of 4 to 8 mg/kg P.O. or I.V. daily, divided q 12 hours.
Seizures in patients who have been receiving phenytoin but have missed one or more doses and have subtherapeutic levels
Adults: 100 to 300 mg I.V., not to exceed 50 mg/minute.
Children: 5 to 7 mg/kg I.V., not to exceed 50 mg/minute. May repeat lower dose in 30 minutes if needed.
Neuritic pain (migraine, trigeminal neuralgia, and Bell's palsy)
Adults: 200 to 600 mg P.O. daily in divided doses.
†*Ventricular arrhythmias unresponsive to lidocaine or procainamide, and arrhythmias induced by cardiac glycosides*
Adults: Loading dosage is 1 g P.O. divided over first 24 hours, followed by 500 mg daily for 2 days, then maintenance dosage 300 mg P.O. daily; 250 mg I.V. over 5 minutes until arrhythmias subside, adverse effects develop, or 1 g has been given. Infusion rate should never exceed 50 mg/minute (slow I.V. push).
Alternate method: 100 mg I.V. q 15 minutes until adverse effects develop, arrhythmias are controlled, or 1 g has been given. Also may administer entire loading dose of 1 g I.V. slowly at 25 mg/minute. Can be diluted in normal saline solution. I.M. dosage is not recommended because of pain and erratic absorption.
Children: 3 to 8 mg/kg P.O. or slow I.V. daily, or 250 mg/m² daily given as single dose or divided in two doses.

†*Treatment of recessive dystrophic epidermolysis bullosa*
Adults: Initially 2 to 3 mg/kg P.O. daily divided b.i.d. Increase dosage at 2- to 3-week intervals to a plasma level of 8 mcg/ml (usual dose: 100 to 300 mg daily).

Pharmacodynamics
- *Anticonvulsant action:* Like other hydantoin derivatives, phenytoin stabilizes neuronal membranes and limits seizure activity by either increasing efflux or decreasing influx of sodium ions across cell membranes in the motor cortex during generation of nerve impulses. Phenytoin exerts its antiarrhythmic effects by normalizing sodium influx to Purkinje's fibers inpatients with digitalis-induced arrhythmias. It is indicated for tonic-clonic (grand mal) and partial seizures.
- *Other actions:* Phenytoin inhibits excessive collagenase activity in patients with epidermolysis bullosa.

Pharmacokinetics
- *Absorption:* Phenytoin is absorbed slowly from the small intestine; absorption is formulation-dependent and bioavailability may differ among products. Extended-release capsules give peak serum concentrations at 4 to 12 hours; prompt-release products peak at 1½ to 3 hours. I.M. doses are absorbed erratically; about 50% to 75% of I.M. dose is absorbed in 24 hours.
- *Distribution:* Phenytoin is distributed widely throughout the body; therapeutic plasma levels are 10 to 20 mcg/ml, although in some patients, they occur at 5 to 10 mcg/ml. Lateral nystagmus may occur at levels above 20 mcg/ml; ataxia usually occurs at levels above 30 mcg/ml; significantly decreased mental capacity occurs at 40 mcg/ml. Phenytoin is about 90% protein-bound, less so in uremic patients.
- *Metabolism:* Phenytoin is metabolized by the liver to inactive metabolites.
- *Excretion:* Phenytoin is excreted in urine and exhibits dose-dependent (zero-order) elimination kinetics; above a certain dosage level, small increases in dosage disproportionately increase serum levels.

Contraindications and precautions
Phenytoin is contraindicated in patients with hypersensitivity to hydantoins or phenacemide; I.V. phenytoin is contraindicated in patients with sinus bradycardia, sinoatrial or atrioventricular block, or Stokes-Adams syndrome.

Phenytoin should be used with caution in patients with acute intermittent porphyria, hepatic or renal dysfunction (especially in uremic patients, who have higher serum drug levels from decreased protein-binding), myocardial insufficiency, or respiratory depression; in elderly or debilitated patients; and in patients taking other hydantoin derivatives.

If a rash appears during phenytoin therapy, drug should be discontinued until cause of rash is determined. If the rash recurs after rechallenge, drug is contraindicated.

Interactions
Phenytoin interacts with many drugs. Diminished therapeutic effects and toxic reactions often are the result of recent changes in drug therapy. Phenytoin's therapeutic effects may be increased by concomitant use with allopurinol, chloramphenicol, cimetidine, diazepam, disulfiram, ethanol (acute), isoniazid, miconazole, phenacemide, phenylbutazone, succinimides, trimeth-

oprim, valproic acid, salicylates, ibuprofen, chlorphen-iramine, or imipramine.

Phenytoin's therapeutic effects may be decreased by barbiturates, carbamazepine, diazoxide, ethanol (chronic), folic acid, theophylline, antacids, antineo-plastics, calcium gluconate, calcium, charcoal, loxap-ine, nitrofurantoin, or pyridoxine. Other drugs that lower seizure threshold (such as antipsychotic agents) may attenuate phenytoin's therapeutic effects.

Phenytoin may decrease the effects of the following drugs by stimulating hepatic metabolism: corticoste-roids, cyclosporine, dicumarol, digitoxin, meperidine, disopyramide, doxycycline, estrogens, haloperidol, methadone, metyrapone, quinidine, oral contracep-tives, dopamine, furosemide, levodopa, or sulfonyl-ureas.

Effects on diagnostic tests
Phenytoin may raise blood glucose levels by inhibiting pancreatic insulin release; it may decrease serum levels of protein-bound iodine and may interfere with the 1-mg dexamethasone suppression test.

Adverse reactions
● CNS: ataxia, slurred speech, confusion, dizziness, insomnia, nervousness, twitching, headache.
● CV: hypotension, *ventricular fibrillation.*
● DERM: scarlatiniform or morbilliform rash; bullous, exfoliative, or purpuric dermatitis; *Stevens-Johnson syndrome;* lupus erythematosus; hirsutism; *toxic epidermal necrolysis;* photosensitivity.
● EENT: nystagmus, diplopia, blurred vision.
● GI: nausea, vomiting, gingival hyperplasia (especially in children).
● HEMA: thrombocytopenia, leukopenia, *agranulocytosis,* pancytopenia, macrocytosis, megaloblastic anemia.
● Hepatic: *toxic hepatitis,* jaundice.
● Local: pain, necrosis, and inflammation at injection site; purple glove syndrome.
● Other: periarteritis nodosa, lymphadenopathy, hyperglycemia, osteomalacia, hypertrichosis.
   Note: Drug should be discontinued if signs of hypersensitivity, hepatotoxicity, or blood dyscrasias occur, or if lymphadenopathy or skin rash occurs.

Overdose and treatment
Early signs of overdose may include drowsiness, nausea, vomiting, nystagmus, ataxia, dysarthria, tremor, and slurred speech; hypotension, respiratory depression, and coma may follow. Death is caused by respiratory and circulatory depression. Estimated lethal dose in adults is 2 to 5 g.

Treat overdose with gastric lavage or emesis and follow with supportive treatment. Carefully monitor vital signs and fluid and electrolyte balance. Forced diuresis is of little or no value. Hemodialysis or peritoneal dialysis may be helpful.

▶ Special considerations
Besides those relevant to all *hydantoin derivatives,* consider the following recommendations.
● Monitoring of serum levels is essential because of dose-dependent excretion.
● Only extended-release capsules are approved for once-daily dosing; all other forms are given in divided doses every 8 to 12 hours.
● Oral or nasogastric feeding may interfere with absorption of oral suspension; separate doses as much

as possible from feedings but no less than 1 hour. During continuous tube feeding, tube should be flushed before and after dose.
● If suspension is used, shake well.
● I.M. administration should be avoided; it is painful and drug absorption is erratic.
● Mix I.V. doses in normal saline solution and use within 1 hour; mixtures with dextrose 5% will precipitate. Do not refrigerate solution; do not mix with other drugs.
● When giving I.V., continuous monitoring of ECG, blood pressure, and respiratory status is essential.
● Abrupt withdrawal may precipitate status epilepticus.
● If using I.V. bolus, use slow (50 mg/minute) I.V. push or constant infusion; too-rapid I.V. injection may cause hypotension and circulatory collapse. Do not use I.V. push in veins on back of hand; larger veins are needed to prevent discoloration associated with purple glove syndrome.
● Phenytoin often is abbreviated as DPH (diphenyl-hydantoin), an older drug name.

Information for the patient
● Tell patient to use same brand of phenytoin consistently. Changing brands may change therapeutic effect.
● Tell patient to take drug with food or milk to minimize GI distress.
● Warn patient not to discontinue drug, except with medical supervision; to avoid hazardous activities that require alertness until CNS effect is determined; and to avoid alcoholic beverages, which can decrease effectiveness of drug and increase adverse reactions.
● Encourage patient to wear a Medic Alert bracelet or necklace.
● Encourage good oral hygiene to minimize overgrowth and sensitivity of gums.

Geriatric use
Elderly patients metabolize and excrete phenytoin slowly; therefore, they may require lower doses.

Pediatric use
Special pediatric-strength suspension is available (30 mg/5 ml). Take extreme care to use correct strength. Do not confuse with adult strength (125 mg/5 ml).

Breast-feeding
Phenytoin is excreted into breast milk. Alternative feeding method is recommended during therapy.

---

physostigmine salicylate
Antilirium

physostigmine sulfate
Eserine, Isopto Eserine

● Pharmacologic classification: cholinesterase inhibitor
● Therapeutic classification: antimuscarinic antidote, antiglaucoma agent
● Pregnancy risk category C

How supplied
Available by prescription only
Injection: 1 mg/ml
Ophthalmic ointment: 0.25%
Ophthalmic solution: 0.25%, 0.5%

Indications, route, and dosage
Tricyclic antidepressant and anticholinergic poisoning
Adults: 0.5 to 2 mg I.M. or I.V. given slowly (not to exceed 1 mg/minute I.V.). Dosage individualized and repeated as necessary.

Children: Not more than 0.5 mg I.V. over at least 1 minute. Dosage may be repeated at 5- to 10-minute intervals to a maximum of 2 mg if no adverse cholinergic signs are present.

Open-angle glaucoma
Adults: Instill 2 drops into eye(s) up to q.i.d., or apply ointment to lower fornix up to t.i.d.

Pharmacodynamics
Antimuscarinic action: Physostigmine competitively blocks acetylcholine hydrolysis by cholinesterase, resulting in acetylcholine accumulation at cholinergic synapses; that antagonizes the muscarinic effects of overdose with antidepressants and anticholinergics. With ophthalmic use, miosis and ciliary muscle contraction increase aqueous humor outflow and decrease intraocular pressure.

Pharmacokinetics
● *Absorption:* Physostigmine is well absorbed when given I.M. or I.V., with effects peaking within 5 minutes. After ophthalmic use, physostigmine may be absorbed orally after passage through the nasolacrimal duct.
● *Distribution:* Physostigmine is distributed widely and crosses the blood-brain barrier.
● *Metabolism:* Cholinesterase hydrolyzes physostigmine relatively quickly. Duration of effect is 1 to 2 hours after I.V. administration, 12 to 36 hours after ophthalmic use.
● *Excretion:* Only a small amount of physostigmine is excreted in urine. Exact mode of excretion is unknown.

Contraindications and precautions
Physostigmine is contraindicated in patients with narrow-angle glaucoma because it may cause pupillary blockage, resulting in increased intraocular pressure; and in patients with known hypersensitivity to cholinesterase inhibitors. Administer cautiously to patients with vagotonia, because they may experience enhanced drug effects; to patients with diabetes, because it may change insulin requirements; to patients with mechanical obstruction of the intestine or urinary tract, because of the drug's stimulatory effect on smooth muscle; to patients with bradycardia and hypotension, because the drug may exacerbate these conditions; and to patients receiving depolarizing neuromuscular blocking agents, because physostigmine may enhance and prolong the effects of such drugs.

Also administer the drug cautiously to patients with epilepsy, because of the drug's possible CNS stimulatory effects; to patients with recent coronary occlusion or cardiac arrhythmias, because of the drug's stimulatory effects on the cardiovascular system; to patients with peptic ulcer disease, because the drug may stimulate gastric acid secretion; and to patients with bronchial asthma, because the drug may precipitate asthma attacks.

Interactions
Concomitant use with succinylcholine may prolong respiratory depression by inhibiting hydrolysis of succinylcholine by plasma esterases. Concomitant use with ganglionic blockers, such as mecamylamine, may crit-

ically decrease blood pressure; this effect is usually preceded by abdominal symptoms. Concomitant use with systemic cholinergic agents may cause additive toxicity.

Effects on diagnostic tests
None reported.

Adverse reactions
● CNS: headache, *convulsions,* confusion, restlessness, hallucinations, muscle twitching, muscle weakness, ataxia, excitability.
● CV: bradycardia, hypotension, cardiac irregularities.
● EENT: blurred vision, conjunctivitis, miosis, ocular burning or stinging, lacrimation, browache, accommodative spasm, eyelid twitching, myopia, retinal detachment, vitreous hemorrhage, conjunctival and ciliary erythema, lens opacities, obstructed nasolacrimal canals, paradoxical increased intraocular pressure, activation of latent iritis or uveitis, iris cysts (usually in children).
● GI: nausea, vomiting, increased gastric and intestinal secretions, epigastric pain, diarrhea, excessive salivation.
● GU: urinary urgency, incontinence.
● Respiratory: increased tracheobronchial secretions, bronchiolar constriction, *bronchospasm.*
● Other: allergic reaction, sweating.
  Note: Drug should be discontinued if hypersensitivity, difficulty breathing, incoordination, restlessness, agitation, or skin rash occurs.

Overdose and treatment
Clinical effects of overdose include headache, nausea, vomiting, diarrhea, blurred vision, miosis, myopia, excessive tearing, bronchospasm, increased bronchial secretions, hypotension, incoordination, excessive sweating, muscle weakness, bradycardia, excessive salivation, restlessness or agitation, and confusion.

Support respiration; bronchial suctioning may be performed. The drug should be discontinued immediately. Atropine may be given to block physostigmine's muscarinic effects. Avoid atropine overdose, because it may cause bronchial plug formation.

▶ Special considerations
Besides those relevant to all *cholinesterase inhibitors,* consider the following recommendations.
● Observe solution for discoloration. Do not use if darkened; contact pharmacist.
● Physostigmine sulfate injection has been used to reverse CNS depression caused by general anesthesia and drug overdose. However, this is an experimental use.

Ophthalmic
● Have patient lie down or tilt his head back to facilitate administration of eye drops.
● Wait at least 5 minutes before administering any other eye drops.
● Gently pinch patient's nasal bridge for 1 to 2 minutes after administering each dose of eye drops to minimize systemic absorption.
● After applying ointment, have patient close eyelids and roll eye.

Information for the patient
Ophthalmic
- Teach patient how to administer ophthalmic ointment or solution.
- Instruct patient not to close his eyes tightly or blink unnecessarily after instilling the ophthalmic solution.
- Warn patient that he may experience blurred vision and difficulty seeing after initial doses.
- Instruct patient to report abdominal cramps, diarrhea, or excessive salivation.
- Remind patient to wait 5 minutes (if using eye drops) or 10 minutes (if using ointment) before using another eye preparation.

Geriatric use
Use caution when administering physostigmine to elderly patients, because they may be more sensitive to the drug's effects.

Breast-feeding
Physostigmine may be excreted in breast milk, resulting in infant toxicity. Breast-feeding women should avoid this drug.

---

pilocarpine hydrochloride
Adsorbocarpine, Akarpine, Almocarpine, I-Pilopine, Isopto Carpine, Minims Pilocarpine*, Miocarpine*, Ocusert Pilo, Pilocar, Pilokair, Pilopine HS

pilocarpine nitrate
P.V. Carpine Liquifilm

- Pharmacologic classification: cholinergic agonist
- Therapeutic classification: miotic
- Pregnancy risk category C

How supplied
Available by prescription only
Pilocarpine hydrochloride
Solution: 0.25%, 0.5%, 1%, 2%, 3%, 4%, 5%, 6%, 8%, 10%
Gel: 4%
Releasing-system insert: 20 mcg/hr, 40 mcg/hr
Pilocarpine nitrate
Solution: 1%, 2%, 4%

Indications, route, and dosage
Chronic open-angle glaucoma; before, or instead of, emergency surgery in acute narrow-angle glaucoma
Adults and children: Instill 1 or 2 drops in eye b.i.d. to q.i.d.; or apply ½" ribbon of 4% gel (Pilopine HS) at h.s.
Alternatively, apply one Ocusert Pilo System (20 or 40 mcg/hour) q 7 days.
Emergency treatment of acute narrow-angle glaucoma
Adults and children: 1 drop of 2% solution q 5 minutes for three to six doses, followed by 1 drop q 1 to 3 hours until pressure is controlled.

Pharmacodynamics
Miotic action: Pilocarpine stimulates cholinergic receptors of the sphincter muscles of the iris, resulting in miosis. It also produces ciliary muscle contraction, resulting in accommodation with deepening of the anterior chamber, and vasodilation of conjunctival vessels of the outflow tract.

Pharmacokinetics
- *Absorption:* Pilocarpine drops act within 10 to 30 minutes, with peak effect at 2 to 4 hours. With the Ocusert Pilo System, 0.3 to 7 mg of pilocarpine are released during the initial 6-hour period; during the remainder of the 1-week insertion period, the release rate is within ± 20% of the rated value. Effect is seen in 1½ to 2 hours and is maintained for the 1-week life of the insertion.
- *Distribution:* Unknown.
- *Metabolism:* Unknown.
- *Excretion:* Duration of effect of pilocarpine drops is 4 to 6 hours.

Contraindications and precautions
Pilocarpine is contraindicated in patients with acute iritis or hypersensitivity to the drug or any of the preparation's components. It should be used cautiously in patients with acute cardiac failure, bronchial asthma, urinary tract obstruction, GI spasm, peptic ulcer, hyperthyroidism, or Parkinson's disease.

Interactions
When used concomitantly, pilocarpine can enhance reductions in intraocular pressure caused by epinephrine derivatives and timolol.
Demecarium, echothiophate, and isoflurophate decrease the pharmacologic effects of pilocarpine.

Effects on diagnostic tests
None reported.

Adverse reactions
- CNS: headache, syncope, tremors.
- CV: flushing, sweating, hypotension, bradycardia, *arrhythmias.*
- Eye: suborbital headache, myopia, burning, itching, ciliary spasm, blurred vision, conjunctival irritation, lacrimation, changes in visual field, brow pain.
- GI: nausea, vomiting, epigastric distress, abdominal cramps, diarrhea, salivation.
- GU: bladder tightness.
- Respiratory: asthma, *bronchospasm.*
Note: Drug should be discontinued if signs of systemic toxicity appear.

Overdose and treatment
Clinical manifestations of overdose include flushing, vomiting, bradycardia, bronchospasm, increased bronchial secretion, sweating, tearing, involuntary urination, hypotension, and tremors. Vomiting is usually spontaneous with accidental ingestion; if not, induce emesis and follow with activated charcoal or a cathartic. Treat dermal exposure by washing the areas twice with water. Use epinephrine to treat the cardiovascular responses. Atropine sulfate is the antidote of choice. Flush the eye with water or saline to treat a local overdose. Doses up to 20 mg are generally considered nontoxic.

▶ **Special considerations**
Drug may be used alone or with mannitol, urea, glycerol, or acetazolamide. It also may be used to counteract effects of mydriatic and cycloplegic agents after surgery or ophthalmoscopic examination and may be used alternately with atropine to break adhesions.

Information for the patient
● Warn patient that vision will be temporarily blurred, that miotic pupil may make surroundings appear dim and reduce peripheral field of vision, and that transient brow ache and myopia are common at first; assure patient that side effects subside 10 to 14 days after therapy begins.
● Instruct patient that if the Ocusert System falls out of the eye during sleep, he should wash hands, then rinse Ocusert in cool tap water and reposition it in the eye. Do not use the insert if it's deformed.
● Tell patient to use caution in night driving and other activities in poor illumination, because miotic pupil diminishes side vision and illumination.
● Stress importance of complying with prescribed medical regimen.
● Reassure patient that side effects will subside.
● Teach patient the correct way to instill drops and to apply light finger pressure on lacrimal sac for 1 minute after administration to minimize systemic absorption.
● Gel should be applied at bedtime because it will cause blurred vision.

---

pimozide
Orap

● Pharmacologic classification: diphenylbutylpiperidine
● Therapeutic classification: antipsychotic
● Pregnancy risk category C

How supplied
Available by prescription only
Tablets: 2 mg

Indications, route, and dosage
Suppression of severe motor and phonic tics in patients with Gilles de la Tourette's syndrome
Adults and children over age 12: Initially, 1 to 2 mg/day in divided doses. Then, increase dosage as needed every other day.
Maintenance dose: From 7 to 16 mg/day. Maximum dosage is 20 mg/day.

Pharmacodynamics
Antipsychotic action: Pimozide's mechanism of action in Gilles de la Tourette's syndrome is unknown: it is thought to exert its effects by postsynaptic and/or presynaptic blockade of CNS dopamine receptors, thus inhibiting dopamine-mediated effects. Pimozide also has anticholinergic, antiemetic, and anxiolytic effects and produces alpha blockade.

Pharmacokinetics
● *Absorption:* Pimozide is absorbed slowly and incompletely from the GI tract; bioavailability is about 50%. Peak plasma levels may occur from 4 to 12 hours (usually in 6 to 8 hours).

● *Distribution:* Pimozide is distributed widely into the body.
● *Metabolism:* Pimozide is metabolized by the liver; a significant first-pass effect exists.
● *Excretion:* About 40% of a given dose is excreted in urine as parent drug and metabolites in 3 to 4 days; about 15% is excreted in feces via the biliary tract within 3 to 6 days.

Contraindications and precautions
Pimozide is contraindicated in patients with known hypersensitivity to phenothiazines, thioxanthenes, haloperidol, and molindone; in patients with any form of mild or severe tic, including those induced by pemoline, methylphenidate, or amphetamines; in patients with arrhythmias because drug may cause ventricular arrhythmias or aggravate existing arrhythmias; in patients with congenital long Q-T syndrome because drug may cause conduction defects and sudden death; and in comatose states and CNS depression because of the risk of additive effects.

Pimozide should be used with extreme caution in patients taking antiarrhythmic drugs, tricyclic antidepressants, or other antipsychotic agents because additive effect may further depress cardiac conduction and prolong Q-T interval, and may induce arrhythmias. Use pimozide cautiously in patients with other cardiac disease (congestive heart failure, angina pectoris, valvular disease, or heart block), encephalitis, Reye's syndrome, hematologic disorders, epilepsy and other seizure disorders, glaucoma, prostatic hypertrophy, urine retention, hepatic or renal dysfunction, and Parkinson's disease because drug may worsen these conditions.

Interactions
Concomitant use of pimozide with quinidine, procainamide, disopyramide and other antiarrhythmics, phenothiazines, other antipsychotics, and antidepressants may further depress cardiac conduction and prolong Q-T interval, resulting in serious arrhythmias.

Concomitant use with anticonvulsants (phenytoin, carbamazepine, or phenobarbital) may induce seizures, even in patients previously stabilized on anticonvulsants; an anticonvulsant dosage increase may be required.

Concomitant use with amphetamines, methylphenidate, or pemoline may induce Tourette-like tic and may exacerbate existing tics.

Concomitant use with CNS depressants, including alcohol, analgesics, barbiturates, narcotics, anxiolytics, parenteral magnesium sulfate, tranquilizers, and general, spinal, or epidural anesthetics may cause oversedation and respiratory depression because of additive CNS depressant effects.

Effects on diagnostic tests
Pimozide causes quinidine-like ECG effects (including prolongation of Q-T interval and flattened T waves).

Adverse reactions
● CNS: parkinsonian symptoms, other extrapyramidal symptoms (dystonia, akathisia, hyperreflexia, opisthotonos, oculogyric crisis), tardive dyskinesia, sedation, headache, *neuroleptic malignant syndrome* (dose-related; fatal *respiratory failure* in over 10% of patients if untreated), *hyperpyrexia. Seizures and sudden death* have occurred with doses above 20 mg/day.
● CV: *ventricular arrhythmias* (rare), ECG changes (prolonged Q-T interval, hypotension).

- EENT: visual disturbances, photophobia.
- GI: dry mouth, constipation, nausea, vomiting, taste changes.
- GU: impotence.
- Other: muscle tightness.

Note: Drug should be discontinued immediately if hypersensitivity or neuroleptic malignant syndrome (marked hyperthermia, extrapyramidal effects, autonomic dysfunction) occurs; if severe extrapyramidal symptoms occur even after dose is lowered; if ventricular arrhythmias occur; or if Q-T interval is prolonged as follows: beyond 0.52 second in adults, beyond 0.47 second in children, or over 25% of patient's original baseline.

When feasible, drug should be withdrawn slowly and gradually; many drug effects persist after withdrawal.

Overdose and treatment
Clinical signs of overdose include severe extrapyramidal reactions, hypotension, respiratory depression, coma, and ECG abnormalities, including prolongation of Q-T interval, inversion or flattening of T waves, and/or new appearance of U waves.

Treat with gastric lavage to remove unabsorbed drug. Maintain blood pressure with I.V. fluids, plasma expanders, or norepinephrine. *Do not use epinephrine.*

Do not induce vomiting because of the potential for aspiration.

Treat extrapyramidal symptoms with parenteral diphenhydramine. Monitor for adverse effects for at least 4 days because of prolonged half-life (55 hours) of drug.

▶ **Special considerations**
- Elderly patients may be at greater risk for adverse cardiovascular effects.
- All patients should have have baseline ECGs before therapy begins and periodic ECGs thereafter to monitor cardiovascular effects.
- Patient's serum potassium level should be maintained within normal range at all times; decreased potassium concentrations increase risk of arrhythmias. Monitor potassium level in patients with diarrhea and those who are taking diuretics.
- Assess patient periodically for abnormal body movement.
- Extrapyramidal reactions develop in approximately 10% to 15% of patients at normal doses. They are especially likely to occur during early days of therapy.
- If excessive restlessness and agitation occur, therapy with a beta blocker, such as propranolol or metoprolol, may be helpful.

Information for the patient
- Inform patient of the risks, signs, and symptoms of dystonic reactions and tardive dyskinesia.
- Advise patient to take pimozide exactly as prescribed, not to double doses for missed doses, not to share drug with others, and not to stop taking it suddenly.
- Explain that pimozide's therapeutic effect may not be apparent for several weeks.
- Urge patient to report unusual effects promptly.
- Tell patient not to take pimozide with alcohol, sleeping medications, or any other drugs that may cause drowsiness without medical approval.
- Suggest using sugarless hard candy or chewing gum, ice chips, or artificial saliva to relieve dry mouth.
- To prevent dizziness at start of therapy, patient should lie down for 30 minutes after taking each dose and should avoid sudden changes in posture, especially when rising to upright position.
- To minimize daytime sedation, suggest taking entire daily dose at bedtime.
- Warn patient to avoid hazardous activities that require alertness until the drug's effects are known.

Geriatric use
Elderly patients are more likely to develop cardiac toxicity and tardive dyskinesia even at normal doses.

Pediatric use
Use and efficacy in children under age 12 are limited. Dosage should be kept at the lowest possible level. Use of the drug in children for any disorder other than Gilles de la Tourette's syndrome is not recommended.

---

pinacidil
Pindac

- **Pharmacologic classification: vasodilator**
- **Therapeutic classification: antihypertensive**
- **Pregnancy risk category B**

How supplied
Available by prescription only
Capsules: 12.5 mg, 25 mg

Indications, route, and dosage
Treatment of hypertension either alone or in combination with a diuretic and/or beta blocker
Adults: Initially, 12.5 mg P.O. b.i.d. If response is inadequate, a diuretic may be added. If response is still inadequate, increase dose of pinacidil to 25 mg. Doses above 25 mg are not recommended because of increased frequency of adverse reactions and little or no benefit to blood pressure response.

Decision to increase dose should be based on peak postdose blood pressure, which usually occurs 2 to 5 hours after dosing.

In mild hypertension, wait 1 to 2 weeks to see full effect of dosage. In elderly patients and in those with renal or hepatic dysfunction, the 12.5 mg dose is usually sufficient. In these patients, a 2- to 3-week interval is recommended before titration of dose.

If necessary, therapy may be stopped abruptly without special consideration. Blood pressure will return to pretreatment levels within several days.

Pharmacodynamics
Antihypertensive action: Pinacidil is a direct-acting arterial vasodilator, reducing diastolic and systolic blood pressure by decreasing peripheral vascular resistance. This effect may be mediated by its ability to modulate potassium ion channels in vascular smooth muscle, which causes increased renin excretion that leads to increased cardiac rate; increased cardiac output, cardiac work, and stroke volume; and fluid retention (manifested as increased plasma volume, peripheral edema, and, sometimes, worsened heart failure and pericardial effusion). Concomitant use of diuretics or beta blockers may reduce or offset these effects.

Pharmacokinetics
● *Absorption:* Pinacidil is completely absorbed after oral administration and provides peak plasma levels at 1 to 3 hours and again at 5 to 7 hours after administration because of its modified release formulation.
● *Distribution:* 60% is plasma protein-bound.
● *Metabolism:* About 20% undergoes first-pass metabolism in the liver. Pinacidil N-oxide is the active metabolite.
● *Excretion:* Within 24 hours, 55% is excreted in urine as other metabolites; 3%, in feces.

Contraindications and precautions
Contraindicated in patients with known hypersensitivity to the drug.

Use with caution in patients with coronary artery disease (CAD) because drug may exacerbate reflex tachycardia and angina. Do not use in patients with symptomatic CAD, recent MI, a history of dissecting aneurysm, significant cerebrovascular disease, or tachyarrhythmia. Use with caution in patients with migraine or other forms of vascular headache because condition may be worsened.

Interactions
Plasma clearance of pinacidil is increased by concomitant therapy with phenobarbital and decreased with cimetidine and probenecid.

Effects on diagnostic tests
Transient asymptomatic abnormalities in liver function tests, including AST (SGOT), ALT (SGPT), alkaline phosphatase, gamma-glutamyltransferase, and bilirubin have been reported, as well as small decreases in hemoglobin, transient symptomatic decreases in neutrophil counts, increases in serum creatinine and BUN levels (transient), and positive antinuclear antibody tests.

Adverse reactions
● CNS: headache, asthenia, malaise.
● CV: ECG changes, palpitations, tachycardia, vasodilation, vascular headache, syncope, orthostatic hypotension, chest pain.
● GI: nausea, diarrhea, dyspepsia, constipation, vomiting, flatulence, gastritis.
● Other: weight gain, fever, edema, hypokalemia, back pain, gout, weight loss.

Overdose and treatment
Hypotension and tachycardia can be expected. Supportive measures, such as volume expansion, vasopressors, and careful hemodynamic monitoring, are recommended. Hemodialysis may not be effective.

▶ Special considerations
● Drug may be discontinued abruptly.
● Abnormalities in liver function tests have been noted most often within first 3 to 4 months of therapy.
● Monitor patients closely – especially elderly patients and those with kidney or liver dysfunction – for signs and symptoms of fluid retention.
● Use capsules intact; they should *not* be opened, crushed, or mixed with foods or liquids for administration. Such usage may result in rapid absorption with excessive hypotension occurring shortly after administration. If this happens, place patient in the supine position, treat with fluids and vasopressor drugs, and provide careful hemodynamic monitoring.

Information for the patient
● Warn patient that dizziness may occur. Advise caution during exercise and any potentially hazardous tasks until extent of adverse effect is known.
● Advise patient to sit or lie down if signs of low blood pressure occur and to notify physician.
● Tell patient to notify physician immediately if substernal chest pain or tightness in chest develops, and if edema or weight gain occurs, especially if accompanied by shortness of breath.
● Advise patient not to open capsules but to take them intact.

Geriatric use
Elderly patients may be more sensitive to the effects of the drug. Dosage adjustments may be necessary.

Pediatric use
Safety and efficacy have not been established.

Breast-feeding
It is unknown if pinacidil is excreted in breast milk. Potential risk of serious adverse reactions in infants must be considered.

---

pindolol
Visken

● Pharmacologic classification: beta-adrenergic blocking agent
● Therapeutic classification: antihypertensive
● Pregnancy risk category B

How supplied
Available by prescription only
Tablets: 5 mg, 10 mg

Indications, route, and dosage
Hypertension
Adults: Initially, 5 mg P.O. b.i.d. increased by 10 mg/day every 3 to 4 weeks up to a maximum of 60 mg/day. Usual dosage is 10 to 30 mg daily, given in two or three divided doses. In some patients, once-daily dosing may be possible.
Angina
Adults: 15 to 40 mg daily P.O. in three or four divided doses.

Pharmacodynamics
Antihypertensive action: The exact mechanism of hypertensive action is unknown. Pindolol does not consistently affect cardiac output or renin release, and its other mechanisms, such as decreased peripheral resistance, probably contribute to its hypotensive effect. Because pindolol has some intrinsic sympathomimetic activity – that is, beta-agonist sympathomimetic activity – it may be useful in patients who develop bradycardia with other beta-blocking agents. It is a nonselective beta-blocking agent, inhibiting both $beta_1$ and $beta_2$ receptors.

Pharmacokinetics
● *Absorption:* After oral administration, pindolol is absorbed rapidly from the GI tract; peak plasma concentrations occur in 1 to 2 hours. Pindolol's effect on the

heart rate usually occurs in 3 hours. Food does not reduce bioavailability but may increase the rate of GI absorption.

• *Distribution:* Pindolol is distributed widely throughout the body and is 40% to 60% protein-bound.

• *Metabolism:* About 60% to 65% of a given dose of pindolol is metabolized by the liver.

• *Excretion:* In adults with normal renal function, 35% to 50% of a given dose of pindolol is excreted unchanged in urine; half-life is about 3 to 4 hours. Pindolol's antihypertensive effect usually persists for 24 hours.

Contraindications and precautions

Pindolol is contraindicated in patients with known hypersensitivity to the drug; and in patients with severe bradycardia, overt cardiac failure, second- or third-degree atrioventricular block, or bronchial asthma because the drug may worsen these conditions.

Pindolol should be used cautiously in patients with impaired hepatic or renal function or coronary insufficiency because beta-adrenergic blockade may precipitate congestive heart failure (CHF); in patients with hyperthyroidism or diabetes mellitus because the drug may mask tachycardia; in patients undergoing general anesthesia because severe hypotension or bradycardia may develop; and in patients with emphysema or other pulmonary disease.

Interactions

Concomitant use with digoxin may transiently decrease serum digoxin level.

Pindolol may potentiate the antihypertensive effects of other antihypertensive agents.

Effects on diagnostic tests

Pindolol may elevate serum transaminase, alkaline phosphatase, lactic dehydrogenase, and uric acid levels.

Adverse reactions

• CNS: insomnia, fatigue, dizziness, nervousness, vivid dreams, hallucinations, lethargy.

• CV: edema, bradycardia, *CHF*, peripheral vascular disease, hypotension.

• DERM: rash.

• EENT: visual disturbances.

• GI: nausea, vomiting, diarrhea.

• Metabolic: hypoglycemia without tachycardia.

• Other: *bronchospasm;* muscle, joint, and chest pain.

   Note: Drug should be discontinued if signs of cardiac failure develop.

Overdose and treatment

Clinical signs of overdose include severe hypotension, bradycardia, heart failure, and bronchospasm.

After acute ingestion, empty stomach by induced emesis or gastric lavage, and give activated charcoal to reduce absorption. Subsequent treatment is usually symptomatic and supportive.

▶ Special considerations

Besides those relevant to all *beta-adrenergic blocking agents,* consider the following recommendation.

• Maximum therapeutic response may not be seen for 2 weeks or more.

Geriatric use

Elderly patients may require lower maintenance doses of pindolol because of increased bioavailability or delayed metabolism; they also may experience enhanced adverse effects. The half-life of pindolol may be increased in elderly patients.

Pediatric use

Safety and efficacy of pindolol in children have not been established; use only if potential benefit outweighs risk.

Breast-feeding

Pindolol passes into breast milk; an alternative feeding method is recommended during therapy.

---

pipecuronium bromide
Arduan

• Pharmacologic classification: nondepolarizing neuromuscular blocking agent
• Therapeutic classification: skeletal muscle relaxant
• Pregnancy risk category C

How supplied

Available by prescription only
Injection: 10 mg/vial

Indications, route, and dosage
To provide skeletal muscle relaxation during surgery as a adjunct to general anesthesia
Adults and children: Dosage is highly individualized. The following doses may serve as a guide, assuming that the patient is not obese and has normal renal function. Initially, doses of 70 to 85 mcg/kg I.V. are used to provide conditions considered ideal for endotracheal intubation and will maintain paralysis for 1 to 2 hours. If succinylcholine is used for endotracheal intubation, initial doses of 50 mcg/kg will provide good relaxation for 45 minutes or more. Maintenance doses of 10 to 15 mcg/kg provide relaxation for about 50 minutes.
Dosage adjustments for patients in renal failure

Creatinine clearance (ml/minute)	Dose (mcg/kg)
100	85
80	70
60	55
40	50

Pharmacodynamics

Muscle relaxant action: Like other nondepolarizing muscle relaxants, pipecuronium competes with acetylcholine for receptor sites at the motor end-plate. Because this action may be antagonized by cholinesterase inhibitors, it is considered a competitive antagonist.

Pharmacokinetics

• *Absorption:* No information is available regarding the use of the drug by any route other than I.V. Maximum onset of action occurs within 5 minutes.

• *Distribution:* Volume of distribution (V_D) is about 0.25

---

liters/kg and increases in patients with renal failure. Other conditions associated with increased V_D (including edema, old age, and cardiovascular disease) may delay onset.

• *Metabolism:* Only about 20% to 40% of an administered dose is metabolized, probably in the liver. One metabolite (3-desacetyl pipecuronium) has about 50% of the neuromuscular blocking activity of the parent drug.

• *Excretion:* Primarily renal. In preliminary studies, the half-life of the drug has been estimated at 1.7 hours; it may increase to 4 hours or more in patients with severe renal disease.

Contraindications and precautions

There are no known contraindications to the use of the drug. However, this drug should be used only under direct medical supervision by personnel familiar with the use of neuromuscular blocking agents and techniques involved in maintaining a patent airway. It should not be used unless facilities and equipment for artificial respiration, mechanical ventilation, oxygen therapy, and intubation and an antagonist are within reach.

Because of the lack of data supporting safety, this drug is not recommended for use in patients requiring prolonged mechanical ventilation in the intensive care unit. It is not recommended before or after use of other nondepolarizing neuromuscular blocking agents. It is also not recommended for use during cesarean section because safety to the neonate has not been established; moreover, this drug's long duration of action exceeds the duration of the procedure.

Because the drug is excreted by the kidneys, use with caution in patients with renal failure. No information is available regarding the use of the drug in patients with hepatic disease.

Patients with myasthenia gravis or myasthenic syndrome (Eaton-Lambert syndrome) are particularly sensitive to the effects of nondepolarizing relaxants. Shorter-acting agents are recommended for use in such patients.

Because the drug has minimal vagolytic action, bradycardia during anesthesia may be common, especially when administered with high doses of opioid narcotics for the induction and maintenance of anesthesia.

A nerve stimulator and train-of-four (T4) monitoring is recommended to document antagonism of neuromuscular blockade and recovery of muscle strength. Before pharmacologic reversal with neostigmine is attempted, some evidence of spontaneous recovery (T4/T1 ratio > 0, or T1 > 10% of control) should be evident. Reversal with edrophonium is not recommended due to its short duration of action in comparison to neostigmine.

Interactions

Concomitant parenteral or intraperitoneal administration of certain antibiotics in high doses has been associated with muscle weakness; this weakness may worsen in the presence of a nondepolarizing neuromuscular blocking agent. These antibiotics include aminoglycosides (kanamycin, neomycin, streptomycin, dihydrostreptomycin, and gentamicin), bacitracin, colistin, polymyxin B, sodium colistimethate, and tetracyclines.

Some volatile inhalational anesthetics may intensify or prolong the action of nondepolarizing neuromuscular blocking agents.

Concomitant use with quinidine may prolong the action of nondepolarizing neuromuscular blocking agents. Use with magnesium salts, such as those used for treatment of toxemia of pregnancy, may enhance and prolong neuromuscular blockade.

Experimental evidence suggests that acid-base balance may influence the actions of pipecuronium. Alkalosis may counteract the paralysis and acidosis may enhance it. Electrolyte disturbances may also influence response.

Pipecuronium may be administered after succinylcholine when the latter is used to facilitate intubation. There is no evidence to support the safe use of pipecuronium before succinylcholine to decrease adverse effects of the latter drug. Concomitant use with other nondepolarizing neuromuscular blocking agents is not recommended.

Effects on diagnostic tests

None reported.

Adverse reactions

• CV: hypotension, bradycardia, hypertension, *myocardial ischemia, cerebrovascular accident,* thrombosis, atrial fibrillation, ventricular extrasystole.
• GU: anuria.
• Metabolic: increased creatinine levels.
• Respiratory: dyspnea, respiratory depression, *respiratory insufficiency or apnea.*
• Other: prolonged muscle weakness.

Overdose and treatment

No cases have been reported. Provide supportive treatment, and ventilate patient as necessary. Closely monitor vital signs.

Antagonists such as neostigmine should not be used until there is some evidence of spontaneous recovery of neuromuscular function. A nerve stimulator is recommended to document antagonism of neuromuscular blockade.

▶ Special considerations

• Because of its prolonged duration of action, pipecuronium is recommended only for procedures that take 90 minutes or longer.
• Dosage should be adjusted to ideal body weight in obese patients.
• Store the powder at room temperature or in the refrigerator (36° to 86° F [2° to 30° C]).
• Reconstitute with 10 ml solution before use to yield a solution of 1 mg/ml. Large volumes of diluent or addition of the drug to a hanging I.V. solution is not recommended.
• When reconstituted with sterile water for injection or other compatible I.V. solutions, such as 0.9% sodium chloride injection, dextrose 5% in water, lactated Ringer's injection, and dextrose 5% in saline, the drug is stable for 24 hours if refrigerated.
• If reconstituted with any solution other than bacteriostatic water for injection, unused portions of the drug should be discarded.
• When reconstituted with bacteriostatic water for injection, the drug is stable for 5 days at room temperature or in the refrigerator. Note that bacteriostatic water contains benzyl alcohol and is not intended for use in neonates.
• Clinical trials have shown that edrophonium 0.5 mg/kg was not as effective as neostigmine 0.04 mg/kg in reversing the effects of pipecuronium. Higher doses of

edrophonium and pyridostigmine have not been studied.

Pediatric use
Not recommended for use in children younger than age 3 months. Limited evidence suggests that children (age 1 to 14 years) under balanced anesthesia or halothane anesthesia may be less sensitive than adults.

Breast-feeding
There is no information regarding the distribution of pipecuronium into breast milk. Use with caution in breast-feeding women.

---

piperacillin sodium
Pipracil

- Pharmacologic classification: extended-spectrum penicillin, acyclaminopenicillin
- Therapeutic classification: antibiotic
- Pregnancy risk category B

How supplied
Available by prescription only
Injection: 2 g, 3 g, 4 g
Infusion: 2 g, 3 g, 4 g
Pharmacy bulk package: 40 g

Indications, route, and dosage
Infections caused by susceptible organisms
Adults and children over age 12: 100 to 300 mg/kg/day divided q 4 to 6 hours I.V. or I.M. Usual dosage is 3 g q 4 hours (18 g/day) and it is usually administered with an aminoglycoside. Maximum daily dosage is usually 24 g. Dosage for children under age 12 has not been established.
Prophylaxis of surgical infections
Adults: 2 g I.V., given 30 to 60 minutes before surgery. Depending on type of surgery, dose may be repeated during surgery and once or twice after surgery according to the manufacturer. However, clinicians strongly discourage this practice.
Dosage in renal failure

DOSAGE IN ADULTS			
Creatinine clearance (ml/min/1.73 m²)	Urinary tract infection uncomplicated	Urinary tract infection complicated	Serious systemic infection
>40	*	*	*
20 to 40	*	3g q 8 hr	4g q 8 hr
<20	3g q 12 hr	3g q 12 hr	4g q 12 hr

*no dosage adjustment necessary

Pharmacodynamics
Antibiotic action: Piperacillin is bactericidal; it adheres to bacterial penicillin-binding proteins, thus inhibiting bacterial cell wall synthesis.

Extended-spectrum penicillins are more resistant to inactivation by certain beta-lactamases, especially those produced by gram-negative organisms, but are still liable to inactivation by certain others. Because of the potential for rapid development of bacterial resistance, it should not be used as a sole agent in the treatment of an infection.

Piperacillin's spectrum of activity includes many gram-negative aerobic and anaerobic bacilli, many gram-positive and gram-negative aerobic cocci, and some gram-positive aerobic and anaerobic bacilli. Piperacillin may be effective against some strains of carbenicillin-resistant and ticarcillin-resistant gram-negative bacilli. Piperacillin is more active against *Pseudomonas aeruginosa* than is mezlocillin and more active against *Enterobacteriaceae* than is azlocillin.

Pharmacokinetics
- *Absorption:* Peak plasma concentrations occur 30 to 50 minutes after an I.M. dose.
- *Distribution:* Piperacillin is distributed widely after parenteral administration. It penetrates minimally into uninflamed meninges and slightly into bone and sputum. Piperacillin is 16% to 22% protein-bound; it crosses the placenta.
- *Metabolism:* Piperacillin is probably not significantly metabolized.
- *Excretion:* Piperacillin is excreted primarily (42% to 90%) in urine by renal tubular secretion and glomerular filtration; it is also excreted in bile and in breast milk. Elimination half-life in adults is about ½ to 1½ hours; in extensive renal impairment, half-life is extended to about 2 to 6 hours; in combined hepatorenal dysfunction, half-life may extend from 11 to 32 hours. Piperacillin is removed by hemodialysis but not by peritoneal dialysis.

Contraindications and precautions
Piperacillin is contraindicated in patients with known hypersensitivity to any other penicillin or to cephalosporins.

Piperacillin should be used cautiously in patients with renal impairment because it is excreted in urine; decreased dosage is required in moderate to severe renal failure. Use with caution in patients with bleeding tendencies, uremia, or hypokolemia.

Interactions
Concomitant use of piperacillin with aminoglycoside antibiotics results in synergistic bactericidal effects against *Pseudomonas aeruginosa, Escherichia coli, Klebsiella, Citrobacter, Enterobacter, Serratia,* and *Proteus mirabilis.* However, the drugs are physically and chemically incompatible and are inactivated when mixed or given together. In vivo inactivation has been reported when aminoglycosides and extended-spectrum penicillins are used concomitantly.

Concomitant use of piperacillin (and other extended-spectrum penicillins) with clavulanic acid also produces a synergistic bactericidal effect against certain beta-lactamase-producing bacteria.

Probenecid blocks tubular secretion of piperacillin, raising serum concentrations of drug.

Large doses of penicillins may interfere with renal tubular secretion of methotrexate, thus delaying elimination and elevating serum concentrations of methotrexate.

Effects on diagnostic tests
Piperacillin may falsely decrease serum aminoglycoside concentrations. Piperacillin may cause hypokalemia and hypernatremia and may prolong prothrombin

---

times; it may also cause transient elevations in liver function studies and transient reductions in red blood cell, white blood cell, and platelet counts.

Piperacillin may cause positive Coombs' tests.

Adverse reactions
● CNS: neuromuscular irritability, headache, dizziness.
● GI: nausea, diarrhea, vomiting.
● GU: *acute interstitial nephritis.*
● HEMA: *bleeding with high doses,* neutropenia, eosinophilia, leukopenia, *thrombocytopenia.*
● Metabolic: *hypokalemia.*
● Local: pain at injection site, vein irritation, phlebitis.
● Other: *hypersensitivity reactions* (edema, fever, chills, rash, pruritus, urticaria, *anaphylaxis*), bacterial and fungal superinfections.

Note: Drug should be discontinued if immediate hypersensitivity reactions occur, if bleeding complications occur, or if severe diarrhea occurs, as this may indicate pseudomembranous colitis.

Overdose and treatment
Clinical signs of overdose include neuromuscular hypersensitivity or seizures resulting from CNS irritation by high drug concentrations. A 4- to 6-hour hemodialysis will remove 10% to 50% of piperacillin.

▶ Special considerations
Besides those relevant to all *penicillins,* consider the following recommendations.
● Piperacillin is almost always used with another antibiotic, such as an aminoglycoside, in life-threatening situations.
● Piperacillin may be more suitable than carbenicillin or ticarcillin for patients on salt-free diets; piperacillin contains only 1.85 mEq of sodium per gram.
● Piperacillin may be administered by direct I.V. injection, given slowly over at least 5 minutes; chest discomfort occurs if injection is given too rapidly.
● Patients with cystic fibrosis are most susceptible to fever or rash from piperacillin.
● Monitor serum electrolytes, especially potassium.
● Monitor neurologic status. High serum levels of this drug may cause seizures.
● Reduced dosage is necessary in patients with creatinine clearance below 40 ml/minute.
● Monitor complete blood count, differential, and platelets. Drug may cause thrombocytopenia. Observe patient carefully for signs of occult bleeding.
● Because piperacillin is dialyzable, patients undergoing hemodialysis may need dosage adjustments.

Geriatric use
Half-life may be prolonged in elderly patients because of impaired renal function.

Pediatric use
Safe use of piperacillin in children under age 12 has not been established.

Breast-feeding
Piperacillin is excreted in breast milk; drug should be used with caution in breast-feeding women.

piperazine citrate
Antepar, Vermizine

● Pharmacologic classification: piperazine
● Therapeutic classification: anthelmintic
● Pregnancy risk category B

How supplied
Available by prescription only
Tablets: 250 mg
Syrup: 500 mg/5 ml

Indications, route, and dosage
Pinworm infections
Adults and children: 65 mg/kg P.O. daily for 7 days. Maximum daily dosage is 2.5 g. Repeat treatment course after 1-week interval in severe infection.
Roundworm infections
Adults: 3.5 g P.O. in single doses for 2 consecutive days.
Children: 75 mg/kg P.O. daily in single doses for 2 consecutive days. Maximum daily dosage is 3.5 g.

Pharmacodynamics
Anthelmintic action: Piperazine blocks the stimulatory effects of acetylcholine at the neuromuscular junction of *Ascaris lumbricoides* (roundworm); it also inhibits succinate production, causing paralysis in the parasite. The mechanism of action against *Enterobius vermicularis* (pinworm) is unknown.

Pharmacokinetics
● *Absorption:* Piperazine is absorbed readily from the GI tract.
● *Distribution:* Distribution of piperazine has not been adequately described.
● *Metabolism:* Piperazine is metabolized partially (25%) by the liver.
● *Excretion:* Most of an administered dose is excreted unchanged in the urine within 24 hours. It is unknown if piperazine is excreted in breast milk.

Contraindications and precautions
Piperazine is contraindicated in patients with known sensitivity to piperazine compounds; in patients with impaired renal or hepatic function; and in patients with seizure disorders because it can exacerbate seizures.

Piperazine should be used with caution in patients with severe malnutrition. Also use cautiously in patients with anemia because drug can cause hemolytic anemia.

Interactions
Concomitant use with chlorpromazine may precipitate seizures; concomitant use with chlorpromazine or other tranquilizers may exaggerate extrapyramidal symptoms. Piperazine antagonizes the effects of pyrantel pamoate.

Effects on diagnostic tests
Piperazine may cause electroencephalogram (EEG) changes, particularly in children; it may also interfere with serum uric acid measurements, leading to falsely low values.

Adverse reactions
● CNS: ataxia, tremors, choreiform movements, muscular weakness, myoclonus, hyporeflexia, paresthesias, *seizures*, sense of detachment, EEG abnormalities, memory defect, headache, vertigo.
● DERM: urticaria, photodermatitis, *erythema multiforme*, purpura, eczematous skin reactions.
● EENT: nystagmus, blurred vision, paralytic strabismus, cataracts with visual impairment, lacrimation, difficulty in focusing, rhinorrhea, cough.
● GI: nausea, vomiting, diarrhea, abdominal cramps.
● HEMA: *hemolytic anemia.*
● Other: arthralgia, fever, *bronchospasm.*
   Note: Drug should be discontinued if significant GI or hypersensitivity reactions occur.

Overdose and treatment
Overdose may cause nausea, vomiting, confusion, weakness, ataxia, seizures, and coma. Treatment includes gastric lavage, followed by activated charcoal and cathartics. Seizures should be managed initially with diazepam; phenytoin or phenobarbital should be reserved for refractory seizures. Monitor fluid and electrolyte balance.

▶ Special considerations
● Piperazine may be taken with food but is most effective when taken on an empty stomach.
● Worm specimens are best obtained in early morning on arising.
● Laxatives, enemas, or dietary restrictions are unnecessary.
● Protect drug from light, air, and moisture.

Information for the patient
● Warn patient not to exceed recommended dosage because of hazard of neurotoxicity at high doses.
● Tell patient to discontinue drug and to report CNS, GI, or hypersensitivity reactions.
● Teach patient and family members personal hygiene measures to prevent reinfection: washing perianal area daily, changing undergarments and bedclothes daily, washing hands and cleaning fingernails before meals and after defecation, and sanitary disposal of feces.
● Explain that transmission can occur by direct or indirect transfer of ova by hands, food, or contaminated articles and that washing clothes in a household washing machine will destroy ova.

Geriatric use
Elderly patients are susceptible to extrapyramidal symptoms.

Pediatric use
Avoid prolonged treatment or repeated treatment in excess of recommended dosage because of hazard of neurotoxicity; therapeutic dosages have caused EEG changes in children.

Breast-feeding
Safety has not been established.

pipobroman
Vercyte

● Pharmacologic classification: alkylating agent
● Therapeutic classification: antineoplastic agent
● Pregnancy risk category D

How supplied
Available by prescription only
Tablets: 25 mg

Indications, route, and dosage
Dosage and indications may vary. Check current literature for recommended protocol.
Polycythemia vera
Adults and children over age 15: 1 mg/kg P.O. daily for 30 days; may increase to 1.5 to 3 mg/kg P.O. daily until hematocrit reduced to 50% to 55%, then 0.1 to 0.2 mg/kg daily maintenance.
Chronic myelocytic leukemia
Adults and children over age 15: 1.5 to 2.5 mg/kg P.O. daily until WBC count drops to 10,000/mm³, then start maintenance 7 mg to 175 mg daily. Stop drug if WBC count falls below 3,000/mm³ or platelets fall below 150,000/mm³.

Pharmacodynamics
Alkylating action: Although classified as an alkylating agent, the exact mechanism of action is unknown.

Pharmacokinetics
● *Absorption:* After oral administration, pipobroman is absorbed readily from the GI tract.
● *Distribution:* Unknown.
● *Metabolism:* Unknown.
● *Excretion:* Unknown.

Contraindications and precautions
Pipobroman is contraindicated in patients with bone marrow depression resulting from X-ray or cytotoxic chemotherapy because of potential for additive bone marrow depression.

Interactions
Use cautiously in patients taking anticoagulants, and monitor for bleeding.

Effects on diagnostic tests
None reported.

Adverse reactions
● DERM: rash.
● GI: nausea, vomiting, abdominal cramps, diarrhea.
● HEMA: leukopenia, anemia, thrombocytopenia.
   Note: Drug should be discontinued if adverse reactions are persistent.

Overdose and treatment
No information available.

▶ Special considerations
● Administer in daily divided doses.
● Before therapy begins and periodically thereafter, liver and kidney function tests should be performed.

• Do complete blood counts once or twice a week and leukocyte counts every other day until desired result is obtained or toxic effects appear.
• Bone marrow studies should be performed before treatment and at time of maximal hematologic response. Bone marrow depression may not occur for 4 weeks or more after initiation of treatment. Leukocyte count is the most reliable index of bone marrow activity, but platelet count is also a helpful guide. Temporarily discontinue treatment if leukocyte count is less than 3,000/mm³ or if platelet count is less than 150,000/mm³. Treatment may be reinstated cautiously once counts rise.
• Dose-dependent anemia frequently develops. Dose reduction and blood transfusions usually reverse the anemia. Anemia caused by a hemolytic process is marked by a rapid drop in hemoglobin, increased bilirubin levels, and reticulocytosis. In this case, the drug should be discontinued.

Information for the patient
• Caution patient to call if nausea, vomiting, diarrhea, abdominal cramps, or skin rash become pronounced.
• Advise patient to use contraceptive measures during therapy.

Pediatric use
Drug is not recommended for children under age 15.

---

pirbuterol acetate
Maxair

• Pharmacologic classification: beta-adrenergic agonist
• Therapeutic classification: bronchodilator
• Pregnancy risk category C

How supplied
Available by prescription only
Inhaler: 0.2 mg per inhalation

Indications, route, and dosage
Prevention and reversal of bronchospasm; asthma
Adults: 1 or 2 inhalations (0.2 to 0.4 mg) repeated every 4 to 6 hours. Not to exceed 12 inhalations daily.

Pharmacodynamics
Bronchodilating action: Pirbuterol stimulates beta$_2$-adrenergic receptors and increases the activity of intracellular adenylate cyclase, and enzyme that catalyzes the conversion of adenosine triphosphate (ATP) to cyclic adenosine monophosphate (cAMP). Elevated cellular cAMP is associated with bronchodilation and inhibition of the cellular release of mediators of immediate hypersensitivity.

Pharmacokinetics
• *Absorption:* Negligible serum levels are achieved after inhalation of the usual dose.
• *Distribution:* Pirbuterol acts locally.
• *Metabolism:* Hepatic.
• *Excretion:* About 50% of an inhaled dose is recovered in the urine as the parent drug and metabolites.

Contraindications and precautions
Contraindicated in patients allergic to pirbuterol or other adrenergics, in patients with digitalis toxicity, and in patients with cardiac arrhythmias associated with tachycardia.
    Beta-adrenergic agonists may cause significant cardiovascular effects, as well as paradoxical bronchospasm in some patients.
    Administer cautiously to patients with a history of exaggerated responses to sympathetic amines, and to patients with a history of convulsive disorders.

Interactions
Propranolol and other beta-adrenergic blocking agents may decrease the bronchodilating effects of beta agonists. Administer cautiously to patients receiving monoamine oxidase (MAO) inhibitors or tricyclic antidepressants, because these agents may enhance the vascular effects of beta-adrenergic agonists.

Effects on diagnostic tests
None reported.

Adverse reactions
• CNS: tremors, nervousness, dizziness, insomnia, headache.
• CV: tachycardia, palpitations, increased blood pressure.
• EENT: drying or irritation of throat.

Overdose and treatment
Anginal pain, hypertension and tachycardia may result from overdose. Treatment is generally supportive. Sedatives or barbiturates may be necessary to counter any adverse CNS effects; cautious use of beta blockers may be useful to counter cardiac effects.

▶ Special considerations
Besides those relevant to all *adrenergics*, consider the following recommendation.
• Do not administer to patients who are receiving other beta-adrenergic bronchodilators.

Information for the patient
• Warn patient not to exceed the recommended maximum dose of 12 inhalations daily. He should seek medical attention if a previously effective dosage does not control symptoms because this may signify a worsening of the disease.
• Tell patient to call promptly if he experiences increased bronchospasm after using the drug.
• Teach patient how to use metered dose inhaler correctly. Have him shake container, exhale through the nose; administer aerosol while inhaling deeply on mouthpiece of inhaler; hold breath for a few seconds, then exhale slowly. Tell him to allow at least 2 minutes between inhalations, and to wait at least 5 minutes before using his steroid inhalant (if he's taking concomitant inhalational corticosteroids).

Pediatric use
Use in children under age 12 is not recommended.

Breast-feeding
It is not known if pirbuterol is excreted in breast milk. Use with caution in breast-feeding women.

---

piroxicam
Apo-piroxicam*, Feldene,
Novopirocam*

- Pharmacologic classification: nonsteroidal anti-inflammatory
- Therapeutic classification: nonnarcotic analgesic, antipyretic, anti-inflammatory
- Pregnancy risk category D

How supplied
Available by prescription only
Capsules: 10 mg, 20 mg

Indications, route, and dosage
Osteoarthritis and rheumatoid arthritis
Adults: 20 mg P.O. once daily. If desired, the dose may be divided.
Elderly patients over age 60: Initial dose should be 10 mg daily.

Pharmacodynamics
Analgesic, antipyretic, and anti-inflammatory actions: The exact mechanisms of action are unknown, but piroxicam is thought to inhibit prostaglandin synthesis.

Pharmacokinetics
- *Absorption:* Piroxicam is absorbed rapidly from the GI tract. The peak effect is seen 3 to 5 hours after dosing. Food delays absorption.
- *Distribution:* Piroxicam is highly protein-bound.
- *Metabolism:* The drug is metabolized in the liver.
- *Excretion:* Piroxicam is excreted in urine. Its long half-life (about 50 hours) allows for once-daily dosing.

Contraindications and precautions
Piroxicam is contraindicated in patients with known hypersensitivity to this drug, and in patients in whom aspirin or other nonsteroidal anti-inflammatory drugs (NSAIDs) induce symptoms of asthma, urticaria, or rhinitis.

Serious GI toxicity, especially ulceration or hemorrhage, can occur at any time in patients on chronic NSAID therapy. Piroxicam should be used cautiously in patients with a history of peptic ulcer disease, angioedema, or cardiac disease, because the drug may worsen these conditions; and in patients with decreased renal function because it may cause a further reduction in renal function.

Patients with known "triad" symptoms (aspirin hypersensitivity, rhinitis/nasal polyps, and asthma) are at high risk of bronchospasm. NSAIDs may mask the signs and symptoms of acute infection (fever, myalgia, erythema); carefully evaluate patients with high risk (such as those with diabetes).

Interactions
Concomitant use of piroxicam with anticoagulants and thrombolytic drugs (coumarin derivatives, heparin, streptokinase, or urokinase) may potentiate anticoagulant effects. Bleeding problems may occur if used with other drugs that inhibit platelet aggregation, such as azlocillin, parenteral carbenicillin, dextran, dipyridamole, mezlocillin, piperacillin, sulfinpyrazone, ticarcillin, valproic acid, cefamandole, cefoperazone, moxalactam, plicamycin, aspirin, salicylates, or other anti-inflammatory agents. Concomitant use with salicylates, anti-inflammatory agents, alcohol, corticotropin, or steroids may cause increased GI adverse effects, including ulceration and hemorrhage. Aspirin may decrease the bioavailability of piroxicam. Because of the influence of prostaglandins on glucose metabolism, concomitant use with insulin on oral hypoglycemic agents may potentiate hypoglycemic effects.

Piroxicam may displace highly protein-bound drugs from binding sites. Toxicity may occur with coumarin derivatives, phenytoin, verapamil, or nifedipine. Increased nephrotoxicity may occur with gold compounds, other anti-inflammatory agents, or acetaminophen. Piroxicam may decrease the renal clearance of methotrexate and lithium. Piroxicam may decrease the effectiveness of antihypertensive agents and diuretics. Concomitant use with diuretics may increase risk of nephrotoxicity.

Effects on diagnostic tests
The physiologic effects of the drug may prolong bleeding time (may persist for 2 weeks after discontinuing drug); increase BUN, creatinine, and potassium levels or prothrombin time; decrease serum glucose (in diabetic patients), hemoglobin, hematocrit, or uric acid levels; and increase liver function test (alkaline phosphatase, lactic dehydrogenase, or transaminase levels).

Adverse reactions
- CNS: headache, drowsiness, malaise, vertigo, dizziness.
- CV: peripheral edema.
- DERM: pruritus, rash, urticaria, bruising, erythema, photosensitivity.
- EENT: blurred vision, tinnitus.
- GI: epigastric distress, nausea, vomiting, *severe GI bleeding*, diarrhea, constipation, anorexia, flatulence, indigestion, occult blood loss.
- GU: hematuria, proteinuria, nephrotoxicity.
- HEMA: prolonged bleeding time, anemia.
- Other: elevated liver enzymes, hepatotoxicity.
  Note: Drug should be discontinued if hypersensitivity or hepatotoxicity occurs.

Overdose and treatment
To treat piroxicam overdose, empty stomach immediately by inducing emesis with ipecac syrup or by gastric lavage. Administer activated charcoal via nasogastric tube. Provide symptomatic and supportive measures (respiratory support and correction of fluid and electrolyte imbalances). Monitor laboratory parameters and vital signs closely.

▶ Special considerations
Besides those relevant to all *NSAIDs*, consider the following recommendations.
- Drug is usually administered as a single dose.
- Adverse skin reactions are more common with piroxicam than with other NSAIDs; photosensitivity reactions are the most common.
- Effectiveness of piroxicam usually is not seen for at least 2 weeks after therapy begins. Evaluate response to drug as evidenced by reduced symptoms.

Information for the patient
- Advise patient to seek medical approval before taking any nonprescription medications.
- Caution patient to avoid hazardous activities requir-

ing alertness until CNS effects are known. Instruct patient in safety measures to prevent injury.
● Instruct patient in signs and symptoms of adverse effects. Tell patient to report them immediately.
● Encourage patient to comply with recommended medical follow-up.

Geriatric use
● Patients over age 60 are more sensitive to the adverse effects of piroxicam. Use with caution.
● Through its effect on renal prostaglandins, piroxicam may cause fluid retention and edema. This may be significant in elderly patients and those with congestive heart failure.

Pediatric use
The safe use of long-term piroxicam in children has not been established.

Breast-feeding
Piroxicam may inhibit lactation. Because piroxicam is distributed into breast milk at 1% of maternal serum concentration, an alternative feeding method should be considered during therapy with piroxicam. Avoid use in breast-feeding women.

PHARMACOLOGIC CLASS

pituitary hormones, posterior

**desmopressin acetate
lypressin
oxytocin
posterior pituitary hormone
vasopressin (antidiuretic hormone)**

In 1954, the structure of antidiuretic hormone (ADH) was determined and its synthesis achieved. The following year, duVigneaud was awarded the Nobel prize for his work. The drugs in this class are used to treat postoperative ileus, diabetes insipidus, and upper GI hemorrhage and to stimulate expulsion of gas before pyelography. Oxytocin is used in labor and delivery.

Pharmacology
Endogenous vasopressin and oxytocin are secreted by the hypothalamus and stored in the posterior pituitary. Vasopressin is found in all mammals except swine. Lypressin, found in swine, is different from vasopressin only by one peptide. Desmopressin, an analog of vasopressin, was synthesized in 1967.

Posterior pituitary preparations have oxytocic and vasopressor activity. Posterior pituitary powder is obtained from the dried posterior lobe of the pituitary of domesticated animals used by humans for food. These drugs increase cyclic $3',5'$-adenosine monophosphate (cAMP), thereby increasing water reabsorption in the kidneys, causing increased urine osmolality and decreased urinary flow rate. Desmopressin also increases Factor VIII activity by causing the release of endogenous Factor VIII from plasma stores. Oxytocin causes contraction of uterine smooth muscle (increasing amplitude and frequency of contractions), and myoepithelial cells surrounding breast alveoli (causing milk ejection).

Clinical indications and actions
Diabetes insipidus
Vasopressin, lypressin, desmopressin, and posterior pituitary hormone are used to control or prevent signs and complications of neurogenic diabetes insipidus. Acting primarily at the renal tubular level, they increase cAMP, which increases water permeability at the renal tubule and collecting duct, causing increased urine osmolality and decreased urinary flow rate.
Postoperative abdominal distention and abdominal radiographic procedures
Vasopressin and posterior pituitary hormone increase peristalsis by directly stimulating smooth muscle contraction in the GI tract.
GI hemorrhage
Vasopressin has been used I.V. or intra-arterially into the superior mesenteric artery to temporarily control bleeding of esophageal varices by directly stimulating capillaries and small arterioles, causing vasoconstriction. Posterior pituitary hormone, I.M. or S.C., also is used as an aid to achieve hemostasis in surgery and in the presence of esophageal varices.
Hemophilia A and von Willebrand's disease
Desmopressin increases Factor VIII activity by releasing endogenous Factor VIII from plasma storage sites.
Induction and augmentation of labor
Oxytocin is used to induce labor in prolonged pregnancies (greater than 42 weeks' gestation) and in complicated term or near-term pregnancies (hypertension, antepartum bleeding, preeclampsia, eclampsia, or premature rupture of membranes in which spontaneous labor does not ensue).

Overview of adverse reactions
Adverse effects of posterior pituitary hormones commonly reflect excessive oxytoxic or vasopressor activity and may include abdominal and uterine smooth muscle cramping, chest pain, and hypertension. *Anaphylaxis* and other hypersensitivity reactions may occur.

▶ Special considerations
● Use with caution in patients with coronary artery insufficiency or hypertensive cardiovascular disease.
● Adjust fluid intake to reduce risk of water intoxication and sodium depletion, especially in young or old patients.
● Overdose may cause oxytocic or vasopressor activity. If patient develops uterine cramps, increased GI activity, fluid retention, or hypertension, withhold drug until effects subside. Furosemide may be used if fluid retention is excessive.
● Some patients may have difficulty measuring and inhaling drug into nostrils. Teach patient correct method of administration.

Representative combinations
None.

plague vaccine

- Pharmacologic classification: vaccine
- Therapeutic classification: bacterial vaccine
- Pregnancy risk category C

How supplied
Available by prescription only
Injection: 2 billion killed plague bacilli (*Yersinia pestis*) per milliliter in 20-ml vials

Indications, route, and dosage
Primary immunization and booster
Adults and children over age 10: 1 ml I.M. followed by 0.2 ml in 4 weeks, then 0.2 ml 6 months after the first dose. Booster dosage is 0.1 to 0.2 ml q 6 months for three doses and thereafter q 1 to 2 years while in endemic area.

Although its efficacy has not been determined, an accelerated adult immunization schedule can be used: three doses of 0.5 ml each, administered at least 1 week apart.
Children age 5 to 10: Three fifths the adult primary or booster dosage.
Children age 1 to 4: Two fifths the adult primary or booster dosage.
Children under age 1: One fifth the adult primary or booster dosage.

Pharmacodynamics
Plague prophylaxis: This vaccine is used to promote active immunity to plague.

Pharmacokinetics
The duration of vaccine-induced immunity appears to be about 6 to 12 months. Booster doses are required to maintain immunity.

Contraindications and precautions
Plague vaccine is contraindicated in patients with acute respiratory or other active infections or immunodeficiency states; in patients allergic to any of the vaccine components (beef, yeast, agar, soybean, casein, and phenol); and in those with previous sensitivity reactions to plague vaccine. Use cautiously in patients with thrombocytopenia or a bleeding disorder because bleeding may occur after I.M. injection.

Interactions
Concomitant use with corticosteroids or other immunosuppressants may impair the immune response to plague vaccine and vaccination may fail to elicit an arbitrary response in these patients. Antibody determinations may be necessary.

Effects on diagnostic tests
None reported.

Adverse reactions
- Local: swelling, induration, and erythema at injection site, sterile abscess.
- Systemic: malaise, headache, asthmatic response, urticaria, fever, lymphadenopathy, *anaphylaxis.*
 Note: The frequency of adverse reactions usually increases with administration of booster doses.

Overdose and treatment
No information available.

▶ Special considerations
- Obtain a thorough history of allergies and reactions to immunizations.
- Epinephrine solution 1:1,000 should be available to treat allergic reactions.
- Before withdrawing the dose, shake the vial until the suspension is uniform.
- The vaccine is a turbid, whitish liquid with a faint odor.
- Deltoid muscle is the preferred I.M. injection site.
- Never administer plague vaccine I.V.
- Store at 2 to 8 C. (36 to 46 F.). Do not freeze. Vaccine is stable at room temperature for 15 days.
- Administer to pregnant women only when a high risk of infection exists. There is no data regarding safety and efficacy during pregnancy.

Information for the patient
- Explain to patient that he will receive three doses of plague vaccine to develop immunity to plague. Thereafter, he will need a booster every 6 months initially, then every 1 to 2 years.
- Tell patient that he may experience pain and inflammation at the injection site and may develop fever, general malaise, headache, swollen lymph nodes, or difficulty breathing. Encourage him to report any distressing adverse reactions.

Breast-feeding
Adverse effects are unknown. Vaccine should be used with caution in breast-feeding women.

plasma protein fraction
Plasmanate, Plasma-Plex, Plasmatein, Protenate

- Pharmacologic classification: blood derivative
- Therapeutic classification: plasma volume expander
- Pregnancy risk category C

How supplied
Available by prescription only
Injection: 5% solution in 50-ml, 250-ml, 500-ml vials

Indications, route, and dosage
Shock
Adults: Varies with patient's condition and response, but usually 250 to 500 ml (12.5 to 25 g protein) I.V., not to exceed 10 ml/minute.
Children: 22 to 33 ml/kg I.V. infused at rate of 5 to 10 ml/minute.
Hypoproteinemia
Adults: 1,000 to 1,500 ml I.V. daily. Maximum infusion rate: 8 ml/minute.

Pharmacodynamics
Plasma-expanding action: Plasma protein fraction supplies colloid to the blood and expands plasma volume. It causes fluid to shift from interstitial spaces into the circulation, and slightly increases plasma protein concentration. It is comprised mostly of albumin, but may

contain up to 17% alpha and beta globulins, and not more than 1% gamma globulin.

Pharmacokinetics
The pharmacokinetics of plasma protein fraction (PPF) are similar to its chief constituent, albumin (approximately 83% to 90%).
● *Absorption:* Albumin is not adequately absorbed from the GI tract.
● *Distribution:* Albumin accounts for approximately 50% of plasma proteins. It is distributed into the intravascular space and extravascular sites, including skin, muscle, and lungs. In patients with reduced circulating blood volumes, hemodilution secondary to albumin administration persists for many hours; in patients with normal blood volume, excess fluid and protein are lost from the intravascular space within a few hours.
● *Metabolism:* Although albumin is synthesized in the liver, the liver is not involved in clearance of albumin from the plasma in healthy individuals.
● *Excretion:* Little is known about albumin excretion in healthy individuals. Administration of albumin decreases hepatic albumin synthesis and increases albumin clearance if plasma oncotic pressure is high. In certain pathologic states, the liver, kidneys, or intestines may provide elimination mechanisms.

Contraindications and precautions
Plasma protein fraction (PPF) is contraindicated in patients with severe anemia or heart failure, in patients undergoing cardiac bypass surgery, and in patients with increased blood volume.

Administer PPF cautiously to patients with hepatic or renal failure, low cardiac reserve, or restricted salt intake.

Interactions
None significant.

Effects on diagnostic tests
PPF slightly increases plasma protein levels.

Adverse reactions
● CNS: headache.
● CV: variable effects on blood pressure after rapid I.V. infusion or after intraarterial administration, *vascular overload after rapid infusion.*
● DERM: erythema, urticaria
● GI: nausea, vomiting, hypersalivation.
● Other: hypersensitivity, (flushing, chills, fever, back pain, dyspnea, chest tightness, *cyanosis, shock*).

Overdose and treatment
Rapid infusion can cause circulatory overload and pulmonary edema. Watch patient for signs of hypervolemia; monitor blood pressure and central venous pressure. Treatment is symptomatic.

▶ Special considerations
● Do not use solution that is cloudy, contains sediment, or has been frozen. Store at room temperature; freezing may break bottle and allow bacterial contamination.
● Use opened solution promptly, discarding unused portion after 4 hours; solution contains no preservatives and becomes unstable.
● One "unit" is usually considered to be 250 ml of the 5% concentration.
● Avoid rapid I.V. infusion. Rate is individualized according to patient's age, condition, and diagnosis. Max-

imum dosage is 250 g/48 hours; do not give faster than 10 ml/minute. Decrease infusion rate to 5 to 8 ml/minute as plasma volume approaches normal.
● Monitor blood pressure frequently; slow or stop infusion if hypotension suddenly occurs. Vital signs should return to normal gradually.
● Observe patient for signs of vascular overload (heart failure, pulmonary edema, widening pulse pressure indicating increased cardiac output) and signs of hemorrhage or shock (after surgery or trauma); be alert for bleeding sites not evident at lower blood pressure.
● Monitor intake and output (watch especially for decreased output), hemoglobin, hematocrit, and serum protein and electrolyte levels to help determine ongoing dosage.
● If patient is dehydrated, give additional fluids either P.O. or I.V.
● Each liter contains 130 to 160 mEq of sodium before dilution with any additional I.V. fluids; a 250-ml container of the 5% concentration contains approximately 33 to 40 mEq sodium.

---

plicamycin (formerly mithramycin)
Mithracin

● Pharmacologic classification: antibiotic antineoplastic (cell cycle-phase nonspecific)
● Therapeutic classification: antineoplastic, hypocalcemic agent
● Pregnancy risk category X

How supplied
Available by prescription only
Injection: 2.5-mg vials

Indications, route, and dosage
Dosage and indications may vary. Check current literature for recommended protocol.
Hypercalcemia
Adults: 15 to 25 mcg/kg I.V. daily over a period of 4 to 6 hours for 3 to 4 days. Repeat at intervals of 1 week as needed.
Testicular cancer
Adults: 25 to 30 mcg/kg I.V. daily over a period of 4 to 6 hours for up to 10 days (based on ideal body weight or actual weight, whichever is less).

Pharmacodynamics
● *Antineoplastic action:* Plicamycin exerts its cytotoxic activity by intercalating between DNA base pairs and also binding to the outside of the DNA molecule. The result is inhibition of DNA-dependent RNA synthesis.
● *Hypocalcemic action:* The exact mechanism by which plicamycin lowers serum calcium levels is unknown. Plicamycin may block the hypercalcemic effect of vitamin D or may inhibit the effect of parathyroid hormone upon osteoclasts, preventing osteolysis. Both mechanisms reduce serum calcium concentrations.

Pharmacokinetics
● *Absorption:* Plicamycin is not administered orally.
● *Distribution:* Plicamycin distributes mainly into the Kupffer's cells of the liver, into renal tubular cells, and along formed bone surfaces. The drug also crosses the

---

blood-brain barrier and achieves appreciable concentrations in the cerebrospinal fluid.
● *Metabolism:* The metabolic fate of plicamycin is unclear.
● *Excretion:* Plicamycin is eliminated primarily through the kidneys.

Contraindications and precautions
Plicamycin is contraindicated in patients with impaired bone marrow function, thrombocytopenia, thrombocytopathy, coagulation disorders, or electrolyte imbalance because it may worsen the symptoms associated with these disorders.

Exercise caution in patients with hepatic and renal dysfunction and in those who have previously received abdominal or mediastinal radiation, because these patients may be more susceptible to the drug's toxic effects.

Interactions
None reported.

Effects on diagnostic tests
Because of drug-induced toxicity, plicamycin therapy may increase serum concentrations of alkaline phosphatase, AST (SGOT), ALT (SGPT), LDH, and bilirubin; it may also increase serum creatinine and BUN levels through nephrotoxicity.

Adverse reactions
● CNS: severe headache, lethargy.
● DERM: periorbital pallor, usually the day before toxic symptoms occur; facial flushing.
● GI: nausea, vomiting, anorexia, diarrhea, stomatitis, metallic taste.
● GU: proteinuria; increased BUN and serum creatinine levels.
● HEMA: *bone marrow depression* (dose-limiting); *thrombocytopenia; bleeding syndrome,* from epistaxis to generalized hemorrhage; depression of clotting factors; *leukopenia.*
● Metabolic: decreased serum calcium, potassium, and phosphorus levels.
● Local: extravasation causes irritation, cellulitis.

Overdose and treatment
Clinical manifestations of overdose include myelosuppression, electrolyte imbalance, and coagulation disorders.

Treatment is usually supportive and includes transfusion of blood components and appropriate symptomatic therapy. Patient's renal and hepatic status should be closely monitored.

▶ Special considerations
● To reconstitute drug, use 4.9 ml of sterile water to give a concentration of 0.5 mg/ml. Reconstitute drug immediately before administration, and discard any unused solution.
● Drug may be further diluted with normal saline solution or dextrose 5% in water (D_5W) to a volume of 1,000 ml and administered as an I.V. infusion over 4 to 6 hours.
● Drug may be administered by I.V. push injection, but this method is discouraged because of the higher incidence and greater severity of GI toxicity. Nausea and vomiting are greatly diminished as the infusion rate is decreased.

● Infusions of plicamycin in 1,000 ml D_5W are stable for up to 24 hours.
● If I.V. infiltrates, infusion should be stopped immediately and ice packs applied before restarting an I.V. in other arm.
● Give antiemetics before administering drug, to reduce nausea.
● Monitor LDH, AST (SGOT), ALT (SGPT), alkaline phosphatase, BUN, creatinine, potassium, calcium, and phosphorus levels.
● Monitor platelet count and prothrombin time before and during therapy.
● Check serum calcium levels. Monitor patient for tetany, carpopedal spasm, Chvostek's sign, and muscle cramps, because a precipitous drop in calcium levels is possible.
● Observe for signs of bleeding. Facial flushing may be an early indicator.
● Therapeutic effect in hypercalcemia may not be seen for 24 to 48 hours; may last 3 to 15 days.
● Avoid drug contact with skin or mucous membranes.
● Store lyophilized powder in refrigerator.

Information for the patient
● Tell patient to use salicylate-free medication for pain relief or fever reduction.
● Tell patient to avoid exposure to people with infections.
● Patient should not receive immunizations during therapy and for several weeks after therapy. Members of the same household should not receive immunizations during the same period.

Breast-feeding
It is not known whether plicamycin distributes into breast milk. However, because of the potential for serious adverse reactions, mutagenicity, and carcinogenicity in the infant, breast-feeding is not recommended.

pneumococcal vaccine, polyvalent
Pneumovax 23, Pnu-Imune 23

● Pharmacologic classification: vaccine
● Therapeutic classification: bacterial vaccine
● Pregnancy risk category C

How supplied
Available by prescription only
Injection: 25 mcg each of 23 polysaccharide isolates of *Streptococcus pneumoniae* per 0.5-ml dose, in 1-ml and 5-ml vials

Indications, route, and dosage
Pneumococcal immunization
Adults and children over age 2: 0.5 ml I.M. or S.C.

Pharmacodynamics
Pneumonia prophylaxis: Pneumococcal vaccine promotes active immunity to infections caused by *S. pneumoniae.*

Pharmacokinetics
Protective antibodies are produced within 3 weeks after injection. The duration of vaccine-induced immunity is at least 5 years in adults.

Contraindications and precautions
Polyvalent pneumococcal vaccine is contraindicated in patients who previously received any polyvalent pneumococcal vaccine and those with a hypersensitivity to any component of the vaccine, such as thimerosal or phenol. Pneumococcal vaccine should not be given to patients with Hodgkin's disease or those who have received extensive chemotherapy or radiation therapy (especially within the last 10 days). Pneumococcal vaccine also is not recommended in patients with an acute respiratory infection or any other active infection. Defer elective immunization during these situations.

Interactions
Concomitant use of pneumococcal vaccine with corticosteroids or other immunosuppressants may impair the immune response to the vaccine; therefore, vaccination should be avoided.

Effects on diagnostic tests
None reported.

Adverse reactions
● Local: soreness, erythema, and induration at injection site in approximately 71% of patients.
● Systemic: low-grade fever (usually subsides within 48 hours), rash, myalgia, arthralgia, *anaphylaxis*, neurologic disorders.

Overdose and treatment
No information available.

▶ Special considerations
● Obtain a thorough history of allergies and reactions to immunizations.
● Persons with asplenia who received the 14-valent vaccine should be revaccinated with the 23-valent vaccine.
● Epinephrine solution 1:1,000 should be available to treat allergic reactions.
● Use the deltoid or midlateral thigh. Do not inject I.V. Avoid intradermal administration because this may cause severe local reactions.
● This vaccine protects against 23 pneumococcal types, accounting for 90% of pneumococcal disease.
● Polyvalent pneumococcal vaccine also may be administered to children to prevent pneumococcal otitis media.
● Candidates for pneumococcal vaccine include persons age 65 and older; adults and children age 2 or older with chronic illness, asplenia, or splenic dysfunction; and those with sickle-cell anemia and HIV infection.
● The vaccine also is recommended for patients awaiting organ transplants, those receiving radiation therapy or cancer chemotherapy, persons in nursing homes and orphanages, and bedridden individuals.
● If different sites and separate syringes are used, pneumococcal vaccine may be administered simultaneously with influenza, DTP, poliovirus, or Hae-mophilus type b polysaccharide vaccines.
● Store at 2° to 8° C. (36° to 46° F.). Reconstitution or dilution is unnecessary.

Information for the patient
● Tell patient to expect redness, soreness, swelling, and pain at the injection site after vaccination. Patient may also develop fever, joint or muscle aches and pains, rash, itching, general weakness, or difficulty breathing.
● Encourage patient to report distressing adverse reactions promptly.
● Advise patient to use acetaminophen to relieve adverse reactions promptly.

Pediatric use
Children under age 2 do not respond satisfactorily to pneumococcal vaccine. The vaccine's safety and efficacy in this group have not been established.

Breast-feeding
It is unknown whether pneumococcal vaccine is distributed into milk. Use with caution in breast-feeding women.

---

podofilox
Condylox

● Pharmacologic classification: antimitotic
● Therapeutic classification: keratolytic
● Pregnancy risk category C

How supplied
Available by prescription only
Topical solution: 0.5% in 95% alcohol; 3.5-ml amber glass bottles

Indications, route, and dosage
Treatment of external genital warts
Adults: Apply q12 hours for 3 consecutive days, and then withhold use for 4 consecutive days. Repeat this 1-week cycle of treatment up to four times until there is no visible wart tissue. If response is incomplete after four treatment weeks, alternative therapy should be considered.
   Apply to warts with supplied cotton-tipped applicator. Touch drug-dampened applicator to wart, applying minimum amount of solution needed to cover wart. Limit treatment to less than 10 cm² of wart tissue and less than 0.5 ml of solution per day. Allow solution to dry before returning opposing skin surfaces to their normal positions. After treatment, carefully dispose of applicator and wash hands.

Pharmacodynamics
Keratolytic action: The exact mechanism of action is unknown. Treatment results in necrosis of visible wart tissue.

Pharmacokinetics
● *Absorption:* Topical application does not result in detectable serum levels.
● *Distribution:* Unknown.
● *Metabolism:* Unknown.
● *Excretion:* Unknown.

Contraindications and precautions
Podofilox is contraindicated in patients with known hypersensitivity or intolerance to the drug or any component of its formulation.

Interactions
None reported.

Adverse reactions
● DERM: burning, pain, inflammation, erosion, itching, tingling, bleeding, tenderness, chafing, malodor, scarring, vesicle formation, dryness and peeling, foreskin irretraction, ulceration.
● Other: painful intercourse, insomnia, dizziness, crusting edema, hematuria, vomiting.

Overdose and treatment
Topically applied podofilox may be absorbed systemically, resulting in nausea, vomiting, fever, diarrhea, bone marrow depression, and oral ulcers. Treat by washing skin free of any remaining drug and follow by symptomatic and supportive measures.

▶ Special considerations
● Toxicity has been reported after systemic use in an investigational protocol for cancer treatment. After five to ten daily I.V. doses of 0.5 to 1 mg/kg, significant, reversible hematologic toxicity has occurred. At lower doses, other toxicities have been reported.
● Reports of burning and pain were more frequent and more severe in women than in men.
● There is no evidence that more frequent application will increase efficacy.

Information for the patient
● Tell patient to use only as directed and not to apply more frequently than prescribed.
● Tell patient to allow solution to dry before returning opposing skin surfaces to their normal positions.
● Instruct patient to use applicator provided, discard after each treatment, and wash hands.
● Tell patient not to refrigerate, freeze, or store drug near excessive heat.
● Advise patient to read information leaflet provided and to avoid smoking during application.

Pediatric use
Safety and efficacy have not been established.

Breast-feeding
It is unknown if podofilox is excreted in breast milk. The risk-to-benefit ratio of therapy must be considered.

poliovirus vaccine, live, oral, trivalent (TOPV, Sabin)
Orimune Trivalent

● Pharmacologic classification: vaccine
● Therapeutic classification: viral vaccine
● Pregnancy risk category C

How supplied
Available by prescription only
Oral vaccine: mixture of three viruses (types 1, 2, and 3), grown in monkey kidney tissue culture, in 0.5-ml single-dose Dispettes

Indications, route, and dosage
Poliovirus immunization (primary series)
Adolescents and older children: Two 0.5-ml doses should be administered 8 weeks apart. Give third 0.5-ml dose 6 to 12 months after second dose.
Infants: 0.5 ml at age 2 months, 4 months, and 18 months. Optional dose may be given at 6 months when substantial risk of exposure exists.
Supplementary: All children entering elementary school (age 4 to 6) who have completed the primary series should receive a single follow-up dose of TOPV. Booster vaccination beyond elementary school is not routinely recommended.
Adults age 18 and over: TOPV should not be given to persons age 18 and over who have not received at least one prior dose of TOPV. Enhanced potency inactivated polio vaccine [eIPV] should be used if polio vaccination is indicated.
 If less than 4 weeks are available before protection is needed, a single dose of TOPV is recommended, followed by IPV later if the person remains at increased risk.
 Persons traveling to countries with endemic or epidemic polio who previously completed a primary series should receive a single follow-up dose of TOPV. This vaccine should not be administered to neonates under age 6 weeks.

Pharmacodynamics
Polio prophylaxis: TOPV promotes immunity to poliomyelitis by inducing humoral and secretory antibodies and antibodies in the lymphatic tissue of the GI tract.

Pharmacokinetics
Antibody response to the vaccine occurs within 7 to 10 days after ingestion and peaks around 21 days. The duration of immunity is thought to be lifelong.

Contraindications and precautions
TOPV is contraindicated in patients with persistent vomiting or diarrhea; in patients with immunodeficiency or infection or those receiving immunosuppressants; in those in a severely debilitated condition; and in patients severely allergic to sorbitol, streptomycin, or neomycin, components of the vaccine. Household contacts of an immunosuppressed child should not receive TOPV.

Interactions
Concomitant use of TOPV with corticosteroids or other immunosuppressants may impair the immune response to the vaccine. Vaccination with TOPV should be deferred until the immunosuppressant is discontinued or, alternatively, inactivated poliovirus vaccine may be used. Immune serum globulin and transfusions of blood or blood products may also interfere with the immune response to poliovirus vaccine. Defer vaccination for 3 months in these situations.

Effects on diagnostic tests
TOPV may temporarily decrease the response to tuberculin skin testing. If a tuberculin test is necessary, administer either before, simultaneously with, or at least 8 weeks after TOPV.

Adverse reactions
Systemic: *paralytic poliomyelitis* (extremely rare, 1 case per 2.6 million doses distributed).

Overdose and treatment
No information available.

▶ Special considerations
• Obtain a thorough history of allergies, especially to antibiotics, and of reactions to immunizations.
• This vaccine is not effective in modifying or preventing existing or incubating poliomyelitis.
• Check the parents' immunization history when they bring in a child for the vaccine; this is an excellent time for parents to receive booster immunizations.
• Adults and immunocompromised persons who have not been vaccinated should receive IPV (Salk) in three doses, given 1 month apart, before other household contacts are immunized with TOPV.
• This vaccine is not for parenteral use. Dose may be administered directly or mixed with distilled water, chlorine-free tap water, simple syrup U.S.P., or milk. It also may be placed on bread, cake, or a sugar cube.
• Keep vaccine frozen until used. It may be refrigerated up to 30 days once thawed, if unopened. Opened vials may be refrigerated up to 7 days.
• Color change from pink to yellow has no effect on the efficacy of the vaccine as long as the vaccine remains clear. Yellow color results from storage at low temperatures.

Information for the patient
• The risk of vaccine-associated paralysis is extremely small for vaccines, susceptible family members, and other close contacts (about 1 case per 2.6 million doses given).
• Encourage patient to report distressing adverse reactions promptly.

Pediatric use
Poliovirus vaccine should not be administered to neonates under age 6 weeks.

Breast-feeding
Breast-feeding does not interfere with successful immunization, hence no interruption in the feeding schedule is necessary.

---

polymyxin B sulfate
Aerosporin

• Pharmacologic classification: polymyxin antibiotic
• Therapeutic classification: antibiotic
• Pregnancy risk category B

How supplied
Available by prescription only
Powder for injection: 500,000-unit vials
Ophthalmic sterile powder for solution: 500,000-unit vials to be reconstituted to 20 to 50 ml

Indications, route, and dosage
Acute urinary tract infections, septicemia, or bacteremia caused by sensitive organisms when other antibiotics are ineffective or contraindicated
Adults and children: 15,000 to 25,000 units/kg daily I.V. infusion, divided q 12 hours; or 25,000 to 30,000 units/kg daily, divided q 4 to 8 hours. I.M. injection not advised because of severe pain at injection site.
Meningitis caused by sensitive Pseudomonas aeruginosa or Haemophilus influenzae when other antibiotics are ineffective or contraindicated
Adults and children over age 2: 50,000 units intrathecally once daily for 3 to 4 days, then 50,000 units every other day for at least 2 weeks after CSF tests are negative and CSF glucose level is normal.
Children under age 2: 20,000 units intrathecally once daily for 3 to 4 days, then 25,000 units every other day for at least 2 weeks after CSF tests are negative and CSF glucose level is normal.
Eye infections caused by sensitive P. aeruginosa
Adults and children: 1 to 3 drops of a solution containing 10,000 to 25,000 units/ml every hour until favorable response occurs. Do not exceed 25,000 units/kg or 2,000,000 units per day.
Dosage in renal failure

Creatinine clearance (ml/min/1.73 m²)	Dosage in adults
>20	75 to 100% of usual dose in 2 divided doses q 12 hr
5 to 20	50% of the usual dose in 2 divided doses q 12 hr
<5	15% of the usual dose of q 12 hr

Pharmacodynamics
Antibacterial action: Polymyxin B sulfate alters permeability of bacterial cytoplasmic membrane. It is bactericidal against many gram-negative organisms and is indicated for sensitive strains of *P. aeruginosa, Enterobacter aerogenes, Klebsiella pneumoniae,* or *Escherichia coli. Proteus, Neisseria,* and gram-positive organisms resist the drug.

Pharmacokinetics
• *Absorption:* Polymyxin B sulfate is not significantly absorbed from GI tract. With I.M. administration, peak serum levels occur in 2 hours.
• *Distribution:* With systemic administration, polymyxin B sulfate is distributed widely except in CSF, aqueous humor, and placental and synovial fluids. Drug is minimally bound to plasma proteins.
• *Metabolism:* Polymyxin B sulfate's metabolism is unknown.
• *Excretion:* About 60% of dose is excreted renally. In patients with normal renal function, plasma half-life is 4 to 6 hours. In patients with creatinine clearance below 10 ml/minute, half-life is 2 to 3 days. There is no appreciable clearance by either hemodiaylsis or peritoneal dialysis.

Contraindications and precautions
Polymyxin B sulfate is contraindicated in patients with known hypersensitivity to the drug.
Polymyxin B sulfate should be administered cautiously to patients with such neuromuscular diseases as myasthenia gravis because drug's neuromuscular blockade may exacerbate symptoms.

Interactions

When used concomitantly, polymyxin B sulfate may prolong, intensify, or reinstate neuromuscular blockade and paralysis induced by neuromuscular blocking agents and some anesthetic agents (for example, gallamine, tubocurarine, succinylcholine, and decamethonium). Concomitant use with other nephrotoxic drugs (such as aminoglycosides, amphotericin B, cisplatin, capreomycin, vancomycin, and methoxyflurane) may increase risk of polymyxin B-induced nephrotoxicity.

Effects on diagnostic tests

Blood urea nitrogen (BUN) and serum creatinine levels may increase during polymyxin B therapy. CSF protein and leukocyte levels may increase during intrathecal polymyxin B therapy.

Adverse reactions

● CNS: dizziness, confusion, irritability, nystagmus, muscle weakness, drowsiness, slurred speech, coma, *seizures*, flushing, headache.
● EENT: eye itching and irritation.
● GU: albuminura, azotemia, hematuria, leukocyturia, cylindruria, *nephrotoxicity*.
● Local: pain at I.M. injection site; phlebitis at I.V. site; eye irritation and conjunctivitis (with ophthalmic preparations); ear itchiness, irritation, and urticaria (with otic preparations).
● Other: hypersensitivity reactions (fever, anaphylaxis), *respiratory paralysis*, neuromuscular blockade, superinfection.
   Note: Drug should be discontinued if nephrotoxicity develops.

Overdose and treatment

Clinical effects of overdose with polymyxin B may include respiratory paralysis that may resist treatment with neostigmine and edrophonium.

   Treatment includes supportive measures until muscle function returns. Calcium chloride may be given. The drug is not dialyzable.

▶ Special considerations

● Obtain culture and sensitivity tests before starting therapy.
● Obtain baseline renal function indices (BUN and serum creatinine levels and urine output), and monitor them during therapy.
● To prepare I.V. infusion, dilute each 500,000-unit vial in 300 to 500 ml dextrose 5% in water; infuse over 60 to 90 minutes. Prepared solution remains stable for 72 hours when refrigerated.
● To prepare I.M. injection, reconstitute according to package instructions and give deep I.M. Procaine 1% may be used as a diluent (unless patient is allergic to procaine).
● To prepare intrathecal injection, add 10 ml of preservative-free sterile saline solution to vial to yield 50,000 units/ml. Withdraw desired dose.
● Ensure adequate fluid intake to maintain urine output at 1,500 ml/day.
● Monitor patient for fever, CNS toxicity, rash, or evidence of renal toxicity.
● Monitor for signs and symptoms of local superinfection.
● If patient is receiving drug concomitantly with neuromuscular blocking agents and certain anesthetic agents (such as gallamine, tubocurarine, succinylcholine, and decamethonium), monitor closely and keep mechanical ventilator available.
● Drug should be administered I.V. only in hospital where patient can be monitored appropriately.
● Patients with renal impairment require reduced dose.
● Patients with meningitis require intrathecal administration to ensure adequate CSF drug levels.

Information for the patient

Encourage patient to report any severe or unusual adverse effects immediately.

---

polythiazide
Renese

● Pharmacologic classification: thiazide diuretic
● Therapeutic classification: diuretic, antihypertensive
● Pregnancy risk category B

How supplied

Available by prescription only
Tablets: 1 mg, 2 mg, 4 mg

Indications, route, and dosage
Hypertension
Adults: 2 to 4 mg P.O. daily.
Edema
Adults: 1 to 4 mg P.O. daily.
Children: 0.02 to 0.08 mg/kg P.O. daily.

Pharmacodynamics

● *Diuretic action:* Polythiazide increases urinary excretion of sodium and water by inhibiting sodium reabsorption in the cortical diluting tubule of the nephron, thus relieving edema.
● *Antihypertensive action:* The exact mechanism of polythiazide's antihypertensive effect is unknown. It may be partially from direct arteriolar vasodilatation and a decrease in total peripheral resistance.

Pharmacokinetics

● *Absorption:* Polythiazide is absorbed from the GI tract.
● *Distribution:* Unknown.
● *Metabolism:* In dogs, about 30% of a polythiazide dose is metabolized by the liver; the percentage metabolized in humans is unknown.
● *Excretion:* Between 60% and 90% of polythiazide and its metabolites are excreted in urine.

Contraindications and precautions

Polythiazide is contraindicated in patients with anuria and in those with known sensitivity to the drug or to other sulfonamide derivatives. Polythiazide should be used cautiously in patients with severe renal disease because it may decrease glomerular filtration rate and precipitate azotemia; in patients with impaired hepatic function or liver disease because electrolyte changes may precipitate coma; and in patients taking digoxin, because hypokalemia may predispose them to digitalis toxicity.

Interactions
Polythiazide potentiates the hypotensive effects of most other antihypertensive drugs; this may be used to therapeutic advantage.

Polythiazide may potentiate hyperglycemic, hypotensive, and hyperuricemic effects of diazoxide, and its hyperglycemic effect may increase insulin or sulfonylurea requirements in diabetic patients.

Polythiazide may reduce renal clearance of lithium, elevating serum lithium levels, and may necessitate a 50% reduction in lithium dosage.

Polythiazide turns urine slightly more alkaline and may decrease urinary excretion of some amines, such as amphetamine and quinidine; alkaline urine may also decrease therapeutic efficacy of methenamine compounds such as methenamine mandelate.

Cholestyramine and colestipol may bind polythiazide, preventing its absorption; give drugs 1 hour apart.

Effects on diagnostic tests
Polythiazide therapy may alter serum electrolyte levels and may increase serum urate, glucose, cholesterol, and triglyceride levels. It also may interfere with tests for parathyroid function and should be discontinued before such tests.

Adverse reactions
● CV: volume depletion and dehydration, orthostatic hypotension, hypercholesterolemia, hypertriglyceridemia.
● DERM: dermatitis, photosensitivity, rash.
● GI: anorexia, nausea, *pancreatitis.*
● HEMA: *aplastic anemia, agranulocytosis,* leukopenia, thrombocytopenia.
● Hepatic: hepatic encephalopathy.
● Metabolic: asymptomatic hyperuricemia; gout; hyperglycemia and impairment of glucose tolerance; fluid and electrolyte imbalances, including hyponatremia, hypochloremia, hypercalcemia, and hypokalemia; metabolic alkalosis.
● Other: hypersensitivity reactions, such as pneumonitis and vasculitis.
Note: Drug should be discontinued if rising BUN and serum creatinine levels indicate renal impairment or if patient shows signs of impending coma.

Overdose and treatment
Clinical signs of overdose include GI irritation and hypermotility, diuresis, and lethargy, which may progress to coma.

Treatment is mainly supportive; monitor and assist respiratory, cardiovascular, and renal function as indicated. Monitor fluid and electrolyte balance. Induce vomiting with ipecac in conscious patient; otherwise, use gastric lavage to avoid aspiration. Do not give cathartics; these promote additional loss of fluids and electrolytes.

▶ Special considerations
Recommendations for use of polythiazide and for care and teaching of the patient during therapy are the same as those for all *thiazide and thiazide-like diuretics.*

Geriatric use
Elderly and debilitated patients require close observation and may require reduced dosages. They are more sensitive to excess diuresis because of age-related changes in cardiovascular and renal function. Excess diuresis promotes orthostatic hypotension, dehydration, hypovolemia, hyponatremia, hypomagnesemia, and hypokalemia.

Breast-feeding
Polythiazide may be distributed in breast milk; its safety and effectiveness in breast-feeding women have not been established.

posterior pituitary hormone
Pituitrin (S)

● Pharmacologic classification: posterior pituitary hormone
● Therapeutic classification: antidiuretic agent, peristaltic stimulant agent, hemostatic agent
● Pregnancy risk category D

How supplied
Available by prescription only
Injection: 1-ml ampules, 20 units/ml
Inhalation: 40 mg/activation

Indications, route, and dosage
To control postoperative ileus; as a surgical aid to achieve hemostasis; to treat diabetes insipidus
Adults: 5 to 20 units S.C. or I.M.; intranasal – individualized dose, repeated t.i.d. or q.i.d.

Pharmacodynamics
● *Antidiuretic action:* Posterior pituitary hormone is used to control or prevent signs and complications of neurogenic diabetes insipidus. Acting primarily at the renal tubular level, posterior pituitary hormone increases cyclic $3',5'$-adenosine monophosphate, which increases water permeability at the renal tubule and collecting duct, resulting in increased urine osmolality and decreased urinary flow rate.
● *Peristaltic stimulant action:* Posterior pituitary hormone induces peristalsis by directly stimulating contraction of smooth muscle in the GI tract.
● *Hemostatic action:* By directly stimulating capillaries and small arterioles, posterior pituitary hormone, administered I.M. or S.C., constricts these vessels to aid in achieving hemostasis during surgery and in the presence of esophageal varices.

Pharmacokinetics
● *Absorption:* Posterior pituitary hormone is well absorbed after I.M., S.C. or inhalation administration.
● *Distribution:* Posterior pituitary hormone probably is distributed throughout the extracellular fluid.
● *Metabolism:* Posterior pituitary hormone is metabolized by the liver and kidneys.
● *Excretion:* Posterior pituitary hormone is excreted by the kidneys.

Contraindications and precautions
Posterior pituitary hormone is contraindicated in patients with known hypersensitivity to the hormone; in epileptic patients because of rapid addition to extracellular water; in those with coronary artery disease, hypertension, cardiovascular disease, or arteriosclerosis because the drug may provoke myocardial infarction; in pregnant patients because injection before

or during labor carries a high risk of inducing severe fetal distress; and in patients with asphyxia neonatorum or uterine rupture.

Drug should be used with caution in patients in shock because the pressor effects of this hormone result from constriction of the vascular bed and increased peripheral resistance. This decreases cardiac output and coronary artery blood flow, thereby augmenting the underlying cause of shock.

Interactions
Concomitant use of posterior pituitary hormone with barbiturates, cyclopropane, or primidone may increase the risk of cardiac arrhythmias and coronary insufficiency. Concomitant use with chlorpropamide, clofibrate, or carbamazepine may potentiate the antidiuretic effect of posterior pituitary hormone. Use with lithium or demeclocycline may reduce the antidiuretic effect.

Effects on diagnostic tests
None reported.

Adverse reactions
- CNS: anxiety, tinnitus, *eclampsia, unconsciousness.*
- CV: chest pain.
- DERM: facial pallor, rash.
- EENT: mydriasis, blindness.
- GI: increased GI motility, abdominal cramps, diarrhea.
- GU: uterine cramps, proteinuria.
- Other: *hypersensitivity reactions, anaphylaxis.*

   Note: Drug should be discontinued if cloudy urine, sudden unexplained loss of eyesight, tinnitus, chest pain, wheezing, or shortness of breath occur.

Overdose and treatment
Posterior pituitary hormone has vasopressor and oxytocic activity. Clinical manifestations include uterine stimulation, hypertensive episodes, drowsiness, listlessness, headache, confusion, anuria, and weight gain. Treatment requires water restriction and temporary withdrawal of the drug. Severe water intoxication may require osmotic diuresis with mannitol, hypertonic dextrose, or urea, either alone or with furosemide.

▶ Special considerations
Besides those relevant to all *posterior pituitary hormones,* consider the following recommendations.
- The preferred route of administration is I.M.
- Inhalation form contains 45 units of antidiuretic activity and a similar amount of oxytocin.
- Posterior pituitary hormone should not be used as an oxytocic agent; high risk of fetal distress exists. Use of posterior pituitary hormone in pregnant patients may cause abortion.
- Initial dose should be given in the evening to observe nighttime antidiuretic effect. Dosage should be increased until a nocturia-free night occurs.
- Monitor fluid intake and output.

Information for the patient
- Teach patient the following inhalation procedure: remove the plastic tip of the inhalator from the body of the blower with a rotary motion; remove the top of the capsule and hold the capsule in an upright position; place the capsule in the body of the inhalator with the open end of the capsule up, then replace the blower tip by a rotary motion; and place the tip in the nostril

and squeeze the rubber bulb once or twice to expel a small portion of the powder into the nasal passage.
- Advise patient to call immediately if chest pain, rash, wheezing, shortness of breath, cloudy urine, loss of eyesight, or ringing or buzzing sounds in ears occur.
- Instruct patient to maintain a record of fluid intake and output.

potassium iodide (KI, SSKI)
Iosat, Pima, Thyro-Block

- Pharmacologic classification: electrolyte
- Therapeutic classification: antihyperthyroid agent, expectorant
- Pregnancy risk category D

How supplied
Available by prescription only
Tablets (enteric-coated): 300 mg
Syrup: 325 mg/5 ml
Solution: 500 mg/15 ml
Saturated solution (SSKI): 1 g/ml
Strong iodine solution (Lugol's solution): iodine 50 mg/ml and potassium iodide 100 mg/ml

Indications, route, and dosage
Expectorant
Adults: 300 to 650 mg t.i.d. or q.i.d.
Children: 60 to 250 mg t.i.d.
Preoperative thyroidectomy
Adults and children: 50 to 250 mg (or one to five drops) SSKI t.i.d.; or 0.1 to 0.3 ml (or three to five drops) Lugol's solution t.i.d.; give drug for 10 to 14 days before surgery.
Nuclear radiation protection and thyrotoxic crisis
Adults and children: 0.13 ml P.O. of SSKI (130 mg) immediately before or after initial exposure will block 90% of radioactive iodine. Same dosage given 3 to 4 hours after exposure will provide 50% block. Drug should be administered for up to 10 days under medical supervision.
Infants under age 1: Half the adult dosage.

   Potassium iodide is used unofficially as an iodine replenisher (adults: 5 to 10 mg daily; children: 1 mg/day) and as an antifungal agent.

Pharmacodynamics
- *Expectorant action:* The exact mechanism of potassium iodide's expectorant effect is unknown; it is believed that potassium iodide reduces viscosity of mucus by increasing respiratory tract secretions.
- *Antihyperthyroid agent action:* Potassium iodide acts directly on the thyroid gland to inhibit synthesis and release of thyroid hormone.

Pharmacokinetics
Absoorption, distribution, metabolism, and excretion have not been reported.

Contraindications and precautions
Potassium iodide is contraindicated in patients hypersensitive to iodides or iodine, and during pregnancy, because abnormal thyroid and goiter may occur. Drug should be used with caution in patients with hyperkalemia, acute bronchitis, or tuberculosis; in children with cystic fibrosis, because they are especially susceptible

to the goitrogenic effects of iodides; and in patients with thyroid disease. Prolonged use of potassium iodide may cause hypothyroidism; goiter may occur in iodide-sensitive hyperthyroid patients.

Interactions
Lithium potentiates both hypothyroid and goitrogenic effects of potassium iodide. Concomitant use with potassium-sparing diuretics or potassium-containing drugs may cause hyperkalemia and subsequent arrhythmia or cardiac arrest.

Effects on diagnostic tests
Potassium iodide may alter the results of thyroid function tests.

Adverse reactions
● DERM: rash.
● GI: nausea, vomiting, epigastric pain.
● Metabolic: goiter, hyperthyroid adenoma, hypothyroidism (with excessive use), collagen disease-like syndrome.
● Prolonged use: chronic iodine poisoning, soreness of mouth, coryza, sneezing, swelling of eyelids.
   Note: Drug should be discontinued if skin rash or signs of acute or chronic poisoning occur; or if patient has abdominal pain, distention, nausea, vomiting, or GI bleeding: enteric-coated tablets reportedly have caused bowel lesions, with possible obstruction, perforation, and hemorrhage.

Overdose and treatment
Acute overdose is rare; angioedema, laryngeal edema, and cutaneous hemorrhages may occur. Treat hyperkalemia immediately; salt and fluid intake help eliminate iodide.

Iodism (chronic iodine poisoning) may follow prolonged use; symptoms include metallic taste, sore mouth, swollen eyelids, sneezing, skin eruptions, nausea, vomiting, epigastric pain, and diarrhea. Discontinue drug and treat supportively.

▶ Special considerations
● Monitor serum potassium levels before and during therapy; patients taking any diuretic, especially potassium-sparing diuretics, are at risk of hyperkalemia.
● Dilute with 180 ml of water, fruit juice, or broth to reduce GI distress and disguise strong, salty metallic taste; advise patient to use a straw to avoid teeth discoloration.
● Store in light-resistant container, because exposure to light liberates traces of free iodine; if crystals develop in solution, dissolve them by placing container in warm water and carefully agitating it.
● Drug may cause flare-up of adolescent acne or other skin rash.
● Sudden withdrawal may precipitate thyroid storm.
● Maintain fluid intake when using drug as an expectorant; adequate hydration encourages optimal expectorant action.

Information for the patient
● Enteric-coated tablets are seldom used because of reports of small-bowel lesions with possible obstruction, perforation, and hemorrhage; when prescribed, give tablet with small amount of water, and tell patient to swallow tablet whole (do not crush or chew) and follow with 240 ml of water or juice.

● Advise patient to drink all of solution prepared and to use a straw to avoid discoloring teeth.
● Review signs of iodism with patient, and instruct patient to report such symptoms, especially abdominal pain, distention, nausea, vomiting, or GI bleeding.
● Caution patient not to use nonprescription drugs without medical approval; many preparations contain iodides and could potentiate drug. For the same reason, patient should discuss ingestion of iodized salt and shellfish.

Geriatric use
Serum potassium determinations may be recommended in elderly patients with renal dysfunction.

Pediatric use
Strong iodine solution is used for treating Graves' disease in neonates (one drop every 8 hours).

Breast-feeding
Potassium iodide should not be used during breast-feeding; drug is secreted in breast milk and may cause skin rash and thyroid suppression in the infant.

---

potassium salts, oral

potassium acetate

potassium bicarbonate
Klor-Con, EF, K-Lyte, Quic-K

potassium chloride
Apo-K★, Cena-K, K-10★, Kalium Durules★, Kaochlor, Kaochlor S-F, Kaon-Cl, Kato, Kay Ciel, KCL★, K-Dur, K-Long★, K-Lor, Klor-10%, Klor-Con, Klor-Con/25, Klorvess, Klotrix, K-Lyte/Cl Powder, K-Tab, Micro-K, Novolente-K★, Potachlor, Potage, Potasalan, Potassine, Roychlor★, Rum-K, Slo-Pot★, Slow-K, Ten-K

potassium gluconate

● Pharmacologic classification: potassium supplement
● Therapeutic classification: therapeutic agent for electrolyte balance
● Pregnancy risk category C

How supplied
Available by prescription only
Sustained-released tablets (chloride): 8 mEq, 10 mEq
Powder: 20 mEq/package
Liquid: 15 mEq/15 ml, 20 mEq/15 ml, 30 mEq/15 ml
Effervescent tablets: 20 mEq, 25 mEq, 50 mEq
Liquid (gluconate): 15 mEq/15 ml, 20 mEq/15ml
Vial: 2 mEq/ml in 20-ml vial (acetate)

Indications, route, and dosage
Hypokalemia
Adults and children: 25-mEq tablet of potassium bicarbonate dissolved in water daily to q.i.d. Use I.V. potassium phosphate when oral replacement is not feasible or when hypokalemia is life-threatening. Dosage up to 20 mEq/hour in concentration of 60 mEq/liter or

less. Further dose based on serum potassium determinations. Total daily dose should not exceed 150 mEq (3 mEq/kg in children).

To treat, give 40 to 100 mEq potassium phosphate orally divided into three to four doses daily; for prevention, 20 mEq daily. Further doses are based on serum potassium level and blood pH. Potassium replacement should be carried out only with ECG monitoring and frequent serum potassium determinations.

Prevention of hypokalemia
Adults and children: Initially, 20 mEq of potassium acetate P.O. daily, in divided doses if needed. Or 10 to 15 mEq of potassium chloride 3 or 4 times a day.

Potassium replacement
Adults and children: Potassium chloride should be diluted in a suitable intravenous solution (not more than 40 mEq/liter) and administered at a rate no greater than 10 to 15 mEq/hr. Total dosage should not exceed 400 mEq/day. Alternatively, potassium replacement should be carried out only with ECG monitoring and frequent serum potassium determinations.

Pharmacodynamics
Potassium replacement action: Potassium, the main cation in body tissue, is necessary for physiological processes such as maintaining intracellular tonicity, maintaining a balance with sodium across cell membranes, transmitting nerve impulses, maintaining cellular metabolism, contracting cardiac and skeletal muscle, maintaining acid-base balance, and maintaining normal renal function.

Pharmacokinetics
• *Absorption:* Potassium is well absorbed from the GI tract. It should be taken with meals and sipped slowly over a 5- to 10-minute period to decrease irritation. Potassium bicarbonate does not correct hypochloremic alkalosis.
• *Distribution:* The normal serum levels of potassium range from 3.8 to 5 mEq/liter. Plasma potassium concentrations up to 7.7 mEq/liter may be normal in neonates. Up to 60 mEq/liter of potassium may be found in gastric secretions and diarrhea fluid.
• *Metabolism:* None significant.
• *Excretion:* Potassium is excreted largely by the kidneys. Small amounts of potassium may be excreted via the skin and intestinal tract, but intestinal potassium usually is reabsorbed. A healthy patient on a potassium-free diet will excrete 40 to 50 mEq of potassium daily.

Contraindications and precautions
Potassium is contraindicated in patients with severe renal impairment, oliguria, anuria, or azotemia (unless patient is hypokalemic); hyperkalemia from any cause; untreated Addison's disease because of the potential for hyperkalemia; acute dehydration; or heat cramps because administration of potassium can worsen these conditions.

Concomitant use of potassium-sparing diuretics is contraindicated, unless patients are routinely monitored.

Administer potassium (particularly I.V. potassium) cautiously in patients with cardiac disease, renal disease, or acidosis; conduct careful analysis of the acid-base balance, and monitor serum electrolytes, ECG, and clinical status of the patient. Acidosis can raise serum potassium levels to the normal range even when total body potassium is reduced.

Interactions
When used concomitantly with potassium, anticholinergics that slow GI motility may increase the chance of GI irritation and ulceration.

Concomitant administration with potassium-containing products may cause hyperkalemia within 1 to 2 days. Potassium is not recommended in digitalized patients with severe or complete heart block because of potential for arrhythmias. Concomitant use of potassium with potassium-sparing diuretics, ACE inhibitors (Captopril), or salt substitutes containing potassium salts can cause severe hyperkalemia.

Effects on diagnostic tests
None reported.

Adverse reactions
Signs of hyperkalemia:
• CNS: paresthesias of the extremities, headache, listlessness, mental confusion, weakness or heaviness of limbs, flaccid paralysis.
• CV: *peripheral vascular collapse with fall in blood pressure, cardiac arrhythmias,* heart block, possible *cardiac arrest,* ECG changes (prolonged P-R interval; wide QRS complex; ST segment depression; tall, tented T waves.) Extremely high plasma concentrations (8 to 11 mEq/liter) may cause death from cardiac depression, arrhythmias, or arrest.
• DERM: cold skin, gray pallor.
• GI: nausea, vomiting, abdominal pain, diarrhea, GI ulcerations (possible stenosis, *hemorrhage,* obstruction, perforation), esophageal ulceration from wax matrix tablets (sustained-release) in patient with enlarged atrium.
• GU: oliguria.
• Local: postinfusion phlebitis.
• Other: soft tissue calcification.

Overdose and treatment
Clinical manifestations of overdose include increased serum potassium concentration and characteristic ECG changes, including tall peaked T waves, depression of ST segment, disappearance of P wave, prolonged QT interval, and widening and slurring of the QRS complex. Late clinical signs include weakness, paralysis of voluntary muscles, respiratory distress, and dysphagia. These may precede severe or fatal cardiac toxicity. Hyperkalemia produces symptoms paradoxically similar to those of hypokalemia.

Treatment of potassium overdose includes discontinuation of the potassium supplement and, if necessary, lavage of the GI tract. In patients with a potassium concentration greater then 6.5 mEq/liter, supportive therapy may include the following interventions (with continuous ECG monitoring):

Infuse 40 to 160 mEq sodium bicarbonate I.V. over a 5-minute interval; repeat in 10 to 15 minutes if ECG abnormalities persist.

Infuse 300 to 500 ml of dextrose 10% to 25% over 1 hour. Insulin (5 to 10 units per 20 grams of dextrose) should be added to the infusion or, ideally, administered as a separate injection.

Patients with absent P waves or broad QRS complex who are not receiving cardiotonic glycosides should immediately be given 0.5 g to 1 g of calcium gluconate or another calcium salt I.V. over a 2-minute period (with continuous ECG monitoring) to antagonize the cardiotoxic effect of the potassium. May be repeated in 1 to 2 minutes if ECG abnormalities persist.

---

*Canada only   †Unlabeled clinical use   Italicized adverse reactions are life-threatening.

To remove potassium from the body, use sodium polystyrene sulfonate resin, hemodialysis, or peritoneal dialysis. Administer potassium-free I.V. fluids when hyperkalemia is associated with water loss.

▶ **Special considerations**
• In patients receiving digitalis, removing potassium too rapidly may result in digitalis toxicity.
• Monitor serum potassium, BUN, and serum creatinine levels; pH; and intake and output.
• Potassium should not be given during immediate postoperative period until urine flow is established.
• Give parenteral potassium by slow infusion only, never by I.V. push or I.M. Dilute I.V. potassium preparations with large volume of parenteral solutions.
• Give oral potassium supplements with extreme caution, because its many forms deliver varying amounts of potassium. Patient may tolerate one product better than another.
• Potassium gluconate does not correct hypokalemic hypochloremic alkalosis.
• Enteric-coated tablets are not recommended because of the potential for GI bleeding and small-bowel ulcerations.
• Tablets in wax matrix sometimes lodge in esophagus and cause ulceration in cardiac patients who have esophageal compression due to enlarged left atrium. In such patients and in those with esophageal or GI stasis or obstruction, use liquid form.
• Often used orally with diuretics that cause potassium excretion. Potassium chloride most useful since diuretics waste chloride ion. Hypokalemic alkalosis treated best with potassium chloride.
• Monitor ECG, pH, serum potassium levels, and other electrolytes during therapy.
• Do not crush sustained-released potassium products.

Information for the patient
• Tell patient potassium is available only with a prescription, because the wrong amount may cause severe reactions.
• Suggest diluting liquid potassium product in at least 4 to 8 oz of water; to take it after meals; and to sip liquid potassium slowly to minimize GI irritation.
• Tell patient to dissolve powder, soluble tablets, or granules completely in at least 4 oz of water or juice, and to allow fizzing to finish before drinking.
• Sustained-release capsules should not be crushed or chewed, but the capsule contents can be opened and sprinkled onto applesauce or other soft food.
• Tell the patient to stop taking the drug immediately and report any of the following reactions: confusion; irregular heartbeat; numbness of feet, fingers or lips; shortness of breath; anxiety, excessive tiredness or weakness of legs; unexplained diarrhea; nausea and vomiting; stomach pain; or bloody or black stools. Such reactions are rare.
• Tell the patient that expelling a whole tablet in the stool (sustained-release tablet) is normal. The body eliminates the shell after absorbing the potassium.
• Warn patient to avoid salt substitutes except when recommended by physician.

Pediatric use
Safety and efficacy for use in children have not been established.

Breast-feeding
Potassium supplements pass into the breast milk. Safety in breast-feeding has not been established; therefore, use potassium only when the benefits to the breast-feeding woman outweigh the risk to the infant.

pralidoxime chloride (2-PAM chloride, pyridine-2-aldoxime methochloride)
Protopam

• Pharmacologic classification: quaternary ammonium oxime
• Therapeutic classification: antidote
• Pregnancy risk category C

How supplied
Available by prescription only
Injection: 1 g/20 ml vial (without diluent or syringe); 1 g/20 ml vial with diluent, syringe, needle, alcohol swab (emergency kit); 600 mg/2 ml auto-injector, parenteral

Indications, route, and dosage
Organophosphate pesticide poisoning
Adults: 1 to 2 g I.V. over 15 to 30 minutes, followed by 500 mg/hr I.V. infusion.
Children: 20 to 40 mg/kg I.V. infusion over 15 to 30 minutes.
Pralidoxime chloride is most effective when administered within 24 hours of exposure. It should be administered with atropine.

Pharmacodynamics
Antidote action: Pralidoxime reactivates cholinesterase that has been inactivated by phosphorylation due to exposure to an organophosphate pesticide or related compound. One of the few drugs that correct a biochemical lesion, pralidoxime acts by removing the phosphoryl group from the active site of the inhibited enzyme, freezing and reactivating acetylcholinesterase. It also directly reacts with and detoxifies the organophosphorous molecule and may also react with cholinesterase to protect it from inhibition.
Cholinesterase reactivation occurs primarily at the neuromuscular junction where pralidoxime exerts its most critical effect – reversal of respiratory paralysis or paralysis of other skeletal muscles. Reactivation also occurs at autonomic effector sites and, to a lesser degree, within the CNS.

Pharmacokinetics
• *Absorption:* Pralidoxime is absorbed variably and incompletely after oral administration, with peak plasma levels in 2 to 3 hours. After I.V. administration, peak plasma levels are reached in 5 to 15 minutes; after I.M., in 10 to 20 minutes.
• *Distribution:* Pralidoxime is distributed throughout the extracellular water; it is not appreciably bound to plasma protein. It does not readily pass into the CNS. Distribution into breast milk is unknown. Therapeutic concentrations are achieved in the eye following subconjunctival injection.
• *Metabolism:* Exact mechanism is unknown, but hepatic metabolism is considered likely.
• *Excretion:* Drug is excreted rapidly in urine as un-

changed drug and metabolite; 80% to 90% of I.V. or I.M. dose is excreted unchanged within 12 hours.

Contraindications and precautions
Use cautiously in patients with myasthenia gravis who are receiving anticholinesterase agents because drug may precipitate a myasthenic crisis; and in patients with impaired renal function because accumulation of drug and metabolites may occur. Reduced dosage may be advisable in these patients.

Interactions
Concurrent use of respiratory or CNS depressants, skeletal muscle relaxants, or drugs that lower the seizure threshold should be avoided in patients with anticholinesterase poisoning. Therefore, avoid the use of morphine, theophylline, aminophylline, succinylcholine, reserpine, phenothiazines, and other respiratory depressants in patients receiving pralidoxime. Use barbiturates with caution to treat convulsions, because barbiturates are potentiated by anticholinesterase.

Effects on diagnostic tests
Elevated AST (SGOT), ALT (SGPT) (return to normal in 2 weeks); transient elevation in creatine phosphokinase levels.

Adverse reactions
- CNS: dizziness, headache, drowsiness.
- CV: tachycardia.
- DERM: maculopapular rash.
- EENT: blurred vision, diplopia, and impaired accommodation.
- GI: nausea.
- Other: hyperventilation, muscular weakness, mild to moderate pain at injection site.
  Note: It is difficult to differentiate the toxic effects of atropine and organophosphates from those of pralidoxime, and the patient's condition will generally mask minor signs and symptoms.

When atropine and pralidoxime are used together, signs of atropinism may occur earlier than expected, especially if the dose of atropine was large and administration of pralidoxime delayed. Excitement, confusion, manic behavior, and muscle rigidity have been reported after recovery of consciousness whether or not pralidoxime was used.

Overdose and treatment
Clinical manifestations of overdose include dizziness, headache, blurred vision, diplopia, impaired accommodation, nausea, and tachycardia. However, these effects may also result from organophosphate toxicity or the use of atropine.

To treat, remove secretions and all contaminated clothing. Administer artificial respiration; maintain airway. Provide supportive therapy as needed, and monitor ECG. After ingested overdose, induce emesis if patient is fully alert. Perform gastric lavage with activated charcoal and sodium sulfate.

▶ Special considerations
- Assess vital signs and insert I.V. line. Use requires close medical supervision, and close observation of the patient for at least 24 hours.
- Reconstitute pralidoxime with 20 ml of sterile water for injection to provide a solution containing 50 mg/ml. For I.V. infusion, dilute calculated dose to a volume of 100 ml with normal saline injection. Use within a few hours.
- Pralidoxime usually is administered by I.V. infusion over 15 to 30 minutes. Rapid administration has produced tachycardia, laryngospasm, muscle rigidity, and transient neuromuscular blockade. Hypertension may also occur, related to dose and rate of infusion; it may be treated by discontinuing the infusion or slowing the rate of infusion. 5 mg of phentolamine I.V. quickly reverses pralidoxime-induced hypertension. Closely monitor blood pressure.
- In patients with pulmonary edema, or when I.V. infusion is not practical, or a more rapid effect is needed, pralidoxime may be given by slow I.V. injection over at least 5 minutes. It may also be given I.M. or S.C.
- Dosage should be reduced in patients with impaired renal function.
- Institute treatment of organophosphate poisoning without waiting for laboratory test results. Draw blood for RBC and cholinesterase levels before giving pralidoxime. Begin pralidoxime and atropine therapy simultaneously. Give 2 to 6 mg of atropine I.V. (I.M. if patient is cyanotic) every 5 to 60 minutes in adults until muscarinic effects (dyspnea, cough, salivation, bronchospasm) subside. Repeat dosage if signs reappear. Maintain some degree of atropinism for at least 48 hours.
- Treatment is most effective when started within the first 24 hours, preferably within a few hours after poisoning. Even severe poisoning may be reversed if drug is given within 48 hours. Monitor effect of therapy by ECG because of possible heart block due to the anticholinesterase. Continued absorption of the anticholinesterase from the lower bowel constitutes new toxic exposure that may require additional doses of pralidoxime every 3 to 8 hours, or over several days.
- After dermal exposure, the patient's clothing should be removed and hair and skin should be washed with sodium bicarbonate, soap, water, or alcohol as soon as possible. While cleaning the patient, caregiver should wear gloves and protective garb to avoid contamination. Patient may need a second washing.
- Pralidoxime is not effective in treating toxic exposure to phosphorous, inorganic phosphates, or organophosphates that do not have anticholinesterase activity.
- Give I.V. sodium thiopental or diazepam if seizures interfere with respiration.
- Subconjunctival injection is currently an unapproved method of administration but has been used to reverse adverse ocular effects resulting from systemic overdose or splashing of an organophosphate agent into the eye.

Information for the patient
Warn patient that mild to moderate pain may occur 20 to 40 minutes after I.M. injection.

Pediatric use
Safety has not been established.

Breast-feeding
It is unknown if drug is distributed into breast milk.

---

pramoxine hydrochloride
Fleet relief, PrameGel, Prax,
ProctoFoam, Tronolane, Tronothane

- Pharmacologic classification: unclassified local anesthetic
- Therapeutic classification: topical local anesthetic
- Pregnancy risk category C

How supplied
Available without a prescription
Cream: 1%
Lotion: 1%
Ointment: 1%
Suppositories: 1%
Aerosol: 1% foam suspension
Gel: 1% gel

Indications, route, and dosage
For temporary relief of pain and itching caused by dermatoses, minor burns
Adults and children: Apply cream, gel or lotion to affected area t.i.d or q.i.d. or as directed.
For temporary relief of pain and itching associated with anogenital pruritus or irritation
Adults and children: Apply aerosol foam to affected area as directed.
For temporary relief of pain and itching caused by hemorrhoids
Adults: Apply cream, ointment, or suppositories up to 5 times daily or as directed; or alternatively, one applicatorful of the foam rectally b.i.d. to q.i.d. and after bowel movements.

Pharmacodynamics
Anesthetic action: Inhibits the conduction of nerve impulses by causing an alteration of cell membrane permeability to ions. This causes a specific anesthetic action on the local nerve cells.

Pharmacokinetics
- *Absorption:* Limited with topical use, unless skin tissue is abraded or drug is applied to mucous membranes.
- *Distribution:* None.
- *Metabolism:* None.
- *Excretion:* None.

Contraindications and precautions
Avoid use over large areas. Do not use in or near the eyes or nose. Pramoxine is contraindicated in patients with known hypersensitivity to the drug.

Interactions
None reported.

Effects on diagnostic tests
None reported.

Adverse reactions
- Local: burning, stinging.
Note: Drug should be discontinued if sensitization, extreme irritation, or redness occurs.

Overdose and treatment
No information available.

▶ Special considerations
- Drug is not recommended for prolonged use. Drug should be discontinued after 4 consecutive weeks of use.
- Drug may be applied with gauze or sprayed directly on skin. Cleanse and thoroughly dry rectal area before applying.

Information for the patient
- Tell patient to wash hands thoroughly before and after use.
- Advise patient to apply drug sparingly, to minimize untoward effects.
- Instruct patient to avoid eating for 1 hour after oral administration. Topical anesthetic action increases risk of aspiration.

Geriatric use
Dosage should be adjusted to patient's age, size, and physical condition.

Pediatric use
Dosage should be adjusted to patient's age, size, and physical condition.

pravastatin sodium
Pravachol

- Pharmacologic classification: HMG-CoA reductase inhibitor
- Therapeutic classification: antilipemic
- Pregnancy risk category X

How supplied
Available by prescription only
Tablets: 10 mg, 20 mg

Indications, route, and dosage
Reduction of low-density lipoprotein and total cholesterol levels in patients with primary hypercholesterolemia (types IIa and IIb)
Adults: Initially, 5 to 10 mg daily h.s. Adjust dosage q 4 weeks based on patient tolerance and response; maximum daily dosage is 40 mg. Most elderly patients respond to a daily dosage of 20 mg or less.

Pharmacodynamics
- *Antilipemic action:* Pravastatin inhibits the enzyme 3-hydroxy-3-methylglutaryl-coenzyme A (HMG-CoA) reductase. This hepatic enzyme is an early (and rate limiting) step in the synthetic pathway of cholesterol.

Pharmacokinetics
- *Absorption:* Pravastatin is rapidly absorbed, with peak plasma levels in 1 to 1½ hours. Average oral absorption is 34%, with absolute bioavailability of 17%. Although food reduces bioavailability, drug effects are the same if drug is taken with or 1 hour before meals.
- *Distribution:* Plasma levels of drug are proportional to dose, but do not necessarily correlate perfectly with lipid-lowering effects. About 50% is bound to plasma proteins. Drug experiences extensive first-pass extrac-

tion, possibly because of an active transport system into hepatocytes.

● *Metabolism:* Drug is metabolized by the liver; at least six metabolites have been identified. Some are active.
● *Excretion:* Pravastatin is excreted by the liver and kidneys.

Contraindications and precautions

Pravastatin is contraindicated in patients with hypersensitivity to the drug and in patients with active liver disease or conditions that have unexplained persistent elevations of serum transaminase. Drug is also contraindicated in pregnant and breast-feeding women and should not be administered to women of childbearing age unless there is no risk of pregnancy.

Liver function tests should be performed frequently at the start of therapy and periodically thereafter.

Clinical evidence of liver dysfunction may occur in up to 1.3% of patients. Persistent elevations of serum transaminase up to three times the upper normal limit may occur; these elevations are not associated with jaundice or other symptoms. Drug should be discontinued and patients monitored closely. A liver biopsy may be performed in patients whose enzyme elevations persist.

Interactions

Concomitant use with immunosuppressive agents (such as cyclosporine), fibric acid derivatives (such as clofibrate or gemfibrozil), high doses of niacin (1 g or more nicotinic acid daily), and erythromycin may increase risk of rhabdomyolysis. Monitor patient closely if concomitant use can't be avoided.

Hepatotoxic drugs or chronic alcohol abuse may increase risk of hepatotoxicity. Concurrent use with cholestyramine or colestipol may decrease plasma levels of pravastatin. Administer pravastatin 1 hour before or 4 hours after these drugs.

Avoid concomitant use with gemfibrozil because it decreases protein-binding and urinary clearance of pravastatin.

Drugs that decrease levels or activity of endogenous steroids (such as cimetidine, spironolactone, ketoconazole) may increase risk of endocrine dysfunction. No intervention appears necessary; take complete drug history in patients who develop endocrine dysfunction.

Effects on diagnostic tests

None reported.

Adverse reactions

● CNS: headache, fatigue, dizziness.
● CV: chest pain.
● DERM: rash.
● GI: vomiting, diarrhea, heartburn, nausea.
● Hepatic: liver dysfunction, elevated serum transaminase levels.
● Other: influenza, localized muscle pain, myalgia, cold, rhinitis, cough.

Overdose and treatment

No information available. Treat symptomatically.

▶ Special considerations

● Drug should be temporarily discontinued in any patient with an acute condition that suggests a developing myopathy or in patients having risk factors that may predispose them to development of renal failure secondary to rhabdomyolysis (including severe acute in-

fection; severe endocrine, metabolic, or electrolyte disorders; hypotension; major surgery; or uncontrolled seizures).

● Watch for signs of myositis. Rarely, myopathy and marked elevations of CPK, possibly leading to rhabdomyolysis and renal failure secondary to myoglobinuria, have been reported.

● Initiate pravastatin only after diet and other nonpharmacologic therapies have proved ineffective. Patients should continue a cholesterol-lowering diet during therapy.

● The recommended dosage should be administered in the evening, preferably at bedtime. Drug may be given without regard to meals.

● Dosage adjustments should be made about every 4 weeks. If cholesterol levels fall below the target range, dosage may be reduced.

Information for the patient

● Teach patient appropriate dietary management (restricting total fat and cholesterol intake), weight control, and exercise. Explain the importance of these interventions in controlling serum lipids.
● Because of drug's possible impact on liver function, advise patient to restrict alcohol intake.
● Tell patient to call if he experiences adverse reactions, particularly muscle aches and pains.

Geriatric use

Maximum effectiveness is usually evident with daily doses of 20 mg or less.

Pediatric use

Safety and efficacy in children under age 18 have not been established.

Breast-feeding

Pravastatin is excreted in breast milk. Women should not breast-feed while taking pravastatin.

---

prazepam
Centrax

● Pharmacologic classification: benzodiazepine
● Therapeutic classification: antianxiety agent
● Controlled substance schedule IV
● Pregnancy risk category D

How supplied

Available by prescription only
Tablets: 10 mg
Capsules: 5 mg, 10 mg, 20 mg

Indications, route, and dosage
Anxiety

Adults: 30 mg P.O. daily in divided doses. Dosage range is 20 to 60 mg/day. May be administered as single daily dose h.s., with an initial dose of 20 mg.

Pharmacodynamics

Anxiolytic and sedative-hypnotic action: Prazepam depresses the CNS at the limbic and subcortical levels of the brain. It produces an antianxiety effect by enhancing the effect of the neurotransmitter gamma-aminobutyric acid (GABA) on its receptor in the ascending reticular activating system, which increases inhibition and blocks both cortical and limbic arousal.

Pharmacokinetics
• *Absorption:* When administered orally, prazepam is well absorbed through the GI tract. Peak levels occur in 2½ to 6 hours. Prazepam undergoes nearly complete first-pass metabolism to desmethyldiazepam after absorption.
• *Distribution:* Prazepam is distributed widely throughout the body. Drug is 85% to 95% protein-bound.
• *Metabolism:* Prazepam is metabolized in the liver to desmethyldiazepam and oxazepam.
• *Excretion:* The metabolites of prazepam are excreted in urine as glucuronide conjugates. The half-life of desmethyldiazepam ranges from 30 to 200 hours, and oxazepam is from 5 to 15 hours.

Contraindications and precautions
Prazepam is contraindicated in patients with known hypersensitivity to the drug; in those with acute narrow-angle glaucoma or untreated open-angle glaucoma, because of the drug's possible anticholinergic effect; in patients in coma, because the drug's hypnotic or hypotensive effect may be prolonged or intensified; and in patients with acute alcohol intoxication who have depressed vital signs, because the drug will worsen CNS depression.

Prazepam should be used cautiously in patients with psychoses, because the drug is rarely beneficial in such patients and may induce paradoxical reactions; in patients with myasthenia gravis or Parkinson's disease, because it may exacerbate the disorder; in patients with impaired renal or hepatic function, which prolongs elimination of the drug; in elderly or debilitated patients, who are usually more sensitive to the drug's CNS effects; and in individuals prone to addiction or drug abuse.

Interactions
Prazepam potentiates the CNS depressant effects of phenothiazines, narcotics, antihistamines, monoamine oxidase inhibitors, barbiturates, alcohol, general anesthetics, and antidepressants.

Concomitant use with cimetidine and possibly disulfiram causes diminished hepatic metabolism of prazepam, which increases its plasma concentration.

Heavy smoking accelerates prazepam's metabolism, thus lowering clinical effectiveness.

Antacids may delay the absorption of prazepam. Prazepam may antagonize levodopa's therapeutic effects.

Effects on diagnostic tests
Prazepam therapy may elevate liver function test results. Minor changes in EEG patterns (usually low-voltage, fast activity) may occur during and after prazepam therapy.

Adverse reactions
• CNS: confusion, depression, drowsiness, lethargy, hangover effect, ataxia, dizziness, syncope, nightmares, fatigue, slurred speech, tremors, vertigo, behavior problems, headache.
• CV: bradycardia, *circulatory collapse,* transient hypotension.
• DERM: rash, urticaria.
• EENT: diplopia, blurred vision, nystagmus.
• GI: constipation, dry mouth, anorexia, nausea, vomiting, abdominal discomfort.

• GU: urinary incontinence or retention.
• Other: *respiratory depression,* dysarthria, hepatic dysfunction, changes in libido.
  Note: Drug should be discontinued if hypersensitivity or the following paradoxical reactions occur: acute hyperexcited state, anxiety, hallucinations, increased muscle spasticity, insomnia, or rage.

Overdose and treatment
Clinical manifestations of overdose include somnolence, confusion, coma, hypoactive reflexes, dyspnea, labored breathing, hypotension, bradycardia, slurred speech, and unsteady gait or impaired coordination.

Support blood pressure and respiration until drug effects subside; monitor vital signs. Flumazenil, a benzodiazepine antagonist, may be useful. Mechanical ventilatory assistance via endotracheal tube may be required to maintain a patent airway and support adequate oxygenation. Use I.V. fluids and vasopressors such as dopamine and phenylephrine to treat hypotension, as needed. If patient is conscious, induce emesis. Use gastric lavage if ingestion was recent, but only if an endotracheal tube is present to prevent aspiration. After emesis or lavage, administer activated charcoal with a cathartic as a single dose. Dialysis is of limited value.

▶ Special considerations
Besides those relevant to all *benzodiazepines,* consider the following recommendations.
• Use lowest possible effective dose. Gradually increase dose as necessary to avoid adverse reactions.
• Lower doses are effective in patients with renal or hepatic dysfunction.
• Monitor hepatic function studies periodically to prevent toxicity.
• Do not discontinue drug suddenly if patient is on long-term therapy.

Information for the patient
• As necessary, teach patient safety measures to prevent injury, such as gradual position changes and supervised ambulation.
• Caution patient to seek medical approval before making any changes in drug regimen.
• Advise patient of the potential for physical and psychological dependence with chronic use.
• Do not discontinue drug suddenly if patient has received long-term therapy.

Geriatric use
• Lower doses usually are effective in elderly patients because of decreased elimination.
• Elderly patients are more susceptible to the CNS depressant effects of prazepam. Use with caution.
• Elderly patients who receive this drug require supervision with ambulation and activities of daily living during initiation of therapy or after an increase in dose.

Pediatric use
• Safe use in patients under age 18 has not been established.
• Closely observe a neonate for withdrawal symptoms if mother took prazepam during pregnancy. Use of prazepam during labor may cause neonatal flaccidity.

Breast-feeding

Prazepam is excreted in breast milk. A breast-fed infant may become sedated, have feeding difficulties, or lose weight. Avoid use in breast-feeding women.

---

praziquantel
Biltricide

- Pharmacologic classification: pyrazinoisoquinoline
- Therapeutic classification: anthelmintic
- Pregnancy risk category B

How supplied

Available by prescription only
Tablets: 600 mg

Indications, route, and dosage
Schistosomiasis

Adults and children age 4 and older: 20 mg/kg P.O. t.i.d. as a 1-day treatment. The interval between doses should be between 4 and 6 hours; however, some clinicians give the drug in two divided doses 4 hours apart.

Pharmacodynamics

Anthelmintic action: Praziquantel appears to increase cell permeability to calcium, causing paralysis of the worms' musculature, dislodgment from mesenteric and pelvic veins, and subsequent death by host tissue reaction. It is effective against all pathogenic *Schistosoma,* including *S. mekongi, S. japonicum, S. mansoni,* and *S. haematobium,* and has some activity against tapeworms.

Pharmacokinetics

- *Absorption:* About 80% of praziquantel is absorbed; peak serum concentrations occur at 1 to 3 hours.
- *Distribution:* Distribution of praziquantel is not well documented; however, CSF levels are approximately 14% to 20% of plasma levels.
- *Metabolism:* Praziquantel undergoes significant first-pass metabolism to hydroxylated metabolites in the liver.
- *Excretion:* Drug and metabolites are excreted primarily in urine. Drug half-life is about 1 to 1½ hours; metabolite half-life is 4 to 5 hours. Drug is excreted in breast milk.

Contraindications and precautions

Praziquantel is contraindicated in patients with known hypersensitivity to the drug and in patients with ocular involvement of schistosomiasis, because destruction of parasites within eyes may cause irreversible ocular damage.

Interactions

None reported.

Effects on diagnostic tests

Praziquantel may increase CSF protein concentrations and serum liver enzyme concentrations.

Adverse reactions

- CNS: *drowsiness, malaise,* headache, dizziness, seizures.
- GI: abdominal discomfort, nausea, vomiting, anorexia, diarrhea.
- Hepatic: minimal increase in liver enzyme levels.
- Other: rise in body temperature, sweating.
  Note: Drug should be discontinued if signs of hypersensitivity or toxicity occur.

Overdose and treatment

Acute overdose has not been reported. Should it occur, a fast-acting laxative would be appropriate treatment.

▶ Special considerations

- Give drug during meals or with food, and follow with water to minimize GI discomfort; tablets are bitter and may cause gagging or vomiting if chewed or incompletely swallowed.
- Adverse effects may be more common and severe in patients with heavy infestation.
- Steroids are sometimes given concomitantly to reduce CNS adverse effects.

Information for the patient

- Tell patient to swallow tablets whole and not to chew or crush them.
- Tell patient that drug may cause drowsiness; patient should not drive or perform other hazardous activities on the day of and the day after treatment.
- Counsel patient to return as requested for post-treatment evaluation of stool specimens, to ensure destruction of parasites.

Pediatric use

Safety has not been established in children under age 4.

Breast-feeding

Drug is excreted in breast milk. Women should refrain from breast-feeding on the day of treatment and for the next 3 days.

---

prazosin hydrochloride
Minipress

- Pharmacologic classification: alpha-adrenergic blocking agent
- Therapeutic classification: antihypertensive
- Pregnancy risk category C

How supplied

Available by prescription only
Capsules: 1 mg, 2 mg, 5 mg

Indications, route, and dosage
Hypertension

Adults: Initially, 1 mg P.O. b.i.d. or t.i.d.; gradually increased to a maximum of 20 mg daily. Usual maintenance dosage is 6 to 15 mg daily in divided doses. If other antihypertensive or diuretics are added to prazosin therapy, reduce dosage of prazosin to 1 or 2 mg t.i.d. and then gradually increase as necessary.

Pharmacodynamics

Antihypertensive action: Prazosin selectively and competitively inhibits alpha-adrenergic receptors, causing arterial and venous dilation, reducing peripheral vascular resistance and blood pressure.

Pharmacokinetics

● *Absorption:* Absorption from the GI tract is variable; antihypertensive effect begins in about 2 hours, peaking in 2 to 4 hours. Full antihypertensive effect may not occur for 4 to 6 weeks.

● *Distribution:* Prazosin is distributed throughout the body and is highly protein-bound (approximately 97%).

● *Metabolism:* Prazosin is metabolized extensively in the liver.

● *Excretion:* Over 90% of a given dose is excreted in feces via bile; remainder is excreted in urine. Plasma half-life is 2 to 4 hours. Antihypertensive effect lasts less than 24 hours.

Contraindications and precautions

Prazosin is contraindicated in patients with known hypersensitivity to the drug.

Drug should be used cautiously in elderly patients, in patients taking other antihypertensive drugs, and in patients with chronic renal failure.

Interactions

Prazosin may potentiate the antihypertensive effects of other antihypertensive agents, including propranolol.

Concomitant use with propranolol and other beta blockers may cause severe hypotension.

Because prazosin is highly bound to plasma proteins, it may interact with other highly protein-bound drugs.

Effects on diagnostic tests

Prazosin alters results of screening tests for pheochromocytoma and causes increases in levels of the urinary metabolite of norepinephrine and vanillylmandelic acid; it may cause positive antinuclear antibody (ANA) titer and liver function test abnormalities. A transient fall in leukocyte count and increased serum uric acid and BUN levels may also occur.

Adverse reactions

● CNS: dizziness, headache, drowsiness, weakness, *first-dose syncope,* depression.
● CV: orthostatic hypotension, palpitations.
● EENT: blurred vision, dry mouth.
● GI: vomiting, diarrhea, abdominal cramps, constipation, nausea.
● GU: priapism, impotence.

Overdose and treatment

Overdose is manifested by hypotension and drowsiness. After acute ingestion, empty stomach by induced emesis or gastric lavage, and give activated charcoal to reduce absorption. Further treatment is usually symptomatic and supportive. Prazosin is not dialyzable.

▶ Special considerations

Besides those relevant to all *alpha-adrenergic blocking agents,* consider the following recommendations.
● First-dose syncope – dizziness, light-headedness, and syncope – may occur within 30 minutes to 1 hour after the initial dose; it may be severe, with loss of consciousness, if initial dose is greater than 2 mg. The effect is transient and may be diminished by giving the drug at bedtime; it is more common during febrile illness and more severe if patient has hyponatremia. Always increase dosage gradually and have patient sit or lie down if he experiences dizziness.
● Prazosin's effect is most pronounced on diastolic blood pressure.
● Prazosin has been used to treat vasospasm asso-

ciated with Raynaud's syndrome. It also has been used with diuretics and cardiac glycosides to treat severe congestive heart failure, to manage the signs and symptoms of pheochromocytoma preoperatively, and to treat ergotamine-induced peripheral ischemia.

Information for the patient

● Teach patient about his disease and therapy, and explain why he must take drug exactly as prescribed, even when feeling well; advise him never to discontinue drug suddenly, because severe rebound hypertension may occur, and to promptly report any malaise or any unusual adverse effects.

● Tell patient to avoid hazardous activities that require mental alertness until tolerance develops to sedation, drowsiness, and other CNS effects; to avoid sudden position changes to minimize orthostatic hypotension; and to use ice chips, candy, or gum to relieve dry mouth.

● Warn patient to seek medical approval before taking nonprescription cold preparations.

Geriatric use

Elderly patients may be more sensitive to hypotensive effects and may require lower doses because of altered drug metabolism.

Pediatric use

Safety and efficacy in children have not been established; use only when potential benefit outweighs risk.

Breast-feeding

Small amounts of prazosin are excreted in breast milk; an alternative feeding method is recommended during therapy.

---

prednisolone (systemic)
Cortalone, Delta-Cortef, Novoprednisolone*, Prelone

prednisolone acetate
Articulose, Deltastab*, Key-Pred, Predaject, Predate, Predcor

prednisolone acetate and prednisolone sodium phosphate

prednisolone sodium phosphate
Codelsol*, Hydeltrasol, Key-Pred SP, Pediapred, Predate-S

prednisolone tebutate
Hydeltra-T.B.A., Metalone T.B.A., Nor-Pred T.B.A., Predate T.B.A., Predcor T.B.A., Predisol T.B.A.

● Pharmacologic classification: glucocorticoid, mineralocorticoid
● Therapeutic classification: anti-inflammatory, immunosuppressant
● Pregnancy risk category C

How supplied
Available by prescription only
Prednisolone
Tablets: 5 mg
Syrup: 15 mg/5 ml

Prednisolone acetate
Injection: 25 mg/ml, 50 mg/ml, 100 mg/ml suspension
Prednisolone acetate and prednisolone sodium phosphate
Injection: 80 mg acetate and 20 mg sodium phosphate/ml suspension
Prednisolone sodium phosphate
Oral liquid: 6.7 mg (5 mg base)/5 ml
Injection: 20 mg/ml solution
Prednisolone tebutate
Injection: 20 mg/ml suspension

Indications, route, and dosage
Severe inflammation or immunosuppression
Adults: 2.5 to 15 mg P.O. b.i.d., t.i.d., or q.i.d.
Children: 0.14 to 2 mg/kg or 4 to 6 mg/m² daily in divided doses.
Prednisolone acetate
Adults: 2 to 30 mg I.M. q 12 hours.
Prednisolone sodium phosphate
Adults: 2 to 30 mg I.M. or I.V. q 12 hours, or into joints, lesions and soft tissue, p.r.n.
Children: 0.04 to 0.25 mg/kg or 1.5 to 7.5 mg/m² I.M. or I.V. daily in divided doses.
Prednisolone tebutate
Adults: 4 to 40 mg into joints and lesions, p.r.n.
Prednisolone acetate and prednisolone sodium phosphate suspension
Adults: 0.25 to 1 ml into joints weekly, p.r.n.

Pharmacodynamics
Anti-inflammatory action: Prednisolone stimulates the synthesis of enzymes needed to decrease the inflammatory response. It suppresses the immune system by reducing activity and volume of the lymphatic system, thus producing lymphocytopenia (primarily of T-lymphocytes), decreasing immunoglobulin and complement concentrations, decreasing passage of immune complexes through basement membranes, and possibly depressing reactivity of tissue to antigen-antibody interactions.

The mineralocorticoids regulate electrolyte homeostasis by acting renally at the distal tubules to enhance the reabsorption of sodium ions (and thus water) from the tubular fluid into the plasma and enhance the excretion of both potassium and hydrogen ions.

Prednisolone is an adrenocorticoid with both glucocorticoid and mineralocorticoid properties. It is a weak mineralocorticoid with only half the potency of hydrocortisone but is a more potent glucocorticoid, having four times the potency of equal weight of hydrocortisone. It is used primarily as an anti-inflammatory agent and an immunosuppressant. It is not used for mineralocorticoid replacement therapy because of the availability of more specific and potent agents.

Prednisolone may be administered orally. Prednisolone sodium phosphate is highly soluble, has a rapid onset and a short duration of action, and may be given I.M. or I.V. Prednisolone acetate and tebutate are suspensions that may be administered by intra-articular, intrasynovial, intrabursal, intralesional, or soft tissue injection. They have a slow onset but a long duration of action. Prednisolone sodium phosphate and prednisolone acetate is a combination product of the rapid-acting phosphate salt and the slightly soluble, slowly released acetate salt. This product provides rapid anti-inflammatory effects with a sustained duration of action. It is a suspension and should not be given I.V. It is particularly useful as an anti-inflammatory agent in intra-articular, intradermal, and intralesional injections.

Pharmacokinetics
● *Absorption:* Prednisolone is absorbed readily after oral administration. After oral and I.V. administration, peak effects occur in about 1 to 2 hours. The acetate and tebutate suspensions for injection have a variable absorption over 24 to 48 hours, depending on whether they are injected into an intra-articular space or a muscle, and on the blood supply to that muscle. Systemic absorption occurs slowly after intra-articular injection.
● *Distribution:* Prednisolone is removed rapidly from the blood and distributed to muscle, liver, skin, intestines, and kidneys. Prednisolone is extensively bound to plasma proteins (transcortin and albumin). Only the unbound portion is active. Adrenocorticoids are distributed into breast milk and through the placenta.
● *Metabolism:* Prednisolone is metabolized in the liver to inactive glucuronide and sulfate metabolites.
● *Excretion:* The inactive metabolites, and small amounts of unmetabolized drug, are excreted in urine. Insignificant quantities of drug are excreted in feces. The biological half-life of prednisolone is 18 to 36 hours.

Contraindications and precautions
Prednisolone is contraindicated in patients with hypersensitivity to ingredients of adrenocorticoid preparations or in those with systemic fungal infections (except in adrenal insufficiency). Patients who are receiving prednisolone should not receive live virus vaccines because prednisolone suppresses the immune response.

Prednisolone should be used with extreme caution in patients with GI ulceration, renal disease, hypertension, osteoporosis, diabetes mellitus, thromboembolic disorders, seizures, myasthenia gravis, congestive heart failure (CHF), tuberculosis, hypoalbuminemia, hypothyroidism, cirrhosis of the liver, emotional instability, psychotic tendencies, hyperlipidemias, glaucoma, or cataracts, because the drug may exacerbate these conditions.

Because adrenocorticoids increase the susceptibility to and mask symptoms of infection, prednisolone should not be used (except in life-threatening situations) in patients with viral or bacterial infections not controlled by anti-infective agents.

Interactions
When used concomitantly, prednisolone rarely may decrease the effects of oral anticoagulants by unknown mechanisms.

Glucocorticoids increase the metabolism of isoniazid and salicylates; they cause hyperglycemia, requiring dosage adjustment of insulin or oral hypoglycemic agents in diabetic patients; and may enhance hypokalemia associated with diuretic or amphotericin B therapy. The hypokalemia may increase the risk of toxicity in patients concurrently receiving digitalis glycosides.

Barbiturates, phenytoin, and rifampin may cause decreased corticosteroid effects because of increased hepatic metabolism. Cholestyramine, colestipol, and antacids decrease prednisolone's effect by adsorbing the corticosteroid, decreasing the amount absorbed.

Concomitant use with estrogens may reduce the metabolism of prednisolone by increasing the concentration of transcortin. The half-life of the corticosteroid is then prolonged because of increased protein binding. Concomitant administration of ulcerogenic drugs such as nonsteroidal anti-inflammatory agents may increase the risk of GI ulceration.

Effects on diagnostic tests
Prednisolone suppresses reactions to skin tests; causes false-negative results in the nitroblue tetrazolium test for systemic bacterial infections; decreases ^{131}I uptake and protein-bound iodine concentrations in thyroid function tests; may increase glucose and cholesterol levels; may decrease serum potassium, calcium, thyroxine, and triiodothyronine levels; and may increase urine glucose and calcium levels.

Adverse reactions
When administered in high doses or for prolonged therapy, prednisolone suppresses release of adrenocorticotropic hormone (ACTH) from the pituitary gland; in turn, the adrenal cortex stops secreting endogenous corticosteroids. The degree and duration of hypothalamic-pituitary-adrenal (HPA) axis suppression produced by the drugs is highly variable among patients and depends on the dose, frequency and time of administration, and duration of glucocorticoid therapy.
● CNS: euphoria, insomnia, headache, psychotic behavior, pseudotumor cerebri, mental changes, nervousness, restlessness.
● CV: CHF, hypertension, edema.
● DERM: delayed healing, acne, skin eruptions, striae.
● EENT: cataracts, glaucoma, thrush.
● GI: peptic ulcer, irritation, increased appetite.
● Immune: immunosuppression, increased susceptibility to infection.
● Metabolic: hypokalemia, sodium retention, fluid retention, weight gain, hyperglycemia, osteoporosis, growth suppression in children.
● Musculoskeletal: muscle atrophy, weakness.
● Other: *pancreatitis*, hirsutism, cushingoid symptoms, withdrawal syndrome (nausea, fatigue, anorexia, dyspnea, hypotension, hypoglycemia, myalgia, arthralgia, fever, dizziness, and fainting). *Sudden withdrawal may be fatal or may exacerbate the underlying disease.* Acute adrenal insufficiency may occur with increased stress (infection, surgery, trauma) or abrupt withdrawal after long-term therapy.

Overdose and treatment
Acute ingestion, even in massive doses, is rarely a clinical problem. Toxic signs and symptoms rarely occur if drug is used for less than 3 weeks, even at large dosage ranges. However, chronic use causes adverse physiologic effects, including suppression of the HPA axis, cushingoid appearance, muscle weakness, and osteoporosis.

▶ Special considerations
Recommendations for use of prednisolone and for care and teaching of patients are the same as those for all *systemic adrenocorticoids.*

Pediatric use
Chronic use of adrenocorticoids or corticotropin may suppress growth and maturation in children and adolescents.

prednisolone acetate (ophthalmic)
AK-Tate, Econopred Ophthalmic, I-Prednicet, Ocu-Pred-A, Predair-A, Pred Forte, Pred Mild Ophthalmic

prednisolone sodium phosphate
AK Pred, Inflamase, Inflamase Mild Ophthalmic, Inflamase Forte, I-Pred, Metreton, Ocu-Pred, Predair, Predsol*

● Pharmacologic classification: corticosteroid
● Therapeutic classification: ophthalmic anti-inflammatory
● Pregnancy risk category C

How supplied
Available by prescription only
Prednisolone acetate
Suspension: 0.12%, 0.125%, 0.25%, 1%
Prednisolone sodium phosphate
Solution: 0.125%, 0.5%, 1%

Indications, route, and dosage
Inflammation of palpebral and bulbar conjunctiva, cornea, and anterior segment of globe
Adults and children: Instill 1 or 2 drops in eye. In severe conditions, may be used hourly, tapering to discontinuation as inflammation subsides. In mild conditions, may be used four to six times daily.

Pharmacodynamics
Anti-inflammatory action: Corticosteroids stimulate the synthesis of enzymes needed to decrease the inflammatory response. Prednisolone, a synthetic corticosteroid, has about four times the anti-inflammatory potency of an equal weight of hydrocortisone. Prednisolone acetate is poorly soluble and therefore has a slower onset of action, but a longer duration of action, when applied in a liquid suspension. The sodium phosphate salt is highly soluble and has a rapid onset but short duration of action.

Pharmacokinetics
● *Absorption:* After ophthalmic administration, prednisolone is absorbed through the aqueous humor. Systemic absorption rarely occurs.
● *Distribution:* After ophthalmic application, prednisolone is distributed throughout the local tissue layers. Any drug that is absorbed into circulation is rapidly removed from the blood and distributed into muscle, liver, skin, intestines, and kidneys.
● *Metabolism:* After ophthalmic administration, corticosteroids are primarily metabolized locally. The small amount that is absorbed into systemic circulation is metabolized primarily in the liver to inactive compounds.
● *Excretion:* Inactive metabolites are excreted by the kidneys, primarily as glucuronides and sulfates, but also as unconjugated products. Small amounts of the metabolites are excreted in feces.

Contraindications and precautions
Prednisolone is contraindicated in patients who are hypersensitive to any component of the preparation; in

patients with fungal infections of the eye; and in patients with acute, untreated purulent bacterial, viral, or fungal ocular infections. It should be used cautiously in patients with corneal abrasions. If a bacterial infection does not respond promptly to appropriate anti-infective therapy, prednisolone should be discontinued and another therapy applied.

Measure intraocular pressure every 2 to 4 weeks for the first 2 months of ophthalmic corticosteroid therapy; if no increase in pressure has occurred, measure about every 1 to 2 months thereafter.

Interactions
None reported.

Effects on diagnostic tests
None reported.

Adverse reactions
● Eye: transient burning or stinging on administration; mydriasis, ptosis, epithelial punctate keratitis, possible corneal or scleral malacia (rare); increased intraocular pressure, thinning of the cornea, interference with corneal wound healing, increased susceptibility to viral or fungal corneal infection, corneal ulceration; glaucoma, cataracts, defects in visual acuity and visual field (with long-term use).
● Systemic: rare, but may occur with excessive doses or long-term use.
Note: Drug should be discontinued if topical application results in local irritation, infection, significant systemic absorption, or hypersensitivity reaction; if visual acuity decreases or visual field is diminished; or if burning, stinging, or watering of eyes does not resolve quickly after administration.

Overdose and treatment
No information available.

▶ Special considerations
Recommendations for use of ophthalmic prednisolone and for care and teaching of patients during therapy are the same as those for all *ophthalmic adrenocorticoids.*

prednisone
Apo-Prednisone*, Meticorten, Novoprednisone*, Orasone, Panasol, Prednicen-M, SK-Prednisone, Winpred*

● Pharmacologic classification: adrenocorticoid
● Therapeutic classification: anti-inflammatory, immunosuppressant
● Pregnancy risk category C

How supplied
Available by prescription only
Tablets: 1 mg, 2.5 mg, 5 mg, 10 mg, 20 mg, 25 mg, 50 mg
Oral solution: 5 mg/ml; 5 mg/5 ml
Syrup: 5 mg/5 ml

Indications, route, and dosage
Severe inflammation or immunosuppression
Adults: 5 to 60 mg P.O. daily in single dose or divided doses. (Maximum daily dose is 250 mg.) Maintenance dose given once daily or every other day. Dosage must be individualized.
Children: 0.14 mg/kg or 4 to 6 mg/m² P.O. daily in divided doses; alternatively, may use the following dosage schedule.
Children age 11 to 18: 20 mg P.O. q.i.d.
Children age 5 to 10: 15 mg P.O. q.i.d.
Children age 18 months to 4 years: 7.5 to 10 mg P.O. q.i.d.
Acute exacerbations of multiple sclerosis
Adults: 200 mg P.O. daily for 1 week, then 80 mg every other day for 1 month.

Pharmacodynamics
● *Immunosuppressant action:* Prednisone stimulates the synthesis of enzymes needed to decrease the inflammatory response. It suppresses the immune system by reducing activity and volume of the lymphatic system, thus producing lymphocytopenia (primarily of T-lymphocytes), decreasing immunoglobulin and complement concentrations, decreasing passage of immune complexes through basement membranes, and possibly by depressing reactivity of tissue to antigen-antibody interactions.
● *Anti-inflammatory action:* Prednisone is one of the intermediate-acting glucocorticoids, with greater glucocorticoid activity than cortisone and hydrocortisone, but less anti-inflammatory activity than betamethasone, dexamethasone, and paramethasone. Prednisone is about four to five times more potent as an anti-inflammatory agent than hydrocortisone, but it has only half the mineralocorticoid activity of an equal weight of hydrocortisone. Prednisone is the oral glucocorticoid of choice for anti-inflammatory or immunosuppressant effects. For those patients who cannot swallow tablets, liquid forms are available. The oral concentrate (5 mg/ml) may be diluted in juice or another flavored diluent or mixed in semisolid food (such as applesauce) before administration.

Pharmacokinetics
● *Absorption:* Prednisone is absorbed readily after oral administration, with peak effects occuring in about 1 to 2 hours.
● *Distribution:* Prednisone is distributed rapidly to muscle, liver, skin, intestines, and kidneys. Prednisone is extensively bound to plasma proteins (transcortin and albumin). Only the unbound portion is active. Adrenocorticoids are distributed into breast milk and through the placenta.
● *Metabolism:* Prednisone is metabolized in the liver to the active metabolite prednisolone, which in turn is then metabolized to inactive glucuronide and sulfate metabolites.
● *Excretion:* The inactive metabolites and small amounts of unmetabolized drug are excreted by the kidneys. Insignificant quantities of drug are also excreted in feces. The biological half-life of prednisone is 18 to 36 hours.

Contraindications and precautions
Prednisone is contraindicated in patients with systemic fungal infections (except in adrenal insufficiency) and in those with hypersensitivity to ingredients of adrenocorticoid preparations. Patients receiving prednisone

---

should not be given live virus vaccines because prednisone suppresses the immune response.

Prednisone should be used with extreme caution in patients with GI ulceration, renal disease, hypertension, osteoporosis, diabetes mellitus, thromboembolic disorders, seizures, myasthenia gravis, congestive heart failure (CHF), tuberculosis, hypoalbuminemia, hypothyroidism, cirrhosis of the liver, emotional instability, psychotic tendencies, hyperlipidemias, glaucoma, or cataracts because the drug may exacerbate these conditions.

Because adrenocorticoids increase the susceptibility to and mask symptoms of infection, prednisone should not be used (except in life-threatening situations) in patients with viral or bacterial infections not controlled by anti-infective agents.

Interactions
Concomitant use of prednisone rarely may decrease the effects of oral anticoagulants by unknown mechanisms.

Prednisone increases the metabolism of isoniazid and salicylates; causes hyperglycemia, requiring dosage adjustment of insulin or oral hypoglycemic agents in diabetic patients; and may enhance hypokalemia associated with diuretic or amphotericin B therapy. The hypokalemia may increase the risk of toxicity in patients concurrently receiving digitalis glycosides.

Barbiturates, phenytoin, and rifampin may cause decreased effects because of increased hepatic metabolism. Cholestyramine, colestipol, and antacids decrease the effect of prednisone by adsorbing the corticosteroid, decreasing the amount absorbed.

Concomitant use with estrogens may reduce the metabolism of prednisone by increasing the concentration of transcortin. The half-life of prednisone is then prolonged because of increased protein binding.

Concomitant administration of ulcerogenic drugs such as nonsteroidal anti-inflammatory agents may increase the risk of GI ulceration.

Effects on diagnostic tests
Prednisone suppresses reactions to skin tests; causes false-negative results in the nitroblue tetrazolium test for systemic bacterial infections; decreases ^{131}I uptake and protein-bound iodine concentrations in thyroid function tests; may increase glucose and cholesterol levels; may decrease serum potassium, calcium, thyroxine, and triiodothyronine levels; and may increase urine glucose and calcium levels.

Adverse reactions
When administered in high doses or for prolonged therapy, prednisone suppresses release of adrenocorticotropic hormone (ACTH) from the pituitary gland. In turn, the adrenal cortex stops secreting endogenous corticosteroids. The degree and duration of hypothalamic-pituitary-adrenal (HPA) axis suppression produced by the drugs is highly variable among patients and depends on the dose, frequency and time of administration, and duration of glucocorticoid therapy.
- CNS: euphoria, insomnia, headache, psychotic behavior, pseudotumor cerebri, mental changes, nervousness, restlessness.
- CV: CHF, hypertension, edema.
- DERM: delayed healing, acne, skin eruptions, striae.
- EENT: cataracts, glaucoma, thrush.
- GI: peptic ulcer, irritation, increased appetite.
- Immune: increased susceptibility to infection.

- Metabolic: hypokalemia, sodium retention, fluid retention, weight gain, hyperglycemia, osteoporosis, growth suppression in children.
- Musculoskeletal: muscle atrophy, weakness.
- Other: *pancreatitis*, hirsutism, cushingoid symptoms, withdrawal syndrome (nausea, fatigue, anorexia, dyspnea, hypotension, hypoglycemia, myalgia, arthralgia, fever, dizziness, and fainting). *Sudden withdrawal may be fatal or may exacerbate the underlying disease.* Acute adrenal insufficiency may occur with increased stress (infection, surgery, trauma) or abrupt withdrawal after long-term therapy.

Overdose and treatment
Acute ingestion, even in massive doses, is rarely a clinical problem. Toxic signs and symptoms rarely occur if drug is used for less than 3 weeks, even at large dosage ranges. However, chronic use causes adverse physiologic effects, including suppression of the HPA axis, cushingoid appearance, muscle weakness, and osteoporosis.

▶ Special considerations
Recommendations for use of prednisone and for care and teaching of patients are the same as those for all *systemic adrenocorticoids.*

Pediatric use
Chronic use of prednisone in children or adolescents may delay growth and maturation.

primaquine phosphate
- Pharmacologic classification: 8-amino-quinoline
- Therapeutic classification: antimalarial
- Pregnancy risk category C

How supplied
Available by prescription only
Tablets: 26.3 mg (15-mg base)
Note: Production of primaquine is temporarily discontinued because a chemical precursor is unavailable. Physicians may obtain drug free of charge from the Centers for Disease Control [(404) 639-3670 Monday to Friday from 8 a.m. to 4:30 p.m. Eastern time] for patients with parasitologically confirmed *Plasmodium vivax* or *P. ovale* who live in the United States or its territories. Because the supply is limited, drug will not be provided for prophylaxis or for *P. falciparum* or *P. malariae* infections, which do not *require* primaquine therapy. Physicians who call must supply parasitologic and clinical data, places and dates of travel to malarious areas, and use of malaria chemoprophylaxis.

Indications, route, and dosage
Radical cure of relapsing vivax malaria, eliminating symptoms and infection completely; and prevention of relapse
Adults: 15 mg (base) P.O. daily for 14 days (26.3-mg tablet equals 15 mg of base), or 79 mg (45-mg base) once a week for 8 weeks.
Children: 0.3 mg (base)/kg/day for 14 days, or 0.9 mg (base)/kg/day once a week for 8 weeks.

Pharmacodynamics
Antimalarial action: Primaquine disrupts the parasitic mitochondria, thereby interrupting metabolic processes requiring energy.

The spectrum of activity includes preerythrocytic and exoerythrocytic forms of *Plasmodium falciparum, P. malariae, P. ovale,* and *P. vivax.* Nifurtimox (Lampit), an investigational agent available from the Centers for Disease Control, is preferred for intracellular parasites.

Pharmacokinetics
● *Absorption:* Primaquine is well absorbed from the GI tract, with peak concentrations occurring at 2 to 6 hours.
● *Distribution:* Primaquine is distributed widely into the liver, lungs, heart, brain, skeletal muscle, and other tissues.
● *Metabolism:* Primaquine is carboxylated rapidly in the liver.
● *Excretion:* Only a small amount of primaquine is excreted unchanged in urine. The plasma half-life is 4 to 10 hours.

Contraindications and precautions
Primaquine is contraindicated in patients receiving quinacrine because of possible additive toxicity. It also is contraindicated in patients predisposed to granulocytopenia and in patients receiving other drugs that might cause hemolysis or bone marrow depression.

Primaquine should be used cautiously in patients who previously have had an idiosyncratic reaction to primaquine and in patients with a history of favism, G6PD deficiency, or NADH methemoglobin reductase deficiency, because hemolytic reactions may occur in these groups. It is contraindicated in patients with lupus erythematosus or rheumatoid arthritis.

Interactions
Quinacrine may potentiate the toxic effects of primaquine. Concomitant use with magnesium and aluminum salts may decrease gastrointestinal absorption.

Effects on diagnostic tests
Decreases or increases in white blood cell counts and decreases in red blood cell counts may occur during primaquine therapy. Methemoglobinemia may occur.

Adverse reactions
● CNS: headache.
● DERM: urticaria.
● EENT: disturbances of visual accommodation.
● GI: nausea, vomiting, epigastric distress, abdominal cramps.
● HEMA: leukopenia, hemolytic anemia in G6PD deficiency, methemoglobinemia in NADH methemoglobin reductase deficiency, leukocytosis, mild anemia, *granulocytopenia, agranulocytosis.*
Note: Drug should be discontinued immediately if urine darkens or if hemoglobin or hematocrit levels fall.

Overdose and treatment
Symptoms of overdose include abdominal distress, vomiting, CNS and cardiovascular disturbances, cyanosis, methemoglobinemia, leukocytosis, leukopenia, and anemia. Treatment is symptomatic.

▶ **Special considerations**
Besides those relevant to all *aminoquinolines,* consider the following recommendations.

● Primaquine is often used with a fast-acting antimalarial, such as chloroquine.
● Before starting therapy, screen patients for possible G6PD deficiency.
● Light-skinned patients taking more than 30 mg daily, dark-skinned patients taking more than 15 mg daily, and patients with severe anemia or suspected sensitivity should have frequent blood studies and urine examinations. A sudden fall in hemoglobin concentrations or erythrocyte or leukocyte counts, or a marked darkening of the urine suggests impending hemolytic reaction.
● All patients should have periodic blood studies and urinalyses to monitor for impending hemolytic reactions.

Information for the patient
● Teach patient the signs and symptoms of adverse reactions and to report them if they occur.
● Advise patient to check urine color at each voiding and to report if urine darkens, becomes tinged with red, or decreases in volume.
● Tell patient to take drug with meals to minimize gastric irritation. Do not take with antacids, which may decrease absorption.
● Advise patient to complete entire course of therapy.

Breast-feeding
Safety has not been established.

primidone
Myidone, Mysoline, Sertan

● Pharmacologic classification: barbiturate analogue
● Therapeutic classification: anticonvulsant
● Pregnancy risk category D

How supplied
Available by prescription only
Tablets: 50 mg, 250 mg
Suspension: 250 mg/5 ml

Indications, route, and dosage
Generalized tonic-clonic seizures, complex-partial (psychomotor) seizures
Adults and children age 8 and over: 250 mg P.O. daily. Increase by 250 mg weekly, up to a maximum of 2 g daily, divided q.i.d.
Children under age 8: 10 to 25 mg/kg P.O. daily, up to a maximum of 1 g daily, divided q.i.d.
Benign familial tremor (essential tremor)
Adults: 750 mg/day divided t.i.d.

Pharmacodynamics
Anticonvulsant action: Primidone acts as a nonspecific CNS depressant used alone or with other anticonvulsants to control refractory tonic-clonic seizures and to treat psychomotor or focal seizures. Mechanism of action is unknown; some activity may be from phenobarbital, an active metabolite.

Pharmacokinetics
● *Absorption:* Primidone is absorbed readily from the GI tract; serum concentrations peak at about 3 hours. Phenobarbital appears in plasma after several days of

continuous therapy; most laboratory assays detect both phenobarbital and primidone. Therapeutic levels are 5 to 12 mcg/ml for primidone and 10 to 30 mcg/ml for phenobarbital.

• *Distribution:* Primidone is distributed widely throughout the body.

• *Metabolism:* Primidone is metabolized slowly by the liver to phenylethylmalonamide (PEMA) and phenobarbital; PEMA is the major metabolite.

• *Excretion:* Primidone is excreted in urine; substantial amounts are excreted in breast milk.

Contraindications and precautions
Primidone is contraindicated in patients with known hypersensitivity to barbiturates; in pregnancy because of hazard of respiratory depression and neonatal coagulation defects; in patients with severe respiratory disease or status asthmaticus because of respiratory depressant effects; in patients with porphyria because of potential for adverse hematologic effects; and in patients with markedly impaired hepatic function because of potential for enhanced hepatic impairment. Use drug with caution in patients taking alcohol and other CNS depressants.

Interactions
Alcohol and other CNS depressants, including narcotic analgesics, cause excessive depression in patients taking primidone. Carbamazepine and phenytoin may decrease effects of primidone and increase its conversion to phenobarbital; monitor serum levels to prevent toxicity.

Effects on diagnostic tests
Primidone may cause abnormalities in liver function test results.

Adverse reactions
• CNS: drowsiness, ataxia, emotional disturbances, vertigo, hyperirritability, fatigue.
• DERM: morbilliform rash, alopecia.
• EENT: diplopia, nystagmus, edema of the eyelids.
• GI: anorexia, nausea, vomiting.
• GU: impotence, polyuria.
• HEMA: leukopenia, eosinophilia.
• Other: edema, thirst.

Note: Drug should be discontinued if signs of hypersensitivity or hepatic dysfunction occur.

Overdose and treatment
Symptoms of overdose resemble those of barbiturate intoxication; they include CNS and respiratory depression, areflexia, oliguria, tachycardia, hypotension, hypothermia, and coma. Shock may occur.

Treat overdose supportively: in conscious patient with intact gag reflex, induce emesis with ipecac; follow in 30 minutes with repeated doses of activated charcoal. Use lavage if emesis is not feasible. Alkalinization of urine and forced diuresis may hasten excretion. Hemodialysis may be necessary. Monitor vital signs and fluid and electrolyte balance.

▶ Special considerations
Besides those relevant to all *barbiturates,* consider the following recommendations.
• Patient should have review of complete blood count and liver function tests every 6 months.
• Abrupt withdrawal of primidone may cause status epilepticus; dosage should be reduced gradually.

• Barbiturates impair ability to perform tasks requiring mental alertness, such as driving a car.

Information for the patient
• Explain rationale for therapy and the potential risks and benefits.
• Teach patient signs and symptoms of adverse reactions.
• Tell patient to avoid alcohol and other sedatives to prevent added CNS depression.
• Tell patient not to discontinue drug or to alter dosage without medical approval.
• Explain that barbiturates may render oral contraceptives ineffective; advise patient to consider a different birth control method.
• Advise patient to avoid hazardous tasks that require mental alertness until degree of sedative effect is determined. Tell the patient that dizziness and incoordination are common at first but will disappear.
• Recommend that patient wear a Medic Alert bracelet or necklace identifying him as having a seizure disorder and listing the drug.

Geriatric use
Reduce dose in elderly patients; they often have decreased renal function.

Pediatric use
Primidone may cause hyperexcitability in children under age 6.

Breast-feeding
Considerable amounts of primidone are excreted in breast milk. Alternative feeding method is recommended during therapy.

---

probenecid
Benemid, Probalan

• Pharmacologic classification: sulfonamide-derivative
• Therapeutic classification: uricosuric agent
• Pregnancy risk category B

How supplied
Available by prescription only
Tablets: 500 mg

Indications, route, and dosage
Adjunct to penicillin therapy
Adults and children over age 14 or weighing more than 50 kg: 500 mg P.O. q.i.d.
Children age 2 to 14 or weighing less than 50 kg: Initially, 25 mg/kg or 1.2 g/m² daily, then 40 mg/kg or 700 mg/m² divided q.i.d.
Single-dose penicillin treatment of gonorrhea
Adults: 1 g P.O. given together with penicillin treatment, or 1 g P.O. 30 minutes before I.M. dose of penicillin.
Hyperuricemia associated with gout
Adults: 250 mg P.O. b.i.d. for 1st week, then 500 mg b.i.d., to maximum of 2 to 3 g daily.

Pharmacodynamics
• *Uricosuric action:* Probenecid competitively inhibits the active reabsorption of uric acid at the proximal con-

---

voluted tubule, thereby increasing urinary excretion of uric acid.

● *Adjunctive action in antibiotic therapy:* Probenecid competitively inhibits secretion of weak organic acids, including penicillins, cephalosporins, and other beta-lactam antibiotics, thereby increasing concentrations of these drugs.

Pharmacokinetics

● *Absorption:* Probenecid is completely absorbed after oral administration; peak serum levels are reached at 2 to 4 hours.
● *Distribution:* Probenecid distributes throughout the body; drug is about 75% protein-bound. CSF levels are about 2% of serum levels.
● *Metabolism:* Probenecid is metabolized in the liver to active metabolites, with some uricosuric effect.
● *Excretion:* Drug and metabolites are excreted in urine; probenecid (but not metabolites) is actively reabsorbed.

Contraindications and precautions

Probenecid is contraindicated in patients with hypersensitivity to the drug and in patients with acute gout, blood dyscrasias, or uric acid kidney stones because it may worsen these conditions.

Probenecid should be used cautiously in patients with a history of peptic ulcer disease; in patients with renal impairment (drug is ineffective if glomerular filtration rate is lower than 30 ml/minute); and in patients with acute intermittent porphyria.

Interactions

Probenecid significantly increases or prolongs effects of penicillins, cephalosporins, and other beta-lactam antibiotics, sulfonamides, and possibly thiopental and ketamine; it enhances hypoglycemic effects of chlorpropamide and other oral sulfonylureas, and increases serum levels (thus increasing risk of toxicity) of dapsone, aminosalicylic acid, methotrexate, and nitrofurantoin.

Probenecid inhibits urinary excretion of weak organic acids; it impairs natriuretic effects of ethacrynic acid, furosemide, and bumetanide; it also decreases excretion of indomethacin and naproxen, permitting use of lower doses.

Diuretics, alcohol, and pyrazinamide decrease uric acid levels of probenecid; increased doses of probenecid may be required. Salicylates inhibit the uricosuric effect of probenecid only in doses that achieve levels of 50 mcg/ml or more; occasional use of low-dose aspirin does not interfere.

Effects on diagnostic tests

Probenecid causes false-positive test results for urinary glucose with tests using cupric sulfate reagent (Benedict's reagent, Clinitest, and Fehling's test); perform tests with glucose oxidase reagent (Clinistix, Tes-Tape) instead.

Adverse reactions

● CNS: headache, dizziness.
● CV: hypotension.
● EENT: sore gums.
● GI: anorexia, nausea, vomiting, gastric distress.
● GU: urinary frequency, renal colic, hematuria, uric acid stones.
● HEMA: leukopenia, *hemolytic or aplastic anemia.*
● Other: hair loss, increased gouty arthritis attacks, fever, sweating, flushing.

Note: Drug should be discontinued if patient shows signs of hypersensitivity reaction, rash, leukopenia, hemolytic anemia, or aplastic anemia.

Overdose and treatment

Clinical signs include nausea, copious vomiting, stupor, coma, and tonic-clonic seizures. Treat supportively, using mechanical ventilation if needed; induce emesis or use gastric lavage, as appropriate. Control seizures with I.V. phenobarbital and phenytoin.

▶ Special considerations

● When used for hyperuricemia associated with gout, probenecid has no analgesic or anti-inflammatory actions, and no effect on acute attacks; start therapy after attack subsides. Because the drug may increase the frequency of acute attacks during the first 6 to 12 months of therapy, prophylactic doses of colchicine or a nonsteroidal anti-inflammatory drug should be administered during the first 3 to 6 months of probenecid therapy.
● Monitor BUN and serum creatinine levels closely; drug is ineffective in severe renal insufficiency.
● Monitor uric acid levels and adjust dose to the lowest dose that maintains normal uric acid levels.
● Give with food, milk, or prescribed antacids to lessen GI upset.
● Maintain adequate hydration with high fluid intake to prevent formation of uric acid stones. Also maintain alkalinization of urine.
● Probenecid has been used in the diagnosis of parkinsonian syndrome and mental depression.

Information for the patient

● Patient should not discontinue drug without medical approval.
● Warn patient not to use drug for pain or inflammation and not to increase dose during gouty attack.
● Tell patient to drink 8 to 10 glasses of fluid daily and to take drug with food to minimize GI upset.
● Warn patient to avoid aspirin and other salicylates, which may antagonize probenecid's uricosuric effect.
● Caution diabetic patients to use Tes-tape, Diastix, or Clinistix for urine glucose testing.

Geriatric use

Lower doses are indicated in elderly patients.

Pediatric use

Drug is contraindicated in children younger than age 2.

Breast-feeding

It unknown whether probenecid is excreted in breast milk. An alternative feeding method is recommended during therapy with probenecid.

---

probucol
Lorelco

- Pharmacologic classification: bis-phenol derivative
- Therapeutic classification: cholesterol lowering agent
- Pregnancy risk category B

How supplied
Available by prescription only
Tablets: 250 mg, 500 mg

Indications, route, and dosage
Primary hypercholesterolemia
Adults: 500 mg P.O. b.i.d. with morning and evening meals. Not recommended for children.

Pharmacodynamics
Antilipemic action: Probucol lowers cholesterol levels (the exact mechanism is unknown), but has little effect on triglycerides. Probucol increases catabolism of low-density lipoproteins and inhibits early stages of cholesterol synthesis. Drug seems to be more effective in patients with mild disease.

Pharmacokinetics
- *Absorption:* GI absorption is limited (2% to 8%) and variable. When taken with food, probucol produces high blood levels and is less variable. Blood levels increase during first 3 to 4 months, then remain constant; clinical response usually occurs in 1 to 3 months.
- *Distribution:* Probucol is lipid-soluble and accumulates slowly in adipose tissue, persisting in fat and blood for at least 6 months after the last dose. Probucol blood level declines by 80% after 6 months; cholesterol-lowering effects disappear well before tissue level decrease.
- *Metabolism:* Unknown.
- *Excretion:* Probucol is eliminated via bile in feces; half-life ranges from 12 hours to over 500 hours, as drug slowly leaches out of fat tissues.

Contraindications and precautions
Probucol is contraindicated in patients with recent or progressive myocardial damage or cardiac dysrhythmia because serious CV toxicity occurs in animals. Although such toxicity has not been reported in humans, ECG monitoring before and during probucol therapy is advised. Probucol also is contraindicated in patients hypersensitive to the drug and in pregnant patients. Patients wishing to conceive should stop drug at least 6 months before attempt and use birth control throughout the waiting period because of persistent blood levels.

Interactions
Concomitant use with clofibrate does not produce additive effect; in some patients, combination decreases high-density lipoprotein cholesterol.

Effects on diagnostic tests
Probucol alters serum levels of bilirubin, glucose, creatine phosphokinase, AST (SGOT), ALT (SGPT), uric acid, and alkaline phosphatase; blood urea nitrogen; and eosinophil, hematocrit, and hemoglobin counts.

Adverse reactions
- CNS: headache, dizziness, insomnia, tinnitus, paresthesia, peripheral neuritis.
- CV: prolonged Q-T interval on ECG.
- DERM: hyperhidrosis, fetid sweat, rash, itching, ecchymoses, petechiae.
- GI: diarrhea, flatulence, abdominal pain, nausea, vomiting, indigestion, GI bleeding.
- HEMA: eosinophilia, thrombocytopenia, decreased hemoglobin and hematocrit levels.
- Other: angioneurotic edema, conjunctivitis, impotence.

Note: Drug should be discontinued if cardiac arrhythmia or prolonged Q-T interval occurs.

Overdose and treatment
No specific data available and no specific antidote for overdose with probucol; drug is not dialyzable. Treatment is symptomatic and supportive.

▶ Special considerations
Do not exceed dosage of 1 g daily. Monitor electrocardiograms before and during drug therapy.

Information for the patient
- Tell patient to take probucol with food to enhance absorption.
- GI adverse reactions usually disappear with continued use. Tell patient to report any adverse reactions that persist.
- Encourage patient to adhere to low-fat diet; drug is not curative.

Pediatric use
Safety and efficacy in children have not been established.

Breast-feeding
Use of probucol during breast-feeding is not recommended; drug is excreted in animal milk. It is unknown whether probucol enters human milk.

procainamide hydrochloride
Procan SR, Promine, Pronestyl, Pronestyl-SR, Rhythmin

- Pharmacologic classification: procaine derivative
- Therapeutic classification: ventricular antiarrhythmic, supraventricular antiarrhythmic
- Pregnancy risk category C

How supplied
Available by prescription only
Tablets: 250 mg, 375 mg, 500 mg; 250 mg, 500 mg, 750 mg, 1 g (extended-release)
Capsules: 250 mg, 375 mg, 500 mg
Injection: 100 mg/ml, 500 mg/ml

Indications, route, and dosage

Premature ventricular contractions; ventricular tachycardia; atrial fibrillation and flutter unresponsive to quinidine; paroxysmal atrial tachycardia

Adults: 100 mg q 5 minutes by slow I.V. push, no faster than 25 to 50 mg/minute, until arrhythmias disappear, adverse effects develop, or 500 mg has been given. When arrhythmias disappear, give continuous infusion of 2 to 6 mg/minute. Usual effective loading dose is 500 to 600 mg. If arrhythmias recur, repeat bolus as above and increase infusion rate. For oral therapy, initiate dosage at 50 mg/kg P.O. in divided doses q 3 hours until therapeutic levels are reached. Once patient is stable, may substitute sustained-release form q 6 hours.

Loading dose for atrial fibrillation or paroxysmal atrial tachycardia

Adults: 1 to 1.25 g P.O. If arrhythmias persist after 1 hour, give additional 750 mg. If no change occurs, give 500 mg to 1 g q 2 hours until arrhythmias disappear or adverse effects occur.

Loading dose for ventricular tachycardia

Adults: 1 g P.O. Maintenance dosage is 50 mg/kg/day given at 3-hour intervals; average is 250 to 500 mg q 4 hours but may require 1 to 1.5 g q 4 to 6 hours.

Note: Sustained-release tablets may be used for maintenance dosing when treating ventricular tachycardia, atrial fibrillation, and paroxysmal atrial tachycardia. Dosage is 500 mg to 1 g q 6 hours.

Pharmacodynamics

Antiarrhythmic action: A Class IA antiarrhythmic agent, procainamide depresses phase 0 of the action potential. It is considered a myocardial depressant because it decreases myocardial excitability and conduction velocity and may depress myocardial contractility. It also possesses anticholinergic activity, which may modify its direct myocardial effects. In therapeutic doses, it reduces conduction velocity in the atria, ventricles, and His-Purkinje system. Its effectiveness in controlling atrial tachyarrhythmias stems from its ability to prolong the effective refractory period (ERP) and increase the action potential duration in the atria, ventricles, and His-Purkinje system. Because ERP prolongation exceeds action potential duration, tissue remains refractory even after returning to resting membrane potential (membrane-stabilizing effect). Procainamide shortens the effective refractory period of the AV node. The drug's anticholinergic action also may increase AV node conductivity. Suppression of automaticity in the His-Purkinje system and ectopic pacemakers accounts for the drug's effectiveness in treating ventricular premature beats. At therapeutic doses, procainamide prolongs the PR and QT intervals (this effect may be used as an index of drug effectiveness and toxicity.) The QRS interval usually is not prolonged beyond normal range; the QT interval is not prolonged to the extent achieved with quinidine.

Procainamide exerts a peripheral vasodilatory effect; with I.V. administration, it may cause hypotension, which limits the administration rate and amount of drug deliverable.

Pharmacokinetics

● *Absorption:* Rate and extent of drug's absorption from the intestines vary; usually, 75% to 95% of an orally administered dose is absorbed. With administration of tablets and capsules, peak plasma levels occur in approximately 1 hour. Extended-release tablets are formulated to provide a sustained and relatively constant rate of release and absorption throughout the small intestine. After the drug's release, extended wax matrix is not absorbed and may appear in feces after 15 minutes to 1 hour. With I.M. injection, onset of action occurs in about 10 to 30 minutes, with peak levels in about 1 hour.

● *Distribution:* Procainamide is distributed widely in most body tissues, including cerebrospinal fluid, liver, spleen, kidneys, lungs, muscles, brain, and heart. Only about 15% binds to plasma proteins. Usual therapeutic range for serum procainamide concentrations is 4 to 8 mcg/ml. Some experts suggest that a range of 10 to 30 mcg/ml for the sum of procainamide and N-acetyl procainamide (NAPA) serum concentrations are therapeutic.

● *Metabolism:* Procainamide is acetylated in the liver to form NAPA. Acetylation rate is determined genetically and affects NAPA formation. (NAPA also exerts antiarrhythmic activity.)

● *Excretion:* Procainamide and NAPA metabolite are excreted in the urine. Procainamide's half-life is about 2½ to 4¾ hours. NAPA's half-life is about 6 hours. In patients with congestive heart failure and/or renal dysfunction, half-life increases; therefore, in such patients, dosage reduction is required to avoid toxicity.

Contraindications and precautions

Procainamide is contraindicated in patients with complete AV block with AV junctional or idioventricular pacemaker without an operative artificial pacemaker, and in patients with prolonged QT interval or QRS duration, because of potential for heart block; in patients with digitalis toxicity, because the drug may further depress conduction, which may result in ventricular asystole or fibrillation; in patients with torsades de pointes, because the drug may exacerbate this arrhythmia; in patients with myasthenia gravis, because the drug may exacerbate muscle weakness; and in patients with hypersensitivity to procainamide or related compounds (such as procaine).

Procainamide should be used with caution in patients with incomplete AV block or bundle branch block, because the drug may further depress conduction; in patients with congestive heart failure, because drug may worsen this condition; and in patients with renal or hepatic dysfunction, because the drug may accumulate, causing toxicity.

Interactions

Concomitant use of procainamide with neuromuscular blocking agents (such as pancuronium bromide, succinylcholine chloride, tubocurarine chloride, gallium triethiodide, metocurine iodide, and decamethonium bromide) may potentiate procainamide drug effects. Concomitant use with anticholinergic agents (such as diphenhydramine, atropine, and tricyclic antidepressants) may cause additive anticholinergic effects.

Concomitant use with cholinergic agents (such as neostigmine and pyridostigmine, which are used to treat myasthenia gravis) may negate the effects of these agents, requiring increased dosage.

Concomitant use with antihypertensives may cause additive hypotensive effects (most common with I.V. procainamide). Concomitant use with other antiarrhythmics may result in additive or antagonistic cardiac effects and with possible additive toxic effects. Concomitant use with cimetidine may result in impaired renal clearance of procainamide and NAPA, with elevated serum drug concentrations. Concomitant use with captopril may cause additive immunosuppression.

Effects on diagnostic tests
Procainamide will invalidate bentiromide test results; discontinue at least 3 days before bentiromide test. Procainamide may alter edrophonium test results; positive ANA titers, positive direct antiglobulin (Coombs') tests, and ECG changes may be seen. The physiologic effects of the drug may result in decreased leukocytes and platelets, and increased bilirubin, LDH, alkaline phosphatase, ALT (SGPT), and AST (SGOT).

Adverse reactions
● CNS: hallucinations, confusion, convulsions, depression.
● CV: severe hypotension, bradycardia, AV block, *ventricular fibrillation* (with parenteral administration).
● DERM: maculopapular rash.
● GI: nausea, vomiting, anorexia, diarrhea, bitter taste.
● HEMA: thrombocytopenia, neutropenia (especially with sustained-release forms), *agranulocytosis, hemolytic anemia,* increased antinuclear antibody (ANA) titer.
● Other: fever, lupus erythematosus syndrome (especially after prolonged administration).
Note: Drug should be discontinued if granulocytopenia or lupus erythematosus syndrome occur, unless drug's benefits outweigh risks.

Overdose and treatment
Clinical effects of overdose include severe hypotension, widening QRS complex, junctional tachycardia, intraventricular conduction delay, ventricular fibrillation, oliguria, confusion and lethargy, and nausea and vomiting.

Treatment involves general supportive measures (including respiratory and cardiovascular support) with hemodynamic and ECG monitoring. After recent ingestion of oral form, gastric lavage, emesis, and activated charcoal may be used to decrease absorption. Phenylephrine or norepinephrine may be used to treat hypotension after adequate hydration has been ensured. Hemodialysis may be effective in removing procainamide and NAPA. A ⅙ molar solution of sodium lactate may reduce procainamide's cardiotoxic effect.

▶ Special considerations
● In treating atrial fibrillation and flutter, ventricular rate may accelerate due to vagolytic effects on the AV node; to prevent this effect, digitalis may be administered before procainamide therapy begins.
● Patients receiving infusions must be attended at all times.
● Infusion pump or microdrip system and timer should be used to monitor infusion precisely.
● Monitor blood pressure and ECG continuously during I.V. administration. Watch for prolonged QT and QRS intervals, heart block, or increased arrhythmias.
● Monitor therapeutic serum levels of procainamide: 3 to 10 mcg/ml (most patients are controlled at 4 to 8 mcg/ml); may exhibit toxicity at levels greater than 16 mcg/ml). Monitor NAPA levels as well; some clinicians feel that procainamide and NAPA levels should be 10 to 30 mcg/ml.
● Baseline and periodic determinations of ANA titers, LE cell preparations, and CBCs may be indicated because procainamide therapy (usually long-term) has been associated with syndrome resembling systemic lupus erythematosus.

● I.V. drug form is more likely to cause adverse cardiac effects, possibly resulting in severe hypotension.
● In prolonged use of oral form, ECGs should be performed occasionally to determine continued need for the drug.

Geriatric use
Elderly patients may require reduced dosage. Because of highly variable metabolism, monitoring of serum levels is recommended.

Pediatric use
Manufacturer has not established dosage guidelines for pediatric patients. For treating arrhythmias, the suggested dosage is 40 to 60 mg/kg of standard tablets or capsules, P.O. daily, given in 4 to 6 divided doses; or 3 to 6 mg/kg I.V. over 5 minutes, followed by a drip of 0.02 to 0.08 mg/kg/minute.

Breast-feeding
Because procainamide and NAPA are distributed into breast milk, alternative feeding method is recommended for women receiving procainamide.

procainamide hydrochloride
Matulane, Natulan*

● Pharmacologic classification: antibiotic antineoplastic (cell cycle-phase specific, S phase)
● Therapeutic classification: antineoplastic
● Pregnancy risk category D

How supplied
Available by prescription only
Capsules: 50 mg

Indications, route, and dosage
Dosage and indications may vary. Check current literature for recommended protocol.
Hodgkin's disease; lymphomas; brain and lung cancer
Adults: 2 to 4 mg/kg/day P.O. in single or divided doses for the first week, followed by 4 to 6 mg/kg/day until response or toxicity occurs. Maintenance dosage is 1 to 2 mg/kg/day.
Children: 50 mg P.O. daily for first week, then 100 mg/m² until response or toxicity occurs. Maintenance dosage is 50 mg P.O. daily after bone marrow recovery.

Pharmacodynamics
Antineoplastic action: The exact mechanism of procarbazine's cytotoxic activity is unknown. The drug appears to have several sites of action; the result is inhibition of DNA, RNA, and protein synthesis. Procarbazine has also been reported to damage DNA directly and to inhibit the mitotic S phase of cell division.

Pharmacokinetics
● *Absorption:* Procarbazine is rapidly and completely absorbed following oral administration.
● *Distribution:* Procarbazine distributes widely into body tissues, with the highest concentrations found in the liver, kidneys, intestinal wall, and skin. The drug crosses the blood-brain barrier.
● *Metabolism:* Procarbazine is extensively metabo-

lized in the liver. Some of the metabolites have cytotoxic activity.
● *Excretion:* Procarbazine and its metabolites are excreted primarily in urine.

Contraindications and precautions
Procarbazine is contraindicated in patients with a history of hypersensitivity to the drug and in patients with poor bone marrow reserve because of potential for serious toxicity.

Drug should be used cautiously in patients with hepatic or renal impairment because of potential for drug accumulation; in those with infections because of decreased immune response; and in those taking concurrent CNS depressants or MAO inhibitors because the drug has MAO-inhibiting activity.

Interactions
Concomitant use of procarbazine with alcohol can cause a disulfiram-like reaction. The mechanism of this interaction is poorly defined. Concomitant use with CNS depressants enhances CNS depression through an additive mechanism; concomitant use with sympathomimetics, tricyclic antidepressants, MAO inhibitors, or tyramine-rich foods can cause a hypertensive crisis, tremors, excitation, and cardiac palpitations through inhibition of MAO by procarbazine. Serum digoxin levels may be decreased. Concomitant use with meperidine may result in severe hypotension and death.

Effects on diagnostic tests
None reported.

Adverse reactions
● CNS: paresthesias, myalgias, arthralgias, fatigue, lethargy, nervousness, depression, insomnia, nightmares, hallucinations, confusion.
● DERM: dermatitis, pruritus, flushing, hyperpigmentation, photosensitivity.
● EENT: retinal hemorrhage, nystagmus, photophobia, diplopia, papilledema, altered hearing abilities.
● GI: nausea, vomiting, anorexia, stomatitis, dry mouth, dysphagia, diarrhea, constipation.
● GU: decreased spermatogenesis, infertility.
● HEMA: *bone marrow depression* (dose-limiting), *pancytopenia, hemolysis,* bleeding tendency, *thrombocytopenia, leukopenia,* anemia.
● Other: chills, fever, pneumonitis, hypotension, reversible alopecia, pleural effusion.
Note: Drug should be discontinued if the following occur: bleeding or bleeding tendencies, stomatitis, diarrhea, paresthesias, neuropathies, confusion, or hypersensitivity.

Overdose and treatment
Clinical manifestations of overdose include myalgia, arthralgia, fever, weakness, dermatitis, alopecia, paresthesias, hallucinations, tremors, convulsions, coma, myelosuppression, nausea, and vomiting.

Treatment is usually supportive and includes transfusion of blood components, antiemetics, antipyretics, and appropriate antianxiety agents.

▶ Special considerations
● Nausea and vomiting may be decreased if taken at bedtime and in divided doses.
● Procarbazine inhibits MAO. Use procarbazine cautiously with MAO inhibitors, tricyclic antidepressants, or tyramine-rich foods.

● Use cautiously in inadequate bone marrow reserve, leukopenia, thrombocytopenia, anemia, and impaired hepatic or renal function.
● Observe for signs of bleeding.
● Store capsules in dry environment.

Information for the patient
● Emphasize importance of continuing medication despite nausea and vomiting.
● Advise patient to call immediately if vomiting occurs shortly after taking dose.
● Warn patient that drowsiness may occur, so patient should avoid hazardous activities that require alertness until drug's effect is established.
● Warn patient not to drink alcoholic beverages while taking this drug.
● Instruct patient to stop medication and call immediately if disulfiram-like reaction occurs (chest pains, rapid or irregular heartbeat, severe headache, stiff neck).
● Tell patient to avoid exposure to people with infections.
● Warn patient to avoid prolonged exposure to the sun because photosensitivity occurs during therapy.
● Tell patient to call if he develops a sore throat or fever or notices any unusual bruising or bleeding.

Pediatric use
Severe reactions, such as tremors, seizures, and coma, have occurred after administration of procarbazine to children.

Breast-feeding
It is not known whether procarbazine distributes into breast milk. However, because of the potential for serious adverse reactions, mutagenicity, and carcinogenicity in the infant, breast-feeding is not recommended.

---

prochlorperazine
Compazine, Stemetil*

prochlorperazine edisylate
Compazine

prochlorperazine maleate
Chlorazine, Compazine, Compazine Spansule, Stemetil*

● Pharmacologic classification: phenothiazine (piperazine derivative)
● Therapeutic classification: antipsychotic, antiemetic, antianxiety agent
● Pregnancy risk category C

How supplied
Available by prescription only
Prochlorperazine maleate
Tablets: 5 mg, 10 mg, 25 mg
Prochlorperazine edisylate
Spansules (sustained-release): 10 mg, 15 mg, 30 mg
Syrup: 1 mg/ml
Injection: 5 mg/ml
Suppositories: 2.5 mg, 5 mg, 25 mg

Indications, route, and dosage
Preoperative nausea control
Adults: 5 to 10 mg I.M. 1 to 2 hours before induction of anesthesia, repeated once in 30 minutes if necessary; or 5 to 10 mg I.V. 15 to 30 minutes before induction of anesthesia, repeated once if necessary; or 20 mg/liter dextrose 5% and sodium chloride 0.9% solution by I.V. infusion, added to infusion 15 to 30 minutes before induction. Maximum parenteral dosage is 40 mg daily.

Severe nausea, vomiting
Adults: 5 to 10 mg P.O. t.i.d. or q.i.d.; or 15 mg of sustained-release form P.O. on arising; or 10 mg of sustained-release form P.O. q 12 hours; or 25 mg rectally b.i.d.; or 5 to 10 mg I.M. injected deeply into upper outer quadrant of gluteal region. Repeat q 3 to 4 hours, p.r.n. May be given I.V. Maximum parenteral dosage is 40 mg daily.

Children weighing 18 to 39 kg: 2.5 mg P.O. or rectally t.i.d.; or 5 mg P.O. or rectally b.i.d.; or 0.132 mg/kg deep I.M. injection. (Control usually obtained with one dose.) Maximum dosage is 15 mg daily.

Children weighing 14 to 17 kg: 2.5 mg P.O. or rectally b.i.d. or t.i.d.; or 0.132 mg/kg deep I.M. injection. (Control usually is obtained with one dose.) Maximum dosage is 10 mg daily.

Children weighing 9 to 13 kg: 2.5 mg P.O. or rectally daily or b.i.d.; or 0.132 mg/kg deep I.M. injection. (Control usually is obtained with one dose.) Maximum dosage is 7.5 mg daily.

Pharmacodynamics
• *Antipsychotic action:* Prochlorperazine is thought to exert its antipsychotic effects by postsynaptic blockade of CNS dopamine receptors, thus inhibiting dopamine-mediated effects.
• *Antiemetic action:* Antiemetic effects are attributed to dopamine receptor blockade in the medullary chemoreceptor trigger zone.

Prochlorperazine has many other central and peripheral effects: it produces alpha and ganglionic blockade and counteracts histamine- and serotonin-mediated activity. Its most prevalent adverse reactions are extrapyramidal. It is used primarily as an antiemetic; it is ineffective against motion sickness.

Pharmacokinetics
• *Absorption:* Rate and extent of absorption vary with administration route: oral tablet absorption is erratic and variable, with onset of action ranging from ½ to 1 hour; oral concentrate absorption is more predictable. I.M. drug is absorbed rapidly.
• *Distribution:* Prochlorperazine is distributed widely into the body, including breast milk. Drug is 91% to 99% protein-bound. Peak effect occurs at 2 to 4 hours; steady-state serum levels are achieved within 4 to 7 days.
• *Metabolism:* Prochlorperazine is metabolized extensively by the liver, but no active metabolites are formed; duration of action is about 3 to 4 hours.
• *Excretion:* Most of drug is excreted in urine via the kidneys; some is excreted in feces via the biliary tract.

Contraindications and precautions
Prochlorperazine is contraindicated in patients with known hypersensitivity to phenothiazines and related compounds, including allergic reactions involving hepatic function; in patients with blood dyscrasias and bone marrow depression; and in patients with disorders accompanied by coma, brain damage, CNS depres-

sion, circulatory collapse, or cerebrovascular disease, because of adverse effects on blood pressure and possible additive CNS depression. It also is contraindicated for use with adrenergic-blocking agents or spinal or epidural anesthetics.

Prochlorperazine should be used cautiously in patients with cardiac disease (arrhythmias, congestive heart failure, angina pectoris, valvular disease, or heart block) because of additive arrhythmic effects; in patients with encephalitis; in patients with Reye's syndrome, head injury, or respiratory disease, because of additive CNS and respiratory depression; in patients with epilepsy and other seizure disorders because of lowered seizure threshold; in patients with glaucoma because of increased intraocular pressure; in patients with prostatic hypertrophy; in patients with urinary retention; in patients with hepatic or renal dysfunction; in patients with Parkinson's disease; in patients with pheochromocytoma because excessive buildup of neurotransmitters may have adverse cardiovascular effects; and in patients with hypocalcemia, which increases the risk of extrapyramidal symptoms.

Interactions
Concomitant use of prochlorperazine with sympathomimetics, including epinephrine, phenylephrine, phenylpropanolamine, and ephedrine (often found in nasal sprays), and with appetite suppressants may decrease their stimulatory and pressor effects and may cause epinephrine reversal (hypotensive response to epinephrine).

Prochlorperazine may inhibit blood pressure response to centrally acting antihypertensive drugs, such as guanethidine, guanabenz, guanadrel, clonidine, methyldopa, and reserpine. Additive effects are likely after concomitant use of prochlorperazine with CNS depressants, including analgesics barbiturates, narcotics, tranquilizers, and anesthetics (general, spinal, or epidural), and parenteral magnesium sulfate (oversedation, respiratory depression, and hypotension); antiarrhythmic agents, quinidine, disopyramide, and procainamide (increased incidence of cardiac arrhythmias and conduction defects); atropine and other anticholinergic drugs, including antidepressants, monoamine oxidase inhibitors, phenothiazines, antihistamines, meperidine, and antiparkinsonian agents (oversedation, paralytic ileus, visual changes, and severe constipation); nitrates (hypotension); and metrizamide (increased risk of convulsions).

Beta-blocking agents may inhibit prochlorperazine metabolism, increasing plasma levels and toxicity.

Concomitant use with propylthiouracil increases risk of agranulocytosis; concomitant use with lithium may result in severe neurologic toxicity with an encephalitis-like syndrome, and in decreased therapeutic response to prochlorperazine.

Pharmacokinetic alterations and subsequent decreased therapeutic response to prochlorperazine may follow concomitant use with phenobarbital (enhanced renal excretion); aluminum- and magnesium-containing antacids and antidiarrheals (decreased absorption); caffeine; or heavy smoking (increased metabolism).

Prochlorperazine may antagonize therapeutic effect of bromocriptine on prolactin secretion; it also may decrease the vasoconstricting effects of high-dose dopamine and may decrease effectiveness and increase toxicity of levodopa (by dopamine blockade). Prochlorperazine may inhibit metabolism and increase toxicity of phenytoin.

Effects on diagnostic tests

Prochlorperazine causes false-positive test results for urinary porphyrins, urobilinogen, amylase, and 5-HIAA, because of darkening of urine by metabolites; it also causes false-positive urine pregnancy results in tests using human chorionic gonadotropin as the indicator.

Prochlorperazine elevates test results for liver enzymes and protein-bound iodine and causes quinidine-like ECG effects.

Adverse reactions

● CNS: extrapyramidal symptoms – dystonia, akathisia, torticollis, tardive dyskinesia (dose-related, long-term therapy), pseudoparkinsonism, *neuroleptic malignant syndrome* (dose-related; fatal *respiratory failure* in over 10% of patients if untreated), dizziness, drowsiness, sedation, headache, exacerbation of psychotic symptoms.
● CV: *asystole*, orthostatic hypotension, tachycardia, dizziness or fainting, arrhythmias, ECG changes, increased anginal pain after I.M. injection.
● EENT: blurred vision, tinnitus, mydriasis, increased intraocular pressure, ocular changes (retinal pigmentary change with long-term use).
● GI: dry mouth, constipation, nausea, vomiting, anorexia, diarrhea.
● GU: urinary retention, gynecomastia, hypermenorrhea, inhibited ejaculation.
● HEMA: transient leukopenia, *agranulocytosis*, thrombocytopenia, anemia (within 30 to 90 days).
● Local: contact dermatitis from concentrate or injectable form, muscle necrosis from I.M. injection.
● Other: hyperprolactinemia, photosensitivity, increased appetite (weight gain), hypersensitivity (rash, urticaria, drug fever, edema, cholestatic jaundice [in 0.1% to 4% of patients within first 30 days]).

After abrupt withdrawal of long-term therapy, gastritis, nausea, vomiting, dizziness, tremors, feeling of heat or cold, sweating, tachycardia, headache, or insomnia may occur.

Note: Drug should be discontinued if hypersensitivity, jaundice, agranulocytosis, neuroleptic malignant syndrome (marked hyperthermia, extrapyramidal effects, autonomic dysfunction) occurs or if severe extrapyramidal symptoms occur even after dose is lowered. Drug should be discontinued 48 hours before and 24 hours after myelography using metrizamide, because of the risk of convulsions. When feasible, drug should be withdrawn slowly and gradually; many drug effects persist after withdrawal.

Overdose and treatment

CNS depression is characterized by deep, unarousable sleep and possible coma, hypotension or hypertension, extrapyramidal symptoms, dystonia, abnormal involuntary muscle movements, agitation, seizures, dysrhythmias, ECG changes, hypothermia or hyperthermia, and autonomic nervous system dysfunction.

Treatment is symptomatic and supportive and includes maintaining vital signs, airway, stable body temperature, and fluid and electrolyte balance.

Do not induce vomiting: drug inhibits cough reflex, and aspiration may occur. Use gastric lavage, then activated charcoal and saline cathartics; dialysis does not help. Regulate body temperature as needed. Treat hypotension with I.V. fluids: *do not give epinephrine.* Treat seizures with parenteral diazepam or barbiturates; dysrhythmias with parenteral phenytoin (1 mg/kg with rate titrated to blood pressure); and extrapyramidal reactions with benztropine or parenteral diphenhydramine 2 mg/kg/minute.

▶ **Special considerations**

Besides those relevant to all *phenothiazines,* consider the following recommendations.
● The liquid and injectable formulations may cause a rash after contact with skin.
● Drug may cause a pink to brown discoloration of urine.
● Prochlorperazine is associated with a high incidence of extrapyramidal effects and in institutionalized mental patients, photosensitivity reactions; patient should avoid exposure to sunlight or heat lamps.
● Oral formulations may cause stomach upset. Administer with food or fluid.
● Dilute the concentrate in 2 to 4 oz of water. The suppository form should be stored in a cool place.
● Give I.V. dose slowly (5 mg/minute). I.M. injection may cause skin necrosis; take care to prevent extravasation. Do not mix with other medications in the syringe. Do not administer subcutaneously.
● Administer I.M. injection deep into the upper outer quadrant of the buttock. Massaging the area after administration may prevent formation of abscesses.
● Solution for injection may be slightly discolored. Do not use if excessively discolored or if a precipitate is evident. Contact pharmacist.
● Monitor patient's blood pressure before and after parenteral administration.
● The sustained-release form should not be given to children.
● Prochlorperazine is ineffective in treating motion sickness.
● Chewing gum, hard candy, or ice may help relieve dry mouth.
● Protect the liquid formulation from light.

Information for the patient

● Explain the risks of dystonic reactions and tardive dyskinesia. Tell patient to report abnormal body movements promptly.
● Tell patient to avoid sun exposure and to wear sunscreen when going outdoors, to prevent photosensitivity reactions. (Note that heat lamps and tanning beds also may cause burning of the skin or skin discoloration.)
● Tell patient to avoid spilling the liquid form. Contact with skin may cause rash and irritation.
● Warn patient to avoid extremely hot or cold baths and exposure to temperature extremes, sunlamps, or tanning beds; drug may cause thermoregulatory changes.
● Advise patient to take the drug exactly as prescribed, not to double doses after missing one, and not to share drug with others.
● Tell patient not to drink alcohol or take other medications that may cause excessive sedation.
● Tell patient to dilute the concentrate in water; explain the dropper technique of measuring dose; teach correct use of suppository.
● Tell patient that hard candy, chewing gum, or ice chips can alleviate dry mouth.
● Urge patient to store this drug safely away from children.
● Tell patient that interactions are possible with many drugs. Warn him to seek medical approval before taking *any* self-prescribed medication.
● Warn patient not to stop taking the drug suddenly

---

and to promptly report difficulty urinating, sore throat, dizziness, or fainting. Reassure patient that most reactions can be relieved by reducing dose.
• Warn patient to avoid hazardous activities that require alertness until the drug's effect is established. Reassure patient that sedative effects subside and become tolerable in several weeks.

Geriatric use
Elderly patients tend to require lower doses, titrated to individual effects. These patients are at greater risk for adverse reactions, especially tardive dyskinesia, other extrapyramidal effects, and hypotension.

Pediatric use
Prochlorperazine is not recommended for patients under age 2 or weighing less than 9 kg.

Breast-feeding
Prochlorperazine may enter breast milk and should be used with caution. Potential benefits to the mother should outweigh potential harm to the infant.

procyclidine hydrochloride
Kemadrin

• Pharmacologic classification: anticholinergic
• Therapeutic classification: antiparkinsonian agent
• Pregnancy risk category C

How supplied
Available by prescription only
Tablets: 5 mg

Indications, route, and dosage
Parkinsonism, muscle rigidity
Adults: Initially, 2.5 mg P.O. t.i.d., after meals. Increase as needed to maximum 60 mg daily.

Procyclidine is also used to relieve extrapyramidal dysfunction that accompanies treatment with phenothiazines and rauwolfia derivatives; drug controls excessive salivation from neuroleptic medications.

Pharmacodynamics
Antiparkinsonian action: Procyclidine blocks central cholinergic receptors, helping to balance cholinergic activity in the basal ganglia. It may also prolong dopamine's effects by blocking dopamine reuptake and storage at central receptor sites.

Pharmacokinetics
• *Absorption:* Procyclidine is absorbed from the GI tract.
• *Distribution:* Procyclidine crosses the blood-brain barrier; little else is known about its distribution.
• *Metabolism:* Exact metabolic fate is unknown.
• *Excretion:* Procyclidine is excreted in the urine as unchanged drug and metabolites.

Contraindications and precautions
Procyclidine is contraindicated in patients with narrow-angle glaucoma, because drug-induced cycloplegia and mydriasis may increase intraocular pressure.

Administer procyclidine cautiously to patients with tachycardia, because drug may block vagal inhibition

of the sinoatrial node pacemaker, thus exacerbating tachycardia; and to patients with urinary retention or prostatic hypertrophy, because drug may exacerbate these conditions.

Interactions
Procyclidine may reduce the antipsychotic effectiveness of haloperidol and phenothiazines, possibly by direct CNS antagonism; concomitant use with phenothiazines also increases the risk of anticholinergic adverse effects. Paralytic ileus may result from concomitant use with phenothiazines or tricyclic antidepressants. Concomitant use with alcohol and other CNS depressants increases procyclidine's sedative effects.

Antacids and antidiarrheals may decrease procyclidine's absorption, thus reducing its effectiveness.

Effects on diagnostic tests
None reported.

Adverse reactions
• CNS: light-headedness, giddiness, nervousness, headache, confusion, muscle weakness, paresthesia, disorientation, memory loss, agitation, delusions, delirium, paranoia, euphoria, excitement, psychoses, depression, heaviness of extremities.
• CV: tachycardia, palpitations.
• DERM: rash, flushing, decreased sweating.
• EENT: blurred vision, mydriasis.
• GI: constipation, dry mouth, nausea, vomiting, epigastric distress.
• GU: urinary hesitancy.
• Other: hypersensitivity.
Note: Drug should be discontinued if hypersensitivity or skin rash develops.

Overdose and treatment
Clinical effects of overdose include central stimulation followed by depression, and such psychotic symptoms as disorientation, confusion, hallucinations, delusions, anxiety, agitation, and restlessness. Peripheral effects may include dilated, nonreactive pupils; blurred vision; flushed, hot, dry skin; dry mucous membranes; dysphagia; decreased or absent bowel sounds; urinary retention; hyperthermia; tachycardia; hypertension; and increased respiration.

Treatment is primarily symptomatic and supportive, as needed. Maintain patent airway. If the patient is alert, induce emesis (or use gastric lavage) and follow with a saline cathartic and activated charcoal to prevent further drug absorption. In severe cases, physostigmine may be administered to block procyclidine's antimuscarinic effects. Give fluids, as needed, to treat shock; diazepam to control psychotic symptoms; and pilocarpine (instilled into the eyes) to relieve mydriasis. If urinary retention develops, catheterization may be necessary.

▶ Special considerations
Besides those relevant to all *anticholinergics,* consider the following recommendations.
• Monitor closely for confusion, disorientation, agitation, hallucinations, and other psychotic symptoms, especially if patient is elderly.
• Give procyclidine with food to decrease adverse GI effects.
• In patients with severe parkinsonism, tremors may increase because drug relieves spasticity.
• When switching from therapy with another drug to

procyclidine, substitution should be made gradually by initiating therapy with procyclidine and increasing dose while gradually decreasing dosage of other drug.

Geriatric use
Administer cautiously to elderly patients; lower doses are indicated.

Breast-feeding
Procyclidine may be excreted in breast milk, possibly resulting in infant toxicity. Breast-feeding women should avoid this drug. Drug may also decrease milk production.

---

progesterone
Bay Progest, Femotrone, Gesterol 50, Progestaject-50, Progestasert, Progestronaq-LA

- Pharmacologic classification: progestin
- Therapeutic classification: progestin, contraceptive
- Pregnancy risk category X

How supplied
Available by prescription only
Injection: 25 mg, 50 mg, and 100 mg/ml (in oil); 25 mg and 50 mg/ml (aqueous)
Intrauterine device: 38 mg (with barium sulfate, dispersed in silicone fluid)

Indications, route, and dosage
Amenorrhea
Adults: 5 to 10 mg I.M. daily for 6 to 8 days.
Dysfunctional uterine bleeding
Adults: 5 to 10 mg I.M. daily for 6 days. Alternatively, a single 50 to 100 mg I.M. dose.
Contraception (as an intrauterine device [IUD])
Adults: Progestasert system inserted into uterine cavity; replaced after 1 year.

Pharmacodynamics
Contraceptive action: Progesterone suppresses ovulation, thickens cervical mucus, and induces sloughing of the endometrium.

Pharmacokinetics
- *Absorption:* Progesterone must be administered parenterally since it is inactivated by the liver after oral administration.
- *Distribution:* Little information available.
- *Metabolism:* Progesterone is reduced to pregnanediol in the liver, then conjugated with glucuronic acid. The plasma half-life of progesterone is very short (several minutes).
- *Excretion:* Glucuronide-conjugated pregnanediol is excreted in urine.

Contraindications and precautions
Progesterone is contraindicated in patients with known hypersensitivity to progestins or a history of thromboembolic disorder, severe hepatic disease, breast cancer, or undiagnosed abnormal vaginal bleeding; and in pregnant or breast-feeding women.

Use cautiously in patients with cardiac or renal disease, epilepsy, migraine, or other conditions that might be aggravated by fluid and electrolyte retention; in diabetic patients because glucose tolerance may occur; or in patients with a history of mental depression because the drug may worsen this condition.

Interactions
Progesterone may cause amenorrhea or galactorrhea, thus interfering with the action of bromocriptine. Concurrent use of these drugs is not recommended. Use IUD with caution in patients receiving anticoagulants.

Effects on diagnostic tests
Pregnanediol excretion may decrease; serum alkaline phosphatase and amino acid levels may increase. Glucose tolerance has been shown to decrease in a small percentage of patients receiving this drug.

Adverse reactions
- CNS: dizziness, headache, lethargy, depression, fatigue.
- CV: thrombophlebitis, *pulmonary embolism,* edema.
- DERM: melasma, rash, acne, hair loss.
- GU: breakthrough bleeding, dysmenorrhea, amenorrhea; cervical erosion or abnormal secretions.
- Hepatic: cholestatic jaundice.
- Metabolic: hyperglycemia, decreased libido.
- Local: pain at injection site.
   Note: Drug should be discontinued if hypersensitivity, thromboembolic or thrombotic disorders, visual disturbances, migraine headache, or severe depression occurs.

Overdose and treatment
No information available.

▶ Special considerations
Besides those relevant to all *progestins,* consider the following recommendations.
- Parenteral form is for I.M. administration only. Inject deep into large muscle mass, preferably the gluteal muscle. Check sites for irritation.
- Large doses of progesterone may cause a moderate catabolic effect and a transient increase in sodium and chloride excretion.

Information for the patient
- Advise patient that withdrawal bleeding usually occurs 2 to 3 days after discontinuing the drug.
- Instruct patient to call promptly if she suspects pregnancy while receiving progestin therapy.

For patient using Progestasert
- Inform patient that bleeding and cramping may occur for a few weeks after insertion.
- Advise patient to call if abnormal or excessive bleeding, severe cramping, abnormal vaginal discharge, fever, or flu-like syndrome occurs.
- Teach patient how to check for proper placement of IUD.
- Tell patient with Progestasert IUD that the progesterone supply is depleted in 1 year and the device must be changed at that time. Pregnancy risk increases after 1 year if patient relies on progesterone-depleted device for contraception.
- Inform patient of side effects, including uterine perforation, increased risk of infection, pelvic inflammatory disease, ectopic pregnancy, abdominal cramping, increased menstrual flow, and expulsion of the device.

Breast-feeding
Progesterone is contraindicated in breast-feeding women.

PHARMACOLOGIC CLASS

progestins

hydroxyprogesterone caproate
medroxyprogesterone acetate
megestrol acetate
norethindrone
norethindrone acetate
norgestrel
progesterone

Progesterone is the endogenous progestin, secreted by the corpus luteum within the female ovary. Several synthetic progesterone derivatives with greater potency or duration of action have been synthesized. Some of these derivatives also possess weak androgenic or estrogenic activity. The progestins are used to treat dysfunctional uterine bleeding and certain cancers. They also are used as contraceptives, either alone or in combination with estrogens.

Pharmacology
Progesterone causes secretory changes in the endometrium, changes in the vaginal epithelium, increases in body temperature, relaxation of uterine smooth muscle, stimulation of growth of breast alveolar tissue, inhibition of gonadotropin release from the pituitary, and withdrawal bleeding (in the presence of estrogens). The synthetic progesterone derivatives have these properties as well.

Clinical indications and actions
Hormonal imbalance, female
Hydroxyprogesterone, medroxyprogesterone, norethindrone, and progesterone are indicated to treat amenorrhea and dysfunctional uterine bleeding resulting from hormonal imbalance. Hydroxyprogesterone also is indicated to produce desquamation and a secretory endometrium.
Endometriosis
Norethindrone and norethindrone acetate are indicated to treat endometriosis.
Carcinoma
Hydroxyprogesterone, medroxyprogesterone, and megestrol are indicated in the adjunctive and palliative treatment of certain types of metastatic tumors. They are not considered primary therapy. See individual agents for specific indications.
Contraception
Norethindrone and norgestrel are approved for use with estrogens or alone as oral contraceptives.

Medroxyprogesterone (parenteral) is not approved for use as a contraceptive in the United States but is used in other countries as a long-acting, effective contraceptive.

Progestins are no longer indicated to detect pregnancy (because of teratogenicity) or to treat threatened or habitual abortion, for which they are not effective.

Overview of adverse reactions
The most common side effect of progestin administration is a change in menstrual bleeding pattern, ranging from spotting or breakthrough bleeding to complete amenorrhea. Breast tenderness and breast secretion may occur. Weight changes, increases in body temperature, edema, nausea, or acne also may occur. Somnolence, insomnia, hirsutism, hair loss, depression, cholestatic jaundice, and rare allergic reactions (ranging from rash to anaphylaxis) also have been reported. A few patients taking parenteral progestins have suffered localized reactions at the injection site.

▶ Special considerations
● Progestins are contraindicated in patients with thromboembolic disorders, breast cancer, undiagnosed abnormal vaginal bleeding, or severe hepatic disease; and in pregnant patients. Use cautiously in patients with diabetes mellitus, cardiac or renal disease, seizure disorder, migraine, or mental depression.
● Food and Drug Administration regulations require that before receiving their first dose, patients read the package insert describing the possible progestin side effects. Provide verbal explanations as well. However, if progestin is being used for antineoplastic effect, patients are not required to receive and read the package insert.
● Give oil injections deep I.M. in gluteal muscles. I.M. injections may be painful; observe injection site for sterile abscess formation.
● Progestins are not indicated for use during breast-feeding.
● Glucose tolerance may be altered in diabetic patients. Monitor patient closely because antidiabetic medication may need to be adjusted.
● Clinical studies in women with benign breast disease or a family history of breast cancer have not confirmed increased risk of breast cancer with use of oral contraceptives including norethindrone or norgestrel.
● When used as an oral contraceptive, progestins are administered daily without interruption, regardless of menstrual cycle. Continuous administration of progestins may alter the patient's menstrual pattern and cause unpredictable bleeding during therapy.
● Use of progestins may lead to gingival bleeding and hyperplasia, which usually starts as gingivitis or gum inflammation.
● A patient who is exposed to progestins during the first 4 months of pregnancy or who becomes pregnant while receiving the drug should be informed of the potential risks to the fetus.

Information for the patient
● Tell patient that GI distress may subside with use (after a few cycles).
● Because oral contraceptive combinations contain progestins, the precautions associated with oral contraceptives should be considered in patients receiving progestins.
● Patients receiving progestins should have a full physical examination, including a gynecologic exam and a Papanicolaou test, every 6 to 12 months.
● Advise patient to discontinue therapy and call immediately if migraine or visual disturbances occur, or if sudden severe headache or vomiting develops.
● Patients should be taught breast self-examination.
● Tell patient to call promptly if period is missed or unusual bleeding occurs; and to call and discontinue drug immediately if pregnancy is suspected.
● Advise patient who misses a dose to take the missed dose as soon as possible or omit it; and not to double doses.
● Advise patient who misses a dose when used as a

---

contraceptive to discontinue the drug and use an alternative contraception method until period begins or pregnancy is ruled out.
● Inform patient that drug may cause possible dental problems (tenderness, swelling, or bleeding of gums). Advise patient to brush and floss teeth, massage gums, and have dentist clean teeth regularly. Patient should check with dentist if there are questions about care of teeth or gums or if tenderness, swelling, or bleeding of gums is noticed.
● Advise patient to use extra care to avoid pregnancy when starting use of drug as an oral contraceptive and for at least 3 months after discontinuing it.
● Advise patient to keep an extra 1-month supply available.
● Tell patient to keep tablets in original container.
● Emphasize the importance of not giving the medication to anyone else.

Representative combinations

Hydroxyprogesterone caproate with estradiol valerate: Hy-Gestradol, Hylutin-Est.

Norethindrone acetate with ethinyl estradiol: Brevicon 21/28, Gestest, Loestrin, Modicon 21/28, Norinyl 1 + 35, Norlestrin, Norquest, Ortho 1/35*, Ortho 7/7/7*, Ortho 10/11*, Ortho-Novum 21/28, 7/7/7, 10/11, Ovcon-35, Ovcon-50, Tri-norinyl; with mestranol: Norinyl 1/50, Norinyl 1 + 80, Norinyl 1/80*, Norinyl 2, Ortho-Novum 0.5*, Ortho-Novum 1/50, Ortho-Novum 1/80, Ortho-Novum 2, Program-20*, Program-40*, Program-80*; with mestranol and ferrous fumarate: Norinyl-1 Fe 28; with ethinyl estradiol and ferrous fumarate: Norlestrin Fe 1/50, 2.5/50.

Norgestrel with ethinyl estradiol: Lo/Ovral, Ovral-Prep, Lo/Ovral, Miss-Ovral*, Ovral.

Progesterone with estradiol benzoate: Pro-Estrone; with estradiol, testosterone and procaine hydrochloride: Hormo-Triad; with estrogenic substance: Profoygen Aqueous; with estrone: Proestrone.

---

promazine hydrochloride
Prozine, Sparine

● Pharmacologic classification: aliphatic phenothiazine
● Therapeutic classification: antipsychotic, antiemetic
● Pregnancy risk category C

How supplied
Available by prescription only
Tablets: 25 mg, 50 mg, 100 mg
Injection: 25 mg, 50 mg/ml

Indications, route, and dosage
Psychosis
Adults: 10 to 200 mg P.O. or I.M. q 4 to 6 hours, up to 1 g daily; in acutely agitated patients, the initial I.M. or I.V. dose is 50 to 150 mg. Dose may be repeated within 5 to 10 minutes if necessary. Give I.V. dose in concentrations no greater than 25 mg/ml.
Children over age 12: 10 to 25 mg P.O. or I.M. q 4 to 6 hours.

Use of doses over 1,000 mg/day has not increased therapeutic effect.

Pharmacodynamics
Antipsychotic action: Promazine is thought to exert its antipsychotic effects by postsynaptic blockade of CNS dopamine receptors, thus inhibiting dopamine-mediated effects; antiemetic effects are attributed to dopamine receptor blockade in the medullary chemoreceptor trigger zone. Promazine has many other central and peripheral effects: it produces both alpha and ganglionic blockade and counteracts histamine- and serotonin-mediated activity. Its most prevalent side effects are antimuscarinic and sedative; it causes fewer extrapyramidal effects than other drugs in this class.

Pharmacokinetics
● *Absorption:* Promazine usually is absorbed well from the GI tract and rapidly following I.M. injection. Onset of effect ranges from 1/2 to 1 hour.
● *Distribution:* Promazine is distributed widely into the body, including breast milk. Peak effect occurs at 2 to 4 hours; steady-state serum level is achieved within 4 to 7 days. Drug is 91% to 99% protein-bound.
● *Metabolism:* Promazine is metabolized extensively by the liver, but no active metabolites are formed.
● *Excretion:* Most of drug is excreted as metabolites in urine; some is excreted in feces via the biliary tract.

Contraindications and precautions
Promazine is contraindicated in patients with known hypersensitivity to phenothiazines and related compounds, including allergic reactions involving hepatic function; in patients with blood dyscrasias and bone marrow depression because of adverse hematologic effects; in patients with disorders accompanied by coma, CNS depression, or in patients with brain damage, because of additive CNS depression; in patients with circulatory collapse or cerebrovascular disease because of adverse effects on blood pressure; and in patients who are receiving adrenergic-blocking agents or spinal or epidural anesthetics, because of potential for excessive hypotensive response.

Promazine should be used cautiously in patients with cardiac disease (arrhythmias, congestive heart failure, angina pectoris, valvular disease, or heart block), encephalitis, Reye's syndrome, head injury, respiratory disease, epilepsy and other seizure disorders, glaucoma, prostatic hypertrophy, urinary retention, hepatic or renal dysfunction, Parkinson's disease, pheochromocytoma, or hypocalcemia. Some oral preparations of promazine contain tartrazine; dyes may cause allergic reaction in aspirin-allergic patients.

Interactions
Concomitant use of promazine with sympathomimetics, including epinephrine, phenylephrine, phenylpropanolamine, and ephedrine (often found in nasal sprays), and with appetite suppressants may decrease their stimulatory and pressor effects.

Promazine may inhibit blood pressure response to centrally acting antihypertensive drugs, such as guanethidine, guanabenz, guanadrel, clonidine, methyldopa, and reserpine. Additive effects are likely after concomitant use of promazine with CNS depressants, including alcohol, analgesics, barbiturates, narcotics, tranquilizers, anesthetics (general, spinal or epidural), and parenteral magnesium sulfate (oversedation, respiratory depression, and hypotension); antiarrhythmic agents, quinidine, disopyramide, and procainamide (increased incidence of cardiac arrhythmias and conduction defects); atropine and other anticholinergic drugs,

---

including antidepressants, monoamine oxidase inhibitors, phenothiazines, antihistamines, meperidine, and antiparkinsonian agents (oversedation, paralytic ileus, visual changes, and severe constipation); nitrates (hypotension); and metrizamide (increased risk of convulsions).

Beta-blocking agents may inhibit promazine metabolism, increasing plasma levels and toxicity.

Concomitant use with propylthiouracil increases risk of agranulocytosis; concomitant use with lithium may result in severe neurologic toxicity with an encephalitis-like syndrome, and in decreased therapeutic response to promazine.

Pharmacokinetic alterations and subsequent decreased therapeutic response to promazine may follow concomitant use with phenobarbital (enhanced renal excretion); aluminum- and magnesium-containing antacids and antidiarrheals (decreased absorption); caffeine; or heavy smoking (increased metabolism).

Promazine may antagonize the therapeutic effect of bromocriptine on prolactin secretion; it also may decrease the vasoconstricting effects of high-dose dopamine and may decrease effectiveness and increase toxicity of levodopa (by dopamine blockade). Promazine may inhibit metabolism and increase toxicity of phenytoin.

Effects on diagnostic tests
Promazine causes false-positive test results for urinary porphyrins, urobilinogen, amylase, and 5-HIAA because of darkening of urine by metabolites; it also causes false-positive urine pregnancy results in tests using human chorionic gonadotropin as the indicator.

Promazine elevates test results for liver enzymes and protein-bound iodine and causes quinidine-like effects on the ECG.

Adverse reactions
● CNS: extrapyramidal symptoms—dystonia, akathisia, torticollis, tardive dyskinesia (usually dose-related with long-term therapy, but it can develop rapidly), sedation, pseudoparkinsonism, drowsiness (frequent), *neuroleptic malignant syndrome* (dose-related; if untreated, fatal *respiratory failure* in over 10% of patients), dizziness, headache, insomnia, exacerbation of psychotic symptoms.
● CV: *asystole*, orthostatic hypotension, tachycardia, dizziness or fainting, arrhythmias, ECG changes, increased anginal pain after I.M. injection.
● EENT: blurred vision, tinnitus, mydriasis, increased intraocular pressure, ocular changes (retinal pigmentary change with long-term use).
● GI: dry mouth, constipation, nausea, vomiting, anorexia, diarrhea.
● GU: urinary retention, gynecomastia, hypermenorrhea, inhibited ejaculation.
● HEMA: transient leukopenia, *agranulocytosis*, thrombocytopenia, anemia (within 30 to 90 days).
● Local: contact dermatitis from injectable form, muscle necrosis from I.M. injection.
● Other: hyperprolactinemia, photosensitivity (high incidence), increased appetite or weight gain, hypersensitivity (rash, urticaria, drug fever, edema, cholestatic jaundice [in 0.1% to 4% of patients within first 30 days]), decreased libido.

After abrupt withdrawal of long-term therapy, gastritis, nausea, vomiting, dizziness, tremors, feeling of heat or cold, sweating, tachycardia, headache, or insomnia may occur.

Note: Drug should be discontinued immediately if any of the following occurs: hypersensitivity, jaundice, agranulocytosis, neuroleptic malignant syndrome (marked hyperthermia, extrapyramidal effects, autonomic dysfunction), or severe extrapyramidal symptoms even after dosage is lowered. Drug should be discontinued 48 hours before and 24 hours after myelography using metrizamide, because of the risk of convulsions. When feasible, drug should be withdrawn slowly and gradually; many drug effects persist after withdrawal.

Overdose and treatment
CNS depression is characterized by deep, unarousable sleep and possible coma, hypotension or hypertension, extrapyramidal symptoms, abnormal involuntary muscle movements, agitation, seizures, arrhythmias, ECG changes, hypothermia or hyperthermia, and autonomic nervous system dysfunction.

Treatment is symptomatic and supportive and includes maintaining vital signs, airway, stable body temperature, and fluid and electrolyte balance.

Do not induce vomiting: drug inhibits cough reflex, and aspiration may occur. Use gastric lavage, then activated charcoal and saline cathartics; dialysis does not help. Regulate body temperature as needed. Treat hypotension with I.V. fluids: *do not give epinephrine.* Treat seizures with parenteral diazepam or barbiturates; dysrhythmias with parenteral phenytoin (1 mg/kg with rate titrated to blood pressure); and extrapyramidal reactions with benztropine or parenteral diphenhydramine 2 mg/kg/minute.

▶ Special considerations
Besides those relevant to all *phenothiazines*, consider the following recommendations.
● Injectable formulations may cause a rash after contact with skin.
● Drug may cause a pink to brown discoloration of the urine.
● Promazine is associated with a high incidence of sedation and orthostatic hypotension.
● Tablets may cause stomach upset. Administer with food or fluid.
● I.V. use is not recommended; however, if it is necessary, drug should be diluted to not more than 25 mg/ml, given slowly with special care to prevent extravasation. I.V. route should be used during surgery or for severe hiccups.
● To prevent photosensitivity reactions, patient should avoid exposure to sunlight or heat lamps.
● Administer I.M. injection deep into the upper outer quadrant of the buttock. Massaging the area after administration may prevent the formation of abscesses. I.M. injection may cause skin necrosis; take care to avoid extravasation. Monitor blood pressure before and after parenteral administration.
● Chewing gum, hard candy, or ice may help relieve dry mouth.
● The injection may be slightly discolored. Do not use if excessively discolored or if a precipitate is evident. Contact pharmacist.
● Protect the liquid formulation from light.

Information for the patient
● Explain the risks of dystonic reactions and tardive dyskinesias, and tell patient to report abnormal body movements promptly.
● Tell patient to avoid sun exposure and to wear sun-

screen when going outdoors, to prevent photosensitivity reactions. (Note that heat lamps and tanning beds also may cause burning of the skin or skin discoloration.)
• Warn patient to avoid extremely hot or cold baths or exposure to temperature extremes, sunlamps, or tanning beds; drug may cause thermoregulatory changes.
• Urge patient to take drug exactly as prescribed; not to double doses for missed doses; not to share drug with others; and not to stop taking the drug suddenly.
• Reassure patient that most adverse reactions can be alleviated by dosage reduction, but tell patient to call promptly if difficulty urinating, sore throat, dizziness, or fainting develops.
• Warn patient to avoid hazardous activities that require alertness until the drug's effect is established. Reassure patient that excessive sedative effects usually subside after several weeks.
• Tell patient to avoid alcohol and other medications that may cause excessive sedation.
• Suggest sugarless hard candy, chewing gum, or ice to relieve dry mouth.
• Store drug safely away from children.
• Tell patient that many drug interactions are possible. Patient should seek medical approval before taking *any* self-prescribed medication.

Geriatric use
Elderly patients tend to require lower dosages, titrated to individual response. Such patients are more likely to develop adverse reactions, especially tardive dyskinesia and other extrapyramidal effects.

Pediatric use
Promazine is not recommended for children under age 12.

Breast-feeding
Promazine enters into breast milk. Potential benefits to the mother should outweigh the potential harm to the infant.

promethazine hydrochloride
Anergan, Baymethazine, Ganphen, Histanil*, K-Phen, Mallergan, Pentazine, Phenameth, Phenazine, Phencen-50, Phenergan, Phenergan Fortis, Phenergan Plain, Phenoject-50, PMS Promethazine*, Prometh, Prorex, Prothazine, Prothazine Plain, Provigan, Remsed, V-Gan

• Pharmacologic classification: phenothiazine derivative
• Therapeutic classification: antiemetic and antivertigo agent; antihistamine (H_1-receptor antagonist); preoperative, postoperative, or obstetric sedative and adjunct to analgesics
• Pregnancy risk category C

How supplied
Available by prescription only
Tablets: 12.5 mg, 25 mg, 50 mg
Syrup: 6.25 mg/5 ml, 10 mg/5 ml, 25 mg/5 ml
Suppositories: 12.5 mg, 25 mg, 50 mg
Injection: 25 mg/ml, 50 mg/ml

Indications, route, and dosage
Motion sickness
Adults: 25 mg P.O. b.i.d.
Children: 12.5 to 25 mg P.O., I.M., or rectally b.i.d.
Nausea
Adults: 12.5 to 25 mg P.O., I.M., or rectally q 4 to 6 hours, p.r.n.
Children: 0.25 to 0.5 mg/kg I.M. or rectally q 4 to 6 hours, p.r.n.
Rhinitis, allergy symptoms
Adults: 12.5 mg P.O. before meals and at bedtime; or 25 mg P.O. at bedtime.
Children: 6.25 to 12.5 mg P.O. t.i.d., or 25 mg P.O. or rectally at bedtime.
Sedation
Adults: 25 to 50 mg P.O. or I.M. at bedtime or p.r.n.
Children: 12.5 to 25 mg P.O., I.M., or rectally at bedtime.
Routine preoperative or postoperative sedation or as an adjunct to analgesics
Adults: 25 to 50 mg I.M., I.V., or P.O.
Children: 12.5 to 25 mg I.M., I.V., or P.O.
Obstetric sedation
25 to 50 mg I.M. or I.V. in early stages of labor, and 25 to 75 mg after labor is established; repeat every 2 to 4 hours, p.r.n. Maximum daily dosage is 100 mg.

Pharmacodynamics
• *Antiemetic and antivertigo action:* The central antimuscarinic actions of antihistamines probably are responsible for their antivertigo and antiemetic effects; promethazine also is believed to inhibit the medullary chemoreceptor trigger zone.
• *Antihistamine action:* Promethazine competes with histamine for the H_1-receptor, thereby suppressing allergic rhinitis and urticaria; drug does not prevent the release of histamine.
• *Sedative action:* CNS depressant mechanism of promethazine is unknown; phenothiazines probably cause sedation by reducing stimuli to the brain-stem reticular system.

Pharmacokinetics
• *Absorption:* Promethazine is well absorbed from the GI tract. Onset begins 20 minutes after oral, rectal, or I.M. administration and within 3 to 5 minutes after I.V. administration. Effects usually last 4 to 6 hours but may persist for 12 hours.
• *Distribution:* Promethazine is distributed widely throughout the body; drug crosses the placenta.
• *Metabolism:* Promethazine is metabolized in the liver.
• *Excretion:* Metabolites are excreted in urine and feces.

Contraindications and precautions
Promethazine is contraindicated in patients with known hypersensitivity to promethazine or other antihistamines or phenothiazines; during asthmatic attacks, because it thickens bronchial secretions; in acutely ill or dehydrated children, because they are at increased risk of dystonias; in patients with bone marrow depression, because it may induce blood dyscrasias; in epilepsy, because it may worsen seizure disorder; in comatose patients; and in neonates.

Like other antihistamines, promethazine has significant anticholinergic effects; it should be used with caution in patients with narrow-angle glaucoma, peptic ulcer, or pyloroduodenal obstruction or urinary bladder obstruction from prostatic hypertrophy or narrowing of the bladder neck. It also should be used with caution in patients with cardiovascular disease or hypertension because of the risk of palpitations, tachycardia, and increased hypertension; in patients with acute or chronic respiratory dysfunction (especially children), because drug may suppress the cough reflex; in patients with hepatic dysfunction; and in children with a history of sleep apnea or a family history of sudden infant death syndrome – the relationship between these conditions and the use of promethazine has not been studied; however, a number of deaths have occurred in children who were given usual dosages of phenothiazine and antihistamines.

Antiemetic action may mask symptoms of undiagnosed diseases, drug overdose, and the ototoxic effects of aspirin – dizziness, vertigo, tinnitus – or other ototoxic drugs.

Interactions
Do not give promethazine concomitantly with epinephrine, because it may result in partial adrenergic blockade, producing further hypotension; or with monoamine oxidase (MAO) inhibitors, which interfere with the detoxification of antihistamines and phenothiazines and thus prolong and intensify their sedative and anticholinergic effects. Additive CNS depression may occur when promethazine is given with other antihistamines or CNS depressants, such as alcohol, barbiturates, tranquilizers, sleeping aids, and antianxiety agents. Promethazine may block the antiparkinsonian action of levodopa.

Effects on diagnostic tests
Promethazine should be discontinued 4 days before diagnostic skin tests, to avoid preventing, reducing, or masking test response. Promethazine may cause hyperglycemia and either false-positive or false-negative pregnancy test results. It also may interfere with blood grouping in the ABO system.

Adverse reactions
● CNS: (especially in the elderly) sedation, confusion, restlessness, tremors, drowsiness, extrapyramidal symptoms (especially in the elderly), dizziness, disorientation, disturbed coordination.
● CV: hypotension, hypertension.
● EENT: transient myopia, nasal congestion, oculogyric crisis.
● GI: anorexia, nausea, vomiting, constipation, dry mouth.
● GU: urinary retention.
● HEMA: leukopenia, *agranulocytosis,* thrombocytopenia.
● Other: photosensitivity, reversible obstructive jaundice.

Overdose and treatment
Clinical manifestations of overdose may include either CNS depression (sedation, reduced mental alertness, apnea, and cardiovascular collapse) or CNS stimulation (insomnia, hallucinations, tremors, or convulsions). Atropine-like symptoms, such as dry mouth, flushed skin, fixed and dilated pupils, and GI symptoms, are common, especially in children.

Empty stomach by gastric lavage; do not induce vomiting. Treat hypotension with vasopressors, and control seizures with diazepam or phenytoin; correct acidosis

and electrolyte imbalance. Urinary acidification promotes excretion of drug. *Do not give stimulants.*

▶ Special considerations
Besides those relevant to all *phenothiazines,* consider the following recommendations.
● Pronounced sedative effects may limit use in some ambulatory patients.
● The 50 mg/ml concentration is for I.M. use only; inject deep into large muscle mass. Do not administer drug subcutaneously; this may cause chemical irritation and necrosis. Drug may be administered I.V., in concentrations not to exceed 25 mg/ml and at a rate not to exceed 25 mg/minute; when using I.V. drip, wrap in aluminum foil to protect drug from light.
● Promethazine and meperidine (Demerol) may be mixed in the same syringe.

Information for the patient
● Warn patient about possible photosensitivity and ways to avoid it.
● When treating motion sickness, tell patient to take first dose 30 to 60 minutes before travel; on succeeding days, he should take dose upon arising and with evening meal.

Geriatric use
Elderly patients are usually more sensitive to adverse effects of antihistamines and are especially likely to experience a greater degree of dizziness, sedation, hyperexcitability, dry mouth, and urinary retention than younger patients. Symptoms usually respond to a decrease in medication dosage.

Pediatric use
Use cautiously in children with respiratory dysfunction. Safety and efficacy in children younger than age 2 have not been established; do not give promethazine to infants under age 3 months.

Breast-feeding
Antihistamines such as promethazine should not be used during breast-feeding. Many of these drugs are secreted in breast milk, exposing the infant to risks of unusual excitability, especially premature infants and other neonates, who may experience convulsions.

---

propafenone hydrochloride
Rythmol

● Pharmacologic classification: sodium channel antagonist
● Therapeutic classification: antiarrhythmic (Class IC)
● Pregnancy risk category C

How supplied
Available by prescription only
Tablets: 150 mg, 300 mg

Indications, route, and dosage
Suppression of documented life-threatening ventricular arrhythmias
Adults: Initially, 150 mg P.O. q 8 hours. Dosage may be increased to 225 mg q 8 hours after 3 or 4 days; if

necessary, increase dosage to 300 mg q 8 hours. Maximum daily dosage is 900 mg.

Dosage in patients with hepatic failure
The manufacturer recommends that the dosage of propafenone in patients with hepatic impairment should be reduced to 20% to 30% of the usual dosage.

Pharmacodynamics
Antiarrhythmic action: Propafenone reduces the inward sodium current in myocardial cells and Purkinje fibers; it also has weak beta-adrenergic blocking effects. It slows the upstroke velocity of the action potential (phase 0 depolarization) and slows conduction in the AV node, His-Purkinje system, and intraventricular conduction system and prolongs the refractory period in the AV node.

Pharmacokinetics
● *Absorption:* Propafenone is well absorbed from the GI tract; absorption is not affected by food. Because of a significant first-pass effect, bioavailability is limited; however, it increases with dosage. Absolute bioavailability is 3.4% with the 150-mg tablet and 10.6% with the 300-mg tablet.
● *Distribution:* Peak plasma levels occur about 3.5 hours after administration.
● *Metabolism:* Hepatic, with a significant first-pass effect. Two active metabolites have been identified: 5-hydroxypropafenone and N-depropylpropafenone. A few patients (10% of all patients and patients receiving quinidine) metabolize the drug more slowly. Little (if any) 5-hydroxypropafenone is present in the plasma.
● *Excretion:* Elimination half-life is 2 to 10 hours in normal metabolizers (about 90% of patients); it can be as long as 10 to 32 hours in slow metabolizers.

Contraindications and precautions
Propafenone is contraindicated in patients with uncontrolled CHF; cardiogenic shock; SA, AV, and intraventricular conduction disorders (such as sick sinus syndrome or AV block) in the absence of an artificial pacemaker; bradycardia; bronchospasm; significant hypotension; symptomatic electrolyte disturbances; and known hypersensitivity to the drug. Patients with bronchospastic disease should not receive this drug because of its beta-adrenergic blocking properties.

Use all Class IC antiarrhythmics cautiously because of an association between other agents within the class and an increased cardiac morbidity and mortality as compared with placebo. The use of this drug should be limited to persons who have life-threatening arrhythmias. Because antiarrhythmic agents can cause new or worsened arrhythmias ranging from worsened premature ventricular contractions (PVCs) to ventricular tachycardia, evaluate the ECG frequently to determine if the continued use of the drug is warranted. Propafenone may alter both the pacing and sensing thresholds of artificial pacemakers. Pacemakers should be monitored and reprogrammed as necessary.

Use cautiously in patients with a history of CHF. Because sympathetic stimulation may be important to continued function of the failing heart, the beta-adrenergic blocking effects of propafenone may be detrimental to these patients.

Because propafenone is extensively metabolized by the liver and excreted by the kidneys, it should be used cautiously in patients with hepatic or renal disease.

Complete blood counts (CBCs) should be performed in patients with unexplained fever or decreased white cell count to rule out the possibility of agranulocytosis or granulocytopenia, especially during the first 3 months of therapy.

Interactions
Concurrent use of quinidine competitively inhibits one of the metabolic pathways for propafenone, thereby increasing its half-life, and is not recommended. Cimetidine may increase the plasma levels of propafenone. Monitor patients closely. Concurrent use of local anesthetics may increase the risk of CNS toxicity.

Propafenone causes a dose-related increase in plasma digoxin levels, ranging from 35% at 450 mg/day to 85% at 900 mg/day. Monitor plasma digoxin levels closely and adjust dosage of digoxin as necessary. In addition, propafenone may increase plasma levels of some beta-adrenergic blocking agents, including propranolol and metoprolol, and of warfarin, resulting in increased prothrombin time. Monitor appropriately.

Effects on diagnostic tests
Although the drug may slow conduction and increase PR interval and QRS duration, ECG changes alone cannot be used to predict plasma concentration or drug efficacy.

Increased liver enzymes have been rarely reported (less than 0.2% of patients). Hematologic abnormalities have also been rarely reported (positive antinuclear antibody titer, decreased CBC, and altered electrolyte levels).

Adverse reactions
● CNS: anorexia, anxiety, ataxia, dizziness, drowsiness, fatigue, headache, insomnia, syncope, tremor, weakness.
● CV: angina, atrial fibrillation, bradycardia, bundle branch block, *CHF*, chest pain, edema, first-degree AV block, hypotension, prolonged QRS, intraventricular conduction delay, palpitations, *proarrhythmic events (ventricular tachycardia, PVCs)*.
● DERM: rash.
● EENT: blurred vision, unusual taste.
● GI: abdominal pain or cramps, constipation, diarrhea, dyspepsia, flatulence, nausea, vomiting, dry mouth.
● Respiratory: dyspnea.
● Other: diaphoresis, joint pain.

Overdose and treatment
Symptoms usually develop within 3 hours of ingestion. Hypotension, somnolence, bradycardia, conduction disturbances, ventricular arrhythmias, and seizures have been reported. Provide supportive treatment and assist respirations as necessary. Rhythm and blood pressure may be controlled with dopamine and isoproterenol; seizures may respond to I.V. diazepam.

▶ Special considerations
Propafenone pharmacokinetics are complex; studies have shown that a three-fold increase in daily dosage (from 300 to 900 mg/day) may produce a ten-fold increase in plasma levels. Dosage must be individualized for each patient.

Information for the patient
Instruct patient to report any signs of infection, such as sore throat, chills, or fever.

Geriatric use
In elderly patients and patients with substantial heart disease, increase dosage more gradually during the initial phase of treatment.

Breast-feeding
It is not known if the drug is excreted in breast milk. Because of the potential for serious toxicity in the infant, consider alternative feeding methods during therapy.

---

propantheline bromide
Norpanth, Pro-Banthine, Propanthel*

- Pharmacologic classification: anticholinergic
- Therapeutic classification: antimuscarinic, gastrointestinal antispasmodic
- Pregnancy risk category C

How supplied
Available by prescription only
Tablets: 7.5 mg, 15 mg

Indications, route, and dosage
Adjunctive treatment of peptic ulcer, irritable bowel syndrome, and other GI disorders; to reduce duodenal motility during diagnostic radiologic procedures
Adults: 15 mg P.O. t.i.d. before meals, and 30 mg h.s. up to 60 mg q.i.d.
Elderly patients: 7.5 mg P.O. t.i.d. before meals.
Children: Antispasmodic dose 2 to 3 mg/kg/day P.O. divided q 4 hours to q 6 hours and h.s. Antisecretory dose 1.5 mg/kg/day P.O. divided q 6 hours to q 8 hours.

Pharmacodynamics
Anticholinergic action: Propantheline competitively blocks acetylcholine's actions at cholinergic neuroeffector sites, decreasing GI motility and inhibiting gastric acid secretion.

Pharmacokinetics
- *Absorption:* Only about 10% to 25% of propantheline is absorbed (absorption varies among patients).
- *Distribution:* Propantheline does not cross the blood-brain barrier; little else is known about its distribution.
- *Metabolism:* Propantheline appears to undergo considerable metabolism in the upper small intestine and liver.
- *Excretion:* Absorbed drug is excreted in urine as metabolites and unchanged drug.

Contraindications and precautions
Propantheline is contraindicated in patients with narrow-angle glaucoma, because drug-induced cycloplegia and mydriasis may increase intraocular pressure; in patients with obstructive uropathy, obstructive GI tract disease, severe ulcerative colitis, myasthenia gravis, paralytic ileus, intestinal atony, or toxic megacolon, because the drug may exacerbate these conditions; and in patients with known hypersensitivity to anticholinergics or bromides.

Administer propantheline cautiously to patients with autonomic neuropathy, hyperthyroidism, coronary artery disease, cardiac arrhythmias, congestive heart failure, or ulcerative colitis, because the drug may exacerbate symptoms of these disorders; to patients with hepatic or renal disease, because toxic accumulation may occur; to patients over age 40, because the drug increases the glaucoma risk; to patients with hiatal hernia associated with reflux esophagitis, because the drug may decrease lower esophageal sphincter tone; and in hot or humid environments, because the drug may predispose the patient to heatstroke.

Interactions
Concurrent administration of antacids decreases oral absorption of anticholinergics. Administer propantheline at least 1 hour before antacids.

Concomitant administration of drugs with anticholinergic effects may cause additive toxicity.

Decreased GI absorption of many drugs has been reported after the use of anticholinergics (for example, levodopa and ketoconazole). Conversely, slowly dissolving digoxin tablets may yield higher serum digoxin levels when administered with anticholinergics.

Use cautiously with oral potassium supplements (especially wax-matrix formulations) because the incidence of potassium-induced GI ulcerations may be increased.

Propantheline may increase atenolol absorption, thereby enhancing atenolol's effects.

Effects on diagnostic tests
None reported.

Adverse reactions
- CNS: headache, insomnia, drowsiness, dizziness, confusion or excitement (in elderly patients), nervousness, weakness.
- CV: palpitations, tachycardia, orthostatic hypotension.
- DERM: urticaria, decreased sweating or anhidrosis, other dermal manifestations.
- EENT: blurred vision, mydriasis, cycloplegia, increased ocular tension, photophobia.
- GI: dry mouth, dysphagia, heartburn, loss of taste, nausea, constipation, vomiting, paralytic ileus, abdominal distention.
- GU: urinary hesitancy and retention, impotence.
- Other: fever, allergic reaction.
Note: Drug should be discontinued if hypersensitivity, urinary retention, confusion or excitement, curarelike symptoms, or skin rash occurs.

Overdose and treatment
Clinical manifestations of overdose include curare-like symptoms and such peripheral effects as headache; dilated, nonreactive pupils; blurred vision; flushed, hot, dry skin; dryness of mucous membranes; dysphagia; decreased or absent bowel sounds; urinary retention; hyperthermia; tachycardia; hypertension; and increased respirations.

Treatment is primarily symptomatic and supportive, as needed. If the patient is alert, induce emesis (or use gastric lavage) and follow with a saline cathartic and activated charcoal to prevent further drug absorption. In severe cases, physostigmine may be administered to block propantheline's antimuscarinic effects. Give fluids, as needed, to treat shock. If urinary retention develops, catheterization may be necessary.

▶ **Special considerations**
Besides those relevant to all *anticholinergics*, consider the following recommendations.

---

*Canada only   †Unlabeled clinical use   Italicized adverse reactions are life-threatening.

• Drug may be used with histamine H_2 receptor to treat Zollinger-Ellison syndrome.
• Propantheline should be titrated until therapeutic effect is obtained or adverse effects become intolerable.

Information for the patient
Instruct patient to swallow tablets whole rather than chewing or crushing them.

Geriatric use
Propantheline should be administered cautiously to elderly patients. Lower doses are recommended.

Breast-feeding
Propantheline may be excreted in breast milk, possibly resulting in infant toxicity. Breast-feeding women should avoid this drug. Propantheline may decrease milk production.

proparacaine hydrochloride
Ak-Taine, Alcaine, Ophthaine
Hydrochloride, Ophthetic Sterile
Ophthalmic Solution

• Pharmacologic classification: local anesthetic
• Therapeutic classification: local anesthetic
• Pregnancy risk category C

How supplied
Available by prescription only
Ophthalmic solution: 0.5%

Indications, route, and dosage
Anesthesia for tonometry, gonioscopy; suture removal from cornea; removal of corneal foreign bodies
Adults and children: Instill 1 or 2 drops of 0.5% solution in eye just before procedure.
Anesthesia for cataract extraction, glaucoma surgery
Adults and children: Instill 1 drop of 0.5% solution in eye every 5 to 10 minutes for 5 to 7 doses.

Pharmacodynamics
Anesthetic action: Produces anesthesia by preventing initiation and transmission of impulse at the nerve cell membrane.

Pharmacokinetics
• *Absorption:* Onset of action is within 20 seconds of instillation.
• *Distribution:* Unknown.
• *Metabolism:* Unknown.
• *Excretion:* Duration of action is 15 to 20 minutes.

Contraindications and precautions
Proparacaine hydrochloride is contraindicated in patients with hypersensitivity to ester-type local anesthetics, para-aminobenzoic acid or its derivatives, or any other ingredient in the preparation. It should be used with caution in patients with cardiac disease or hyperthyroidism.

Interactions
None reported.

Effects on diagnostic tests
Proparacaine hydrochloride therapy may inhibit the growth of organisms on cultures for detection of infection.

Adverse reactions
• Eye: occasional conjunctival congestion or hemorrhage, transient pain, pupil dilation, cycloplegic effect, softening and erosion of the corneal epilthelium, hyperallergenic corneal reaction.
• Other: hypersensitivity, allergic contact dermatitis.
   Note: Drug should be discontinued if symptoms of hypersensitivity occur.

Overdose and treatment
Clinical manifestations of overdose are extremely rare with ophthalmic administration. Clinical manifestations are CNS stimulation (such as alertness, agitation), followed by depression.
   Ocular overexposure should be treated by irrigation with warm water for at least 15 minutes.

▶ Special considerations
• Proparacaine is the topical ophthalmic anesthetic of choice in diagnostic and minor surgical procedures.
• Drug is not for long-term use; may delay wound healing.
• Do not use discolored solution; store in tightly closed original container.
• Ophthaine brand packaging resembles that of Hemoccult in size and shape; check label carefully.

Information for the patient
• Warn patient not to rub or touch eye while cornea is anesthetized; this may cause corneal abrasion and greater discomfort when anesthesia wears off; advise use of a protective eye patch after procedures.
• Explain that corneal pain in abrasion is relieved only temporarily by the application of proparacaine hydrochloride.
• Tell patient local irritation or stinging may occur several hours after instillation of proparacaine.

Geriatric use
May need to reduce dosage in elderly, debilitated patients.

propofol
Diprivan

• Pharmacologic classification: phenol derivative
• Therapeutic classification: anesthetic
• Pregnancy risk category B

How supplied
Available by prescription only
Injection: 10 mg/ml in 20-ml ampules

Indications, route, and dosage
Induction of anesthesia
Adults: Doses must be individualized according to patient's condition and age. Most patients classified as

American Society of Anesthesiologists (ASA) Physical Status category (PS) I or II under age 55 require 2 to 2.5 mg/kg I.V. The drug is usually administered in a 40-mg bolus q 10 seconds until the desired response is obtained.

Elderly, debilitated, or hypovolemic patients or patients in ASA PS III or IV should receive half of the usual induction dose (20-mg bolus q 10 seconds).

Maintenance of anesthesia

Adults: Propofol may be given as a variable rate infusion, titrated to clinical effect. Most patients may be maintained with 0.1 to 0.2 mg/kg/minute (6 to 12 mg/kg/hour).

Elderly, debilitated, or hypovolemic patients or patients in ASA PS III or IV should receive half of the usual maintenance dose (0.05 to 0.1 mg/kg/minute or 3 to 6 mg/kg/hour).

Pharmacodynamics

Anesthetic action: Propofol produces a dose-dependent CNS depression similar to benzodiazepines and barbiturates. However, it can be used to maintain anesthesia through careful titration of infusion rate.

Pharmacokinetics

● *Absorption:* Propofol must be administered I.V.
● *Distribution:* The drug has a biphasic distribution phase; the rapid distribution has a half-life of 1.8 to 8.3 minutes; the slower phase has a half-life of 34 to 64 minutes.
● *Metabolism:* Drug is metabolized within liver and tissues. Metabolites are not fully characterized.
● *Excretion:* Drug is excreted through the kidneys. However, termination of drug action is probably caused by redistribution out of the CNS as well as metabolism. Terminal elimination half-life ranges from 5 to 12 hours.

Contraindications and precautions

Propofol is contraindicated in patients hypersensitive to propofol or any components of the emulsion, including soybean oil, egg lecithin, and glycerol. Because the drug is administered as an emulsion, administer with caution to patients with a disorder of lipid metabolism (such as pancreatitis, primary hyperlipoproteinemia, and diabetic hyperlipidemia). Use cautiously in elderly or debilitated patients and in those with circulatory disorders. Although the hemodynamic effects of the drug can vary, its major effect in patients maintaining spontaneous ventilation is arterial hypotension (arterial pressure can decrease as much as 30%) with little or no change in heart rate and cardiac output. However, significant depression of cardiac output may occur in patients undergoing assisted or controlled positive pressure ventilation.

Propofol is not recommended for use in obstetric anesthesia because the safety to the fetus has not been established. It is also not recommended for use in patients with increased intracranial pressure or impaired cerebral circulation because the reduction in systemic arterial pressure caused by the drug may substantially reduce cerebral perfusion pressure.

Propofol should be administered under direct medical supervision by persons familiar with airway management and the administration of I.V. anesthetics.

Patients receiving propofol should be closely monitored for signs of significant hypotension or bradycardia. Treatment may include increased rate of fluid administration, pressor agents, elevation of lower extremities, or atropine. Apnea may occur during induction and may persist for longer than 60 seconds. Ventilatory support may be required.

Interactions

Concomitant use of inhalational anesthetics (such as enflurane, isoflurane, and halothane) or supplemental anesthetics (such as nitrous oxide and opiates) may be expected to enhance the anesthetic and CV actions of propofol. Use with opiate analgesics or sedatives may intensify the reduction of systolic, diastolic, mean arterial pressure, and cardiac output and may decrease induction dose requirements.

Propofol should not be mixed with other drugs or blood products. If it is to be diluted before infusion, use only dextrose 5% in water and do not dilute to a concentration less than 2 mg/ml. After dilution, drug appears to be more stable in glass containers than plastic.

Effects on diagnostic tests

None reported.

Adverse reactions

● CNS: movement, headache, dizziness, twitching, clonic/myoclonic movement.
● CV: hypotension, bradycardia, hypertension.
● DERM: flushing.
● GI: nausea, vomiting, abdominal cramping.
● Respiratory: apnea, cough, hiccups.
● Local: injection site burning/stinging, pain, tingling or numbness, coldness.
● Other: fever.

Overdose and treatment

Specific information not available. However, treatment of overdosage may include support of respiration and administration of fluids, pressor agents, and anticholinergics as indicated.

▶ Special considerations

● Propofol has no vagolytic activity. Premedication with anticholinergics such as glycopyrrolate or atropine may help manage potential increases in vagal tone caused by other drugs or surgical manipulations.
● When administered into a running I.V. catheter, propofol emulsion is compatible with dextrose 5% in water, lactated Ringer's injection, lactated Ringers and 5% dextrose injection, 5% dextrose and 0.45% sodium chloride injection, and 5% dextrose and 0.2% sodium chloride injection.
● Propofol emulsion should be stored above 40° F. (4° C.) and below 72° F. (22° C.). Refrigeration is not recommended.

Geriatric use

Pharmacokinetics of propofol are not influenced by chronic hepatic cirrhosis, chronic renal failure, or gender.

Pediatric use

Safe use in children has not been established.

Breast-feeding

Because propofol is excreted in breast milk, drug is not recommended for use in breast-feeding women.

propoxyphene hydrochloride
Darvon, Dolene, Doxaphene, Novopropoxyn*, Profene

propoxyphene napsylate
Darvon-N, Doloxene*

- Pharmacologic classification: opioid
- Therapeutic classification: analgesic
- Controlled substance schedule IV
- Pregnancy risk category C

How supplied
Available by prescription only
Propoxyphene hydrochloride
Capsules: 32 mg, 65 mg
Tablets: 65 mg
Propoxyphene napsylate
Capsules: 50 mg, 100 mg
Suspension: 50 mg/5 ml
Tablets: 50 mg, 100 mg

Indications, route, and dosage
Mild to moderate pain
Adults: 65 mg (hydrochloride) P.O. q 4 hours, p.r.n., or 100 mg (napsylate) P.O. q 4 hours, p.r.n.

Pharmacodynamics
Analgesic action: Propoxyphene exerts its analgesic effect via opiate agonist activity and alters the patient's response to painful stimuli, particularly mild to moderate pain.

Pharmacokinetics
- *Absorption:* After oral administration, propoxyphene is absorbed primarily in the upper small intestine. Equimolar doses of the hydrochloride and napsylate salts provide similar plasma concentrations. The onset of analgesia occurs in 20 to 60 minutes, and peak analgesic effects occur at 2 to 2½ hours.
- *Distribution:* Propoxyphene enters the CSF. It is assumed that it crosses the placental barrier; however, placental fluid and fetal blood concentrations have not been determined.
- *Metabolism:* Propoxyphene is degraded mainly in the liver; about one quarter of a dose is metabolized to norpropoxyphene, an active metabolite.
- *Excretion:* The drug is excreted in the urine. Duration of effect is 4 to 6 hours.

Contraindications and precautions
Propoxyphene is contraindicated in patients with known hypersensitivity to the drug or to methadone.

Administer propoxyphene with extreme caution to patients with supraventricular arrhythmias; avoid, or administer drug with extreme caution to patients with head injury or increased intracranial pressure, because drug obscures neurologic parameters; and during pregnancy and labor, because drug readily crosses placenta (premature infants are especially sensitive to respiratory and CNS depressant effects).

Administer propoxyphene cautiously to patients with renal or hepatic dysfunction, because drug accumulation or prolonged duration of action may occur; to patients with pulmonary disease (asthma, chronic obstructive pulmonary disease), because drug depresses respiration and suppresses cough reflex; to patients undergoing biliary tract surgery, because drug may cause biliary spasm; to patients with convulsive disorders, because drug may precipitate seizures; to elderly or debilitated patients, who are more sensitive to both therapeutic and adverse drug effects; and to patients prone to physical or psychic addiction, because of the high risk of addiction to this drug.

Propoxyphene is not recommended for use in suicidal or addiction-prone patients.

Interactions
Comcomitant use with carbamazepine will increase carbamazepine's effects. (Monitor serum carbamazepine levels.) Propoxyphene may inhibit the metabolism of antidepressants, such as doxepin, necessitating a lower dose of antidepressant.

Reduced doses of propoxyphene are usually needed when given concomitantly with other CNS depressants (narcotic analgesics, general anesthetics, antihistamines, phenothiazines, barbiturates, benzodiazepines, sedative-hypnotics, antidepressants and muscle relaxants) to avoid potentiation of adverse effects (respiratory depression, sedation, hypotension).

Concurrent use with cimetidine may enhance respiratory and CNS depression, resulting in confusion, disorientation, apnea, or seizures.

Ingestion of alcohol will significantly potentiate the CNS depressant effects of propoxyphene.

Use propoxyphene with caution with drugs that are highly metabolized in the liver (rifampin, phenytoin, and digitoxin), because accumulation of either drug may occur. Withdrawal symptoms may result if used together.

Patients who develop physical dependence on propoxyphene may experience acute withdrawal syndrome when given a single dose of an antagonist. Use with caution and monitor closely.

Severe cardiovascular depression may result from concomitant use with general anesthetics.

Effects on diagnostic tests
Propoxyphene may cause false decrease in test for urinary steroid excretion.

Adverse reactions
- CNS: dizziness, sedation, dysphoria, euphoria, headache, light-headedness, weakness.
- DERM: rashes.
- GI: abdominal pain, nausea, vomiting, constipation.
- Other: minor visual disturbances, liver dysfunction.
  Note: Drug should be discontinued if hypersensitivity, seizures, or cardiac arrhythmias occur.

Overdose and treatment
The most common signs and symptoms of overdose are CNS depression, respiratory depression, and miosis (pinpoint pupils). Others include hypotension, bradycardia, hypothermia, shock, apnea, cardiopulmonary arrest, circulatory collapse, pulmonary edema, and convulsions.

Propoxyphene is known to cause ECG changes (prolonged QRS complex) and nephrogenic diabetes insipidus in acute toxic doses. Death from an acute overdose is most likely to occur within the first hour. Signs and symptoms of overdose with propoxyphene combination products may include salicylism from aspirin or acetaminophen toxicity.

To treat an acute overdose, first establish adequate

respiratory exchange via a patent airway and ventilation as needed; administer a narcotic antagonist (naloxone) to reverse respiratory depression. (Because the duration of action of propoxyphene is longer than naloxone, repeated dosing is necessary.) Do not give naloxone in the absence of clinically significant respiratory or cardiovascular depression. Monitor vital signs closely.

If the patient presents within 2 hours of ingestion of an oral overdose, empty the stomach immediately by inducing emesis (ipecac syrup) or gastric lavage. Use caution to avoid any risk of aspiration. Administer activated charcoal via nasogastric tube for further removal of the drug in an oral overdose.

Provide symptomatic and supportive treatment (continued respiratory support, correction of fluid or electrolyte imbalance). Anticonvulsants may be needed; monitor laboratory parameters, vital signs, and neurologic status closely. Dialysis may be helpful in the treatment of overdose with propoxyphene combination products containing aspirin or acetaminophen.

▶ **Special considerations**
Besides those relevant to all *opioids*, consider the following recommendations.
● Propoxyphene may obscure the signs and symptoms of an acute abdominal condition or worsen gallbladder pain.
● Propoxyphene should not be prescribed for maintenance purposes in narcotic addiction.
● Propoxyphene can be considered a mild narcotic analgesic, but pain relief is equivalent to aspirin.

Information for the patient
● Warn patient not to exceed recommended dosage.
● Tell the patient to avoid use of alcohol because it will cause additive CNS depressant effects.
● Warn patient of the additive depressant effect which can occur if this drug must be prescribed for patients whose medical conditions require use of sedatives, tranquilizers, muscle relaxants, antidepressants, or other CNS-depressant drugs.

Geriatric use
Lower doses are usually indicated for elderly patients, because they may be more sensitive to the therapeutic and adverse effects of the drug.

Breast-feeding
Propoxyphene is excreted in breast milk; it should be used with caution in breast-feeding women.

propranolol
Inderal, Inderal LA

● Pharmacologic classification: beta-adrenergic blocking agent
● Therapeutic classification: antihypertensive, antianginal, antiarrhythmic, adjunctive therapy of migraine, adjunctive therapy of myocardial infarction (MI)
● Pregnancy risk category C

How supplied
Available by prescription only
Tablets: 10 mg, 20 mg, 40 mg, 60 mg, 80 mg, 90 mg
Injection: 1 mg/ml

Capsules (extended-release): 80 mg, 120 mg, 160 mg

Indications, route, and dosage
Hypertension
Adults: Initially, 80 mg P.O. daily in two to four divided doses or the sustained-release form once daily. Increase at 3- to 7-day intervals to maximum daily dose of 640 mg. Usual maintenance dosage is 160 to 480 mg daily.
Management of angina pectoris
Adults: 10 to 20 mg t.i.d. or q.i.d., or one 80-mg sustained-release capsule daily. Dosage may be increased at 7- to 10-day intervals. The average optimum dosage is 160 to 240 mg daily.
Supraventricular, ventricular, and atrial arrhythmias; tachyarrhythmias caused by excessive catecholamine action during anesthesia, hyperthyroidism, and pheochromocytoma
Adults: 1 to 3 mg I.V. diluted in 50 ml dextrose 5% in water (D_5W) or normal saline solution infused slowly, not to exceed 1 mg/minute. After 3 mg have been infused, another dose may be given in 2 minutes; subsequent doses no sooner than q 4 hours. Usual maintenance dosage is 10 to 80 mg P.O. t.i.d. or q.i.d.
Prevention of frequent, severe, uncontrollable, or disabling migraine or vascular headache
Adults: Initially, 80 mg daily in divided doses or one sustained-release capsule once daily. Usual maintenance dosage is 160 to 240 mg daily, divided t.i.d. or q.i.d.
To reduce mortality after MI
Adults: 180 to 240 mg P.O. daily in divided doses. Usually administered in three to four doses daily, beginning 5 to 21 days after infarct.
†*Adjunctive treatment of anxiety*
Adults: 10 to 80 mg P.O. 1 hour before anxiety-provoking activity
†*Treatment of essential, familial, or senile movement tremors*
Adults: 40 mg P.O. t.i.d. or q.i.d., as tolerated and needed.
†*Adjunctive treatment of thyrotoxicosis*
Adults: 10 to 40 mg P.O. t.i.d. or q.i.d., as tolerated and needed.

Pharmacodynamics
● *Antihypertensive action:* Exact mechanism of propranolol's antihypertensive effect is unknown; drug may reduce blood pressure by blocking adrenergic receptors (thus decreasing cardiac output), by decreasing sympathetic outflow from the CNS, and by suppressing renin release.
● *Antianginal action:* Propranolol decreases myocardial oxygen consumption by blocking catecholamine access to beta-adrenergic receptors, thus relieving angina.
● *Antiarrhythmic action:* Propranolol decreases heart rate and prevents exercise-induced increases in heart rate. It also decreases myocardial contractility, cardiac output, and sinoatrial and atrioventricular (AV) nodal conduction velocity.
● *Migraine prophylactic action:* The migraine-preventive effect of propranolol is thought to result from inhibition of vasodilation.
● *MI prophylactic action:* The exact mechanism by which propranolol decreases mortality after MI is unknown.

COMPARING ANTIHYPERTENSIVE DRUGS

DRUG	PLASMA VOLUME	PLASMA RENIN ACTIVITY	PERIPHERAL RESISTANCE	DURATION
Peripherally acting drugs				
guanadrel	Moderate increase	Unknown	Moderate decrease	4 to 14 hours
guanethidine	Moderate increase	Moderate decrease	Moderate decrease or no change	24 to 48 hours
prazosin	Slight increase	Moderate decrease	Moderate decrease	< 24 hours
reserpine	Moderate increase	Moderate decrease	Moderate decrease	6 to 24 hours
terazosin	Slight increase	Unknown	Moderate decrease	24 hours
Centrally acting drugs				
clonidine	Slight increase	Moderate decrease	Moderate decrease	12 to 24 hours
guanabenz	No change	Moderate decrease	Moderate decrease	6 to 12 hours
methyldopa	Moderate increase	Moderate decrease	Moderate decrease	12 to 24 hours
Beta-adrenergic blockers				
acebutolol	Unknown	Unknown	Slight decrease	24 to 30 hours
atenolol	Slight decrease or no change	Moderate decrease	Moderate decrease	> 24 hours
metoprolol	Slight decrease or no change	Moderate decrease	Moderate decrease or no change	13 to 24 hours
nadolol	Slight decrease or no change	Moderate decrease	No change	17 to 24 hours
pindolol	Unknown	No change	Moderate decrease	> 24 hours
propranolol	Slight decrease or no change	Moderate decrease	No change	8 to 12 hours
timolol	Slight decrease or no change	Moderate decrease	No change	12 hours

Pharmacokinetics
● *Absorption:* Propranolol is absorbed almost completely from the GI tract. Absorption is enhanced when given with food. Peak plasma concentrations occur 60 to 90 minutes after administration of regular-release tablets. After I.V. administration, peak concentrations occur in about 1 minute, with virtually immediate onset of action.
● *Distribution:* Propranolol is distributed widely throughout the body; drug is more than 90% protein-bound.
● *Metabolism:* Hepatic metabolism is almost total; oral dosage form undergoes extensive first-pass metabolism.
● *Excretion:* Approximately 96% to 99% of a given dose of propranolol is excreted in urine as metabolites; re-

mainder is excreted in feces as unchanged drug and metabolites. Biological half-life is about 4 hours.

Contraindications and precautions
Propranolol is contraindicated in patients with known hypersensitivity to the drug; in patients with overt cardiac failure, sinus bradycardia, second- or third-degree AV block, bronchial asthma, cardiogenic shock, and Raynaud's syndrome, because drug may worsen these conditions.

Propranolol should be used cautiously in patients with coronary insufficiency because beta-adrenergic blockade may precipitate congestive heart failure (CHF); in patients with pulmonary disease; in patients with diabetes mellitus, hypoglycemia, or hyperthyroidism because propranolol may mask tachycardia (it does

*Canada only   †Unlabeled clinical use   Italicized adverse reactions are life-threatening.

not mask dizziness and sweating caused by hypoglycemia); and in patients with impaired hepatic function. Propranolol may also mask common signs of shock.

Interactions

Concomitant use with cardiac glycosides potentiates bradycardia and myocardial depressant effects of propranolol; cimetidine may decrease clearance of propranolol via inhibition of hepatic metabolism, and thus also enhance its beta-blocking effects.

Propranolol may potentiate antihypertensive effects of other antihypertensive agents, especially catecholamine-depleting agents such as reserpine.

Propranolol may antagonize beta-adrenergic stimulating effects of sympathomimetic agents such as isoproterenol and of monoamine oxidase inhibitors; use with epinephrine cause severe vasoconstriction.

Atropine, tricyclic antidepressants, and other drugs with anticholinergic effects may antagonize propranolol-induced bradycardia; nonsteroidal anti-inflammatory drugs may antagonize its hypotensive effects.

High doses of propranolol may potentiate neuromuscular blocking effect of tubocurarine and related compounds.

Concomitant use with insulin or hypoglycemic agents can alter dosage requirements in previously stable diabetic patients.

Effects on diagnostic tests

Propranolol may elevate serum transaminase, alkaline phosphatase, and lactic dehydrogenase levels, and may elevate BUN levels in patients with severe heart disease.

Adverse reactions

- CNS: fatigue, lethargy, vivid dreams, hallucinations.
- CV: bradycardia, hypotension, *CHF*, peripheral vascular disease.
- DERM: rash.
- GI: nausea, vomiting, diarrhea.
- GU: impotence
- Metabolic: hypoglycemia without tachycardia.
- Other: *bronchospasm*, fever, arthralgia.
  Note: Drug should be discontinued if signs of heart failure or bronchospasm develop.

Overdose and treatment

Clinical signs of overdose include severe hypotension, bradycardia, heart failure, and bronchospasm.

After acute ingestion, induce emesis or empty stomach by gastric lavage; follow with activated charcoal to reduce absorption, and administer symptomatic and supportive care. Treat bradycardia with atropine (0.25 to 1 mg); if no response, administer isoproterenol cautiously. Treat cardiac failure with digitalis and diuretics, and hypotension with vasopressors: epinephrine is preferred. Treat bronchospasm with isoproterenol and aminophylline.

▶ Special considerations

Besides those relevant to all *beta-adrenergic blocking agents*, consider the following recommendations.
- After prolonged atrial fibrillation, restoration of normal sinus rhythm may dislodge thrombi from atrial wall, resulting in thromboembolism; anticoagulation is often advised before procedure.
- Propranolol also has been used to treat aggression and rage, stage fright, recurrent GI bleeding in cirrhotic patients, and menopausal symptoms.

- Propranolol should never be administered as an adjunct in the treatment of pheochromocytoma unless the patient is pre-treated with alpha-adrenergic blocking agents.

Information for the patient

Advise patient to take drug with meals because food increases absorption.

Geriatric use

Elderly patients may require lower maintenance doses of propranolol because of increased bioavailability or delayed metabolism; they also may experience enhanced adverse effects.

Pediatric use

Safety and efficacy of propranolol in children have not been established; use only if potential benefit outweighs risk.

Breast-feeding

Propranolol is distributed into breast milk; an alternative feeding method is recommended during therapy.

---

propylthiouracil (PTU)
Propyl-Thyracil★

- Pharmacologic classification: thyroid hormone antagonist
- Therapeutic classification: antihyperthyroid agent
- Pregnancy risk category D

How supplied

Available by prescription only
Tablets: 50 mg

Indications, route, and dosage
Hyperthyroidism

Adults: 100 mg P.O. t.i.d.; up to 300 mg q 8 hours have been used in severe cases. Continue until patient is euthyroid, then start maintenance dose of 100 mg daily to t.i.d.

Neonates and children: 5 to 7 mg/kg P.O. daily in divided doses q 8 hours. Alternatively, give according to age.
Children age 6 to 10: 50 to 150 mg P.O. daily in divided doses q 8 hours.
Children over age 10: 100 mg P.O. t.i.d. Continue until patient is euthyroid, then start maintenance dosage of 25 mg t.i.d. to 100 mg b.i.d.

Preparation for thyroidectomy

Adults and children: Same dosage as for hyperthyroidism; then iodine may be added 10 days before surgery.

Thyrotoxic crisis

Adults and children: Same dosage as for hyperthyroidism, with concomitant iodine therapy and propranolol.

Pharmacodynamics

Antithyroid action: Used to treat hyperthyroidism, PTU inhibits synthesis of thyroid hormone by interfering with the incorporation of iodine into thyroglobulin; it also inhibits the formation of iodothyronine. Besides blocking hormone synthesis, it also inhibits the peripheral deiodination of thyroxine to triiodothyronine (liothyronine). Clinical effects become evident only when the preformed hormone is depleted and circulating hormone levels decline.

As preparation for thyroidectomy, PTU inhibits synthesis of the thyroid hormone and causes a euthyroid state, reducing surgical problems during thyroidectomy; as a result, the mortality for a single-stage thyroidectomy is low. Iodide reduces the vascularity of the gland and makes it less friable.

Used in treating thyrotoxic crisis, PTU inhibits peripheral deiodination of thyroxine to triiodothyronine. Theoretically, it is preferred over methimazole in thyroid storm because of its peripheral action.

Pharmacokinetics
• *Absorption:* PTU is absorbed rapidly and readily (about 80%) from the GI tract. Peak levels occur at 1 to 1½ hours.
• *Distribution:* PTU appears to be concentrated in the thyroid gland. PTU readily crosses the placenta and is distributed into breast milk. It is 75% to 80% protein-bound.
• *Metabolism:* PTU is metabolized rapidly in the liver.
• *Excretion:* About 35% of a dose is excreted in urine. Half-life is 1 to 2 hours in patients with normal renal function and 8½ hours in anuric patients.

Contraindications and precautions
PTU is contraindicated in patients with hypersensitivity to the drug. It should be used with caution in patients over age 40, because of an increased risk of agranulocytosis, and in patients receiving other agents known to cause agranulocytosis or those with infection or hepatic dysfunction.

Interactions
Concomitant use of PTU with adrenocorticoids or ACTH may require a dosage adjustment of the steroid when thyroid status changes. Concomitant use with bone marrow depressant agents increases the risk of agranulocytosis; use with hepatotoxic agents increases the risk of hepatotoxicity; use with iodinated glycerol, lithium, or potassium iodide may potentiate hypothyroid effects.

Effects on diagnostic tests
PTU therapy alters selenomethionine (^{75}Se) levels and prothrombin time; it also alters AST (SGOT), ALT (SGPT), and lactic dehydrogenase levels, as well as liothyronine uptake.

Adverse reactions
• CNS: headache, drowsiness, vertigo, depression, paresthesias.
• DERM: rash, urticaria, discoloration, pruritus, lupus-like syndrome, *exfoliative dermatitis.*
• GI: diarrhea, nausea, vomiting, epigastric distress, sialadenopathy (appear to be dose-related).
• HEMA: *agranulocytosis,* leukopenia, granulocytopenia, thrombocytopenia (appear to be dose-related).
• Hepatic: *jaundice, hepatitis.*
• Renal: nephritis.
• Other: arthralgia, myalgia, salivary gland enlargement, loss of taste, drug fever, lymphadenopathy, hair loss, edema.
    Note: Drug should be discontinued at the first sign of hepatotoxicity or if the patient develops signs of agranulocytosis, pancytopenia, hepatitis (fever, swelling of cervical lymph nodes), or exfoliative dermatitis.

Overdose and treatment
Clinical manifestations of overdose include nausea, vomiting, epigastric distress, fever, headache, arthralgia, pruritus, edema, and pancytopenia.

Treatment includes withdrawal of the drug in the presence of agranulocytosis, pancytopenia, hepatitis, fever, or exfoliative dermatitis. For depression of bone marrow, treatment may require antibiotics and transfusions of fresh whole blood. For hepatitis, treatment includes rest, adequate diet, and symptomatic support, including analgesics, gastric lavage, I.V. fluids, and mild sedation.

▶ **Special considerations**
Besides those relevant to all *thyroid hormone antagonists,* consider the following recommendations.
• Best response occurs when drug is administered around the clock and given at the same time each day in respect to meals.
• A beta blocker, usually propranolol, commonly is given to manage the peripheral signs of hyperthyroidism, which are primarily cardiac-related (tachycardia).
• Observe for signs of hypothyroidism (mental depression; cold intolerance; hard, nonpitting edema; hair loss).
• Therapy should be discontinued if patient develops severe rash or enlarged cervical lymph nodes.

Information for the patient
• Warn patient to avoid using self-prescribed cough medicines; many contain iodine.
• Suggest taking drug with meals to reduce GI side effects.
• Instruct patient to store drug in a light-resistant container. Warn patient not to store medication in the bathroom; heat and humidity may cause the drug to deteriorate.
• Tell patient to promptly report fever, sore throat, malaise, unusual bleeding, yellowing of eyes, nausea, or vomiting.
• Advise patient to have medical review of thyroid status before undergoing surgery (including dental surgery).
• Teach patient how to recognize the signs of hyperthyroidism and hypothyroidism and what to do if they occur.

Breast-feeding
Because PTU is excreted in breast milk, breast-feeding should be avoided during treatment with this hormone. However, if breast-feeding is necessary, PTU is the preferred antithyroid agent.

---

protamine sulfate

• Pharmacologic classification: antidote
• Therapeutic classification: heparin antagonist
• Pregnancy risk category C

How supplied
Available by prescription only
Injection: 50-mg vial, 250-mg vial, requiring reconstitution

Indications, route, and dosage
Heparin overdose
Adults and children: Dosage based on venous blood coagulation studies, usually 1 mg for each 90 units of heparin derived from lung tissue or 1 mg for each 115 units of heparin derived from intestinal mucosa. Give by slow I.V. injection over 1 to 3 minutes. Maximum dosage: 50 mg in any 10-minute period.

Pharmacodynamics
Heparin antagonism: Protamine has weak anticoagulant activity; however, when given in the presence of heparin, it forms a salt that neutralizes anticoagulant effects of both drugs.

Pharmacokinetics
• *Absorption:* Heparin-neutralizing effect of protamine occurs within 30 to 60 seconds.
• *Distribution:* Not applicable.
• *Metabolism:* Fate of the heparin-protamine complex is unknown; however, it appears to be partially degraded, with release of some heparin.
• *Excretion:* Protamine's binding action lasts about 2 hours.

Contraindications and precautions
Administer protamine cautiously to patients allergic to fish; protamine is derived from sperm of salmon and other fish.

Watch for spontaneous bleeding (heparin rebound), especially in patients undergoing dialysis and patients who have had cardiac surgery.

Interactions
None significant.

Effects on diagnostic tests
Drug shortens heparin-prolonged partial thromboplastin time.

Adverse reactions
• CV: sudden fall in blood pressure, bradycardia.
• Other: transitory flushing, feeling of warmth, dyspnea, bleeding, heparin rebound, hypersensitivity.

Overdose and treatment
No information available.

▶ Special considerations
• Check for possible fish allergy.
• Do not mix protamine with any other medication.
• Reconstitute powder by adding 5 ml sterile water to 50-mg vial (25 ml to 250-mg vial); discard unused solution.
• Slow I.V. administration (over 1 to 3 minutes) decreases adverse effects; have antishock equipment available.
• Monitor patient continually, and check vital signs frequently; blood pressure may fall suddenly.
• Dosage is based upon blood coagulation studies, as well as on route of administration of heparin and time elapsed since heparin was administered.

Information for the patient
Advise patient that he may experience transitory flushing or feel warm after I.V. administration.

---

protriptyline hydrochloride
Triptil, Vivactil

• Pharmacologic classification: tricyclic antidepressant
• Therapeutic classification: antidepressant
• Pregnancy risk category C

How supplied
Available by prescription only
Tablets: 5 mg, 10 mg

Indications, route, and dosage
Depression
Adults: 15 to 40 mg P.O. daily in divided doses, increasing gradually to a maximum of 60 mg/day.

Pharmacodynamics
Antidepressant action: Protriptyline is thought to exert its antidepressant effects by inhibiting reuptake of norepinephrine and serotonin in CNS nerve terminals (presynaptic neurons), which results in increased concentrations of these neurotransmitters in the synaptic cleft. Protriptyline inhibits reuptake of serotonin and norepinephrine equally. Protriptyline has CNS stimulatory effects and may be most useful in treating withdrawn, depressed patients.

Pharmacokinetics
• *Absorption:* Protriptyline is absorbed slowly from the GI tract after oral administration. Peak plasma levels occur in 24 to 30 hours.
• *Distribution:* Protriptyline is distributed widely into the body. Drug is 90% protein-bound. Proposed therapeutic drug levels range from 70 to 170 ng/ml. Steady-state plasma levels and peak therapeutic effect are achieved within 2 weeks.
• *Metabolism:* Protriptyline is metabolized by the liver; a significant first-pass effect may account for variability of serum concentrations in different patients taking the same dosage.
• *Excretion:* Most of drug is excreted slowly in urine; some is excreted in feces via the biliary tract. About 50% of a given dose is excreted as metabolites within 16 days.

Contraindications and precautions
Protriptyline is contraindicated in patients with known hypersensitivity to tricyclic antidepressants, trazodone, and related compounds; in the acute recovery phase of myocardial infarction (MI) because of potential for cardiac arrhythmias; in coma or severe respiratory depression because of additive CNS depression; and during or within 14 days of therapy with monoamine oxidase inhibitors because this combination may result in hypertensive response.

Protriptyline should be used cautiously in patients with other cardiac disease (arrhythmias, congestive heart failure [CHF], angina pectoris, valvular disease, or heart block) because of additive antiarrhythmic effects; in patients with respiratory disorders because of additive respiratory depression; in patients with alcoholism, epilepsy, and other seizure disorders, or during scheduled electroconvulsive therapy because drug lowers seizure threshold; in patients with bipolar disease because drug may induce or worsen manic phase;

---

in patients with glaucoma; in patients with hyperthyroidism or in patients taking thyroid replacement; in patients with Type I and Type II diabetes; in patients with prostatic hypertrophy, paralytic ileus, or urinary retention because drug may worsen these conditions; in patients with hepatic or renal dysfunction because diminished metabolism and excretion cause drug to accumulate; in patients with Parkinson's disease because drug may exacerbate tremors, expecially at high doses; and in patients undergoing surgery with general anesthesia, because of increased sensitivity to cardiac effects of general anesthetics or pressor agents.

Interactions

Concomitant use of protriptyline with sympathomimetics, including epinephrine, phenylephrine, phenylpropanolamine, and ephedrine (often found in nasal sprays), may increase blood pressure; use with warfarin may increase prothrombin time and cause bleeding. Concomitant use with thyroid medication, pimozide, and antiarrhythmic agents (quinidine, disopyramide, procainamide) may increase incidence of cardiac arrhythmias and conduction defects.

Protriptyline may decrease hypotensive effects of centrally acting antihypertensive drugs, such as guanethidine, guanabenz, guanadrel, clonidine, methyldopa, and reserpine.

Concomitant use with disulfiram or ethchlorvynol may cause delirium.

Additive effects are likely after concomitant use of protriptyline with CNS depressants, including alcohol, analgesics, barbiturates, narcotics, tranquilizers, and anesthetics (oversedation); atropine and other anticholinergic drugs, including phenothiazines, antihistamines, meperidine, and antiparkinsonian agents (oversedation, paralytic ileus, visual changes, and severe constipation); and metrizamide (increased risk of convulsions).

Barbiturates and heavy smoking induce protriptyline metabolism and decrease therapeutic efficacy; phenothiazines and haloperidol decrease protriptyline's metabolism, decreasing its therapeutic efficacy; methylphenidate, cimetidine, oral contraceptives, propoxyphene, and beta blockers may inhibit protriptyline metabolism, increasing plasma levels and toxicity.

Effects on diagnostic tests

Protriptyline may prolong conduction time (elongation of Q-T and PR intervals, flattened T waves on ECG); it also may elevate liver enzyme levels, decrease white blood cell counts, and decrease or increase serum glucose levels.

Adverse reactions

● CNS: drowsiness, dizziness, sedation, excitation, tremors, weakness, headache, nervousness, seizures, peripheral neuropathy, extrapyramidal symptoms, anxiety, vivid dreams, confusion (more marked in elderly patients), decreased libido.
● CV: orthostatic hypotension, tachycardia, *arrhythmias, MI, stroke, heart block, CHF,* palpitations, hypertension, ECG changes.
● EENT: blurred vision, tinnitus, mydriasis, increased intraocular pressure.
● GI: dry mouth, constipation, nausea, vomiting, anorexia, diarrhea, paralytic ileus, jaundice.
● GU: urinary retention.
● Other: sweating, photosensitivity, hypersensitivity (rash, urticaria, drug fever, edema).

After abrupt withdrawal of long-term therapy, nausea, headache, and malaise (does not indicate addiction) may occur.

Note: Drug should be discontinued (not abruptly) if signs of hypersensitivity occur, such as urinary retention, extreme dry mouth, skin rash, excessive sedation, seizures, tachycardia, sore throat, fever, or jaundice.

Overdose and treatment

The first 12 hours after acute ingestion are a stimulatory phase characterized by excessive anticholinergic activity (agitation, irritation, confusion, hallucinations, parkinsonian symptoms, seizures, urinary retention, dry mucous membranes, pupillary dilation, constipation, and ileus). This is followed by CNS depressant effects, including hypothermia, decreased or absent reflexes, sedation, hypotension, cyanosis, and cardiac irregularities, including tachycardia, conduction disturbances, and quinidine-like effects on the ECG.

Severity of overdose is best indicated by prolongation of QRS complex beyond 100 ms, which usually represents a serum level in excess of 1,000 ng/ml; serum levels are usually not helpful. Metabolic acidosis may follow hypotension, hypoventilation, and convulsions.

Treatment is symptomatic and supportive, including maintaining airway, stable body temperature, and fluid and electrolyte balance. Induce emesis if gag reflex is intact; follow with gastric lavage and activated charcoal to prevent further absorption. Dialysis is usually ineffective. Treat seizures with parenteral diazepam or phenytoin; arrhythmias with parenteral phenytoin or lidocaine; and acidosis with sodium bicarbonate. *Do not give barbiturates;* these may enhance CNS and respiratory depressant effects.

▶ Special considerations

Besides those relevant to all *tricyclic antidepressants,* consider the following recommendations.
● Consider the inherent risk of suicide until significant improvement of depressive state occurs. High-risk patients should have close supervision during initial drug therapy. To reduce risk of suicidal overdose, prescribe the smallest quantity of tablets consistent with good management.
● Protriptyline has a stimulatory effect on the CNS and may be better suited for withdrawn patients. It also has less sedative effect and a lower incidence of orthostatic hypotension.
● Protriptyline should be withdrawn gradually over a period of a few weeks; never abruptly.
● The drug should be discontinued at least 48 hours before surgical procedures.
● Chewing gum, hard candy, or ice chips may alleviate dry mouth.

Information for the patient

● Explain that patient may not experience full effects of the drug for up to 4 weeks or longer after therapy begins.
● Tell patient to take the medication exactly as prescribed, not to double doses for missed doses, and to avoid alcoholic beverages while taking this drug.
● Warn patient that drug may cause stimulation or dizziness. Patient should avoid hazardous activities that require alertness until the drug's full effects are known.
● Tell patient not to share drug with others and to store it safely away from children.
● Suggest taking protriptyline with food or milk if it

---

*Canada only   †Unlabeled clinical use   Italicized adverse reactions are life-threatening.

causes stomach upset and relieving dry mouth with chewing gum or sugarless candy.
• To prevent dizziness or fainting at start of therapy, patient should lie down for about 30 minutes after taking each dose and should avoid sudden postural changes, especially when rising to upright position.
• Advise patient not to stop taking drug suddenly; to report adverse effects promptly, especially confusion, movement disorders, rapid heartbeat, dizziness, fainting, or difficulty urinating.
• To relieve insomnia with this drug, patient should take dose as early in the day as possible.
• Tell patient to store drug safely away from children.

Geriatric use
Elderly patients are more sensitive to therapeutic effects and more prone to adverse cardiac effects.

Pediatric use
Protriptyline is not recommended for children under age 12.

Breast-feeding
Protriptyline may be excreted in breast milk. The potential benefit to the mother should outweigh the possible adverse effects in the infant.

---

pseudoephedrine hydrochloride
pseudoephedrine sulfate
Afrinol, Cenafed, Decofed, Dorcol, Myfedrine, NeoFed, Novafed, PediaCare, Pseudogest, Sudafed, Sinufed

• Pharmacologic classification: adrenergic
• Therapeutic classification: decongestant
• Pregnancy risk category B

How supplied
Available without prescription
Oral solution: 15 mg/5 ml, 30 mg/5 ml, 7.5 mg/0.8 ml
Tablets: 30 mg, 60 mg
Capsules (extended-release): 120 mg

Indications, route, and dosage
Nasal and eustachian tube decongestant
Adults and children age 12 and over: 60 mg P.O. q 4 to 6 hours. Maximum dosage, 240 mg daily, or 120 mg P.O. extended-release tablet q 12 hours.
Children age 6 to 11: Administer 30 mg P.O. q 4 to 6 hours. Maximum dosage, 120 mg daily.
Children age 2 to 5: 15 mg P.O. q 4 to 6 hours. Maximum dosage, 60 mg/day, or 4 mg/kg or 125 mg/m² P.O. divided q.i.d.

Pharmacodynamics
Decongestant action: Pseudoephedrine directly stimulates alpha-adrenergic receptors of respiratory mucosa to produce vasoconstriction; shrinkage of swollen nasal mucous membranes; reduction of tissue hyperemia, edema, and nasal congestion; an increase in airway (nasal) patency and drainage of sinus excretions; and opening of obstructed eustachian tube. Relaxation of bronchial smooth muscle may result from direct stimulation of beta-adrenergic receptors. Mild CNS stimulation may also occur.

Pharmacokinetics
• *Absorption:* Nasal decongestion occurs within 30 minutes and persists 4 to 6 hours after oral dose of 60-mg tablet or oral solution. Effects persist 8 hours after 60-mg dose and up to 12 hours after 120-mg dose of extended-release form.
• *Distribution:* Pseudoephedrine is widely distributed throughout the body.
• *Metabolism:* Pseudoephedrine is incompletely metabolized in liver by N-demethylation to inactive compounds.
• *Excretion:* 55% to 75% of a dose is excreted unchanged in urine; remainder is excreted as unchanged drug and metabolites.

Contraindications and precautions
Pseudoephedrine is contraindicated in patients with hypersensitivity to the drug and to other sympathomimetics, severe hypertension, or severe coronary artery disease and in those taking monoamine oxidase (MAO) inhibitors because of the potential for severe adverse cardiovascular effects.
Administer cautiously to patients with hyperthyroidism, diabetes, ischemic heart disease, elevated intraocular pressure, or prostatic hypertrophy, because the drug may worsen these conditions.

Interactions
Concomitant use with other sympathomimetics may produce additive effects and toxicity; with reserpine, methyldopa, mecamylamine, and *Veratrum* alkaloids, may reduce their antihypertensive effects.
Beta blockers may increase pressor effects of pseudoephedrine. Tricyclic antidepressants may antagonize effects of pseudoephedrine. MAO inhibitors potentiate pressor effects of pseudoephedrine.

Effects on diagnostic tests
None reported.

Adverse reactions
• CNS: nervousness, excitability, restlessness, dizziness, weakness, insomnia, headache, drowsiness, lightheadedness, fear, anxiety, tremor, hallucinations, *seizures.*
• CV: *cardiovascular collapse,* tachycardia, *palpitations,* arrhythmias.
• GI: nausea, vomiting, anorexia, dry mouth.
• Other: pallor, respiratory difficulty, dysuria.
Note: Drug should be discontinued if hypersensitivity, cardiac arrhythmias, or hypertension occurs.

Overdose and treatment
Clinical manifestations of overdose include exaggeration of common adverse reactions, particularly seizures, cardiac arrhythmias, and nausea and vomiting.
Treatment may include an emetic and gastric lavage within 4 hours of ingestion. Charcoal is effective only if administered within 1 hour, unless extended-release form was used. If renal function is adequate, forced diuresis will increase elimination. Do not force diuresis in severe overdose. Monitor vital signs, cardiac state, and electrolyte levels. I.V. propranolol may control cardiac toxicity; I.V. diazepam may be helpful to manage delirium or convulsions; dilute potassium chloride solutions (I.V.) may be given for hypokalemia.

▶ **Special considerations**
Besides those relevant to all *adrenergics*, consider the following recommendations.
● Administer last daily dose several hours before bedtime to minimize insomnia.
● If symptoms persist longer than 5 days or fever is present, reevaluate therapy.
● Observe patient for complaints of headache or dizziness; monitor blood pressure.

Information for the patient
● If patient finds swallowing medication difficult, suggest opening capsules and mixing contents with applesauce, jelly, honey, or syrup. Mixture must be swallowed without chewing.
● Dry mouth may occur. Suggest using ice chips, sugarless gum, or hard candy for relief.
● Instruct patient to take missed dose if remembered within 1 hour. If beyond 1 hour, patient should skip and resume regular schedule and should not double dose.
● Tell patient to store drug away from heat and light (not in bathroom medicine cabinet) and safely out of reach of children.
● Caution patient that many nonprescription preparations may contain sympathomimetics, which can cause additive, hazardous reactions.
● Advise patient to take last dose at least 2 to 3 hours before bedtime to avoid insomnia.

Geriatric use
Elderly patients may be sensitive to effects of drug; lower dose may be needed. Overdosage may cause hallucinations, CNS depression, seizures, and death in patients over age 60. Use extended-release preparations with caution in elderly patients.

Pediatric use
Extended-release preparations should not be administered to patients under age 12.

Breast-feeding
Because drug may be distributed into breast milk, breast-feeding women should avoid using this drug; infant may be susceptible to drug effects.

---

psyllium
Cillium, Fiberall, Hydrocil Instant, Konsyl, Konsyl-D, Metamucil, Mucilose, Naturacil, Perdiem Plain, Reguloid, Serutan, Siblin, Syllact, V-Lax

● Pharmacologic classification: adsorbent
● Therapeutic classification: bulk laxative
● Pregnancy risk category C

How supplied
Available without prescription
Powder: 3.3 g/tsp, 3.4 g/tsp, 3.5 g/tsp, 4.94 g/tsp
Effervescent powder: 3.4 g/packet, 3.7 g/packet
Granules: 2.5 g/tsp, 4.03 g/tsp
Chewable pieces: 1.7 g/piece
Wafers: 3.4 g/wafer

Indications, route, and dosage
Constipation, bowel management, irritable bowel syndrome
Adults: 1 to 2 rounded tsp P.O. in full glass of liquid daily, b.i.d. or t.i.d., followed by second glass of liquid; or 1 packet P.O. dissolved in water daily, b.i.d., or t.i.d.
Children over age 6: 1 level tsp P.O. in ½ glass of liquid h.s.

Pharmacodynamics
Laxative action: Psyllium adsorbs water in the gut; it also serves as a source of indigestible fiber, increasing stool bulk and moisture, thus stimulating peristaltic activity and bowel evacuation.

Pharmacokinetics
● *Absorption:* None; onset of action varies from 12 hours to 3 days.
● *Distribution:* Psyllium is distributed locally in the gut.
● *Metabolism:* None.
● *Excretion:* Psyllium is excreted in feces.

Contraindications and precautions
Psyllium is contraindicated in patients with abdominal pain, fecal impaction, or intestinal obstruction or ulceration, because the drug may worsen these symptoms or conditions.
Effervescent powder should be used with caution in patients requiring sodium restriction because of the drug's high sodium content. Sugar-free drug preparations should be used with caution in patients who must restrict phenylalanine intake; these products may contain aspartame, which the GI tract metabolizes to phenylalanine.

Interactions
Psyllium may adsorb oral medications, such as anticoagulants, digitalis glycosides, and salicylates.

Effects on diagnostic tests
None reported.

Adverse reactions
● GI: abdominal cramps (especially in severe constipation); diarrhea; nausea; vomiting; esophageal or intestinal obstruction in patients with esophageal stricture or if powder form is used without water.
Note: Drug should be discontinued if abdominal pain develops.

Overdose and treatment
No cases of overdose have been reported; probable clinical effects include abdominal pain and diarrhea.

▶ **Special considerations**
● Before administering drug, add at least 8 oz (240 ml) of water or juice and stir for a few seconds (improves drug's taste). Have patient drink mixture immediately to prevent it from congealing, then have him drink another glass of fluid.
● Separate administration of psyllium and oral anticoagulants, digitalis glycosides, and salicylates by at least 2 hours.
● Drug may reduce appetite if administered before meals.
● Psyllium and other bulk laxatives most closely mimic natural bowel function and do not cause laxative dependence; they are especially useful for patients with postpartum constipation or diverticular disease, for de-

---

bilitated patients, for irritable bowel syndrome, and for chronic laxative users.

• Give diabetic patients a sugar- and sodium-free psyllium product.

Information for the patient

• Warn patient not to swallow drug in dry form; he should mix it with at least 8 oz of fluid, stir briefly, drink immediately (to prevent mixture from congealing), and follow it with another 8 oz of fluid.

• Explain that drug may reduce appetite if taken before meals; recommend taking drug 2 hours after meals and any other oral medication.

• Advise diabetic patients and those with restricted sodium or sugar intake to avoid psyllium products containing salt or sugar. Advise patients who must restrict phenylalanine intake to avoid psyllium products containing aspartame.

Breast-feeding

Because the drug is not absorbed, it presumably is safe for use in breast-feeding women.

---

pyrantel pamoate
Antiminth, Combantrin*

• Pharmacologic classification: pyrimidine derivative
• Therapeutic classification: anthelmintic
• Pregnancy risk category C

How supplied
Available by prescription only
Oral suspension: 50 mg/ml

Indications, route, and dosage
Roundworm and pinworm infections
Adults and children over age 2: Single dose of 11 mg/kg P.O. Maximum dosage is 1 g. For pinworm infection, dosage should be repeated in 2 weeks.

Pharmacodynamics
Anthelmintic action: Pyrantel causes the release of acetylcholine and inhibits cholinesterases, paralyzing the worms. It is active against *Enterobius vermicularis*, *Ascaris lumbricoides*, *Ancylostoma duodenale*, *Necator americanus*, and *Trichostrongylus orientalis*.

Pharmacokinetics
• *Absorption:* Pyrantel pamoate is absorbed poorly; peak concentrations occur in 1 to 3 hours.
• *Distribution:* Little is known about the distribution of pyrantel pamoate.
• *Metabolism:* The small amount of absorbed drug is metabolized partially in the liver.
• *Excretion:* Over 50% of an oral dose of pyrantel pamoate is excreted unchanged in feces; about 7% is excreted in urine as unchanged drug or known metabolites. It is unknown if pyrantel pamoate is excreted in urine.

Contraindications and precautions
Pyrantel pamoate is contraindicated in patients with known hypersensitivity to the drug. It should be used with caution in malnourished or anemic patients and in patients with hepatic disease because it may cause transient elevations in liver function tests.

Interactions
Pyrantel pamoate antagonizes the effects of piperazine.

Effects on diagnostic tests
Pyrantel pamoate may cause transient elevations of liver function tests.

Adverse reactions
• CNS: headache, dizziness, drowsiness, insomnia.
• DERM: rashes.
• GI: anorexia, nausea, vomiting, gastralgia, cramps, diarrhea, tenesmus.
• Hepatic: transient SGOT level elevation.
• Other: fever, weakness.
   Note: Drug should be discontinued if signs of hypersensitivity or toxicity occur.

Overdose and treatment
Treatment of overdose is largely supportive, particularly of cardiovascular and respiratory functions. After recent ingestion (within 4 hours), empty stomach by induced emesis or gastric lavage. Follow with activated charcoal to decrease absorption. Osmotic cathartics may be helpful.

▶ **Special considerations**
• Shake suspension well before measuring, to ensure accurate dosage.
• Drug may be given with milk, fruit juice, or food.
• Laxatives, enemas, or dietary restrictions are unnecessary.
• Protect drug from light.
• Treat all family members.

Information for the patient
• Tell patient to wash perianal area daily and to change undergarments and bedclothes daily.

• To help prevent reinfection, instruct patient and family members in personal hygiene, including sanitary disposal of feces and hand washing and nail cleaning after defecation and before handling, preparing, or eating food.

• Explain routes of transmission and tell patient to encourage other household members and suspected contacts to be tested and, if necessary, treated.

Pediatric use
Safety and efficacy for children under age 2 have not been established.

Breast-feeding
Safety has not been established.

---

pyrazinamide
PMS-Pyrazinamide*, Tebrazid*

- Pharmacologic classification: synthetic pyrazine analogue of nicotinamide
- Therapeutic classification: antituberculosis agent
- Pregnancy risk category C

How supplied
Available by prescription only
Tablets: 500 mg

Indications, route, and dosage
Adjunctive treatment of tuberculosis (when primary and secondary antitubercular drugs cannot be used or have failed)
Adults: 20 to 35 mg/kg P.O. daily, in one or more doses. Maximum dosage is 3 g daily. Lower dosage is recommended in decreased renal function.

Pharmacodynamics
Antibiotic action: The mechanism of action of pyrazinamide is unknown; drug may be bactericidal or bacteriostatic depending on organism susceptibility and drug concentration at infection site. Pyrazinamide is active only against *Mycobacterium tuberculosis.* Pyrazinamide is considered adjunctive in tuberculosis therapy and is given with other drugs to prevent or delay development of resistance to pyrazinamide by *M. tuberculosis.*

Pharmacokinetics
- *Absorption:* Pyrazinamide is absorbed well after oral administration; peak serum levels occur 2 hours after an oral dose.
- *Distribution:* Pyrazinamide is distributed widely into body tissues and fluids, including lungs, liver, and CSF; drug is 50% protein-bound. It is not known if pyrazinamide crosses the placenta.
- *Metabolism:* Pyrazinamide is hydrolyzed in the liver; some hydrolysis occurs in stomach.
- *Excretion:* Pyrazinamide is excreted almost completely in urine by glomerular filtration. It is not known if pyrazinamide is excreted in breast milk. Elimination half-life in adults is 9 to 10 hours. Half-life is prolonged in renal and hepatic impairment.

Contraindications and precautions
Pyrazinamide is contraindicated in patients with known hypersensitivity to pyrazinamide and in patients with severe hepatic disease.

Pyrazinamide should be used cautiously in patients with acute intermittent porphyria, decreased renal function, diabetes, or a history of peptic ulcer disease or gout.

Interactions
None reported.

Effects on diagnostic tests
Pyrazinamide may interfere with urine ketone determinations. The drug's systemic effects may temporarily decrease 17-ketosteroid levels; it may increase protein-bound iodine and urate levels and results of liver enzyme tests.

Adverse reactions
- CNS: neuromuscular blockade.
- DERM: maculopapular rash, photosensitivity (skin turns reddish-brown).
- GI: anorexia, nausea, vomiting.
- GU: dysuria.
- HEMA: sideroblastic anemia, possible bleeding tendency due to thrombocytopenia.
- Hepatic: *hepatitis,* jaundice.
- Metabolic: interference with control in diabetes mellitus, hyperuricemia.
- Other: malaise, fever, arthralgia, porphyria.

Note: Drug should be discontinued if patient shows signs of hypersensitivity reactions or hepatic damage.

Overdose and treatment
No specific recommendations are available. Treatment is supportive. After recent ingestion (4 hours or less), empty stomach by induced emesis or gastric lavage. Follow with activated charcoal to decrease absorption.

▶ Special considerations
- Monitor liver function, especially enzyme and bilirubin levels, and renal function, especially serum uric acid levels, before therapy and thereafter at 2- to 4-week intervals; observe patient for signs of liver damage or decreased renal function.
- In a patient with diabetes mellitus, pyrazinamide therapy may hinder stabilization of serum glucose levels.
- Pyrazinamide frequently elevates serum uric acid levels. Although usually asymptomatic, a uricosuric agent, such as probenecid or allopurinol, may be necessary.

Information for the patient
- Explain disease process and rationale for long-term therapy.
- Teach signs and symptoms of hypersensitivity and other adverse reactions, and emphasize need to report them; urge patient to report *any* unusual reactions, especially signs of gout.
- Be sure patient understands how and when to take drugs; urge patient to complete entire prescribed regimen, to comply with instructions for around-the-clock dosage, and to keep follow-up appointments.
- Tell patient to keep fluid intake at 2 quarts (about 2 liters)/day; explain need for good hydration to prevent renal damage.

Geriatric use
Because elderly patients commonly have diminished renal function, which decreases drug excretion, pyrazinamide should be used with caution.

Pediatric use
Not recommended for use in children.

Breast-feeding
Safety in breast-feeding women has not been established. Alternative feeding method is recommended during therapy.

pyridostigmine bromide
Mestinon, Regonol

- Pharmacologic classification: cholinesterase inhibitor
- Therapeutic classification: muscle stimulant
- Pregnancy risk category C

How supplied
Available by prescription only
Tablets: 60 mg
Tablets (timed-release): 180 mg
Syrup: 60 mg/5 ml
Injection: 5 mg/ml in 2-ml ampule or 5-ml vial

Indications, route, and dosage
Curariform antagonist (postoperatively)
Adults: 10 to 30 mg I.V. preceded by atropine sulfate 0.6 to 1.2 mg I.V.
Myasthenia gravis
Adults: 60 to 180 mg P.O. b.i.d. or q.i.d. Usual dose 600 mg daily, but higher doses may be needed (up to 1,500 mg daily). Give ⅓₀ of oral dose I.M. or I.V. Dosage must be adjusted for each patient, depending on response and tolerance of adverse effects.
Children: 1 to 2 mg/kg P.O. q 3 to 4 hours while awake.
Neonates of myasthenic mothers: 0.05 to 0.15 mg/kg I.M.

Pharmacodynamics
Muscle stimulant action: Pyridostigmine blocks acetylcholine's hydrolysis by cholinesterase, resulting in acetylcholine accumulation at cholinergic synapses, increasing stimulation of cholinergic receptors at the myoneural junction.

Pharmacokinetics
- *Absorption:* Pyridostigmine is poorly absorbed from the GI tract. Onset of action usually occurs 30 to 45 minutes after oral administration, 2 to 5 minutes after I.V., and 15 minutes after I.M.
- *Distribution:* Little is known about pyridostigmine's distribution; however, drug may cross the placenta, especially when administered in large doses.
- *Metabolism:* Exact metabolic fate is unknown. Duration of effect is usually 3 to 6 hours after oral dose and 2 to 3 hours after I.V. dose, depending on patient's physical and emotional status and disease severity. Pyridostigmine is not hydrolyzed by cholinesterase.
- *Excretion:* Drug and metabolites are excreted in urine.

Contraindications and precautions
Pyridostigmine is contraindicated in patients with intestinal or urinary tract obstruction because of its stimulatory effect on smooth muscle and in patients with bradycardia, because drug may exacerbate this condition.

Administer pyridostigmine with extreme caution to patients with bronchial asthma, because it may precipitate asthma attacks. Administer pyridostigmine cautiously in patients with epilepsy, because the drug may cause CNS stimulation; to patients with vagotonia, hyperthyroidism, or cardiac arrhythmias, because the drug may exacerbate these conditions; and to patients with peptic ulcer disease, because the drug may increase gastric acid secretion.

Interactions
Concomitant use with procainamide or quinidine may reverse pyridostigmine's cholinergic effect on muscle. Corticosteroids may decrease pyridostigmine's cholinergic effect; when corticosteroids are stopped, this effect may increase, possibly affecting muscle strength.

Concomitant use with succinylcholine may result in prolonged respiratory depression from plasma esterase inhibition, delaying succinylcholine hydrolysis. Concomitant use with ganglionic blockers, such as mecamylamine, may critically decrease blood pressure; effect is usually preceded by abdominal symptoms. Magnesium has a direct depressant effect on skeletal muscle and may antagonize pyridostigmine's beneficial effects.

Effects on diagnostic tests
None reported.

Adverse reactions
- CNS: headache (with high doses), fasciculations, *convulsions.*
- CV: bradycardia, hypotension (rare).
- DERM: rash, excessive sweating.
- EENT: miosis.
- GI: abdominal cramps, nausea, vomiting, diarrhea, excessive salivation.
- Other: thrombophlebitis (with I.V. administration), *bronchospasm,* bronchoconstriction, increased bronchial secretions, weakness, muscle cramps.
  Note: Drug should be discontinued if hypersensitivity, headache, convulsions, difficulty breathing, skin rash, or paralysis occurs.

Overdose and treatment
Clinical effects of overdose include nausea, vomiting, diarrhea, blurred vision, miosis, excessive tearing, bronchospasm, increased bronchial secretions, hypotension, incoordination, excessive sweating, muscle weakness, cramps, fasciculations, paralysis, bradycardia or tachycardia, excessive salivation, and restlessness or agitation.

Support respiration; bronchial suctioning may be performed. The drug should be discontinued immediately. Atropine may be given to block pyridostigmine's muscarinic effects; however, it will not counter skeletal muscle paralysis. Avoid atropine overdose, because it may lead to bronchial plug formation.

▶ Special considerations
Besides those relevant to all *cholinesterase inhibitors,* consider the following recommendations.
- If muscle weakness is severe, determine if this effect stems from drug toxicity or exacerbation of myasthenia gravis. A test dose of edrophonium I.V. will aggravate drug-induced weakness but will temporarily relieve weakness that results from the disease.
- Avoid giving large pyridostigmine doses to patients with decreased GI motility, because toxicity may result once motility has been restored.
- Give pyridostigmine with food or milk to reduce the risk of muscarinic adverse effects.
- When indicated, consider providing bedside supply of tablets hospitalized patients may take themselves. Many patients with long-standing, stabilized disease insist on this.

● Stop all other cholinergic drugs during pyridostigmine therapy to avoid additive toxicity.
● Patients may develop resistance to this drug.

Information for the patient
● When administering pyridostigmine to patient with myasthenia gravis, stress the importance of taking the drug exactly as ordered, on time, and in evenly spaced doses.
● If patient is taking sustained-release tablets, explain how these work and instruct him to take them at the same time each day and to swallow these tablets whole rather than crushing them.
● Teach patient how to evaluate muscle strength; instruct him to observe changes in muscle strength and to report muscle cramps, rash, or fatigue.

Breast-feeding
Pyridostigmine may be excreted in breast milk, possibly resulting in infant toxicity. The woman's clinical status will determine whether she should discontinue breast-feeding or stop use of the drug.

---

pyridoxine hydrochloride (vitamin B₆)
Beesix, Hexa-Betalin, Nestrex

● Pharmacologic classification: water-soluble vitamin
● Therapeutic classification: nutritional supplement
● Pregnancy risk category A (C if > recommended daily allowance [RDA])

How supplied
Available by prescription only
Injection: 10-ml vial (100 mg/ml), 30-ml vial (100 mg/ml), 10-ml vial (100 mg/ml, with 1.5% benzyl alcohol), 30-ml vial (100 mg/ml, with 1.5% benzyl alcohol), 10-ml vial (100 mg/ml, with 0.5% chlorobutanol), 1-ml vial (100 mg/ml)
Available without prescription
Tablets: 10 mg, 25 mg, 50 mg, 100 mg, 200 mg, 250 mg, 500 mg, 500 mg timed-release

Indications, route, and dosage
Recommended daily allowance (RDA)
Neonates and infants to age 6 months: 0.3 mg daily.
Infants age 6 months to 1 year: 0.6 mg daily.
Children age 1 to 3 years: 1 mg daily.
Children age 4 to 6 years: 1.1 mg daily.
Children age 7 to 10 years: 1.4 mg daily.
Females age 11 to 14 years: 1.4 mg daily.
Females age 15 to 18 years: 1.5 mg daily.
Females age 19 and older: 1.6 mg daily.
Females during pregnancy: 2.2 mg daily.
Lactating women: 2.1 mg daily.
Males age 11 to 14 years: 1.7 mg daily.
Males age 15 and over: 2 mg daily.
Dietary vitamin B₆ deficiency
Adults: 2.5 to 10 mg P.O., I.M., or I.V. daily for 3 weeks, then 2 to 5 mg daily as a supplement to a proper diet.
Children: 100 mg P.O., I.M., or I.V. to correct deficiency, then an adequate diet with supplementary RDA doses to prevent recurrence.

Seizures related to vitamin B₆ deficiency or dependency
Adults and children: 100 mg I.M. or I.V. in single dose.
Vitamin B₆-responsive anemias or dependency syndrome (inborn errors of metabolism)
Adults: 100 to 200 mg P.O., I.M., or I.V. daily for 3 weeks then 2.5 to 100 mg daily until symptoms subside; then 50 mg daily for life.
Children: 100 mg I.M. or I.V., then 2 to 10 mg I.M. or 10 to 100 mg P.O. daily.
Prevention of vitamin B₆ deficiency during isoniazid therapy
Adults: 25 to 50 mg P.O. daily.
Children: 0.5 to 1.5 mg P.O. daily.
Infants: 0.1 to 0.5 mg P.O. daily.
If neurologic symptoms develop in pediatric patients, increase dosage as necessary.
Treatment of vitamin B₆ deficiency secondary to isoniazid
Adults: 100 mg P.O. daily for 3 weeks, then 50 mg daily.
Children: Titrate dosages.

Pharmacodynamics
Metabolic action: Natural vitamin B₆ contained in plant and animal foodstuffs is converted to physiologically active forms of vitamin B₆, pyridoxal phosphate and pyridoxamine phosphate. Exogenous forms of the vitamin are metabolized in humans. Vitamin B₆ acts as a coenzyme in protein, carbohydrate, and fat metabolism and participates in the decarboxylation of amino acids in protein metabolism. Vitamin B₆ also helps convert tryptophan to niacin or serotonin as well as the deamination, transamination, and transsulfuration of amino acids. Finally, vitamin B₆ is responsible for the breakdown of glycogen to glucose-1-phosphate in carbohydrate metabolism. The total adult body store consists of 16 to 27 mg of pyridoxine. The need for pyridoxine increases with the amount of protein in the diet.

Pharmacokinetics
● *Absorption:* After oral administration, pyridoxine and its substituents are absorbed readily from the GI tract. GI absorption may be diminished in patients with malabsorption syndromes or following gastric resection. Normal serum levels of pyridoxine are 30 to 80 ng/ml.
● *Distribution:* Pyridoxine is stored mainly in the liver. The total body store is approximately 16 to 27 mg. Pyridoxal and pyridoxal phosphate are the most common forms found in the blood and are highly protein-bound. Pyridoxal crosses the placenta; fetal plasma concentrations are five times greater than maternal plasma concentrations. After maternal intake of 2.5 to 5 mg/day of pyridoxine, the concentration of the vitamin in breast milk is approximately 240 ng/ml.
● *Metabolism:* Pyridoxine is degraded to 4-pyridoxic acid in the liver.
● *Excretion:* In erythrocytes, pyridoxine is converted to pyridoxal phosphate, and pyridoxamine to pyridoxamine phosphate. The phosphorylated form of pyridoxine is transaminated to pyridoxal and pyridoxamine, which is phosphorylated rapidly. The conversion of pyridoxine phosphate to pyridoxal phosphate requires riboflavin. Biological half-life is 15 to 20 days.

Contraindications and precautions
Pyridoxine is contraindicated in patients with a history of pyridoxine sensitivity. Pyridoxine should not be administered I.V. to patients with heart disease. An in-

---

adequate diet may cause multiple vitamin deficiencies; proper nutrition is important. Pyridoxine-dependent seizures in infants may result from the use of large doses of pyridoxine during pregnancy.

Interactions
Pyridoxine reverses the therapeutic effects of levodopa by accelerating peripheral metabolism. Concomitant use of pyridoxine with phenobarbital or phenytoin may cause a 50% decrease in serum concentrations of these anticonvulsants. Isoniazid, cycloserine, penicillamine, hydralazine, and oral contraceptives may increase pyridoxine requirements.

Effects on diagnostic tests
Pyridoxine therapy alters determinations for urobilinogen in the spot test using Ehrlich's reagent, resulting in a false-positive reaction.

Adverse reactions
● CNS: paresthesias, headache, somnolence, *seizures* (with I.V. administration), sensory neuropathic syndrome.
● GI: nausea.
● Local: burning or stinging at I.M. or S.C. site.
● Other: allergic reactions.

Overdose and treatment
Clinical manifestations of overdose include: ataxia and severe sensory neuropathy after chronic consumption of high daily doses of pyridoxine (2 to 6 g). These neurologic deficits usually resolve after pyridoxine is discontinued.

▶ Special considerations
● Prepare a dietary history. A single vitamin deficiency is unusual; lack of one vitamin often indicates a deficiency of others.
● Monitor protein intake; excessive protein intake increases pyridoxine requirements.
● A dosage of 25 mg/kg/day is well-tolerated. Adults consuming 200 mg/day for 33 days and on a normal dietary intake develop vitamin B_6 dependency.
● Do not mix with sodium bicarbonate in the same syringe.
● Patients receiving levodopa shouldn't take pyridoxine in dosages greater than 5 mg/day.
● To treat seizures and coma from isoniazid overdose, dosage equals dosage of isoniazid.
● Store in a tight, light-resistant container.
● Do not use injection solution if it contains precipitate. Slight darkening is acceptable.
● Pyridoxine is sometimes of value for treating nausea and vomiting during pregnancy.

Information for the patient
Teach the patient about dietary sources of vitamin B_6, such as yeast, wheat germ, liver, whole-grain cereals, bananas, and legumes.

Pediatric use
● Safety and efficacy have not been established.
● The use of large doses of pyridoxine during pregnancy has been implicated in pyridoxine-dependency seizures in neonates.

Breast-feeding
It is unknown whether this drug is excreted in breast milk. Use caution when administering to breast-feeding

women. Pyridoxine may inhibit lactation by suppression of prolactin.

pyrimethamine
Daraprim

● Pharmacologic classification: aminopyrimidine derivative [folic acid antagonist]
● Therapeutic classification: antimalarial
● Pregnancy risk category C

How supplied
Available by prescription only
Tablets: 25 mg of pyrimethamine

Indications, route, and dosage
Malaria prophylaxis and transmission control
Adults and children over age 10: 25 mg P.O. weekly.
Children ages 4 to 10: 12.5 mg P.O. weekly.
Children under age 4: 6.25 mg P.O. weekly.
Dosage should be continued for all age-groups for at least 10 weeks after leaving endemic areas.
Acute attacks of malaria
Not recommended alone in nonimmune persons; use with faster-acting antimalarials, such as chloroquine, for 2 days to initiate transmission control and suppressive cure. For chloroquine-resistant strain, administer with sulfonamides, and possibly quinine.
Adults and children over age 15: 25 mg P.O. daily for 2 days.
Children under age 15: 12.5 mg P.O. daily for 2 days.
Toxoplasmosis
Adults: 25 mg P.O. daily for 3 to 4 weeks, with sulfadiazine 2 to 8 g P.O. daily in three or four divided doses.
†Children: 2 mg/kg/day P.O. (maximum daily dosage is 25 mg) in divided doses q 12 hours for 3 days, then 1 mg/kg/day P.O. for 4 weeks. Administer with sulfadoxine 100 to 200 mg P.O. daily in divided doses.

Pharmacodynamics
Antimalarial action: Pyrimethamine inhibits the reduction of dihydrofolate to tetrahydrofolate, thereby blocking folic acid metabolism needed for survival of susceptible organisms. This mechanism is distinct from sulfonamide-induced folic acid antagonism. Pyrimethamine is active against the asexual erythrocytic forms of susceptible plasmodia and against *Toxoplasma gondii.*

Pharmacokinetics
● *Absorption:* Pyrimethamine is well absorbed from the intestinal tract; peak serum concentrations occur within 2 hours.
● *Distribution:* Pyrimethamine is distributed to the kidneys, liver, spleen, and lungs; it is approximately 80% bound to plasma proteins.
● *Metabolism:* Pyrimethamine is metabolized to several unidentified compounds.
● *Excretion:* Pyrimethamine is excreted in the urine and in breast milk; elimination half-life is 2 to 6 days. Its half-life is not changed in end-stage renal disease.

Contraindications and precautions
Pyrimethamine is contraindicated in patients with megaloblastic anemia from folate deficiency, because it is a folate antagonist, and in patients with known hypersensitivity to the drug. Pyrimethamine also is contra-

indicated in chloroquine-resistant malaria and should be used with caution after therapy with chloroquine. The drug should be used with caution in patients with G6PD deficiency because it may induce hemolytic anemia.

Initial dosage for toxoplasmosis in patients with seizure disorders should be lowered to avoid CNS toxicity. Concomitant use with sulfadoxine is contraindicated in patients with porphyria and should be used with caution in patients with impaired hepatic or renal function, severe allergy, bronchial asthma, or G6PD deficiency.

Interactions

Pyrimethamine and sulfonamides act synergistically against some organisms, because each inhibits folic acid synthesis at a different level.

Pyrimethamine and sulfadoxine should not be given concomitantly with other sulfonamides or with cotrimoxazole because of additive adverse effects. Concomitant use with para-aminobenzoic acid and folic acid reduces the antitoxoplasmic effects of pyrimethamine and may require higher dosage of the latter drug.

Effects on diagnostic tests

Pyrimethamine therapy may decrease white blood cell, red blood cell, and platelet counts.

Adverse reactions

● CNS: stimulation and *seizures* (acute toxicity), ataxia, tremors.
● DERM: rashes, *erythema multiforme (Stevens-Johnson syndrome), toxic epidermal necrolysis.*
● GI: anorexia, vomiting, diarrhea, atrophic glossitis, abdominal cramps.
● HEMA: *agranulocytosis, aplastic anemia,* megaloblastic anemia, bone marrow suppression, leukopenia, thrombocytopenia, pancytopenia.
Note: Drug should be discontinued or dosage reduced if signs of folic acid or folinic acid deficiency develop. Parenteral folinic acid (leucovorin) may be given (up to 9 mg I.M. daily for 3 days) until blood counts are restored to normal.

Overdose and treatment

Overdose is marked by anorexia, vomiting, and CNS stimulation, including seizures. Megaloblastic anemia, thrombocytopenia, leukopenia, glossitis, and crystalluria may also occur.

Treatment of overdose consists of gastric lavage followed by a cathartic; barbiturates may help to control seizures. Leucovorin (folinic acid) in a dosage of 3 to 9 mg daily for 3 days or longer is used to restore decreased platelet or leukocyte counts.

▶ Special considerations

● No longer considered a first-line antimalarial agent. Other antimalarial drugs (mefloquine, chloroquine, sulfadoxine) are generally preferred.
● Give with meals to minimize GI distress.
● Monitor complete blood counts, including platelet counts twice a week.
● Monitor patient for signs of folate deficiency or bleeding when platelet count is low; if abnormalities appear, decrease dosage or discontinue drug. Leucovorin (folinic acid) may be prescribed to raise blood counts during reduced dosage or after drug is discontinued.
● When pyrimethamine with sulfadoxine (Fansidar) is used prophylactically, the first dose should be given 1 or 2 days before travel to an area where malaria is endemic.
● Use Fansidar in patients with febrile illness.
● Because severe reactions may occur, pyrimethamine with sulfadoxine should be given only to patients traveling to areas where chloroquine-resistant malaria is prevalent and only if traveler will be in such areas longer than 3 weeks.

Information for the patient

● Teach patient how to recognize signs and symptoms of adverse blood reactions; tell patient to report them immediately. Teach emergency measures to control overt bleeding.
● Teach patient signs and symptoms of folate deficiency.
● Counsel patient about need to report any adverse effects and to keep follow-up medical appointments.
● Keep drug out of reach of children.

Pediatric use

May be used with caution in children.

Breast-feeding

Pyrimethamine with sulfadoxine is contraindicated in breast-feeding women because it contains a sulfonamide.

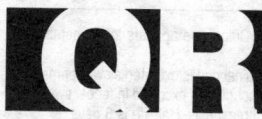

quazepam
Doral

- Pharmacologic classification: benzodiazepine
- Therapeutic classification: hypnotic
- Controlled substance schedule IV
- Pregnancy risk category X

How supplied
Available by prescription only
Tablets: 7.5 mg, 15 mg

Indications, route, and dosage
Insomnia
Adults: 15 mg P.O. h.s. Some patients may respond to lower doses. Decrease dosage in elderly patients to 7.5 mg P.O. h.s. after 2 days of therapy.

Pharmacodynamics
Hypnotic action: Quazepam acts on the limbic system and thalamus of the CNS by binding to specific benzodiazepine receptors responsible for inducing sleep.

Pharmacokinetics
- *Absorption:* Quazepam is well absorbed from the GI tract. Peak plasma levels of about 15 ng/ml occur within 2 hours.
- *Distribution:* Steady-state plasma levels of the parent drug appear after 7 days of once-daily administration. The drug is more than 95% bound to plasma proteins.
- *Metabolism:* Hepatic; two active metabolites have been identified.
- *Excretion:* 31% appears in the urine and 23% appears in the feces over a 5-day period. Only a trace amount of unchanged drug appears in the urine. The mean elimination half-life of the parent drug and 2-oxoquazepam, a metabolite, is 39 hours; of N-desalkyl-2-oxoquazepam, 733 hours.

Contraindications and precautions
Quazepam is contraindicated in patients allergic to the drug or other benzodiazepines, in pregnant patients, and in those with suspected or established sleep apnea. Patients who receive prolonged therapy with benzodiazepines may experience withdrawal symptoms if the drug is suddenly withdrawn (possibly after 6 weeks of continuous therapy).

Interactions
Concomitant use with alcohol, CNS depressants including antihistamines, opiate analgesics, and other benzodiazepines causes increased CNS depression.

Effects on diagnostic tests
None reported.

Adverse reactions
- CNS: fatigue, dizziness, daytime drowsiness, headache.

Overdose and treatment
Although not specifically reported for quazepam, overdose with other benzodiazepines has produced somnolence, confusion, and coma.

General supportive measures, including gastric lavage and support of respirations, should be employed. Flumazenil, a specific benzodiazepine antagonist, may be useful. Metaraminol or levarterenol may be used to treat hypotension.

▶ Special considerations
- Prevent hoarding or self-overdosing by hospitalized patients who are depressed, suicidal, or known drug abusers.
- Avoid prolonged administration. In patients who have received prolonged therapy, avoid abrupt discontinuation of drug to prevent withdrawal symptoms.

Information for the patient
- Warn the patient about the possible excessive depressant effects that can occur with ingestion of alcohol. Additive effects can occur if alcohol is consumed on the day after the use of the drug.
- Warn patients to avoid activities that require alertness, such as driving a car, until the adverse CNS effects of the drug are known.
- Tell patients not to increase the dosage on their own and to call if they feel that the drug is no longer effective.

Geriatric use
- The elimination half-life of the parent drug and of the metabolite 2-oxoquazepam are the same in elderly patients. However, the elimination half-life of N-desalkyl-2-oxoquazepam is twice that of young adults.
- Elderly patients should have assistance with walking and other activities until the adverse CNS effects of the drug are known.

Pediatric use
Safety and efficacy in children under age 18 have not been established.

Breast-feeding
Because the drug and its metabolites are excreted in breast milk, breast-feeding is not recommended during therapy.

---

*Canada only   †Unlabeled clinical use   Italicized adverse reactions are life-threatening.

926 QUINACRINE HYDROCHLORIDE

quinacrine hydrochloride
Atabrine hydrochloride

- Pharmacologic classification: acridine derivative
- Therapeutic classification: anthelmintic, antiprotozoal, antimalarial
- Pregnancy risk category C

How supplied
Available by prescription only
Tablets: 100 mg

Indications, route, and dosage
Treatment of giardiasis in patients who cannot take furazolidone or metronidazole
Adults: 300 mg P.O. in three divided doses for 5 to 7 days.
Children: 6 mg/kg P.O. daily given in three divided doses after meals for 5 days. Maximum dosage is 300 mg/day. If necessary, the dosage may be repeated in 2 weeks.
Tapeworm (beef, pork, and fish) infections
Adults and children over age 14: Four doses of 200 mg given 10 minutes apart (800 mg total).
Children ages 11 to 14: 600 mg as a total dosage, administered in three or four divided doses, 10 minutes apart.
Children ages 5 to 10: 400 mg as a total dosage, administered in three or four divided doses, 10 minutes apart.
Malaria
Adults and children over age 8: 200 mg with 1 g sodium bicarbonate q 6 hours for five doses, then 100 mg t.i.d. for 6 days.
Children ages 4 to 8: 200 mg t.i.d. for 1 day, then 100 mg q 12 hours for 6 days.
Children ages 1 to 4: 100 mg t.i.d. for 1 day, then 100 mg once daily for 6 days.
Malaria suppression
Adults: 100 mg daily for 1 to 3 months.
Children: 50 mg daily for 1 to 3 months.

Pharmacodynamics
- *Antiprotozoal action:* Mechanism of action is unknown.
- *Anthelmintic and antimalarial actions:* Quinacrine intercalates into the parasite's DNA, inhibiting replication and protein synthesis. It is active against *Giardia lamblia, Diphyllobothrium latum, Dipylidium caninum, Hymenolepis diminuta, H. nana, Taenia saginata,* and *T. solium.* It also is active against asexual forms of *Plasmodium malariae, P. vivax,* and *P. falciparum.*
- Metronidazole and similar nitroimidazole compounds have generally replaced quinacrine in the treatment of giardiasis because they are less toxic and more effective. Some clinicians consider quinacrine obsolete for the treatment of malaria and tapeworm.

Pharmacokinetics
- *Absorption:* Quinacrine is absorbed readily; peak serum concentrations usually occur within 8 hours.
- *Distribution:* Quinacrine is distributed widely to tissues, especially into the pancreas, lungs, liver, spleen, bone marrow, erythrocytes, and skeletal muscle; it crosses the placenta. The drug is highly protein-bound.

- *Metabolism:* Quinacrine appears to be metabolized slowly.
- *Excretion:* Quinacrine is excreted slowly, primarily in urine; small amounts are excreted in feces, sweat, saliva, bile, and breast milk. Half-life is 5 days.

Contraindications and precautions
Quinacrine is contraindicated in patients taking primaquine. It should be used with caution in patients with severe cardiac disease or G6PD deficiency; in patients with severe renal disease because the drug accumulates; in patients with hepatic or alcoholic illness or in those taking hepatotoxic drugs, because it concentrates in the liver; in patients with psoriasis or porphyria because it may exacerbate these conditions; and in psychotic patients because it can cause psychosis. Quinacrine also should be used with caution in patients over age 60 and in infants under age 1.

Interactions
Quinacrine increases primaquine's plasma concentrations to potentially toxic levels. Quinacrine may inhibit alcohol dehydrogenase. Patients should avoid alcohol ingestion during therapy with quinacrine because it may result in disulfiram-like reaction.

Quinacrine potentiates the toxicity of antimalarial agents structurally related to primaquine and should not be used concomitantly.

Effects on diagnostic tests
Quinacrine may cause falsely elevated cortisol concentrations in urine and plasma. It also produces a deep yellow discoloration of acid urine.

Adverse reactions
- CNS: headache, dizziness, nervousness, vertigo, mood shifts, nightmares, *seizures,* transient psychosis.
- DERM: pleomorphic skin eruptions, yellow skin, *exfoliative dermatitis,* contact dermatitis.
- EENT: corneal damage with long-term therapy.
- GI: diarrhea, anorexia, nausea, abdominal cramps, vomiting.
- GU: deep-yellow urine.
  Note: Drug should be discontinued if signs of hypersensitivity or toxicity occur.

Overdose and treatment
Clinical signs of overdose include restlessness, psychic stimulation, seizures, nausea, vomiting, abdominal cramps, diarrhea, hypotension, arrhythmias, and yellow skin.

To treat overdose, perform gastric lavage. Symptomatic treatment may include diazepam to control initial seizures, phenytoin to control refractory seizures, and respiratory and vasopressor support as needed. After the acute phase, forced fluids and urinary acidification may help.

▶ Special considerations
- Give quinacrine after meals with a large glass of water, tea, or fruit juice to reduce GI irritation. Honey or jam may disguise bitter taste. Concomitant sodium bicarbonate may reduce nausea and vomiting associated with large doses.
- Patient should have a bland, nonfat, semisolid diet for 24 hours before treatment and should fast after the evening meal before treatment.
- Patient should have a saline cathartic and cleansing enema before treatment to reduce amount of stool for

examination; the cathartic should be repeated 1 to 2 hours after ingestion of drug, to expel worm.

● Collect all stool expelled for 48 hours after treatment; examine stool for worm's attachment organ, which will be stained yellow by drug. Worm usually passes in 4 to 10 hours after treatment.

● Patient should have regular CBCs and ophthalmoscopic examinations during prolonged treatment to detect adverse effects.

● Be alert for signs of drug-induced behavioral changes and psychosis, which may last up to 4 weeks after drug is discontinued.

Information for the patient
● Explain that the drug temporarily will turn skin and urine yellow – it is not jaundice.

● Explain that the drug turns some patients' ears, nasal cartilage, and fingernail beds a bluish gray, resembling cyanosis; it usually disappears about 2 weeks after drug is discontinued.

● Teach patient the signs and symptoms of adverse reactions. Tell patient to report them immediately.

● Advise patient to have follow-up stool examinations for 3 to 6 months to ensure elimination of worm.

● Warn patient to store drug out of reach of children.

Geriatric use
Use with caution in patients over age 60, especially in those with a history of psychosis.

Pediatric use
Use with caution in infants under age 1.

Breast-feeding
Safety has not been established; small amounts of drug are excreted in breast milk.

---

quinapril hydrochloride
Accupril

● Pharmacologic classification: angiotensin-converting enzyme (ACE) inhibitor
● Therapeutic classification: antihypertensive
● Pregnancy risk category D

How supplied
Available by prescription only
Tablets: 5 mg, 10 mg, 20 mg, 40 mg

Indications, route, and dosage
Hypertension
Adults: Initially, 10 mg P.O. daily. Adjust dosage based on response at intervals of about 2 weeks. Most patients are controlled at 20, 40, or 80 mg daily, as a single dose or in two divided doses.
Hypertension in patients receiving diuretics
Adults: Initially, 5 mg P.O. daily. Adjust dosage based on response.

Pharmacodynamics
Antihypertensive action: Quinapril and its active metabolite, quinaprilat, inhibit ACE, preventing pulmonary conversion of angiotensin I to angiotensin II, a potent vasoconstrictor. Reduced formation of angiotensin II decreases peripheral arterial resistance, decreases al-

dosterone secretion, reduces sodium and water retention, and lowers blood pressure. Quinapril also has antihypertensive activity in patients with low-renin hypertension.

Pharmacokinetics
● *Absorption:* At least 60% of drug is absorbed; peak plasma levels are seen within 1 hour. Rate and extent of absorption are decreased 25% to 30% when drug is administered during a high-fat meal.
● *Distribution:* About 97% of drug and active metabolite are bound to plasma proteins.
● *Metabolism:* About 38% of an oral dose is deesterified in the liver to quinalaprilat, the active metabolite.
● *Excretion:* Primarily excreted in the urine; terminal elimination half-life is about 25 hours.

Contraindications and precautions
Quinapril is contraindicated in patients with hypersensitivity to ACE inhibitors or with a history of angioedema. It is also contraindicated during pregnancy because ACE inhibitors can cause fetal or neonatal injury or death. When pregnancy is detected, ACE inhibitors should be discontinued as soon as possible.

Use cautiously in patients with impaired renal or hepatic function and in situations conducive to development of hyperkalemia, including use of potassium-sparing diuretics, renal insufficiency, diabetes mellitus, potassium supplementation, and use of potassium-containing sodium substitutes.

Interactions
Potassium-sparing diuretics and potassium supplements may increase risk of hyperkalemia. Avoid concomitant use.

Increased serum lithium levels and lithium toxicity have been reported when used concurrently with ACE inhibitors.

Diuretics and other antihypertensives increase risk of excessive hypotension. Discontinue diuretic or lower dose of quinapril as needed.

Each tablet of quinapril contains magnesium carbonate and magnesium stearate. Concomitant administration of quinapril with tetracycline significantly impairs absorption of tetracycline.

Effects on diagnostic tests
In clinical trials, up to 2% of patients exhibited elevated serum potassium levels.

Adverse reactions
● CNS: somnolence, vertigo, syncope, nervousness, depression.
● CV: palpitations, vasodilation, tachycardia, *heart failure, hyperkalemia, MI, hypertensive crisis, CVA,* angina, orthostatic hypotension, cardiac rhythm disturbances.
● DERM: sweating, pruritus, *exfoliative dermatitis,* photosensitivity.
● EENT: cough, dry mouth or throat.
● GI: abdominal pain, constipation, GI hemorrhage, *pancreatitis.*
● Other: back pain, malaise, elevated liver enzymes.

Overdose and treatment
No data are available regarding overdosage in humans. Animal studies suggest that the most likely symptom would be hypotension.

Peritoneal dialysis or hemodialysis would not be ben-

---

eficial; no data are available to support use of certain physiologic maneuvers, such as acidification of urine. Treat symptomatically. Infusions of 0.9% sodium chloride solution have been suggested to treat hypotension.

▶ **Special considerations**
● Blood pressure measurements should be made when drug levels are at their peak (2 to 6 hours after dosing) and at their trough (just before a dose) to verify adequate blood pressure control.
● Because concurrent administration with diuretics is associated with risk of excessive hypotension, diuretic therapy should be discontinued 2 to 3 days before start of quinapril, if possible. If quinapril alone does not adequately control blood pressure, a diuretic may be carefully added to the regimen.
● Like other ACE inhibitors, drug may cause a dry, persistent, tickling cough; it is reversible when therapy is discontinued.
● Assess renal and hepatic function before and periodically throughout therapy. Also monitor CBC and serum potassium levels.

Information for the patient
● Tell patient that drug should be taken on an empty stomach because meals, particularly high-fat meals, can impair absorption.
● Tell patient to immediately report any signs or symptoms of angioedema: swelling of face, eyes, lips, tongue, or difficulty in breathing. If any of these occur, patient should stop taking drug until after physician has reenlisted therapy.
● Warn patient that he may feel light-headed, especially during the first few days of therapy. Tell him to arise slowly to minimize this effect and to report persistent or severe symptoms. If syncope (fainting) occurs, patient should stop taking the drug and call immediately.
● Inadequate fluid intake, vomiting, diarrhea, and excessive perspiration can lead to light-headedness and syncope. Patient should take care in hot weather and during periods of exercise to avoid dehydration and overheating.
● Tell patient not to use sodium substitutes because they contain potassium and can cause hyperkalemia.
● Tell patient to report immediately any signs of infection (sore throat, fever) or of easy bruising or bleeding. Other ACE inhibitors have been associated with development of agranulocytosis and neutropenia.

Geriatric use
Elderly patients have demonstrated higher peak plasma levels and slower elimination of drug; these changes were related to decreased renal function that often occurs in elderly patients. No overall differences in safety or efficacy have been seen in elderly patients.

Pediatric use
Safety and efficacy in children have not been established.

Breast-feeding
It is unknown if drug is excreted in breast milk. Use with caution in breast-feeding women.

quinestrol
Estrovis

● Pharmacologic classification: estrogen
● Therapeutic classification: estrogen replacement
● Pregnancy risk category X

How supplied
Available by prescription only
Tablets: 100 mcg

Indications, route, and dosage
Moderate to severe vasomotor symptoms in menopause; atrophic vaginitis, kraurosis vulvae, female hypogonadism, ovariectomy, and ovarian failure
Adults: 100-mcg tablet once daily for 7 days, followed by 100 mcg/week as maintenance dosage, beginning 2 weeks after start of treatment. Dosage may be increased to 200 mcg/week.

Pharmacodynamics
Estrogenic action: Quinestrol mimics the action of endogenous estrogen in treating female hypogonadism, menopausal symptoms, and atrophic vaginitis.

Pharmacokinetics
Pharmacokinetics of quinestrol are not well described.

Contraindications and precautions
Quinestrol is contraindicated in patients with thrombophlebitis or thromboembolism because it may induce thromboembolic disease; in patients with estrogen-responsive carcinoma (breast or genital tract cancer); because it may increase tumor growth; in patients with undiagnosed abnormal genital bleeding; and in pregnant or breast-feeding women.

Quinestrol should be administered cautiously to patients with disorders that may be aggravated by fluid and electrolyte accumulation, such as asthma, seizure disorders, migraine, or cardiac, renal, or hepatic dysfunction. Carefully monitor female patients who have breast nodules, fibrocystic breast disease, or a family history of breast cancer. Because of the risk of thromboembolism, therapy with this drug should be discontinued at least 1 week before elective surgical procedures associated with an increased incidence of thromboembolism.

Interactions
Concomitant administration of drugs that induce hepatic metabolism, such as rifampin, barbiturates, primidone, carbamazepine, and phenytoin, may result in decreased estrogenic effects from a given dose. These drugs are known to accelerate the rate of metabolism of certain other agents.

In patients with diabetes, this agent increases blood glucose levels, necessitating dosage adjustment of insulin or oral hypoglycemic drugs.

Quinestrol has the potential to decrease the effects of warfarin-type anticoagulants. Patients receiving this drug concurrently with an adrenocorticosteroid or adrenocorticotropic hormone are at greater risk for fluid and electrolyte accumulation.

Effects on diagnostic tests

Quinestrol increases sulfobromophthalein retention, prothrombin time and clotting Factors VII to X, and norepinephrine-induced platelet aggregability. Increases in thyroid-binding globulin concentration may occur, resulting in increased total thyroid concentrations (measured by protein-bound iodine or total thyroxine) and decreased uptake of free triiodothyronine resin. Serum folate, pyridoxine, and antithrombin III concentrations may decrease; triglyceride, glucose, cortisol, and phospholipid levels may increase. Glucose tolerance may be impaired. Pregnanediol excretion may decrease.

Adverse reactions

● CNS: headache, dizziness, chorea, migraine, depression, libido changes.
● CV: thrombophlebitis; *thromboembolism;* hypertension; edema; *increased risk of stroke, pulmonary embolism, and myocardial infarction.*
● DERM: melasma, urticaria, acne, seborrhea, oily skin, hirsutism or hair loss, chloasma, *erythema multiforme.*
● EENT: worsening of myopia or astigmatism, intolerance of contact lenses.
● GI: nausea, vomiting, abdominal cramps, bloating, diarrhea, constipation, anorexia, increased appetite, excessive thirst, weight changes.
● GU: breakthrough bleeding, altered menstrual flow, dysmenorrhea, amenorrhea, cervical erosion or abnormal secretions, enlargement of uterine fibromas, vaginal candidiasis.
● Hepatic: cholestatic jaundice.
● Metabolic: hyperglycemia, hypercalcemia, folic acid deficiency.
● Other: leg cramps, purpura, breast changes (tenderness, enlargement, secretions).

Overdose and treatment

No information available.

▶ Special considerations

Recommendations for administration of quinestrol and for care and teaching of the patient during therapy are the same as those for all *estrogens.*

Breast-feeding

Estrogens decrease milk volume in breast-feeding women. It is not known if the drug is excreted in breast milk. Use with caution.

---

quinethazone
Aquamox*, Hydromox

● Pharmacologic classification: quinazoline derivative (thiazide-like) diuretic
● Therapeutic classification: diuretic, antihypertensive
● Pregnancy risk category D

How supplied

Available by prescription only
Tablets: 50 mg

Indications, route, and dosage
Edema

Adults: 50 to 100 mg P.O. daily or 50 mg P.O. b.i.d. Occasionally, up to 150 to 200 mg P.O. daily may be needed.

Pharmacodynamics

● *Diuretic action:* Quinethazone increases urinary excretion of sodium and water by inhibiting sodium reabsorption in the cortical diluting tubule of the nephron, thus relieving edema.
● *Antihypertensive action:* The exact mechanism of quinethazone's antihypertensive effect is unknown; it may act by direct arteriolar vasodilatation. Quinethazone also reduces total body sodium and total peripheral resistance.

Pharmacokinetics

Quinethazone is well absorbed from the GI tract after oral administration. Limited data are available on quinethazone's other pharmacokinetic parameters.

Contraindications and precautions

Quinethazone is contraindicated in patients with anuria and in those with known sensitivity to the drug.

Quinethazone should be used cautiously in patients with severe renal disease because it may decrease glomerular filtration rate and precipitate azotemia; in patients with impaired hepatic function or liver disease because electrolyte changes may precipitate coma; and in patients taking digoxin, because hypokalemia may predispose them to digitalis toxicity.

Interactions

Quinethazone potentiates the hypotensive effects of most other antihypertensive drugs; this may be used to therapeutic advantage.

Quinethazone may potentiate hyperglycemic, hypotensive, and hyperuricemic effects of diazoxide, and its hyperglycemic effect may increase insulin or sulfonylurea requirements in diabetic patients.

Quinethazone may reduce renal clearance of lithium, elevating serum lithium levels, and may necessitate a 50% reduction in lithium dosage.

Quinethazone turns urine slightly more alkaline and may decrease urinary excretion of some amines, such as amphetamine and quinidine; alkaline urine also may decrease therapeutic efficacy of methenamine compounds, such as methenamine mandelate.

Cholestyramine and colestipol may bind quinethazone, preventing its absorption; give drugs 1 hour apart.

Effects on diagnostic tests

Quinethazone therapy may alter serum electrolyte levels and may increase serum urate, glucose, cholesterol, and triglyceride levels.

Quinethazone may interfere with tests for parathyroid function and should be discontinued before such tests.

Adverse reactions

● CV: volume depletion and dehydration, orthostatic hypotension, hypercholesterolemia, hypertriglyceridemia.
● DERM: dermatitis, photosensitivity, rash.
● GI: anorexia, nausea, pancreatitis.
● HEMA: *aplastic anemia, agranulocytosis,* leukopenia, thrombocytopenia.
● Hepatic: *hepatic encephalopathy.*
● Metabolic: asymptomatic hyperuricemia; gout; hy-

---

perglycemia and impairment of glucose tolerance; fluid and electrolyte imbalances, including hyponatremia, hypochloremia, hypercalcemia, and hypokalemia; metabolic alkalosis.
• Other: hypersensitivity reactions, such as pneumonitis and vasculitis.
Note: Drug should be discontinued if rising BUN and serum creatinine levels indicate renal impairment or if patient shows signs of impending coma.

Overdose and treatment
Clinical signs of overdose include GI irritation and hypermotility, diuresis, and lethargy, which may progress to coma.
Treatment is mainly supportive; monitor and assist respiratory, cardiovascular, and renal function as indicated. Monitor fluid and electrolyte balance. For recent ingestion (less than 4 hours), induce vomiting with ipecac in conscious patient; otherwise, use gastric lavage to avoid aspiration. Do not give cathartics; these promote additional loss of fluids and electrolytes.

▶ Special considerations
Recommendations for use of quinethazone and for care and teaching of the patient during therapy are the same as those for all *thiazide and thiazide-like diuretics.*

Geriatric use
Elderly and debilitated patients require close observation and may require reduced dosages. They are more sensitive to excess diuresis because of age-related changes in cardiovascular and renal function. Excess diuresis promotes orthostatic hypotension, dehydration, hypovolemia, hyponatremia, hypomagnesemia, and hypokalemia.

Pediatric use
Safety and effectiveness have not been established.

Breast-feeding
Quinethazone may be distributed in breast milk; its safety and effectiveness in breast-feeding women have not been established.

---

quinidine gluconate
Duraquin, Quinaglute Dura-Tabs, Quinalan, Quinate

quinidine polygalacturonate
Cardioquin

quinidine sulfate
Apo-Quinidine★, Cin-Quin, Novoquinidin, Quinidex Extentabs, Quinora

- Pharmacologic classification: cinchona alkaloid
- Therapeutic classification: ventricular antiarrhythmic, supraventricular antiarrhythmic, atrial antitachyarrhythmic
- Pregnancy risk category C

How supplied
Available by prescription only
Tablets: 325 mg★ (gluconate); 324 mg, 330 mg (ex-

tended-release, polygalacturonate); 100 mg, 200 mg, 300 mg (sulfate); 300 mg (extended-release, sulfate)
Capsules: 300 mg (sulfate)
Injection: 80 mg/ml (gluconate); 200 mg/ml (sulfate); 190 mg/ml★

Indications, route, and dosage
Atrial flutter or fibrillation
Adults: 200 mg of quinidine sulfate or equivalent base P.O. q 2 to 3 hours for five to eight doses with subsequent daily increases until sinus rhythm is restored or toxic effects develop. Administer quinidine only after digitalization, to avoid increasing AV conduction. Maximum dosage is 3 to 4 g daily.

Paroxysmal supraventricular tachycardia
Adults: 400 to 600 mg I.M. of gluconate q 2 to 3 hours until toxic effects develop or dysrhythmia subsides.

Premature atrial and ventricular contractions, paroxysmal atrioventricular junctional rhythm or atrial and ventricular tachycardia, maintenance of cardioversion
Adults: Give test dose of 50 to 200 mg P.O., then monitor vital signs before beginning therapy: 200 to 400 mg of quinidine sulfate or equivalent base P.O. q 4 to 6 hours; or initially, 600 mg of quinidine gluconate I.M., then up to 400 mg q 2 hours, p.r.n.; or 800 mg of quinidine gluconate I.V. diluted in 40 ml of dextrose 5% in water, infused at 16 mg (1 ml)/minute. Alternately, give 600 mg of quinidine sulfate in extended-release form, or 324 to 648 mg of quinidine gluconate in extended-release form, every 8 to 12 hours.
Children: Give test dose of 2 mg/kg, then 3 to 6 mg/kg P.O. q 2 to 3 hours for five doses daily.

†Malaria (when quinine dihydrochloride is unavailable)
Adults: Administer quinidine gluconate by continuous I.V. infusion. Loading dose 10 mg/kg infused over 1 hr, followed by maintenance infusion of 20 mcg/kg/minute for 72 hours. Contact the CDC Malaria Branch for protocol instructions for recommendations at (404) 488-4046 (weekdays) or (404) 639-2888 (evenings, weekends, holidays), if using this regimen.

Pharmacodynamics
Antiarrhythmic action: A Class IA antiarrhythmic, quinidine depresses phase O of the action potential. It is considered a myocardial depressant because it decreases myocardial excitability and conduction velocity and may depress myocardial contractility. It also exerts anticholinergic activity, which may modify its direct myocardial effects. In therapeutic doses, quinidine reduces conduction velocity in the atria, ventricles, and His-Purkinje system. It helps control atrial tachyarrhythmias by prolonging the effective refractory period (ERP) and increasing the action potential duration in the atria, ventricles, and His-Purkinje system. Because ERP prolongation exceeds action potential duration, tissue remains refractory even after returning to resting membrane potential (membrane-stabilizing effect). Quinidine shortens the effective refractory period of the AV node. Because quinidine's anticholinergic action also may increase AV node conductivity, digitalis should be administered for atrial tachyarrhythmias before quinidine therapy begins, to prevent ventricular tachyarrhythmias. Quinidine also suppresses automaticity in the His-Purkinje system and ectopic pacemakers, making it useful in treating ventricular premature beats. At therapeutic doses, quinidine prolongs the QRS duration and

---

Q-T interval; these ECG effects may be used as an index of drug effectiveness and toxicity.

Pharmacokinetics

• *Absorption:* Although all quinidine salts are well absorbed from the GI tract, serum drug levels vary greatly among individuals. Onset of action of quinidine sulfate is from 1 to 3 hours. For extended-release forms, onset of action may be slightly slower but duration of effect is longer, because this drug delivery system allows longer than usual dosing intervals. Peak plasma levels occur in 3 to 4 hours for quinidine gluconate and 6 hours for quinidine polygalacturonate.

• *Distribution:* Quinidine is well distributed in all tissues except the brain. It concentrates in the heart, liver, kidneys, and skeletal muscle. Distribution volume decreases in patients with congestive heart failure, possibly requiring reduction in maintenance dosage. Approximately 80% of drug is bound to plasma proteins; the unbound (active) fraction may increase in patients with hypoalbuminemia from various causes, including hepatic insufficiency. Usual therapeutic serum levels depend on assay method and ranges as follows:

—Specific assay (EMIT, HPLC, fluorescence polarization): 2 to 5 mcg/ml.
—Nonspecific assay (fluorometric): 4 to 8 mcg/ml.

• *Metabolism:* About 60% to 80% of drug is metabolized in the liver to two metabolites that may have some pharmacologic activity.

• *Excretion:* Approximately 10% to 30% of an administered dose is excreted in the urine within 24 hours as unchanged drug. Urine acidification increases quinidine excretion; alkalinization decreases excretion. Most of an administered dose is eliminated in the urine as metabolites; elimination half-life ranges from 5 to 12 hours (usual half-life is about 6½ hours). Duration of effect ranges from 6 to 8 hours.

Contraindications and precautions

Quinidine is contraindicated in patients with complete AV block with an AV junctional or idioventricular pacemaker, because of potential for asystole; in patients with intraventricular conduction defects (especially with prolonged QT interval or QRS duration, or digitalis toxicity manifested by arrhythmias or AV conduction disorders), because quinidine in therapeutic concentration increases the QT interval and QRS duration through AV node and His-Purkinje effects; because further prolongation would be detrimental in these conditions; and because complete heart block, ventricular tachycardia, ventricular fibrillation, or asystole may result.

Quinidine is contraindicated in patients with myasthenia gravis, because the drug's anticholinergic effects may exacerbate muscle weakness; and in patients with hypersensitivity to quinidine or related compounds.

Use quinidine with caution in patients with incomplete AV block, because complete heart block may occur; in patients with congestive heart failure, because the drug's direct myocardial depressant effect may worsen heart failure; in patients with hypotension, because the drug causes alpha blockade, which exacerbates hypotension (especially when given I.V.); in patients with renal and hepatic dysfunction because toxic drug accumulation may result; and in patients with asthma, muscle weakness, or infection with fever, because these conditions may mask hypersensitivity reactions to the drug.

Interactions

Concomitant use of quinidine with hypotensive agents may cause additive hypotensive effects (mainly when administered I.V.); with phenothiazines or reserpine, it may cause additive cardiac depressant effects.

Concomitant use with digoxin or digitoxin may cause increased (possibly toxic) serum digoxin levels. (Some experts recommend a 50% reduction in digoxin dosage when quinidine therapy is initiated, with subsequent monitoring of serum concentrations.)

Concomitant use with anticonvulsants (such as phenytoin and phenobarbital) increases the rate of quinidine metabolism; this leads to decreased quinidine levels. Concomitant use with coumarin may potentiate coumarin's anticoagulant effect, possibly leading to hypoprothrombinemic hemorrhage.

When used concomitantly, cholinergic agents may fail to terminate paroxysmal supraventricular tachycardia, because quinidine antagonizes cholinergics' vagal excitation effect on the atria and AV node. Also, quinidine's anticholinergic effects may negate the effects of such anticholinesterase drugs as neostigmine and pyridostigmine, when these agents are used to treat myasthenia gravis.

Concomitant use with anticholinergic agents may lead to additive anticholinergic effects. Concomitant use with neuromuscular blocking agents (such as pancuronium bromide, succinylcholine chloride, tubocurarine chloride, gallium triethiodide, metocurine iodide, and decamethonium bromide) may potentiate anticholinergic effects. Use of quinidine should be avoided immediately after use of these agents; if quinidine must be used, respiratory support may be needed.

Concomitant use with thiazide diuretics, some antacids, and sodium bicarbonate may decrease quinidine elimination when urine pH increases, requiring close monitoring of therapy.

Concomitant use with rifampin may increase quinidine metabolism and decrease serum quinidine levels, possibly necessitating dosage adjustment when rifampin therapy is initiated or discontinued.

Concomitant use with nifedipine may result in decreased quinidine levels. Concomitant use with verapamil may result in significant hypotension in some patients with hypertrophic cardiomyopathy.

Concomitant use with other antiarrhythmic agents (such as amiodarone, lidocaine, phenytoin, procainamide, or propranolol) may cause additive or antagonistic cardiac effects and additive toxic effects. For example, concurrent use of quinidine and other antiarrhythmics that increase the QT interval may further prolong the QT interval and lead to Torsades de Pointes tachycardia.

Effects on diagnostic tests

None reported.

Adverse reactions

• CNS: vertigo, headache, light-headedness, confusion, restlessness, cold sweat, pallor, fainting, dementia.

• CV: premature ventricular contractions, severe hypotension, SA and AV block, *ventricular fibrillation, ventricular tachycardia*, aggravated congestive heart failure, ECG changes (particularly widening QRS complex, notched P waves, widened QT interval, and ST segment depression), *Torsades de Pointes tachycardia*.

• DERM: rash, petechial hemorrhage of buccal mucosa, pruritus.

- EENT: tinnitus, excessive salivation, blurred vision.
- GI: diarrhea, nausea, vomiting, anorexia, abdominal pain.
- HEMA: hemolytic anemia, thrombocytopenia, *agranulocytosis*.
- Hepatic: hepatotoxicity, including granulomatous hepatitis.
- Other: angioedema, acute asthmatic attack, *respiratory arrest*, fever, cinchonism, lupus erythematosus syndrome.

Note: Drug should be discontinued if the following problems develop: blood dyscrasias; hepatic dysfunction; renal dysfunction; syncope; cardiotoxicity, including conduction defects (25% widening of QRS complex); ventricular tachycardia or flutter; frequent premature ventricular contractions; or complete AV block.

Overdose and treatment
The most serious clinical effects of overdose include severe hypotension, ventricular arrhythmias (including Torsades de Pointes), and seizures. QRS complexes and QT and PR intervals may be prolonged, and ataxia, anuria, respiratory distress, irritability, and hallucinations may develop. If ingestion was recent, gastric lavage, emesis, and activated charcoal may be used to decrease absorption. Urine acidification may be used to help increase quinidine elimination.

Treatment involves general supportive measures (including cardiovascular and respiratory support) with hemodynamic and ECG monitoring. Metaraminol or norepinephrine may be used to reverse hypotension (after adequate hydration has been ensured). CNS depressants should be avoided, because CNS depression may occur, possibly with seizures. Cardiac pacing may be necessary. Isoproterenol and/or ventricular pacing possibly may be used to treat Torsades de Pointes tachycardia.

I.V. infusion of 1/6 molar sodium lactate solution reduces quinidine's cardiotoxic effect. Hemodialysis, although rarely warranted, also may be effective.

▶ **Special considerations**
- When drug is used to treat atrial tachyarrhythmias, ventricular rate may be accelerated from drug's anticholinergic effects on AV node. This can be prevented by previous treatment with digitalis.
- Because conversion of chronic atrial fibrillation may be associated with embolism, anticoagulant should be administered before quinidine therapy begins.
- Check apical pulse rate, blood pressure, and ECG tracing, before starting therapy.
- I.V. route is generally avoided because of the potential for severe hypotension; it should be used to treat acute arrhythmias only.
- Never use discolored (brownish) quinidine solution.
- For maintenance, give only by oral or I.M. route. Dosage requirements vary. Some patients may require drug q 4 hours, others q 6 hours. Titrate dose by both clinical response and blood levels.
- When changing administration route, alter dosage to compensate for variations in quinidine base content.
- Dosage should be decreased in patients with congestive heart failure and hepatic disease.
- Monitor ECG, especially when large doses of the drug are being administered.
- Monitor liver function tests during first 4 to 8 weeks of therapy.
- Drug may increase toxicity of digitalis derivatives.

Use with caution in patients who are receiving digitalis. Monitor digoxin levels.
- GI side effects, especially diarrhea, are signs of toxicity. Check quinidine blood levels; suspect toxicity when they exceed 8 mcg/ml. GI symptoms may be minimized by giving drug with meals.
- Lidocaine may be effective in treating quinidine-induced arrhythmias, because it increases AV conduction.
- Quinidine may cause hemolysis in patients with G6PD deficiency.
- Quinidine is hemodializable. Dosage adjustment may be necessary in patients undergoing dialysis.
- The amount of quinidine in the various salt forms varies as shown below:
  – Gluconate: 62% quinidine (324 mg of gluconate, 250 mg sulfate)
  – Polygalacturonate: 60% quinidine (275 mg polygalacturonate, 200 mg sulfate)
  – Sulfate: 83% quinidine. The sulfate form is considered the standard dosage preparation.
- Quinidine gluconate is reported to be as or more active in vitro against *Plasmodium falciparum* than quinine dihydrochloride. Since the latter drug is only available through the CDC, quinidine gluconate may be useful in the treatment of severe malaria when delay of therapy may be life-threatening. The current CDC protocol involves follow-up treatment with either tetracycline or sulfadoxine and pyrimethamine.

Information for the patient
Instruct patient to report any skin rash, fever, unusual bleeding, bruising, ringing in ears, or visual disturbance.

Geriatric use
Dosage reduction may be necessary in elderly patients. Because of highly variable metabolism, serum level monitoring is advised.

Breast-feeding
Because drug is excreted in breast milk, alternative feeding method is recommended during therapy with quinine.

---

quinine sulfate
Quinaminoph, Quinamm, Quine, Quinite

- Pharmacologic classification: cinchona alkaloid
- Therapeutic classification: antimalarial, skeletal muscle relaxant
- Pregnancy risk category X

How supplied
Available by prescription and without prescription
Capsules: 130 mg, 195 mg, 200 mg, 260 mg, 300 mg, 325 mg
Tablets: 260 mg, 325 mg

Indications, route, and dosage
Malaria (chloroquine-resistant)
Adults: 650 mg P.O. q 8 hours for 10 days, with 25 mg pyrimethamine q 12 hours for 3 days and with 500 mg sulfadiazine q.i.d. for 5 days.

Children: 25 mg/kg/day divided into three doses for 10 days.

I.V. quinine is available from the CDC for the treatment of severe malaria with coma.

Nocturnal leg cramps
Adults: 200 to 300 mg P.O. at bedtime.

Dosage in renal failure

Creatinine clearance (ml/min/ 1.73 m²)	Percent of usual dose	Interval
≥ 50	100	q 8 hours
10 to 50	75	q 8 to 12 hours
< 10	30 to 50	q 24 hours

Pharmacodynamics
- *Antimalarial action:* Quinine intercalates into DNA, disrupting the parasite's replication and transcription; it also depresses its oxygen uptake and carbohydrate metabolism. It is active against the asexual erythrocytic forms of *Plasmodium falciparum, P. malariae, P. ovale,* and *P. vivax* and is used for chloroquine-resistant malaria.
- *Skeletal muscle relaxant effects:* Quinine increases the refractory period, decreases excitability of the motor endplate, and affects calcium distribution within muscle fibers.

Pharmacokinetics
- *Absorption:* Quinine is absorbed almost completely; peak serum concentrations occur at 1 to 3 hours.
- *Distribution:* Quinine is distributed widely into the liver, lungs, kidneys, and spleen; CSF levels reach 2% to 5% of serum levels. Quinine is about 70% bound to plasma proteins and readily crosses the placenta.
- *Metabolism:* Quinine is metabolized in the liver.
- *Excretion:* Less than 5% of a single dose is excreted unchanged in the urine; small amounts of metabolites appear in the feces, gastric juice, bile, saliva, and breast milk. Half-life is 4 to 21 hours in healthy or convalescing persons; it is longer in patients with malaria. Urine acidification hastens elimination.

Contraindications and precautions
Quinine is contraindicated in pregnant patients and in patients with known hypersensitivity to the drug, G6PD deficiency, optic neuritis, or tinnitus; and in patients with a history of blackwater fever or of thrombocytopenic purpura associated with previous quinine ingestion.

Quinine should be used with caution in patients with cardiac arrhythmias and in those taking sodium bicarbonate concomitantly.

Interactions
Quinine may increase plasma levels of digoxin and digitoxin. It may potentiate the effects of neuromuscular blocking agents, and it may potentiate the action of warfarin by depressing synthesis of vitamin K-dependent clotting factors.

Concomitant use of aluminum-containing antacids may delay or decrease absorption of quinine. Concomitant use of sodium bicarbonate or acetazolamide may increase absorption of quinine by decreasing urinary excretion.

Effects on diagnostic tests
Quinine may decrease platelet and red blood cell counts. It also may cause hypoglycemia and false elevations of urinary catecholamines and may interfere with 17-hydroxycorticosteroid and 17-ketogenic steroid tests.

Adverse reactions
- CNS: severe headache, apprehension, excitement, confusion, delirium, syncope, hypothermia, *seizures* (with toxic doses).
- CV: hypotension, *cardiovascular collapse* with overdosage of rapid I.V. administration, conduction disturbances.
- DERM: rashes, pruritus.
- EENT: altered color perception, photophobia, blurred vision, night blindness, amblyopia, scotoma, diplopia, mydriasis, optic atrophy, tinnitus, impaired hearing.
- GI: epigastric distress, diarrhea, nausea, vomiting.
- GU: renal tubular damage, anuria.
- HEMA: *hemolytic anemia, thrombocytopenia, agranulocytosis,* hypoprothrombinemia.
- Local: thrombosis at infusion site.
- Other: asthma, flushing, fever, facial edema, dyspnea, vertigo, hypoglycemia.
  Note: Drug should be discontinued if signs of hypersensitivity or toxicity occur.

Overdose and treatment
Signs of overdose include tinnitus, vertigo, headache, fever, rash, cardiovascular effects, GI distress (including vomiting), blindness, apprehension, confusion, and seizures.

Treatment includes gastric lavage followed by supportive measures, which may include fluid and electrolyte replacement, artificial respiration, and stabilization of blood pressure and renal function.

Anaphylactic reactions may require epinephrine, corticosteroids, or antihistamines. Urinary acidification may increase elimination of quinine but will also augment renal obstruction. Hemodialysis or hemoperfusion may be helpful. Vasodilator therapy or stellate blockage may relieve visual disturbances.

▶ Special considerations
- Administer quinine after meals to minimize gastric distress; do not crush tablets, as drug irritates gastric mucosa.
- Discontinue drug if signs of idiosyncrasy or toxicity occur.
- Serum concentrations of 10 mg/ml or more may confirm toxicity as the cause of tinnitus or hearing loss.
- Quinine is no longer used for acute malarial attack by *Plasmodium vivax* or for suppression of malaria from resistant organisms.
- Parenteral form may be obtained from Centers for Disease Control when oral therapy is unfeasible; administer by slow infusion (over 1 hour), and monitor I.V. sites and patient for adverse effects.

Information for the patient
- Teach patient about adverse reactions and the need to report these immediately – especially tinnitus and hearing impairment.
- Tell patient to avoid concomitant use of aluminum-containing antacids because these may alter drug absorption.
- Patient should keep drug out of reach of children.

Geriatric use
Use with caution in patients with conduction disturbances.

Breast-feeding
If a breast-feeding woman is to receive quinine, the infant should be evaluated for possible G6PD deficiency before therapy.

rabies immune globulin, human (RIG)
Hyperab, Imogam Rabies Immune Globulin

- Pharmacologic classification: immune serum
- Therapeutic classification: rabies prophylaxis agent
- Pregnancy risk category B

How supplied
Available by prescription only
Injection: 150 IU/ml in 2-ml and 10-ml vials

Indications, route, and dosage
Rabies exposure
Adults and children: 20 IU/kg at time of first dose of rabies vaccine. Use half dose to infiltrate wound area. Give remainder I.M. Don't give rabies vaccine and RIG in same syringe or at same site.

Pharmacodynamics
Postexposure rabies prophylaxis: RIG provides passive immunity to rabies.

Pharmacokinetics
- Absorption: After slow I.M. absorption, rabies antibody appears in serum within 24 hours and peaks within 2 to 13 days.
- Distribution: RIG probably crosses the placenta and distributes into breast milk.
- Metabolism: No information is available.
- Excretion: The serum half-life for rabies antibody titer is reportedly about 24 days.

Contraindications and precautions
RIG is contraindicated in patients with known hypersensitivity to thimerosal, a component of this immune serum.

Interactions
Concomitant use of this product with corticosteroids and immunosuppressant agents may interfere with the immune response to RIG. Whenever possible, avoid using these agents during the postexposure immunization period. Because antirabies serum may partially suppress the antibody response to rabies vaccine, use only the recommended dose of antirabies vaccine. Also, RIG may interfere with the immune response to live virus vaccine and rubella virus vaccine. Do not administer live virus vaccines within 3 months after administration of RIG.

Effects on diagnostic tests
None reported.

Adverse reactions
- Local: pain, redness, and induration at injection site.
- Systemic: slight fever, headache, malaise, angioedema, nephrotic syndrome, anaphylaxis.

Overdose and treatment
No information available.

▶ Special considerations
- Obtain a thorough history of the animal bite, allergies, and reactions to immunizations.
- Epinephrine solution 1:1,000 should be available to treat allergic reactions.
- Repeated doses of RIG should not be given after rabies vaccine is started.
- Do not administer more than 5 ml I.M. at one injection site; divide I.M. doses greater than 5 ml and administer them at different sites.
- Do not confuse this drug with rabies vaccine, which is a suspension of attenuated or killed microorganisms used to confer active immunity. These two drugs are often given together prophylactically after exposure to known or suspected rabid animals.
- Because rabies can be fatal if untreated, the use of RIG during pregnancy appears justified. No fetal risk from RIG use has been reported to date.
- Ask patient when he received his last tetanus immunization because a booster may be indicated.
- Patients previously immunized with a tissue culture-derived rabies vaccine and those who have confirmed adequate rabies antibody titers should receive only the vaccine.
- RIG has not been associated with an increased frequency of acquired immunodeficiency syndrome. The immune globulin is devoid of human immunodeficiency virus (HIV). Immune globulin recipients do not develop antibodies to HIV.
- Store between 2° to 8° C (36° to 46° F). Do not freeze.

Information for the patient
- Explain to patient that the body needs about a week to develop immunity to rabies after the vaccine is administered. Therefore, patients receive RIG to provide antibodies in their blood for immediate protection against rabies.
- Reactions to antirabies serum may occur up to 12 days after this product is administered. Encourage patient to report skin changes, difficulty breathing, or headache.
- Patient also may experience some local pain, swelling, and tenderness at the injection site. Recommend acetaminophen to alleviate these minor effects.

Breast-feeding
RIG's safety in breast-feeding women has not been established. RIG probably distributes into breast milk. An alternative feeding method is recommended.

---

rabies vaccine, human diploid cell (HDCV)
Imovax Rabies I.D. Vaccine (inactivated whole virus), Imovax Rabies Vaccine

- Pharmacologic classification: vaccine
- Therapeutic classification: viral vaccine
- Pregnancy risk category C

How supplied
Available by prescription only
Intramuscular injection: 2.5 IU of rabies antigen/ml, in single-dose vial with diluent
Intradermal injection: 0.25 IU rabies antigen per dose

Indications, route, and dosage
Preexposure prophylaxis immunization for persons in high-risk groups
Adults and children: Three 0.1-ml injections intradermally or three 1-ml injections I.M. Give first dose on day 0 (the first day vaccination), second dose on day 7, and third dose on either day 21 or 28.
Booster: Persons exposed to rabies virus at their workplace should have antibody titers checked every 6 months. Those persons with continued risk of exposure should have antibody titers checked every 2 years. When the titers are inadequate, administer a booster dose.
Intradermal vaccine
Primary postexposure dosage: Five 1-ml doses I.M. on each of days 3, 7, 14, and 28 (in conjunction with rabies immune globulin on day 0). A sixth dose may be given on day 90.
Previously immunized postexposure dosage: Two 1-ml doses I.M.; one immediately and one 3 days later (without concomitant rabies immune globulin).

Pharmacodynamics
Rabies prophylaxis: This vaccine promotes active immunity to rabies.

Pharmacokinetics
After intradermal injection, rabies antibodies appear in the serum within 7 to 10 days and peak at 30 to 60 days. Vaccine-induced immunity persists for about 1 year.

Contraindications and precautions
Rabies vaccine for preexposure prophylaxis should be postponed in patients with febrile illness. Use cautiously in persons with a history of hypersensitivity to neomycin or phenolsulfonphthalein, components of the vaccine.

Interactions
Concomitant use of rabies vaccine with corticosteroids or immunosuppressants may interfere with the development of active immunity to rabies vaccine. Avoid its use in this situation whenever possible.

Effects on diagnostic tests
None reported.

Adverse reactions
- Local: pain, erythema, swelling, or itching at injection site.
- Systemic: headache, nausea, abdominal pain, myalgia, dizziness, fever, diarrhea, *anaphylaxis*, immune complex-like reactions.

Overdose and treatment
No information available.

▶ Special considerations
- Obtain a thorough history of allergies, especially to antibiotics, and of reactions to immunizations.
- Epinephrine solution 1:1,000 should be available to treat allergic reactions.
- I.M. injections should be made in the deltoid or upper outer quadrant of the gluteus muscle in adults. In infants and children, use the midlateral aspect of the thigh.
- Reconstitute with diluent provided. Gently shake the vial until the vaccine is completely dissolved.
- Store at 2° to 8° C (36° to 46° F). Do not freeze.

Information for the patient
- Tell patient what to expect after vaccination: pain, swelling, and itching at the injection site as well as headache, stomach upset, or fever.
- Recommend acetaminophen to alleviate headache, fever, and muscle aches.

Breast-feeding
It is not known if HDCV distributes into breast milk or if transmission to breast-feeding infant presents risk. Breast-feeding women should choose an alternative feeding method.

radioactive iodine (sodium iodide) 131I
Iodotope Therapeutic, Sodium Iodide 131I Therapeutic

- Pharmacologic classification: thyroid hormone antagonist
- Therapeutic classification: antihyperthyroid agent
- Pregnancy risk category X

How supplied
Available by prescription only
All radioactivity concentrations are determined at the time of calibration; 131I has a physical half-life of about 8 days.
Iodotope Therapeutic
Capsules: Radioactivity range is 1 to 50 mCi/capsule at time of calibration.
Oral solution: Radioactivity concentration is 7.05 mCi/ml at time of calibration; in vials containing approximately 7, 14, 28, 70, or 106 mCi at time of calibration.
Sodium Iodide 131I Therapeutic
Capsules: Radioactivity range is 0.8 to 100 mCi/capsule.
Oral solution: Radioactivity range is 3.5 to 150 mCi/vial.

Indications, route, and dosage
Hyperthyroidism
Adults: Usual dose is 4 to 10 mCi P.O. Dose based on estimated weight of thyroid gland and thyroid uptake. Treatment may be repeated after 6 weeks, according to serum thyroxine levels.

Thyroid cancer
Adults: 50 to 150 mCi P.O. Dose based on estimated malignant thyroid tissue and metastatic tissue as determined by total body scan. Dose may be repeated according to clinical status.

Pharmacodynamics
Antithyroid action: ^{131}I is accumulated and retained by the thyroid, thus allowing radioactivity to selectively damage or destroy thyroidal tissue. Thyroid localization of the radioiodine allows thyroid uptake testing and thyroid imaging.

^{131}I is trapped rapidly by the thyroid and deposited in the colloid of the follicles. Its radioactive decay emits beta rays that originate within the follicle and act almost exclusively on the parenchymal cells of the thyroid, with little damage to surrounding tissue. However, with large doses of ^{131}I, the characteristic cytotoxic action of ionizing radiation occurs.

Pharmacokinetics
● *Absorption:* ^{131}I is absorbed readily from the GI tract.
● *Distribution:* ^{131}I is distributed into the extracellular fluid. It is selectively concentrated and bound to tyrosyl residues of thyroglobulin in the thyroid gland. It is also concentrated in the stomach, choroid plexus, salivary glands, and lactating breast.
● *Metabolism:* ^{131}I is converted readily to protein-bound iodine by the thyroid.
● *Excretion:* ^{131}I is excreted by the kidneys with a half-life of 138 days; however, its effective radioactive half-life is 7.6 days. Onset of action occurs in approximately 2 to 4 weeks, with peak effects noted within 2 to 4 months.

Contraindications and precautions
^{131}I is contraindicated in patients with preexisting vomiting and diarrhea, in breast-feeding or pregnant patients, or in those who wish to become pregnant.

Discontinuation of antithyroid therapy in a severely hyperthyroid patient is recommended for 3 to 4 days before administration of ^{131}I.

Interactions
Concomitant use of ^{131}I will be affected by recent intake of stable iodine and the use of thyroid or antithyroid drugs. Concomitant use with antineoplastic agents may increase bone marrow depression, requiring dosage reduction of these agents.

Effects on diagnostic tests
^{131}I therapy alters ^{131}I thyroid uptake and protein-bound iodine levels.

Adverse reactions
● EENT: feeling of fullness in neck, metallic taste, "radiation mumps," sore throat, cough after 3rd day of treatment.
● Endocrine: hypothyroidism, radiation thyroiditis.
● HEMA: *hematopoietic system depression, bone marrow depression, acute leukemia,* anemia, *blood dyscrasias,* leukopenia, thrombocytopenia.
● Other: radiation sickness (nausea, vomiting), increase in clinical symptoms, acute thyroid crisis, severe sialoadenitis, chromosomal abnormalities, increased risk of developing *leukemia* later in life after sufficient ^{131}I dose for thyroid ablation after cancer surgery, temporary hair loss 2 to 3 months after treatment.

Note: Drug should be discontinued if symptoms of agranulocytosis or hypothyroidism occur.

Overdose and treatment
In the unlikely event of an acute overdose, clinical manifestations include hypersensitivity reactions, which may be life-threatening (for example, angioedema or laryngeal edema).

Acute allergic reaction requires administering epinephrine 1:1,000 (0.01 ml/kg, to a maximum of 0.5 ml) S.C. or I.M., repeated every 15 minutes if needed, and diphenhydramine (25 to 50 mg) I.V., I.M., or P.O.

▶ Special considerations
● Radioactive iodine is contraindicated in pregnancy and breast-feeding unless used to treat thyroid cancer.
● Presence of food may delay absorption. Patient should fast overnight before administration.
● All antithyroid medications, thyroid preparations, and iodine-containing preparations should be discontinued 1 week before ^{131}I dose, or patient may receive thyroid-stimulating hormone for 3 days before ^{131}I dose.
● When treating women of childbearing age, give dose during menstruation or within 7 days after menstruation.
● After therapy for hyperthyroidism, patient should not resume antithyroid drugs but should continue propranolol or other drugs used to treat symptoms of hyperthyroidism until onset of full ^{131}I effect (usually several weeks).
● Monitor thyroid function with serum thyroxine levels.
● After a dose of ^{131}I for hyperthyroidism, patient's urine and saliva are slightly radioactive for 6 to 8 hours. Institute full radiation precautions during this time. Instruct patient to use appropriate disposal methods when coughing and expectorating.
● After a dose of ^{131}I for thyroid cancer, patient's urine, saliva, and perspiration remain radioactive for 3 days. Patient should be isolated and should use disposable eating utensils and linens.
● Instruct patient to save all urine in lead containers for 24 to 48 hours so amount of radioactive material excreted can be determined
● Do not allow pregnant staff members to care for patient.
● Patient should drink as much fluid as possible for 48 hours after drug administration to facilitate excretion.
● Caregivers should limit contact with patient to 30 minutes per shift per person the 1st day, then increase contact time to 1 hour on 2nd day and longer on 3rd day.

Information for the patient
● Advise patient to call for further recommendations before undergoing surgery (including dental surgery).
● Warn patient who is discharged less than 7 days after ^{131}I dose for thyroid cancer to avoid close, prolonged contact with small children (for example, holding children on lap).
● Instruct patient not to sleep in same room with spouse for 7 days after treatment because of an increased risk of thyroid cancer in persons exposed to ^{131}I.
● Patient may use the same bathroom facilities as rest of family.

Geriatric use
Patients with severe thyrotoxic cardiac disease should be given antithyroid agents, or beta blockers, or both for 4 to 6 weeks before radioactive iodine treatment to

---

reduce possible aggravation of the condition by radiation thyroiditis.

Pediatric use
Radioactive iodine is not recommended for persons under age 30, unless circumstances preclude other treatments.

Breast-feeding
Radioactive iodine is excreted in breast milk, reaching or exceeding maternal plasma levels; therefore, patient should not breast-feed during treatment.

---

ramipril
Altace

- Pharmacologic classification: angiotensin-converting enzyme inhibitor
- Therapeutic classification: antihypertensive
- Pregnancy risk category D

How supplied
Available by prescription only
Capsules: 1.25 mg, 2.5 mg, 5 mg, 10 mg

Indications, route, and dosage
Treatment of hypertension either alone or in combination with thiazide diuretics
Adults: Initially, 2.5 mg P.O. daily in patients not receiving concomitant diuretic therapy. Adjust dose based on blood pressure response. Usual maintenance dosage is 2.5 to 20 mg daily as a single dose or in two equal doses.

In patients receiving diuretic therapy, symptomatic hypotension may occur. To minimize this, discontinue diuretic, if possible, 2 to 3 days before starting ramipril. When this is not possible, initial dose of ramipril should be 1.25 mg.

In patients with renal impairment as characterized by creatinine clearance below 40 ml/min/1.73 m² (serum creatinine above 2.5 mg/dl), the recommended initial dose is 1.25 mg daily, titrating upward to a maximum dose of 5 mg based on blood pressure response.

Pharmacodynamics
Antihypertensive action: Ramipril and its active metabolite, ramiprilat, inhibits angiotensin-converting enzyme (ACE), preventing pulmonary conversion of angiotensin I to angiotensin II, a potent vasoconstrictor. Reduced formation of angiotensin II decreases peripheral arterial resistance and, in turn, decreases aldosterone secretion, reduces sodium and water retention, and lowers blood pressure. Ramipril also has antihypertensive activity in patients with low-renin hypertension.

Pharmacokinetics
Absorption: 50% to 60% is absorbed after oral administration with peak concentrations reached within 1 hour. Peak plasma levels of ramiprilat are achieved in 2 to 4 hours.
- *Distribution:* Ramipril is 73% serum protein-bound; ramiprilat, 58%.
- *Metabolism:* Ramipril is almost completely metabolized to ramiprilat, which has six times more ACE inhibitory effects than the parent drug.

- *Excretion:* 60% is excreted in urine; 40%, in feces. Less than 2% of administered dose is excreted in urine as unchanged drug.

Contraindications and precautions
Ramipril is contraindicated in patients with known hypersensitivity to the drug or with a history of angioneurotic edema. Use with caution in patients with impaired renal or hepatic function and in situations conducive to development of hyperkalemia, including use of potassium-sparing diuretics, renal insufficiency, diabetes mellitus, potassium supplementation, and use of potassium-containing sodium substitutes.

Interactions
Concurrent use of potassium-sparing diuretics or potassium supplements may result in hyperkalemia. Increased serum lithium levels and lithium toxicity have been reported with concomitant use. Excessive hypotension may result with concomitant use of diuretics; discontinue diuretic or lower dosage of ramipril as needed.

Effects on diagnostic tests
Transient increases in BUN and creatinine levels, decreases in hemoglobin and hematocrit, and elevations of liver enzymes, serum bilirubin, uric acid, and blood glucose levels have been reported.

Adverse reactions
- CNS: headache, dizziness, anxiety, amnesia, seizures, depression, insomnia, nervousness, neuralgia, neuropathy, paresthesia, somnolence, tremor, vertigo, asthenia.
- CV: symptomatic hypotension, syncope, angina, *arrhythmia,* chest pain, palpitations, *MI.*
- DERM: hypersensitivity reactions, rash, dermatitis, pruritus, photosensitivity, purpura.
- EENT: epistaxis.
- GI: nausea, vomiting, abdominal pain, anorexia, constipation, diarrhea, dry mouth, dyspepsia, dysphagia, gastroenteritis, increased salivation, taste disturbance.
- GU: impotence.
- Respiratory: dry, persistent, tickling, nonproductive cough; dyspnea.
- Other: angioedema, arthralgia, arthritis, edema, increased sweating, malaise, myalgia, weight gain.

Overdose and treatment
The most common manifestation is expected to be hypotension. No cases of overdose have been reported; specific management of ramipril overdose has not been established. Provide supportive care.

▶ Special considerations
- Diuretic therapy should be discontinued 2 to 3 days before the start of ramipril therapy, if possible, to decrease potential for excessive hypotensive response.
- Like other ACE inhibitors, ramipril may cause dry, persistent, tickling, nonproductive cough. This effect is reversible when therapy is discontinued.
- Assess renal and hepatic function before and periodically throughout therapy.
- Bioavailability is not affected by food.
- No interactions with digoxin, antacid, or anticoagulant therapy have been reported.
- There are no apparent age, sex, or weight-related differences in effect.
- Monitor serum potassium levels.

Information for the patient
● Tell patient to report any signs or symptoms of angioedema to physician immediately: swelling of face, eyes, lips, tongue, or difficulty in breathing. If any of these occur, patient should stop taking drug until physician has been consulted.
● Warn patient that light-headedness can occur, especially during first few days of therapy. Patient should change positions slowly to minimize hypotensive effect and should report such symptoms to physician. If syncope (fainting) occurs, patient should stop drug immediately and call physician.
● Warn patient that inadequate fluid intake, vomiting, diarrhea, or excessive perspiration can lead to light-headedness and syncope. Advise caution in excessive heat and during exercise.
● Tell patient to avoid using sodium substitutes containing potassium unless recommended by physician.
● Tell patient to report immediately any signs of infection, such as sore throat or fever.

Geriatric use
No age-related differences in efficacy or safety have been observed.

Pediatric use
Safety and efficacy have not been established.

Breast-feeding
Ramipril should not be administered to breast-feeding women.

---

ranitidine
Zantac

● Pharmacologic classification: histamine₂-receptor antagonist
● Therapeutic classification: antiulcer agent
● Pregnancy risk category B

How supplied
Available by prescription only
Tablets: 150 mg, 300 mg
Injection: 25 mg/ml
Oral solution: 75 mg/5 ml

Indications, route, and dosage
Duodenal and gastric ulcer (short-term treatment); pathologic hypersecretory conditions, such as Zollinger-Ellison syndrome
Adults: 150 mg P.O. b.i.d. or 300 mg h.s. Doses up to 6.3 g/day may be prescribed in patients with Zollinger-Ellison syndrome.
　Drug also may be administered parenterally: 50 mg I.V. or I.M. q 6 to 8 hours.
Maintenance therapy in duodenal ulcer
Adults: 150 mg P.O. h.s.
Prophylaxis of stress ulcer
Adults: Continuous I.V. infusion of 150 mg in 250 ml compatible solution delivered at a rate of 6.25 mg/hour using an infusion pump.
Gastroesophageal reflux disease (GERD)
Adults: 150 mg P.O. b.i.d.

Pharmacodynamics
Antiulcer action: Ranitidine competitively inhibits histamine's action at H_2-receptors in gastric parietal cells. This reduces basal and nocturnal gastric acid secretion, as well as that caused by histamine, food, amino acids, insulin, and pentagastrin.

Pharmacokinetics
● *Absorption:* Approximately 50% to 60% of an oral dose is absorbed; food does not significantly affect absorption. After I.M. injection, drug is absorbed rapidly from parenteral sites.
● *Distribution:* Ranitidine is distributed to many body tissues and appears in CSF and breast milk. Drug is about 10% to 19% protein-bound.
● *Metabolism:* Ranitidine is metabolized in the liver.
● *Excretion:* Ranitidine is excreted in urine and feces. Half-life is 2 to 3 hours.

Contraindications and precautions
Ranitidine is contraindicated in patients with ranitidine allergy. Use drug cautiously in patients with impaired hepatic function; dosage adjustment may be necessary in patients with impaired renal function.

Interactions
Antacids decrease ranitidine absorption; separate drugs by at least 1 hour. Concomitant use decreases absorption of diazepam. Use with glipizide may increase hypoglycemic effect; dosage adjustment of glipizide may be necessary. Drug may decrease renal clearance of procainamide and may interfere with clearance of warfarin.

Effects on diagnostic tests
Ranitidine may cause false-positive results in urine protein tests using Multistix.
　Ranitidine may increase serum creatinine, lactic dehydrogenase, alkaline phosphatase, AST (SGOT), ALT (SGPT), and total bilirubin levels. Drug may decrease white blood cell, red blood cell, and platelet counts.

Adverse reactions
● CNS: malaise, dizziness, insomnia, vertigo, reversible confusion, agitation, hallucinations.
● DERM: rash.
● GI: constipation, nausea, abdominal pain.
● HEMA (rare): reversible leukopenia, granulocytopenia, *agranulocytosis,* thrombocytopenia.
● Local: itching and burning at injection site.

Overdose and treatment
No cases of overdose have been reported. However, treatment would involve emesis or gastric lavage and supportive measures as needed. Hemodialysis will remove ranitidine.

▶ Special considerations
● When administering I.V. push, dilute to a total volume of 20 ml and inject over a period of 5 minutes. No dilution necessary when administering I.M. May also be administered by intermittent I.V. infusion. Dilute 50 mg ranitidine in 100 ml of dextrose 5% in water and infuse over 15 to 20 minutes.
● Patients with impaired renal function may require dosage adjustment.
● Dialysis removes ranitidine; administer drug after treatment.

---

*Canada only　　　　†Unlabeled clinical use　　　　Italicized adverse reactions are life-threatening.

Information for the patient
● Instruct patient to take drug as directed, even after pain subsides, to ensure proper healing.
● If patient is taking a single daily dose, advise him to take it at bedtime.

Geriatric use
Elderly patients may experience more adverse reactions because of reduced renal clearance. Debilitated patients may experience reversible confusion, agitation, depression, and hallucinations.

Breast-feeding
Ranitidine is excreted in breast milk; use it cautiously in breast-feeding women.

rauwolfia alkaloids

alseroxylon
deserpidine
rauwolfia
rescinnamine
reserpine

Therapeutic use of rauwolfia alkaloids can be traced to primitive Hindu medicine, when extracts of *Rauwolfia serpentina* root were given for such diverse conditions as snakebite, hypertension, and insanity. Not until the mid-1950s were these agents recognized by Western cultures as therapeutically useful in hypertension and psychosis. Over the past several years, they have been replaced by newer agents that are better tolerated by most patients and usually have fewer adverse effects.

Pharmacology
Rauwolfia alkaloids deplete catecholamine and serotonin stores in many body organs, including the brain and adrenal medulla. They also decrease catecholamine uptake by peripheral adrenergic neurons.

Clinical indications and actions
Hypertension
All available rauwolfia alkaloids are used to treat hypertension. The exact mechanism of their antihypertensive effect is unknown but is believed due primarily to blockade of peripheral adrenergic neurons. Continuous therapy causes venous dilation, decreasing venous return and thus decreasing cardiac output. Blood pressure decreases on the average about 10 mm|Hg; maximal antihypertensive response occurs in 3 to 6 weeks and may persist for over a week after withdrawal of the drug.

†Psychoses
All rauwolfia alkaloids except rescinnamine are used for symptomatic treatment of agitated psychotic states such as schizophrenia. The antipsychotic, or tranquilizing, effect of these agents is thought to be subsequent to depleted CNS serotonin and catecholamines. These agents have largely been replaced by other drugs but are still used in patients who are also hypertensive or who cannot tolerate other antipsychotic agents.

Overview of adverse reactions
Therapeutic doses of rauwolfia alkaloids may cause drowsiness, fatigue, lethargy, depression, bradycardia, and nasal congestion. Excessively large doses may cause a parkinsonian syndrome and other extrapyramidal reactions. Coma, respiratory depression, and hypothermia may be associated with toxic levels of the drugs.

▶ Special considerations
● Monitor pulse and blood pressure frequently; monitor closely for signs of depression.
● Depression may develop as long as 2 to 8 months after initiation of therapy.
● Give drugs with meals or milk to minimize gastric irritation.
● Keep in mind that drug effects are cumulative.
● Monitor fluid intake and output; check for weight gain.
● If patient is scheduled for surgery, notify anesthesiologist that patient is taking rauwolfia alkaloid.

Information for the patient
● Teach patient about his disease and therapy, and explain why he must take drug exactly as prescribed, even when feeling well; advise him never to discontinue drug suddenly.
● Explain adverse effects, and advise patient to report any unusual effects, especially symptoms of depression (nightmares, despondency, insomnia, loss of appetite).
● Explain that orthostatic hypotension can be minimized by avoiding sudden position changes and hot showers; that dry mouth can be relieved by sugarless gum, hard candy, or ice chips; and that taking drug with meals or milk will minimize gastric irritation.
● Advise patient to promptly report pregnancy or weight gain that exceeds 5 lb (2.25 kg) per week.
● Warn patient to seek medical approval before taking nonprescription cold preparations.

Geriatric use
Lower dose may be necessary because of decreased drug clearance in elderly patients.

Pediatric use
The safety and efficacy of rauwolfia alkaloids in children have not been established; use only if potential benefit outweighs risk.

Breast-feeding
Rauwolfia alkaloids are distributed into breast milk; administer drugs cautiously to breast-feeding women.

Representative combinations
Deserpidine with methyclothiazide: Enduronyl; with hydrochlorothiazide: Oreticyl.

Rauwolfia with bendroflumethiazide and potassium chloride: Rautrax-N; with veratrum viride: Rauverat; with veratrum viride, rutin, and mannitol hexanitrate: Rauver-tin; with bendroflumethiazide: Rauzide; with phenobarbital: Raudilan PB.

Reserpine with methyclothiazide: Diutensen-R; with chlorthalidone: Demi-Regroton, Regroton; with chlorothiazide: Diupres; with hydrochlorothiazide and hydralazine: Harbolin, Hydroserpine plus, SER-AP-ES, Serapine, Serpahyde, Thia-Serpa-Zine, Unipres; with quinethazone: Hydromox-R; with hydrochlorothiazide: Hydropres, Hydroserp, Hydroserpine, Hydrotensin 50, Mallopress; with trichlormethiazide: Metatensin, Naquival; with polythiazide: Renese-R; with hydroflumethiazide: Salutensin.

rauwolfia
Raudixin, Rauval, Rauverid, Wolfina

- Pharmacologic classification: rauwolfia alkaloid, peripherally acting adrenergic-blocking agent
- Therapeutic classification: antihypertensive
- Pregnancy risk category C

How supplied
Available by prescription only
Tablets: 50 mg, 100 mg

Indications, route, and dosage
Mild to moderate hypertension
Adults: Initially, 200 to 400 mg P.O. daily as a single dose or in two divided doses. Maintenance dosage is 300 mg/day.

Note: Some clinicians recommend an initial dose of 50 mg P.O. daily and a maintenance dose of 100 mg/day.

Pharmacodynamics
Antihypertensive action: The exact antihypertensive mechanism is unknown; however, it is thought to result from peripheral adrenergic blockade and possibly CNS effects. Rauwolfia depletes catecholamine and serotonin stores in many organs and decreases catecholamine uptake by adrenergic neurons.

Pharmacokinetics
- *Absorption:* Orally administered rauwolfia is believed to be absorbed rapidly; however, full antihypertensive effects do not occur for 2 to 3 weeks.
- *Distribution:* Rauwolfia appears to be distributed widely into the body; high concentrations are found in adipose tissue.
- *Metabolism:* Rauwolfia is metabolized extensively to inactive compounds.
- *Excretion:* Rauwolfia is excreted slowly as unchanged drug and metabolites in urine and feces. Antihypertensive effects may persist for several days to weeks after chronic therapy is discontinued.

Contraindications and precautions
Rauwolfia is contraindicated in patients with known hypersensitivity to the drug; in patients receiving electroconvulsive therapy, because cerebral depletion of serotonin and catecholamine stores may predispose the patient to convulsions and extrapyramidal reactions; and in patients with mental depression, ulcerative colitis, or peptic ulcer disease, because the drug may exacerbate these conditions.

Rauwolfia should be used cautiously in patients with epilepsy or impaired renal function, because the drug may worsen these conditions.

Interactions
Rauwolfia may potentiate the antihypertensive effects of diuretics or other antihypertensive agents and the depressant effects of alcohol and CNS depressants. Rauwolfia may diminish the effects of levodopa.

Concomitant use with cardiac glycosides may increase the risk of cardiac arrhythmia in some patients; with methotrimeprazine may result in increased orthostatic hypotension; with monoamine oxidase inhibitors may cause excitability and antagonize the antihypertensive effects of rauwolfia.

Effects on diagnostic tests
Rauwolfia therapy alters detection of urine corticosteroids by colorimetric assay and may interfere with excretion of urine catecholamines and vanillylmandelic acid.

Adverse reactions
- CNS: mental confusion, depression, drowsiness, nervousness, paradoxical anxiety, nightmares, sedation, headache, extrapyramidal symptoms.
- CV: orthostatic hypotension, bradycardia, syncope, *arrhythmias.*
- DERM: pruritus, rash.
- EENT: dry mouth, nasal stuffiness, glaucoma.
- GI: hypersecretion of gastric acid, nausea, vomiting, diarrhea.
- Other: impotence, weight gain.
Note: Drug should be discontinued if patient shows signs of drug-induced mental depression.

Overdose and treatment
Signs of overdose include hypotension, bradycardia, CNS depression, coma, respiratory depression, hypothermia, diarrhea, vomiting, skin flushing, miosis, leg pain, and tremors.

After acute ingestion, empty the stomach by induced emesis or gastric lavage; follow with a saline cathartic. Subsequent treatment is usually symptomatic and supportive. Because effects of rauwolfia are prolonged, the patient should be observed closely for at least 72 hours.

▶ Special considerations
Besides those relevant to all *rauwolfia alkaloids,* consider the following recommendation.
- Some preparations contain tartrazine. Patients who are allergic to aspirin show signs of cross-sensitivity.

Geriatric use
Lower dosages may be necessary because of decreased drug clearance in elderly patients. Use with caution in elderly patients with severe cardiac or cerebrovascular disease.

Pediatric use
The safety and efficacy of rauwolfia in children have not been established; use only if potential benefit outweighs risk.

Breast-feeding
Rauwolfia is distributed into breast milk. Because of the potential adverse reactions in breast-feeding infants, an alternative feeding method is recommended during therapy.

rescinnamine
Moderil

- Pharmacologic classification: rauwolfia alkaloid, peripherally acting adrenergic blocking agent
- Therapeutic classification: antihypertensive
- Pregnancy risk category C

How supplied
Available by prescription only
Tablets: 0.25 mg, 0.5 mg

Indications, route, and dosage
Mild to moderate hypertension
Adults: Initially, 1 mg P.O. daily in single dose or divided into two doses. *Maintenance dose:* 0.5 mg/day.
Note: Some clinicians recommend an initial dose of 0.25 mg P.O. daily and a maintenance dose of 2 mg/day.

Pharmacodynamics
Antihypertensive action: The exact mechanism is unknown; however, rescinnamine's antihypertensive effect is thought to result from peripheral adrenergic blockade and possibly CNS effects. Rescinnamine depletes catecholamine and serotonin stores in many organs and decreases catecholamine uptake by adrenergic neurons.

Pharmacokinetics
- *Absorption:* Orally administered rescinnamine is believed to be absorbed rapidly; however, maximum antihypertensive effect does not occur for at least 2 to 3 weeks.
- *Distribution:* Rescinnamine appears to be distributed widely in the body; high concentrations are found in adipose tissue.
- *Metabolism:* Rescinnamine is metabolized extensively to inactive compounds.
- *Excretion:* Rescinnamine is excreted slowly as unchanged drug and metabolites in urine and feces. Antihypertensive effects may persist for several days to weeks after discontinuation of chronic therapy.

Contraindications and precautions
Rescinnamine is contraindicated in patients with known hypersensitivity to the drug; in patients receiving electroconvulsive therapy, because cerebral depletion of serotonin and catecholamines may predispose patient to convulsions and extrapyramidal reactions; and in patients with depression, ulcerative colitis, gallstones, or active peptic ulcer disease, because the drug may exacerbate these conditions.

Rescinnamine should be used cautiously in patients with renal insufficiency or epilepsy because the drug may worsen these conditions.

Interactions
Rescinnamine may potentiate antihypertensive effects of diuretics or other antihypertensive agents, and depressant effects of alcohol and CNS depressants. Rescinnamine may diminish the effects of levodopa.

Concomitant use with quinidine or cardiac glycosides may increase the risk of cardiac arrhythmias in some patients; with monoamine oxidase inhibitors may cause excitability and antagonize the hypotensive effects of rescinnamine; with methotrimeprazine may result in increased orthostatic hypotension.

Effects on diagnostic tests
Rescinnamine therapy alters the detection of urinary corticosteroids by colorimetric assay and may interfere with excretion of urinary catecholamines and vanillylmandelic acid.

Adverse reactions
- CNS: mental confusion, depression, drowsiness, coma, nervousness, anxiety, nightmares, sedation, parkinsonism.
- CV: orthostatic hypotension, bradycardia, syncope, *arrhythmias.*
- DERM: pruritus, rash.
- EENT: dry mouth, nasal stuffiness, glaucoma, miosis.
- GI: hypersecretion of gastric acid, nausea, vomiting, diarrhea.
- Other: impotence, weight gain, respiratory depression, hypothermia, leg pain, tremors.
Note: Drug should be discontinued if patient shows signs of drug-induced mental depression.

Overdose and treatment
Signs of overdose include hypotension, bradycardia, CNS depression, coma, respiratory depression, hypothermia, diarrhea, vomiting, skin flushing, miosis, leg pain, and tremors.

After acute ingestion, empty stomach by induced emesis or gastric lavage, and follow with a saline cathartic. Subsequent treatment is usually symptomatic and supportive. Because effects of rescinnamine are prolonged, closely observe the patient for at least 72 hours.

▶ Special considerations
Besides those relevant to all *rauwolfia alkaloids*, consider the following recommendations.
- Drowsiness and dizziness are common in early therapy; patient may require assistance with ambulation.
- Some preparations contain tartrazine. Patients who are allergic to aspirin often show signs of crosssensitivity.

Geriatric use
Lower dose may be necessary because of decreased drug clearance in elderly patients.

Pediatric use
The safety and efficacy of rescinnamine in children have not been established; use only if potential benefit outweighs risk.

Breast-feeding
Rescinnamine is distributed into breast milk. Because of the potential for adverse reactions, an alternative feeding method is recommended during therapy.

---

reserpine
Sandril, Serpalan, Serpanray, Serpasil,
Serpate, Zepine

- Pharmacologic classification: rauwolfia
alkaloid, peripherally acting anti-adrenergic agent
- Therapeutic classification: antihypertensive, antipsychotic
- Pregnancy risk category C

How supplied
Available by prescription only
Tablets: 0.1 mg, 0.25 mg, 1 mg

Indications, route, and dosage
Mild to moderate essential hypertension
Adults: Initially, 0.5 mg P.O. in a single daily dose or
divided into two doses daily.
Maintenance dose: 0.25 mg/day.
  Note: Some clinicians recommend an initial dose of
0.1 mg/day.
Antipsychotic therapy
Adults: 0.1 to 1 mg P.O. daily.

Pharmacodynamics
- *Antihypertensive action:* The exact mechanism is unknown; however, it is thought to result from peripheral
adrenergic blockade and possibly CNS effects. Reserpine depletes catecholamine and serotonin stores
in many organs and decreases catecholamine uptake
by adrenergic neurons.
- *Antipsychotic action:* Reserpine depletes brain stores
of serotonin and catecholamines, producing a tranquilizing effect.

Pharmacokinetics
- *Absorption:* Orally administered reserpine is believed
to be absorbed rapidly; however, maximum antihypertensive effect does not occur for at least 2 to 3 weeks.
- *Distribution:* Reserpine appears to be distributed
widely in the body; high concentrations are found in
adipose tissue.
- *Metabolism:* Reserpine is metabolized extensively to
inactive compounds.
- *Excretion:* Reserpine is excreted slowly as unchanged drug and metabolites in urine and feces. Antihypertensive effects may persist for several days to
weeks after discontinuation of chronic therapy. Mean
half-life is 33 hours.

Contraindications and precautions
Reserpine is contraindicated in patients with known
hypersensitivity to the drug; in patients receiving electroconvulsive therapy, because cerebral depletion of
serotonin and catecholamines may predispose patient
to convulsions and extrapyramidal reactions; and in
patients with mental depression, ulcerative colitis, or
peptic ulcer disease, because drug may exacerbate
these conditions.
  Reserpine should be used cautiously in patients with
epilepsy or impaired renal function because the drug
may worsen these conditions.

Interactions
Reserpine may potentiate antihypertensive effects of
diuretics or other antihypertensive agents, and depressant effects of alcohol and CNS depressants.
  Reserpine may diminish the effects of levodopa.
  Concomitant use with quinidine and cardiac glycosides may increase the risk of arrhythmias in some
patients; with methotrimeprazine may result in increased orthostatic hypotension; with monoamine oxidase inhibitors may cause excitability and antagonize
the hypotensive effects of reserpine.

Effects on diagnostic tests
Reserpine therapy alters the detection of urinary corticosteroids by colorimetric assay and may interfere
with excretion of urinary catecholamines and vanillylmandelic acid.

Adverse reactions
- CNS: mental confusion, depression, drowsiness, nervousness, paradoxical anxiety, nightmares, extrapyramidal symptoms, sedation.
- CV: orthostatic hypotension, bradycardia, syncope,
arrhythmias.
- DERM: pruritus, skin flushing, rash.
- EENT: dry mouth, nasal stuffiness, glaucoma, miosis,
uveitis, optic atrophy, conjunctival injection.
- GI: hyperacidity, nausea, vomiting, diarrhea.
- GU: dysuria, impotence.
- Other: dyspnea, hypothermia, leg pain, weight gain.
  Note: Drug should be discontinued if signs of drug-induced mental depression develop.

Overdose and treatment
Signs of overdose include hypotension, bradycardia,
CNS depression, coma, respiratory depression, hypothermia, diarrhea, vomiting, skin flushing, miosis, leg
pain, and tremors.
  After acute ingestion, induce emesis if patient is conscious and not convulsing, or use gastric lavage; follow
with a saline cathartic. Subsequent treatment is usually
symptomatic and supportive. Because effects of reserpine are prolonged, the patient should be closely
observed for at least 72 hours.

▶ Special considerations
Besides those relevant to all *rauwolfia alkaloids*, consider the following recommendations.
- Drowsiness and dizziness are common in early therapy; patient should have assistance with ambulation.
- Tell patient to report pregnancy promptly.

Geriatric use
Lower dose may be necessary because of decreased
drug clearance in elderly patients.

Pediatric use
The safety and efficacy of reserpine in children have
not been established; use only if potential benefit outweighs risk.

Breast-feeding
Reserpine is distributed into breast milk. Because of
the potential for adverse reactions in breast-fed infants,
an alternative feeding method is recommended during
therapy.

Rh$_o$ (D) immune globulin, human
Gamulin Rh, HypRh$_o$-D, Rhesonativ, Rh$_o$GAM

Rh$_o$ (D) immune globulin, microdose
HypRh$_o$-D Mini-Dose, MICRh$_o$GAM, Mini-Gamulin Rh

- Pharmacologic classification: immune serum
- Therapeutic classification: Anti-Rh$_o$ (D)-positive prophylaxis agent
- Pregnancy risk category C

How supplied
Available by prescription only
Injection: 300 mcg of Rh$_o$ (D) immune globulin/vial (standard dose); 50 mcg of Rh$_o$ (D) immune globulin/vial (microdose)

Indications, route, and dosage
Rh-positive exposure (full-term pregnancy or termination of pregnancy beyond 13 weeks of gestation)
Administer 1 vial I.M. for each 15 ml of estimated fetal packed red blood cell (RBC) volume entering the woman's blood, as determined by a modified Kleihauer-Betke technique to determine the fetal packed RBC volume. The usual (standard) dose after delivery of a full-term infant is 1 vial; it must be given within 72 hours after delivery or miscarriage.

If Rh$_o$ (D) immune globulin is indicated before delivery, 1 vial (standard dose) should be administered at approximately 28 weeks of gestation and a second vial within 72 hours of delivery.
Transfusion accidents
Premenopausal women: Consult blood bank or transfusion unit at once. The number of vials (standard dose) to administer is calculated via the following formula:

$$\text{Number of vials} = \frac{\text{volume of whole blood transfused}}{15} \times \text{donor unit Hct}$$

Dose must be given within 72 hours.
Termination of pregnancy (spontaneous or induced abortion or ectopic pregnancy) up to 13 weeks of gestation
Women: 1 vial of microdose immune globulin I.M.; ideally, should be given within 3 hours but may be given up to 72 hours after abortion or miscarriage.
Amniocentesis or abdominal trauma during pregnancy
Women: Dosage varies, depending on the extent of estimated fetomaternal hemorrhage.

Pharmacodynamics
Rh reaction prophylaxis: Rh$_o$ (D) immune globulin suppresses the active antibody response and formation of anti-Rh$_o$ (D) in Rh$_o$ (D)-negative or D^u-negative individuals exposed to Rh-positive blood. It provides passive immunity to women exposed to Rh$_o$-positive fetal blood during pregnancy. It prevents formation of maternal antibodies (active immunity), which prevents hemolytic disease of the Rh-positive newborn in a subsequent pregnancy.

Pharmacokinetics
No information available.

Contraindications and precautions
Human Rh$_o$ (D) immune globulin is contraindicated in Rh$_o$ (D)-positive or D^u-positive patients; in those previously immunized to Rh$_o$ (D) blood factor; and in patients with known hypersensitivity to thimerosal, a component of this immune serum. Rhesonativ is preservative-free and should be used for individuals sensitive to thimerosal.

Interactions
Rh$_o$ (D) immune globulin may interfere with the immune response to live virus vaccines, for example, those for measles, mumps, and rubella. Do not administer live virus vaccines within 3 months after administration of Rh$_o$ (D) immune globulin. If postpartum women receive both Rh$_o$ (D) immune globulin and rubella virus vaccine within a 3-month period, serologic tests should be performed 6 to 8 weeks after vaccination to confirm seroconversion.

Effects on diagnostic tests
None reported.

Adverse reactions
- Local: discomfort at injection site.
- Systemic: slight fever or *anaphylaxis*.

Overdose and treatment
No information available.

▶ Special considerations
- Obtain a thorough history of allergies and reactions to immunizations.
- Epinephrine solution 1:1,000 should be available to treat allergic reactions.
- Immediately after delivery, send a sample of the infant's cord blood to laboratory for type and cross match and direct antiglobulin test. Infant must be Rh$_o$ (D)-positive or D^u-positive. Confirm that mother is Rh$_o$ (D)-negative and D^u-negative.
- For best results, Rh$_o$ (D) immune globulin must be administered within 72 hours of Rh-incompatible delivery, spontaneous or induced abortion, or transfusion.
- The microdose formulation is recommended for use after every spontaneous or induced abortion up to 12 weeks' gestation unless the mother is Rh$_o$ (D)-positive or D^u-positive, the mother has Rh antibodies, or the father or fetus is Rh-negative.
- Administer I.M. in the deltoid muscle. Do not give I.V.
- Rh$_o$ (D) immune globulin has not been associated with an increased frequency of acquired immunodeficiency syndrome (AIDS). The immune globulin is devoid of human immunodeficiency virus (HIV). Immune globulin recipients do not develop antibodies to HIV.
- Store between 2° to 8° C. (36° to 46° F.). Do not freeze.
- To reconstitute, inject the diluent down the inside of the vial. Swirl slowly for 20 seconds and let stand for 1 minute. Swirl again if not completely dissolved. Avoid foaming, which delays dissolution.

Information for the patient
● Inform patient that she is receiving this product because her blood has been exposed to the Rh-positive factor. Tell the postpartum patient that her body will naturally develop antibodies to destroy this factor which could threaten any future Rh-positive pregnancy.
● Tell patient there is no known risk of infection with the AIDS virus after receiving this medication.
● Tell patient what to expect after vaccination: some local pain, swelling, and tenderness at the injection site. Recommend acetaminophen to ease minor discomfort.
● Tell patient to report headache, skin changes, or difficulty breathing.

Breast-feeding
Immune globulins are distributed into breast milk. Their safety in breast-feeding has not been established.

---

ribavirin
Virazole

● Pharmacologic classification: synthetic nucleoside
● Therapeutic classification: antiviral agent
● Pregnancy risk category X

How supplied
Available by prescription only
Powder to be reconstituted for inhalation: 6 g in 100-ml glass vial

Indications, route, and dosage
Treatment of hospitalized infants and young children infected by respiratory syncytial virus (RSV)
Infants and young children: Solution in concentration of 20 mg/ml delivered via the Viratek Small Particle Aerosol Generator (SPAG-2) results in a mist with a concentration of 190 mcg/liter. Treatment is carried out for 12 to 18 hours/day for at least 3, and no more than 7, days with a flow rate of 12.5 liters of mist per minute.

Pharmacodynamics
Antiviral action: Drug action probably involves inhibition of ribonucleic acid (RNA) and deoxyribonucleic acid (DNA) synthesis, inhibition of RNA polymerase, and interference with completion of viral polypeptide coat.

Pharmacokinetics
● *Absorption:* Some ribavirin is absorbed systemically.
● *Distribution:* Ribavirin concentrates in bronchial secretions; plasma levels are subtherapeutic for plaque inhibition.
● *Metabolism:* Ribavirin is metabolized to 1,2,4-triazole-3-carboxamide (deribosylated ribavirin).
● *Excretion:* Most of dose is excreted renally. First phase of plasma half-life is 9½ hours; second phase has extended half-life of 40 hours (from slow drug release from red blood cell binding sites).

Contraindications and precautions
Ribavirin is contraindicated in pregnant women and those who might become pregnant during therapy because of drug's potentially teratogenic or embryocidal effects.

Ribavirin should be administered with extreme caution to patients requiring ventilatory assistance because drug may precipitate in ventilatory apparatus, impairing ventilation.

Interactions
None reported.

Effects on diagnostic tests
None reported.

Adverse reactions
● CV: *cardiac arrest,* hypotension.
● HEMA: anemia, reticulocytosis.
● Respiratory: *worsening respiratory status,* bacterial pneumonia, apnea, pneumothorax, ventilator dependency.
● Other: rash, conjunctivitis.

Overdose and treatment
Unknown in humans; high doses in animals have produced GI symptoms.

▶ Special considerations
● Ribavirin aerosol is indicated only for lower respiratory tract infection caused by RSV. (Although treatment may begin before test results are available, RSV infection must eventually be confirmed.)
● Administer ribavirin aerosol only by SPAG-2. Do not use any other aerosol-generating device.
● To prepare drug, reconstitute solution with USP sterile water for injection or inhalation, then transfer aseptically to sterile 500-ml Erlenmeyer flask. Dilute further with sterile water to 300 ml to yield final concentration of 20 mg/ml. Solution remains stable for 24 hours at room temperature.
● Do not use bacteriostatic water (or any other water containing antimicrobial agent) to reconstitute drug.
● Discard unused solution in SPAG-2 unit before adding newly reconstituted solution. Solution should be changed at least every 24 hours.
● Monitor ventilator-dependent patients carefully because drug may precipitate in ventilatory apparatus.
● Drug is most useful for infants with most severe RSV form – typically premature infants and those with underlying disorders, such as cardiopulmonary disease. (Most other infants and children with RSV infection do not require treatment because disease is self-limiting.)
● Drug therapy must be accompanied by appropriate respiratory and fluid therapy.

---

riboflavin (vitamin B₂)

● Pharmacologic classification: water-soluble vitamin
● Therapeutic classification: vitamin B complex vitamin
● Pregnancy category A (C if > recommended daily allowance [RDA])

How supplied
Available without prescription, as appropriate
Tablets: 5 mg, 10 mg, 25 mg, 50 mg, 100 mg, 250 mg
Tablets (sugar-free): 50 mg, 100 mg

Indications, route, and dosage
Riboflavin deficiency or adjunct to thiamine treatment for polyneuritis or cheilosis secondary to pellagra

Adults and children over age 12: 5 to 50 mg P.O., S.C., I.M., or I.V. daily, depending on severity.
Children under age 12: 2 to 10 mg P.O., S.C., I.M., or I.V. daily, depending on severity.
For maintenance, increase nutritional intake and supplement with vitamin B complex.

Pharmacodynamics
Metabolic action: Riboflavin, a coenzyme, functions in the forms of flavin adenine dinucleotide (FAD) and flavin mononucleotide (FMN) and plays a vital metabolic role in numerous tissue respiration systems. FAD and FMN act as hydrogen-carrier molecules for several flavoproteins involved in intermediary metabolism. Riboflavin is also directly involved in maintaining erythrocyte integrity.

Riboflavin deficiency causes a clinical syndrome with the following symptoms: cheilosis, angular stomatitis, glossitis, keratitis, scrotal skin changes, ocular changes, and seborrheic dermatitis. In severe deficiency, normochromic, normocytic anemia and neuropathy may occur. Clinical signs may become evident after 3 to 8 months of inadequate riboflavin intake. Administration of riboflavin reverses signs of deficiency. Riboflavin deficiency rarely occurs alone and is often associated with deficiency of other B vitamins and protein.

Pharmacokinetics
● *Absorption:* Although riboflavin is absorbed readily from the GI tract, the extent of absorption is limited. Absorption occurs at a specialized segment of the mucosa; riboflavin absorption is limited by the duration of the drug's contact with this area. Before being absorbed, riboflavin-5-phosphate is rapidly dephosphorylated in the GI lumen. GI absorption increases when the drug is administered with food and decreases when hepatitis, cirrhosis, biliary obstruction, or probenecid administration is present.
● *Distribution:* FAD and FMN are distributed widely to body tissues. Free riboflavin is present in the retina. Riboflavin is stored in limited amounts in the liver, spleen, kidneys, and heart, mainly in the form of FAD. FAD and FMN are approximately 60% protein-bound in blood. Riboflavin crosses the placenta, and breast milk contains about 400 ng/ml.
● *Metabolism:* Riboflavin is metabolized in the liver.
● *Excretion:* After a single oral dose or I.M. administration, the biologic half-life is approximately 66 to 84 minutes in healthy individuals. Riboflavin is metabolized to FMN in erythrocytes, GI mucosal cells, and the liver; FMN is converted to FAD in the liver. Approximately 9% of the drug is excreted unchanged in the urine after normal ingestion. Excretion involves renal tubular secretion and glomerular filtration. The amount renally excreted unchanged is directly proportional to the dose. Removal of riboflavin by hemodialysis is slower than by natural renal excretion.

Contraindications and precautions
None reported.

Interactions
Concomitant use of riboflavin with propantheline bromide delays the absorption rate of riboflavin but increases the total amount absorbed. If the patient is using oral contraceptives, riboflavin's dose may need to be increased.

Effects on diagnostic tests
Riboflavin therapy alters urinalysis based on spectrophotometry or color reactions. Large doses of the drug result in bright yellow urine. Riboflavin produces fluorescent substances in urine and plasma, which can falsely elevate fluorometric determinations of catecholamines and urobilinogen.

Adverse reactions
GU: bright yellow urine with high doses.

Overdose and treatment
No information available.

▶ Special considerations
● The RDA of riboflavin is 0.4 to 1.8 mg/day in children, 1.2 to 1.7 mg/day in adults, and 1.6 to 1.8 mg/day in pregnant and lactating women.
● Give the oral preparation of riboflavin with food to increase absorption.
● Obtain a dietary history because other vitamin deficiencies may coexist.

Information for the patient
● Inform the patient that riboflavin may cause a yellow discoloration of the urine.
● Teach the patient about good dietary sources of riboflavin, such as whole-grain cereals and green vegetables. Liver, kidney, heart, eggs, and dairy products are also dietary sources but may not be appropriate, depending on the patient's serum cholesterol and triglyceride levels.
● Tell the patient to store riboflavin in a tight, light-resistant container.

Breast-feeding
Riboflavin crosses the placenta; during pregnancy and lactation, riboflavin requirements are increased. Increased food intake during this time usually provides adequate amounts of the vitamin. The National Research Council recommends daily intake of 1.8 mg/day during the first 6 months of breast-feeding.

---

rifampin
Rifadin, Rimactane

● Pharmacologic classification: semisynthetic rifamycin B derivative (macrocyclic antibiotic)
● Therapeutic classification: antituberculosis agent
● Pregnancy risk category C

How supplied
Available by prescription only
Capsules: 150 mg, 300 mg
Kit: 60 capsules, 300 mg
Injection: 600 mg/vial

Indications, route, and dosage
Primary treatment in pulmonary tuberculosis
Adults: 600 mg P.O. daily single dose 1 hour before or 2 hours after meals.

Children over age 5: 10 to 20 mg/kg P.O. daily single dose 1 hour before or 2 hours after meals. Maximum dose is 600 mg daily. Concomitant administration of other effective antitubercular drugs is recommended.
Asymptomatic meningococcal carriers
Adults: 600 mg P.O. b.i.d. for 2 days.
Children ages 1 to 10: 10 mg/kg P.O. b.i.d. for 2 days.
Infants ages 3 months to 1 year: 5 mg/kg P.O. b.i.d. for 2 days.
  Note: Reduce dosage in liver dysfunction.
Prophylaxis of Haemophilus influenzae type B
Adults and children: 20 mg/kg (up to 600 mg) once daily for 4 consecutive days.
†*Staphylococcus aureus and* S. epidermidis
Adults: 150 to 300 mg P.O. q.i.d. usually used in combination with other agents.

Pharmacodynamics
Antibiotic action: Rifampin impairs ribonucleic acid (RNA) synthesis by inhibiting deoxyribonucleic acid-dependent RNA polymerase. Rifampin may be bacteriostatic or bactericidal, depending on organism susceptibility and drug concentration at infection site.
  Rifampin acts against *Mycobacterium tuberculosis, M. bovis, M. marinum, M. kansasii,* some strains of *M. fortuitum, M. avium,* and *M. intracellulare,* and many gram-positive and some gram-negative bacteria. Resistance to rifampin by *M. tuberculosis* can develop rapidly; rifampin is usually given with other antituberculosis drugs to prevent or delay resistance.

Pharmacokinetics
● *Absorption:* Rifampin is absorbed completely from the GI tract after oral administration; peak serum concentrations occur 1 to 4 hours after ingestion. Food delays absorption.
● *Distribution:* Rifampin is distributed widely into body tissues and fluids, including ascitic, pleural, seminal, and cerebrospinal fluids, tears, and saliva; and into liver, prostate, lungs, and bone. Rifampin crosses the placenta; it is 84% to 91% protein-bound.
● *Metabolism:* Rifampin is metabolized extensively in the liver by deacetylation. The drug undergoes interohepatic circulation.
● *Excretion:* Rifampin undergoes enterohepatic circulation, and drug and metabolite are excreted primarily in bile; drug, but not metabolite, is reabsorbed. From 6% to 30% of rifampin and metabolite appear unchanged in urine in 24 hours; about 60% is excreted in feces. Some drug is excreted in breast milk. Plasma half-life in adults is 1½ to 5 hours; serum levels rise in obstructive jaundice. Dosage adjustment is not necessary for patients with renal failure.
  Rifampin is not removed by either hemodialysis or peritoneal dialysis.

Contraindications and precautions
Rifampin is contraindicated in patients with known hypersensitivity to any rifamycin. Use rifampin with caution and at reduced dosages in patients with hepatic disease or alcoholism and in patients taking other hepatotoxic drugs.

Interactions
Rifampin-induced enzyme activity may accelerate metabolic conversion of isoniazid (INH) to hepatotoxic metabolites, increasing hazard of INH hepatotoxicity.
  Concomitant use of para-aminosalicylate may decrease oral absorption of rifampin, lowering serum con-

centrations; administer drugs 8 to 12 hours apart. Rifampin-induced hepatic microsomal enzymes inactivate the following drugs: beta blockers, barbiturates, methadone, oral sulfonylureas, corticosteroids, digitalis derivatives, oral contraceptives and anticoagulants, chloramphenicol, disopyramide, quinidine, phenytoin, tocainide, verapamil, estrogens, dapsone, cyclosporine, and clofibrate; decreased serum concentrations of those drugs require dosage adjustments.
  Daily use of alcohol while using rifampin may increase risk of hepatotoxicity.

Effects on diagnostic tests
Rifampin alters standard serum folate and vitamin B_{12} assays. The drug's systemic effects may cause asymptomatic elevation of liver function tests (14%) and serum uric acid and may reduce vitamin D levels.
  Rifampin may cause temporary retention of sulfobromophthalein in the liver excretion test; it may also interfere with contrast material in gallbladder studies and urinalysis based on spectrophotometry.

Adverse reactions
● CNS: headache, fatigue, drowsiness, ataxia, dizziness, mental confusion, generalized numbness.
● DERM: pruritus, urticaria, rash, red-orange discoloration of skin.
● EENT: visual disturbances, conjunctivitis.
● GI: epigastric distress, anorexia, nausea, vomiting, abdominal pain, diarrhea, flatulence, sore mouth and tongue, *pseudomembranous colitis,* red-orange discoloration of feces.
● GU: red-orange discoloration of urine.
● HEMA: *thrombocytopenia,* transient leukopenia, *hemolytic anemia.*
● Hepatic: *serious hepatotoxicity as well as transient abnormalities in liver function tests.*
● Metabolic: hyperuricemia.
● Other: flu-like syndrome; red-orange discoloration of sweat and tears.
  Note: Drug should be discontinued if patient shows signs of hypersensitivity reactions or hepatotoxicity or if severe diarrhea indicates pseudomembranous colitis.

Overdose and treatment
Signs of overdose include lethargy, nausea, and vomiting; hepatotoxicity from massive overdose includes hepatomegaly, jaundice, elevated liver function studies and bilirubin levels, and loss of consciousness. Red-orange discoloration of the skin, urine, sweat, saliva, tears, and feces may occur.
  Treat by gastric lavage, followed by activated charcoal; if necessary, force diuresis. Perform bile drainage if hepatic dysfunction persists beyond 24 to 48 hours.

▶ Special considerations
● Give drug 1 hour before or 2 hours after meals for maximum absorption; capsule contents may be mixed with food or fluid to enhance swallowing.
● Obtain specimens for culture and sensitivity testing before first dose but do not delay therapy; repeat periodically to detect drug resistance.
● Observe patient for adverse reactions and monitor hematologic, renal and liver function studies, and serum electrolytes to minimize toxicity. Watch for signs of hepatic impairment (anorexia, fatigue, malaise, jaundice, dark urine, liver tenderness).
● Increased liver enzyme activity inactivates certain

---

drugs (especially warfarin, corticosteroids, and oral hypoglycemics), requiring dosage adjustments.
• Prepared I.V. admixtures are stable for 24 hours at room temperature.

Information for the patient
• Explain disease process and rationale for long-term therapy.
• Teach signs and symptoms of hypersensitivity and other adverse reactions, and emphasize need to call if these occur; urge patient to report *any* unusual reactions.
• Tell patient to take rifampin on an empty stomach, at least 1 hour before or 2 hours after a meal. If GI irritation occurs, patient may need to take drug with food.
• Urge patient to comply with prescribed regimen, not to miss doses, and not to discontinue drug without medical approval. Explain importance of follow-up appointments.
• Encourage patient to report promptly any flu-like symptoms, weakness, sore throat, loss of appetite, unusual bruising, rash, itching, tea-colored urine, clay-colored stools, or yellow discoloration of eyes or skin.
• Explain that drug turns all body fluids red-orange color; advise patient of possible permanent stains on clothes and soft contact lenses.
• Advise oral contraceptive users to substitute other methods; rifampin inactivates such drugs and may alter menstrual patterns.

Geriatric use
Usual dose in elderly and debilitated patients is 10 mg/kg once a day.

Pediatric use
Safety in children under age 5 has not been established.

Breast-feeding
Rifampin may be excreted in breast milk. Use with caution in breast-feeding women.

Ringer's injection

• Pharmacologic classification: electrolyte solution
• Therapeutic classification: electrolyte and fluid replenishment
• Pregnancy risk category C

How supplied
Available by prescription only
Injection: 250 ml, 500 ml, 1,000 ml

Indications, route, and dosage
Fluid and electrolyte replacement
Adults and children: Dose highly individualized according to patient's size and clinical condition, but usually 1.5 to 3 liters (2% to 6% body weight) infused I.V. over 18 to 24 hours.

Pharmacodynamics
Fluid and electrolyte replacement: Ringer's injection replaces fluid and supplies important electrolytes: sodium 147 mEq/liter, potassium 4 mEq/liter, calcium 4.5 mEq/liter, and chloride 155.5 mEq/liter. However, clinically, the addition of potassium and calcium only slightly increases the therapeutic value of an isotonic sodium chloride solution. Neither potassium nor calcium is present in sufficient concentration in Ringer's injection to correct a deficit of these ions adequately. As with sodium chloride injection, large volumes of Ringer's injection usually cause minimal distortion of cation composition of the extracellular fluid. However, either solution may alter the acid-base balance.

Pharmacokinetics
• *Absorption:* Given by direct I.V. infusion.
• *Distribution:* Widely distributed.
• *Metabolism:* None significant.
• *Excretion:* Excreted primarily in urine, with minor excretion in feces.

Contraindications and precautions
Ringer's injection is contraindicated in renal failure, except as an emergency volume expander. Use with caution in renal dysfunction, congestive heart failure, circulatory insufficiency, hypoproteinemia, or pulmonary edema.

Interactions
Several drugs, as well as packed red blood cells, are incompatible with Ringer's solution. Consult specialized references for further information.

Effects on diagnostic tests
None reported.

Adverse reactions
• CV: fluid overload.
• Other: hypernatremia, hyperkalemia, hypercalcemia, hyperchloremia.

Overdose and treatment
If overinfusion occurs, stopping infusion is usually sufficient treatment. In some cases, a loop diuretic, such as furosemide, may be necessary to increase the rate of fluid and electrolyte elimination. Dialysis may be needed in renal failure.

▶ **Special considerations**
Monitor for acid-base imbalance when large volume of solution is infused. Ringer's injection is a colorless, odorless solution with a salty taste and a pH between 5.0 and 7.5.

Ringer's injection, lactated

• Pharmacologic classification: electrolyte-carbohydrate solution
• Therapeutic classification: electrolyte and fluid replenishment
• Pregnancy risk category C

How supplied
Available by prescription only
Injection: 250 ml, 500 ml, 1,000 ml

Indications, route, and dosage
Fluid and electrolyte replacement
Adults and children: Dose highly individualized, but usually 1.5 to 3 liters (2% to 6% body weight) infused I.V. over 18 to 24 hours.

This solution approximates the contents of the blood more closely than Ringer's injection does; however, additional electrolytes may have to be added to meet the patient's needs. Specific formulations of I.V. solutions are frequently preferred to this premixed formulation. The lactate has an alkalinizing effect in the body, requiring 1 to 2 hours to be fully effective.

Pharmacodynamics
Fluid and electrolyte replacement: Ringer's injection (lactated) replaces fluid and supplies important electrolytes: sodium 130 mEq/liter, potassium 4 mEq/liter, calcium 3 mEq/liter, chloride 109.7 mEq/liter, and lactate 28 mEq/liter. However, clinically, the addition of potassium and calcium only slightly increases the therapeutic value of an isotonic sodium chloride solution. Neither potassium nor calcium is present in sufficient concentration in Ringer's injection (lactated) to correct a deficit of these ions. As with sodium chloride injection, large volumes of Ringer's injection (lactated) usually cause minimal distortion of cation composition of the extracellular fluid. However, either solution may alter the acid-base balance.

Ringer's injection (lactated) may be used for its alkalinizing effect, because the lactate is ultimately metabolized to bicarbonate. In persons with normal cellular oxidative activity, the alkalinizing effect will be fully realized in 1 to 2 hours.

Pharmacokinetics
● *Absorption:* Given by direct I.V. infusion.
● *Distribution:* Ringer's injection (lactated) is distributed widely.
● *Metabolism:* None significant for electrolytes. Lactate is oxidized to bicarbonate.
● *Excretion:* Ringer's injection (lactated) is excreted primarily in urine, with minor excretion in feces.

Contraindications and precautions
Ringer's injection (lactated) is contraindicated in patients with renal failure, except as a volume expander in hypovolemic emergencies; and in patients with lactic acidosis because of the lactate content. Use cautiously in patients with renal dysfunction, congestive heart failure, circulatory insufficiency, hypoproteinemia, or pulmonary edema because of potential for fluid overload.

Interactions
Several drugs, as well as packed red blood cells, are incompatible with Ringer's injection (lactated). Consult specialized references for further information.

Effects on diagnostic tests
None reported.

Adverse reactions
● CV: fluid overload.
● Other: hypernatremia, hyperkalemia, hypercalcemia, hyperchloremia.

Overdose and treatment
If overinfusion occurs, stopping infusion is usually sufficient treatment. Dialysis may be needed in renal failure. Monitor blood acid-base balance.

▶ Special considerations
● The solution is colorless and odorless with a salty taste and a pH between 6.0 and 7.5. The absence of bicarbonate from the solution stabilizes the calcium,

which may precipitate as calcium bicarbonate. It contains no antibacterial agent.
● Monitor for acid-base imbalance when large volume of solution is infused.

---

ritodrine hydrochloride
Yutopar

● Pharmacologic classification: beta-receptor agonist
● Therapeutic classification: adjunctive agent in suppression of preterm labor
● Pregnancy risk category B

How supplied
Available by prescription only
Injection: ampule 10 mg/ml, 15 mg/ml
Tablet: 10 mg

Indications, route, and dosage
Management of preterm labor
Adults: Initially, 50 to 100 mcg (0.05 to 0.1 mg)/minute I.V. infusion; increased every 10 minutes as necessary in increments of 50 mcg (0.05 mg) to effective dose (usually 150 to 350 mcg [0.15 to 0.35 mg]/minute).
Oral maintenance: 1 tablet (10 mg) may be given approximately 30 minutes before termination of I.V. therapy, then 10 mg q 2 hours for 24 hours. Thereafter, dose is 10 to 20 mg q 4 to 6 hours. Maximum dosage is 120 mg daily.

Pharmacodynamics
Tocolytic action: Ritodrine is a beta-receptor agonist that exerts a preferential effect on beta$_2$-adrenergic receptors (such as uterine smooth muscle). Stimulation of the beta$_2$-receptors inhibits contractility of the uterine smooth muscle. Ritodrine also may act to affect directly the interaction between actin and myosin in muscle to decrease the intensity and frequency of contractions.

Pharmacokinetics
● *Absorption:* Ritodrine is 30% absorbed by the oral route and 100% by the I.V. route. Food may inhibit the absorption and effectiveness of oral ritodrine.
● *Distribution:* Peak ritodrine serum levels are 5 to 15 ng/ml after an oral dose and 32 to 50 ng/ml after an I.V. dose. The I.V. dose is distributed to the tissues within 6 to 9 minutes.
● *Metabolism:* Ritodrine is metabolized in the liver, primarily to inactive sulfate and glucuronide conjugates.
● *Excretion:* About 70% to 90% of an oral or I.V. dose of ritodrine is excreted in urine in 10 to 12 hours as unchanged drug and its conjugates. Ritodrine can be removed by dialysis.

Contraindications and precautions
Ritodrine is contraindicated before the 20th week or after the 36th week of pregnancy; in patients with antepartum hemorrhage, preeclampsia or eclampsia, intrauterine infection, fetal death, chorioamnionitis, or conditions in which continuation of the pregnancy is hazardous; in those with maternal cardiac disease, pulmonary hypertension, uncontrolled cervical dilation, or maternal diabetes mellitus, because the drug may exacerbate these conditions; in patients with medical conditions that would be seriously affected by the drug,

such as hypovolemia, cardiac arrhythmias associated with tachycardia or digitalis intoxication, and uncontrolled hypertension or bronchial asthma already treated with betamimetics or steroids; and in patients with known hypersensitivity to any component of the preparation.

Interactions
Concomitant use of ritodrine with corticosteroids may produce additive diabetogenic effects, pulmonary edema, and possibly death in mother. Discontinue drugs if pulmonary edema occurs. Monitor patient closely during concurrent use.

Concomitant use with beta blockers (propranolol) may inhibit ritodrine's action. Avoid concurrent administration.

Use with sympathomimetic amines may produce an additive effect (especially cardiovascular). Use together with caution.

Concurrent use with magnesium sulfate, diazoxide, or meperidine may potentiate cardiovascular effects. Use with atropine may worsen hypertension.

Effects on diagnostic tests
I.V. administration of ritodrine elevates the plasma insulin and glucose levels and decreases plasma potassium concentrations (values usually return to normal within 24 hours after drug is stopped).

Adverse reactions
With I.V. administration:
● CNS: nervousness, jitteriness, tremor, anxiety, headache, malaise, emotional upset.
● CV: dose-related alterations in blood pressure, chest pain, palpitations, dyspnea, *pulmonary edema,* tachycardia, ECG changes, altered maternal and fetal heart rates.
● GI: nausea, vomiting, constipation, diarrhea, epigastric distress, bloating.
● Metabolic: hyperglycemia in mother and neonate, hypokalemia, ketoacidosis.
● Other: *anaphylactic shock,* erythema, sweating, chills, drowsiness, weakness, hemolytic icterus, glycosuria, lactic acidosis.
With oral administration:
● CNS: headache, tremor, nervousness, jitteriness, hyperventilation.
● CV: palpitations, increase in maternal but not fetal heart rate.
● DERM: rash.
● GI: nausea, vomiting.
Note: Drug should be discontinued if pulmonary edema occurs.

Overdose and treatment
Overdose produces symptoms similar to those of excessive beta-adrenergic stimulation (maternal and fetal tachycardia, palpitations, cardiac arrhythmia, hypotension, nervousness, tremor, nausea, and vomiting).

Treat I.V. overdose by stopping infusion and administering appropriate beta-adrenergic blocking agent (such as propranolol) as an antidote. Treat oral overdose by emptying stomach and administering activated charcoal. Subsequent treatment is supportive and symptomatic.

▶ **Special considerations**
● Because cardiovascular responses are common, especially during I.V. administration, cardiovascular effects—including maternal pulse rate and blood pressure and fetal heart rate—must be closely monitored. A maternal tachycardia of over 140 beats/minute or persistent respiratory rate of over 20 breaths/minute may be signs of impending pulmonary edema.
● Monitor blood glucose concentrations during ritodrine infusions, especially in mothers predisposed to diabetes mellitus.
● Discontinue drug if pulmonary edema occurs.
● Monitor the amount of I.V. fluid administered, to prevent circulatory overload.
● Do not use ritodrine I.V. if solution is discolored or contains a precipitate. Do not use more than 48 hours after preparation.
● Control infusion rate by use of a microdrip chamber I.V. infusion set or an infusion control device.
● Prepare I.V. solution by diluting 150 mg ritodrine in 500 ml of dextrose 5% injection, 10% Dextran 40 in sodium chloride injection, 10% invert sugar solution, Ringer's injection, or Hartmann's solution to produce a solution containing 300 mcg (0.3 mg) of ritodrine per milliliter.
● Place patient in left lateral recumbent position to reduce risk of hypotension.
● Ritodrine may uncover previously unknown cardiac pathology. Sinus bradycardia may follow drug withdrawal.
● Maternal tachycardia or decreased diastolic blood pressure usually reverses with a dosage reduction but requires discontinuation of the drug in 1% of patients.

Information for the patient
● Caution patient not to stop taking the drug without medical approval.
● Advise patient to keep scheduled follow-up appointments and to report any adverse reactions promptly.

rubella and mumps virus vaccine, live
Biavax II

● Pharmacologic classification: vaccine
● Therapeutic classification: viral vaccine
● Pregnancy risk category X

How supplied
Available by prescription only
Injection: single-dose vial containing not less than 1,000 $TCID_{50}$ (tissue culture infective doses) of the Wistar RA 27/3 rubella virus (propagated in human diploid cell culture) and not less than 5,000 $TCID_{50}$ of the Jeryl Lynn mumps strain (grown in chick embryo cell culture)

Indications, route, and dosage
Rubella (German measles) and mumps immunization
Adults and children over age 1: 1 vial (1,000 units) S.C. in outer aspect of the upper arm.

Pharmacodynamics
Live rubella and mumps prophylaxis: This vaccine promotes active immunity to rubella and mumps by inducing production of antibodies.

Pharmacokinetics
Antibodies are usually detectable within 2 to 6 weeks. The duration of vaccine-induced immunity is expected to be lifelong.

Contraindications and precautions
Live rubella and mumps virus vaccine is contraindicated in patients with a history of anaphylactic reactions to neomycin, a trace component of the vaccine, and eggs; in patients with generalized cancers, cancers of or affecting the bone marrow or lymphatic systems, or primary immunodeficiency states; in pregnant patients; and in those receiving adrenocorticotropic hormone, corticosteroids (except in patients receiving corticosteroids as replacement therapy, for example, for Addison's disease), irradiation, or other immunosuppressant therapy. Patients with leukemia whose therapy has been terminated for at least 3 months may receive live rubella and mumps virus vaccine.

Interactions
Concomitant use of rubella and mumps vaccine with immune serum globulin or transfusions of blood and blood products may impair the immune response to the vaccine. Defer vaccination for 3 months in these situations.

The administration of immunosuppressive agents may interfere with the response to the vaccine.

Effects on diagnostic tests
Rubella and mumps vaccine temporarily may decrease the response to tuberculin skin testing. Should a tuberculin skin test be necessary, administer it either before or simultaneously with rubella and mumps vaccine.

Adverse reactions
● Local: pain, erythema, and induration at injection site.
● Systemic: fever, rash, urticaria, arthralgia; very rarely: regional lymphadenopathy, parotitis, orchitis, malaise, arthritis, polyneuritis, thrombocytopenic purpura, *anaphylaxis.*

Overdose and treatment
No information available.

▶ Special considerations
● Obtain a thorough history of allergies (especially to antibiotics, eggs, chicken, or chicken feathers) and of reactions to immunizations.
● Patients with a history of anaphylactoid reactions to egg ingestion should have skin testing performed first to assess vaccine sensitivity (against a control of normal saline solution in the opposite arm). Administer intradermal or scratch test with a 1:10 dilution. Read results after 5 to 30 minutes. *Positive reaction:* wheal with or without pseudopodia and surrounding erythema.
● Epinephrine solution 1:1,000 should be available to treat allergic reactions.
● Rubella and mumps vaccine should not be given less than 1 month before or after immunization with other live virus vaccines—except for monovalent or trivalent live poliovirus vaccine or live, attenuated measles virus vaccine, which may be administered simultaneously.
● Use only the diluent supplied. Discard reconstituted vaccine after 8 hours.
● Inject S.C. (not I.M.) into the outer aspect of the upper arm.
● Revaccination or booster is not required if patient

was previously vaccinated at age 1 or older; however, there is no conclusive evidence of an increased risk of adverse reactions for persons who are already immune when vaccinated.
● Women who have rubella antibody titers of 1:8 or greater (by hemagglutination inhibition) need not be vaccinated with the rubella vaccine component.
● The vaccine will not offer protection when given after exposure to natural rubella or mumps, but there is no evidence that it would be harmful.
● Although rubella vaccine administration should be deferred in patients with febrile illness, the vaccine may be administered to susceptible children with mild illness, such as upper respiratory infection.
● According to Centers for Disease Control recommendations, measles, mumps, and rubella (MMR) is the preferred vaccine.
● Women who are not immune to rubella are at risk of congenital rubella injury to the fetus if exposed to it during pregnancy.
● Store at 2° to 8° C (36° to 46° F) and protect from light. Solution may be used if red, pink, or yellow, but it must be clear.

Information for the patient
● Tell patient what to expect after vaccination: tingling sensations in the extremities or joint aches and pains that may resemble arthritis, beginning several days to several weeks after vaccination. These symptoms usually resolve within 1 week. Patient also may have pain and inflammation at the injection site and low-grade fever, rash, or breathing difficulties. Encourage patient to report distressing adverse reactions.
● Recommend acetaminophen to relieve fever or other minor discomfort.
● Tell female patients of childbearing age to avoid pregnancy for 3 months after immunization. Provide contraceptive information if necessary.

Pediatric use
Live rubella and mumps virus vaccine is not recommended for children under age 1 because retained maternal antibodies may interfere with the immune response.

Breast-feeding
No data are available regarding mumps vaccine in breast-feeding women. Some reports have demonstrated transfer of rubella virus or virus antigen into breast milk in approximately 68% of patients. Few adverse effects have been associated with breast-feeding after immunization with rubella-containing vaccines. Therefore, breast-feeding women may be immunized with the rubella vaccine component if necessary.

---

rubella virus vaccine, live, attenuated
Meruvax II

● Pharmacologic classification: vaccine
● Therapeutic classification: viral vaccine
● Pregnancy risk category X

How supplied
Available by prescription only
Injection: single-dose vial containing not less than 1,000

TCID$_{50}$ (tissue culture infective doses) of the Wistar RA 27/3 strain of rubella virus propagated in human diploid cell culture

Indications, route, and dosage
Rubella (German measles) immunization
Adults and children over age 1: 1 vial (1,000 units) S.C.

Pharmacodynamics
Rubella prophylaxis: This vaccine promotes active immunity to rubella by inducing production of antibodies.

Pharmacokinetics
Antibodies are usually detectable 2 to 6 weeks after injection. The duration of vaccine-induced immunity is expected to be lifelong.

Contraindications and precautions
The U.S. Public Health Service Immunization Practices Advisory Committee and the Centers for Disease Control state that the use of rubella virus vaccine is contraindicated during pregnancy because of the theoretical, albeit small, risk of congenital rubella syndrome. Patients should avoid pregnancy for 3 months after vaccination.

Live, attenuated rubella virus vaccine also is contraindicated in patients with a history of anaphylactic reactions to neomycin, a trace component of the vaccine; in patients with generalized cancers, cancer of or affecting the bone marrow or lymphatic system, or primary immunodeficiency states; and in those receiving adrenocorticotropic hormone, corticosteroids (except in patients receiving corticosteroids as replacement therapy, for example, for Addison's disease), irradiation, or other immunosuppressant therapy. Patients with leukemia whose therapy has been terminated for at least 3 months may receive live rubella virus vaccine.

Interactions
Concomitant use of rubella vaccine with immune serum globulin or transfusions of blood and blood products may impair the immune response to the vaccine. If possible, defer vaccination for 3 months in these situations.

Effects on diagnostic tests
Rubella vaccine may temporarily decrease response to tuberculin skin testing. If a tuberculin test is necessary, administer it either before, simultaneously with, or at least 8 weeks after rubella vaccine.

Adverse reactions
● Local: pain, erythema, and induration at injection site.
● Systemic: arthralgia (in about 40% of patients), fever, urticaria, rash, sore throat, headache, regional lymphadenopathy; very rarely: *thrombocytopenic purpura, arthritis, paresthesia, polyneuritis, anaphylaxis.*

Overdose and treatment
No information available.

▶ Special considerations
● Obtain a thorough history of allergies, especially to antibiotics, and of reactions to immunizations.
● Epinephrine solution 1:1,000 should be available to treat allergic reactions.
● Rubella vaccine should not be given less than 1 month before or after immunization with other live virus vaccines – except for monovalent or trivalent live poliovirus

vaccine; live, attenuated measles virus vaccine; or live mumps virus vaccine, which may be administered simultaneously.
● Do not inject I.M. Inject S.C. into the outer aspect of the upper arm.
● Use only diluent supplied. Discard 8 hours after reconstituting.
● Store at 2° to 8° C (36° to 46° F), and protect from light. Solution may be used if red, pink, or yellow, but it must be clear.
● The vaccine will not offer protection when given after exposure to natural rubella, although there is no evidence that it would be harmful.
● Revaccination or a booster dose is not required if patient was previously vaccinated at age 1 or older; however, there is no conclusive evidence of an increased risk of adverse reactions for persons who are already immune when revaccinated.
● Although rubella vaccine administration should be deferred in patients with febrile illness, it may be administered to susceptible children with mild illnesses, such as upper respiratory infection.
● Women who are not immune to rubella are at risk of congenital rubella injury to the fetus if exposed to rubella during pregnancy.
● Women who have rubella antibody titers of 1:8 or greater (by hemagglutination inhibition) need not be vaccinated with rubella virus vaccine.

Information for the patient
● Tell patient what to expect: tingling sensations in the extremities or joint aches and pains that may resemble arthritis, beginning several days to several weeks after vaccination. The symptoms usually resolve within 1 week. Patient also may have pain and inflammation at the injection site and low-grade fever, rash, or breathing difficulties. Encourage patient to report distressing reactions.
● Recommend acetaminophen to relieve fever or other minor discomfort after vaccination.
● Tell women of childbearing age to avoid pregnancy for 3 months after rubella immunization. Provide contraceptive information if necessary.

Pediatric use
Live, attenuated rubella virus vaccine is not recommended for children under age 1 because retained maternal antibodies may impair the immune response.

Breast-feeding
Although early studies failed to show evidence of the attenuated rubella virus in breast milk, subsequent reports showed transfer of rubella virus or virus antigen into breast milk in approximately 68% of patients. Few adverse effects have been associated with breast-feeding after immunization with rubella-containing vaccines. The risk-benefit ratio suggests that breast-feeding women may be immunized if necessary.

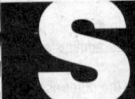

salicylates

aspirin
choline magnesium trisalicylate
choline salicylate
magnesium salicylate
salicylamide
salsalate
sodium salicylate
sodium thiosalicylate

Salicylates provide temporary relief of mild to moderate pain, especially pain associated with inflammation. Widely prescribed, these drugs are the standard of comparison and evaluation for other nonnarcotic analgesics, nonsteroidal anti-inflammatory drugs, and antipyretic drugs.

Pharmacology
Salicylates produce analgesic, anti-inflammatory, and antipyretic effects through action of the salicylate moiety; dissociation or hydrolysis to salicylic acid is not required for pharmacologic effects.

Salicylates may act peripherally by inhibiting the enzyme cyclo-oxygenase, thus decreasing formation of the prostaglandins involved in pain and inflammation. These prostaglandins appear to sensitize pain receptors to mechanical stimulation or to other chemical mediators. These drugs may also act centrally, possibly in the hypothalamus. The anti-inflammatory action of the salicylates, also related to prostaglandin inhibition, may contribute to their analgesic effect. The exact mechanism of the latter effect is unknown.

Salicylates lower body temperature principally by inhibiting synthesis and release of the prostaglandins that mediate the effect of endogenous pyrogens on the hypothalamus. Also, salicylates produce a centrally mediated dilation of peripheral blood vessels, enhancing heat dissipation and sweating. Salicylates rarely decrease body temperature in afebrile patients.

Clinical indications and actions
Salicylates are used principally for the symptomatic relief of mild to moderate pain, inflammation, and fever.
Pain
Salicylates are most effective in treating low-intensity pain of headache, arthralgia, myalgia, and neuralgia. They may also relieve mild to moderate pain from dental and surgical procedures, dysmenorrhea, and rheumatic fever.
Inflammation
Salicylates are commonly used for initial long-term treatment of rheumatoid arthritis, juvenile arthritis, and osteoarthritis. It is important to note that in rheumatoid conditions, these agents offer only symptomatic relief, reducing pain, stiffness, swelling, and tenderness. They do not reverse or arrest the disease process.

Fever
Use of salicylates in fever is nonspecific and does not influence the course of the underlying disease.

Overview of adverse reactions
Adverse reactions to salicylates involve mainly the GI tract, particularly gastric mucosa. Also, adverse GI reactions occur more frequently when aspirin is used than with other salicylates. Most common symptoms are dyspepsia, heartburn, epigastric distress, nausea, and abdominal pain. GI reactions usually occur in the first few days of therapy, often subside with continuous treatment, and can be minimized by administering salicylates with meals or food, antacids, or 8 oz of water or milk. The incidence and severity of GI bleeding are exposure related.

Chronic salicylate intoxication (salicylism) may occur with prolonged therapy, at high doses. Signs and symptoms include tinnitus, hearing loss, hepatotoxicity, moderate to severe noncardiogenic edema, and adverse renal effects.

Salicylate-induced bronchospasm, with or without urticaria and angioedema, may occur in patients with hypersensitivity to these drugs, particularly those with the "triad" of aspirin sensitivity, rhinitis/nasal polyps, and asthma. A significant incidence of cross-reactivity has been observed with tartrazine; 5% of allergic patients also exhibit cross-sensitivity with acetaminophen.

▶ Special considerations
● Use salicylates with caution in patients with a history of GI disease (especially peptic ulcer disease), increased risk of GI bleeding, or decreased renal function.
● Administer non-enteric-coated tablets with food or after meals to minimize gastric upset.
● Tablets may be chewed, broken, or crumbled and administered with food or fluids to aid swallowing. Uncoated plain aspirin tablets allowed to remain in contact with mucous membranes of the mouth and aspirin chewing gum have produced mucosal erosions and mouth ulcerations.
● Do not crush enteric-coated tablets.
● Patient should take a full glass of water or milk with salicylates to ensure passage into stomach. Patient should sit up for 15 to 30 minutes after taking salicylates to prevent lodging of salicylate in esophagus.
● Administer antacids, if prescribed, with salicylates except enteric-coated forms. Separate doses of antacids and enteric-coated salicylates by 1 to 2 hours to ensure adequate absorption.
● Monitor vital signs frequently, especially temperature.
● Salicylates may mask the signs and symptoms of acute infection (fever, myalgia, erythema); carefully evaluate patients at risk for infections, such as those with diabetes.
● Monitor CBC; platelets; prothrombin times; and BUN, serum creatinine, and liver function studies periodically during salicylate therapy to detect abnormalities.
● Assess hearing function before and periodically during therapy to prevent ototoxicity.

• Assess level of pain and inflammation before initiation of therapy. Evaluate effectiveness of therapy as evidenced by relief of these symptoms.

• Assess for signs and symptoms of potential hemorrhage, such as petechiae, bruising, coffee ground vomitus, and black tarry stools.

• If fever or illness causes fluid depletion, dosage should be reduced.

Information for the patient

• Tell the patient to take tablet or capsule forms of medication with 8 oz of water and not to lie down for 15 to 30 minutes after swallowing the drug.

• Tell patient to take the medication 30 minutes before or 2 hours after meals, or with food or milk if gastric irritation occurs.

• Explain that taking the drug as directed is necessary to achieve the desired effect; 2 to 4 weeks of treatment may be needed before benefit is seen.

• Advise patients on chronic salicylate therapy to arrange for monitoring of laboratory parameters, especially BUN, serum creatinine, liver function tests, CBC, and prothrombin times.

• Warn patients with current or history of rectal bleeding to avoid using salicylate suppositories. The latter must be retained in the rectum for at least 1 hour and could cause irritation and bleeding.

• Warn patients who could become pregnant to avoid the use of all salicylates. Pregnant patients should avoid all salicylates, especially during the third trimester, when prostaglandin inhibition can adversely affect fetal cardiovascular development.

• Advise patient to avoid taking aspirin-containing medications or NSAIDs such as ibuprofen without medical approval.

• Warn patient that use of alcoholic beverages with salicylates may cause increased GI irritation and possibly GI bleeding.

• Tell patient to take a missed dose as soon as he remembers, unless it is almost time for next dose; then skip the missed dose and return to regular schedule.

• Tell patient not to take these medications for more than 10 consecutive days unless otherwise directed.

Geriatric use

• Patients over age 60 may be more susceptible to the toxic effects of salicylates because of possible impaired renal function.

• The effects of salicylates on renal prostaglandins may cause fluid retention and edema, a significant disadvantage in elderly patients, especially those with congestive heart failure.

Pediatric use

• Children may be more susceptible to toxic effects of salicylates. Use with caution.

• Because of epidemiologic association with Reye's syndrome, the Centers for Disease Control recommend that children with chicken pox or flulike symptoms not be given salicylates.

• Do not use long-term salicylate therapy in children under age 14; safety of this use has not been established.

• Generally, children should not take salicylates more than five times or for more than 5 days.

Breast-feeding

Salicylates are distributed into breast milk and should be avoided during breast-feeding.

Representative combinations

Aspirin with magnesium hydroxide and aluminum hydroxide: Buff A, Buffadyne; with caffeine: Accutrate, Acotin, Alsidol, Anacin, Asafen, C-2, CP-2, 812, Instantine, Major-cin, Neo-Tigol, Nervine, P.A.C. revised formula Paradol, 217; with phenacetin (acetophenetidin) and caffeine: APC, Pan-APC, Aspodyne; with phenacetin, caffeine, and phenolphthalein: Phenodyne, Gelsodyne; with butabarbital: Axotal; with caffeine and butabarbital: Fiorinal, Marnal, Buff-A-Comp; with phenobarbital: Aspirbar; with acetaminophen, salicylamide, and caffeine: S.A.C., Saleto, Salocal; with meprobomate: Epromate, Equagesic, Equazine M, Meprogesic Q, Micrainin.

Salicylamide with aspirin and caffeine: Anodynos; with acetaminophen: Arthrol; with calcium succinate, phenobarbital, and vitamin C: Calsuxaphen; with phenacetin, caffeine, ascorbic acid, phenylphrine hydrochloride, and chlorpheniramine maleate: Genaid; with phenacetin, caffeine, ascorbic acid, phenylephrine hydrochloride, chlorpheniramine maleate, and dextromethorphan: Centuss; with phenacetin and chlorpheniramine maleate: Chlorphen.

Salicylic acid with sulfur: Sebulex, Fostex Medicated Cleansing, Meted.

See also: Opioids

---

salsalate
Arthra-G, Disalcid, Mono-Gesic

• Pharmacologic classification: salicylate
• Therapeutic classification: nonnarcotic analgesic, antipyretic, anti-inflammatory
• Pregnancy risk category C

How supplied
Available by prescription only
Capsules: 500 mg
Tablets: 500 mg, 750 mg

Indications, route, and dosage
Minor pain or fever, arthritis
Adults: 3 g P.O. daily, divided b.i.d., t.i.d., or q.i.d., p.r.n.

Pharmacodynamics
• *Analgesic action:* Salsalate produces analgesia by an ill-defined effect on the hypothalamus (central action) and by blocking generation of pain impulses (peripheral action). The peripheral action may involve inhibition of prostaglandin synthesis.

• *Anti-inflammatory action:* Drug probably exerts its anti-inflammatory effect by inhibiting prostaglandin synthesis; it may also inhibit the synthesis or action of other mediators of inflammation.

• *Antipyretic action:* Drug relieves fever by acting on the hypothalamic heat-regulating center to produce peripheral vasodilation. This increases peripheral blood supply and promotes sweating, which leads to loss of heat and to cooling by evaporation.

Pharmacokinetics
• *Absorption:* Salsalate is absorbed rapidly and completely from the GI tract, chiefly the small intestine. Peak effect occurs at 2 hours.

• *Distribution:* Salsalate is distributed widely to most

---

body fluids and tissues. Protein-binding varies from 75% to 90%; it is concentration-dependent and decreases as serum concentrations increase.

● *Metabolism:* Salsalate is hydrolyzed in the liver, plasma, blood, and GI mucosa to salicylic acid.
● *Excretion:* Metabolite and parent drug are excreted in urine.

Contraindications and precautions

Salsalate is contraindicated in patients with known hypersensitivity to aspirin or other nonsteroidal anti-inflammatory drugs (NSAIDs); and in the presence of GI ulcer or GI bleeding because drug may irritate GI tract. It should be used cautiously in patients with hypoprothrombinemia, vitamin K deficiency, and bleeding disorders, because of the potential for bleeding problems.

Patients with known "triad" symptoms (aspirin hypersensitivity, rhinitis/nasal polyps, and asthma) are at high risk of cross-sensitivity to salicylates with precipitation of bronchospasm.

Interactions

Concomitant use of salsalate with drugs that are highly protein-bound (phenytoin, sulfonylureas, warfarin) may cause displacement of either drug, and adverse effects. Monitor therapy closely for both drugs. Concomitant use with other GI-irritating drugs (steroids, antibiotics, other NSAIDs) may potentiate adverse GI effects of salsalate. Use together with caution.

Ammonium chloride and other urine acidifiers, as well as probenecid and sulfinpyrazone, increase salsalate blood levels; monitor for salsalate toxicity. Antacids in high doses, and other urine alkalizers, decrease salsalate blood levels; monitor for decreased salicylate effect. Corticosteroids enhance salsalate elimination. Food and antacids delay and decrease absorption of salsalate.

Effects on diagnostic tests

Doses of 1 to 8 g/day or more may cause false-positive copper sulfate uric test results or false-negative enzymatic uric sugar test results. False elevations of serum uric acid tests may result. Salsalate may interfere with the Gerhardt test for uric aceto-acetic acid. Increases or decreases of urine vanillylmandelic acid (VMA) may occur. Physiologic effects of the drug may increase serum AST (SGOT), prothrombin time, and T_3 resin uptake; the drug may decrease uric phenolsulfonphthalein concentrations, serum T_3 and T_4 concentrations, serum potassium levels, and serum cholesterol levels. Increases or decreases in serum uric acid levels may be seen.

Adverse reactions

● DERM: rash, bruising.
● EENT: tinnitus and hearing loss.
● GI: nausea, vomiting, GI distress, occult bleeding.
● Other: hypersensitivity manifested by *anaphylaxis* or asthma, abnormal liver function tests, *hepatitis*.

Note: Drug should be discontinued if hypersensitivity, hepatotoxicity, or salicylism occurs.

Overdose and treatment

Clinical manifestations of overdose, which include metabolic acidosis with respiratory alkalosis, hyperpnea, and tachypnea, are caused by increased CO_2 production and direct stimulation of the respiratory center.

To treat salsalate overdose, empty stomach immediately by inducing emesis with ipecac syrup or by gastric lavage. Administer activated charcoal via nasogastric tube. Provide symptomatic and supportive measures (respiratory support and correction of fluid and electrolyte imbalances). Monitor laboratory parameters and vital signs closely. Alkaline diuresis may enhance renal excretion.

▶ Special considerations

Besides those relevant to all *salicylates,* consider the following recommendations.
● Drug is not absorbed until it reaches the small intestine.
● Monitor patient's serum laboratory tests.
● Do not administer salsalate with any alcohol-containing products. May cause increased GI irritation and possibly GI bleeding.
● Store tightly closed in a cool, dry place away from light.

Information for the patient
● Instruct patient to follow prescribed regimen.
● Warn patient to avoid concurrent use of alcohol when taking salsalate.
● Advise patient to report any adverse reactions.
● Instruct patient to keep medication out of children's reach.

Geriatric use
● Patients over age 60 are more sensitive to the adverse effects of salsalate.
● Because of its effect on renal prostaglandins, salsalate may cause fluid retention and edema. This may be significant in elderly patients, especially those with congestive heart failure.

Pediatric use
Safe use in children has not been established.

Breast-feeding
Safety has not been established. Avoid use in breast-feeding women.

---

sargramostim (granulocyte macrophage-colony stimulating factor, GM-CSF)
Leukine, Prokine

● Pharmacologic classification: biologic response modifier
● Therapeutic classification: colony stimulating factor
● Pregnancy risk category C

How supplied
Available by prescription only
Injection (preservative-free): 250 mcg, 500 mcg (as lyophilized powder) in single-dose vials

---

Indications, route, and dosage
Acceleration of hematopoietic reconstitution after autologous bone marrow transplantation in patients with non-Hodgkin's lymphoma, acute lymphoblastic leukemia, or Hodgkin's disease undergoing autologous bone marrow transplantation (BMT)

Adults: 250 mcg/m² daily for 21 consecutive days given as a 2-hour I.V. infusion daily beginning 2 to 4 hours after the bone marrow transplant. Do not administer within 24 hours of last dose of chemotherapy or within 12 hours after the last dose of radiotherapy because of the potential sensitivity of rapidly dividing progenitor cells to cytotoxic chemotherapeutic or radiologic therapies.

Reduce dosage by half or temporarily discontinue if severe adverse reactions occur. Therapy may be resumed when reaction abates. If blast cells appear or increase to 10% or more of the WBC count or if progression of the underlying disease occurs, discontinue therapy. If absolute neutrophil count is above 20,000 cells/mm³ or if WBC counts are above 50,000 cells/mm³, therapy should be discontinued temporarily and the dose reduced by half.

Bone marrow transplantation failure or engraftment delay
Adults: 250 mcg/m² daily for 14 days as a 2-hour I.V. infusion. The same course may be repeated after 7 days off therapy if engraftment has not occurred. A third course of 500 mcg/m² daily for 14 days may be given after another 7 days off therapy if engraftment has not occurred.

Pharmacodynamics
Sargramostim is a 127-amino acid glycoprotein manufactured by recombinant DNA technology in a yeast expression system. It differs from the natural human granulocyte-macrophage colony stimulating factor by substitution of leucine for arginine at position 23. The carbohydrate moiety may also be different. Sargramostim induces cellular responses by binding to specific receptors on cell surfaces of target cells. Blood counts return to normal or baseline levels within 3 to 7 days after stopping treatment.

Pharmacokinetics
• *Absorption:* Blood levels are detected within 5 minutes after I.V. administration; peak levels, within 2 hours.
• *Distribution:* Bound to specific receptors on target cells.
• *Metabolism:* Undetermined.
• *Excretion:* Unknown.

Contraindications and precautions
Sargramostim is contraindicated in patients with excessive leukemic myeloid blasts in bone marrow or peripheral blood and in patients with known hypersensitivity to the drug, any of its components, or yeast-derived products. Use with caution in patients with pre-existing cardiac disease, hypoxia, preexisting fluid retention, pulmonary infiltrates, CHF, or impaired renal or hepatic function, as these conditions may be exacerbated.

Interactions
Lithium and corticosteroids should be used with caution because they may potentiate sargramostim's myeloproliferative effects.

Effects on diagnostic tests
No interference reported. Since hematopoiesis is stimulated, effects on CBC and differential blood counts will be noted.

Adverse reactions
• CNS: malaise, CNS disorder, asthenia.
• CV: *blood dyscrasias,* hemorrhage.
• DERM: alopecia, rash.
• GI: nausea, vomiting, diarrhea, anorexia, hemorrhage, stomatitis, liver damage.
• GU: urinary tract disorder, abnormal kidney function.
• Respiratory: dyspnea.
• Other: fever, edema, peripheral edema, *sepsis.*

Overdose and treatment
Doses up to 16 times the recommended dose have been administered with the following reversible adverse reactions: WBC counts up to 200,000/mm³, dyspnea, malaise, nausea, fever, rash, sinus tachycardia, headache, and chills. The maximum dose that can be administered safely has yet to be determined. If overdose is suspected, monitor WBC count increase and respiratory symptoms.

▶ Special considerations
• Stimulation of marrow precursors may result in rapid rise of WBC count; biweekly monitoring of CBC with differential, including examination for blast cells, is recommended.
• Transient rashes and local injection site reactions may occur; no serious allergic or anaphylactic reactions have been reported.
• Sargramostim can act as a growth factor for any tumor type, particularly myeloid malignancies.
• Unlabeled indications include use to increase WBC counts in patients with myelodysplastic syndromes and in acquired immunodeficiency syndrome patients on zidovudine; to decrease nadir of leukopenia secondary to myelosuppressive chemotherapy; to decrease myelosuppression in preleukemic patients; to correct neutropenia in aplastic anemia; and to decrease transplant-associated organ system damage, particularly of the liver and kidneys.
• Sargramostim is effective in accelerating myeloid recovery in patients receiving bone marrow purged from monoclonal antibodies.
• The effect of sargramostim may be limited in patients who have received extensive radiotherapy to hematopoietic sites for treatment of primary disease in the abdomen or chest or have been exposed to multiple agents (alkylating agents, anthracycline antibiotics, antimetabolites) before autologous BMT.
• Refrigerate the sterile powder, the reconstituted solution, and the diluted solution for injection. Do not freeze or shake. Do not use after expiration date.
• To prepare, reconstitute with 1 ml sterile water for injection. Do not reenter or reuse the single-dose vial. Discard any unused portion. Direct stream of sterile water against side of vial and *gently swirl* contents to minimize foaming. Avoid excessive or vigorous agitation or shaking. Dilute in 0.9% sodium chloride. If final concentration is below 10 mcg/ml, add albumin (human) at a final concentration of 0.1% to the saline *before* addition of sargramostim to prevent adsorption to components of the delivery system. For a final concentration of 0.1% human albumin, add 1 mg human albumin/ml sodium chloride. Administer as soon as possible after admixture, as sargramostim has no preservative, and

within 6 hours of reconstitution or dilution. Do not add other medications to infusion solution without compatibility and stability data. Discard any unused solution after 6 hours.

● Refrigerate the sterile powder, the reconstituted solution, and the diluted solution for injection. Do not freeze or shake. Do not use after expiration date.

Pediatric use
Safety and efficacy have not been established; however, available data suggest that no differences in toxicity exist. The type and frequency of adverse reactions were comparable to those seen in adults.

Breast-feeding
It is unknown if sargramostim is excreted in breast milk; use with caution.

---

scopolamine
Transderm Scōp, Transderm V*

scopolamine hydrobromide
Isopto Hyoscine, Triptone

- Pharmacologic classification: anticholinergic
- Therapeutic classification: antimuscarinic, antiemetic/antivertigo agent, antiparkinsonian agent, cycloplegic mydriatic
- Pregnancy risk category C

How supplied
Available by prescription only
Transdermal patch: 1.5 mg
Injection: 0.3, 0.4, 0.5, 0.86, and 1 mg/ml in 1-ml vials and ampules; 0.86 mg/ml in 0.5-ml ampules
Ophthalmic solution: 0.25%

Indications, route, and dosage
Antimuscarinic; adjunct to anesthesia
Adults: 0.3 to 0.6 I.M. or I.V. as a single dose.
Children over age 8 to 12 years: 300 mcg I.M. or I.V.
Children over age 3 to 8 years: 200 mcg I.M. or I.V.
Children age 8 months to 3 years: 150 mcg I.M. or I.V.
Infants age 4 to 7 months: 100 mcg I.M. or I.V.
Prevention of nausea and vomiting associated with motion sickness
Adults: 1 transdermal patch designed to deliver 0.5 mg/day over 3 days (72 hours), applied to the skin behind the ear at least 4 hours before the antiemetic is required.
Not recommended for children.
Postencephalitic parkinsonism and other spastic states
Adults: 0.3 to 0.6 S.C., I.M., or I.V. (with suitable dilution) t.i.d. to q.i.d.
Children: 0.006 mg/kg S.C. t.i.d. to q.i.d.; or 0.2 mg/m².
Infants age 4 to 7 months: 0.1 mg I.M. or S.C.
Cycloplegic refraction
Adults: 1 to 2 drops 0.25% solution in eye 1 hour before refraction.
Children: 1 drop 0.25% solution b.i.d. for 2 days before refraction.
Iritis, uveitis
Adults: 1 to 2 drops of 0.25% solution daily, b.i.d., or t.i.d.

Pharmacodynamics
Scopolamine's main therapeutic effects involve antimuscarinic, antiemetic, antiparkinsonian, and mydriatic activities.

● *Antimuscarinic action:* Scopolamine inhibits acetylcholine's muscarinic actions on autonomic effectors, resulting in decreased secretions and GI motility; it also blocks vagal inhibition of the sinoatrial node.
● *Antiemetic action:* Although its exact mechanism of action is unknown, scopolamine may affect neural pathways affecting the vestibular input to the CNS originating in the labyrinth of the ear, thereby inhibiting nausea and vomiting in patients with motion sickness.
● *Antiparkinsonian action:* Scopolamine blocks central cholinergic receptors, helping to balance cholinergic activity in the basal ganglia. It may also prolong dopamine's effects by blocking dopamine reuptake and storage at central receptor sites.
● *Mydriatic action:* Scopolamine competitively blocks acetylcholine at cholinergic neuroeffector sites, antagonizing acetylcholine's effects on the sphincter muscle and ciliary body, thereby producing mydriasis and cycloplegia; these effects are used to produce cycloplegic refraction and pupil dilation to treat preoperative and postoperative iridocyclitis.

Pharmacokinetics
● *Absorption:* Scopolamine is well absorbed percutaneously from behind the ear; antiemetic effects begin several hours after application. Scopolamine is well absorbed from the GI tract. It is absorbed rapidly when administered I.M. or S.C. Effects occur 15 to 30 minutes after I.M. or S.C. administration. Systemic scopolamine absorption may occur from drug passage through the nasolacrimal duct. Ophthalmic mydriatic effect peaks at 20 to 30 minutes after administration; cycloplegic effects peak 30 to 60 minutes after administration.
● *Distribution:* Scopolamine is distributed widely throughout body tissues. It crosses the placenta and probably the blood-brain barrier.
● *Metabolism:* Scopolamine is probably metabolized completely in the liver; however, its exact metabolic fate is unknown. Mydriatic and cycloplegic effects persist for 3 to 7 days.
● *Excretion:* Scopolamine is probably excreted in urine as metabolites.

Contraindications and precautions
Scopolamine is contraindicated in patients with glaucoma or a tendency toward glaucoma, because drug-induced cycloplegia and mydriasis may increase intraocular pressure; and in patients with obstructive uropathy, obstructive GI tract disease, asthma, chronic pulmonary disease, myasthenia gravis, paralytic ileus, intestinal atony, or toxic megacolon, because the drug may exacerbate these conditions.

Administer scopolamine cautiously to patients with autonomic neuropathy, hyperthyroidism, coronary artery disease, congestive heart failure, hypertension, or ulcerative colitis, because the drug may exacerbate these conditions; to patients with hepatic or renal disease, because toxic accumulation may occur; to patients with cardiac arrhythmias, because the drug may block vagal inhibition of the sinoatrial node pacemaker, worsening the arrhythmia; to patients with hiatal hernia associated with reflux esophagitis, because this drug may decrease lower esophageal sphincter tone; to patients over age 40, because the drug increases the glaucoma risk; to young children, because they may

---

be more sensitive to drug effects; and to patients with known hypersensitivity to belladonna alkaloids.

Interactions

Concomitant use of scopolamine with CNS depressants (alcohol, tranquilizers, and sedative-hypnotics) may increase CNS depression.

Concurrent administration of antacids decreases oral absorption of anticholinergics. Administer scopolamine at least 1 hour before antacids.

Concomitant administration of drugs with anticholinergic effects may cause additive toxicity.

Decreased GI absorption of many drugs has been reported after the use of anticholinergics (for example, levodopa and ketoconazole). Conversely, slowly dissolving digoxin tablets may yield higher serum digoxin levels when administered with anticholinergics.

Use cautiously with oral potassium supplements (especially wax-matrix formulations) because the incidence of potassium-induced GI ulcerations may be increased.

Effects on diagnostic tests

None reported.

Adverse reactions

● CNS: headache, disorientation, restlessness, drowsiness, irritability, dizziness, hallucinations, memory disturbances, confusion, violent behavior, amnesia, unconsciousness, spastic extremities.
● CV: palpitations, tachycardia, paradoxical bradycardia.
● DERM: flushing, dryness, rash, erythema.
● EENT: dilated pupils; blurred vision; photophobia; cycloplegia; increased intraocular pressure; dry, itchy, or red eyes; acute narrow-angle glaucoma; ocular congestion (prolonged use).
● GI: constipation, dry mouth, dysphagia, nausea, vomiting, epigastric distress.
● GU: dysuria.
● Other: bronchial plug formation, fever, respiratory depression.
  Note: Drug should be discontinued if urinary retention, confusion, difficulty breathing, hypersensitivity, or eye pain occurs.

Overdose and treatment

Clinical effects of overdose include excitability, seizures, CNS stimulation followed by depression, and such psychotic symptoms as disorientation, confusion, hallucinations, delusions, anxiety, agitation, and restlessness. Peripheral effects include dilated, nonreactive pupils; blurred vision; flushed, hot, dry skin; dryness of mucous membranes; dysphagia; decreased or absent bowel sounds; urinary retention; hyperthermia; tachycardia; hypertension; and increased respiration.

Treatment is primarily symptomatic and supportive, as needed. Maintain patent airway. If patient is awake and alert, induce emesis (or use gastric lavage) and follow with a saline cathartic and activated charcoal to prevent further drug absorption. In severe cases, physostigmine may be administered to block scopolamine's antimuscarinic effects. Give fluids, as needed, to treat shock; diazepam to control psychotic symptoms; and pilocarpine (instilled into the eyes) to relieve mydriasis. If urinary retention develops, catheterization may be necessary. Mild symptoms will be transient and disappear after removing patch.

▶ Special considerations

Besides those relevant to all *anticholinergics*, consider the following recommendations.
● Therapeutic doses may produce amnesia, drowsiness, and euphoria (desired effects for use as an adjunct to anesthesia. As necessary, reorient patient.
● Some patients (especially the elderly) may experience transient excitement or disorientation.

Transdermal
● Transdermal patch releases controlled therapeutic dose.
● Withdrawal symptoms (such as nausea, vomiting, headache, dizziness, and equilibrium disturbances) may occur if the transdermal system is used longer than 72 hours.
● To apply transdermal patch, first wash and dry hands thoroughly, then apply patch on dry skin behind patient's ear.

Ophthalmic
● Apply pressure to the lacrimal sac for 1 minute after instillation to reduce the risk of systemic drug absorption.
● Have patient lie down, tilt his head back, or look at ceiling to aid instillation.

Information for the patient
Transdermal
● Inform patient that he can obtain literature on transdermal patch from pharmacist.
● Caution patient to wash his hands after applying transdermal patch – particularly before touching the eye (scopolamine may cause pupil dilation).
● To ensure optimal effectiveness, advise patient to apply transdermal patch the night before a planned trip. Patch becomes effective after 4 hours and lasts 72 hours.
● After removing patch, patient should discard it, then thoroughly wash hands and application site.

Ophthalmic
● Instruct patient to apply pressure to bridge of nose for about 1 minute after instillation.
● Advise patient not to close eyes tightly or blink for about 1 minute after instillation.

Geriatric use

Use caution when administering scopolamine to elderly patients. Lower doses are indicated.

Breast-feeding

Scopolamine may be excreted in breast milk, possibly resulting in infant toxicity. Breast-feeding women should avoid this drug. Drug may decrease milk production.

---

secobarbital sodium
Novosecobarb*, Seconal

- Pharmacologic classification: barbiturate
- Therapeutic classification: sedative-hypnotic, anticonvulsant
- Controlled substance schedule II (suppositories are schedule III)
- Pregnancy risk category D

How supplied
Available by prescription only
Injection: 50 mg/ml in 1-ml and 2-ml disposable syringe; 50 mg/ml in 20-ml vial
Capsules: 50 mg, 100 mg
Tablets: 100 mg
Rectal suppositories: 200 mg

Indications, route, and dosage
Preoperative sedation
Adults: 200 to 300 mg P.O. 1 to 2 hours before surgery.
Children: 50 to 100 mg P.O. or 4 to 5 mg/kg rectally 1 to 2 hours before surgery.
Insomnia
Adults: 100 to 200 mg P.O. or I.M.
Children: 3 to 5 mg/kg I.M., not to exceed 100 mg, with no more than 5 ml injected in any one site. Or 4 to 5 mg/kg rectally.
Acute tetanus convulsion
Adults and children: 5.5 mg/kg I.M. or slow I.V., repeated q 3 to 4 hours, if needed; I.V. injection rate not to exceed 50 mg/15 seconds.
Acute psychotic agitation
Adults: Initially, 50 mg/minute I.V. up to 250 mg I.V.; additional doses given cautiously after 5 minutes if desired response is not obtained. Not to exceed 500 mg total.
Status epilepticus
Adults and children: 250 to 350 mg I.M. or I.V.

Pharmacodynamics
Sedative-hypnotic action: Secobarbital acts throughout the CNS as a nonselective depressant with a rapid onset of action and short duration of action. Particularly sensitive to this drug is the reticular activating system, which controls CNS arousal. Secobarbital decreases both presynaptic and postsynaptic membrane excitability by facilitating the action of gamma-aminobutyric acid (GABA). The exact cellular site and mechanism(s) of action are unknown.

Pharmacokinetics
- *Absorption:* After oral administration, 90% of secobarbital is absorbed rapidly. After rectal administration, secobarbital is nearly 100% absorbed. Peak serum concentration after oral or rectal administration occurs between 2 and 4 hours. The onset of action is rapid, occurring within 15 minutes when administered orally. Peak effects are seen 15 to 30 minutes after oral and rectal administration, 7 to 10 minutes after I.M. administration, and 1 to 3 minutes after I.V. administration. Concentrations of 1 to 5 mcg/ml are needed to produce sedation; 5 to 15 mcg/ml are needed for hypnosis. Hypnosis lasts for 1 to 4 hours after oral doses of 100 to 150 mg.
- *Distribution:* Secobarbital is distributed rapidly throughout body tissues and fluids; approximately 30% to 45% is protein-bound.
- *Metabolism:* Secobarbital is oxidized in the liver to inactive metabolites. Duration of action is 3 to 4 hours.
- *Excretion:* 95% of a secobarbital dose is eliminated as glucuronide conjugates and other metabolites in urine.

Contraindications and precautions
Secobarbital is contraindicated in patients with known hypersensitivity to barbiturates and in patients with bronchopneumonia, status asthmaticus, or other severe respiratory distress because of the potential for respiratory depression. Secobarbital should not be used in patients who are depressed or have suicidal ideation, because the drug can worsen depression; in patients with uncontrolled acute or chronic pain, because exacerbation of pain and paradoxical excitement can occur; and in patients with porphyria, because this drug can trigger symptoms of this disease.

Secobarbital should be used cautiously in patients who must perform hazardous tasks requiring mental alertness, because the drug causes drowsiness. Administer parenteral phenobarbital slowly and with extreme caution to patients with hypotension or severe pulmonary or cardiovascular disease because of potential adverse hemodynamic effects. Because tolerance and physical or psychological dependence may occur, prolonged use of high doses should be avoided.

Prenatal exposure to barbiturates is associated with an increased incidence of fetal abnormalities, and possibly brain tumors. Use of barbiturates in the third trimester may be associated with physical dependence in neonates. Risk-benefit must be considered.

Interactions
Secobarbital may add to or potentiate CNS and respiratory depressant effects of other sedative-hypnotics, antihistamines, narcotics, antidepressants, tranquilizers, and alcohol.

Secobarbital enhances the enzymatic degradation of warfarin and other oral anticoagulants; patients may require increased doses of the anticoagulant. Drug also enhances hepatic metabolism of some drugs, including digitoxin (not digoxin), corticosteroids, oral contraceptives and other estrogens, theophylline and other xanthines, and doxycycline. Secobarbital impairs the effectiveness of griseofulvin by decreasing absorption from the GI tract.

Valproic acid, phenytoin, disulfiram, and monoamine oxidase inhibitors decrease the metabolism of secobarbital and can increase its toxicity. Rifampin may decrease secobarbital levels by increasing metabolism.

Effects on diagnostic tests
Secobarbital may cause a false-positive phentolamine test. The physiologic effects of the drug may impair the absorption of cyanocobalamin C_o57; it may decrease serum bilirubin concentrations in neonates, epileptic patients, and in patients with congenital nonhemolytic unconjugated hyperbilirubinemia. EEG patterns show a change in low-voltage, fast activity; changes persist for a time after discontinuation of therapy.

Adverse reactions
- *CNS:* drowsiness, lethargy, vertigo, headache, CNS depression, paradoxical excitement, confusion and agitation (especially in elderly patients), rebound insom-

nia, increased dreams or nightmares, possibly seizures (after acute withdrawal or reduction in dosage).
- CV: hypotension (after rapid I.V. administration), bradycardia, *circulatory collapse.*
- DERM: urticaria, rash, *exfoliative dermatitis, Stevens-Johnson syndrome.*
- EENT: miosis.
- GI: nausea, vomiting, diarrhea, constipation.
- Local: thrombophlebitis, pain and possible tissue damage at site of extravascular injection.
- Other: *respiratory depression,* laryngospasm, *bronchospasm.* Reported vitamin K deficiency and bleeding have occurred in newborns of mothers treated during pregnancy. Hyperalgesia may occur with low doses or in patients with chronic pain.

Note: Drug should be discontinued if hypersensitivity reaction, profound CNS or respiratory depression, or skin eruption occurs.

Overdose and treatment
Clinical manifestations of overdose include unsteady gait, slurred speech, sustained nystagmus, somnolence, confusion, respiratory depression, pulmonary edema, areflexia, and coma. Typical shock syndrome with tachycardia and hypotension, jaundice, hypothermia followed by fever, and oliguria may occur.

Maintain and support ventilation and pulmonary function as necessary; support cardiac function and circulation with vasopressors and I.V. fluids as needed. If patient is conscious and gag reflex is intact, induce emesis (if ingestion was recent) by administering ipecac syrup. If emesis is contraindicated, perform gastric lavage while a cuffed endotracheal tube is in place to prevent aspiration. Follow with administration of activated charcoal or saline cathartic. Measure intake and output, vital signs, and laboratory parameters; maintain body temperature. Patient should be rolled from side to side every 30 minutes to avoid pulmonary congestion.

Alkalinization of urine may be helpful in removing drug from the body; hemodialysis may be useful in severe overdose.

▶ Special considerations
Besides those relevant to all *barbiturates,* consider the following recommendations.
- Use I.V. route of administration only in emergencies or when other routes are unavailable.
- Dilute secobarbital injection with sterile water for injection solution, 0.9% sodium chloride injection, or Ringer's injection solution. Total I.V. dose should not exceed 500 mg. Do not use if solution is discolored or if a precipitate forms.
- Avoid I.V. administration at a rate greater than 50 mg/ 15 seconds to prevent hypotension and respiratory depression. Have emergency resuscitative equipment on hand.
- Administer I.M. dose deep into large muscle mass to prevent tissue injury.
- Store rectal suppositories in refrigerator. To ensure accurate dosage, do not divide suppository.
- Secobarbital sodium injection, diluted with lukewarm tap water to a concentration of 10 to 15 mg/ml, may be administered rectally in children. A cleansing enema should be administered before secobarbital enema.
- Monitor hepatic and renal studies frequently to prevent possible toxicity.

Information for the patient
Emphasize the danger of combining this drug with alcohol. An excessive depressive effect is possible even if the drug is taken the evening before ingestion of alcohol.

Geriatric use
Elderly patients are more susceptible to effects of secobarbital and usually require lower doses. Confusion, disorientation, and excitability may occur in elderly patients.

Pediatric use
Secobarbital may cause paradoxical excitement in children; use cautiously.

Breast-feeding
Secobarbital passes into breast milk; do not administer to breast-feeding women.

---

selegiline hydrochloride (L-deprenyl hydrochloride)
Eldepryl

- Pharmacologic classification: MAO inhibitor
- Therapeutic classification: antiparkinsonian agent
- Pregnancy risk category C

How supplied
Available by prescription only
Tablets: 5 mg

Indications, route, and dosage
Adjunctive treatment to carbidopa-levodopa in the management of the symptoms associated with Parkinson's disease
Adults: 10 mg P.O. daily, taken as 5 mg at breakfast and 5 mg at lunch. After 2 or 3 days of therapy, begin gradual decrease of carbidopa-levodopa dosage.

Pharmacodynamics
Antiparkinsonian action: Probably acts by selectively inhibiting MAO type B (found mostly in the brain). At higher-than-recommended doses, it is a nonselective inhibitor of MAO, including MAO type A found in the GI tract. It may also directly increase dopaminergic activity by decreasing the reuptake of dopamine into nerve cells. It has pharmacologically active metabolites (amphetamine and methamphetamine) that may contribute to this effect.

Pharmacokinetics
- *Absorption:* Little is known about the absorption of selegiline.
- *Distribution:* After a single dose, plasma levels are below detectable levels (less than 10 ng/ml).
- *Metabolism:* Three metabolites have been detected in the serum and urine: N-desmethyldeprenyl, amphetamine, and methamphetamine.
- *Excretion:* 45% of the drug appears as a metabolite in the urine after 48 hours.

Contraindications and precautions
Selegiline is contraindicated in patients hypersensitive to the drug.

Some patients may experience an exacerbation of levodopa-induced adverse effects (including GI or CNS disturbances). Such effects may be ameliorated by decreasing the dosage of carbidopa-levodopa.

Interactions
Concomitant use with adrenergic agents may increase the pressor response, particularly in patients who have taken an overdose of selegiline.

Effects on diagnostic tests
None reported.

Adverse reactions
● CNS: dizziness, increased tremor, chorea, loss of balance, restlessness, blepharospasm, increased bradykinesia, facial grimace, stiff neck, dyskinesia, syncope, behavioral changes, tiredness, involuntary movements, increased apraxia, headache.
● CV: orthostatic hypotension, hypertension, hypotension, arrhythmias, palpitations, new or increased anginal pain, tachycardia, peripheral edema.
● DERM: rash, hair loss, sweating.
● GI: nausea, vomiting, constipation, weight loss, anorexia or poor appetite, dysphagia, diarrhea, heartburn, dry mouth, taste disturbance.
● GU: slow urination, transient nocturia, prostatic hypertrophy, urinary hesitancy, urinary frequency, urine retention.
● Other: malaise, sexual dysfunction.

Overdose and treatment
Limited experience with overdosage suggests that symptoms may include hypotension and psychomotor agitation. Because selegiline becomes a nonselective MAO inhibitor in high doses, consider the possibility of symptoms of MAO inhibitor poisoning: drowsiness, dizziness, hyperactivity, agitation, seizures, coma, hypertension, hypotension, cardiac conduction disturbances, and CV collapse. These symptoms may not develop immediately after ingestion (delays of 12 hours or more are possible).

Provide supportive treatment and closely monitor the patient for worsening of symptoms. Emesis or lavage may be helpful in the early stages of overdose treatment. Avoid phenothiazine derivatives and CNS stimulants; adrenergic agents may provoke an exaggerated response. Diazepam may be useful in treating seizures.

▶ Special considerations
In some patients who experience an increase of adverse reactions associated with levodopa (including muscle twitches), reduction of carbidopa-levodopa is necessary. Most of these patients require a carbidopa-levodopa dosage reduction of 10% to 30%.

Information for the patient
● Advise patient not to take more than 10 mg daily. There is no evidence that higher dosage improves efficacy and it may increase adverse reactions.
● Warn patients to move about cautiously at the start of therapy because they may experience dizziness, which can cause them to fall.
● Because the drug is an MAO inhibitor, tell patients about the possibility of an interaction with tyramine-containing foods. They should immediately report any

signs or symptoms of hypertension, including severe headache. Reportedly, however, this interaction does not occur at the recommended dosage; at 10 mg daily the drug inhibits only MAO type B. Therefore, dietary restrictions appear unnecessary, provided the patient does not exceed the recommended dose.
● Emphasize the danger of combining this drug with alcohol. An excessive depressant effect is possible even if the drug is taken the evening before ingestion of alcohol.

Breast-feeding
It is not known if the drug is excreted in breast milk. Use with caution in breast-feeding women.

sermorelin acetate
Geref

● Pharmacologic classification: polypeptide
● Therapeutic classification: growth hormone releasing hormone (GHRH)
● Pregnancy risk category C

How supplied
Available by prescription only
Powder for injection: 50 mcg/ampule

Indications, route, and dosage
Diagnostic aid to determine the pituitary gland's ability to secrete growth hormone
Adults and children: 1 mcg/kg as a single I.V. injection.

Pharmacodynamics
Growth hormone releasing action: Sermorelin mimics the aminoterminal segment of the naturally occurring human GH.

Pharmacokinetics
Unknown.

Contraindications and precautions
Sermorelin is contraindicated in patients with hypersensitivity to the drug or any components of the formulation.

Although hypersensitivity reactions have been reported with the administration of other polypeptide hormones, none have been reported with sermorelin. About 25% of patients develop antibody formation with prolonged use, but no symptomatic allergic reactions have been reported.

Interactions
Don't perform the test in patients receiving drugs that alter the pituitary secretion of somatotropin, such as corticosteroids, insulin, and cyclo-oxygenase inhibitors (for example, aspirin, acetaminophen, or NSAIDs).

Somatotropin levels may be elevated by clonidine, levodopa, or insulin-induced hypoglycemia.

Response to the drug may be blunted in hypothyroid patients, in patients receiving antithyroid drugs such as propylthiouracil, and in those receiving anticholinergics.

Effects on diagnostic tests
In clinical trials, GH peak plasma levels of 28 ± 15 ng/ml occur at 30 ± 27 minutes after the injection.

Adverse reactions
● CNS: headache.
● GI: nausea.
● Local: pain, redness, or swelling at the injection site.
● Other: transient warmth or flushing of the face, unusual taste in the mouth, antibody formation, paleness, tightness in the chest.

Overdose and treatment
Other GNRH analogues have caused changes in heart rate and blood pressure. Cardiovascular collapse is possible but hasn't been reported. Treat symptomatically.

▶ Special considerations
● Discontinue GH therapy 1 week before the test.
● One ampule contains 50 mcg of drug, which is sufficient to test a 110-lb (50-kg) subject. Larger subjects will require the use of multiple ampules. Reconstitute each ampule with a minimum of 0.5 ml of the supplied diluent.
● Venous blood samples for GH determinations should be drawn 15 minutes before and immediately before injection. Administer bolus injection (1 mcg/kg I.V.) and follow with a 3-ml saline flush. Venous samples for GH determinations should also be drawn at 15-minute intervals after injection (15 minutes, 30 minutes, 45 minutes, and 60 minutes).
● Baseline GH levels are generally low (< 4 ng/ml). Provocative tests such as sermorelin are useful in determining that the pituitary somatotroph can respond. However, a normal response won't rule out GH deficiency if the deficit is caused by hypothalamic dysfunction. This test is most easily interpreted if patient has had a subnormal response to conventional provocative testing (such as clonidine, levodopa, or arginine) and a normal response to sermorelin, suggesting that the cause of GH deficiency is hypothalamic dysfunction. Abnormal results from both conventional tests and sermorelin can't locate the dysfunction.

Information for the patient
Be sure patient understands that the test must be performed in the morning after an overnight fast. He should take nothing by mouth after midnight.

Geriatric use
An age-related decline in responsiveness to GHRH hasn't been fully characterized.

Breast-feeding
It is unknown if drug is excreted in breast milk. Use with caution in breast-feeding women.

senna
Black Draught, Fletcher's Castoria, Genna, Gentlax-B, Gentle Nature, Nytilax, Senexon, Senokot, Senolax, X-Prep

● Pharmacologic classification: anthraquinone derivative
● Therapeutic classification: stimulant laxative
● Pregnancy risk category C

How supplied
Available without prescription
Tablets: 187 mg, 217 mg, 600 mg
Granules: 326 mg/tsp, 1.65 g/½ tsp
Suppositories: 652 mg
Syrup: 218 mg/5 ml

Indications, route, and dosage
Acute constipation, preparation for bowel examination
Black Draught tablets
Adults: 2 tablets or ¼ to ½ level tsp of granules mixed with water. Not recommended for children.
Other preparations
Adults: Usual dose is two tablets, 1 tsp of granules dissolved in water, or 10 to 15 ml of syrup h.s.; not to exceed four tablets b.i.d. or 2 tsp of granules b.i.d.
   X-Prep liquid is used solely as a single dose for preradiographic bowel evacuation. Give 20 mg powder dissolved in juice or 75 ml liquid between 2 p.m. and 4 p.m. on day before procedure. Dose may be divided for elderly or debilitated patients.
Children over 27 kg: One tablet, ½ tsp of granules dissolved in water, or ½ suppository h.s.
Children under 27 kg: Follow manufacturer's recommendation.

Pharmacodynamics
Laxative action: Senna has a local irritant effect on the colon, which promotes peristalsis and bowel evacuation. It also enhances intestinal fluid accumulation, thereby increasing the stool's moisture content.

Pharmacokinetics
● *Absorption:* Senna is absorbed minimally. With oral administration, laxative effect occurs in 6 to 10 hours; with suppository administration, laxative effect occurs in 30 minutes to 2 hours.
● *Distribution:* Senna may be distributed in bile, saliva, the colonic mucosa, and breast milk.
● *Metabolism:* Absorbed portion is metabolized in the liver.
● *Excretion:* Unabsorbed senna is excreted mainly in feces; absorbed drug is excreted in urine and feces.

Contraindications and precautions
Senna is contraindicated in patients with fluid and electrolyte disturbances, appendicitis, abdominal pain, nausea or vomiting, fecal impaction, or intestinal obstruction or perforation, because the drug may worsen these conditions or symptoms.

Interactions
None reported.

Effects on diagnostic tests

In the phenolsulfonphthalein excretion test, senna may turn urine pink to red, red to violet, or red to brown.

Adverse reactions

● GI: nausea; vomiting; diarrhea; loss of normal bowel function in excessive use; abdominal cramps, especially in severe constipation; malabsorption of nutrients; "cathartic colon" (syndrome resembling ulcerative colitis radiologically) in chronic misuse; constipation after catharsis; yellow or yellow-green cast feces; diarrhea in breast-feeding infants of mothers on senna; darkened pigmentation of rectal mucosa in long-term use (usually reversible within 4 to 12 months after stopping drug).
● GU: red-pink discoloration in alkaline urine; yellow-brown color in acidic urine.
● Metabolic: hypokalemia, protein enteropathy, electrolyte imbalance in excessive use.
● Other: laxative dependence in long-term or excessive use.

Note: Drug should be discontinued if abdominal pain develops.

Overdose and treatment

No information available.

▶ Special considerations

● When administering X-Prep, limit patient's diet to clear liquids to ensure adequate evacuation.
● Protect drug from excessive heat or light.

Information for the patient

● Warn patient that drug may turn urine pink, red, violet, or brown, depending on urinary pH.
● Tell patient that bowel movement may have a yellow or yellow-green cast.

Geriatric use

Elderly persons often overuse laxatives and may be more prone to laxative dependency.

Pediatric use

Senna and other stimulant laxatives usually are not used in children.

Breast-feeding

Senna enters breast milk; diarrhea has been reported in breast-feeding infants.

sertraline hydrochloride
Zoloft

● Pharmacologic classification: serotonin uptake inhibitor
● Therapeutic classification: antidepressant
● Pregnancy risk category B

How supplied

Available by prescription only
Tablets: 50 mg, 100 mg

Indications, route, and dosage
Depression; obsessive-compulsive disorder

Adults: 50 mg P.O. daily. Adjust dosage as needed and tolerated; clinical trials involved dosage of 50 to 200 mg daily. Dosage adjustments should be made at intervals of no less than 1 week.

Pharmacodynamics

Antidepressant action: Sertraline probably acts by blocking the reuptake of serotonin (5-hydroxytryptamine; 5-HT) into presynaptic neurons in the CNS, prolonging the action of 5-HT.

Pharmacokinetics

● *Absorption:* Sertraline is well absorbed after oral administration; absorption rate and extent is enhanced when taken with food. Peak serum levels occur between 4.5 and 8.4 hours after a dose.
● *Distribution:* In vitro studies indicate that drug is highly protein-bound (>98%).
● *Metabolism:* Metabolism is probably hepatic; drug undergoes significant first-pass metabolism. N-desmethylsertraline is substantially less active than the parent compound.
● *Excretion:* Drug is excreted mostly as metabolites in the urine and feces. Mean elimination half-life is 26 hours. Steady-state levels are reached within 1 week of daily dosing in young, healthy patients.

Contraindications and precautions

Sertraline is contraindicated in patients with hypersensitivity to the drug and with or within 14 days of taking an MAO inhibitor.

Because drug is extensively metabolized in the liver, use with caution in patients with hepatic impairment. Also use with caution in patients with seizure disorders, a history of drug abuse, and suicidal ideation. Because the possibility of suicide is inherent in depressed patients, provide close supervision during initiation of drug therapy. Prescriptions for the drug should limit the supply of tablets to reduce the risk of overdose.

Mania or hypomania occurred in a few (0.4%) patients during clinical trials. Like other antidepressants, drug can also activate mania in patients with major affective disorders.

Interactions

Clearance of diazepam and tolbutamide are decreased by sertraline. Clinical significance is unknown; however, monitor patient for increased drug effects.

Concomitant use with MAO inhibitors may cause serious mental status changes, hyperthermia, autonomic instability, rapid fluctuations of vital signs, delirium, coma, and death. Don't administer with or within 14 days after discontinuing an MAO inhibitor. Allow 14 days after discontinuing sertraline before starting an MAO inhibitor.

Warfarin and other highly protein-bound drugs may cause interactions, increasing the plasma levels of sertraline or the other highly bound drug. Small (8%) increases in prothrombin time have occurred with concomitant use of warfarin. Monitor closely.

Effects on diagnostic tests

Minor changes in several laboratory values have occurred in patients taking sertraline. Elevated serum transaminase levels (AST [SGOT], ALT [SGPT]) have occurred, usually within the first 9 weeks of therapy; values returned to normal after discontinuing drug. Minor increases in serum cholesterol and triglycerides and minor decreases in uric acid have been seen. Clinical significance is unknown.

Adverse reactions
● CNS: headache, tremor, dizziness, insomnia, somnolence, syncope, paresthesia, hypoesthesia, hyperesthesia, twitching, hypertonia, confusion, ataxia, abnormal coordination or gait, nystagmus, vertigo, hyperkinesia, hypokinesia, mania.
● CV: palpitations, chest pain, postural hypotension, hypertension, hypotension, edema, peripheral ischemia, tachycardia.
● DERM: rash, acne, pruritus, erythematous or maculopapular rash, dry skin, cold or clammy skin, flushing.
● GI: dry mouth, nausea, diarrhea, loose stools, dyspepsia, vomiting, flatulence, anorexia, abdominal pain, increased appetite, dysphagia.
● Other: increased sweating, male sexual dysfunction, myalgia.

Overdose and treatment
Clinical experience with sertraline overdosage is limited. Treatment is supportive. Establish an airway and maintain adequate ventilation. Because recent studies question the value of forced emesis or lavage, consider the use of activated charcoal in sorbitol to bind any drug in the GI tract.

There is no specific antidote for sertraline. Monitor vital signs closely. Because drug has a large volume of distribution, hemodialysis, peritoneal dialysis, or forced diuresis probably aren't useful.

▶ Special considerations
Patients who respond during the first 8 weeks of therapy will probably continue to respond to drug, although there are limited studies of drug in depressed patients for periods longer than 16 weeks. If patients are continued on drug for prolonged therapy, periodically monitor the effectiveness of drug. It is unknown if periodic dosage adjustments are necessary to maintain effectiveness.

Information for the patient
● Sertraline should be taken once daily, either in the morning or evening. It may be taken with or without food.
● Although problems haven't been reported to date, advise patient to avoid the use of alcohol while taking this drug and to check with the physician or pharmacist before taking any OTC medication.
● Although problems haven't been reported to date, advise patient to use caution when performing hazardous tasks that require alertness, such as driving and operating heavy machinery. Drugs that influence the CNS may impair judgment.

Geriatric use
Plasma clearance of the drug is slower in elderly patients. Studies indicate that it may take 2 to 3 weeks of daily dosing before steady-state levels are reached.

Pediatric use
Safety and efficacy have not been established.

Breast-feeding
It is unknown if drug is excreted in breast milk. Use with caution in breast-feeding women.

silver nitrate, silver nitrate 1%
Dey Drops Silver Nitrate

● Pharmacologic classification: heavy metal (silver compound)
● Therapeutic classification: ophthalmic antiseptic; topical cauterizing agent
● Pregnancy risk category C (1%)

How supplied
Available by prescription only
Ophthalmic solution: 1%
Topical ointment: 10%
Topical solution: 10%, 25%, 50%

Indications, route, and dosage
Prevention of gonorrheal ophthalmia neonatorum
Neonates: Cleanse lids thoroughly; instill 2 drops of 1% solution into lower conjunctival sac of each eye and ensure that solution contacts the entire conjunctival sac for 30 seconds or longer.
To treat indolent wounds, destroy exuberant granulations, freshen the edges of ulcers and fissures, provide styptic action, and treat vesicular bullous or aphthous lesions
Adults: Apply ointment on a pad to lesion for 5 days; or a cotton applicator dipped in solution to affected area two to three times a week for 2 to 3 weeks.

Pharmacodynamics
● *Antiseptic action:* Liberated silver ions precipitate bacterial proteins, resulting in germicidal activity. Drug is effective mainly in preventing gonorrheal ophthalmia neonatorum.
● *Cauterizing action:* Denatures protein, producing a caustic or corrosive effect.

Pharmacokinetics
● *Absorption:* Silver nitrate isn't readily absorbed from mucous membranes or other tissues.
● *Distribution:* Unknown.
● *Metabolism:* Unknown.
● *Excretion:* Unknown.

Contraindications and precautions
Silver nitrate is contraindicated in patients with hypersensitivity to the preparation or any of its components. For ophthalmic use, the 1% solution is considered optimal but still must be used with caution, because cauterization of the cornea and blindness may result, especially with repeated applications.

Solution should not be applied to wounds, cuts, or broken skin.

Interactions
Silver nitrate is incompatible with thimerosal, benzalkonium chloride, halogenated acids or salts, alkalies, and phosphates.

Effects on diagnostic tests
None reported.

Adverse reactions
● DERM: argyria (permanent silver discoloration of the skin) with prolonged use.

● Eye: periorbital edema, temporary staining of lids and surrounding tissue, conjunctivitis (with concentrations of 1% or greater); mild chemical conjunctivitis may follow prophylaxis in neonates, but rarely persists beyond 24 hours.

Note: Drug should be discontinued if redness or irritation occurs (topical).

Overdose and treatment
Clinical manifestations of overdose are extremely rare with ophthalmic use.

Toxicity is highly dependent on the concentration of silver nitrate and extent of exposure. Oral overdose would be treated by dilution with 4 to 8 oz of water. To remove the chemical, administer sodium chloride (10 g/liter) by lavage in order to precipitate silver chloride. Activated charcoal or a cathartic can be used. Treat eye overexposure initially by irrigation with tepid water for at least 15 minutes. Treat dermal overexposure by washing with soap and water twice. Dizziness, seizures, mucous membrane irritation, nausea, vomiting, stomachache and diarrhea, methemoglobinemia, dermatitis, rash, and hypochloremia with associated hyponatremia may occur. Treat seizures with diazepam. Depending on the extent of exposure, evaluate for methemoglobinemia; treat with methylene blue.

▶ Special considerations
● Silver nitrate is bacteriostatic, germicidal, and astringent.
● Do not use repeatedly.
● If solution stronger than 1% is accidentally used in eye, promptly irrigate with isotonic sodium chloride to prevent eye irritation.
● Solution may stain skin and utensils. Handle drug carefully.
● Instillation may be briefly delayed to allow neonate to bond with mother; however, application should occur within 1 hour after delivery. Instillation at birth is required by law in most states; do not irrigate eyes after instillation. Store wax ampules away from light and heat.
● Do not use solution if it is discolored or contains a precipitate.
● Topical use of solutions greater than 1% concentration may cause burns. Avoid contact with skin and eyes. If accidental contact with skin occurs, flush with water for at least 15 minutes; for accidental contact with eyes, irrigate with sterile water or normal saline immediately.
● Silver nitrate pencils must be moistened with water before use.
● In low concentrations (0.125% to 0.5%) as a wet dressing, silver nitrate is used as a local anti-infective to treat burn patients and in skin wounds or ulcers.
● Drug may be painful when administered topically in higher concentrations.

Information for the patient
● Explain that preparations may stain skin and clothing. Teach parents that silver nitrate may discolor neonate's eyelids temporarily.
● Inform parents that instillation at birth is required by law in most states.

silver protein, mild
Argyrol S.S.

● Pharmacologic classification: heavy metal (silver compound)
● Therapeutic classification: antiseptic
● Pregnancy risk category C

How supplied
Available by prescription only
Topical (ophthalmic solution): 20%

Available without prescription
Topical solution: 10%

Indications, route, and dosage
Topical application for inflammation of eye, ear, nose, throat, rectum, urethra, and vagina
Adults and children: Apply p.r.n. as a 10% or 20% solution.

Pharmacodynamics
Antiseptic action: Silver protein stains and coagulates mucus and inhibits the growth of both gram-positive and gram-negative organisms. When instilled in the eye before ophthalmic surgery, removal of stained material may reduce incidence of postoperative infection.

Pharmacokinetics
Unknown.

Contraindications and precautions
Silver protein is contraindicated in patients with hypersensitivity to any component of the preparation. It is not recommended for prolonged use.

Interactions
When used concomitantly with sulfacetamide, silver protein may result in precipitates.

Effects on diagnostic tests
None reported.

Adverse reactions
● DERM: argyria (permanent discoloration of skin and conjunctiva) with long-term use.
● Eye: chemical conjunctivitis.

Overdose and treatment
Clinical manifestations of ingested overdose include argyria (blue-gray discoloration of the skin, mucous membranes, and eyes), neuropathies, severe gastroenteritis, blindness. Because some silver salts may be corrosive, do not induce emesis. Sodium chloride may be administered by gastric lavage to remove the drug. Treat ocular exposure by flushing the eye for 15 minutes with warm water.

▶ Special considerations
● Store drug in amber glass bottles; protect from light.
● Do not use if drug is discolored or contains a precipitate.
● Prolonged use should be avoided.

Information for the patient
- Demonstrate correct application and proper storage.
- Caution patient against long-term use.

silver sulfadiazine
Flint SSD, Silvadene, SSD AF

- Pharmacologic classification: synthetic anti-infective
- Therapeutic classification: topical antibacterial
- Pregnancy risk category B

How supplied
Available by prescription only
Cream: 1%

Indications, route, and dosage
Adjunct in the prevention and treatment of wound infection for second- and third-degree burns
Adults and children: Apply 1/16" (16 mm) thickness of ointment to cleansed and debrided burn wound daily. Reapply if accidentally removed.

Pharmacodynamics
Antibacterial action: Acts on bacterial cell membrane and bacterial cell wall. Silver sulfadiazine has a broad spectrum of activity, including gram-negative and gram-positive organisms.

Pharmacokinetics
- *Absorption:* Limited with topical use.
- *Distribution:* None.
- *Metabolism:* None.
- *Excretion:* Silver sulfadiazine is excreted in the urine.

Contraindications and precautions
Silver sulfadiazine is contraindicated in pregnant women near term and in premature infants because drug has produced kernicterus in neonates. Do not use on women of childbearing age unless benefits outweigh the possibility of fetal damage.

Silver sulfadiazine should be used cautiously in patients with known hypersensitivity to the drug. The possibility of cross-hypersensitivity with other sulfonamides should be kept in mind. It should be used cautiously in patients with impaired hepatic or renal function.

Interactions
Collagenase, papain, and sutilains may be inactivated if used concurrently.

Effects on diagnostic tests
If used on extensive areas of body surface, systemic absorption may result in a decreased neutrophil count, indicating a reversible leukopenia.

Adverse reactions
- Local: pain, burning, rash, itching.
- Other: reversible leukopenia.
Note: Drug should be discontinued if sensitization develops.

Overdose and treatment
To treat local overapplication, discontinue drug and cleanse area thoroughly.

▶ Special considerations
- Avoid contacting drug with eyes and mucous membranes.
- Apply drug with a sterile gloved hand. The burned area should be covered with cream at all times.
- Daily bathing is an aid in debridement of burn patients.
- Continue treatment until site is healed or is ready for skin grafting.
- Monitor for signs of fungal superinfection.
- Delayed eschar separation may result when drug is used.
- Monitor CBCs, serum sulfadiazine levels, urine for crystalluria, calculi formation.

Information for the patient
- Teach patient about wound care.
- Advise patient that silver sulfadiazine does not stain the skin.
- Teach patient proper application.
- Warn patient of potential photosensitivity.

Pediatric use
Silver sulfadiazine is contraindicated in premature infants or infants younger than age 2 months.

Breast-feeding
Breast-feeding should be avoided during and for several days after treatment with silver sulfadiazine.

simethicone
Gas-X, Mylicon, Phazyme, Silain

- Pharmacologic classification: dispersant
- Therapeutic classification: antiflatulent
- Pregnancy risk category C

How supplied
Available without prescription
Tablets: 40 mg, 50 mg, 60 mg, 80 mg, 95 mg, 125 mg
Capsules: 40 mg/0.6 ml

Indications, route, and dosage
Flatulence, functional gastric bloating
Adults and children over age 12: 40 to 125 mg after each meal and h.s.

Pharmacodynamics
Antiflatulent action: Simethicone acts as a defoaming agent by decreasing the surface tension of gas bubbles, thereby preventing the formation of mucus-coated gas bubbles.

Pharmacokinetics
- *Absorption:* None.
- *Distribution:* None.
- *Metabolism:* None.
- *Excretion:* Simethicone is excreted in feces.

Contraindications and precautions
None reported.

Interactions

Simethicone may decrease the effectiveness of alginic acid.

Effects on diagnostic tests

None reported.

Adverse reactions

None reported.

Overdose and treatment

No information available.

▶ **Special considerations**

Simethicone is found in many combination antacid products.

Information for the patient

Tell patient to chew tablets thoroughly or to shake suspension well before using.

Pediatric use

Simethicone is not recommended as treatment for infant colic; it has limited use in children.

---

simvastatin

Zocor

- Pharmacologic classification: HMG-CoA reductase inhibitor
- Therapeutic classification: antilipemic, cholesterol-lowering agent
- Pregnancy risk category X

How supplied

Available by prescription only
Tablets: 5 mg, 10 mg, 20 mg, 40 mg

Indications, route, and dosage

Reduction of low-density lipoprotein (LDL) and total cholesterol levels in patients with primary hypercholesterolemia (types IIa and IIb)

Adults: Initially, 5 to 10 mg daily in the evening. Adjust dosage q 4 weeks based on patient tolerance and response; maximum daily dosage is 40 mg.

Dosage adjustment for patients in renal failure

Patients with mild to moderate renal insufficiency should take the usual daily dose. Patients with severe renal impairment should start therapy with 5 mg P.O. daily and should be closely monitored.

Pharmacodynamics

Antilipemic action: Simvastatin inhibits the enzyme 3-hydroxy-3-methylglutaryl-coenzyme A (HMG-CoA) reductase. This hepatic enzyme is an early (and rate limiting) step in the synthetic pathway of cholesterol.

Pharmacokinetics

- *Absorption:* Simvastatin is readily absorbed; however, extensive hepatic extraction limits the plasma availability of active inhibitors to 5% of a dose or less. Individual absorption varies considerably.
- *Distribution:* Parent drug and active metabolites are over 95% bound to plasma proteins.

- *Metabolism:* Hydrolysis occurs in the plasma; at least three major metabolites have been identified.
- *Excretion:* Excretion is primarily in bile.

Contraindications and precautions

Simvastatin is contraindicated in patients with hypersensitivity to the drug and in patients with active liver disease or other conditions associated with persistent elevations of serum transaminase levels. Simvastatin is also contraindicated in pregnant and breast-feeding women and should not be administered to women of childbearing age unless there is no risk of pregnancy.

Clinical evidence of liver dysfunction may occur in up to 1% of patients. Persistent elevations of serum transaminase levels to three times the upper normal limit may occur. These elevations aren't associated with jaundice or other symptoms. If liver enzyme levels rise, drug should be discontinued and patients monitored closely; if elevated levels persist after discontinuation of drug, a liver biopsy may be performed.

Watch for signs of myositis. Rarely, myopathy and marked elevations of CPK, possibly leading to rhabdomyolysis and renal failure secondary to myoglobinuria, have been reported.

Drug should be temporarily discontinued in any patient with an acute condition that suggests a developing myopathy or in a patient with risk factors that may predispose to development of renal failure secondary to rhabdomyolysis (including severe acute infection; severe endocrine, metabolic, or electrolyte disorders; hypotension; major surgery; or uncontrolled seizures).

Interactions

Concomitant use with immunosuppressive agents (such as cyclosporine), fibric acid derivatives (such as clofibrate or gemfibrozil), high doses of niacin (nicotinic acid; 1 g or more daily), or erythromycin may increase the risk of rhabdomyolysis. Monitor patient closely if concomitant use can't be avoided. Limit daily dosage of simvastatin to 10 mg if patient must take cyclosporine.

Patients taking hepatotoxic drugs and those who chronically abuse alcohol may be at increased risk for hepatotoxicity.

Simvastatin may slightly elevate digoxin levels. Closely monitor plasma digoxin levels at the start of simvastatin therapy.

Simvastatin may slightly enhance the anticoagulant effect of warfarin. Monitor prothrombin time at the start of therapy and during dosage adjustment.

Drugs that decrease the levels or activity of endogenous steroids (such as cimetidine, spironolactone, and ketoconazole) may increase the risk of developing endocrine dysfunction. No intervention appears necessary; take complete drug history in patients who develop endocrine dysfunction.

Effects on diagnostic tests

As an expected pharmacologic effect, simvastatin will reduce total plasma cholesterol, very low-density lipoprotein (VLDL), and LDL and may variably increase high-density lipoprotein (HDL). The ratios of total cholesterol to HDL, total cholesterol to LDL, and LDL to HDL are reduced. Modest decreases in triglycerides may also occur.

Toxic effects of the drug may be evident by marked, persistent elevations of serum transaminases. During clinical trials, about 5% of patients had asymptomatic, marked elevations in the non-cardiac fraction of CPK.

Adverse reactions

- CNS: headache.
- GI: abdominal pain, constipation, diarrhea, dyspepsia, flatulence, nausea.
- Hepatic: marked elevations of serum transaminase, hepatotoxicity.
- Other: asthenia, upper respiratory infection.

Overdose and treatment

There has been no experience with simvastatin overdosage in humans. No specific antidote is known. Treat symptomatically.

▶ Special considerations

- Dosage adjustments should be made about every 4 weeks. If the cholesterol levels falls below the target range, dosage may be reduced.
- Liver function tests should be performed frequently at the start of therapy and periodically thereafter.
- Initiate simvastatin only after diet and other non-pharmacologic therapies have proved ineffective. Patients should continue a cholesterol-lowering diet during therapy.

Information for the patient

- Tell patient that drug should be taken in the evening and may be taken without regard to meals.
- Because of drug's possible impact on liver function, advise patient to restrict alcohol intake.
- Tell patient to report any adverse reactions, particularly muscle aches and pains.
- Explain the importance of controlling serum lipids to cardiovascular health. Teach appropriate dietary management (restricting total fat and cholesterol intake), weight control, and exercise.

Geriatric use

Most elderly patients respond to daily dosage of 20 mg or less.

Pediatric use

Safety and efficacy have not been established.

Breast-feeding

It is unknown if drug is excreted in breast milk. Because of the risk to infants, women should not breast-feed while taking this drug.

---

sodium benzoate-sodium phenylacetate
Ucephan

- Pharmacologic classification: enzyme substrates
- Therapeutic classification: urea cycle enzymopathy (UCE) treatment adjunct
- Pregnancy risk category C

How supplied

Available by prescription only
Solution: 10 g sodium benzoate and 10 g sodium phenylacetate per 100 ml

Indications, route, and dosage
Prevention or treatment of hyperammonemia in patients with urea cycle enzymopathy

Children: 2.5 ml/kg P.O. daily in three to six equally divided doses. Total daily dose should not exceed 100 ml.

Pharmacodynamics

Ammonia-reducing action: Sodium benzoate and sodium phenylacetate activate metabolic pathways that are ineffective in patients with urea cycle enzymopathies, resulting in decreasing ammonia formation.

Pharmacokinetics

- Absorption: Preliminary data from adult volunteers indicate that peak plasma levels occur in about 1 hour after oral administration.
- Distribution: Not fully characterized.
- Metabolism: Occurs in the liver and kidneys.
- Excretion: Rapid and nearly completely excreted by the kidneys in 24 hours.

Contraindications and precautions

Contraindicated in patients with hypersensitivity to sodium benzoate or sodium phenylacetate. Use cautiously in neonates with hyperbilirubinemia. Benzoic acid may compete with bilirubin for binding sites on serum albumin.

Not intended as sole therapy for patients with urea cycle enzymopathies. Most effective when used with dietary modification (low-protein diet) and amino acid supplementation.

Interactions

By competing with transport systems within the kidney, penicillin and probenecid may impair renal excretion of conjugated metabolites.

Effects on diagnostic tests

None reported.

Adverse reactions

GI: nausea and vomiting.

Overdose and treatment

Few cases have been reported. Patients became irritable and experienced vomiting when a three-fold increase in dosage was administered. Full recovery was obtained in 24 hours without treatment.

Treatment should be supportive. Observe for metabolic acidosis and circulatory collapse. Hemodialysis or peritoneal dialysis may be beneficial.

▶ Special considerations

- Dilute each dose in 4 to 8 oz of infant's formula or milk and administer with meals. Inspect the mixture for compatibility if other liquids are used. The drug may precipitate in some solutions (especially acidic solutions like fruit juice) depending upon concentration and pH.
- Carefully measure the required dose because the stock solution is very concentrated (10 g of sodium benzoate and 10 g of sodium phenylacetate per 100 ml).
- Benzoic acid is structurally similar to salicylates. Watch for side effects associated with salicylates, including mild respiratory alkalosis or exacerbation of peptic ulcers.

Information for the patient
Tell parents or caregiver to avoid getting the solution on skin or clothing. The drug has a lingering odor that may be offensive.

Breast-feeding
It is not known if the drug is excreted in breast milk. Use with caution in breast-feeding women.

sodium bicarbonate
Neut, Soda Mint

- Pharmacologic classification: alkalizing agent
- Therapeutic classification: systemic and urinary alkalinizer, systemic hydrogen ion buffer, oral antacid
- Pregnancy risk category C

How supplied
Available by prescription only
Injection: 4% (2.4 mEq/5 ml), 4.2% (5 mEq/10 ml), 5% (297.5 mEq/500 ml), 7.5% (8.92 mEq/10 ml and 44.6 mEq/50 ml), 8.4% (10 mEq/10 ml and 50 mEq/50 ml)

Available without prescription
Tablets: 300 mg, 325 mg, 600 mg, 650 mg

Indications, route, and dosage
Adjunct to advanced cardiac life support
Adults and children over age 2: Although no longer routinely recommended, 1 mEq/kg I.V. bolus of a 7.5% or 8.4% solution followed by 0.5 mEq/kg every 10 minutes depending on blood gas values. Further doses are based on subsequent blood gas values. If blood gas values are unavailable, use 0.5 mEq/kg q 10 minutes until spontaneous circulation returns.
Infants to age 2: 1 mEq/kg I.V. bolus of a 4.2% solution. Dose may be repeated every 10 minutes depending on blood gas values. Dosage not to exceed 8 mEq/kg daily.
Metabolic acidosis
Adults and children: Dose depends on blood CO_2 content, pH, and patient's clinical condition. Generally, 2 to 5 mEq/kg I.V. infused over 4 to 8 hours.
Urinary alkalization
Adults: 48 mEq (4 g) P.O. followed by 12 to 24 mEq (1 to 2 g) every 4 hours.
Children: 1 to 10 mEq (84 to 840 mg) per kg daily.
Antacid
Adults: 300 mg to 2 g P.O. one to four times daily.

Pharmacodynamics
- *Alkalizing buffering action:* Sodium bicarbonate is an alkalinizing agent that dissociates to provide bicarbonate ion. Bicarbonate in excess of that needed to buffer hydrogen ions causes systemic alkalinization and, when excreted, urinary alkalinization as well.
- *Oral antacid:* Taken orally, sodium bicarbonate neutralizes stomach acid by the above mechanism.

Pharmacokinetics
- *Absorption:* Sodium bicarbonate is well absorbed after oral administration as sodium ion and bicarbonate.
- *Distribution:* Bicarbonate occurs naturally and is confined to the systemic circulation.
- *Metabolism:* None.

- *Excretion:* Bicarbonate is filtered and reabsorbed by the kidney; less than 1% of filtered bicarbonate is excreted.

Contraindications and precautions
Sodium bicarbonate is contraindicated in patients with metabolic or respiratory alkalosis; in patients with hypochloremic alkalosis from diuretics, vomiting, or nasogastric suction; and in patients with hypocalcemia because alkalosis may produce tetany.

Sodium bicarbonate should be used cautiously in patients with congestive heart failure (CHF), pulmonary disease, ascites, or other fluid-retaining states because of the large sodium load; in patients with potassium depletion because alkalosis may lower serum potassium levels, predisposing the patient to cardiac arrhythmias; and in neonates and children under age 2 because rapid injection of hypertonic sodium may cause hypernatremia.

Sodium bicarbonate is contraindicated for prolonged therapy because it may cause sodium overload or metabolic acidosis.

Interactions
If urinary alkalinization occurs, sodium bicarbonate increases half-life of quinidine, amphetamines, ephedrine, and pseudoephedrine, and it increases urinary excretion of tetracyclines, salicylates, chlorpropamide, and lithium. Use with corticosteroids may increase sodium retention.

Effects on diagnostic tests
Sodium bicarbonate therapy may alter serum electrolyte levels and may increase serum lactate levels.

Adverse reactions
- CNS: altered consciousness, obtundation (hypernatremia), tremors.
- CV: fluid retention, *worsening heart failure.*
- GI: bloating and flatulence after oral use, cramps.
- GU: renal calculi.
- Metabolic: alkalosis, hypernatremia, hypercholemia, hyperosmolarity.
- Local: pain and tissue necrosis after I.V. extravasation.
   Note: Drug should be discontinued if metabolic alkalosis occurs.

Overdose and treatment
Clinical signs of overdose include depressed consciousness and obtundation from hypernatremia, tetany from hypocalcemia, cardiac arrhythmias from hypokalemia, and seizures from alkalosis. Correct fluid, electrolyte, and pH abnormalities. Monitor vital signs and fluid and electrolytes closely.

▶ Special considerations
- Monitor vital signs regularly; when drug is used as urinary alkalinizer, monitor urine pH.
- Avoid extravasation of I.V. solutions. Addition of calcium salts may cause precipitate; bicarbonate may inactivate catecholamines in solution (epinephrine, phenylephrine, and dopamine).
- Discourage use as an oral antacid because of hazardous excessive systemic absorption.
- Assess patient for milk-alkali syndrome if drug use is long-term.

---

*Canada only   †Unlabeled clinical use   Italicized adverse reactions are life-threatening.

Information for the patient
● Advise patient to avoid chronic use as oral antacid, and recommend nonabsorbable antacids.
● If patient takes an oral dosage form, tell patient to take drug 1 hour before or 2 hours after enteric-coated medications, because drug may cause enteric-coated products to dissolve in the stomach.

Geriatric use
Elderly patients with CHF or other fluid-retaining conditions are at greater risk for increased fluid retention; therefore, drug should be used with caution.

Pediatric use
Avoid rapid infusion (10 ml/minute) of hypertonic solutions in children under age 2.

Breast-feeding
Sodium bicarbonate is safe for cautious use during breast-feeding.

sodium cellulose phosphate
Calcibind

● Pharmacologic classification: ion exchange resin
● Therapeutic classification: antiurolithic
● Pregnancy risk category C

How supplied
Available by prescription only
Powder: 2.5-g packets or 300-g bulk. Inorganic phosphate content approximately 34%; sodium content approximately 11%.

Indications, route, and dosage
Absorptive hypercalciuria Type I; prophylaxis of calcium renal calculi
Adults: 15 g P.O. daily (5 g with each meal) in patients with urinary calcium greater than 300 mg/day. When urinary calcium declines to less than 150 mg/day, reduce dosage to 10 g/day (5 g with dinner, 2.5 g with two remaining meals).

In patients with a urinary excretion between 200 mg and 300 mg/day, the usual dosage is 10 g/day (divided among three daily meals). Mix commercially available sodium cellulose phosphate with about 100 to 300 ml of juice, water, or soft drink, and ingest within 30 minutes of a meal.

Pharmacodynamics
Antiurolithic action: Sodium cellulose phosphate is a cation-exchange resin that releases sodium in exchange for divalent cations in the intestine to form a nonabsorbable complex. Sodium cellulose phosphate is used as an adjunct to dietary restriction in the management of absorptive Type I hypercalciuria to reduce renal calculus formation. When given orally with meals, sodium cellulose phosphate binds dietary and secreted calcium and reduces urinary calcium by approximately 50 mg/5 g sodium cellulose phosphate. It also binds dietary magnesium and lowers urinary magnesium. Oral magnesium supplementation may be given separately.

Pharmacokinetics
● *Absorption:* Sodium cellulose phosphate is not absorbed from the GI tract.
● *Distribution:* None significant.
● *Metabolism:* Sodium cellulose phosphate undergoes partial (7% to 30%) hydrolysis in the intestine, which causes release of phosphorus ions. The resin undergoes cationic modification in the intestine, exchanging calcium and magnesium for sodium.
● *Excretion:* The nonabsorbable cationically modified resin and unchanged resin are excreted in feces.

Contraindications and precautions
Sodium cellulose phosphate is contraindicated in patients with primary or secondary hyperthyroidism, including renal hypercalciuria (renal calcium leak); hypomagnesemic states (serum magnesium less than 1.5 mg/dl); bone disease (such as osteoporosis, osteomalacia, and osteitis); hypocalcemic states (such as hypoparathyroidism and intestinal malabsorption); normal or low intestinal absorption and renal excretion of calcium; and enteric hyperoxaluria.

Use with caution to avoid parathyroid bone disease caused by inhibiting intestinal calcium absorption. When used in patients with Type I hypercalciuria, dosage should be just sufficient to restore normal calcium absorption.

Use sodium cellulose phosphate with caution, if at all, in patients with congestive heart failure or ascites. Safe use in pregnancy has not been established.

Use sodium cellulose phosphate only while monitoring serum calcium, magnesium, copper, zinc, iron, parathyroid hormone, and complete blood count every 3 to 6 months. Hyperoxaluria and hypomagnesiuria may negate the beneficial effects of hypocalciuria on new stone formation.

Interactions
Concomitant use with magnesium-containing products may bind drug. Separate doses by at least 1 hour. Use with ascorbic acid may decrease the effectiveness of the sodium cellulose phosphate in preventing stone formation.

Effects on diagnostic tests
None reported.

Adverse reactions
● GI: dyspepsia, nausea, diarrhea.
● GU: hyperoxaluria, hypomagnesiuria.
● Other: acute arthralgia.

Overdose and treatment
Remove the excess drug from the stomach by lavage. Subsequent management is supportive.

▶ Special considerations
● Recommended only for the type of absorptive hypercalciuria in which both intestinal calcium absorption and urinary calcium remain abnormally high even with a calcium-restricted diet. When administered inappropriately, it can cause hypocalciuria, which could stimulate parathyroid function and lead to parathyroid bone disease.
● Patients should maintain a calcium-restricted diet and avoid all dairy products (such as milk, cheese, ice cream, and yogurt).
● Patients taking sodium cellulose phosphate may de-

velop hyperoxaluria and hypomagnesiuria, which predispose to stone formation.
● Because of the difficulty involved in managing sodium cellulose phosphate therapy, many physicians treat hypercalciuria with a low-calcium diet, high fluid intake, and thiazides.

Information for the patient
● Advise patient to restrict dietary intake of oxalate (found in spinach, rhubarb, chocolate, brewed tea).
● Avoid vitamin C because it can increase urinary oxalate.
● Encourage fluid intake. Urine output should be at least 2 liters/day.
● Patient can mix the powder in fruit juice, water, or a soft drink and take it with meals.
● Encourage a low-sodium diet. Tell patient to avoid adding salt at the table.
● Advise patient to report any unusual or allergic reaction to sodium cellulose phosphate; any low-salt, low-sugar, or other special diet; and allergy to any substance, such as foods, sulfites or other preservatives, or dyes.

Pediatric use
Sodium cellulose phosphate is not recommended in children age 16 or younger, because they have a higher dietary calcium requirement.

Breast-feeding
Because calcium is needed in infant development, sodium cellulose phosphate should be used in breast-feeding women only when clearly needed.

---

sodium chloride
Slo-Salt, Thermotab

● Pharmacologic classification: electrolyte
● Therapeutic classification: sodium and chloride replacement
● Pregnancy risk category C

How supplied
Available by prescription only
Injection: 0.45% sodium chloride 500 ml, 1,000 ml; 0.9% sodium chloride 50 ml, 100 ml, 150 ml, 250 ml, 500 ml, 1,000 ml; 3% sodium chloride 500 ml; 5% sodium chloride 500 ml

Available without a prescription
Tablets: 250 mg, 650 mg
Tablets (slow-release): 600 mg
Tablets (enteric-coated): 1 g

Indications, route, and dosage
Water and electrolyte replacement in hyponatremia from electrolyte loss or severe sodium chloride depletion
Adults and children: For severe hyponatremia (serum sodium level below 120 mEq/ml), give 400 ml of 3% or 5% solutions I.V., with no more than 100 ml being administered over a 1-hour period.

To correct sodium depletion of isotonic proportions, infuse 0.9% sodium chloride (2% to 6% of body weight) I.V. over 18 to 24 hours; 0.9% sodium chloride also is used as a priming fluid for hemodialysis procedures

and to initiate and terminate blood transfusions. The usual oral replacement dosage of sodium chloride is 1 to 2 g t.i.d.

Hypotonic solutions (usually 0.45% containing 77 mEq sodium and chloride per liter) are usually given I.V. with dextrose solutions for maintenance therapy for 1 to 3 days in patients unable to take fluid and nutrients orally and are administered without dextrose in the management of hyperosmolar diabetes mellitus.
Management of "heat cramps" and heat prostration from excessive perspiration during exposure to high temperatures
Adults: Give 1 g orally with a full glass of water 1 to 10 times daily. Do not exceed 4.8 g/day. A solution of 3 to 4 g of sodium chloride and 1.5 to 2 g of sodium bicarbonate per liter also is acceptable for oral use if patient cannot tolerate solid foods.

Sodium chloride solution is also used as a vehicle for drugs. The pharmacy may admix compatible drugs in sodium chloride for infusion.

Pharmacodynamics
Electrolyte replacement: Sodium chloride solution replaces deficiencies of the sodium and chloride ions in the blood plasma.

Pharmacokinetics
● *Absorption:* Oral and parenteral sodium chloride are absorbed readily.
● *Distribution:* Sodium chloride is distributed widely.
● *Metabolism:* None significant.
● *Excretion:* Sodium and chloride are eliminated primarily in urine, but also in the sweat, tears, and saliva.

Contraindications and precautions
The 3% and 5% sodium chloride solutions are contraindicated in the presence of elevated, normal, or only slightly decreased plasma sodium and chloride concentrations. They should be given slowly in small volumes (200 to 400 ml) because of the danger of hypervolemia caused by water flowing from the intercellular space to the hyperosmolar plasma.

Use 0.9% sodium chloride cautiously in patients with congestive heart failure (CHF), renal failure, cirrhotic and nephrotic disease, or hypoproteinemia. Use cautiously in patients receiving corticosteroids or corticotropin.

Infusion of isotonic (0.9%) sodium chloride during or immediately after surgery may result in excessive sodium retention. Infusion of a potassium-free solution may cause hypokalemia.

Pediatric patients (especially neonates) should not receive sodium chloride with benzyl alcohol as preservative (antimicrobial agent), nor should solution be used to flush I.V. catheters in neonates. Administration of sodium chloride with benzyl alcohol has caused deaths that were preceded by metabolic acidosis, CNS depression, respiratory distress progressing to gasping respiration, hypotension, renal failure, and, occasionally, seizures and intracranial hemorrhage.

Interactions
None reported.

Effects on diagnostic tests
None reported.

Adverse reactions
• CNS: irritability, restlessness, weakness, muscular twitching, headache, dizziness, obtundation with possible coma.
• CV: aggravation of CHF; hypervolemia; edema; hypertension, tachycardia, and fluid accumulation.
• HEMA: hyperosmolarity with confusion, stupor, or coma.
• Metabolic: hypernatremia and aggravation of existing acidosis with excessive infusion; severe electrolyte disturbance, loss of potassium. Excessive infusion of chloride may cause the loss of bicarbonate ions, causing acidification of the blood.
• Respiratory: *pulmonary edema* (if too much is given or rate of administration is too rapid); *respiratory arrest.*
• Other: Contaminated I.V. solutions may cause fever, infection at the infusion site, and extravasation.

Overdose and treatment
Sodium chloride overdose causes serious electrolyte disturbances. Oral ingestion of large quantities irritates the GI mucosa and may cause nausea and vomiting, diarrhea, and abdominal cramps.

Treatment of oral overdose consists of emptying the stomach, giving magnesium sulfate as a cathartic, and supportive therapy. Provide airway and ventilation if necessary. Excessive I.V. administration requires discontinuation of sodium chloride infusion.

▶ Special considerations
• Use concentrated solutions (3% and 5%) only for correcting severe sodium deficits (sodium level below 120 mEq/ml). The solutions should be infused very slowly and with caution to avoid pulmonary edema. Patient should be observed constantly.
• Concentrated solutions (3.5 and 4 mEq/ml) are available for addition to parenteral nutrition solutions.
• Monitor changes in fluid balance, serum electrolyte disturbances, and acid-base imbalances.
• Monitor for hypokalemia with administration of potassium-free solutions.
• Sodium chloride 0.9% may be used in managing extreme dilution of hyponatremia and hypochloremia resulting from administration of sodium-free fluids during fluid and electrolyte therapy, and in managing extreme dilution of extracellular fluid after excessive water intake (for example, after multiple enemas).

sodium fluoride
ACT, Fluorigard, Fluorinse, Fluoritabs, Flura, Flura-Drops, Flura-Loz, Gel II, Karidium, Karigel, Karigel-N, Listermint with Fluoride, Luride, Luride Lozi-Tabs, Luride-SF Lozi-Tabs, Pediaflor, Phos-Flur, Point Two, PreviDent, Thera-Flur, Thera-Flur-N

• Pharmacologic classification: trace mineral
• Therapeutic classification: dental caries prophylactic
• Pregnancy risk category C

How supplied
Available without prescription
Rinse: 0.01% (180 ml, 260 ml, 540 ml, 720 ml); 0.02% (180 ml, 300 ml, 360 ml, 480 ml)

Available by prescription only
Tablets: 0.5 mg, 1 mg (sugar-free)
Tablets (chewable): 0.25 mg (sugar-free)
Drops: 0.125 mg/drop (30 ml), 0.125 mg/drop (60 ml, sugar-free), 0.25 mg/drop (19 ml), 0.25 mg/drop (24 ml, sugar-free), 0.5 mg/ml (50 ml)
Rinse: 0.02% (250 ml, 480 ml, 500 ml), 0.09% (250 ml, 480 ml), 0.09% (480 ml, sugar-free)
Gel: 0.5% (24 g, 30 g, 60 g, 120 g, 125 g, 130 g), 0.5% sugar-free (250 g), 1.23% (480 g)
Gel drops: 0.5% (24 ml, 60 ml)

Indications, route, and dosage
Aid in the prevention of dental caries
Oral
Children over age 3: 1 mg daily.
Children to age 3: 0.5 mg daily.
Note: If fluoride in the drinking water is < 0.3 ppm, use dosage listed; if fluoride content is 0.3 to 0.7 ppm, use one-half of this dosage; if fluoride content is > 0.7 ppm, do not use.
Topical
Adults and children over age 12: 10 ml of 0.02% rinse. Use once daily after thoroughly brushing teeth and rinsing mouth. Rinse around and between teeth for 1 minute, then spit out.
Children age 6 to 12: 5 ml of 0.2% solution.

Pharmacodynamics
Dental caries prophylactic action: Sodium fluoride acts systemically before tooth eruption and topically afterward by increasing tooth resistance to acid dissolution, by promoting remineralization, and by inhibiting the cariogenic microbial process. Acidulation provides greater topical fluoride uptake by dental enamel than neutral solutions. When topical fluoride is applied to hypersensitive exposed dentin, the formation of insoluble materials within the dentinal tubules blocks transmission of painful stimuli.

Pharmacokinetics
• *Absorption:* Sodium fluoride is absorbed readily and almost completely from the GI tract. A large amount of an oral dose may be absorbed in the stomach, and the rate of absorption may depend on the gastric pH. Oral fluoride absorption may be decreased by simultaneous

ingestion of aluminum or magnesium hydroxide. Simultaneous ingestion of calcium also may decrease absorption of large doses. Normal total plasma fluoride concentrations range from 0.14 to 0.19 mcg/ml.
• *Distribution:* Sodium fluoride is stored in bones and developing teeth after absorption. Skeletal tissue also has a high storage capacity for fluoride ions. Because of the storage-mobilization mechanism in skeletal tissue, a constant fluoride supply may be provided. Although teeth have a small mass, they also serve as storage sites. Fluoride deposited in teeth is not released readily. Fluoride has been found in all organs and tissues with a low accumulation in noncalcified tissues. Fluoride is distributed into sweat, tears, hair, and saliva. Fluoride crosses the placenta and is distributed into breast milk. Fluoride concentrations in milk range from approximately 0.05 to 0.13 ppm and remain fairly constant.
• *Metabolism:* None.
• *Excretion:* Fluoride is excreted rapidly, mainly in the urine. About 90% of fluoride is filtered by the glomerulus and reabsorbed by the renal tubules.

Contraindications and precautions
Sodium fluoride is contraindicated in patients with hypersensitivity to the fluoride ion and when the fluoride content of drinking water exceeds 0.7 ppm. Patients on a low-sodium or sodium-free diet should avoid sodium fluoride. If the fluoride content of drinking water is 0.3 ppm or more, 1-mg tablets or rinse must not be used in children under age 3. The 1-mg rinse should not be used in children under age 6 because young children cannot perform the necessary rinse correctly. Some formulations contain tartrazine, which may precipitate allergic reaction in certain individuals.

Interactions
Incompatibility of systemic fluoride with dairy foods has reportedly caused calcium fluoride formation.

Concomitant use with magnesium or aluminum hydroxide may impair the absorption of sodium fluoride.

Effects on diagnostic tests
None reported.

Adverse reactions
• CNS: headaches, weakness.
• DERM: hypersensitivity reactions, such as atopic dermatitis, eczema, and urticaria.
• GI: gastric distress.
• Other: mottling of tooth enamel with chronic overdose.

Overdose and treatment
In children, acute ingestion of 10 to 20 mg of sodium fluoride may cause excessive salivation and GI disturbances; 500 mg may be fatal. GI disturbances include salivation, nausea, abdominal pain, vomiting, and diarrhea. CNS disturbances include CNS irritability, paresthesias, tetany, hyperactive reflexes, seizures, and respiratory or cardiac failure (from the calcium-binding effect of fluoride). Hypoglycemia and hypocalcemia are frequent laboratory findings.

By using gastric lavage with 1% to 5% calcium chloride solution, the fluoride may be precipitated. Administer glucose I.V. in saline solution; parenteral calcium administration maybe indicated for tetany. Adequate urine output should be maintained.

▶ Special considerations
• Recommended doses are currently under study. Some evidence suggests that considerably less fluoride is needed for adequate supplementation.
• Review dietary history with the family. A diet that includes large amounts of fish, mineral water, and tea provides approximately 5 mg/day of fluoride.
• Fluoride supplementation must be continuous from infancy to age 14 to be effective.
• Tablets can be dissolved in the mouth, chewed, swallowed whole, added to drinking water or fruit juice, or added to water in infant formula or other foods.
• Drops may be administered orally undiluted or added to fluids or food.
• Sodium fluoride may be preferred to stannous fluoride to avoid staining tooth surfaces. Neutral sodium fluoride may also be preferred to acidulated fluoride to avoid dulling of porcelain and ceramic restorations.
• Prolonged intake of drinking water containing a fluoride ion concentration of 4 to 8 ppm may result in increased density of bone mineral and fluoride osteosclerosis.
• An oral sodium fluoride dose of 40 to 65 mg/day has resulted in adverse rheumatic effects.
• Used investigationally to treat osteoporosis.

Information for the patient
• Tell patient that sodium fluoride tablets and drops should be taken with meals. Milk and other dairy products may decrease the absorption of sodium fluoride tablets; patient should avoid simultaneous ingestion.
• Advise patient that rinses and gels are most effective if used immediately after brushing or flossing and taken just before retiring to bed.
• Tell patient to expectorate – and not swallow – any excess liquid or gel.
• Warn patient not to eat, drink, or rinse his mouth for 15 to 30 minutes after application. Tell him to use a plastic container – not glass – to dilute drops or rinse, because the fluoride interacts with glass.
• Encourage patient to notify his dentist if mottling of teeth occurs.
• Advise patient that if he has a change in the water supply or if he moves to another area, he should contact his dentist because excessive fluoride causes mottled tooth enamel. Patients using private wells should have water tested for fluoride.
• Warn parents to treat fluoride tablets as a drug and to keep them away from children.

Pediatric use
• Young children usually cannot perform the rinse process necessary with oral solutions.
• Because prolonged ingestion or improper techniques may result in dental fluorosis and osseous changes, the dosage must be carefully adjusted according to the amount of fluoride ion in drinking water.

Breast-feeding
Very little sodium fluoride is distributed into breast milk. The fluoride concentrations in breast milk increase only when daily intake exceeds 1.5 mg.

sodium lactate

- Pharmacologic classification: alkalinizing agent
- Therapeutic classification: systemic alkalizer
- Pregnancy risk category C

How supplied
Available by prescription only
Injection: ⅙ molar solution
Injection for preparations of I.V. admixtures: 2.5 mEq/ml

Indications, route, and dosage
To alkalinize urine
Adults: 30 ml of a ⅙ molar solution/kg of body weight given in divided doses over 24 hours P.O.
Mild to moderate metabolic acidosis
Adults and children: Dosage is highly individualized and depends on the severity of the acidosis and the patient's age, weight, and clinical condition, and on laboratory determinants. The following formula is used to determine sodium lactate dosage for administration by I.V. infusion.

$$\text{Dose in ml of } \frac{1}{6} \text{ molar solution} = (60 - \text{plasma } CO_2) \times (0.8 \times \text{body weight in lb})$$

Pharmacodynamics
Alkalizing action: Sodium lactate is metabolized in the liver, producing bicarbonate, the primary extracellular alkalotic buffer for the body's acid-base system, and glycogen. The simultaneous removal of lactate and hydrogen ion during metabolism also produces alkalinization.

Pharmacokinetics
- *Absorption:* Not applicable.
- *Distribution:* Lactate ion occurs naturally throughout the human body.
- *Metabolism:* Lactate is metabolized in the liver to glycogen.
- *Excretion:* None.

Contraindications and precautions
Sodium lactate is contraindicated in patients with lactic acidosis, which impairs lactate metabolism and prevents formation of bicarbonate; in patients with metabolic, systemic, or respiratory alkalosis; and in patients with hypernatremia because the drug may worsen these conditions.

Sodium lactate should be used cautiously in patients with congestive heart failure (CHF) or other edematous or sodium-retaining states; in patients with oliguria or anuria; and in patients receiving corticosteroids or corticotropin, because of its sodium content.

Interactions
Sodium lactate is physically incompatible with sodium bicarbonate solutions.

Effects on diagnostic tests
None reported.

Adverse reactions
- CV: excess fluid retention, worsening heart failure.
- Other: metabolic alkalosis.
  Note: Drug should be discontinued if adverse effects occur.

Overdose and treatment
Clinical manifestations of overdose include tetany from hypocalcemia, seizures from alkalosis, and cardiac arrhythmias from hypokalemia. Correct fluid, electrolyte, and pH abnormalities. Monitor vital signs and fluid status closely.

▶ Special considerations
- Assess electrolyte, fluid, and acid-base status throughout infusion to prevent alkalosis.
- Monitor injection site for infiltration or extravasation or both.
- The drug should not be used to treat severe metabolic acidosis because the production of bicarbonate from lactate may take 1 to 2 hours.
- I.V. infusion rate should not exceed 300 ml/hour.

Geriatric use
Drug should be used with caution in elderly patients with CHF and other fluid- and sodium-retaining states.

Pediatric use
Drug is safe to use in children; lower doses are usually indicated.

Breast-feeding
Drug is safe in breast-feeding women.

sodium phosphates
(sodium phosphate and sodium biphosphate)
Fleet Phospho-Soda

- Pharmacologic classification: acid salt
- Therapeutic classification: saline laxative
- Pregnancy risk category C

How supplied
Available without prescription
Solution: 18 g sodium phosphate and 48 g sodium biphosphate/100 ml

Indications, route, and dosage
Constipation
Adults: 20 to 30 ml solution mixed with 4 oz (120 ml) cold water.
Children: 5 to 15 ml solution mixed with 4 oz cold water.

Pharmacodynamics
Laxative action: Sodium phosphate and sodium biphosphate exert an osmotic effect in the small intestine by drawing water into the intestinal lumen, producing distention that promotes peristalsis and bowel evacuation.

Pharmacokinetics
- *Absorption:* About 1% to 20% of an oral dose of sodium and phosphate is absorbed. With oral administration, action begins in 3 to 6 hours.
- *Distribution:* Unknown.

- *Metabolism:* Unknown.
- *Excretion:* Unknown; probably in feces and urine.

Contraindications and precautions

Sodium phosphate and sodium biphosphate are contraindicated in patients with fluid and electrolyte disturbances, impaired renal function, edema, or congestive heart failure and in other patients required to limit sodium intake; and in patients with appendicitis, abdominal pain, nausea or vomiting, fecal impaction, or intestinal obstruction or perforation, because the drug may worsen the symptoms of these disorders.

Drugs should be used cautiously in patients with large hemorrhoids or anal excoriation because of the potential for irritation.

Interactions

Concomitant administration of drug with antacids may cause inactivation of both.

Effects on diagnostic tests

None reported.

Adverse reactions

- GI: abdominal cramps, nausea (rare).
- Metabolic: fluid and electrolyte disturbances (hypernatremia, hyperphosphatemia) in chronic use.
- Other: laxative dependence in long-term use.
  Note: Drug should be discontinued if abdominal pain develops.

Overdose and treatment

No information available; probable clinical effects include abdominal pain and diarrhea.

▶ Special considerations

- Dilute drug with water before giving orally (add 30 ml of drug to 120 ml of water). Follow drug administration with full glass of water.
- Monitor serum electrolyte levels; when drug is given as saline laxative, up to 10% of sodium content may be absorbed.
- Drug is not routinely used to treat constipation but is commonly used to evacuate the bowel.

Information for the patient

- Instruct patient on how to mix the drug and on dosage schedule.
- Warn patient that frequent or prolonged use of drug may lead to laxative dependence.

---

sodium polystyrene sulfonate
Kayexalate, SPS

- Pharmacologic classification: cation-exchange resin
- Therapeutic classification: potassium-removing resin
- Pregnancy risk category C

How supplied

Available by prescription only
Oral powder: 1.25 g/5 ml suspension
Rectal: 1.25 g/5 ml suspension

Indications, route, and dosage
Hyperkalemia
Adults: 15 g P.O. daily to q.i.d. in water or sorbitol. Alternatively, 30 to 50 g p.r.n. as a retention enema.

Pharmacodynamics
Potassium-removing action: Sodium polystyrene sulfonate releases sodium in exchange for other cations such as potassium.

Pharmacokinetics
- *Absorption:* Sodium polystyrene sulfonate is not absorbed. The onset of action varies from hours to days.
- *Distribution:* None.
- *Metabolism:* None.
- *Excretion:* Drug is excreted unchanged in feces.

Contraindications and precautions

Use sodium polystyrene sulfonate cautiously in patients whose sodium intake must be restricted.

Interactions

When used concomitantly, magnesium- and calcium-containing antacids are bound by the resin, possibly causing metabolic alkalosis in patients with renal impairment.

Effects on diagnostic tests

Sodium polystyrene sulfonate therapy may alter serum magnesium and calcium levels.

Adverse reactions

- GI: anorexia, nausea, vomiting, constipation, fecal impaction (in elderly patients), gastric irritation, diarrhea (with sorbitol emulsion).
- Other: electrolyte imbalances, ECG abnormalities, hypokalemia, sodium retention.
  Note: Drug should be discontinued if hypokalemia occurs.

Overdose and treatment

Clinical manifestations of overdose include signs and symptoms of hypokalemia (irritability, confusion, cardiac arrhythmias, ECG changes, severe muscle weakness, and sometimes paralysis) and digitalis toxicity in digitalized patients. Drug may be discontinued or dose lowered when serum potassium level falls to the 4 to 5 mEq/liter range.

▶ Special considerations

- For oral administration: mix resin only with water or sorbitol; never mix with orange juice (high K^+ content).
- Chill oral suspension to increase palatability; do not heat because that inactivates the resin.
- The rectal route is recommended when vomiting, P.O. restrictions, or upper GI tract problems are present.
- Fecal impaction can be prevented in elderly patients by administering resin rectally. Cleansing enema should precede rectal administration.
- For rectal administration, mix polystyrene resin only with water and sorbitol for rectal use. Do not use other vehicles (that is, mineral oil) for rectal administration, to prevent impactions. Ion exchange requires aqueous medium. Sorbitol content prevents impaction. Prepare rectal dose at room temperature. Stir emulsion gently during administration.
- Monitor serum potassium at least once daily. Watch for other signs of hypokalemia.
- Monitor for symptoms of other electrolyte deficien-

---

cies (magnesium, calcium) because drug is nonselective. Monitor serum calcium determination in patients receiving sodium polystyrene therapy for more than 3 days. Supplementary calcium may be needed.
● Constipation is more likely to occur when drug is given with concurrent phosphate binders (such as aluminum hydroxide). Monitor patient's bowel habits.
● If hyperkalemia is severe, more drastic modalities should be added; for example, dextrose 50% with regular insulin I.V. push. Do not depend solely on polystyrene resin to lower serum potassium levels in severe hyperkalemia.

Information for the patient
● Instruct patient in the importance of following a prescribed low-potassium diet.
● Explain necessity of retaining enema to patient. Retention for 6 to 10 hours is ideal, but 30 to 60 minutes is acceptable.

Geriatric use
Fecal impaction is more likely in elderly patients.

Pediatric use
Adjust dosage based upon a calculation of 1 mEq of potassium bound for each 1 g of resin.

Breast-feeding
No problems have been reported.

---

sodium salicylate
Uracel

● Pharmacologic classification: salicylate
● Therapeutic classification: nonnarcotic analgesic, antipyretic, anti-inflammatory
● Pregnancy risk category C

How supplied
Available without prescription
Tablets: 325 mg, 650 mg
Tablets (enteric-coated): 325 mg, 650 mg

Available by prescription only
Injection: 1 g/10 ml for dilution

Indications, route, and dosage
Minor pain or fever
Adults and children over age 12: 325 to 650 mg P.O. q 4 hours, p.r.n., or 500 mg slow I.V. infusion over 4 to 8 hours. Maximum dosage is 1 g daily.
Children age 2 to 11: 25 to 50 mg/kg or 1.5 g/m² P.O. in four or six divided doses. Dosage in children age 2 or younger must be individualized.
Rheumatoid arthritis, osteoarthritis, or other inflammatory conditions
Adults: 3.6 to 5.4 g P.O. daily in divided doses.
Children: 80 to 100 mg/kg P.O. daily in divided doses.

Pharmacodynamics
● *Analgesic action:* Sodium salicylate produces analgesia by an ill-defined effect on the hypothalamus (central action) and by blocking generation of pain impulses (peripheral action). The peripheral action may involve inhibition of prostaglandin synthesis.
● *Anti-inflammatory action:* The drug exerts its anti-inflammatory effect by inhibiting prostaglandin synthesis; it may also inhibit the synthesis or action of other mediators of inflammation.
● *Antipyretic action:* The drug relieves fever by acting on the hypothalamic heat-regulating center to produce peripheral vasodilation. This increases peripheral blood supply and promotes sweating, which leads to loss of heat and to cooling by evaporation.

Pharmacokinetics
● *Absorption:* Sodium salicylate is absorbed rapidly and completely from the GI tract.
● *Distribution:* Sodium salicylate is distributed widely into most body tissues and fluids. Protein-binding is concentration-dependent, varies from 75% to 90%, and decreases as serum concentrations increase. Severe toxic side effects may occur at serum concentrations greater than 400 mcg/ml. Therapeutic blood salicylate concentrations for arthritis are 20 to 30 mg/100 ml.
● *Metabolism:* Sodium salicylate is hydrolyzed in the liver.
● *Excretion:* Metabolites are excreted in urine.

Contraindications and precautions
Sodium salicylate is contraindicated in patients with GI ulcer, GI bleeding, or known hypersensitivity to the drug or other nonsteroidal anti-inflammatory drugs (NSAIDs).

Sodium salicylate should be used cautiously in patients with renal impairment, hypoprothrombinemia, vitamin K deficiency, and bleeding disorders; and in patients with congestive heart failure (CHF) and hypertension because of the drug's sodium content.

Patients with known "triad" symptoms (aspirin hypersensitivity, rhinitis/nasal polyps, and asthma) are at high risk of cross-sensitivity to salicylates with precipitation of bronchospasm.

Interactions
Concomitant use of sodium salicylate with drugs that are highly protein-bound (phenytoin, sulfonylureas, warfarin) may cause displacement of either drug, and adverse effects. Monitor therapy closely for both drugs. Concomitant use of other GI-irritating drugs (steroids, antibiotics, other NSAIDs) may potentiate the adverse GI effects of sodium salicylate. Use together with caution.

Ammonium chloride and other urine acidifiers increase sodium salicylate blood levels; monitor for sodium salicylate toxicity. Antacids in high doses, and other urine alkalizers, decrease sodium salicylate blood levels; monitor for decreased sodium salicylate effect. Corticosteroids enhance sodium salicylate elimination. Food and antacids delay and decrease absorption of sodium salicylate.

Effects on diagnostic tests
False-positive urine glucose test results may occur if the copper sulfate method is used in patients undergoing high-dose (2.4 mg/day) therapy; false-negative results may occur in these patients if the glucose oxidase method is used. Sodium salicylate may interfere with urinary vanillylmandelic acid determination or the Gerhardt test for urine aceto-acetic acid. False increases in serum uric acid may occur.

Adverse reactions
● DERM: rash, bruising.
● EENT: tinnitus and hearing loss.
● GI: nausea, vomiting, GI distress, occult bleeding.

• Local: thrombophlebitis (from I.V. use); extravasation of injection may cause sloughing of tissue.
• Other: hypersensitivity manifested by *anaphylaxis* or asthma, elevated liver function tests, *hepatitis*.
   Note: Drug should be discontinued if hypersensitivity, hepatotoxicity, or salicylism occurs.

Overdose and treatment
Clinical manifestations of overdose, including respiratory alkalosis, hyperpnea, and tachypnea, are caused by increased CO_2 production and direct stimulation of the respiratory center.
   To treat sodium salicylate overdose, empty stomach immediately by inducing emesis with ipecac syrup or by gastric lavage. Administer activated charcoal (most effective if given within 2 hours of ingestion) by nasogastric tube. Provide symptomatic and supportive measures (respiratory support and correction of fluid and electrolyte imbalances). Monitor laboratory parameters and vital signs closely. Alkalinization of urine may enhance excretion.

▶ Special considerations
Besides those relevant to all *salicylates,* consider the following recommendations.
• Each gram of sodium salicylate contains 6.25 mEq of sodium and should be avoided in sodium-restricted patients. Monitor patient for signs and symptoms of fluid retention.
• Do not crush enteric-coated tablet or administer with antacid.
• Dilute injectable formulation in 1 liter 0.9% normal saline or lactated Ringer's solution.
• Administer I.V. dose slowly over 4 to 8 hours to prevent possible thrombophlebitis.
• Check I.V. site for signs of phlebitis and extravasation.
• Monitor serum salicylate levels, especially when administering I.V., to avoid possible toxicity.
• Do not administer sodium salicylate with mineral acids or ferric salts. They are incompatible.
• Store in tightly closed container away from light. Medication turns pink when exposed to light.

Information for the patient
• Instruct patient to follow prescribed regimen. Caution him not to change prescribed drug regimen without medical approval.
• Advise patient to report adverse reactions, especially bleeding or changes in hearing.
• Tell patient not to self-administer drug for longer than 10 days.

Geriatric use
• Patients over age 60 are more sensitive to the adverse effects of sodium salicylate.
• Because of its effect on renal prostaglandins, sodium salicylate may cause fluid retention and edema. This may be significant in elderly patients and those with CHF.

Pediatric use
• Dosage of sodium salicylate for children under age 2 must be individualized.
• Because of epidemiologic association with Reye's syndrome, the Centers for Disease Control recommend that children with chicken pox or flulike symptoms not be given salicylates.
• Do not use long-term salicylate therapy in children

under age 14; safety of this use has not been established.

Breast-feeding
Salicylates are distributed into breast milk. Avoid use in breast-feeding women.

sodium thiosalicylate
Arthrolate, Thiocyl, Thiosal, Tusal

• Pharmacologic classification: salicylate
• Therapeutic classification: nonnarcotic analgesic, antipyretic, anti-inflammatory
• Pregnancy risk category C

How supplied
Available by prescription only
Injection: 50 mg/2 ml ampules, 30-ml vials

Indications, route, and dosage
Mild pain
Adults: 50 to 100 mg I.M. or by slow I.V. infusion daily or every other day.
Rheumatic fever
Adults: 100 to 150 mg I.M. or by slow I.V. infusion q 4 to 6 hours for 3 days, then 100 mg b.i.d. until asymptomatic.
Acute gouty arthritis
Adults: 100 mg I.M. or by slow I.V. infusion q 3 to 4 hours for 2 days, then 100 mg daily until patient is asymptomatic.

Pharmacodynamics
• *Analgesic action:* Sodium thiosalicylate is structurally related to aspirin. It may produce analgesia by an ill-defined effect on the hypothalamus (central action) and by blocking generation of pain impulses (peripheral action). The peripheral action may involve inhibition of prostaglandin synthesis.
• *Anti-inflammatory action:* The drug may exert its anti-inflammatory effect by inhibiting prostaglandin synthesis; it may also inhibit the synthesis or action of other mediators of inflammation.
• *Antipyretic action:* The drug may relieve fever by acting on the hypothalamic heat-regulating center to produce peripheral vasodilation. This increases peripheral blood supply and promotes sweating, which leads to loss of heat and to cooling by evaporation.

Pharmacokinetics
• *Absorption:* The drug is well-absorbed with parenteral administration.
• *Distribution, metabolism,* and *excretion* have not been described.

Contraindications and precautions
Sodium thiosalicylate is contraindicated in patients with known hypersensitivity to aspirin or other NSAIDs and in the presence of GI ulcer or GI bleeding. Because of the drug's sodium content, it should be used cautiously in patients with congestive heart failure (CHF) and hypertension.
   Patients with known "triad" symptoms (aspirin hypersensitivity, rhinitis/nasal polyps, and asthma) are at high risk for cross-sensitivity to salicylates and NSAIDs with precipitation of bronchospasm.

Interactions
Concomitant use of sodium thiosalicylate with drugs that are highly protein-bound (phenytoin, sulfonylureas, warfarin) may cause displacement of either drug, and adverse effects. Monitor therapy closely for both drugs. Concomitant use with other GI-irritant drugs (steroids, antibiotics, other NSAIDs) may potentiate the adverse GI effects of sodium thiosalicylate. Use together with caution. Ammonium chloride and other urine acidifiers increase sodium thiosalicylate blood levels; monitor for salicylate toxicity. Corticosteroids enhance sodium thiosalicylate elimination; monitor for decreased salicylate effect.

Effects on diagnostic tests
Sodium thiosalicylate may increase serum levels of AST (SGOT), ALT (SGPT), alkaline phosphatase, and bilirubin.

Adverse reactions
● DERM: rash, bruising, pain at injection site, tissue sloughing, extravasation.
● EENT: tinnitus and hearing loss.
● GI: nausea, vomiting, GI distress, occult bleeding.
● Other: hypersensitivity manifested by *anaphylaxis* or asthma, abnormal liver function tests, hepatitis.
  Note: Drug should be discontinued if hypersensitivity or hepatotoxicity occurs.

Overdose and treatment
Clinical manifestations of overdose, including metabolic acidosis with respiratory alkalosis, hyperpnea, and tachypnea, are caused by increased CO_2 production and direct stimulation of the respiratory center.

Treat overdose of sodium thiosalicylate with symptomatic and supportive measures (respiratory support and correction of fluid and electrolyte imbalances). Monitor laboratory parameters and vital signs closely. Alkalinization of urine may enhance renal excretion.

▶ Special considerations
Besides those relevant to all *salicylates*, consider the following recommendations.
● I.M. administration is preferred. Administer deep into large muscle mass (gluteus maximus or midlateral thigh). Alternate injection sites.
● Sodium thiosalicylate may be given by slow I.V. injection into large vein. Monitor I.V. site closely for signs of infiltration, phlebitis, or extravasation.
● Monitor serum salicylate level, especially if giving by I.V. route, to prevent possible complications.
● With sodium thiosalicylate therapy, laboratory indices, especially BUN, serum creatinine, CBC, and liver function tests, should be monitored periodically.
● Assess patient for signs and symptoms of fluid retention such as weight gain, edema, reduced urine output, and shortness of breath.

Information for the patient
● Instruct patient to report any discomfort at injection or I.V. site.
● Tell patient to report any increase in symptoms.

Geriatric use
● Patients over age 60 are more sensitive to the adverse effects of sodium thiosalicylate.
● Because of its effect on renal prostaglandins, this drug may cause fluid retention and edema. This may

be significant in elderly patients, especially those with CHF.

Pediatric use
● Because of epidemiologic association with Reye's syndrome, the Centers for Disease Control recommends that children with chicken pox or flulike symptoms should not be given salicylates.
● Febrile, dehydrated children can develop toxicity rapidly.
● The safety of long-term sodium thiosalicylate use in children under age 14 has not been established.

Breast-feeding
Salicylates are distributed into breast milk. Safe use in breast-feeding women has not been established.

somatrem
Protropin

● Pharmacologic classification: anterior pituitary hormone
● Therapeutic classification: human growth hormone

How supplied
Available by prescription only
Injectable lyophilized powder: 5 mg (10 IU)/vial

Indications, route, and dosage
Long-term treatment of growth failure from lack of adequate endogenous growth hormone secretion
Children (prepuberty): Up to 0.1 mg/kg I.M. three times weekly. Some clinicians consider it is equally effective if given subcutaneously and more effective if given daily at doses of 0.05 mg/kg.

Pharmacodynamics
Growth-stimulating action: Somatrem is a purified polypeptide hormone of recombinant DNA origin containing a sequence of 192 amino acids identical to the naturally occurring human growth hormone (plus methionine). Somatrem stimulates growth of linear bone, skeletal muscle, and organs and increases red blood cell mass by stimulating erythropoietin. Most actions are mediated through somatomedins (liver-synthesized hormones).

Pharmacokinetics
● *Absorption:* Somatrem is given by I.M. injection.
● *Distribution:* Not fully understood.
● *Metabolism:* Approximately 90% of a dose is metabolized in the liver.
● *Excretion:* Approximately 0.1% of a dose is excreted in urine unchanged. The half-life is 20 to 30 minutes; however, its tissue effects are long-lasting.

Contraindications and precautions
Somatrem is contraindicated in patients with known hypersensitivity to the drug or to benzyl alcohol, closed epiphyses (because the drug stimulates bone growth), or an intracranial lesion actively growing within the previous 12 months.

The drug's diabetogenic action requires that it be used cautiously in patients with a family history of dia-

---

betes. Untreated hypothyroidism may interfere with growth response to somatrem.

Interactions
Concomitant use of somatrem with adrenocorticoids, glucocorticoids, or corticotropin may inhibit growth response. Concomitant use of somatrem with anabolic steroids, androgens, estrogens, or thyroid hormones may accelerate epiphyseal maturation.

Effects on diagnostic tests
Somatrem therapy alters glucose tolerance test (reduced with high doses) and total protein and thyroid function tests (thyroxine-binding capacity and radioactive iodine uptake may be decreased).

Adverse reactions
● Endocrine: hypothyroidism, hyperglycemia.
● Local: pain and swelling at injection site.
● Other: antibody to growth hormone.
   Note: Drug should be discontinued if patient reaches mature adult height; patient's epiphyses close; or patient shows evidence of recurrent intracranial tumor growth.

Overdose and treatment
Clinical manifestations of overdose include gigantism in children and acromegalic features, organ enlargement, diabetes mellitus, atherosclerosis, and hypertension in patients who are not growth hormone deficient. The drug should be discontinued in such situations.

▶ Special considerations
● To prepare the solution, inject the bacteriostatic water for injection (supplied) into the vial containing the drug. Then swirl the vial with a gentle rotary motion until the contents are completely dissolved. *Do not shake the vial.*
● After reconstitution, vial solution should be clear. Do not inject if the solution is cloudy or contains any particles.
● Store reconstituted vial in refrigerator. Must be used within 7 days.
● Be sure to check the expiration date.
● Observe patient for signs of glucose intolerance.
● Monitor thyroid function tests for development of hypothyroidism.

Information for the patient
● Emphasize to parents the importance of regular follow-up visits.
● Advise parents to seek medical approval before administering any other medication.

spectinomycin hydrochloride
Trobicin

● Pharmacologic classification: aminocyclitol
● Therapeutic classification: antibiotic
● Pregnancy risk category C

How supplied
Available by prescription only
Injection: 2-g vial with 3.2-ml diluent; 4-g vial with 6.2-ml diluent

Indications, route, and dosage
Uncomplicated gonorrhea in patients who cannot take ceftriaxone
Adults: 2 to 4 g I.M. single dose injected deeply into upper outer quadrant of the buttocks.
Disseminated gonorrhea
Adults: 2 g I.M. b.i.d. for 3 to 7 days. Inject deeply into upper outer quadrant of the buttocks.

Pharmacodynamics
Antibacterial action: Bacteriostatic effect results from binding of drug to 30S ribosomal subunits, thus inhibiting protein synthesis. Although drug is effective against many gram-positive and gram-negative organisms, it is used mostly against penicillin-resistant *Neisseria gonorrhoeae.*

Pharmacokinetics
● *Absorption:* Spectinomycin is not absorbed orally. I.M. injection results in rapid absorption; peak concentrations occur in 1 and 2 hours for 2-g and 4-g doses, respectively.
● *Distribution:* Spectinomycin's distribution is largely unknown.
● *Metabolism:* Spectinomycin's metabolism is unknown.
● *Excretion:* Most of dose is excreted unchanged in the urine. Elimination half-life ranges from 1 to 3 hours. Drug dosage is unchanged in renal failure.

Contraindications and precautions
Spectinomycin is contraindicated in patients with known hypersensitivity to the drug.
   Spectinomycin should be administered cautiously to patients with strong history of drug allergies.

Interactions
None reported.

Effects on diagnostic tests
BUN, AST (SGOT), and serum alkaline phosphatase levels increase, and hemoglobin, hematocrit, and creatinine clearance levels decrease during spectinomycin therapy.

Adverse reactions
● CNS: insomnia, dizziness.
● DERM: urticaria, rash, pruritus.
● GI: nausea, vomiting.
● GU: decreased urine output.
● Local: pain at injection site.
● Other: fever, chills.

Overdose and treatment
No information available.

▶ **Special considerations**
● Obtain culture and sensitivity tests before starting therapy.
● Drug is usually reserved for patients with penicillin-resistant gonorrhea strains or for whom other drugs are contraindicated. Ceftriaxone is considered the drug of choice for uncomplicated gonorrhea.
● To prepare drug, add supplied diluent to vial and shake until completely dissolved. Use reconstituted solution within 24 hours.
● Inject deep I.M. into upper outer quadrant of gluteal muscle. Give 2-g dose at single site; divide 4-g dose into two equal injections and give at two sites.
● Drug is ineffective against syphilis and may mask symptoms of incubating syphilis infection.
● Lack of response to drug usually results from reinfection.

Information for the patient
Tell patients that sexual partners must be treated.

Pediatric use
Because its safety in infants and children has not been established, drug is not first choice in treating these patients. A single dose of 40 mg/kg is recommended by the Centers for Disease Control.

Breast-feeding
Because researchers do not know if spectinomycin is excreted in breast milk, alternative feeding method is recommended during therapy with spectinomycin.

---

spironolactone
Aldactone

● Pharmacologic classification: potassium-sparing diuretic
● Therapeutic classification: management of edema; antihypertensive; diagnosis of primary hyperaldosteronism; treatment of diuretic-induced hypokalemia
● Pregnancy risk category C

How supplied
Available by prescription only
Tablets: 25 mg, 50 mg, 100 mg

Indications, route, and dosage
Edema
Adults: 25 to 200 mg P.O. daily in divided doses.
Children: Initially, 3.3 mg/kg or 60 mg/m² P.O. daily in divided doses.
Hypertension
Adults: 50 to 100 mg P.O. daily in divided doses.
Diuretic-induced hypokalemia
Adults: 25 to 100 mg P.O. daily when oral potassium supplements are considered inappropriate.
†*Detection of primary hyperaldosteronism*
Adults: 400 mg P.O. daily for 4 days (short test) or for 3 to 4 weeks (long test). If hypokalemia and hypertension are corrected, a presumptive diagnosis of primary hyperaldosteronism is made.

Pharmacodynamics
● *Diuretic and potassium-sparing action:* Spironolactone competitively inhibits aldosterone effects on the distal renal tubules, increasing sodium and water excretion and decreasing potassium excretion.
Spironolactone is used to treat edema associated with excessive aldosterone secretion, such as that associated with hepatic cirrhosis, nephrotic syndrome, and congestive heart failure. It is also used to treat diuretic-induced hypokalemia.
● *Antihypertensive action:* The mechanism of action is unknown; spironolactone may block the effect of aldosterone on arteriolar smooth muscle.
● *Diagnosis of primary hyperaldosteronism:* Spironolactone inhibits the effects of aldosterone; therefore, correction of hypokalemia and hypertension is presumptive evidence of primary hyperaldosteronism.

Pharmacokinetics
● *Absorption:* About 90% of spironolactone is absorbed after oral administration. Onset of action is gradual; maximum effect occurs on 3rd day of therapy.
● *Distribution:* Spironolactone and its major metabolite, canrenone, are more than 90% plasma protein-bound.
● *Metabolism:* Spironolactone is metabolized rapidly and extensively to canrenone, its major active metabolite.
● *Excretion:* Canrenone and other metabolites are excreted primarily in urine, and a small amount is excreted in feces via the biliary tract; half-life of canrenone is 13 to 24 hours.

Contraindications and precautions
Spironolactone is contraindicated in patients with serum potassium levels above 5.5 mEq/liter; in patients who are receiving other potassium-sparing diuretics or potassium supplements because these drugs conserve potassium and can cause severe hyperkalemia in such patients; and in patients with anuria, acute or chronic renal insufficiency, or diabetic nephropathy because of risk of hyperkalemia; and in patients with known hypersensitivity to the drug.
Spironolactone should be used cautiously in patients with severe hepatic insufficiency because electrolyte imbalance may precipitate hepatic encephalopathy and in patients with diabetes, who are at increased risk of hyperkalemia.

Interactions
Spironolactone may potentiate the hypotensive effects of other antihypertensive agents; this may be used to therapeutic advantage.
Spironolactone increases the risk of hyperkalemia when administered with other potassium-sparing diuretics, angiotensin-converting enzyme inhibitors (captopril or enalapril), potassium supplements, potassium-containing medications (parenteral penicillin G), or salt substitutes.
Nonsteroidal anti-inflammatory agents, such as indomethacin or ibuprofen, may impair renal function and thus affect potassium excretion. Aspirin may slightly decrease the clinical response to spironolactone.

Effects on diagnostic tests
Spironolactone therapy alters fluorometric determinations of plasma and urinary 17-hydroxycorticosteroid levels and may cause false elevations on radioimmunoassay of serum digoxin.

Adverse reactions
- CNS: headache.
- DERM: urticaria.
- GI: anorexia, nausea, diarrhea.
- Metabolic: hyperkalemia, dehydration, hyponatremia, transient rise in BUN level, acidosis.
- Other: gynecomastia in males, breast soreness and menstrual disturbances in females.

Overdose and treatment
Clinical signs of overdose are consistent with dehydration and electrolyte disturbance.

Treatment is supportive and symptomatic. In acute ingestion, empty stomach by emesis or lavage. In severe hyperkalemia (> 6.5 mEq/liter), reduce serum potassium levels with I.V. sodium bicarbonate or glucose with insulin. A cation exchange resin, sodium polystyrene sulfonate (Kayexalate), given orally or as a retention enema, may also reduce serum potassium levels.

▶ Special considerations
Besides those relevant to all *potassium-sparing diuretics,* consider the following recommendations.
- Give drug with meals to enhance absorption.
- Diuretic effect may be delayed 2 to 3 days if drug is used alone; maximum antihypertensive effect may be delayed 2 to 3 weeks.
- Protect drug from light.
- Adverse reactions are related to dosage levels and duration of therapy and usually disappear with withdrawal of the drug; however, gynecomastia may not.
- Spironolactone is antiandrogenic and has been used to treat hirsutism in dosages of 200 mg/day.
- Unnecessary use of spironolactone should be avoided. This drug has been shown to induce tumors in laboratory animals.

Information for the patient
- Explain that maximal diuresis may not occur until the 3rd day of therapy and that diuresis may continue for 2 to 3 days after drug is withdrawn.
- Instruct patient to report mental confusion or lethargy immediately.
- Explain that adverse reactions usually disappear after drug is discontinued; gynecomastia, however, may persist.
- Caution patient to avoid such hazardous activities as driving until response to drug is known.

Geriatric use
Elderly patients are more susceptible to diuretic effects and may require lower doses to prevent excessive diuresis.

Pediatric use
When administering spironolactone to children, crush tablets and administer them in cherry syrup as an oral suspension.

Breast-feeding
Spironolactone's safety during breast-feeding has not been established. Canrenone, a metabolite, is distributed into breast milk. Alternative feeding method is recommended during therapy with spironolactone.

stanozolol
Winstrol

- Pharmacologic classification: anabolic steroid
- Therapeutic classification: angioedema prophylactic
- Controlled substance schedule III
- Pregnancy risk category X

How supplied
Available by prescription only
Tablets: 2 mg

Indications, route, and dosage
Prevention of hereditary angioedema
Adults: Initially, 2 mg P.O. t.i.d. to 4 mg q.i.d. for 5 days. Reduce dosage after favorable response at 1- to 3-month intervals to maintenance dose of 2 mg daily.
Children age 6 to 12: Up to 2 mg P.O. daily administered only during an attack.
Children up to age 6: 1 mg P.O. daily administered only during an attack.

Dosage for continuous treatment is highly individualized.

Pharmacodynamics
Angioedema prophylactic action: Stanozolol increases the concentration of C1 esterase inhibitor in patients with hereditary angioedema. This leads to an increased level of the C4 component of complement, which may be deficient in these patients, thus decreasing the number and severity of attacks of this disorder.

Pharmacokinetics
Stanozolol is metabolized by the liver. Its pharmacokinetics are otherwise poorly described.

Contraindications and precautions
Stanozolol is contraindicated in patients with severe renal or cardiac disease, which may be worsened by the fluid and electrolyte retention this drug may cause; in patients with hepatic disease because impaired elimination may cause toxic accumulation of the drug; in male patients with breast cancer, benign prostatic hypertrophy with obstruction, or undiagnosed abnormal genital bleeding because this drug can stimulate the growth of cancerous breast or prostate tissue in males; and in pregnant women because animal studies have shown that administration of anabolic steroids during pregnancy causes masculinization of the fetus. Because of its hypercholesterolemic effects, stanozolol should be administered cautiously in patients with a history of coronary artery disease.

Interactions
In patients with diabetes, decreased blood glucose levels require adjustment of insulin or oral hypoglycemic drug dosage.

Stanozolol may potentiate the effects of warfarin-type anticoagulants, prolonging prothrombin time. Use with adrenocorticosteroids or adrenocorticotropic hormone results in increased potential for fluid and electrolyte retention.

Effects on diagnostic tests
Stanozolol may cause abnormal results of fasting plasma glucose, glucose tolerance, and metyrapone tests. It may increase sulfobromophthalein retention. Thyroid function test results (protein-bound iodine, radioactive iodine uptake, thyroid-binding capacity) and 17-ketosteroid levels may decrease. Liver function test results, prothrombin time (especially in patients receiving anticoagulant therapy), and serum creatinine levels may be elevated. Because of this agent's anabolic activity, serum sodium, potassium, calcium, phosphate, and cholesterol levels may all rise.

Adverse reactions
● Androgenic: *in females:* deepening of voice, clitoral enlargement, changes in libido; *in males:* prepubertal – premature epiphyseal closure, priapism, phallic enlargement; postpubertal – testicular atrophy, oligospermia, decreased ejaculatory volume, impotence, gynecomastia, epididymitis.
● CNS: headache, mental depression.
● CV: edema.
● DERM: acne, oily skin, hirsutism, flushing, sweating.
● GI: gastroenteritis, nausea, vomiting, diarrhea, constipation, change in appetite, weight gain.
● GU: bladder irritability, vaginitis, menstrual irregularities.
● Hepatic: reversible jaundice, hepatotoxicity.
● Other: hypercalcemia.
  Note: Drug should be discontinued if hypercalcemia, edema, hypersensitivity reaction, priapism, or excessive sexual stimulation occurs or if virilization occurs in females.

Overdose and treatment
No information available.

▶ **Special considerations**
Besides those relevant to all *anabolic steroids,* consider the following recommendations.
● Smaller doses (2 mg b.i.d.) may be used in females to minimize virilization. Routinely monitor for side effects.
● Check serum cholesterol level in cardiac patients. These patients also should be on salt-restricted diets.
● Stanozolol has been used investigationally to increase hemoglobin levels in patient with aplastic anemia.

Geriatric use
Observe elderly male patients for the development of prostatic hypertrophy.

Pediatric use
Use with extreme caution to prevent premature sexual maturation and epiphyseal closure. Long-term therapy in children is not recommended.

Breast-feeding
It is not known if stanozolol is excreted in breast milk. Because of the risk to the infant, alternative feeding methods are recommended.

streptokinase
Kabikinase, Streptase

● Pharmacologic classification: plasminogen activator
● Therapeutic classification: thrombolytic enzyme
● Pregnancy risk category C

How supplied
Available by prescription only
Injection: 250,000 IU, 600,000 IU, 750,000 IU in vials for reconstitution

Indications, route, and dosage
Lysis of coronary artery thrombi after acute myocardial infarction (MI)
Adults: 1,500,000 IU by I.V. infusion over 60 minutes; intracoronary loading dose of 20,000 IU via coronary catheter, followed by a maintenance dose of 2,000 IU/minute for 60 minutes as an infusion.
Arteriovenous cannula occlusion
Adults: 250,000 IU in 2 ml I.V. solution by I.V. infusion pump into each occluded limb of the cannula over 25 to 35 minutes. Clamp off cannula for 2 hours; then aspirate contents of cannula, flush with saline solution, and reconnect.
Venous thrombosis, pulmonary embolism, and arterial thrombosis and embolism
Adults: Loading dose of 250,000 IU I.V. infusion over 30 minutes. Sustaining dose: 100,000 IU/hour I.V. infusion for 72 hours for deep vein thrombosis and 100,000 IU/hour over 24 to 72 hours by I.V. infusion pump for pulmonary embolism.

Pharmacodynamics
Thrombolytic action: Streptokinase promotes thrombolysis by activating plasminogen in two steps: 1) plasminogen and streptokinase form a complex, exposing plasminogen-activating site; and 2) cleavage of peptide bond converts plasminogen to plasmin.
  In treatment of acute MI, streptokinase prevents primary or secondary thrombus formation in microcirculation surrounding the necrotic area.

Pharmacokinetics
● *Absorption:* Plasminogen activation begins promptly after infusion or instillation of streptokinase; adequate activation of fibrinolytic system occurs in 3 to 4 hours.
● *Distribution:* Streptokinase does not cross placenta, but antibodies do.
● *Metabolism:* Insignificant.
● *Excretion:* Streptokinase is removed from circulation by antibodies and reticuloendothelial system. Half-life is biphasic: Initially it is 18 minutes (from antibody action) and then extends up to 83 minutes. Anticoagulant effect may persist for 12 to 24 hours after infusion is discontinued.

Contraindications and precautions
Streptokinase is contraindicated in patients with ulcerative wounds, active internal bleeding, recent trauma with possible internal injuries, visceral or intracranial malignancy, ulcerative colitis, diverticulitis, severe hypertension, acute or chronic hepatic or renal insufficiency, uncontrolled hypocoagulation, chronic pulmo-

nary disease with cavitation, subacute bacterial endocarditis or rheumatic valvular disease, recent cerebral embolism, thrombosis or hemorrhage, and diabetic hemorrhagic retinopathy, because excessive bleeding may occur.

Administer streptokinase with extreme caution during pregnancy or 10 days postpartum and for 10 days after any intracranial, intraspinal, or intraarterial diagnostic procedure or any surgery, including liver or kidney biopsy, lumbar puncture, thoracentesis, paracentesis, or extensive or multiple cutdowns. Use reasonable caution when treating patients with arterial emboli originating from left side of heart because of risk of cerebral infarction.

Interactions
Concomitant use with anticoagulants may cause hemorrhage; heparin must be stopped and its effects allowed to diminish. It may also be necessary to reverse effects of oral anticoagulants before beginning therapy. Concomitant use with aspirin, indomethacin, phenylbutazone, or other drugs affecting platelet activity increases risk of bleeding; do not use together.

Aminocaproic acid inhibits streptokinase-induced activation of plasminogen.

Effects on diagnostic tests
Streptokinase increases thrombin time, activated partial thromboplastin time, and prothrombin time; drug sometimes moderately decreases hematocrit.

Adverse reactions
● CV: transient lowering or elevation of blood pressure, reperfusion atrial or *ventricular arrhythmias.*
● DERM: urticaria, ecchymosis.
● EENT: periorbital edema, gum bleeding.
● GI: nausea.
● HEMA: *spontaneous bleeding,* prolonged systemic hypocoagulability, bleeding or oozing from percutaneous trauma site.
● Local: phlebitis at injection site.
● Other: hypersensitivity, fever, *anaphylaxis,* musculoskeletal pain, minor breathing difficulty, *bronchospasm,* angioneurotic edema, hematuria.
  Note: Drug should be discontinued if allergic reaction or severe bleeding occurs.

Overdose and treatment
Clinical manifestations of overdose include signs of potentially serious bleeding: bleeding gums, epistaxis, hematoma, spontaneous ecchymoses, oozing at catheter site, increased pulse, and pain from internal bleeding. Discontinue drug and restart when bleeding stops.

▶ Special considerations
Besides those relevant to all *thrombolytic enzymes,* consider the following recommendations.
● Reconstitute vial with 5 ml normal saline injection, and further dilute to 45 ml; roll gently to mix. *Do not shake.* Use immediately; refrigerate remainder and discard after 24 hours. Store powder at room temperature.
● Rate of I.V. infusion depends on thrombin time and streptokinase resistance; higher loading dose may be necessary in patients with recent streptococcal infection or recent treatment with streptokinase, to compensate for antibody drug neutralization.
● Therapy need not be discontinued for minor allergic reactions that can be treated with antihistamines or corticosteroids; about one third of patients experience

a slight temperature elevation, and some have chills. Symptomatic treatment with acetaminophen (but not aspirin or other salicylates) is indicated if temperature reaches 104° F. (40° C.). Patients may be pretreated with corticosteroids, repeating doses during therapy, to minimize pyrogenic or allergic reactions.
● If minor bleeding can be controlled by local pressure, do not decrease dose, because that makes more plasminogen available for conversion to plasmin.
● Antibodies to streptokinase can persist for 3 to 6 months or longer after the initial dose; if further thrombolytic therapy is needed, consider urokinase.

Geriatric use
Patients age 75 or older have a greater risk of cerebral hemorrhage, because they are more apt to have pre-existing cerebrovascular disease.

---

streptomycin sulfate

● Pharmacologic classification: aminoglycoside
● Therapeutic classification: antibiotic
● Pregnancy risk category D

How supplied
Available by prescription only
Injection: 400 mg/ml, 500 mg/ml, 1-g vial, 5-g vial

Indications, route, and dosage
Primary and adjunctive treatment in tuberculosis
Adults with normal renal function: 1 g I.M. daily for 2 to 3 months, then 1 g two or three times a week. Inject deeply into upper outer quadrant of buttocks.
Children with normal renal function: 20 mg/kg I.M. daily in divided doses injected deeply into large muscle mass. Give concurrently with other antitubercular agents, but *not* with capreomycin, and continue until sputum specimen becomes negative.
Enterococcal endocarditis
Adults: 1 g I.M. q 12 hours for 2 weeks, then 500 mg I.M. q 12 hours for 4 weeks with penicillin.
Tularemia
Adults: 1 to 2 g I.M. daily in divided doses injected deep into upper outer quadrant of buttocks. Continue until patient is afebrile for 5 to 7 days.
Dosage in renal failure
Adults and children: Initial dosage is same as for those with normal renal function. Subsequent doses and frequency determined by renal function study results and blood serum concentrations; keep peak serum levels between 5 and 25 mcg/ml, and trough levels below 5 mcg/ml. Patients with a creatinine clearance > 50 ml/min usually can tolerate the drug daily; if creatinine clearance is 10 to 50 ml/min, administration interval is increased to every 24 to 72 hours. Patients with a creatinine clearance < 10 ml/min may require 72 to 96 hours between doses.

Pharmacodynamics
Antibiotic action: Streptomycin is bactericidal; it binds directly to the 30S ribosomal subunit, thus inhibiting bacterial protein synthesis. Its spectrum of activity includes many aerobic gram-negative organisms and some aerobic gram-positive organisms. Streptomycin

---

is generally less active against many gram-negative organisms than is tobramycin, gentamicin, amikacin, or netilmicin. Streptomycin is also active against *Mycobacterium* and *Brucella.*

Pharmacokinetics

• *Absorption:* Streptomycin is absorbed poorly after oral administration and usually is given parenterally; peak serum concentrations occur 1 to 2 hours after I.M. administration.

• *Distribution:* Streptomycin is distributed widely after parenteral administration; intraocular penetration is poor. CSF penetration is low, even in patients with inflamed meninges. Streptomycin crosses the placenta; it is 36% protein-bound.

• *Metabolism:* Not metabolized.

• *Excretion:* Streptomycin is excreted primarily in urine by glomerular filtration; small amounts may be excreted in bile and breast milk. Elimination half-life in adults is 2 to 3 hours. In severe renal damage, half-life may extend to 110 hours.

Contraindications and precautions

Streptomycin is contraindicated in patients with known hypersensitivity to streptomycin or any other aminoglycoside.

Streptomycin should be used cautiously in patients with decreased renal function; in patients with tinnitus, vertigo, and high-frequency hearing loss who are susceptible to ototoxicity; in patients with dehydration, myasthenia gravis, parkinsonism, and hypocalcemia; in neonates and other infants; and in elderly patients.

Interactions

Concomitant use with the following drugs may increase the hazard of nephrotoxicity, ototoxicity, and neurotoxicity: methoxyflurane, polymyxin B, vancomycin, capreomycin, cisplatin, cephalosporins, amphotericin B, and other aminoglycosides; hazard of ototoxicity is also increased during use with ethacrynic acid, furosemide, bumetanide, urea, or mannitol. Dimenhydrinate and other antiemetic and antivertigo drugs may mask streptomycin-induced ototoxicity.

Concomitant use with penicillins results in synergistic bactericidal effect against *Pseudomonas aeruginosa, Escherichia coli, Klebsiella, Citrobacter, Enterobacter, Serratia,* and *Proteus mirabilis;* however, the drugs are physically and chemically incompatible and are inactivated when mixed or given together. In vivo inactivation has been reported when aminoglycosides and penicillins are used concomitantly.

Streptomycin may potentiate neuromuscular blockade from general anesthetics or neuromuscular blocking agents such as succinylcholine and tubocurarine.

Effects on diagnostic tests

Streptomycin may cause false-positive reaction in copper sulfate test for urine glucose (Benedict's reagent or Clinitest).

Streptomycin-induced nephrotoxicity may elevate levels of blood urea nitrogen, nonprotein nitrogen, or serum creatinine levels and increase urinary excretion of casts.

Adverse reactions

• CNS: headache, lethargy.
• EENT: ototoxicity (tinnitus, vertigo, hearing loss).
• GI: diarrhea.

• GU: some nephrotoxicity (less frequent than with other aminoglycosides).
• HEMA: transient agranulocytosis.
• Local: pain, irritation, and sterile abscesses at injection site.
• Other: hypersensitivity reactions (rash, fever, urticaria, angioneurotic edema, *anaphylaxis*), bacterial and fungal superinfection, *neuromuscular blockade.*

Note: Drug should be discontinued if patient shows signs of ototoxicity, nephrotoxicity, or hypersensitivity, or if severe diarrhea indicates pseudomembranous colitis.

Overdose and treatment

Clinical signs of overdose include ototoxicity, nephrotoxicity, and neuromuscular toxicity. Remove drug by hemodialysis or peritoneal dialysis. Treatment with calcium salts or anticholinesterases reverses neuromuscular blockade.

▶ Special considerations

Besides those relevant to all *aminoglycosides,* consider the following recommendations.

• Protect hands when preparing drug; drug irritates skin.

• In primary tuberculosis therapy, discontinue streptomycin when sputum test is negative.

• Because streptomycin is dialyzable, patients undergoing hemodialysis may need dosage adjustments.

---

streptozocin
Zanosar

• Pharmacologic classification: alkylating agent, nitrosourea (cell cycle-phase nonspecific)
• Therapeutic classification: antineoplastic
• Pregnancy risk category C

How supplied

Available by prescription only
Injection: 1-g vials

Indications, route, and dosage

Dosage and indications may vary. Check current literature for recommended protocol.
Metastatic islet cell carcinoma of the pancreas, colon cancer, exocrine pancreatic tumors, carcinoid tumors
Adults and children: 500 mg/m² I.V. for 5 consecutive days q 4 to 6 weeks until maximum benefit or toxicity is observed. Alternatively, 1,000 mg/m² at weekly intervals for the first 2 weeks, increased to a maximum single dose of 1,500 mg/m². Usual course of therapy is 4 to 6 weeks.

Pharmacodynamics

Antineoplastic action: Streptozocin exerts its cytotoxic activity by selectively inhibiting DNA synthesis. The drug also causes cross-linking of DNA strands through an alkylation mechanism.

Pharmacokinetics

• *Absorption:* Streptozocin is not active orally; drug must be given intravenously.
• *Distribution:* After an I.V. dose, streptozocin and its

---

metabolites distribute mainly into the liver, kidneys, intestines, and pancreas. The drug has not been shown to cross the blood-brain barrier; however, its metabolites achieve concentrations in the cerebrospinal fluid equivalent to the concentration in the plasma.

● *Metabolism:* Streptozocin is extensively metabolized in the liver and kidneys.

● *Excretion:* The elimination of streptozocin from the plasma is biphasic, with an initial half-life of 5 minutes and a terminal phase half-life of 35 to 40 minutes. The plasma half-life of the metabolites is longer than that of the parent drug. The drug and its metabolites are excreted primarily in urine. A small amount of a dose may also be excreted in expired air.

Contraindications and precautions
No contraindications have been reported for streptozocin.

Drug should be used cautiously in patients with renal or hepatic dysfunction or hematologic compromise. Dosage adjustments are necessary.

Interactions
When used concomitantly, other nephrotoxic drugs may potentiate the nephrotoxicity caused by streptozocin. Concomitant use with doxorubicin prolongs the elimination half-life of doxorubicin and requires reduced dosage of doxorubicin. Concurrent use with phenytoin may decrease the effects of streptozocin on the pancreas.

Effects on diagnostic tests
Streptozocin therapy may decrease serum albumin and increase liver function test values; these increases are a sign of hepatotoxicity. BUN and serum creatinine levels may be increased, indicating nephrotoxicity. The drug may decrease blood glucose levels because of a sudden release of insulin.

Adverse reactions
● CNS: lethargy, confusion.
● GI: nausea and vomiting (dose-limiting), diarrhea.
● HEMA: *leukopenia, thrombocytopenia,* anemia.
● Hepatic: elevated liver enzymes, liver dysfunction.
● Local: sloughing, severe irritation if extravasation occurs.
● Metabolic: hyperglycemia, hypoglycemia.
● Renal: renal toxicity (evidenced by azotemia, glycosuria, and renal tubular acidosis), mild proteinuria.

Overdose and treatment
Clinical manifestations of overdose include myelosuppression, nausea, and vomiting.

Treatment is usually supportive and includes transfusion of blood components and antiemetics.

▶ Special considerations
Besides those relevant to all *alkylating agents,* consider the following recommendations.
● To reconstitute drug, use 9.5 ml of normal saline injection to yield a concentration of 100 mg/ml.
● It is best to use streptozocin within 12 hours of reconstitution. The reconstituted solution is a golden color that changes to dark brown upon decomposition.
● The product contains no preservatives and is not intended as a multiple-dose vial.
● Drug may be administered by rapid I.V. push injection.
● Drug may be further diluted in 10 to 200 ml of dextrose 5% in water to infuse over 10 to 15 minutes. It can also be infused over 6 hours.

● Gloves should be worn to protect the skin from contact during preparation or administration. If contact occurs, solution should be washed off immediately with soap and water. Follow recommended procedures for the safe preparation, administration, and disposal of chemotherapeutic agents.
● Extravasation may cause ulceration and tissue necrosis.
● Phenytoin may be administered concomitantly to protect pancreatic beta cells from cytotoxicity.
● Keep dextrose 50% at bedside because of risk of hypoglycemia from sudden release of insulin.
● Nausea and vomiting occur in almost all patients within 1 to 4 hours. Make sure patient is being treated with an antiemetic.
● Mild proteinuria is one of the first signs of renal toxicity and may require dosage reduction.
● Urine should be tested regularly for protein and glucose.
● Monitor CBC and liver function studies at least weekly.
● Use cautiously in patients with preexisting renal and hepatic disease.
● Renal toxicity resulting from streptozocin therapy is dose related and cumulative. Monitor renal function before and after each course of therapy. Obtain urinalysis, BUN levels, and creatinine clearance before therapy and at least weekly during drug administration. Continue weekly monitoring for 4 weeks after each course.

Information for the patient
● Encourage adequate fluid intake to increase urine output and reduce potential for renal toxicity.
● Remind diabetic patients that intensive monitoring of blood glucose levels is necessary.
● Tell patient to report any symptoms of anemia, infection, or bleeding immediately.

Breast-feeding
It is not known whether streptozocin distributes into breast milk. However, because of the potential for serious adverse reactions, mutagenicity, and carcinogenicity in the infant, breast-feeding is not recommended.

succimer
Chemet

● Pharmacologic classification: heavy metal
● Therapeutic classification: chelating agent
● Pregnancy risk category C

How supplied
Available by prescription only
Capsules: 100 mg

Indications, route, and dosage
Treatment of lead poisoning in children with blood lead levels above 45 mcg/dl
Children: Initially, 10 mg/kg or 350 mg/m² P.O. q 8 hours for 5 days. Higher starting doses are not recommended. Frequency of administration may be reduced to 10 mg/kg or 350 mg/m² q 12 hours for an additional 2 weeks of therapy. A course of treatment lasts 19 days and repeated courses may be necessary if indicated by

weekly monitoring of blood lead levels. A minimum of 2 weeks between courses is recommended unless blood lead concentrations mandate more prompt action.

SUCCIMER PEDIATRIC DOSING CHART			
WEIGHT			
Lb	Kg	DOSE (mg)	No. of Capsules
18 to 35	8 to 15	100	1
36 to 55	16 to 23	200	2
56 to 75	24 to 34	300	3
76 to 100	35 to 44	400	4
> 100	> 45	500	5

Dose is to be administered q 8 hours for 5 days, followed by same dose at q 12 hours for 14 days.

Pharmacodynamics
Antidote action: Succimer forms water-soluble chelates and increases the urinary excretion of lead.

Pharmacokinetics
● *Absorption:* Rapid but variable absorption after oral administration; peak blood levels in 1 to 2 hours.
● *Distribution:* Unknown.
● *Metabolism:* Rapidly and extensively metabolized.
● *Excretion:* 39% in feces as nonabsorbed drug; 9%, in urine; 1%, as carbon dioxide from the lungs. Approximately 90% of absorbed drug is excreted in urine.

Contraindications and precautions
Succimer is contraindicated in patients with known hypersensitivity or previous allergic reaction to the drug.
Use with caution in patients with renal dysfunction.

Interactions
Concurrent administration of succimer with other chelating agents is not recommended.

Effects on diagnostic tests
False-positive results for ketones in urine using nitroprusside reagents (Ketostix) and false decreased levels of serum uric acid and CPK have been reported. Transient mild elevations of serum transaminase levels have also been observed.

Adverse reactions
● CNS: drowsiness, dizziness, sensory motor neuropathy, sleepiness, paresthesia, headache.
● CV: *arrhythmias.*
● DERM: papular rash, herpetic rash, mucocutaneous eruptions, pruritus.
● EENT: ears plugged, cloudy film in eyes, otitis media, rhinorrhea, nasal congestion, watery eyes.
● GI: nausea, vomiting, diarrhea, loss of appetite, abdominal cramps, hemorrhoidal symptoms, metallic taste in mouth, loose stools.
● GU: decreased urination, difficulty voiding, proteinuria.
● HEMA: increased platelet count, intermittent eosinophilia.
● Respiratory: sore throat, cough, head cold.
● Other: leg pain; kneecap pain; back, stomach, rib, or flank pain; flulike symptoms; moniliasis; elevated levels of AST (SGOT), ALT (SGPT), alkaline phosphatase, and serum cholesterol.

Overdose and treatment
No cases of overdose have been reported. In cases of acute overdose, induce vomiting with ipecac syrup or perform gastric lavage, followed by administration of activated charcoal slurry and appropriate supportive therapy.

▶ Special considerations
● Identification and abatement of lead sources in child's environment is critical to successful therapy. Chelation therapy is not a substitute for preventing further exposure and should not be used to permit continued exposure.
● Patients who have received ethylenediaminetetra-acetic acid with or without dimercaprol may use succimer as subsequent therapy after an interval of 4 weeks. Use with other chelating agents concurrently is not recommended.
● Monitor serum transaminase levels before and at least weekly during therapy. Patients with a history of liver disease should be monitored more closely.
● The possiblity of allergic or other mucocutaneous reactions must be considered each time the drug is used, including the initial course.
● Elevated blood lead levels and associated symptoms may return rapidly after drug is discontinued because of redistribution of lead from bone to soft tissues and blood. Monitor patients at least once weekly for rebound blood lead levels.
● The severity of lead intoxication should be used as a guide for more frequent blood lead monitoring. This is measured by the initial blood lead level and the rate and degree of rebound of blood lead.
● Succimer is not indicated for prophylaxis of lead poisoning.

Information for the patient
● Instruct parents to maintain adequate fluid intake.
● Tell parents to consult physician if rash occurs.
● Urge parents to identify and remove source of lead in environment.
● Tell parents to store capsules at room temperature, out of children's reach.

Pediatric use
For young children who cannot swallow capsules, succimer capsule may be opened and sprinkled on a small amount of soft food or medicated beads from the capsules may be poured onto a spoon and followed with a fruit drink.

PHARMACOLOGIC CLASS

succinimide derivatives

ethosuximide
methsuximide
phensuximide

Succinimides, of which ethosuximide is the prototype, are similar in ring structure to hydantoins. They evolved from an attempt to synthesize less toxic oxazolidine-dione derivatives.

Pharmacology
Like the oxazolidinediones, succinimides elevate the seizure threshold in the basal ganglia and cerebral cortex and attenuate the synaptic response to repetitive

stimulation. They do not affect post-tetanic potentiation. These drugs suppress the characteristic spike-and-wave pattern of the EEG seen with absence seizures.

Clinical indications and actions
Convulsive disorders
Succinimides are used primarily to control absence seizures; they are used with other anticonvulsants when absence seizures are accompanied by other forms of epilepsy. Ethosuximide is the drug of choice; phensuximide is both the least effective and least toxic of this class. Methsuximide is used to control absence seizures refractory to other anticonvulsants. A beneficial therapeutic effect has been noted in patients with myoclonus and partial seizures with complex symptomatology.

Overview of adverse reactions
Most common adverse effects from succinimides involve the CNS and include drowsiness, headache, and blurred vision. Other adverse effects include acute dermatologic reactions (Stevens-Johnson syndrome), blood dyscrasias, renal dysfunction, and systemic lupus erythematosus. Drug should be used with caution in patients with acute intermittent porphyria.

▶ Special considerations
● Succinimides are contraindicated in patients with known hypersensitivity to succinimides; they should be used with caution in patients with hepatic or renal dysfunction.
● Monitor baseline liver and renal function studies and blood studies; repeat complete blood counts every 3 months and urinalysis and liver function tests every 6 months.
● Observe patient closely for dermatologic reactions at initiation of therapy.
● Monitor closely for signs of hypersensitivity or adverse reactions: skin rash, sore throat, joint pain, unexplained fever, or unusual bleeding or bruising.
● Succinimide anticonvulsants should not be discontinued abruptly.
● Succinimides add to CNS depressant effects of alcohol, narcotics, anxiolytics, antidepressants, and tranquilizers.
● Carefully follow manufacturer's directions for reconstitution, storage, and administration of all preparations.

Information for the patient
● Tell patient not to use alcohol while taking drug; it may decrease drug's effectiveness and increase CNS adverse effects.
● Advise patient to avoid hazardous tasks that require mental alertness until degree of sedative effect is determined.
● Tell patient to take oral drug with food if GI distress occurs.
● Teach patient signs and symptoms of hypersensitivity, liver dysfunction, and blood dyscrasias and advise patient to report them promptly. Also tell patient to call immediately if pregnancy occurs.
● Warn patient never to discontinue drug or to change dosage without medical approval.
● Encourage patient to wear a Medic Alert bracelet or necklace, listing drug and seizure disorder, while taking anticonvulsants.
● Inform patient to protect capsules from excessive heat, such as in a closed car or near a heat source.

Geriatric use
Use anticonvulsant drugs with caution. Elderly patients metabolize and excrete all drugs slowly and may obtain therapeutic effect from lower doses.

Pediatric use
Use with caution in children.

Breast-feeding
It is unknown whether succinimide anticonvulsants are excreted in breast milk; women should discontinue breast-feeding while taking these drugs.

Representative combinations
None.

---

succinylcholine chloride (suxamethonium chloride)
Anectine, Anectine Flo-Pack, Quelicin, Sucostrin

● Pharmacologic classification: depolarizing neuromuscular blocking agent
● Therapeutic classification: skeletal muscle relaxant
● Pregnancy risk category C

How supplied
Available by prescription only
Injection: 20 mg/ml, 50 mg/ml, 100 mg/ml (parenteral); 100 mg, 500 mg, 1 g (sterile for I.V. infusion)

Indications, route, and dosage
To induce skeletal muscle relaxation; facilitate intubation, ventilation, or orthopedic manipulations; and lessen muscle contractions in induced convulsions
Dosage depends on the anesthetic used, patient's needs, and response. Doses are representative and must be adjusted. Paralysis is induced after inducing hypnosis with thiopental or other appropriate agent.
Adults: For short procedures, 0.6 mg/kg (range 0.3 to 1.1 mg/kg) I.V. over 10 to 30 seconds; additional doses may be given if needed. For long procedures, 2.5 mg/minute (range 0.5 to 10 mg/minute) continuous I.V. infusion, or alternatively, 0.3 to 1.1 mg/kg by intermittent I.V. injection, followed by additional doses of 0.04 to 0.07 mg/kg as needed. Total dosage should not exceed 250 mg. If administered I.M., usual dose is 2.5 to 4 mg/kg, not to exceed 150 mg.
Children: 1 to 2 mg/kg I.V. or 2.5 to 4 mg/kg I.M. Maximum I.M. or I.V. dosage 150 mg.

Pharmacodynamics
Skeletal muscle relaxant action: Similar to acetylcholine (ACh), succinylcholine produces depolarization of the motor end-plate at the myoneural junction. The drug has a high affinity for ACh receptor sites and is resistant to acetylcholinesterase, thus producing a more prolonged depolarization at the motor end-plate. It also possesses histamine-releasing properties and reportedly stimulates the cardiac vagus and sympathetic ganglia.

A transient increase in intraocular pressure occurs immediately after injection and may persist after the onset of complete paralysis.

Pharmacokinetics

• *Absorption:* After I.V. administration, succinylcholine has a rapid onset of action (30 seconds), reaches its peak within 1 minute, and persists for 2 to 3 minutes, gradually dissipating within 10 minutes. After I.M. administration, the onset occurs within 2 to 3 minutes and persists for 10 to 30 minutes.

• *Distribution:* After I.V. administration, it is distributed in extracellular fluid and rapidly reaches its site of action. It crosses the placenta.

• *Metabolism:* Occurs rapidly by plasma pseudocholinesterase.

• *Excretion:* About 10% is excreted unchanged in urine.

Contraindications and precautions

Succinylcholine is contraindicated in patients with known hypersensitivity to the drug, or genetic disorders of plasma pseudocholinesterase, because of the potential for impaired metabolism; in patients with personal or family history of malignant hyperthermia, because drug may induce the disorder; with myopathies associated with elevated serum creatine kinase values, because the drug may exacerbate the damage associated with the disease; and in patients with narrow-angle glaucoma or penetrating eye injuries, because the drug elevates intraocular pressure.

Succinylcholine should be used with extreme caution in patients with low plasma pseudocholinesterase and in those recovering from severe trauma. It also should be used with caution in patients with electrolyte imbalances; in those receiving quinidine or cardiac glycosides; in patients with preexisting hyperkalemia, paraplegia, extensive or severe burns, extensive denervation of skeletal muscle from disease or injury; in patients who have had a stroke; in degenerative or dystrophic neuromuscular disease, because the drug may raise potassium levels; and during ocular surgery, because the drug increases intraocular pressure.

Use in pregnancy is appropriate only when clearly needed. Pregnant patients have lower levels of pseudocholinesterase, which may prolong the action of drug.

Interactions

Concomitant use with aminoglycoside antibiotics (including amikacin, gentamicin, kanamycin, neomycin, streptomycin), polymyxin antibiotics (polymyxin B sulfate, colistin), clindamycin, lincomycin, general anesthetics, local anesthetics, antimalarial agents, cholinesterase inhibitors (echothiophate, demecarium, isoflurophate), cyclophosphamide, oral contraceptives, nondepolarizing neuromuscular blocking agents, parenteral magnesium salts, lithium, phenelzine, hexafluorenium, quinidine, quinine, pancuronium, phenothiazines, thiotepa, and exposure to neurotoxic insecticides enhance or prolong succinylcholine's neuromuscular blocking effects. Use these drugs cautiously during surgical and postoperative periods.

Concomitant use with cardiac glycosides produces possible cardiac arrhythmias. Use together cautiously.

Effects on diagnostic tests

Use of succinylcholine may increase serum potassium concentrations.

Adverse reactions

• CV: transient bradycardia, tachycardia, hypertension, hypotension, *arrhythmias, sinus arrest.*
• EENT: increased intraocular pressure.

• Other: *prolonged respiratory depression, apnea,* wheezing or troubled breathing, *malignant hyperthermia,* muscle fasciculation, postoperative muscle pain, myoglobinemia, excessive salivation, myoglobinuria, rash, tachyphylaxis (after repeated doses).

Overdose and treatment

Clinical manifestations of overdose include apnea or prolonged muscle paralysis, which may be treated with controlled respiration. Use a peripheral nerve stimulator to monitor effects and degree of blockade.

▶ Special considerations

• Succinylcholine is the drug of choice for short procedures (less than 3 minutes) and for orthopedic manipulations; use caution in fractures or dislocations.
• Duration of action is prolonged to 20 minutes with continuous I.V. infusion or when given with hexafluorenium bromide.
• Some clinicians advocate pretreating adult patients with tubocurarine (3 to 6 mg) to minimize muscle fasciculations.
• Repeated fractional doses of succinylcholine alone are not advised; they may cause reduced response or prolonged apnea.
• Monitor baseline electrolyte determinations and vital signs (check respirations every 5 to 10 minutes during infusion).
• Keep airway clear. Have emergency respiratory support (endotracheal equipment, ventilator, oxygen, atropine, neostigmine) on hand.
• Store injectable form in refrigerator. Store powder form at room temperature and keep tightly closed. Use immediately after reconstitution.
• Do not mix with alkaline solutions (thiopental, sodium bicarbonate, barbiturates).
• Administration requires direct medical supervision by trained anesthesia personnel.
• Usually administered I.V., succinylcholine may be administered I.M. if suitable vein is inaccessible. Give deep I.M., preferably high into the deltoid muscle.
• Tachyphylaxis may occur.

Information for the patient

Reassure patient that postoperative stiffness is normal and will soon subside. Monitor for residual muscle weakness.

Geriatric use

Use with caution in elderly patients.

Pediatric use

Children may require larger doses of succinylcholine.

Breast-feeding

It is unknown whether drug is excreted in breast milk. Use with caution in breast-feeding women.

---

sucralfate
Carafate

- Pharmacologic classification: pepsin inhibitor
- Therapeutic classification: antiulcer agent
- Pregnancy risk category B

How supplied
Available by prescription only
Tablets: 1 g

Indications, route, and dosage
Short-term (up to 8 weeks) treatment of duodenal ulcer
Adults: 1 g P.O. q.i.d. 1 hour before meals and h.s.
Maintenance therapy of duodenal ulcer
Adults: 1 g P.O. b.i.d.

Pharmacodynamics
Antiulcer action: Sucralfate has a unique mechanism of action. The drug adheres to proteins at the ulcer site, forming a protective coating against gastric acid, pepsin, and bile salts. It also inhibits pepsin, exhibits a cytoprotective effect, and forms a viscous, adhesive barrier on the surface of the intact intestinal mucosa and stomach.

Pharmacokinetics
- *Absorption:* Only about 3% to 5% of a dose is absorbed. Drug activity is not related to the amount absorbed.
- *Distribution:* Sucralfate acts locally, at the ulcer site. Absorbed drug is distributed to many body tissues, including the liver and kidneys.
- *Metabolism:* None.
- *Excretion:* About 90% of a dose is excreted in feces; absorbed drug is excreted unchanged in urine. Duration of effect is 5 hours.

Contraindications and precautions
Sucralfate is contraindicated in patients with sucralfate allergy.

Interactions
Sucralfate decreases absorption of tetracycline, quinolones, phenytoin, digoxin, quinidine, cimetidine, ranitidine, theophylline, and fat-soluble vitamins A, D, E, and K. Antacids may decrease binding of drug to gastroduodenal mucosa, impairing effectiveness. Separate dosing of sucralfate and antacids by 2 hours.

Effects on diagnostic tests
None reported.

Adverse reactions
- CNS: dizziness, drowsiness, vertigo.
- GI: constipation (most common), diarrhea, nausea, dry mouth, gastric discomfort, indigestion.
- Other: rash, pruritus, back pain.
  Note: Drug should be discontinued if abdominal pain develops.

Overdose and treatment
No information available.

▶ Special considerations
- Sucralfate may inhibit absorption of other drugs. Schedule other medications 2 hours before or after sucralfate.
- Sucralfate is poorly water-soluble. For administration by nasogastric tube, have pharmacist prepare water-sorbitol suspension of sucralfate. Alternatively, place tablet in 60-ml syringe; add 20 ml water. Let stand with tip up for about 5 minutes, occasionally shaking gently. A suspension will form that may be administered from the syringe. After administration, tube should be flushed several times to ensure that the patient receives the entire dose.
- Patients who have difficulty swallowing tablet may place it in 15 to 30 ml of water at room temperature, allow it to disintegrate, and then ingest the resulting suspension. This is particularly useful for patient with esophagitis and painful swallowing.
- Monitor patient for constipation.
- Therapy exceeding 8 weeks is not recommended.
- Some experts believe that 2 g given b.i.d. are as effective as standard regimen.
- Drug treats ulcers as effectively as histamine₂-receptor antagonists.

Information for the patient
- Remind patient to take the drug on an empty stomach and to take sucralfate at least 1 hour before meals.
- Advise patient to continue taking drug as directed, even after pain begins to subside, to ensure adequate healing.
- Tell patient that he may take an antacid 30 minutes before or 2 hours after sucralfate.
- Warn patient not to take drug longer than 8 weeks.

Breast-feeding
Drug's risks to breast-feeding infants must be weighed against benefits.

sufentanil citrate
Sufenta

- Pharmacologic classification: opioid
- Therapeutic classification: analgesic, adjunct to anesthesia, anesthetic
- Controlled substance schedule II
- Pregnancy risk category C (D for prolonged use or use of high doses at term)

How supplied
Available by prescription only
Injection: 50 mcg/ml

Indications, route, and dosage
Adjunct to general anesthetic
Adults: 1 to 8 mcg/kg I.V. administered with nitrous oxide and oxygen.
Primary anesthetic
Adults: 8 to 30 mcg/kg I.V. administered with 100% oxygen and a muscle relaxant.

Pharmacodynamics
Analgesic action: Sufentanil has a high affinity for the opiate receptors with an agonistic effect to provide analgesia. It is also used as an adjunct to anesthesia or

---

as a primary anesthetic because of its potent CNS depressant effects.

Pharmacokinetics
• *Absorption:* After I.V. administration, sufentanil has a more rapid onset of action (1½ to 3 minutes) than does morphine or fentanyl.
• *Distribution:* The drug is highly lipophilic and is rapidly and extensively distributed in animals. It is highly protein-bound (> 90%) and redistributed rapidly.
• *Metabolism:* Sufentanil appears to be metabolized mainly in the liver and small intestine. Relatively little accumulation occurs. It has an elimination half-life of about 2.5 hours.
• *Excretion:* Sufentanil and its metabolites are excreted primarily in urine.

Contraindications and precautions
Sufentanil is contraindicated in patients with known hypersensitivity to the drug or any phenylpiperidine opiate (alfentanil, diphenoxylate, fentanyl, or meperidine).

Administer sufentanil with extreme caution to patients with supraventricular arrhythmias; avoid, or administer drug with extreme caution to patients with head injury or increased intracranial pressure, because drug obscures neurologic parameters; and during pregnancy and labor, because drug readily crosses placenta (premature infants are especially sensitive to the drug's respiratory and CNS depressant effects).

Administer sufentanil cautiously to patients with renal or hepatic dysfunction, because drug accumulation or prolonged duration of action may occur; to patients with pulmonary disease (asthma, chronic obstructive pulmonary disease), because drug depresses respiration and suppresses cough reflex; to patients undergoing biliary tract surgery, because drug may cause biliary spasm; to patients with convulsive disorders, because drug may precipitate seizures; to elderly or debilitated patients, who are more sensitive to both therapeutic and adverse drug effects; and to patients prone to physical or psychic addiction, because of the high risk of abuse potential.

Interactions
Concomitant use with other CNS depressants (narcotic analgesics, general anesthetics, antihistamines, phenothiazines, barbiturates, benzodiazepines, sedative-hypnotics, tricyclic antidepressants, alcohol, and muscle relaxants) potentiates drug's respiratory and CNS depression, sedation, and hypotensive effects. Concomitant use with cimetidine may also increase respiratory and CNS depression, causing confusion, disorientation, apnea, or seizures. Reduced dosage of sufentanil is usually necessary.

Drug accumulation and enhanced effects may result from concomitant use with other drugs that are extensively metabolized in the liver (rifampin, phenytoin, and digitoxin); combined use with anticholinergics may cause paralytic ileus.

Patients who become physically dependent on this drug may experience acute withdrawal syndrome if given high doses of a narcotic agonist-antagonist or a single dose of an antagonist.

Severe cardiovascular depression may result from the concomitant use of sufentanil with general anesthetics. If beta blockers have been used preoperatively, decrease dose of sufentanil. Nitrous oxide may produce cardiovascular depression when given with high doses of sufentanil.

The vagolytic effects of pancuronium may produce a dose-dependent elevation in heart rate during sufentanil and oxygen anesthesia; use moderate doses of pancuronium or a less vagolytic neuromuscular blocking agent; the vagolytic effect of pancuronium may be reduced in patients administered nitrous oxide with sufentanil.

Sufentanil may produce muscle rigidity involving all the skeletal muscles (incidence and severity are dose-related). Choose a neuromuscular blocking agent appropriate for the patient's cardiovascular status.

Effects on diagnostic tests
Sufentanil may increase plasma amylase and lipase and serum prolactin levels.

Adverse reactions
• CNS: chills.
• CV: tachycardia, bradycardia, chest wall rigidity, hypertension, hypotension.
• DERM: pruritus, erythema.
• GI: nausea, vomiting.
• Other: *respiratory depression* (common), skeletal muscle rigidity (common), apnea, *bronchospasm*, intraoperative muscle movement.
  Note: Drug should be discontinued if hypersensitivity, seizures, or life-threatening cardiac arrhythmias occur.

Overdose and treatment
To date, there is no clinical experience with acute overdose of sufentanil, but signs and symptoms are expected to be similar to those occurring with other opioids, with less cardiovascular toxicity. The most common signs and symptoms of acute opiate overdose are CNS depression, respiratory depression, and miosis (pinpoint pupils). Other acute toxic effects include hypotension, bradycardia, hypothermia, shock, apnea, cardiopulmonary arrest, circulatory collapse, pulmonary edema, and convulsions.

To treat acute overdose, first establish adequate respiratory exchange via a patent airway and ventilation as needed; administer a narcotic antagonist (naloxone) to reverse respiratory depression. (Because the duration of action of sufentanil is longer than that of naloxone, repeated naloxone dosing is necessary.) Do not give naloxone unless the patient has clinically significant respiratory or cardiovascular depression. Monitor vital signs closely.

Provide symptomatic and supportive treatment (continued respiratory support, correction of fluid or electrolyte imbalance). Monitor laboratory parameters, vital signs, and neurologic status closely.

▶ Special considerations
Besides those relevant to all *opioids,* consider the following recommendations.
• Sufentanil should only be administered by persons specifically trained in the use of I.V. anesthetics.
• When used at doses greater than 8 mcg/kg, postoperative mechanical ventilation and observation are essential because of extended postoperative respiratory depression.
• Compared to fentanyl, sufentanil has a more rapid onset and shorter duration of action.
• High doses can produce muscle rigidity. This effect can be reversed by administration of neuromuscular blocking agents.
• In patients weighing more than 20% above ideal body

---

weight, determine the sufentanil dosage on the basis of ideal body weight.

Geriatric use
Lower doses are usually indicated for elderly patients, who may be more sensitive to the therapeutic and adverse effects of the drug.

Pediatric use
The safety and efficacy of sufentanil in children under age 2 has been documented in only a limited number of patients (who were undergoing cardiovascular surgery).

sulconazole nitrate
Exelderm

- Pharmacologic classification: imidazole derivative
- Therapeutic classification: antifungal agent
- Pregnancy risk category C

How supplied
Available by prescription only
Cream: 1%
Topical solution: 1%

Indications, route, and dosage
Treatment of tinea cruris and tinea corporis caused by Trichophyton mentagrophytes, Epidermophyton floccosum, *and* Microsporum canis; *treatment of tinea versicolor caused by* Malassezia furfur
Adults: Massage a small amount of solution or cream into affected area daily to b.i.d.

Pharmacodynamics
Antifungal action: Mechanism is unknown. Drug is an imidazole derivative that inhibits the growth of both fungi and yeast.

Pharmacokinetics
Unknown.

Contraindications and precautions
Sulconazole is contraindicated in patients hypersensitive to any component of the product.

Interactions
None reported.

Effects on diagnostic tests
None reported.

Adverse reactions
- Local: itching, burning, stinging.

Overdose and treatment
No information available.

▶ Special considerations
Clinical improvement usually is noted within a week, with symptomatic relief in just a few days. Treatment should continue for at least 3 weeks. If no improvement

after 4 weeks, diagnosis should be reconsidered. Efficacy has not been proven in tinea pedis (athlete's foot).

Information for the patient
- Tell patient that, if irritation develops during treatment, he should discontinue drug and report the irritation.
- Explain to patient that he should continue therapy for the full course to prevent recurrence.
- Tell patient to avoid drug contact with the eyes and to wash hands thoroughly after applying.

Breast-feeding
It is not known if the drug appears in breast milk. Use with caution in breast-feeding women.

sulfacetamide sodium
AK-Sulf Forte, AK-Sulf Ointment, Bleph-10 S.O.P., Cetamide, Isopto Cetamide, Sodium Sulamyd 10%, Sodium Sulamyd 30%, Sulamyd, Sulf-10, Sulfair 15, Sulfex*, Sulten-10

- Pharmacologic classification: sulfonamide
- Therapeutic classification: antibiotic
- Pregnancy risk category C

How supplied
Available by prescription only
Ophthalmic solution: 10%, 15%, 30%
Ophthalmic ointment: 10%

Indications, route, and dosage
Inclusion conjunctivitis, corneal ulcers, trachoma, prophylaxis to ocular infection
Adults and children: Instill 1 or 2 drops of 10% solution into lower conjunctival sac q 2 to 3 hours during day, less often at night; or instill 1 or 2 drops of 15% solution into lower conjunctival sac q 1 to 2 hours initially, increasing interval as condition responds; or instill 1 drop of 30% solution into lower conjunctival sac q 2 hours. Instill ½" to 1" of 10% ointment into conjunctival sac q.i.d. and at bedtime. May use ointment at night along with drops during the day.

Pharmacodynamics
Antibiotic action: Sulfonamides act by inhibiting the uptake of para-aminobenzoic acid, which is required in the synthesis of folic acid needed for bacterial growth.

Pharmacokinetics
- *Absorption:* Sulfonamides aren't readily absorbed from mucous membranes.
- *Distribution:* Unknown.
- *Metabolism:* Unknown.
- *Excretion:* Unknown.

Contraindications and precautions
Sulfacetamide is contraindicated in patients with known or suspected sensitivity to sulfonamides or to any ingredients of the preparation. It should be used with caution to avoid overgrowth of nonsusceptible organisms during prolonged therapy. Use of the drug in children under age 2 months isn't recommended by the manufacturers.

Interactions
Tetracaine or other local anesthetics that are para-aminobenzoic acid derivatives may decrease the antibacterial activity of sulfacetamide. Concomitant use of silver preparations or gentamicin sulfate ophthalmic solution is not recommended.

Sulfonamides are inactivated by para-aminobenzoic acid present in purulent exudates.

Effects on diagnostic tests
None reported.

Adverse reactions
● Eye: blurred vision, transient burning and stinging, hyperemia, epithelial keratitis.
● Other: hypersensitivity (including itching or burning), headache, overgrowth of nonsusceptible organisms, Stevens-Johnson syndrome (rare), sensitivity to light, systemic lupus erythematosus.

Note: Drug should be discontinued if any signs of sensitivity occur.

Overdose and treatment
No information available.

▶ Special considerations
● Drug has largely been replaced by antibiotics for treating major infections, but it is still used in minor ocular infections.
● Purulent exudate interferes with sulfacetamide action; remove as much as possible from lids before instilling sulfacetamide.
● Warn patient that eye drop burns slightly.
● Warn patient not to touch tip of tube or dropper to eye or surrounding tissue.
● Store in tightly closed, light-resistant container away from heat and light; do not use discolored (dark brown) solution.

Information for the patient
● Teach patient how to instill drops correctly.
● Warn patient not to touch tip of tube or dropper to eye or surrounding tissue.
● Tell patient to watch for signs of sensitivity, such as itching lids or constant burning, and to report these immediately.
● Explain that eye drops may burn slightly.
● Tell patient to avoid sharing washcloths and towels with family members.
● Advise patient to wait for 10 minutes before using another eye preparation.

Pediatric use
Use of the drug in children under age 2 months is not recommended.

Breast-feeding
Although orally ingested sulfonamides have been reported to be excreted in low concentrations in breast milk, no data are available concerning ophthalmic sulfacetamide.

sulfadiazine
Microsulfon

● Pharmacologic classification: sulfonamide
● Therapeutic classification: antibiotic
● Pregnancy risk category B (D at term)

How supplied
Available by prescription only
Tablets: 500 mg

Indications, route, and dosage
Urinary tract infection
Adults: Initially, 2 to 4 g P.O.; then 500 mg to 1 g P.O. q 6 hours.
Children: Initially, 75 mg/kg or 2 g/m² P.O.; then 150 mg/kg or 4 g/m² P.O. in four to six divided doses daily. Maximum daily dose is 6 g.
Rheumatic fever prophylaxis, as an alternative to penicillin
Children weighing more than 30 kg: 1 g P.O. daily.
Children weighing less than 30 kg: 500 mg P.O. daily.
Adjunctive treatment in toxoplasmosis
Adults: 4 g P.O. in divided doses q 6 hours for 3 to 4 weeks and up to 6 months or longer in patients with acquired immunodeficiency syndrome; given with pyrimethamine 25 mg P.O. daily.
Children: 100 mg/kg P.O. in divided doses q 6 hours for 3 to 4 weeks; given with pyrimethamine 2 mg/kg daily for 3 days, then 1 mg/kg daily for 3 to 4 weeks.
Uncomplicated attacks of malaria
Adults: 500 mg P.O. q.i.d. for 5 days.
Children: 25 to 50 mg/kg P.O. q.i.d. for 5 days.

Pharmacodynamics
Antibacterial action: Sulfadiazine is bacteriostatic. It inhibits formation of dihydrofolic acid from para-aminobenzoic acid (PABA), thus preventing bacterial cell synthesis of essential nucleic acids. It acts synergistically with agents such as trimethoprim that block folic acid synthesis at a later stage, thus delaying or preventing bacterial resistance.

Sulfadiazine is active against many gram-positive bacteria, *Chlamydia trachomatis,* many Enterobacteriaceae, and some strains of *Toxoplasma gondii* and *Plasmodium falciparum.*

Pharmacokinetics
● *Absorption:* Sulfadiazine is absorbed from the GI tract after oral administration; peak serum levels occur at 2 hours.
● *Distribution:* Sulfadiazine is distributed widely into most body tissues and fluids, including synovial, pleural, amniotic, prostatic, peritoneal, and seminal fluids; CSF penetration is poor. Sulfadiazine crosses the placenta; it is 32% to 56% protein-bound.
● *Metabolism:* Sulfadiazine is metabolized partially in the liver.
● *Excretion:* Both unchanged drug and metabolites are excreted primarily in urine by glomerular filtration and, to a lesser extent, renal tubular secretion; some drug is excreted in breast milk. Urine solubility of unchanged drug increases as urine pH increases.

Contraindications and precautions

Sulfonamides are contraindicated in patients with known hypersensitivity to sulfonamides or to any other drug containing sulfur (e.g., thiazides, furosemide, or oral sulfonylureas); and in patients with severe renal or hepatic dysfunction, or porphyria; during pregnancy at term, and during lactation; and in infants under age 2 months.

Administer sulfadiazine with caution to patients with mild to moderate renal or hepatic impairment, urinary obstruction (because of the risk of drug accumulation), severe allergies, asthma, blood dyscrasias, or glucose-6-phosphate dehydrogenase deficiency.

Interactions

Sulfadiazine may inhibit hepatic metabolism of oral anticoagulants, displacing them from binding sites and enhancing anticoagulant effects.

Concomitant use with PABA antagonizes effects of sulfonamides; with oral hypoglycemics (sulfonylureas) enhances their hypoglycemic effects, probably by displacing sulfonylureas from protein-binding sites; with either trimethoprim or pyrimethamine (folic acid antagonists with different mechanisms of action) results in synergistic antibacterial effects and delays or prevents bacterial resistance.

Concomitant use of urine acidifying agents (ammonium chloride or ascorbic acid) or methenamine decreases sulfonamide solubility, which increases risk of crystalluria.

Effects on diagnostic tests

Sulfadiazine alters urine glucose tests utilizing cupric sulfate (Benedict's reagent or Clinitest). Sulfadiazine may elevate liver function test results; it may decrease serum levels of erythrocytes, platelets, or leukocytes.

Adverse reactions

- CNS: headache, mental depression, *seizures*, hallucinations.
- DERM: *erythema multiforme (Stevens-Johnson syndrome)*, generalized skin eruption, epidermal necrolysis, *exfoliative dermatitis*, photosensitivity, urticaria, pruritus.
- GI: nausea, vomiting, diarrhea, abdominal pain, anorexia, stomatitis.
- GU: toxic nephrosis with oliguria and anuria, crystalluria, hematuria.
- HEMA: *agranulocytosis, aplastic anemia,* megaloblastic anemia, thrombocytopenia, leukopenia, hemolytic anemia.
- Hepatic: jaundice.
- Local: irritation, extravasation.
- Other: hypersensitivity, serum sickness, drug fever, *anaphylaxis,* bacterial and fungal superinfection.

Note: Drug should be discontinued if signs of toxicity or hypersensitivity occur; if hematologic abnormalities are accompanied by sore throat, pallor, fever, jaundice, purpura, or weakness; if crystalluria is accompanied by renal colic, hematuria, oliguria, proteinuria, urinary obstruction, urolithiasis, increased BUN levels, or anuria; or if severe diarrhea indicates pseudomembranous colitis.

Overdose and treatment

Clinical signs of overdose include dizziness, drowsiness, headache, unconsciousness, anorexia, abdominal pain, nausea, and vomiting. More severe complications, including hemolytic anemia, agranulocytosis, dermatitis, acidosis, sensitivity reactions, and jaundice, may be fatal.

Treatment includes gastric lavage, if ingestion has occurred within the preceding 4 hours followed by correction of acidosis, forced fluids, and urinary alkalinization to enhance solubility and excretion. Treatment of renal failure as well as transfusion of appropriate blood products (in severe hematologic toxicity) may be required.

▶ **Special considerations**

Besides those relevant to all *sulfonamides,* consider the following recommendation.

- Sulfadiazine is a less soluble sulfonamide; therefore, it is more likely to cause crystalluria. Avoid concomitant use of urine acidifiers and ensure adequate fluid intake. If you can't ensure adequate fluid intake, recommend sodium bicarbonate to reduce risk of crystalluria.

Pediatric use

Sulfadiazine is contraindicated in children younger than age 2 months.

Breast-feeding

Sulfadiazine is excreted in breast milk and should not be used in breast-feeding women.

sulfamethizole
Thiosulfil-Forte

- Pharmacologic classification: sulfonamide
- Therapeutic classification: antibiotic
- Pregnancy risk category B (D at term)

How supplied

Available by prescription only
Tablets: 500 mg

Indications, route, and dosage

Urinary tract infections
Adults: Initially, 0.5 to 1 g P.O. t.i.d. to q.i.d.
Children and infants over age 2 months: 30 to 45 mg/kg P.O. daily in four equally divided doses.
Lymphogranuloma venereum (genital, inguinal, or anorectal infection)
Adults: 1 g daily for at least 2 weeks.

Pharmacodynamics

Antibacterial action: Sulfamethizole is bacteriostatic. It acts by inhibiting formation of dihydrofolic acid from para-aminobenzoic acid (PABA), thus preventing bacterial cell synthesis of essential nucleic acids.

Sulfamethizole's spectrum of action includes *Escherichia coli, Klebsiella, Enterobacter, Staphylococcus aureus,* and *Proteus mirabilis* and *vulgaris.*

Pharmacokinetics

- *Absorption:* Sulfamethizole is absorbed from the GI tract after oral administration; peak serum levels occur after 2 hours.
- *Distribution:* Sulfamethizole is distributed into CSF and crosses the placenta; it is 90% protein-bound.
- *Metabolism:* Sulfamethizole is metabolized partially in the liver.
- *Excretion:* Both unchanged drug and metabolites are excreted primarily in urine by glomerular filtration and,

to a lesser extent, renal tubular secretion; some drug is excreted in breast milk. Urinary solubility of unchanged drug increases as urine pH increases.

Contraindications and precautions
Sulfamethizole is contraindicated in patients with known hypersensitivity to sulfonamides or to any other drug containing sulfur (for example, thiazides, furosemide, or oral sulfonylureas); in patients with severe renal or hepatic dysfunction, or porphyria; during pregnancy, at term, and during lactation; and in infants under age 2 months.

Administer sulfamethizole cautiously in patients with mild to moderate renal or hepatic impairment, urinary obstruction (because of the risk of drug accumulation), severe allergies, asthma, blood dyscrasias, and glucose-6-phosphate dehydrogenase deficiency.

Interactions
Sulfamethizole may inhibit hepatic metabolism of oral anticoagulants, displacing them from binding sites and enhancing anticoagulant effects; it may also inhibit metabolism of phenytoin, enhancing effects of phenytoin.

Concomitant use with PABA antagonizes sulfonamide effects; with oral sulfonylureas enhances their hypoglycemic effects, probably by displacing sulfonylureas from protein-binding sites; with either trimethoprim or pyrimethamine (folic acid antagonists with different mechanisms of action) results in synergistic antibacterial effects and delays or prevents bacterial resistance; and with phenytoin inhibits phenytoin metabolism and leads to elevated serum levels of the anticonvulsant drug.

Concomitant use of urine acidifying agents (ammonium chloride, or ascorbic acid) or methenamine decreases sulfonamide solubility, thus increasing risk of crystalluria.

Effects on diagnostic tests
Sulfamethizole alters results of urine glucose tests utilizing cupric sulfate (Benedict's reagent or Clinitest).

Sulfamethizole may elevate liver function test results; it may decrease serum levels of erythrocytes, platelets, or leukocytes.

Adverse reactions
● CNS: headache, mental depression, *seizures*, hallucinations.
● DERM: *erythema multiforme (Stevens-Johnson syndrome)*, generalized skin eruption, epidermal necrolysis, *exfoliative dermatitis*, photosensitivity, urticaria, pruritus.
● GI: nausea, vomiting, diarrhea, abdominal pain, anorexia, stomatitis.
● GU: toxic nephrosis with oliguria and anuria, crystalluria, hematuria.
● HEMA: *agranulocytosis, aplastic anemia,* megaloblastic anemia, thrombocytopenia, leukopenia, hemolytic anemia.
● Hepatic: jaundice.
● Other: hypersensitivity, serum sickness, drug fever, *anaphylaxis,* bacterial and fungal superinfection.
Note: Drug should be discontinued if signs of toxicity or hypersensitivity occur; if hematologic abnormalities are accompanied by sore throat, pallor, fever, jaundice, purpura, or weakness; if crystalluria is accompanied by renal colic, hematuria, oliguria, proteinuria, urinary obstruction, urolithiasis, increased BUN levels, or anuria;

or if severe diarrhea indicates pseudomembranous colitis.

Overdose and treatment
Clinical signs of overdose include dizziness, drowsiness, headache, unconsciousness, anorexia, abdominal pain, nausea, and vomiting. More severe complications, including hemolytic anemia, agranulocytosis, dermatitis, acidosis, sensitivity reactions, and jaundice, may be fatal.

Treat by gastric lavage, if ingestion has occurred within the preceding 4 hours, followed by correction of acidosis, forced fluids, and urinary alkalinization to enhance solubility and excretion. Treatment of renal failure and transfusion of appropriate blood products (in severe hematologic toxicity) may be required.

▶ **Special considerations**
Besides those relevant to all *sulfonamides,* consider the following recommendation.
● During treatment with combinations of sulfamethizole and phenazopyridine, the drug colors urine red-orange. Do not mistake this for hematuria.

Information for the patient
Tell the patient receiving a combination product containing pherazopyridine (such as Urobiotic-250) that the drug normally turns urine red-orange and can stain fabrics and soft contact lenses.

Pediatric use
Sulfamethizole is contraindicated in children younger than age 2 months.

Breast-feeding
Sulfamethizole is excreted in breast milk and should not be used in breast-feeding women.

---

sulfamethoxazole
Gamazole, Gantanol, Gantanol DS, Methanoxanol

● Pharmacologic classification: sulfonamide
● Therapeutic classification: antibiotic
● Pregnancy risk category B (D at term)

How supplied
Available by prescription only
Tablets: 500 mg, 1,000 mg
Suspension: 500 mg/5 ml

Indications, route, and dosage
Urinary tract and systemic infections
Adults: Initially, 2 g P.O.; then 1 g P.O. b.i.d., up to t.i.d. for severe infections.
Children and infants over age 2 months: Initially, 50 to 60 mg/kg P.O., then 25 to 30 mg/kg b.i.d. Maximum dosage should not exceed 75 mg/kg daily.
Lymphogranuloma venereum (genital, inguinal, or anorectal infection)
Adults: 1 g P.O. b.i.d. for at least 2 weeks.

Pharmacodynamics
Antibacterial action: Sulfamethoxazole is bacteriostatic. It acts by inhibiting formation of dihydrofolic acid from para-aminobenzoic acid (PABA), thus preventing

---

bacterial cell synthesis of essential nucleic acids. It acts synergistically with agents such as trimethoprim that block folic acid synthesis at a later stage, thus delaying or preventing bacterial resistance.

Sulfamethoxazole's spectrum of action includes some gram-positive bacteria, *Chlamydia trachomatis,* many Enterobacteriaceae, and some strains of *Toxoplasma* and *Plasmodium.*

Pharmacokinetics
● *Absorption:* Sulfamethoxazole is absorbed from the GI tract after oral administration; peak serum levels occur at 2 hours.
● *Distribution:* Sulfamethoxazole is distributed widely into most body tissues and fluids, including cerebrospinal, synovial, pleural, amniotic, prostatic, peritoneal, and seminal fluids. Sulfamethoxazole crosses the placenta; it is 50% to 70% protein-bound.
● *Metabolism:* Sulfamethoxazole is metabolized partially in the liver.
● *Excretion:* Both unchanged drug and metabolites are excreted primarily in urine by glomerular filtration and, to a lesser extent, renal tubular secretion; some drug is excreted in breast milk. Urinary solubility of unchanged drug increases as urine pH increases. Plasma half-life in patients with normal renal function is 7 to 12 hours.

Contraindications and precautions
Sulfamethoxazole is contraindicated in patients with known hypersensitivity to sulfonamides or to any other drug containing sulfur (for example, thiazides, furosemide, or oral sulfonylureas); in patients with severe renal or hepatic dysfunction, or porphyria; during pregnancy at term, and during lactation; and in infants under age 2 months.

Administer sulfonamides with caution to patients with mild to moderate renal or hepatic impairment, urinary obstruction (because of the risk of drug accumulation), severe allergies, asthma, blood dyscrasias, or glucose-6-phosphate dehydrogenase deficiency.

Interactions
Sulfamethoxazole may inhibit hepatic metabolism of oral anticoagulants, displacing them from binding sites and enhancing anticoagulant effects. Concomitant use with PABA antagonizes sulfonamide effects; with oral hypoglycemics (sulfonylureas) enhances their hypoglycemic effects, probably by displacing sulfonylureas from protein-binding sites; and with either trimethoprim or pyrimethamine (folic acid antagonists with different mechanisms of action) results in synergistic antibacterial effects and delays or prevents bacterial resistance.

Concomitant use of urine acidifying agents (ammonium chloride or ascorbic acid) decreases urine pH and sulfonamide solubility, thus increasing risk of crystalluria.

Effects on diagnostic tests
Sulfamethoxazole alters results of urine glucose tests utilizing cupric sulfate (Benedict's reagent or Clinitest).

Sulfamethoxazole may elevate liver function test results; it may decrease serum levels of erythrocytes, platelets, or leukocytes.

Adverse reactions
● CNS: headache, mental depression, *seizures,* hallucinations.

● DERM: *erythema multiforme (Stevens-Johnson syndrome),* generalized skin eruption, epidermal necrolysis, *exfoliative dermatitis,* photosensitivity, urticaria, pruritus.
● GI: nausea, vomiting, diarrhea, abdominal pain, anorexia, stomatitis.
● GU: toxic nephrosis with oliguria and anuria, crystalluria, hematuria.
● HEMA: *agranulocytosis, aplastic anemia,* megaloblastic anemia, thrombocytopenia, leukopenia, hemolytic anemia.
● Hepatic: jaundice.
● Other: hypersensitivity, serum sickness, drug fever, *anaphylaxis,* bacterial and fungal superinfection.
Note: Drug should be discontinued if signs of toxicity or hypersensitivity occur; if hematologic abnormalities are accompanied by sore throat, pallor, fever, jaundice, purpura, or weakness; if crystalluria is accompanied by renal colic, hematuria, oliguria, proteinuria, urinary obstruction, urolithiasis, increased BUN levels, or anuria; or if severe diarrhea indicates pseudomembranous colitis.

Overdose and treatment
Clinical signs of overdose include dizziness, drowsiness, headache, unconsciousness, anorexia, abdominal pain, nausea, and vomiting. More severe complications, including hemolytic anemia, agranulocytosis, dermatitis, acidosis, sensitivity reactions, and jaundice, may be fatal.

Treat by gastric lavage, if ingestion has occurred within the preceding 4 hours, followed by correction of acidosis, forced fluids, and urinary alkalinization to enhance solubility and excretion. Treatment of renal failure and transfusion of appropriate blood products (in severe hematologic toxicity) may be required.

▶ Special considerations
Recommendations for administration, preparation and storage, and care and teaching of the patient during therapy with sulfamethoxazole are those common to all *sulfonamides.*

Pediatric use
Sulfamethoxazole is contraindicated in children younger than age 2 months.

Breast-feeding
Sulfamethoxazole is excreted in breast milk and should not be administered to breast-feeding women.

sulfasalazine
Azaline, Azaline EC, Azulfidine, Azulfidine En-tabs, Salazopyrin*, S.A.S.-500

● Pharmacologic classification: sulfonamide
● Therapeutic classification: antibiotic
● Pregnancy risk category B (D at term)

How supplied
Available by prescription only
Tablets: 500 mg with or without enteric coating
Suspension: 250 mg/5 ml

Indications, route, and dosage
Mild to moderate ulcerative colitis, adjunctive therapy in severe ulcerative colitis

Adults: Initially, 3 to 4 g P.O. daily in evenly divided doses. Maintenance dose is 1.5 to 2 g P.O. daily in divided doses q 6 hours. May need to start with 1 to 2 g initially, with a gradual increase in dose to minimize adverse reactions.

Children over age 2: Initially, 40 to 60 mg/kg P.O. daily, divided into three to six doses; then 30 mg/kg daily in four doses. May need to start at lower dose if gastrointestinal intolerance occurs.

Pharmacodynamics
Antibacterial action: The exact mechanism of action of sulfasalazine in ulcerative colitis is unknown; it is believed to be a pro-drug metabolized by intestinal flora in the colon. One metabolite (5-amino salicylic acid or mesalamine) is responsible for the anti-inflammatory effect; the other metabolite (sulfapyridine) may be responsible for some adverse effects.

Pharmacokinetics
• *Absorption:* Sulfasalazine is absorbed poorly from the GI tract after oral administration; about 80% is transported to the colon where intestinal flora metabolize the drug to its active ingredients, sulfapyridine (antibacterial) and 5-aminosalicylic acid (anti-inflammatory), which exert their effects locally. Sulfapyridine is absorbed from the colon, but 5-aminosalicylic acid is not.
• *Distribution:* Human data on sulfasalazine distribution is lacking; animal studies have identified drug and metabolites in sera, liver, and intestinal walls. Parent drug and both metabolites cross the placenta.
• *Metabolism:* Sulfasalazine is cleaved by intestinal flora in the colon.
• *Excretion:* Systemically absorbed sulfasalazine is excreted chiefly in urine; some parent drug and metabolites are excreted in breast milk. Plasma half-life is about 6 to 8 hours.

Contraindications and precautions
Like all sulfonamides, sulfasalazine is contraindicated in patients with known hypersensitivity to sulfonamides or to any other drug containing sulfur (for example, thiazides, furosemide, or oral sulfonylureas) in patients with known hypersensitivity to salicylates; in patients with severe renal or hepatic dysfunction, or porphyria; during pregnancy, at term, and during lactation; and in infants and children under age 2. Sulfasalazine is also contraindicated in patients with intestinal or urinary tract obstructions because of the risk of local GI irritation and of crystalluria.

Administer sulfonamides with caution to patients with mild to moderate renal or hepatic impairment, severe allergies, asthma, blood dyscrasias, or glucose-6-phosphate dehydrogenase deficiency.

Interactions
Sulfasalazine may inhibit hepatic metabolism of oral anticoagulants, displacing them from binding sites and enhancing anticoagulant effects.

Concomitant use with oral hypoglycemics (sulfonylureas) enhances hypoglycemic effects, probably by displacing sulfonylureas from protein-binding sites.

Sulfasalazine may reduce GI absorption of digoxin and folic acid.

Concomitant use of urine acidifying agents (ammonium chloride, ascorbic acid) decreases urine pH and sulfonamide solubility, thus increasing risk of crystalluria. Concomitant use with antibiotics that alter intestinal flora may interfere with conversion of sulfasalazine to sulfapyridine and 5-aminosalicylic acid, decreasing its effectiveness.

Concomitant use of antacids may cause premature dissolution of enteric-coated tablets (which are designed to dissolve in the intestines), thus increasing systemic absorption and hazard of toxicity.

Effects on diagnostic tests
Sulfasalazine alters results of urine glucose tests utilizing cupric sulfate (Benedict's reagent or Clinitest).

Sulfasalazine may elevate liver function test results; it may decrease serum levels of erythrocytes, platelets, or leukocytes.

Adverse reactions
• CNS: headache, mental depression, *seizures*, hallucinations, tinnitus.
• DERM: *erythema multiforme (Stevens-Johnson syndrome)*, generalized skin eruption, *epidermal necrolysis, exfoliative dermatitis*, photosensitivity, urticaria, pruritus.
• GI: nausea, vomiting, diarrhea, abdominal pain, anorexia, stomatitis.
• GU: toxic nephrosis with oliguria and anuria, crystalluria, hematuria, oligospermia, infertility.
• HEMA: *agranulocytosis, aplastic anemia*, megaloblastic anemia, thrombocytopenia, leukopenia, hemolytic anemia.
• Hepatic: jaundice.
• Other: hypersensitivity, serum sickness, drug fever, *anaphylaxis*, bacterial and fungal superinfection.
   Note: Drug should be discontinued if signs of toxicity or hypersensitivity occur; if hematologic abnormalities are accompanied by sore throat, pallor, fever, jaundice, purpura, or weakness; if crystalluria is accompanied by renal colic, hematuria, oliguria, proteinuria, urinary obstruction, urolithiasis, increased BUN levels, or anuria; if severe diarrhea indicates pseudomembranous colitis; if severe nausea, vomiting, or diarrhea persists.

Overdose and treatment
Clinical signs of overdose include dizziness, drowsiness, headache, unconsciousness, anorexia, abdominal pain, nausea, and vomiting. More severe complications, including hemolytic anemia, agranulocytosis, dermatitis, acidosis, sensitivity reactions, and jaundice, may be fatal.

Treat by gastric lavage, if ingestion has occurred within the preceding 4 hours, followed by correction of acidosis, forced fluids, and urinary alkalinization to enhance solubility and excretion. Treatment of renal failure and transfusion of appropriate blood products (in severe hematologic toxicity) may be required.

▶ Special considerations
Besides those relevant to all *sulfonamides*, consider the following recommendations.
• Most adverse effects from sulfasalazine involve the GI tract; minimize reactions and facilitate absorption by spacing doses evenly and administering drug after food.
• Drug colors urine orange-yellow. The patient's skin may also turn orange-yellow.
• Do not administer antacids concomitantly with enteric-coated sulfasalazine; they may alter absorption.

Information for the patient
● Tell patient that sulfasalazine normally turns urine orange-yellow. Warn patient that skin may also turn orange-yellow.
● Advise patient not to take antacids simultaneously with sulfasalazine.
● Advise patient to take drug after meals to reduce GI distress and to facilitate passage into intestines.

Pediatric use
Sulfasalazine is contraindicated in patients younger than age 2 months.

Breast-feeding
Sulfasalazine is excreted in breast milk and should not be administered to breast-feeding women.

---

sulfinpyrazone
Anturane, Aprazone

● Pharmacologic classification: uricosuric agent
● Therapeutic classification: renal tubular-blocking agent, platelet aggregation inhibitor
● Pregnancy risk category C

How supplied
Available by prescription only
Tablets: 100 mg
Capsules: 200 mg

Indications, route, and dosage
Chronic gouty arthritis and intermittent gouty arthritis, or hyperuricemia associated with gout
Adults: Initially, 200 to 400 mg P.O. daily in two divided doses, gradually increasing to maintenance dosage in 1 week. Maintenance dosage is 400 mg P.O. daily in two divided doses; may increase to 800 mg daily or decrease to 200 mg daily.
†**Prophylaxis of thromboembolic disorders, including angina, myocardial infarction, transient (cerebral) ischemic attacks, and in patients with prosthetic heart valves**
Adults: 600 to 800 mg daily in divided doses to decrease platelet aggregation.

Pharmacodynamics
Uricosuric action: Sulfinpyrazone competitively inhibits renal tubule reabsorption of uric acid. Sulfinpyrazone inhibits prostaglandin synthesis, thereby preventing platelet aggregation.

Pharmacokinetics
● *Absorption:* Sulfinpyrazone is absorbed completely after oral administration; peak plasma levels occur in 2 hours. Effects usually last 4 to 6 hours but may persist up to 10 hours.
● *Distribution:* Sulfinpyrazone is 98% to 99% protein-bound.
● *Metabolism:* Sulfinpyrazone is metabolized rapidly in the liver.
● *Excretion:* Sulfinpyrazone and its metabolites are eliminated in urine; about 50% is excreted unchanged.

Contraindications and precautions
Sulfinpyrazone is contraindicated in patients with hypersensitivity to the drug or to other prazolone derivatives, such as phenylbutazone; in patients with active peptic ulcer disease, gouty nephropathy, bone-marrow depression, or azotemia; in patients with elevated uric acid levels from radiation, chemotherapy, or myeloproliferative disease; or in patients with history of an acute attack (within 2 weeks).
Sulfinpyrazone should be used cautiously in patients with a history of peptic ulcer disease and in patients with impaired renal or hepatic function, because drug may worsen these conditions.

Interactions
Sulfinpyrazone decreases renal tubular secretion of penicillin, other beta-lactam antibiotics, nitrofurantoin, and sulfonylureas. Reduced excretion of nitrofurantoin decreases sulfinpyrazone's efficacy in urinary tract infections and increases systemic toxicity; decreased excretion of sulfonylureas may cause hypoglycemia. Sulfinpyrazone may potentiate effects of oral hypoglycemic agents, such as sulfonylureas.
Sulfinpyrazone decreases the metabolism of warfarin, enhancing its hypoprothrombinemic effect and the risk of bleeding; increased bleeding in these patients also may result from sulfinpyrazone's anti-platelet effect.
Most diuretics, pyrazinamide, alcohol, and diazoxide increase serum uric acid and thus increase sulfinpyrazone dosage requirements.
Salicylates block sulfinpyrazone's uricosuric effects only in high doses; small occasional doses usually do not interact significantly.
Cholestyramine decreases absorption of sulfinpyrazone; sulfinpyrazone should be taken 1 hour before or 4 to 6 hours after cholestyramine. Probenecid inhibits renal excretion of sulfinpyrazone.

Effects on diagnostic tests
Drug decreases urinary excretion of aminohippuric acid and phenolsulfonphthalein and may alter renal function test results.

Adverse reactions
● CNS: dizziness, vertigo, tinnitus, ataxia.
● GI: nausea, dyspepsia, abdominal pain, blood loss, reactivation of peptic ulcer.
● GU: renal colic, hematuria, uric acid stones.
● HEMA: anemia, leukopenia, *agranulocytosis*, thrombocytopenia.
● Other: rash.
Note: Drug should be discontinued if hypersensitivity, reactivation of peptic ulcer disease, leukopenia, thrombocytopenia, or granulocytopenia occurs.

Overdose and treatment
Clinical signs of overdose include nausea, vomiting, epigastric pain, ataxia, labored breathing, seizures, and coma. Treat supportively; induce emesis or use gastric lavage as appropriate. Treat seizures with diazepam or phenytoin or both.

▶ Special considerations
● Sulfinpyrazone does not accumulate and tolerance to it does not develop; it is suitable for long-term use.
● Sulfinpyrazone has no analgesic or anti-inflammatory actions and no effect on acute peptic ulcer attacks; start therapy after attack subsides.

• Monitor renal function and CBC routinely.
• Monitor serum uric acid levels and adjust dosage accordingly.
• Give with food, milk, or prescribed antacids to lessen GI upset.
• Sulfinpyrazone is used investigationally to increase platelet survival time, to treat thromboembolic phenomena, and to prevent myocardial infarction recurrence.
• Maintain adequate hydration with high fluid intake to prevent formation of uric acid kidney stones.

Information for the patient
• Explain that gouty attacks may increase during the first 6 to 12 months of therapy; patient should not discontinue drug without medical approval.
• Encourage patient to comply with dosage regimen and to keep scheduled follow-up visits.
• Tell patient to drink 8 to 10 glasses of fluid each day and take drug with food to minimize GI upset; warn patient to avoid alcoholic beverages, which decrease sulfinpyrazone's therapeutic effect.

Geriatric use
Elderly patients are more likely to have glomerular filtration rates below 50 ml/minute; sulfinpyrazone may be ineffective.

Breast-feeding
Safety has not been established. An alternative feeding method is recommended during therapy.

---

sulfisoxazole
Gantrisin

sulfisoxazole diolamine
Gantrisin Ophthalmic Ointment,
Gantrisin Ophthalmic Solution

• Pharmacologic classification: sulfonamide
• Therapeutic classification: antibiotic
• Pregnancy risk category B (D at term)

How supplied
Available by prescription only
Tablets: 500 mg
Liquid: 500 mg/5 ml
Ophthalmic ointment: 4%
Ophthalmic solution: 4%

Indications, route, and dosage
Urinary tract and systemic infections
Adults: Initially, 2 to 4 g P.O. then 4 to 8 g P.O. daily in divided doses q 4 to 6 hours.
Children and infants over age 2 months: Initially, 75 mg/kg P.O., then 150 mg/kg (or 4 g/m²) P.O. daily in divided doses q 4 to 6 hours. Maximum dose should not exceed 6 g/24 hours.
Lymphogranuloma venereum (genital, inguinal, or anorectal infection)
Adults: 500 mg to 1 g q.i.d. for 3 weeks.
Conjunctivitis, corneal ulcer, superficial ocular infections; adjunct in systemic treatment of trachoma
Adults: 2 to 3 drops in eye three or more times daily or small ribbon of ointment in lower conjunctival sac one to three times daily and h.s.

Pharmacodynamics
Antibacterial action: Sulfisoxazole is bacteriostatic. It acts by inhibiting formation of dihydrofolic acid from para-aminobenzoic acid (PABA), thus preventing bacterial cell synthesis of essential nucleic acids. It acts synergistically with folic acid antagonists such as trimethoprim, that block folic acid synthesis at a later stage, thus delaying or preventing bacterial resistance.
Sulfisoxazole is active against some gram-positive bacteria, *Chlamydia trachomatis,* many Enterobacteriaceae, and some strains of *Toxoplasma* and *Plasmodium.*

Pharmacokinetics
• *Absorption:* Sulfisoxazole is absorbed readily from the GI tract after oral administration; peak serum levels occur at 2 to 4 hours.
• *Distribution:* Sulfisoxazole is distributed into extracellular compartments; CSF penetration is 8% to 57% in uninflamed meninges. Sulfisoxazole crosses the placenta; it is 85% protein-bound.
• *Metabolism:* Sulfisoxazole is metabolized partially in the liver.
• *Excretion:* Both unchanged drug and metabolites are excreted primarily in urine by glomerular filtration and, to a lesser extent, renal tubular secretion; some drug is excreted in breast milk. Urinary solubility of unchanged drug increases as urine pH increases. Plasma half-life in patients with normal renal function is about 4½ to 8 hours.

Contraindications and precautions
Sulfisoxazole is contraindicated in patients with known hypersensitivity to sulfonamides or to any other drug containing sulfur (for example, thiazides, furosemide, or oral hypoglycemics); in patients with severe renal or hepatic dysfunction, or porphyria; during pregnancy, at term, and during lactation; and in infants under age 2 months.
Administer sulfonamides with caution to patients with mild to moderate renal or hepatic impairment, urinary obstruction (because of hazard of drug accumulation), severe allergies, asthma, blood dyscrasias, or glucose-6-phosphate dehydrogenase deficiency.
Ophthalmic preparations are incompatible with silver preparations. Corneal healing may be impaired with ophthalmic ointment. Nonsusceptible organisms and fungi may proliferate. Para-aminobenzoic acid, present in purulent exudate, will inactivate sulfonamides.

Interactions
Sulfisoxazole may inhibit hepatic metabolism of oral anticoagulants, displacing them from binding sites and exaggerating anticoagulant effects. Concomitant use with PABA antagonizes effects of sulfonamides; with oral hypoglycemics (sulfonylureas) enhances hypoglycemic effects, probably by displacing sulfonylureas from protein-binding sites; with either trimethoprim or pyrimethamine (folic acid antagonists with different mechanisms of action) results in synergistic antibacterial effects and delays or prevents bacterial resistance.
Concomitant use of urine acidifying agents (ammonium chloride, ascorbic acid) decreases urine pH and sulfonamide solubility, thus increasing risk of crystalluria.

Effects on diagnostic tests
Sulfisoxazole alters results of urine glucose tests utilizing cupric sulfate (Benedict's reagent or Clinitest).

---

*Canada only   †Unlabeled clinical use   Italicized adverse reactions are life-threatening.

Sulfisoxazole may elevate liver function test results; it may decrease serum levels of erythrocytes, platelets, or leukocytes.

Adverse reactions
● CNS: headache, mental depression, *seizures*, hallucinations.
● DERM: *erythema multiforme (Stevens-Johnson syndrome)*, generalized skin eruption, *epidermal necrolysis, exfoliative dermatitis*, photosensitivity, urticaria, pruritus.
● GI: nausea, vomiting, diarrhea, abdominal pain, anorexia, stomatitis.
● GU: toxic nephrosis with oliguria and anuria, crystalluria, hematuria.
● HEMA: *agranulocytosis, aplastic anemia*, megaloblastic anemia, thrombocytopenia, leukopenia, hemolytic anemia.
● Hepatic: jaundice.
● Other: hypersensitivity, serum sickness, drug fever, *anaphylaxis*, bacterial and fungal superinfection.

Note: Drug should be discontinued if signs of toxicity or hypersensitivity occur; if hematologic abnormalities are accompanied by sore throat, pallor, fever, jaundice, purpura, or weakness; if crystalluria is accompanied by renal colic, hematuria, oliguria, proteinuria, urinary obstruction, urolithiasis, increased BUN levels, or anuria; or if severe diarrhea indicates pseudomembranous colitis.

Overdose and treatment
Clinical signs of overdose include dizziness, drowsiness, headache, unconsciousness, anorexia, abdominal pain, nausea, and vomiting. More severe complications, including hemolytic anemia, agranulocytosis, dermatitis, acidosis, sensitivity reactions, and jaundice, may be fatal.

Treatment requires gastric lavage, if ingestion has occurred within the preceding 4 hours, followed by correction of acidosis, and forced fluids and urinary alkalinization to enhance solubility and excretion. Treatment of renal failure and transfusion of appropriate blood products (in severe hematologic toxicity) may be required.

▶ Special considerations
Besides those relevant to all *sulfonamides*, consider the following recommendations.
● Sulfisoxazole-pyrimethamine is used to treat toxoplasmosis.

Information for the patient
● Tell patient to drink 8 oz of water with each oral dose and to take drug on an empty stomach.
● Tell patient to finish prescribed medication.
● Teach patient how to use ophthalmic preparations. Warn patient not to touch tip of dropper or tube to any surface.
● Warn patient that ophthalmic ointment may cause blurred vision immediately after application. Tell patient to gently close eyes and keep closed for 1 to 2 minutes.

Pediatric use
Sulfisoxazole is contraindicated in children younger than age 2 months.

Breast-feeding
Sulfisoxazole is excreted in breast milk and should not be administered to breast-feeding women.

PHARMACOLOGIC CLASS

sulfonamides

co-trimoxazole (trimethoprim-sulfamethoxazole)
sulfacetamide
sulfadiazine
sulfamethizole
sulfamethoxazole
sulfasalazine
sulfisoxazole

Sulfonamides were the first effective drugs used to treat systemic bacterial infections. The prototype, sulfanilamide, was discovered in 1908 and first used clinically in 1933. Since then, many derivatives have been synthesized, and many therapeutic milestones have been reached, including improved solubility of sulfonamides in urine (which reduces renal toxicity) and discovery of the advantages of combinations such as triple sulfa and, especially, of combined trimethoprim and sulfamethoxazole (co-trimoxazole). Development of other major antibiotics has reduced the clinical impact of sulfonamides; however, introduction of the combination agent co-trimoxazole has increased their usefulness in certain infections.

Pharmacology
Sulfonamides are bacteriostatic. Their mechanism of action correlates directly with the structural similarities they share with para-aminobenzoic acid (PABA). They inhibit biosynthesis of folic acid, which is needed for cell growth; susceptible bacteria are those that synthesize folic acid.

Sulfonamides are well absorbed from the GI tract after oral administration, except for sulfasalazine, which is absorbed minimally by the oral route. Sulfonamides are distributed widely into tissues and fluids, including pleural, peritoneal, synovial, and ocular fluids; some, including sulfisoxazole, penetrate CSF. Sulfonamides readily cross the placenta and are found in low concentrations in breast milk. Sulfonamides are metabolized by the liver and the parent drug and metabolites are excreted in urine by glomerular filtration. Hemodialysis removes both sulfamethoxazole and sulfisoxazole, but peritoneal dialysis removes only sulfisoxazole.

Clinical indications and actions
Bacterial infections
When first introduced, sulfonamides were active against many gram-positive and gram-negative organisms; over time, many bacteria have become resistant. Currently, sulfonamides are active against some strains of staphylococci, streptococci, *Nocardia asteroides* and *brasiliensis, Clostridium tetani* and *perfringens, Bacillus anthracis, Escherichia coli*, and *Neisseria gonorrhoeae* and *meningitidis*. Resistance to sulfonamides is common if therapy continues beyond 2 weeks; resistance to one sulfonamide usually means cross-resistance to others.

Sulfonamides are used to treat urinary tract infections caused by *E. coli, Proteus mirabilis* and *vulgaris, Klebsiella, Enterobacter*, and *Staphylococcus aureus*, and genital lesions caused by *Haemophilus ducreyi* (chancroid). They are the drugs of choice in nocardiosis, usually with surgical drainage and/or combined with other antibiotics, including ampicillin, erythromycin, cycloserine, or minocycline. Sulfonamides also are used to treat otitis media and may be used as alternative therapy to tetracyclines against *Chlamydia trachomatis* (lymphogranuloma venereum). Sulfadiazine is used to eradicate meningococci from the nasopharynx of carriers of *N. meningitidis*.

Co-trimoxazole is used to treat infections of the urinary tract, respiratory tract, and ear; to treat chronic bacterial prostatitis; and to prevent recurrent urinary tract infection in women, and "traveler's diarrhea."

Parasitic infections

Sulfonamides combined with pyrimethamine are used to treat toxoplasmosis; certain sulfonamides are combined with quinine and pyrimethamine to treat chloroquine-resistant *Plasmodium falciparum* malaria.

Co-trimoxazole is also used to treat *Pneumocystis carinii* pneumonia.

Inflammations

Sulfasalazine, used to treat inflammatory bowel disease, is cleaved in the intestine to sulfapyridine and 5-aminosalicylic acid.

Overview of adverse reactions

Sulfonamides cause adverse reactions affecting many organs and systems. Many are considered caused by hypersensitivity, including the following: rash, fever, pruritus, erythema multiforme, erythema nodosum, Stevens-Johnson syndrome, Lyell's syndrome, exfoliative dermatitis, photosensitivity, joint pain, conjunctivitis, leukopenia, and bronchospasm. Hematologic reactions include granulocytopenia, thrombocytopenia, agranulocytosis, hypoprothrombinemia, and, in glucose-6-phosphate dehydrogenase (G6PD) deficiency, hemolytic anemia. Renal effects usually result from crystalluria (precipitation of the sulfonamide in the renal system). GI reactions include anorexia, stomatitis, pancreatitis, diarrhea, and folic acid malabsorption. Oral therapy commonly causes nausea and vomiting. Hepatotoxicity and CNS reactions (dizziness, confusion, headache, ataxia, drowsiness, and insomnia) are rare.

▶ Special considerations

● Assess patient's history of allergies; do not give a sulfonamide to any patient with a history of hypersensitivity reactions to sulfonamides or to any other drug containing sulfur (such as thiazides, furosemide, and oral sulfonylureas).

● Sulfonamides are also contraindicated in patients with severe renal or hepatic dysfunction, or porphyria; during pregnancy at term and during breast-feeding. Sulfonamides may cause kernicterus in infants, because they displace bilirubin at the binding site, cross the placenta, and are excreted in breast milk. Infants under age 2 months should receive sulfonamides only if there is no therapeutic alternative.

● Administer sulfonamides with caution to patients with the following conditions: mild to moderate renal or hepatic impairment; urinary obstruction, because of the risk of drug accumulation; severe allergies; asthma; blood dyscrasias; or G6PD deficiency.

● Monitor continuously for possible hypersensitivity reactions or other untoward effects; patients with acquired immunodeficiency syndrome have a much higher incidence of adverse reactions.

● Obtain results of cultures and sensitivity tests before first dose, but therapy may begin before laboratory tests are complete; check test results periodically to assess drug efficacy. Monitor urine cultures, complete blood counts, and urinalysis before and during therapy.

● Monitor patients on long-term therapy for possible superinfection, especially elderly and debilitated patients and others receiving immunosuppressants or radiation therapy.

● Sulfonamides may interact with other drugs and may alter test results; consult individual drug entries for possible test interactions.

Administration

● Give oral dosage with full glass (8 oz [240 ml]) of water, and force fluids to 3,000 to 4,000 ml/day; patient's urine output should be at least 1,500 ml/day.

● Always consult manufacturer's directions for reconstitution, dilution, and storage of drugs; check expiration dates.

● Give oral sulfonamide at least 1 hour before or 2 hours after meals for maximum absorption.

● Shake oral suspensions well before administering to ensure correct dosage.

Information for the patient

● Teach signs and symptoms of hypersensitivity and other adverse reactions, and emphasize need to report these; specifically urge patient to report bloody urine, difficult breathing, rash, fever, chills, or severe fatigue.

● Teach signs and symptoms of bacterial and fungal superinfection to elderly and debilitated patients and others with low resistance from immunosuppressants or irradiation; emphasize need to report them.

● Advise diabetic patients that sulfonamides may increase effects of oral hypoglycemic and not to monitor urine glucose levels with Clinitest; sulfonamides alter results of tests utilizing cupric sulfate.

● Advise patient to avoid exposure to direct sunlight because of risk of photosensitivity reaction.

● Tell patient to take oral drug with a full glass of water and to drink at least 3,000 to 4,000 ml of water daily; explain that tablet may be crushed and swallowed with water to ensure maximal absorption.

● Be sure patient understands how and when to take drugs; urge patient to complete entire prescribed regimen, to comply with instructions for around-the-clock dosage, and to keep follow-up appointments.

● Teach patient to check expiration date of drug and how to store drug, and to discard unused drug.

Geriatric use

Use with caution; elderly patients are susceptible to bacterial and fungal superinfection, are at greater risk of folate deficiency anemia after sulfonamide therapy, and commonly are at greater risk of renal and hematologic effects because of diminished renal function.

Pediatric use

● Sulfonamides are contraindicated in infants under age 2 months, unless there is no therapeutic alternative.

● Give sulfonamides with caution to children with fragile X chromosome associated with mental retardation, because they are vulnerable to psychomotor depression from folate depletion.

Breast-feeding

Sulfonamides are contraindicated during pregnancy at term and during lactation; they displace bilirubin at the binding site and may cause kernicterus in neonates; they cross the placenta and are excreted in breast milk.

Representative combinations

Sulfadiazine with sulfamerazine: Dia-Mer-Sulfonamides, Cetazine, Chemozine, Cherasulfa, Gelazine,

Lantrisol, Quadettes, Quad-Rumoid, Sul-Trio, Terfonyl, Triosulfon, Triple-Sulfa; with sulfamerazine and sulfacetamide: Acet-Dia-Mer-Sulfonamides, Coco-Diazine, Chero-Trisulfa; with sulfamerazine and sulfathiazole: Dia-Mer-Sulfonamides.

Sulfamethizole with sulfacetamide and phenazopyridine: Triurisil, Urotrol; with phenazopyridine and oxytetracycline: Azotrex, Urobiotic; with sulfathiazole, sulfacetamide, sulfabenzamide, and urea: Triple Sulfa, Sulfa-gyn, V.V.S., Trysul, Gyne-Sulf, Sultrin, Femguard.

Sulfamethoxazole with phenazopyridine hydrochloride: Azo Gantanol, Azo Sulfamethoxazole; with trimethoprim: Apo-Sulfatrim*, Bactrim, Cotrim, Co-trimoxazole, Novotrimel*, Protrin*, Roubac*, Septra, SMZ-TMP.

Sulfisoxazole with phenylazodiaminopyridine hydrochloride: Azo-sulfisoxazole, Azo-Sulfizin, Velmatrol-A; with aminacrine hydrochloride and allantoin: Cantri, Vagilia; with erythromycin ethyl succinate: Pediazole; with phenazopyridine hydrochloride: Azo-Gantrisin, Azo-Soxazole, ·Axo-Sulfisoxazole, Azo-Urizole, Barazole-Azo, Thiosulfil-A, Thiosulfil-A Forte, Rosoxol-Azo, Suldiazo.

PHARMACOLOGIC CLASS

sulfonylureas

acetohexamide
chlorpropamide
glipizide
glyburide
tolazamide
tolbutamide

In 1942, a sulfonamide, an antibacterial agent, was discovered to have hypoglycemic effects. Subsequent experiments showed that this drug did not exert similar effects in pancreatectomized animals. Later, tolbutamide was introduced and soon became popular for managing certain diabetic patients. Sulfonylureas are useful only in patients with mild to moderately severe non-insulin-dependent diabetes mellitus (type II) (NIDDM). These drugs can be used only in patients with functioning beta cells of the pancreas.

Pharmacology

The sulfonylurea hypoglycemic agents are sulfonamide derivatives that exert no antibacterial activity.

Sulfonylureas lower blood glucose levels by stimulating insulin release from the pancreas. These agents work only in the presence of functioning beta cells in the islet tissue of the pancreas. After prolonged administration, they produce hypoglycemia through significant extrapancreatic effects, including reduction of hepatic glucose production and enhanced peripheral sensitivity to insulin. The latter may result from an increase in the number of insulin receptors or from changes in events after insulin binding.

The sulfonylureas are divided into first-generation agents (acetohexamide, chlorpropamide, tolbutamide, and tolazamide) and second-generation agents (glyburide and glipizide). Although their mechanisms of action are similar, the second-generation agents carry a more lipophilic side chain, are more potent, and cause fewer adverse reactions. Clinically, their most important differences are their durations of action.

Clinical indications and actions
Diabetes mellitus, non-insulin-dependent
Sulfonylureas are used to manage mild to moderately severe, stable, nonketotic NIDDM that cannot be controlled by diet alone. Sulfonylureas stimulate insulin release from the pancreas. After long-term therapy, extrapancreatic hypoglycemic effects include reduced hepatic glucose production, an increased number of insulin receptors, and changes in insulin binding.

Neurogenic diabetes insipidus
Although an unlabeled indication, chlorpropamide has been used in selected patients to treat neurogenic diabetes insipidus. The drug appears to potentiate the effect of minimal levels of antidiuretic hormone.

Overview of adverse reactions
Dose-related side effects, which are usually not serious and respond to decreased dosage, include headache, nausea, vomiting, anorexia, heartburn, weakness, and paresthesia. Hypoglycemia may follow excessive dosage, increased exercise, decreased food intake, or consumption of alcohol. Signs and symptoms of overdose include anxiety, chills, cold sweats, confusion, cool pale skin, difficulty in concentration, drowsiness, excessive hunger, headache, nausea, nervousness, rapid heartbeat, shakiness, unsteady gait, weakness, and unusual fatigue. Administration of oral hypoglycemics has been associated with increased cardiovascular mortality compared with treatment by diet alone or diet plus insulin, according to a long-term prospective clinical trial conducted by the University Group Diabetes Program.

▶ Special considerations
● Sulfonylureas should be administered 30 minutes before the morning meal for once-daily dosing, or 30 minutes before the morning and evening meals for twice-daily dosing.
● These agents are contraindicated in treating juvenile-onset, brittle, or severe diabetes; diabetes mellitus adequately controlled by diet; and maturity-onset diabetes complicated by ketosis, acidosis, diabetic coma, Raynaud's gangrene, renal or hepatic impairment, or thyroid or other endocrine dysfunction. Use cautiously in patients with sulfonamide hypersensitivity.
● Sulfonylurea hypoglycemic agents should not be used during pregnancy because of prolonged, severe hypoglycemia lasting from 4 to 10 days in neonates born to mothers taking these drugs. Also, use of insulin permits more rigid control of blood glucose levels, which should reduce the incidence of congenital abnormalities, mortality, and morbidity caused by abnormal glucose levels.
● Monitor patients transferring from insulin therapy to a sulfonylurea agent for urine glucose and ketones at least t.i.d. before meals; emphasize the need for testing a double-voided specimen. Patients may require hospitalization during such changes in therapy.
● Patients transferring from another sulfonylurea (except chlorpropamide) usually need no transition period.
● NIDDM patients may require insulin therapy during periods of increased stress, such as infection, fever, surgery, or trauma. Monitor patients closely for hyperglycemia in these situations.

Information for the patient
● Teach patients about the nature of their disease.
● Emphasize the importance of following therapeutic regimen and adhering to specific diet, weight reduction, exercise, and personal hygiene recommendations. Pa-

---

*Canada only   †Unlabeled clinical use   Italicized adverse reactions are life-threatening.

COMPARING ORAL HYPOGLYCEMICS

Typically, sulfonylureas have similar actions and produce similar effects. They differ mainly in duration of action and dosage.

SULFONYLUREAS	USUAL DAILY DOSAGE	ONSET	ACTION PEAK	DURATION
First generation				
acetohexamide (Dymelor)	500 mg once daily or b.i.d.	1 hr	2 hr	12 to 24 hr
chlorpropamide (Diabenase)	250 mg once daily	1 hr	3 to 6 hr	60 hr
tolazamide (Tolinase)	250 mg once daily or b.i.d.	4 to 6 hr	6 to 10 hr	12 to 24 hr
tolbutamide (Orinase)	1,000 mg b.i.d. or t.i.d.	½ to 1 hr	4 to 8 hr	6 to 12 hr
Second generation				
glipizide (Glucotrol)	5 mg once daily	1 to 1½ hr	2 to 3 hr	10 to 24 hr
glyburide (Diaβeta)	5 mg once daily	2 hr	3 to 4 hr	24 hr

tients also should know how to avoid infections, how to test for glycosuria and ketonuria, and how to recognize signs and symptoms of hypoglycemia (fatigue, excessive hunger, profuse sweating, and numbness of extremities) and hyperglycemia (excessive thirst or urination and excessive urine glucose or ketones).
• Be sure patients know that therapy relieves symptoms but does not cure the disease.
• Discourage patients from consuming moderate to large amounts of alcohol while taking sulfonylureas; disulfiram-type reactions are possible.

Geriatric use
• Elderly patients and those with renal insufficiency may be more sensitive to these agents because of decreased metabolism and excretion. They usually require lower dosages and should be closely monitored.
• Hypoglycemia may be more difficult to recognize in elderly patients, although it usually causes neurologic symptoms in such patients. Agents with prolonged duration of action should be avoided in elderly patients.

Pediatric use
Oral hypoglycemic agents are not effective in insulin-dependent (type I, juvenile-onset) diabetes mellitus.

Breast-feeding
Oral hypoglycemics are excreted in breast milk in minimal amounts and may cause hypoglycemia in the breast-feeding infant.

Representative combinations
None.

sulindac
Clinoril

• Pharmacologic classification: nonsteroidal anti-inflammatory
• Therapeutic classification: nonnarcotic analgesic, antipyretic, anti-inflammatory
• Pregnancy risk category B (D in third trimester)

How supplied
Available by prescription only
Tablets: 150 mg, 200 mg

Indications, route, and dosage
Osteoarthritis, rheumatoid arthritis, ankylosing spondylitis
Adults: 150 mg P.O. b.i.d. initially; may increase to 200 mg P.O. b.i.d.
Acute subacromial bursitis or supraspinatus tendinitis, acute gouty arthritis
Adults: 200 mg P.O. b.i.d. for 7 to 14 days. Dose may be reduced as symptoms subside.

Pharmacodynamics
Analgesic, antipyretic, and anti-inflammatory actions:
Mechanisms of action are unknown but thought to inhibit prostaglandin synthesis.

Pharmacokinetics
• *Absorption:* Sulindac is absorbed rapidly and completely from the GI tract.
• *Distribution:* The drug is highly protein-bound.
• *Metabolism:* Sulindac is inactive and is metabolized hepatically to the active sulfide metabolite.
• *Excretion:* The drug is excreted in urine. The half-life

---

of the parent drug is about 8 hours; the half-life of the active metabolite is about 16 hours.

Contraindications and precautions
Sulindac is contraindicated in patients with known hypersensitivity to it and in patients in whom aspirin or other nonsteroidal anti-inflammatory drugs (NSAIDs) induce symptoms of asthma, urticaria, or rhinitis.

Serious GI toxicity, especially ulceration and hemorrhage, can occur at any time in patients on chronic NSAID therapy. Sulindac should be used cautiously in patients with a history of GI bleeding, hepatic or renal disease, cardiac decompensation, or hypertension.

Patients with known "triad" symptoms (aspirin hypersensitivity, rhinitis/nasal polyps, and asthma) are at high risk of cross-sensitivity to sulindac with precipitation of bronchospasm.

The signs and symptoms of acute infection (fever, myalgias, erythema) may be masked by the use of sulindac. Evaluate patients with high infection risk (such as those with diabetes) carefully.

Interactions
When used concomitantly, anticoagulants and thrombolytic drugs may be potentiated by the platelet-inhibiting effect of sulindac. Concomitant use of sulindac with highly protein-bound drugs (phenytoin, sulfonylureas, warfarin) may cause displacement of either drug, and adverse effects. Monitor therapy closely for both drugs. Concomitant use with other GI-irritating drugs (such as steroids, antibiotics, NSAIDs) may potentiate the adverse GI effects of sulindac. Use together with caution.

Antacids and food delay and decrease the absorption of sulindac. NSAIDs are known to decrease renal clearance of lithium carbonate, thus increasing lithium serum levels and risks of adverse effects. Dimethylsulfoxide (DMSO) may interact with sulindac, causing decreased plasma levels of the active sulfide metabolite. Peripheral neuropathies have also been reported with this combination. Diflunisal and aspirin are known to cause decreased plasma levels of the active sulfide metabolite. Probenecid increases plasma levels of sulindac and its inactive sulfane metabolite; sulindac may decrease the uricosuric effect of probenecid.

Effects on diagnostic tests
The physiologic effect of the drug may result in increased bleeding time; increased BUN, serum creatinine, and potassium levels; and increased serum alkaline phosphatase and serum transaminase concentrations.

Adverse reactions
- CNS: headache, dizziness, nervousness.
- CV: edema, congestive heart failure (CHF), palpitations.
- DERM: pruritus, rash.
- EENT: tinnitus, transient visual disturbances, epistaxis, dry mouth, bitter taste, photosensitivity.
- GI: nausea, vomiting, epigastric distress, occult blood loss, bleeding, diarrhea, anorexia, constipation.
- GU: flank pain, nephrotoxicity, hematuria.
- HEMA: prolonged bleeding time, *aplastic anemia*, thrombocytopenia, hemolytic anemia.
- Other: elevated liver enzymes, severe hepatic reactions.

Note: Drug should be discontinued if hypersensitivity, hepatotoxicity, rash, or pruritus occurs.

Overdose and treatment
Clinical manifestations of overdose include dizziness, drowsiness, mental confusion, disorientation, lethargy, paresthesias, numbness, vomiting, gastric irritation, nausea, abdominal pain, headache, stupor, coma, and hypotension.

To treat overdose of sulindac, empty stomach immediately by inducing emesis with ipecac syrup or by gastric lavage. Administer activated charcoal via nasogastric tube. Provide symptomatic and supportive measures (respiratory support and correction of fluid and electrolyte imbalances). Dialysis is thought to be of minimal value because sulindac is highly protein-bound. Monitor laboratory parameters and vital signs closely.

▶ Special considerations
Besides those relevant to all *NSAIDs*, consider the following recommendations.
- Sulindac is the safest NSAID for patients with mild renal impairment. It is also less likely to cause further renal toxicity.
- Assess cardiopulmonary status frequently. Monitor vital signs, especially heart rate and blood pressure, to detect any abnormalities.
- Assess fluid balance status. Monitor intake and output and daily weight. Observe for presence and amount of edema.
- Impose safety measures to prevent injury, such as raised side rails and supervised ambulation.
- Symptomatic improvement may take 7 days or longer. Evaluate patient's response as evidenced by a reduction in symptoms.

Information for the patient
- Caution patient to avoid use of nonprescription medications unless medically approved.
- Teach patient how to recognize signs and symptoms of possible adverse reactions; instruct patient to report them.
- Instruct patient to check weight two or three times weekly and to report any weight gain of 3 pounds or more within 1 week.
- Because drug causes sodium retention, advise patient to report edema and have blood pressure checked routinely.
- Instruct patient in safety measures; advise patient to avoid hazardous activities that require alertness until CNS effects of the drug are known.

Geriatric use
- Patients over age 60 are more sensitive to the adverse effects of sulindac. Use with caution.
- Because of its effect on renal prostaglandins, sulindac may cause fluid retention and edema. This may be significant in elderly patients and those with CHF.

Pediatric use
The safety of long-term sulindac use in children has not been established.

Breast-feeding
Safe use has not been established. Avoid use of sulindac in breast-feeding women.

---

suprofen
Profenal

- Pharmacologic classification: phenyl-kanoic acid derivative; nonsteroidal anti-inflammatory
- Therapeutic classification: ophthalmic anti-inflammatory
- Pregnancy risk category C

How supplied
Available by prescription only
Ophthalmic solution: 1%

Indications, route, and dosage
Inhibition of intraoperative miosis
Adults: Instill 2 drops into the conjunctival sac q 4 hours the day before surgery. On the day of surgery, instill 2 drops 3 hours, 2 hours, and 1 hour before surgery.

Pharmacodynamics
Anti-inflammatory action: Suprofen inhibits the action of cyclo-oxygenase, an enzyme responsible for the synthesis of prostaglandins. Prostaglandins are mediators of the inflammatory response and also cause miosis.

Pharmacokinetics
- *Absorption:* Some drug is absorbed systemically; detailed pharmacokinetic information is unknown.

Contraindications and precautions
Suprofen is contraindicated in patients with hypersensitivity to any component of the formulation and in patients with epithelial herpes simplex keratitis.

Because of the risk of cross sensitivity, use cautiously in patients who have experienced hypersensitivity reactions to other NSAIDs or aspirin. Also use cautiously in patients with bleeding disorders.

Interactions
Acetylcholine and carbachol may be ineffective in patients treated with suprofen.

Effects on diagnostic tests
None reported.

Adverse reactions
- EENT: transient stinging and burning upon instillation, discomfort, itching, redness, iritis, pain, chemosis, photophobia, irritation, punctate epithelial staining.
- Other: allergy.

Overdose and treatment
Overdosage usually will not cause symptoms. Oral ingestion of drug may be treated by drinking fluids to dilute.

▶ Special considerations
Store away from heat in a dark, tightly closed container; protect drug from freezing.

Information for the patient
- Teach patient not to touch dropper to eye.
- Advise patient to discard drug when no longer needed.

Pediatric use
Safety and efficacy have not been established.

Breast-feeding
After systemic administration, drug is excreted in breast milk. Because of the risk of serious adverse effects to the infant, do not administer to breast-feeding women.

sutilains
Travase

- Pharmacologic classification: topical proteolytic enzyme
- Therapeutic classification: topical debriding agent
- Pregnancy risk category D

How supplied
Available by prescription only
Ointment: 82,000 Casein units/g

Indications, route, and dosage
Debridement of major burns, decubitus ulcers, ulcers in peripheral vascular disease and incisional, traumatic, and pyogenic wounds
Adults and children: After cleansing and moistening wound area, apply thinly to area, extending ¼″ to ½″ beyond area to be debrided. Cover with loose, wet dressing t.i.d. or q.i.d.

Pharmacodynamics
Proteolytic action: Sutilains converts denatured proteins found in necrotic tissue and exudates to peptides and amino acids.

Pharmacokinetics
- *Absorption:* Limited with topical use.
- *Distribution:* None.
- *Metabolism:* None.
- *Excretion:* None.

Contraindications and precautions
Sutilains is contraindicated for use on wounds communicating with major body cavities or those containing exposed major nerves or nerve tissue; on fungating neoplastic ulcers; and in pregnant women and women of childbearing age. Sutilains should be used with caution near the eyes or mucous membranes. Avoid applying the drug to more than 10% to 15% of the burned area at one time.

Interactions
Concomitant use with detergents and anti-infectives, such as benzalkonium chloride, hexachlorophene, and nitrofurazone iron, and with metallic compounds, such as thimerosal and silver nitrate, may decrease activity of sutilains.

Effects on diagnostic tests
None reported.

Adverse reactions
- Local: pain, paresthesias, bleeding, and transient dermatitis.
  Note: Drug should be discontinued if sensitization

develops or if bleeding or dermatitis occurs at wound site.

Overdose and treatment
If drug accidentally contacts eyes, flush eyes repeatedly with large amounts of normal saline solution or sterile water.

▶ Special considerations
● Maintain strict aseptic conditions when applying drug.
● Cleanse area with normal saline solution or water before applying the drug. Wound area should be well moistened before applying sutilains.
● Concomitant systemic or topical antibiotic therapy or prophylaxis may be necessary because the proteolytic action of sutilains produces an excellent growth medium for bacteria if sepsis has occurred; if topical, apply sutilains first.
● Refrigerate ointment at 36.6° to 50° F (2° to 10° C).
● Maximal effect usually is achieved in 5 to 7 days for burns and wounds and in 8 to 12 days for decubital and peripheral vascular ulcers.

Information for the patient
Instruct patient in correct use of ointment.

Breast-feeding
Drug should be avoided in breast-feeding women.

tamoxifen citrate
Nolvadex, Nolvadex-D*, Tamofen*

- Pharmacologic classification: nonsteroidal antiestrogen
- Therapeutic classification: antineoplastic
- Pregnancy risk category D

How supplied
Available by prescription only
Tablets: 10 mg
Tablets (enteric coated)*: 20 mg

Indications, route, and dosage
Dosage and indications may vary. Check current literature for recommended protocol.
Advanced postmenopausal breast cancer
Adults: 10 to 20 mg P.O. b.i.d.

Pharmacodynamics
Antineoplastic action: The exact mechanism of action is unclear. Tamoxifen may exert its cytotoxic action by blocking estrogen receptors within tumor cells which require estrogen to thrive. The estrogen receptor-tamoxifen complex may be translocated into the nucleus of the tumor cell, where it inhibits DNA synthesis.

Pharmacokinetics
- *Absorption:* Tamoxifen appears to be well absorbed across the GI tract after oral administration.
- *Distribution:* Tamoxifen is distributed widely into total body water.
- *Metabolism:* Tamoxifen is metabolized extensively in the liver to several metabolites.
- *Excretion:* Tamoxifen and its metabolites are excreted primarily in feces, mostly as metabolites. The drug has a distribution phase half-life of 7 to 14 hours. Secondary peak plasma levels occur 4 days after a dose, probably because of enterohepatic circulation. The half-life of the terminal elimination phase is more than 7 days.

Contraindications and precautions
Tamoxifen is contraindicated in the first 4 months of pregnancy because of the potential for fetal harm.

Interactions
None reported.

Effects on diagnostic tests
Tamoxifen therapy may increase concentrations of serum calcium. This effect usually occurs in patients with bone metastases.

Adverse reactions
- CNS: headache, dizziness, depression, confusion.
- CV: thrombosis.
- DERM: rash, photosensitivity.
- EENT: blurred vision, decreased visual acuity, corneal changes.
- GI: nausea, vomiting, anorexia.
- GU: vaginal discharge and bleeding.
- HEMA: transient fall in WBC or platelet counts.
- Metabolic: hypercalcemia.
- Other: temporary bone or tumor pain, hot flashes, brief exacerbation of pain from osseous metastases.

Overdose and treatment
No information available.

▶ Special considerations
- Initial adverse reactions (increased bone pain) may mimic a "disease-flare."
- Hot flashes may be relieved by administration of Bellergal-S tablets.
- Analgesics are indicated to relieve pain.
- Adverse reactions are usually minor and well tolerated. They can usually be controlled by dosage reduction.
- Use cautiously in preexisting leukopenia and thrombocytopenia.
- Monitor WBC and platelet counts.
- Monitor serum calcium levels. Drug may compound hypercalcemia related to bone metastases.
- Tamoxifen acts as an antiestrogen. Best results occur in patients with positive estrogen receptors.
- Drug is also used to treat breast cancer in males; advanced ovarian cancer in women; and metastatic melanoma (in combination therapy).

Information for the patient
- Emphasize importance of continuing medication despite nausea and vomiting.
- Tell patient to call promptly if vomiting occurs shortly after a dose is taken.
- Reassure patient that acute exacerbation of bone pain during tamoxifen therapy usually indicates drug will produce good response.

Breast-feeding
It is not known whether tamoxifen distributes into breast milk. However, because of the potential for serious adverse reactions and carcinogenicity in the infant, breast-feeding is not recommended.

temazepam
Razepam, Restoril, Temaz

- Pharmacologic classification: benzodi-azepine
- Therapeutic classification: sedative-hypnotic
- Controlled substance schedule IV
- Pregnancy risk category X

How supplied
Available by prescription only
Capsules: 15 mg, 30 mg

Indications, route, and dosage
Insomnia
Adults: 15 to 30 mg P.O. 30 minutes before bedtime.
Adults over age 65: 15 mg P.O. h.s.

Pharmacodynamics
Sedative-hypnotic action: Temazepam depresses the CNS at the limbic and subcortical levels of the brain.It produces a sedative-hypnotic effect by potentiating the effect of the neurotransmitter gamma-aminobutyric acid (GABA) on its receptor in the ascending reticular activating system, which increases inhibition and blocks both cortical and limbic arousal.

Pharmacokinetics
- *Absorption:* When administered orally, temazepam is well absorbed through the GI tract. Peak levels occur in 1 to 3 hours. Onset of action occurs at 30 to 60 minutes.
- *Distribution:* Temazepam is distributed widely throughout the body. Drug is 98% protein-bound.
- *Metabolism:* Temazepam is metabolized in the liver primarily to inactive metabolites.
- *Excretion:* The metabolites of temazepam are excreted in urine as glucuronide conjugates. The half-life of temazepam ranges from 10 to 17 hours.

Contraindications and precautions
Temazepam is contraindicated in patients with known hypersensitivity to the drug; in patients with acute narrow-angle glaucoma or untreated open-angle glaucoma because of the drug's possible anticholinergic effect; in patients in coma, because the drug's hypnotic or hypotensive effect may be prolonged or intensified; in patients with acute alcohol intoxication who have depressed vital signs, because the drug will worsen CNS depression; and in pregnant patients. Do not use in patients with a history of drug abuse or suicidal tendencies.

Temazepam should be used cautiously in patients with psychoses, because the drug is rarely beneficial in such patients and may induce paradoxical reactions; in patients with myasthenia gravis, Parkinson's disease, or chronic obstructive pulmonary disease, because it may exacerbate these disorders; in patients with impaired hepatic or renal function, which prolongs elimination of the drug; in elderly or debilitated patients, who are usually more sensitive to the drug's CNS effects.

Interactions
Temazepam potentiates the CNS depressant effects of phenothiazines, narcotics, antihistamines, monoamine oxidase inhibitors, barbiturates, alcohol, general anesthetics, and antidepressants.

Concomitant use with cimetidine and possibly disulfiram causes diminished hepatic metabolism of temazepam, which increases its plasma concentration.

Heavy smoking accelerates temazepam metabolism, thus lowering clinical effectiveness.

Benzodiazepines block the therapeutic effects of levodopa.

Temazepam may decrease plasma levels of haloperidol.

Effects on diagnostic tests
Temazepam therapy may increase liver function test results. Minor changes in EEG patterns, usually low-voltage, fast activity, may occur during and after temazepam therapy.

Adverse reactions
- CNS: confusion, depression, drowsiness, lethargy, hangover effect, ataxia, dizziness, syncope, nightmares, fatigue, slurred speech, tremors, vertigo, nervousness, irritability, daytime sedation, headache.
- CV: palpitations, tachycardia, hypotension (rare).
- DERM: rash, urticaria.
- EENT: diplopia, blurred vision, nystagmus.
- GI: constipation, dry mouth, taste alterations, nausea, vomiting, abdominal discomfort, anorexia, diarrhea.
- GU: urinary incontinence or retention.
- Other: *respiratory depression,* dysarthria, hepatic dysfunction, changes in libido.
  Note: Drug should be discontinued if hypersensitivity or the following paradoxical reactions occur: acute hyperexcited state, anxiety, hallucinations, increased muscle spasticity, insomnia, or rage.

Overdose and treatment
Clinical manifestations of overdose include somnolence, confusion, hypoactive or absent reflexes, dyspnea, labored breathing, hypotension, bradycardia, slurred speech, unsteady gait or impaired coordination, and, ultimately, coma.

Support blood pressure and respiration until drug effects subside; monitor vital signs. Mechanical ventilatory assistance via endotracheal tube may be required to maintain a patent airway and support adequate oxygenation. Flumazenil, a specific benzodiazepine antagonist, may be useful. Use I.V. fluids and vasopressors such as dopamine and phenylephrine to treat hypotension as needed. If patient is conscious, induce emesis. Use gastric lavage if ingestion was recent, but only if an endotracheal tube is present to prevent aspiration. After emesis or lavage, administer activated charcoal with a cathartic as a single dose. Do not use barbiturates if excitation occurs. Dialysis is of limited value.

▶ Special considerations
Besides those relevant to all *benzodiazepines,* consider the following recommendations.
- Evaluate the patient for the cause of the insomnia, which is frequently a symptom of an underlying disorder, such as depression.
- Useful for patients who have difficulty falling asleep or who awaken frequently in the night.

• Prolonged use not recommended, however, this drug has proven effective for up to 4 weeks of continuous use.
• Remove all potential safety hazards, such as cigarettes, from patient's reach.
• Impose safety measures, such as call bell within reach, and side rails raised, to prevent possible injury.
• Monitor hepatic function studies to prevent toxicity; lower doses are indicated in patients with hepatic dysfunction.
• After long-term use, withdraw the drug slowly (over 6 to 12 weeks).
• Store in a cool, dry place away from light.

Information for the patient
• Instruct patient to seek medical approval before making any changes in medication regimen.
• As necessary, teach patient safety measures to prevent injury, such as gradual position changes and supervised ambulation.
• Advise patient of the potential for physical and psychological dependence with chronic use.

Geriatric use
• Elderly patients are more susceptible to the CNS depressant effects of temazepam. Use with caution.
• Lower doses are usually effective in elderly patients because of decreased elimination.
• Elderly patients who receive this drug require supervision with ambulation and activities of daily living during initiation of therapy or after an increase in dose.

Pediatric use
Safe use in patients under age 18 has not been established.

Breast-feeding
Temazepam is excreted in breast milk. A breast-fed infant may become sedated, have feeding difficulties, or lose weight. Avoid use in breast-feeding women.

---

teniposide (VM-26)
Vumon*

• Pharmacologic classification: podophyllotoxin (cell cycle-phase specific, G2 and late S phase)
• Therapeutic classification: antineoplastic
• Pregnancy risk category D

How supplied
Available only through investigational protocols
Injection: 50 mg/5 ml ampules

Indications, route, and dosage
Dosage and indications may vary. Check current literature for recommended protocol.
†*Hodgkin's and non-Hodgkin's lymphomas, acute lymphocytic leukemia, bladder carcinoma*
Adults: 50 to 100 mg/m² I.V. once or twice weekly for 4 to 6 weeks, or 40 to 50 mg/m² I.V. daily for 5 days, repeated q 3 to 4 weeks.
Children: 130 mg/m²/week, increasing to 150 mg/m² after 3 weeks and to 180 mg/m² after 6 weeks.

†*Neuroblastoma*
Adults: 130 to 180 mg/m²/day once a week.

Pharmacodynamics
Antineoplastic action: Teniposide exerts its cytotoxic activity as a mitotic spindle poison, resulting in a reversible metaphase arrest and an irreversible blockade of cell cycle traverse by impairment of cellular respiration and energy production.

Pharmacokinetics
• *Absorption:* Teniposide is not administered orally.
• *Distribution:* Teniposide distributes mainly into the liver, kidneys, small intestine, and adrenals. The drug is highly bound to plasma proteins. Teniposide crosses the blood-brain barrier to a limited extent.
• *Metabolism:* Teniposide is metabolized extensively in the liver.
• *Excretion:* Approximately 40% of a dose is eliminated through the kidneys as unchanged drug or metabolites. The elimination of teniposide from the plasma is described as triphasic, with half-lives of 45 minutes, 4 hours, and 20 hours for the initial, secondary, and terminal phases, respectively.

Contraindications and precautions
Teniposide is contraindicated in patients with hypersensitivity to podophyllum or semisynthetic podophyllotoxin derivatives.

Interactions
None reported.

Effects on diagnostic tests
Teniposide therapy may increase blood and urine concentrations of uric acid.

Adverse reactions
• CV: hypotension from rapid infusion.
• GI: nausea and vomiting, diarrhea.
• HEMA: *bone marrow depression* (dose-limiting), *leukopenia, thrombocytopenia, pancytopenia.*
• Local: chemical thrombophlebitis.
• Other: alopecia (rare), *anaphylaxis* (rare), *bronchospasm.*

Overdose and treatment
Clinical manifestations of overdose include myelosuppression, nausea, and vomiting.
Treatment is usually supportive and includes transfusion of blood components, antiemetics, and antibiotics for infections that may develop.

▶ Special considerations
• Teniposide is currently an investigational drug within the United States. Information concerning its availability may be obtained by calling 1-800-4-CANCER.
• Dilute with at least 5 equal volumes (preferably 10 to 20 volumes) of normal saline solution for I.V. infusion. Normal saline solution is preferred because of the high incidence of precipitation with dextrose 5% in water. Discard cloudy solutions.
• Solutions containing 0.5 to 2 mg/ml are stable for 4 hours. Solutions containing 0.1 to 0.2 mg/ml are stable for 6 hours.
• Should not be administered through a membrane-type in-line filter because the diluent may dissolve the filter.
• Administer I.V. infusion over at least 45 minutes to

---

prevent hypotension. Avoid I.V. push because of increased risk of hypotension.
• Dosage should be decreased in patients with renal or hepatic insufficiency.
• Monitor for chemical phlebitis at injection site.
• Have diphenhydramine, hydrocortisone, epinephrine, and airway available in case of an anaphylactic reaction.
• Monitor blood pressure before infusion and at 30-minute intervals during infusion. If systolic blood pressure falls below 90 mm Hg, stop infusion.
• Monitor CBC. Observe patient for signs of bone marrow depression.
• Drug may be given by local bladder instillation to treat bladder cancer.

Information for the patient
• Encourage adequate fluid intake to increase urine output and facilitate excretion of uric acid.
• Tell patient to avoid exposure to people with infections.
• Advise patient that hair should grow back after treatment is discontinued.
• Tell patient to call promptly if he develops a sore throat or fever or notices unusual bruising or bleeding.

Breast-feeding
It is not known whether teniposide distributes into breast milk. However, because of the risk of serious adverse reactions, mutagenicity, and carcinogenicity in the infant, breast-feeding is not recommended.

terazosin hydrochloride
Hytrin

• Pharmacologic classification: selective alpha$_1$ blocker
• Therapeutic classification: antihypertensive
• Pregnancy risk category C

How supplied
Available by prescription only
Tablets: 1 mg, 2 mg, 5 mg

Indications, route, and dosage
Mild to moderate hypertension
Adults: Initially, 1 mg at bedtime. Adjust dose and schedule according to patient response. Recommended range: 1 to 5 mg daily or divided b.i.d.
   If therapy is discontinued for several days or longer, reinstitute using the initial dosing regimen of 1 mg at bedtime. Slowly increase dose until desired blood pressure is attained. Doses over 20 mg do not appear to further affect blood pressure.

Pharmacodynamics
Antihypertensive action: Terazosin reduces blood pressure by selectively inhibiting alpha$_1$ receptors in vascular smooth muscle and thus reducing peripheral vascular resistance. Due to its selectivity for alpha$_1$ receptors, heart rate increases minimally. Significant decreases in serum cholesterol, low density lipoprotein (LDL), and very low density lipoprotein (VLDL) cholesterol fractions occur during therapy; the significance of

these changes is unknown, as is the mechanism by which they occur.
   Terazosin administration does not significantly alter potassium or glucose levels; it has been used successfully with diuretics, beta blockers, and a combination of other antihypertensive regimens.

Pharmacokinetics
• *Absorption:* Terazosin is absorbed rapidly after oral administration, reaching peak plasma concentrations in 1 to 2 hours. Approximately 90% of the oral dose is bioavailable; ingestion of food does not appear to alter bioavailability.
• *Distribution:* About 90% to 94% is plasma protein-bound.
• *Metabolism:* The drug is metabolized in the liver. The pharmacokinetics of terazosin do not appear to be affected by hypertension, congestive heart failure, or age.
• *Excretion:* About 40% is excreted in urine, 60% in feces, mostly as metabolites. Up to 30% may be excreted unchanged. Elimination half-life is approximately 12 hours.

Contraindications and precautions
Terazosin is contraindicated in patients with known hypersensitivity to the drug.

Interactions
None reported.

Effects on diagnostic tests
Terazosin therapy causes small but significant decreases in hematocrit, hemoglobin, white blood cells, total protein, and albumin; the magnitude of these decreases has not been shown to worsen with time, suggesting the possibility of hemodilution.

Adverse reactions
• CNS: dizziness, headache, nervousness, paresthesia, somnolence.
• CV: palpitations, tachycardia, postural hypotension, syncope.
• EENT: blurred vision, nasal congestion, sinusitis.
• GI: nausea.
• GU: impotence, decreased libido.
• Other: dyspnea, asthenia, back pain, peripheral edema, weight gain.

Overdose and treatment
Clinical signs of overdose are exaggerated adverse reactions, particularly hypotension and shock. In case of overdose, treatment is symptomatic and supportive. Dialysis may not be helpful, as drug is highly protein-bound.

▶ Special considerations
Besides those relevant to all *alpha-adrenergic blocking agents,* consider the following recommendation.
• Terazosin can cause marked hypotension, especially postural hypotension, and syncope with the first dose or during the first few days of therapy. A similar response occurs if therapy is interrupted for more than a few doses.

Information for the patient
• Caution patient to avoid hazardous tasks that require alertness for 12 hours after first dose, when dose is first increased, or when restarting dose after interruption of therapy.

• Caution patient to rise carefully and slowly from sitting and supine positions and to report dizziness, lightheadedness, or palpitations. Dosage adjustment may be necessary.

terbutaline sulfate
Brethine, Bricanyl

• Pharmacologic classification: adrenergic (beta₂ agonist)
• Therapeutic classification: bronchodilator, premature labor inhibitor (tocolytic)
• Pregnancy risk category B

How supplied
Available by prescription only
Tablets: 2.5 mg, 5 mg
Aerosol inhaler: 200 mcg/metered spray
Injection: 1 mg/ml parenteral

Indications, route, and dosage
Relief of bronchospasm in patients with reversible obstructive airway disease
Adults and children over age 12: Administer 5 mg P.O. t.i.d. at 6-hour intervals. Maximum dosage, 15 mg daily. If adverse reactions occur or for children ages 12 to 15, dosage may be reduced to 2.5 mg P.O. t.i.d.; maximum 7.5 mg daily. Alternatively, 0.25 mg S.C. may be repeated in 15 to 30 minutes; maximum, 0.5 mg q 4 hours. Alternatively, 2 inhalations q 4 to 6 hours with 1 minute elapsing between inhalations.
†*Premature labor*
Adults: Initially, 10 mcg/minute I.V. Titrate to a maximum dose of 80 mcg/minute. Maintain I.V. dosage at minimum effective dose for 4 hours. Maintenance therapy until term: 2.5 mg P.O. q 4 to 6 hours.

Pharmacodynamics
• *Bronchodilator action:* Terbutaline acts directly on beta₂-adrenergic receptors to relax bronchial smooth muscle, relieving bronchospasm and reducing airway resistance. Cardiac and CNS stimulation may occur with high doses.
• *Tocolytic action:* When used in premature labor, relaxes uterine smooth muscle, which inhibits uterine contractions.

Pharmacokinetics
• *Absorption:* 33% to 50% of an oral dose is absorbed through the GI tract. Onset of action occurs within 30 minutes, peaks within 2 to 3 hours, and persists for 4 to 8 hours. After S.C. injection, onset occurs within 15 minutes, peaks within 30 to 60 minutes, and persists for 1½ to 4 hours. After oral inhalation, onset of action occurs within 5 to 30 minutes, peaks within 1 to 2 hours, and persists for 3 to 4 hours.
• *Distribution:* Widely distributed throughout the body.
• *Metabolism:* Partially metabolized in liver to inactive compounds.
• *Excretion:* After parenteral administration, 60% is excreted unchanged in urine, 3% in feces via bile, and the remainder in urine as metabolites. After oral administration, most drug is excreted as metabolites.

Contraindications and precautions
Terbutaline is contraindicated in patients with known hypersensitivity to the drug or to other sympathomimetics. It should be used with caution in patients with diabetes, hypertension, hyperthyroidism, or cardiac disease (especially when associated with arrhythmias).

Interactions
When used concomitantly with other sympathomimetics, terbutaline may potentiate adverse cardiovascular effects of the other drugs; however, as an aerosol bronchodilator (adrenergic stimulator type), concomitant use may relieve acute bronchospasm in patients on long-term oral terbutaline therapy.
Beta blockers may antagonize bronchodilating effects of terbutaline. Use of monoamine oxidase inhibitors within 14 days of terbutaline or the concomitant use of tricyclic antidepressants may potentiate terbutaline's effects on the vascular system.

Effects on diagnostic tests
Terbutaline may reduce the sensitivity of spirometry for diagnosis of bronchospasm.

Adverse reactions
• CNS: nervousness, tremors, dizziness, headache, anxiety, restlessness, lethargy, vertigo, drowsiness, insomnia.
• CV: increased heart rate, palpitations, tachycardia, *arrhythmias,* increased blood pressure, angina, ECG changes.
• GI: nausea, vomiting, digestive disorders.
• Other: bronchoconstriction, sweating, tinnitus, dyspnea, wheezing, unusual taste, drying or irritation of oropharynx.
Note: Drug should be discontinued if hypersensitivity or bronchoconstriction occurs.

Overdose and treatment
Clinical manifestations of overdose include exaggeration of common adverse reactions, particularly arrhythmias, seizures, nausea, and vomiting. Treatment requires supportive measures. If patient is conscious and ingestion was recent, induce emesis and follow with gastric lavage. If patient is comatose, after endotracheal tube is in place with cuff inflated, perform gastric lavage; then administer activated charcoal to reduce drug absorption. Maintain adequate airway, provide cardiac and respiratory support, and monitor vital signs closely.

▶ Special considerations
Besides those relevant to all *adrenergics,* consider the following recommendations.
• Protect injection solution from light. Do not use if discolored.
• Double-check dosage: oral is 2.5 mg, whereas S.C. is 0.25 mg. *Note:* A decimal error can be fatal.
• Give S.C. injection in lateral deltoid area.
• Cardiovascular effects are more likely with S.C. route and when patient has arrhythmias. Check pulse rate and blood pressure before each dose, and monitor for any changes from baseline.
• Most adverse reactions are transient; however, tachycardia may persist for a relatively long time.
• Patient may use tablets and aerosol concomitantly. Carefully monitor patient for toxicity.
• Aerosol terbutaline produces minimal cardiac stimulation and tremors.

---

*Canada only　　　†Unlabeled clinical use　　　Italicized adverse reactions are life-threatening.

● When drug is used for tocolytic therapy, monitor patient for cardiovascular effects including tachycardia for 12 hours after discontinuation of the drug. Monitor intake and output; fluid restriction may be necessary. Muscle tremor is common but may subside with continued use.

● Monitor neonate for hypoglycemia if the mother used terbutaline during pregnancy.

Information for the patient
● Instruct patient taking oral terbutaline on how to take pulse rate and to call if pulse varies significantly from baseline.

● Instruct patient to avoid simultaneous administration with adrenocorticoid aerosol. Separate administration time by 15 minutes.

● Demonstrate and give patient instructions on proper use of inhaler: Shake canister thoroughly to activate; place mouthpiece well into mouth, aimed at back of throat. Close lips and teeth around mouthpiece. Exhale through nose as completely as possible, then inhale through mouth slowly and deeply while actuating the nebulizer to release dose. Hold breath 10 seconds (count "1-100, 2-100, 3-100," until "10-100" is reached); remove mouthpiece, and then exhale slowly.

● Warn patient not to puncture aerosol terbutaline container. Contents are under pressure. Instruct the patient not to store it near heat or open flame or to expose it to temperatures above 120° F. (48.9° C.), which may burst the container. Tell him that cans should not be discarded into a fire or incinerator and that they should be stored out of children's reach.

● Advise patient to take a missed dose within 1 hour. After 1 hour, he should skip dose and resume regular schedule. He shouldn't double dose.

● Instruct the patient to use terbutaline only as directed. If the drug produces no relief or his condition worsens, he should call promptly.

● Warn patient not to use nonprescription drugs without medical approval. Many cold and allergy remedies contain a sympathomimetic agent that may be harmful when combined with terbutaline.

● Advise patient to report decreased effectiveness. Excessive or prolonged use of aerosol form can lead to tolerance.

Geriatric use
Lower dose may be required because elderly patients are more sensitive to the drug's effects.

Pediatric use
Not recommended for use in children under age 12.

Breast-feeding
The drug is distributed into breast milk, but in minute amounts. Use the drug with caution in breast-feeding women.

terconazole
Terazol 3, Terazol 7

● Pharmacologic classification: triazole derivative
● Therapeutic classification: antifungal
● Pregnancy risk category C

How supplied
Available by prescription only
Vaginal cream: 0.4%, 0.8%; in 45-g tubes with applicator
Vaginal suppositories: 80 mg

Indications, route, and dosage
Local treatment of vulvovaginal candidiasis (moniliasis)
Adults: 1 full application (5 g) intravaginally h.s. for 7 consecutive days. Alternatively, insert 1 suppository vaginally h.s. for 3 consecutive days.

Pharmacodynamics
Exact mechanism of action is unknown. Terconazole may disrupt fungal cell membrane permeability.

Pharmacokinetics
● *Absorption:* Minimal; absorption may range from 5% to 16%.
● *Distribution:* Effect is mainly local.
● *Metabolism:* Unknown.
● *Excretion:* Elimination of terconazole has not been described.

Contraindications and precautions
Terconazole is contraindicated in patients who are allergic to the drug or to any of its components. If irritation or sensitization occurs, drug should be discontinued. If patient does not respond to terconazole therapy, repeat microbiological studies to confirm diagnosis.

Interactions
None reported.

Effects on diagnostic tests
None reported.

Adverse reactions
CNS: headache.
Local: itching, burning, irritation.

Overdose and treatment
No information available.

▶ Special considerations
● Drug is only effective against vulvovaginitis caused by *Candida.* Diagnosis should be confirmed by cultures or potassium hydroxide (KOH) smears.
● A persistent infection may be caused by reinfection. Evaluate patient for possible sources.
● Intractable candidiasis may be a sign of diabetes mellitus. Perform blood and urine glucose determinations to rule out undiagnosed diabetes mellitus.

Information for the patient
● Instruct patient to insert cream high into the vagina.
● Tell patient to complete full course of therapy, and to

use it continuously, even during menstrual period. The therapeutic effect of terconazole is not affected by menstruation.
● Tell patient to report if drug causes burning or irritation.
● Patient should refrain from sexual intercourse or advise partner to use a condom to avoid reinfection.
● Advise patient to use a sanitary napkin to prevent staining of clothing.

Breast-feeding
Safety is not established. Breast-feeding is not recommended during therapy with terconazole.

---

terfenadine
Seldane

● Pharmacologic classification: butyrophenone derivative
● Therapeutic classification: antihistamine (H_1-receptor antagonist)
● Pregnancy risk category C

How supplied
Available by prescription only
Tablets: 60 mg

Indications, route, and dosage
Rhinitis, allergy symptoms
Adults and children age 12 or older: 60 mg P.O. q 8 to 12 hours.
Children age 6 to 12: 30 to 60 mg P.O. b.i.d.
Children age 3 to 5: 15 mg P.O. b.i.d.

Pharmacodynamics
Antihistamine action: Antihistamines compete with histamine for histamine H_1-receptor sites on the smooth muscle of the bronchi, GI tract, uterus, and large blood vessels; by binding to cellular receptors, they prevent access of histamine and suppress histamine-induced allergic symptoms, even though they do not prevent its release.

Pharmacokinetics
● *Absorption:* Terfenadine is well absorbed from the GI tract; after a 60-mg dose, action begins within 1 to 2 hours and peaks in 3 to 6 hours.
● *Distribution:* Terfenadine is distributed mainly into the lungs, liver, GI tract, spleen, and bile; lower concentrations have been detected in the blood, kidneys, and heart. Terfenadine is extensively (97%) protein-bound; it does not cross the blood-brain barrier, and it is unknown if the drug crosses the placenta or is distributed into breast milk. Plasma half-life of terfenadine is 3½ hours.
● *Metabolism:* Terfenadine is metabolized almost completely in the GI tract and liver (first-pass effect).
● *Excretion:* Terfenadine's elimination half-life is about 16 to 23 hours. Only 1% of drug is excreted unchanged; about 60% of drug and metabolites is excreted in feces, with the remaining 40% excreted in urine.

Contraindications and precautions
Terfenadine is contraindicated in patients with known hypersensitivity to the drug. It should be used with caution in patients with asthma or other lower respiratory diseases, because its mild anticholinergic effects might aggravate these conditions.

Interactions
Unlike other antihistamines, terfenadine has minimal anticholinergic activity and does not potentiate the CNS effects of alcohol, antianxiety agents, or other CNS depressants. Erythromycin, itraconazole, or ketoconazole may decrease the hepatic metabolism of terfenadine, leading to increased terfenadine serum levels and possible toxicity.

Effects on diagnostic tests
Terfenadine should be discontinued 2 days before using diagnostic skin tests, to prevent masking of test response.

Adverse reactions
● CNS: fatigue, dizziness, headache.
● EENT: dry mouth and throat, nasal stuffiness.
● GI: nausea, abdominal distress, cholestatic jaundice.

Overdose and treatment
Symptoms of overdose include mild headache, nausea, and confusion. One patient who ingested 56 tablets (3,360 mg) of Seldane developed ventricular dysrhythmia progressing to fibrillation; he responded well to defibrillation and lidocaine. Because the potential for cardiac arrhythmias exists, continue cardiac monitoring for at least 24 hours.
   Treat overdose by inducing emesis with ipecac syrup (in conscious patient), followed by activated charcoal to absorb any excess drug that may have remained in the stomach. Use gastric lavage if the patient is unconscious or if induction of vomiting fails. It is unknown if terfenadine is dialyzable.

▶ Special considerations
Besides those relevant to all *antihistamines,* consider the following recommendations.
● Drug may have drying effect in patients with asthma or other lower airway disease; keep patient well hydrated.
● Terfenadine does not cause drowsiness and sedation associated with other antihistamines because it does not cross the blood-brain barrier; anticholinergic and antiserotonin effects are mild.

Information for the patient
● Instruct patient not to exceed prescribed dosage and to take the drug only when needed.
● Tell patient to store the drug in a tightly sealed container away from heat and direct sunlight.

Pediatric use
Although its safety has not been established in children under age 12, terfenadine has been used in children age 3 to 12.

Breast-feeding
Antihistamines such as terfenadine should not be used during breast-feeding. Many of these drugs are secreted in breast milk, exposing the infant to risks of unusual excitability; premature infants are at particular risk for seizures.

---

terpin hydrate

- Pharmacologic classification: aliphatic alcohol
- Therapeutic classification: expectorant
- Pregnancy risk category C

How supplied
Available without prescription
Elixir: 85 mg/5 ml (43% alcohol)

Indications, route, and dosage
Excessive bronchial secretions
Adults: 5 to 10 ml of elixir P.O. q 4 to 6 hours.

Pharmacodynamics
Expectorant action: Terpin hydrate probably reduces viscosity of thick secretions by increasing respiratory tract secretions via direct stimulation of lower respiratory tract secretory glands.

Pharmacokinetics
Unknown.

Contraindications and precautions
Drug is contraindicated in patients with peptic ulcer. It is not recommended in children under age 12, because of its high alcohol content. It should be used with caution in patients taking other CNS depressants and during pregnancy; alcohol crosses the placental barrier, and excessive use may cause congenital anomalies from its high alcohol content.

Interactions
Concomitant use with CNS depressants may result in added sedation and CNS depression; elixir contains 43% alcohol. Disulfiram, metronidazole, and the sulfonylureas inhibit alcohol dehydrogenase – the enzyme that catalyzes alcohol detoxification; because of its high alcohol content, concomitant use of terpin hydrate elixir with these drugs may result in a disulfiram reaction: respiratory depression, cardiac arrhythmias, cardiovascular collapse, MI, seizures, unconsciousness, and sudden death.

Effects on diagnostic tests
None reported.

Adverse reactions
- CNS: sedation.
- GI: nausea, vomiting.

Overdose and treatment
No information available.

▶ **Special considerations**
Monitor cough and frequency.

Information for the patient
- Instruct patient to take only the amount prescribed at the designated time, with a glass of water to help loosen mucus; warn patient to take it with some food to avoid epigastric distress.
- Instruct patient to notify physician if cough persists after 7 days of therapy or if high fever, skin rash, continuing headache, or sore throat is present with cough.

- Explain risks of high alcohol content. Tell patient to avoid use of alcohol or other CNS depressants during therapy.

Geriatric use
Elderly patients should use the drug with caution because of their greater susceptibility to depressant effects of alcohol.

Pediatric use
Terpin hydrate is not recommended for use in children under age 12 because of its alcohol content.

Breast-feeding
Terpin hydrate should not be used during breast-feeding; alcohol is secreted into breast milk.

testolactone
Teslac

- Pharmacologic classification: androgen
- Therapeutic classification: antineoplastic
- Pregnancy risk category C

How supplied
Available by prescription only
Tablets: 50 mg

Indications, route, and dosage
Dosage and indications may vary. Check current literature for recommended protocol.
Advanced postmenopausal breast cancer
Adults: 250 mg P.O. q.i.d.

Pharmacodynamics
Antineoplastic action: The exact mechanism of action is unclear. Testolactone's cytotoxic activity may result from depressed ovarian function that follows inhibition of pituitary gonadotropin synthesis or prevention of steroid action on tumor cell, which the cell requires for survival.

Pharmacokinetics
- *Absorption:* Testolactone is well absorbed across the GI tract after oral administration.
- *Distribution:* Testolactone is widely distributed into total body water.
- *Metabolism:* Testolactone is extensively metabolized in the liver.
- *Excretion:* Testolactone and its metabolites are excreted primarily in urine.

Contraindications and precautions
Testolactone is contraindicated in the treatment of breast cancer in males and in premenopausal women because of the potential for adverse hormonal effects.
   Use cautiously in patients with hypercalcemia and cardiovascular disease.

Interactions
None reported.

Effects on diagnostic tests
Testolactone therapy may increase concentrations of serum calcium, urinary creatinine, and urinary 17-ketosteroids.

Adverse reactions
- CNS: paresthesias.
- CV: hypertension, orthostasis.
- DERM: maculopapular rash, erythema.
- GI: nausea, vomiting, anorexia, glossitis, diarrhea.
- Metabolic: hypercalcemia.
- Other: edema, hot flashes.

Overdose and treatment
No information available.

▶ Special considerations
- Adequate trial is 3 months. Reassure patient that therapeutic response isn't immediate.
- Monitor fluids and electrolytes, especially calcium levels.
- Immobilized patients are prone to hypercalcemia. Exercise may prevent it. Force fluids to aid calcium excretion.
- Treat hypercalcemia with generous hydration; obtain calcium levels before and during therapy.
- Higher-than-recommended doses do not increase incidence of remission.
- Drug does not cause virilization when used at recommended doses.

Information for the patient
- Emphasize importance of continuing medication despite nausea and vomiting.
- Tell patient to call promptly if vomiting occurs shortly after a dose is taken.

Breast-feeding
It is not known whether testolactone distributes into breast milk. However, because of the risk of serious adverse reactions in the infant, breast-feeding is not recommended.

---

testosterone
Andro 100, Andronaq-50, Histerone, Testaqua, Testoject-50

testosterone cypionate
Andro-Cyp 100, Andro-Cyp 200, Andronate, dep Andro 100, dep Andro 200, Depo-Testosterone, Duratest, Testa-C, Testoject LA

testosterone enanthate
Andro L.A. 200, Andryl, Delatestryl, Everone, Testone L.A., Testrin-P.A.

testosterone propionate
Testex

- Pharmacologic classification: androgen
- Therapeutic classification: androgen replacement, antineoplastic
- Controlled substance schedule III
- Pregnancy risk category X

How supplied
Available by prescription only
Testosterone
Injection (aqueous suspension): 25 mg/ml, 50 mg/ml, 100 mg/ml

Testosterone cypionate (in oil)
Injection: 50 mg/ml, 100 mg/ml, 200 mg/ml
Testosterone enanthate (in oil)
Injection: 100 mg/ml, 200 mg/ml
Testosterone propionate (in oil)
Injection: 25 mg/ml, 50 mg/ml, 100 mg/ml

Indications, route, and dosage
Male hypogonadism
Testosterone or testosterone propionate
Adults: 10 to 25 mg I.M. two or three times weekly.
Testosterone cypionate or enanthate
Adults: 50 to 400 mg I.M. q 2 to 4 weeks.
Delayed puberty in males
Testosterone or testosterone propionate
Children: 12.5 to 25 mg I.M. two or three times weekly for up to 6 months.
Testosterone cypionate or enanthate
Children: 25 to 200 mg I.M. q 2 to 4 weeks for up to 6 months.
Postpartum breast pain and engorgement
Testosterone or testosterone propionate
Adults: 25 to 50 mg I.M. daily for 3 to 4 days.
Inoperable breast cancer
Testosterone or testosterone propionate
Adults: 50 to 100 mg I.M. three times weekly.
Testosterone cypionate or enanthate
Adults: 200 to 400 mg q 2 to 4 weeks.

Pharmacodynamics
- Androgenic action: Testosterone is the endogenous androgen that stimulates receptors in androgen-responsive organs and tissues to promote growth and development of male sexual organs and secondary sexual characteristics.
- Antineoplastic action: Testosterone exerts inhibitory, antiestrogenic effects on hormone-responsive breast tumors and metastases.

Pharmacokinetics
- Absorption: Testosterone and its esters must be administered parenterally because they are inactivated rapidly by the liver when given orally. The onset of action of testosterone's cypionate and enanthate esters is somewhat slower than that of testosterone itself.
- Distribution: Testosterone is normally 98% to 99% plasma protein-bound, primarily to the testosterone-estradiol binding globulin.
- Metabolism: Testosterone is metabolized to several 17-ketosteroids by two main pathways in the liver. A large portion of these metabolites then form glucuronide and sulfate conjugates. The plasma half-life of testosterone ranges from 10 to 100 minutes. The cypionate and enanthate esters of testosterone have longer durations of action than testosterone.
- Excretion: Very little unchanged testosterone appears in urine or feces. Approximately 90% of metabolized testosterone is excreted in urine in the form of sulfate and glucuronide conjugates.

Contraindications and precautions
Testosterone is contraindicated in patients with severe renal or cardiac disease, which may be worsened by the fluid and electrolyte retention caused by this drug; in patients with hepatic disease because impaired elimination of the drug may cause toxic accumulation; in male patients with prostatic or breast cancer, benign prostatic hypertrophy with obstruction, or undiagnosed abnormal genital bleeding because the drug can stim-

late the growth of cancerous breast or prostate tissue; and in pregnant or breast-feeding women because animal studies have shown that administration of androgens during pregnancy causes masculinization of the fetus.

Interactions
In patients with diabetes, decreased blood glucose levels may require adjustment of insulin or oral hypoglycemic drug dosage.

Testosterone may potentiate the effects of warfarin-type anticoagulants, prolonging prothrombin time. Concurrent administration with oxyphenbutazone may increase serum oxyphenbutazone concentrations.

Effects on diagnostic tests
Testosterone may cause abnormal results of glucose tolerance tests. Thyroid function test results (protein-bound iodine, radioactive iodine uptake, thyroid-binding capacity) and serum 17-ketosteroid levels may decrease. Liver function test results, prothrombin time (especially in patients on anticoagulant therapy), and serum creatinine levels may be elevated. Because of the anabolic activity of testosterone, increases may occur in serum sodium, potassium, calcium, phosphate, and cholesterol levels.

Adverse reactions
● Androgenic *in females:* deepening of voice, clitoral enlargement, changes in libido; *in males:* prepubertal – premature epiphyseal closure, priapism, phallic enlargement; postpubertal – testicular atrophy, oligospermia, decreased ejaculatory volume, impotence, gynecomastia, epididymitis.
● CNS: headache, anxiety, mental depression, generalized paresthesias.
● CV: edema.
● DERM: acne, oily skin, hirsutism, flushing, sweating, male pattern baldness.
● GI: gastroenteritis, nausea, vomiting, diarrhea, constipation, change in appetite, weight gain.
● GU: bladder irritability, vaginitis, menstrual irregularities
● HEMA: polycythemia; suppression of clotting factors II, V, VII, and X.
● Hepatic: cholestatic hepatitis, jaundice.
● Local: pain, induration, irritation at injection site; postinjection furunculosis, edema.
● Other: hypercalcemia, *hepatocellular cancer* (with long-term use).
Note: Drug should be discontinued if hypercalcemia, edema, hypersensitivity reaction, priapism, or excessive sexual stimulation develops or if virilization occurs in females.

Overdose and treatment
No information available.

▶ Special considerations
Besides those relevant to all *androgens,* consider the following recommendations.
● When used to treat male hypogonadism, initiate therapy with full therapeutic doses and taper according to patient tolerance and response. Administering long-acting esters (enanthate or cypionate) at intervals greater than every 2 to 3 weeks may cause hormone levels to fall below those found in normal adults.
● Carefully observe female patients for signs of excessive virilization. If possible, discontinue therapy at

the first sign of virilization because some adverse effects (deepening of voice, clitoral enlargement) are irreversible. Patients with metastatic breast cancer should have regular determinations of serum calcium levels to avoid serious hypercalcemia.
● Inject deeply I.M., preferably into a large muscle mass such as the upper outer quadrant of the gluteal muscle.
● Testosterone enanthate has been used for postmenopausal osteoporosis and to stimulate erythropoiesis.
● Solutions of long-acting esters (enanthate and cypionate) may become cloudy if a wet needle is used to draw up the solution. This will not affect potency.
● Warming (to room temperature) and shaking vial will help redissolve crystals that have formed after storage.

Information for the patient
● Explain to female patient that virilization may occur. Tell patient to report androgenic effects immediately. Stopping drug will prevent further androgenic changes but will probably not reverse those already present.
● Tell females to report menstrual irregularities; discontinue therapy pending determination of the cause.
● Advise male patient to report too frequent or persistent penile erections.
● Advise patients to report persistent GI distress, diarrhea, or the onset of jaundice.

Geriatric use
Observe elderly male patients for the development of prostatic hypertrophy. Development of symptomatic prostatic hypertrophy or prostatic carcinoma mandates the discontinuation of the drug.

Pediatric use
Use with extreme caution in children, to avoid precocious puberty and premature closure of the epiphyses. X-ray examinations every 6 months are recommended to assess skeletal maturation.

Breast-feeding
Distribution into breast milk is unknown. An alternative feeding method is recommended because of potential for severe adverse effects of androgens on the infant.

---

tetanus antitoxin (TAT), equine

● Pharmacologic classification: antitoxin
● Therapeutic classification: tetanus antitoxin
● Pregnancy risk category D

How supplied
Available by prescription only
Injection: not less than 400 units/ml in 1,500-unit and 20,000-unit vials

Indications, route, and dosage
Indicated for tetanus prophylaxis or treatment only when human tetanus immune globulin is unavailable.
Tetanus prophylaxis
Adults and children over 65 lb (30 kg): 3,000 to 5,000 units I.M. or S.C.
Adults and children under 65 lb (30 kg): 1,500 units I.M. or S.C.

Tetanus treatment
Adults and children: 10,000 to 20,000 units injected into wound. Give additional 40,000 to 100,000 units I.V. Administer adsorbed tetanus toxoid at same time but at different sites and with a different syringe, because toxoid neutralization may occur.

Pharmacodynamics
Antitoxin action: TAT neutralizes and binds toxin.

Pharmacokinetics
No information is available.

Contraindications and precautions
Use TAT with caution in patients allergic to equine-derived preparations.

Interactions
No significant interactions have been reported.

Effects on diagnostic tests
None reported.

Adverse reactions
● Local: pain, numbness, or skin eruptions at or near injection site.
● Systemic: joint pain, *difficulty breathing,* hypersensitivity, *anaphylaxis,* serum sickness.
   Note: Drug should be discontinued if severe systemic reactions occur.

Overdose and treatment
No information available.

▶ Special considerations
● Obtain a thorough patient history of allergies, especially to horses and horse immune serum, and of previous reactions to immunizations.
● Test patient for sensitivity (against a control of normal saline solution in the other arm) before administration. Give 0.1 ml of a 1:100 dilution of antitoxin in 0.9% normal saline solution intradermally (0.05 ml of a 1:1,000 dilution in patients with a history of allergy).
● Epinephrine solution 1:1,000 should be available to treat allergic reactions.
● Use only when human tetanus immune globulin is not available.
● A preventive dose should be given to those with dirty wounds who have had three or fewer injections of tetanus toxoid and who have tetanus-prone injuries more than 24 hours old.
● Protection from TAT lasts approximately 15 days; duration of protection may be shorter in those who received a recent injection of a product derived from a horse.
● Because this product is derived from an animal source (that is, horses), patient may have anaphylactic reactions, such as rash, joint swelling or pain, fever, serum sickness, or difficulty breathing. Monitor patient closely and treat with medication, as ordered, if these effects occur.
● Store TAT between 2° and 8° C (36° to 46° F).

Information for the patient
Tell patient that he may experience pain, numbness, or rash at or near the injection site.

Breast-feeding
Patient should discontinue breast-feeding temporarily until effects of the toxin subside and if symptoms of serum sickness develop.

---

tetanus immune globulin, human (TIG)
Hyper-Tet

● Pharmacologic classification: immune serum
● Therapeutic classification: tetanus prophylaxis agent
● Pregnancy risk category B

How supplied
Available by prescription only
Injection: 250 units per vial or syringe

Indications, route, and dosage
Tetanus exposure
Adults and children: 250 to 500 units I.M.
Tetanus treatment
Adults and children: Single doses of 3,000 to 6,000 units have been used. Optimal dosage schedules not established. Don't give at same site as toxoid.

Pharmacodynamics
Antitetanus action: TIG provides passive immunity to tetanus. Antibodies remain at effective levels for 3 weeks or longer. TIG protects the patient for the incubation period of most tetanus cases.

Pharmacokinetics
● *Absorption:* Slow.
● *Distribution:* No information is available.
● *Metabolism:* No information is available.
● *Excretion:* The serum half-life of TIG is approximately 28 days.

Contraindications and precautions
TIG should be used with caution in patients with known hypersensitivity to thimerosal, a component of this preparation.

Interactions
None reported.

Effects on diagnostic tests
None reported.

Adverse reactions
● Local: pain, tenderness, stiffness, and erythema at injection site.
● Systemic: slight fever, hives, *angioedema, anaphylaxis.*

Overdose and treatment
No information available.

▶ Special considerations
● Obtain a thorough history of injury, tetanus immunizations, last tetanus toxoid injection, allergies, and reactions to immunizations.
● Epinephrine solution 1:1,000 should be available to treat allergic reactions.

● For wound management, use TIG for prophylaxis in patients with dirty wounds if patient has had fewer than three previous tetanus toxoid injections, or if the immunization history is unknown or uncertain.

● Thoroughly cleanse and remove all foreign matter and necrotic tissue from wound.

● Immune globulin (gamma globulin) should only be given when TIG is not available.

● Do not confuse this drug with tetanus toxoid, which should be given at the same time (but at different sites) to produce active immunization.

● Administer I.M. in the deltoid muscle for adults and in the anterolateral thigh for infants and small children. Do not inject I.V.

● Tetanus risks severe morbidity and mortality in both mother and fetus if untreated. No fetal risk from the use of immune globulin has been reported to date.

● TIG has not been associated with an increased frequency of acquired immunodeficiency syndrome (AIDS). The immune globulin is devoid of human immunodeficiency virus (HIV). Immune globulin recipients do not develop antibodies to HIV.

● Store between 2° and 8° C (36° and 46° F). Do not freeze.

Information for the patient

● Available data indicate that TIG administration does not cause AIDS or hepatitis.

● Tell patient that he may experience some local pain, swelling, and tenderness at the injection site. Recommend acetaminophen to alleviate these minor effects.

● Encourage patient to report headache, skin changes, or difficulty breathing.

Breast-feeding

It is unknown whether TIG is distributed into breast milk. Use with caution in breast-feeding women.

tetanus toxoid, adsorbed

tetanus toxoid, fluid

● Pharmacologic classification: toxoid
● Therapeutic classification: tetanus prophylaxis agent
● Pregnancy risk category C

How supplied

Available by prescription only
Adsorbed toxoid
Injection: 5 to 10 Lf units of inactivated tetanus/0.5-ml dose, in 0.5-ml syringes and 5-ml vials
Fluid toxoid
Injection: 4 to 5 Lf units of inactivated tetanus/0.5-ml dose, in 0.5-ml syringes and 7.5-ml vials

Indications, route, and dosage

Primary immunization (adsorbed formulation)
Adults and children: 0.5 ml I.M. 4 to 6 weeks apart for two doses, then a third dose 1 year after the second dose. Booster dosage is 0.5 ml I.M. every 10 years.
Primary immunization (fluid formulation)
Adults and children: 0.5 ml I.M. or S.C. 4 to 8 weeks apart for three doses, then a fourth dose 6 to 12 months

after the third dose. Booster dosage is 0.5 ml I.M. or S.C. every 10 years.
Tetanus prophylaxis in wound management
Adults and children: In patients with history of primary immunization and booster less than 10 years ago and a clean wound—no tetanus toxoid is required. In patients with history of primary immunization and booster more than 10 years ago and a clean wound—give 0.5 ml of adsorbed tetanus toxoid I.M. All patients with a dirty (tetanus-prone) wound and a history of primary immunization or booster more than 5 years before should receive a booster dose of adsorbed tetanus toxoid I.M. In patients with incomplete or unknown history of immunization—give 0.5 ml adsorbed tetanus toxoid I.M. and complete primary immunization. In patients with no history of primary immunization—initiate primary immunization.

Concurrent use of tetanus immune globulin depends on primary immunization history, the type of wound (tetanus-prone), and care received for the wound. (See the "Tetanus immune globulin" entry for more information.)

Pharmacodynamics

Tetanus prophylaxis: Tetanus toxoid promotes active immunity by inducing production of tetanus antitoxin.

Pharmacokinetics

● *Absorption:* Slow. Fluid formulation provides quicker booster effect.
● *Distribution:* Unknown.
● *Metabolism:* Unknown.
● *Excretion:* Unknown. Active immunity usually persists for 10 years. Adsorbed tetanus toxoid usually produces more persistent antitoxin titers than fluid tetanus toxoid.

Contraindications and precautions

Tetanus toxoid is contraindicated in patients with a history of neurologic or severe hypersensitivity reaction following a previous dose.

Interactions

Concomitant use with chloramphenicol, corticosteroids, or immunosuppressants theoretically may impair the immune response to tetanus toxoid. Avoid elective immunization under these circumstances.

Effects on diagnostic tests

None reported.

Adverse reactions

● Local: stinging, edema, erythema, pain, induration; nodule may develop and last for several weeks.
● Systemic: slight fever, chills, malaise, arthralgia, myalgia, flushing, urticaria, pruritus, tachycardia, *hypotension,* neurologic disorders, *anaphylaxis,* Arthus-like reaction.

Overdose and treatment

No information available.

▶ Special considerations

● Obtain a thorough history of allergies and reactions to immunizations.
● Epinephrine solution 1:1,000 should be available to treat allergic reactions.
● Determine tetanus immunization status and date of last tetanus immunization.
● The preferred I.M. injection site is the deltoid or mid-

lateral thigh in adults and children and the midlateral thigh in infants.
• Preferably, tetanus immunization should be completed and maintained using multiple antigen preparations appropriate for the patient's age, such as DTP, DT, or Td.
• Shake vial vigorously to ensure a uniform suspension before withdrawing the dose.
• Do not confuse this drug with tetanus immune globulin.
• These toxoids are used to prevent, not treat, tetanus infections.
• Store at 2° to 8° C (36° to 46° F). Do not freeze.

Information for the patient
• Tell patient what to expect after immunization: discomfort at the injection site and a nodule that may develop there and persist for several weeks. Patient also may develop fever, general malaise, or body aches and pains. Recommend acetaminophen to alleviate these effects.
• Instruct patient not to use hot or cold compresses at the injection site because this may increase the severity of the local reaction.
• Encourage patient to report distressing adverse reactions.
• Tell patient that immunization requires a series of injections. Stress the importance of keeping scheduled appointments for subsequent doses.

Breast-feeding
It is unknown whether tetanus toxoid is distributed into breast milk. Use with caution in breast-feeding women.

---

tetracycline hydrochloride
Achromycin, Cefracycline*, Cyclopar, Medicycline*, Neo-Tetrine*, Novotetra*, Panmycin, Retet-s, Robitet, SK-Tetracycline, Sumycin, Tetracyn, Tetralean*, Tetrex, Topicycline (topical)

• Pharmacologic classification: tetracycline
• Therapeutic classification: antibiotic
• Pregnancy risk category D

How supplied
Available by prescription only
Capsules: 100 mg, 250 mg, 500 mg
Tablets: 250 mg, 500 mg
Suspension: 125 mg/5 ml, 250 mg/5 ml
Injectable: 100 mg, 250 mg, 500 mg
Topical: 2.2-mg/ml solution, 3% ointment

Indications, route, and dosage
Infections caused by sensitive organisms
Adults: 250 to 500 mg P.O. q 6 hours; 250 mg I.M. daily or 150 mg I.M. q 12 hours; or 250 to 500 mg I.V. q 8 to 12 hours (I.M. and I.V. hydrochloride salt only).
Children over age 8: 25 to 50 mg/kg P.O. daily, divided q 6 hours; 15 to 25 mg/kg daily (maximum 250 mg) I.M. in single dose or divided q 8 to 12 hours; or 20 to 30 mg/kg/day I.V. in divided doses q 12 hours.
Uncomplicated urethral, endocervical, or rectal infection
Adults: 500 mg P.O. q.i.d. for at least 7 days.

Brucellosis
Adults: 500 mg P.O. q 6 hours for 3 weeks with streptomycin 1 g I.M. q 12 hours week 1 and daily week 2.
Gonorrhea in patients sensitive to penicillin
Adults: Initially, 1.5 g P.O.; then 500 mg q 6 hours for 7 days.
Syphilis in nonpregnant patients sensitive to penicillin
Adults: 500 mg P.O., q.i.d. for 14 days.
Acne
Adults and adolescents: Initially, 250 mg P.O. q 6 hours; then 125 to 500 mg P.O. daily or every other day, apply topical ointment generously to affected areas b.i.d. until skin is thoroughly wet.
Shigellosis
Adults: 2.5 g P.O. in 1 dose.
Lymphogranuloma venereum
Adults: 500 mg P.O. q.i.d. for 21 days.
Superficial ocular infections and inclusion conjunctivitis
Adults and children: Instill 1 to 2 drops of ophthalmic solution in eye b.i.d., q.i.d., or more often, depending on severity of infection.
Trachoma
Adults and children: Instill 2 drops of ophthalmic solution in each eye b.i.d., t.i.d., or q.i.d. Continue for 1 to 2 months or longer, or use 1% ointment t.i.d. or q.i.d. for 30 days.
Prophylaxis of ophthalmia neonatorum
Neonates: 1 to 2 drops of ophthalmic solution into each eye shortly after delivery.
Infection prophylaxis in minor skin abrasions and treatment of superficial infections caused by susceptible organisms
Adults and children: Apply topical ointment to infected area one to five times daily.

Pharmacodynamics
Antibacterial action: Tetracycline is bacteriostatic; it binds reversibly to ribosomal subunits, thus inhibiting bacterial protein synthesis. Its spectrum of action includes many gram-negative and gram-positive organisms, *Mycoplasma, Rickettsia, Chlamydia,* and spirochetes.
It is useful against brucellosis, glanders, mycoplasma pneumonia infections (some clinicians prefer erthromycin), leptospirosis, early stages of Lyme disease, rikettsial infections (such as Rocky Mountain spotted fever, Q fever, and typhus fever) and chlamydial infections. It is an alternative to penicillin for *Neisseria gonorrhoeae,* but because of a high level of resistance in the United States, other alternative agents should be considered.

Pharmacokinetics
• *Absorption:* Tetracycline is 75% to 80% absorbed after oral administration; peak serum levels occur at 2 to 4 hours. Food or milk products significantly reduce oral absorption.
• *Distribution:* Tetracycline is distributed widely into body tissues and fluids, including synovial, pleural, prostatic, and seminal fluids, bronchial secretions, saliva, and aqueous humor; CSF penetration is poor. Tetracycline crosses the placenta; it is 20% to 67% protein-bound.
• *Metabolism:* Tetracycline is not metabolized.
• *Excretion:* Tetracycline is excreted primarily unchanged in urine by glomerular filtration; plasma half-life is 6 to 12 hours in adults with normal renal function.

Some drug is excreted in breast milk. Only minimal amounts of tetracycline are removed by hemodialysis or peritoneal dialysis.

Contraindications and precautions
Tetracycline is contraindicated in patients with known hypersensitivity to any tetracycline; during the second half of pregnancy; and in children under age 8 because of the risk of permanent discoloration of teeth, enamel defects, and retardation of bone growth.

Drug should be used cautiously in patients with decreased renal function because it may elevate BUN levels and exacerbate renal dysfunction; and in patients apt to be exposed to direct sunlight or ultraviolet light, because of the risk of photosensitivity reactions.

Interactions
Tetracycline absorption may be decreased by antacids containing aluminum, calcium, or magnesium and laxatives containing magnesium because of chelation, and by food and dairy products, oral iron, and sodium bicarbonate.

Tetracycline may antagonize bactericidal effects of penicillin, inhibiting cell growth from bacteriostatic action; administer penicillin 2 to 3 hours before tetracycline.

Concomitant use of tetracycline increases the risk of nephrotoxicity from methoxyflurane.

Concomitant use of tetracycline necessitates lowered dosage of oral anticoagulants because of enhanced effects, and lowered dosage of digoxin because of increased bioavailability.

Effects on diagnostic tests
Tetracycline causes false-negative results in urine tests using glucose oxidase reagent (Clinistix or Tes-Tape), and false elevations in fluorometric tests for urinary catecholamines.

Tetracycline may elevate BUN levels in patients with decreased renal function.

Adverse reactions
● CNS: dizziness, headache, intracranial hypertension.
● CV: pericarditis.
● DERM: maculopapular and erythematous rashes, urticaria, photosensitivity, increased pigmentation, discolored nails and teeth. With topical use: temporary stinging or burning on application, slight yellowing of treated skin (especially in persons of fair complexion), severe dermatitis, fluorescence of treated skin under black light.
● EENT: sore throat, glossitis, dysphagia, eye itching (with ophthalmic use).
● GI: anorexia, epigastric distress, nausea, vomiting, diarrhea, stomatitis, enterocolitis, inflammatory lesions in anogenital region.
● GU: reversible nephrotoxicity (Fanconi's syndrome) with *outdated* tetracycline.
● HEMA: neutropenia, eosinophilia.
● Hepatic: hepatotoxicity with large doses given I.V.
● Metabolic: increased BUN level.
● Local: irritation after I.M. injection, thrombophlebitis.
● Other: bacterial and fungal superinfection.
   Note: Drug should be discontinued if signs of toxicity or hypersensitivity, progressive renal dysfunction, or superinfection occur; if erythema follows exposure to sunlight or ultraviolet light; or if severe diarrhea indicates pseudomembranous colitis.

Overdose and treatment
Clinical signs of overdose are usually limited to GI tract; give antacids or empty stomach by gastric lavage if ingestion occurs within the preceding 4 hours.

▶ Special considerations
Besides those relevant to all *tetracyclines,* consider the following recommendations.
● Tetracycline may be administered by intracavitary instillation (chest tube) as a pleural sclerosing agent in malignant pleural effusion.
Parenteral use
● Discard I.M. solutions after 24 hours because they deteriorate. Exception: Discard Achromycin solution in 12 hours.
● Inject I.M. dose deeply into large muscle. Warn patient that it may be painful. Rotate sites. I.M. preparations in many cases contain a local anesthetic; ask patient about hypersensitivity to local anesthetics.
● Watch for overgrowth of nonsusceptible organisms. Assess patient for signs of bacterial and fungal superinfection. Check patient's tongue for signs of monilia infection. Stress good oral hygiene. Stop drug if superinfection occurs. Carefully monitor patient's vital signs, especially temperature.
● Monitor for diarrhea, which may result from local irritation or superinfection.
● For I.V. use, reconstitute 100 mg and 250 mg of powder for injection with 5 ml of sterile water; with 10 ml for 500 mg. Further dilute in 100 to 1,000 ml volume of dextrose 5% in 0.9% saline solution. Refrigerate diluted solution and use within 24 hours. Exception: Use Achromycin solution immediately. Infuse over 2 hours.
● Do not mix tetracycline solution with any other I.V. additive; may cause drug inactivation or interaction.
● For I.M. use, reconstitute 100 mg powder for injection with 2 ml sterile water for injection. Concentration will be 50 mg/ml. Amount of diluent for 250 mg injection varies according to brand. Check with pharmacy or follow manufacturer's instructions.
Ophthalmic use
● For prophylaxis of ophthalmia neonatorum, apply ointment no later than 1 hour after birth.
● Apply light finger-pressure on lacrimal sac for 1 minute after drops are instilled.
● Always wash hands before and after applying solution.
● Cleanse eye area of excessive exudate before application.
● Store in tightly closed, light-resistant container.
Topical use
● Discontinue if no improvement or condition worsens.
● To control the rate of flow, increase or decrease pressure of applicator against skin.
● Avoid contact with eyes, nose, and mouth.
● Solution should be used within 2 months.

Information for the patient
● Warn patient to avoid sharing washcloths and towels with family members.
● Tell patient to watch for signs of sensitivity, such as itching lids or constant burning. Patient who develops such signs should stop drug and call immediately.
● Show patient how to instill. Stress importance of compliance with recommended therapy.
● Warn patient not to touch tip of dropper to eye or surrounding tissue.
● Tell patient not to share medication with others.
● Patient may continue normal use of cosmetics.

● Explain that floating plug in bottle of topical tetracycline is an inert and harmless result of proper reconstitution of the preparation and should not be removed.
● Tell patient stinging may occur but will resolve quickly, and that drug may stain clothing.

Pediatric use
Tetracycline should not be used in children younger than age 9.

Breast-feeding
Tetracycline is excreted in breast milk and should not be used in breast-feeding women.

PHARMACOLOGIC CLASS

tetracyclines

demeclocycline hydrochloride
doxycycline hyclate
methacycline sulfate
minocycline hydrochloride
oxytetracycline hydrochloride
tetracycline hydrochloride

Tetracycline antibiotics were discovered during the random screening of soil samples for antibiotic-producing microorganisms. The prototype, chlortetracycline, was discovered in 1948; tetracycline was developed in 1952. Structural modifications that enhanced both antibacterial activity and pharmacokinetic parameters led to development of doxycycline in 1966 and minocycline in 1972.

Usually well-tolerated with few adverse effects, tetracyclines have an unusually broad spectrum of antibacterial activity, including gram-negative and gram-positive anaerobic and aerobic bacteria, *Chlamydia*, and protozoa; longer-acting tetracyclines have enhanced activity against *Chlamydia* and *Legionella*.

Demeclocycline has a higher incidence of severe photosensitivity reactions; also, because of its renal effects, it is rarely prescribed for clinical use, although it is used investigationally to treat the syndrome of inappropriate antidiuretic hormone (SIADH) secretion.

Pharmacology
Tetracyclines are bacteriostatic but may be bactericidal against certain organisms. They bind reversibly to 30S and 50S ribosomal subunits, inhibiting bacterial protein synthesis. Bacterial resistance to tetracyclines is usually mediated by plasmids (R-factor resistance), which decrease bacterial cell wall permeability; this is the most important cause of resistance by staphylococci, streptococci, most aerobic gram-negative organisms, and *Pseudomonas aeruginosa*. With two exceptions, cross-resistance occurs with all tetracyclines; doxycycline is active against *Bacteroides fragilis*, and minocycline is active against *Staphylococcus aureus*.

Tetracyclines attack many common pathogens as well as some less common ones; they are not antifungal or antiviral.

Susceptible gram-positive organisms include *Bacillus anthracis*, *Actinomyces israelii*, *Clostridium perfringens*, *C. tetani*, *Listeria monocytogenes*, and *Nocardia*. Initial but transient activity exists against staphylococci and streptococci; infections caused by these organisms are usually treated with other drugs.

Susceptible gram-negative organisms include *Neisseria meningitidis*, *Pasteurella multocida*, *Legionella pneumophila*, *Brucella*, *Vibrio cholerae*, *Yersinia enterocolitica*, *Y. pestis*, *Bordetella pertussis*, *Haemophilus influenzae*, *H. ducreyi*, *Campylobacter fetus*, *Shigella*, and many other common pathogens.

Other susceptible organisms include *Rickettsia akari*, *R. typhi*, *R. prowazekii*, *R. tsutsugamushi*, *Coxiella burnetii*, *Chlamydia trachomatis*, *C. psittaci*, *Mycoplasma pneumoniae*, *M. hominis*, *Leptospira*, *Treponema pallidum*, *T. pertenue*, and *Borrelia recurrentis*.

Tetracyclines are absorbed systemically after oral administration, chiefly from the duodenum; with the exception of doxycycline and minocycline, absorption is decreased by food, milk, and divalent and trivalent cations. Oral absorption of tetracyclines is affected by chelation with certain minerals such as calcium (doxycycline is least involved); chelation causes tetracyclines to localize in bones and teeth. Because of hepatotoxicity and thrombophlebitis, only doxycycline and, to a lesser extent, minocycline, are used I.V.

Tetracyclines are distributed widely into body tissues and fluid, but CSF penetration is minimal; lipid-soluble minocycline and doxycycline are better able to penetrate fluids and tissues; all tetracyclines cross the placenta.

Tetracyclines are excreted primarily in urine, chiefly by glomerular filtration; some drug is excreted in breast milk, and some inactivated drug is excreted in feces. Unlike other tetracyclines, minocycline undergoes enterohepatic circulation and is excreted in feces.

Oxytetracycline is moderately hemodialyzable; other tetracyclines are removed only minimally by hemodialysis or peritoneal dialysis.

Clinical indications and actions
Bacterial, antiprotozoal, rickettsial, and fungal infections
Tetracyclines are used as first-line therapy for chlamydial infections and are the drugs of choice for lymphogranuloma venereum, nonlymphogranuloma venereum strains of *C. trachomatis* in sexually transmitted diseases (STDs), psittacosis, and nongonococcal urethritis if the primary pathogen is probably *M. hominis* or *C. trachomatis*. They are also the drugs of choice for rickettsial infections (Rocky Mountain spotted fever, scrub and endemic typhus, rickettsial pox, and Q fever) and brucellosis. Tetracyclines also are used to treat infections caused by *Campylobacter*, mycoplasma pneumonia (after Legionnaire's disease is ruled out), pertussis, and cholera (in United States only).

Tetracyclines are second-line drugs in therapy of syphilis, actinomycosis, listeriosis, chancroid, and infections caused by *Pasteurella multocida* and *Yersinia pestis*. They also provide economical prophylaxis in chronic pulmonary disease.

Tetracyclines are used orally to treat inflammatory acne vulgaris, topically for mild to moderate inflammatory acne, and as eye drops for superficial eye infections, inclusion conjunctivitis, and prophylaxis of ophthalmia neonatorum.

Individual tetracyclines are more effective against certain species or strains of a particular organism.
†Diuretic agent in SIADH
Demeclocycline causes diuresis by blocking ADH-induced reabsorption of water in the distal convoluted tubules and collecting ducts of the kidney.

Sclerosing agent

Parenteral tetracycline hydrochloride has been administered by intracavitary injection as a sclerosing agent in pleural or pericardial effusion.

Overview of adverse reactions

The most common adverse effects of tetracyclines involve the GI tract and are dose related; among them are anorexia; flatulence; nausea; vomiting; bulky, loose stools; epigastric burning; and abdominal discomfort.

Hypersensitivity reactions are infrequent; they manifest as urticaria, rash, pruritus, eosinophilia, and exfoliative dermatitis.

Photosensitivity reactions (exaggerated response to sunlight) may be severe; they are most common with demeclocycline, rare with minocycline.

Renal effects are minor and include occasional elevations in BUN levels (without rise in serum creatinine level) and a reversible diabetes insipidus syndrome (reported only with demeclocycline); renal failure has been attributed to Fanconi's syndrome after use of outdated tetracycline.

Rare adverse effects include hepatotoxicity (most commonly in pregnant women receiving more than 2 g/day I.V.), and leukocytosis, thrombocytopenia, hemolytic anemia, leukopenia, neutropenia, and atypical lymphocytes. There have also been reports of vaginal candidiasis, microscopic thyroid discoloration (after chronic use), light-headedness, dizziness, drowsiness, vein irritation (after I.V. use), and permanent discoloration of teeth, in children under age 8.

▶ Special considerations

● Assess patient's allergic history; do not give any tetracycline antibiotic to a patient with a history of hypersensitivity reactions to any other tetracycline; monitor patient continuously for this and other adverse reactions.
● Obtain results of cultures and sensitivity tests before first dose, but do not delay therapy; check cultures periodically to assess drug efficacy.
● Monitor vital signs, electrolytes, and renal function studies before and during therapy.
● Check expiration dates. Outdated tetracyclines may cause nephrotoxicity.
● Monitor for bacterial and fungal superinfection, especially in elderly, debilitated, and other patients who are receiving immunosuppressants or radiation therapy; watch especially for oral candidiasis. If symptoms occur, discontinue drug.
● Tetracyclines may interfere with certain laboratory tests; consult individual drug entry.

Administration

● Give oral tetracyclines 1 hour before or 2 hours after meals for maximum absorption; do not give with food, milk or other dairy products, sodium bicarbonate, iron compounds, or antacids, which may impair absorption.
● Give water with and after oral drug to facilitate passage to stomach, because incomplete swallowing can cause severe esophageal irritation; do not administer within 1 hour of bedtime, to prevent esophageal reflux.
● Always follow manufacturer's directions for reconstitution and storage; keep product refrigerated and away from light.
● Avoid I.V. use of drug in patients with decreased renal function.
● I.V. use of tetracyclines in pregnancy or in patients with renal impairment, especially when dosage exceeds 2 g/day, can cause hepatic failure.
● Monitor I.V. injection sites and rotate routinely to minimize local irritation. I.V. administration may cause severe phlebitis.

Information for the patient

● Explain disease process and rationale for therapy.
● Teach signs and symptoms of adverse reactions, and emphasize need to report these promptly; urge patient to report *any* unusual effects.
● Teach signs and symptoms of bacterial and fungal superinfection to elderly and debilitated patients and others with low resistance from immunosuppressants or irradiation.
● Advise patient to avoid direct exposure to sunlight and to use a sunscreen to help prevent photosensitivity reactions.
● Tell patient to take oral tetracyclines with a full glass of water (to facilitate passage to the stomach), 1 hour before or 2 hours after meals for maximum absorption, and not less than 1 hour before bedtime (to prevent irritation from esophageal reflux).
● Emphasize that taking the drug with food, milk or other dairy products, sodium bicarbonate, or iron compounds may interfere with absorption. Tell patient to take antacids 3 hours after tetracycline.
● Emphasize importance of completing prescribed regimen exactly as ordered and keeping follow-up appointments.
● Tell patient to check expiration dates and discard any expired drug.

Geriatric use

Some elderly patients have decreased esophageal motility; administer tetracyclines with caution and monitor for local irritation from slowly passing oral dosage forms. Elderly patients are also more susceptible to superinfection.

Pediatric use

Children age 8 and under should not receive tetracyclines unless there is no alternative. Tetracyclines can cause permanent discoloration of teeth, enamel hypoplasia, and a reversible decrease in bone calcification.

Reversible decreases in bone calcification have been reported in infants.

Breast-feeding

Tetracyclines are excreted in breast milk; when possible, they should be avoided by breast-feeding women.

Representative combinations

Oxytetracycline with sulfamethizole and phenazopyridine: Azotrex, Urobiotic; with nystatin: Comycin; with hydrocortisone: Terra-cortril; with polymyxin B sulfate: Terramycin Hydrochloride with Polymyxin B, Terramycin topical ointment.

Tetracycline hydrochloride with nystatin: Comycin, Tetrastatin; with amphotericin B: Mysteclin F; with citric acid: Achromycin V.

Note: Drug should be discontinued if symptoms of systemic absorption occur.

tetrahydrozoline hydrochloride
Collyrium Fresh, Murine Plus, Ocu-Drop, Soothe, Tyzine, Tyzine Pediatric, Visine

- Pharmacologic classification: sympathomimetic agent
- Therapeutic classification: vasoconstrictor, decongestant
- Pregnancy risk category C

How supplied
Available without prescription.
Ophthalmic solution: 0.05%

Available by prescription only
Nasal solution: 0.05%, 0.1%

Indications, route, and dosage
Nasal congestion
Adults and children over age 6: Apply 2 to 4 drops of 0.1% solution or spray to nasal mucosa q 4 to 6 hours, p.r.n.
Children ages 2 to 6: Apply 2 or 3 drops of 0.05% solution to nasal mucosa q 4 to 6 hours, p.r.n.
Conjunctival congestion
Adults: 1 or 2 drops in each eye b.i.d. to q.i.d.

Pharmacodynamics
Decongestant action: In ocular use, it produces vasoconstriction by local adrenergic action on the blood vessels of the conjunctiva. After nasal application, drug acts on alpha-adrenergic receptors in the nasal mucosa to produce constriction, thereby decreasing blood flow and nasal congestion.

Pharmacokinetics
Unknown.

Contraindications and precautions
Tetrahydrozoline is contraindicated in patients with narrow-angle glaucoma, because it may increase intraocular pressure; in those receiving MAO inhibitors, because it may precipitate a hypertensive crisis; and in those hypersensitive to any component of the preparation. It should be used cautiously in patients with hyperthyroidism, hypertension, heart disease, or diabetes mellitus.

Interactions
When used concomitantly with MAO inhibitors, tetrahydrozoline may cause an increased adrenergic response and hypertensive crisis.

Effects on diagnostic tests
None reported.

Adverse reactions
- CNS: drowsiness, *CNS depression*, dizziness, headache, insomnia tremor, *seizures*, anxiety, hallucinations, weakness, prolonged psychosis, insomnia.
- CV: hypertension, palpation, sweating, *arrhythmias*.
- EENT: transient burning, stinging, or dryness of mucosa; sneezing; rebound nasal congestion with excessive or long-term use.
- Eye: blurred vision, pupillary dilation, irritation, tearing, photophobia.

Overdose and treatment
Clinical manifestations of accidental overdose include bradycardia, decreased body temperature, shocklike hypotension, apnea, drowsiness, CNS depression, and coma.

Because of rapid onset of sedation, emesis is not recommended in therapy unless given early.

Activated charcoal or gastric lavage may be used initially. Monitor vital signs and ECG. Treat seizures with I.V. diazepam.

▶ Special considerations
- Excessive use of either preparation may cause rebound effect.
- Drug should not be used for more than 5 days.

Information for the patient
- Teach patient how to instill ophthalmic or nasal medication and tell him not to share drug with other family members.
- Advise patient not to exceed recommended dosage, and to use only when needed.
- Tell patient to remove contact lenses before using.

Geriatric use
Do not use in elderly patients to treat redness and inflammation, which may represent more serious eye conditions. Use in glaucoma requires close medical supervision.

Pediatric use
The 0.1% nasal solution is contraindicated in children younger than age 6. All use is contraindicated in children younger than age 2.

theophylline
Aerolate, Bronkodyl, Constant-T, Elixophyllin, Quibron-T*, Slo-bid, Slo-Phyllin, Somophyllin-T, Sustaire, Theobid, Theoclear, Theo-Dur, Theolair, Theophyl, Theospan-SR, Theo-24, Theovent, Uniphyl

theophylline sodium glycinate
Synophylate

- Pharmacologic classification: xanthine derivative
- Therapeutic classification: bronchodilator
- Pregnancy risk category C

How supplied
Available by prescription only
Capsules: 50 mg, 100 mg, 200 mg, 250 mg
Capsules (extended-release): 50 mg, 60 mg, 65 mg, 75 mg, 100 mg, 125 mg, 130 mg, 200 mg, 250 mg, 260 mg, 300 mg
Elixir: 27 mg/5 ml, 50 mg/5 ml
Oral solution: 27 mg/5 ml, 53 mg/5 ml
Oral suspension: 100 mg/5 ml
Syrup: 27 mg/5 ml, 50 mg/5 ml
Tablets: 100 mg, 125 mg, 200 mg, 225 mg, 250 mg, 300 mg

---

*Canada only   †Unlabeled clinical use   Italicized adverse reactions are life-threatening.

Tablets (chewable): 100 mg
Tablets (extended-release): 100 mg, 200 mg, 250 mg, 300 mg, 400 mg, 500 mg
Theophylline
Dextrose 5% injection: 200 mg in 50 ml or 100 ml; 400 mg in 100 ml, 250 ml, 500 ml, or 1,000 ml; 800 mg in 500 ml or 1,000 ml
Theophylline sodium glycinate
Elixir: 110 mg/5 ml (equivalent to 55 mg anhydrous theophylline per 5 ml)

Indications, route, and dosage
Symptomatic relief of bronchospasm in patients not currently receiving theophylline who require rapid relief of acute symptoms
Loading dose: 6 mg/kg anhydrous theophylline, then—
Adults (nonsmokers): 3 mg/kg q 6 hours for two doses; then 3 mg/kg q 8 hours.
Otherwise-healthy adult smokers: 3 mg/kg q 4 hours for three doses; then 3 mg/kg q 6 hours.
Older adults with cor pulmonale: 2 mg/kg q 6 hours for two doses; then 2 mg/kg q 8 hours.
Adults with CHF: 2 mg/kg q 8 hours for two doses; then 1 to 2 mg/kg q 12 hours.
Children age 9 to 16: 3 mg/kg q 4 hours for three doses; then 3 mg/kg q 6 hours.
Children age 6 months to 9 years: 4 mg/kg q 4 hours for three doses; then 4 mg/kg q 6 hours.
Neonates and children under age 6 months: Dosage is highly individualized.
Loading dose: 1 mg/kg for each 2 mcg/ml increase in theophylline concentration; then—
Infants age 8 weeks to 6 months: 1 to 3 mg/kg q 6 hours.
Infants age 4 to 8 weeks: 1 to 2 mg/kg q 8 hours.
Infants up to age 4 weeks: 1 to 2 mg/kg q 12 hours.
Premature infants (under 40 weeks' gestational age): 1 mg/kg q 12 hours.
Parenteral theophylline for patients not currently receiving theophylline
Loading dose: 4.7 mg/kg I.V. slowly; then maintenance infusion.
Adults (nonsmokers): 0.55 mg/kg/hour for 12 hours, then 0.39 mg/kg/hour.
Otherwise-healthy adult smokers: 0.79 mg/kg/hour for 12 hours; then 0.63 mg/kg/hour.
Older adults with cor pulmonale: 0.47 mg/kg/hour for 12 hours; then 0.24 mg/kg/hour.
Adults with CHF or liver disease: 0.39 mg/kg/hour for 12 hours; then 0.08 to 0.16 mg/kg/hour.
Children age 9 to 16: 0.79 mg/kg/hour for 12 hours; then 0.63 mg/kg/hour.
Children age 6 months to 9 years: 0.95 mg/kg/hour for 12 hours; then 0.79 mg/kg/hour.
Switch to oral theophylline as soon as patient shows adequate improvement.
Symptomatic relief of bronchospasm in patients currently receiving theophylline
Adults and children: Each 0.5 mg/kg I.V. or P.O. (loading dose) will increase plasma levels by 1 mcg/ml. Ideally, dose is based upon current theophylline level. In emergency situations, some clinicians recommend a 2.5 mg/kg P.O. dose of rapidly absorbed form if no obvious signs of theophylline toxicity are present.
Prophylaxis of bronchial asthma, bronchospasm of chronic bronchitis and emphysema
Adults and children: 16 mg/kg P.O. daily anhydrous theophylline divided q 6 or 8 hours; do not exceed 400 mg/day. Increase dose at 2- to 3-day intervals to maximum daily dose.
Adults: 13 mg/kg P.O. or 900 mg P.O. daily in divided doses.
Children age 12 to 16: 18 mg/kg P.O. daily in divided doses.
Children age 9 to 12: 20 mg/kg P.O. daily in divided doses.
Children under age 9: 24 mg/kg P.O. daily in divided doses.
Note: Dosage individualization is required. Use peak plasma and trough levels to estimate dose. Therapeutic range is 10 to 20 mcg/ml. All doses are based upon theophylline anhydrous and lean body weight.

Pharmacodynamics
Bronchodilator action: Drug may act by inhibiting phosphodiesterase, elevating cellular cyclic AMP levels, or antagonizing adenosine receptors in the bronchi, resulting in relaxation of the smooth muscle.
Drug also increases sensitivity of the medullary respiratory center to CO_2, to reduce apneic episodes. It also prevents muscle fatigue, especially that of the diaphragm.

Pharmacokinetics
● *Absorption:* Drug is well absorbed. Rate and onset of action depend upon the dosage form; food may further alter rate of absorption.
● *Distribution:* Drug is distributed throughout the extracellular fluids; equilibrium between fluid and tissues occurs within an hour of an I.V. loading dose. Therapeutic plasma levels are 10 to 20 mcg/ml, but many patients respond to lower levels.
● *Metabolism:* Theophylline is metabolized in the liver to inactive compounds. Half-life is 7 to 9 hours in adults, 4 to 5 hours in smokers, 20 to 30 hours in premature infants, and 3 to 5 hours in children.
● *Excretion:* Approximately 10% of the dose is excreted in urine unchanged. The other metabolites include 1,3 dimethyluric acid, 1 methyluric acid, and 3-methylxanthine.

Contraindications and precautions
Theophylline is contraindicated in patients with hypersensitivity to xanthines. Use cautiously in patients with compromised cardiac or circulatory function, diabetes, glaucoma, hypertension, hyperthyroidism, peptic ulcer, or gastroesophageal reflux.

Interactions
When used concomitantly, theophylline increases the excretion of lithium. Also, cimetidine, allopurinol (high dose), propranolol, erythromycin, and troleandomycin may cause an increase in serum concentrations of theophylline by decreasing the hepatic clearance. Barbiturates and phenytoin enhance hepatic metabolism of theophylline, decreasing plasma levels. Beta-adrenergic blockers exert an antagonistic pharmacologic effect.

Effects on diagnostic tests
Theophylline increases plasma-free fatty acids and urinary catecholamines. Depending on assay used, theophylline levels may be falsely elevated in the presence of furosemide, phenylbutazone, probenecid, theobromine, caffeine, tea, chocolate, cola beverages, and acetaminophen.

---

*Canada only   †Unlabeled clinical use   Italicized adverse reactions are life-threatening.

Adverse reactions
- CNS: irritability, restlessness, headache, insomnia, dizziness, *seizures*, depression.
- CV: palpitations, hypotension, sinus tachycardia, *ventricular tachycardia and other life-threatening arrhythmias*, extrasystoles, *circulatory failure*.
- GI: nausea, vomiting, epigastric pain, loss of appetite, diarrhea.
- Respiratory: tachypnea, *respiratory arrest*.
- Other: fever, flushing, urinary retention, hyperglycemia.

Note: Drug should be discontinued if any adverse reaction intensifies; this signals impending overdose.

Overdose and treatment
Clinical manifestations of overdose include nausea, vomiting, insomnia, irritability, tachycardia, extrasystoles, tachypnea, or tonic/clonic seizures. The onset of toxicity may be sudden and severe, with arrhythmias and seizures as the first signs. Induce emesis except in convulsing patients, then use activated charcoal and cathartics. Treat arrhythmias with lidocaine and seizures with I.V. diazepam; support respiratory and cardiovascular systems.

▶ Special considerations
- Do not crush extended-release tablets. Some capsules are formulated to be opened and sprinkled on food.
- Monitor vital signs and observe for signs and symptoms of toxicity.
- Serum theophylline measurements are recommended for patients receiving long-term therapy. Ideally, levels should be between 10 and 20 mcg/ml. Check every 6 months. If levels are less than 10 mcg/ml, increase dose by about 25% each day. If levels are 20 to 25 mcg/ml, decrease dose by about 10% each day. If levels are 25 to 30 mcg/ml, skip next dose and decrease by 25% each day. If levels are over 30 mcg/ml, skip next two doses and decrease by 50% each day. Repeat serum level determination.

Information for the patient
- Instruct patient regarding medications and dosage schedule; if a dose is missed, take as soon as possible, but do not double up on doses.
- Advise patient to take drug at regular intervals as instructed, around the clock.
- Advise patient of the adverse effects and possible signs of toxicity.
- Tell patient to avoid excessive use of xanthine-containing foods and beverages.
- Warn elderly patients of dizziness, a common reaction at start of therapy.
- If GI upset occurs with liquid preparations or non-sustained release forms, take with food.

Pediatric use
Use with caution in neonates. Children usually require higher doses (on a mg/kg basis) than adults. Maximum recommended doses are 24 mg/kg/day in children younger than age 9; 20 mg/kg/day in children age 9 to 12; 18 mg/kg/day in children age 12 to 16; 13 mg/kg/day or 900 mg (whichever is less) in children age 16 or older.

Breast-feeding
Drug is excreted in breast milk and may cause irritability, insomnia, or fretfulness in the breast-fed infant.

thiabendazole
Mintezol

- Pharmacologic classification: benzimidazole
- Therapeutic classification: anthelmintic
- Pregnancy risk category C

How supplied
Available by prescription only
Tablets (chewable): 500 mg
Oral suspension: 500 mg/5 ml

Indications, route, and dosage
Systemic infections with pinworm, roundworm, threadworm, whipworm, cutaneous larva migrans, and trichinosis
Adults and children: 25 mg/kg P.O. q 12 hours for 2 successive days. Maximum dosage is 3 g daily.
Cutaneous infestations with larva migrans (creeping eruption)
Adults and children: 25 mg/kg P.O. b.i.d. for 2 to 5 days. Maximum dosage is 3 g daily. If lesions persist after 2 days, repeat course.
Pinworm—two doses daily for 1 day; repeat in 7 days.
Roundworm, threadworm, and whipworm—two doses daily for 2 successive days.
Trichinosis—two doses daily for 2 to 4 successive days.

Pharmacodynamics
Anthelmintic action: Thiabendazole kills susceptible helminths by inhibiting fumarate reductase. It is the drug of choice for *Strongyloides stercoralis* (threadworm) infections and may be useful in disseminated strongyloidiasis. It is also preferred for oral and topical therapy of *Ancylostoma braziliense*, *Toxocara canis*, and *T. cati*. It has shown activity in certain other nematode infections, but other agents are preferred for the treatment of ascariasis, tricuriasis, uncinariasis, and enterobiasis.

Pharmacokinetics
- *Absorption:* Thiabendazole is absorbed readily; peak serum concentrations occur at 1 to 2 hours.
- *Distribution:* Little is known about the distribution of thiabendazole.
- *Metabolism:* Thiabendazole is metabolized almost completely by hydroxylation and conjugation.
- *Excretion:* Approximately 90% of a thiabendazole dose is excreted in urine as metabolites within 48 hours; about 5% is excreted in feces.

Contraindications and precautions
Thiabendazole is contraindicated in patients with known hypersensitivity to the drug. It should be used with caution in patients with compromised renal or hepatic function, in patients with malnutrition or anemia, and in patients in whom vomiting would be hazardous.

Interactions
Thiabendazole may inhibit the metabolism of aminophylline; concomitant use raises theophylline levels.

Effects on diagnostic tests
Transient elevations of AST (SGOT) levels have been reported.

---

*Canada only   †Unlabeled clinical use   Italicized adverse reactions are life-threatening.

Adverse reactions
- CNS: impaired mental alertness, impaired physical coordination, drowsiness, giddiness, headache, dizziness.
- DERM: rash, pruritus, *erythema multiforme*.
- GI: anorexia, nausea, vomiting, diarrhea, epigastric distress.
- GU: enuresis, malodorous urine.
- Other: lymphadenopathy, fever, flushing, chills.
  Note: Drug should be discontinued if hypersensitivity reactions occur.

Overdose and treatment
Signs of overdose may include visual disturbances and altered mental status. Treatment includes induced emesis or gastric lavage if ingested within 4 hours, followed by supportive and symptomatic treatment.

▶ Special considerations
- Give drug after meals; shake suspension well to ensure accurate dosages.
- Drug may be given with milk, fruit juice, or food.
- Laxatives, enemas, and dietary restrictions are unnecessary.
- Assess patient and review laboratory reports for signs of anemia, dehydration, or malnutrition before starting therapy.
- Monitor patient for adverse reactions, which usually occur 3 to 4 hours after drug is administered. Adverse effects are usually mild and related to dosage and duration of therapy.

Information for the patient
- Warn patient that drug causes drowsiness or dizziness. Tell patient to avoid driving or other hazardous activities during therapy.
- Teach patient the signs of hypersensitivity and to call immediately if they occur.
- Tell patient to wash perianal area daily and to change undergarments and bedclothes daily.
- To help prevent reinfection, instruct patient and family members in personal hygiene, including sanitary disposal of feces and hand washing and nail cleaning after defecation and before handling, preparing, or eating food.
- Explain routes of transmission, and encourage other household members and suspected contacts to be tested and, if necessary, treated.

Breast-feeding
Safety has not been established.

---

thiamine hydrochloride (vitamin B₁)
Biamine

- Pharmacologic classification: water-soluble vitamin
- Therapeutic classification: nutritional supplement
- Pregnancy risk category A (C if > recommended daily allowance [RDA])

How supplied
Available by prescription only
Injection: 1-ml ampules (100 mg/ml), 1-ml vials (100 mg/ml), 2-ml vials (100 mg/ml), 10-ml vials (100 mg/ml), 30-ml vials (100 mg/ml), 30-ml vials (200 mg/ml), 30-ml vials (100 mg/ml, with 0.5% chlorobutanol)

Available without a prescription
Tablets: 5 mg, 10 mg, 25 mg, 50 mg, 100 mg, 250 mg, 500 mg

Indications, route, and dosage
Beriberi
Adults: 10 to 500 mg, depending on severity, I.M. t.i.d. for 2 weeks, followed by dietary correction and multivitamin supplement containing 5 to 10 mg thiamine daily for 1 month.
Children: 10 to 50 mg, depending on severity, I.M. daily for several weeks with adequate dietary intake.
Anemia secondary to thiamine deficiency; polyneuritis secondary to alcoholism, pregnancy, or pellagra
Adults: 100 mg P.O. daily.
Children: 10 to 50 mg P.O. daily in divided doses.
Wernicke's encephalopathy
Adults: Initially, 100 mg I.V., followed by 50 to 100 mg I.M. or I.V. daily.
"Wet beriberi" with myocardial failure
Adults and children: 100 to 500 mg I.V. for emergency treatment.

Pharmacodynamics
Metabolic action: Exogenous thiamine is required for carbohydrate metabolism. Thiamine combines with adenosine triphosphate to form thiamine pyrophosphate, a coenzyme in carbohydrate metabolism and transketolation reactions. This coenzyme is also necessary in the hexose monophosphate shunt during pentose utilization. One sign of thiamine deficiency is an increase in pyruvic acid. The body's need for thiamine is greater when the carbohydrate content of the diet is high. Within 3 weeks of total absence of dietary thiamine, significant vitamin depletion can occur. Thiamine deficiency can cause beriberi.

Pharmacokinetics
- *Absorption:* Thiamine is absorbed readily after oral administration of small doses; after oral administration of a large dose, the total amount absorbed is limited to 4 to 8 mg. In alcoholics and in patients with cirrhosis or malabsorption, GI absorption of thiamine is decreased. When thiamine is given with meals, its GI rate of absorption decreases, but total absorption remains the same. After I.M. administration, thiamine is absorbed rapidly and completely.
- *Distribution:* Thiamine is distributed widely into body tissues. When intake exceeds the minimal requirements, tissue stores become saturated. About 100 to 200 mcg/day of thiamine is distributed into the milk of breast-feeding women on a normal diet.
- *Metabolism:* Thiamine is metabolized in the liver.
- *Excretion:* Excess thiamine is excreted in the urine. After administration of large doses (more than 10 mg), both unchanged thiamine and metabolites are excreted in urine after tissue stores become saturated.

Contraindications and precautions
Thiamine is contraindicated in patients with suspected vitamin B₁ sensitivity; an intradermal test dose is recommended before parenteral administration. Thiamine is contraindicated in patients hypersensitive to the drug or to any ingredient in thiamine preparations. Thiamine-

deficient patients may experience a sudden onset or worsening of Wernicke's encephalopathy (nystagmus, bilateral sixth nerve palsy, ataxia, and confusion) after I.V. glucose administration; in suspected thiamine deficiency, administer thiamine before a glucose load is given.

Interactions
Concomitant use of thiamine with neuromuscular blocking agents may enhance the latter's effects.

Thiamine may not be used in combination with alkaline solutions (such as carbonates, citrates, or bicarbonates); thiamine is unstable in neutral or alkaline solutions.

Effects on diagnostic tests
Thiamine therapy may produce false-positive results in the phosphotungstate method for determination of uric acid and in the urine spot tests with Ehrlich's reagent for urobilinogen.

Large doses of thiamine interfere with the Schack and Waxler spectrophotometric determination of serum theophylline concentrations.

Adverse reactions
• CNS: restlessness.
• CV: hypotension after rapid I.V. injection, angioneurotic edema, cyanosis.
• DERM: feeling of warmth, pruritus, urticaria, sweating.
• EENT: *tightness of throat* (allergic reaction).
• GI: nausea, hemorrhage, diarrhea.
• Local: pain at I.M. injection site.
• Other: anaphylactic reactions, weakness, *pulmonary edema*, *death*.

Overdose and treatment
Very large doses of thiamine administered parenterally may produce neuromuscular and ganglionic blockade and neurologic symptoms. Treatment is supportive.

▶ Special considerations
• The RDA of thiamine is as follows:
Neonates and infants up to age 6 months: 0.3 mg daily.
Infants age 6 months to 1 year: 0.4 mg daily.
Children age 1 to 3: 0.7 mg daily.
Children age 4 to 6: 0.9 mg daily.
Children age 7 to 10: 1 mg daily.
Males age 11 to 14: 1.3 mg daily.
Males age 15 to 50: 1.5 mg daily.
Males age 51 and over: 1.2 mg daily.
Females age 11 to 50: 1.1 mg daily.
Females age 51 and over: 1 mg daily.
Pregnant women: 1.5 mg daily.
Lactating women: 1 to 6 mg daily.
• Give intradermal skin test before I.V. thiamine administration if sensitivity is suspected, because anaphylaxis can occur. Keep epinephrine available when administering large parenteral doses.
• I.M. injection may be painful. Rotate injection sites and apply cold compresses to ease discomfort.
• Accurate dietary history is important during vitamin replacement therapy. Help patient develop a practical plan for adequate nutrition.
• Total absence of dietary thiamine can produce a deficiency state in about 3 weeks.
• Subclinical deficiency of thiamine or other B vitamins is common in patients who are poor, are chronic alcoholics, follow fad diets, or are pregnant.

• Store in light-resistant, nonmetallic container.

Information for the patient
Inform patient about dietary sources of thiamine such as yeast, pork, beef, liver, whole grains, peas, and beans.

Breast-feeding
Thiamine (in amounts that do not exceed the RDA) is safe to use in breast-feeding women. It is secreted into breast milk and fulfills a nutritional requirement of the infant.

---

thiamylal sodium
Surital

• Pharmacologic classification: barbiturate
• Therapeutic classification: I.V. anesthetic
• Controlled substance schedule III
• Pregnancy risk category C

How supplied
Available by prescription only
Injection: 1-g steri-vials, 5-g amps and vials, 10-g vials

Indications, route, and dosage
General anesthetic for short-term procedures
Adults and children: Dosage is highly individualized according to response. Initial injection of 3 to 6 ml of a 2.5% solution is usually sufficient for short periods of anesthesia; the rate of injection during induction should be 1 ml/5 seconds. A 0.3% solution may be used for continuous drip maintenance.

Pharmacodynamics
Anesthetic action: Thiamylal produces anesthesia by direct depression of the polysynaptic midbrain reticular activating system. Thiamylal decreases presynaptic (via decreased neurotransmitter release) and postsynaptic excitation. These effects may be subsequent to increased γ-aminobutyric acid (GABA) levels, enhancement of GABA's effects, or a direct effect on GABA receptor sites.

Pharmacokinetics
• *Absorption:* Thiamylal is given only I.V.; peak brain concentrations are reached in 10 to 20 seconds. Depth of anesthesia may increase for up to 40 seconds. Consciousness returns in 20 to 30 minutes.
• *Distribution:* Thiamylal distributes throughout the body; highest initial concentration occurs in vascular areas of the brain, primarily gray matter; drug is 80% protein-bound. Redistribution of the drug is primarily responsible for its short duration of action.
• *Metabolism:* Thiamylal is metabolized extensively in the liver.
• *Excretion:* Unchanged thiamylal is not excreted in significant amounts; duration of action depends on tissue redistribution.

Contraindications and precautions
Thiamylal is contraindicated in patients with acute intermittent or variegate porphyria but not in other porphyrias; in patients with known hypersensitivity to the

---

drug; and whenever general anesthesia is contraindicated.

Drug should be used cautiously in patients with respiratory, cardiac, circulatory, renal, or hepatic dysfunction; severe anemia; shock; myxedema; and status asthmaticus (use *extreme* caution), because drug may worsen these conditions.

Interactions
Thiamylal may potentiate or add to the CNS depressant effects of sedatives, hypnotics, antihistamines, narcotics, phenothiazines, benzodiazepines, and alcohol.

Effects on diagnostic tests
Thiamylal causes dose-dependent alteration in EEG patterns.

Adverse reactions
● CNS: anxiety, restlessness, retrograde amnesia, and prolonged somnolence.
● CV: hypotension, tachycardia, peripheral vascular collapse, *myocardial depression, arrhythmias.*
● GI: nausea and vomiting.
● Respiratory: *respiratory depression, apnea,* laryngospasm, *bronchospasm.*
● Local: pain, swelling, ulceration and necrosis on extravasation (unlikely at concentrations under 2.5%).
● Other: gangrene after intraarterial injection, allergic reactions, coughing, sneezing, shivering, local irritation.
Note: Drug should be discontinued if peripheral vascular collapse, respiratory arrest, or hypersensitivity occurs.

Overdose and treatment
Clinical signs of overdose include respiratory depression, respiratory arrest, hypotension, and shock. Treat supportively, using mechanical ventilation if needed; give I.V. fluids or vasopressors (dopamine, phenylephrine) for hypotension. Monitor vital signs closely.

▶ Special considerations
A small test dose (2 ml of 2.5% solution) may be used to assess tolerance or unusual sensitivity.

Geriatric use
Lower doses may be indicated.

Pediatric use
Use cautiously.

---

thioguanine (6-thioguanine, 6-TG)
Lanvis*, Thioguanine Tabloid

● Pharmacologic classification: antimetabolite (cell cycle-phase specific, S phase)
● Therapeutic classification: antineoplastic
● Pregnancy risk category D

How supplied
Available by prescription only
Tablets (scored): 40 mg

Indications, route, and dosage
Dosage and indications may vary. Check current literature for recommended protocol.
Acute lymphoblastic and myelogenous leukemia, chronic granulocytic leukemia
Adults and children: Initially, 2 mg/kg daily P.O. (usually calculated to nearest 20 mg) or 75 to 100 mg/m²/day P.O.; then, if no toxic effects occur, increase gradually over 3 to 4 weeks to 3 mg/kg/day. Maintenance dosage is 2 to 3 mg/kg/day P.O. or 100 mg/m²/day P.O.

Pharmacodynamics
Antineoplastic action: Thioguanine requires conversion intracellularly to its active form to exert its cytotoxic activity. Acting as a false metabolite, thioguanine inhibits purine synthesis. Cross-resistance exists between mercaptopurine and thioguanine.

Pharmacokinetics
● *Absorption:* After an oral dose, the absorption of thioguanine is incomplete and variable. The average bioavailability is 30%.
● *Distribution:* Thioguanine distributes well into bone marrow cells. The drug does not cross the blood-brain barrier to any appreciable extent.
● *Metabolism:* Thioguanine is extensively metabolized to a less active form in the liver and other tissues.
● *Excretion:* Plasma concentrations of thioguanine decrease in a biphasic manner, with a half-life of 15 minutes in the initial phase and 11 hours in the terminal phase. Thioguanine is excreted in the urine, mainly as metabolites.

Contraindications and precautions
Thioguanine is contraindicated in patients with a history of resistance to previous therapy with the drug. Use with caution in renal or hepatic dysfunction because of the potential for drug accumulation.

Interactions
None reported.

Effects on diagnostic tests
Thioguanine therapy may increase blood and urine levels of uric acid.

Adverse reactions
● GI: nausea, vomiting, stomatitis, diarrhea, anorexia.
● HEMA: *bone marrow depression* (dose-limiting), *leukopenia,* anemia, *thrombocytopenia* (occurs slowly over 2 to 4 weeks).
● Hepatic: hepatotoxicity, jaundice.
● Metabolic: hyperuricemia.
Note: Drug should be discontinued if jaundice occurs.

Overdose and treatment
Clinical manifestations of overdose include myelosuppression, nausea, vomiting, malaise, hypertension, and diaphoresis.
Treatment is usually supportive and includes transfusion of blood components and antiemetics. Induction of emesis may be helpful if performed soon after ingestion.

▶ Special considerations
● Total daily dosage can be given at one time.
● Give dose between meals to facilitate complete absorption.

● Dose modification may be required in renal or hepatic dysfunction.

● Monitor serum uric acid levels. Use oral hydration to prevent uric acid nephropathy. Alkalinize urine if serum uric acid levels are elevated.

● Stop drug if hepatotoxicity or hepatic tenderness occurs. Watch for jaundice; may reverse if drug stopped promptly.

● Do CBC daily during induction, then weekly during maintenance therapy.

● Drug is sometimes ordered as 6-thioguanine.

● Avoid all I.M. injections when platelet count is below 100,000/mm³.

Information for the patient

● Emphasize importance of continuing medication despite nausea and vomiting.

● Tell patient to call promptly if vomiting occurs shortly after a dose is taken.

● Encourage adequate fluid intake to increase urine output and facilitate excretion of uric acid.

● Advise avoiding exposure to people with infections.

Breast-feeding

It is not known whether thioguanine distributes into breast milk. However, because of the risk of serious adverse reactions, mutagenicity, and carcinogenicity in the infant, breast-feeding is not recommended.

---

thiopental sodium
Pentothal

● Pharmacologic classification: barbiturate
● Therapeutic classification: I.V. anesthetic
● Controlled substance schedule III
● Pregnancy risk category C

How supplied

Available by prescription only

Injection: 250-mg, 400-mg, and 500-mg syringes; 500-mg and 1-g vials with diluent; 1-g (2.5%), 2.5-g (2.5%), 5-g (2.5%), 2.5-g (2%), and 5-g (2%) kits

Rectal suspension: 2-g disposable syringe (400 mg/g of suspension)

Indications, route, and dosage

General anesthetic for short-term procedures

Adults and children: 2 to 3 ml 2.5% solution (50 to 75 mg) administered I.V. at intervals of 20 to 40 seconds, depending on reaction. Dose may be repeated with caution, if necessary. When thiopental sodium is the sole anesthetic agent, anesthesia can be maintained by small repeated doses as ordered or as a continuous I.V. infusion in a 0.2% to 0.4% concentration. Some clinicians advocate a bolus of 3 to 4 mg/kg for adults (2 to 3 mg/kg for children and elderly patients) as an induction dose.

Convulsive states following anesthesia

75 to 125 mg (3 to 5 ml of 2.5% solution) I.V.

Basal anesthesia by rectal administration

Adults and children: Administer up to 1 g/22.5 kg (50 lb) of body weight. Maximum dosage is 1 to 1.5 g (for children weighing 34 kg [75 lb] or more) and 3 to 4 g (for adults weighing 91 kg [200 lb] or more).

Preanesthetic sedation by rectal administration

Adults and children: The average dose is 1 g/34 kg (75 lb) or about 29.4 mg/kg.

Pharmacodynamics

Anesthetic action: Thiopental produces anesthesia by direct depression of the polysynaptic midbrain reticular activating system. Thiopental decreases presynaptic (via decreased neurotransmitter release) and postsynaptic excitation. These effects may be subsequent to increased γ-aminobutyric acid (GABA) levels, enhancement of GABA's effects, or a direct effect on GABA receptor sites.

Pharmacokinetics

● *Absorption:* Thiopental is given only I.V.; peak brain concentrations are reached in 10 to 20 seconds. Depth of anesthesia may increase for up to 40 seconds. Consciousness returns in 20 to 30 minutes.

● *Distribution:* Thiopental distributes throughout the body; highest initial concentration occurs in vascular areas of the brain, primarily gray matter; drug is 80% protein-bound. Redistribution of the drug is primarily responsible for its short duration of action.

● *Metabolism:* Thiopental is metabolized extensively but slowly in the liver.

● *Excretion:* Unchanged thiopental is not excreted in significant amounts; duration of action depends on tissue redistribution.

Contraindications and precautions

Thiopental is contraindicated in patients with acute intermittent or variegate porphyria but not in other porphyrias; in patients with known hypersensitivity to the drug; and whenever general anesthesia is contraindicated.

Drug should be used cautiously in patients with respiratory, cardiac, circulatory, renal, or hepatic dysfunction; severe anemia; shock; myxedema; and status asthmaticus (use *extreme* caution), because drug may worsen these conditions.

Interactions

Thiopental may potentiate or add to the CNS depressant effects of sedatives, hypnotics, antihistamines, narcotics, phenothiazines, benzodiazepines, and alcohol.

Effects on diagnostic tests

Thiopental causes dose-dependent alteration in EEG patterns.

Adverse reactions

● CNS: anxiety, restlessness, retrograde amnesia, and prolonged somnolence.

● CV: hypotension, tachycardia, peripheral vascular collapse, *myocardial depression, arrhythmias.*

● GI: nausea and vomiting.

● Respiratory: *respiratory depression, apnea,* laryngospasm, *bronchospasm.*

● Local: pain, swelling, ulceration and necrosis on extravasation (unlikely at concentrations under 2.5%).

● Other: gangrene after intraarterial injection, allergic reactions, hiccups, coughing, sneezing, shivering, local irritation.

Note: Drug should be discontinued if peripheral vascular collapse, respiratory arrest, or hypersensitivity occurs.

---

*Canada only   †Unlabeled clinical use   Italicized adverse reactions are life-threatening.

Overdose and treatment
Clinical signs of overdose include respiratory depression, respiratory arrest, hypotension, and shock. Treat supportively, using mechanical ventilation if needed; give I.V. fluids or vasopressors (dopamine, phenylephrine) for hypotension. Monitor vital signs closely.

▶ Special considerations
● Solutions of succinylcholine, tubocurarine, or atropine should not be mixed with thiopental but can be given to the patient concomitantly.
● A small test dose (25 to 75 mg) may be administered to assess tolerance or unusual sensitivity.

Geriatric use
Lower doses may be indicated.

Pediatric use
Use cautiously.

thioridazine
Mellaril-S

thioridazine hydrochloride
Apo-Thioridazine*, Mellaril, Millazine, Novoridazine*, PMS Thioridazine*

● Pharmacologic classification: phenothiazine (piperidine derivative)
● Therapeutic classification: antipsychotic
● Pregnancy risk category C

How supplied
Available by prescription only
Tablets: 10 mg, 15 mg, 25 mg, 50 mg, 100 mg, 150 mg, 200 mg
Syrup: 10 mg/5 ml
Oral concentrate: 30 mg/ml, 100 mg/ml (3% to 4.2% alcohol)
Suspension: 25 mg/5 ml, 100 mg/5 ml

Indications, route, and dosage
Psychosis
Adults: Initially, 50 to 100 mg P.O. t.i.d., with gradual increments up to 800 mg daily in divided doses, if needed. Dosage varies.
Adults over age 65: Initial dose is 25 mg t.i.d.
Dysthymic disorder (neurotic depression), alcohol withdrawal, dementia in geriatric patients, behavioral problems in children
Adults: Initially, 25 mg P.O. t.i.d. Maintenance dosage is 20 to 200 mg daily.
Children over age 2: Usually, 1 mg/kg/day P.O. in divided doses.

Pharmacodynamics
Antipsychotic action: Thioridazine is thought to exert its antipsychotic effects by postsynaptic blockade of CNS dopamine receptors, thereby inhibiting dopamine-mediated effects.

Thioridazine has many other central and peripheral effects: it produces both alpha and ganglionic blockade and counteracts histamine- and serotonin-mediated activity. Its most prevalent adverse reactions are antimuscarinic and sedative; it causes fewer extrapyramidal effects than other antipsychotics.

Pharmacokinetics
● *Absorption:* Rate and extent of absorption vary with administration route: oral tablet absorption is erratic and variable, with onset ranging from ½ to 1 hour. Oral concentrates and syrups are much more predictable.
● *Distribution:* Thioridazine is distributed widely into the body, including breast milk. Peak effects occur at 2 to 4 hours; steady-state serum level is achieved within 4 to 7 days. Drug is 91% to 99% protein-bound.
● *Metabolism:* Thioridazine is metabolized extensively by the liver and forms the active metabolite mesoridazine; duration of action is 4 to 6 hours.
● *Excretion:* Most of drug is excreted as metabolites in urine; some is excreted in feces via the biliary tract.

Contraindications and precautions
Thioridazine is contraindicated in patients with known hypersensitivity to phenothiazines and related compounds, including allergic reactions involving hepatic function; in patients with blood dyscrasias or bone marrow depression (adverse hematologic effects); in patients with disorders accompanied by coma, brain damage, CNS depression, circulatory collapse, or cerebrovascular disease (additive CNS depression and adverse effects on blood pressure); and in patients receiving adrenergic-blocking agents or spinal or epidural anesthetics (excessive respiratory, cardiac, and CNS depression).

Thioridazine should be used cautiously in patients with cardiac disease (arrhythmias, CHF, angina pectoris, valvular disease, or heart block), encephalitis, Reye's syndrome, head injury, respiratory disease, epilepsy and other seizure disorders, glaucoma, prostatic hypertrophy, urinary retention, Parkinson's disease, and pheochromocytoma, because drug may exacerbate these conditions; and in hypocalcemia, because it increases the risk of extrapyramidal reactions.

Interactions
Concomitant use of thioridazine with sympathomimetics, including epinephrine, phenylephrine, phenylpropanolamine, and ephedrine (often found in nasal sprays), and with appetite suppressants may decrease their stimulatory and pressor effects. Thioridazine may cause epinephrine reversal.

Thioridazine may inhibit blood pressure response to centrally acting antihypertensive drugs, such as guanethidine, guanabenz, guanadrel, clonidine, methyldopa, and reserpine. Additive effects are likely after concomitant use of thioridazine with CNS depressants, including alcohol, analgesics, barbiturates, narcotics, tranquilizers, anesthetics (general, spinal, or epidural), and parenteral magnesium sulfate (oversedation, respiratory depression, and hypotension); antiarrhythmic agents, including quinidine, disopyramide, and procainamide (increased incidence of cardiac arrhythmias and conduction defects); atropine and other anticholinergic drugs, including antidepressants, MAO inhibitors, phenothiazines, antihistamines, meperidine, and antiparkinsonian agents (oversedation, paralytic ileus, visual changes, and severe constipation); nitrates (hypotension); and metrizamide (increased risk of seizures).

Beta-blocking agents may inhibit thioridazine metabolism, increasing plasma levels and toxicity.

Concomitant use with propylthiouracil increases risk of agranulocytosis; concomitant use with lithium may result in severe neurologic toxicity with an encephalitis-

---

like syndrome and in decreased therapeutic response to thioridazine.

Pharmacokinetic alterations and subsequent decreased therapeutic response to thioridazine may follow concomitant use with phenobarbital (enhanced renal excretion); aluminum- and magnesium-containing antacids and antidiarrheals (decreased absorption); caffeine; or heavy smoking (increased metabolism).

Thioridazine may antagonize therapeutic effect of bromocriptine on prolactin secretion; it also may decrease the vasoconstricting effects of high-dose dopamine and may decrease effectiveness and increase toxicity of levodopa (by dopamine blockade). Thioridazine may inhibit metabolism and increase toxicity of phenytoin.

Effects on diagnostic tests

Thioridazine causes false-positive test results for urinary porphyrins, urobilinogen, amylase, and 5-HIAA, because of darkening of urine by metabolites; it also causes false-positive urine pregnancy results in tests using human chorionic gonadotropin as the indicator.

Thioridazine elevates test results for liver enzymes and protein-bound iodine and causes quinidine-like effects on the ECG.

Adverse reactions

● CNS: extrapyramidal symptoms – dystonia, akathisia, torticollis, tardive dyskinesia (usually dose-related with long-term therapy, but it can develop rapidly), sedation (high incidence), pseudoparkinsonism, drowsiness (frequent), *neuroleptic malignant syndrome* (dose-related; if untreated, fatal *respiratory failure* in over 20% of patients), dizziness, headache, insomnia, exacerbation of psychotic symptoms.
● CV: *asystole*, orthostatic hypotension (high incidence), tachycardia, dizziness or fainting, *arrhythmias*, ECG changes, increased anginal pain after I.M. injection.
● EENT: blurred vision, tinnitus, mydriasis, increased intraocular pressure, ocular changes (retinal pigmentary change with long-term use).
● GI: dry mouth, constipation, nausea, vomiting, anorexia, diarrhea.
● GU: urinary retention, gynecomastia, hypermenorrhea, inhibited ejaculation.
● HEMA: transient leukopenia, *agranulocytosis*, thrombocytopenia, anemia (within 30 to 90 days).
● Local: contact dermatitis from concentrate or injectable form, muscle necrosis from I.M. injection.
● Other: hyperprolactinemia, photosensitivity (high incidence), increased appetite or weight gain, hypersensitivity (rash, urticaria, drug fever, edema, cholestatic jaundice [in 0.1% to 4% of patients within first 30 days]) decreased libido.

After abrupt withdrawal of long-term therapy, gastritis, nausea, vomiting, dizziness, tremors, feeling of heat or cold, sweating, tachycardia, headache, or insomnia may occur.

Note: Drug should be discontinued if any of the following occur: hypersensitivity, jaundice, agranulocytosis, neuroleptic malignant syndrome (marked hyperthermia, extrapyramidal effects, autonomic dysfunction), or severe extrapyramidal symptoms even after dose is lowered. Drug should be discontinued 48 hours before and 24 hours after myelography using metrizamide, because of the risk of seizures. When feasible, drug should be withdrawn slowly and gradually; many drug effects persist after withdrawal.

Overdose and treatment

CNS depression is characterized by deep, unarousable sleep and possible coma, hypotension or hypertension, extrapyramidal symptoms, abnormal involuntary muscle movements, agitation, seizures, arrhythmias, ECG changes, hypothermia or hyperthermia, and autonomic nervous system dysfunction.

Treatment is symptomatic and supportive and includes maintaining vital signs, airway, stable body temperature, and fluid and electrolyte balance.

Do not induce vomiting: drug inhibits cough reflex, and aspiration may occur. Use gastric lavage, then activated charcoal and saline cathartics; dialysis does not help. Regulate body temperature as needed. Treat hypotension with I.V. fluids: *do not give epinephrine.* Treat seizures with parenteral diazepam or barbiturates; arrhythmias with parenteral phenytoin (1 mg/kg with rate titrated to blood pressure); and extrapyramidal reactions with benztropine or parenteral diphenhydramine 2 mg/kg/minute. Contact local or regional poison information center for specific instructions.

▶ Special considerations

Besides those relevant to all *phenothiazines,* consider the following recommendations.
● Doses greater than 300 mg/day are usually reserved for adults with severe psychosis. Do *not* exceed 800 mg daily because of ophthalmic toxicity.
● Liquid and injectable formulations may cause a rash if skin contact occurs.
● Drug causes pink to brown discoloration of patient's urine.
● Thioridazine is associated with a high incidence of sedation, anticholinergic effects, orthostatic hypotension, photosensitivity reactions, and delayed or absent ejaculation. It has the lowest potential for extrapyramidal reactions of all phenothiazines.
● Oral formulations may cause stomach upset. Administer with food or fluid.
● Check patient regularly for abnormal body movements (at least once every 6 months).
● Concentrate must be diluted in 2 to 4 oz of liquid, preferably water, carbonated drinks, fruit juice, tomato juice, milk, or pudding.
● All liquid formulations must be protected from light.

Information for the patient

● Explain the risks of dystonic reactions and tardive dyskinesia, and tell patient to report any abnormal body movements.
● Tell patient to avoid sun exposure and to wear sunscreen when going outdoors, to prevent photosensitivity reactions. (Note that heat lamps and tanning beds also may cause burning of the skin or skin discoloration.)
● Warn patient not to spill the liquid on the skin; rash and irritation may result.
● Warn patient to avoid extremely hot or cold baths or exposure to temperature extremes, sunlamps, or tanning beds; drug may cause thermoregulatory changes.
● Advise patient to take the drug exactly as prescribed and not to double doses for missed doses.
● Explain that many drug interactions are possible. Patient should seek medical approval before taking *any* self-prescribed medication.
● Tell patient not to stop taking the drug suddenly; most adverse reactions may be relieved by dosage reduction. However, patient should call promptly if difficulty uri-

nating, sore throat, dizziness or fainting, or any visual changes develop.
● Warn patient to avoid hazardous activities that require alertness until the drug's effect is established. Reassure patient that excessive sedation usually subsides after several weeks.
● Tell patient not to drink alcohol or take other medications that may cause excessive sedation.
● Explain which fluids are appropriate for diluting the concentrate and the dropper technique of measuring dose.
● Suggest sugarless gum or candy, ice chips, or artificial saliva to relieve dry mouth.
● Tell patient to store drug safely away from children.

Geriatric use
Elderly patients tend to require lower dosages, titrated to individual response. Such patients also are more likely to develop adverse reactions, especially tardive dyskinesia and other extrapyramidal effects.

Pediatric use
Thioridazine is not recommended for patients under age 2. For patients over age 2, dosage is 1 mg/kg/day in divided doses.

Breast-feeding
Thioridazine may enter breast milk. Potential benefits to the mother should outweigh the potential harm to the infant.

thiotepa

● Pharmacologic classification: alkylating agent (cell cycle-phase nonspecific)
● Therapeutic classification: antineoplastic
● Pregnancy risk category D

How supplied
Available by prescription only
Injection: 15-mg vials

Indications, route, and dosage
Dosage and indications may vary. Check current literature for recommended protocol.
Breast, lung, and ovarian cancer; Hodgkin's disease; lymphomas
Adults and children age 12 and over: 0.2 mg/kg I.V. daily for 5 days, repeated q 2 to 4 weeks; or 0.3 to 0.4 mg/kg I.V. q 1 to 4 weeks.
Bladder tumor
Adults and children age 12 and over: 30 to 60 ml of a 1 mg/ml solution (thiotepa in distilled water) instilled in bladder once weekly for 4 weeks.
Neoplastic effusions
Adults and children age 12 and over: 0.6 to 0.8 mg/kg intracavity or intratumor q 1 to 4 weeks.

Pharmacodynamics
Antineoplastic action: Thiotepa exerts its cytotoxic activity as an alkylating agent, cross-linking strands of DNA and RNA and inhibiting protein synthesis, resulting in cell death.

Pharmacokinetics
● Absorption: The absorption of thiotepa across the GI tract is incomplete. Absorption from the bladder is variable, ranging from 10% to 100% of an instilled dose. Absorption is increased by certain pathologic conditions. Intramuscular and pleural membrane absorption of thiotepa is also variable.
● Distribution: Thiotepa crosses the blood-brain barrier.
● Metabolism: Thiotepa is metabolized extensively in the liver.
● Excretion: Thiotepa and its metabolites are excreted in urine.

Contraindications and precautions
Thiotepa is contraindicated in patients with a history of hypersensitivity to the drug and in patients with pre-existing hepatic, renal, or bone marrow impairment, because of the potential for additive toxicity.

Interactions
When used concomitantly, thiotepa may cause prolonged respirations and apnea in patients receiving succinylcholine. Thiotepa appears to inhibit the activity of pseudocholinesterase, the enzyme that deactivates succinylcholine. Use succinylcholine with extreme caution in patients receiving thiotepa.

Effects on diagnostic tests
Thiotepa therapy may increase blood and urine levels of uric acid and decrease plasma pseudocholinesterase concentrations.

Adverse reactions
● CNS: dizziness.
● DERM: hives, rash.
● GI: nausea, vomiting, anorexia.
● GU: amenorrhea, decreased spermatogenesis.
● HEMA: bone marrow depression (dose-limiting), leukopenia (begins within 5 to 30 days), thrombocytopenia, neutropenia, anemia.
● Metabolic: hyperuricemia.
● Local: intense pain at administration site.
● Other: headache, fever, tightness of throat.
  Note: Drug should be discontinued if leukocyte or platelet count drops rapidly.

Overdose and treatment
Clinical manifestations of overdose include nausea, vomiting, and precipitation of uric acid in the renal tubules.
  Treatment is usually supportive and includes transfusion of blood components, antiemetics, hydration, and allopurinol.

▶ Special considerations
Besides those relevant to all alkylating agents, consider the following recommendations.
● To reconstitute drug, use 1.5 ml of sterile water for injection to yield a concentration of 10 mg/ml. The solution is clear to slightly opaque.
● A 1 mg/ml solution is considered isotonic.
● Use only sterile water for injection to reconstitute. Refrigerated solution is stable 5 days.
● Refrigerate dry powder; protect from light.
● Drug can be given by all parenteral routes, including direct injection into the tumor.
● Stop drug or decrease dosage if WBC count falls

---

below 4,000/mm³ or if platelet count falls below 150,000/mm³.

● Drug may be mixed with procaine 2% or epinephrine 1:1,000, or both, for local use.

● Drug may be further diluted to larger volumes with normal saline solution, dextrose 5% in water, or lactated Ringer's solution for administration by I.V. infusion, intracavitary injection, or perfusion therapy.

● Withhold fluids for 8 to 10 hours before bladder instillation. Instill 60 ml of drug into bladder by catheter; ask patient to retain solution for 2 hours. Volume may be reduced to 30 ml if discomfort is too great. Reposition patient every 15 minutes for maximum area contact.

● To prevent hyperuricemia with resulting uric acid nephropathy, allopurinol may be given; keep patient well hydrated. Monitor uric acid.

● Monitor CBC weekly for at least 3 weeks after last dose. Warn patient to report even mild infections.

● Use cautiously in bone marrow depression and renal or hepatic dysfunction.

● Avoid all I.M. injections when platelet count is below 100,000/mm³.

● Anticoagulants and aspirin products should be used cautiously. Watch closely for signs of bleeding. Instruct patient to avoid nonprescription products containing aspirin.

● Toxicity may be delayed and prolonged because drug binds to tissues and stays in body several hours.

● GU adverse reactions are reversible in 6 to 8 months.

Information for the patient
● Encourage patient to maintain an adequate fluid intake to facilitate the excretion of uric acid.

● Tell patient to avoid exposure to people with infections.

● Advise patient that hair should grow back after therapy has ended.

● Tell patient to call if he has a sore throat or fever or notices any unusual bruising or bleeding.

Breast-feeding
It is not known whether thiotepa distributes into breast milk. However, because of the risk of serious adverse reactions, mutagenicity, and carcinogenicity in the infant, breast-feeding is not recommended.

---

thiothixene
thiothixene hydrochloride
Navane

● Pharmacologic classification: thioxanthene
● Therapeutic classification: antipsychotic
● Pregnancy risk category C

How supplied
Available by prescription only
Capsules: 1 mg, 2 mg, 5 mg, 10 mg, 20 mg
Oral concentrate: 5 mg/ml (7% alcohol)
Injection: 2 mg, 5 mg/ml

Indications, route, and dosage
Acute agitation
Adults: 4 mg I.M. b.i.d. to q.i.d.; maximum dosage is 30 mg I.M. daily. Change to P.O. form as soon as possible; I.M. dosage form is irritating.

Mild-to-moderate psychosis
Adults: Initially, 2 mg P.O. t.i.d.; may increase gradually to 15 mg daily.
Severe psychosis
Adults: Initially, 5 mg P.O. b.i.d.; may increase gradually to 15 to 30 mg daily. Maximum recommended daily dosage is 60 mg.

Pharmacodynamics
Antipsychotic action: Thiothixene is thought to exert its antipsychotic effects by postsynaptic blockade of CNS dopamine receptors, thereby inhibiting dopamine-mediated effects.

Thiothixene has many other central and peripheral effects: it also acts as an alpha-blocking agent. Its most prominent adverse reactions are extrapyramidal.

Pharmacokinetics
● *Absorption:* Absorption is rapid; I.M. onset of action is 10 to 30 minutes.
● *Distribution:* Thiothixene is distributed widely into the body. Peak effects occur at 1 to 6 hours after I.M. administration; drug is 91% to 99% protein-bound.
● *Metabolism:* Metabolism of thiothixene is minimal.
● *Excretion:* Most of drug is excreted as parent drug in feces via the biliary tract.

Contraindications and precautions
Thiothixene is contraindicated in patients with known hypersensitivity to thioxanthenes, phenothiazines, and related compounds, including that evidenced by jaundice and other allergic symptoms; in patients with blood dyscrasias and bone marrow depression (adverse hematologic effects); and in patients with disorders accompanied by coma, brain damage, CNS depression, circulatory collapse, or cerebrovascular disease (additive CNS depression and adverse effects on blood pressure).

Thiothixene should be used cautiously in patients with cardiac disease (arrhythmias, CHF, angina pectoris, valvular disease, or heart block), encephalitis, Reye's syndrome, head injury, respiratory disease, epilepsy and other seizure disorders, glaucoma, prostatic hypertrophy, urinary retention, Parkinson's disease, or pheochromocytoma, because it may exacerbate these conditions; in patients with hypocalcemia because it increases the risk of extrapyramidal reactions; and in patients with hepatic or renal impairment because diminished metabolism and excretion cause drug to accumulate.

Interactions
Concomitant use of thiothixene with sympathomimetics, including epinephrine, phenylephrine, phenylpropanolamine, and ephedrine (often found in nasal sprays) and with appetite suppressants may decrease their stimulatory and pressor effects. Thiothixene may cause epinephrine reversal; patients taking thiothixene may experience a decrease in blood pressure when epinephrine is used as a pressor agent.

Thiothixene may inhibit blood pressure response to centrally acting antihypertensive drugs, such as guanethidine, guanabenz, guanadrel, clonidine, methyldopa, and reserpine. Additive effects are likely after concomitant use of thiothixene with CNS depressants, including alcohol, analgesics, barbiturates, narcotics, tranquilizers, anesthetics (general, spinal, or epidural) and parenteral magnesium sulfate (oversedation, respiratory depression, and hypotension); antiarrhythmic

---

agents, including quinidine, disopyramide, and procainamide (increased incidence of cardiac arrhythmias and conduction defects); atropine and other anticholinergic drugs, including antidepressants, MAO inhibitors, phenothiazines, antihistamines, meperidine, and antiparkinsonian agents (oversedation, paralytic ileus, visual changes, and severe constipation); nitrates (hypotension); and metrizamide (increased risk of seizures).

Beta-blocking agents may inhibit thiothixene metabolism, increasing plasma levels and toxicity.

Concomitant use with propylthiouracil increases risk of agranulocytosis; concomitant use with lithium may result in severe neurologic toxicity with an encephalitis-like syndrome and in decreased therapeutic response to thiothixene.

Pharmacokinetic alterations and subsequent decreased therapeutic response to thiothixene may follow concomitant use with phenobarbital (enhanced renal excretion); aluminum- and magnesium-containing antacids and antidiarrheals (decreased absorption); caffeine; or heavy smoking (increased metabolism).

Thiothixene may antagonize therapeutic effect of bromocriptine on prolactin secretion; it may also decrease the vasoconstricting effects of high-dose dopamine and may decrease effectiveness and increase toxicity of levodopa (by dopamine blockade). Thiothixene may inhibit metabolism and increase toxicity of phenytoin.

Effects on diagnostic tests

Thiothixene causes false-positive test results for urinary porphyrins, urobilinogen, amylase, and 5-HIAA because of darkening of urine by metabolites; it also causes false-positive urine pregnancy results in tests using human chorionic gonadotropin as the indicator.

Thiothixene elevates test results for liver enzymes and protein-bound iodine and causes quinidine-like effects on the ECG.

Adverse reactions

● CNS: extrapyramidal symptoms – dystonia, akathisia, torticollis, tardive dyskinesia (dose-related, long-term therapy), sedation, pseudoparkinsonism, drowsiness (frequent), *neuroleptic malignant syndrome* (dose-related; if untreated, fatal *respiratory failure* in over 10% of patients), dizziness, headache, insomnia, exacerbation of psychotic symptoms.
● CV: *asystole*, orthostatic hypotension, tachycardia, dizziness or fainting, *arrhythmias*, ECG changes, increased anginal pain after I.M. injection.
● EENT: blurred vision, tinnitus, mydriasis, increased intraocular pressure, ocular changes (retinal pigmentary change with long-term use).
● GI: dry mouth, constipation, nausea, vomiting, anorexia, diarrhea.
● GU: urinary retention, gynecomastia, hypermenorrhea, inhibited ejaculation.
● HEMA: transient leukopenia, *agranulocytosis*, thrombocytopenia, anemia (within 30 to 90 days).
● Local: contact dermatitis from concentrate or injectable form, muscle necrosis from I.M. injection.
● Other: hyperprolactinemia, photosensitivity, increased appetite or weight gain, hypersensitivity (rash, urticaria, drug fever, edema, cholestatic jaundice [in 0.1% to 4% of patients within first 30 days]), decreased libido.

After abrupt withdrawal of long-term therapy, gastritis, nausea, vomiting, dizziness, tremors, feeling of heat or cold, sweating, tachycardia, headache, or insomnia may occur.

Note: Drug should be discontinued if any of the following occur: hypersensitivity, jaundice, agranulocytosis, neuroleptic malignant syndrome (marked hyperthermia, extrapyramidal effects, autonomic dysfunction), or severe extrapyramidal symptoms even after dose is lowered. Drug should be discontinued 48 hours before and 24 hours after myelography using metrizamide, because of risk of seizures. When feasible, drug should be withdrawn slowly and gradually; many drug effects persist after withdrawal.

Overdose and treatment

CNS depression is characterized by deep, unarousable sleep and possible coma, hypotension or hypertension, extrapyramidal symptoms, abnormal involuntary muscle movements, agitation, seizures, arrhythmias, ECG changes, hypothermia or hyperthermia, and autonomic nervous system dysfunction.

Treatment is symptomatic and supportive and includes maintaining vital signs, airway, stable body temperature, and fluid and electrolyte balance.

Do not induce vomiting: drug inhibits cough reflex, and aspiration may occur. Use gastric lavage, then activated charcoal and saline cathartics; dialysis does not help. Regulate body temperature as needed. Treat hypotension with I.V. fluids: *do not give epinephrine.* Seizures may be treated with parenteral diazepam or barbiturates; arrhythmias with parenteral phenytoin (1 mg/kg with rate titrated to blood pressure); and extrapyramidal reactions with benztropine or parenteral diphenhydramine 2 mg/kg/minute.

▶ Special considerations

● Liquid and injectable formulations may cause a rash if skin contact occurs.
● Thiothixene is associated with a high incidence of extrapyramidal effects.
● Oral formulations may cause stomach upset. Administer with food or fluid.
● Check patient regularly for abnormal body movements (at least once every 6 months).
● Dilute the concentrate in 2 to 4 oz of liquid, preferably water, carbonated drinks, fruit juice, tomato juice, milk, or pudding.
● Photosensitivity reactions may occur; patient should avoid exposure to sunlight or heat lamps.
● Administer I.M. injection deep into upper outer quadrant of the buttock. Massaging the area after administration may prevent formation of abscesses. I.M. injection may cause skin necrosis; do not extravasate, or give I.V.
● Solution for injection may be slightly discolored. Do not use if excessively discolored or if a precipitate is evident. Contact pharmacist.
● Monitor blood pressure before and after parenteral administration.
● Shake concentrate before administration.
● Chewing sugarless gum or hard candy as well as ice may help relieve dry mouth.
● Drug is stable after reconstitution for 48 hours at room temperature.
● Protect liquid formulation from light.

Information for the patient

● Explain the risks of dystonic reactions and tardive dyskinesia, and tell patient to report any abnormal body movements.

• Tell patient to avoid sun exposure and to wear sunscreen when going outdoors, to prevent photosensitivity reactions. (Note that heat lamps and tanning beds also may cause burning of the skin or skin discoloration.)

• Tell patient not to spill the liquid. Contact with skin may cause rash and irritation.

• Warn patient to avoid extremely hot or cold baths or exposure to temperature extremes, sunlamps, or tanning beds; drug may cause thermoregulatory changes.

• Tell patient to take drug exactly as prescribed; not to double doses for missed doses; and not to share drug with others.

• Explain that many drug interactions are possible. Patient should seek medical approval before taking *any* self-prescribed medication.

• Patient should become tolerant to the drug's sedative effects in several weeks.

• Tell patient not to stop taking the drug suddenly; most adverse reactions may be relieved by reducing the dosage. However, patient should call if difficulty urinating, sore throat, dizziness, or fainting develops.

• Warn patient against hazardous activities that require alertness until the drug's effect is established. Reassure patient that sedation usually subsides after several weeks.

• Tell patient not to drink alcohol or take other medications that may cause excessive sedation.

• Explain which fluids are appropriate for diluting the concentrate and the dropper technique of measuring dose.

• Tell patient that sugarless hard candy, chewing gum, or ice can alleviate dry mouth.

• Tell patient to shake concentrate before administration.

• Store drug safely away from children.

Geriatric use
Elderly patients tend to require lower dosages, titrated to individual response. Such patients also are more likely to develop adverse reactions, especially tardive dyskinesia and other extrapyramidal effects.

Pediatric use
Drug is not recommended for children under age 12.

---

thrombin
Thrombinar, Thrombogen, Thrombostat

• Pharmacologic classification: enzyme
• Therapeutic classification: topical hemostatic
• Pregnancy risk category C

How supplied
Available by prescription only
Powder: 1,000-, 5,000-, 10,000-, 20,000-, and 50,000-unit vials
Kit: 20,000-unit with sprayer assembly

Indications, route, and dosage
Bleeding from parenchymatous tissue, cancellous bone, dental sockets, during nasal and laryngeal surgery, and in plastic surgery and skin-grafting procedures
Adults: Apply 100 units/ml of sterile isotonic saline solution or sterile distilled water to area where clotting needed (or may apply dry powder in bone surgery); in major bleeding, apply 1,000 to 2,000 units/ml sterile isotonic saline solution. Sponge blood from area before application, but avoid sponging area after application.
GI hemorrhage
Adults: Give 2 ounces (60 ml) of milk, followed by 2 ounces of milk containing 10,000 to 20,000 units thrombin. Repeat t.i.d. for 4 to 5 days or until bleeding is controlled.

Pharmacodynamics
Hemostatic action: Thrombin catalyzes the conversion of fibrinogen to fibrin, one of the last stages of clot formation.

Pharmacokinetics
Not applicable.

Contraindications and precautions
Thrombin is contraindicated in patients with hypersensitivity to thrombin or to bovine products. Do not inject thrombin or allow it to enter large blood vessels; death may result from severe intravascular clotting.

Interactions
None significant.

Effects on diagnostic tests
None reported.

Adverse reactions
• Systemic: hypersensitivity, fever, *intravascular clotting* (could cause death if thrombin enters large vessels).

Overdose and treatment
No information available.

▶ Special considerations
• Keep refrigerated until ready to use, and use as soon as possible after reconstitution; if several hours will elapse, refrigerate or freeze solution. Discard solutions prepared with preservative-free diluent within 4 hours and those with preservative after 48 hours. May be used with absorbable gelatin sponge, but not oxidized cellulose. Check label before using.
• Obtain patient history of reactions to thrombin or bovine products.
• Observe patient for hypersensitivity reaction after administering.
• Be certain patient with GI hemorrhage drinks all pretherapy milk and milk-thrombin solution as ordered; gastric acid will decrease thrombin activity unless neutralized. Thrombin activity is also decreased by alkali, heat, and heavy metals.
• Contents of a 5,000-unit vial dissolved in 5 ml saline solution are capable of clotting an equal volume of blood in less than 1 second, or 1,000 ml in less than a minute.

Information for the patient
Advise patients taking drug for GI hemorrhage to drink all prescribed milk and milk-thrombin solution.

---

thrombolytic enzymes

alteplase
anistreplase
streptokinase
urokinase

When a thrombus obstructs a blood vessel, permanent damage to the ischemic area may occur before the body can dissolve the clot. Thrombolytic agents were developed in the hope that speeding lysis of the clot would prevent permanent ischemic damage. Thrombolytic activity attributable to streptokinase was described in 1933; this compound's effects have since been studied on various kinds of clots. It is not clear whether such agents significantly reduce thrombosis-induced ischemic damage in all situations for which the drugs are currently used.

Pharmacology
Streptokinase is a protein-like substance produced by group C beta-hemolytic streptococci; urokinase is an enzyme isolated from human kidney tissue cultures. Alteplase is a tissue-type plasminogen activator synthesized by recombinant DNA technology. Anistreplase is anisoylated streptokinase-plasminogen activated complex (APSAC); it is a fibrinolytic enzyme (plasminogen) plus activator complex (streptokinase) with the activator temporarily blocked by an anisoyl group. Thrombolytic enzymes act chiefly by converting plasminogen to plasmin; in contrast, anticoagulants act by preventing thrombi from developing. Thrombolytics are more likely to produce clinical bleeding than are oral anticoagulants.

Clinical indications and actions
Thrombosis, thromboembolism
Alteplase, streptokinase, and urokinase are used to treat acute pulmonary thromboembolism; streptokinase and urokinase are used to treat deep vein thrombosis, acute arterial thromboembolism, or acute coronary arterial thrombosis and to clear arteriovenous cannula occlusion and venous catheter obstruction. Anistreplase is used, with alteplase, streptokinase, and urokinase, to manage acute myocardial infarction. These agents are administered in an attempt to lyse coronary artery thrombi, which may result in improved ventricular function and decreased risk of CHF.

Overview of adverse reactions
Adverse reactions to these agents are essentially an extension of their actions; hemorrhage is the most common adverse effect. These agents cause bleeding twice as often as does heparin, and, although both may cause allergic reactions, streptokinase is more likely to do so than urokinase. Information regarding hypersensitivity to alteplase is limited.

▶ Special considerations
● Thrombolytic therapy requires medical supervision with continuous clinical and laboratory monitoring; patient must be on complete bed rest.
● Thrombolytics act only on fibrin clots, not those formed by a precipitated drug.
● Follow instructions for reconstitution precisely and pass solution through a filter 0.45 microns or smaller to remove any filaments in the solution; do not use dextran concomitantly, because it can interfere with coagulation as well as blood typing and cross matching.
● Obtain pretherapy baseline determinations of thrombin time, activated partial thromboplastin time, prothrombin time (PT), hematocrit, and platelet count for subsequent blood monitoring. Monitor laboratory studies on a flowsheet in patient's chart. During systemic thrombolytic therapy, as in pulmonary embolism or venous thrombosis, PT or thrombin time after 4 hours of therapy should be approximately twice the pretreatment value.
● Keep venipuncture sites to a minimum; apply pressure dressings for at least 15 minutes, to prevent bleeding and hematoma. For arterial puncture (except intracoronary), use upper extremities, which are more accessible for pressure dressings; apply pressure for at least 30 minutes after arterial puncture.
● Administer drugs by infusion pump to ensure accuracy; I.M. injections are contraindicated during therapy because of increased risk of bleeding at the injection site.
● Check vital signs frequently. Monitor for blood pressure alterations in excess of 25 mm Hg and any change in cardiac rhythm; check pulses, color, and sensitivity of extremities every hour; monitor for excessive bleeding every 15 minutes for first hour, every 30 minutes for second through eighth hours; then at least once every 8 hours. Stop therapy if bleeding is evident; pretreatment with heparin or drugs affecting platelets increases risk.
● Monitor for hypersensitivity as well as hemorrhage: keep available typed and cross matched packed red blood cells and whole blood, aminocaproic acid to treat bleeding, and corticosteroids to treat allergic reactions.
● Keep involved extremity in straight alignment to prevent bleeding from infusion site. Establish precautions to prevent injury and avoid unnecessary handling of patient, because bruising is likely.
● At end of infusion, flush remaining dose from pump tubing with I.V. 5% dextrose or normal saline solution.
● Continuous heparin infusion usually is started within 1 hour after stopping thrombolytic; before starting, be sure thrombin time or activated partial thromboplastin time is less than twice normal. Heparin does not require a loading dose.
● Before using thrombolytic to clear an occluded catheter, try to gently aspirate or flush with heparinized saline solution. Avoid forcible flushing or vigorous suction, which could rupture the catheter or expel the clot into the circulation.

Information for the patient
● Explain rationale for treatment and procedure, and necessity for bed rest.
● Ask patient to be alert for signs of bleeding.
● When using these drugs to clear catheter, instruct patient to exhale and hold breath at any time catheter is not connected, to prevent air entering the open catheter.

Geriatric use
Patients age 75 or older are at greater risk of cerebral hemorrhage, because they are more apt to have pre-existing cerebrovascular disease.

Pediatric use
Safe use in children has not been established.

COMPARING THROMBOLYTIC ENZYMES

Thrombolytic enzymes dissolve clots by accelerating the formation of plasmin by activated plasminogen. Plasminogen activators, found in most tissues and body fluids, help plasminogen (an inactive enzyme) convert to plasmin (an active enzyme), which dissolves the clot.

Two thrombolytic enzymes—streptokinase and urokinase—have been widely used; two enzymes—tissue plasminogen activator (TPA or alteplase) and anistreplase—have recently been added to current use. Doses of these enzymes may vary according to the patient's condition.

DRUG	ACTION	INITIAL DOSE	MAINTENANCE THERAPY
alteplase	Directly converts plasminogen to plasmin	I.V. bolus: 6 to 10 mg over 1 to 2 min	I.V. infusion: 50 to 54 mg/hr over 1st hour; 20 mg (20 ml)/hr over next 2 hr, then discontinue
anistreplase	Directly converts plasminogen to plasmin	I.V. push: 30 units over 2 to 3 min	Not necessary
streptokinase	Indirectly activates plasminogen, which converts to plasmin	Intracoronary bolus: 15,000 to 20,000 IU I.V. bolus: none needed	Intracoronary infusion: 2,000 to 4,000 IU/min over 60 min I.V. infusion: 1,500,000 units over 60 min
urokinase	Directly converts plasminogen to plasmin	Intracoronary bolus: none needed	Intracoronary infusion: 2,000 units/lb/hr (4,400 units/kg/hr); rate of 15 ml of solution/hr for total of 12 hr (total volume shouldn't exceed 200 ml)

Breast-feeding
Safe use during breast-feeding has not been established.

Representative combinations
None.

---

thyroglobulin
Proloid

- Pharmacologic classification: thyroid hormone
- Therapeutic classification: thyroid agent
- Pregnancy risk category A

How supplied
Available by prescription only
Tablets: 32 mg, 65 mg, 100 mg, 130 mg, 200 mg

Indications, route, and dosage
Cretinism and juvenile hypothyroidism (not a first line agent)
Children over age 1: Dosage may approach adult dosage (60 to 180 mg P.O. daily), depending on response. Children age 4 to 12 months: 60 to 80 mg P.O. daily. Children age 1 to 4 months: Initially, 15 to 30 mg P.O. daily, increased at 2-week intervals. Usual maintenance dosage is 30 to 45 mg P.O. daily.

Hypothyroidism or myxedema (not a first line agent)
Adults: Initially, 15 to 30 mg P.O. daily, increased by 15 to 30 mg at 2-week intervals until desired response is obtained. Usual maintenance dosage is 60 to 200 mg P.O. daily, as a single dose.
Adults over age 65: Initially, 7.5 to 15 mg P.O. daily; the dosage is doubled at 6- to 8-week intervals until desired response is obtained.

Pharmacodynamics
Thyrotropic action: Thyroglobulin affects protein and carbohydrate metabolism, promotes gluconeogenesis, increases the utilization and mobilization of glycogen stores, stimulates protein synthesis, and regulates cell growth and differentiation. The major effect of thyroglobulin is to increase the metabolic rate of tissue.

Pharmacokinetics
- Absorption: Thyroglobulin is absorbed from the GI tract.
- Distribution: Not fully understood. It is highly protein-bound.
- Metabolism: Not fully understood.
- Excretion: Not fully understood.

Contraindications and precautions
Thyroglobulin is contraindicated in patients with hypersensitivity to beef or pork and in patients with thyrotoxicosis, acute myocardial infarction, and uncorrected adrenal insufficiency because thyroid hormones increase tissue metabolic demands. Thyroglobulin is also contraindicated for treating obesity because it is

---

ineffective and can cause life-threatening adverse reactions.

Thyroglobulin should be used cautiously in patients with angina or other cardiovascular disease because of the risk of increased metabolic demands; in patients with diabetes mellitus because of reduced glucose tolerance; in patients with malabsorption states; and in patients with long-standing hypothyroidism or myxedema because these patients may be more sensitive to the effects of thyroid hormones.

Interactions
Concomitant use of thyroglobulin with an adrenocorticoid or corticotropin changes thyroid status and may require dosage changes of thyroid, adrenocorticoid, or corticotropin. Concomitant use with an anticoagulant may alter the anticoagulant's effects, requiring an increase in thyroglobulin dosage. Concomitant use with tricyclic antidepressants or sympathomimetics may increase the effects of these medications or of thyroglobulin, possibly leading to coronary insufficiency or cardiac arrhythmias.

Use with oral antidiabetic agents or insulin may affect the dosage requirements of these agents. Estrogens, which increase serum thyroxine-binding globulin levels, raise thyroid hormone requirements. Hepatic enzyme inducers (such as phenytoin) may increase hepatic degradation of levothyroxine and raise dosage requirements of levothyroxine. Concomitant use with somatrem may accelerate epiphyseal maturation. I.V. phenytoin may release free thyroid. Cholestyramine or colestipol may impair absorption.

Effects on diagnostic tests
Thyroglobulin alters ^{131}I thyroid uptake, protein-bound iodine levels, and liothyronine uptake.

Adverse reactions
● CNS: nervousness, insomnia, tremor.
● CV: *tachycardia*, palpitations, *arrhythmias*, angina pectoris, hypertension, elevated pulse pressure, *cardiac arrest*.
● GI: change in appetite, nausea, diarrhea.
● Other: headache, leg cramps, weight loss, sweating, heat intolerance, allergic skin reactions, fever, menstrual irregularities.
  Note: Drug should be discontinued if patient develops signs of allergic reaction or hyperthyroidism.

Overdose and treatment
Clinical manifestations of overdose include signs and symptoms of hyperthyroidism, including weight loss, increased appetite, palpitations, nervousness, diarrhea, abdominal cramps, sweating, tachycardia, increased pulse and blood pressure, angina, cardiac arrhythmias, tremor, headache, insomnia, heat intolerance, fever, and menstrual irregularities.

Overdose treatment requires reduction of GI absorption and efforts to counteract central and peripheral effects, primarily sympathetic. Use gastric lavage or induce emesis (follow with activated charcoal, up to 4 hours after ingestion). If the patient is comatose or is having seizures, inflate cuff on endotracheal tube to prevent aspiration. Treatment may include oxygen and artificial ventilation, as needed to support respiration. It should also include appropriate measures to treat congestive heart failure and control fever, hypoglycemia, and fluid loss. Propranolol may be used to combat many of the effects of increased sympathetic

activity. Thyroid therapy should be withdrawn gradually over 2 to 6 days, then resumed at a lower dose.

▶ Special considerations
Besides those relevant to all *thyroid hormones*, consider these recommendations.
● Variable hormonal content of commercial preparations may produce fluctuations of liothyronine and levothyroxine.
● Monitor patient's pulse rate and blood pressure.
● Prescribe as morning dose to prevent insomnia.

Information for the patient
● Advise patient to report headache, diarrhea, nervousness, excessive sweating, heat intolerance, chest pain, increased pulse rate, or palpitations.
● Encourage patient to take daily dose at the same time each day, preferably in the morning to avoid insomnia.
● Tell patient not to store medication in warm, humid areas such as the bathroom to prevent deterioration of the drug.

Geriatric use
Elderly patients are more sensitive to thyroglobulin's effects. In patients over age 60, initial dosage should be 25% lower than usual recommended dosage.

Pediatric use
Partial hair loss may occur during the first few months of therapy. Reassure child and parents that this is temporary.

Breast-feeding
Minimal amounts of this drug are excreted in breast milk. Use with caution in breast-feeding women.

PHARMACOLOGIC CLASS

thyroid hormones

levothyroxine sodium (T_4)
liothyronine sodium (T_3)
liotrix
thyroglobulin
thyroid USP (desiccated)
thyrotropin (TSH)

The thyroid gland was first described by Wharton in 1656. In 1891, Murray was the first to treat hypothyroidism by injecting an extract of the thyroid gland. The next year, the extract was found to be effective orally. Thyroid hormones are now used for treating hypothyroidism (myxedema and cretinism), nontoxic goiter, and (with antithyroid drugs) thyrotoxicosis and as a diagnostic aid.

Thyroid hormone synthesis is regulated by thyroid-stimulating hormone (TSH) secreted by the anterior pituitary. TSH secretion is controlled by a feedback mechanism and by thyrotropin-releasing hormone (TRH) from the hypothalamus. Thyroid hormone, which contains triiodothyronine (T_3) and thyroxine (T_4), is stored in the thyroid as thyroglobulin. The amounts of T_3 and T_4 released into circulation are regulated by TSH. T_4 is the major component of normal secretions of the thyroid gland and is the major determinant of normal thyroid function. A major portion of T_3 (about 80%) is derived from T_4 by deiodination in peripheral tissues. Approximately 35% of secreted T_4 is mono-deiodinated peripherally to T_3. In normal human thyroid tissue, the T_4:T_3 ratio ranges from 10:1 to 15:1; in a hyperthyroid patient, the ratio is about 5:1.

Pharmacology

Thyroid hormones include natural (thyroid USP and thyroglobulin) and synthetic (levothyroxine, liothyronine, and liotrix) derivatives. The thyroid hormones have catabolic and anabolic effects and influence normal metabolism, growth, and development. Thyroid hormones influence every organ system and are vital to normal central nervous system (CNS) function.

TSH increases iodine uptake by the thyroid and increases formation and release of thyroid hormone. TSH is isolated from bovine anterior pituitary glands.

Clinical indications and actions
Hypothyroidism (myxedema, cretinism, or replacement therapy)

All drugs in this class (except TSH) are used to treat hypothyroidism but the drug of choice is levothyroxine (T_4). Dessicated thyroid is rarely used today. These hormones affect protein and carbohydrate metabolism, promote gluconeogenesis, increase the utilization and mobilization of glycogen stores, stimulate protein synthesis, and regulate cell growth and differentiation. The major effect of exogenous thyroid hormones is to increase the metabolic rate of tissue.

Nontoxic goiter

Levothyroxine, liotrix, liothyronine, and thyroid USP are used to suppress TSH secretion in the management of simple goiter.

Diagnostic uses

Liothyronine is used in the T_3 suppression test to differentiate suspected hyperthyroidism from euthyroidism in patients with borderline or high ^{131}I uptake values. TSH increases iodine uptake by the thyroid and increases formation and release of thyroid hormone.

Thyrotoxicosis

Levothyroxine, liotrix, and thyroid USP are used with antithyroid agents to prevent goitrogenesis and hypothyroidism.

Because thyroid hormones have wide-ranging metabolic effects and are potentially dangerous, they are not indicated for relief of vague symptoms, such as mental and physical sluggishness, irritability, depression, nervousness and ill-defined pains; to treat obesity in patients with normal thyroid function; to treat metabolic insufficiency not associated with thyroid insufficiency; or to treat menstrual disorders or male infertility not associated with hypothyroidism.

Overview of adverse reactions

Adverse reactions to thyroid hormones are extensions of their pharmacologic properties. Signs of overdose include nervousness, insomnia, tremor, tachycardia, palpitations, nausea, headache, fever, and sweating.

▶ Special considerations

● Thyroid hormone dosage varies widely among patients. Treatment should start at the lowest level, titrating to higher doses according to patient's symptoms and laboratory data, until euthyroid state is reached.
● Thyroid hormones should be administered at the same time each day. Morning dosage is preferred to prevent insomnia.
● Monitor pulse rate and blood pressure.

● Monitor prothrombin time; patients taking anticoagulants usually require lower doses.
● Signs of thyrotoxicosis or inadequate dosage therapy include diarrhea, fever, irritability, listlessness, rapid heartbeat, vomiting, or weakness.

Information for the patient

Advise patient to call at once if signs or symptoms of overdose (chest pain, palpitations, sweating, nervousness) or of aggravated cardiovascular disease (chest pain, dyspnea, or tachycardia) occur.

Geriatric use

In patients over age 60, initial hormone replacement dosage should be 25% less than the usual recommended starting dosage.

Pediatric use

During first few months of therapy, children may suffer partial hair loss. Reassure child and parents that this is temporary.

Breast-feeding

Minimal amounts of exogenous thyroid hormones are excreted in breast milk. However, problems have not been reported in breast-feeding infants.

Representative combinations

Thyroid dessicated powder with vitamin B_1, vitamin B_2, vitamin B_6, and niacinamide: Henydin-M, Hendyin-R. *Thyroid* with iodized calcium and peptone: Thycal.

PHARMACOLOGIC CLASS

thyroid hormone antagonists

methimazole
propylthiouracil (PTU)
radioactive iodine (^{131}I)

Studies on the developmental mechanism of goiter began in the 1920s. Two goitrogens were found in the 1940s that were the prototypes of two different classes of thyroid hormones, one of which contains the thioureylene moiety. These drugs are useful in treating hyperthyroidism, as in long-term therapy (methimazole, PTU, or ^{131}I), or in preparation for thyroidectomy (PTU and methimazole). They also are used to treat thyroid carcinoma (^{131}I) and thyrotoxic crisis (methimazole and PTU).

Pharmacology

Methimazole and PTU, of the thioureylene class of antithyroid drugs, inhibit oxidation of iodine in the thyroid gland by blocking iodine's ability to combine with tyrosine to form thyroxine. PTU also inhibits the peripheral conversion of thyroxine (T_4) to triiodothyronine (T_3). PTU is theoretically preferred over methimazole in thyroid storm because of its peripheral activity.

^{131}I is deposited rapidly into the colloid of the follicles of the thyroid gland. The beta rays originate within the follicle and destroy parenchymal cells of the thyroid but very little surrounding tissue.

Clinical indications and actions
Hyperthyroidism

Thyroid hormone antagonists inhibit the synthesis of thyroid hormone by interfering with the incorporation of iodine into thyroglobulin. These drugs also inhibit the formation of iodothyronine. Clinical effects of these drugs become evident only when the preformed hormone is depleted and circulating hormone levels decline. PTU, besides blocking hormone synthesis, inhibits the peripheral deiodination of levothyroxine to liothyronine.

Preparation for thyroidectomy
By inhibiting synthesis of thyroid hormone and causing a euthyroid state, these drugs help reduce surgical problems during thyroidectomy; as a result, the mortality for a single-stage thyroidectomy is very low. Iodine reduces the vascularity of the gland and makes it less friable. Sodium iodide or potassium iodide also exert long-term antagonism to the release of preformed thyroid hormones and can be used if the patient needs surgery but is allergic to either methimazole or propylthiouracil.

Thyrotoxic crisis
PTU inhibits peripheral deiodination of levothyroxine to liothyronine.

Thyroid carcinoma
^{131}I is trapped rapidly by the thyroid and deposited in the colloid of the follicles. The destructive beta rays originate within the follicle and act almost exclusively on the parenchymal cells of the thyroid, with little damage to surrounding tissue. However, with large doses of ^{131}I, characteristic cytotoxic effects of ionizing radiation occur.

Overview of adverse reactions
Therapeutic doses can cause fever, chills, sore throat, weakness, backache, swelling of feet, joint pain, and unusual bleeding or bruising. Toxic doses can cause constipation, cold intolerance, dry puffy skin, headache, sleepiness, muscle aches, and unusual weight gain.

▶ Special considerations
● Signs and symptoms of overdose or hypothyroidism include mental depression; changes in menstrual periods; cold intolerance; constipation; dry, puffy skin; headache; listlessness; muscle aches; nausea; vomiting; weakness; fatigue; hard, non-pitting edema; and unusual weight gain.
● Watch for signs of hypothyroidism. Monitor serum TSH as a sensitive indicator of thyroid hormone levels. Dosage adjustment may be required.
● Signs of thyrotoxicosis or inadequate thyroid suppression include diarrhea, fever, irritability, listlessness, rapid heartbeat, vomiting, and weakness.
● Thyroid hormone antagonists should be used cautiously with careful thyroid function monitoring in pregnant patients. Pregnant patients may require less drug as pregnancy progresses. Thyroid hormones may be added to regimen. These drugs may be discontinued during the last few weeks of pregnancy.
● Treatment with antithyroid drugs requires complete blood counts periodically to detect impending leukopenia, thrombocytopenia, or agranulocytosis.
● Drug should be discontinued if patient develops severe rash or enlarged cervical lymph nodes.

Information for the patient
● Advise patient to call immediately if sore throat, fever, or mouth sores occur (possible signs of developing agranulocytosis, which may not be detected by periodic blood cell counts because it can develop so rapidly). Patient should also report immediately any skin eruptions (sign of hypersensitivity).

● Suggest that patient take the drug with meals to reduce GI side effects.

Breast-feeding
Methimazole and PTU are excreted in breast milk. Patients should avoid breast-feeding during treatment with thyroid hormone antagonists.

Representative combinations
None.

---

thyroid USP (desiccated)
Armour Thyroid, Dathroid, Delcoid, S-P-T, Thermoloid, Thyrar, Thyrocrine, Thyroid Strong, Thyro-teric

● Pharmacologic classification: thyroid hormone
● Therapeutic classification: thyroid agent
● Pregnancy risk category A

How supplied
Available by prescription only
Tablets: 15 mg, 30 mg, 60 mg, 65 mg, 90 mg, 120 mg, 130 mg, 180 mg, 240 mg, 300 mg (Armour Thyroid)
Tablets (bovine): 30 mg, 60 mg, 120 mg (Thyrar)
Tablets (enteric-coated): 60 mg, 120 mg
Strong tablets (contains 0.3% iodine): 30 mg, 60 mg, 120 mg, 180 mg

Indications, route, and dosage
Adult hypothyroidism
Adults: Initially, 60 mg P.O. daily, increased by 60 mg q 30 days until desired response is achieved. Usual maintenance dosage is 60 to 180 mg P.O. daily as a single dosage.
Adults over age 65: 7.5 to 15 mg P.O. daily; dosage is doubled at 6- to 8-week intervals.
Adult myxedema
Adults: 15 mg P.O. daily; dosage may be doubled q 2 weeks to a maximum of 120 mg.
Cretinism and juvenile hypothyroidism
Children over age 1: Dosage may approach adult dosage (60 to 180 mg daily), depending on response.
Children age 4 to 12 months: 30 to 60 mg P.O. daily.
Children age 1 to 4 months: Initially, 15 to 30 mg P.O. daily, increased at 2-week intervals. Usual maintenance dosage is 30 to 45 mg P.O. daily.

Pharmacodynamics
Thyrotropic action: Thyroid USP affects protein and carbohydrate metabolism, promotes gluconeogenesis, increases the utilization and mobilization of glycogen stores, stimulates protein synthesis, and regulates cell growth and differentiation. The major effect of thyroid is to increase the metabolic rate of tissue.

Pharmacokinetics
● *Absorption:* Thyroid USP is absorbed from the GI tract.
● *Distribution:* Not fully understood. Thyroid USP is highly protein-bound.
● *Metabolism:* Not fully understood.
● *Excretion:* Not fully understood.

Contraindications and precautions

Thyroid USP is contraindicated in patients with hypersensitivity to beef or pork and in those with thyrotoxicosis, acute myocardial infarction, or uncorrected adrenal insufficiency (thyroid increases tissue metabolic demands). Thyroid USP also is contraindicated for treating obesity because it is ineffective and can cause life-threatening adverse reactions.

Thyroid USP should be used cautiously in patients with angina or other cardiovascular disease because of the risk of increased metabolic demands; in patients with diabetes mellitus because of reduced glucose tolerance; in patients with malabsorption states; and in patients with chronic hypothyroidism or myxedema because these patients may be more sensitive to the effects of thyroid.

Interactions

Concomitant use of thyroid USP with adrenocorticoids or corticotropin causes changes in thyroid status, and changes in thyroid dosages may require adrenocorticoid or corticotropin dosage changes as well. Concomitant use with anticoagulants may alter anticoagulant effect; an increased thyroid USP dosage may necessitate a lower anticoagulant dose.

Use with tricyclic antidepressants or sympathomimetics may increase the effects of these medications or of thyroid USP, possibly leading to coronary insufficiency or cardiac arrhythmias. Use with oral antidiabetic agents or insulin may affect dosage requirements of these agents. Estrogens, which increase serum thyroxine-binding globulin levels, raise thyroid USP requirements.

Hepatic enzyme inducers (for example, phenytoin) may increase hepatic degradation of levothyroxine, causing increased dosage requirements of levothyroxine. Concomitant use with somatrem may accelerate epiphyseal maturation. I.V. phenytoin may release free thyroid from thyroglobulin. Cholestyramine and colestipol may decrease absorption.

Effects on diagnostic tests

Thyroid USP therapy alters ^{131}I thyroid uptake, protein-bound iodine levels, and liothyronine uptake.

Adverse reactions

● CNS: nervousness, insomnia, tremor.
● CV: *tachycardia*, palpitations, *arrhythmias*, angina pectoris, hypertension, widened pulse pressure, *cardiac arrest.*
● GI: change in appetite, nausea, diarrhea.
● Other: headache, leg cramps, weight loss, sweating, heat intolerance, allergic skin reactions, fever, menstrual irregularities.

Note: Drug should be discontinued if patient develops allergic reaction or signs of hyperthyroidism.

Overdose and treatment

Clinical manifestations of overdose include signs and symptoms of hyperthyroidism, including weight loss, increased appetite, palpitations, nervousness, diarrhea, abdominal cramps, sweating, tachycardia, increased pulse and blood pressure, angina, cardiac arrhythmias, tremor, headache, insomnia, heat intolerance, fever, and menstrual irregularities.

Treatment requires reduction of GI absorption and efforts to counteract central and peripheral effects, primarily sympathetic activity. Use gastric lavage or induce emesis (followed with activated charcoal, if less than 4 hours after ingestion). If the patient is comatose or is having seizures, inflate cuff on endotracheal tube to prevent aspiration. Treatment may include oxygen and artificial ventilation to support respiration. It also should include appropriate measures to treat CHF and control fever, hypoglycemia, and fluid loss. Propranolol may be used to combat many of the effects of increased sympathetic activity. Thyroid USP therapy should be withdrawn gradually over 2 to 6 days, then resumed at a lower dose.

▶ Special considerations

Besides those relevant to all *thyroid hormones*, consider these recommendations.
● Levothyroxine is considered the drug of choice for thyroid hormone supplementation.
● Commercial preparations may have variable hormonal content and produce fluctuating liothyronine and levothyroxine levels. Because of this variability the use of thyroid has decreased considerably.
● Monitor patient's pulse rate and blood pressure. Thyroid may exert a greater incidence of cardiovascular adverse effects.
● In children, sleeping pulse rate and basal morning temperature are guides to treatment.
● Enteric-coated tablets give unreliable absorption.

Information for the patient

● Encourage patient to take daily dose at the same time each day, preferably in the morning to avoid insomnia.
● Advise patient to call if headache, diarrhea, nervousness, excessive sweating, heat intolerance, chest pain, increased pulse rate, or palpitations occur.
● Tell patient not to store this medication in warm, humid areas such as the bathroom to prevent deterioration of the drug.

Geriatric use

Elderly patients are more sensitive to thyroid effects. In patients over age 60, initial dosage should be 25% lower than usual recommended dosage.

Pediatric use

Partial hair loss may occur during the first few months of therapy. Reassure child and parents that this is temporary.

Breast-feeding

Minimal amounts of this drug are excreted in breast milk. Use with caution in breast-feeding women.

thyrotropin (thyroid-stimulating hormone, or TSH)
Thytropar

● Pharmacologic classification: anterior pituitary hormone
● Therapeutic classification: thyrotropic hormone
● Pregnancy risk category C

How supplied

Available by prescription only
Powder for injection: 10 units (IU)/vial

Indications, route, and dosage
Diagnosis of thyroid cancer remnant with [131]I
after surgery
Adults and children: 10 units I.M. or S.C. for 3 to 7 days.
Differential diagnosis of primary and second-
ary hypothyroidism
Adults and children: 10 units I.M. or S.C. for 1 to 3 days.
In protein-bound iodine or [131]I *uptake determi-*
nations for differential diagnosis of sub-clinical
hypothyroidism or low thyroid reserve
Adults and children: 10 units I.M. or S.C.
Therapy for thyroid carcinoma (local or meta-
static) with [131]I
Adults and children: 10 units I.M. or S.C. for 3 to 8 days.
To determine thyroid status of patient receiv-
ing thyroid
Adults and children: 10 units I.M. or S.C. for 1 to 3 days.

Pharmacodynamics
Thyrotropic action: Thyrotropin produces increased up-take of iodine by the thyroid and increased formation and release of thyroid hormone.

Pharmacokinetics
● *Absorption:* Onset occurs within minutes after injection.
● *Distribution:* Concentrated primarily in the thyroid gland.
● *Metabolism:* Not fully understood.
● *Excretion:* Not fully understood.

Contraindications and precautions
Thyrotropin is contraindicated in patients with hypersensitivity to the drug, recent myocardial infarction, or untreated Addison's disease.
   Drug should be used cautiously in patients with angina, hypertension, or heart failure, because of the risk of sudden metabolic demands; and in patients with adrenocortical insufficiency or hypopituitarism, because thyrotropin administration can provoke acute adrenocortical crisis.

Interactions
None reported.

Effects on diagnostic tests
Thyrotropin therapy alters ^{131}I thyroid uptake.

Adverse reactions
● CNS: headache, fainting.
● CV: *tachycardia, atrial fibrillation,* angina pectoris, *CHF, hypotension.*
● GI: nausea, vomiting.
● GU: urinary frequency.
● Other: thyroid hyperplasia (large doses), fever, menstrual irregularities, allergic reactions (postinjection flare, urticaria, *anaphylaxis,* wheezing, tightness of throat).
   Note: Drug should be discontinued if hypersensitivity reaction occurs.

Overdose and treatment
Clinical manifestations of overdose include headache, irritability, nervousness, sweating, tachycardia, increased GI motility, and menstrual irregularities. Angina or congestive heart failure may be aggravated. Shock may develop.
   Treatment includes administering propranolol (or another beta blocker) to treat adrenergic effects of hyperthyroidism. Recommended adult dosage of pro-

pranolol is 1 mg/dose over at least 1 minute, repeated every 2 to 5 minutes (to a maximum of 5 mg). Dosage in children is 0.01 to 0.1 mg/kg over 10 minutes (to a maximum of 1 mg). Monitor blood pressure and cardiac function. Exchange transfusions may be beneficial in acute overdose. Diuresis and dialysis are not effective.

▶ Special considerations
Besides those relevant to all *thyroid hormones,* consider these recommendations.
● Thyrotropin may cause thyroid hyperplasia.
● Three-day dosage schedule may be used in long-standing pituitary myxedema or with prolonged use of thyroid medication.

Information for the patient
Warn patient to call immediately if he experiences itching, redness, or swelling at the injection site; skin rash; tightness of throat or wheezing; chest pain; irritability; nervousness; rapid heartbeat; shortness of breath; or unusual sweating.

---

ticarcillin disodium
Ticar

● Pharmacologic classification: extended-spectrum penicillin, alpha-carboxypenicillin
● Therapeutic classification: antibiotic
● Pregnancy risk category B

How supplied
Available by prescription only
Injection: 1 g, 3 g, 6 g
Pharmacy bulk package: 20 g, 30 g
I.V. infusion: 3 g

Indications, route, and dosage
Serious infections caused by susceptible
organisms
Adults: 200 to 300 mg/kg I.V. or I.M. daily, divided into doses given q 3, 4, or 6 hours.
Children under 40 kg: 200 to 300 mg/kg I.V. or I.M. daily, divided into doses given q 4 to 6 hours.
Dosage in renal failure

Creatinine clearance (ml/min/1.73 m²)	Dosage in adults
>60	3 g I.V. q 4 hours
30 to 60	2 g I.V. q 4 hours
10 to 30	2 g I.V. q 8 hours
<10 with hepatic failure	2 g I.V. q 24 hours or 1 g I.V. q 12 hours
Patients on hemodialysis	2 g I.V. q 12 hours with 3 g I.V. after each treatment
Patients on peritoneal dialysis	3 g I.V. q 12 hours

Pharmacodynamics
Antibiotic action: Ticarcillin is bactericidal; it adheres to bacterial penicillin-binding proteins, thus inhibiting bac-

---

terial cell wall synthesis. Extended-spectrum penicillins are more resistant to inactivation by certain beta-lactamases, especially those produced by gram-negative organisms, but are still liable to inactivation by certain others.

Ticarcillin's spectrum of activity includes many gram-negative aerobic and anaerobic bacilli, many gram-positive and gram-negative aerobic cocci, and some gram-positive aerobic and anaerobic bacilli. Ticarcillin may be effective against some strains of carbenicillin-resistant gram-negative bacilli.

Ticarcillin is often more active (by weight) against *Pseudomonas aeruginosa* than is carbenicillin. Its primary use is in combination with an aminoglycoside to treat *P. aeruginosa* infections.

When ticarcillin is used alone, resistance develops rapidly. It is almost always used with other antibiotics (such as aminoglycosides).

Pharmacokinetics

● *Absorption:* Peak plasma concentrations occur 30 to 75 minutes after an I.M. dose.
● *Distribution:* Ticarcillin disodium is distributed widely. It penetrates minimally into CSF with uninflamed meninges. Ticarcillin crosses the placenta; it is 45% to 65% protein-bound.
● *Metabolism:* About 13% of a dose is metabolized by hydrolysis to inactive compounds.
● *Excretion:* Ticarcillin is excreted primarily (80% to 93%) in urine by renal tubular secretion and glomerular filteration; it is also excreted in bile and breast milk. Elimination half-life in adults is about 1 hour; in severe renal impairment, half-life is extended to about 3 hours. Ticarcillin sodium is removed by hemodialysis but not by peritoneal dialysis.

Contraindications and precautions

Ticarcillin is contraindicated in patients with known hypersensitivity to any other penicillin or to cephalosporins.

Ticarcillin should be used cautiously in patients with renal impairment because it is excreted in urine; decreased dosage is required in moderate to severe renal failure. Use cautiously in patients with bleeding tendencies, hypokalemia, or sodium restriction.

Interactions

Concomitant use with aminoglycoside antibiotics results in synergistic bactericidal effects against *Pseudomonas aeruginosa, Escherichia coli, Klebsiella, Citrobacter, Enterobacter, Serratia,* and *Proteus mirabilis.* However, the drugs are physically and chemically incompatible and are inactivated when mixed or given together.

Concomitant use of ticarcillin (and other extended-spectrum penicillins) with clavulanic acid also produces a synergistic bactericidal effect against certain beta-lactamase-producing bacteria.

Probenecid blocks renal tubular secretion of ticarcillin, raising ticarcillin's serum concentrations.

Large doses of penicillins may interfere with renal tubular secretion of methotrexate, thus delaying elimination and elevating serum concentrations of methotrexate.

Effects on diagnostic tests

Ticarcillin alters tests for urinary or serum proteins; it interferes with turbidimetric methods that use sulfosalicylic acid, trichloroacetic acid, acetic acid, or nitric acid. Ticarcillin does not interfere with tests using bromophenol blue (Albustix, Albutest, MultiStix).

Ticarcillin may falsely decrease serum aminoglycoside concentrations. Systemic effects of ticarcillin may cause positive Coombs' test, hypokalemia and hypernatremia, and may prolong prothrombin times (PTs); it may also cause transient elevations in liver function studies and transient reductions in red blood cell, white blood cell, and platelet counts.

Adverse reactions

● CNS: neuromuscular irritability, seizures.
● GI: nausea, diarrhea, vomiting, *pseudomembranous colitis.*
● GU: *acute interstitial nephritis.*
● HEMA: leukopenia, neutropenia, eosinophilia, *thrombocytopenia, hemolytic anemia, bleeding at high doses.*
● Metabolic: *hypokalemia.*
● Local: pain at injection site, vein irritation, phlebitis.
● Other: *hypersensitivity reactions* (rash, pruritus, urticaria, chills, fever, edema, *anaphylaxis*), bacterial and fungal superinfection.

Note: Drug should be discontinued if immediate hypersensitivity reactions occur, if bleeding complications occur, or if severe diarrhea occurs, as this may indicate pseudomembranous colitis.

Overdose and treatment

Clinical signs of overdose include neuromuscular hypersensitivity or seizures resulting from CNS irritation by high drug concentrations. Ticarcillin can be removed by hemodialysis.

▶ Special considerations

Besides those relevant to all *penicillins,* consider the following recommendations.
● Ticarcillin is almost always used with another antibiotic, such as an aminoglycoside, in life-threatening situations.
● Ticarcillin contains 5.2 mEq of sodium per gram of drug. Use with caution in patients who require sodium restriction.
● Monitor serum electrolytes to prevent hypokalemia and hypernatremia.
● Monitor neurologic status. High concentrations may cause seizures.
● Check complete blood count, differential, PT, and partial thromboplastin time. Drug may cause thrombocytopenia. Watch for signs of bleeding.
● Because ticarcillin is dialyzable, patients undergoing hemodialysis may need dosage adjustments.

Geriatric use

Half-life may be prolonged in elderly patients because of impaired renal function.

Pediatric use

Ticarcillin reconstituted for I.M. use with bacteriostatic water for injection containing benzyl alcohol should not be used in neonates because of toxicity.

Breast-feeding

Ticarcillin is excreted in breast milk; drug should be used cautiously in breast-feeding women.

---

ticarcillin disodium/clavulanate potassium
Timentin

- Pharmacologic classification: extended-spectrum penicillin, beta-lactamase inhibitor
- Therapeutic classification: antibiotic
- Pregnancy risk category B

How supplied
Available by prescription only
Injection: 3 g ticarcillin and 100 mg clavulanic acid

Indications, route, and dosage
Infections of the lower respiratory tract, urinary tract, bones and joints, skin and skin structure, and septicemia when caused by susceptible organisms
Adults: 3.1 g (contains 3 g ticarcillin and 0.1 g clavulanate potassium) diluted in 50 to 100 ml dextrose 5% and water, sodium chloride, or lactated Ringer's injection and administered by I.V. infusion over 30 minutes q 4 to 6 hours.
Dosage in renal failure
Loading dose: 3.1 g (3 g ticarcillin with 100 mg clavulanate)

Creatinine clearance (ml/min/1.73 m²)	Dosage in adults
> 60	3.1 g I.V. q 4 hours
30 to 60	2 g I.V. q 4 hours
10 to 30	2 g I.V. q 8 hours
< 10	2 g I.V. q 12 hours
< 10 with hepatic failure	2 g I.V. q 24 hours
Patients on hemodialysis	2 g I.V. q 12 hours, then 3.1 g after treatment
Patients on peritoneal dialysis	3.1 g I.V. q 12 hours

Pharmacodynamics
Antibiotic action: Ticarcillin is bactericidal; it adheres to bacterial penicillin-binding proteins, thus inhibiting bacterial cell wall synthesis. Extended-spectrum penicillins are more resistant to inactivation by certain beta-lactamases, especially those produced by gram-negative organisms, but are still liable to inactivation by certain others.

Clavulanic acid has only weak antibacterial activity and does not affect the action of ticarcillin. However, clavulanic acid has a beta-lactam ring and is structurally similar to penicillin and cephalosporins; it binds irreversibly with certain beta-lactamases, preventing inactivation of ticarcillin and broadening its bactericidal spectrum.

Ticarcillin's spectrum of activity includes many gram-negative aerobic and anaerobic bacilli, many gram-positive and gram-negative aerobic cocci, and some gram-positive aerobic and anaerobic bacilli. The combination of ticarcillin and clavulanate potassium is also effective against many beta-lactamase-producing strains, including *Staphylococcus aureus*, *Haemophilus influenzae*, *Neisseria gonorrhoeae*, *Escherichia coli*, *Klebsiella*, *Providencia*, and *Bacteroides fragilis*, but not *Pseudomonas aeruginosa*.

Pharmacokinetics
- *Absorption:* Ticarcillin disodium/calvulanate potassium is only administered intravenously; peak plasma concentration occurs immediately after infusion is complete.
- *Distribution:* Ticarcillin disodium is distributed widely. It penetrates minimally into CSF with uninflamed meninges; clavulanic acid penetrates into pleural fluid, lungs, and peritoneal fluid.

Ticarcillin sodium achieves high concentrations in urine. Protein-binding is 45% to 65% for ticarcillin and 22% to 30% for clavulanic acid; both cross the placenta.
- *Metabolism:* About 13% of a ticarcillin dose is metabolized by hydrolysis to inactive compounds; clavulanic acid is thought to undergo extensive metabolism, but its fate is as yet unknown.
- *Excretion:* Ticarcillin is excreted primarily (83% to 90%) in urine by renal tubular secretion and glomerular filtration; it is also excreted in bile and in breast milk. Clavulanate's metabolites are excreted in urine by glomerular filtration and in breast milk. Elimination half-life of ticarcillin in adults is about 1 hour and that of clavulanate is about 1 hour; in severe renal impairment, ticarcillin's half-life is extended to about 3 hours and that of clavulanate to about 4½ hours. Both drugs are removed by hemodialysis but only slightly by peritoneal dialysis.

Contraindications and precautions
Ticarcillin/clavulanate potassium is contraindicated in patients with known hypersensitivity to any other penicillin or to cephalosporins.

Ticarcillin/clavulanate potassium should be used with caution in patients with renal impairment because it is excreted in urine; decreased dosage is required in moderate to severe renal failure.

Interactions
Concomitant use of ticarcillin and clavulanate potassium with aminoglycoside antibiotics results in synergistic bactericidal effects against *Pseudomonas aeruginosa*, *Escherichia coli*, *Klebsiella*, *Citrobacter*, *Enterobacter*, *Serratia*, and *Proteus mirabilis*. However, the drugs are physically and chemically incompatible and are inactivated when mixed or given together. In vivo inactivation has been reported when aminoglycosides and extended-spectrum penicillins are used concomitantly.

Probenecid blocks tubular secretion of ticarcillin, raising its serum concentration; it has no effect on clavulanate.

Large doses of penicillin may interfere with renal tubular secretion of methotrexate, thus delaying elimination and elevating serum concentrations of methotrexate.

Effects on diagnostic tests
Ticarcillin/clavulanate potassium alters tests for urinary or serum proteins; it interferes with turbidimetric methods that use sulfosalicylic acid, trichloroacetic acid, acetic acid, or nitric acid. Ticarcillin/clavulanate potassium does not interfere with tests using bromophenol blue (Albustix, Albutest, MultiStix). Ticarcillin/clavulan-

ate potassium may falsely decrease serum aminoglycoside concentration.

Systemic effects of ticarcillin/clavulanate potassium may cause positive Coombs' test, hypokalemia, and hypernatremia and may prolong prothrombin times; it may also cause transient elevations in liver function studies and transient reductions in red blood cell, white blood cell, and platelet counts.

Adverse reactions
- CNS: neuromuscular irritability, *seizures.*
- GI: nausea, diarrhea, vomiting, *pseudomembranous colitis.*
- HEMA: leukopenia, neutropenia, eosinophilia, *thrombocytopenia, hemolytic anemia,* bleeding at high doses.
- Metabolic: *hypokalemia.*
- Local: pain at injection site, vein irritation, phlebitis.
- Other: hypersensitivity reactions (rash, pruritus, urticaria, chills, fever, edema, *anaphylaxis*), bacterial and fungal superinfection.

Note: Drug should be discontinued if immediate hypersensitivity reactions occur, if bleeding complications occur, or if severe diarrhea occurs, as this may indicate pseudomembranous colitis.

Overdose and treatment
Clinical signs of overdose include neuromuscular hypersensitivity or seizures; ticarcillin and clavulanate potassium can be removed by hemodialysis.

▶ Special considerations
Besides those relevant to all *penicillins*, consider the following recommendations.
- Ticarcillin/clavulanate potassium is almost always used with another antibiotic, such as an aminoglycoside, in life-threatening situations.
- Ticarcillin contains 5.2 mEq of sodium per gram of drug. Use with caution in patients with sodium restriction.
- Monitor serum electrolytes. Observe for signs of hypernatremia and hypokalemia.
- Monitor neurologic status. High blood levels may cause seizures.
- Because ticarcillin/clavulanate potassium is dialyzable, patients undergoing hemodialysis may need dosage adjustments.

Geriatric use
Half-life may be prolonged in elderly patients because of impaired renal function.

Breast-feeding
Ticarcillin and clavulanate potassium are excreted in breast milk; they should be used with caution in breast-feeding women.

ticlopidine hydrochloride
Ticlid

- Pharmacologic classification: platelet aggregation inhibitor
- Therapeutic classification: antithrombotic agent
- Pregnancy risk category B

How supplied
Available by prescription only
Tablets (film-coated): 250 mg

Indications, route, and dosage
To reduce the risk of thrombotic stroke in patients with a history of stroke or who have experienced stroke precursors
Adults: 250 mg P.O. b.i.d. with meals.

Pharmacodynamics
Antithrombotic action: Ticlopidine blocks adenosine diphosphate-induced platelet-fibrinogen and platelet-platelet binding.

Pharmacokinetics
- *Absorption:* Ticlopidine is rapidly and extensively (>80%) absorbed after oral administration; peak plasma levels occur within 2 hours. Absorption is enhanced by food.
- *Distribution:* Drug is 98% bound to serum proteins and lipoproteins.
- *Metabolism:* Drug is extensively metabolized by the liver. Over 20 metabolites have been identified; it is unknown if the parent drug or active metabolites are responsible for pharmacologic activity.
- *Excretion:* 60% of drug is excreted in the urine and 23% in the feces; only trace amounts of intact drug are found in the urine.

Contraindications and precautions
Ticlopidine is contraindicated in patients with hypersensitivity to the drug; in patients with hematopoietic disorders, such as neutropenia, thrombocytopenia, or disorders of hemostasis; in patients with active pathologic bleeding, such as peptic ulcer or active intracranial bleeding; and in those with severe liver impairment.

Use cautiously and with close monitoring of CBC and WBC differentials. Moderate to severe neutropenia and agranulocytosis have occurred in patients taking ticlopidine, usually within the first 3 weeks to 3 months of therapy; therefore, CBC and WBC differential determinations must be made beginning the second week of therapy and repeated every 2 weeks until the end of the third month of therapy. Increase the frequency of such tests in any patient showing signs of declining neutrophil count or a count that is 30% less than baseline.

Thrombocytopenia has occurred rarely. Drug should be discontinued in patients with platelet counts of 80,000 cells/mm³ or less.

Interactions
Concurrent use with antacids decreases plasma levels of ticlopidine; separate administration times by at least 2 hours. Use with aspirin potentiates aspirin's effects on platelets; avoid concomitant use. Use with cimeti-

dine decreases clearance of ticlopidine and increases risk of toxicity; avoid concomitant use. Use with digoxin causes slightly decreased serum digoxin levels; monitor serum digoxin levels. Use with theophylline causes decreased theophylline clearance and increased risk of toxicity; monitor closely and adjust theophylline dosage as indicated.

Effects on diagnostic tests
Pharmacologic effects of drug result in prolonged bleeding time. Toxic effects are evident in a decreased neutrophil or platelet count and elevated liver function tests. A positive antinuclear antibody titer has been reported rarely.

Adverse reactions
● CNS: dizziness, anorexia.
● CV: *vasculitis.*
● DERM: rash, purpura, pruritus, ecchymosis, maculopapular rash, urticaria, thrombocytopenic thrombotic purpura.
● EENT: epistaxis, conjunctival hemorrhage.
● GI: diarrhea, nausea, dyspepsia, vomiting, flatulence, GI pain, GI bleeding.
● GU: hematuria, *nephrotic syndrome.*
● HEMA: neutropenia, *pancytopenia, hemolytic anemia, immune thrombocytopenia,* increased serum cholesterol levels.
● Hepatic: hepatitis, cholestatic jaundice.
● Respiratory: *allergic pneumonitis.*
● Other: *allergic reactions,* postoperative bleeding, *systemic lupus, serum sickness, arthropathy, myositis, hyponatremia, peripheral neuropathy.*

Overdose and treatment
Only one case of overdosage has been reported. The patient, who ingested over 6 g of drug, showed increased bleeding time and increased ALT (SGPT) levels. The patient recovered with supportive therapy alone.

Special considerations
● If ticlopidine is being substituted for a fibrinolytic or anticoagulant drug, discontinue the previous drug before starting ticlopidine therapy.
● Patients scheduled for elective surgery should discontinue drug 10 to 14 days before the procedure.
● If necessary, methylprednisolone 20 mg I.V. has been shown to normalize the bleeding time within 2 hours. Platelet transfusions may also be necessary.
● After the first 3 months of therapy, CBC and WBC differential determinations need to be performed only in patients showing signs of infection.
● Perform baseline liver function tests and repeat whenever liver dysfunction is suspected. Monitor closely, especially during the first 4 months of treatment.
● Ticlopidine has been used investigationally for many conditions, including intermittent claudication, chronic arterial occlusion, subarachnoid hemorrhage, primary glomerulonephritis, and sickle cell disease. When used preoperatively, it may decrease incidence of graft occlusion in patients receiving coronary artery bypass grafts and reduce severity of decreased platelet count in patients receiving extracorporeal hemoperfusion during open heart surgery.

Information for the patient
● A patient information leaflet is available that discusses safe use of drug.

● Tell patient to take drug with meals. Taking the drug with food substantially increases bioavailability and improves GI tolerance.
● Be sure that patient understands the need to report for regular blood tests. Neutropenia can result in an increased risk of infection. Tell patient to immediately report any signs of infection, such as fever, chills, or sore throat.
● The patient should also immediately report yellow skin or sclera, severe or persistent diarrhea, skin rashes, subcutaneous bleeding, light-colored stools, or dark urine.
● Make sure patient understands that drug prolongs bleeding time. Tell him to report any unusual bleeding and to inform dentists and other physicians that he is taking ticlopidine.
● Warn patient to avoid aspirin and aspirin-containing products, which may also prolong bleeding. Because many OTC medications contain aspirin, patient should not take them without first checking with the physician or pharmacist.

Pediatric use
Safety and efficacy in children under age 18 have not been established.

Breast-feeding
Drug has been found in breast milk in animal studies; it is unknown if drug is excreted in human breast milk. Breast-feeding is not recommended.

timolol maleate
Blocadren, Timoptic

● Pharmacologic classification: beta-adrenergic blocking agent
● Therapeutic classification: antihypertensive agent, adjunct in myocardial infarction (MI); anti-glaucoma agent
● Pregnancy risk category C

How supplied
Available by prescription only
Tablets: 5 mg, 10 mg, 20 mg
Ophthalmic solution: 0.25%, 0.5%

Indications, route, and dosage
Hypertension
Adults: Initially, 10 mg P.O. b.i.d. Usual daily maintenance dosage is 20 to 40 mg. Maximum daily dosage is 60 mg.
To reduce the risk of cardiovascular mortality and reinfarction after MI
Adults: 10 mg P.O. b.i.d. initiated within 1 to 4 weeks after infarction.
Angina
Adults: 15 to 45 mg P.O. daily given in three divided doses.
Glaucoma
Adults: 1 drop of 0.25% or 0.5% solution to the conjunctiva one or two times a day.

Pharmacodynamics
● *Antihypertensive action:* The exact mechanism of timolol's antihypertensive effect is unknown. Timolol may reduce blood pressure by blocking adrenergic recep-

tors (thus decreasing cardiac output), by decreasing sympathetic outflow from the CNS, and by suppressing renin release.

• *MI prophylactic action:* The exact mechanism by which timolol decreases mortality after MI is unknown. Timolol produces a negative chronotropic and inotropic activity. This decrease in heart rate and myocardial contractility results in reduced myocardial oxygen consumption.

• *Antiglaucoma action:* Timolol's beta-blocking action decreases the production of aqueous humor, thereby decreasing intraocular pressure.

Pharmacokinetics
• *Absorption:* About 90% of an oral dose of timolol is absorbed from the GI tract; peak plasma concentration occurs in 1 to 2 hours.
• *Distribution:* After oral administration, timolol is distributed throughout the body; depending on assay method, drug is 10% to 60% protein-bound.
• *Metabolism:* About 80% of a given dose of timolol is metabolized in the liver to inactive metabolites.
• *Excretion:* Timolol and its metabolites are excreted primarily in urine; half-life is approximately 4 hours. After topical application to the eye, timolol's effects last up to 24 hours.

Contraindications and precautions
Timolol is contraindicated in patients with known hypersensitivity to the drug; in patients with severe bradycardia, overt cardiac failure, second- or third-degree atrioventricular block, or cardiogenic shock, because the drug may worsen these conditions; and in patients with bronchial asthma, allergic bronchospasm, or severe chronic obstructive pulmonary disease.

Timolol should be used cautiously in patients with impaired hepatic or renal function because of potential for impaired metabolism and excretion; in patients with cardiomyopathy because beta-adrenergic blockade may precipitate CHF; in patients with diabetes mellitus because it may mask some signs of hypoglycemia; and in patients with emphysema or other pulmonary disease because the drug may inhibit bronchodilating effects of endogenous catecholamines.

Interactions
When used as an antihypertensive, timolol may potentiate antihypertensive effects of other antihypertensive agents; its antihypertensive effects may be antagonized by nonsteroidal anti-inflammatory agents. Patients receiving ophthalmic or oral timolol may experience excessive hypotension when administered general anesthetics or fentanyl. Timolol may antagonize the effects of xanthines or beta-adrenergic stimulants. Cardiac arrhythmias may occur if used with calcium channel blocking agents or digitalis glycosides. Timolol may increase the plasma concentration of phenothiazines.

Effects on diagnostic tests
Timolol therapy may slightly increase BUN, serum potassium, uric acid, and blood glucose levels and may slightly decrease hemoglobin and hematocrit levels.

Adverse reactions
• CNS: fatigue, lethargy, vivid dreams.
• CV: *bradycardia, hypotension, CHF,* peripheral vascular disease, cold extremities.
• DERM: rash.

• GI: nausea, vomiting, diarrhea.
• GU: impotence.
• Metabolic: hypoglycemia without tachycardia.
• Other: wheezing, dyspnea, increased airway resistance, *bronchospasm,* fever.
   Note: Drug should be discontinued if signs of heart failure or bronchospasm develop.

Overdose and treatment
Clinical signs of overdose include severe hypotension, bradycardia, heart failure, and bronchospasm.

After acute ingestion, empty stomach by induced emesis or gastric lavage, and give activated charcoal to reduce absorption. Subsequent treatment is usually symptomatic and supportive.

▶ Special considerations
Besides those relevant to all *beta-adrenergic blocking agents,* consider the following recommendations.
• Dosage adjustment may be necessary for a patient with renal or hepatic impairment.
• Patients receiving ophthalmic timolol may need to discontinue the drug 48 hours before surgery because systemic absorption of the drug does occur. However, this practice remains controversial.

Information for the patient
For ophthalmic form of timolol, teach patient proper method of eye drop administration. Warn patient not to touch dropper to eye or surrounding tissue; lightly press lacrimal sac with finger after administration to decrease systemic absorption.

Geriatric use
Elderly patients may require lower oral maintenance dosages of timolol because of increased bioavailability or delayed metabolism; they also may experience enhanced adverse effects. Use with caution because half-life may be prolonged in elderly patients.

Pediatric use
Safety and efficacy of timolol in children have not been established; use only if potential benefit outweighs risk.

Breast-feeding
Timolol is distributed into breast milk. Because of the potential for serious adverse reactions in breast-fed infants, an alternative feeding method is recommended during therapy.

tioconazole
Vagistat

• Pharmacologic classification: imidazole derivative
• Therapeutic classification: antifungal
• Pregnancy risk category C

How supplied
Available by prescription only
Vaginal ointment: 6.5%

Indications, route, and dosage
Treatment of vulvovaginal candidiasis
Adults: Insert 1 applicatorful (about 4.6 g) intravaginally h.s.

Pharmacodynamics
Antifungal action: A fungicidal imidazole that alters cell wall permeability.

Pharmacokinetics
- *Absorption:* Negligible.
- *Distribution:* Unknown.
- *Metabolism:* Unknown.
- *Excretion:* Unknown.

Contraindications and precautions
Tioconazole is contraindicated in patients hypersensitive to the drug. Patients should discontinue use of the drug if irritation occurs.

Resistant infections could result from reinfection. Evaluate patients with persistent infections for sources of reinfection.

Note that intractable candidiasis may be a sign of diabetes mellitus. If patient does not respond to therapy, urine and blood glucose tests should be performed.

Effects on diagnostic tests
None reported.

Adverse reactions
- GU: burning, itching, discharge, vulvar edema and swelling, irritation.

Overdose and treatment
No information available.

▶ Special considerations
Because this drug is useful only for candidal vulvovaginitis, the diagnosis should be confirmed by potassium hydroxide smears or cultures before treatment with tioconazole.

Information for the patient
- Review correct use of the drug with the patient. Patient should insert drug high into the vagina. Detailed instructions for the patient are available with the product.
- Tell patient to avoid sexual intercourse during therapy or advise partner to use a condom to prevent reinfection.
- Warn patient to open applicator just before using the product to avoid contamination.
- Tell patient to watch for and report irritation or sensitivity.
- Emphasize to the patient the need to continue therapy for the full course, even if symptoms have improved, and during menstrual period.
- Advise the patient to use a sanitary napkin to avoid staining of clothing.

tiopronin
Thiola

- Pharmacologic classification: thiol compound
- Therapeutic classification: cystine-solubilizing agent
- Pregnancy risk category C

How supplied
Available by prescription only
Tablets: 100 mg

Indications, route, and dosage
Prevention of urinary cystine stone formation in patients with severe homozygous cystinuria (urinary cystine excretion exceeding 500 mg daily) unresponsive to other therapies
Adults: 800 mg P.O. daily, divided t.i.d. initially, then adjust dosage to control urinary cystine levels. Usual dosage is 1,000 mg daily in divided doses.
Children age 9 and over: 15 mg/kg P.O. daily, divided t.i.d.

Pharmacodynamics
Cystine solubilizing action: Tiopronin undergoes a thiol-disulfide exchange with cystine in the urine. This complex is water soluble, increases cystine solubility, and prevents the formation of urinary cystine stones.

Pharmacokinetics
- *Absorption:* Rapidly absorbed after oral administration.
- *Distribution:* Not fully characterized.
- *Metabolism:* Not fully characterized.
- *Excretion:* Up to 48% of a dose appears in the urine after 4 hours; 78% after 3 days.

Contraindications and precautions
Contraindicated in patients with a history of agranulocytosis, aplastic anemia, or thrombocytopenia after receiving tiopronin.

Rare complications to watch for include Goodpasture's syndrome (evidenced by abnormal urinary findings, pulmonary infiltrates, and hemoptysis), myasthenic syndrome (evidenced by severe muscle weakness), and the development of pemphigus-like reactions (evidenced by bullous skin eruptions). These complications have been noted during penicillamine therapy.

Drug fever may develop, especially during the first month of therapy. Discontinue drug until fever subsides, then therapy will probably be reinstituted at lower doses.

Skin rashes have been noted with tiopronin therapy. A generalized rash with mild pruritus that develops in the first few months of therapy may be well controlled with antihistamines, and disappears after discontinuing the drug. A less common rash that appears after at least 6 months of therapy appears on the trunk of the body and is accompanied by intense pruritus. This form of rash disappears slowly after discontinuing the drug.

Proteinuria, at times sufficiently severe to cause nephrotic syndrome, may develop from membranous glomerulopathy. Monitor closely.

---

*Canada only   †Unlabeled clinical use   Italicized adverse reactions are life-threatening.

Interactions
None reported.

Effects on diagnostic tests
None reported.

Adverse reactions
- DERM: rash, pruritus, wrinkling, friability.
- EENT: hypogeusia.
- Other: drug fever, lupus erythematosus-like reaction.

Overdose and treatment
No information available.

▶ **Special considerations**
- Dosage is usually adjusted to keep urinary cystine levels below 250 mg/liter.
- Conservative measures to treat cystinuria should be attempted before tiopronin is administered. Patients should drink at least 3 liters of fluid daily, including at least two 8-oz glasses of water at each meal and at bedtime. Patient's urine output should be at least 2 liters daily, and urine pH should be at least 6.5. Excessive alkalization of urine may precipitate calcium stones. Urine pH should not exceed 7.
- Some clinicians prefer to use penicillamine for cystinuria therapy, but patients may not tolerate it well. Studies indicate about two-thirds of patients who cannot tolerate penicillamine will tolerate tiopronin.
- Several clinical tests are recommended at 3- to 6-month intervals during treatment, including: complete blood count, platelet counts, hemoglobin, serum albumin, liver function tests, 24-hour urinary protein, and routine urinalysis.
- Urinary cystine should be monitored frequently during the first 6 months of treatment (to assess dosage level) and then at least every 6 months.
- An annual abdominal X-ray (KUB) is advised to assess for the presence of stones.

Information for the patient
- Tell patient to report any signs or symptoms of hematologic abnormalities, including fever, sore throat, bleeding or bruising, or chills. Blood dyscrasias have been reported in patients receiving other drugs for cystinuria.
- Whenever possible, tiopronin should be administered at least 1 hour before or 2 hours after meals.
- The patient should report any taste alterations. Hypogeusia may develop as a result of trace metal chelation by the drug.

Pediatric use
Safety and effectiveness in children under age 9 have not been established.

Breast-feeding
Breast-feeding is not recommended. The drug may be excreted in breast milk, and it may be hazardous to neonates and infants.

tobramycin

tobramycin ophthalmic
Tobrex

tobramycin sulfate
Nebcin

- Pharmacologic classification: aminoglycoside
- Therapeutic classification: antibiotic
- Pregnancy risk category D

How supplied
Available by prescription only
Injection: 40 mg/ml, 10 mg/ml (pediatric)
Ophthalmic solution: 0.3%
Ophthalmic ointment: 0.3%

Indications, route, and dosage
Serious infections caused by sensitive Escherichia coli, Proteus, Klebsiella, Enterobacter, Serratia, Staphylococcus aureus, Pseudomonas, Citrobacter, and Providencia
Adults and children with normal renal function: 3 mg/kg I.M. or I.V. daily, divided q 8 hours. Up to 5 mg/kg I.M. or I.V. daily, divided q 6 to 8 hours for life-threatening infections.
Neonates under 1 week: Up to 4 mg/kg I.M. or I.V. daily, divided q 12 hours. For I.V. use, dilute in 50 to 100 ml normal saline solution or dextrose 5% in water for adults and in less volume for children. Infuse over 20 to 60 minutes.
Patients with impaired renal function: Initial dosage is same as for those with normal renal function. Subsequent doses and frequency determined by renal function study results and blood levels; keep peak serum concentrations between 4 and 10 mcg/ml, and trough serum concentrations between 1 and 2 mcg/ml.
Treatment of external ocular infection caused by susceptible gram-negative bacteria
Adults and children: In mild to moderate infections, instill 1 or 2 drops into affected eye q 4 hours. In severe infections, instill 2 drops into the affected eye hourly.
Dosage in renal failure
Several methods have been used to calculate tobramycin dosage in renal failure.

After a 1 mg/kg loading dose, adjust subsequent dosage by reducing doses administered at 8-hour intervals or by prolonging the interval between normal doses. Both of these methods are useful when serum levels of tobramycin cannot be measured directly. They are based on either creatinine clearance (preferred) or serum creatinine because these values correlate with the half-life of tobramycin.

To calculate reduced dosage for 8-hour intervals, use available nomograms; or, if the patient's steady-state serum creatinine values are known, divide the normally recommended dose by the patient's serum creatinine value. To determine frequency in hours for normal dosage (if creatinine clearance rate is not available), divide the normal dose by the patient's serum creatinine value. Dosage schedules derived from either method require careful clinical and laboratory observations of the patient and should be adjusted as appropriate. These methods of calculation may be misleading in elderly patients and those with severe wasting; neither should be used when dialysis is performed.

Hemodialysis removes 50% of a dose in 6 hours. In anephric patients maintained by dialysis, 1.5 to 2 mg/ kg after each dialysis usually maintains therapeutic, nontoxic serum levels. Patients receiving peritoneal dialysis twice a week should receive a 1.5 to 2 mg/kg loading dose followed by 1 mg/kg every 3 days. Those receiving dialysis every 2 days should receive a 1.5 mg/kg loading dose after the first dialysis and 0.75 mg/ kg after each subsequent dialysis.

Pharmacodynamics

Antibiotic action: Tobramycin is bactericidal; it binds directly to the 30S ribosomal subunit, thereby inhibiting bacterial protein synthesis. Its spectrum of activity includes many aerobic gram-negative organisms, including most strains of *Pseudomonas aeruginosa* and some aerobic gram-positive organisms. Tobramycin may act against some bacterial strains resistant to other aminoglycosides; many strains resistant to tobramycin are susceptible to amikacin, gentamicin, or netilmicin.

Pharmacokinetics

● *Absorption:* Tobramycin is absorbed poorly after oral administration and usually is given parenterally; peak serum concentrations occur 30 to 90 minutes after I.M. administration.
● *Distribution:* Tobramycin is distributed widely after parenteral administration; intraocular penetration is poor. CSF penetration is low, even in patients with inflamed meninges. Protein binding is minimal. Tobramycin crosses the placenta.
● *Metabolism:* Not metabolized.
● *Excretion:* Tobramycin is excreted primarily in urine by glomerular filteration; small amounts may be excreted in bile and breast milk. Elimination half-life in adults is 2 to 3 hours. In severe renal damage, half-life may extend to 24 to 60 hours.

Contraindications and precautions

Tobramycin is contraindicated in patients with known hypersensitivity to tobramycin or any other aminoglycoside.

Tobramycin should be used cautiously in patients with decreased renal function; in patients with tinnitus, vertigo, and high-frequency hearing loss who are susceptible to ototoxicity; in patients with dehydration, myasthenia gravis, parkinsonism, and hypocalcemia; in neonates and other infants; and in elderly patients.

Interactions

Concomitant use with the following drugs may increase the hazard of nephrotoxicity, ototoxicity, and neurotoxicity: methoxyflurane, polymyxin B, vancomycin, capreomycin, cisplatin, cephalosporins, amphotericin B, and other aminoglycosides; hazard of ototoxicity is also increased during use with ethacrynic acid, furosemide, bumetanide, urea, or mannitol. Dimenhydrinate and other antiemetic and antivertigo drugs may mask tobramycin-induced ototoxicity.

Concomitant use with penicillin results in a synergistic bactericidal effect against *P. aeruginosa, E. coli, Klebsiella, Citrobacter, Enterobacter, Serratia,* and *Proteus mirabilis.* However, the drugs are physically and chemically incompatible and are inactivated when mixed or given together. In vivo inactivation has been reported when aminoglycosides and penicillins are used concomitantly.

Tobramycin may potentiate neuromuscular blockade from general anesthetics or neuromuscular blocking agents such as succinylcholine and tubocurarine.

Effects on diagnostic tests

Tobramycin may elevate BUN, nonprotein nitrogen, or serum creatinine levels and increase urinary excretion of casts.

Adverse reactions

● CNS: headache, lethargy, *neuromuscular blockade with respiratory depression.*
● EENT: ototoxicity (tinnitus, vertigo, hearing loss); with ophthalmic use, burning or stinging on instillation, lid itching or lid swelling.
● GI: diarrhea.
● GU: *nephrotoxicity* (cells or casts in the urine, oliguria, proteinuria, decreased creatinine clearance, increased BUN, serum creatinine, and nonprotein nitrogen levels).
● Other: hypersensitivity reactions (eosinophilia, fever, rash, urticaria, pruritus), bacterial or fungal superinfection.
Note: Drug should be discontinued if signs of ototoxicity, nephrotoxicity, or hypersensitivity occur.

Overdose and treatment

Clinical signs of overdose include ototoxicity, nephrotoxicity, and neuromuscular toxicity. Remove drug by hemodialysis or peritoneal dialysis. Treatment with calcium salts or anticholinesterases reverses neuromuscular blockade.

▶ Special considerations

Besides those relevant to all *aminoglycosides,* consider the following recommendations.
● Some studies suggest tobramycin may be less nephrotoxic than gentamicin.
● Discontinue ophthalmic preparation if keratitis, erythema, lacrimation, edema, or lid itching occurs.
● Because tobramycin is dialyzable, patients undergoing hemodialysis may need dosage adjustments.

---

tocainide hydrochloride
Tonocard

● Pharmacologic classification: local anesthetic (amide type)
● Therapeutic classification: ventricular antiarrhythmic
● Pregnancy risk category C

How supplied

Available by prescription only
Tablets: 400 mg, 600 mg

Indications, route, and dosage
Suppression of symptomatic ventricular arrhythmias, including frequent premature ventricular tachycardia
Adults: Initially, 400 mg P.O. q 8 hours. Usual dosage is between 1,200 and 1,800 mg/day, divided into three doses.

Pharmacodynamics

Antiarrhythmic action: Tocainide is structurally similar to lidocaine and possesses similar electrophysiologic and hemodynamic effects. A Class IB antiarrhythmic, it suppresses automaticity and shortens the effective refractory period and action potential duration of His-Purkinje fibers and suppresses spontaneous ventricular depolarization during diastole. Conductive atrial tissue and AV conduction are not affected significantly at therapeutic concentrations. Unlike quinidine and procainamide, tocainide does not significantly alter hemodynamics when administered in usual doses. Tocainide exerts its effects on the conduction system, causing inhibition of reentry mechanisms and cessation of ventricular arrhythmias; these effects may be more pronounced in ischemic tissue. Tocainide does not cause a significant negative inotropic effect. Its direct cardiac effects are less potent than those of lidocaine.

Pharmacokinetics

● *Absorption:* Tocainide is rapidly and completely absorbed from the gastrointestinal tract; unlike lidocaine, it undergoes negligible first-pass effect in the liver. Peak serum levels occur in 30 minutes to 2 hours after oral administration. Bioavailability is nearly 100%.
● *Distribution:* Tocainide's distribution is only partially known. However, it appears to be distributed widely and apparently crosses the blood-brain barrier and placenta in animals (however, it is less lipophilic than lidocaine). Only about 10% to 20% of the drug is bound to plasma protein.
● *Metabolism:* Tocainide is metabolized apparently in the liver to inactive metabolites.
● *Excretion:* Tocainide is excreted in the urine as unchanged drug and inactive metabolites. About 30% to 50% of an orally administered dose is excreted in the urine as metabolites. Elimination half-life is approximately 11 to 23 hours, with an initial biphasic plasma concentration decline similar to that of lidocaine's. Half-life may be prolonged in patients with renal or hepatic insufficiency. Urine alkalinization may decrease substantially the amount of unchanged drug excreted in the urine.

Contraindications and precautions

Tocainide is contraindicated in patients with second- or third-degree heart block who do not have an artificial pacemaker, because the drug may further decrease conduction; and in patients with hypersensitivity to amide-type anesthetic agents, including lidocaine. Tocainide appears to have less effect on conduction than quinidine and procainamide.

Tocainide should be used with caution in patients with congestive heart failure, because the drug has a mild negative inotropic action and may slightly increase systemic vascular resistance, thereby exacerbating heart failure; in patients with atrial flutter or ventricular fibrillation, because the drug may accelerate the ventricular rate; in patients with preexisting bone marrow failure or cytopenia, because the drug may cause adverse hematologic effects; and in patients with severe renal or hepatic dysfunction, because the drug may accumulate and cause toxicity.

Interactions

When used concomitantly with other antiarrhythmics, tocainide may cause additive, synergistic, or antagonistic effects. (Concomitant use with lidocaine may cause CNS toxicity.) Concomitant use with metoprolol may cause additive effects on cardiac index, left ventricular function, and pulmonary wedge pressure, necessitating monitoring for decreased myocardial contractility and bradycardia.

Effects on diagnostic tests

None reported.

Adverse reactions

● CNS: light-headedness, tremors, restlessness, paresthesias, confusion, dizziness.
● CV: hypotension, conduction disturbances, *CHF, arrhythmias.*
● DERM: rash.
● EENT: blurred vision.
● GI: nausea, vomiting, epigastric pain, constipation, diarrhea, anorexia.
● HEMA: aplastic anemia, *agranulocytosis.*
● Respiratory: cough, wheezing, dyspnea, *pulmonary fibrosis.*
Note: Drug should be discontinued if signs or symptoms of adverse hematologic, pulmonary, or cardiac effects (including worsening CHF or cardiac conductivity, despite adequate therapy or without external pacing) occur.

Overdose and treatment

Clinical effects of overdose include extensions of common adverse reactions, particularly those associated with the CNS and GI tract.

Treatment generally involves symptomatic and supportive care. In acute overdose, gastric emptying should be performed via emesis induction or gastric lavage. Respiratory depression necessitates immediate attention and maintenance of a patent airway with ventilatory assistance, if required. Convulsions may be treated with small incremental doses of a benzodiazepine, such as diazepam, or a short or ultrashort-acting barbiturate, such as pentobarbital or thiopental.

▶ Special considerations

● Use cautiously in patients with hepatic or renal impairment; such patients may be treated effectively with a lower dose.
● Monitor blood levels; therapeutic levels range from 4 to 10 mcg/ml.
● Monitor periodic blood counts.
● Observe patient for tremors – a possible sign that maximum safe dosage has been reached.
● Adverse reactions are generally mild, transient, and reversible with dosage reduction. Gastrointestinal reactions may be minimized by administering drug with food.
● Drug is considered an oral lidocaine and may be used to ease transition from I.V. lidocaine to oral antiarrhythmic therapy.

Information for the patient

Instruct patient to report any unusual bleeding or bruising; signs of infection, such as fever, sore throat, stomatitis, or chills; or pulmonary symptoms, such as cough, wheezing, or exertional dyspnea.

Geriatric use

● Drug should be used with caution in elderly patients; increased serum drug levels and toxicity are more likely. Monitor patients carefully.
● Elderly patients are more likely to experience dizziness and should have assistance while walking.

Breast-feeding
Safety has not been established. Alternative feeding method is recommended during therapy with tocainide.

tolazamide
Ronase, Tolinase

- Pharmacologic classification: sulfonylurea
- Therapeutic classification: antidiabetic agent
- Pregnancy risk category D

How supplied
Available by prescription only
Tablets: 100 mg, 250 mg, 500 mg

Indications, route, and dosage
Adjunct to diet to lower blood glucose levels in patients with non-insulin-dependent diabetes mellitus (Type II)
Adults: Initially, 100 mg P.O. daily with breakfast if fasting blood sugar (FBS) is under 200 mg/dl; or 250 mg if FBS is over 200 mg/dl. May adjust dosage at weekly intervals by 100 to 250 mg. Maximum dosage is 500 mg b.i.d. before meals.
Adults over age 65: 100 mg once daily.
To change from insulin to oral therapy
If insulin dosage is under 20 units daily, insulin may be stopped and oral therapy started at 100 mg P.O. daily with breakfast. If insulin dosage is 20 to 40 units daily, insulin may be stopped and oral therapy started at 250 mg P.O. daily with breakfast. If insulin dosage is over 40 units daily, decrease insulin dosage by 50% and start oral therapy at 250 mg P.O. daily with breakfast. Increase dosages as above.

EQUIVALENT DOSAGE OF ORAL HYPOGLYCEMIC AGENTS

Hypoglycemic agents	Dosage	Dosage tolazamide
acetohexamide	250 mg/day	100 mg/day
chlorpropamide	250 mg/day	250 mg/day
tolbutamide	1 g/day or less	100 mg/day
	1 g/day or more	250 mg/day

Pharmacodynamics
Antidiabetic action: Tolazamide lowers blood glucose levels by stimulating insulin release from functioning beta cells of the pancreas. After prolonged administration, the drug's hypoglycemic effects appear to reflect extrapancreatic effects, possibly including reduction of basal hepatic glucose production and enhanced peripheral sensitivity to insulin. The latter may result from an increase in the number of insulin receptors or to changes in events subsequent to insulin binding.

Pharmacokinetics
- *Absorption:* Tolazamide is absorbed slowly but well from the GI tract. Onset of action occurs within 4 to 6 hours, with maximum hypoglycemic effect within 10 hours.
- *Distribution:* Tolazamide probably is distributed into the extracellular fluid.
- *Metabolism:* Tolazamide is metabolized to several mildly active metabolites.
- *Excretion:* Tolazamide is excreted in urine primarily as metabolites, with small amounts excreted as unchanged drug. The duration of action is 12 to 24 hours; half-life is 7 hours.

Contraindications and precautions
Tolazamide is contraindicated in patients with known hypersensitivity to sulfonylureas or thiazides and in patients with nonfunctioning pancreatic beta cells. It should not be used in patients with burns, acidosis, diabetic coma, severe infection, ketosis, or severe trauma or in those who are undergoing major surgery, because such conditions of severe physiologic stress require insulin for adequate blood glucose control.
Tolazamide should be used cautiously in patients with hepatic or renal insufficiency because of the important roles of the liver in metabolism and the kidneys in elimination; and in patients with impaired adrenal, pituitary, and thyroid function.

Interactions
Concomitant use of tolazamide with alcohol may produce a disulfiram-like reaction consisting of nausea, vomiting, abdominal cramps, and headaches. Concomitant use with anticoagulants may increase plasma levels of both drugs and, after continued therapy, may reduce the plasma levels and anticoagulant effects. Use with chloramphenicol, guanethidine, insulin, monoamine oxidase inhibitors, probenecid, salicylates, or sulfonamides may enhance the hypoglycemic effect by displacing tolazamide from its protein-binding sites.
Concomitant use with beta-adrenergic blocking agents (including ophthalmics) may increase the risk of hypoglycemia, mask its symptoms (rising pulse rate and blood pressure), and prolong it by blocking gluconeogenesis. Use with drugs that may increase blood glucose levels (adrenocorticoids, glucocorticoids, amphetamines, baclofen, corticotropin, epinephrine, ethacrynic acid, furosemide, phenytoin, thiazide diuretics, triamterene, and thyroid hormones) may require dosage adjustments.
Because smoking increases corticosteroid release, smokers may require higher doses of tolazamide.

Effects on diagnostic tests
Tolazamide therapy alters alkaline phosphatase and cholesterol levels.

Adverse reactions
- CNS: weakness, paresthesias, lethargy, confusion.
- DERM: eczema, pruritus, erythema, urticaria, facial flushing, morbilliform or maculopapular eruptions.
- GI: cholestatic jaundice, nausea, epigastric fullness, heartburn, diarrhea.
- HEMA: leukopenia, thrombocytopenia, mild anemia, *agranulocytosis.*
- Metabolic: hypoglycemia.
- Other: hypersensitivity reactions.
Note: Drug should be discontinued if signs or symptoms of hypersensitivity, including jaundice, skin eruptions, blood dyscrasias, and severe diarrhea, occur or if serial and progressive increases in serum alkaline phosphatase levels occur.

Overdose and treatment

Clinical manifestations of overdose include low blood glucose levels, tingling of lips and tongue, hunger, nausea, decreased cerebral function (lethargy, yawning, confusion, agitation, nervousness), increased sympathetic activity (tachycardia, sweating, tremor), and ultimately, seizures, stupor, and coma.

Mild hypoglycemia, without loss of consciousness or neurologic findings, responds to treatment with oral glucose and dosage adjustments. If the patient loses consciousness or develops neurologic findings, he should receive rapid injection of dextrose 50%, followed by a continuous infusion of dextrose 10% at a rate to maintain blood glucose levels greater than 100 mg/dl. Monitor for 24 to 48 hours.

▶ Special considerations

Besides those relevant to all *sulfonylureas,* consider the following recommendations.
● To avoid GI intolerance for those patients receiving dosages of 500 mg/day or more and to improve control of hyperglycemia, divided doses are recommended; these are given before the morning and evening meals.
● Tablets may be crushed to ease administration.
● Elderly, debilitated, or malnourished patients and those with impaired renal or hepatic function usually require a lower initial dosage.
● When substituting tolazamide for chlorpropamide therapy, monitor patient closely for 1 week because of chlorpropamide's prolonged retention in the body.
● Use with caution in women of childbearing age. Tolazamide is not recommended for treatment of diabetes associated with pregnancy.
● Oral hypoglycemic agents have been associated with an increased risk of cardiovascular mortality as compared to diet or diet and insulin therapy.

Information for the patient

● Emphasize to patient the importance of following prescribed diet, exercise, and medical regimen.
● Advise patient to take medication at the same time each day. Tell patient that, if a dose is missed, it should be taken immediately, unless it is almost time to take the next dose. Patient should not take double doses.
● Warn patient to avoid alcohol while taking tolazamide. Remind him that many foods and nonprescription medications contain alcohol. Alcohol in moderate to large amounts will cause a disulfiram-like reaction.
● Encourage patient to wear a Medic Alert bracelet or necklace.
● Recommend that patient take the medication with food, if it causes GI upset.
● Teach patient how to monitor blood glucose, urine glucose, and ketone levels, as prescribed.
● Teach patient how to recognize the signs and symptoms of hypoglycemia and hyperglycemia and what to do if they occur.

Geriatric use

● Elderly patients may be more sensitive to the effects of this medication because of reduced metabolism and elimination.
● Hypoglycemia causes more neurologic symptoms in elderly patients.
● Elderly patients usually require a lower initial dosage.

Pediatric use

Tolazamide is ineffective in insulin-dependent (Type I, juvenile-onset) diabetes.

Breast-feeding

Because of the risk of hypoglycemia in the breast-fed infant, a decision should be made to discontinue the drug or to discontinue breast-feeding.

---

tolazoline hydrochloride
Priscoline

● Pharmacologic classification: peripheral vasodilator, alpha-adrenergic blocking agent
● Therapeutic classification: antihypertensive
● Pregnancy risk category C

How supplied

Available by prescription only
Injection: 25 mg/ml in 10-ml vials

Indications, route, and dosage
Persistent pulmonary vasoconstriction and hypertension of the newborn (persistent fetal circulation)
Initially, 1 to 2 mg/kg I.V. via a scalp vein over 10 minutes, followed by an I.V. infusion of 1 to 2 mg/kg/hour.

Pharmacodynamics

Antihypertensive action: Tolazoline, by direct relaxation of vascular smooth muscle, causes peripheral vasodilation and decreased peripheral resistance. Tolazoline inhibits responses to adrenergic stimuli by competitively blocking alpha-adrenergic receptors; however, at usual doses, this effect is relatively transient and incomplete.

Pharmacokinetics

● *Absorption:* Tolazoline is absorbed rapidly and almost completely after parenteral administration.
● *Distribution:* Tolazoline concentrates primarily in kidneys and liver.
● *Metabolism:* None.
● *Excretion:* Tolazoline is excreted in urine, primarily as unchanged drug; half-life is inversely related to urine output and can range from 1.5 to 41 hours.

Contraindications and precautions

Tolazoline is contraindicated in patients with known hypersensitivity to the drug and in patients with known or suspected coronary artery disease or after a cerebrovascular accident.

Tolazoline should be used cautiously in patients with gastritis or peptic ulcer disease because the drug can stimulate gastric secretion; and in patients with mitral stenosis because the drug can increase or decrease pulmonary artery pressure and total pulmonary resistance. Tolazoline may activate stress ulcers.

Interactions

Tolazoline may cause a disulfiram-type reaction after alcohol ingestion because of the accumulation of acetaldehyde.

Concomitant use with epinephrine or norepinephrine may cause "epinephrine reversal"—a paradoxical decrease in blood pressure followed by exaggerated rebound hypertension.

---

*Canada only   †Unlabeled clinical use   Italicized adverse reactions are life-threatening.

Effects on diagnostic tests
None reported.

Adverse reactions
- CNS: headache, dizziness, sweating.
- CV: *orthostatic hypotension, tachycardia, arrhythmias, pulmonary hemorrhage, marked hypertension,* shock.
- DERM: flushing, increased pilomotor activity.
- GI: nausea, vomiting, diarrhea, hepatitis.
- GU: oliguria, hematuria.
- HEMA: thrombocytopenia, *agranulocytosis.*

Overdose and treatment
Clinical manifestations of overdose include flushing, hypotension, and shock.

Treat overdose symptomatically and supportively; if vasopressor is necessary, use ephedrine, which has both central and peripheral actions. Avoid epinephrine or norepinephrine because epinephrine reversal may occur from the alpha-blocking effects of tolazoline.

▶ Special considerations
- Keeping patient warm increases drug's effect.
- Monitor blood pH for acidosis, which may reduce drug's effect.
- Tolazoline has been used in adults as a provocative test for glaucoma; intraarterially to improve vascular visualization during angiography; as a diagnostic agent to distinguish between vasospastic or obstructive components of occlusive peripheral vascular disease; and as adjunctive therapy in the treatment of peripheral vascular disorders.

Information for the patient
Advise patient's family of treatment required.

Pediatric use
- Drug is indicated for neonatal hypertension and pulmonary vasoconstriction.
- Pretreatment of infants with antacids may prevent GI bleeding.

tolbutamide
Apo-Tolbutamide*, Mobenol*, Novobutamide*, Oramide, Orinase, SK-Tolbutamide

- Pharmacologic classification: sulfonylurea
- Therapeutic classification: antidiabetic agent
- Pregnancy risk category D

How supplied
Available by prescription only
Tablets: 250 mg, 500 mg

Indications, route, and dosage
Stable, maturity-onset nonketotic diabetes mellitus uncontrolled by diet alone and previously untreated
Adults: Initially, 1 to 2 g P.O. daily as single dose or divided b.i.d. or t.i.d. May adjust dosage to maximum of 3 g daily.

To change from insulin to oral therapy
If insulin dosage is under 20 units daily, insulin may be stopped and oral therapy started at 1 to 2 g daily. If insulin dosage is 20 to 40 units daily, insulin dosage is reduced 30% to 50% and oral therapy started as above. If insulin dosage is over 40 units daily, insulin dosage is decreased 20% and oral therapy started as above. Further reductions in insulin dosage are based on patient's response to oral therapy.

Pharmacodynamics
Antidiabetic action: Tolbutamide lowers blood glucose levels by stimulating insulin release from functioning beta cells of the pancreas. After prolonged administration, the drug's hypoglycemic effects appear to reflect extrapancreatic effects, possibly including reduction of basal hepatic glucose production and enhanced peripheral sensitivity to insulin. The latter may result from an increase in the number of insulin receptors or from changes in events subsequent to insulin binding.

Pharmacokinetics
- *Absorption:* Tolbutamide is absorbed readily from the GI tract. Onset of action occurs within 1 hour. The maximum hypoglycemic activity occurs within 8 hours.
- *Distribution:* Tolbutamide probably is distributed into the extracellular fluid. It is 95% protein-bound.
- *Metabolism:* Tolbutamide is metabolized in the liver to inactive metabolites.
- *Excretion:* Tolbutamide and its metabolites are excreted in urine and feces. The duration of action is 6 to 12 hours. Half-life is 4 to 5 hours.

Contraindications and precautions
Tolbutamide is contraindicated in patients with known hypersensitivity to sulfonylureas or thiazides and in patients with nonfunctioning pancreatic beta cells. It should not be used in patients with burns, acidosis, diabetic coma, severe infection, ketosis, or severe trauma or in those who require major surgery, because such conditions of physiologic stress require insulin for adequate control of glucose levels.

Tolbutamide should be used cautiously in patients with hepatic or renal insufficiency because of the important roles of the liver in metabolism and the kidneys in elimination; and in patients with impaired adrenal, pituitary, or thyroid function.

Interactions
Concomitant use of tolbutamide with alcohol may produce a disulfiram-like reaction consisting of nausea, vomiting, abdominal cramps, and headaches. Concomitant use with anticoagulants may increase plasma levels of both drugs and, after continued therapy, may reduce plasma levels and anticoagulant effect. Use with chloramphenicol, guanethidine, insulin, monoamine oxidase inhibitors, probenecid, salicylates, or sulfonamides may enhance the hypoglycemic effect by displacing tolbutamide from its protein-binding sites. Concomitant use with beta-adrenergic blocking agents (including ophthalmics) may increase the risk of hypoglycemia by masking its developing symptoms, such as rising pulse rate and blood pressure, and may prolong hypoglycemia by blocking gluconeogenesis.

Use with drugs that may increase blood glucose levels (adrenocorticoids, glucocorticoids, amphetamines, baclofen, corticotropin, epinephrine, ethacrynic acid, furosemide, phenytoin, thiazide diuretics, triamterene, and thyroid hormones) may require dosage adjustments.

Because smoking increases corticosteroid release, smokers may require higher doses of tolbutamide.

Effects on diagnostic tests
Tolbutamide therapy alters alkaline phosphatase, bilirubin, cholesterol, total protein, and urine porphyrins and protein levels; it also alters cephalin flocculation (thymol turbidity) and ^{131}I thyroid uptake.

Adverse reactions
● CNS: weakness, paresthesias.
● DERM: eczema, pruritus, erythema, urticaria, facial flushing, morbilliform or maculopapular eruptions.
● GI: cholestatic jaundice, nausea, epigastric fullness, heartburn.
● HEMA: leukopenia, thrombocytopenia, mild anemia, *agranulocytosis.*
● Metabolic: hypoglycemia, dilutional hyponatremia.
● Other: *hypersensitivity reactions.*
Note: Drug should be discontinued if signs or symptoms of hypersensitivity, including jaundice, skin eruptions, blood dyscrasias, and severe diarrhea, occur or if serial and progressive increases in serum alkaline phosphatase levels occur.

Overdose and treatment
Clinical manifestations of overdose include low blood glucose levels, tingling of lips and tongue, hunger, nausea, decreased cerebral function (lethargy, yawning, confusion, agitation, nervousness), increased sympathetic activity (tachycardia, sweating, tremor), and ultimately, seizures, stupor, and coma.

Mild hypoglycemia, without loss of consciousness or neurologic findings, responds to treatment with oral glucose and dosage adjustments. If patient loses consciousness or develops neurologic findings, the patient should receive rapid injection of dextrose 50%, followed by a continuous infusion of dextrose 10% at a rate to maintain blood glucose levels greater than 100 mg/dl. Monitor for 24 to 48 hours.

▶ Special considerations
Besides those relevant to all *sulfonylureas,* consider the following recommendations.
● Elderly or debilitated patients and those with impaired renal or hepatic function usually require a lower initial dosage.
● Tablets may be crushed for ease of administration.
● Physiologic stress (for example, resulting from infection) may cause loss of blood glucose control.
● To avoid GI intolerance for those patients on larger doses and to improve control of hyperglycemia, divided doses given before the morning and evening meals are recommended.
● Patients should avoid taking tolbutamide at bedtime because of the potential for nocturnal hypoglycemia.
● Use with caution in women of childbearing age. Tolbutamide is not recommended for treatment of diabetes associated with pregnancy.
● Oral hypoglycemic agents have been associated with an increased risk of cardiovascular mortality as compared to diet or diet and insulin therapy.

Information for the patient
● Emphasize to patient the importance of following prescribed diet, exercise, and medical regimen.

● Instruct patient to take the medication at the same time each day.
● Inform patient that, if a dose is missed, it should be taken immediately, unless it's almost time to take the next dose. Patient should not take double doses.
● Advise patient to avoid alcohol while taking tolbutamide. Remind him that many foods and nonprescription medications contain alcohol.
● Encourage patient to wear a Medic Alert bracelet or necklace.
● Suggest that patient take the medication with food if it causes GI upset.
● Teach patient how to monitor blood glucose, urine glucose, and ketone levels, as prescribed.
● Teach patient how to recognize the signs and symptoms of hypoglycemia and hyperglycemia and what to do if they occur.

Geriatric use
● Elderly patients may be more sensitive to the effects of this medication because of reduced metabolism and elimination.
● Hypoglycemia causes more neurologic symptoms in elderly patients.
● Elderly patients usually require a lower initial dosage.

Pediatric use
Tolbutamide is ineffective in insulin-dependent (Type I, juvenile-onset) diabetes.

Breast-feeding
Tolbutamide is excreted in breast milk. Because of the risk of hypoglycemia in the breast-fed infant, a decision should be made to discontinue the drug or to discontinue breast-feeding.

---

tolmetin sodium
Tolectin, Tolectin DS

● Pharmacologic classification: nonsteroidal anti-inflammatory
● Therapeutic classification: nonnarcotic analgesic, antipyretic, anti-inflammatory
● Pregnancy risk category C (D in third trimester)

How supplied
Available by prescription only
Tablets: 200 mg
Tablets (coated): 600 mg
Capsules: 400 mg

Indications, route, and dosage
Rheumatoid arthritis and osteoarthritis, juvenile rheumatoid arthritis
Adults: 400 mg P.O. t.i.d. or q.i.d. Maximum dosage is 2 g/day.
Children age 2 or older: 15 to 30 mg/kg/day in three or four divided doses.

Pharmacodynamics
Anti-inflammatory, analgesic, and antipyretic actions: Mechanisms of action are unknown; the drug is thought to inhibit prostaglandin synthesis.

Pharmacokinetics
● *Absorption:* Drug is absorbed rapidly from the GI tract.
● *Distribution:* Drug is highly protein-bound.
● *Metabolism:* Tolmetin is metabolized in the liver.
● *Excretion:* Tolmetin is excreted in urine.

Contraindications and precautions
Tolmetin is contraindicated in patients with known hypersensitivity to tolmetin or zomepirac, or in patients in whom aspirin or other nonsteroidal anti-inflammatory drugs (NSAIDs) induce symptoms of asthma, urticaria, or rhinitis.

Serious GI toxicity, especially ulceration or hemorrhage, can occur at any time in patients on chronic NSAID therapy. Tolmetin should be used cautiously in patients with a history of GI bleeding or GI ulcer because the drug may irritate the GI tract; in patients with renal disease because the drug may be nephrotoxic; or in patients with cardiac disease because it may cause peripheral edema, sodium retention, and hypertension.

Patients with known "triad" symptoms (aspirin hypersensitivity, rhinitis/nasal polyps, and asthma) are at high risk of cross-sensitivity to tolmetin with precipitation of bronchospasm.

The signs and symptoms of acute infection (fever, myalgias, erythema) may be masked by the use of tolmetin. Evaluate patients with high infection risk (such as those with diabetes) carefully.

Interactions
When used concomitantly, anticoagulants and thrombolytic drugs may be potentiated by the platelet-inhibiting effect of tolmetin. Concomitant use of tolmetin with highly protein-bound drugs (for example, phenytoin, sulfonylureas, warfarin) may cause displacement of either drug and adverse effects. Monitor therapy closely for both drugs. Concomitant use with other GI-irritating drugs (such as steroids, antibiotics, NSAIDs) may potentiate the adverse GI effects of tolmetin. Use with caution.

Antacids and food delay and decrease the absorption of tolmetin. NSAIDs are known to decrease renal clearance of lithium carbonate, thus increasing lithium serum levels and risks of adverse effects. Concomitant use of tolmetin and aspirin may decrease plasma levels of tolmetin.

Effects on diagnostic tests
Tolmetin falsely elevates results of urinary protein assays (pseudoproteinuria) in tests using sulfosalicylic acid (not reagent strips like Albustix or Unistix). The physiologic effects of the drug may result in an increased bleeding time; increased BUN, serum potassium, and serum transaminase levels; and decreased hemoglobin and hematocrit levels.

Adverse reactions
● CNS: headache, drowsiness, dizziness.
● CV: hypertension, *CHF*.
● DERM: pruritus, rash, urticaria.
● EENT: tinnitus, visual disturbances.
● GI: epigastric distress, nausea, occult blood loss, diarrhea, constipation, GI bleeding.
● GU: nephrotoxicity, hematuria, urinary tract infection, pseudoproteinuria.
● HEMA: prolonged bleeding time, leukopenia, *hemolytic anemia*.
● Other: sodium retention, edema, *hepatotoxicity*.

Note: Drug should be discontinued if hypersensitivity or signs and symptoms of hepatic or renal toxicity occur.

Overdose and treatment
Clinical manifestations of overdose include dizziness, drowsiness, mental confusion, lethargy.

To treat tolmetin overdose, empty stomach immediately by inducing emesis or by gastric lavage followed by administration of activated charcoal. Provide symptomatic and supportive measures (respiratory support and correction of fluid and electrolyte imbalances). Monitor laboratory parameters and vital signs closely. Alkalinization of urine via sodium bicarbonate ingestion may enhance renal excretion of tolmetin.

▶ Special considerations
Besides those relevant to all *NSAIDs,* consider the following recommendations.
● Assess cardiopulmonary status closely. Tolmetin may cause sodium retention. Monitor vital signs closely, especially heart rate and blood pressure.
● Assess renal function periodically during therapy; monitor intake and output and daily weight.
● Monitor for presence and amount of edema.
● Therapeutic effect usually occurs within a few days to 1 week of therapy. Evaluate patient's response to drug as evidenced by relief of symptoms.

Information for the patient
● Explain that therapeutic effects may occur in 1 week but could take 2 to 4 weeks.
● Advise patient to avoid use of nonprescription medications unless medically approved. Warn patient not to take sodium bicarbonate, which may decrease effectiveness of drug.
● Instruct patient to follow prescribed regimen and recommended schedule of follow-up.
● Advise patient to report any signs of edema; encourage routine check of blood pressure.
● Instruct patient to routinely check weight and to report any significant gain of 3 pounds or more within 1 week.
● Instruct patient in safety measures to prevent injury.

Geriatric use
● Patients over age 60 are more sensitive to the adverse effects of tolmetin.
● Because of its effect on renal prostaglandin, tolmetin may cause fluid retention and edema. This may be significant in elderly patients and in those with CHF.

Pediatric use
The safe use of tolmetin in children under age 2 has not been established.

Breast-feeding
Because small quantities of tolmetin are secreted in breast milk, avoid use in breast-feeding women.

---

tranylcypromine sulfate
Parnate

- Pharmacologic classification: monoamine oxidase inhibitor
- Therapeutic classification: antidepressant
- Pregnancy risk category C

How supplied
Available by prescription only
Tablets: 10 mg

Indications, route, and dosage
Severe depression, †panic disorder

Adults: 10 mg P.O. b.i.d. Increase in 10 mg/day increments every 1 to 3 weeks. Usual effective dose is 30 mg/day in divided doses; maximum dose is 60 mg/day.

During electroconvulsive therapy, maintain current dosage; reduce to 10 mg daily thereafter.

Therapeutic effects of tranylcypromine begin earlier than those of other MAO inhibitors – 7 to 10 days vs. 21 to 30 days; MAO activity also returns to pretreatment values more rapidly.

Pharmacodynamics
Antidepressant action: Endogenous depression is thought to result from low CNS concentrations of neurotransmitters, including norepinephrine and serotonin. Tranylcypromine acts by inhibiting effects of MAO, an enzyme that normally inactivates amine-containing substances, thus increasing concentration and activity of these agents.

Pharmacokinetics
- *Absorption:* Tranylcypromine is absorbed rapidly and completely from the GI tract. Peak serum levels occur at 1 to 3 hours; onset of therapeutic activity may not occur for 3 to 4 weeks.
- *Distribution:* Tranylcypromine's distribution is not fully understood. Dosage adjustments are determined by therapeutic response and adverse reaction profile.
- *Metabolism:* Tranylcypromine is metabolized in the liver.
- *Excretion:* Tranylcypromine is excreted primarily in urine within 24 hours; some drug is excreted in feces via the biliary tract. Half-life is 2½ hours (relatively short); enzyme inhibition is prolonged and unrelated to half-life.

Contraindications and precautions
Tranylcypromine is contraindicated in patients with uncontrolled hypertension, because it may precipitate hypertensive crisis; and in patients with seizure disorders because it lowers the seizure threshold, even in patients controlled on anticonvulsant therapy.

Tranylcypromine should be used cautiously in patients with angina pectoris and other cardiovascular disease, diabetes Types I and II, Parkinson's disease and other motor disorders, hyperthyroidism, pheochromocytoma (drug may worsen these conditions); in patients with renal or hepatic insufficiency (reduced metabolism and excretion may cause drug to accumulate); and in patients with manic-depressive illness (drug may provoke or worsen manic phase; reduce dosage during manic phase).

Interactions
Concomitant use of tranylcypromine with amphetamines, ephedrine, phenylephrine, phenylpropanolamine, or related drugs may result in serious cardiovascular toxicity; most nonprescription cold, hay fever, and weight-reduction products contain these drugs. Circulatory collapse and death have occurred after administration of meperidine. Concomitant use with disulfiram may cause tachycardia, flushing, or palpitations.

Concomitant use with general or spinal anesthetics, which are normally metabolized by MAO, may cause severe hypotension and excessive CNS depression. Tranylcypromine should be discontinued for at least 1 week before using these agents.

Tranylcypromine decreases effectiveness of local anesthetics (such as procaine and lidocaine), resulting in poor nerve block. Cocaine or local anesthetics containing vasoconstrictors should be avoided. Use cautiously and in reduced dosage with alcohol, barbiturates and other sedatives, narcotics, and dextromethorphan. Wait at least 2 weeks before switching to tricyclic antidepressants.

Effects on diagnostic tests
Tranylcypromine therapy elevates liver function tests and urinary catecholamine levels.

Adverse reactions
- CNS: changed libido, dizziness, vertigo, headache, overactivity, hyperreflexia, tremors, muscle twitching, mania, jitters, confusion, memory impairment, fatigue, agitation, nervousness.
- CV: orthostatic hypotension, *arrhythmias*, paradoxical hypertension, palpitations, tachycardia, *fatal intracranial hemorrhage during hypertensive crisis.*
- EENT: blurred vision.
- GI: dry mouth, anorexia, nausea, diarrhea, constipation, abdominal pain.
- GU: impotence, urine retention, dysuria, discolored urine.
- Hepatic: jaundice.
- Other: hypersensitivity (rash), peripheral edema, sweating, weight changes, chills.

Note: Drug should be discontinued if patient develops signs of hypersensitivity, severe headache, palpitations, or fainting spells (which could indicate impending hypertensive crisis).

Overdose and treatment
Signs and symptoms of tranylcypromine overdose include exacerbations of adverse reactions or an exaggerated response to normal pharmacologic activity; such signs and symptoms become apparent slowly (24 to 48 hours) and may persist for up to 2 weeks. Agitation, flushing, tachycardia, hypotension, hypertension, palpitations, increased motor activity, twitching, increased deep tendon reflexes, seizures, hyperpyrexia, cardiorespiratory arrest, or coma may occur. Deaths have occurred with doses of 350 mg.

Treat symptomatically and supportively: give 5 to 10 mg of phentolamine I.V. push for hypertensive crisis; treat seizures, agitation, or tremors with I.V. diazepam, tachycardia with beta-blockers, and fever with cooling blankets. Monitor vital signs and fluid and electrolyte balance. Sympathomimetics (such as norepinephrine and phenylephrine) are contraindicated in hypotension because of MAO inhibitors.

▶ **Special considerations**

Besides those relevant to all *MAO inhibitors*, consider the following recommendations.

● Consider the inherent risk of suicide until significant improvement of depressive state occurs. High-risk patients should have close supervision during initial drug therapy. To reduce risk of suicidal overdose, prescribe the smallest quantity of tablets consistent with good management.

● To prevent dizziness induced by orthostatic blood pressure changes, patient should lie down after taking the drug and avoid abrupt postural changes, especially when arising.

● Tranylcypromine has a more rapid onset of antidepressant effect as compared with other MAO inhibitors (7 to 10 days vs. 21 to 30 days). MAO activity also returns rapidly to pretreatment values.

Information for the patient

● Warn patient to avoid taking alcohol and other CNS depressants or any self-prescribed medications such as cold, hay fever, or diet preparations without medical approval.

● To minimize daytime sedation, patient can take medication at bedtime.

● Explain that many foods and beverages containing tyramine or tryptophan, such as wines, beer, cheeses, preserved fruits, meats, and vegetables, may interact with this drug. Patient can usually obtain list of foods to avoid from the hospital dietary department or pharmacy.

● Tell patient to avoid hazardous activities that require alertness until the full effect of the drug on the CNS is known.

● Tell patient to take drug exactly as prescribed, not to double dose if a dose is missed, and not to stop taking the drug abruptly. Patient should promptly report any adverse reactions. Dosage reduction can relieve most adverse reactions.

● Advise patient to store drug safely away from children.

Geriatric use

Drug is not recommended for patients over age 60.

Pediatric use

Drug is not recommended for patients under age 16.

Breast-feeding

Safety has not been established. Drug should be used with caution.

---

trazodone hydrochloride
Desyrel, Trialodine

● Pharmacologic classification: triazolo-pyridine derivative
● Therapeutic classification: antidepressant
● Pregnancy risk category C

How supplied

Available by prescription only
Tablets: 50 mg, 100 mg, 150 mg

Indications, route, and dosage
Depression

Adults: Initial dosage is 150 mg daily in divided doses, which can be increased by 50 mg/day q 3 to 4 days. Average dosage ranges from 150 mg to 400 mg/day. Maximum dosage is 400 mg/day in outpatients; 600 mg/day in hospitalized patients.

Pharmacodynamics

Antidepressant action: Trazodone is thought to exert its antidepressant effects by inhibiting reuptake of norepinephrine and serotonin in CNS nerve terminals (presynaptic neurons), which results in increased concentration and enhanced activity of these neurotransmitters in the synaptic cleft. Trazodone shares some properties with tricyclic antidepressants: it has antihistaminic, alpha-blocking, analgesic, and sedative effects, and relaxant effects on skeletal muscle. Unlike tricyclic antidepressants, however, trazodone counteracts the pressor effects of norepinephrine, has limited effects on the cardiovascular system, and in particular, has no direct quinidine-like effects on cardiac tissue; it also causes relatively fewer anticholinergic effects. Trazodone has been used in patients with alcohol dependence to decrease tremors and to alleviate anxiety and depression. Adverse reactions are somewhat dose-related; incidence increases with higher dosage levels.

Pharmacokinetics

● *Absorption:* Trazodone is well absorbed from the GI tract after oral administration. Peak effect occurs in 1 hour. Concomitant ingestion of food delays absorption, extends peak effect of drug to 2 hours, and increases amount of drug absorbed by 20%.

● *Distribution:* Trazodone is distributed widely in the body; it does not concentrate in any particular tissue, but small amounts may appear in breast milk. Drug is 90% protein-bound. Proposed therapeutic drug levels have not been established. Steady-state plasma levels are reached in 3 to 7 days, and onset of therapeutic activity occurs in 7 days.

● *Metabolism:* Trazodone is metabolized by the liver; over 75% of metabolites are excreted within 3 days.

● *Excretion:* Majority of drug (75%) is excreted in urine; the rest is excreted in feces via the biliary tract.

Contraindications and precautions

Trazodone is contraindicated in patients with known hypersensitivity to tricyclic antidepressants, trazodone, and related compounds; and in the acute recovery phase of myocardial infarction (MI). It should be used with great caution in patients with other cardiac disease (arrhythmias, CHF, angina pectoris, valvular disease, or heart block) because similar drugs have adversely affected cardiac function.

Trazodone should be used cautiously in patients with priapism or ejaculatory disorders because drug may cause or exacerbate such disorders; surgical correction is necessary (and not always successful) in as many as 30% of patients who experience priapism or prolonged, painful erections. It also should be used with caution in patients receiving electroconvulsive therapy and in patients with hepatic or renal dysfunction.

Interactions

Additive effects are likely after concomitant use of trazodone with antihypertensive drugs, such as guanethidine, guanabenz, guanadrel, clonidine, methyldopa, and reserpine (hypotension); and with CNS depressants, such as alcohol, analgesics, barbiturates, narcotics, tranquilizers, and anesthetics (oversedation).

Trazodone may increase serum levels of phenytoin and digoxin.

Effects on diagnostic tests

Trazodone may prolong conduction time (elongation of Q-T and PR intervals, flattened T waves on ECG); it also may elevate liver function tests, decrease white blood cells counts, and alter serum glucose levels.

Adverse reactions

● CNS: drowsiness, dizziness, sedation (in 20% to 50% of patients), anxiety, tremors, weakness, headache, nervousness, fatigue, vivid dreams and nightmares, confusion, anger, hostility, impaired speech, peripheral neuropathies.
● CV: orthostatic hypotension, tachycardia, *arrhythmias, MI, stroke, heart block, CHF,* palpitations, hypertension, shortness of breath, fainting.
● EENT: blurred vision, tinnitus, mydriasis, increased intraocular pressure.
● GI: dry mouth (in 15% to 30% of patients), constipation, nausea, vomiting, anorexia, bad taste in mouth.
● GU: urinary retention, priapism possibly leading to impotence, retrograde ejaculation, amenorrhea, hematuria.
● Other: sweating, hypersensitivity (rash, urticaria, drug fever, edema).

Note: Drug should be discontinued (not abruptly) if signs of hypersensitivity occur or if urinary retention, hematuria, extreme dry mouth, rash, excessive sedation, seizures, tachycardia or other arrhythmias, fainting spells, or priapism or other sexual dysfunction occurs.

Overdose and treatment

The most common signs and symptoms of trazodone overdose are drowsiness and vomiting; other signs and symptoms include orthostatic hypotension, tachycardia, headache, shortness of breath, dry mouth, and incontinence. Coma may occur.

Treatment is symptomatic and supportive and includes maintaining airway, stable vital signs, and fluid and electrolyte balance. Induce emesis if gag reflex is intact; follow with gastric lavage (begin with lavage if emesis is unfeasible) and activated charcoal to prevent further absorption. Forced diuresis may aid elimination. Dialysis is usually ineffective.

▶ Special considerations

● Consider the inherent risk of suicide until significant improvement of depressive state occurs. High-risk patients should have close supervision during initial drug therapy. To reduce risk of suicidal overdose, prescribe the smallest quantity of tablets consistent with good management.
● Administering trazodone with food helps to prevent GI upset and increases absorption by 20%.
● Adverse effects appear more frequently when dosages exceed 300 mg/day.
● 150-mg tablet may be broken on the scoring to obtain doses of 50, 75, or 100 mg.
● Tolerance to adverse effects (especially sedative effects) usually develops after 1 to 2 weeks of treatment.
● Trazodone has been used in alcohol dependence to decrease tremors and relieve anxiety and depression. Dosages range from 50 to 75 mg daily.
● This drug has fewer adverse cardiac and anticholinergic effects than tricyclic antidepressants.

● Drug may cause prolonged painful erections that may require surgical correction. Consider carefully before prescribing for male patients, especially those who are sexually active.
● Trazodone should not be withdrawn abruptly. However, it should be discontinued at least 48 hours before surgical procedures.
● Sugarless chewing gum or hard candy or ice may relieve dry mouth.
● Hypotension may occur; monitor blood pressure.

Information for the patient
● Tell patient that full effects of the drug may not become apparent for up to 2 weeks after therapy begins.
● Tell patient to take drug exactly as prescribed and not to double dose for missed ones, not to share drug with others, and not to discontinue drug abruptly.
● Inform patient that drug may cause drowsiness or dizziness; instruct patient not to drive or participate in other activities that require mental alertness until the full effects of the drug are known.
● Tell patient to avoid alcoholic beverages or medicinal elixirs while taking this drug.
● Warn patient to store drug safely away from children.
● Suggest taking drug with food or milk if it causes stomach upset.
● To prevent dizziness, patient should lie down for about 30 minutes after taking the medication and avoid sudden postural change, especially rising to upright position.
● Suggest sugarless chewing gum or sugarless hard candy to relieve dry mouth.
● Advise patient to report any unusual effects immediately and to report prolonged, painful erections, sexual dysfunction, dizziness, fainting, or rapid heartbeat. Patients should regard involuntary erection lasting over 1 hour as a medical emergency.

Geriatric use
Elderly patients usually require lower initial dosages; they are more likely to develop adverse reactions. However, it may be preferred in elderly patients because it has fewer adverse cardiac effects.

Pediatric use
Drug is not recommended for patients under age 18.

tretinoin
Retin-A

● Pharmacologic classification: vitamin A derivative
● Therapeutic classification: antiacne agent
● Pregnancy risk category B

How supplied
Available by prescription only
Cream: 0.025%, 0.05%, 0.1%
Gel: 0.025%, 0.01%
Solution: 0.05%

Indications, route, and dosage
Acne vulgaris (especially grades I, II, and III)
Adults and children: Cleanse affected area and lightly apply solution once daily at bedtime or as directed.

†Treatment of photodamaged skin (wrinkles)
Adults: 0.025% or 0.05% solution or 0.025% to 0.1% cream applied daily for at least 4 months.

Pharmacodynamics
Antiacne action: Mechanism of action of tretinoin has not been determined; however, it appears that tretinoin acts as a follicular epithelium irritant, preventing horny cells from sticking together and therefore inhibiting the formation of additional comedones.

Pharmacokinetics
● *Absorption:* Limited with topical use.
● *Distribution:* None.
● *Metabolism:* None.
● *Excretion:* Minimal amount is excreted in the urine.

Contraindications and precautions
Tretinoin is contraindicated in patients with known hypersensitivity to vitamin A/retinoic acid. It should be used cautiously in patients with eczema. Avoid contact of drug with eyes, mouth, angles of the nose, mucous membranes, or open wounds. Use of topical preparations containing high concentrations of alcohol, menthol, spices, or lime should be avoided, as they may cause skin irritation. Avoid use of medicated cosmetics on treated skin.

Interactions
Concomitant use with the following topical agents should be undertaken with caution because of the possibility of interactions: sulfur, resorcinol, benzoyl peroxide, or salicylic acid.

Effects on diagnostic tests
None reported.

Adverse reactions
● Local: peeling, erythema, blisters, crusting, hyperpigmentation and hypopigmentation, contact dermatitis.
 Note: Drug should be discontinued if sensitization or extreme redness and blistering of skin occurs.

Overdose and treatment
No information available. Discontinue use and rinse area thoroughly.

▶ Special considerations
● Make sure that patient knows how to use medication and is aware of time required for clinical effect; therapeutic effect normally occurs in 2 to 3 weeks but may take 6 weeks or more. Relapses generally occur within 3 to 6 weeks of stopping medication.
● Patients who cannot or will not minimize sun exposure should not use this medication.

Information for the patient
● Advise sparing application to thoroughly clean, dry skin, to minimize irritation; to wash face with mild soap no more than 1 or 2 times a day. Stress importance of thorough removal of dirt and make-up before application and of hand washing after each use, but warn against use of strong, medicated, or perfumed cosmetics, soaps, or skin cleansers.
● Explain that application of the medication may cause a temporary feeling of warmth. If discomfort occurs, tell patient to decrease amount, but not to discontinue medication.
● Stress that initial exacerbation of inflammatory lesions is common and that redness and scaling (usually occurring in 7 to 10 days) are normal skin responses; these disappear when medication is decreased or discontinued.
● If severe local irritation develops, advise patient to stop drug temporarily and readjust dosage when irritation or inflammation subsides.
● Caution patient to keep exposure to sunlight or ultraviolet rays to a minimum and, if sunburned, to delay therapy until sunburn fades. If patient cannot avoid exposure to sunlight, recommend use of #15 or higher sunscreen and protective clothing.

---

triamcinolone (systemic)
Aristocort, Kenacort, Ledercort*

triamcinolone acetonide
Kenalog, Kenalone, Triam-A

triamcinolone diacetate
Amcort, Aristocort, Aristocort Forte, Aristocort Intralesional, Articulose LA, Cenocort Forte, Cinalone, Kenacort, Triam-Forte, Triamolone, Tristoject

triamcinolone hexacetonide
Aristospan Intra-articular, Aristospan Intralesional

● Pharmacologic classification: glucocorticoid
● Therapeutic classification: anti-inflammatory, immunosuppressant
● Pregnancy risk category C

How supplied
Available by prescription only
Triamcinolone
Tablets: 1 mg, 2 mg, 4 mg, 8 mg
Syrup: 2 mg/ml, 4 mg/ml
Triamcinolone acetonide
Injection: 10 mg/ml, 40 mg/ml suspension
Triamcinolone diacetate
Injection: 25 mg/ml, 40 mg/ml suspension
Triamcinolone hexacetonide
Injection: 5 mg/ml, 20 mg/ml suspension

Indications, route, and dosage
Adrenal insufficiency
Triamcinolone
Adults: 4 to 12 mg P.O. daily, in a single dose or divided.
Children: 117 mcg/kg or 3.3 mg/m² P.O. daily, in a single dose or divided.
Severe inflammation or immunosuppression
Triamcinolone
Adults: 4 to 60 mg P.O. daily, in a single dose or divided.
Children: 416 mcg to 1.7 mg/kg or 12.5 to 50 mg/m² P.O. daily, in a single dose or divided.
Triamcinolone acetonide
Adults: 40 to 80 mg I.M. q 4 weeks; or 2.5 to 15 mg intra-articularly; or up to 1 mg intralesionally as needed.
Children over age 6: 40 mg I.M. q 4 weeks; or 2.5 to 15 mg intra-articularly as needed.

Triamcinolone diacetate
Adults: 40 mg I.M. once a week; or 3 to 40 mg intra-articularly, intrasynovially, or intralesionally q 1 to 8 weeks.
Children over age 6: 40 mg I.M. once a week.

Triamcinolone hexacetonide
Adults: 2 to 20 mg intra-articularly q 3 to 4 weeks as needed; or up to 0.5 mg intralesionally per square inch of skin.

Pharmacodynamics
Anti-inflammatory action: Triamcinolone stimulates the synthesis of enzymes needed to decrease the inflammatory response. It suppresses the immune system by reducing activity and volume of the lymphatic system, thus producing lymphocytopenia (primarily of T-lymphocytes), decreases immunoglobulin and complement concentrations, decreases passage of immune complexes through basement membranes, and possibly depresses reactivity of tissue to antigen-antibody interactions.

Triamcinolone is an intermediate-acting glucocorticoid. The addition of a fluorine group in the molecule increases the anti-inflammatory activity, which is five times more potent than an equal weight of hydrocortisone. It has essentially no mineralocorticoid activity.

Triamcinolone may be administered orally. The diacetate and acetonide salts may be administered by I.M., intra-articular, intrasynovial, intralesional or sublesional, and soft-tissue injection. The diacetate suspension is slightly soluble, providing a prompt onset of action and a longer duration of effect (1 to 2 weeks). Triamcinolone acetonide is relatively insoluble and slowly absorbed. Its extended duration of action lasts for several weeks. Triamcinolone hexacetonide is relatively insoluble, is absorbed slowly, and has a prolonged action of 3 to 4 weeks. Do not administer any of the parenteral suspensions intravenously.

Pharmacokinetics
• *Absorption:* Triamcinolone is absorbed readily after oral administration. After oral and I.V. administration, peak effects occur in about 1 to 2 hours. The suspensions for injection have variable onset and duration of action, depending on whether they are injected into an intra-articular space or a muscle, and on the blood supply to that muscle.
• *Distribution:* Triamcinolone is removed rapidly from the blood and distributed to muscle, liver, skin, intestines, and kidneys. Triamcinolone is extensively bound to plasma proteins (transcortin and albumin). Only the unbound portion is active. Adrenocorticoids are distributed into breast milk and through the placenta.
• *Metabolism:* Triamcinolone is metabolized in the liver to inactive glucuronide and sulfate metabolites.
• *Excretion:* The inactive metabolites and small amounts of unmetabolized drug are excreted by the kidneys. Insignificant quantities of drug are also excreted in feces. The biologic half-life of triamcinolone is 18 to 36 hours.

Contraindications and precautions
Triamcinolone is contraindicated in patients with hypersensitivity to ingredients of adrenocorticoid preparations and in patients with systemic fungal infections (except in adrenal insufficiency). Patients receiving triamcinolone should not be given live virus vaccines because triamcinolone suppresses the immune response.

Triamcinolone should be used with extreme caution in patients with GI ulceration, renal disease, hypertension, osteoporosis, diabetes mellitus, thromboembolic disorders, seizures, myasthenia gravis, CHF, tuberculosis, hypoalbuminemia, hypothyroidism, cirrhosis of the liver, emotional instability, psychotic tendencies, hyperlipidemias, glaucoma, or cataracts because the drug may exacerbate these conditions.

Because adrenocorticoids increase susceptibility to and mask symptoms of infection, triamcinolone should not be used (except in life-threatening situations) in patients with viral infections or bacterial infections not controlled by anti-infective agents.

Interactions
When used concomitantly, triamcinolone rarely may decrease the effects of oral anticoagulants.

Glucocorticoids increase the metabolism of isoniazid and salicylates; cause hyperglycemia, requiring dosage adjustment of insulin or oral hypoglycemic agents in diabetic patients; and may enhance hypokalemia associated with diuretic or amphotericin B therapy. The hypokalemia may increase the risk of toxicity in patients concurrently receiving digitalis glycosides.

Barbiturates, phenytoin, and rifampin may cause decreased corticosteroid effects because of increased hepatic metabolism. Cholestyramine, colestipol, and antacids decrease triamcinolone's effect by adsorbing the corticosteroid, decreasing the amount absorbed.

Concomitant use with estrogens may reduce the metabolism of triamcinolone by increasing the concentration of transcortin. The half-life of the corticosteroid is then prolonged because of increased protein-binding. Concomitant administration of ulcerogenic drugs, such as nonsteroidal anti-inflammatory agents, may increase the risk of GI ulceration.

Effects on diagnostic tests
Triamcinolone suppresses reactions to skin tests; causes false-negative results in the nitroblue tetrazolium test for systemic bacterial infections; decreases ^{131}I uptake and protein-bound iodine concentrations in thyroid function tests; may increase glucose and cholesterol levels; may decrease serum potassium, calcium, thyroxine, and triiodothyronine levels; and may increase urine glucose and calcium levels.

Adverse reactions
When administered in high doses or for prolonged therapy, triamcinolone suppresses release of adrenocorticotropic hormone (ACTH) from the pituitary gland; in turn, the adrenal cortex stops secreting endogenous corticosteroids. The degree and duration of hypothalamic-pituitary-adrenal (HPA) axis suppression produced by the drugs is highly variable among patients and depends on the dose, frequency, and time of administration, and duration of glucocorticoid therapy.
• CNS: euphoria, insomnia, headache, psychotic behavior, pseudotumor cerebri, mental changes, nervousness, restlessness.
• CV: *CHF,* hypertension, edema.
• DERM: delayed healing, acne, skin eruptions, striae.
• EENT: cataracts, glaucoma, thrush.
• GI: peptic ulcer, irritation, increased appetite.
• Immune: immunosuppression, increased susceptibility to infection.
• Metabolic: hypokalemia, sodium retention, fluid retention, weight gain, hyperglycemia, osteoporosis, growth suppression in children.
• Musculoskeletal: muscle atrophy, weakness.

● Other: *pancreatitis*, hirsutism, cushingoid symptoms, withdrawal syndrome (nausea, fatigue, anorexia, dyspnea, hypotension, hypoglycemia, myalgia, arthralgia, fever, dizziness, and fainting). *Sudden withdrawal may exacerbate the underlying disease or may be fatal.* Acute adrenal insufficiency may occur with increased stress (infection, surgery, trauma) or abrupt withdrawal after long-term therapy.

Overdose and treatment

Acute ingestion, even in massive doses, is rarely a clinical problem. Toxic signs and symptoms rarely occur if the drug is used for less than 3 weeks, even at large doses. However, chronic use causes adverse physiologic effects, including suppression of the HPA axis, cushingoid appearance, muscle weakness, and osteoporosis.

▶ Special considerations

Recommendations for use of triamcinolone and for care and teaching of patients during therapy are the same as those for all *systemic adrenocorticoids*.

Pediatric use

Chronic use of adrenocorticoids or corticotropin in children and adolescents may delay growth and maturation.

triamcinolone acetonide (oral inhalant)
Azmacort

● Pharmacologic classification: glucocorticoid
● Therapeutic classification: anti-inflammatory, antiasthmatic
● Pregnancy risk category D

How supplied

Available by prescription only
Oral inhalation aerosol: 100 mcg/metered spray, 240 doses/inhaler

Indications, route, and dosage
Steroid-dependent asthma

Adults: 2 inhalations t.i.d. to q.i.d. Maximum dosage is 16 inhalations daily.
Children age 6 to 12: 1 or 2 inhalations t.i.d. to q.i.d. Maximum dosage is 12 inhalations daily.

Pharmacodynamics

Anti-inflammatory action: Glucocorticoids stimulate the synthesis of enzymes needed to decrease the inflammatory response. Triamcinolone acetonide is used as an oral inhalant to treat bronchial asthma in patients who require corticosteroids to control symptoms.

Pharmacokinetics

● *Absorption:* Systemic absorption from the lungs is similar to that observed from oral administration. Peak levels are attained in 1 to 2 hours.
● *Distribution:* After oral inhalation, 10% to 25% of the drug is distributed to the lungs. The remainder is swallowed or deposited within the mouth.
● *Metabolism:* Triamcinolone is metabolized mainly by the liver. Some drug that reaches the lungs may be metabolized locally.

● *Excretion:* The major portion of a dose is eliminated in feces. The biologic half-life of triamcinolone is 18 to 36 hours.

Contraindications and precautions

Triamcinolone inhalant is contraindicated in patients with acute status asthmaticus or a hypersensitivity to any component of the preparation.

Drug should be used with caution in patients receiving systemic corticosteroids because of increased risk of hypothalamic-pituitary-adrenal axis suppression; when substituting inhalant for oral systemic therapy (because withdrawal symptoms may occur); and in patients with tuberculosis, healing nasal septal ulcers, oral or nasal surgery or trauma, or bacterial, fungal, or viral respiratory infection.

Interactions
None reported.

Effects on diagnostic tests
None reported.

Adverse reactions
● EENT: flushing, rash, dry mouth, hoarseness, irritation of the tongue or throat, impaired sense of taste.
● Immune: suppression of immune response; fungal overgrowth and infection of the nose, mouth, or throat.
 Note: Drug should be discontinued if no improvement is evident after 3 weeks or if an oral infection develops.

Overdose and treatment
No information available.

▶ Special considerations

Recommendations for use of triamcinolone and for care and teaching of patients during therapy are the same as those for all *inhalant adrenocorticoids*.

triamcinolone acetonide (topical)
Adcortyl*, Adcortyl in Orabase*, Aristocort, Flutex, Kenalog, Kenalog in Orabase, Triacet, Triaderm*, Trianide*

● Pharmacologic classification: topical adrenocorticoid
● Therapeutic classification: anti-inflammatory
● Pregnancy risk category C

How supplied

Available by prescription only
Cream, ointment: 0.025%, 0.1%, 0.5%
Lotion: 0.025%, 0.1%
Aerosol: 0.2 mg/2-second spray
Paste: 0.1%

Indications, route, and dosage
Inflammation of corticosteroid-responsive dermatoses

Adults and children: Apply cream, ointment, or lotion sparingly once daily to q.i.d. Apply aerosol by spraying affected area for about 2 seconds from a distance of 3" to 6" (7.5 to 15 cm) t.i.d. or q.i.d. Apply paste to oral lesions by pressing a small amount into lesion without

---

rubbing until thin film develops. Apply two or three times daily after meals and at bedtime.

Pharmacodynamics

Anti-inflammatory action: Glucocorticoids stimulate the synthesis of enzymes needed to decrease the inflammatory response. Triamcinolone acetonide is a synthetic fluorinated corticosteroid. The 0.5% cream and ointment are recommended only for dermatoses refractory to treatment with lower concentrations.

Pharmacokinetics

● *Absorption:* Drug absorption depends on the potency of the preparation, the amount applied, and the nature of the skin at the application site. It ranges from about 1% in areas with a thick stratum corneum (such as the palms, soles, elbows, and knees) to as high as 36% in areas of the thinnest stratum corneum (face, eyelids, and genitals). Absorption increases in areas of skin damage, inflammation, or occlusion. Some systemic absorption of steroids occurs, especially through the oral mucosa.
● *Distribution:* After topical application, triamcinolone is distributed throughout the local skin layer. Any drug absorbed into circulation is rapidly distributed into muscle, liver, skin, intestines, and kidneys.
● *Metabolism:* After topical administration, triamcinolone is metabolized primarily in the skin. The small amount that is absorbed into systemic circulation is metabolized primarily in the liver to inactive compounds.
● *Excretion:* Inactive metabolites are excreted by the kidneys, primarily as glucuronides and sulfates, but also as unconjugated products. Small amounts of the metabolites are also excreted in feces.

Contraindications and precautions

Triamcinolone is contraindicated in patients who are hypersensitive to any component of the preparation. It should be used cautiously in patients with viral, fungal, or tubercular skin lesions. It should also be used with extreme caution in patients with impaired circulation because the drug may increase the risk of skin ulceration.

Interactions

None reported.

Effects on diagnostic tests

None reported.

Adverse reactions

● Local: burning, itching, irritation, dryness, folliculitis, hypertrichosis, acneiform eruptions, hypopigmentation, perioral dermatitis, allergic contact dermatitis, maceration, secondary infection, atrophy, striae, miliaria.

Significant systemic absorption may produce the following effects.
● CNS: euphoria, insomnia, headache, psychotic behavior, pseudotumor cerebri, mental changes, nervousness, restlessness.
● CV: congestive heart failure, hypertension, edema.
● EENT: cataracts, glaucoma, thrush.
● GI: peptic ulcer, irritation, increased appetite.
● Immune: immunosuppression, increased susceptibility to infection.
● Metabolic: hypokalemia, sodium retention, fluid retention, weight gain, hyperglycemia, osteoporosis, growth suppression in children.

● Musculoskeletal: muscle atrophy.
● Other: withdrawal syndrome (nausea, fatigue, anorexia, dyspnea, hypotension, hypoglycemia, myalgia, arthralgia, fever, dizziness, and fainting).
Note: Drug should be discontinued if local irritation, infection, systemic absorption, or hypersensitivity reaction occurs.

Overdose and treatment

No information available.

▶ Special considerations

Recommendations for use of triamcinolone, for care and teaching of patients during therapy, and for use in elderly patients, children, and breast-feeding women are the same as those for all *topical adrenocorticoids.*

triamterene
Dyrenium

● Pharmacologic classification: potassium-sparing diuretic
● Therapeutic classification: diuretic
● Pregnancy risk category B

How supplied

Available by prescription only
Capsules: 50 mg, 100 mg

Indications, route, and dosage

Diuresis

Adults: Initially, 100 mg P.O. b.i.d. after meals. Total daily dosage should not exceed 300 mg.

Pharmacodynamics

Diuretic action: Triamterene acts directly on the distal renal tubules to inhibit sodium reabsorption and potassium excretion, reducing the potassium loss associated with other diuretic therapy.

Triamterene is commonly used with other more effective diuretics to treat edema associated with excessive aldosterone secretion, hepatic cirrhosis, nephrotic syndrome, and congestive heart failure.

Pharmacokinetics

● *Absorption:* Triamterene is absorbed rapidly after oral administration, but the extent varies. Diuresis usually begins in 2 to 4 hours. Diuretic effect may be delayed 2 to 3 days if drug is used alone; maximum antihypertensive effect may be delayed 2 to 3 weeks.
● *Distribution:* Triamterene is about 67% protein-bound.
● *Metabolism:* Triamterene is metabolized by hydroxylation and sulfation.
● *Excretion:* Triamterene and its metabolites are excreted in urine; half-life of triamterene is 100 to 150 minutes.

Contraindications and precautions

Triamterene is contraindicated in patients with serum potassium levels above 5.5 mEq/liter; in patients who are receiving other potassium-sparing diuretics or potassium supplements because of the potential for hyperkalemia; in patients with anuria, acute or chronic renal insufficiency, or diabetic nephropathy because drug may worsen the signs and symptoms of these conditions; or in patients with known hypersensitivity to the drug.

Triamterene should be used cautiously in patients with severe hepatic insufficiency because electrolyte imbalance may precipitate hepatic encephalopathy, and in patients with diabetes, who are at increased risk of hyperkalemia.

Interactions
Triamterene may potentiate the hypotensive effects of other antihypertensive agents; this may be used to therapeutic advantage.

Triamterene increases the hazard of hyperkalemia when administered with other potassium-sparing diuretics, angiotensin-converting enzyme inhibitors (captopril or enalapril), potassium supplements, potassium-containing medications (parenteral penicillin G), or salt substitutes.

Nonsteroidal anti-inflammatory agents, such as indomethacin or ibuprofen, may alter renal function and thus affect potassium excretion. Diuretics may decrease lithium clearance.

Effects on diagnostic tests
Triamterene therapy may interfere with enzyme assays that use fluorometry, such as serum quinidine determinations.

Adverse reactions
● CNS: dizziness.
● CV: hypotension.
● DERM: photosensitivity, rash.
● EENT: sore throat.
● GI: dry mouth, nausea, vomiting.
● HEMA: megaloblastic anemia related to low folic acid levels.
● Metabolic: *hyperkalemia,* dehydration, hyponatremia, transient rise in BUN levels, acidosis.
● Other: *anaphylaxis,* muscle cramps.
Note: Drug should be discontinued if hyperkalemia occurs.

Overdose and treatment
Clinical signs include those indicative of dehydration and electrolyte disturbance.

Treatment is supportive and symptomatic. For recent ingestion (less than 4 hours), empty stomach by induced emesis or gastric lavage. In severe hyperkalemia (> 6.5 mEq/liter), reduce serum potassium levels with I.V. sodium bicarbonate or glucose with insulin. A cation exchange resin, sodium polystyrene sulfonate (Kayexalate), given orally or as a retention enema, may also reduce serum potassium levels.

▶ Special considerations
Recommendations for the use of triamterene and for care and teaching of the patient during therapy are the same as those for all *potassium-sparing diuretics.*

Geriatric use
Elderly and debilitated patients require close observation because they are more susceptible to drug-induced diuresis and hyperkalemia. Reduced dosages may be indicated.

Pediatric use
Use triamterene with caution; children are more susceptible to hyperkalemia.

Breast-feeding
Triamterene may be excreted in breast milk; safety during breast-feeding has not been established.

---

triazolam
Halcion

● Pharmacologic classification: benzodiazepine
● Therapeutic classification: sedative-hypnotic
● Controlled substance schedule IV
● Pregnancy risk category X

How supplied
Available by prescription only
Tablets: 0.125 mg, 0.25 mg

Indications, route, and dosage
Insomnia
Adults: 0.125 to 0.25 mg P.O. h.s.
Adults over age 65: 0.125 mg P.O. h.s. May give up to 0.25 mg.

Pharmacodynamics
Sedative-hypnotic action: Triazolam depresses the CNS at the limbic and subcortical levels of the brain. It produces a sedative-hypnotic effect by potentiating the effect of the neurotransmitter gamma-aminobutyric acid (GABA) on its receptor in the ascending reticular activating system, which increases inhibition and blocks both cortical and limbic arousal.

Pharmacokinetics
● *Absorption:* When administered orally, triazolam is well absorbed through the GI tract. Peak levels occur in 1 to 2 hours. Onset of action occurs at 15 to 30 minutes.
● *Distribution:* Triazolam is distributed widely throughout the body. Drug is 90% protein-bound.
● *Metabolism:* Triazolam is metabolized in the liver primarily to inactive metabolites.
● *Excretion:* The metabolites of triazolam are excreted in urine. The half-life of triazolam ranges from approximately 1½ to 5½ hours.

Contraindications and precautions
Triazolam is contraindicated in patients with known hypersensitivity to the drug; in patients with acute narrow-angle glaucoma or untreated open-angle glaucoma, because of the drug's possible anticholinergic effect; in patients in coma, because the drug's hypnotic or hypotensive effect may be prolonged or intensified; in pregnant patients, because it may be fetotoxic; and in patients with acute alcohol intoxication who have depressed vital signs, because the drug will worsen CNS depression.

Triazolam should be used cautiously in patients with psychoses, because the drug is rarely beneficial in such patients and may induce paradoxical reactions; in patients with myasthenia gravis or Parkinson's disease, because it may exacerbate the disorder; in patients with impaired hepatic function, which prolongs elimination of the drug; in elderly or debilitated patients, who are usually more sensitive to the drug's CNS effects; and in individuals prone to addiction or drug abuse.

Interactions

Triazolam potentiates the CNS depressant effects of phenothiazines, narcotics, antihistamines, MAO inhibitors, barbiturates, alcohol, general anesthetics, and antidepressants. Enhanced amnestic effects have been reported when combined with alcohol (even in small amounts).

Concomitant use with cimetidine and possibly disulfiram causes diminished hepatic metabolism of triazolam, which increases its plasma concentration.

Heavy smoking accelerates triazolam metabolism, thus lowering clinical effectiveness.

Benzodiazepines may decrease the therapeutic effects of levodopa.

Triazolam may decrease serum levels of haloperidol.

Effects on diagnostic tests

Triazolam therapy may elevate liver function test results. Minor changes in EEG patterns, usually low-voltage, fast activity, may occur during and after triazolam therapy.

Adverse reactions

● CNS: confusion, depression, drowsiness, lethargy, hangover effect, ataxia, dizziness, syncope, nightmares, fatigue, slurred speech, tremors, vertigo, headache, light-headedness, amnesia.
● CV: palpitations, chest pains, hypotension (rare).
● DERM: rash, pruritus, urticaria.
● EENT: diplopia, blurred vision, nystagmus.
● GI: constipation, salivation changes, alterations in taste, anorexia, nausea, vomiting, abdominal discomfort.
● GU: urinary incontinence or retention.
● Other: *respiratory depression,* dysarthria, hepatic dysfunction, changes in libido.
Note: Drug should be discontinued if hypersensitivity or the following paradoxical reactions occur: acute hyperexcited state, anxiety, hallucinations, increased muscle spasticity, insomnia, or rage.

Overdose and treatment

Clinical manifestations of overdose include somnolence, confusion, hypoactive reflexes, dyspnea, labored breathing, hypotension, bradycardia, slurred speech, unsteady gait or impaired coordination, and, ultimately, coma.

Support blood pressure and respiration until drug effects subside; monitor vital signs. Flumazenil, a specific benzodiazepine antagonist, may be useful. Mechanical ventilatory assistance via endotracheal tube may be required to maintain a patent airway and support adequate oxygenation. Use I.V. fluids and vasopressors such as dopamine and phenylephrine to treat hypotension as needed. If patient is conscious, induce emesis. Use gastric lavage if ingestion was recent, but only if an endotracheal tube is present to prevent aspiration. After emesis or lavage, administer activated charcoal with a cathartic as a single dose. Do not use barbiturates if excitation occurs. Dialysis is of limited value.

▶ Special considerations

Besides those relevant to all *benzodiazepines,* consider the following recommendations.
● Monitor hepatic function studies to prevent toxicity.
● Onset of sedation or hypnosis is rapid; patient should be in bed when taking triazolam.
● Store in a cool, dry place away from light.

Information for the patient

● Instruct patient not to take any nonprescription drugs or to change medication regimen without medical approval.
● As necessary, teach safety measures to prevent injury, such as gradual position changes.
● Suggest other measures to promote sleep, such as warm drinks and quiet music, not drinking alcohol near bedtime, regular exercise, and maintaining a regular sleep pattern.
● Advise patient that rebound insomnia may occur after stopping the drug.
● To prevent falls, encourage safety precautions at start of therapy.
● Advise patient of the potential for physical and psychological dependence.

Geriatric use

● Elderly patients are more susceptible to CNS depressant effects of triazolam. Use with caution.
● Lower doses are usually effective in elderly patients because of decreased clearance.
● Elderly patients who receive triazolam require supervision with ambulation and activities of daily living during initiation of therapy or after an increase in dose.

Pediatric use

Safe use in patients under age 18 has not been established.

Breast-feeding

Triazolam is excreted in breast milk. A breast-fed infant may become sedated, have feeding difficulties, or lose weight. Avoid use in breast-feeding women.

---

trichlormethiazide
Diurese, Metahydrin, Naqua, Trichlorex

● Pharmacologic classification: thiazide diuretic
● Therapeutic classification: diuretic, antihypertensive
● Pregnancy risk category B

How supplied

Available by prescription only
Tablets: 2 mg, 4 mg

Indications, route, and dosage
Edema
Adults: 1 to 4 mg P.O. daily or in two divided doses.
Children over age 6 months: 0.07 mg/kg P.O. daily or in two divided doses.
Hypertension
Adults: 2 to 4 mg P.O. daily.
Children over age 6 months: 0.07 mg/kg P.O. daily or in two divided doses.

Pharmacodynamics

● *Diuretic action:* Trichlormethiazide increases urinary excretion of sodium and water by inhibiting sodium reabsorption in the cortical diluting tubule of the nephron, thereby relieving edema.
● *Antihypertensive action:* The exact mechanism of trichlormethiazide's antihypertensive effect is unknown; it may result from direct arteriolar vasodilation. Tri-

---

chlormethiazide also reduces total body sodium and total peripheral resistance.

Pharmacokinetics
Trichlormethiazide is absorbed from the GI tract after oral administration. Limited data are available on other pharmacokinetic parameters; the drug appears to be primarily excreted unchanged in urine.

Contraindications and precautions
Trichlormethiazide is contraindicated in patients with anuria and in those with known hypersensitivity to the drug or to other sulfonamide derivatives. Trichlormethiazide should be used cautiously in patients with severe renal disease because it may decrease glomerular filtration rate and precipitate azotemia; in patients with impaired hepatic function or liver disease because electrolyte alterations may induce hepatic coma; and in patients taking digoxin because hypokalemia may predispose them to digitalis toxicity.

Metahydrin and Trichlorex contain tartrazine, which may cause allergic reactions, including bronchospasm, in asthmatic and aspirin-sensitive patients.

Interactions
Trichlormethiazide potentiates the hypotensive effects of most other antihypertensive drugs; this may be used to therapeutic advantage.

Trichlormethiazide may potentiate hyperglycemic, hypotensive, and hyperuricemic effects of diazoxide, and its hyperglycemic effect may increase insulin or sulfonylurea requirements in diabetic patients.

Trichlormethiazide may reduce renal clearance of lithium, elevating serum lithium levels, and may necessitate reduction in lithium dosage by 50%.

Trichlormethiazide turns urine slightly more alkaline and may decrease urinary excretion of some amines, such as amphetamine and quinidine; alkaline urine also may decrease therapeutic efficacy of methenamine compounds such as methenamine mandelate.

Cholestyramine and colestipol may bind trichlormethiazide, preventing its absorption; give drugs 1 hour apart.

Effects on diagnostic tests
Trichlormethiazide therapy may alter serum electrolyte levels and may increase serum urate, glucose, cholesterol, and triglyceride levels. It also may interfere with tests for parathyroid function and should be discontinued before such tests.

Adverse reactions
● CV: volume depletion and dehydration, orthostatic hypotension, hypercholesterolemia, hypertriglyceridemia.
● DERM: dermatitis, photosensitivity, rash.
● GI: anorexia, nausea, *pancreatitis.*
● HEMA: *aplastic anemia, agranulocytosis,* leukopenia, thrombocytopenia.
● Hepatic: hepatic encephalopathy.
● Metabolic: asymptomatic hyperuricemia; gout; hyperglycemia and impairment of glucose tolerance; fluid and electrolyte imbalances, including hyponatremia, hypochloremia, hypercalcemia, and hypokalemia; metabolic alkalosis.
● Other: hypersensitivity reactions, such as pneumonitis and vasculitis.
Note: Drug should be discontinued if rising BUN and

serum creatinine levels indicate renal impairment or if patient shows signs of impending coma.

Overdose and treatment
Clinical signs of overdose include GI irritation and hypermotility, diuresis, and lethargy, which may progress to coma.

Treatment is mainly supportive; monitor and assist respiratory, cardiovascular, and renal function as indicated. Monitor fluid and electrolyte balance. For recent ingestion (within 4 hours), induce vomiting with ipecac in conscious patient; otherwise, use gastric lavage to avoid aspiration. Do not give cathartics; these promote additional loss of fluids and electrolytes.

▶ Special considerations
Recommendations for the use of trichlormethiazide and for care and teaching of the patient during therapy are the same as those for all *thiazide and thiazide-like diuretics.*

Geriatric use
Elderly and debilitated patients require close observation and may require reduced dosages. They are more sensitive to excess diuresis because of age-related changes in cardiovascular and renal function. Excess diuresis promotes orthostatic hypotension, dehydration leading to hypovolemia, hyponatremia, hypomagnesemia, and hypokalemia.

Breast-feeding
Trichlormethiazide may be distributed in breast milk; its safety and effectiveness in breast-feeding women have not been established.

PHARMACOLOGIC CLASS

tricyclic antidepressants

**amitriptyline hydrochloride
amoxapine
clomipramine hydrochloride
desipramine hydrochloride
doxepin hydrochloride
imipramine hydrochloride
imipramine pamoate
maprotiline hydrochloride
nortriptyline hydrochloride
protriptyline hydrochloride
trimipramine maleate**

The inherent mood-elevating activity of tricyclic antidepressants (TCAs) was discovered during research with iminodibenzyl, a compound originally investigated for sedative, analgesic, antihistaminic, and antiparkinsonian effects. Clinical trials in 1958 with the class prototype, imipramine, found no antipsychotic activity, but clearly demonstrated marked mood-elevating effects.

Pharmacology
Although the precise mechanism of their CNS effects is not established, tricyclic antidepressants may exert their effects by inhibiting reuptake of the neurotransmitters norepinephrine and serotonin in CNS nerve terminals (presynaptic neurons), resulting in increased concentration and enhanced activity of neurotransmitters in the synaptic cleft. TCAs also have antihistaminic,

sedative, anticholinergic, vasodilatory, and quinidine-like effects; the drugs are structurally similar to phenothiazines and share similar adverse reactions.

Individual TCAs differ somewhat in their degree of CNS inhibitory effect. The tertiary amines (amitriptyline, doxepin, imipramine, and trimipramine) exert greater sedative effects; tertiary amines and protriptyline have more profound effects on cardiac conduction, whereas desipramine has the least anticholinergic activity. All of the currently available TCAs have equal clinical efficacy when given in equivalent therapeutic doses; choice of specific therapy is determined primarily by pharmacokinetic properties and the patient's adverse reaction profile. Patients may respond to some TCAs and not others; if a patient does not respond to one drug, another should be tried.

Clinical indications and actions
Depression
TCAs are used to treat major depression and dysthymic disorder. Depressed patients who are also anxious are helped most by the more sedating agents— doxepin, imipramine, and trimipramine. Protriptyline has a stimulant effect that evokes a favorable response in withdrawn depressed patients; only maprotiline has Food and Drug Administration approval for use in depression mixed with anxiety.
Obsessive-compulsive disorder (OCD)
Clomipramine is used in the treatment of OCD.
Enuresis
Imipramine is used to treat enuresis in children over age 6.
Severe, chronic pain
TCAs, especially amitriptyline, desipramine, doxepin, imipramine, and nortriptyline, are useful in the management of severe chronic pain.

Overview of adverse reactions
Adverse reactions to TCAs are similar to those seen with phenothiazine antipsychotic agents, including varying degrees of sedation, anticholinergic effects, and orthostatic hypotension. The tertiary amines have the strongest sedative effects; tolerance to these effects usually develops in a few weeks. Protriptyline has the least sedative effect (and may be stimulatory), but shares with the tertiary amines the most pronounced effects on blood pressure and cardiac tissue. Maprotiline and amoxapine are most likely to cause seizures, especially in overdose situations. Desipramine has a greater margin of safety in patients with prostatic hypertrophy, paralytic ileus, glaucoma, and urinary retention, because of its relatively low level of anticholinergic activity.

▶ Special considerations
● TCAs impair ability to perform tasks requiring mental alertness, such as driving a car.
● Check vital signs regularly for decreased blood pressure or tachycardia; observe patient carefully for other adverse reactions and report changes. Check ECG in patients over age 40 before initiating therapy. Consider having patient take the first dose in the office to allow close observation for adverse reactions.
● Check for anticholinergic adverse reactions (urine retention or constipation), which may require dosage reduction.
● Caregiver should be sure patient swallows each dose of drug when given; as depressed patients begin to improve, they may hoard pills for suicide attempt.

● Observe patients for mood changes to monitor progress; benefits may not be apparent for several (3 to 6) weeks.
● Do not withdraw full dose of drug abruptly; gradually reduce dosage over a period of weeks to avoid rebound effect or other adverse reactions.
● Carefully follow manufacturer's instructions for reconstitution, dilution, and storage of drugs.
● Investigational uses include treating peptic ulcer, migraine prophylaxis, and allergy. Potential toxicity has, to date, outweighed most advantages.
● Because suicidal overdosage with tricyclic antidepressants is commonly fatal, prescribe only small amounts. If possible, entrust a reliable family member with the medication and warn him to store drug safely away from children.

Information for the patient
● Explain rationale for therapy and anticipated risks and benefits; also explain that full therapeutic effect may not occur for several weeks.
● Teach signs and symptoms of adverse reactions and the importance of reporting any that occur.
● Tell patient to avoid beverages and drugs containing alcohol and not to take any other drug (including nonprescription products) without medical approval.
● Teach patient how and when to take drug, not to increase dosage without medical approval, and never to discontinue drug abruptly.
● Advise patient to lie down for 30 minutes after first dose and to rise slowly to prevent orthostatic hypotension.
● Advise taking drug with milk or food to minimize GI distress; suggest taking full dose at bedtime if daytime sedation is troublesome.
● Urge diabetic patients to monitor blood sugar, as drug may alter insulin needs.
● Advise patient to avoid tasks that require mental alertness until full effect of drug is determined.
● Warn patient that excessive exposure to sunlight, heat lamps, or tanning beds may cause burn and abnormal hyperpigmentation.
● Recommend sugarless gum or hard candy, artificial saliva, or ice chips to relieve dry mouth.
● Advise patient that unpleasant side effects (except dry mouth) generally diminish over time.

Geriatric use
Lower doses are indicated in geriatric patients, because they are more sensitive to both therapeutic and adverse effects of TCAs. Recommended starting dosage is 25 mg P.O. t.i.d.

Pediatric use
TCAs are not recommended for children under age 12.

Breast-feeding
Safety in breast-feeding has not been established.

Representative combinations
Amitriptyline hydrochloride with perphenazine: Etrafon, Triavil; with chlordiazepoxide: Limbitrol.

---

trientine hydrochloride
Cuprid

- Pharmacologic classification: chelating agent
- Therapeutic classification: heavy metal antagonist
- Pregnancy risk category C

How supplied
Available by prescription only
Capsules: 250 mg

Indications, route, and dosage
Wilson's disease in patients who are intolerant of penicillamine
Adults: 750 to 1,250 mg in doses divided b.i.d. to q.i.d. Maximum dosage is 2 g/day.
Children under age 12: 500 to 750 mg in doses divided b.i.d. to q.i.d. Maximum dosage is 1,500 mg/day.

Pharmacodynamics
Chelating action: Trientine forms a soluble complex with free serum copper that is renally excreted, removing excess copper.

Pharmacokinetics
- *Absorption:* Trientine is well absorbed after oral administration.
- *Distribution:* Unknown.
- *Metabolism:* None.
- *Excretion:* Drug is excreted in urine as unchanged drug or a trientine-copper complex.

Contraindications and precautions
Trientine is contraindicated in patients with known or suspected hypersensitivity to the drug; it is not intended for use in patients with rheumatoid arthritis, biliary cirrhosis, or cystinuria.

Drug should be used with caution in patients who have or are at risk for iron deficiency, because trientine also chelates iron; and in patients with idiopathic or penicillamine-induced systemic lupus erythematosus (SLE), because trientine may reactivate the disease.

Interactions
Concomitant ingestion of trientine with mineral supplements, especially iron, reduces absorption of the drug.

Effects on diagnostic tests
None reported.

Adverse reactions
- DERM: dermatitis.
- EENT: bronchitis, asthma.
- Other: SLE, iron deficiency anemia.
  Note: Drug should be discontinued if SLE or hypersensitivity occurs.

Overdose and treatment
Data on effects of overdose are unavailable. Treat symptomatically.

▶ **Special considerations**
- Drug is designed for use only in patients unable to tolerate penicillamine, which remains the standard therapy for Wilson's disease.
- Daily dosage may be increased if clinical response is inadequate or free serum copper level remains above 20 mcg/dl.
- Observe patient for any signs or symptoms of hypersensitivity, such as asthma, fever, or skin eruptions; monitor all patients for iron deficiency anemia.
- For optimal therapeutic effect, give drug 1 hour before or 2 hours after meals and at least 1 hour apart from any other drug, food, or milk.

Information for the patient
- Explain disease process and rationale for therapy, stress importance of compliance with low-copper diet and follow-up visits.
- Tell patient how and when to take drug; especially advise patient to swallow capsule whole (do not open or chew), and to drink full glass (8 oz) of water with each dose.
- Advise patient to check for fever nightly for the first month of treatment and to report any signs, such as fever or skin eruption.
- Explain that trientine causes contact dermatitis; after accidental contact, flood with water promptly.

Pediatric use
Safety and efficacy in children have not been established; drug should be used with caution.

Breast-feeding
It is unknown whether the drug crosses into breast milk. Use with caution in breast-feeding women.

triethanolamine polypeptide oleate-condensate
Cerumenex

- Pharmacologic classification: oleic acid derivative
- Therapeutic classification: cerumenolytic
- Pregnancy risk category C

How supplied
Available by prescription only
Otic solution: 10% in 6- and 12-ml bottle with dropper

Indications, route, and dosage
Impacted cerumen
Adults and children: Fill ear canal with solution, and insert cotton plug. After 15 to 30 minutes, flush ear with warm water. Do not expose ear canal to solution for more than 30 minutes.

Pharmacodynamics
Cerumenolytic action: Emulsifies and disperses accumulated cerumen.

Pharmacokinetics
Unknown.

Contraindications and precautions
Triethanolamine is contraindicated in patients who have an untoward reaction to triethanolamine polypeptide

oleate, a perforated eardrum, or a history of otitis media. It should be used with caution in patients with a history of dermatologic idiosyncrasies and allergic reactions.

Interactions
None reported.

Effects on diagnostic tests
None reported.

Adverse reactions
● DERM: dermatitis, ranging from mild redness and itching of the external ear canal to a severe reaction involving the external ear and surrounding tissue (generally lasts 2 to 10 days).
● Ear: erythema, pruritus.
Note: Drug should be discontinued if dermatitis reaction occurs.

Overdose and treatment
Clinical manifestations of overdose include vomiting and diarrhea which, if protracted, may lead to fluid and electrolyte abnormalities. Evaluate patient for oral burns. Spontaneous emesis frequently occurs; if it does not, it is unlikely that significant ingestion has occurred. Activated charcoal or a cathartic are unnecessary.

Ocular exposure may result in transient eye irritation but usually no permanent damage. Treat eye exposure by irrigation with large amounts of tepid water for at least 15 minutes. Treat dermal exposure by washing the exposed area.

▶ Special considerations
● To determine allergic potential, do patch test: place 1 drop of drug on inner forearm, then cover with small bandage; read in 24 hours. If any reaction (redness, swelling) occurs, do not use drug.
● Moisten cotton plug with medication before insertion.
● Keep container tightly closed and away from moisture.
● Avoid touching ear with dropper.

Information for the patient
● Advise patient not to use drops more often than prescribed and to avoid touching the ear with the dropper.
● Teach patient correct application and storage.

---

trifluoperazine hydrochloride
Apo-Trifluoperazine★, Novoflurazine★, Solazine★, Stelazine, Suprazine, Terfluzine★

● Pharmacologic classification: phenothiazine (piperazine derivative)
● Therapeutic classification: antipsychotic, antiemetic
● Pregnancy risk category C

How supplied
Available by prescription only
Tablets (regular and film-coated): 1 mg, 2 mg, 5 mg, 10 mg
Oral concentrate: 10 mg/ml
Injection: 2 mg/ml

Indications, route, and dosage
Anxiety states
Adults: 1 to 2 mg P.O. b.i.d.
Schizophrenia and other psychotic disorders
Adults: For outpatients, 1 to 2 mg P.O. b.i.d., increased as needed. For hospitalized patients, 2 to 5 mg P.O. b.i.d.; may increase gradually to 40 mg daily. For I.M. injection, 1 to 2 mg q 4 to 6 hours, p.r.n.
Children age 6 to 12 (hospitalized or under close supervision): 1 mg P.O. daily or b.i.d.; may increase gradually to 15 mg daily.

Pharmacodynamics
Antipsychotic action: Trifluoperazine is thought to exert its antipsychotic effects by postsynaptic blockade of CNS dopamine receptors, thereby inhibiting dopamine-mediated effects; antiemetic effects are attributed to dopamine receptor blockade in the medullary chemoreceptor trigger zone. Trifluoperazine has many other central and peripheral effects; it produces alpha and ganglionic blockade and counteracts histamine- and serotonin-mediated activity. Its most prevalent adverse reactions are extrapyramidal; it has less sedative and autonomic activity than aliphatic and piperidine phenothiazines.

Pharmacokinetics
● *Absorption:* Rate and extent of absorption vary with route of administration: oral tablet absorption is erratic and variable, with onset of action ranging from ½ to 1 hour; oral concentrate absorption is much more predictable. I.M. drug is absorbed rapidly.
● *Distribution:* Trifluoperazine is distributed widely in the body, including breast milk. Drug is 91% to 99% protein-bound. Peak effect occurs in 2 to 4 hours; steady-state serum levels are achieved within 4 to 7 days.
● *Metabolism:* Trifluoperazine is metabolized extensively by the liver, but no active metabolites are formed; duration of action is about 4 to 6 hours.
● *Excretion:* Most of drug is excreted in urine via the kidneys; some is excreted in feces via the biliary tract.

Contraindications and precautions
Trifluoperazine is contraindicated in patients with known hypersensitivity to phenothiazines and related compounds, including allergic reactions involving hepatic function; in patients with blood dyscrasias and bone marrow depression (adverse hematologic effects); in patients with disorders accompanied by coma, brain damage, CNS depression, circulatory collapse, or cerebrovascular disease (additive CNS depression and adverse blood pressure effects); and in patients taking adrenergic-blocking agents or spinal or epidural anesthetics (excessive respiratory, cardiac, and CNS depression).

Trifluoperazine should be used with caution in patients with cardiac disease (arrhythmias, CHF, angina pectoris, valvular disease, or heart block); encephalitis; Reye's syndrome; head injury; respiratory disease; epilepsy and other seizure disorders; glaucoma; prostatic hypertrophy; urinary retention; Parkinson's disease and pheochromocytoma, because it may exacerbate these conditions; in patients with hypocalcemia because it increases the risk of extrapyramidal reactions; and in patients with hepatic or renal dysfunction (diminished metabolism and excretion cause the drug to accumulate).

Interactions

Concomitant use of trifluoperazine with sympathomimetics, including epinephrine, phenylephrine, phenylpropanolamine, and ephedrine (often found in nasal sprays), and appetite suppressants may decrease their stimulatory and pressor effects. Using epinephrine as a pressor agent in patients taking trifluoperazine may result in epinephrine reversal or further lowering of blood pressure.

Trifluoperazine may inhibit blood pressure response to centrally acting antihypertensive drugs, such as guanethidine, guanabenz, guanadrel, clonidine, methyldopa, and reserpine. Additive effects are likely after concomitant use of trifluoperazine with CNS depressants, including alcohol, analgesics, barbiturates, narcotics, tranquilizers, anesthetics (general, spinal, epidural), and parenteral magnesium sulfate (oversedation, respiratory depression, and hypotension); antiarrhythmic agents, quinidine, disopyramide, and procainamide (increased incidence of cardiac arrhythmias and conduction defects); atropine and other anticholinergic drugs, including antidepressants, monoamine oxidase inhibitors, phenothiazines, antihistamines, meperidine, and antiparkinsonian agents (oversedation, paralytic ileus, visual changes, and severe constipation); nitrates (hypotension); and metrizamide (increased risk of seizures).

Beta-blocking agents may inhibit trifluoperazine metabolism, increasing plasma levels and toxicity.

Concomitant use of trifluoperazine with propylthiouracil increases risk of agranulocytosis; concomitant use with lithium may result in severe neurologic toxicity with an encephalitis-like syndrome and in decreased therapeutic response to trifluoperazine.

Pharmacokinetic alterations and subsequent decreased therapeutic response to trifluoperazine may follow concomitant use with phenobarbital (enhanced renal excretion), aluminum and magnesium-containing antacids and antidiarrheals (decreased absorption), caffeine, and heavy smoking (increased metabolism).

Trifluoperazine may antagonize therapeutic effect of bromocriptine on prolactin secretion; it also may decrease the vasoconstricting effects of high-dose dopamine and may decrease effectiveness and increase toxicity of levodopa (by dopamine blockade). Trifluoperazine may inhibit metabolism and increase toxicity of phenytoin.

Effects on diagnostic tests

Trifluoperazine causes false-positive test results for urine porphyrins, urobilinogen, amylase, and 5-HIAA levels from darkening of urine by metabolites; it also causes false-positive urine pregnancy results in tests using human chorionic gonadotropin as the indicator.

Trifluoperazine elevates tests for liver function and protein-bound iodine and causes quinidine-like effects on the ECG.

Adverse reactions

● CNS: extrapyramidal symptoms (dystonia, akathisia, torticollis, tardive dyskinesia, sedation (low incidence), pseudoparkinsonism, drowsiness (frequent), *neuroleptic malignant syndrome* (dose-related; fatal *respiratory failure* in over 10% of patients if untreated), dizziness, headache, insomnia, exacerbation of psychotic symptoms.
● CV: *asystole*, orthostatic hypotension, tachycardia, dizziness or fainting, *arrhythmias*, ECG changes, increased anginal pain after I.M. injection.
● EENT: blurred vision, tinnitus, mydriasis, increased intraocular pressure, ocular changes (retinal pigmentary change with long-term use).
● GI: dry mouth, constipation, nausea, vomiting, anorexia, diarrhea.
● GU: urinary retention, gynecomastia, hypermenorrhea, inhibited ejaculation.
● HEMA: transient leukopenia, *agranulocytosis*, thrombocytopenia, anemia (within 30 to 90 days).
● Local: contact dermatitis from concentrate or injection, muscle necrosis from I.M. injection.
● Other: hyperprolactinemia, photosensitivity, increased appetite or weight gain, hypersensitivity (rash, urticaria, drug fever, edema, cholestatic jaundice [0.1% to 4% in first 30 days]), decreased libido.

After abrupt withdrawal of long-term therapy, gastritis, nausea, vomiting, dizziness, tremors, feeling of heat or cold, sweating, tachycardia, headache, or insomnia may occur.

Note: Drug should be discontinued immediately if any of the following occur: hypersensitivity, jaundice, agranulocytosis, neuroleptic malignant syndrome (marked hyperthermia, extrapyramidal effects, autonomic dysfunction), severe extrapyramidal symptoms even after dosage is lowered. Drug should be discontinued 48 hours before and 24 hours after myelography using metrizamide, because of risk of seizures. When feasible, drug should be withdrawn slowly and gradually; many drug effects persist after withdrawal.

Overdose and treatment

CNS depression is characterized by deep, unarousable sleep and possible coma, hypotension or hypertension, extrapyramidal symptoms, dystonia, abnormal involuntary muscle movements, agitation, seizures, arrhythmias, ECG changes, hypothermia or hyperthermia, and autonomic nervous system dysfunction.

Treatment is symptomatic and supportive and includes maintaining vital signs, airway, stable body temperature, and fluid and electrolyte balance.

Do not induce vomiting: drug inhibits cough reflex, and aspiration may occur. Use gastric lavage, then activated charcoal and saline cathartics; dialysis is usually ineffective. Regulate body temperature as needed. Treat hypotension with I.V. fluids: *do not give epinephrine.* Treat seizures with parenteral diazepam or barbiturates; arrhythmias with parenteral phenytoin (1 mg/kg with rate titrated to blood pressure); extrapyramidal reactions with benztropine or parenteral diphenhydramine 2 mg/kg/minute.

▶ Special considerations

Besides those relevant to all *phenothiazines,* consider the following recommendations.
● Other agents, such as benzodiazepines, are preferred for the treatment of anxiety. When drug is given for anxiety, do not exceed 6 mg daily for longer than 12 weeks. Some clinicians recommend against use of this drug for anything but psychosis.
● Administer I.M. injection deep in the upper outer quadrant of the buttock. Massaging the area after administration may prevent formation of abscesses. I.M. injection may cause skin necrosis; do not extravasate.
● Solution for injection may be slightly discolored. Do not use if excessively discolored or a precipitate is evident. Contact pharmacist.
● Monitor blood pressure before and after parenteral administration.
● Shake concentrate before administration.

- Chewing sugarless gum or hard candy or ice may help relieve dry mouth.
- Worsening anginal pain has been reported in patients receiving trifluoperazine; however, ECG reactions are less frequent with this drug than with other phenothiazines.
- Liquid and injectable formulations may cause a rash after contact with skin.
- Drug may cause pink to brown discoloration of urine.
- Trifluoperazine is associated with a high incidence of extrapyramidal symptoms and photosensitivity reactions. Patient should avoid exposure to sunlight or heat lamps.
- Monitor regularly for abnormal movements (at least once every 6 months).
- Oral formulations may cause stomach upset. Administer with food or fluid.
- Concentrate must be diluted in 2 to 4 oz of liquid, preferably water, carbonated drinks, fruit juice, tomato juice, milk, or pudding.
- Protect the liquid formulation from light.

Information for the patient

- Explain the risks of dystonic reactions, akathisia, and tardive dyskinesia, and tell patient to report abnormal body movements.
- Explain that many drug interactions are possible. Patient should seek medical approval before taking any self-prescribed medication.
- Tell patient that any adverse reactions may be alleviated by a dosage reduction. Patient should report difficulty urinating, sore throat, dizziness, or fainting; male patients should be warned about inhibited ejaculation.
- Warn patient against hazardous activities that require alertness until the effect of the drug is established. Reassure patient that sedative effects usually subside in several weeks.
- Tell patient to avoid sun exposure and wear sunscreen when going outdoors, to prevent photosensitivity reactions. (Explain that heat lamps and tanning beds also may cause burning of the skin or skin discoloration.)
- Warn patient to avoid extremely hot or cold baths and exposure to temperature extremes, sunlamps, and tanning beds; drug may cause thermoregulatory changes.
- Tell patient to take drug exactly as prescribed, and not to double dose for missed doses, stop taking the drug abruptly, or share drug with others.
- Advise patient to store medication in a safe place, away from children.
- Tell patient to avoid alcohol and other medications that may cause excessive sedation.
- Suggest sugarless candy or gum, ice chips, or artificial saliva to relieve dry mouth.

Geriatric use

Elderly patients tend to require lower doses, titrated to effects. Such patients also are more likely to develop adverse effects, especially tardive dyskinesia and other extrapyramidal effects and hypotension.

Pediatric use

Drug is not recommended for children under age 6.

Breast-feeding

Trifluoperazine may enter breast milk. Potential benefits to the mother should outweigh the potential harm to the infant.

---

trifluridine
Viroptic

- **Pharmacologic classification:** fluorinated pyrimidine nucleoside
- **Therapeutic classification:** antiviral agent
- **Pregnancy risk category C**

How supplied

Available by prescription only
Ophthalmic solution: 1%

Indications, route, and dosage
Primary keratoconjunctivitis and recurrent epithelial keratitis caused by herpes simplex virus types I and II

Adults: 1 drop instilled into the affected eye q 2 hours while patient is awake, to a maximum of 9 drops daily until reepithelialization of the corneal ulcer occurs; then, 1 drop q 4 hours (minimum of 5 drops daily) for an additional 7 days.

Pharmacodynamics

Antiviral action: The exact mechanism of action is unknown, but the drug appears to interfere with DNA synthesis, preventing viral cell replication; it is active against herpes simplex virus types I and II and vaccinia virus.

Pharmacokinetics

- *Absorption:* Intraocular penetration occurs after topical administration. Inflammation may enhance penetration.
- *Distribution:* Unknown.
- *Metabolism:* Unknown.
- *Excretion:* Half-life of trifluridine is approximately 12 to 18 minutes.

Contraindications and precautions

Trifluridine is contraindicated in patients with hypersensitivity reactions or chemical intolerance to trifluridine. It should be used with caution during long-term therapy; the possibility of viral resistance after multiple exposures must be considered.

Interactions
None reported.

Effects on diagnostic tests
None reported.

Adverse reactions
Eye: burning, stinging, irritation, tearing, edema of eyelids, hyperemia, superficial punctate keratopathy, epithelial keratopathy, stromal edema, keratitis sicca, increased intraocular pressure.

Overdose and treatment
The toxicity of ingested trifluridine is unknown; if large quantities are ingested, use general measures, such

---

as emesis, lavage, or a cathartic, to remove drug from the GI tract. Treat dermal exposure by washing the area with soap and water. Observe the patient closely for possible signs and symptoms.

▶ **Special considerations**
● Consider another form of therapy if improvement does not occur after 7 days, or complete re-epithelialization after 14 days' treatment.
● Trifluridine shouldn't be used more than 21 consecutive days because of potential ocular toxicity.
● Keep drug refrigerated; gradually bring drug to room temperature before use.
● Reassure patient that mild local irritation of the conjunctiva and cornea that occurs when solution is instilled is usually temporary.
● Warn patient not to exceed the recommended dosage and frequency of administration.
● Caution patient to call if improvement is not seen in 7 days or if condition worsens or irritation occurs.

---

trihexyphenidyl hydrochloride
Aparkane*, Aphen, Apo-Trihex*, Artane, Artane Sequels, Novohexidyl*, Tremin, Trihexane, Trihexidyl, Trihexy-2, Trihexy-5

● Pharmacologic classification: anticholinergic
● Therapeutic classification: antiparkinsonian agent
● Pregnancy risk category C

How supplied
Available by prescription only
Tablets: 2 mg, 5 mg
Capsules (sustained-release): 5 mg
Elixir: 2 mg/5 ml

Indications, route, and dosage
Drug-induced parkinsonism
Adults: 1 mg P.O. 1st day, 2 mg 2nd day, then increase 2 mg every 3 to 5 days until total of 6 to 10 mg is given daily. Usually given t.i.d. with meals and, if needed, q.i.d. (last dose should be before bedtime). Postencephalitic parkinsonism may require 12 to 15 mg total daily dosage.

Pharmacodynamics
Antiparkinsonian action: Trihexyphenidyl blocks central cholinergic receptors, helping to balance cholinergic activity in the basal ganglia. It may also prolong dopamine's effects by blocking dopamine reuptake and storage at central receptor sites.

Pharmacokinetics
● *Absorption:* Trihexyphenidyl is rapidly absorbed after oral administration. Onset of action occurs within 1 hour.
● *Distribution:* Trihexyphenidyl crosses the blood-brain barrier; little else is known about its distribution.
● *Metabolism:* Exact metabolic fate is unknown. Duration of effect is 6 to 12 hours.
● *Excretion:* Trihexyphenidyl is excreted in the urine as unchanged drug and metabolites.

Contraindications and precautions
Trihexyphenidyl is contraindicated in patients with a history of sensitivity to the drug. Administer trihexyphenidyl cautiously to patients with narrow-angle glaucoma, because drug-induced cycloplegia and mydriasis may increase intraocular pressure; to patients with cardiac disorders, arteriosclerosis, renal disorders, hepatic disorders, hypertension, obstructive GI or genitourinary tract disease, or suspected prostatic hypertrophy, because the drug may exacerbate these conditions.

Interactions
Concomitant use with amantadine may amplify trihexyphenidyl's anticholinergic adverse effects, causing confusion and hallucinations. Concomitant use with haloperidol or phenothiazines may decrease the antipsychotic effectiveness of these drugs, possibly from direct CNS antagonism; concomitant phenothiazine use also increases the risk of anticholinergic adverse effects.

Concomitant use with CNS depressants, such as tranquilizers, sedative-hypnotics, and alcohol, increases trihexyphenidyl's sedative effects. When used with levodopa, dosage of both drugs may need adjustment because of synergistic anticholinergic effects and possible enhanced gastrointestinal metabolism of levodopa from reduced gastric motility and delayed gastric emptying. Antacids and antidiarrheals may decrease trihexyphenidyl's absorption.

Effects on diagnostic tests
None reported.

Adverse reactions
● CNS: nervousness, dizziness, headache, restlessness, hallucinations, insomnia, confusion and excitement (in elderly).
● CV: tachycardia, palpitations, orthostatic hypotension.
● EENT: blurred vision, mydriasis, increased intraocular pressure, photophobia.
● GI: constipation, dry mouth, nausea, vomiting, heartburn, dysphagia, abdominal distention.
● GU: urinary hesitancy or retention.
Note: Drug should be discontinued if hypersensitivity, hallucinations, delusions, or urinary retention occur.

Overdose and treatment
Clinical effects of overdose include central stimulation followed by depression, with such psychotic symptoms as disorientation, confusion, hallucinations, delusions, anxiety, agitation, and restlessness. Peripheral effects may include dilated, nonreactive pupils; blurred vision; flushed, dry, hot skin; dry mucous membranes; dysphagia; decreased or absent bowel sounds; urinary retention; hyperthermia; headache; tachycardia; hypertension; and increased respiration.

Treatment is primarily symptomatic and supportive, as needed. Maintain patent airway. If the patient is alert, induce emesis (or use gastric lavage) and follow with saline cathartic and activated charcoal to prevent further drug absorption. In severe cases, physostigmine may be administered to block trihexyphenidyl's antimuscarinic effects. Give fluids, as needed, to treat shock; diazepam to control psychotic symptoms; and pilocarpine (instilled into the eyes) to relieve mydriasis. If urinary retention occurs, catheterization may be necessary.

▶ **Special considerations**
Besides those relevant to all *anticholinergics*, consider the following recommendations.
● Store trihexyphenidyl in tight containers.
● Monitor patient for urinary hesitancy.
● Arrange for gonioscopic evaluation and close intraocular pressure monitoring, especially in patients over age 40.
● Patients may develop tolerance to this drug, necessitating higher doses.

Geriatric use
Use caution when administering trihexyphenidyl to elderly patients. Lower doses are indicated.

Breast-feeding
Trihexyphenidyl may be excreted in breast milk, possibly resulting in infant toxicity. Breast-feeding women should avoid this drug. Drug may also decrease milk production.

trimeprazine tartrate
Panectyl*, Temaril

● Pharmacologic classification: phenothiazine-derivative antihistamine
● Therapeutic classification: antipruritic
● Pregnancy risk category C

How supplied
Available by prescription only
Tablets: 2.5 mg
Spansule capsules (sustained-release): 5 mg
Syrup: 2.5 mg/5 ml (5.7% alcohol)

Indications, route, and dosage
Pruritus
Adults and children age 12 and older: 2.5 mg P.O. q.i.d.; or (timed-release) 5 mg P.O. q 12 hours.
Children age 6 to 11: One Spansule capsule (5 mg) daily. Spansule capsules are not recommended for children under age 6.
Children age 3 to 5: 2.5 mg P.O. at bedtime or t.i.d., p.r.n.
Children age 6 months to 2 years: 1.25 mg P.O. at bedtime or t.i.d., p.r.n.

Pharmacodynamics
Antipruritic action: Antihistamines compete for histamine H_1-receptor sites by binding to cellular receptors; they prevent access of histamine and suppress histamine-induced allergic symptoms, even though they do not prevent its release.

Pharmacokinetics
● *Absorption:* Well absorbed. After oral administration, onset of action in 15 to 60 minutes with peak effect in 1 to 2 hours and duration of 3 to 6 hours.
● *Metabolism:* Hepatic biotransformation.
● *Distribution:* Unknown.
● *Excretion:* Renal.

Contraindications and precautions
Trimeprazine is contraindicated in patients with known hypersensitivity to trimeprazine or to phenothiazines; during acute asthma attacks, because it thickens bronchial secretions; in acutely ill or dehydrated children, because they are at increased risk of developing dystonias; in patients with bone marrow depression, because the drug may exacerbate this syndrome; in patients with epilepsy, because the drug may increase the incidence of seizures; and in comatose patients and newborns.

Because of its significant anticholinergic activity, trimeprazine should be used with caution in patients with narrow-angle glaucoma; in those with pyloroduodenal obstruction or urinary bladder obstruction from prostatic hypertrophy or narrowing of the bladder neck; in patients with cardiovascular disease or hypertension, because of the hazard of palpitations and tachycardia; and in patients with acute or chronic respiratory dysfunction (especially children) because trimeprazine may suppress the cough reflex.

It also should be used with caution in children with a history of sleep apnea or a family history of sudden infant death syndrome. The relationship between these conditions and trimeprazine has not been studied; however, death has occurred in children given usual doses of phenothiazine antihistamines.

Interactions
MAO inhibitors interfere with the detoxification of antihistamines and phenothiazines and thus prolong and intensify their central depressant and anticholinergic effects; added sedation and CNS depression may occur when trimeprazine is used concomitantly with other CNS depressants, including alcohol, barbiturates, tranquilizers, sleeping aids, and antianxiety agents. Concomitant use with beta blockers and antihypertensives produces additive effects of both drugs.

Phenothiazines potentiate the CNS depressant and analgesic effect of narcotics; the phenothiazine activity of trimeprazine is potentiated by oral contraceptives, progesterone, reserpine, and nylidrin hydrochloride.

Do not give epinephrine to reverse trimeprazine-induced hypotension; partial adrenergic blockade may cause further hypotension. Trimeprazine blocks dopamine receptors and inhibits the antiparkinsonian effect of levodopa.

Effects on diagnostic tests
Trimeprazine should be discontinued 4 days before diagnostic skin tests, to avoid preventing, reducing, or masking positive test response. Trimeprazine may cause false-positive or false-negative urine pregnancy test results.

Adverse reactions
● CNS: drowsiness, dizziness, confusion, headache, restlessness, tremors, irritability, insomnia, extrapyramidal symptoms (especially at high doses), muscular weakness, disturbed coordination, increased appetite, paradoxical excitation.
● CV: postural hypotension, reflex tachycardia, palpitations, ECG changes.
● DERM: urticaria, rash, photosensitivity, systemic lupus erythematosus-like syndrome.
● GI: anorexia, nausea, vomiting, constipation, dry mouth and throat.
● GU: urinary frequency, urinary retention, gynecomastia, decreased libido, inhibition of ejaculation.
● HEMA: *agranulocytosis*, leukopenia.
● Metabolic: hyperprolactinemia.
● Respiratory: chest tightness, wheezing, thickened bronchial secretions.

• Long-term therapy: skin hyperpigmentation; ocular changes, including corneal opacities and impaired vision.

Overdose and treatment
Clinical manifestations of overdose may include either CNS depression (sedation, reduced mental alertness, apnea, and cardiovascular collapse) or CNS stimulation (insomnia, hallucinations, tremors, or seizures). Anticholinergic symptoms, such as dry mouth, flushed skin, fixed and dilated pupils, and GI symptoms, are common, especially in children. The manufacturer warns against inducing emesis because dystonic reaction of head and neck may result in aspiration of vomitus. Use gastric lavage followed by activated charcoal. Treat hypotension with vasopressors, and control seizures with diazepam or phenytoin I.V. *Do not give stimulants.*

▶ Special considerations
Besides those relevant to all *antihistamines*, consider the following recommendations.
• Increased requirements for riboflavin may occur.
• Patients on prolonged therapy should be monitored periodically for cardiovascular, hematologic, and hepatic function and for neurologic or ophthalmologic effects.

Information for the patient
• Warn patient about risk of photosensitivity; recommend sunscreen, and advise patient to report skin reactions immediately.
• Instruct patient to store drug in a tightly closed container away from direct sunlight and heat.

Geriatric use
Elderly patients may experience more frequent and severe adverse effects with this drug than with other antihistamines because of its phenothiazine structure. Elderly patients are usually more sensitive to adverse effects of antihistamines and are especially likely to experience a greater degree of dizziness, sedation, hyperexcitability, dry mouth, and urinary retention than younger patients. Symptoms usually respond to a decrease in dosage.

Pediatric use
Drug is contraindicated for use in neonates; infants and children under age 6 may experience paradoxical hyperexcitability.

Breast-feeding
Antihistamines such as trimeprazine should not be used during breast-feeding. Many of these drugs are secreted in breast milk, exposing the infant to risks of unusual excitability; premature infants are at particular risk for seizures.

---

trimethadione
Tridione

• Pharmacologic classification: oxazolidinedione derivative
• Therapeutic classification: anticonvulsant
• Pregnancy risk category D

How supplied
Available by prescription only
Tablets (chewable): 150 mg
Capsules: 300 mg
Solution: 40 mg/ml

Indications, route, and dosage
Refractory absence seizures
Adults: Initially, 300 mg P.O. t.i.d.; may increase by 300 mg weekly, up to 600 mg P.O. q.i.d.
Children: 20 to 50 mg/kg P.O. daily, divided q 6 to 8 hours. Usual maintenance dosage is 40 mg/kg or 1 g/m^2 P.O. daily in divided doses t.i.d. or q.i.d., not to exceed 900 mg/day.

Pharmacodynamics
Anticonvulsant action: Trimethadione raises the threshold for cortical seizures but does not modify the seizure pattern. It decreases projection of focal activity and reduces both repetitive spinal cord transmission and spike-and-wave patterns of absence seizures.

Pharmacokinetics
• *Absorption:* Trimethadione is well and rapidly absorbed from the GI tract. Peak plasma concentrations occur in 30 minutes to 2 hours.
• *Distribution:* Trimethadione is distributed widely throughout the body; protein-binding is insignificant.
• *Metabolism:* Trimethadione is metabolized in the liver to an active metabolite.
• *Excretion:* Trimethadione is excreted slowly in urine.

Contraindications and precautions
Trimethadione is contraindicated in patients with known hypersensitivity to oxazolidinedione derivatives and in patients with renal or hepatic dysfunction. It should be used with caution in patients with severe blood dyscrasias, acute intermittent porphyria, or diseases of the retina or optic nerve. If a rash occurs, drug should be withdrawn immediately.
Anticonvulsants have been associated with an increased incidence of birth defects. Trimethadione may cause fetal harm and is contraindicated during pregnancy.

Interactions
Concomitant use of trimethadione and mephenytoin or phenacemide may result in a high incidence of toxicity; such combinations should be avoided.

Effects on diagnostic tests
Trimethadione may elevate liver function test results.

Adverse reactions
• CNS: drowsiness, ataxia, fatigue, malaise, insomnia, dizziness, headache, paresthesias, irritability.
• CV: hypertension, hypotension.

- DERM: acneiform and morbilliform rash, *exfoliative dermatitis,* erythema multiforme, petechiae, alopecia.
- EENT: hemeralopia, diplopia, photophobia, epistaxis, retinal hemorrhage.
- GI: nausea, vomiting, anorexia, abdominal pain, bleeding gums.
- GU: nephrosis, albuminuria, vaginal bleeding.
- HEMA: neutropenia, leukopenia, eosinophilia, thrombocytopenia, pancytopenia, *agranulocytosis, hypoplastic and aplastic anemia.*
- Hepatic: abnormal liver function test results.
- Other: lymphadenopathy.

    Note: Drug should be discontinued if signs of hypersensitivity, any rash (even acneiform), or unusual skin lesions occur; if scotomata occur; if neutrophil count falls to or below 2,500/mm³; if any of the following signs of blood dyscrasia occur: joint pain, fever, sore throat, or unusual bleeding or bruising; if patient has persistent or increasing albuminuria; if jaundice or other signs of hepatic dysfunction occur; or if syndromes resembling systemic lupus erythematosus, malignant lymphoma, or myasthenia gravis occur.

Overdose and treatment
Symptoms of overdose include nausea, drowsiness, ataxia, and visual disturbances; coma may follow massive overdose. Treat overdose by immediate gastric lavage or emesis, with supportive measures. Monitor vital signs and fluid and electrolyte balance carefully. Alkalinization of urine may hasten renal excretion. Monitor blood counts and hepatic and renal function after recovery.

▶ Special considerations
- Trimethadione should not be withdrawn abruptly; this can precipitate absence seizures.
- Monitor complete blood counts, urinalysis, and liver enzyme levels periodically during therapy.
- Triamethadione should be used only for absence seizures refractory to other anticonvulsants (such as ethosuximide). It is not effective for other types of seizure disorders and may precipitate a tonic-clonic seizure.

Information for the patient
- Advise patient that follow-up laboratory tests are essential.
- Advise women of childbearing age to use an effective form of contraception and call promptly if pregnancy is suspected.
- Tell patient to avoid ingesting alcoholic beverages.
- Tell patient to take drug with food or milk if GI upset occurs.
- Advise patient to wear a Medic Alert bracelet or necklace indicating medication use and identifying him as a patient with a seizure disorder.
- Explain that the drug may cause sensitivity to bright light. Sunscreens and protective clothing may be necessary.
- Warn that the drug may cause drowsiness or blurred vision. Patient should avoid hazardous tasks that require mental alertness until response to drug is determined.
- Advise patient to report the following: visual disturbances, excessive drowsiness, dizziness, sore throat, fever, unusual bleeding or bruising, or skin rash.
- Inform patient that hemeralopia (day blindness) may be relieved by wearing dark glasses.

Breast-feeding
Safety in breast-feeding has not been established. Alternative feeding method is recommended during therapy.

trimethaphan camsylate
Arfonad

- Pharmacologic classification: ganglionic blocking agent
- Therapeutic classification: antihypertensive
- Pregnancy risk category C

How supplied
Available by prescription only
Injection: 50 mg/ml in 10-ml ampules

Indications, route, and dosage
Severe hypertension and hypertensive emergencies
Adults: 500 mg (10 ml) diluted in 500 ml dextrose 5% in water to yield concentration of 1 mg/ml I.V. Start I.V. drip at 0.5 to 1 mg/minute and titrate to achieve desired response.
Hypertension associated with acute dissecting aortic aneurysms
Adults: Initial infusion rate is 1 to 2 mg/minute, titrated to maintain a systolic blood pressure of 100 to 120 mm Hg.
Controlled hypotension during surgery
Adults: Initially, I.V. infusion at a rate of 3 to 4 mg/minute (usual range is 0.3 to 6 mg/minute), titrated to desired response.

Pharmacodynamics
Antihypertensive action: Trimethaphan blocks transmission of impulses at sympathetic and parasympathetic ganglia, causing vasodilation, increased peripheral blood flow, and decreased blood pressure.

Pharmacokinetics
- *Absorption:* Blood pressure decreases almost immediately after I.V. administration. Drug's antihypertensive effect is reversed within 10 to 30 minutes after I.V. infusion is stopped.
- *Distribution:* Distribution pattern of trimethaphan is unknown; drug crosses placenta.
- *Metabolism:* Trimethaphan may be metabolized by pseudocholinesterase.
- *Excretion:* Trimethaphan is excreted by the kidneys.

Contraindications and precautions
Trimethaphan is contraindicated in patients with known hypersensitivity to the drug; in patients with anemia, hypovolemia, shock, asphyxia, or respiratory insufficiency because hypotension may worsen these conditions.

Trimethaphan should be used cautiously in atopic patients because drug may cause histamine release; and in patients with arteriosclerosis, cardiac disease, hepatic or renal dysfunction, degenerative CNS disease, Addison's disease, or diabetes mellitus because drug may exacerbate these conditions.

Trimethaphan also should be administered cautiously to patients receiving corticosteroids.

Avoid trimethaphan during pregnancy. Pregnant women are sensitized to ganglionic blocking agents. Drug-induced hypotension may have serious adverse fetal effects. The drug crosses the placenta and may cause meconium ileus in the fetus because it decreases fetal GI motility.

Interactions
Trimethaphan may potentiate antihypertensive effects of other antihypertensive agents; additive antihypertensive effects may occur when trimethaphan is used concomitantly with anesthetics or procainamide.

Large doses of trimethaphan may prolong the effects of neuromuscular blocking agents such as tubocurarine.

Effects on diagnostic tests
None reported.

Adverse reactions
● CNS: dilated pupils, extreme weakness.
● CV: severe orthostatic hypotension, tachycardia.
● GI: anorexia, nausea, vomiting, dry mouth.
● GU: urinary retention.
● Other: respiratory depression.
  Note: Drug should be discontinued if excessive hypotension occurs.

Overdose and treatment
Overdose is manifested primarily by excessive hypotension. Treatment is usually supportive and symptomatic. Use vasopressors if necessary.

▶ Special considerations
● Drug-induced pupillary dilation should not be confused with that caused by anoxia or related to depth of anesthesia.
● Tachyphylaxis to trimethaphan may develop within 24 to 72 hours.
● May be necessary to elevate head of bed (not to exceed 30 degrees) for maximal effect and to avoid cerebral anoxia.
● Monitor blood pressure at least every 2 minutes until stable, then at least every 5 minutes to ensure adequacy of dose.
● Monitor closely for respiratory distress, especially if large doses are given; provide oxygen during infusion.
● Use an infusion pump to administer drug slowly and precisely.
● When used to produce controlled hypotension during surgery, discontinue drug before wound closure to allow blood pressure to return to normal.
● Monitor fluid intake and output, because trimethaphan may decrease renal blood flow.
● Induced hypotension may have serious consequences for the fetus.

Information for the patient
● Advise patient to report adverse effects.
● Advise patient about positioning considerations (for example, head-up position) needed during trimethaphan infusion.

Geriatric use
Administer with extreme caution to elderly patients. Elderly patients usually require smaller doses.

Pediatric use
Administer with extreme caution to children.

trimethobenzamide hydrochloride
Tegamide, T-Gen, Ticon, Tigan, Tiject-20

● Pharmacologic classification: ethanol-amine-related antihistamine
● Therapeutic classification: antiemetic
● Pregnancy risk category C

How supplied
Available by prescription only
Capsules: 100 mg, 250 mg
Suppositories: 100 mg, 200 mg
Injection: 100 mg/ml

Indications, route, and dosage
Nausea and vomiting (treatment)
Adults: 250 mg P.O. t.i.d. or q.i.d.; or 200 mg I.M. or rectally t.i.d. or q.i.d.
Children 13.6 to 45 kg: 100 to 200 mg P.O. or rectally t.i.d. or q.i.d.
Children under 13.6 kg: 100 mg rectally t.i.d. or q.i.d.

Pharmacodynamics
Antiemetic action: Trimethobenzamide is a weak antihistamine with limited antiemetic properties. Its exact mechanism of action is unknown. Drug effects may occur in the brain's chemoreceptor trigger zone; however, the drug apparently does not inhibit direct impulses to the vomiting center.

Pharmacokinetics
● *Absorption:* Approximately 60% of an oral dose is absorbed. After oral administration, action begins in 10 to 40 minutes; after I.M. administration, in 15 to 35 minutes.
● *Distribution:* Unknown.
● *Metabolism:* Approximately 50% to 70% of a dose is metabolized, probably in the liver.
● *Excretion:* Drug is excreted in urine and feces. After oral administration, duration of effect is 3 to 4 hours; after I.M. administration, 2 to 3 hours.

Contraindications and precautions
Trimethobenzamide is contraindicated in patients with hypersensitivity to this drug, benzocaine, or other local anesthetics. The injectable form is contraindicated in children; suppositories are contraindicated in neonates and premature infants. Some clinicians consider the use of centrally acting antiemetics a contributing factor in the development of Reye's syndrome.

Trimethobenzamide should be used cautiously in patients with acute febrile illness, encephalitis, Reye's syndrome, encephalopathy, gastroenteritis, dehydration, or electrolyte imbalance, because the drug may mask the symptoms of these conditions.

Antiemetic effect may mask signs of overdose of toxic agents, intestinal obstruction, brain tumor, or other conditions. Antiemetics should not be the sole therapy of severe emesis. Restoration of fluid and electrolyte balance and relief of the underlying disease process are critical.

Interactions
Alcohol and other CNS depressants, including tricyclic antidepressants, antihypertensives, phenothiazines, and belladonna alkaloids, may increase trimethobenzamide toxicity.

Effects on diagnostic tests
None reported.

Adverse reactions
● CNS: drowsiness, dizziness (at high doses), headache, *seizures, coma*, depression, opisthotonos.
● CV: hypotension.
● GI: diarrhea, hepatotoxicity, jaundice, exacerbation of preexisting nausea (at high doses).
● Other: hypersensitivity reactions; parkinsonian-like symptoms; pain, burning, stinging, erythema, swelling at injection site; muscle cramps.
  Note: Drug should be discontinued if CNS or hypersensitivity reactions occur.

Overdose and treatment
Signs and symptoms of overdose may include severe neurologic reactions such as opisthotonos, seizures, coma, and extrapyramidal reactions. Discontinue the drug and provide supportive care.

▶ Special considerations
● Give I.M. dose by deep injection into upper outer gluteal quadrant to minimize pain and local irritation.
● Record frequency and volume of vomiting; observe patient for signs and symptoms of dehydration.
● Drug may be less effective against severe vomiting than other agents.
● Drug has little or no value in treating motion sickness.

Information for the patient
● Warn patient to avoid hazardous activities that require alertness, because drug may cause drowsiness, and to avoid consuming alcohol to prevent additive sedations.
● Instruct patient to report persistent vomiting.
● If patient is using suppositories, instruct him to remove foil and, if necessary, to moisten suppository with water for 10 to 30 seconds before inserting; tell him to store suppositories in refrigerator.

Geriatric use
Use drug with caution in elderly patients because they may be more susceptible to adverse CNS effects.

Pediatric use
Use drug with caution in children. Do not administer to children with viral illness because drug may contribute to development of Reye's syndrome.

trimethoprim
Proloprim, Trimpex

● Pharmacologic classification: synthetic folate antagonist
● Therapeutic classification: antibiotic
● Pregnancy risk category C

How supplied
Available by prescription only
Tablets: 100 mg, 200 mg

Indications, route, and dosage
Treatment of uncomplicated urinary tract infections
Adults: 100 mg P.O. q 12 hours for 10 days. Not recommended for children under age 12.
Prophylaxis of chronic and recurrent urinary tract infections
Adults: 100 mg P.O. h.s. for 6 weeks to 6 months.
Dosage in renal failure
In patients with a creatinine clearance of 10 to 50 ml/minute, increase dosage interval to every 18 hours. If creatinine clearance is less than 10 ml/minute, administer every 24 hours.

Pharmacodynamics
Antibacterial action: By interfering with action of dihydrofolate reductase, drug inhibits bacterial synthesis of folic acid. Drug is effective against many gram-positive and gram-negative organisms, including most Enterobacteriaceae organisms (except *Pseudomonas*), *Proteus mirabilis, Klebsiella,* and *Escherichia coli.*
  Trimethoprim is usually bactericidal.

Pharmacokinetics
● *Absorption:* Trimethoprim is absorbed quickly and completely, reaching peak serum levels in 1 to 4 hours.
● *Distribution:* Trimethoprim is distributed widely. Approximately 42% to 46% of dose is plasma protein-bound.
● *Metabolism:* Less than 20% of dose is metabolized in the liver.
● *Excretion:* Most of dose is excreted in the urine via filtration and secretion. In patients with normal renal function, elimination half-life is 8 to 11 hours; in patients with impaired renal function, half-life is prolonged.

Contraindications and precautions
Trimethoprim is contraindicated in patients who are hypersensitive to the drug and in patients with megaloblastic anemia resulting from folate deficiency because drug may worsen this condition. It is not recommended in patients with creatinine clearance below 15 ml/minute because of potential for increased renal toxicity.
  Trimethoprim should be administered cautiously to patients with renal or hepatic dysfunction because drug accumulation may occur and cause dose-related toxic effects.

Interactions
When used concomitantly, trimethoprim may inhibit phenytoin metabolism, causing increased serum phenytoin levels.

Effects on diagnostic tests
Liver enzyme levels and renal function indices (blood urea nitrogen and serum creatinine levels) may increase during trimethoprim therapy.

Adverse reactions
● DERM: rash, pruritus, *exfoliative dermatitis.*
● GI: epigastric distress, nausea, vomiting, glossitis.
● HEMA: thrombocytopenia, leukopenia, megaloblastic anemia, methemoglobinemia.
● Other: fever.
Note: Drug should be discontinued if signs or symptoms of blood dyscrasias develop.

Overdose and treatment
Clinical effects of acute overdose include nausea, vomiting, dizziness, headache, confusion, and bone marrow depression. Treatment includes gastric lavage and supportive measures. Urine may be acidified to enhance drug elimination.

Clinical effects of chronic toxicity caused by prolonged high-dose therapy include bone marrow depression, leukopenia, thrombocytopenia, and megaloblastic anemia. Treatment includes drug discontinuation and administration of leucovorin – 3 to 6 mg I.M. daily for 3 days or 5 to 15 mg P.O. daily until normal hematopoiesis returns.

▶ Special considerations
● Obtain culture and sensitivity tests before starting therapy.
● Usually used with other antibiotics (especially sulfamethoxazole) because resistance develops rapidly when trimethoprim is used alone.
● If patient is receiving drug concomitantly with phenytoin, monitor serum phenytoin levels.
● Advanced age, malnourishment, pregnancy, debilitation, renal impairment, and prolonged high-dose therapy increase risk of hematologic toxicity, as does concomitant therapy with folate antagonistic drugs (such as phenytoin).
● Sore throat, fever, pallor, and purpura may be early signs of serious blood disorders. Monitor blood counts regularly.

Information for the patient
● Instruct patient to continue taking drug as directed, until it is gone, even if he feels better.
● Advise patient to report signs of blood disorders (sore throat, fever, pallor, and purpura) immediately.

Geriatric use
Elderly patients may be more susceptible to hematologic toxicity.

Pediatric use
Safety in children under age 2 months has not been established; effectiveness in children under age 12 has not been established.

Breast-feeding
Drug is excreted in breast milk; alternative feeding method is recommended during therapy with trimethoprim.

trimetrexate glucuronate

● Pharmacologic classification: dihydrofolate reductase inhibitor
● Therapeutic classification: antimicrobial/antineoplastic
● Pregnancy risk category C

How supplied
Information about use of trimetrexate under the treatment IND available from Warner-Lambert at (800) 426-7527 (outside Michigan) or (800) 833-0014 (inside Michigan) from 8 a.m.-8 p.m., EST, Monday to Friday.
Injection: 25-mg vials

Indications, route, and dosage
Trimetrexate glucuronate is an investigational drug that is available for hospital use in treatment of qualifying patients with *Pneumocystis carinii* pneumonia and who have exhibited serious (severe or life-threatening) intolerance to both co-trimoxazole and pentamidine.

Under the treatment protocol, patients are eligible to receive trimetrexate if they have an unequivocal diagnosis of *P. carinii* pneumonia; are human immunodeficiency virus (HIV)-positive by enzyme-linked immunosorbent assay (ELISA), HIV culture, and/or p24 core antigenemia (p24 *gag* proteinemia); have experienced a serious and/or life-threatening adverse reaction to conventional antipneumocystis therapy (such as co-trimoxazole or pentamidine); and are 12 years of age or older. If laboratory confirmation of HIV infection has not been made prior to request for treatment use of trimetrexate, a history of high-risk behavior for HIV infection (for example, homosexual or bisexual male, I.V. drug abuser, recipient of HIV-positive blood product, or sexual partner of an individual in one of these groups) will suffice.
Adults: Dosage and indication will vary with protocol. 30 mg/m² I.V. bolus daily for 21 days, administered with leucovorin (20 mg/m² I.V. or P.O. daily).

Pharmacodynamics
Dihydrofolate reductase inhibiting action: In vitro, the affinity of trimetrexate for pneumocystis dihydrofolate reductase is about 1,500 times that of trimethoprim. Unlike methotrexate, trimetrexate is highly lipophilic and is passively taken up by and concentrated in protozoan cells.

Pharmacokinetics
● *Absorption:* No data are currently available regarding oral bioavailability.
● *Distribution:* Trimetrexate distributes rapidly after I.V. administration.
● *Metabolism:* Trimetrexate is probably metabolized by the liver; at least two metabolites (one active) have been identified.
● *Excretion:* Trimetrexate is excreted in bile and urine.

Contraindications and precautions
Because of the risk of potentially lethal trimetrexate-induced toxicity (myelosuppression) secondary to the drug's inhibition of dihydrofolate reductase, concomitant leucovorin therapy is essential in patients receiving trimetrexate. Other potentially myelosuppressive (including zidovudine) or nephrotoxic therapy should be

---

discontinued during trimetrexate therapy but can be resumed as soon as treatment with trimetrexate and leucovorin is complete.

Interactions
None reported.

Effects on diagnostic tests
Information not available.

Adverse reactions
● DERM: rash.
● GI: mucositis, stomatitis, nausea, vomiting, diarrhea.
● HEMA: *neutropenia, thrombocytopenia.*
● Metabolic: liver function test abnormalities.
● Other: *hepatotoxicity, peripheral neuropathy, fever.*

Overdose and treatment
Although no overdose information is available clinical effects are expected to be similar to methotrexate.

Methotrexate overdose produces myelosuppression, anemia, nausea, vomiting, dermatitis, alopecia, and melena.

Specific treatment information is unavailable, but calcium levocovorin would probably serve as an appropriate treatment. Contact the manufacturer (Warner-Lambert) for further information.

▶ Special considerations
● Avoid I.M. injections in patient with thrombocytopenia.
● Store intact vials in refrigerator.
● Incompatible with chloride-containing solutions (including normal saline). Only dextrose 5% in water is recommended for infusions.
● Dosage adjustments may be necessary in patients with altered hepatic or renal function.
● Leucovorin should be continued for 72 hours after the last dose of trimetrexate.

---

trimipramine maleate
Surmontil

● Pharmacologic classification: tricyclic antidepressant
● Therapeutic classification: antidepressant, antianxiety agent
● Pregnancy risk category C

How supplied
Available by prescription only
Capsules: 25 mg, 50 mg, 100 mg

Indications, route, and dosage
Depression
Adults: 75 mg/day in divided doses, increased to 200 mg/day. Dosages over 300 mg/day are not recommended.
Enuresis
Children over age 6: Initial dose is 25 mg P.O. 1 hour before bedtime; if no response occurs, increase dose to 50 mg in children under age 12, and to 75 mg in children over age 12. Do not give more than 200 mg in a single dose.

Pharmacodynamics
Trimipramine is thought to exert its antidepressant effects by equally inhibiting reuptake of norepinephrine and serotonin in CNS nerve terminals (presynaptic neurons), which results in increased concentration and enhanced activity of these neurotransmitters in the synaptic cleft. Trimipramine also has anxiolytic effects and inhibits gastric acid secretion.

Pharmacokinetics
● *Absorption:* Trimipramine is absorbed rapidly from the GI tract after oral administration.
● *Distribution:* Trimipramine is distributed widely in the body. Drug is 90% protein-bound. Peak effect occurs in 2 hours; steady state within 7 days.
● *Metabolism:* Trimipramine is metabolized by the liver; a significant first-pass effect may explain variability of serum levels in different patients taking the same dosage.
● *Excretion:* Most of drug is excreted in urine; some is excreted in feces via the biliary tract.

Contraindications and precautions
Trimipramine is contraindicated in patients with known hypersensitivity to tricyclic antidepressants, trazodone, and related compounds; in the acute recovery phase of myocardial infarction (MI) because drug depresses cardiac function and causes dysrhythmia; in patients in coma or severe respiratory depression (additive CNS and respiratory depression); and during or within 14 days of therapy with monoamine oxidase inhibitors.

Trimipramine should be used cautiously in patients with other cardiac disease (arrhythmias, CHF, angina pectoris, valvular disease, or heart block), respiratory disorders, seizure disorders, scheduled electroconvulsive therapy, bipolar disease, glaucoma, hyperthyroidism, and parkinsonism; in patients taking thyroid replacement; in patients with diabetes Types I and II; in patients with prostatic hypertrophy, paralytic ileus, or urinary retention, because drug may worsen these conditions; in patients with hepatic or renal dysfunction because diminished metabolism and excretion causes the drug to accumulate; and in patients undergoing surgery using general anesthesia because drug may increase cardiac sensitivity to the effects of general anesthetics or pressor agents.

Interactions
Concomitant use of trimipramine with sympathomimetics, including epinephrine, phenylephrine, phenylpropanolamine, and ephedrine (often found in nasal sprays) may increase blood pressure; use with warfarin may increase prothrombin time and cause bleeding.

Concomitant use with thyroid medication, pimozide, and antiarrhythmic agents (quinidine, disopyramide, procainamide) may increase incidence of cardiac arrhythmias and conduction defects.

Trimipramine may decrease hypotensive effects of centrally acting antihypertensive drugs, such as guanethidine, guanabenz, guanadrel, clonidine, methyldopa, and reserpine.

Concomitant use with disulfiram or ethchlorvynol may cause delirium and tachycardia.

Additive effects are likely after concomitant use of trimipramine with CNS depressants, including alcohol, analgesics, barbiturates, narcotics, tranquilizers, and anesthetics (oversedation); atropine and other anticholinergic drugs, including phenothiazines, antihistamines, meperidine, and antiparkinsonian agents (oversedation, paralytic ileus, visual changes, and severe

---

constipation); and metrizamide (increased risk of seizures).

Barbiturates and heavy smoking induce trimipramine metabolism and decrease therapeutic efficacy; phenothiazines and haloperidol decrease its metabolism, decreasing therapeutic efficacy; methylphenidate, cimetidine, oral contraceptives, propoxyphene, and beta blockers may inhibit trimipramine metabolism, increasing plasma levels and toxicity.

Effects on diagnostic tests

Trimipramine may prolong conduction time (elongation of Q-T and PR intervals, flattened T waves on ECG); it also may elevate liver function test levels, decrease white blood cell counts, and alter serum glucose levels. Trimipramine may alter prothrombin time.

Adverse reactions

● CNS: drowsiness, dizziness, sedation, excitation, tremors, weakness, headache, nervousness, *seizures*, peripheral neuropathy, extrapyramidal symptoms, anxiety, vivid dreams, confusion (more marked in elderly patients), decreased libido.
● CV: orthostatic hypotension, tachycardia, *arrhythmias, MI, stroke, heart block, CHF,* palpitations, hypertension, ECG changes.
● EENT: blurred vision, tinnitus, mydriasis, increased intraocular pressure.
● GI: dry mouth, constipation, nausea, vomiting, anorexia, diarrhea, paralytic ileus, jaundice.
● GU: urinary retention.
● Other: sweating, photosensitivity, hypersensitivity (rash, urticaria, drug fever, edema).

After abrupt withdrawal of long-term therapy, nausea, headache, malaise (does not indicate addiction) may occur.

Note: Drug should be discontinued (not abruptly) if signs of hypersensitivity occur; dosage adjustment or discontinuation may be required if any of the following occur: urinary retention, extreme dry mouth, skin rash, excessive sedation, seizures, tachycardia, sore throat, fever, or jaundice.

Overdose and treatment

The first 12 hours after acute ingestion are a stimulatory phase characterized by excessive anticholinergic activity (agitation, irritation, confusion, hallucinations, parkinsonism symptoms, seizure, urinary retention, dry mucous membranes, pupillary dilatation, constipation, and ileus). This is followed by CNS depressant effects, including hypothermia, decreased or absent reflexes, sedation, hypotension, cyanosis, and cardiac irregularities (including tachycardia, conduction disturbances, and quinidine-like effects on the ECG).

Severity of overdose is best indicated by prolongation of QRS interval beyond 100 msec, which usually represents a serum level in excess of 1,000 ng/ml; serum levels are generally not helpful. Metabolic acidosis may follow hypotension, hypoventilation, and seizures.

Treatment is symptomatic and supportive and includes maintaining airway, stable body temperature, and fluid and electrolyte balance. Induce emesis with ipecac if patient is conscious; follow with gastric lavage and activated charcoal to prevent further absorption. Dialysis is of little use. Treat seizures with parenteral diazepam or phenytoin; arrhythmias with parenteral phenytoin or lidocaine; and acidosis with sodium bicarbonate. *Do not give barbiturates* – these may enhance CNS and respiratory depressant effects.

▶ Special considerations

Besides those relevant to all *tricyclic antidepressants*, consider the following recommendations.
● Consider the inherent risk of suicide until significant improvement of depressive state occurs. High-risk patients should have close supervision during initial drug therapy. To reduce risk of suicidal overdose, prescribe the smallest quantity of capsules consistent with good management.
● The full dosage may be given at bedtime to help offset daytime sedation.
● Trimipramine also has been used to decrease gastric acid secretion in peptic ulcer disease. The safety and efficacy of trimipramine maleate in peptic ulcer disease has not been established.
● Watch for bleeding because the drug may cause alterations in prothrombin time.
● The drug should not be withdrawn abruptly. However, it should be discontinued at least 48 hours before surgical procedures.
● Tolerance generally develops to the sedative effects of this drug.

Information for the patient

● Advise patient to take full dosage at bedtime to minimize daytime sedation.
● Explain that full effects of the drug may not become apparent for up to 4 to 6 weeks after therapy begins.
● Tell patient to take the drug exactly as prescribed; not to double doses for missed ones; not to discontinue drug suddenly; and not to share drug with others.
● Warn patient that drug may cause drowsiness or dizziness. Patient should avoid hazardous activities that require alertness until the full effects of the drug are known.
● Warn patient not to drink alcoholic beverages or medicinal elixirs while taking this drug.
● Tell patient to store drug safely away from children.
● Suggest taking drug with food or milk if it causes stomach upset and to ease dry mouth with sugarless chewing gum, hard candy, or ice.
● To prevent dizziness, advise patient to lie down for about 30 minutes after each dose and to avoid abrupt postural changes, especially when rising to an upright position.
● Tell patient to report adverse reactions promptly, especially confusion, movement disorders, rapid heartbeat, dizziness, fainting, or difficulty urinating.

Geriatric use

Recommended starting dose for elderly patients is 25 mg. Such patients may be more vulnerable to adverse cardiac effects.

tripelennamine citrate
PBZ

tripelennamine hydrochloride
PBZ, PBZ-SR, Pelamine

- Pharmacologic classification: ethylene-diamine-derivative antihistamine
- Therapeutic classification: antihistamine (H_1-receptor antagonist)
- Pregnancy risk category B

How supplied
Available with or without prescription
Tablets: 25 mg, 50 mg tripelennamine hydrochloride
Tablets (extended-release): 50 mg, 100 mg tripelennamine hydrochloride
Elixir: 37.5 mg/5 ml tripelennamine citrate; 37.5 mg tripelennamine citrate equal 25 mg tripelennamine hydrochloride
Topical cream: 2%

Indications, route, and dosage
Rhinitis, allergy symptoms, allergic reactions to blood or plasma, adjunct to epinephrine in anaphylaxis
Adults: 25 to 50 mg P.O. q 4 to 6 hours; or (timed-release) 50 to 100 mg P.O. b.i.d. or t.i.d. Maximum dosage is 600 mg daily.
Infants and children: 5 mg/kg or 150 mg/m² daily in four to six divided doses. Do not use timed-release tablets in children.
Pruritus, minor burns, insect bites, sunburn, skin irritations
Adults and children: Apply topical cream t.i.d. or q.i.d.
Drug dosages are based on tripelennamine hydrochloride (tablets only); dosage of tripelennamine citrate (elixir only) is about 1½ times that of tripelennamine hydrochloride; 5 mg tripelennamine hydrochloride equals 7.5 mg tripelennamine citrate.

Pharmacodynamics
Antihistamine action: Tripelennamine competes with histamine for the H_1-receptor, thereby ameliorating histamine effects in target tissues; drug does not prevent the release of histamine.

Pharmacokinetics
Tripelennamine is well absorbed; distribution, metabolism, and excretion have not been reported.

Contraindications and precautions
Tripelennamine is contraindicated in patients with known hypersensitivity to this drug or antihistamines with a similar chemical structure, such as pyrilamine; in neonates, other infants, and breast-feeding women, because young children may be more susceptible to the toxic effects of antihistamines; during asthma attacks because it thickens bronchial secretions; and in patients who have taken MAO inhibitors within the preceding 2 weeks.
Because of significant anticholinergic effects, tripelennamine should be used with caution in patients with narrow-angle glaucoma; in those with pyloroduodenal obstruction or urinary bladder obstruction from prostatic hypertrophy or narrowing of the bladder neck; and

in patients with cardiovascular disease or hypertension, because drug may cause palpitations.

Interactions
MAO inhibitors interfere with the detoxification of antihistamines and phenothiazines, and thus prolong and intensify their central depressant and anticholinergic effects; additive CNS depression and sedation may occur when tripelennamine is administered with other CNS depressants, such as alcohol, barbiturates, tranquilizers, sleeping aids, or antianxiety agents.

Effects on diagnostic tests
Tripelennamine should be discontinued 4 days before diagnostic skin tests, to avoid preventing, reducing, or masking test response.

Adverse reactions
- CNS: drowsiness, dizziness, confusion, vertigo, tinnitus, fatigue, disturbed coordination, paresthesias, euphoria, nervousness, restlessness, tremors, irritability, insomnia.
- CV: mild hypertension, hypotension, palpitations, chest tightness.
- DERM: rash, urticaria, photosensitivity.
- EENT: diplopia, blurred vision, dry nose and throat.
- GI: anorexia, diarrhea, constipation, nausea, vomiting.
- GU: urinary frequency or retention.
- HEMA: leukopenia, agranulocytosis, hemolytic anemia.
- Respiratory: thickened bronchial secretions.
- Topical: sensitization.

Overdose and treatment
Clinical manifestations of overdose may include either CNS depression (sedation, reduced mental alertness, apnea, and cardiovascular collapse) or CNS stimulation (insomnia, hallucinations, tremors, or seizures). Anticholinergic symptoms, such as dry mouth, flushed skin, fixed and dilated pupils, and GI symptoms, are common, especially in children; children also may experience fever, excitement, ataxia, and athetosis.
Treat overdose by inducing emesis with ipecac syrup (in conscious patient), followed by activated charcoal to reduce further drug absorption. Use gastric lavage if patient is unconscious or ipecac fails. Treat hypotension with vasopressors, and control seizures with diazepam, phenytoin, or short-acting barbiturates. *Do not give stimulants.*

▶ Special considerations
Besides those relevant to all *antihistamines*, consider the following recommendations.
- Be alert to change in drug dosage when substituting elixir for tablets, or vice versa.
- Give extended-release tablets whole; do not crush.

Geriatric use
Elderly patients are usually more sensitive to adverse effects of antihistamines and are especially likely to experience a greater degree of dizziness, sedation, hyperexcitability, dry mouth, and urinary retention than younger patients. Symptoms usually respond to a decrease in medication dosage.

Pediatric use
Safe use in neonates and premature infants is not established. Other infants and children under age 6 may experience paradoxical hyperexcitability.

Breast-feeding
Antihistamines such as tripelennamine should not be used during breast-feeding. Many of these drugs are secreted in breast milk, exposing the infant to risks of unusual excitability; premature infants are at particular risk for seizures.

triprolidine hydrochloride
Actidil, Myidyl

- Pharmacologic classification: alkylamine antihistamine derivative
- Therapeutic classification: antihistamine (H₁-receptor antagonist)
- Pregnancy risk category B

How supplied
Available with or without prescription
Tablets: 2.5 mg
Syrup: 1.25 mg/5 ml

Indications, route, and dosage
Colds and allergy symptoms
Adults and children age 12 and older: 2.5 mg P.O. q 4 to 6 hours; maximum daily dosage is 10 mg.
Children age 6 to 11: 1.25 mg q 4 to 6 hours; maximum daily dosage is 5 mg.
Children age 4 to 5: 0.9 mg q 6 to 8 hours; maximum daily dosage is 3.75 mg.
Children age 2 to 3: 0.6 mg every 6 to 8 hours; maximum daily dosage is 2.5 mg.
Children age 4 months to 1 year: 0.3 mg every 6 to 8 hours; maximum daily dosage is 1.25 mg.

Pharmacodynamics
Antihistamine action: Antihistamines compete with histamine for histamine H₁-receptor sites on the smooth muscle of the bronchi, GI tract, uterus, and large blood vessels; by binding to cellular receptors, they prevent access of histamine and suppress histamine-induced allergic symptoms, even though they do not prevent its release.

Pharmacokinetics
- *Absorption:* Triprolidine is well absorbed from the GI tract; it has a rapid onset of action, with peak effects occurring in about 3½ hours, and a duration of about 12 hours.
- *Distribution:* Triprolidine's distribution is not fully known; drug is distributed to the lungs, spleen, and kidneys.
- *Metabolism:* Triprolidine is metabolized by the liver.
- *Excretion:* Triprolidine's half-life is about 2 to 6 hours.

Contraindications and precautions
Triprolidine is contraindicated in patients with known hypersensitivity to this drug or other antihistamines with similar chemical structures (brompheniramine, chlorpheniramine, and dexchlorpheniramine); during asthma attacks, because triprolidine thickens bronchial secretions; and in patients who have taken MAO inhibitors within the previous 2 weeks.

Triprolidine should be used with caution in patients with narrow-angle glaucoma; in those with pyloroduodenal obstruction or urinary bladder obstruction from prostatic hypertrophy or narrowing of the bladder neck, because of their marked anticholinergic effects; in patients with cardiovascular disease, hypertension, or hyperthyroidism, because of the risk of palpitations and tachycardia; and in patients with renal disease, diabetes, bronchial asthma, urinary retention, or stenosing peptic ulcers.

Pregnant women should avoid triprolidine, especially in the third trimester, as should nursing women; although most antihistamines have not been studied in such patients, seizures and other severe reactions have occurred in neonates, especially premature infants.

Interactions
MAO inhibitors interfere with the detoxification of antihistamines and thus prolong and intensify their central depressant and anticholinergic effects; added CNS depression may occur when triprolidine is given concomitantly with other CNS depressants, such as alcohol, barbiturates, tranquilizers, sleeping aids, and antianxiety agents.

Triprolidine may diminish the effects of sulfonylureas and may partially counteract the anticoagulant effects of heparin.

Effects on diagnostic tests
Discontinue triprolidine 4 days before diagnostic skin tests; antihistamines can prevent, reduce, or mask positive skin response to the test.

Adverse reactions
- CNS: (especially in elderly patients) drowsiness, dizziness, restlessness, insomnia, stimulation.
- DERM: urticaria, rash.
- EENT: dry nose and throat.
- GI: anorexia, diarrhea, constipation, nausea, vomiting, dry mouth.
- GU: urinary frequency or retention.
- Respiratory: thick bronchial secretions.

Overdose and treatment
Clinical manifestations of overdose may include either CNS depression (sedation, reduced mental alertness, apnea, and cardiovascular collapse) or CNS stimulation (insomnia, hallucinations, tremors, or seizures). Anticholinergic symptoms, such as dry mouth, flushed skin, fixed and dilated pupils, and GI symptoms, are common, especially in children.

Treat overdose by inducing emesis with ipecac syrup (in conscious patient), followed by activated charcoal to reduce further drug absorption. Use gastric lavage if patient is unconscious or ipecac fails. Treat hypotension with vasopressors, and control seizures with diazepam or phenytoin. *Do not give stimulants.*

▶ Special considerations
Besides those relevant to all *antihistamines,* consider the following recommendation.
- Triprolidine has a low incidence of drowsiness.

Information for the patient
Recommendations for patient teaching are the same as those for all antihistamines.

Geriatric use

Elderly patients are usually more sensitive to adverse effects of antihistamines and are especially likely to experience a greater degree of dizziness, sedation, hyperexcitability, dry mouth, and urinary retention than younger patients. Symptoms usually respond to a decrease in medication dosage.

Pediatric use

Drug is not indicated for use in premature or newborn infants; infants and children under age 6 may experience paradoxical hyperexcitability.

Breast-feeding

Antihistamines such as triprolidine should not be used during breast-feeding. Many of these drugs are secreted in breast milk, exposing the infant to risks of unusual excitability; premature infants are at particular risk for seizures.

troleandomycin
TAO

- Pharmacologic classification: macrolide antibiotic
- Therapeutic classification: antibiotic
- Pregnancy risk category C

How supplied

Available by prescription only
Capsules: 250 mg
Suspension: 125 mg/ml

Indications, route, and dosage
Pneumonia or respiratory tract infection caused by sensitive pneumococci or group A beta-hemolytic streptococci
Adults: 250 to 500 mg P.O. q 6 hours.
Children: 25 to 40 mg/kg/day in divided doses q 6 hours.

Pharmacodynamics

Antibacterial action: Drug inhibits bacterial protein synthesis by binding to 50S ribosomal subunit. It produces bacteriostatic effects on susceptible bacteria, including gram-positive cocci and bacilli and a few gram-negative organisms *(Haemophilus influenzae, Neisseria gonorrhoeae,* and *N. meningitidis).*

Pharmacokinetics

- *Absorption:* Troleandomycin is absorbed rapidly but incompletely. Peak serum levels occur in approximately 2 hours.
- *Distribution:* Troleandomycin is distributed widely to body fluids, except to CSF.
- *Metabolism:* Troleandomycin is metabolized in the liver.
- *Excretion:* Troleandomycin is excreted in the bile, feces, and urine (10% to 25%).

Contraindications and precautions

Troleandomycin is contraindicated in patients with known hypersensitivity to the drug.

Troleandomycin should be administered cautiously to patients with hepatic dysfunction because it may cause allergic cholestatic hepatitis, manifested by jaundice, right upper abdominal quadrant pain, fever, nausea and vomiting, leukocytosis, and eosinophilia.

Interactions

When used concomitantly, troleandomycin may decrease clearance of theophylline, carbamazepine, and methylprednisolone, possibly causing toxicity. (Clinical significance of decreased clearance of methylprednisolone is somewhat questionable; however, some clinicians recommend lower doses of the steroid.) Concomitant use with ergotamine may precipitate severe ischemic reactions and peripheral vasospasms. Concomitant use with oral contraceptives may cause marked cholestatic jaundice.

Effects on diagnostic tests

Liver function test results may show increased enzyme levels, and eosinophilia and leukocytosis may occur during troleandomycin therapy.

Adverse reactions

- DERM: urticaria, rash.
- GI: abdominal cramps, vomiting, diarrhea, discomfort.
- Hepatic: cholestatic jaundice.
- Other: *anaphylaxis.*
  Note: Drug should be discontinued if liver function test values increase or if signs or symptoms of cholestatic hepatitis develop.

Overdose and treatment

No information available.

▶ Special considerations

- Obtain culture and sensitivity tests before starting therapy.
- If patient is receiving drug concomitantly with theophylline or carbamazepine, closely monitor serum theophylline or carbamazepine levels and assess patient frequently for signs and symptoms of theophylline or carbamazepine toxicity.
- Patient receiving drug concomitantly with methylprednisolone may require reduced methylprednisolone dose.
- Monitor total serum bilirubin and AST (SGOT), ALT (SGPT), and serum alkaline phosphatase levels.
- Repeated courses of therapy or therapy exceeding 2 weeks may lead to allergic cholestatic hepatitis, as indicated by jaundice, right upper abdominal quadrant pain, fever, nausea, vomiting, eosinophilia, and leukocytosis.

Information for the patient

- Instruct patient to continue taking drug as directed, even if he feels better.
- For best absorption, advise patient to take drug on an empty stomach 1 hour before or 2 hours after meals, with full glass of water.
- Instruct patient to report abdominal pain or nausea immediately.

---

tromethamine
Tham, Tham-E

- Pharmacologic classification: sodium-free organic amine
- Therapeutic classification: systemic alkalinizer
- Pregnancy risk category C

How supplied
Available by prescription only
Injection: 36 g, 36 mg/ml (18 g/500 ml)

Indications, route, and dosage
Correction of metabolic acidosis (associated with cardiac bypass surgery or with cardiac arrest)
Dosage depends on base deficit. Calculate as follows: ml of 0.3 molar tromethamine solution required = body wt in kg × body deficit in mEq/liter. Total dosage should be administered over at least 1 hour and should not exceed 500 mg/kg for an adult. Total dosage should be administered over at least 1 hour and should not exceed 500 mg/kg for an adult.

The usual dose of a 0.3 molar solution (3.6 to 10.8 g of tromethamine) may be administered into a large peripheral vein. If the chest is open, 55 to 165 ml of a 0.3 molar solution (2 to 6 g of tromethamine) has also been injected into the ventricular cavity (*not into the cardiac muscle*).

For systemic acidosis during cardiac bypass surgery, the usual single dose of a 0.3 molar solution is 9 ml/kg (324 mg/kg of tromethamine) or about 500 ml (18 g of tromethamine) for most adults.
To titrate the excess acidity of stored blood used to prime the pump-oxygenator during cardiac bypass surgery
Add 14 to 70 ml of 0.3 molar solution to each 500 ml of blood, depending on the pH of the blood.

Pharmacodynamics
Systemic alkalinizing action: Tromethamine, as a weak base, acts as a proton acceptor to prevent or correct acidosis; drug reduces hydrogen ion concentration. It also acts as a weak osmotic diuretic, increasing the flow of alkaline urine.

Pharmacokinetics
- *Absorption:* Absorption is immediate because tromethamine is available for I.V. use only.
- *Distribution:* At pH of 7.4, about 25% of drug is unionized; this portion may enter cells to neutralize acidic ions of intracellular fluid.
- *Metabolism:* None.
- *Excretion:* Tromethamine is rapidly excreted renally as the bicarbonate salt.

Contraindications and precautions
Tromethamine is contraindicated in patients with uremia or anuria, because of renal excretion; in patients with chronic respiratory acidosis, because it decreases serum carbon dioxide levels and may cause respiratory failure; in pregnant patients; or when used longer than 24 hours, except in life-threatening emergencies.

Drug should be used with caution in neonates and other infants, and in patients with renal disease and poor urinary output, because drug may accumulate in patients with decreased renal function.

Interactions
Concomitant use with other respiratory or CNS depressants may cause cumulative respiratory depression.

Effects on diagnostic tests
Tromethamine alters serum electrolyte levels. Transient decreases in blood glucose concentrations may occur.

Adverse reactions
- CNS: *respiratory depression.*
- Local: tissue irritation, chemical phlebitis, venospasm, I.V. thrombophlebitis.
- Other: hypoglycemia, severe hepatic necrosis in newborns and infants (with 1.2 molar solution), hydropic degeneration of hepatic and renal tubular cells (with a 1.5 molar solution).
  Note: Drug should be discontinued if signs of hypersensitivity, severe hypoglycemia, or respiratory depression occur, or if infusion extravasates.

Overdose and treatment
Clinical signs of overdose include respiratory or systemic alkalosis, cardiac arrhythmias secondary to hypokalemia, respiratory depression, and hypoglycemia. Discontinue drug and correct pH; use decreased ventilation and systemic acidifiers if necessary. Treat hypokalemia cautiously with potassium (serum potassium levels will rise with correction of alkalosis), and hypoglycemia with I.V. glucose as needed.

► Special considerations
- Monitor vital signs, blood pH levels, carbon dioxide tension, and bicarbonate, glucose, and electrolyte levels before, during, and after infusion.
- Tromethamine should be administered by slow I.V. into the largest antecubital vein or via a large needle, indwelling catheter, or pump-oxygenator. Infusion site should be checked frequently to avoid extravasation of solution and prevent tissue damage. If extravasation occurs, aspirate as much fluid as possible. Infiltrating area with 1% procaine hydrochloride to which hyaluronidase has been added may aid in extravasation and venospasm. Local injection of phentolamine can be used to reverse venospasm.

Geriatric use
Patients with severe renal dysfunction or chronic respiratory acidosis are at increased risk with tromethamine; drug should be used with caution.

Pediatric use
Drug should be used with caution; severe hepatic necrosis has occurred in infants and neonates after administration of a 1.2 molar solution through the umbilical vein.

tropicamide
Mydriacyl

- Pharmacologic classification: anticholinergic agent
- Therapeutic classification: cycloplegic, mydriatic

How supplied
Available by prescription only
Ophthalmic solution: 0.5%, 1%

Indications, route, and dosage
Cycloplegic refractions
Adults and children: Instill 1 or 2 drops of 0.5 to 1% solution in each eye; repeat in 5 minutes.
Fundus examinations
Adults and children: Instill 1 or 2 drops of 0.5% to 1% solution in each eye 15 to 20 minutes before examination. May repeat q 30 minutes if necessary.

Physician should apply light finger pressure on lacrimal sac for 1 minute after instillation to minimize systemic absorption.

Pharmacodynamics
Mydriatic action: Anticholinergic action prevents the sphincter muscle of the iris and the muscle of the ciliary body from responding to cholinergic stimulation, producing pupillary dilation (mydriasis) and paralysis of accommodation (cycloplegia).

Pharmacokinetics
- *Absorption:* Peak effect usually occurs in 20 to 40 minutes.
- *Distribution:* Unknown.
- *Metabolism:* Unknown.
- *Excretion:* Recovery from cycloplegic and mydriatic effects usually occurs in about 6 hours.

Contraindications and precautions
Tropicamide is contraindicated in patients with narrow-angle glaucoma and in patients hypersensitive to any component of the preparation. Drug should be used with caution in patients in whom increased intraocular pressure may occur; and in children, because of increased risk of cardiovascular and CNS effects.

Interactions
None significant.

Effects on diagnostic tests
None reported.

Adverse reactions
- CNS: ataxia, behavioral disturbances in children.
- DERM: dryness, flushing.
- ENT: nose and throat dryness.
- Eye: transient stinging, increased intraocular pressure, blurred vision, photophobia.
- Other: fever.
  Note: Drug should be discontinued if behavioral disturbances occur.

Overdose and treatment
Clinical manifestations of overdose include dry, flushed skin; dry mouth; dilated pupils; delirium; hallucination; tachycardia; and decreased bowel sounds. Treat accidental ingestion with emesis or activated charcoal. Use physostigmine to antagonize tropicamide's anticholinergic activity in severe toxicity and propranolol to treat symptomatic tachyarrhythmias unresponsive to physostigmine.

▶ Special considerations
Tropicamide is the shortest-acting cycloplegic, but its mydriatic effect is greater than its cycloplegic effect.

Information for the patient
- Advise patient to protect eyes from bright illumination for comfort.
- Instruct patient to wait 5 minutes before using another eye preparation.

Geriatric use
Drug should be used with caution in the elderly to avoid triggering undiagnosed narrow-angle glaucoma.

Pediatric use
Infants and small children may be especially susceptible to CNS disturbances from systemic absorption. Psychotic reactions, behavioral disturbances, and cardiopulmonary collapse have been reported in children.

Breast-feeding
No data available; however, tropicamide should be used with extreme caution during breast-feeding because of the potential for CNS and cardiopulmonary effects in infants.

tuberculosis skin test antigens

tuberculin purified protein derivative (PPD)
Aplisol, Tubersol

tuberculin cutaneous multiple-puncture device
Aplitest (PPD), Mono-Vacc Test (Old Tuberculin), Sclavo-Test (PPD), Tine Test (Old Tuberculin), Tine Test (PPD)

- Pharmacologic classification: *Mycobacterium tuberculosis* and *Mycobacterium bovis* antigen
- Therapeutic classification: diagnostic skin test antigen
- Pregnancy risk category C

How supplied
Available by prescription only
Tuberculin PPD
Injection (intradermal): 1 tuberculin unit/0.1 ml, 5 tuberculin units/0.1 ml, 250 tuberculin units/0.1 ml
Tuberculin cutaneous multiple-puncture device
Test: 25 devices/pack

Indications, route, and dosage
Diagnosis of tuberculosis; evaluation of immunocompetence in patients with cancer or malnutrition
Adults and children: Intradermal injection of 5 tuberculin units/0.1 ml.

A single-use, multiple-puncture device is used for determining tuberculin sensitivity. All multiple-puncture tests are equivalent to or more potent than 5 tuberculin units of PPD.

Adults and children: Apply the unit firmly and without any twisting to the upper one-third of the forearm for approximately 3 seconds; this will ensure stabilizing the dried tuberculin B in the tissue lymph. Exert enough pressure to ensure that all four tines have entered the skin of the test area and a circular depression is visible.

Pharmacodynamics

- *Diagnosis of tuberculosis:* Administration to a patient with a natural infection with *M. tuberculosis* usually results in sensitivity to tuberculin and a delayed hypersensitivity reaction (after administration of old tuberculin or PPD). The cell-mediated immune reaction to tuberculin in tuberculin-sensitive individuals, which results mainly from cellular infiltrates of the skin's dermis, usually causes local edema.
- *Evaluation of immunocompetence in patients with cancer or malnutrition:* PPD is given intradermally with three or more antigens to detect anergy. The absence of an immune response to the test. The reaction may not be evident. Injection into a site subject to excessive exposure to sunlight may cause a false-negative reaction.

Pharmacokinetics

- *Absorption:* When PPD is injected intradermally, or a multiple-puncture device is used, a delayed hypersensitivity reaction is evident in 5 to 6 hours and peaks in 48 to 72 hours.
- *Distribution:* Injection must be given intradermally or skin puncture; a subcutaneous injection invalidates the test.
- *Metabolism:* Not applicable.
- *Excretion:* Not applicable.

Contraindications and precautions

Severe reactions to tuberculin PPD are rare and usually result from extreme sensitivity to the tuberculin.

Inadvertent subcutaneous administration of PPD may result in a febrile reaction in highly sensitized patients. Old tubercular lesions are not activated by administration of PPD.

Interactions

When PPD antigen is used 4 to 6 weeks after immunization with live or inactivated viral vaccines, the reaction to tuberculin may be suppressed. False-negative reactions may also occur if test is used in patients receiving systemic corticosteroids or aminocaproic acid.

Topical alcohol theoretically may inactivate the PPD antigen and invalidate the test.

Effects on diagnostic tests

None reported.

Adverse reactions

- Local: pain, pruritus, vesiculation, ulceration, necrosis may occur in some tuberculin-sensitive patients.
- Other: hypersensitivity (immediate reaction may occur at the test site in the form of a wheal or flare that lasts less than a day; this should not interfere with the PPD test reading at 48 to 72 hours), *anaphylaxis*, Arthus reaction.

Overdose and treatment

No information available.

▶ Special considerations

Tuberculin PPD

- Obtain a history of allergies and previous skin test reactions before administration of the test.
- Epinephrine 1:1,000 should be available to treat rare anaphylactic reaction.
- Intradermal injection should produce a bleb 6 to 10 mm in diameter on skin. If bleb does not appear, retest at a site at least 5 cm from the initial site.
- Read test in 48 to 72 hours. An induration of 10 mm or greater is a significant reaction in patients who are not suspected to have tuberculosis and who have not been exposed to active tuberculosis. An induration of 5 mm or greater is significant in patients with AIDS, or in patients suspected to have tuberculosis or who have recently been exposed to active tuberculosis. The amount of induration at the site, not the erythema, determines the significance of the reaction.

For either test, keep a record of the administration technique, manufacturer and tuberculin lot number, date and location of administration, date test is read, and the size of the induration in millimeters.

Multiple-puncture device

- Obtain history of allergies, especially to acacia (contained in the Tine Test as stabilizer), and reactions to skin tests.
- Report all known cases of tuberculosis to appropriate public health agency.
- Reaction may be depressed in patients with malnutrition, immunosuppression, or miliary tuberculosis.
- Interpretation: Read test at 48 to 72 hours. Measure the size of the largest induration in millimeters. A large reaction may cause the area around the puncture site to be indistinguishable.

Positive reaction: If vesiculation is present, the test may be interpreted as positive if induration is greater than 2 mm, but consider further diagnostic procedures.

Negative reaction: Induration is less than 2 mm. There is no reason to retest the patient unless the person is a contact of a patient with tuberculosis or there is clinical evidence of the disease.

Diagnosis of tuberculosis: PPD administration to a patient with a natural infection with *Mycobacterium tuberculosis* usually results in sensitivity to tuberculin and a delayed hypersensitivity reaction after administration of old tuberculin or PPD. The cell-mediated immune reaction to tuberculin in tuberculin-sensitive individuals is seen as erythema and induration, which mainly results from cellular infiltrates of the skin's dermis; usually causes local edema.

Diagnosis of immunocompetence in patients with such conditions as cancer or malnutrition: PPD is given intradermally with three or more antigens (such as Multitest CMI) to detect anergy.

- No evidence to date of adverse effects to fetus. Benefits of test are thought to outweigh the potential risk to the fetus.

Information for the patient

- Advise patient to report any unusual side effects. Explain that the induration will disappear in a few days.
- Reinforce the benefits of treatment if test is positive for tuberculosis.

Geriatric use
Elderly patients not having a cell-mediated immune reaction to the test may be anergic or they may test negative.

Breast-feeding
There appears to be no risk to breast-feeding infants.

tubocurarine chloride
Tubarine*

- Pharmacologic classification: nondepolarizing neuromuscular blocking agent
- Therapeutic classification: skeletal muscle relaxant
- Pregnancy risk category C

How supplied
Available by prescription only
Injection: 3 mg/ml parenteral

Indications, route, and dosage
Adjunct to general anesthesia to induce skeletal muscle relaxation, facilitate intubation, and reduce fractures and dislocations
Dose depends on anesthetic used, individual needs, and response. Doses listed are representative and must be adjusted. Dosage may be calculated on the basis of 0.165 mg/kg.
Adults: Initially, 6 to 9 mg I.V. or I.M., followed by 3 to 4.5 mg in 3 to 5 minutes if needed. Additional doses of 3 mg may be given if needed during prolonged anesthesia.
To assist with mechanical ventilation
Adults: Initially, 0.0165 mg/kg I.V. or I.M. (average 1 mg), then adjust subsequent doses to patient's response.
To weaken muscle contractions in pharmacologically or electrically induced seizures
Adults: Initially, 0.165 mg/kg I.V. or I.M. slowly. As a precaution, 3 mg less than the calculated dose should be administered initially.
Diagnosis of myasthenia gravis
Adults: Single I.V. or I.M. dose of 0.004 to 0.033 mg/kg.

Pharmacodynamics
Skeletal muscle relaxant action: Tubocurarine prevents acetylcholine from binding to receptors on motor endplate, thus blocking depolarization. Tubocurarine has histamine-releasing and ganglionic-blocking properties and is usually antagonized by anticholinesterase agents.

Pharmacokinetics
- *Absorption:* After I.V. injection, onset of muscle relaxation is rapid and peaks within 2 to 5 minutes. Duration is dose-related; effects usually begin to subside in 20 to 30 minutes. Paralysis may persist for 25 to 90 minutes. Subsequent doses have longer durations. After I.M. injection, the onset of paralysis is unpredictable (10 to 25 minutes); duration is dose-related.
- *Distribution:* After I.V. injection, tubocurarine is distributed in extracellular fluid and rapidly reaches its site of action. After tissue compartment is saturated, the drug may persist in tissues for up to 24 hours; 40% to 45% is bound to plasma proteins, mainly globulins.

- *Metabolism:* Tubocurarine undergoes N-demethylation in the liver.
- *Excretion:* Approximately 33% to 75% of a dose is excreted unchanged in urine in 24 hours; up to 11% is excreted in bile.

Contraindications and precautions
Tubocurarine is contraindicated in patients with known hypersensitivity to the drug and in whom histamine release may be hazardous and in patients with known sensitivity to sulfites.
   Administer cautiously to patients with bronchogenic carcinoma; cardiovascular, renal, hepatic, or pulmonary function impairment; dehydration or electrolyte imbalance; hyperthermia; hypothermia; hypotension; myasthenia gravis; shock; and in those with known sensitivity to sulfites.

Interactions
Concomitant use with aminoglycoside antibiotics, clindamycin, lincomycin, polymyxin antibiotics, general anesthetics, local anesthetics, beta-adrenergic blockers, calcium salts, trimethaphan, furosemide, parenteral magnesium salts, depolarizing neuromuscular blocking agents, other nondepolarizing neuromuscular blocking agents, quinidine or quinine, thiazide diuretics, or other potassium-depleting drugs may enhance or prolong tubocurarine-induced neuromuscular blockade.
   Respiratory depressant effects may be increased by opioid analgesics, quinidine, and quinine.

Effects on diagnostic tests
None significant.

Adverse reactions
- CV: hypotension.
- GI: increased salivation, decreased GI motility and tone.
- Other: wheezing or troubled breathing, *bronchospasm, respiratory depression to point of apnea*, hypersensitivity, residual muscle weakness.
   Note: Drug should be discontinued if hypersensitivity or cardiovascular collapse occurs.

Overdose and treatment
Clinical manifestations of overdose include apnea or prolonged muscle paralysis, which can be treated with controlled ventilation. Use a peripheral nerve stimulator to monitor effects and to determine nature and degree of blockade. Anticholinesterase agents may antagonize tubocurarine. Atropine given before or concurrently with the antagonist will counteract its muscarinic effects.

▶ Special considerations
- The margin of safety between therapeutic dose and dose causing respiratory paralysis is small.
- Monitor respirations closely for early symptoms of paralysis.
- Allow effects of succinylcholine to subside before giving tubocurarine.
- Measure and record intake and output.
- Decrease dose if inhalation anesthetics are used.
- Use only fresh solution. Discard if discolored.
- Do not mix with barbiturates or other alkaline solutions in same syringe.
- I.V. administration requires direct medical supervision. Drug should be given I.V. slowly over 60 to 90 seconds or I.M. by deep injection in deltoid muscle. Tubocurarine is usually administered by I.V. injection,

---

but if patient's veins are inaccessible, drug may be given I.M. in same dosage as given I.V.
● Assess baseline tests of renal function and serum electrolyte levels before drug administration. Electrolyte imbalance (particularly potassium and magnesium) can potentiate drug's effects.
● Keep airway clear. Have emergency respiratory support equipment handy.
● Be prepared for endotracheal intubation, suction, or assisted or controlled respiration with oxygen administration. Have available atropine and the antagonists neostigmine or edrophonium (cholinesterase inhibitors). A nerve stimulator may be used to evaluate recovery from neuromuscular blockade.
● Muscle paralysis follows drug administration in sequence: jaw muscles, levator eyelid muscles and other muscles of head and neck, limbs, intercostals and diaphragm, abdomen, trunk. Facial and diaphragm muscles recover first, then legs, arms, shoulder girdle, trunk, larynx, hands, feet, pharynx. Muscle function is usually restored within 90 minutes. Patient may find speech difficult until muscles of head and neck recover.
● Monitor blood pressure, vital signs, and airway until patient recovers from drug effects. Ganglionic blockade (hypotension), histamine liberation (increased salivation, bronchospasm), and neuromuscular blockade (respiratory depression) are known effects of tubocurarine.
● After neuromuscular blockade dissipates, watch for residual muscle weakness.
● Renal dysfunction prolongs drug action. Peristaltic action may be suppressed. Check for bowel sounds.
● Test of myasthenia gravis is considered positive if drug exaggerates muscle weakness.
● Drug does not affect consciousness or relieve pain; assess patient's need for analgesic or sedative.

Geriatric use
Administer cautiously to elderly patients.

Pediatric use
Administer cautiously to children.

Breast-feeding
It is unknown whether drug is excreted in breast milk. Use with caution in breast-feeding women.

typhoid vaccine

● Pharmacologic classification: vaccine
● Therapeutic classification: bacterial vaccine
● Pregnancy risk category C

How supplied
Available by prescription only
Oral vaccine: enteric-coated capsules of 2 to 6 × 10⁹ colony-forming units of viable *Salmonella typhi* Ty-21a and 5 to 10 × 10⁹ bacterial cells of nonviable *S. typhi* Ty-21a
Injection: suspension of killed Ty-2 strain of *S. typhi;* provides 8 units/ml in 5-ml, 10-ml, and 20-ml vials

Indications, route, and dosage
Primary immunization (exposure to typhoid carrier or foreign travel planned to area endemic for typhoid fever)
Parenteral
Adults and children over age 9: 0.5 ml S.C.; repeat in 4 or more weeks.
Children age 6 months to 9 years: 0.25 ml S.C.; repeat in 4 or more weeks.
Booster
Adults and children over age 10: 0.5 ml S.C. or 0.1 ml intradermally q 3 years.
Children 6 months to 10 years: 0.25 ml S.C. or 0.1 ml intradermally q 3 years.
Oral
Adults and children over age 6: Primary immunization – 1 capsule on alternate days (for example, days 1, 3, 5, 7) for four doses. Booster – Repeat primary immunization regimen q 5 years.

Pharmacodynamics
Typhoid fever prophylaxis: This vaccine promotes active immunity to typhoid fever in 70% to 90% of patients vaccinated.

Pharmacokinetics
The duration of vaccine-induced immunity is at least 2 years.

Contraindications and precautions
Typhoid vaccine is contraindicated in patients with acute respiratory or other active infections or with previous severe systemic or allergic reactions to typhoid vaccine or phenol. Do not inject I.V. Do not inject typhoid vaccine inactivated with acetone (U.S. government military issue only) intradermally.

Do not administer to patients with congenital or acquired immunodeficient states, including treatment with immunosuppressive and antimitotic drugs.

Interactions
Concomitant use of typhoid vaccine with corticosteroids or immunosuppressants may impair the immune response to this vaccine. Sulfonamides and other antiinfectives active against *S. typhi* may inhibit multiplication of the bacterial strain from the live attenuated oral vaccine, which may prevent the development of a protective immune response.

Effects on diagnostic tests
None reported.

Adverse reactions
● Local: swelling, pain, erythema, inflammation,tenderness.
● Systemic: fever, malaise, headache, nausea, myalgia, *anaphylaxis.*

Overdose and treatment
No information available.

▶ Special considerations
● Obtain a thorough history of allergies and reactions to immunizations.
● Epinephrine solution 1:1,000 should be available to treat allergic reactions.
● Shake vial thoroughly before withdrawing dose.
● Store injection at 36° to 50° F (2° to 10° C). Do not freeze.

● Store oral capsules at 36° to 46° F (2° to 8° C).

Information for the patient
● Tell patient what to expect after vaccination:pain and inflammation at the injection site, fever, malaise, headache, nausea, or difficulty breathing. These reactions occur in most patients within 24 hours and may persist for 1 to 2 days. Recommend acetaminophen for fever.
● Encourage patient to report adverse reactions.
● Patients traveling to an area where typhoid fever is endemic should select their food and water carefully. Vaccination is not a substitute for careful selection of food.
● Not all recipients of typhoid vaccine will be fully protected. Travelers should take all necessary precautions to avoid infection.
● It's essential that all four doses of oral vaccine be taken at the prescribed alternate-day interval to obtain a maximal protective immune response.
● The patient should take oral vaccine capsule about 1 hour before a meal with a cold or lukewarm (not exceeding body temperature) drink, and should swallow the capsule as soon as possible after placement in the mouth. Remind him that he should not chew the capsule.

Pediatric use
Parenteral typhoid vaccine is not indicated for children under age 6 months. Oral typhoid vaccine is not indicated for children under age 6 years.

Breast-feeding
It is unknown whether typhoid vaccine is distributed into breast milk. Use with caution in breast-feeding women.

UVW

uracil mustard

- Pharmacologic classification: alkylating agent (cell cycle-phase nonspecific)
- Therapeutic classification: antineoplastic
- Pregnancy risk category D

How supplied
Available by prescription only
Capsules: 1 mg

Indications, route, and dosage
Dosage and indications may vary. Check current literature for recommended protocol.
Chronic lymphocytic and myelocytic leukemia; Hodgkin's disease; non-Hodgkin's lymphomas of the histiocytic and lymphocytic types; reticulum cell sarcoma; lymphomas; mycosis fungoides; polycythemia vera; ovarian, cervical, and lung cancer
Adults: 1 to 2 mg P.O. daily for 3 months or until desired response or toxicity occurs; maintenance dosage is 1 mg daily for 3 out of 4 weeks until optimum response or relapse occurs. Alternatively, 3 to 5 mg P.O. for 7 days, not to exceed total dose of 0.5 mg/kg, followed by 1 mg daily until response occurs, then 1 mg daily 3 out of 4 weeks; or 0.15 mg/kg P.O. once weekly for 4 weeks.
Children: 0.3 mg/kg P.O. weekly for 4 weeks.
Thrombocytosis
Adults: 1 to 2 mg P.O. daily for 14 days.

Pharmacodynamics
Antineoplastic action: Uracil mustard exerts its cytotoxic activity by cross-linking strands of DNA, interfering with DNA and RNA replication and disrupting normal nucleic acid function, resulting in cell death.

Pharmacokinetics
- *Absorption:* In animal studies, uracil mustard is absorbed quickly but incompletely after oral administration.
- *Distribution:* Unknown.
- *Metabolism:* Unknown.
- *Excretion:* In studies using dogs, elimination of uracil mustard from the plasma is rapid, with no drug detected 2 hours after administration. Less than 1% of a dose is excreted unchanged in urine.

Contraindications and precautions
Uracil mustard is contraindicated in patients with a history of hypersensitivity to tartrazine, a dye contained in the capsules. The incidence of hypersensitivity is low, but it seems to occur frequently in patients allergic to aspirin.
Drug should be used cautiously in patients whose bone marrow shows infiltration with malignant cells, because hematopoietic toxicity may be increased.

Interactions
None reported.

Effects on diagnostic tests
Uracil mustard therapy may increase blood and urine uric acid levels.

Adverse reactions
- CNS: irritability, nervousness, mental cloudiness, depression.
- DERM: pruritus, dermatitis, hyperpigmentation
- GI: nausea, vomiting, diarrhea, epigastric distress, abdominal pain, anorexia.
- HEMA: *bone-marrow depression* (dose-limiting), *thrombocytopenia, leukopenia,* anemia.
- Metabolic: hyperuricemia.
- Other: alopecia.

Overdose and treatment
Clinical manifestations of overdose include myelosuppression, nausea, and vomiting.
Treatment is usually supportive and includes antiemetics and transfusion of blood components.

▶ Special considerations
Besides those relevant to all *alkylating agents*, consider the following recommendations.
- Give at bedtime to reduce nausea.
- Drug is usually not administered until 2 or 3 weeks after the maximum effect of previous drugs is reached or until radiation effects are evident.
- Watch for signs of ecchymoses, easy bruising, and petechiae.
- To prevent hyperuricemia and resulting uric acid nephropathy, allopurinol can be given; keep patient hydrated. Monitor uric acid levels.
- Monitor platelet count regularly. Perform a CBC one to two times weekly for 4 weeks, then 4 weeks after stopping drug.
- Avoid all I.M. injections when platelet count is below 100,000/mm³.
- Anticoagulants and aspirin products should be used cautiously. Watch closely for signs of bleeding. Instruct patient to avoid nonprescription products containing aspirin.
- Dose modification may be required in severe thrombocytopenia, aplastic anemia or leukopenia, or acute leukemia.

Information for the patient
- Emphasize the importance of continuing the medication despite nausea and vomiting.
- Tell patient to call immediately if vomiting occurs shortly after taking a dose, if he develops a sore throat or fever, or if he notices unusual bruising or bleeding.
- Encourage adequate fluid intake to increase urine output and facilitate excretion of uric acid. Patient should void frequently.
- Tell patient that hair growth should resume after treatment has ended.
- Advise patient to avoid exposure to people with infections.

---

*Canada only   †Unlabeled clinical use   Italicized adverse reactions are life-threatening.

Breast-feeding

It is not known whether uracil mustard distributes into breast milk. However, because of the risk of serious adverse reactions, mutagenicity, and carcinogenicity in the infant, breast-feeding is not recommended.

urea (carbamide)
Ureaphil

- Pharmacologic classification: carbonic acid salt
- Therapeutic classification: osmotic diuretic
- Pregnancy risk category C

How supplied
Available by prescription only
Injectable: 40-g vial

Indications, route, and dosage
Reduction of intracranial or intraocular pressure
Adults: 1 to 1.5 g/kg as a 30% solution given by slow I.V. infusion over 1 to 2½ hours.
Children over age 2: 0.5 to 1.5 g/kg by slow I.V. infusion.
Children under age 2: As little as 0.1 g/kg by slow I.V. infusion may be given. Maximum dosage is 4 ml/minute.
   Maximum daily adult dosage is 120 g. To prepare 135 ml of 30% solution, mix contents of a 40-g vial of urea with 105 ml of dextrose 5% or 10% in water or with 10% invert sugar in water. Each milliliter of 30% solution provides 300 mg of urea.
Diuresis
Adults: 20 g P.O. two to five times daily.
Children: 800 mg/kg P.O. daily, divided every 8 hours.

Pharmacodynamics
Diuretic action: Urea elevates plasma osmolality, enhancing the flow of water into extracellular fluid, such as blood, and reducing intracranial and intraocular pressure.

Pharmacokinetics
- *Absorption:* I.V. urea produces diuresis and maximal reduction of intraocular and intracranial pressure within 1 to 2 hours; even though drug is administered I.V., it is hydrolyzed and absorbed from the GI tract.
- *Distribution:* Urea distributes into intracellular and extracellular fluid, including lymph, bile, and cerebrospinal fluid.
- *Metabolism:* Urea is hydrolyzed in the GI tract by bacterial uridase.
- *Excretion:* Urea is excreted by the kidneys.

Contraindications and precautions
Urea is contraindicated in patients with severely impaired renal function because it is excreted in urine; marked dehydration follows volume depletion and liver failure.

Interactions
Urea may enhance renal excretion of lithium and lower serum lithium levels.

Effects on diagnostic tests
Urea therapy alters electrolyte balance.

Adverse reactions
- CNS: headache.
- CV: tachycardia, *CHF, pulmonary edema.*
- GI: nausea, vomiting.
- Metabolic: sodium and potassium depletion.
- Local: irritation or necrotic sloughing may occur with extravasation.
   Note: Drug should be discontinued if BUN level rises above 75 mg/dl or if diuresis does not occur within 1 to 2 hours.

Overdose and treatment
Clinical signs of overdose include polyuria, cellular dehydration, hypotension, and cardiovascular collapse. Discontinue infusion and institute supportive measures.

▶ Special considerations
Besides those relevant to all *osmotic diuretics,* consider the following recommendations.
- Avoid rapid I.V. infusion, which may cause hemolysis or increased capillary bleeding. Also avoid extravasation, which may cause reactions ranging from mild irritation to necrosis.
- Do not administer through the same infusion line as blood.
- Do not infuse into leg veins; this may cause phlebitis or thrombosis, especially in elderly patients.
- Watch for hyponatremia or hypokalemia (muscle weakness, lethargy); such signs may indicate electrolyte depletion before serum levels are reduced.
- Maintain adequate hydration; monitor fluid and electrolyte balance.
- In renal disease, monitor BUN levels frequently.
- Indwelling urethral catheter should be used in comatose patients to ensure bladder emptying. Use of an hourly urometer collection bag facilitates accurate measurement of urine output.
- If satisfactory diuresis does not occur in 6 to 12 hours, urea should be discontinued and renal function reevaluated.
- Use only freshly reconstituted urea for I.V. infusion; solution turns to ammonia when left standing. Use within minutes of reconstitution.
- Urea has been used orally on an investigational basis for migraine prophylaxis, acute sickle-cell crisis prevention, and the correction of syndrome of inappropriate antidiuretic hormone (SIADH).
- Mix with carbonated beverages, jelly, or jam to disguise unpleasant flavor.

Geriatric use
Elderly or debilitated patients will require close observation and may require lower dosages. Excessive diuresis promotes rapid dehydration and hypovolemia, hypokalemia, and hyponatremia.

Breast-feeding
Safety has not been established.

---

urokinase
Abbokinase, Abbokinase Open-Cath, Ukidan*

- Pharmacologic classification: thrombolytic enzyme
- Therapeutic classification: thrombolytic enzyme
- Pregnancy risk category B

How supplied
Injection: 5,000 IU/ml unit-dose vial; 250,000-IU vial

Indications, route, and dosage
Lysis of acute massive pulmonary emboli and of pulmonary emboli accompanied by unstable hemodynamics
Adults: For I.V. infusion only by constant infusion pump; priming dose: 4,400 IU/kg over 10 minutes, followed with 4,400 IU/kg hourly.
Coronary artery thrombosis
Adults: 6,000 IU/minute of urokinase intraarterial via a coronary artery catheter until artery is maximally opened, usually within 15 to 30 minutes; however, drug has been administered for up to 2 hours. Average total dose is 500,000 IU.
Venous catheter occlusion
Adults: Instill 5,000 IU into occluded line.

Pharmacodynamics
Thrombolytic action: Urokinase promotes thrombolysis by directly activating conversion of plasminogen to plasmin.

Pharmacokinetics
- *Absorption:* Urokinase is not absorbed from GI tract; plasminogen activation begins promptly after infusion or instillation; adequate activation of fibrinolytic system occurs in 3 to 4 hours.
- *Distribution:* Urokinase is rapidly cleared from circulation; most drug accumulates in kidney and liver.
- *Metabolism:* Urokinase is rapidly metabolized by the liver.
- *Excretion:* Small amount is eliminated in urine and bile. Half-life is 10 to 20 minutes; longer in patients with hepatic dysfunction. Anticoagulant effect may persist for 12 to 24 hours after the infusion is discontinued.

Contraindications and precautions
Urokinase is contraindicated in patients with ulcerative wounds, active internal bleeding and recent trauma with possible internal injuries, pregnancy and first 10 days postpartum, ulcerative colitis, diverticulitis, severe hypertension, acute or chronic hepatic or renal insufficiency, uncontrolled hypocoagulation, chronic pulmonary disease with cavitation, subacute bacterial endocarditis or rheumatic valvular disease and recent cerebral embolism, thrombosis or hemorrhage, or diabetic hemorrhagic retinopathy, because of the potential for excessive bleeding.

Administer urokinase with extreme caution for 10 days after intracranial, intraspinal, or intraarterial diagnostic procedure or after any surgery, including liver or kidney biopsy, lumbar puncture, thoracentesis, paracentesis, or extensive or multiple cutdowns.

Interactions
Concomitant use with anticoagulants may cause hemorrhage; heparin must be stopped and its effects allowed to diminish. It may also be necessary to reverse effects of oral anticoagulants before beginning therapy. Concomitant use with aspirin, indomethacin, phenylbutazone, or other drugs affecting platelet activity increases risk of bleeding; *do not use together.*

Aminocaproic acid inhibits urokinase-induced activation of plasminogen.

Effects on diagnostic tests
Urokinase increases thrombin time, activated partial thromboplastin time, and prothrombin time; drug sometimes moderately decreases hematocrit.

Adverse reactions
- CV: transient lowering or elevation of blood pressure, *reperfusion atrial or ventricular arrhythmias.*
- DERM: urticaria, ecchymosis.
- EENT: periorbital edema, gum bleeding.
- GI: nausea.
- HEMA: spontaneous bleeding, prolonged systemic hypocoagulability, bleeding or oozing from percutaneous trauma sites, low hematocrit.
- Local: phlebitis at injection site.
- Other: hypersensitivity (not as often as with streptokinase), *anaphylaxis,* musculoskeletal pain, bronchospasm, hematuria.

 Note: Drug should be discontinued if allergic reaction or severe bleeding occurs.

Overdose and treatment
Clinical manifestations of overdose include signs of potentially serious bleeding: bleeding gums, epistaxis, hematoma, spontaneous ecchymoses, oozing at catheter site, increased pulse, and pain from internal bleeding. Discontinue drug and restart when bleeding stops.

▶ Special considerations
Besides those relevant to all *thrombolytic enzymes,* consider the following recommendation.
- To reconstitute I.V. solution, add 5.2 ml sterile water for injection; dilute further with normal saline injection or 5% dextrose injection before infusion. Don't use bacteriostatic water, which contains preservatives. A catheter-clearing product is available in a Univial, containing 5,000 IU urokinase with the proper diluent. Discard unused portion; product contains no preservatives.

Geriatric use
Patients age 75 or older have a greater risk of cerebral hemorrhage, because they are more apt to have preexisting cerebrovascular disease.

ursodiol (ursodeoxycholic acid)
Actigall

- Pharmacologic classification: bile acid
- Therapeutic classification: gallstone solubilizing agent
- Pregnancy risk category B

How supplied
Available by prescription only
Capsules: 300 mg

Indications, route, and dosage
Dissolution of radiolucent gallbladder stones; to increase the flow of bile in patients with bile duct prosthesis or stents
Adults: 8 to 10 mg/kg/day given in two or three divided doses.

Ursodiol is indicated for patients with radiolucent, noncalcified, gallbladder stones smaller than 20 mm in greatest diameter in whom elective cholecystectomy is not feasible because of increased surgical risk related to systemic disease, advanced age, or idiosyncratic reaction to anesthesia; or because the patient has refused surgery.

Pharmacodynamics
Gallstone dissolving action: Ursodiol, an agent intended for dissolution of radiolucent gallstones, is a naturally occurring bile acid found in small quantities in normal human bile and in larger quantities in the biles of certain species of bears. Ursodiol suppresses hepatic synthesis and secretion of cholesterol and also inhibits intestinal absorption of cholesterol. It has little inhibitory effect on synthesis and secretion into bile of endogenous bile acids and does not appear to affect phospholipid secretion into bile.

Ursodiol also appears to solubilize cholesterol.

Pharmacokinetics
- *Absorption:* About 90% of a therapeutic dose of ursodiol is absorbed in the small bowel after oral administration.
- *Distribution:* After absorption, ursodiol enters the portal vein and is extracted from portal blood by the liver ("first pass" effect) where it is conjugated with either glycine or taurine and is then secreted into the hepatic bile ducts. Ursodiol in bile is concentrated in the gallbladder and expelled into the duodenum via the gallbladder bile via the cystic and common ducts by gallbladder contractions provoked by physiologic responses to eating.

Small quantities of ursodiol appear in the systemic circulation.
- *Metabolism:* Ursodiol is metabolized by the liver. A small portion of orally administered drug undergoes bacterial degradation with each cycle of enterohepatic circulation. Ursodiol can be both oxidized and reduced, yielding either 7-keto-lithocholic acid or lithocholic acid, respectively.
- *Excretion:* Very small amounts are excreted in the urine.

Free ursodiol, 7-keto-lithocholic acid, and lithocholic acid are relatively insoluble in aqueous media, and larger proportions of these compounds are excreted via the feces. 80% of lithocholic acid formed in the small bowel is excreted in the feces; the 20% that is absorbed is sulfated in the liver to relatively insoluble lithocholyl conjugates which are excreted into bile and lost in feces. Absorbed 7-keto-lithocholic acid is stereospecifically reduced in the liver to chenodiol. Reabsorbed free ursodiol is reconjugated by the liver.

Contraindications and precautions
Ursodiol is contraindicated in patients with calcified cholesterol stones, radiopaque stones, or radiolucent bile pigment stones because it will not dissolve such stones. Ursodiol should not be used in patients with compelling reasons for cholecystectomy including unremitting acute cholecystitis, cholangitis, biliary obstruction, gallstone pancreatitis, or biliary-gastrointestinal fistula; in patients with allergy to bile acids; or in those with chronic liver disease.

A nonfunctioning (nonvisualizing) gallbladder by oral cholecystogram before therapy is not a contraindication to ursodiol therapy. However, gallbladder nonvisualization developing during ursodiol treatment predicts failure of complete stone dissolution and requires discontinuation of therapy.

Ursodiol therapy has not been associated with liver damage. Lithocholic acid, a naturally occurring bile acid and metabolite of ursodiol, is known to be a liver-toxic metabolite. This bile acid is formed in the gut from ursodiol less efficiently and in smaller amounts than that seen from chenodiol. Lithocholic acid is detoxified in the liver by sulfation and although man appears to be an efficient sulfater, it is possible that some patients may have a congenital or acquired deficiency in sulfation, thereby predisposing them to lithocholate-induced liver damage. Therefore, measure AST (SGOT) and ALT (SGPT) at the initiation of therapy, after 1 and 3 months of therapy, and every 6 months thereafter.

Patients with significant abnormalities in liver tests at any point should be monitored frequently; evaluate carefully for worsening gallstone disease, which in the controlled clinical trials has been the only identified cause of significant liver test abnormality. Discontinue therapy with ursodiol if increased levels persist.

Interactions
Concurrent use of estrogens, oral contraceptives, and clofibrate (and perhaps other lipid-lowering drugs) that increase hepatic cholesterol secretion and encourage cholesterol gallstone formation may counteract the effectiveness of ursodiol. Aluminum-based antacids adsorb bile acids in vitro and interfere with the action of ursodiol by reducing its absorption. Cholestyramine and colestipol may interfere with the action of ursodiol by reducing its absorption.

Effects on diagnostic tests
None reported.

Adverse reactions
- DERM: exacerbation of preexisting psoriasis, pruritus, rash, urticaria, dry skin, sweating, hair thinning.
- GI: diarrhea (< 1%) at doses of 8 to 10 mg/kg/day, nausea, vomiting, dyspepsia, metallic taste, abdominal pain, biliary pain, cholecystitis, constipation, stomatitis, flatulence.
- Other: headache, fatigue, anxiety, depression, sleep disorder, arthralgia, myalgia, back pain, cough, rhinitis.

Overdose and treatment

The most likely manifestation of severe overdose with ursodiol would probably be diarrhea. Treatment includes symptomatic and supportive measures.

▶ Special considerations

● Gallbladder stone dissolution with ursodiol treatment requires months of therapy. Complete dissolution may not occur, and recurrence of stones is possible within 5 years in up to 50% of patients. Carefully select patients for therapy, and consider alternative therapies. Safety of use of ursodiol beyond 24 months is not established.

● Monitor gallstone response. Obtain ultrasound images of the gallbladder at 6-month intervals for the first year of ursodiol therapy. If gallstones appear to have dissolved, continue therapy and confirm dissolution on a repeat ultrasound within 1 to 3 months. Most patients who achieve complete stone dissolution show partial or complete dissolution at the first on-treatment re-evaluation. If partial stone dissolution does not occur by 12 months, eventual dissolution is unlikely.

● Partial stone dissolution occurring within 6 months of therapy appears to be associated with a > 70% chance of eventual complete stone dissolution with further treatment; partial dissolution within 1 year of therapy indicates a 40% probability of complete dissolution.

● Consider that some patients may never require therapy. Patients with silent or minimally symptomatic stones develop moderate to severe symptoms or gallstone complications at a rate between 2% and 6% per year; 7% to 27% in 5 years. The rate is higher for patients already having symptoms.

● Cholecystectomy offers immediate and permanent stone removal but carries a high risk in some patients.

● Surgical risk varies as a function of age and the presence of other disease. About 5% of cholecystectomized patients have residual symptoms of retained common duct stones.

Geriatric use

Age, sex, weight, degree of obesity, and serum cholesterol level are not related to the chance of stone dissolution with ursodiol.

Pediatric use

Safety and efficacy for use of ursodiol in children have not been established.

Breast-feeding

It is not known whether ursodiol is excreted in breast milk. Use with caution in breast-feeding women.

valproic acid
Depakene

divalproex sodium
Depakote

● Pharmacologic classification: carboxylic acid derivative
● Therapeutic classification: anticonvulsant
● Pregnancy risk category D

How supplied

Available by prescription only

Valproic acid
Capsules: 250 mg
Syrup: 250 mg/ml

Divalproex sodium
Tablets (enteric-coated): 125 mg, 250 mg, 500 mg
Capsules: 125 mg

Indications, route, and dosage
Simple and complex absence seizures and mixed seizure types; investigationally in tonic-clonic seizures

Adults and children: Initially, 15 mg/kg P.O. daily, divided b.i.d. or t.i.d.; may increase by 5 to 10 mg/kg daily at weekly intervals up to a maximum of 60 mg/kg daily, divided b.i.d. or t.i.d. The b.i.d. dosage is recommended for the enteric-coated tablets.

Note: Dosages of divalproex sodium (Depakote) are expressed as valproic acid.

Pharmacodynamics

Anticonvulsant action: Valproic acid's mechanism of action is unknown; effects may be from increased brain levels of gamma-aminobutyric acid (GABA), an inhibitory transmitter. Valproic acid also may decrease GABA's enzymatic catabolism. Onset of therapeutic effects may require a week or more. Valproic acid may be used with other anticonvulsants.

Pharmacokinetics

● Absorption: Valproate sodium and divalproex sodium quickly convert to valproic acid after administration of oral dose; peak plasma concentrations occur in 1 to 4 hours (with uncoated tablets) and 3 to 5 hours (with enteric-coated tablets); bioavailability of drug is same for both dosage forms.
● Distribution: Valproic acid is distributed rapidly throughout the body; drug is 80% to 95% protein-bound.
● Metabolism: Valproic acid is metabolized by the liver.
● Excretion: Valproic acid is excreted in urine; some drug is excreted in feces and exhaled air. Breast milk levels are 1% to 10% of serum levels.

Contraindications and precautions

Valproic acid is contraindicated in patients with known hypersensitivity to valproic acid and in patients with a history of hepatic disease because valproic acid may be hepatotoxic. It should be used with caution in patients taking oral anticoagulants or multiple anticonvulsants. Patients with congenital metabolic or seizure disorders with mental retardation, especially in children under age 2, appear to be at increased risk of adverse effects.

Interactions
Valproic acid may potentiate effects of monoamine oxidase (MAO) inhibitors and other CNS antidepressants and of oral anticoagulants. Besides additive sedative effects, valproic acid increases serum levels of primidone and phenobarbital; such combinations may cause excessive somnolence and require careful monitoring. Concomitant use with clonazepam may cause absence seizures and should be avoided.

Effects on diagnostic tests
Valproic acid may cause false-positive test results for urinary ketones; it also may cause abnormalities in liver function test results.

Adverse reactions
Because drug usually is used with other anticonvulsants, the adverse reactions reported may not be caused by valproic acid alone.
● CNS: sedation, emotional upset, depression, psychosis, aggression, hyperactivity, behavioral deterioration, muscle weakness, tremors, ataxia, headache, hallucinations.
● EENT: stomatitis, hypersalivation, nystagmus, diplopia, scotomata.
● GI: nausea, vomiting, indigestion, diarrhea, abdominal cramps, constipation, increased appetite and weight gain, anorexia, pancreatitis.
Note: Lower incidence of GI effects occurs with divalproex.
● HEMA: inhibited platelet aggregation, *thrombocytopenia, increased bleeding time.*
● Hepatic: enzyme level elevations, *toxic hepatitis.*
● Metabolic: elevated serum ammonia levels.
● Other: alopecia, enuresis, curling or waving hair.
Note: Drug should be discontinued if signs of hypersensitivity, hepatic dysfunction (markedly elevated liver enzyme levels or jaundice), or coagulation abnormalities (bruising or hemorrhage) occur.

Overdose and treatment
Symptoms of overdose include somnolence and coma. Treat overdose supportively: maintain adequate urinary output, and monitor vital signs and fluid and electrolyte balance carefully. Naloxone reverses CNS and respiratory depression but also may reverse anticonvulsant effects of valproic acid. Valproic acid is not dialyzable.

▶ **Special considerations**
● Patient should have review of liver function, platelet counts, and prothrombin times at baseline and at monthly intervals – especially during first 6 months.
● Therapeutic range is 50 to 100 mcg/ml.
● Drug should not be withdrawn abruptly.
● Tremors may indicate need for dosage reduction.
● Administer drug with food to minimize GI irritation. Enteric-coated formulation may be better tolerated.

Information for the patient
● Advise patient not to discontinue drug suddenly, not to alter dosage without medical approval, and to consult pharmacist before changing brand or using generic drug as therapeutic effect may change.
● Tell patient to swallow tablets or capsules whole to avoid local mucosal irritation and, if necessary, to take with food but not carbonated beverages because tablet may dissolve before swallowing, causing irritation and unpleasant taste.
● Tell patient not to use alcohol while taking drug; it

may decrease drug's effectiveness and may increase CNS adverse effects.
● Advise patient to avoid tasks that require mental alertness until degree of CNS sedative effect is determined. Drug may cause drowsiness and dizziness.
● Teach patient signs and symptoms of hypersensitivity and adverse effects and the need to report them.
● Encourage patient to wear a Medic Alert bracelet or necklace, listing drug and seizure disorders, while taking anticonvulsants.

Geriatric use
Elderly patients eliminate drug more slowly; lower dosages are recommended.

Pediatric use
Valproic acid is not recommended for use in children under age 2; this age-group is at highest risk of adverse effects. Reportedly, hyperexcitability and aggressiveness have occurred in a few children.

Breast-feeding
Valproic acid appears in breast milk in concentration levels from 1% to 10% of serum concentrations. Alternate feeding method is recommended during therapy.

vancomycin
Vancocin

● Pharmacologic classification: glycopeptide
● Therapeutic classification: antibiotic
● Pregnancy risk category C

How supplied
Available by prescription only
Capsules: 125 mg, 250 mg
Powder for oral solution: 1-g, 10-g bottles
Powder for injection: 500-mg, 1-g, 5-g vials; 10-g pharmacy bulk package

Indications, route, and dosage
Severe staphylococcal infections when other antibiotics are ineffective or contraindicated
Adults: 500 mg I.V. q 6 hours, or 1 g q 12 hours.
Children: 40 mg/kg I.V. daily, divided q 6 hours.
Neonates: 10 mg/kg I.V. daily, divided q 6 to 12 hours.
Antibiotic-associated pseudomembranous and staphylococcal enterocolitis
Adults: 125 to 500 mg P.O. q 6 hours for 7 to 10 days.
Children: 40 mg/kg P.O. daily, divided q 6 hours. Do not exceed 2 g/day in children.
Endocarditis prophylaxis for dental, GI, biliary, and genitourinary instrumentation procedures; surgical prophylaxis in patients allergic to penicillin
Adults: 1 g I.V., given slowly over 1 hour, starting 1 hour before procedure. In high-risk patients, dose may be repeated in 8 to 12 hours.
Children: 20 mg/kg, if child weighs less than 27 kg; adult dose, if child weighs more than 27 kg. In high-risk patients, dose may be repeated in 8 to 12 hours.
Dosage in renal failure
Dosage and/or frequency of administration should be modified according to degree of renal impairment, severity of infection, and susceptibility of the causative

organism. Dosage should be based upon serum concentrations of drug.

The recommended initial dose is 15 mg/kg. Subsequent doses should be adjusted as needed. Some clinicians use the following schedule:

Serum creatinine level	Dosage in adults
< 1.5 mg/100 ml	1 g q 12 hr
1.5 to 5 mg/100 ml	1 g q 3 to 6 days
> 5 mg/100 ml	1 g q 10 to 14 days

Pharmacodynamics
Antibacterial action: Vancomycin is bactericidal by hindering cell-wall synthesis and blocking glycopeptide polymerization. Its spectrum of activity includes many gram-positive organisms, including those resistant to other antibiotics. It is useful for *Staphylococcus epidermidis* and methicillin-resistant *S. aureus*. It is also useful for penicillin-resistant *S. pneumococcus*.

Pharmacokinetics
● *Absorption:* Minimal systemic absorption occurs when vancomycin is administered orally. (However, drug may accumulate in patients with colitis or renal failure.)
● *Distribution:* Vancomycin is distributed widely in body fluids, including pericardial, pleural, ascitic, synovial, and placental fluid. It will achieve therapeutic levels in CSF in patients with inflamed meninges. Therapeutic drug levels are 18 to 26 mcg/ml for 2-hour, postinfusion peaks; 5 to 10 mcg/ml for preinfusion troughs (however, these values may vary, depending on laboratory and sampling time).
● *Metabolism:* Vancomycin's metabolism is unknown.
● *Excretion:* When administered parenterally, vancomycin is excreted renally, mainly by filtration. When administered orally, drug is excreted in feces. In patients with normal renal function, plasma half-life is 6 hours; in patients with creatinine clearance ranging from 10 to 30 ml/minute, plasma half-life is about 32 hours; if creatinine clearance is below 10 ml/minute, plasma half-life is 146 hours.

Contraindications and precautions
Vancomycin is contraindicated in patients with known hypersensitivity to the drug.

Vancomycin should be administered cautiously to patients with hearing loss because of its ototoxic effect (especially at high serum levels).

Interactions
When used concomitantly, vancomycin may have additive nephrotoxic effects with other nephrotoxic drugs such as aminoglycosides, polymyxin B, colistin, amphotericin B, capreomycin, methoxyflurane, and cisplatin.

Effects on diagnostic tests
Blood urea nitrogen (BUN) and serum creatinine levels may increase, and neutropenia and eosinophilia may occur during vancomycin therapy.

Adverse reactions
● DERM: rash.
● EENT: tinnitus, ototoxicity.
● GI: nausea and vomiting.
● GU: nephrotoxicity.
● HEMA: neutropenia, eosinophilia.

● Local: phlebitis, pain at I.V. site.
● Other: anaphylaxis; fever; chills; hypotension; flushing; maculopapular rash on face, neck, trunk, and upper extremities (from overly rapid infusion).
Note: Drug should be discontinued if hypersensitivity develops. Do not confuse hypersensitivity with maculopapular rash.

Overdose and treatment
No information available.

▶ Special considerations
● Obtain culture and sensitivity tests before starting therapy (unless drug is being used for prophylaxis).
● To prepare drug for oral administration, reconstitute as directed in manufacturer's instructions. Reconstituted solution remains stable for 2 weeks when refrigerated.
● To prepare drug for I.V. injection, reconstitute 500-mg or 1-g vial with 10 ml of sterile water for injection, to yield 50 mg/ml or 100 mg/ml, respectively. Withdraw desired dose and further dilute to 100 to 250 ml with normal saline solution or 5% dextrose in water. Infuse over at least 60 minutes to avoid adverse effects related to rapid infusion rate. Reconstituted solution remains stable for 96 hours when refrigerated.
● Do not give I.M. because drug is highly irritating.
● Monitor blood counts and BUN, serum creatinine, and drug levels.
● If patient develops maculopapular rash on face, neck, trunk, and upper extremities, slow infusion rate.
● If patient has preexisting auditory dysfunction or requires prolonged therapy, auditory function tests may be indicated before and during therapy.
● Hemodialysis and peritoneal dialysis remove only minimal drug amounts. Patients receiving these treatments require usual dose only once every 5 to 7 days.

Information for the patient
● If patient is receiving drug orally, remind him to continue taking it as directed, even if he feels better.
● Advise patient not to take antidiarrheal agents concomitantly with drug except as prescribed.
● Instruct patient to call promptly if he develops ringing in the ears.

Geriatric use
Elderly patients may be more susceptible to drug's ototoxic effects. Monitor serum levels closely.

Breast-feeding
Drug effects in breast-feeding infants are unknown.

varicella-zoster immune globulin (VZIG)

● Pharmacologic classification: immune serum
● Therapeutic classification: varicella-zoster prophylaxis agent
● Pregnancy risk category C

How supplied
Available by prescription only
Injection: 10% to 18% solution of the globulin fraction

of human plasma containing 125 units of varicella-zoster virus antibody (volume is about 1.25 ml)

Indications, route, and dosage
Passive immunization of susceptible patients, primarily immunocompromised patients after exposure to varicella (chicken pox or herpes zoster)
Adults and children: 125 units per 10 kg of body weight I.M., to a maximum of 625 units. Higher doses may be needed in immunocompromised adults.

Pharmacodynamics
Postexposure prophylaxis: This agent provides passive immunity to varicella-zoster virus.

Pharmacokinetics
After I.M. absorption, the persistence of antibodies is unknown, but protection should last at least 3 weeks. Protection is sufficient to prevent or lessen the severity of varicella infections.

Contraindications and precautions
VZIG should be used with caution in patients with known hypersensitivity to thimerosal, a component of this immune serum.

Interactions
Concomitant use of VZIG with corticosteroids or immunosuppressants may interfere with the immune response to this immune globulin. Whenever possible, avoid using these agents during the postexposure immunization period.

Also, VZIG may interfere with the immune response to live virus vaccines (for example, those for measles, mumps, and rubella). Do not administer live virus vaccines within 3 months after or 2 weeks before administering VZIG. If it becomes necessary to administer VZIG and a live virus vaccine concomitantly, confirm seroconversion with follow-up serologic testing.

Effects on diagnostic tests
None reported.

Adverse reactions
● Local: discomfort and rash at injection site.
● Systemic: gastrointestinal distress, malaise, headache, *respiratory distress, anaphylaxis, angioneurotic edema.*

Overdose and treatment
No information available.

▶ Special considerations
● Obtain a thorough history of allergies and reactions to immunizations.
● Epinephrine solution 1:1,000 should be available to treat allergic reactions.
● VZIG is recommended primarily for immunodeficient patients under age 15 and certain infants exposed in utero, although use in other patients (especially immunocompromised patients of any age, normal adults, pregnant women, and premature and full-term infants) should be considered on a case-by-case basis. It is not routinely recommended for use in immunocompetent pregnant women because chicken pox is much less severe than in immunosuppressed patients. Moreover, it will not protect the fetus.

● Although usually used only in children under age 15, VZIG may be administered to adults if necessary.
● Administer only by deep I.M. injection. Never administer I.V. Use the gluteal muscle in infants and small children and the deltoid or anterolateral thigh in adults and larger children.
● For maximum benefit, administer VZIG within 96 hours of presumed exposure.
● Store unopened vials between 2° and 8° C. (36° and 46° F.). Do not freeze.

Information for the patient
● Explain to patient that his chances of getting AIDS or hepatitis from VZIG are very small.
● Tell patient that he may experience some local pain, swelling, and tenderness at the injection site. Recommend acetaminophen to alleviate these minor effects.
● Encourage patient to report severe reactions.

Breast-feeding
It is unknown whether VZIG is distributed into breast milk. Use cautiously in breast feeding-women.

---

vasopressin (antidiuretic hormone [ADH])
Pitressin Synthetic

● Pharmacologic classification: posterior pituitary hormone
● Therapeutic classification: antidiuretic hormone, peristaltic stimulant, hemostatic agent
● Pregnancy risk category B

How supplied
Available by prescription only
Injection: 0.5-ml and 1-ml ampules, 20 units/ml

Indications, route, and dosage
Nonnephrogenic, nonpsychogenic diabetes insipidus
Adults: 5 to 10 units I.M. or S.C. b.i.d. to q.i.d., p.r.n.; or intranasally (spray or cotton balls) in individualized doses, based on response.
Children: 2.5 to 10 units I.M. or S.C. b.i.d. to q.i.d., p.r.n.; or intranasally (spray or cotton balls) in individualized doses.
Postoperative abdominal distention
Adults: 5 units I.M. initially, then q 3 to 4 hours, increasing dosage to 10 units, if needed. Reduce dosage for children proportionately.
To expel gas before abdominal X-ray
Adults: Inject 10 units S.C. at 2 hours, then again at 30 minutes before X-ray. Enema before first dose may also help to eliminate gas.
Upper GI tract hemorrhage
Adults: 0.2 to 0.4 units/minute I.V. or 0.1 to 0.5 units/minute intraarterially.

Pharmacodynamics
● *Antidiuretic action:* Vasopressin is used as an antidiuretic to control or prevent signs and complications of neurogenic diabetes insipidus. Acting primarily at the renal tubular level, vasopressin increases cyclic 3′,5′-adenosine monophosphate, which increases water per-

meability at the renal tubule and collecting duct, resulting in increased urine osmolality and decreased urinary flow rate.
● *Peristaltic stimulant action:* Used to treat postoperative abdominal distention and to facilitate abdominal radiographic procedures, vasopressin induces peristalsis by directly stimulating contraction of smooth muscle in the GI tract.
● *Hemostatic action:* In patients with GI hemorrhage, vasopressin, administered I.V. or intraarterially into the superior mesenteric artery, controls bleeding of esophageal varices by directly stimulating vasoconstriction of capillaries and small arterioles.

Pharmacokinetics
● *Absorption:* Vasopressin is destroyed by trypsin in the GI tract and must be administered intranasally or parenterally.
● *Distribution:* Vasopressin is distributed throughout the extracellular space, with no evidence of protein-binding.
● *Metabolism:* Most of a dose is destroyed rapidly in the liver and kidneys.
● *Excretion:* Approximately 5% of an S.C. dose of vasopressin is excreted unchanged in urine after 4 hours. Duration of action after I.M. or S.C. administration is 2 to 8 hours. Half-life is 10 to 20 minutes.

Contraindications and precautions
Vasopressin is contraindicated in patients with chronic nephritis accompanied by nitrogen retention or hypersensitivity to the drug.

It should be used with caution in patients with seizure disorders, migraines, asthma, or heart failure (because rapid addition of extracellular water may be hazardous) and in those with vascular disease, angina pectoris, coronary thrombosis, or arteriosclerosis (because large doses may precipitate myocardial infarction). Preoperative and postoperative polyuric patients may have considerably reduced hormone requirements.

Interactions
Concomitant use of vasopressin with carbamazepine, chlorpropamide, or clofibrate may potentiate vasopressin's antidiuretic effect; use with demeclocycline, lithium, norepinephrine, epinephrine, heparin, or alcohol may decrease antidiuretic effect.

Effects on diagnostic tests
None reported.

Adverse reactions
● CNS: tremor, dizziness, headache.
● CV: angina in patients with vascular disease, vasoconstriction. Large doses may cause hypertension, ECG changes. With intraarterial infusion: *bradycardia, cardiac arrhythmias, pulmonary edema.*
● DERM: circumoral pallor.
● GI: abdominal cramps, nausea, vomiting, diarrhea, intestinal hyperactivity.
● GU: uterine cramps, anuria.
● Other: water intoxication (drowsiness, listlessness, headache, confusion, weight gain), hypersensitivity reactions (urticaria, angioneurotic edema, *bronchoconstriction,* fever, rash, wheezing, dyspnea, *anaphylaxis*), sweating.
Note: Drug should be discontinued if signs or symptoms of anaphylaxis, hypersensitivity, or water intoxication occur.

Overdose and treatment
Clinical manifestations of overdose include drowsiness, listlessness, headache, confusion, anuria, and weight gain (water intoxication). Treatment requires water restriction and temporary withdrawal of vasopressin until polyuria occurs. Severe water intoxication may require osmotic diuresis with mannitol, hypertonic dextrose, or urea, either alone or with furosemide.

▶ **Special considerations**
Besides those relevant to all *posterior pituitary hormones,* consider the following recommendations.
● Establish baseline vital signs and intake and output ratio at the initiation of therapy.
● Monitor patient's blood pressure twice daily. Watch for excessively elevated blood pressure or lack of response to drug, which may be indicated by hypotension. Also monitor fluid intake and output and daily weights.
● Question the patient with abdominal distention about passage of flatus and stool.
● A rectal tube will facilitate gas expulsion after vasopressin injection.
● Observe for signs of early water intoxication – drowsiness, listlessness, headache, confusion, and weight gain – to prevent seizures, coma, and death.
● Never inject during first stage of labor; this may cause ruptured uterus.
● Use extreme caution to avoid extravasation because of the risk of necrosis and gangrene.

Information for the patient
● Tell patient to drink one or two glasses of water with each dose of vasopressin. This reduces the adverse reactions of unusual paleness, nausea, abdominal cramps, and vomiting.
● Teach patient how to maintain a fluid intake and output record.
● Show patient how to check the expiration date.
● Tell patient to call immediately if any of the following symptoms occur: chest pain, confusion, fever, hives, skin rash, headache, problems with urination, seizures, weight gain, unusual drowsiness, wheezing, trouble with breathing, or swelling of face, hands, feet, or mouth.
● Encourage patient to rotate injection sites.

Geriatric use
Elderly patients show increased sensitivity to the effects of vasopressin. Use with caution.

Pediatric use
Children show increased sensitivity to the effects of vasopressin. Use with caution.

vecuronium bromide
Norcuron

● Pharmacologic classification: nondepolarizing neuromuscular blocking agent
● Therapeutic classification: skeletal muscle relaxant
● Pregnancy risk category C

How supplied
Available by prescription only
Injection: 10 mg

Indications, route, and dosage
Adjunct to anesthesia, to facilitate intubation, and to provide skeletal muscle relaxation during surgery or mechanical ventilation
Dose depends on anesthetic used, individual needs, and response. Doses are representative and must be adjusted.
Adults and children age 10 and over: Initially, 0.08 to 0.10 mg/kg I.V. bolus. Higher initial doses (up to 0.3 mg/kg) may be used for rapid onset. Maintenance doses of 0.010 to 0.015 mg/kg within 25 to 40 minutes of initial dose should be administered during prolonged surgical procedures. Maintenance doses may be given q 12 to 15 minutes in patients receiving balanced anesthetic.

Pharmacodynamics
Skeletal muscle relaxant action: Vecuronium prevents acetylcholine from binding to receptors on motor end-plate, thus blocking depolarization. Vecuronium exhibits minimal cardiovascular effects and does not appear to alter heart rate or rhythm, systolic or diastolic blood pressure, cardiac output, systemic vascular resistance, or mean arterial pressure. It has little or no histamine-releasing properties.

Pharmacokinetics
● *Absorption:* After I.V. administration of 0.08 to 0.1 mg/kg, onset of action occurs within 1 minute; action peaks at 3 to 5 minutes. The duration is about 25 to 40 minutes depending on anesthetic used, dose, and number of doses given.
● *Distribution:* After I.V. administration, vecuronium is distributed in extracellular fluid and rapidly reaches its site of action. It is 60% to 90% plasma protein-bound. The volume of distribution is decreased in children under age 1 and may be decreased in elderly patients.
● *Metabolism:* Vecuronium undergoes rapid and extensive hepatic metabolism.
● *Excretion:* Vecuronium and its metabolites appear to be primarily excreted in feces by biliary elimination; drug and its metabolites are also excreted in urine.

Contraindications and precautions
Vecuronium is contraindicated in patients with known hypersensitivity to the drug. Administer with extreme caution to patients with myasthenia gravis, neuromuscular diseases, or bronchogenic carcinoma because of the potential for prolonged neuromuscular blockade; and to patients with severe electrolyte disorders or dehydration. Administer cautiously to elderly or debilitated patients and those with cardiovascular, hepatic, pulmonary, or renal function impairment or in pregnant women receiving magnesium sulfate because lower doses may be required. In severely obese patients, maintenance of airway and ventilation support may require special attention.

Interactions
Concomitant use with aminoglycosides, clindamycin, lincomycin, polymyxin antibiotics, furosemide, parenteral magnesium salts, depolarizing neuromuscular blocking agents, other nondepolarizing neuromuscular blocking agents, quinidine or quinine, thiazide diuretics, other potassium-depleting drugs, and general anesthetics (decrease dose by 15%, especially with enflurane and isoflurane) may increase vecuronium-induced neuromuscular blockade. Concomitant use with anticholinesterase agents may also antagonize effects of

vecuronium. Concomitant use with narcotic (opioid) analgesics may increase central respiratory depression.

Effects on diagnostic tests
None significant.

Adverse reactions
● CV: minimal and transient effects.
● Other: skeletal muscle weakness or paralysis; respiratory insufficiency; *respiratory paralysis; prolonged, dose-related apnea; malignant hyperthermia.*

Overdose and treatment
Clinical manifestations of overdose include prolonged duration of neuromuscular blockade, skeletal muscle weakness, decreased respiratory reserve, low tidal volume, and apnea. Treatment is supportive and symptomatic. Keep airway clear and maintain adequate ventilation.

Use peripheral nerve stimulator to determine and monitor the degree of blockade. Give anticholinesterase agent (edrophonium, neostigmine, or pyridostigmine) to reverse neuromuscular blockade and atropine or glycopyrrolate to overcome muscarinic effects.

▶ Special considerations
● Administer by rapid I.V. injection or I.V. infusion. Do not give I.M.
● Reconstitute using 5 ml of sterile water for injection (provided by manufacturer) to produce a solution containing 2 mg/ml.
● Do not mix in same syringe or give through same needle as barbiturates or other alkaline solutions.
● Protect solution from light.
● After reconstitution, solution should be stored in refrigerator or at room temperature not exceeding 86° F. (30° C.). Do not use if discolored. Discard unused portion after 24 hours.
● Have emergency respiratory support equipment immediately available.
● Assess baseline serum electrolyte levels, acid-base balance, and renal and hepatic function before administration.
● Peripheral nerve stimulator may be used to identify residual paralysis during recovery and is especially useful during administration to high-risk patients.
● After procedure, monitor vital signs at least every 15 minutes until patient is stable, then every ½ hour for the next 2 hours. Monitor airway and pattern of respirations until patient has recovered from drug effects. Anticipate problems with ventilation in obese patients and those with myasthenia gravis or other neuromuscular disease.
● Evaluate recovery from neuromuscular blockade by checking strength of hard grip, ability to breathe naturally, to take deep breaths and cough, to keep eyes open, and to lift head keeping mouth closed.
● Drug does not relieve pain or affect consciousness; if indicated, assess need for analgesic or sedative.

Geriatric use
Administer cautiously to elderly patients.

Pediatric use
Safety and efficacy have not been established in infants under age 7 weeks. Infants age 7 weeks to 1 year are more sensitive to neuromuscular blocking effects; less frequent administration may be necessary. Higher doses may be needed in children age 1 to 9.

Breast-feeding
It is unknown if vercuronium is excreted in breast milk. Use with caution in breast-feeding women.

---

verapamil hydrochloride
Calan, Calan SR, Isoptin, Isoptin SR, Verelan

- Pharmacologic classification: calcium channel blocker
- Therapeutic classification: antianginal, antihypertensive, antiarrhythmic
- Pregnancy risk category C

How supplied
Available by prescription only
Tablets: 80 mg, 120 mg
Tablets (extended-release): 180 mg, 240 mg
Capsules (extended-release): 120 mg, 180 mg, 240 mg
Injection: 2.5 mg/ml

Indications, route, and dosage
Management of Prinzmetal's or variant angina or unstable or chronic, stable angina pectoris
Adults: Initial dose of 80 mg P.O., every 6 to 8 hours. Dosage may be increased at weekly intervals. Some patients may require up to 480 mg daily.
Supraventricular tachyarrhythmias
Adults: 0.075 to 0.15 mg/kg (5 to 10 mg) I.V. push over 2 minutes. If no response occurs, give a second dose of 10 mg (0.15 mg/kg) 15 to 30 minutes after the initial dose.
Children age 1 to 15: 0.1 to 0.3 mg/kg (2 to 5 mg) as I.V. bolus over 2 minutes. Dose should not exceed 5 mg. Dose may be repeated in 30 minutes if no response occurs (should not exceed 10 mg).
Children under age 1: 0.1 to 0.2 mg/kg (0.75 to 2 mg) as I.V. bolus over 2 minutes. Dose may be repeated in 30 minutes if no response occurs.
Prevention of recurrent paroxysmal supraventricular tachycardia
Adults: 240 to 480 mg P.O. daily in three to four divided doses.
Control of ventricular rate in digitalized patients with chronic atrial flutter and/or fibrillation
Adults: 240 to 320 mg P.O. daily in three to four divided doses.
Hypertension
Adults: Usual starting dose is 80 mg P.O. t.i.d., or 1 240-mg sustained-release tablet or capsule daily in the morning. Dosage may be increased at weekly intervals. For patients taking sustained-release tablets, dosage may be increased in 120-mg increments, with second dose added in the evening. Elderly or patients of smaller stature may initiate therapy at 120 mg P.O. b.i.d.

Initiate therapy with sustained-release capsules at 120 mg daily in the morning. Adjust dosage based on clinical effectiveness 24 hours after dosing. Increase by 120 mg daily until a maximum dose of 480 mg daily is given. Sustained-release capsules should be given only once daily. Anithypertensive effects are usually seen within the first week of therapy. Most patients respond to 240 mg daily.

Pharmacodynamics
- *Antianginal action:* Verapamil manages unstable and chronic stable angina by reducing afterload, both at rest and with exercise, thereby decreasing oxygen consumption. It also decreases myocardial oxygen demand and cardiac work by exerting a negative inotropic effect, reducing heart rate, relieving coronary artery spasm (via coronary artery vasodilation), and dilating peripheral vessels. The net result of these effects is relief of angina-related ischemia and pain. In patients with Prinzmetal's variant angina, verapamil inhibits coronary artery spasm, resulting in increased myocardial oxygen delivery.
- *Antihypertensive action:* Verapamil reduces blood pressure mainly by dilating peripheral vessels. Its negative inotropic effect blocks reflex mechanisms that lead to increased blood pressure.
- *Antiarrhythmic action:* Verapamil's combined effects on the SA and AV nodes help manage arrhythmias. The drug's primary effect is on the AV node; slowed conduction reduces the ventricular rate in atrial tachyarrhythmias and blocks reentry paths in paroxysmal supraventricular arrhythmias.

Pharmacokinetics
- *Absorption:* Verapamil is absorbed rapidly and completely from the GI tract after oral administration; however, only about 20% to 35% of the drug reaches systemic circulation because of first-pass effect. When administered orally, peak effects occur within 1 to 2 hours with conventional tablets and within 4 to 8 hours with sustained-release preparations. When administered I.V., effects occur within minutes after injection and usually persist about 30 to 60 minutes (although they may last up to 6 hours). Therapeutic serum levels are 80 to 300 ng/ml.
- *Distribution:* Steady-state distribution volume in healthy adults ranges from about 4.5 to 7 liters/kg but may increase to 12 liters/kg in patients with hepatic cirrhosis. Approximately 90% of circulating drug is bound to plasma proteins.
- *Metabolism:* Verapamil is metabolized in the liver.
- *Excretion:* Verapamil is excreted in the urine as unchanged drug and active metabolites. Elimination half-life is normally 6 to 12 hours and increases to as much as 16 hours in patients with hepatic cirrhosis. In infants, elimination half-life may be 5 to 7 hours.

Contraindications and precautions
Verapamil is contraindicated in patients with severe hypotension (systolic blood pressure below 90 mm Hg) or cardiogenic shock, because of the drug's hypotensive effect; in patients with second- or third-degree AV block or sick sinus syndrome (unless a functioning artificial ventricular pacemaker is in place), because of the drug's effects on the cardiac conduction system; in patients with severe left ventricular dysfunction (indicated by pulmonary wedge pressure above 20 mm Hg and left ventricular ejection fraction below 20%), unless heart failure results from supraventricular tachycardia, because the drug may worsen the condition; in patients with ventricular dysfunction or AV abnormalities who are receiving beta-adrenergic blockers, because of the drug's negative inotropic effect and inhibition of the cardiac conduction system; and in patients with known hypersensitivity to the drug.

All verapamil forms should be used with caution in patients with moderately severe ventricular dysfunction or heart failure, because the drug may precipitate or

---

worsen the condition; in patients with hypertrophic cardiomyopathy, because the drug may cause serious and sometimes fatal adverse cardiovascular effects (such as pulmonary edema, hypotension, heart block, or sinus arrest); in patients with hepatic or renal impairment, because the drug may accumulate (generally, the dose should be reduced and the patient carefully monitored); in patients with sick sinus syndrome or atrial flutter or fibrillation with an accessory bypass tract (such as Wolff-Parkinson-White or Lown-Ganong-Levine syndrome), because the drug may precipitate life-threatening adverse effects (for example, ventricular fibrillation or cardiac arrest); in patients with wide-complex ventricular tachycardia, because the drug may cause marked hemodynamic deterioration and ventricular fibrillation; and in patients receiving the drug I.V., because of possible adverse hemodynamic effects (hypotension) and adverse ECG effects (such as bradycardia and heart block).

Interactions

Concomitant use of verapamil with beta blockers may cause additive effects leading to congestive heart failure, conduction disturbances, arrhythmias, and hypotension, especially if high beta-blocker doses are used, if the drugs are administered I.V., or if the patient has moderately severe to severe congestive heart failure, severe cardiomyopathy, or recent myocardial infarction.

Concomitant use of oral verapamil with digoxin may increase serum digoxin concentration by 50% to 75% during the 1st week of therapy. Concomitant use with antihypertensives may lead to combined antihypertensive effects, resulting in clinically significant hypotension. Concomitant use with drugs that attenuate alpha-adrenergic response (such as prazosin and methyldopa) may cause excessive blood pressure reduction. Concomitant use with disopyramide may cause combined negative inotropic effects; with quinidine to treat hypertrophic cardiomyopathy, may cause excessive hypotension; with carbamazepine, may cause increased serum carbamazepine levels and subsequent toxicity; with rifampin, may substantially reduce verapamil's oral bioavailability.

Effects on diagnostic tests

None reported.

Adverse reactions

- CNS: dizziness, headache, fatigue.
- CV: transient hypotension, *heart failure*, bradycardia, AV block, *ventricular asystole*, peripheral edema.
- GI: constipation, nausea (primarily with oral form).
- Hepatic: elevated liver enzyme levels.
  Note: Drug should be discontinued if systolic pressure falls below 90 mm Hg, if heart failure worsens, or if arrhythmias, hemodynamically significant bradycardia, or second- or third-degree heart block occurs.

Overdose and treatment

Clinical effects of overdose are primarily extensions of adverse reactions. Heart block, asystole, and hypotension are the most serious reactions and require immediate attention.

Treatment may include administering I.V. isoproterenol, norepinephrine, epinephrine, atropine, or calcium gluconate in usual doses. Adequate hydration should be ensured.

In patients with hypertrophic cardiomyopathy, alpha-adrenergic agents, including methoxamine, phenylephrine, and metaraminol, should be used to maintain blood pressure. (Isoproterenol and norepinephrine should be avoided.) Inotropic agents, including dobutamine and dopamine, may be used if necessary.

If severe conduction disturbances, such as heart block and asystole, occur with hypotension that does not respond to drug therapy, cardiac pacing should be initiated immediately, with cardiopulmonary resuscitation measures as indicated.

In patients with Wolff-Parkinson-White or Lown-Ganong-Levine syndrome and a rapid ventricular rate caused by hemodynamically significant antegrade conduction, synchronized cardioversion may be used. Lidocaine and/or procainamide may be used as adjuncts.

▶ Special considerations

- If verapamil is initiated in patient receiving carbamazepine, a 40% to 50% reduction in carbamazepine dosage may be necessary. Monitor patient closely for signs of toxicity.
- Reduce dosage in patients with renal or hepatic impairment.
- If patient is receiving I.V. verapamil, monitor ECG continuously.
- If verapamil is added to therapy of patient receiving digoxin, digoxin dose should be reduced by half with subsequent monitoring of serum digoxin levels.
- During long-term combination therapy involving verapamil and digoxin, monitor ECG periodically to observe for AV block and bradycardia, because of drugs' possible additive effects on the AV node.
- Obtain periodic liver function tests.
- Patients with severely compromised cardiac function and those receiving beta blockers should receive lower verapamil doses. Monitor these patients closely.
- Discontinue disopyramide 48 hours before starting verapamil therapy and do not reinstitute until 24 hours after verapamil has been discontinued.
- Generic sustained-release verapamil tablets may be substituted only for Isoptin SR and Calan SR, not Verelan capsules. The capsule formulation should be given only once daily. When using sustained-release tablets, doses over 240 mg should be given b.i.d.

Information for the patient

- Urge patient to report signs of CHF, such as swelling of hands and feet or shortness of breath.
- Urge patient who is receiving nitrate therapy while verapamil dose is being titrated to comply with prescribed therapy.

Geriatric use

Elderly patients may require lower doses. In elderly patients, administer I.V. doses over at least 3 minutes to minimize the risk of adverse effects.

Pediatric use

Currently, only the I.V. form is indicated for use in pediatric patients to treat supraventricular tachyarrhythmias.

Breast-feeding

Verapamil is excreted in breast milk. To avoid possible adverse effects in infants, breast-feeding should be discontinued during verapamil therapy.

vidarabine monohydrate
(adenine arabinoside)
Vira-A

- Pharmacologic classification: purine nucleoside
- Therapeutic classification: antiviral agent
- Pregnancy risk category C

How supplied
Available by prescription only
Concentrate for I.V. infusion: 200 mg/ml in 5-ml vial (equivalent to 187.4 mg vidarabine)
Ophthalmic ointment: 3% in 3.5-g tube (equivalent to 2.8% vidarabine)

Indications, route, and dosage
Herpes simplex virus encephalitis
Adults and children (including neonates): 15 mg/kg daily for 10 days. Slowly infuse the total daily dosage by I.V. infusion at a constant rate over a 12- to 24-hour period. Avoid rapid or bolus injection.
Herpes zoster in immunocompromised patient
Adults and children: 10 mg/kg I.V. daily for 5 days at constant rate over 12 to 24 hours/day.
Acute keratoconjunctivitis and recurrent epithelial keratitis caused by herpes simplex virus Types I and II
Adults and children: Administer ½" (1.3 cm) ointment into lower conjunctival sac five times daily at 3-hour intervals.
Dosage in renal failure
Adults: Dosage should be reduced by at least 25% in patients with creatinine clearance < 10 ml/min.

Pharmacodynamics
Antiviral action: Vidarabine is an adenine analog. Its exact mechanism of action is unknown; presumably it involves inhibition of deoxyribonucleic acid (DNA) polymerase and viral replication by incorporation into viral DNA.

Pharmacokinetics
- *Absorption:* Vidarabine is absorbed poorly when administered orally, I.M., or S.C. I.V. administration results in rapid deamination to the active metabolite, arabinosyl-hypoxanthine.
- *Distribution:* Vidarabine and arabinosyl-hypoxanthine, its active metabolite, are distributed widely in body tissues and fluids. CSF concentration equals about 30% of serum levels. Parent compound is 20% to 30% plasma protein-bound; arabinosyl-hypoxanthine is 1% to 3% plasma protein-bound.
- *Metabolism:* Vidarabine is metabolized into the active metabolite arabinosyl-hypoxanthine.
- *Excretion:* Both parent compound and active metabolite are excreted primarily by the kidneys. Half-lives of parent compound and active metabolite are 1½ and 3½ hours, respectively.

Contraindications and precautions
Vidarabine is contraindicated in patients with known hypersensitivity to the drug.
   Vidarabine should be administered cautiously to patients with hepatic or renal dysfunction because they may be more susceptible to dose-related adverse effects, and to patients with restricted fluid intake because they may not tolerate the large fluid volumes needed for drug administration.

Interactions
When used concomitantly, vidarabine may inhibit theophylline metabolism, increasing the risk of theophylline toxicity. Concomitant use with allopurinol may inhibit vidarabine metabolism, causing tremor, anemia, nausea, pain, or pruritus.

Effects on diagnostic tests
AST (SGOT) and serum bilirubin levels may increase, and leukocyte, platelet, reticulocyte, hemoglobin, and hematocrit values may decrease during vidarabine therapy.

Adverse reactions
- CNS: tremor, dizziness, hallucinations, confusion, psychosis, ataxia, coma (especially in patients in renal failure)
- DERM: pruritus, rash.
- EENT (with ophthalmic application): lacrimation, foreign body sensation, conjunctival injection, burning, irritation, superficial keratitis, pain, photophobia, punctal occlusion, sensitivity.
- GI: anorexia, nausea, vomiting, diarrhea.
- HEMA: anemia, neutropenia, thrombocytopenia.
- Hepatic: elevated AST (SGOT) and bilirubin levels.
- Local: pain at injection site.
- Other: weight loss.

Overdose and treatment
Clinical effects of overdose may reflect fluid overload and potential risk of heart failure caused by volume of fluid needed to administer drug. Carefully monitor renal, hepatic, and hematologic status in patient who received excessive dose.

▶ **Special considerations**
- Drug proves effective only if patient has at least minimal immunocompetence.
- Definitive diagnosis of herpes simplex conjunctivitis should be made before administration of ophthalmic form.
- Drug reduces mortality from herpes simplex encephalitis from 70% to 28%. However, no evidence suggests that drug is effective against encephalitis caused by other viruses.
- Do not give I.M. or S.C. because drug is poorly and unreliably absorbed by these routes.
- To prepare I.V. infusion, shake vial well to achieve uniform suspension before transferring to I.V. solution container. Examine vial for uniformity. Use at least 1 liter for every 450 mg of drug (every milligram requires at least 2.22 ml of I.V. fluid). Infuse drug via continuous drip over 12 to 24 hours. Avoid rapid or bolus injection. Use I.V. in-line filter (0.45 microns or smaller).
- To facilitate dissolution, warm solution to 95° to 104° F. (35° to 40° C.). Once in solution, vidarabine remains stable at room temperature for 48 hours. Do not refrigerate diluted solution.
- Any crystalloid solution may be used to prepare I.V. drug. Do not use biologic (blood) or colloidal (albumin) fluids.
- If patient is receiving drug concomitantly with theophylline, monitor serum theophylline levels and observe for signs and symptoms of theophylline toxicity.

Information for the patient

• Warn patient who is receiving ophthalmic ointment not to exceed recommended frequency or duration of therapy. Instruct him to wash hands before and after applying ointment, and warn him against allowing tip of tube to touch eye or surrounding area.

• Advise patient to wear sunglasses if photosensitivity occurs.

• Advise patient to store ophthalmic ointment in tightly sealed, light-resistant container.

---

vinblastine sulfate (VLB)
Velban, Velbe*

• Pharmacologic classification: vinca alkaloid (cell cycle-phase specific, M phase)
• Therapeutic classification: antineoplastic
• Pregnancy risk category D

How supplied
Available by prescription only
Injection: 10-mg vials (lyophilized powder), 10 mg/10 ml vials

Indications, route, and dosage
Dosage and indications may vary. Check current literature for recommended protocol.
Breast or testicular cancer, Hodgkin's and non-Hodgkin's lymphomas, choriocarcinoma, lymphosarcoma, neuroblastoma, lung cancer, mycosis fungoides, histiocytosis, Kaposi's sarcoma
Adults: 0.1 mg/kg or 3.7 mg/m² I.V. weekly or q 2 weeks. May be increased in weekly increments of 50 mcg/kg or 1.8 to 1.9 mg/m² to maximum dose of 0.5 mg/kg or 18.5 mg/m² I.V. weekly, according to response. Dose should not be repeated if WBC count falls below 4,000/mm³.
Children: 2.5 mg/m² I.V. as a single dose every week, increased weekly in increments of 1.25 mg/m² to a maximum of 7.5 mg/m².

Pharmacodynamics
Antineoplastic action: Vinblastine exerts its cytotoxic activity by arresting the cell cycle in the metaphase portion of cell division, resulting in a blockade of mitosis. The drug also inhibits DNA-dependent RNA synthesis and interferes with amino acid metabolism, inhibiting purine synthesis.

Pharmacokinetics
• *Absorption:* Vinblastine is absorbed unpredictably across the GI tract after oral administration, which is why it must be given I.V.
• *Distribution:* Vinblastine is distributed widely into body tissues. The drug crosses the blood-brain barrier but does not achieve therapeutic concentrations in the CSF.
• *Metabolism:* Vinblastine is metabolized partially in the liver to an active metabolite.
• *Excretion:* Vinblastine is excreted primarily in bile as unchanged drug. A smaller portion is excreted in urine. The plasma elimination of vinblastine is described as triphasic, with half-lives of 35 minutes, 53 minutes, and 19 hours for the alpha, beta, and terminal phases, respectively.

Contraindications and precautions
Vinblastine is contraindicated in patients with severe leukopenia or bacterial infections because treatment with myelosuppressive drugs such as vinblastine causes an increased frequency of infections. Instruct patients to report any symptoms of sore throat and fever and of unusual bruising or bleeding. Leukocyte, erythrocyte, and platelet counts, and hemoglobin should be monitored weekly during therapy. Vinblastine can impair fertility. Aspermia has occurred after treatment with vinblastine.

Interactions
Concomitant use of vinblastine increases the effect of methotrexate by increasing cellular uptake of methotrexate. This interaction allows a lower dose of methotrexate, reducing the potential for methotrexate toxicity.

Effects on diagnostic tests
Vinblastine therapy may increase blood and urine concentrations of uric acid.

Adverse reactions
• CNS: depression, paresthesias, peripheral neuropathy and neuritis, numbness, loss of deep tendon reflexes, muscle pain and weakness.
• DERM: dermatitis, vesiculation.
• EENT: pharyngitis.
• GI: nausea, vomiting, stomatitis, ulcer, bleeding, constipation, ileus, anorexia, weight loss, abdominal pain.
• GU: oligospermia, aspermia, urinary retention.
• HEMA: *bone marrow depression* (dose-limiting), *leukopenia* (nadir on days 4 to 10 and lasts another 7 to 14 days), *thrombocytopenia.*
• Local: irritation, phlebitis, cellulitis, necrosis if I.V. extravasates.
• Other: acute *bronchospasm,* reversible alopecia in 5% to 10% of patients, pain in tumor site, low fever.
   Note: Drug should be discontinued if patient develops stomatitis.

Overdose and treatment
Clinical manifestations of overdose include stomatitis, ileus, mental depression, paresthesias, loss of deep reflexes, permanent CNS damage, and myelosuppression.
   Treatment is usually supportive and includes transfusion of blood components and appropriate symptomatic therapy.

▶ Special considerations
Besides those relevant to all *vinca alkaloids,* consider the following recommendations.
• To reconstitute drug, use 10 ml of preserved normal saline injection to yield a concentration of 1 mg/ml.
• Drug may be administered by I.V. push injection over 1 minute into the tubing of a freely flowing I.V. infusion.
• Dilution into larger volume is not recommended for infusion into peripheral veins. This method increases risk of extravasation. Drug may be administered as an I.V. infusion through a central venous catheter.
• Give an antiemetic before administering drug, to reduce nausea.
• Do not administer more frequently than every 7 days to allow review of effect on leukocytes before administration of next dose. Leukopenia may develop.
• Reduced dosage may be required in patients with liver disease.
• After administering, monitor for life-threatening acute

---

bronchospasm reaction. This reaction is most likely to occur in a patient who is also receiving mitomycin.

• Prevent uric acid nephropathy with generous oral fluid intake and administration of allopurinol.

• Treat extravasation with liberal injection of hyaluronidase into the site, followed by warm compresses to minimize the spread of the reaction. (Some clinicians treat extravasation with cold compresses.) Prepare hyaluronidase by adding 3 ml of normal saline solution to the 150-unit vial.

• Give laxatives as needed. Stool softeners may be used prophylactically.

• Do not confuse vinblastine with vincristine or the investigational agent vindesine.

• Drug is less neurotoxic than vincristine.

Information for the patient
• Encourage adequate fluid intake to increase urine output and facilitate excretion of uric acid.

• Reassure patient that therapeutic response is not immediate. Adequate trial is 12 weeks.

• Advise patient to avoid exposure to people with infections.

• Reassure patient that hair should grow back after treatment has ended.

Geriatric use
Patients with cachexia or ulceration of the skin (which is more common in elderly patients) may be more susceptible to the leukopenic effect of this drug.

Breast-feeding
It is not known whether vinblastine distributes into breast milk. However, because of the risk of serious adverse reactions, mutagenicity, and carcinogenicity in infants, breast-feeding is not recommended.

PHARMACOLOGIC CLASS

vinca alkaloids

vinblastine
vincristine
vindesine

The vinca alkaloids are isolates of the periwinkle plant (*Vinca rosea*), which has a history of use in folk medicine. However, this plant's therapeutic effects were not studied scientifically until 1945. In 1958, several isolates from the periwinkle plant were identified. Vinblastine and vincristine are now available commercially; vindesine is still being studied investigationally. Although vinca alkaloids are similar chemically, their individual profiles of clinical activity and toxicity vary.

Pharmacology
The exact mechanism of cytotoxicity of the vinca alkaloids is unclear. However, it appears that these agents arrest cells in the metaphase portion of cell division by crystallizing the microtubular spindle proteins. Therefore, the vinca alkaloids are considered to be cell cycle-phase specific to the M phase. At higher concentrations, the vinca alkaloids may inhibit nucleic acid and protein synthesis. There appears to be no cross resistance among the drugs in this class. The therapeutic activity and toxicity of the vincas seems to be related to their ability to enter different cell types.

Clinical indications and actions
Lymphomas and other carcinomas
The vinca alkaloids have shown clinical efficacy in a variety of tumor types. All three are effective in treating Hodgkin's and non-Hodgkin's lymphomas, and carcinoma of the breast. Vincristine and vindesine are effective against acute lymphocytic and myelogenous leukemia; they also have been used successfully in small-cell cancer of the lung. Vincristine and vinblastine are effective against neuroblastomas. Vinblastine is used to treat testicular tumors and choriocarcinoma. Vincristine is effective against rhabdomyosarcoma and Wilms' tumor.

Accepted indications are changing as continuing research reveals new indications, combination regimens, and dosing schedules.

Overview of adverse reactions
The dose-limiting toxicity of vinblastine and vindesine is bone marrow depression evident by leukopenia, which occurs 4 to 10 days after a dose, with recovery within 10 to 21 days. Neurotoxicity is the dose-limiting toxicity of vincristine, clinically manifested as peripheral neuropathy, with loss of deep tendon reflex, weakness, vocal cord paralysis, and paralytic ileus.

The vinca alkaloids can cause life-threatening acute bronchospasm. They are potent vesicants and can cause severe tissue necrosis if extravasated.

▶ Special considerations
• Take special care to avoid extravasation. Treatment of extravasation includes liberal injection of hyaluronidase into the site, followed by warm compresses to minimize the spread of the reaction. Prepare hyaluronidase by adding 3 ml of normal saline injection to the 150-unit vial.

• Monitor patients closely for acute bronchospasm reaction and have supportive treatment readily available.

• Prevent uric acid nephropathy with generous oral fluid intake and administration of allopurinol.

• The agents in this class have similiar names. Do not confuse one drug for another.

Pediatric use
No specific recommendations available.

Geriatric use
Elderly patients may be more sensitive to the neurotoxic and myelosuppressive effects of vinca alkaloids.

Breast-feeding
It is unknown whether the vinca alkaloids distribute into breast milk. However, because of the risk of serious adverse reactions, mutagenicity, and carcinogenicity in the infant, breast-feeding is not recommended.

Representative combinations
None.

---

vincristine sulfate
Oncovin

- Pharmacologic classification: vinca alkaloid (cell cycle-phase specific, M phase)
- Therapeutic classification: antineoplastic
- Pregnancy risk category D

How supplied
Available by prescription only
Injection: 1 mg/1 ml, 2 mg/2 ml, 5 mg/5 ml multiple-dose vials; 1 mg/1 ml, 2 mg/2 ml preservative-free vials

Indications, route, and dosage
Dosage and indications may vary. Check current literature for recommended protocol.
Acute lymphoblastic and other leukemias; Hodgkin's disease; lymphosarcoma; reticulum cell, osteogenic, and other sarcomas; neuroblastoma; rhabdomyosarcoma; Wilms' tumor; lung and breast cancer
Adults: 10 to 30 mcg/kg I.V. or 0.4 to 1.4 mg/m² I.V. weekly.
Children: 1.5 to 2 mg/m² I.V. weekly. Maximum single dose (adults and children) is 2 mg.
Children under 10 kg or < 1 m²: 0.05 mg/kg once weekly.

Pharmacodynamics
Antineoplastic action: Vincristine exerts its cytotoxic activity by arresting the cell cycle in the metaphase portion of cell division, resulting in a blockade of mitosis. The drug also inhibits DNA-dependent RNA synthesis and interferes with amino acid metabolites, inhibiting purine synthesis.

Pharmacokinetics
- *Absorption:* Vincristine is absorbed unpredictably across the GI tract after oral administration and therefore must be given I.V.
- *Distribution:* Vincristine is rapidly and widely distributed into body tissues and is bound to erythrocytes and platelets. The drug crosses the blood-brain barrier but does not achieve therapeutic concentrations in the cerebrospinal fluid.
- *Metabolism:* Vincristine is extensively metabolized in the liver.
- *Excretion:* Vincristine and its metabolites are primarily excreted into bile. A smaller portion is eliminated through the kidneys. The plasma elimination of vincristine is described as triphasic, with half-lives of about 4 minutes, 2¼ hours, and 85 hours for the distribution, second, and terminal phases, respectively.

Contraindications and precautions
Vincristine is contraindicated in patients with the demyelinating form of Charcot-Marie-Tooth syndrome because of the drug's neurotoxic effects. It's also contraindicated in patients with hepatic failure and in those receiving radiation through ports that include the liver.
Treatment with myelosuppressive drugs such as vincristine causes an increased frequency of infections. Patient should call if sore throat or fever develops. Use with caution in patients with preexisting neuromuscular disease, closely monitoring for neurotoxicity. Also use cautiously in patients receiving other neurotoxic drugs. Leukocyte count and hemoglobin should be checked before each dose of vincristine. Use cautiously in patients with jaundice or hepatic dysfunction.

Interactions
Concomitant use of vincristine increases the therapeutic effect of methotrexate. This interaction may be used to therapeutic advantage; it allows a lower dose of methotrexate, reducing the potential for methotrexate toxicity. Concomitant use with other neurotoxic drugs increases neurotoxicity through an additive effect.
Asparaginase decreases the hepatic clearance of vincristine. Calcium channel blockers enhance vincristine accumulation in cells. Concomitant use with digoxin decreases digoxin levels; monitor serum digoxin levels. Use with mitomycin may possibly increase the frequency of bronchospasm and acute pulmonary reactions.

Effects on diagnostic tests
Vincristine therapy may increase blood and urine concentrations of uric acid and serum potassium.

Adverse reactions
- CNS: neurotoxicity (dose-limiting), peripheral neuropathy, sensory loss, deep tendon reflex loss, paresthesias, wristdrop and footdrop, ataxia, cranial nerve palsies (headache, jaw pain, hoarseness, vocal cord paralysis, visual disturbances), muscle weakness and cramps, depression, agitation, insomnia; some neurotoxicities may be permanent.
- EENT: diplopia, optic and extraocular neuropathy, ptosis.
- GI: constipation, cramps, ileus that mimics surgical abdomen, nausea, vomiting, anorexia, stomatitis, weight loss, dysphagia, *intestinal necrosis.*
- GU: urinary retention.
- HEMA: rapidly reversible mild anemia and *leukopenia.*
- Local: severe local reaction when extravasated, phlebitis, cellulitis.
- Other: *acute bronchospasm,* reversible alopecia (in up to 71% of patients), syndrome of inappropriate antidiuretic hormone.

Overdose and treatment
Clinical manifestations of overdose include alopecia, myelosuppression, paresthesias, neuritic pain, motor difficulties, loss of deep tendon reflexes, nausea, vomiting, and ileus.
Treatment is usually supportive and includes transfusion of blood components, antiemetics, enemas for ileus, phenobarbital for convulsions, and other appropriate symptomatic therapy. Administration of calcium leucovorin at a dosage of 15 mg I.V. q 3 hours for 24 hours, then q 6 hours for 48 hours may help protect cells from the toxic effects of vincristine.

▶ Special considerations
Besides those relevant to all *vinca alkaloids,* consider the following recommendations.
- Drug may be administered by I.V. push injection over 1 minute into the tubing of a freely flowing I.V. infusion.
- Dilution into larger volumes is not recommended for infusion into peripheral veins; this method increases risk of extravasation. Drug may be administered as an I.V. infusion through a central venous catheter.

● Necrosis may result from extravasation. Manufacturer recommends treatment with cold compresses and prompt administration of 150 units of intradermal hyaluronidase, sodium bicarbonate, and local injection of hydrocortisone, or a combination of these treatments. However, some clinicians prefer to treat extravasation only with warm compresses.

● After administering, monitor for life-threatening bronchospasm reaction. It is most likely to occur in a patient who is also receiving mitomycin.

● Because of potential for neurotoxicity, do not give drug more than once a week. Children are more resistant to neurotoxicity than adults. Neurotoxicity is dose-related and usually reversible; reduce dose if symptoms of neurotoxicity develop.

● Monitor for neurotoxicity by checking for depression of Achilles tendon reflex, numbness, tingling, footdrop or wristdrop, difficulty in walking, ataxia, and slapping gait. Also check ability to walk on heels. Patient should have support during walking.

● Prevent uric acid nephropathy with generous oral fluid intake and administration of allopurinol. Alkalinization of urine may be required if serum uric acid concentration is increased.

● Monitor bowel function. Patient should have stool softener, laxative, or water before dosing. Constipation may be an early sign of neurotoxicity.

● Patients with obstructive jaundice or liver disease should receive a reduced dosage.

● Be extremely careful to avoid confusing vincristine with vinblastine or the investigational agent vindesine.

● Vials of 5 mg are for multiple-dose use only. Do not administer entire vial to patient as single dose.

● Drug may cause inappropriate ADH secretion. Treatment requires fluid restriction and a loop diuretic.

Information for the patient
● Encourage adequate fluid intake to increase urine output and facilitate excretion of uric acid.

● Tell patient to call regarding use of laxatives if constipation or stomach pain occurs.

● Assure patient that hair growth should resume after treatment is discontinued.

Geriatric use
Elderly patients who are weak or bedridden may be more susceptible to neurotoxic effects.

Breast-feeding
It is not known whether vincristine distributes into breast milk. However, because of the risk of serious adverse reactions, mutagenicity, and carcinogenicity in the infant, breast-feeding is not recommended.

vitamins

Fat-soluble
vitamin A₁ (retinol)
vitamin A₂ (dehydroretinol)
vitamin A acid (retinoic acid)
provitamin A (carotene)
vitamin D
vitamin D₂ (ergocalciferol)
vitamin D₃ (cholecalciferol)
vitamin E
tocopherol and tocotrienols: alpha, beta, gamma, delta
vitamin K (menadione, phytonadione)

Water-soluble
vitamin B₁ (thiamine)
vitamin B₂ (riboflavin)
vitamin B₃ (niacin)
vitamin B₅ (pantothenic acid)
vitamin B₆ (pyridoxine)
vitamin B₉ (folic acid, folacin)
vitamin B₁₂ (cyanocobalamin)
vitamin C (ascorbic acid)
biotin

Vitamins are chemically unrelated organic compounds which are required for normal growth and maintenance of metabolic functions. Since the body is unable to synthesize many vitamins, it must obtain them from exogenous sources. Vitamins do not furnish energy and are not essential building blocks for the body; however, they are essential for the transformation of energy and for the regulation of metabolic processes.

Vitamins are classified as fat-soluble or water-soluble, and the Food and Nutrition Board of the National Research Council determines the recommended dietary allowances (RDAs) for each. These allowances represent amounts that will provide adequate nutrition in most healthy persons; they are not minimum requirements. Note that a diet which includes ample intake of the four basic food groups will provide sufficient quantities of vitamins. If needed, vitamins should be used as an adjunct to a regular diet and not as a food substitute.

Controversy has existed for years over the vitamin issue. Some argue that vitamin supplementation is unnecessary; some recommend moderate supplementation for everyone; still others advocate the use of megavitamins. The public should be warned against self-medication with vitamins, as the safety and efficacy of their chronic use for relief of mild or self-limiting conditions has not been established.

Pharmacology
Vitamins are available as single drugs or in combination with several other vitamins with or without minerals, trace elements, iron, fluoride, or other nutritional supplements. Frequently, diets deficient in one vitamin are also deficient in other vitamins of similar dietary source. Malabsorption syndromes also affect the usage of several vitamins as do certain disease states which increase metabolic rates. Therefore, multiple vitamin therapy may prove rational and useful in these situations.

RECOMMENDED DAILY ALLOWANCES FOR ADULTS AGES 23 TO 50

VITAMIN	MALES	FEMALES	PREGNANT FEMALES	LACTATING FEMALES*
A	1,000 mcg	800 mcg	800 mcg	1,300 mcg
B_1	1.5 mg	1.1 mg	1.5 mg	1.6 mg
B_2	1.7 mg	1.3 mg	1.6 mg	1.8 mg
B_6	2 mg	1.6 mg	2.2 mg	2.1 mg
B_{12}	2 mcg	2 mcg	2.2 mcg	2.6 mcg
C	60 mg	60 mg	70 mg	95 mg
D	200 IU	200 IU	400 IU	400 IU
E	10 IU	8 IU	10 IU	12 IU
K	80 mcg	65 mcg	65 mcg	65 mcg
Folic acid	200 mcg	180 mcg	400 mcg	280 mcg
Niacin	19 mg	15 mg	17 mg	20 mg

*first 6 months

Fat-soluble vitamins are absorbed with dietary fats and stored in the body in moderate amounts. They are not normally excreted in urine. Chronic ingestion of therapeutic amounts can result in excessive build-up of these agents and lead to toxicity.

Water-soluble vitamins are not stored in the body in any appreciable amounts and are excreted in urine. These agents seldom cause toxicity in patients with normal renal function.

Both fat-soluble and water-soluble vitamins are essential for the maintenance of normal structure and normal metabolic functions of the body.

Clinical indications and actions
Vitamin deficiency or malabsorption; conditions of metabolic stress
Vitamin supplementation is required when deficiencies exist, in malabsorption syndrome, in hypermetabolic disease states, during pregnancy and lactation, and in the elderly, alcoholics, or dieters. Multiple vitamins may be indicated for patients taking oral contraceptives, estrogens, prolonged antibiotic therapy, isoniazid, or for patients receiving prolonged I.V. hyperalimentation (IVH).

Persons with increased metabolic requirements, such as infants, and those suffering severe injury, trauma, major surgery, or severe infection also require supplementation. Prolonged diarrhea, severe GI disorders, malignancy, surgical removal or sections of GI tract, obstructive jaundice, cystic fibrosis, and other conditions leading to reduced or poor absorption are included indications for multiple vitamin therapy. Refer to individual agents for specific indications.

Overview of adverse reactions
The most frequent adverse reactions seen with both types of vitamins include nausea, vomiting, diarrhea, tiredness, weakness, headache, loss of appetite, skin rash, and itching.

▶ Special considerations
● Monitoring may be required. See specific vitamin entries for details.
● Vitamins containing iron may cause constipation and black, tarry stools.
● Excessive fluoride supplements can result in hypocalcemia and tetany.
● Give with food or milk or after meals to reduce GI distress associated with vitamin therapy.
● Vitamins are not food substitutes. Stress the importance of adequate dietary intake of four basic food groups.

Information for the patient
● Stress the importance of adequate dietary intake of four basic food groups. Vitamins are not food substitutes.
● Tell the patient to take vitamins only as directed, not to exceed recommended daily allowance, and to take with food, milk, or after meals to reduce chance of stomach upset.
● Store vitamins away from heat and light, and out of small children's reach.
● Warn patients that vitamins with iron may cause constipation and black tarry stools.
● Tell the patient to read all label directions. Warn them not to take large doses unless prescribed.
● Liquid vitamins may be mixed with food or juice.
● Advise the patient not to refer to vitamins or other drugs as candy. Children should be taught that vitamins and other drugs cannot be taken indiscriminately.

Geriatric use
No specific recommendations available.

Pediatric use
Recommended daily allowances vary with age. Excessive amounts of vitamins, particularly in neonates, may be toxic.

---

*Canada only   †Unlabeled clinical use   Italicized adverse reactions are life-threatening.

Breast-feeding
Recommended daily allowances may be increased in breast-feeding women.

Representative combinations
The following list includes selected combinations that are available only by prescription.

B vitamins (oral) niacin (B_3), pantothenic acid (B_5), pyridoxine (B_6), and cyanocobalamin (B_{12}), with folic acid (B_9), iron, manganese, zinc, and 13% alcohol: Megaton Elixir; with thiamine (B_1), riboflavin (B_2), ferric pyrophosphate, and 15% alcohol: Senilizol Elixir; with thiamine (B_1), riboflavin (B_2), ascorbic acid, and folic acid: Berocca, B Plex, Strovite, BC with folic acid; with thiamine (B_1), riboflavin (B_2), ascorbic acid, folic acid, and biotin: Nephrocaps.

B vitamins (parenteral) thiamine (B_1) and cyanocobalamin (B_{12}): Bexibee injection; with riboflavin (B_2), niacin (B_3), pantothenic acid (B_5), pyridoxine (B_6), and ascorbic acid: Becomject/C, Kay Plex, Vicam, Scorbex/12.

Multivitamins (oral) vitamins A, D, E, thiamine (B_1), riboflavin (B_2), niacin (B_3), pantothenic acid (B_5), pyridoxine (B_6), cyanocobalamin (B_{12}), and ascorbic acid: Theracebrin, Al-Vite; vitamins E, thiamine (B_1), riboflavin (B_2), niacin (B_3), pantothenic acid (B_5), pyridoxine (B_6), cyanocobalamin (B_{12}), ascorbic acid, and folic acid: Cefol Filmtabs; vitamins E, thiamine (B_1), niacin (B_3), pyridoxine (B_6), cyanocobalamin (B_{12}), ascorbic acid, folic acid, and iron: Vicef; vitamins A, E, thiamine (B_1), riboflavin (B_2), niacin (B_3), pantothenic acid (B_5), pyridoxine (B_6), cyanocobalamin (B_{12}), ascorbic acid, folic acid, iron, iodine, and calcium: Eldec.

Multivitamins (parenteral) vitamins A, D, E, thiamine (B_1), riboflavin (B_2), thiamine (B_3), pantothenic acid (B_5), pyridoxine (B_6), cyanocobalamin (B_{12}), ascorbic acid, biotin, and folic acid: Berocca parenteral nutrition, MVI, MVC.

Multivitamins with fluoride (oral) vitamins A, D, thiamine (B_1), riboflavin (B_2), niacin (B_3), pantothenic acid (B_5), pyridoxine (B_6), cyanocobalamin (B_{12}), ascorbic acid, folic acid, and fluoride: Aldeflor, Polyvitamins with fluoride, Mulvidren, Polytabs-F; vitamins A, D, E, thiamine (B_1), riboflavin (B_2), niacin (B_3), pyridoxine (B_6), cyanocobalamin (B_{12}), ascorbic acid, folic acid, and fluoride: Poly-Vi-Flor, Florvite, Vidaylin F.

vitamin A (retinol)
Aquasol A

- Pharmacologic classification: fat-soluble vitamin
- Therapeutic classification: vitamin
- Pregnancy risk category A (X if > recommended daily allowance [RDA])

How supplied
Available by prescription only
Tablets: 10,000 IU
Capsules: 25,000 IU, 50,000 IU
Injection: 2-ml vials (50,000 IU/ml with 0.5% chlorobutanol, polysorbate 80, butylated hydroxyanisol, and butylated hydroxytoluene)

Available without prescription, as appropriate
Drops: 30 ml with dropper (5,000 IU/0.1 ml)
Capsules: 10,000 IU

Indications, route, and dosage
Severe vitamin A deficiency with xerophthalmia
Adults and children over age 8: 500,000 IU P.O. daily for 3 days, then 50,000 IU P.O. daily for 14 days, then maintenance dosage of 10,000 to 20,000 IU P.O. daily for 2 months, followed by adequate dietary nutrition and RDA vitamin A supplements.
Severe vitamin A deficiency
Adults and children over age 8: 100,000 IU P.O. or I.M. daily for 3 days, then 50,000 IU P.O. or I.M. daily for 14 days, then maintenance dosage of 10,000 to 20,000 IU P.O. daily for 2 months, followed by adequate dietary nutrition and RDA vitamin A supplements.
Children age 1 to 8: 17,500 to 35,000 IU I.M. daily for 10 days.
Infants under age 1: 7,500 to 15,000 IU I.M. daily for 10 days.
Maintenance only
Children age 4 to 8: 15,000 IU I.M. daily for 2 months, then adequate dietary nutrition and RDA vitamin A supplements.
Children under age 4: 10,000 IU I.M. daily for 2 months, then adequate dietary nutrition and RDA vitamin A supplements.
Note: The RDA for vitamin A is as follows:

Infants		
age 6 to 12 months	375 RE	1,875 IU
birth to 6 months	375 RE	1,875 IU
Children		
age 7 to 10	700 RE	3,300 IU
age 4 to 6	500 RE	2,500 IU
age 1 to 3	400 RE	2,000 IU
Males		
age 11 and over	1,000 RE	5,000 IU
Females		
age 11 and over	800 RE	4,000 IU
Pregnant	+ 200 RE	+ 1,000 IU
Lactating	+ 400 RE	+ 2,000 IU
RE = retinol equivalents		

Pharmacodynamics
Metabolic action: One IU of vitamin A is equivalent to 0.3 mcg of retinol or 0.6 mcg of beta-carotene. Beta-carotene, or provitamin, A yields retinol after absorption from the intestinal tract.

Retinol's combination with opsin, the red pigment in the retina, helps form rhodopsin, which is necessary for visual adaptation to darkness. Vitamin A prevents growth retardation and preserves the integrity of the epithelial cells. Vitamin A deficiency is characterized by nyctalopia (night blindness), keratomalacia (necrosis of the cornea), keratinization and drying of the skin, low resistance to infection, growth retardation, bone thickening, diminished cortical steroid production, and fetal malformations.

Pharmacokinetics
- *Absorption:* In normal doses, vitamin A is absorbed readily and completely if fat absorption is normal. Larger doses, or regular doses in patients with fat malabsorp-

---

tion, low protein intake, or hepatic or pancreatic disease, may be absorbed incompletely. Because vitamin A is fat-soluble, absorption requires bile salts, pancreatic lipase, and dietary fat.

• *Distribution:* Vitamin A is stored (primarily as palmitate) in Kupffer's cells of the liver. Normal adult liver stores are sufficient to provide vitamin A requirements for 2 years. Lesser amounts of retinyl palmitate are stored in the kidneys, lungs, adrenal glands, retinas, and intraperitoneal fat. Vitamin A circulates bound to a specific alpha$_1$ protein, retinol-binding protein (RBP). Blood level assays may not reflect liver storage of vitamin A because serum levels depend partly on circulating RBP. Liver storage should be adequate before discontinuing therapy. Vitamin A is distributed into breast milk. It does not readily cross the placenta.

• *Metabolism:* Vitamin A is metabolized in the liver.

• *Excretion:* Retinol (fat-soluble) is conjugated with glucuronic acid and then further metabolized to retinal and retinoic acid. Retinoic acid is excreted in feces via biliary elimination. Retinal, retinoic acid, and other water-soluble metabolites are excreted in urine and feces. Normally, no unchanged retinol is excreted in urine, except in patients with pneumonia or chronic nephritis.

Contraindications and precautions

Vitamin A is contraindicated in patients with hypervitaminosis A and in those with sensitivity to vitamin A or other ingredients in commercially available preparations. Intravenous use is contraindicated because it may cause fatal anaphylaxis.

Vitamin A intake from fortified foods, dietary supplements, self-prescribed drugs, and prescription drug sources should be evaluated. Prolonged administration of dosages that exceed 25,000 IU/day requires close supervision.

The efficacy of large systemic doses of vitamin A in treating acne has not been established; this use should be avoided because of the potential for toxicity. Topical vitamin A acid (tretinoin) is useful in treating acne.

Interactions

Concomitant use of vitamin A with oral contraceptives significantly increases the vitamin's plasma levels.

Prolonged use of mineral oil may interfere with the intestinal absorption of vitamin A.

Concomitant use with cholestyramine may decrease the absorption of vitamin A by decreasing bile acids and preventing the micellar phase in the GI lumen. Daily vitamin A supplements have been recommended during long-term cholestyramine therapy.

Use with neomycin may decrease vitamin A absorption.

Large doses of vitamin A may interfere with the hypoprothrombinemic effect of warfarin.

Because of the potential for additive adverse effects, patients receiving retinoids (such as etretinate or isotretinoin) should avoid concomitant use of vitamin A.

Effects on diagnostic tests

Vitamin A therapy may falsely increase serum cholesterol level readings by interfering with the Zlatkis-Zak reaction. Vitamin A has also been reported to falsely elevate bilirubin determinations.

Adverse reactions

Adverse reactions are usually seen only with toxicity (hypervitaminosis A).

• CNS: irritability, headache, *increased intracranial pressure,* fatigue, lethargy, malaise.

• DERM: alopecia; drying, cracking, scaling skin; pruritus; lip fissures; *massive desquamation;* increased pigmentation.

• EENT: miosis, papilledema, exophthalmos.

• GI: anorexia, epigastric pain, diarrhea, vomiting.

• GU: hypomenorrhea.

• HEMA: hypoplastic anemia, leukopenia.

• Hepatic: jaundice, hepatomegaly.

• Metabolic: hypercalcemia.

• Other: night sweating; skeletal – slow growth, decalcification of bone, fractures, hyperostosis, painful periostitis, premature closure of epiphyses, migratory arthralgia, cortical thickening over the radius and tibia, bulging fontanelles, splenomegaly. Fatal *anaphylaxis* has been reported after I.V. use.

Overdose and treatment

In cases of acute toxicity, increased intracranial pressure develops within 8 to 12 hours; cutaneous desquamation follows in a few days. Toxicity can follow a single dose of 25,000 IU/kg, which in infants would represent about 75,000 IU and in adults over 2 million IU.

Chronic toxicity results from administration of 4,000 IU/kg for 6 to 15 months. In infants (age 3 to 6 months) this would represent about 18,500 IU/day for 1 to 3 months; in adults, 1 million IU/day for 3 days, 50,000 IU/day for more than 18 months, or 500,000 IU/day for 2 months.

To treat toxicity, discontinue vitamin A administration if hypercalcemia persists, and administer I.V. saline solution, prednisone, and calcitonin, if indicated. Perform liver function tests to detect possible liver damage.

▶ Special considerations

• Safety of amounts exceeding 6,000 IU/day during pregnancy is not known.

• In any dietary deficiency, multiple vitamin deficiency should be suspected.

• Give vitamin A concurrently with bile salts to patients with malabsorption caused by inadequate bile secretion.

• Vitamin A given by I.V. push is contraindicated because it can cause anaphylaxis and death.

• Use special water-miscible form of vitamin A when adding to large parenteral volumes.

Information for the patient

• Explain to patient that he must avoid prolonged use of mineral oil while taking this drug because mineral oil reduces vitamin A absorption in the intestine.

• Tell patient not to exceed recommended dosage.

• Tell patient to report promptly any symptoms of overdose (nausea, vomiting, anorexia, malaise, drying or cracking of skin or lips, irritability, headache, or loss of hair) and to discontinue the drug immediately when such symptoms occur.

• Teach patient to consume adequate protein, vitamin E, and zinc, which, along with bile, are necessary for vitamin A absorption.

• Tell patient to store vitamin A in a tight, light-resistant container.

Geriatric use

Liquid preparations are available to give by nasogastric tube.

Pediatric use
Liquid preparations may be mixed with fruit juice or cereal.

Breast-feeding
Vitamin A is distributed into breast milk. The RDA of vitamin A for lactating women in the United States is 1,200 retinol equivalents. Unless the maternal diet is grossly inadequate, infants can usually obtain sufficient vitamin A from breast-feeding. The effect of large maternal dosages of vitamin A on breast-feeding infants is unknown.

vitamin E (alpha tocopherol)
Aquasol E, CEN-E, E-Ferol, E-Ferol Succinate, Eprolin Gelseals, Epsilan-M, E-Vital, Pheryl-E 400, Tocopher-Caps, Vita-Plus E, Viterra E

- Pharmacologic classification: fat-soluble vitamin
- Therapeutic classification: vitamin
- Pregnancy risk category A (C if > recommended daily allowance [RDA])

How available
Available without prescription, as appropriate
Oral solution: 50 IU/ml
Capsules: 50 IU, 100 IU, 200 IU, 400 IU, 600 IU, 1,000 IU
Tablets: 100 IU, 200 IU, 400 IU, 500 IU, 600 IU, 1,000 IU
Tablets (chewable): 100 IU, 200 IU, 400 IU

Indications, route, and dosage
Vitamin E deficiency in premature infants and in patients with impaired fat absorption (including patients with cystic fibrosis); biliary atresia
Adults: 60 to 75 IU, depending on severity, P.O. or I.M. daily. Maximum dosage is 300 IU/day.
Children: 1 mg equivalent/0.6 g of dietary unsaturated fat P.O. or I.M. daily.
Premature neonates: 5 units P.O. daily.
Full-term neonates: 5 units P.O. per liter of formula.
   Note: The RDA for vitamin E is as follows:
Infants: 0 to 6 months – 4 TE.
Children: 6 months to 1 year – 6 TE.
1 to 3 years – 9 TE.
4 to 10 years – 10 TE.
Males: over 11 years – 15 TE.
Females: over 11 years – 12 TE.
Pregnant women: 15 TE.
Lactating women (0 to 6 months): 18 TE;
(over 6 months): 16 TE.
   TE is alpha tocopherol equivalent (equal to 1 mg d-alpha-tocopherol or 1.49 IU).

Pharmacodynamics
Nutritional action: As a dietary supplement, the exact biochemical mechanism is unclear, although it is believed to act as an antioxidant. Vitamin E protects cell membranes, vitamin A, vitamin C (ascorbic acid), and polyunsaturated fatty acids from oxidation. It also may act as a cofactor in enzyme systems, and some evidence exists that it decreases platelet aggregation.

Pharmacokinetics
- *Absorption:* GI absorption depends on the presence of bile. Only 20% to 60% of the vitamin obtained from dietary sources is absorbed. As dosage increases, the fraction of vitamin E absorbed decreases.
- *Distribution:* Vitamin E is distributed to all tissues and is stored in adipose tissue.
- *Metabolism:* Vitamin E is metabolized in the liver by glucuronidation.
- *Excretion:* Vitamin E is excreted primarily in bile. Some enterohepatic circulation may occur. Small amounts of the metabolites are excreted in urine.

Contraindications and precautions
Vitamin E is usually nontoxic. A complex and potentially fatal syndrome has occurred in several premature infants who received I.V. therapy with vitamin E; however, this form of the drug is no longer available.

Interactions
Concomitant use of vitamin E with mineral oil, colestipol, cholestyramine, or sucralfate may increase vitamin E requirements.
   Vitamin E may have anti-vitamin K effects; patients receiving oral anticoagulants may be at risk for hemorrhage after large doses of vitamin E.

Effects on diagnostic tests
None reported.

Adverse reactions
None reported.

Overdose and treatment
Clinical manifestations of overdose include a possible increase in blood pressure. Treatment is generally supportive.

▶ Special considerations
- Give concurrently with bile salts if patient has malabsorption caused by lack of bile.
- Vitamin E has been used investigationally to prevent retrolental fibroplasia and bronchopulmonary dysplasia in neonates, to prevent periventricular hemorrhage in premature infants, and to decrease the severity of hemolytic anemia in infants.

Information for the patient
- Inform patient about dietary sources of vitamin E, such as vegetable oil, green leafy vegetables, nuts, wheat germ, eggs, meat, liver, dairy products, and cereals.
- Tell patient to store vitamin E in a tight, light-resistant container.

---

vitamin K derivatives

menadiol sodium diphosphate
Synkayvite

phytonadione
AquaMEPHYTON, Konakion,
Mephyton

- Pharmacologic classification: vitamin K
- Therapeutic classification: blood coagulation modifier
- Pregnancy risk category C (X if used in third trimester or near term)

How supplied
All products available by prescription only
Menadiol sodium diphosphate
Tablets: 5 mg
Injection: 5 mg/ml, 10 mg/ml, 37.5 mg/ml
Phytonadione
Tablets: 5 mg
Injection (aqueous colloidal solution): 2 mg/ml, 10 mg/ml
Injection (aqueous dispersion): 2 mg/ml, 10 mg/ml

Indications, route, and dosage
Hypoprothrombinemia secondary to vitamin K malabsorption or drug therapy, or when oral administration is desired and bile secretion is inadequate
Adults: 5 to 10 mg menadiol sodium diphosphate or phytonadione P.O. daily or 5 to 15 mg menadiol sodium diphosphate I.M. once or twice daily, or titrated to patient's requirements.
Hypoprothrombinemia secondary to vitamin K malabsorption, drug therapy, or excess vitamin A
Adults: 2 to 25 mg phytonadione P.O. or parenterally, repeated and increased up to 50 mg, if necessary.
Children: 5 to 10 mg P.O. or parenterally.
Infants: 2 mg P.O. or parenterally. I.V. injection rate for children and infants should not exceed 3 mg/m²/minute or a total of 5 mg.
Hypoprothrombinemia secondary to effect of oral anticoagulants
Adults: 2.5 to 10 mg phytonadione P.O., S.C., or I.M., based on prothrombin time, repeated, if necessary, 12 to 48 hours after oral dose or 6 to 8 hours after parenteral dose. In emergency, give 10 to 50 mg slow I.V., rate not to exceed 1 mg/minute, repeated every 6 to 8 hours, as needed.
Prevention of hemorrhagic disease in neonates
Neonates: 0.5 to 1 mg phytonadione S.C. or I.M. immediately after birth, repeated in 6 to 8 hours, if needed, especially if mother received oral anticoagulants or long-term anticonvulsant therapy during pregnancy.
Differentiation between hepatocellular disease or biliary obstruction as source of hypoprothrombinemia
Adults and children: 10 mg phytonadione I.M. or S.C.
Prevention of hypoprothrombinemia related to vitamin K deficiency in long-term parenteral nutrition
Adults: 5 to 10 mg phytonadione S.C. or I.M. weekly.
Children: 2 to 5 mg S.C. or I.M. weekly.

Prevention of hypoprothrombinemia in infants receiving less than 0.1 mg/liter vitamin K in breast milk or milk substitutes
Infants: 1 mg phytonadione S.C. or I.M. monthly.
  Note: The RDA for Vitamin K is as follows:
Infants: age 0 to 6 months – 5 mcg.
Children: 6 months to 1 year – 10 mcg.
1 to 3 years – 15 mcg.
4 to 6 years – 20 mcg.
7 to 10 years – 30 mcg.
Males: 11 to 14 years – 45 mcg.
15 to 18 years – 65 mcg.
19 to 24 years – 70 mcg.
over 24 years – 80 mcg.
Females: 11 to 14 years – 45 mcg.
15 to 18 years – 55 mcg.
19 to 24 years – 60 mcg.
over age 24 – 65 mcg.
Pregnant or lactating women – 65 mcg.

Pharmacodynamics
Coagulation modifying action: Vitamin K is a lipid-soluble vitamin that promotes hepatic formation of active prothrombin and several other coagulation factors.

Phytonadione (vitamin K_1) is a synthetic form of vitamin K, and is also lipid-soluble; menadiol sodium diphosphate (vitamin K_4) is a water-soluble derivative converted in the body to menadione (vitamin K_3), which has activity similar to naturally occurring vitamin K.

Vitamin K does not counteract the action of heparin.

Pharmacokinetics
- *Absorption:* Phytonadione requires the presence of bile salts for GI tract absorption; menadiol sodium diphosphate can be absorbed in the absence of bile salts. Once absorbed, vitamin K enters the blood directly. Onset of action after I.V. injection is more rapid, but of shorter duration, than that occurring after S.C. or I.M. injection.
- *Distribution:* Vitamin K concentrates in the liver. Action of parenteral phytonadione begins in 1 to 2 hours; hemorrhage is usually controlled within 3 to 6 hours, and normal prothrombin levels are achieved in 12 to 14 hours. Oral phytonadione begins to act within 6 to 10 hours; parenteral menadiol sodium diphosphate begins to act in 8 to 24 hours.
- *Metabolism:* Vitamin K is metabolized rapidly by the liver; little tissue accumulation occurs.
- *Excretion:* Data are limited. High concentrations occur in feces; however, intestinal bacteria can synthesize vitamin K.

Contraindications and precautions
Vitamin K is contraindicated in patients hypersensitive to any of its analogues; and during the last few weeks of pregnancy or labor, because menadiol sodium diphosphate has caused toxic reactions in neonates. Menadiol sodium diphosphate is contraindicated in infants.

Administer vitamin K cautiously to patients with impaired hepatic function, because large doses may further decrease hepatic function. Menadiol sodium diphosphate may induce erythrocyte hemolysis in patients with glucose-6-phosphate dehydrogenase deficiency.

Interactions
Broad-spectrum antibiotics (especially cefoperazone, moxalactam, cefamandole, and cefotetan) may inter-

---

fere with the actions of vitamin K, producing hypoprothrombinemia.

Mineral oil inhibits absorption of oral vitamin K; give drugs at well-spaced intervals, and monitor result.

Vitamin K antagonizes the effects of oral anticoagulants; patients receiving these agents should take vitamin K *only* for severe hypoprothrombinemia.

Effects on diagnostic tests
Phytonadione can falsely elevate urine steroid levels.

Adverse reactions
- CNS: headache, dizziness, convulsive movements.
- CV: transient hypotension after I.V. administration, rapid weak pulse, *cardiac arrhythmias.*
- DERM: allergic rash, pruritus, urticaria, eruptions on repeated injections, sweating, flushing, erythema.
- GI: nausea, vomiting.
- Local: pain, swelling, hematoma at injection site.
- Other: *bronchospasm*, dyspnea, cramp-like pain, *anaphylaxis and anaphylactoid reactions* (usually after rapid I.V. administration).
- Neonates: hyperbilirubinemia, *fatal kernicterus, severe hemolytic anemia.*

Note: Drug should be discontinued if allergic or severe CNS reactions appear.

Overdose and treatment
Excessive doses of vitamin K may cause hepatic dysfunction in adults; in neonates and premature infants, large doses may cause hemolytic anemia, kernicterus, and death. Treatment is supportive.

▶ Special considerations
- Check particular product for approved routes of administration.
- Administration of menadiol sodium diphosphate I.V. push should not exceed rate of 1 mg/minute.
- If severity of condition warrants I.V. infusion, mix with normal saline, dextrose 5% in water, or dextrose 5% in normal saline solution. Monitor for flushing, weakness, tachycardia, and hypotension; shock may follow. Deaths have occurred.
- Monitor prothrombin time to determine effectiveness.
- Monitor patient response, and watch for adverse effects; failure to respond to vitamin K may indicate coagulation defects or irreversible hepatic damage.
- Excessive use of vitamin K may temporarily defeat oral anticoagulant therapy; higher doses of oral anticoagulant or interim use of heparin may be required.
- Phytonadione for hemorrhagic disease in infants causes fewer adverse reactions than do other vitamin K analogues; phytonadione is the vitamin K analogue of choice to treat an oral anticoagulant overdose.
- Patients receiving phytonadione who have bile deficiency require concomitant use of bile salts to ensure adequate absorption.

Information for the patient
- For patients receiving oral form, explain rationale for drug therapy; stress importance of complying with medical regimen and keeping follow-up appointments. Tell patient to take a missed dose as soon as possible, but not if it is almost time for next dose, and to report missed doses.
- Warn patient to avoid taking nonprescription products containing aspirin, other salicylates, or drugs that may interact with the anticoagulant, causing an increase or

decrease in action of drug, and to seek medical approval before stopping or starting any medication.
- Advise patient not to substantially alter daily intake of leafy green vegetables (asparagus, broccoli, cabbage, lettuce, turnip greens, spinach, or watercress) or of fish, pork or beef liver, green tea, or tomatoes; these foods contain vitamin K, and widely varying daily intake may alter anticoagulant effect.
- Instruct patients to tell every physician and dentist that they are taking this drug.

Pediatric use
In prophylaxis and treatment of hemorrhagic disease of the newborn, phytonadione has a greater margin of safety than menadiol sodium diphosphate.

Breast-feeding
Vitamin K is not excreted in breast milk. No clinical problems have been associated with its use during breast-feeding.

---

warfarin sodium
Coumadin, Panwarfin, Sofarin

- Pharmacologic classification: coumarin derivative
- Therapeutic classification: anticoagulant
- Pregnancy risk category D

How supplied
Available by prescription only
Tablets: 2 mg, 2.5 mg, 5 mg, 7.5 mg, 10 mg
Injection: 50 mg/vial

Indications, route, and dosage
Pulmonary emboli; deep vein thrombosis, myocardial infarction, rheumatic heart disease with heart valve damage, atrial arrhythmias
Adults: 10 to 15 mg P.O. for 3 days; then daily prothrombin times (PT) are used to establish optimal dose. Usual maintenance dosage is 2 to 10 mg P.O. daily. Also available for I.M. or I.V. use; reconstitute with 2 ml sterile water to make 25 mg/ml solution for injection.

Pharmacodynamics
Anticoagulant action: Warfarin inhibits vitamin K-dependent activation of clotting factors II, VII, IX, and X, which are formed in the liver; it has no direct effect on established thrombi and cannot reverse ischemic tissue damage. However, warfarin may prevent additional clot formation, extension of formed clots, and secondary complications of thrombosis.

Pharmacokinetics
- *Absorption:* Warfarin is rapidly and completely absorbed from the GI tract.
- *Distribution:* Warfarin is highly bound to plasma protein, especially albumin; drug crosses placenta but does not appear to accumulate in breast milk.
- *Metabolism:* Warfarin is hydroxylated by liver into inactive metabolites.
- *Excretion:* Metabolites are reabsorbed from bile and excreted in urine. Half-life of parent drug is 1 to 3 days. Because therapeutic effect is relatively more dependent on clotting factor depletion (Factor X has half-life of 40

---

hours), PT will not peak for 1½ to 3 days despite use of a loading dose. Duration of action is 2 to 5 days – more closely reflecting drug's half-life.

Contraindications and precautions
Warfarin is contraindicated in patients with bleeding or hemorrhagic tendencies caused by open wounds, visceral cancer, GI ulcers, severe hepatic or renal disease, severe or uncontrolled hypertension (diastolic pressure over 110 mm Hg), subacute bacterial endocarditis, or vitamin K deficiency, or after recent brain, eye, or spinal cord surgery, because excessive bleeding can occur.

Administer warfarin cautiously to patients with diverticulitis, colitis, mild to moderate hypertension, or mild to moderate hepatic or renal disease; during lactation; to patients with any drainage tubes; in conjunction with regional or lumbar block anesthesia; or to patients with any condition that increases risk of hemorrhage.

Interactions
Oral anticoagulants interact with many drugs; thus, any change in drug regimen, including use of nonprescription compounds, requires careful monitoring. The most significant interactions follow.

Concomitant use with amiodarone, anabolic steroids, chloramphenicol, metronidazole, cimetidine, clofibrate, dextrothyroxine and other thyroid preparations, salicylates, streptokinase, urokinase, disulfiram, or sulfonamides markedly increases warfarin's anticoagulant effect; *avoid concomitant use.*

Concomitant use with ethacrynic acid, indomethacin, mefenamic acid, phenylbutazone, or sulfinpyrazone increases warfarin's anticoagulant effect and causes severe GI irritation (may be ulcerogenic); *avoid concomitant use when possible.*

Concomitant use with allopurinol, moxalactam, cefoperazone, cefamandole, cefotetan, danazol, diflunisal, erythromycin, glucagon, heparin, miconazole, quinidine, sulindac, or vitamin E increases warfarin's anticoagulant effects. Monitor carefully.

Concomitant use with glutethimide or rifampin causes decreased anticoagulant effect of major significance and should be avoided. Barbiturates may inhibit anticoagulant effect for several weeks after barbiturate withdrawal, and fatal hemorrhage can occur after cessation of barbiturate effect; if barbiturates are withdrawn, reduce anticoagulant dose.

Concomitant use with carbamazepine, oral contraceptives, corticosteroids, ethchlorvynol, griseofulvin, and vitamin K may cause decreased anticoagulant effect; monitor carefully. Cholestyramine decreases warfarin's anticoagulant effect when used close together; administer 6 hours after warfarin.

Concomitant use with chloral hydrate may increase or decrease warfarin's anticoagulant effect; monitor therapy carefully and avoid when possible. Acute alcohol intoxication increases warfarin's anticoagulant effect, and chronic alcohol abuse decreases anticoagulant effect but may predispose patient to bleeding problems.

Effects on diagnostic tests
Warfarin prolongs both PT and partial thromboplastin time; it may enhance uric acid excretion, elevate serum transaminase levels, increase lactic dehydrogenase activity, and cause false-negative serum theophylline levels.

Adverse reactions
● DERM: dermatitis, urticaria, rash, necrosis, petechiae, alopecia, ecchymoses.
● GI: paralytic ileus and intestinal obstruction (caused by hemorrhage), diarrhea, vomiting, cramps, nausea, melena, hematemesis.
● GU: excessive uterine bleeding.
● HEMA: *hemorrhage with excessive dosage,* leukopenia.
● Other: fever, hemoptysis, burning sensation of feet.
Note: Drug should be discontinued if patient shows any sign of bleeding or allergic tendencies, or shows signs of necrosis of the skin or other tissues.

Overdose and treatment
Clinical manifestations of overdose vary with severity and may include internal or external bleeding or skin necrosis of fat-rich areas, but most common sign is hematuria. Excessive prolongation of PT or minor bleeding mandates withdrawal of therapy; withholding one or two doses may be adequate in some cases. Treatment to control bleeding may include oral or I.V. phytonadione (vitamin K₁) and, in severe hemorrhage, fresh frozen plasma or whole blood. Use of phytonadione may interfere with subsequent oral anticoagulant therapy.

▶ **Special considerations**
Besides those relevant to all *coumarin derivatives,* consider the following recommendations.
● After reconstitution, warfarin injection may be stored for several days at 4° C. (39.2° F.). Store drug in light-resistant containers.
● Discard solution that contains a precipitate.

Geriatric use
Elderly patients are more susceptible to effects of anticoagulants and are at increased risk of hemorrhage; this may be caused by altered hemostatic mechanisms or age-related deterioration of hepatic and renal functions.

Pediatric use
Infants, especially neonates, may be more susceptible to anticoagulants because of vitamin K deficiency.

Breast-feeding
Women should avoid breast-feeding during anticoagulant therapy if possible; oral anticoagulants appear in breast milk and may cause coagulation problems in the infant. Some recent evidence suggests that these quantities may be insufficient to cause clinical problems; however, more data are needed.

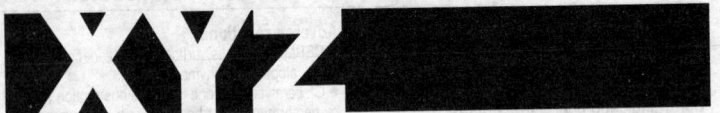

xanthine derivatives

aminophylline
caffeine
dyphylline
oxtriphylline
theophylline

The xanthines have been used in beverages for their stimulant action for many centuries. Theophylline and its salts and analogs were first found to relax smooth muscle. These drugs have extensive therapeutic use, especially in management of chronic respiratory disorders. Numerous dosage forms are available to assist in patient compliance and help control the toxicities associated with these agents.

Pharmacology
The xanthines (caffeine, theobromine, and theophylline) are structurally related; they directly relax smooth muscle, stimulate the CNS, induce diuresis, increase gastric acid secretion, inhibit uterine contractions, and have weak inotropic and chronotropic effects on the heart. Of these agents, theophylline exerts the greatest effect on smooth muscle. The action of xanthine derivatives is not totally mediated by inhibition of phosphodiesterase; current data suggest that inhibition of adenosine receptors, or other as yet unidentified mechanisms, is responsible for the therapeutic effects of these drugs. Their physiologic effect is a relaxation of all smooth muscle, with respiratory smooth muscle the most sensitive to this effect at nontoxic doses.

Clinical indications and actions
Treatment of respiratory disorders
Xanthines are indicated in the symptomatic treatment of asthma and bronchospasm associated with emphysema and chronic bronchitis. By relaxing the smooth muscle of the respiratory tract, they increase air flow and vital capacity. Additionally, they slow the onset of diaphragmatic fatigue and stimulate the respiratory center in the CNS.

Overview of adverse reactions
The xanthines stimulate the CNS and heart while relaxing smooth muscle. This produces such reactions as hypotension, palpitations, arrhythmias, restlessness, irritability, nausea, vomiting, urinary retention, and headache. Adverse effects are dose-related, except for hypersensitivity, and can be controlled by dosage adjustment and monitored via serum levels.

▶ Special considerations
● Many dosage forms and agents are available; it is important to select the form that offers maximum potential for patient compliance and minimal toxicity to the individual. Timed-release preparations may not be crushed or chewed.
● Dosage should be calculated from lean body weight, because theophylline does not distribute into fatty tissue.
● Individuals metabolize theophylline at different rates, and metabolism is influenced by many factors, including age and life-style (smoking).
● Daily dosage may need to be adjusted in patients with congestive heart failure, hepatic disease, or in elderly patients. Monitor carefully, using blood levels.
● Oxtriphylline, aminophylline, and theophylline all release theophylline in the blood; theophylline blood levels are used to monitor therapy.
● Dyphylline is a theophylline analog, and special blood tests are used to monitor dyphylline therapy.

Representative combinations
Dyphylline with chlorpheniramine maleate, guaifenesin, dextromethorphan hydrobromide and phenylephrine: Dilor-G. *Oxtriphylline* with guaifenesin: Brondecon. *Theophylline* with phenobarbital: Bronkolixir, Bronkotab, with ephedrine and phenobarbital: Quadrinal,

---

COMPARING XANTHINE DERIVATIVES
The table below compares the varying theophylline content of several common xanthine derivatives. (Dyphylline is not included because although it has the same pharmacologic action as theophylline, it is a chemical derivative and not a true theophylline salt.)

DRUG	APPROXIMATE THEOPHYLLINE CONTENT	EQUIVALENT DOSE
theophylline anhydrous	100%	100 mg
theophylline monohydrate	90.7% ($\pm 1.1\%$)	110 mg
aminophylline anhydrous	85.7% ($\pm 1.7\%$)	116 mg
aminophylline dehydrate	78.9% ($\pm 1.6\%$)	127 mg
oxytriphylline	63.6% ($\pm 1.9\%$)	156 mg
theophylline sodium glycinate	45.9% ($\pm 1.4\%$)	217 mg

---

*Canada only   †Unlabeled clinical use   Italicized adverse reactions are life-threatening.

Azma-Aid, Phedral, Primatene "P" Formula, Tedral, Tedrigen, Theofedral; with guaifenesin: Asbron G, Quibron; with hydroxyzine hydrochloride and ephedrine: Marax, Marax D.F.

xylometazoline hydrochloride
Chlorohist-LA, Neo-Spray Long Acting, Neo-Synephrine II, Otrivin, Sinutab*, Sustaine*

- Pharmacologic classification: sympathomimetic
- Therapeutic classifications: decongestant, vasoconstrictor
- Pregnancy risk category C

How supplied
Available without prescription
Nasal drops: 0.05%, 0.1% (pediatric use)
Nasal spray: 0.1%

Indications, route, and dosage
Nasal congestion
Adults and children over age 12: Apply 2 or 3 drops or sprays of 0.1% solution to nasal mucosa q 8 to 10 hours, not to exceed three times in 24 hours.
Infants and children age 6 months to 12 years: Apply 2 or 3 drops or 1 spray of 0.05% solution to nasal mucosa q 8 to 10 hours, not to exceed three times in 24 hours.
Infants under age 6 months: 1 drop of 0.05% solution in each nostril q 6 hours as needed under direction of physician.

Pharmacodynamics
Decongestant action: Acts on alpha-adrenergic receptors in nasal mucosa to produce constriction, thereby decreasing blood flow and nasal congestion.

Pharmacokinetics
Unknown.

Contraindications and precautions
Xylometazoline is contraindicated in patients with narrow-angle glaucoma, because the drug may increase intraocular pressure; in patients receiving tricyclic antidepressants, because of the potential for adverse cardiovascular effects; and in those hypersensitive to any components of the preparation.

Xylometazoline should be used with caution in patients with hyperthyroidism, cardiac disease, hypertension, diabetes mellitus, or advanced arteriosclerosis.

Interactions
When used concomitantly with tricyclic antidepressants, xylometazoline may potentiate the pressor effects of tricyclic antidepressants if significant systemic absorption occurs.

Effects on diagnostic tests
None reported.

Adverse reactions
- CNS: headache, drowsiness, dizziness, insomnia, tremor, psychological disturbances, seizures, CNS depression, weakness, hallucinations, prolonged psychosis.
- EENT: blurred vision, ocular irritation, tearing, photophobia, rebound nasal congestion or irritation with excessive or long-term use, transient burning, stinging, dryness or ulceration of nasal mucosa, sneezing.
- Other: dysuria, orofacial dystonia, pallor, sweating.
  Note: Drug should be discontinued if symptoms of systemic toxicity occur.

Overdose and treatment
Clinical manifestations of overdose include somnolence, sedation, sweating, CNS depression with hypertension, bradycardia, decreased cardiac output, rebound hypotension, cardiovascular collapse, depressed respirations, coma.

Because of rapid onset of sedation, emesis is not recommended in therapy unless given early. Activated charcoal or gastric lavage may be used initially. Monitor vital signs and ECG. Treat seizures with I.V. diazepam.

▶ Special considerations
- Monitor carefully for adverse effects in patients with cardiovascular disease, diabetes mellitus, or hyperthyroidism.
- Nasal spray is less likely to cause systemic absorption and is more effective if 3 to 5 minutes elapse between sprays and nose is cleared before next spray.

Information for the patient
- Patient should understand that this drug should only be used for short-term relief of symptoms, no longer than 3 to 5 days.
- Teach patient how to use correctly. Have patient hold head upright and sniff spray briskly. Only one person should use dropper bottle or nasal spray.
- Caution patient not to exceed recommended dosage, in order to avoid rebound congestion.
- Tell patient to report insomnia, dizziness, weakness, tremor, or irregular heartbeat.

Geriatric use
Drug should be used with caution in elderly patients with cardiac disease, diabetes mellitus, or poorly controlled hypertension.

Pediatric use
Children may be prone to greater systemic absorption, with resultant increase in side effects.

yellow fever vaccine
YF-VAX

- Pharmacologic classification: vaccine
- Therapeutic classification: viral vaccine
- Pregnancy risk category D

How supplied
Available by prescription only
Injection: live, attenuated 17D yellow fever virus in 1-dose and 5-dose vials, with diluent; supplied only to designated yellow fever vaccination centers authorized to issue yellow fever vaccination certificates

---

*Canada only   †Unlabeled clinical use   Italicized adverse reactions are life-threatening.

Indications, route, and dosage
Primary vaccination
Adults and children over age 6 months: 0.5 ml deep S.C. Booster dosage is 0.5 ml S.C. q 10 years.

Pharmacodynamics
Yellow fever prophylaxis: This vaccine promotes active immunity to yellow fever.

Pharmacokinetics
Immunity usually develops within 7 to 10 days and lasts for 10 years or longer.

Contraindications and precautions
Yellow fever vaccine is contraindicated in patients with a sensitivity to egg or chick embryo protein and those with acute febrile illness or immunosuppression. Serious adverse reactions (such as encephalitis) occur more frequently in children under age 4 months. If possible, delay vaccination until age 9 months.

Interactions
Concomitant use of yellow fever vaccine with corticosteroids or other immunosuppressants may impair the immune response to the vaccine. Vaccination should be deferred for 2 months after a blood or plasma transfusion.

Administration of yellow fever and cholera vaccines simultaneously or 1 to 3 weeks apart may result in lower than normal antibody responses to both vaccines.

Effects on diagnostic tests
None reported.

Adverse reactions
● Local: swelling, pain, and inflammation.
● Systemic: fever, malaise (occurring 7 to 14 days after vaccination in approximately 10% of patients), myalgia and headache (in about 2% to 5% of patients), *anaphylaxis, encephalitis (only demonstrated in infants and children).*

Overdose and treatment
No information available.

▶ Special considerations
● Obtain a thorough history of allergies, especially to eggs, and of reactions to immunizations.
● Epinephrine solution 1:1,000 should be available to treat allergic reactions.
● Yellow fever vaccine should not be given less than 1 month before or after immunization with other live virus vaccines except for live, attenuated measles virus vaccine; BCG vaccine and hepatitis B vaccine may also be given concurrently.
● Whenever possible, cholera and yellow fever vaccines should be administered at least 3 weeks apart, but they may be administered simultaneously if time constraints require it.
● Usage in pregnancy: Because of the theoretical risk of maternal-fetal transmission of infection through vaccination, yellow fever vaccine should not be given to pregnant women unless they are at high risk of exposure in an epidemic focus. There are no data that exhibit teratogenicity, or ill effects in the fetus following maternal immunization.
● Reconstitute vaccine only with diluent provided. Follow package insert carefully for reconstitution directions. Swirl and agitate reconstituted vial but do not

shake vigorously to avoid foaming of the suspension. Use vaccine within 60 minutes of preparation.
● Unreconstituted vials must be stored between −30° to 5° C (−22° to 41° F). Do not use unless shipping case contains some dry ice upon arrival.
● Discard unused reconstituted vaccine.

Information for the patient
● Tell patient what to expect after vaccination: some pain or swelling at the injection site and fever or general malaise. Recommend acetaminophen to alleviate fever.
● Encourage patient to report adverse reactions.
● Inform patient about the need for revaccination in 10 years to maintain his traveler's vaccination certificate.

Pediatric use
Vaccine should never be given to children under 4 months of age. Vaccination of children 4 to 9 months of age may be necessary in high-risk areas or when travel to high-risk areas cannot be postponed and a high level of protection against mosquito exposure is not feasible.

Breast-feeding
It is unknown whether this vaccine is distributed into breast milk. Use with caution in breast-feeding women.

zalcitabine (dideoxycytidine, ddC)
Hivid

● Pharmacologic classification: nucleoside analogue
● Therapeutic classification: antiviral agent
● Pregnancy risk category C

How supplied
Available by prescription only
Tablets (film-coated): 0.375 mg, 0.75 mg

Indications, route, and dosage
Patients with advanced human immunodeficiency virus (HIV) infection (CD4 count below 300 cells/mm³) who have demonstrated significant clinical or immunologic deterioration
Adults 30 kg and over: 0.75 mg P.O. q 8 hours. Must be taken with zidovudine 200 mg P.O. q 8 hours.
Dosage adjustments in adults with renal failure

Creatinine clearance	Dose
>40 ml/minute	0.75 mg P.O. q 8 hours
10 to 40 ml/minute	0.75 mg P.O. q 12 hours
<10 ml/minute	0.75 mg P.O. q 24 hours

Pharmacodynamics
Antiviral action: Zalcitabine is active against HIV. Within cells, it is converted by cellular enzymes into its active metabolite, dideoxycytidine 5'-triphosphate (ddCTP).

It inhibits the replication of HIV by blocking viral DNA synthesis. The drug inhibits reverse transcriptase by acting as an alternative for the enzyme's substrate, deoxycytidine triphosphate (dCTP).

Pharmacokinetics
● *Absorption:* Mean absolute bioavailability is above 80%; administering drug with food decreases the rate and extent of absorption.
● *Distribution:* Steady-state volume of distribution is 0.534 ± 0.127 liters/kg. Drug enters the CNS.
● *Metabolism:* Drug doesn't appear to undergo significant hepatic metabolism; phosphorylation to the active form occurs within cells.
● *Excretion:* Excretion is primarily by the kidneys; about 70% of a dose appears in urine within 24 hours. Mean elimination half-life is 2 hours.

Contraindications and precautions
Zalcitabine is contraindicated in patients with hypersensitivity to the drug or any component of the formulation. Because peripheral neuropathy is a major toxic effect, use with extreme caution in patients with preexisting peripheral neuropathy. No data exists regarding toxicity in these patients because clinical trials excluded patients with peripheral neuropathy.

Pancreatitis, although uncommon, has been fatal in patients receiving zalcitabine. In patients receiving zalcitabine alone, incidence was less than 1%. Use with caution in patients with a history of pancreatitis.

Other drug-related toxicities include esophageal ulcers, cardiomyopathy, CHF, allergic reactions, and anaphylactoid reactions.

Patients with renal impairment (creatinine clearance below 55 ml/minute) may be at increased risk for drug toxicity. Dosage adjustments are necessary in moderate to severe renal failure.

In clinical trials, the drug regimen (zalcitabine plus zidovudine) exacerbated hepatic dysfunction in patients with preexisting liver impairment.

Interactions
Concomitant use with drugs that cause peripheral neuropathy (such as chloramphenicol, cisplatin, dapsone, disulfiram, ethionamide, glutethimide, gold salts, hydralazine, iodoquinol, isoniazid, metronidazole, nitrofurantoin, phenytoin, ribavirin, and vincristine) may increase risk of peripheral neuropathy.

Drugs that may impair renal function may also increase risk of zalcitabine-induced adverse effects; these drugs include aminoglycosides, amphotericin, and foscarnet. Concomitant use with pentamidine is not recommended because of the risk of pancreatitis.

Effects on diagnostic tests
Toxic effects of the drug may cause abnormalities in several laboratory tests, including CBC, leukocyte count, reticulocyte count, granulocyte count, hemoglobin, platelet count, AST (SGOT), ALT (SGPT), or alkaline phosphatase.

Adverse reactions
Note: Limited data are available regarding drug toxicity. Consult current literature for more details.
● CNS: peripheral neuropathy, headache.
● DERM: pruritus, night sweats; erythematous, maculopapular, or follicular rash.
● EENT: pharyngitis.

● GI: nausea, vomiting, diarrhea, abdominal pain, anorexia, constipation, stomatitis.
● Other: myalgia, arthralgia, fatigue, fever, rigors, chest pain, weight increase, *pancreatitis*.

Overdose and treatment
There is little experience with acute overdosage. It's unknown if drug is dialyzable. Treat symptomatically.

During early clinical trials, patients exposed chronically to doses about six times higher than the current recommended dosage experienced peripheral neuropathy within 10 weeks; patients exposed to twice the recommended dosage experienced peripheral neuropathy within 12 weeks.

▶ Special considerations
● If zalcitabine is discontinued because of toxicity, patient should resume the recommended dosage for zidovudine alone, which is 100 mg q 4 hours.
● If patient experiences symptoms that suggest peripheral neuropathy, drug should be discontinued if symptoms are bilateral and persist beyond 72 hours. If these symptoms persist or worsen beyond 1 week, drug should be permanently discontinued; however, if all findings relevant to peripheral neuropathy have resolved to minor symptoms, drug may be reintroduced at 0.375 mg P.O. q 8 hours.
● In clinical trials in which zalcitabine was the only treatment, peripheral neuropathy occurred in 17% to 31% of patients. The peripheral neuropathy seen with zalcitabine therapy is a sensorimotor neuropathy, initially characterized by numbness and burning in the extremities. If drug is not withdrawn, symptoms can progress to sharp, shooting pain or severe, continuous burning pain requiring narcotic analgesics and may or may not be reversible.
● Women of childbearing age should use an effective contraceptive while taking this drug.

Information for the patient
● Make sure patient understands that drug doesn't cure HIV infection and that he can still transmit HIV. Opportunistic infections may continue to occur despite use of drug. Review safe sex practices with the patient.
● Make sure patient understands that drug may cause peripheral neuropathy and life-threatening pancreatitis. Review the signs and symptoms of these reactions, and instruct patient to call immediately if any appear.

Pediatric use
Safety and efficacy in children under age 13 have not been established.

Breast-feeding
It is unknown if drug is excreted in breast milk. Because of the risk of transmitting the virus, HIV-positive women should not breast-feed.

zidovudine (AZT)
Retrovir

- Pharmacologic classification: thymidine analogue
- Therapeutic classification: antiviral agent
- Pregnancy risk category C

How supplied
Capsules: 100 mg
Syrup: 50 mg/5 ml
Injection: 10 mg/ml

Indications, route, and dosage
Symptomatic human immunodeficiency virus (HIV), acquired immunodeficiency syndrome (AIDS), or advanced AIDS-related complex (ARC)
Adults: 200 mg P.O. q 4 hours. After 1 month, reduce dosage to 100 mg q 4 hours while awake (500 mg daily). Or administer by I.V. infusion. Give 1 to 2 mg I.V. infused over 1 hour at a constant rate q 4 hours.
Asymptomatic HIV infection (CD4 count below 500/mm³)
Adults: 100 mg P.O. q 4 hours while awake (500 mg daily).
Children age 3 months to 12 years: 180 mg/m² q 6 hours or 720 mg/m² daily in divided doses q 6 hours. Do not exceed 200 mg q 6 hours.

Pharmacodynamics
Antiviral action: Zidovudine is converted intracellularly to an active triphosphate compound that inhibits reverse transcriptase (an enzyme essential for retroviral DNA synthesis), thereby inhibiting viral replication. When used in vitro, drug inhibits certain other viruses and bacteria; however, this has undetermined clinical significance.

Pharmacokinetics
- *Absorption:* Zidovudine is absorbed rapidly from the GI tract. Average systemic bioavailability is 65% of dose (drug undergoes first-pass metabolism).
- *Distribution:* Preliminary data reveal good CSF penetration. Approximately 36% of zidovudine dose is plasma protein-bound.
- *Metabolism:* Zidovudine is metabolized rapidly to an inactive compound.
- *Excretion:* Parent drug and metabolite are excreted by glomerular filtration and tubular secretion in the kidneys. Urine recovery of parent drug and metabolite is 14% and 74%, respectively. Elimination half-lives of these compounds equal 1 hour.

Contraindications and precautions
Zidovudine should be administered with extreme caution to patients with compromised bone marrow function. Significant anemia may occur after 2 to 6 weeks of therapy, possibly necessitating dosage adjustment, drug discontinuation, epoetin alfa therapy, or transfusions.

Interactions
When used concomitantly with drugs that are nephrotoxic or that affect bone marrow function or formation of bone marrow elements (such as dapsone, pentamidine, amphotericin B, flucytosine, vincristine, vinblastine, doxorubicin, and interferon), zidovudine may increase the risk of drug toxicity. Concomitant use with probenecid may impair elimination of zidovudine.

Effects on diagnostic tests
Zidovudine may cause depression of formed elements (erythrocytes, leukocytes, and platelets) in peripheral blood.

Adverse reactions
- CNS: headache, malaise, dizziness, paresthesia.
- GI: nausea, vomiting, anorexia.
- HEMA: *anemia, granulocytopenia, thrombocytopenia.*
- Other: myalgia.
  Note: Temporarily discontinue zidovudine if marked anemia, as indicated by hemoglobin level below 7.5 mg/dl (or reduction by more than 25% of baseline value), or granulocytopenia (granulocyte count less than 750/mm³, or reduction by more than 50% of baseline value) occurs.

Overdose and treatment
No information available.

▶ Special considerations
- The optimum duration of treatment, as well as the dosage for optimum effectiveness and minimum toxicity, is not yet known.
- Monitor complete blood count and platelet count at least every 2 weeks. Dosage may be discontinued or reduced if hematologic toxicity occurs.
- The I.V. dosage equivalent to 100 mg P.O. q 4 hours is approximately 1 mg/kg I.V. q 4 hours.
- Because zidovudine frequently causes a low red blood cell count, advise patients that they may need blood transfusions or epoetin alfa therapy during treatment.
- Observe patient for signs and symptoms of opportunistic infection (including pneumonia, meningitis, and sepsis).
- Store undiluted injection, capsules, and syrup at room temperature (77° F [25° C]); protect from light. Dilute I.V. form to less than 4 mg/ml with dextrose 5% in water before administering. Do not mix with protein-containing solutions. To minimize potential for microbial contamination, administer within 8 hours of mixing if left at room temperature or within 24 hours if refrigerated (36° to 46° F [2° to 8° C]).
- Drug does not cure HIV infection or AIDS but may reduce morbidity resulting from opportunistic infections and thus prolong the patient's life.

Information for the patient
- Teach patient about his disease, ways to prevent disease transmission, rationale for drug therapy, and drug's limitations.
- Teach patient about proper drug administration. When the drug must be taken every 4 hours around the clock, explain the importance of maintaining an adequate blood level and suggest ways to avoid missing doses, such as using an alarm clock.
- Inform patient about the importance of follow-up medical visits to evaluate for adverse effects and to monitor clinical status.
- Instruct patient how to recognize adverse drug effects and to report these immediately.

- Warn patient not to take any other drugs for AIDS (especially from the "street") without medical approval.
- Make sure patient understands that zidovudine therapy does not reduce his ability to transmit HIV infection.

Breast-feeding
To avoid transmitting HIV to the infant, HIV-positive women should not breast-feed.

zinc
Medizinc, Orazinc, Scrip Zinc, Verazine, Zinc 15, Zinc 220, Zincate, Zinkaps-220

zinc sulfate (ophthalmic)
Eye-Sed Ophthalmic, Op-Thal-Zin

- Pharmacologic classification: trace element; miscellaneous anti-infective
- Therapeutic classification: nutritional supplement; topical anti-infective
- Pregnancy risk category C

How supplied
Available by prescription only
Injection: 10 ml (1 mg/ml), 30 ml (1 mg/ml with 0.9% benzyl alcohol), 5 ml (5 mg/ml); 10 ml (5 mg/ml), 50 ml (1 mg/ml)
Tablets: 220 mg (50 mg zinc)
Capsules: 220 mg (50 mg zinc)

Available without prescription, as appropriate
Tablets: 110 mg (25 mg zinc), 200 mg (47 mg zinc)
Capsules: 110 mg (25 mg zinc), 220 mg (50 mg zinc)
Solution: 15 ml (0.217%)

Indications, route, and dosage
Zinc deficiency; adjunct in ulcers, acne, ear granulomata, rheumatoid arthritis, hypogeusia, anosmia; vitamin A therapy, and acrodermatitis enteropathica
Adults: 200 to 220 mg P.O. t.i.d. (equivalent to 135 to 150 mg elemental zinc daily, 9 to 10 times the adult RDA of 15 mg daily).
Children: Dosage not established. RDA is 0.3 mg/kg/day.
For relief of minor eye irritation
Adults: 1 to 2 drops ophthalmic solution into the eye b.i.d. to q.i.d. Patients are advised to report irritation that persists for more than 3 days.

Pharmacodynamics
Metabolic action: Zinc serves as a cofactor for more than 70 different enzymes. It facilitates wound healing, normal growth rates, and normal skin hydration and helps maintain the senses of taste and smell.

Adequate zinc provides normal growth and tissue repair. In patients receiving total parenteral nutrition with low plasma levels of zinc, dermatitis has been followed by alopecia. Zinc is an integral part of many enzymes important to carbohydrate and protein mobilization of retinal-binding protein.

Zinc sulfate ophthalmic solution exhibits astringent and weak antiseptic activity, which may result from precipitation of protein by the zinc ion and by clearing

mucus from the outer surface of the eye. This drug has no decongestant action and produces mild vasodilation.

Pharmacokinetics
- *Absorption:* Zinc sulfate is absorbed poorly from the GI tract; only 20% to 30% of dietary zinc is absorbed. After administration, zinc resides in muscle, bone, skin, kidney, liver, pancreas, retina, prostate, and, particularly, red and white blood cells. Zinc binds to plasma albumin, alpha-2 macroglobulin, and some plasma amino acids including histidine, cysteine, threonine, glycine, and asparagine.
- *Distribution:* Major zinc stores are in the skeletal muscle, skin, bone, and pancreas.
- *Metabolism:* Zinc is a cofactor in many enzymatic reactions. It is required for the synthesis and mobilization of retinal binding protein.
- *Excretion:* After parenteral administration, 90% of zinc is excreted in the stool, urine, and sweat. After oral use, the major route of excretion is secretion into the duodenum and jejunum. Small amounts are also excreted in the urine (0.3 to 0.5 mg/day) and in sweat (1.5 mg/day).

Contraindications and precautions
Parenteral use of zinc sulfate is contraindicated in patients with renal failure or biliary obstruction (and requires caution in all patients) because metals may accumulate; zinc plasma levels must be determined frequently. In renal dysfunction or GI malfunction, trace metal supplements may need to be reduced, adjusted, or omitted. Hypersensitivity may result.

Administering copper in the absence of zinc or administering zinc in the absence of copper may result in decreased serum levels of either element. When only one trace element is needed, it should be added separately and serum levels monitored closely. To avoid overdose, administer multiple trace elements only when clearly needed. In patients with extreme vomiting or diarrhea, extreme amounts of trace elements replacement may be needed.

Interactions
Concomitant use of oral zinc sulfate with tetracycline will impair antibiotic absorption. When zinc sulfate ophthalmic solution is used with sodium borate, precipitation of zinc borate may occur; glycerin may prevent this interaction. Zinc sulfate ophthalmic solution has a dehydrating effect on methylcellulose suspensions, causing precipitation of methylcellulose. Zinc sulfate ophthalmic solution may also precipitate acacia and certain proteins.

Effects on diagnostic tests
None reported.

Adverse reactions
- CNS: restlessness.
- DERM: rash.
- GI: distress and irritation, nausea, vomiting with high doses, gastric ulceration, diarrhea.
- Other: dehydration.

Overdose and treatment
Clinical manifestations of severe toxicity include hypotension, pulmonary edema, diarrhea, vomiting, jaundice, and oliguria. Dosage must be discontinued and support measures begun.

▶ Special considerations

● Results may not appear for 6 to 8 weeks in zinc-depleted patients.
● Zinc decreases the absorption of tetracyclines.
● Monitor for severe vomiting and dehydration, which may indicate overdose.
● Calcium supplements may confer a protective effect against zinc toxicity.
● Because of the potential for infusion phlebitis and tissue irritation, an undiluted direct injection must not be administered into a peripheral vein.
● Do not exceed prescribed dosage of oral zinc; if oral zinc is administered in single 2-g doses, emesis will occur.
● If ophthalmic use causes increasing irritation, patient should discontinue use.

Information for the patient

● Tell patient not to take zinc with dairy products, which can reduce zinc absorption.
● Teach patient how to instill ophthalmic solution and to prevent contamination. Tell him to avoid contacting the lip of the container with any other surface and to tightly close the container after each use.
● Warn patient about self-medication with zinc sulfate ophthalmic solution, which should not continue longer than 3 days. Patient should report increased irritation or redness which may be signs of a serious ocular condition.
● Warn patient that GI upset may occur after oral administration but may be diminished if zinc is taken with food. Patients must avoid foods high in calcium, phosphorus, or phytate during zinc therapy.

Investigational drugs

amsacrine (m-AMSA, acridinyl anisidide)
Amekrin, Amsidyl

- Pharmacologic classification: alkylating agent
- Therapeutic classification: antineoplastic

How supplied
Injection: 50 mg/ml in 2-ml ampules

Indications, route, and dosage
Refractory acute myelogenous leukemia
Adults and children: Induction dose is 450 to 600 mg/m² I.V. (using a central vein) over 3 to 5 days. Induction is repeated after bone marrow recovery.

Adverse reactions
- CV: sinus tachycardia, atrial fibrillation, ventricular fibrillation.
- DERM: alopecia, rash.
- GI: nausea, vomiting, stomatitis, diarrhea.
- HEMA: pancytopenia, bone marrow depression.
- Other: pyrexia, injection site irritation.

▶ Special considerations
Information is based on current literature. Dosage, indications, and adverse reaction profile can change with additional clinical experience.
- Amsacrine is a bone marrow suppressant. Repeated doses should not be administered until hematologic parameters have adequately recovered. Close monitoring of bone marrow function is recommended.
- Patient should be reminded to promptly report signs and symptoms of an infection (such as fever or sore throat) or any unusual bruising or bleeding.
- Amsacrine is supplied with lactic acid diluent. Follow manufacturer's directions to prepare solution for injection. To mix a solution containing 5 mg/ml amsacrine, withdraw 1.5 ml amsacrine from the ampule and mix with 13.5 ml lactic acid. Use a glass syringe. The resulting solution is red. Add to at least 500 ml of dextrose 5% in water and administer by infusion into central vein over 30 to 90 minutes.
- Do not use a membrane-type in-line filter because the solution may dissolve the filter.
- Amsacrine is incompatible with saline solutions. Use only dextrose 5% in water for administration.
- Dosage should be reduced by 25% to 50% in patients with moderate to severe renal or hepatic impairment.
- Inform the patient that the drug may discolor the urine red or orange.
- Infusion into peripheral veins may cause severe irritation and necrosis.

antiendotoxin monoclonal antibodies
E5, HA-1A

- Pharmacological classification: antibody
- Therapeutic classification: immunotherapeutic agent

Indications, route, and dosage
Life-threatening gram-negative sepsis
Adults: 100 mg HA-1A by I. V. bolus as a single dose. Or 2 mg/kg E5 by I.V. infusion; repeat in 24 hours. All information is based on current literature.

Pharmacodynamics
Immunotherapeutic action: These synthetic antibodies neutralize endotoxin, a lipopolysaccharide found in the outer membrane of gram-negative bacteria that is associated with significant morbidity and mortality in patients experiencing septic shock. E5 is a murine IgM antibody derived from murine (mouse) cells; HA-1A is derived from a human cell line.

Adverse reactions
- DERM: hives.
- CV: hypotension.
- Other: *anaphylactoid reactions,* facial flushing.

▶ Special considerations
All information based upon current literature. Dosage, indications, adverse effect profile can change with additional clinical experience.
- Antiendotoxin monoclonal antibody therapy is expected to be very expensive. Careful patient selection is essential to optimize therapy.
- Criteria for the diagnosis of sepsis must be developed. Early clinical studies have included fever (above 101° F [38° C]) or hypothermia (below 96° F [36° C]); heart rate over 90 beats/minute; tachypnea, with a respiratory rate of 20 or more breaths/minute; hypotension, with a systolic blood pressure under 90 mm Hg despite adequate fluid challenge; arterial hypoxemia; unexplained metabolic acidosis; acute renal failure; sudden vascular resistance. Other criteria include presence of a known or suspected site of gram-negative infusion, WBC count above 12,000/mm³ or below 3,000/mm³, or a positive blood culture for a gram-negative rod within the previous 48 hours.

---

domperidone
Motilium

- Pharmacologic classification: dopamine antagonist
- Therapeutic classification: antiemetic

How supplied
Tablets: 10 mg

Indications, route, and dosage
Symptomatic treatment of upper GI motility disorders associated with gastric and diabetic gastroparesis; prevention of nausea and vomiting caused by antiparkinsonian medications
Adults: 10 mg P.O. t.i.d. to q.i.d. 30 minutes before meals and h.s. Maximum dose is 20 mg P.O. q.i.d.

Pharmacodynamics
Antiemetic action: Domperidone blocks dopamine receptors in the chemoreceptor trigger zone. In the GI tract, the drug enhances motility in the stomach and small intestine.

Adverse reactions
- CNS: headache.
- DERM: rash.
- GI: dry mouth.
- Other: galactorrhea, gynecomastia, menstrual irregularities.

▶ Special considerations
Information is based on current literature. Dosage, indications, and adverse reaction profile can change with additional clinical experience.
- Domperidone is contraindicated in patients hypersensitive to the drug and in patients with mechanical obstruction of the GI tract or GI hemorrhage.
- Parenteral domperidone has been tested as an antiemetic for patients undergoing chemotherapy. Doses up to 1 mg/kg have been effective and well tolerated.
- The drug causes enhanced GI motility and promotes gastric emptying. It may alter the absorption of other orally administered drugs.

enoxacin
Comprecin

- Pharmacologic classification: fluoroquinolone quinoline
- Therapeutic classification: antibiotic

How supplied
Tablets: 200 mg, 300 mg, 400 mg

Indications, route and dosage
Mild to moderate urinary tract infections
Adults: 200 mg P.O. b.i.d. for 5 days.
Complicated to severe urinary tract infections
Adults: 400 mg P.O. b.i.d. for 14 days.

Skin and skin-structure infections
Adults: 400 mg P.O. b.i.d. for 7 to 14 days.
Uncomplicated genital tract infections (urethral or endocervical gonorrhea caused by susceptible strains of Neisseria gonorrhoeae)
Adults: 400 mg P.O. for one dose.

Adverse reactions
- CNS: headache, insomnia, tremor, restlessness.
- GI: nausea, vomiting, diarrhea.

▶ Special considerations
Information is based on current literature. Dosage, indications, and adverse reaction profile can change with additional clinical experience.
- Be aware of potential drug interactions. Do not administer with antacids containing aluminum or magnesium because these cations will inhibit enoxacin absorption. Limited evidence suggests that concomitant use of NSAIDs may increase the risk of seizures. Enoxacin will decrease the clearance of xanthines, including theophylline and caffeine.
- Do not use in children under age 18 or in pregnant women. Fluoroquinolones have been associated with the development of arthropathy in juvenile animals.
- Dehydration, alkaline urine, or high doses of fluoroquinolones have been associated with crystalluria.
- Use with caution in patients with a history of seizures or severe cerebral arteriosclerosis. Fluoroquinolones have been associated with seizures in certain predisposed individuals.
- Photosensitivity and skin rashes have been reported with other fluoroquinolones. Tell patient to use a sunscreen when outdoors and to avoid unnecessary exposure to sunlight.

ketotifen fumarate
Globofil, Ketasma, Zaditen

- Pharmacologic classification: antihistamine
- Therapeutic classification: antiasthmatic

How supplied
Tablets: 1 mg
Elixir: 1 mg/5 ml

Indications, route, and dosage
Prophylaxis of asthma; treatment of allergic rhinitis and conjunctivitis
Adults: 1 mg P.O. b.i.d. with food. Dosage may be increased to 2 mg b.i.d. as needed and tolerated.

Pharmacodynamics
Antiasthmatic action: Ketotifen stabilizes mast cells in a manner similar to cromolyn sodium. It has other pharmacologic effects, including antihistamine, phosphodiesterase-inhibiting, calcium channel blocking, and $beta_2$ agonist effects, which contribute to its usefulness in the treatment of asthma.

Adverse reactions
- CNS: sedation, tiredness, dizziness, headache.
- GI: dry mouth, nausea.
- Other: increased appetite and weight gain, exacerbation of asthma, bronchospasm.

▶ **Special considerations**
Information is based on current literature. Dosage, indications, and adverse reaction profile can change with additional clinical experience.
● Long-term therapy with ketotifen, as with cromolyn, improves its usefulness in the prophylaxis of asthma. Patients taking the drug for 3 months or more report alleviation of symptoms. The drug should not be used during an acute asthmatic attack.
● Patients should avoid driving and other hazardous activities that require alertness until the adverse CNS effects of the drug are known.

loracarbef
Lorabid

● Pharmacologic classification: cephalosporin
● Therapeutic classification: antibiotic

How supplied
Capsules: 200 mg
Oral suspension: 100 mg/5 ml, 200 mg/5 ml

Indications, route and dosage
Otitis media. respiratory tract, sinus, and urinary tract infections
Adults: 200 mg P O. b.i.d. for 7 days.

Pharmacodynamics
Antibiotic action: Loracarbef inhibits cell wall formation in dividing bacteria. Bactericidal.

Contraindications and precautions
Loracarbef is contraindicated in patients with severe hypersensitivity reaction to penicillins, cephalosporins, or other beta-lactam antibiotics.

Adverse reactions
● CNS: headache.
● GI: diarrhea, loose stools, abdominal pain.
● Other: rash, superinfection.

▶ **Special considerations**
All information is based on current literature. Indications, dosage, and adverse effect profile can change with additional clinical experience.
● Drug has shown in vitro activity against various organisms, including *Haemophilus influenzae, Moraxella (Branhamella) catarrhalis, Escherichia coli, Klebsiella* species, *Proteus mirabilis, Citrobacter diversus,* non-Penicillin-resistant streptococcus pneumoniae, non-methicillin-resistant *Staphylococcus aureus,* and pathogenic *Neisseria* species.
● Monitor patient for the development of superinfection. Most antibitics can cause pseudomembranous colitis; patients with severe or persistant diarrhea should have stool cultures performed to detect presence of the suspected causative organism, *Clostridium difficile.*

nedocromil sodium
Tilade

● Pharmacologic classification: cromolyn derivative
● Therapeutic classification: antiasthmatic agent

How supplied
Inhaler: 2 mg per metered dose

Indications, route, and dosage
Prophylaxis of asthma
Adults: 2 inhalations b.i.d. to q.i.d.

Pharmacodynamics
Antiasthmatic action: Inhibits activation and mediator release from inflammatory cells, including mast cells.

Adverse reactions
● CNS: headache, dizziness.
● EENT: unpleasant taste.
● GI: nausea, vomiting.

▶ **Special considerations**
Information is based on current literature. Dosage, indications, and adverse reaction profile can change with additional clinical experience.
● Drug should not be used during an acute asthmatic attack. Beneficial effects stem from long-term use.
● Limited evidence suggests that drug may have some anti-inflammatory properties. Patients have been able to reduce the use of bronchodilators and corticosteroids without increasing asthmatic symptoms.

taxol

● Pharmacologic classification: derivative of *Taxus brevifolia*
● Therapeutic classification: antineoplastic

How supplied
Injection: 6 mg/ml in 5-ml vials

Indications, route. and dosage
Ovarian cancer
Adults: 135 mg/m² by continuous I.V. infusion over 24 hours. Repeat q 3 weeks until response is seen.
Non-small-cell lung cancer
Adults: 200 mg/m² by continuous I.V infusion over 24 hours Repeat q 3 weeks.

Pharmacodynamics
Antineoplastic action: A derivative of the western yew evergreen tree *Taxus brevifolia,* taxol blocks cell in the G2 and M phase of the cell cycle by blocking mitosis. Drug appears to enhance the assembly of cellular microtubules and prevent their depolymerization.

Contraindications and precautions
Hematologic toxicity limits dosage. Patients who have received substantial chemotherapy or radiation before

treatment with taxol may require lower doses of drug because pretreatment may enhance toxicity.

Adverse reactions
- CNS: headache, fatigue, peripheral neuropathy.
- CV: bradycardia.
- GI: diarrhea, nausea, vomiting, mucositis.
- HEMA: *neutropenia, thrombocytopenia, leukemia.*
- Other: alopecia, arthralgia, myalgia, fever, taste perversion, hypersensitivity reactions (dyspnea, *bronchospasm,* hypotension, urticaria and erythematous rashes).

▶ **Special considerations**
All information is based on current literature. Dosage, indications, and adverse effects can change with additional clinical experience.
- Most adverse reactions are dose related. Neutropenia is significant but transient (less than 10 days in clinical trials). In one study, all patients developed complete alopecia.
- Hypersensitivity reactions are minimized by infusing the drug over 24 hours and pretreating the patient with antihistamines or corticosteroids. These adverse reactions may be caused by polyoxyethylated castor oil (Cremophor EL), the vehicle for the drug.
- Drug is in extremely short supply; 25,000 lb of tree bark yields only 1 kg of drug, and most patients need 1.2 to 1.5 kg for full course of therapy. Several alternatives are being investigated, including both naturally occurring and synthetic derivatives of the drug, synthetic cultures of the tree, and taxotere, an extract of the needles of the tree.

---

tenoxicam
Tilcotil

- Pharmacologic classification: nonsteroidal anti-inflammatory drug (NSAID), oxicam derivative
- Therapeutic category: anti-inflammatory agent

How supplied
Tablets: 10 mg

Indications, route, and dosage
Symptomatic management of painful inflammatory disorders such as rheumatoid arthritis, osteoarthritis, or ankylosing spondylitis
Adults: Initially, 10 mg P.O. daily. If no relief after 2 weeks, increase dosage to 20 mg/day. Dosage over 20 mg/day is associated with increased incidence of adverse reactions.

Pharmacodynamics
Anti-inflammatory action: Inhibits the production of prostaglandins, known mediators of inflammation.

Adverse reactions
- CNS: headache, dizziness.
- DERM: erythema, urticaria, pruritus.
- GI: epigastritis, nausea, vomiting.
- HEMA: prolonged bleeding time.

▶ **Special considerations**
Information is based on current literature. Dosage, indications, and adverse reaction profile can change with additional clinical experience.
- Like other NSAIDs, the drug may mask some signs of infection, including fever and pain.
- Use with caution in patients with compromised renal or cardiac function. Because of their actions on renal prostaglandins, other NSAIDs can impair renal function.
- NSAIDs can cause GI bleeding, sometimes without warning, especially during prolonged use. Be sure to review the early warning signs of GI bleeding with the patient.
- Tenoxicam is highly (> 99%) bound to plasma proteins. The potential for interactions with other highly protein-bound drugs exists.

---

vindesine sulfate
Eldisine*

- Pharmacologic classification: vinca alkaloid
- Therapeutic classification: antineoplastic

How supplied
Injection: 5 mg, 10 mg ampules

Indications, route, and dosage
Acute lymphocytic leukemia, breast cancer, malignant melanoma, lymphosarcoma, non-small-cell lung carcinoma
Adults: 3 to 4 mg/m² I.V. q 7 to 14 days. Some protocols have used a continuous I.V. infusion of 1.2 to 1.5 mg/m² daily for 5 days, repeated q 3 weeks.

Pharmacodynamics
Antineoplastic action: Blocks cell proliferation by preventing cell division. Arrests mitosis in metaphase.

Adverse reactions
- CNS: paresthesias, decreased deep tendon reflexes, muscle weakness.
- HEMA: leukopenia, thrombocytopenia.
- Local: thrombophlebitis, necrosis with extravasation.
- Other: bronchospasm, alopecia, fever.

▶ **Special considerations**
Information is based on current literature. Dosage, indications, and adverse reaction profile can change with additional clinical experience.
- Continuous infusion by peripheral I.V. line is not recommended. Central venous catheter should be used.
- Bronchospasm appears more likely in patients also receiving mitomycin.
- Drug is stable for 30 days in refrigerator when reconstituted with supplied diluent. Dilute in normal saline.
- Avoid extravasation because vindesine is a vesicant. Flush peripheral lines with 10 ml normal saline before injection to ensure vein patency. Flush line with an additional 10 ml after injection to remove residual drug.

Appendices, selected references, and index

CANCER CHEMOTHERAPY: ACRONYMS AND PROTOCOLS

ACRONYM & INDICATION	DRUG		DOSAGE
	GENERIC NAME	TRADE NAME	
AA (Leukemia — AML, induction)	cytarabine (ARA-C)	Cytosar-U	100 mg/m² daily by continuous I.V. infusion for 7 to 10 days
	doxorubicin	Adriamycin	30 mg/m² I.V., days 1 to 3
ABVD (Hodgkin's lymphoma)	doxorubicin	Adriamycin	25 mg/m² I.V., days 1 and 15
	bleomycin	Blenoxane	10 units/m² I.V., days 1 and 15
	vinblastine	Velban	6 mg/m² I.V., days 1 and 15
	dacarbazine	DTIC-Dome	375 mg/m² I.V., days 1 and 15 *Repeat cycle q 28 days.*
AC (Multiple myeloma)	doxorubicin	Adriamycin	30 mg/m² I.V., day 1
	carmustine	BiCNU	30 mg/m² I.V., day 1 *Repeat cycle q 21 to 28 days.*
AC (Bony sarcoma)	doxorubicin	Adriamycin	75 to 90 mg/m² by 96-hour continuous I.V. infusion
	cisplatin	Platinol	90 to 120 mg/m² IA or I.V., day 6 *Repeat cycle q 28 days.*
AFM (Breast cancer)	doxorubicin	Adriamycin	25 mg/m² by continuous I.V. infusion, days 1 to 3
	fluorouracil (5-FU)	Adrucil	400 mg/m² I.V., days 1 to 5
	methotrexate sodium	Folex	250 mg/m² I.V., day 18
	leucovorin calcium	Wellcovorin	15 mg/m² P.O. q 6 hours, days 19 to 20 *Repeat cycle q 21 days for four cycles.*
AP (Ovarian cancer, epithelial)	doxorubicin	Adriamycin	50 to 60 mg/m² I.V., day 1
	cisplatin	Platinol	50 to 60 mg/m² I.V., day 1 *Repeat cycle q 21 days.*
APE (Gastric cancer)	doxorubicin	Adriamycin	20 mg/m² I.V. daily, days 1 and 7
	cisplatin	Platinol	40 mg/m² I.V. daily, days 2 and 8
	etoposide (VP-16)	VePesid	120 mg/m² I.V. daily, days 4, 5, and 6 *Repeat cycle q 21 days.*
ASHAP (Non-Hodgkin's lymphoma)	doxorubicin	Adriamycin	10 mg/m² daily by continuous I.V. infusion, days 1 to 4
	cisplatin	Platinol	25 mg/m² daily by continuous I.V. infusion days 1 to 4
	cytarabine (ARA-C)	Cytosar-U	1,500 mg/m² I.V. immediately after completion of doxorubicin and cisplatin therapy
	methylprednisolone	Solu-Medrol	500 mg I.V. daily, days 1 to 5 *Repeat cycle q 21 to 25 days.*
BACON (Non-small cell lung cancer)	bleomycin	Blenoxane	30 units I.V. q 6 weeks, day 2
	doxorubicin	Adriamycin	40 mg/m² I.V. q 4 weeks, day 1
	lomustine (CCNU)	CeeNU	65 mg/m² P.O. q 8 weeks, day 1
	vincristine	Oncovin	0.75 to 1 mg/m² I.V. q 6 weeks, day 2
	mechlorethamine (nitrogen mustard)	Mustargen	8 mg/m² I.V. q 4 weeks, day 1

CANCER CHEMOTHERAPY: ACRONYMS AND PROTOCOLS *(continued)*

ACRONYM & INDICATION	DRUG		DOSAGE
	GENERIC NAME	TRADE NAME	
BACOP (Non-Hodgkin's lymphoma)	bleomycin	Blenoxane	5 units/m² I.V. daily, days 15 and 22
	doxorubicin	Adriamycin	25 mg/m² I.V., days 1 and 8
	cyclophosphamide	Cytoxan	650 mg/m² I.V., days 1 and 8
	vincristine	Oncovin	1.4 mg/m² (2 mg maximum) I.V., days 1 and 8
	prednisone	Deltasone	60 mg/m² P.O., days 15 to 28 *Repeat cycle q 28 days.*
BCP (Multiple myeloma)	carmustine	BiCNU	75 mg/m² I.V., day 1
	cyclophosphamide	Cytoxan	400 mg/m² I.V., day 1
	prednisone	Deltasone	75 mg P.O., days 1 to 7 *Repeat cycle q 28 days.*
BEP (Genitourinary cancer)	bleomycin	Blenoxane	30 units I.V., days 2, 9, and 16
	etoposide (VP-16)	VePesid	100 mg/m², days 1 to 5
	cisplatin	Platinol	20 mg/m² I.V., days 1 to 5
BHD (Malignant melanoma)	carmustine	BiCNU	100 to 150 mg/m² I.V. q 6 weeks
	hydroxyurea	Hydrea	1,480 mg/m² P.O. q 3 weeks, days 1 to 5
	dacarbazine	DTIC-Dome	100 to 150 mg/m² I.V. q 3 weeks, days 1 to 5
CAF (Breast cancer)	cyclophosphamide	Cytoxan	100 mg/m² P.O., days 1 to 14
	doxorubicin	Adriamycin	30 mg/m² I.V., days 1 and 8
	fluorouracil (5-FU)	Adrucil	400 to 500 mg/m² I.V., days 1 and 8 *Repeat cycle q 28 days.*
CAMP (Non-small cell lung cancer)	cyclophosphamide	Cytoxan	300 mg/m² I.V. days 1 and 8
	doxorubicin	Adriamycin	20 mg/m² I.V., days 1 and 8
	methotrexate sodium	Folex	15 mg/m² I.V., days 1 and 8
	procarbazine	Matulane	100 mg/m² P.O., days 1 to 10 *Repeat cycle q 28 days.*
CAP (Genitourinary cancer)	cisplatin	Platinol	60 mg/m² I.V., day 1
	doxorubicin	Adriamycin	40 mg/m² I.V., day 1
	cyclophosphamide	Cytoxan	400 mg/m² I.V., day 1 *Repeat cycle q 21 days.*
CAP (Non-small cell lung cancer)	cyclophosphamide	Cytoxan	400 mg/m² I.V., day 1
	doxorubicin	Adriamycin	40 mg/m² I.V., day 1
	cisplatin	Platinol	60 mg/m² I.V., day 1 *Repeat cycle q 28 days.*

(continued)

CANCER CHEMOTHERAPY: ACRONYMS AND PROTOCOLS *(continued)*

ACRONYM & INDICATION	DRUG		DOSAGE
	GENERIC NAME	**TRADE NAME**	
CAV (Small-cell lung cancer)	cyclophosphamide	Cytoxan	750 mg/m² I.V., day 1
	doxorubicin	Adriamycin	50 mg/m² I.V., day 1
	vincristine	Oncovin	2 mg/m² I.V., day 1 *Repeat cycle q 3 weeks.*
CAVe (Hodgkin's lymphoma)	lomustine (CCNU)	CeeNU	100 mg/m² I.V., day 1
	doxorubicin	Adriamycin	60 mg/m² I.V., day 1
	vinblastine	Velban	5 mg/m² I.V., day 1 *Repeat cycle q 6 weeks.*
CD (DC) (Leukemia— ANLL, consolidation)	cytarabine (ARA-C)	Cytosar-U	3,000 mg/m² I.V. q 12 hours for 6 days
	daunorubicin (DNR)	Cerubidine	30 mg/m² I.V. daily for 3 days, after cytarabine therapy
CDC (Ovarian cancer, epithelial)	carboplatin	Paraplatin	300 mg/m² I.V., day 1
	doxorubicin	Adriamycin	40 mg/m² I.V., day 1
	cyclophosphamide	Cytoxan	500 mg/m² I.V., day 1 *Repeat cycle q 28 days.*
CF (Head and neck cancer)	cisplatin	Platinol	100 mg/m² I.V., day 1
	fluorouracil (5-FU)	Adrucil	1,000 mg/m² daily by continuous I.V. infusion, days 1 to 5 *Repeat cycle q 21 to 28 days.*
CFL (Head and neck cancer)	cisplatin	Platinol	100 mg/m² I.V., day 1
	fluorouracil (5-FU)	Adrucil	600 to 800 mg/m² daily by continuous I.V. infusion, days 1 to 5
	leucovorin calcium	Wellcovorin	200 to 300 mg/m² I.V. daily, days 1 to 5 *Repeat cycle q 21 days.*
CFM (Breast cancer)	cyclophosphamide	Cytoxan	500 mg/m² I.V., day 1
	fluorouracil (5-FU)	Adrucil	500 mg/m² I.V., day 1
	mitoxantrone	Novantrone	10 mg/m² I.V., day 1 *Repeat cycle q 21 days.*
CFPT (Breast cancer)	cyclophosphamide	Cytoxan	150 mg/m² I.V., days 1 to 5
	fluorouracil (5-FU)	Adrucil	300 mg/m² I.V., days 1 to 5
	prednisone	Deltasone	10 mg P.O. t.i.d. for first 7 days of each course
	tamoxifen	Nolvadex	10 mg P.O. b.i.d. (continue daily through all courses) *Repeat cycle q 6 weeks.*
CHAP (Ovarian cancer, epithelial)	cyclophosphamide	Cytoxan	300 to 500 mg/m² I.V., day 1
	altretamine	Hexalen	150 mg/m² mg/m² P.O., days 1 to 7
	doxorubicin	Adriamycin	30 to 50 mg/m² I.V., day 1
	cisplatin	Platinol	50 mg/m² I.V., day 1 *Repeat cycle q 28 days.*

CANCER CHEMOTHERAPY: ACRONYMS AND PROTOCOLS *(continued)*

ACRONYM & INDICATION	DRUG		DOSAGE
	GENERIC NAME	TRADE NAME	
CHOP (Non-Hodgkin's lymphoma)	cyclophospha-mide	Cytoxan	750 mg/m² I.V., day 1
	doxorubicin	Adriamycin	50 mg/m² I.V., day 1
	vincristine	Oncovin	1.4 mg/m² (2 mg maximum) I.V., day 1
	prednisone	Deltasone	100 mg/m² P.O., days 1 to 5 *Repeat cycle q 21 days.*
CHOP-Bleo (Non-Hodgkin's lymphoma)	cyclophospha-mide	Cytoxan	750 mg/m² I.V., day 1
	doxorubicin	Adriamycin	50 mg/m² I.V., day 1
	vincristine	Oncovin	2 mg I.V., days 1 and 5
	prednisone	Deltasone	100 mg P.O., days 1 to 5
	bleomycin	Blenoxane	15 units I.V., days 1 and 5 *Repeat cycle q 21 days.*
CISCA (Genitourinary cancer)	cyclophospha-mide	Cytoxan	650 mg/m² I.V., day 1
	doxorubicin	Adriamycin	50 mg/m² I.V., day 1
	cisplatin	Platinol	70 to 100 mg/m² I.V., day 2 *Repeat cycle q 21 to 28 days.*
CMF (Breast cancer)	cyclophospha-mide	Cytoxan	100 mg/m² P.O., days 1 to 14 or 400 to 600 mg/m² I.V., day 1
	methotrexate	Folex	40 to 60 mg/m² I.V., days 1 and 8
	fluorouracil (5-FU)	Adrucil	400 to 600 mg/m² I.V., days 1 and 8 *Repeat cycle q 28 days.*
CMFVP (Cooper's) (Breast cancer)	cyclophospha-mide	Cytoxan	2 to 2.5 mg/kg P.O. daily for 9 months
	methotrexate	Folex	0.7 mg/kg/week I.V. for 8 weeks, then every other week for 7 months
	fluorouracil (5-FU)	Adrucil	12 mg/kg/week I.V. for 8 weeks, then weekly for 7 months
	vincristine	Oncovin	0.035 mg/kg (2 mg/week maximum) I.V. for 5 weeks, then once monthly
	prednisone	Deltasone	0.75 mg/kg P.O. daily, days 1 to 10, then taper over next 40 days and discontinue
CMFVP (SWOG) (Breast cancer)	cyclophospha-mide	Cytoxan	60 mg/m² P.O. daily for 1 year
	methotrexate	Folex	15 mg/m² I.V. weekly for 1 year
	fluorouracil (5-FU)	Adrucil	300 mg/m² I.V. weekly for 1 year
	vincristine	Oncovin	0.625 mg/m² I.V. weekly for 1 year
	prednisone	Deltasone	30 mg/m² P.O., days 1 to 14; 20 mg/m², days 15 to 28; 10 mg/m², days 29 to 42 *Repeat cycle q 28 days.*

(continued)

CANCER CHEMOTHERAPY: ACRONYMS AND PROTOCOLS *(continued)*

ACRONYM & INDICATION	DRUG		DOSAGE
	GENERIC NAME	TRADE NAME	
COAP (Leukemia—AML, induction)	cyclophosphamide	Cytoxan	100 mg/m^2 I.V. or P.O., days 1 to 5
	vincristine	Oncovin	2 mg/m^2 I.V., day 1
	cytarabine (ARA-C)	Cytosar-U	100 mg/m^2 I.V., days 1 to 5
	prednisone	Deltasone	100 mg P.O., days 1 to 5
COB (Head and neck cancer)	cisplatin	Platinol	100 mg/m^2 I.V., day 1
	vincristine	Oncovin	1 mg I.V., days 2 and 5
	bleomycin	Blenoxane	30 units daily by continuous I.V. infusion, days 2 to 5 *Repeat cycle q 21 days.*
COMLA (Non-Hodgkin's lymphoma)	cyclophosphamide	Cytoxan	1,500 mg/m^2 I.V., day 1
	vincristine	Oncovin	1.4 mg/m^2 (2.5 mg maximum) I.V., days 1, 8, and 15
	methotrexate	Folex	120 mg/m^2 I.V., days 22, 29, 36, 43, 50, 57, 64, and 71
	leucovorin calcium	Wellcovorin	25 mg/m^2 P.O. q 6 hours for four doses, beginning 24 hours after methotrexate dose
	cytarabine (ARA-C)	Cytosar-U	300 mg/m^2 I.V., days 22, 29, 36, 43, 50, 57, 64, and 71 *Repeat cycle q 21 days.*
COP (Non-Hodgkin's lymphoma)	cyclophosphamide	Cytoxan	800 to 1,000 mg/m^2 I.V., day 1
	vincristine	Oncovin	1.4 mg/m^2 (2 mg maximum) I.V., day 1
	prednisone	Deltasone	60 mg/m^2 P.O., days 1 to 5 *Repeat cycle q 21 days.*
COP-BLAM (Non-Hodgkin's lymphoma)	cyclophosphamide	Cytoxan	400 mg/m^2 I.V., day 1
	vincristine	Oncovin	1 mg/m^2 I.V., day 1
	prednisone	Deltasone	40 mg/m^2 P.O., days 1 to 10
	bleomycin	Blenoxane	15 mg I.V., day 14
	doxorubicin	Adriamycin	40 mg/m^2, day 1
	procarbazine	Matulane	100 mg/m^2, days 1 to 10 *Repeat cycle q 21 days*
COPE (Small-cell lung cancer)	cyclophosphamide	Cytoxan	750 mg/m^2 I.V., day 1
	cisplatin	Platinol	20 mg/m^2 I.V., days 1 to 3
	etoposide (VP-16)	VePesid	100 mg/m^2 I.V., days 1 to 3
	vincristine	Oncovin	2 mg/m^2 I.V., day 3 *Repeat cycle q 21 days.*

CANCER CHEMOTHERAPY: ACRONYMS AND PROTOCOLS (continued)

ACRONYM & INDICATION	DRUG		DOSAGE
	GENERIC NAME	TRADE NAME	
COPP (Non-Hodgkin's lymphoma)	cyclophospha-mide	Cytoxan	400 to 650 mg/m² I.V., days 1 and 8
	vincristine	Oncovin	1.4 to 1.5 mg/m² (2 mg maximum) I.V., days 1 and 8
	procarbazine	Matulane	100 mg/m² P.O., days 1 to 10 or 1 to 14
	prednisone	Deltasone	40 mg/m² P.O., days 1 to 14 *Repeat cycle q 28 days.*
CP (Ovarian cancer, epithelial)	cyclophospha-mide	Cytoxan	1,000 mg/m² I.V., day 1
	cisplatin	Platinol	50 to 60 mg/m² I.V., day 1 *Repeat cycle q 21 days.*
CV (Small-cell lung cancer)	cisplatin	Platinol	50 mg/m² I.V., day 1
	etoposide (VP-16)	VePesid	60 mg/m² I.V., days 1 to 5 *Repeat cycle q 21 to 28 days.*
CV (Non-small cell lung cancer)	cisplatin	Platinol	60 to 80 mg/m² I.V., day 1
	etoposide (VP-16)	VePesid	120 mg/m² I.V., days 4, 6, and 8 *Repeat cycle q 21 to 28 days.*
CVEB (Genitourinary cancer)	cisplatin	Platinol	40 mg/m² I.V., days 1 to 5
	vinblastine	Velban	7.5 mg/m² I.V., day 1
	etoposide (VP-16)	VePesid	100 mg/m² I.V., days 1 to 5
	bleomycin	Blenoxane	30 units I.V. weekly *Repeat cycle q 21 days.*
CVI (VIC) (Non-small cell lung cancer)	carboplatin	Paraplatin	300 mg/m² I.V., day 1
	etoposide (VP-16)	VePesid	60 to 100 mg/m² I.V., day 1
	ifosfamide	Ifex	1.5 g/m² I.V., days 1, 3, and 5
	mesna	Mesnex	Uroprotection at 20% of ifosfamide dose, given immediately before and at 4 and 8 hours after ifosfamide infusion *Repeat cycle q 28 days.*
CVP (Leukemia— CLL, blast crisis)	cyclophospha-mide	Cytoxan	300 mg/m² P.O., days 1 to 5
	vincristine	Oncovin	1.4 mg/m² (2 mg maximum) I.V., day 1
	prednisone	Deltasone	100 mg/m² P.O., days 1 to 5 *Repeat cycle q 21 days.*
CVP (Non-Hodgkin's lymphoma)	cyclophospha-mide	Cytoxan	400 mg/m² P.O., days 1 to 5
	vincristine	Oncovin	1.4 mg/m² (2 mg maximum) I.V., day 1
	prednisone	Deltasone	100 mg/m² P.O., days 1 to 5 *Repeat cycle q 21 days.*

(continued)

CANCER CHEMOTHERAPY: ACRONYMS AND PROTOCOLS (continued)

ACRONYM & INDICATION	DRUG		DOSAGE
	GENERIC NAME	TRADE NAME	
CVPP (Hodgkin's lymphoma)	lomustine (CCNU)	CeeNU	75 mg/m^2 P.O., day 1
	vinblastine	Velban	4 mg/m^2 I.V., days 1 and 8
	procarbazine	Matulane	100 mg/m^2 P.O., days 1 to 14
	prednisone	Deltasone	30 mg/m^2 P.O., days 1 to 14 (cycles 1 and 4 only) *Repeat cycle q 28 days.*
CYADIC (Soft-tissue sarcoma)	cyclophosphamide	Cytoxan	600 mg/m^2 I.V., day 1
	doxorubicin	Adriamycin	15 mg/m^2 daily by continuous I.V. infusion, on days 1 to 4
	dacarbazine	DTIC-Dome	250 mg/m^2 daily by continuous I.V. infusion, on days 1 to 4
CYVADIC (Bony sarcoma)	cyclophosphamide	Cytoxan	600 mg/m^2 I.V., day 1
	vincristine	Oncovin	1.4 mg/m^2 (2 mg maximum) I.V. weekly for 6 weeks, then on day 1 of future cycles
	doxorubicin	Adriamycin	15 mg/m^2 daily by continuous I.V. infusion, days 1 to 4
	dacarbazine	DTIC-Dome	250 mg/m^2 I.V. daily by continuous I.V. infusion, days 1 to 4 *Repeat cycle q 21 to 28 days.*
CYVADIC (Soft-tissue sarcoma)	cyclophosphamide	Cytoxan	500 mg/m^2 I.V., day 1
	vincristine	Oncovin	1.4 mg/m^2 (2 mg maximum) I.V., days 1 and 5
	doxorubicin	Adriamycin	50 mg/m^2 I.V., day 1
	dacarbazine	DTIC-Dome	250 mg/m^2 I.V., days 1 to 5 *Repeat cycle q 21 days.*
DC (Pediatric AML, induction)	daunorubicin (DNR)	Cerubidine	45 to 60 mg/m^2 I.V., days 1 to 3
	cytarabine (ARA-C)	Cytosar-U	100 mg/m^2 I.V. or S.C. q 12 hours for 5 to 7 days
DCPM (Pediatric AML, induction)	daunorubicin (DNR)	Cerubidine	25 mg/m^2 I.V., day 1
	cytarabine (ARA-C)	Cytosar-U	80 mg/m^2 I.V., days 1 to 3
	prednisone	Deltasone	40 mg/m^2 P.O. daily
	mercaptopurine (6-MP)	Purinethol	100 mg/m^2 P.O. daily
DCT (Leukemia— ANLL, induction)	daunorubicin (DNR)	Cerubidine	60 mg/m^2 I.V., days 1 to 3
	cytarabine (ARA-C)	Cytosar-U	200 mg/m^2 daily by continuous I.V. infusion, days 1 to 5
	thioguanine (6-TG)		100 mg/m^2 P.O. q 12 hours, days 1 to 5

CANCER CHEMOTHERAPY: ACRONYMS AND PROTOCOLS (continued)

ACRONYM & INDICATION	DRUG		DOSAGE
	GENERIC NAME	TRADE NAME	
DHAP (Hodgkin's lymphoma)	dexamethasone	Decadron	40 mg P.O. or I.V., days 1 to 4
	cisplatin	Platinol	100 mg/m² by continuous I.V. infusion, day 1
	cytarabine (ARA-C)	Cytosar-U	2 g/m² I.V. q 12 hours for two doses, day 2 *Repeat cycle q 3 to 4 weeks.*
DTIC-ACTD (Malignant melanoma)	dacarbazine	DTIC-Dome	750 mg/m² I.V., day 1
	dactinomycin (actinomycin D)	Cosmegen	1 mg/m² I.V., day 1 *Repeat cycle q 28 days.*
DVP (Leukemia— ALL, induction)	daunorubicin (DNR)	Cerubidine	45 mg/m² I.V., days 1, 2, 3, and 4
	vincristine	Oncovin	2 mg/m² (2 mg maximum) I.V. weekly for 4 weeks
	prednisone	Deltasone	45 mg/m² P.O., for 28 to 35 days
ESHAP (Non-Hodgkin's lymphoma)	etoposide (VP-16)	VePesid	40 mg/m² by continuous I.V. infusion, days 1 to 4
	cisplatin	Platinol	25 mg/m² daily by continuous I.V. infusion, days 1 to 4
	cytarabine (ARA-C)	Cytosar-U	2 g/m² I.V. immediately after completion of etoposide and cisplatin therapy
	methylprednisolone	Solu-Medrol	500 mg I.V. daily, days 1 to 4 *Repeat cycle q 21 to 28 days.*
EVA (Hodgkin's lymphoma)	etoposide (VP-16)	VePesid	100 mg/m² I.V., days 1 to 3
	vinblastine	Velban	6 mg/m² I.V., day 1
	doxorubicin	Adriamycin	50 mg/m² I.V., day 1 *Repeat cycle q 28 days.*
FAC (CAF) (Breast cancer)	fluorouracil (5-FU)	Adrucil	500 mg/m² I.V., days 1 and 8
	doxorubicin	Adriamycin	50 mg/m² I.V., day 1
	cyclophosphamide	Cytoxan	500 mg/m² I.V., day 1 *Repeat cycle q 21 days.*
FAM (Colon cancer; gastric cancer)	fluorouracil (5-FU)	Adrucil	600 mg/m² I.V., days 1, 8, 29, and 36
	doxorubicin	Adriamycin	30 mg/m² I.V., days 1 and 29
	mitomycin (mitomycin C)	Mutamycin	10 mg/m² I.V., day 1 *Repeat cycle q 8 weeks.*
FAM (Non-small cell lung cancer)	fluorouracil (5-FU)	Adrucil	600 mg/m² I.V., days 1, 8, 28, and 36
	doxorubicin	Adriamycin	30 mg/m² I.V., days 1 and 28
	mitomycin (mitomycin C)	Mutamycin	10 mg/m² I.V., day 1 *Repeat cycle q 8 weeks.*

(continued)

CANCER CHEMOTHERAPY: ACRONYMS AND PROTOCOLS *(continued)*

ACRONYM & INDICATION	DRUG		DOSAGE
	GENERIC NAME	**TRADE NAME**	
FAM (Pancreatic cancer)	fluorouracil (5-FU)	Adrucil	600 mg/m^2 I.V., days 1, 8, 29, and 36
	doxorubicin	Adriamycin	30 mg/m^2 I.V., days 1 and 29
	mitomycin (mitomycin C)	Mutamycin	10 mg/m^2 I.V., day 1 *Repeat cycle q 2 weeks.*
FAME (Gastric cancer)	fluorouracil (5-FU)	Adrucil	350 mg/m^2 I.V., days 1 to 5 and 36 to 40
	doxorubicin	Adriamycin	40 mg/m^2 I.V., days 1 and 36
	semustine	methyl CCNU	150 mg/m^2 P.O., day 1 *Repeat cycle q 10 weeks.*
FCE (Gastric cancer)	fluorouracil (5-FU)	Adrucil	900 mg/m^2 daily by continuous I.V. infusion, days 1 to 5
	cisplatin	Platinol	20 mg/m^2 I.V., days 1 to 5
	etoposide (VP-16)	VePesid	90 mg/m^2 I.V., days 1, 3, and 5 *Repeat cycle q 21 days.*
F-CL (Colon cancer)	fluorouracil (5-FU)	Adrucil	370 to 400 mg/m^2 I.V., days 1 to 5
	leucovorin calcium	Wellcovorin	200 mg/m^2 daily I.V., days 1 to 5, beginning 15 minutes before fluorouracil infusion *Repeat cycle q 21 days.*
5+2 (Leukemia— ANLL, consolidation)	cytarabine (ARA-C)	Cytosar-U	100 mg/m^2 I.V. q 12 hours for 6 days
	daunorubicin (DNR)	Cerubidine	45 mg/m^2 I.V., days 1 and 2
FL (Genitourinary cancer)	flutamide	Eulexin	250 mg P.O. t.i.d.
	leuprolide acetate	Lupron	1 mg S.C., daily
FL (Genitourinary cancer, alternate regimen)	flutamide	Eulexin	250 mg P.O. t.i.d.
	leuprolide acetate	Lupron Depot	7.5 mg I.M. q 28 days
FLe (Colon cancer)	levamisole	Ergamisol	50 mg P.O. t.i.d. for 3 days, repeated q 2 weeks for 1 year
	fluorouracil (5-FU)	Adrucil	450 mg/m^2 I.V. for 5 days, then, after a pause of 4 weeks, 450 mg/m^2 I.V. weekly for 48 weeks
FMS (Pancreatic cancer)	fluorouracil (5-FU)	Adrucil	600 mg/m^2 I.V., days 1, 8, 29, and 36
	mitomycin (mitomycin C)	Mutamycin	10 mg/m^2 I.V., day 1
	streptozocin	Zanosar	1 g/m^2 I.V., days 1, 8, 29, and 36 *Repeat cycle q 8 weeks.*
FMV (Colon cancer)	fluorouracil (5-FU)	Adrucil	10 mg/kg daily, I.V. days 1 to 5
	semustine	methyl CCNU	175 mg/m^2 P.O., day 1
	vincristine	Oncovin	1 mg/m^2 (2 mg maximum) I.V., day 1 *Repeat cycle q 35 days.*

CANCER CHEMOTHERAPY: ACRONYMS AND PROTOCOLS (continued)

ACRONYM & INDICATION	DRUG		DOSAGE
	GENERIC NAME	TRADE NAME	
HDMTX High-dose methotrexate (Bony sarcoma)	methotrexate	Folex	12 g/m^2 I.V. (20 g maximum)
	leucovorin calcium	Wellcovorin	15 mg I.V. or P.O. q 6 hours for 10 doses, beginning 24 hours after methotrexate dose (serum methotrexate levels must be monitored) *Repeat cycle q 4 to 16 weeks.*
Hexa-CAF (Ovarian cancer, epithelial)	altretamine	Hexalen	150 mg/m^2 P.O., days 1 to 14
	cyclophosphamide	Cytoxan	150 mg/m^2 P.O., days 1 to 14
	methotrexate	Folex	40 mg/m^2, days 1 and 8
	fluorouracil (5-FU)	Adrucil	600 mg/m^2 I.V., days 1 and 8 *Repeat cycle q 28 days.*
IMF (Breast cancer)	ifosfamide	Ifex	1.5 g/m^2 I.V., days 1 and 8
	mesna	Mesnex	Uroprotection I.V. at 20% of ifosfamide dose, given immediately before and at 4 and 8 hours after ifosfamide infusion
	methotrexate	Folex	40 mg/m^2 I.V., days 1 and 8
	fluorouracil (5-FU)	Adrucil	600 mg/m^2 I.V., days 1 and 8 *Repeat cycle q 28 days.*
L-VAM (Genitourinary cancer)	leuprolide acetate	Lupron	1 mg S.C. daily
	vinblastine	Velban	1.5 mg/m^2 daily by continuous I.V. infusion, days 2 to 7
	doxorubicin	Adriamycin	50 mg/m^2 I.V. by 24-hour continuous infusion, day 1
	mitomycin (mitomycin C)	Mutamycin	10 mg/m^2 I.V., day 2 *Repeat VAM cycle q 28 days.*
MAID (Bony sarcoma)	mesna	Mesnex	Uroprotection 1.5 g/m^2 by continuous I.V. infusion, days 1 to 4
	doxorubicin	Adriamycin	15 mg/m^2 by continuous I.V. infusion, days 1 to 3
	ifosfamide	Ifex	1.5 g/m^2 by continuous I.V. infusion, days 1 to 3
	dacarbazine	DTIC-Dome	250 mg/m^2 by continuous I.V. infusion, days 1 to 3 *Repeat cycle q 21 to 28 days.*
MAP (Head and neck cancer)	mitomycin (mitomycin C)	Mutamycin	8 mg/m^2 I.V., day 1
	doxorubicin	Adriamycin	40 mg/m^2 I.V., day 1
	cisplatin	Platinol	60 mg/m^2 I.V., day 1 *Repeat cycle q 28 days.*

(continued)

CANCER CHEMOTHERAPY: ACRONYMS AND PROTOCOLS (continued)

ACRONYM & INDICATION	DRUG		DOSAGE
	GENERIC NAME	TRADE NAME	
m-BACOD (Non-Hodgkin's lymphoma)	bleomycin	Blenoxane	4 units/m² I.V., day 1
	doxorubicin	Adriamycin	45 mg/m² I.V., day 1
	cyclophosphamide	Cytoxan	600 mg/m² I.V., day 1
	vincristine	Oncovin	1 mg/m² I.V., day 1
	dexamethasone	Decadron	6 mg/m², days 1 to 5
	methotrexate	Folex	200 mg/m² I.V., days 8 and 15
	leucovorin calcium	Wellcovorin	10 mg/m² P.O. q 6 hours for eight doses, beginning 24 hours after methotrexate dose *Repeat cycle q 21 days.*
m-BACOS (Non-Hodgkin's lymphoma)	doxorubicin	Adriamycin	50 mg/m² by continuous I.V. infusion over 24 hours, day 1
	vincristine	Oncovin	1.4 mg/m² (2 mg maximum) I.V., day 1
	bleomycin	Blenoxane	10 units/m² I.V., day 1
	cyclophosphamide	Cytoxan	750 mg/m² I.V., day 1
	methotrexate	Folex	1 g/m² I.V., day 2
	leucovorin calcium	Wellcovorin	15 mg P.O. q 6 hours for eight doses, starting 24 hours after methotrexate dose *Repeat cycle q 21 to 25 days.*
MBC (Head and neck cancer)	methotrexate	Folex	40 mg/m² I.M. or I.V., days 1 and 15
	bleomycin	Blenoxane	10 units I.M. or I.V. weekly
	cisplatin	Platinol	50 mg/m² I.V., day 1 *Repeat cycle q 21 days.*
MC (Leukemias— ANLL, consolidation)	mitoxantrone	Novantrone	12 mg/m² I.V. daily, days 1 and 2
	cytarabine (ARA-C)	Cytosar-U	100 mg/m² daily by continuous I.V. infusion, days 1 to 5 *Repeat cycle.*
MC (Leukemias— ANLL, induction)	mitoxantrone	Novantrone	12 mg/m² I.V., days 1 to 3 and 17 to 18
	cytarabine (ARA-C)	Cytosar-U	100 mg/m² daily by continuous I.V. infusion, days 1 to 7 and 17 to 21
MF (Head and neck cancer)	methotrexate	Folex	125 to 150 mg/m² I.V., day 1
	fluorouracil (5-FU)	Adrucil	600 mg/m² I.V., day 1, beginning 1 hour after methotrexate dose
	leucovorin calcium	Wellcovorin	10 mg/m² I.V. or P.O. q 6 hours for five doses, beginning 24 hours after methotrexate dose *Repeat cycle weekly.*

CANCER CHEMOTHERAPY: ACRONYMS AND PROTOCOLS *(continued)*

ACRONYM & INDICATION	DRUG		DOSAGE
	GENERIC NAME	TRADE NAME	
MM (Leukemia — ALL, maintenance)	mercaptopurine (6-MP)	Purinethol	50 mg/m² P.O. daily
	methotrexate	Folex	20 mg/m² P.O. or I.V. weekly
MOP (Pediatric brain tumors)	mechlorethamine (nitrogen mustard)	Mustargen	6 mg/m² I.V., days 1 and 8
	vincristine	Oncovin	1.4 mg/m² (2 mg maximum) I.V., days 1 and 8
	procarbazine	Matulane	100 mg/m² P.O. days 1 to 14 *Repeat cycle q 28 days.*
MOPP (Hodgkin's lymphoma)	mechlorethamine (nitrogen mustard)	Mustargen	6 mg/m² I.V., days 1 and 8
	vincristine	Oncovin	1.4 mg/m² (2 mg maximum) I.V., days 1 and 8
	procarbazine	Matulane	100 mg/m² P.O., days 1 to 14
	prednisone	Deltasone	40 mg/m² P.O., days 1 to 14 *Repeat cycle q 28 days.*
MP (Multiple myeloma)	melphalan (L-phenylalanine mustard)	Alkeran	8 mg/m² P.O., days 1 to 4
	prednisone	Deltasone	40 mg/m² P.O., days 1 to 7 *Repeat cycle q 28 days.*
m-PFL (Genitourinary cancer)	methotrexate	Folex	60 mg/m², day 1
	cisplatin	Platinol	25 mg/m² by continuous I.V. infusion, days 2 to 6
	fluorouracil (5-FU)	Adrucil	800 mg/ml by continuous I.V. infusion, days 2 to 6
	leucovorin calcium	Wellcovorin	500 mg/m² by continuous I.V. infusion, days 2 to 6 *Repeat cycle q 28 days for four cycles.*
M-2 (Multiple myeloma)	vincristine	Oncovin	0.03 mg/kg (2 mg maximum) I.V., day 1
	carmustine	BiCNU	0.5 mg/kg I.V., day 1
	cyclophosphamide	Cytoxan	10 mg/kg I.V, day 1
	melphalan (L-phenylalanine mustard)	Alkeran	0.25 mg/kg P.O., days 1 to 14
	prednisone	Deltasone	1 mg/kg/daily on days 1 to 7, then taper over next 14 days *Repeat cycle q 35 days.*
MV (Leukemia — AML, induction)	mitoxantrone	Novantrone	10 mg/m² I.V. daily, days 1 to 5
	etoposide (VP-16)	VePesid	100 mg/m² I.V. days 1 to 3

(continued)

CANCER CHEMOTHERAPY: ACRONYMS AND PROTOCOLS (continued)

ACRONYM & INDICATION	DRUG		DOSAGE
	GENERIC NAME	TRADE NAME	
MVAC (Genitourinary cancer)	methotrexate	Folex	30 mg/m² I.V., days 1, 15, and 22
	vinblastine	Velban	3 mg/m² I.V., days 2, 15, and 22
	doxorubicin	Adriamycin	30 mg/m² I.V., day 2
	cisplatin	Platinol	70 mg/m² I.V., day 2 *Repeat cycle q 28 days.*
MVPP (Hodgkin's lymphoma)	mechlorethamine (nitrogen mustard)	Mustargen	6 mg/m² I.V., days 1 and 8
	vinblastine	Velban	6 mg/m² I.V., days 1 and 8
	procarbazine	Matulane	100 mg/m² P.O., days 1 to 14
	prednisone	Deltasone	40 mg/m² P.O., days 1 to 14 *Repeat cycle q 42 days for six cycles.*
PCV (Pediatric brain tumors)	procarbazine	Matulane	60 mg/m² P.O., days 18 to 21
	lomustine (CCNU)	CeeNU	110 mg/m² P.O., day 1
	vincristine	Oncovin	1.4 mg/m² (2 mg maximum), days 8 and 29 *Repeat cycle q 6 to 8 weeks.*
PFL (Head and neck cancer)	cisplatin	Platinol	25 mg/m² daily by continuous I.V. infusion, days 1 to 5
	fluorouracil (5-FU)	Adrucil	800 mg/m² daily by continuous I.V. infusion, days 2 to 6
	leucovorin calcium	Wellcovorin	500 mg/m² daily by continuous I.V. infusion, days 1 to 6 *Repeat cycle q 28 days.*
ProMACE (Non-Hodgkin's lymphoma)	prednisone	Deltasone	60 mg/m² P.O., days 1 to 14
	methotrexate	Folex	1.5 g/m² I.V., day 14
	leucovorin calcium	Wellcovorin	50 mg/m² I.V. q 6 hours for five doses, beginning 24 hours after methotrexate dose
	doxorubicin	Adriamycin	25 mg/m² I.V., days 1 and 8
	cyclophosphamide	Cytoxan	650 mg/m² I.V., days 1 and 8
	etoposide (VP-16)	VePesid	120 mg/m² I.V., days 1 and 8 *Repeat ProMACE cycle q 28 days; MOPP therapy to begin after the required number of ProMACE cycles are completed.*
ProMACE/ cytaBOM (Non-Hodgkin's lymphoma)	cyclophosphamide	Cytoxan	650 mg/m² I.V., day 1
	doxorubicin	Adriamycin	25 mg/m² I.V., day 1
	etoposide (VP-16)	VePesid	120 mg/m² I.V., day 1
	prednisone	Deltasone	60 mg/m² P.O., days 1 to 14
	cytarabine (ARA-C)	Cytosar-U	300 mg/m² I.V., day 8
	bleomycin	Blenoxane	5 mg/m² I.V., day 8

CANCER CHEMOTHERAPY: ACRONYMS AND PROTOCOLS *(continued)*

ACRONYM & INDICATION	DRUG		DOSAGE
	GENERIC NAME	TRADE NAME	
ProMACE/ cytaBOM (Non-Hodgkin's lymphoma) *(continued)*	vincristine	Oncovin	1.4 mg/m² I.V., day 8
	methotrexate	Folex	120 mg/m² I.V., day 8
	leucovorin calcium	Wellcovorin	25 mg/m² P.O. q 6 hours for four doses *Repeat cycle q 28 days.*
(pulse) VAC (Soft-tissue sarcoma)	vincristine	Oncovin	1.5 g/m² (2 mg maximum) I.V., day 1 or weekly starting on day 1
	dactinomycin (actinomycin D)	Cosmegen	0.4 mg/m² I.V., day 1
	cyclophosphamide	Cytoxan	1,000 mg/m² I.V., day 1 *Repeat cycle q 3 to 4 weeks.*
7 + 3 (A + D) (Leukemias — AML, induction)	cytarabine (ARA-C)	Cytosar-U	100 or 200 mg/m² by continuous I.V. infusion, days 1 to 7
	daunorubicin (ADR)	Cerubidine	45 mg/m² I.V., days 1 to 3
TC (Leukemia — ANLL, maintenance)	thioguanine (6-TG)		40 mg/m² P.O. q 12 hours weekly for eight doses, days 1 to 4
	cytarabine (ARA-C)	Cytosar-U	60 mg/m² S.C. weekly, day 5
VAB (Genitourinary cancer)	vinblastine	Velban	4 mg/m² I.V., day 1
	dactinomycin (actinomycin D)	Cosmegen	1 mg/m² I.V., day 1
	bleomycin	Blenoxane	30 units I.V. push, then 20 units/m² daily by continuous I.V. infusion, days 1 to 3
	cisplatin	Platinol	120 mg/m² I.V., day 4
	cyclophosphamide	Cytoxan	600 mg/m² I.V., day 1 *Repeat cycle q 21 days.*
VAC (Small-cell lung cancer)	vincristine	Oncovin	2 mg I.V., day 1
	doxorubicin	Adriamycin	50 mg/m² I.V., day 1
	cyclophosphamide	Cytoxan	750 mg/m² I.V., day 1 *Repeat cycle q 21 days for four cycles.*
VAC (Germ-cell ovarian cancer)	vincristine	Oncovin	1.2 to 1.5 mg/m² (2 mg maximum) I.V. weekly for 10 to 12 weeks, or q 2 weeks for 12 doses
	dactinomycin (actinomycin D)	Cosmegen	0.3 to 0.4 mg/m² I.V., days 1 to 5
	cyclophosphamide	Cytoxan	150 mg/m² I.V., days 1 to 5 *Repeat cycle q 28 days.*
VAD (Multiple myeloma)	vincristine	Oncovin	0.4 mg daily by continuous I.V. infusion, days 1 to 4
	doxorubicin	Adriamycin	9 to 10 mg/m² daily by continuous I.V. infusion, days 1 to 4
	dexamethasone	Decadron	40 mg P.O. on days 1 to 4, 9 to 12, and 17 to 20 *Repeat cycle q 25 to 35 days.*

(continued)

CANCER CHEMOTHERAPY: ACRONYMS AND PROTOCOLS (continued)

ACRONYM & INDICATION	DRUG		DOSAGE
	GENERIC NAME	**TRADE NAME**	
VAP (VP + A) (Pediatric ALL, induction)	vincristine	Oncovin	1.5 to 2 mg/m² (2 mg maximum) I.V. weekly for 4 weeks
	asparaginase	Elspar	10,000 units I.M., days 1 and 8 (other doses include 6,000 units/m² I.M. for 3 days/week or 25,000 units/m²)
	prednisone	Deltasone	40 mg/m² P.O., days 1 to 28, then taper over 7 days
VATH (Breast cancer)	vinblastine	Velban	4.5 mg/m² I.V., day 1
	doxorubicin	Adriamycin	45 mg/m² I.V., day 1
	thiotepa	Thiotepa	12 mg/m² I.V., day 1 *Repeat cycle q 21 days.*
	fluoxymesterone	Halotestin	30 mg P.O. (continue daily through all courses)
VB (Genitourinary cancer)	vinblastine	Velban	3 to 4 mg/m² I.V., day 1
	methotrexate	Folex	30 to 40 mg/m² I.V., day 1 *Repeat cycle weekly.*
VBAP (Multiple myeloma)	vincristine	Oncovin	1 mg I.V., day 1
	carmustine	BiCNU	30 mg/m² I.V., day 1
	doxorubicin	Adriamycin	30 mg/m² I.V., day 1
	prednisone	Deltasone	100 mg P.O., days 1 to 4 *Repeat cycle q 21 days.*
VBC (Malignant melanoma)	vinblastine	Velban	6 mg/m² I.V., days 1 and 2
	bleomycin	Blenoxane	15 units/m² by continuous I.V. infusion, days 1 to 5
	cisplatin	Platinol	50 mg/m² I.V., day 5 *Repeat cycle q 28 days.*
VBP (Genitourinary cancer)	vinblastine	Velban	6 mg/m² I.V., days 1 and 2
	bleomycin	Blenoxane	30 units I.V., weekly
	cisplatin	Platinol	20 mg/m² I.V., days 1 to 5 *Repeat cycle q 21 to 28 days.*
VC (Small-cell lung cancer)	etoposide (VP-16)	VePesid	100 to 200 mg/m² I.V., days 1 to 3
	carboplatin	Paraplatin	50 to 125 mg/m² I.V., days 1 to 3 *Repeat cycle q 28 days.*
VCAP (Multiple myeloma)	vincristine	Oncovin	1 mg I.V., day 1
	cyclophosphamide	Cytoxan	100 mg/m² P.O., days 1 to 4
	doxorubicin	Adriamycin	25 mg/m² I.V., day 2
	prednisone	Deltasone	60 mg/m² P.O., days 1 to 4 *Repeat cycle q 28 days.*
VDP (Malignant melanoma)	vinblastine	Velban	5 mg/m² I.V., days 1 and 2
	dacarbazine	DTIC-Dome	150 mg/m² I.V., days 1 to 5
	cisplatin	Platinol	75 mg/m² I.V., day 5 *Repeat cycle q 21 to 28 days.*
VIP (Genitourinary cancer)	vinblastine	Velban	0.11 mg/kg I.V., days 1 and 2

ANTIBIOTICS: EFFICACY AGAINST SUSCEPTIBLE PATHOGENS

The following charts provide a ready reference to in vivo activity when the infecting organism has been identified. Empiric therapy often demands a powerful broad-spectrum antibiotic, in contrast to therapy designed to attack a specific invader. However, antimicrobial susceptibility testing should be routinely performed to ensure that an organism is indeed susceptible to the selected antibiotic.

KEY

1 Drug of choice as determined by comparative clinical efficacy or experience, susceptibility patterns, toxicity, cost, and practice patterns. In CNS infections, check package insert.

2 Alternative drug as determined by clinical practice, drug allergy, toxicity, and cost.

3 Drug with a low level of activity against this organism; variable or limited efficacy.

U Effective for treating urinary tract infections.

G Effective for GI infections.

☐ (Blank). Not indicated for this organism, or no information available for clinical evaluation.

NOTES TO CHARTS

A Cephalosporins, imipenem, and beta-lactamase inhibition combinations are not effective.

B Use penicillin or ampicillin plus an aminoglycoside for serious systemic infections due to enterococci.

C Antitoxin is primary therapy; antimicrobials are used only to decrease toxin production and to prevent a carrier state.

D Use ampicillin or penicillin with or without gentamicin. Preferred for bactericidal action.

E Spectinomycin is active against penicillin-resistant strains; however, resistance to this agent has been reported.

F *Citrobacter freundii* and *C. diversus* often have significantly different antibiotic sensitivity patterns. Speciation and susceptibility testing are particularly important.

G Use a tetracycline or chloramphenicol with or without streptomycin.

H For *Haemophilus influenzae* resistant to ampicillin, possible choices include chloramphenicol, a second- or third-generation cephalosporin, or trimethoprim-sulfamethoxazole, or a beta-lactamase-inhibitor combination agent.

I Combination therapy with an aminoglycoside and an antipseudomonal penicillin is warranted for serious systemic infections. Monotherapy with ceftazidime, cefoperazone, imipenem, or ciprofloxacin may be adequate in selected clinical settings.

J Vancomycin is effective orally only. Metronidazole is effective both orally and parenterally.

K *Bacteroides bivius, B. distasonis, B. melaninogenicus, B. ovatus, B. thetaiotaomicron, B. uniformis.*

L Isoniazid and rifampin are drugs of choice. However, nontubercular mycobacterial infections may require treatment with as many as five antibiotics.

M Tetracyclines are drugs of choice. Erythromycin and newer macrolides are alternatives.

N Contraindicated in children under age 18.

O The quinolones are currently not indicated for the treatment of meningitis.

P Norfloxacin is currently FDA-approved only for the treatment of urinary tract infections; however, clinical use includes treatment of susceptible prostatitis, gonorrhea, and infectious diarrhea and prophylactic bowel decontamination during neutropenia.

Q Drug often used as co-drug to maximize bactericidal action or reduce resistance. Also indicated for prophylaxis or eradication of selected carrier states.

R Tetracycline hydrochloride is preferred for most indications. Doxycycline is recommended for renal failure patients with infections outside the urinary tract for which a tetracycline is indicated. Tetracyclines are not recommended for pregnant women, infants, or children under age 8. A tetracycline class disk may be used to test susceptibility. However, minocycline may be effective against some strains of bacteria (for example, *Acinetobacter*, Enterobacteriaceae, and *Staphylococcus aureus*) resistant to other tetracyclines. No currently available tetracycline should be used in meningitis. Minocycline, rifampin, or ciprofloxacin is effective in the treatment of asymptomatic carriers of *Neisseria meningitidis* to eliminate meningococci from the nasopharynx.

S These agents are used in combination with aminoglycosides. This negates the minimal efficacy differences.

Adapted with permission from *Pharmacy Practice News*, October 1992.

AMINOGLYCOSIDES AND OTHER ANTIBIOTICS

Column groups: GRAM-POSITIVE AEROBES — Cocci (columns 1–12), Bacilli (columns 13–16); GRAM-NEGATIVE AEROBES — Cocci (columns 17–19), Enteric bacilli (columns 20–32).

Columns:
1. S. aureus (non-penicillinase)
2. S. aureus (penicillinase-producing)
3. S. aureus (methicillin-resistant[A])
4. S. epidermidis (non-penicillinase)
5. S. epidermidis (penicillinase-prod.)
6. S. epidermidis (methicillin-resistant[A])
7. Strep. group A (Strep. pyogenes)
8. Strep. group B
9. Strep. group D (enterococcal[B])
10. Strep. group D (nonenterococcal)
11. Strep. pneumoniae
12. Strep. viridans
13. Bacillus anthracis
14. Corynebacterium diphtheriae[C]
15. Corynebacterium jeikeium
16. Listeria monocytogenes[D]
17. Moraxella catarrhalis (Branhamella)
18. Neisseria gonorrhoeae[E]
19. Neisseria meningitidis
20. Citrobacter sp.[F]
21. Enterobacter sp.
22. Escherichia coli
23. Klebsiella pneumoniae
24. Morganella morganii
25. Proteus mirabilis
26. Proteus vulgaris
27. Providencia stuartii
28. Salmonella sp.
29. Salmonella typhi
30. Serratia sp.
31. Shigella sp.
32. Yersinia enterocolitica

	1	2	3	4	5	6	7	8	9	10	11	12	13	14	15	16	17	18	19	20	21	22	23	24	25	26	27	28	29	30	31	32
AMINOGLYCOSIDES																																
AMIKACIN									3	3					2	2				1	1	2	2	2	2	2	1		1			2
GENTAMICIN	3	3	2	3	2	2			1	3					2	2				1	1	2	2	2	2	2	2	3	3	1	3	2
NETILMICIN															2	2				1	1	2	2	2	2	2	2	3	3	1	3	2
STREPTOMYCIN									2	3																						
TOBRAMYCIN	3	3		3						3					2	2				1	1	2	2	2	2	2	2	3	3	2		2
OTHER ANTIBIOTICS																																
CHLORAMPHENICOL											2						2		2									2	1		2	
CLINDAMYCIN	2	2		2	2		2	2			3	2	3	3																		
ERYTHROMYCIN	2	2					2	2	3		2		2	1	2	2	2	3	3													
METRONIDAZOLE																																
RIFAMPIN[G]	2	2	2	2	2	2										3			3													
SULFONAMIDES																			3	U	U	U	U	U	U			2			2	
TETRACYCLINES[N,R]	3	3						2			2	2	2			2	2	2	2	3		3	3	3	2	2					2	2
TRIMETHOPRIM-SULFAMETHOXAZOLE	2	2	2	2	2	2												1	1	2	2	2	2	2	2	1	2	1	1	2	2	1
VANCOMYCIN	2	2	1	2	2	1	2	2	2	2	2	2						1														
UTI AGENTS																																
CARBENICILLIN INDANYL	U						U	U	U											U	U	U		U	U	U	U				U	
NITROFURANTOIN	U						U	U	U											U	U	U	U									

Column groups across the top of the table:

- **GRAM-NEGATIVE AEROBES** (Other bacilli): Acinetobacter sp.; Aeromonas hydrophila; Bordetella pertussis; Brucella sp.[G]; Campylobacter jejuni; Francisella tularensis[G]; Gardnerella vaginalis; Haemophilus ducreyi; Haemophilus influenzae[H]; Legionella pneumophila; Pasteurella multocida; Pseudomonas aeruginosa[I]; Pseudomonas cepacia; Pseudomonas mallei[S]; Pseudomonas maltophilia; Streptobacillus moniliformis; Vibrio cholerae; Yersinia pestis
- **ANAEROBES — Gram-positive**: Clostridium difficile[J]; Clostridium perfringens; Clostridium tetani; Peptococcus sp.; Peptostreptococcus sp.
- **ANAEROBES — Gram-negative**: Bacteroides fragilis; Bacteroides sp.[K]; Fusobacterium sp.
- **Acid-fast**: M. avium-intracellulare[L]; M. tuberculosis[L]
- **Actinomycetes**: Actinomyces israelii; Nocardia sp.
- **Chlamydia**: Chlamydia psittaci[M]; Chlamydia trachomatis[M]
- **Mycoplasma**: Mycoplasma pneumoniae[M]; Ureaplasma urealyticum[M]
- **Rickettsia**: Rickettsia sp.
- **Spirochetes**: Borrelia burgdorferi; Borrelia recurrentis; Leptospira sp.; Treponema pallidum

Acinetobacter sp.	Aeromonas hydrophila	Bordetella pertussis	Brucella sp.[G]	Campylobacter jejuni	Francisella tularensis[G]	Gardnerella vaginalis	Haemophilus ducreyi	Haemophilus influenzae[H]	Legionella pneumophila	Pasteurella multocida	Pseudomonas aeruginosa[I]	Pseudomonas cepacia	Pseudomonas mallei[S]	Pseudomonas maltophilia	Streptobacillus moniliformis	Vibrio cholerae	Yersinia pestis	Clostridium difficile[J]	Clostridium perfringens	Clostridium tetani	Peptococcus sp.	Peptostreptococcus sp.	Bacteroides fragilis	Bacteroides sp.[K]	Fusobacterium sp.	M. avium-intracellulare[L]	M. tuberculosis[L]	Actinomyces israelii	Nocardia sp.	Chlamydia psittaci[M]	Chlamydia trachomatis[M]	Mycoplasma pneumoniae[M]	Ureaplasma urealyticum[M]	Rickettsia sp.	Borrelia burgdorferi	Borrelia recurrentis	Leptospira sp.	Treponema pallidum
1	1			2	1		2			1	2	2	2		2											2	3		2									
1	1		2	2	1		2			1	2	2	2		2												3		2									
2	2			2	1		2			1	2	2	2		2														2									
		1		1											1													2	2									
1	2			2	1		2			1	2	2	2		2														2									
	2		1	2	2			2		2		2		2			2	2	2	2	2	2	2				3		2						2		2	
			2															2	2	2	2	2	2	2			3											
			1		1				1			1	3								3	3	3	3					2	1	1	1		2	1			3
						1											1	2	2	3	3	1	1	1															
					1				2				2															1	3										
2	3	1	2	2			2	2		2				2		1	2		3	2	2	2	2	3	2			2	2	1	1	1	2	1	1	1	2	2
1	2	2			1	2					1		1		2														1									
																	1																					
U																	U																					

CEPHALOSPORINS AND QUINOLONES

Key
(*) first generation
(†) second generation
(**) third generation

Column groupings: Columns 1–16 are **GRAM-POSITIVE AEROBES** (1–12 = Cocci, 13–16 = Bacilli); columns 17–32 are **GRAM-NEGATIVE AEROBES** (17–19 = Cocci, 20–32 = Enteric bacilli).

CEPHALOSPORINS

Drug	S. aureus (non-penicillinase)	S. aureus (penicillinase-producing)	S. aureus (methicillin-resistant[A])	S. epidermidis (non-penicillinase)	S. epidermidis (penicillinase-prod.)	S. epidermidis (methicillin-resistant[A])	Strep. group A (Strep. pyogenes)	Strep. group B	Strep. group D (enterococcal[B])	Strep. group D (nonenterococcal)	Strep. pneumoniae	Strep. viridans	Bacillus anthracis	Corynebacterium diphtheriae[C]	Corynebacterium jeikeium	Listeria monocytogenes[D]	Moraxella catarrhalis (Branhamella)	Neisseria gonorrhoeae[E]	Neisseria meningitidis	Citrobacter sp.[F]	Enterobacter sp.	Escherichia coli	Klebsiella pneumoniae	Morganella morganii	Proteus mirabilis	Proteus vulgaris	Providencia stuartii	Salmonella sp.	Salmonella typhi	Serratia sp.	Shigella sp.	Yersinia enterocolitica
CEFADROXIL (*)	1	1		1	1		2	2		2	2	2										2	2		2							
CEFAZOLIN (*)	1	1		1	1		2	2		2	2	2										1	1		1							
CEPHALEXIN (*)	1	1		1	1		2	2		2	2	2										2	2		2							
CEPHALOTHIN (*)	1	1		1	1		2	2		2	2	2										1	1		1							
CEPHAPIRIN (*)	1	1		1	1		2	2		2	2	2										1	1		1							
CEPHRADINE (*)	1	1		1	1		2	2		2	2	2										1	1		1							
CEFACLOR (†)	2	2		2	2		2	2		2	2	2					2	2				1	1		2							
CEFAMANDOLE (†)	2	2		2	2		2	2		2	2	2					2	2				1	1		2							
CEFMETAZOLE (†)	2	2		3	3		2	2		2	2	2					2	1				1	1	2	2	2	1			2		2
CEFONICID (†)	3	3		3	3		2	2		2	2	2					2	2				1	1		2							
CEFOTETAN (†)	3	3		3	3		2	2		2	2	2					2	1				1	1	2	2	2	1			1		2
CEFOXITIN (†)	2	2		3	3		2	2		2	2	2					2	1				1	1	3	2	2	1			3		
CEFUROXIME (†)	2	2		2	2		2	2		2	2	2					2	1	2			1	1		2							
CEFUROXIME AXETIL (†)	2	2		2	2		2	2		2	2	2					2	2				1	1		2							
CEFIXIME (**)							2	2		2	2	2					1	1		2	1	1	3	1	1	1				2		
CEFOPERAZONE (**)	2	2		3	3		2	2		2	2	2					2	1		1	2	1	1	1	2	1	1			2	1	
CEFOTAXIME (**)	2	2		2	2		2	2		2	2	2					1	1	2	1	2	1	1	1	2	1	1	1				2
CEFPROZIL (**)	2	2		2			2	2		3	2	2					2	2				U	3		2							
CEFTAZIDIME (**)	3	3		3	3		2	3		2	3	2					2	1		1	2	1	1	1	2	1	1			1		
CEFTIZOXIME (**)	2	2		2	2		2	2		2	2	2					1	1	2	1	2	1	1	1	2	1	1	1				2
CEFTRIAXONE (**)	2	2		2	2		2	2		2	2	3					1	1	2	1	2	1	1	1	2	1	1	2	1			2
LORACARBEF (**)	2	3		2	3		2	2		2	2	2					1	1				1	1		2							

QUINOLONES

Drug	S. aureus (non-penicillinase)	S. aureus (penicillinase-producing)	S. aureus (methicillin-resistant[A])	S. epidermidis (non-penicillinase)	S. epidermidis (penicillinase-prod.)	S. epidermidis (methicillin-resistant[A])	Strep. group A (Strep. pyogenes)	Strep. group B	Strep. group D (enterococcal[B])	Strep. group D (nonenterococcal)	Strep. pneumoniae	Strep. viridans	Bacillus anthracis	Corynebacterium diphtheriae[C]	Corynebacterium jeikeium	Listeria monocytogenes[D]	Moraxella catarrhalis (Branhamella)	Neisseria gonorrhoeae[E]	Neisseria meningitidis	Citrobacter sp.[F]	Enterobacter sp.	Escherichia coli	Klebsiella pneumoniae	Morganella morganii	Proteus mirabilis	Proteus vulgaris	Providencia stuartii	Salmonella sp.	Salmonella typhi	Serratia sp.	Shigella sp.	Yersinia enterocolitica
CIPROFLOXACIN[N,O]	2	2	2	2	2	2	3	3	3	3	3	3				2	2	2	2	1	1	1	1	1	1	1	1	1	1	2	1	2
LOMEFLOXACIN[N]	2	2	2	2	2	2	3	3	3	3	3	3			3	3	2	2	2	3	1	1	1	1	1	1	3	2	1	1	1	2
NORFLOXACIN[N,O,P]	U	U	U	U	U	U	U			U	U	U						U		U	U	G	U	U	U	U	U	U	G	U	G	G
OFLOXACIN[N,O]	2	2	2	2	2	2	3	3	3	3	3	3				2	2	2	2	1	1	1	1	1	1	1	1	1	1	2	1	2

GRAM-NEGATIVE AEROBES																		ANAEROBES								Acid-fast		Actinomycetes		Chlamydia		Mycoplasma		Rickettsia	Spirochetes			
Other bacilli																		Gram-positive					Gram-negative															
Acinetobacter sp.	Aeromonas hydrophila	Bordetella pertussis	Brucella sp.[G]	Campylobacter jejuni	Francisella tularensis[G]	Gardnerella vaginalis	Haemophilus ducreyi	Haemophilus influenzae[H]	Legionella pneumophila	Pasteurella multocida	Pseudomonas aeruginosa[I]	Pseudomonas cepacia	Pseudomonas mallei[G]	Pseudomonas maltophilia	Streptobacillus moniliformis	Vibrio cholerae	Yersinia pestis	Clostridium difficile[J]	Clostridium perfringens	Clostridium tetani	Peptococcus sp.	Peptostreptococcus sp.	Bacteroides fragilis	Bacteroides sp.[K]	Fusobacterium sp.	M. avium-intracellulare[L]	M. tuberculosis[L]	Actinomyces israelii	Nocardia sp.	Chlamydia psittaci[M]	Chlamydia trachomatis[M]	Mycoplasma pneumoniae[M]	Ureaplasma urealyticum[M]	Rickettsia sp.	Borrelia burgdorferi	Borrelia recurrentis	Leptospira sp.	Treponema pallidum
								2																														
								2		2										2	2	2																
								2																														
								2		2																												
								2		2																												
								2																														
								2																														
								2		2																												
	2							2		2									2	2	2	2	2	2	2													
								2																														
	2							2		2									2	2	2	2	2	3	2													
	3							2		2									2	2	2	2	2	2	2													
	2							1											2	2	2	2																
								2		2																												
								1																														
3	2							1		2	2	2		2					3	3	3	3																
3	1						2	1		1	3								2	2	2	2	3	3	3				2						1			
								2																														
2	2							1			1	2		2					3	3	3	3																
3	1							1		2	U								2	2	2	2	3	3	3													
3	1						1	1		2	3																								1			3
								2																														
2	1		1	1		2	1	1	2	2	2	3		2		2										2	3				3	3	3	3				
3	1		1	1		3	1	1	2	2	3	3		3		2											3				3	3	3					
	G			G							U	U																					U					
2	1		1	1		2	1	1	2	2	2	3		2		2										2	3				2	3	3	3				

PENICILLINS AND RELATED ANTIBIOTICS

Column groups: **GRAM-POSITIVE AEROBES** — Cocci (columns 1–12), Bacilli (columns 13–16); **GRAM-NEGATIVE AEROBES** — Cocci (columns 17–19), Enteric bacilli (columns 20–32).

Drug	S. aureus (non-penicillinase)	S. aureus (penicillinase-producing)	S. aureus (methicillin-resistant)[A]	S. epidermidis (non-penicillinase)	S. epidermidis (penicillinase-prod.)	S. epidermidis (methicillin-resistant)[A]	Strep. group A (Strep. pyogenes)	Strep. group B	Strep. group D (enterococcal)[B]	Strep. group D (nonenterococcal)	Strep. pneumoniae	Strep. viridans	Bacillus anthracis	Corynebacterium diphtheriae[C]	Corynebacterium jeikeium	Listeria monocytogenes[D]	Moraxella catarrhalis (Branhamella)	Neisseria gonorrhoeae[E]	Neisseria meningitidis	Citrobacter sp.[F]	Enterobacter sp.	Escherichia coli	Klebsiella pneumoniae	Morganella morganii	Proteus mirabilis	Proteus vulgaris	Providencia stuartii	Salmonella sp.	Salmonella typhi	Serratia sp.	Shigella sp.	Yersinia enterocolitica
β-LACTAMASE-SUSCEPTIBLE (Nonantipseudomonal)																																
AMOXICILLIN	2			2			2	1	2	2	2							1	2			2			1			1	2			
AMPICILLIN	2			2			2	1	1	2	2	2				1		1	2			2			1			1	2			2
BACAMPICILLIN	2			2			2	1	2	2	2								3			2			1			1	2			
PENICILLIN G	1			1			1	1	1	1	1	1	1	2				1	1													
PENICILLIN V	1			1			1	1	2	1	1	1	1	2			3															
β-LACTAMASE-SUSCEPTIBLE (Antipseudomonal)																																
AZLOCILLIN																																
MEZLOCILLIN	3			3			2	1	2	3	2	3							2		2	2	2	2	2	2	2			2		
PIPERACILLIN	3			3			2	1	2	3	2	3							2		2	2	2	2	2	2	2			2		
TICARCILLIN	3			3			2	2		3	2	3							2			2		2	2	2	2			2		
β-LACTAMASE-RESISTANT (Antistaphylococcal)																																
CLOXACILLIN	2	1		2	1		3				3																					
DICLOXACILLIN	2	1		2	1		3				3																					
METHICILLIN	2	1		2	1		3				3																					
NAFCILLIN	2	1		2	1		3				3																					
OXACILLIN	2	1		2	1		3				3																					
β-LACTAMASE-RESISTANT (Others)																																
AMOXICILLIN/ CLAVULANATE	2	2	3	2	2	3	2	1	3	2	2	2				2	1	1	2			2	2		2			1	2			
AMPICILLIN/ SULBACTAM	2	2	3	2	2	3	2	2	2	2	2	2				2	1	1	2			2	2	2	2			1	2			2
TICARCILLIN/ CLAVULANATE	2	2		3	2		2	2		3	2	3					2	2	2			2	2	2	2	2	2			2		
AZTREONAM																			2	2	2	2	2	2	2	2	2			2		
IMIPENEM/ CILASTATIN	2	2	3	2	2	3	2		2		2						2	2	3	1	1	2	2	1	2	1	1			2		

	GRAM-NEGATIVE AEROBES — Other bacilli																		ANAEROBES — Gram-positive					ANAEROBES — Gram-negative			Acid-fast		Actinomycetes		Chlamydia		Mycoplasma		Rickettsia	Spirochetes			
	Acinetobacter sp.	Aeromonas hydrophila	Bordetella pertussis	Brucella sp.[G]	Campylobacter jejuni	Francisella tularensis[G]	Gardnerella vaginalis	Haemophilus ducreyi	Haemophilus influenzae[H]	Legionella pneumophila	Pasteurella multocida	Pseudomonas aeruginosa[I]	Pseudomonas cepacia	Pseudomonas mallei[G]	Pseudomonas maltophilia	Streptobacillus moniliformis	Vibrio cholerae	Yersinia pestis	Clostridium difficile[J]	Clostridium perfringens	Clostridium tetani	Peptococcus sp.	Peptostreptococcus sp.	Bacteroides fragilis	Bacteroides sp.[K]	Fusobacterium sp.	M. avium-intracellulare[L]	M. tuberculosis[J]	Actinomyces israelii	Nocardia sp.	Chlamydia psittaci[M]	Chlamydia trachomatis[M]	Mycoplasma pneumoniae[M]	Ureaplasma urealyticum[M]	Rickettsia sp.	Borrelia burgdorferi	Borrelia recurrentis	Leptospira sp.	Treponema pallidum
			2		2	1														2	2																		
			2	2	2	1														2	2										1	2							
			2		2	1														2	2																		
											1						1		1	1	1	1			1				1							1	2	1	1
											1						1		1	1	1	1			1				1							1	2	1	1
	2										1																												
	2											3		2	1				2	2	2	2	2	3														
	2											3			1				2	2	2	2	2	3														
	2											3		2	1				2	2	2	2	2	3	2													
		2					2	2	1		2		2							2	2	2	2															
	3										1								2	2	2	2	1	1	1													
	2										2	2	2		2				2	2	2	2	1	1	2													
	3	2									2		2																										
	1	2			2						2		2						2	2	2	2	1	1	1				2									

ORPHAN DRUGS AND BIOLOGICALS

As defined by the Orphan Drug Act, an orphan drug is one that is useful for the diagnosis, treatment, or prevention of a rare disease or disorder. This act defines a rare disease as one that affects fewer than 200,000 persons in the United States, or one for which the expected sales will not recover the cost of developing and making the drug available. The following list includes the drugs and biologicals that have received orphan drug designation.*

GENERIC NAME	TRADE NAME	DESIGNATED USE
Drugs		
aconiazide	Not established	Treatment of tuberculosis.
adenosine	Not established	Treatment of brain tumors.
allopurinol	Zyloprim	For use in the ex vivo preservation of cadaveric kidneys for transplantation.
allopurinol riboside	Not established	Treatment of cutaneous and visceral leishmaniasis and Chagas' disease.
anagrelide	Not established	Treatment of polycythemia vera and thrombocytosis in chronic myelogenous leukemia.
antiepilepsirine	Not established	Treatment of refractory generalized tonic-clonic seizures.
antipyrine	Not established	Antipyrine test as an index of hepatic drug-metabolizing capacity.
AS-101	Not established	Treatment of AIDS.
3′ azido-2, 3′dideoxyuridine	Not established	Treatment of AIDS.
bacitracin zinc	Altracin	Treatment of antibiotic-associated pseudomembranous enterocolitis caused by toxins A and B from *Clostridium difficile*.
baclofen (intrathecal)	Lioresal	Treatment of intractable spasticity caused by spinal cord injury or multiple sclerosis.
bethanidine sulfate	Not established	Prevention or treatment of primary ventricular fibrillation.
BMY-45622	Not established	Treatment of ovarian cancer.
bromhexine	Not established	Treatment of keratoconjunctivitis sicca in patients with Sjögren's syndrome.
BW B759U	Not established	Treatment of severe human CMV infections in specific immunosuppressed patient populations (for example, bone marrow transplant, AIDS).
BW 12C	Not established	Treatment of sickle cell disease crisis.
566C80	Not established	Treatment of *Pneumocystis carinii* pneumonia in patients with AIDS.
calcitonin salmon nasal spray	Miacalcin Nasal Spray	Treatment of symptomatic Paget's disease of bone (osteitis deformans).
calcium carbonate	Calcium Carbonate/600	Treatment of hyperphosphatemia in patients with end-stage renal disease.
calcium gluconate gel 2.5%	H-F Gel	Emergency topical treatment of hydrogen fluoride (hydrofluoric acid) burns.
carbovir	Not established	Treatment of AIDS and symptomatic HIV infection.

ORPHAN DRUGS AND BIOLOGICALS (continued)

GENERIC NAME	TRADE NAME	DESIGNATED USE
Drugs (continued)		
ceramide trihexosidase/ alpha galactosidase A	Not established	Treatment of Fabry's disease.
cetiedil citrate	Not established	Treatment of sickle cell disease crisis.
chlorhexidine gluconate mouthrinse	Peridex	Amelioration of oral mucositis associated with cytoreductive therapy used in conditioning patients for bone marrow transplantation therapy.
2-chlorodeoxyadenosine	Not established	Treatment of chronic lymphocytic leukemia and hairy-cell leukemia.
2-chloro-2'-deoxyadenosine	Not established	Treatment of acute myeloid leukemia.
citric acid, glucono-delta-lactone, and magnesium carbonate	Renacidin	Treatment of apatite or struvite renal or bladder calculi.
copolymer 1 (COP 1)	Not established	Treatment of multiple sclerosis.
cyproterone acetate	Androcur, Cyproteron	Treatment of severe hirsutism.
cysteamine hydrochloride (2-aminoethanethiol)	Not established	Treatment of nephropathic cystinosis.
decitabine (5-AZA-2'-deoxycytidine; DAC)	Not established	Treatment of acute leukemias.
defibrotide	Not established	Treatment of thrombotic thrombocytopenic purpura.
deslorelin	Somagard	Treatment of central precocious puberty.
dextran and deferoxamine	Bio-Rescue	Treatment of acute iron poisoning.
dextran sulfate aerosol inhalation	Uendex	Adjunctive treatment of cystic fibrosis.
dextran sulfate sodium (UA001)	Not established	Treatment of AIDS.
3,4-diaminopyridine	Not established	Treatment of Eaton-Lambert (myasthenic) syndrome.
diaziquone	Not established	Treatment of primary brain malignancies (grades III to IV astrocytomas).
2'-3'-dideoxyadenosine	Not established	Treatment of AIDS.
2'-3'-dideoxycytidine	Not established	Treatment of AIDS.
2'-3'-dideoxyinosine	Not established	Treatment of AIDS.
diethyldithiocarbamate (DTC)	Imuthiol	Treatment of AIDS.

(continued)

ORPHAN DRUGS AND BIOLOGICALS (continued)

GENERIC NAME	TRADE NAME	DESIGNATED USE
Drugs (continued)		
dihematoporphyrin ethers	Photofrin II	Photodynamic treatment of primary or recurrent obstructive esophageal carcinoma; treatment of transitional cell carcinoma of the bladder.
2,3-dimercaptosuccinic acid (DMSA)	Not established	Treatment of lead poisoning in children.
dimethyl sulfoxide (DMSO)	Sclerosol	Treatment of cutaneous manifestations of scleroderma.
disodium clodronate tetrahydrate	Bonefos	Treatment of bone resorption caused by malignancy.
disodium silibinin dih-emisuccinate	Legalon Sil	Treatment of hepatic intoxication by *Amanita phalloides* (mushroom poisoning).
D,L-sotalol hydrochloride	Not established	Treatment of life-threatening ventricular tachyarrhythmias.
dynamine	Not established	Treatment of Eaton-Lambert (myasthenic) syndrome.
enisoprost	Not established	Adjunctive treatment (with cyclosporine) to reduce rejection and decrease cyclosporine nephrotoxicity in transplant recipients.
epidermal growth factor (human)	Not established	Acceleration of corneal epithelial regeneration and healing of stromal incisions from corneal transplant surgery; use in the acceleration of corneal epithelial regeneration and the healing of stromal tissue in the condition of nonhealing corneal defects; and promotion of cutaneous wound healing in extreme burn treatment protocols.
epoprostenol	Cyclo-Prostin	Replacement of heparin in patients requiring hemodialysis and who are at increased risk for hemorrhage.
epoprostenol, prostacyclin, PGI_2, PGX	Flolan	Replacement of heparin in patients requiring hemodialysis and who are at increased risk for hemorrhage and treatment of pulmonary hypertension.
ethiofos	Ethyol	Adjunctive therapy (chemoprotective agent) with cisplatin or cyclophosphamide in the treatment of malignant melanoma or ovarian carcinoma.
fatty acid solution, short chain	Not established	Treatment of ulcerative colitis (active phase) with involvement restricted to the left side of the colon.
felbamate	Not established	Treatment of Lennox-Gastaut syndrome.
fibronectin (plasma derived)	Not established	Treatment of corneal ulcers or epithelial defects refractory to conventional therapy.
flumecinol	Zixoryn	Hyberbilirubinemia in neonates unresponsive to phototherapy.
flunarizine	Sibelium	Treatment of alternating hemiplegia.
fosphenytoin	Not established	Acute treatment of status epilepticus.
gangliosides (sodium salts)	Cronassial	Treatment of retinitis pigmentosa.

ORPHAN DRUGS AND BIOLOGICALS (continued)

GENERIC NAME	TRADE NAME	DESIGNATED USE
Drugs (continued)		
gentamicin-impregnated PMMA beads on surgical wire	Septopal	Treatment of chronic osteomyelitis.
gossypol	Not established	Treatment of adrenal cortex cancer.
guanethidine monosulfate	Ismelin I.V.	Treatment of moderate to severe reflex sympathetic dystrophy and causalgia.
HPA-23	Not established	Treatment of AIDS.
human growth hormone releasing factor	Not established	Treatment of children with growth failure caused by lack of endogenous growth hormone secretion.
hydroxycobalamin/sodium thiosulfate	Not established	Treatment of severe acute cyanide poisoning.
iloprost	Not established	Treatment of heparin-induced thrombocytopenia and Raynaud's phenomenon secondary to systemic sclerosis.
inosine pranobex	Isoprinosine	Treatment of subacute sclerosing panencephalitis.
iodine ^{131}I 6B-iodomethyl-19-norcholesterol	Not established	Adrenocortical imaging.
iodine ^{131}I iodobenzylguanidine	Not established	Diagnostic adjunct in patients with pheochromocytoma.
leupeptin	Not established	Adjunctive treatment of microsurgical nerve repair.
levocabastine hydrochloride	Not established	Treatment of vernal keratoconjunctivitis.
LHRH [(des-gly^{10})-d-tri^8-Pro^9-n-ethylamide]	Not established	Treatment of central precocious puberty.
L-5 hydroxytryp-tophan (L-5-HTP)	Not established	Treatment of postanoxic intention myoclonus.
L-leucine, L-isoleucine, and L-valine	Not established	Treatment of amyotrophic lateral sclerosis.
L-leucovorin	Isovorin	Palliative treatment (with fluorouracil) of metastatic adenocarcinoma of the colon and rectum.
L-threonine	Threostat	Treatment of amyotropic lateral sclerosis.
luteinizing hormone-releasing hormone (GnRH)	Not established	Induction of ovulation in women with hypothalamic amenorrhea due to a deficiency or absence in the quantity or pulse pattern of endogenous GnRH secretion.
lysine acetylsalicylate	Aspegic	Treatment of pain and fever associated with sickle cell disease crisis.
mazindol	Sanorex	Treatment of Duchenne muscular dystrophy.
methotrexate with laurocapram	Not established	Treatment of mycosis fungoides.

(continued)

ORPHAN DRUGS AND BIOLOGICALS *(continued)*

GENERIC NAME	TRADE NAME	DESIGNATED USE
Drugs *(continued)*		
4-methylpyrazole (4-MP)	Not established	Treatment of poisoning from methanol, ethylene glycol, 2-methoxy-ethanol, or 2-butoxyethanol.
mitodrine hydrochloride	Midamine	Treatment of idiopathic orthostatic hypotension.
mitolactol (dibromodulcitol, DBD)	Not established	Treatment of invasive cervical carcinoma.
n-acetylprocainamide (NAPA)	Not established	Adjunctive treatment of ventricular fibrillation in patients with automatic implantable cardioverter defibrillators.
NG-29	Somatrel	Assessment of pituitary function in children with suspected growth hormone deficiency.
ofloxacin ophthalmic solution	Not established	Treatment of bacterial corneal ulcers.
ovine corticotropin-releasing hormone (oCRH)	Not established	To differentiate pituitary and ectopic production of corticotropin in patients with corticotropin-dependent Cushing's syndrome.
PEG-adenosine deaminase (PEG-ADA)	Imudon	Enzyme replacement therapy for ADA deficiency in patients with severe combined immunodeficiency.
phosphocysteamine	Not established	Treatment of cystinosis.
physostigmine salicylate	Antilirium	Friedreich's and other inherited ataxias.
piracetam	Nootropil	Treatment of myoclonus.
piritrexim isethionate	Not established	Treatment of infections caused by *Pneumocystis carinii, Toxoplasma gondii,* and *Mycobacterium avium-intracellulare.*
poloxamer 188	Rheoth Rx Copolymer	Treatment of sickle cell disease crisis and severe burns.
poloxamer 331	Protox	Initial treatment of toxoplasmosis in patients with AIDS.
polymer implant containing carmustine	Biodel	Localized treatment of recurrent malignant melanoma in the brain.
potassium citrate	Urocit-K	Prevention of calcium renal stones in patients with hypocitraturia, avoidance of calcium stone formation in patients with uric lithiasis, and prevention of uric acid nephrolithiasis.
potassium citrate and citric acid	Polycitra-K	Dissolution and control of uric acid and cystine calculi in the urinary tract.
PR-122 (redox-phenytoin)	Not established	Emergency treatment of status epilepticus.
PR-225 (redox acyclovir)	Not established	Treatment of herpes simplex encephalitis in patients with AIDS.
PR-239 (redox penicillin G)	Not established	Treatment of neurosyphilis associated with AIDS.

ORPHAN DRUGS AND BIOLOGICALS *(continued)*

GENERIC NAME	TRADE NAME	DESIGNATED USE
Drugs *(continued)*		
PR-320 (molecusol-car-bamazepine)	Not established	Emergency treatment of status epilepticus.
prednimustine	Sterecyt	Treatment of non-Hodgkin's lymphomas.
propamidine isethionate 0.1%	Brolene Eye Drops	Treatment of *Acanthamoeba* keratitis.
protirelin (TRH)	Thymone	Treatment of amyotrophic lateral sclerosis.
quinacrine hydrochloride	Not established	Prevention of recurrence of pneumothorax in patients at high risk for recurrence, for example, those with cystic fibrosis.
rifabutin	Not established	Prevention and treatment of *Mycobacterium avium* complex disease in patients with low CD4 counts.
rifampin, isoniazid, pyrazinamide	Rifater	Short-course treatment of tuberculosis.
secalciferol (24, 25 dihydroxycholecalciferol)	Not established	Treatment of uremic osteodystrophy.
sermorelin acetate	Geref	Treatment of idiopathic growth hormone deficiency in children and ovulatory failure in women who fail to respond to clomiphene or gonadotropin.
sodium dichloroacetate	Not established	Treatment of homozygous familial hypercholesterolemia and congenital lactic acidosis.
sodium monomercaptoundecahydro-closo-dodeca-borate	Borolife	Treatment of gliobastoma multiforme as an alternative to conventional photon therapy.
sodium oxybate (sodium gamma hydroxybutyrate)	Not established	Treatment of narcolepsy and the auxiliary symptoms of cataplexy, sleep paralysis, hypnagogic hallucinations, and automatic behavior.
sodium tetradecyl sulfate	Sotradecol	Treatment of bleeding esophageal varices.
spiramycin	Rovamycine	Symptomatic relief and parasitic cure of chronic cryptosporidosis in patients with immunodeficiency.
superoxide dismutase (recombinant, human)	Not established	Protection of donor organ tissue from damage or injury mediated by oxygen-derived free radicals that are generated during the necessary periods of ischemia (hypoxia) and especially reperfusion and anoxia associated with the operative procedure; prevention of bronchopulmonary dysplasia in premature neonates (under 1,500 g).
T4 endonuclease V, liposome encapsulated	T4N5 Liposomes	Prevention of skin abnormalities such as cutaneous neoplasms in patients with xeroderma pigmentosum.
teniposide (VM-26)	Not established	Treatment of refractory childhood acute lymphocytic leukemia.

(continued)

ORPHAN DRUGS AND BIOLOGICALS (continued)

GENERIC NAME	TRADE NAME	DESIGNATED USE
Drugs (continued)		
teriparatide	Parathar	To aid diagnosis in patients with clinical and laboratory evidence of hypocalcemia due to either hypoparathyroidism or pseudohypoparathyroidism.
terlipressin	Glypressin	Treatment of bleeding esophageal varices.
thalidomide	Not established	Prevention and treatment of graft-versus-host disease in patients receiving bone marrow transplant; treatment and maintenance of reactional lepromatous leprosy.
thymoxamine hydrochloride	Not established	Reversal of phenylephrine-induced mydriasis in patients who have narrow anterior angles and are at risk for developing an acute attack of angle-closure glaucoma after mydriasis.
tocophersolan oral solution (vitamin E, d-alpha tocopheryl polylene glycol-1000 succinate, TPGS)	Not established	Treatment of vitamin E deficiency in patients with malabsorption caused by prolonged cholestatic hepatobiliary disease.
tranexamic acid	Cyklokapron	Treatment of hereditary angioneurotic edema, patients undergoing prostatectomy where there is hemorrhage or risk of hemorrhage from increased fibrinolysis or fibrinogenolysis, and patients with congenital coagulopathies who are undergoing surgical procedures, such as dental extractions.
tretinoin	Not established	Treatment of squamous metaplasia of the ocular surface epithelia (conjunctiva and/or cornea) with mucous deficiency and keratinization.
triptorelin pamoate	Decapeptyl Injection	Palliative treatment of advanced ovarian carcinoma of epithelial origin.
troleandomycin	Not established	Adjunctive treatment of severe steroid-dependent asthma.
urofollitropin	Metrodin	Induction of ovulation in patients with polycystic ovarian disease who have an elevated luteinizing hormone to follicle-stimulating hormone and who have failed to respond to adequate clomiphene therapy.
viloxazine hydrochloride	Catatrol	Treatment of narcolepsy and cataplexy.
zinc acetate	Not established	Treatment of Wilson's disease.
Biologicals		
alpha-1-antitrypsin (recombinant DNA origin)	Not established	Supplementation therapy for alpha-1-antitrypsin deficiency in the ZZ phenotype population.
ancrod	Arvin	Treatment of heparin-induced thrombosis or thrombocytopenia.
anticytomegalovirus monoclonal antibodies	Not established	Prevention or treatment of CMV infection in patients with AIDS, and in organ transplant or bone marrow transplant recipients.

ORPHAN DRUGS AND BIOLOGICALS (continued)

GENERIC NAME	TRADE NAME	DESIGNATED USE
Biologicals (continued)		
antihemophilic factor (recombinant DNA origin)	Not established	Prophylaxis and treatment of bleeding in patients with hemophilia A.
antimelanoma antibody XMMME-001-RTA	Not established	Treatment of Stage III melanoma not amenable to surgical resection.
anti-TAP-72 immunotoxin	Xomazyme-791	Treatment of metastatic colorectal cancer adenocarcinoma.
benzylpenicillin, benzylpenicilloic acid, and benzylpenilloic acid	Pre-Pen/MDM	For assessing the risk of administering penicillin when it's the drug of choice in adults who have a history of clinical hypersensitivity.
botulism immune globulin	Not established.	Treatment of infant botulism.
bovine colostrum	Not established	Treatment of AIDS-related diarrhea.
CD4, human recombinant soluble	Receptin	Treatment of AIDS.
CD4, human truncated-369 AA polypeptide (recombinant CHO cells)	Soluble T4	Treatment of AIDS.
CD4 immunoglobulin G (recombinant human)	Not established	Treatment of AIDS.
CD-45 monoclonal antibodies	Not established	Prevention of rejection of human organ transplants.
CD5-T lymphocyte Immunotoxin	Xomazyme-H65	Ex vivo treatment to eliminate mature T cells from potential bone marrow grafts, in vivo treatment of bone marrow recipients to prevent graft rejection and graft-versus-host disease (GVHD), and treatment of GVHD and/or rejection in patients who have received bone marrow transplants.
chimeric M-T412 (human-murine) IgG monoclonal anti-CD4	Not established	Treatment of multiple sclerosis.
C1-inhibitor	C1-inhibitor (human) vapor treated, Immuno	Prevention or treatment of acute attacks of angioedema.
deoxyribonuclease, recombinant human	rhDNase	To reduce the viscosity of mucus secretions and enhance airway clearance in patients with cystic fibrosis.
disaccharide tripeptide glycerol dipalmitoyl	Immther	Treatment of hepatic and pulmonary metastases in patients with colorectal adenocarcinoma.
epoetin beta (recombinant-human)	Marogen	Treatment of anemia associated with end-stage renal disease.
factor VIIa (recombinant, DNA origin)	Not established	Treatment of von Willebrand's disease and of patients with hemophilia A and B with and without antibodies against factor VIII and IX.

(continued)

ORPHAN DRUGS AND BIOLOGICALS (continued)

GENERIC NAME	TRADE NAME	DESIGNATED USE
Biologicals (continued)		
factor XIII	Fibrogammin	Congenital factor XIII deficiency.
fibronectin (human plasma derived)	Not established	Treatment of epithelial defects or nonhealing corneal ulcers unresponsive to conventional therapy.
group B streptococcus immune globulin	Not established	Treatment of disseminated group B streptococcus infection in neonates.
heme arginate	Normosang	Treatment of acute, symptomatic porphyria.
hemin	Panhematin	Amelioration of recurrent attacks of acute intermittent porphyria temporally related to the menstrual cycle in susceptible women and similar symptoms that occur in other patients with acute intermittent porphyria, porphyria variegata, and hereditary coproporphyria.
human IgM monoclonal antibody (C-58) to cytomegalovirus (CMV)	Centovir	Prophylaxis and treatment of CMV infections in bone marrow transplant recipients.
human immunodeficiency virus (HIV-1) immune globulin (human) I.V.	Not established	Treatment of AIDS.
human monoclonal antibody against hepatitis B virus	Not established	Prophylaxis against reinfection with hepatitis B in patients undergoing liver transplant secondary to end-stage chronic hepatitis B infection.
human T-lymphotropic virus type III gp160 antigens, recombinant vaccine, alum absorbed	VaxSyn HIV-1	Treatment of AIDS.
interferon beta (recombinant, human)	Betaseron	Treatment of AIDS and multiple sclerosis.
interleukin-1 alpha (recombinant, human)	Not established	Promotion of graft acceptance in patients undergoing bone marrow transplant.
interleukin-3 (recombinant, human)	Not established	Promotion of erythropoiesis in patients with congenital pure cell aplasia (Diamond-Blackfan anemia).
iodine 131I Lym-1 monoclonal antibody	Not established	Treatment of B-cell lymphoma.
iodine 131I murine monoclonal antibody to human alpha-fetoprotein	AFP-I 131	Treatment of hepatocellular carcinoma, hepatoblastoma, and alpha-fetoprotein-producing germ cell tumors.
iodine 131I murine monoclonal antibody to human chorionic gonadotropin	hCG-I 131	Treatment of human chorionic gonadotropin-producing tumors, including germ cell and trophoblastic cell tumors.
iodine 131I murine monoclonal antibody IgG2a to B cell	LL-2-I 131	Treatment of B-cell leukemia and lymphoma.

ORPHAN DRUGS AND BIOLOGICALS (continued)

GENERIC NAME	TRADE NAME	DESIGNATED USE
Biologicals (continued)		
lactobin	Lactobin	Treatment of refractory diarrhea associated with AIDS.
melanoma vaccine	Melaccine	Treatment of melanoma (stage III or IV).
monoclonal antibodies (murine or human) recognizing B-cell lymphoma idiotypes	Not established	Treatment of B-cell lymphoma.
monoclonal antibodies PM-81 and AML-2-23	Not established	Treatment of patients with acute myelogenous leukemia undergoing bone marrow transplant.
monoclonal antibody 17-1A	Panorex	Treatment of pancreatic cancer.
monoclonal antibody PM-81	Not established	Adjunctive treatment of acute myelogenous leukemia.
monoclonal factor IX	Not established	Treatment of hemophilia B.
mucoid exopolysaccharide Pseudomonas hyperimmune globulin	MEPIG	Prevention or treatment of Pseudomonas aeruginosa pulmonary infections in patients with cystic fibrosis.
myelin	Not established	Treatment of multiple sclerosis.
PEG-interleukin 2	Not established	Treatment of immunodeficiencies associated with T-cell defects.
PEG-L-asparaginase	Not established	Treatment of acute lymphocytic leukemia.
pentastarch	Pentaspan	Adjunctive use in leukapheresis, to improve the harvesting and increase the yield of leukocytes by centrifugal means.
poly I:poly C12U	Ampligen	Treatment of renal cell carcinoma.
polyribonucleotide	Ampligen	Treatment of AIDS.
respiratory syncytial virus imune globulin (human)	Hyperimmune RSV	Prophylaxis and treatment of respiratory syncytial virus infections in hospitalized infants and children.
ricin (blocked) conjugated murine monoclonal antibody (anti-B4) to B cell (CD19)	Not established	Treatment of B-cell leukemia and B-cell lymphoma.
ricin (blocked) conjugated murine monoclonal antibody (anti-My^9) to myeloid cells (CD-33)	Anti-My^9-bR	Treatment of myeloid leukemias.
ricin (blocked) conjugated murine monoclonal antibody (N901)	Not established	Treatment of small-cell lung cancer.
secretory leukocyte protease inhibitor, recombinant	Not established	Treatment of congenital deficiency of alpha-1-antitrypsin; treatment of cystic fibrosis.
septomonab	anti-J5mAb; Centoxin	Treatment of endotoxin shock in patients with gram-negative bacteremia.

(continued)

ORPHAN DRUGS AND BIOLOGICALS *(continued)*		
GENERIC NAME	**TRADE NAME**	**DESIGNATED USE**
Biologicals *(continued)*		
Serratia marcescens extract (ribosomes and lipid vesicles)	ImuVert	Treatment of primary brain malignancies.
ST1-RTA immunotoxin (SR 44163)	Not established	Prevention of acute graft-versus-host disease in allogenic bone marrow transplantation and treatment of patients with B-chronic lymphocytic leukemia.
teceleukin	Not established	Treatment of metastatic malignant melanoma (with interferon alfa-2a).
thymosin alpha-1	Not established	Adjunctive treatment of active chronic hepatitis B.
trisaccharides A and B	Not established	Treatment of moderate to severe clinical forms of hemolytic disease of the newborn arising from placental transfer of antibodies against blood group substances A and B; use in ABO-incompatible solid organ transplantation, including kidney, heart, liver, and pancreas; and treatment of moderate to very severe clinical forms of transfusion reactions arising from ABO-incompatible transfusion of blood, blood products, and blood derivatives.

US PDI, vol. 1, 12th ed. (Appendix V), 1-59, 1992.

TABLE OF EQUIVALENTS

Frequently used equivalents in the metric system

Metric Weight		Metric Volume	
1 gram (g)	= 0.001 kilogram (kg or Kg)	1 liter (L)	= 0.001 kiloliter (kl or Kl)
	= 0.01 hectogram (hg or Hg)		= 0.01 hectoliter (hl or Hl)
	= 0.1 decagram (dag or Dg)		= 0.1 decaliter (dal or Dl)
	= 10 decigrams (dg)		= 10 deciliters (dl)
	= 100 centigrams (cg)		= 100 centiliters (cl)
	= 1,000 milligrams (mg)		= 1,000 milliliters (ml)*

Frequently used equivalents in the apothecary system

Apothecary Weight		Apothecary Volume	
20 grains (gr)	= 1 scruple (3)	60 minims (♏)†	= 1 fluidram (f3)
3 scruples	= 1 dram (3)	8 fluidrams	= 1 fluidounce (f3)
8 drams	= 1 ounce (3)	16 fluidounces	= 1 pint (pt)
12 ounces	= 1 pound (b)	2 pints	= 1 quart (qt)
		4 quarts	= 1 gallon (gal)

Approximate metric and apothecary weight equivalents

Metric	Apothecary	Metric	Apothecary
1 gram (g)	= 15 grains	0.05 g (50 mg)	= ¾ grain
(1,000 mg)			
0.6 g (600 mg)	= 10 grains	0.03 g (30 mg)	= ½ grain
0.5 g (500 mg)	= 7½ grains	0.015 g (15 mg)	= ¼ grain
0.3 g (300 mg)	= 5 grains	0.001 g (1 mg)	= 1/60 grain
0.2 g (200 mg)	= 3 grains	0.6 mg	= 1/100 grain
0.1 g (100 mg)	= 1½ grains	0.5 mg	= 1/120 grain
0.06 g (60 mg)	= 1 grain	0.4 mg	= 1/150 grain

Approximate household, apothecary, and metric volume equivalents

Household	Apothecary	Metric
1 teaspoon (t or tsp)	= 1 fluidram (f3)	= 4 or 5 ml‡
1 tablespoon (T or tbs)	= ½ fluidounce (f3)	= 15 ml
2 tablespoons	= 1 fluidounce	= 30 ml
1 measuring cupful	= 8 fluidounces	= 240 ml
1 pint (pt)	= 16 fluidounces	= 473 ml
1 quart (qt)	= 32 fluidounces	= 946 ml
1 gallon (gal)	= 128 fluidounces	= 3,785 ml

*1 ml = 1 cubic centimeter (cc); however, ml is the preferred measurement term today

†A minim is *almost equal* to a drop. When a drug is prescribed in minims, it is best to measure it in minims. The minim is measured with a minim glass; a drop, with a medicine dropper.

‡Although the fluidram is approximately 4 ml, in prescriptions it is considered equivalent to the teaspoon (which is 5 ml).

ANTIDOTES TO POISONING OR OVERDOSE

The chart below summarizes the major uses and dosage recommendations for selected antidotes. For more information, contact your local poison information center.

ANTIDOTE	TYPE OF POISONING OR OVERDOSE	GENERAL CONSIDERATIONS
acetylcysteine (Mucomyst) *Adults:* 140 mg/kg P.O. diluted in soft drinks, juice, or water. Follow loading dose with 17 additional doses of 70 mg/kg q 4 hours (repeat if dose is vomited within 1 hour).	acetaminophen	• Activated charcoal will adsorb the antidote if both are present in the gut. If charcoal is used, it must be aspirated before the antidote is given.
activated charcoal (Actidose-Aqua, LiquiChar) *Adults and children:* 5 to 10 times the weight of the ingested poison. Minimum dose is 20 to 30 g (½ cup of lightly packed powder) in 250 ml of water to make a slurry; repeat as soon as possible. Most adults can tolerate doses of 120 g.	All oral poisonings except those caused by iron, cyanide, organic solvents, mineral acids, or corrosive agents	• Repeated doses may not provide additional benefit unless the poison undergoes enterohepatic recycling. • Activated charcoal may adsorb other orally administered antidotes (such as acetylcysteine).
amyl nitrite inhalants (Step I) *Adults:* Inhale for 30 seconds for every 1 to 2 minutes. **sodium nitrite** (Step II) *Adults:* 300 mg in 10-ml solution given I.V. over 2 to 4 minutes (repeat once if symptoms reappear). *Children:* Depends on hemoglobin level. **sodium thiosulfate** (Step III) *Adults:* 12.5 g in 50-ml solution given I.V. over 10 minutes (if symptoms reappear, give sodium nitrite again in half the original dose). *Children:* Depends on hemoglobin level.	cyanide	• Nitrites cause vasodilation. Hypotension is a common adverse reaction.
atropine sulfate *Adults:* 2 to 5 mg I.V. for pesticides (may repeat every 10 to 30 minutes until signs of atropinization appear). *Children:* 0.05 mg/kg for pesticides (may repeat every 10 to 30 minutes until signs of atropinization appear).	anticholinesterase substances, organophosphate pesticides, carbamate pesticides	• Large doses (2 to 2,000 mg over several hours to several days) may be required to maintain full atropinization. • Sudden cessation of atropine may cause pulmonary edema. • Maintain adequate ventilation to prevent cardiac arrhythmias.
calcium disodium edetate (Calcium Disodium Versenate, EDTA) *Adults:* 75 mg/kg/day deep I.M. or slow I.V. infusion given in three to six divided doses for up to 5 days	iron, lead, mercury, copper, nickel, zinc, cadmium, cobalt	• EDTA should not be started until all lead has been removed from the gut. • Rapid injection may precipitate renal failure.
deferoxamine mesylate (Desferal) *Adults and children:* 1,000 mg I.M. or I.V. initially, then 500 mg q 4 hours for two doses. Subsequent doses of 500 mg q 4 to 12 hours may be given; maximum dosage 6,000 mg daily.	heavy metals, iron	• Renal excretion of compound will cause the urine to turn pink.
digoxin immune Fab (Digibind) *Adults:* Depends on amount of digoxin or digitoxin to be neutralized. If unable to determine dosage using manufacturer-supplied dosage formulas, 800 mg I.V. may be infused over 30 minutes.	digoxin, digitoxin	• Use is reserved for severe overdose only. • If cardiac arrest seems imminent, administer dose as a bolus injection. • Monitor serum potassium levels carefully for hyperkalemia or hypokalemia. • Monitor cardiac rate and rhythm.

ANTIDOTES TO POISONING OR OVERDOSE (continued)

ANTIDOTE	TYPE OF POISONING OR OVERDOSE	GENERAL CONSIDERATIONS
dimercaprol (BAL) *Adults:* 3 to 5 mg/kg deep I.M. q 4 hours for 2 days; q 4 to 6 hours for 2 more days; then q 4 to 12 hours up to 12 more days.	mercury, arsenic, gold	• Dimercaprol must be administered promptly to be effective. • It is contraindicated with iron poisoning. • Use requires that patient has adequate renal and hepatic function to excrete toxins.
flumazenil (Mazicon) *Adults:* Initially, give 0.2 mg I.V. over 15 seconds. If patient does not reach the desired level of consciousness after 30 seconds, administer 0.3 mg over 30 seconds. If response is inadequate, give 0.5 mg over 30 seconds; repeat doses of 0.5 mg at 1-minute intervals until 3 mg has been given.	benzodiazepines	• Most patients respond to cumulative doses between 1 and 3 mg; in rare instances, patients who partially respond after 3 mg may require more. Do not give more than 5 mg over a 5-minute period initially, and do not give more than 3 mg/hour. • Use with caution in cases of mixed overdose. Seizures or arrhythmias can develop.
naloxone hydrochloride (Narcan) *Adults:* 0.4 to 0.8 mg I.V. bolus to reverse the narcotic effect (may need to repeat dose every 20 to 60 minutes to maintain reversal). *Children:* 0.01 mg/kg I.V. bolus.	opiates: morphine, heroin, methadone, meperidine, oxycodone	• Time of action is shorter than that of narcotic; therefore, observe patient for recurring narcosis (loss of consciousness or depressed respirations). Repeat doses or a continuous infusion may be necessary.
D-penicillamine (Cuprimine) *Adults:* 250 mg P.O. q.i.d. for up to 5 days. Do not exceed 40 mg/kg/ day. *Children:* 24 to 50 mg/kg P.O. q.i.d.	lead, iron, mercury, copper	• D-penicillamine should be used in patients with minimal signs and symptoms and positive serum lead levels.
physostigmine salicylate (Antilirium) *Adults:* 2 mg I.V. slowly over 2 to 3 minutes (repeat with a 1-mg to 2-mg dose in 20 minutes if symptoms are still present; repeat with a 1-mg to 4-mg dose if life-threatening symptoms reappear). *Children:* 0.5 mg slow I.V. over 2 to 3 minutes (repeat within 5 minutes if symptoms recur); maximum dosage is 2 mg	anticholinergics; tricyclics (amitriptyline, atropine); plants (jimsonweed, some mushroom species, black nightshade); antihistamines	• Use is reserved for severe poisoning (coma, hallucinations, delirium, tachycardia, arrhythmias, and hypertension). • Rapid I.V. injection may cause bradycardia and hypersalivation with respiratory difficulties and convulsions. • Physostigmine can produce a cholinergic crisis. If so, atropine should be used as an antidote.
pralidoxime chloride (Pralidoxime Chloride, Protopam Chloride) *Adults:* 1 g I.V. at 0.5 g/minute or diluted in 250 ml normal saline solution and given over 30 minutes (repeat in three intervals 8 to 12 hours apart if muscle weakness persists). *Children:* 25 to 50 mg/kg I.V. (may repeat in 8- to 12-hour intervals).	organophosphate pesticides	• Effective if given up to 36 hours after exposure. • Pesticide absorption is possible through the skin — wash patient and remove contaminated clothing, or symptoms may reappear within 48 to 72 hours. • Drug has no anticholinergic effects.
protamine sulfate *Adults:* 5 ml of a 1% solution slow I.V. over 10 minutes (give 1 to 1.25 mg protamine for each 100 units of heparin consumed).	heparin	• Maximum dosage is 50 mg (as a single dose).
vitamin K analogue (AquaMEPHYTON) *Adults:* 10 mg I.M. for large ingestions (can be given P.O. if patient is not vomiting). *Children:* 1 to 5 mg I.M.	warfarin	• Fresh whole blood may be necessary to stop bleeding.

TOPICAL AGENTS

DRUG	INDICATIONS AND DOSAGE
Acne preparations	
benzoyl peroxide (Clearasil, Loroxide, Oxy-5, Oxy-10, Xerac)	*Acne:* Apply once daily to q.i.d., depending on tolerance and effect.
sulfur (Acne-Aid*, Bensulfoid, Fostex, Liquimat, P and S, Postacne*, Transact, Xerac, Xseb)	*Acne, ringworm, psoriasis, seborrheic dermatitis, chigger infestation, scabies, favus, staphylococcal folliculitis:* Apply to affected areas b.i.d., t.i.d., or as directed.
Antibacterials and antifungals	
alcohol, ethyl and isopropyl	*To disinfect skin, instruments, and ampules:* Disinfect as needed. Isopropyl alcohol is superior to ethyl alcohol as an anti-infective (70%). *Antipyresis:* Apply 25% solution. *Anhidrosis:* Apply 50% solution p.r.n.
carbol-fuchsin solution (Castaderm, Castallani Paint, Castel Minus, Castel Plus)	*Tinea, dermatophytosis fungal skin infections:* Apply liberally once or twice daily.
hydrogen peroxide	*Cleansing wounds:* Use 1.5% to 3% solution, p.r.n. *Mouthwash for necrotizing ulcerative gingivitis:* Gargle with 3% solution, p.r.n. *Cleansing douche:* Use 2% solution q.i.d., p.r.n.
iodochlorhydroxyquin (Clioquinol, Torofor, Vioform)	*Inflamed skin conditions, including eczema, athlete's foot, and other fungal infections; cutaneous or mucocutaneous monilial infections:* Apply a thin layer b.i.d. or t.i.d., or as directed. Continue for 1 week after clinical cure.
potassium permanganate	*Topical antiseptic:* Apply 1:10,000 to 1:500 solution.
salicyclic acid (Calicyclic, Compound W, Derma-Soft Creme, Freezone, Gordofilm, Hydrisalic, Keralyt, Occlusal, Off-Ezy, Salacid, Salonil, Wart-Off)	*Superficial fungal infections, acne, psoriasis, seborrheic dermatitis, other scaling dermatoses, hyperkeratosis, calluses, warts:* Apply to affected area and place under occlusion at night.

*Available in Canada only

ACTION	SPECIAL CONSIDERATIONS
Heals and prevents acne through antibacterial and keratolytic actions.	• Avoid use around eyes and mucous membranes. • Apply small amount initially to determine tolerance. • May bleach clothing or skin.
Controls acne through antibacterial and keratolytic actions.	• Avoid use around eyes and mucous membranes. • Wash and dry skin before applying. • Massage into skin until absorbed. • May cause discoloration of red, blonde, or white hair. • Do not use with other topical medication. • Transient tingling sensation may occur on application.
Antibacterial effect through reduction of surface tension of bacterial cell walls, inhibiting bacterial growth. Also antipyretic and astringent effects.	• Avoid contact with eyes and mucous membranes. • Contraindicated in patients taking disulfiram if used over large surface area. • Do not apply to open wounds.
Topical fungicide through disruption of protein synthesis in fungal cell metabolism.	• Do not use in patients with dermatitis or inflammation on or around area of application. • Cleanse skin before application. • Do not use in eyes. • Stains skin and clothing; let dry before contact with clothing or linen. • May be toxic if ingested or with prolonged use. • Store in airtight, light-resistant container. • Discontinue if no improvement in 1 week. • Perform a patch test to prevent contact dermatitis.
Antibacterial effect through oxidation.	• Do not instill into closed body cavities or abscesses because gas generated cannot escape. • Store in tightly capped, dark container in cool, dry place. • Do not confuse with peroxide (6% to 20%) used for bleaching hair.
Topical fungicide.	• Do not use in iodine-sensitive patients or patients with tuberculosis or viral exanthems. • Cleanse skin before application. Stains skin, hair, and clothing. • Do not use in eyes. • Not effective in fungal infections of the hair and nails.
Strong oxidizing agent with disinfectant and deodorizing properties, and both antifungal and antibacterial actions.	• Solutions greater than 1:5,000 are irritating to skin. • Do not insert into vagina. • Dilutions of 1:1,000 in water may be used to cleanse wounds. • Dilutions of 1:4,000 in water may be used as a gargle or mouthwash. • A solution of 0.02% may be used for gastric lavage in treatment of poisoning. • Repeated use may cause corrosive burns.
Causes desquamation of cornified epithelium by increasing hydration.	• Avoid use on eyes and mucous membranes. • Do not use in aspirin-sensitive patients. • Apply emollient such as petrolatum to surrounding skin for protection. • Do not use on birth marks, moles, or areas with hair follicle involvement. • Wash off thoroughly in the morning, after overnight applications.

(continued)

TOPICAL AGENTS *(continued)*

DRUG	INDICATIONS AND DOSAGE

Antibacterials and antifungals *(continued)*

tolnaftate
(Aftate, Footwork, Fungatin, Genaspor, NP-27, Tinactin, Zeasorb)

Superficial fungal infections of the skin; infections due to common pathogenic fungi; tinea pedis; tinea cruris; tinea corporis; tinea manuum: Apply ¼" to ½" ribbon of cream or 3 drops of lotion to cover area of one hand; same amount of cream or 3 drops of lotion to cover the toes and interdigital webs of one foot. Apply and massage gently into skin b.i.d. for 2 weeks, or up to 6 weeks.

undecylenic acid, zinc undecylenate
(Caldesene, Desenex, Ting, Decylenes, Cruex, Quinsana Plus, Undoguent, Kool Foot)

Athlete's foot and ringworm of the body except nails and hairy areas: Apply b.i.d. to thoroughly cleansed area for at least 2 weeks.

Antiseptics and germicidals

benzalkonium chloride
(Benza, Germicin, Spensomide, Zephiran)

Preoperative disinfection of unbroken skin: Apply 1:750 tincture or spray.
Disinfection of mucous membranes and denuded skin: Apply 1:10,000 to 1:5,000 aqueous solution.
Irrigation of vagina: Instill 1:5,000 to 1:2,000 aqueous solution.
Irrigation of deep infected wounds: Instill 1:20,000 to 1:3,000 aqueous solution.
Preservation of metallic instruments, ampules, thermometers, and rubber articles: Wipe with or soak objects in 1:5,000 to 1:750 solution.
Disinfection of operating room equipment: Wipe with 1:5,000 solution.

chlorhexidine gluconate
(Hibiclens, Hibistat, Peridex)

Surgical hand scrub, hand wash, hand rinse, skin wound cleanser: Use p.r.n.
Gingivitis: Use 0.12% strength (Peridex oral rinse), p.r.n.

hexachlorophene
(pHisoHex, pHisoScrub, Septisol, Septsoft)

Surgical scrub, bacteriostatic skin cleanser: Use p.r.n. in 0.25% to 3% concentrations.

iodine
(Sepp)

Preoperative disinfection of skin (small wounds and abraded areas): Apply p.r.n.

povidone-iodine
(Acu-dyne, Betadine, Biodine, Efodine, Frepp, Iodex, Isodine, Operand, Pharmadine, Polydine, Proviodine*, Sepp)

Preoperative skin preparation and scrub; germicide for surface wounds; postoperative application to incisions; prophylactic application to urinary meatus of catheterized patients; miscellaneous disinfection: Apply p.r.n., or use as scrub p.r.n.

Astringents

calamine

Astringent and protectant; itching, poison ivy and poison oak, non-poisonous insect bites, mild sunburn, minor skin irritations: Apply p.r.n., t.i.d., or q.i.d.

*Available in Canada only

ACTION	SPECIAL CONSIDERATIONS
Fungicidal action against superficial skin infections, possibly through distortion of hyphae structure and stunting of mycelial growth.	• Do not use around eyes. • Not effective for nail and scalp infections. • Cleanse skin thoroughly before application. • Use powder form for adjunct therapy only. • Patients should wear loose-fitting cotton clothing and well-ventilated shoes.
Antifungal, antibacterial action.	• Do not use around eyes or on mucous membranes or puncture wounds. • Cleanse skin thoroughly before application. • Use powder form for adjunct therapy only. • Patients should wear loose-fitting cotton clothing and well-ventilated shoes.
Cationic surface action producing bacteriostatic or bacteriocidal effect depending on the concentration used.	• Do not use with occlusive dressings or packs. • Use only in proper diluted strength for each use. • Inactivated by anionic compounds such as soap. • Rinse area thoroughly after each application. • Skin inflammation and irritation may require lower concentration or discontinuation.
Persistent antimicrobial effect against gram-negative and gram-positive bacteria.	• Avoid contact with eyes, ears, and mucous membranes. • May cause deafness if drug enters middle ear. • Rinse well if drug enters eyes or ears.
Bacteriostatic effect against staphylococci and other gram-positive bacteria, probably due to inhibition of bacterial membrane-bound enzymes.	• Do not use on broken skin, skin lesions, burns, wounds, or under occlusive dressings to prevent increased absorption and neurotoxicity. • Do not use around eyes or mucous membranes. • Use for at least 3 days preoperatively for optimum effect. • Rinse thoroughly after use. • Do not apply alcohol to skin after use. • Do not use in infants; use cautiously in children. • May be toxic if ingested.
Germicidal effect against bacteria, fungi, and viruses, probably due to disruption of microorganism proteins.	• Cleanse area before applying. • Do not cover after application to avoid skin irritation. • Iodine stains skin and clothing. • Do not use in or around eyes or mucous membranes. • Toxic if ingested; sodium thiosulfate is antidote.
Germicidal effect against bacteria, fungi, and viruses; has same action as iodine without its irritating effects.	• Contraindicated in known sensitivity to iodine. • Do not use around eyes; do not use full-strength solution on mucous membranes. • May stain skin and mucous membranes.
Antipruritic and astringent activity through drying effect.	• Avoid use on eyes and mucous membranes. • Do not apply to raw, oozing areas. • Cleanse and dry affected area well before each application.

(continued)

TOPICAL AGENTS (continued)

DRUG	INDICATIONS AND DOSAGE
Astringents (continued)	
hamamelis water, witch hazel (Mediconet, Tucks)	*Anal discomfort, itching, burning, minor external hemorrhoidal or outer vaginal discomfort, diaper rash:* Apply t.i.d. or q.i.d.
Emollients	
oatmeal (Aveeno Colloidal)	*Emollient and demulcent; local irritation:* Use as a lotion; 1 level tablespoon to a cup of warm water. *Skin irritation, pruritus, common dermatoses, sunburn, dry skin:* Adults: 1 packet in tub of warm water. Children: 1 to 2 rounded tablespoons in 3″ to 4″ (8 to 10 cm) of bath water. Infants: 2 or 3 level teaspoons, depending on size of bath.
petrolatum (Vaseline)	*Dry rough skin; temporary relief of discomfort due to sunburn, windburn, or any drying of epithelial tissue:* Topical protection and emollience: use alone or with other drugs, apply p.r.n.
Keratolytics	
podophyllum resin (Pod-Ben 25, Podoben, Pudofin)	*Venereal warts:* Apply podophyllum resin preparation to the lesion, cover with waxed paper, and bandage. Leave covered for 4 to 6 hours, then wash lesion to remove medication. Repeat at weekly intervals, if indicated. *Multiple superficial epitheliomatosis and keratosis:* Apply daily with applicator and allow to dry. Remove necrotic tissue before each application.
resorcinol, resorcinol monoacetate (Acnomel, BiCozene)	*Acute eczema, urticaria, and other inflammatory skin diseases (1% or 2% concentration in alcohol); acne or seborrhea (5% lotion or 10% soap liniment for scalp); chronic eczema, psoriasis (2% to 10% ointment); acne scarring (45% peeling paste):* Apply b.i.d. to t.i.d.
Protectants	
collodion, flexible collodion	*Protectant; vehicle for other medicinal agents; sealant for small wounds:* Apply to dry skin, p.r.n., or use flexible collodion when a flexible noncontracting film is desired.
compound benzoin tincture	*Demulcent and protectant (cutaneous ulcers, bedsores, cracked nipples, fissures of lips and anus):* Apply locally once daily or b.i.d.
zinc gelatin (Dome-Paste, Unna's Boot, Unna's Powder)	*Protectant (lesions or injuries of lower legs or arms):* Wrap the wet bandage in place and retain for about 1 week. Dome-Paste, in 3″ and 4″ (8 to 10 cm) bandages, can be applied directly to arm or leg.

*Available in Canada only

ACTION	SPECIAL CONSIDERATIONS
Soothing, cooling effect of superficial irritation through astringent action.	• Avoid use around eyes. • Cleanse area before use.
Soothing, protective, and cleansing effects through mild absorptive and surfactant action.	• Avoid use in eyes. • Avoid use on acutely inflamed areas. • Blend product in warm water, not hot. • Soak at least 20 minutes. • May cause bath surfaces to become slippery.
Protective and emollient effect through formation of moisture barrier, increasing the natural retention of moisture.	• Avoid use in eyes. • May stain clothing. • May cause body surfaces to become slippery. • Apply sparingly; is not absorbed, so coating is all that is necessary.
Caustic and erosive action due to disruption of cell division of the epithelium.	• Avoid eye contact. • May be toxic if applied to large surface area or applied too frequently. • Should not be used in pregnant women. • Wash hands thoroughly after applying. • Protect surrounding area with petrolatum. • Wash off thoroughly with soap and water after prescribed time period. • May cause abnormal pigmentation.
Has keratolytic effect as well as antipruritic, bactericidal, and fungicidal effects.	• Avoid use on eyes and mucous membranes. • May cause excessive dryness, peeling, and irritation of skin; decrease use.
Protects wounds from the environment by forming an occlusive seal and excluding air.	• Do not use on deep or puncture wounds; may promote growth of anaerobic bacteria. • Avoid use on eyes and mucous membranes. • May be painful on application or cause dry skin. • Use alcohol or acetone as solvent for removal.
Protects skin from external environment by coating action.	• Avoid contact with eyes and mucous membranes. • Cleanse and dry area before application. • Useful in protection of skin from adhesive.
Protects skin by forming occlusive barrier.	• Avoid contact with eyes and mucous membranes. • Watch for signs of infection; may promote growth of anaerobic bacteria. • Retain for 1 to 2 weeks, remove by soaking in warm water. • Remove all traces of previous application before reapplication. • Apply with nap of hair to avoid folliculitis. • Do not use with constrictive bandage. Warn patient not to shower or bathe with gel on.

(continued)

TOPICAL AGENTS (continued)

DRUG	INDICATIONS AND DOSAGE
Wet dresssings/soaks	
aluminum acetate, aluminum sulfate (Bluboro Powder, Burow's solution, Domeboro powder, Pedi-Boro Soak Paks)	*Mild skin irritation from exposure to soaps, detergents, chemicals, diaper rash, acne, scaly skin, eczema:* Apply p.r.n. *Skin inflammation, insect bites, poison ivy or other contact dermatoses, swelling, athlete's foot:* Mix powder or tablet with 1 pint of lukewarm tap water and apply to loose dressing every 15 to 30 minutes for 48 hours.
sulfurated lime solution (Vlemasque, Vlem-Dome, Vleminckx's solution)	*Acne vulgaris, seborrhea:* Dilute 1 packet in 1 pint hot water and apply as hot dressing for 15 to 20 minutes daily. Or apply as a mask to affected, dry areas, and rinse away with warm water after 15 to 20 minutes once daily. *Generalized furunculosis:* Add 30 to 60 ml solution to bath water.
Miscellaneous agents	
benzyl benzoate	*Treatment of scabies:* Apply 28% lotion to entire body surface after bathing and towel drying, let dry, then apply second layer and rinse off in 24 to 48 hours. May repeat in 7 to 10 days if necessary. *Treatment of pediculosis capitis and Anthrius pubis:* Rub into hairy areas, remove with soap and water 12 to 24 hours later. May repeat in 1 week if necessary.
hydroquinone (Eldoquin, Esoterica, Porcelana, Solaquin Forte)	*Treatment of hyperpigmentation in conditions such as freckling, inactive chloasma, lentigo, photosensitization:* Apply uniformly to desired area b.i.d., until desired depigmentation occurs, then as needed to maintain depigmentation.
methyl salicylate (Ben-Gay, Icy Hot Balm/Cream, Deep Heating Rub)	*Counterirritant (minor pains of osteoarthritis, rheumatism, sprains, muscle and tendon soreness and tightness, lumbago, sciatica):* Apply with gentle massage several times daily for adults. Not recommended for children.
para-aminobenzoic acid (PABA) (Pabanol)	*Topical protectant; sunburn protection, sun-sensitive skin, slow tanning:* Apply evenly to skin indoors before exposure to sun. Do not apply to wet skin. Reapply after swimming. Not recommended for infants.
selenium sulfide (Exsel, Selsun, Selsun Blue)	*Treatment of tinea versicolor:* Massage into affected area; leave on for 10 minutes; rinse. Apply daily for 7 days. *Dandruff, seborrheic scalp dermatitis:* Massage 1 to 2 teaspoonfuls into wet scalp. Leave on for 2 to 3 minutes. Rinse thoroughly, and repeat application. Apply twice weekly for at least 2 weeks.

*Available in Canada only

ACTION	SPECIAL CONSIDERATIONS
Reduces friction and provides soothing relief through astringent action.	• Avoid use around eyes and mucous membranes. • Do not apply under occlusive dressings. • Discontinue if irritation occurs.
Sublimed sulfur products are germicidal through oxidation of the sulfur ion.	• Avoid use around eyes. • Contraindicated in sulfur-sensitive patients. • Do not use with other acne preparations; may cause excessive drying of skin. • May discolor jewelry and other metals.
Scabicidal and pediculocidal action through unknown mechanism.	• Avoid use near eyes and on mucous membranes. • Less toxic than lindane, drug may be used in children, infants, and pregnant women. • Do not apply to inflamed, weeping surfaces. • Patients should bathe with soap and water before application and remove crusts and scales. • Patients should wash their clothing and linens in hot water.
Depigmenting action.	• Avoid use near eyes and on broken skin. • Perform patch test before use to test for hypersensivity. • Sunscreen and protective clothing should be used during and after depigmentation to prevent repigmentation. • Should not be used in children and pregnant women. • May be toxic if ingested.
Acts as counterirritant, replacing pain perception with another sensation that blocks pain temporarily.	• Avoid use around eyes, on mucous membranes, or on broken skin. • May be toxic if ingested. • Do not use with heating pad or hot water. • Avoid use in patients allergic to salicylates.
Provides sun-screening action by absorbing ultraviolet rays.	• Avoid use in eyes and on mucous membranes. • May discolor clothing. • Must be reapplied if rubbed or rinsed off.
Antiseborrheic effect through cytostatic action on epithelial cells, which inhibits corneocyte production.	• Avoid use in eyes and on mucous membranes or inflamed areas. • May damage jewelry. • Should not be used in pregnant women. • May discolor hair or cause increased hair loss.

SELECTED DRUG LEVELS IN CONVENTIONAL AND S.I. UNITS

DRUG	CONVENTIONAL VALUES	CONVERSION FACTOR (CONVENTIONAL→S.I.)	S.I. UNITS
acetaminophen (P)			
toxic	>5 mg/dl	66.16	>330 μmol/L
carbamazepine (P)			
therapeutic	4 to 10 mg/liter	4.233	17 to 42 μmol/L
chlordiazepoxide (P)			
therapeutic	0.5 to 5 mg/liter	3.336	2 to 17 μmol/L
toxic	>10 mg/liter		>33 μmol/L
chlorpromazine (P)			
therapeutic	50 to 300 ng/ml	3.136	150 to 950 nmol/L
chlorpropamide (P)			
therapeutic	75 to 250 mg/liter	3.613	270 to 900 μmol/L
diazepam (P)			
therapeutic	0.10 to 0.25 mg/liter	3,512.0	350 to 900 nmol/L
toxic	>1.0 mg/liter		>3,510 nmol/L
dicumarol (P)			
therapeutic	8 to 30 mg/liter	2.974	25 to 90 μmol/L
digoxin (P)			
therapeutic	0.5 to 2.2 ng/ml	1.281	0.6 to 2.8 nmol/L
toxic	>2.5 ng/ml		>3.2 nmol/L
disopyramide (P)			
therapeutic	2 to 6 ng/liter	2.946	6 to 18 μmol/L
epinephrine (P)			
therapeutic	31 to 95 pg/ml (at rest for 15 min)	5.458	170 to 520 pmol/L
epinephrine (U)	<10 mcg/24 hr	5.458	<55 nmol/day
ethanol (P)			
legal limit (driving)	<80 mg/dl	0.2171	<17 mmol/L
toxic	>100 mg/dl		>22 mmol/L
ethosuximide (P)			
therapeutic	40 to 110 mg/liter	7.084	280 to 780 μmol/L
gold (S)			
therapeutic	300 to 800 mcg/dl	0.05077	15 to 40 μmol/L
insulin (P, S)			
therapeutic	(P) 5 to 20 mcg/ml	7.175	35 to 145 pmol/L
	(S) 0.20 to 0.84 mcg/ml	172.2	35 to 145 pmol/L
isoniazid (P)			
therapeutic	<2 mg/liter	7.291	<15 μmol/L
toxic	>3 mg/liter		>22 μmol/L
lidocaine (P)			
therapeutic	1 to 5 mg/liter	4.267	4.5 to 21.5 μmol/L
lithium ion (S)			
therapeutic	0.5 to 1.5 mEq/liter	1.0	0.5 to 1.5 mmol/L
meprobamate (P)			
therapeutic	<20 mg/liter	4.582	<90 μmol/L
toxic	>40 mg/liter		>180 μmol/L

KEY: (B) Blood   (P) Plasma   (S) Serum   (U) Urine

SELECTED DRUG LEVELS IN CONVENTIONAL AND S.I. UNITS *(continued)*

DRUG	CONVENTIONAL VALUES	CONVERSION FACTOR (CONVENTIONAL→S.I.)	S.I. UNITS
methotrexate (S) toxic	> 2.3 mg/liter	2.2	> 5.0 μmol/L
methsuximide (as desmethylsuximide) (P) therapeutic	10 to 40 mg/liter	5.285	50 to 210 μmol/L
nitroprusside (as thiocyanate) (P) toxic	10 mg/dl	0.1722	1.7 mmol/L
nortriptyline (P) therapeutic	25 to 200 ng/ml	3.797	90 to 760 nmol/L
pentobarbital (P) therapeutic	20 to 40 mg/liter	4.419	90 to 170 μmol/L
phenobarbital (P) therapeutic	2 to 5 mg/dl	43.06	85 to 215 μmol/L
phensuximide (P) therapeutic	4 to 8 mg/liter	5.285	20 to 40 μmol/L
phenytoin (P) therapeutic	10 to 20 mg/liter	3.964	40 to 80 μmol/L
phenytoin (P) toxic	> 30 mg/liter		> 120 μmol/L
primidone (P) therapeutic	6 to 10 mg/liter	4.582	25 to 46 μmol/L
primidone (P) toxic	> 10 mg/liter		46 μmol/L
procainamide (P) therapeutic	4 to 8 mg/liter	4.249	17 to 34 μmol/L
procainamide (P) toxic	> 12 mg/liter		> 50 μmol/L
propoxyphene (P) toxic	> 2 mg/liter	2.946	> 5.9 μmol/L
propranolol (P) therapeutic	50 to 200 ng/ml	3.856	190 to 770 nmol/L
quinidine (P) therapeutic	1.5 to 3 mg/liter	3.082	4.6 to 9.2 μmol/L
quinidine (P) toxic	> 6 mg/liter		> 18.5 μmol/L
salicylate (salicylic acid) (S) toxic	> 20 mg/dl	0.0724	> 1.45 mmol/L
sulfonamides (as sulfanilamide) (B) therapeutic	10 to 15 mg/dl	58.07	580 to 870 μmol/L
theophylline (P) therapeutic	10 to 20 mg/liter	5.55	55 to 110 μmol/L
warfarin (P) therapeutic	1 to 3 mg/liter	3.243	3.3 to 9.8 μmol/L

KEY: (B) Blood   (P) Plasma   (S) Serum   (U) Urine

Selected references

AHFS Drug Information '91. Bethesda, Md.: American Society of Hospital Pharmacists, 1991.

Badewitz-Dodd, L.H., et al., eds. *MIMS Annual 1991,* 15th ed. Crows Nest, NSW, Australia: IMS Publishing, 1991.

Bennett, W.M., et al. *Drug Prescribing in Renal Failure.* Philadelphia: American College of Physicians, 1987.

Bhatt, D.R., et al., eds. *Neonatal Drug Formulary.* Covina, Calif.: California Perinatal Association, 1988.

Billups, N., ed. *American Drug Index,* 35th ed. Philadelphia: J.B. Lippincott Co., 1991.

Briggs, G., et al. *Drugs in Pregnancy and Lactation: A Reference Guide to Fetal and Neonatal Risk,* 3rd ed. Baltimore: Williams & Wilkins Co., 1990.

Compendium of Pharmaceuticals and Specialties, 26th ed. Ottawa, Canada: Canadian Pharmaceutical Association, 1991.

Dorland's Illustrated Medical Dictionary, 27th ed. Philadelphia: W.B. Saunders Co., 1988.

Drug Interaction Facts. St. Louis: J.B. Lippincott Co. (Facts and Comparisons Division), 1989.

Facts and Comparisons. St. Louis: J.B. Lippincott Co. (Facts and Comparisons Division), 1991.

Fleeger, C.A., et al., eds. *USAN 1992 and the USP Dictionary of Drug Names.* Rockville, Md.: The United States Pharmacopeial Convention, 1991.

Gilman, A., et al., eds. *Goodman and Gilman's The Pharmacological Basis of Therapeutics,* 8th ed. New York: Pergamon Press, 1990.

Guide for adult immunization, ACP Task Force on Adult Immunization and Infectious Diseases Society of America. Philadelphia: America College of Physicians, 1991.

Haddad, L.M., and Winchester, J. *Clinical Management of Poisoning & Drug Overdose.* Philadelphia: W.B. Saunders Co., 1983.

Handbook of Nonprescription Drugs, 9th ed. Washington, D.C.: American Pharmaceutical Association, 1990.

Handbook of Pediatric Drug Therapy. Springhouse, Pa.: Springhouse Corp., 1991.

Hansten, P., and Horn, J.R. *Drug Interactions,* 7th ed. Philadelphia: Lea and Febiger, 1990.

Knoben, J. E., and Anderson, P.O. *Handbook of Clinical Drug Data,* 6th ed. Hamilton, Ill.: Drug Intelligence Publications, Inc., 1988.

The Merck Manual of Diagnosis and Therapy, 15th ed. Rahway, N.J.: Merck & Co., Inc., 1987.

Nelson, J.D. *1990-1991 Pocketbook of Pediatric Antimicrobial Therapy,* 9th ed. Baltimore: Williams & Wilkins Co., 1991.

Peter, G., ed. *Report of the Committee on Infectious Diseases.* Elk Grove Village, Ill.: American Academy of Pediatrics, 1986.

Pharmacy Law Digest. St. Louis: J.B. Lippincott Co. (Facts and Comparisons Division), 1987.

Physician's Desk Reference, 45th ed. Oradell, N.J.: Medical Economics Books, 1991.

Physician's Desk Reference for Nonprescription Drugs, 12th ed. Oradell, N.J.: Medical Economics Books, 1991.

Physician's Desk Reference for Ophthalmology, 19th ed. Oradell, N.J.: Medical Economics Books 1991.

Rakel, R. E., ed. *Conn's Current Therapy 1991.* Philadelphia: W.B. Saunders Co., 1991.

Reynolds, J.E.F., et al., eds. *Martindale: The Extra Pharmacopeia,* 29th ed. London: The Pharmaceutical Press, 1989.

Rowe, P. C., ed. *The Harriet Lane Handbook,* 11th ed. Chicago: Year Book Medical Publishers, 1987.

Speight, T. *Avery's Drug Treatment,* 3rd ed. Baltimore: Williams & Wilkins Co., 1987.

Trissel, L. *Handbook of Injectable Drugs,* 6th ed. Bethesda, Md.: American Society of Hospital Pharmacists, 1990.

United States Pharmacopeia Dispensing Information (USP DI). Rockville, Md.: United States Pharmacopeial Convention, Inc., 1992.

Wilson, J.D., et al., eds. *Harrison's Principles of Internal Medicine.* New York: McGraw-Hill, Inc. 1991.

Index

B

t refers to table